Pediatric Clinical Practice Guidelines & Policies

• •

A Compendium of Evidence-based Research for Pediatric Practice

19th Edition

American Academy of Pediatrics
345 Park Blvd
Itasca, IL 60143
www.aap.org

The American Academy of Pediatrics is an organization of 67,000 primary care pediatricians, pediatric medical subspecialists, and pediatric surgical specialists dedicated to the health, safety, and well-being of infants, children, adolescents, and young adults.

The recommendations in this publication do not indicate an exclusive course of treatment or serve as a standard of medical care. Variations, taking into account individual circumstances, may be appropriate.

Products are mentioned for informational purposes only. Inclusion in this publication does not imply endorsement by the American Academy of Pediatrics.

Every effort has been made to ensure that the drug selection and dosage set forth in this publication are in accordance with the current recommendations and practice at the time of publication. It is the responsibility of the health care professional to check the package insert of each drug for any change in indications and dosage and for added warnings and precautions.

This publication has been developed by the American Academy of Pediatrics. The authors, editors, and contributors are expert authorities in the field of pediatrics. No commercial involvement of any kind has been solicited or accepted in the development of the content of this publication.

Printed in the United States of America

9-5/0618
MA0906
ISBN: 978-1-61002-293-4
eBook: 978-1-61002-294-1
ISSN: 1942-2024

INTRODUCTION TO
PEDIATRIC CLINICAL PRACTICE GUIDELINES & POLICIES: A COMPENDIUM OF EVIDENCE-BASED RESEARCH FOR PEDIATRIC PRACTICE

Clinical practice guidelines have long provided physicians with evidence-based decision-making tools for managing common pediatric conditions. Policy statements issued and endorsed by the American Academy of Pediatrics (AAP) are developed to provide physicians with a quick reference guide to the AAP position on child health care issues. We have combined these 2 authoritative resources into 1 comprehensive manual/eBook resource to provide easy access to important clinical and policy information.

This manual contains
- Clinical practice guidelines from the AAP, plus related recommendation summaries, *ICD-10-CM* coding information, and AAP patient education handouts
- Clinical practice guidelines endorsed by the AAP, including abstracts where applicable
- Policy statements, clinical reports, and technical reports issued or endorsed through December 2018, including abstracts where applicable
- Full text of all 2018 AAP policy statements, clinical reports, and technical reports
  The eBook, which is available via the code on the inside cover of this manual, builds on content of the manual and points to the full text of all AAP
- Clinical practice guidelines
- Policy statements
- Clinical reports
- Technical reports
- Endorsed clinical practice guidelines and policies

For easy reference within this publication, dates when AAP clinical practice guidelines, policy statements, clinical reports, and technical reports first appeared in the AAP journal *Pediatrics* are provided. In 2009, the online version of *Pediatrics* at http://pediatrics.aappublications.org became the official journal of record; therefore, date of online publication is given for policies from 2010 to present.

Additional information about AAP policy can be found in a variety of professional publications such as

Guidelines for Air and Ground Transport of Neonatal and Pediatric Patients, 4th Edition

Pediatric Nutrition, 7th Edition

Guidelines for Perinatal Care, 8th Edition

Pediatric Environmental Health, 4th Edition

Care of the Young Athlete, 2nd Edition

Red Book®, 31st Edition, and *Red Book® Online* (http://redbook.solutions.aap.org)

To order these and other pediatric resources, please call 866/843-2271 or visit http://shop.aap.org/books.

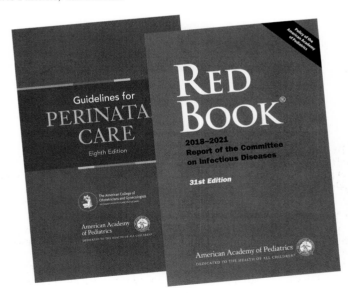

AMERICAN ACADEMY OF PEDIATRICS

The American Academy of Pediatrics (AAP) and its member pediatricians dedicate their efforts and resources to the health, safety, and well-being of infants, children, adolescents, and young adults. The AAP has approximately 67,000 members in the United States, Canada, and Latin America. Members include pediatricians, pediatric medical subspecialists, and pediatric surgical specialists.

Core Values. *We believe*
- In the inherent worth of all children; they are our most enduring and vulnerable legacy.
- Children deserve optimal health and the highest quality health care.
- Pediatricians, pediatric medical subspecialists, and pediatric surgical specialists are the best qualified to provide child health care.
- Multidisciplinary teams including patients and families are integral to delivering the highest quality health care.

The AAP is the organization to advance child health and well-being and the profession of pediatrics.

Vision. Children have optimal health and well-being and are valued by society. American Academy of Pediatrics members practice the highest quality health care and experience professional satisfaction and personal well-being.

Mission. The mission of the AAP is to attain optimal physical, mental, and social health and well-being for all infants, children, adolescents, and young adults. To accomplish this mission, the AAP shall support the professional needs of its members.

Table of Contents

PPI
AAP Partnership for Policy Implementation   See Appendix 1.

SECTION 5

CURRENT POLICIES FROM THE AMERICAN ACADEMY OF PEDIATRICS

PPI
AAP Partnership for Policy Implementation   See Appendix 1.

SECTION 6

ENDORSED POLICIES

APPENDIX 1

**PPI: AAP PARTNERSHIP FOR POLICY
IMPLEMENTATION**

APPENDIX 2

**AMERICAN ACADEMY OF PEDIATRICS
ACRONYMS**

SECTION 1

Clinical Practice Guidelines
From the American Academy of Pediatrics
• • • • • • • • • • • • • • • • • • • •

- ### *Clinical Practice Guidelines*
  EVIDENCE-BASED DECISION-MAKING TOOLS FOR MANAGING COMMON PEDIATRIC CONDITIONS

- ### *Quick Reference Tools*
  TOOLS FOR IMPLEMENTING AMERICAN ACADEMY OF PEDIATRICS GUIDELINES IN YOUR
  PRACTICE AND AT THE POINT OF CARE

FOREWORD

To promote the practice of evidence-based medicine and to improve the health outcomes of children, the American Academy of Pediatrics (AAP) provides physicians with evidence-based guidelines for managing common pediatric conditions. The AAP has established an organizational process and methodology for the development, implementation, and improvement of these clinical practice guidelines.

The evidence-based approach to developing clinical practice guidelines begins by systematically reviewing and synthesizing the literature to provide the scientific basis for guideline recommendations. Clinical practice guideline teams with stakeholder representation systematically develop recommendations by carefully considering the evidence, risk, benefits, and patient and caregiver preferences. Each clinical practice guideline undergoes a thorough peer-review process before publication. The AAP supports efforts to implement the recommendations into practice and to evaluate whether they are leading to improved outcomes. Each clinical practice guideline is periodically reviewed to ensure that it is based on the most current data available.

American Academy of Pediatrics clinical practice guidelines are designed to provide physicians with an analytic framework for evaluating and treating common pediatric conditions and are not intended as an exclusive course of treatment or standard of care. The AAP recognizes circumstances in which there is a lack of definitive data and relies on expert consensus in cases in which data do not exist. American Academy of Pediatrics clinical practice guidelines allow for flexibility and adaptability at the local and patient levels to address unique circumstances and should not replace sound clinical judgment.

This section contains clinical practice guidelines, technical reports, and technical report summaries developed and published by the AAP. Each one contains a summary of data reviewed, results of data analysis, complete evidence tables, and a bibliography of articles included in the review. Clinical practice guidelines will continually be added to this compendium as they are released or updated.

If you have any questions about current or future clinical practice guidelines, please contact Kymika Okechukwu, senior manager of evidence-based medicine initiatives at the AAP, at 630/626-6317 or via email at kokechukwu@aap.org.

To order copies of patient education resources that accompany each guideline, please call the AAP at 866/843-2271 or visit http://shop.aap.org/books.

Joel Tieder, MD, MPH, FAAP
Chairperson, Council on Quality Improvement and Patient Safety

ADHD: Clinical Practice Guideline for the Diagnosis, Evaluation, and Treatment of Attention-Deficit/Hyperactivity Disorder in Children and Adolescents

- *Clinical Practice Guideline*

  - *PPI: AAP Partnership for Policy Implementation*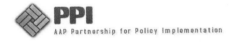
    See Appendix 1 for more information.

CLINICAL PRACTICE GUIDELINE

ADHD: Clinical Practice Guideline for the Diagnosis, Evaluation, and Treatment of Attention-Deficit/ Hyperactivity Disorder in Children and Adolescents

SUBCOMMITTEE ON ATTENTION-DEFICIT/HYPERACTIVITY DISORDER, STEERING COMMITTEE ON QUALITY IMPROVEMENT AND MANAGEMENT

KEY WORDS
attention-deficit/hyperactivity disorder, children, adolescents, preschool, behavioral therapy, medication

ABBREVIATIONS
AAP—American Academy of Pediatrics
ADHD—attention-deficit/hyperactivity disorder
DSM-PC—*Diagnostic and Statistical Manual for Primary Care*
CDC—Centers for Disease Control and Prevention
FDA—Food and Drug Administration
DSM-IV—*Diagnostic and Statistical Manual of Mental Disorders, Fourth Edition*
MTA—Multimodal Therapy of ADHD

www.pediatrics.org/cgi/doi/10.1542/peds.2011-2654

doi:10.1542/peds.2011-2654

All clinical practice guidelines from the American Academy of Pediatrics automatically expire 5 years after publication unless reaffirmed, revised, or retired at or before that time.

PEDIATRICS (ISSN Numbers: Print, 0031-4005; Online, 1098-4275).

abstract

Attention-deficit/hyperactivity disorder (ADHD) is the most common neurobehavioral disorder of childhood and can profoundly affect the academic achievement, well-being, and social interactions of children; the American Academy of Pediatrics first published clinical recommendations for the diagnosis and evaluation of ADHD in children in 2000; recommendations for treatment followed in 2001. *Pediatrics* 2011;128: 1007–1022

Summary of key action statements:

1. The primary care clinician should initiate an evaluation for ADHD for any child 4 through 18 years of age who presents with academic or behavioral problems and symptoms of inattention, hyperactivity, or impulsivity (quality of evidence B/strong recommendation).

2. To make a diagnosis of ADHD, the primary care clinician should determine that *Diagnostic and Statistical Manual of Mental Disorders, Fourth Edition* criteria have been met (including documentation of impairment in more than 1 major setting); information should be obtained primarily from reports from parents or guardians, teachers, and other school and mental health clinicians involved in the child's care. The primary care clinician should also rule out any alternative cause (quality of evidence B/strong recommendation).

3. In the evaluation of a child for ADHD, the primary care clinician should include assessment for other conditions that might coexist with ADHD, including emotional or behavioral (eg, anxiety, depressive, oppositional defiant, and conduct disorders), developmental (eg, learning and language disorders or other neurodevelopmental disorders), and physical (eg, tics, sleep apnea) conditions (quality of evidence B/strong recommendation).

4. The primary care clinician should recognize ADHD as a chronic condition and, therefore, consider children and adolescents with ADHD as children and youth with special health care needs. Management of children and youth with special health care needs should follow the principles of the chronic care model and the medical home (quality of evidence B/strong recommendation).

5. Recommendations for treatment of children and youth with ADHD vary depending on the patient's age:

   a. For *preschool-aged children (4–5 years of age)*, the primary care clinician should prescribe evidence-based parent- and/or teacher-administered behavior therapy as the first line of treatment (quality of evidence A/strong recommendation) and may prescribe methylphenidate if the behavior interventions do not provide significant improvement and there is moderate-to-severe continuing disturbance in the child's function. In areas where evidence-based behavioral treatments are not available, the clinician needs to weigh the risks of starting medication at an early age against the harm of delaying diagnosis and treatment (quality of evidence B/recommendation).

   b. For *elementary school–aged children (6–11 years of age)*, the primary care clinician should prescribe US Food and Drug Administration–approved medications for ADHD (quality of evidence A/strong recommendation) and/or evidence-based parent- and/or teacher-administered behavior therapy as treatment for ADHD, preferably both (quality of evidence B/strong recommendation). The evidence is particularly strong for stimulant medications and sufficient but less strong for atomoxetine, extended-release guanfacine, and extended-release clonidine (in that order) (quality of evidence A/strong recommendation). The school environment, program, or placement is a part of any treatment plan.

   c. For *adolescents (12–18 years of age)*, the primary care clinician

should prescribe Food and Drug Administration–approved medications for ADHD with the assent of the adolescent (quality of evidence A/strong recommendation) and may prescribe behavior therapy as treatment for ADHD (quality of evidence C/recommendation), preferably both.

6. The primary care clinician should titrate doses of medication for ADHD to achieve maximum benefit with minimum adverse effects (quality of evidence B/strong recommendation).

INTRODUCTION

This document updates and replaces 2 previously published clinical guidelines from the American Academy of Pediatrics (AAP) on the diagnosis and treatment of attention-deficit/hyperactivity disorder (ADHD) in children: "Clinical Practice Guideline: Diagnosis and Evaluation of the Child With Attention-Deficit/Hyperactivity Disorder" (2000)[1] and "Clinical Practice Guideline: Treatment of the School-aged Child With Attention-Deficit/Hyperactivity Disorder" (2001).[2] Since these guidelines were published, new information and evidence regarding the diagnosis and treatment of ADHD has become available. Surveys conducted before and after the publication of the previous guidelines have also provided insight into pediatricians' attitudes and practices regarding ADHD. On the basis of an increased understanding regarding ADHD and the challenges it raises for children and families and as a source for clinicians seeking to diagnose and treat children, this guideline pays particular attention to a number of areas.

Expanded Age Range

The previous guidelines addressed diagnosis and treatment of ADHD in chil-

dren 6 through 12 years of age. There is now emerging evidence to expand the age range of the recommendations to include preschool-aged children and adolescents. This guideline addresses the diagnosis and treatment of ADHD in children 4 through 18 years of age, and attention is brought to special circumstances or concerns in particular age groups when appropriate.

Expanded Scope

Behavioral interventions might help families of children with hyperactive/impulsive behaviors that do not meet full diagnostic criteria for ADHD. Guidance regarding the diagnosis of problem-level concerns in children based on the *Diagnostic and Statistical Manual for Primary Care* (DSM-PC), *Child and Adolescent Version*,[3] as well as suggestions for treatment and care of children and families with problem-level concerns, are provided here. The current DSM-PC was published in 1996 and, therefore, is not consistent with intervening changes to *International Classification of Diseases, Ninth Revision, Clinical Modification* (ICD-9-CM). Although this version of the DSM-PC should not be used as a definitive source for diagnostic codes related to ADHD and comorbid conditions, it certainly may continue to be used as a resource for enriching the understanding of ADHD manifestations. The DSM-PC will be revised when both the DSM-V and ICD-10 are available for use.

A Process of Care for Diagnosis and Treatment

This guideline and process-of-care algorithm (see Supplemental Fig 2 and Supplemental Appendix) recognizes evaluation, diagnosis, and treatment as a continuous process and provides recommendations for both the guideline and the algorithm in this single publication. In addition to the formal recommendations for assessment, diagnosis, and treatment, this guideline provides a single algorithm to guide the clinical process.

Integration With the Task Force on Mental Health

This guideline fits into the broader mission of the AAP Task Force on Mental Health and its efforts to provide a base from which primary care providers can develop alliances with families, work to prevent mental health conditions and identify them early, and collaborate with mental health clinicians.

The diagnosis and management of ADHD in children and youth has been particularly challenging for primary care clinicians because of the limited payment provided for what requires more time than most of the other conditions they typically address. The procedures recommended in this guideline necessitate spending more time with patients and families, developing a system of contacts with school and other personnel, and providing continuous, coordinated care, all of which is time demanding. In addition, relegating mental health conditions exclusively to mental health clinicians also is not a viable solution for many clinicians, because in many areas access to mental health clinicians to whom they can refer patients is limited. Access in many areas is also limited to psychologists when further assessment of cognitive issues is required and not available through the education system because of restrictions from third-party payers in paying for the evaluations on the basis of them being educational and not health related.

Cultural differences in the diagnosis and treatment of ADHD are an important issue, as they are for all pediatric conditions. Because the diagnosis and treatment of ADHD depends to a great extent on family and teacher perceptions, these issues might be even more prominent an issue for ADHD. Specific cultural issues are beyond the scope of this guideline but are important to consider.

METHODOLOGY

As with the 2 previously published clinical guidelines, the AAP collaborated with several organizations to develop a working subcommittee that represented a wide range of primary care and subspecialty groups. The subcommittee included primary care pediatricians, developmental-behavioral pediatricians, and representatives from the American Academy of Child and Adolescent Psychiatry, the Child Neurology Society, the Society for Pediatric Psychology, the National Association of School Psychologists, the Society for Developmental and Behavioral Pediatrics, the American Academy of Family Physicians, and Children and Adults With Attention-Deficit/Hyperactivity Disorder (CHADD), as well as an epidemiologist from the Centers for Disease Control and Prevention (CDC).

This group met over a 2-year period, during which it reviewed the changes in practice that have occurred and issues that have been identified since the previous guidelines were published. Delay in completing the process led to further conference calls and extended the years of literature reviewed in order to remain as current as possible. The AAP funded the development of this guideline; potential financial conflicts of the participants were identified and taken into consideration in the deliberations. The guideline will be reviewed and/or revised in 5 years unless new evidence emerges that warrants revision sooner.

The subcommittee developed a series of research questions to direct an extensive evidence-based review in partnership with the CDC and the University of Oklahoma Health Sciences Center. The diagnostic review was conducted by the CDC, and the evidence was evaluated in a combined effort of the AAP, CDC, and University of Oklahoma Health Sciences Center staff. The treatment-related evidence relied on a recent evidence review by the Agency for Healthcare Research and Quality and was supplemented by evidence identified through the CDC review.

The diagnostic issues were focused on 5 areas:

1. ADHD prevalence—specifically: (a) What percentage of the general US population aged 21 years or younger has ADHD? (b) What percentage of patients presenting at pediatricians' or family physicians' offices in the United States meet diagnostic criteria for ADHD?

2. Co-occurring mental disorders—of people with ADHD, what percentage has 1 or more of the following co-occurring conditions: sleep disorders, learning disabilities, depression, anxiety, conduct disorder, and oppositional defiant disorder?

3. What are the functional impairments of children and youth diagnosed with ADHD? Specifically, in what domains and to what degree do youth with ADHD demonstrate impairments in functional domains, including peer relations, academic performance, adaptive skills, and family functioning?

4. Do behavior rating scales remain the standard of care in assessing the diagnostic criteria for ADHD?

5. What is the prevalence of abnormal findings on selected medical screening tests commonly recommended as standard components of an evaluation of a child with suspected ADHD? How accurate are these tests in the diagnosis of ADHD compared with a reference standard (ie, what are the psychometric properties of these tests)?

The treatment issues were focused on 3 areas:

1. What new information is available

regarding the long-term efficacy and safety of medications approved by the US Food and Drug Administration (FDA) for the treatment of ADHD (stimulants and nonstimulants), and specifically, what information is available about the efficacy and safety of these medications in preschool-aged and adolescent patients?

2. What evidence is available about the long-term efficacy and safety of psychosocial interventions (behavioral modification) for the treatment of ADHD for children, and specifically, what information is available about the efficacy and safety of these interventions in preschool-aged and adolescent patients?

3. Are there any additional therapies that reach the level of consideration as evidence based?

Evidence-Review Process for Diagnosis

A multilevel, systematic approach was taken to identify the literature that built the evidence base for both diagnosis and treatment. To increase the likelihood that relevant articles were included in the final evidence base, the reviewers first conducted a scoping review of the literature by systematically searching literature using relevant key words and then summarized the primary findings of articles that met standard inclusion criteria. The reviewers then created evidence tables that were reviewed by content-area experts who were best able to identify articles that might have been missed through the scoping review. Articles that were missed were reviewed carefully to determine where the abstraction methodology failed, and adjustments to the search strategy were made as required (see technical report to be published). Finally, although published literature reviews did not contribute directly to the evidence

base, the articles included in review articles were cross-referenced with the final evidence tables to ensure that all relevant articles were included in the final evidence tables.

For the scoping review, articles were abstracted in a stratified fashion from 3 article-retrieval systems that provided access to articles in the domains of medicine, psychology, and education: PubMed (www.ncbi.nlm.nih.gov/sites/entrez), PsycINFO (www.apa.org/pubs/databases/psycinfo/index.aspx), and ERIC (www.eric.ed.gov). English-language, peer-reviewed articles published between 1998 and 2009 were queried in the 3 search engines. Key words were selected with the intent of including all possible articles that might have been relevant to 1 or more of the questions of interest (see the technical report to be published). The primary abstraction included the following terms: "attention deficit hyperactivity disorder" or "attention deficit disorder" or "hyperkinesis" and "child." A second, independent abstraction was conducted to identify articles related to medical screening tests for ADHD. For this abstraction, the same search terms were used as in the previous procedure along with the additional condition term "behavioral problems" to allow for the inclusion of studies of youth that sought to diagnose ADHD by using medical screening tests. Abstractions were conducted in parallel fashion across each of the 3 databases; the results from each abstraction (complete reference, abstract, and key words) were exported and compiled into a common reference database using EndNote 10.0.[4] References were subsequently and systematically deduplicated by using the software's deduplication procedure. References for books, chapters, and theses were also deleted from the library. Once a deduplicated library was developed, the semifinal

database of 8267 references was reviewed for inclusion on the basis of inclusion criteria listed in the technical report. Included articles were then pulled in their entirety, the inclusion criteria were reconfirmed, and then the study findings were summarized in evidence tables. The articles included in relevant review articles were revisited to ensure their inclusion in the final evidence base. The evidence tables were then presented to the committee for expert review.

Evidence-Review Process for Treatment

In addition to this systematic review, for treatment we used the review from the Agency for Healthcare Research and Quality (AHRQ) Effective Healthcare Program "Attention Deficit Hyperactivity Disorder: Effectiveness of Treatment in At-Risk Preschoolers; Long-term Effectiveness in All Ages; and Variability in Prevalence, Diagnosis, and Treatment."[5] This review addressed a number of key questions for the committee, including the efficacy of medications and behavioral interventions for preschoolers, children, and adolescents. Evidence identified through the systematic evidence review for diagnosis was also used as a secondary data source to supplement the evidence presented in the AHRQ report. The draft practice guidelines were developed by consensus of the committee regarding the evidence. It was decided to create 2 separate components. The guideline recommendations were based on clear characterization of the evidence. The second component is a practice-of-care algorithm (see Supplemental Fig 2) that provides considerably more detail about how to implement the guidelines but is, necessarily, based less on available evidence and more on consensus of the committee members. When data were lacking, particularly in the

Evidence Quality	Preponderance of Benefit or Harm	Balance of Benefit and Harm
A. Well-designed RCTs or diagnostic studies on relevant population	Strong recommendation	
B. RCTs or diagnostic studies with minor limitations; overwhelmingly consistent evidence from observational studies		Option
C. Observational studies (case-control and cohort design)	Recommendation	
D. Expert opinion, case reports, reasoning from first principles	Option	No Rec
X. Exceptional situations in which validating studies cannot be performed and there is a clear preponderance of benefit or harm	Strong recommendation / Recommendation	

FIGURE 1
Integrating evidence-quality appraisal with an assessment of the anticipated balance between benefits and harms if a policy is conducted leads to designation of a policy as a strong recommendation, recommendation, option, or no recommendation. The evidence is discussed in more detail in a technical report that will follow in a later publication. RCT indicates randomized controlled trial; Rec, recommendation.

process-of-care algorithmic portion of the guidelines, a combination of evidence and expert consensus was used. Action statements labeled "strong recommendation" or "recommendation" were based on high- to moderate-quality scientific evidence and a preponderance of benefit over harm.[6] Option-level action statements were based on lesser-quality or limited data and expert consensus or high-quality evidence with a balance between benefits and harms. These clinical options are interventions that a reasonable health care provider might or might not wish to implement in his or her practice. The quality of evidence supporting each recommendation and the strength of each recommendation were assessed by the committee member most experienced in epidemiology and graded according to AAP policy (Fig 1).[6]

The guidelines and process-of-care algorithm underwent extensive peer review by committees, sections, councils, and task forces within the AAP; numerous outside organizations; and other individuals identified by the subcommittee. Liaisons to the subcommittee also were invited to distribute the draft to entities within their organizations. The re-

sulting comments were compiled and reviewed by the chairperson, and relevant changes were incorporated into the draft, which was then reviewed by the full committee.

ABOUT THIS GUIDELINE

Key Action Statements

In light of the concerns highlighted previously and informed by the available evidence, the AAP has developed 6 action statements for the evaluation, diagnosis, and treatment of ADHD in children. These action statements provide for consistent and quality care for children and families with concerns about or symptoms that suggest attention disorders or problems.

Context

This guideline is intended to be integrated with the broader algorithms developed as part of the mission of the AAP Task Force on Mental Health.[7]

Implementation: A Process-of-Care Algorithm

The AAP recognizes the challenge of instituting practice changes and adopting new recommendations for care. To address the need, a process-of-care algorithm has been devel-

oped and has been used in the revision of the AAP ADHD toolkit.

Implementation: Preparing the Practice

Full implementation of the action statements described in this guideline and the process-of-care algorithm might require changes in office procedures and/or preparatory efforts to identify community resources. The section titled "Preparing the Practice" in the process-of-care algorithm and further information can be found in the supplement to the Task Force on Mental Health report.[7] It is important to document all aspects of the diagnostic and treatment procedures in the patients' records. Use of rating scales for the diagnosis of ADHD and assessment for comorbid conditions and as a method for monitoring treatment as described in the process algorithm (see Supplemental Fig 2), as well as information provided to parents such as management plans, can help facilitate a clinician's accurate documentation of his or her process.

Note

The AAP acknowledges that some primary care clinicians might not be confident of their ability to successfully diagnose and treat ADHD in a child because of the child's age, coexisting conditions, or other concerns. At any point at which a clinician feels that he or she is not adequately trained or is uncertain about making a diagnosis or continuing with treatment, a referral to a pediatric or mental health subspecialist should be made. If a diagnosis of ADHD or other condition is made by a subspecialist, the primary care clinician should develop a management strategy with the subspecialist that ensures that the child will continue to receive appropriate care consistent with a medical home model wherein the pediatrician partners with parents so that both health and mental health needs are integrated.

KEY ACTION STATEMENTS FOR THE EVALUATION, DIAGNOSIS, TREATMENT, AND MONITORING OF ADHD IN CHILDREN AND ADOLESCENTS

Action statement 1: The primary care clinician should initiate an evaluation for ADHD for any child 4 through 18 years of age who presents with academic or behavioral problems and symptoms of inattention, hyperactivity, or impulsivity (quality of evidence B/strong recommendation).

Evidence Profile

- **Aggregate evidence quality:** B.
- **Benefits:** In a considerable number of children, ADHD goes undiagnosed. Primary care clinicians' systematic identification of children with these problems will likely decrease the rate of undiagnosed and untreated ADHD in children.
- **Harms/risks/costs:** Children in whom ADHD is inappropriately diagnosed might be labeled inappropriately, or another condition might be missed, and they might receive treatments that will not benefit them.
- **Benefits-harms assessment:** The high prevalence of ADHD and limited mental health resources require primary care pediatricians to play a significant role in the care of their patients with ADHD so that children with this condition receive the appropriate diagnosis and treatment. Treatments available have shown good evidence of efficacy, and lack of treatment results in a risk for impaired outcomes.
- **Value judgments:** The committee considered the requirements for establishing the diagnosis, the prevalence of ADHD, and the efficacy and adverse effects of treatment as well as the long-term outcomes.

- **Role of patient preferences:** Success with treatment depends on patient and family preference, which has to be taken into account.
- **Exclusions:** None.
- **Intentional vagueness:** The limits between what can be handled by a primary care clinician and what should be referred to a subspecialist because of the varying degrees of skills among primary care clinicians.
- **Strength: strong recommendation.**

The basis for this recommendation is essentially unchanged from that in the previous guideline. ADHD is the most common neurobehavioral disorder in children and occurs in approximately 8% of children and youth[8–10]; the number of children with this condition is far greater than can be managed by the mental health system. There is now increased evidence that appropriate diagnosis can be provided for preschool-aged children[11] (4–5 years of age) and for adolescents.[12]

Action statement 2: To make a diagnosis of ADHD, the primary care clinician should determine that *Diagnostic and Statistical Manual of Mental Disorders, Fourth Edition* (DSM-IV-TR) criteria have been met (including documentation of impairment in more than 1 major setting), and information should be obtained primarily from reports from parents or guardians, teachers, and other school and mental health clinicians involved in the child's care. The primary care clinician should also rule out any alternative cause (quality of evidence B/strong recommendation).

Evidence Profile

- **Aggregate evidence quality:** B.
- **Benefits:** The use of DSM-IV criteria has lead to more uniform categorization of the condition across professional disciplines.

- **Harms/risks/costs:** The DSM-IV system does not specifically provide for developmental-level differences and might lead to some misdiagnoses.
- **Benefits-harms assessment:** The benefits far outweigh the harm.
- **Value judgments:** The committee took into consideration the importance of coordination between pediatric and mental health services.
- **Role of patient preferences:** Although there is some stigma associated with mental disorder diagnoses resulting in some families preferring other diagnoses, the need for better clarity in diagnoses was felt to outweigh this preference.
- **Exclusions:** None.
- **Intentional vagueness:** None.
- **Strength: strong recommendation.**

As with the findings in the previous guideline, the DSM-IV criteria continue to be the criteria best supported by evidence and consensus. Developed through several iterations by the American Psychiatric Association, the DSM-IV criteria were created through use of consensus and an expanding research foundation.[13] The DSM-IV system is used by professionals in psychiatry, psychology, health care systems, and primary care. Use of DSM-IV criteria, in addition to having the best evidence to date for criteria for ADHD, also affords the best method for communication across clinicians and is established with third-party payers. The criteria are under review for the development of the DSM-V, but these changes will not be available until at least 1 year after the publication of this current guideline. The diagnostic criteria have not changed since the previous guideline and are presented in Supplemental Table 2. An anticipated change in the DSM-V is increasing the age limit for when ADHD needs to have first presented from 7 to 12 years.[14]

Special Circumstances: Preschool-aged Children (4–5 Years Old)

There is evidence that the diagnostic criteria for ADHD can be applied to preschool-aged children; however, the subtypes detailed in the DSM-IV might not be valid for this population.[15–21] A review of the literature, including the multisite study of the efficacy of methylphenidate in preschool-aged children, revealed that the criteria could appropriately identify children with the condition.[11] However, there are added challenges in determining the presence of key symptoms. Preschool-aged children are not likely to have a separate observer if they do not attend a preschool or child care program, and even if they do attend, staff in those programs might be less qualified than certified teachers to provide accurate observations. Here, too, focused checklists can help physicians in the diagnostic evaluation, although only the Conners Comprehensive Behavior Rating Scales and the ADHD Rating Scale IV are DSM-IV–based scales that have been validated in preschool-aged children.[22]

When there are concerns about the availability or quality of nonparent observations of a child's behavior, physicians may recommend that parents complete a parent-training program before confirming an ADHD diagnosis for preschool-aged children and consider placement in a qualified preschool program if they have not done so already. Information can be obtained from parents and teachers through the use of validated DSM-IV–based ADHD rating scales. The parent-training program must include helping parents develop age-appropriate developmental expectations and specific management skills for problem behaviors. The clinician may obtain reports from the parenting class instructor about the parents' ability to manage their children, and if the children are

in programs in which they are directly observed, instructors can report information about the core symptoms and function of the child directly. Qualified preschool programs include programs such as Head Start or other public prekindergarten programs. Preschool-aged children who display significant emotional or behavioral concerns might also qualify for Early Childhood Special Education services through their local school districts, and the evaluators for these programs and/or Early Childhood Special Education teachers might be excellent reporters of core symptoms.

Special Circumstances: Adolescents

Obtaining teacher reports for adolescents might be more challenging, because many adolescents will have multiple teachers. Likewise, parents might have less opportunity to observe their adolescent's behaviors than they had when their children were younger. Adolescents' reports of their own behaviors often differ from those of other observers, because they tend to minimize their own problematic behaviors.[23–25] Adolescents are less likely to exhibit overt hyperactive behavior. Despite the difficulties, clinicians need to try to obtain (with agreement from the adolescent) information from at least 2 teachers as well as information from other sources such as coaches, school guidance counselors, or leaders of community activities in which the adolescent participates. In addition, it is unusual for adolescents with behavioral/attention problems not to have been previously given a diagnosis of ADHD. Therefore, it is important to establish the younger manifestations of the condition that were missed and to strongly consider substance use, depression, and anxiety as alternative or co-occurring diagnoses. Adolescents with ADHD, especially when untreated, are at greater risk of substance abuse.[26] In addition, the risks of

mood and anxiety disorders and risky sexual behaviors increase during adolescence.[12]

Special Circumstances: Inattention or Hyperactivity/Impulsivity (Problem Level)

Teachers, parents, and child health professionals typically encounter children with behaviors relating to activity level, impulsivity, and inattention who might not fully meet DSM-IV criteria. The DSM-PC[3] provides a guide to the more common behaviors seen in pediatrics. The manual describes common variations in behavior as well as more problematic behaviors at levels of less impairment than those specified in the DSM-IV.

The behavioral descriptions of the DSM-PC have not yet been tested in community studies to determine the prevalence or severity of developmental variations and problems in the areas of inattention, hyperactivity, or impulsivity. They do, however, provide guidance to clinicians regarding elements of treatment for children with problems with mild-to-moderate inattention, hyperactivity, or impulsivity. The DSM-PC also considers environmental influences on a child's behavior and provides information on differential diagnosis with a developmental perspective.

Action statement 3: In the evaluation of a child for ADHD, the primary care clinician should include assessment for other conditions that might coexist with ADHD, including emotional or behavioral (eg, anxiety, depressive, oppositional defiant, and conduct disorders), developmental (eg, learning and language disorders or other neurodevelopmental disorders), and physical (eg, tics, sleep apnea) conditions (quality of evidence B/strong recommendation).

Evidence Profile

- **Aggregate evidence quality:** B.
- **Benefits:** Identifying coexisting conditions is important for developing the most appropriate treatment plan.
- **Harms/risks/costs:** The major risk is misdiagnosing the conditions and providing inappropriate care.
- **Benefits-harms assessment:** There is a preponderance of benefit over harm.
- **Value judgments:** The committee members took into consideration the common occurrence of coexisting conditions and the importance of addressing them in making this recommendation.
- **Role of patient preferences:** None.
- **Exclusions:** None.
- **Intentional vagueness:** None.
- **Strength: strong recommendation.**

A variety of other behavioral, developmental, and physical conditions can coexist in children who are evaluated for ADHD. These conditions include, but are not limited to, learning problems, language disorder, disruptive behavior, anxiety, mood disorders, tic disorders, seizures, developmental coordination disorder, or sleep disorders.[23,24,27–38] In some cases, the presence of a coexisting condition will alter the treatment of ADHD. The primary care clinician might benefit from additional support and guidance or might need to refer a child with ADHD and coexisting conditions, such as severe mood or anxiety disorders, to subspecialists for assessment and management. The subspecialists could include child psychiatrists, developmental-behavioral pediatricians, neurodevelopmental disability physicians, child neurologists, or child or school psychologists.

Given the likelihood that another condition exists, primary care clinicians should conduct assessments that determine or at least identify the risk of coexisting conditions. Through its Task Force on Mental Health, the AAP has developed algorithms and a toolkit[39] for assessing and treating (or comanaging) the most common developmental disorders and mental health concerns in children. These resources might be useful in assessing children who are being evaluated for ADHD. Payment for evaluation and treatment must cover the fixed and variable costs of providing the services, as noted in the AAP policy statement "Scope of Health Care Benefits for Children From Birth Through Age 26.[40]

Special Circumstances: Adolescents

Clinicians should assess adolescent patients with newly diagnosed ADHD for symptoms and signs of substance abuse; when these signs and symptoms are found, evaluation and treatment for addiction should precede treatment for ADHD, if possible, or careful treatment for ADHD can begin if necessary.[25]

Action statement 4: The primary care clinician should recognize ADHD as a chronic condition and, therefore, consider children and adolescents with ADHD as children and youth with special health care needs. Management of children and youth with special health care needs should follow the principles of the chronic care model and the medical home (quality of evidence B/strong recommendation).

Evidence Profile

- **Aggregate evidence quality:** B.
- **Benefits:** The recommendation describes the coordinated services most appropriate for managing the condition.
- **Harms/risks/costs:** Providing the services might be more costly.
- **Benefits-harms assessment:** There is a preponderance of benefit over harm.
- **Value judgments:** The committee members considered the value of medical home services when deciding to make this recommendation.
- **Role of patient preferences:** Family preference in how these services are provided is an important consideration.
- **Exclusions:** None.
- **Intentional vagueness:** None.
- **Strength: strong recommendation.**

As in the previous guideline, this recommendation is based on the evidence that ADHD continues to cause symptoms and dysfunction in many children who have the condition over long periods of time, even into adulthood, and that the treatments available address symptoms and function but are usually not curative. Although the chronic illness model has not been specifically studied in children and youth with ADHD, it has been effective for other chronic conditions such as asthma,[23] and the medical home model has been accepted as the preferred standard of care.[41] The management process is also helped by encouraging strong family-school partnerships.[42]

Longitudinal studies have found that, frequently, treatments are not sustained despite the fact that long-term outcomes for children with ADHD indicate that they are at greater risk of significant problems if they discontinue treatment.[43] Because a number of parents of children with ADHD also have ADHD, extra support might be necessary to help those parents provide medication on a consistent basis and institute a consistent behavioral program. The medical home and chronic illness approach is provided in the process algorithm (Supplemental Fig 2). An important process in ongoing care is bidirectional communication with teachers and other school and mental health clinicians involved in the child's care as well as with parents and patients.

Special Circumstances: Inattention or Hyperactivity/Impulsivity (Problem Level)

Children with inattention or hyperactivity/impulsivity at the problem level (DSM-PC) and their families might also benefit from the same chronic illness and medical home principles.

Action statement 5: Recommendations for treatment of children and youth with ADHD vary depending on the patient's age.

Action statement 5a: For *preschoolaged children (4–5 years of age)*, the primary care clinician should prescribe evidence-based parent- and/or teacher-administered behavior therapy as the first line of treatment (quality of evidence A/strong recommendation) and may prescribe methylphenidate if the behavior interventions do not provide significant improvement and there is moderate-to-severe continuing disturbance in the child's function. In areas in which evidence-based behavioral treatments are not available, the clinician needs to weigh the risks of starting medication at an early age against the harm of delaying diagnosis and treatment (quality of evidence B/recommendation).

Evidence Profile

- **Aggregate evidence quality:** A for behavior; B for methylphenidate.
- **Benefits:** Both behavior therapy and methylphenidate have been demonstrated to reduce behaviors associated with ADHD and improve function.
- **Harms/risks/costs:** Both therapies increase the cost of care, and behavior therapy requires a higher level of family involvement, whereas methylphenidate has some potential adverse effects.
- **Benefits-harms assessment:** Given the risks of untreated ADHD, the benefits outweigh the risks.
- **Value judgments:** The committee mem-

bers included the effects of untreated ADHD when deciding to make this recommendation.

- **Role of patient preferences:** Family preference is essential in determining the treatment plan.
- **Exclusions:** None.
- **Intentional vagueness:** None.
- **Strength: strong recommendation.**

Action statement 5b: For *elementary school-aged children (6–11 years of age)*, the primary care clinician should prescribe FDA-approved medications for ADHD (quality of evidence A/strong recommendation) and/or evidence-based parent- and/or teacher-administered behavior therapy as treatment for ADHD, preferably both (quality of evidence B/strong recommendation). The evidence is particularly strong for stimulant medications and sufficient but less strong for atomoxetine, extended-release guanfacine, and extended-release clonidine (in that order) (quality of evidence A/strong recommendation). The school environment, program, or placement is a part of any treatment plan.

Evidence Profile

- **Aggregate evidence quality:** A for treatment with FDA-approved medications; B for behavior therapy.
- **Benefits:** Both behavior therapy and FDA-approved medications have been demonstrated to reduce behaviors associated with ADHD and improve function.
- **Harms/risks/costs:** Both therapies increase the cost of care, and behavior therapy requires a higher level of family involvement, whereas FDA-approved medications have some potential adverse effects.
- **Benefits-harms assessment:** Given the risks of untreated ADHD, the benefits outweigh the risks.
- **Value judgments:** The committee members included the effects of untreated

ADHD when deciding to make this recommendation.

- **Role of patient preferences:** Family preference, including patient preference, is essential in determining the treatment plan.
- **Exclusions:** None.
- **Intentional vagueness:** None.
- **Strength: strong recommendation.**

Action statement 5c: For *adolescents (12–18 years of age)*, the primary care clinician should prescribe FDA-approved medications for ADHD with the assent of the adolescent (quality of evidence A/strong recommendation) and may prescribe behavior therapy as treatment for ADHD (quality of evidence C/recommendation), preferably both.

Evidence Profile

- **Aggregate evidence quality:** A for medications; C for behavior therapy.
- **Benefits:** Both behavior therapy and FDA-approved medications have been demonstrated to reduce behaviors associated with ADHD and improve function.
- **Harms/risks/costs:** Both therapies increase the cost of care, and behavior therapy requires a higher level of family involvement, whereas FDA-approved medications have some potential adverse effects.
- **Benefits-harms assessment:** Given the risks of untreated ADHD, the benefits outweigh the risks.
- **Value judgments:** The committee members included the effects of untreated ADHD when deciding to make this recommendation.
- **Role of patient preferences:** Family preference, including patient preference, is essential in determining the treatment plan.
- **Exclusions:** None.
- **Intentional vagueness:** None.
- **Strength: strong recommendation/ recommendation.**

Medication

Similar to the recommendations from the previous guideline, stimulant medications are highly effective for most children in reducing core symptoms of ADHD.[44] One selective norepinephrine-reuptake inhibitor (atomoxetine[45,46]) and 2 selective α_2-adrenergic agonists (extended-release guanfacine[47,48] and extended-release clonidine[49]) have also demonstrated efficacy in reducing core symptoms. Because norepinephrine-reuptake inhibitors and α_2-adrenergic agonists are newer, the evidence base that supports them—although adequate for FDA approval—is considerably smaller than that for stimulants. None of them have been approved for use in preschool-aged children. Compared with stimulant medications that have an effect size [effect size = (treatment mean − control mean)/control SD] of approximately 1.0,[50] the effects of the nonstimulants are slightly weaker; atomoxetine has an effect size of approximately 0.7, and extended-release guanfacine and extended-release clonidine also have effect sizes of approximately 0.7.

The accompanying process-of-care algorithm provides a list of the currently available FDA-approved medications for ADHD (Supplemental Table 3). Characteristics of each medication are provided to help guide the clinician's choice in prescribing medication.

As was identified in the previous guideline, the most common stimulant adverse effects are appetite loss, abdominal pain, headaches, and sleep disturbance. The results of the Multimodal Therapy of ADHD (MTA) study revealed a more persistent effect of stimulants on decreasing growth velocity than have most previous studies, particularly when children were on higher and more consistently administered doses. The effects diminished by the third year of treatment, but no compensatory rebound effects were found.[51] However, diminished growth was in the range of 1 to 2 cm. An uncommon additional significant adverse effect of stimulants is the occurrence of hallucinations and other psychotic symptoms.[52] Although concerns have been raised about the rare occurrence of sudden cardiac death among children using stimulant medications,[53] sudden death in children on stimulant medication is extremely rare, and evidence is conflicting as to whether stimulant medications increase the risk of sudden death.[54–56] It is important to expand the history to include specific cardiac symptoms, Wolf-Parkinson-White syndrome, sudden death in the family, hypertrophic cardiomyopathy, and long QT syndrome. Preschool-aged children might experience increased mood lability and dysphoria.[57] For the nonstimulant atomoxetine, the adverse effects include initial somnolence and gastrointestinal tract symptoms, particularly if the dosage is increased too rapidly; decrease in appetite; increase in suicidal thoughts (less common); and hepatitis (rare). For the nonstimulant α_2-adrenergic agonists extended-release guanfacine and extended-release clonidine, adverse effects include somnolence and dry mouth.

Only 2 medications have evidence to support their use as adjunctive therapy with stimulant medications sufficient to achieve FDA approval: extended-release guanfacine[26] and extended-release clonidine. Other medications have been used in combination off-label, but there is currently only anecdotal evidence for their safety or efficacy, so their use cannot be recommended at this time.

Special Circumstances: Preschool-aged Children

A number of special circumstances support the recommendation to initiate ADHD treatment in preschool-aged children (ages 4–5 years) with behavioral therapy alone first.[57] These circumstances include:

- The multisite study of methylphenidate[57] was limited to preschool-aged children who had moderate-to-severe dysfunction.

- The study also found that many children (ages 4–5 years) experience improvements in symptoms with behavior therapy alone, and the overall evidence for behavior therapy in preschool-aged children is strong.

- Behavioral programs for children 4 to 5 years of age typically run in the form of group parent-training programs and, although not always compensated by health insurance, have a lower cost. The process algorithm (see Supplemental pages s15-16) contains criteria for the clinician to use in assessing the quality of the behavioral therapy. In addition, programs such as Head Start and Children and Adults With Attention Deficit Hyperactivity Disorder (CHADD) (www.chadd.org) might provide some behavioral supports.

Many young children with ADHD might still require medication to achieve maximum improvement, and medication is not contraindicated for children 4 through 5 years of age. However, only 1 multisite study has carefully assessed medication use in preschool-aged children. Other considerations in the recommendation about treating children 4 to 5 years of age with stimulant medications include:

- The study was limited to preschool-aged children who had moderate-to-severe dysfunction.

- Research has found that a number of young children (4–5 years of age) experience improvements in symptoms with behavior therapy alone.

- There are concerns about the possible effects on growth during this rapid growth period of preschool-aged children.

- There has been limited information about and experience with the effects of stimulant medication in children between the ages of 4 and 5 years.

Here, the criteria for enrollment (and, therefore, medication use) included measures of severity that distinguished treated children from the larger group of preschool-aged children with ADHD. Thus, before initiating medications, the physician should assess the severity of the child's ADHD. Given current data, only those preschool-aged children with ADHD who have moderate-to-severe dysfunction should be considered for medication. Criteria for this level of severity, based on the multisite-study results,[57] are (1) symptoms that have persisted for at least 9 months, (2) dysfunction that is manifested in both the home and other settings such as preschool or child care, and (3) dysfunction that has not responded adequately to behavior therapy. The decision to consider initiating medication at this age depends in part on the clinician's assessment of the estimated developmental impairment, safety risks, or consequences for school or social participation that could ensue if medications are not initiated. It is often helpful to consult with a mental health specialist who has had specific experience with preschool-aged children if possible.

Dextroamphetamine is the only medication approved by the FDA for use in children younger than 6 years of age. This approval, however, was based on less stringent criteria in force when the medication was approved rather than on empirical evidence of its safety and efficacy in this age group. Most of the evidence for the safety and efficacy of treating preschool-aged children with stimulant medications has been

from methylphenidate.[57] Methylphenidate evidence consists of 1 multisite study of 165 children and 10 other smaller single-site studies that included from 11 to 59 children (total of 269 children); 7 of the 10 single-site studies found significant efficacy. It must be noted that although there is moderate evidence that methylphenidate is safe and efficacious in preschool-aged children, its use in this age group remains off-label. Although the use of dextroamphetamine is on-label, the insufficient evidence for its safety and efficacy in this age group does not make it possible to recommend at this time.

If children do not experience adequate symptom improvement with behavior therapy, medication can be prescribed, as described previously. Evidence suggests that the rate of metabolizing stimulant medication is slower in children 4 through 5 years of age, so they should be given a lower dose to start, and the dose can be increased in smaller increments. Maximum doses have not been adequately studied.[57]

Special Circumstances: Adolescents

As noted previously, before beginning medication treatment for adolescents with newly diagnosed ADHD, clinicians should assess these patients for symptoms of substance abuse. When substance use is identified, assessment when off the abusive substances should precede treatment for ADHD (see the Task Force on Mental Health report[7]). Diversion of ADHD medication (use for other than its intended medical purposes) is also a special concern among adolescents[58]; clinicians should monitor symptoms and prescription-refill requests for signs of misuse or diversion of ADHD medication and consider prescribing medications with no abuse potential, such as atomoxetine (Strattera [Ely Lilly Co, Indianapolis, IN]) and

extended-release guanfacine (Intuniv [Shire US Inc, Wayne, PA]) or extended-release clonidine (Kapvay [Shionogi Inc, Florham Park, NJ]) (which are not stimulants) or stimulant medications with less abuse potential, such as lisdexamfetamine (Vyvanse [Shire US Inc]), dermal methylphenidate (Daytrana [Noven Therapeutics, LLC, Miami, FL]), or OROS methylphenidate (Concerta [Janssen Pharmaceuticals, Inc, Titusville, NJ]). Because lisdexamfetamine is dextroamphetamine, which contains an additional lysine molecule, it is only activated after ingestion, when it is metabolized by erythrocyte cells to dexamphetamine. The other preparations make extraction of the stimulant medication more difficult.

Given the inherent risks of driving by adolescents with ADHD, special concern should be taken to provide medication coverage for symptom control while driving. Longer-acting or late-afternoon, short-acting medications might be helpful in this regard.[59]

Special Circumstances: Inattention or Hyperactivity/Impulsivity (Problem Level)

Medication is not appropriate for children whose symptoms do not meet DSM-IV criteria for diagnosis of ADHD, although behavior therapy does not require a specific diagnosis, and many of the efficacy studies have included children without specific mental behavioral disorders.

Behavior Therapy

Behavior therapy represents a broad set of specific interventions that have a common goal of modifying the physical and social environment to alter or change behavior. Behavior therapy usually is implemented by training parents in specific techniques that improve their abilities to modify and

TABLE 1 Evidence-Based Behavioral Treatments for ADHD

Intervention Type	Description	Typical Outcome(s)	Median Effect Size[a]
Behavioral parent training (BPT)	Behavior-modification principles provided to parents for implementation in home settings	Improved compliance with parental commands; improved parental understanding of behavioral principles; high levels of parental satisfaction with treatment	0.55
Behavioral classroom management	Behavior-modification principles provided to teachers for implementation in classroom settings	Improved attention to instruction; improved compliance with classroom rules; decreased disruptive behavior; improved work productivity	0.61
Behavioral peer interventions (BPI)[b]	Interventions focused on peer interactions/relationships; these are often group-based interventions provided weekly and include clinic-based social-skills training used either alone or concurrently with behavioral parent training and/or medication	Office-based interventions have produced minimal effects; interventions have been of questionable social validity; some studies of BPI combined with clinic-based BPT found positive effects on parent ratings of ADHD symptoms; no differences on social functioning or parent ratings of social behavior have been revealed	

[a] Effect size = (treatment median − control median)/control SD.

[b] The effect size for behavioral peer interventions is not reported, because the effect sizes for these studies represent outcomes associated with combined interventions. A lower effect size means that they have less of an effect. The effect sizes found are considered moderate.

Adapted from Pelham W, Fabiano GA. *J Clin Child Adolesc Psychol.* 2008;37(1):184–214.

shape their child's behavior and to improve the child's ability to regulate his or her own behavior. The training involves techniques to more effectively provide rewards when their child demonstrates the desired behavior (eg, positive reinforcement), learn what behaviors can be reduced or eliminated by using planned ignoring as an active strategy (or using praising and ignoring in combination), or provide appropriate consequences or punishments when their child fails to meet the goals (eg, punishment). There is a need to consistently apply rewards and consequences as tasks are achieved and then to gradually increase the expectations for each task as they are mastered to shape behaviors. Although behavior therapy shares a set of principles, individual programs introduce different techniques and strategies to achieve the same ends.

Table 1 lists the major behavioral intervention approaches that have been demonstrated to be evidence based for the management of ADHD in 3 different types of settings. The table is based on 22 studies, each completed between 1997 and 2006.

Evidence for the effectiveness of behavior therapy in children with ADHD is derived from a variety of studies[60–62] and an Agency for Healthcare Research and Quality review.[5] The diversity of interventions and outcome measures makes meta-analysis of the effects of behavior therapy alone or in association with medications challenging. The long-term positive effects of behavior therapy have yet to be determined. Ongoing adherence to a behavior program might be important; therefore, implementing a chronic care model for child health might contribute to the long-term effects.[63]

Study results have indicated positive effects of behavior therapy when combined with medications. Most studies that compared behavior therapy to stimulants found a much stronger effect on ADHD core symptoms from stimulants than from behavior therapy. The MTA study found that combined treatment (behavior therapy and stimulant medication) was not significantly more efficacious than treatment with medication alone for the core symptoms of ADHD after correction for multiple tests in the primary analysis.[64] However, a secondary analysis of a combined measure of parent and teacher ratings of ADHD symptoms revealed a significant advantage for the combination with a small effect size of $d = 0.26$.[65] However, the same study also found that the combined treatment compared with medication alone did offer greater improvements on academic and conduct measures when ADHD coexisted with anxiety and when children lived in low socioeconomic environments. In addition, parents and teachers of children who were receiving combined therapy were significantly more satisfied with the treatment plan. Finally, the combination of medication management and behavior therapy allowed for the use of lower dosages of stimulants, which possibly reduced the risk of adverse effects.[66]

School Programming and Supports

Behavior therapy programs coordinating efforts at school as well as home might enhance the effects. School programs can provide classroom adaptations, such as preferred seating, modified work assignments, and test modifications (to the location at which it is administered and time allotted for taking the test), as well as behavior plans as part of a 504 Rehabilitation Act Plan or special education Individualized Education Program (IEP) under the "other health impairment" designation as part of the Individuals With

Disability Education Act (IDEA).[67] It is helpful for clinicians to be aware of the eligibility criteria in their state and school district to advise families of their options. Youths documented to have ADHD can also get permission to take college-readiness tests in an untimed manner by following appropriate documentation guidelines.[68]

The effect of coexisting conditions on ADHD treatment is variable. In some cases, treatment of the ADHD resolves the coexisting condition. For example, treatment of ADHD might resolve oppositional defiant disorder or anxiety.[68] However, sometimes the co-occurring condition might require treatment that is in addition to the treatment for ADHD. Some coexisting conditions can be treated in the primary care setting, but others will require referral and co-management with a subspecialist.

Action statement 6: Primary care clinicians should titrate doses of medication for ADHD to achieve maximum benefit with minimum adverse effects (quality of evidence B/strong recommendation).

Evidence Profile

- **Aggregate evidence quality:** B.
- **Benefits:** The optimal dose of medication is required to reduce core symptoms to or as close to the levels of children without ADHD.
- **Harms/risks/costs:** Higher levels of medication increase the chances of adverse effects.
- **Benefits-harms assessment:** The importance of adequately treating ADHD outweighs the risk of adverse effects.
- **Value judgments:** The committee members included the effects of untreated ADHD when deciding to make this recommendation.
- **Role of patient preferences:** The families' preferences and comfort need to be taken into consideration in developing a titration plan.
- **Exclusions:** None.

- **Intentional vagueness:** None.
- **Strength: strong recommendation.**

The findings from the MTA study suggested that more than 70% of children and youth with ADHD respond to one of the stimulant medications at an optimal dose when a systematic trial is used.[65] Children in the MTA who were treated in the community with care as usual from whomever they chose or to whom they had access received lower doses of stimulants with less frequent monitoring and had less optimal results.[65] Because stimulants might produce positive but suboptimal effects at a low dose in some children and youth, titration to maximum doses that control symptoms without adverse effects is recommended instead of titration strictly on a milligram-per-kilogram basis.

Education of parents is an important component in the chronic illness model to ensure their cooperation in efforts to reach appropriate titration (remembering that the parents themselves might be challenged significantly by ADHD).[69,70] The primary care clinician should alert parents and children that changing medication dose and occasionally changing a medication might be necessary for optimal medication management, that the process might require a few months to achieve optimal success, and that medication efficacy should be systematically monitored at regular intervals.

Because stimulant medication effects are seen immediately, trials of different doses of stimulants can be accomplished in a relatively short time period. Stimulant medications can be effectively titrated on a 3- to 7-day basis.[65]

It is important to note that by the 3-year follow-up of 14-month MTA interventions (optimal medications management, optimal behavioral management, the combination of the 2, or community treatment), all differences among the initial 4 groups were no longer present. After the initial 14-month intervention, the children no longer received the careful monthly monitoring provided by the study and went back to receiving care from their community providers. Their medications and doses varied, and a number of them were no longer taking medication. In children still on medication, the growth deceleration was only seen for the first 2 years and was in the range of 1 to 2 cm.

CONCLUSION

Evidence continues to be fairly clear with regard to the legitimacy of the diagnosis of ADHD and the appropriate diagnostic criteria and procedures required to establish a diagnosis, identify co-occurring conditions, and treat effectively with both behavioral and pharmacologic interventions. However, the steps required to sustain appropriate treatments and achieve successful long-term outcomes still remain a challenge. To provide more detailed information about how the recommendations of this guideline can be accomplished, a more detailed but less strongly evidence-based algorithm is provided as a companion article.

AREAS FOR FUTURE RESEARCH

Some specific research topics pertinent to the diagnosis and treatment of ADHD or developmental variations or problems in children and adolescents in primary care to be explored include:

- identification or development of reliable instruments suitable to use in primary care to assess the nature or degree of functional impairment in children/adolescents with ADHD and monitor improvement over time;
- study of medications and other therapies used clinically but not approved by the FDA for ADHD, such as

electroencephalographic biofeedback;

- determination of the optimal schedule for monitoring children/adolescents with ADHD, including factors for adjusting that schedule according to age, symptom severity, and progress reports;

- evaluation of the effectiveness of various school-based interventions;

- comparisons of medication use and effectiveness in different ages, including both harms and benefits;

- development of methods to involve parents and children/adolescents in their own care and improve adherence to both behavior and medication treatments;

- standardized and documented tools that will help primary care providers in identifying coexisting conditions;

- development and determination of effective electronic and Web-based systems to help gather information to diagnose and monitor children with ADHD;

- improved systems of communication with schools and mental health professionals, as well as other community agencies, to provide effective collaborative care;

- evidence for optimal monitoring by

some aspects of severity, disability, or impairment; and

- long-term outcomes of children first identified with ADHD as preschool-aged children.

SUBCOMMITTEE ON ATTENTION DEFICIT HYPERACTIVITY DISORDER (OVERSIGHT BY THE STEERING COMMITTEE ON QUALITY IMPROVEMENT AND MANAGEMENT, 2005–2011)

WRITING COMMITTEE

Mark Wolraich, MD, Chair – *(periodic consultant to Shire, Eli Lilly, Shinogi, and Next Wave Pharmaceuticals)*

Lawrence Brown, MD – *(neurologist; AAP Section on Neurology; Child Neurology Society) (Safety Monitoring Board for Best Pharmaceuticals for Children Act for National Institutes of Health)*

Ronald T. Brown, PhD – *(child psychologist; Society for Pediatric Psychology) (no conflicts)*

George DuPaul, PhD – *(school psychologist; National Association of School Psychologists) (participated in clinical trial on Vyvanse effects on college students with ADHD, funded by Shire; published 2 books on ADHD and receives royalties)*

Marian Earls, MD – *(general pediatrician with QI expertise, developmental and behavioral pediatrician) (no conflicts)*

Heidi M. Feldman, MD, PhD – *(developmental and behavioral pediatrician; Society for Developmental and Behavioral Pediatricians) (no conflicts)*

Theodore G. Ganiats, MD – *(family physician; American Academy of Family Physicians) (no conflicts)*

Beth Kaplanek, RN, BSN – *(parent advocate, Children and Adults With Attention Deficit Hyperactivity Disorder [CHADD]) (no conflicts)*

Bruce Meyer, MD – *(general pediatrician) (no conflicts)*

James Perrin, MD – *(general pediatrician; AAP Mental Health Task Force, AAP Council on Children With Disabilities) (consultant to Pfizer not related to ADHD)*

Karen Pierce, MD – *(child psychiatrist; American Academy of Child and Adolescent Psychiatry) (no conflicts)*

Michael Reiff, MD – *(developmental and behavioral pediatrician; AAP Section on Developmental and Behavioral Pediatrics) (no conflicts)*

Martin T. Stein, MD – *(developmental and behavioral pediatrician; AAP Section on Developmental and Behavioral Pediatrics) (no conflicts)*

Susanna Visser, MS – *(epidemiologist) (no conflicts)*

CONSULTANT

Melissa Capers, MA, MFA – *(medical writer) (no conflicts)*

STAFF

Caryn Davidson, MA

ACKNOWLEDGMENTS

This guideline was developed with support from the Partnership for Policy Implementation (PPI) initiative. Physicians trained in medical informatics were involved with formatting the algorithm and helping to keep the key action statements actionable, decidable, and executable.

REFERENCES

1. American Academy of Pediatrics, Committee on Quality Improvement and Subcommittee on Attention-Deficit/Hyperactivity Disorder. Clinical practice guideline: diagnosis and evaluation of the child with attention-deficit/hyperactivity disorder. *Pediatrics.* 2000;105(5):1158–1170

2. American Academy of Pediatrics, Subcommittee on Attention-Deficit/Hyperactivity Disorder, Committee on Quality Improvement. Clinical practice guideline: treatment of the school-aged child with attention-deficit/hyperactivity disorder. *Pediatrics.* 2001;108(4):1033–1044

3. Wolraich ML, Felice ME, Drotar DD. *The Classification of Child and Adolescent Mental Conditions in Primary Care: Diagnostic and Statistical Manual for Primary Care (DSM-PC), Child and Adolescent Version.* Elk Grove, IL: American Academy of Pediatrics; 1996

4. *EndNote* [computer program]. 10th ed. Carlsbad, CA: Thompson Reuters; 2009

5. Charach A, Dashti B, Carson P, Booker L, Lim CG, Lillie E, Yeung E, Ma J, Raina P, Schachar R. *Attention Deficit Hyperactivity Disorder: Effectiveness of Treatment in At-Risk Preschoolers; Long-term Effectiveness in All Ages; and Variability in Prevalence, Diagnosis, and Treatment.* Comparative Effectiveness Review No. 44. (Prepared by the McMaster University Evidence-based Practice Center under Contract No. MME2202 290-02-0020.) AHRQ Publication No. 12-EHC003-EF. Rockville, MD: Agency for Healthcare Research and Quality. October 2011.

6. American Academy of Pediatrics, Steering Committee on Quality Improvement. Classifying recommendations for clinical practice guidelines. *Pediatrics.* 2004;114(3):874–877

7. Foy JM; American Academy of Pediatrics Task Force on Mental Health. Enhancing pediatric mental health care: report from the American Academy of Pediatrics Task Force on Mental Health. Introduction. *Pediatrics.* 2010;125(suppl 3)S69–S174

8. Visser SN, Lesesne CA, Perou R. National estimates and factors associated with medication treatment for childhood

attention-deficit/hyperactivity disorder. *Pediatrics*. 2007;119(suppl 1):S99–S106

9. Centers for Disease Control and Prevention. Mental health in the United States: prevalence of diagnosis and medication treatment for attention-deficit/hyperactivity disorder—United States, 2003. *MMWR Morb Mortal Wkly Rep*. 2005; 54(34):842–847

10. Centers for Disease Control and Prevention. Increasing prevalence of parent-reported attention deficit/hyperactivity disorder among children: United States, 2003–2007. *MMWR Morb Mortal Wkly Rep*. 2010;59(44): 1439–1443

11. Egger HL, Kondo D, Angold A. The epidemiology and diagnostic issues in preschool attention-deficit/hyperactivity disorder. *Infant Young Child*. 2006;19(2):109–122

12. Wolraich ML, Wibbelsman CJ, Brown TE, et al. Attention-deficit/hyperactivity disorder among adolescents: a review of the diagnosis, treatment, and clinical implications. *Pediatrics*. 2005;115(6):1734–1746

13. American Psychiatric Association. *Diagnostic and Statistical Manual of Mental Disorders, 4th ed, Text Revision (DSM-IV-TR)*. Washington, DC: American Psychiatric Association; 2000

14. American Psychiatric Association. Diagnostic criteria for attention deficit/hyperactivity disorder. Available at: www.dsm5.org/ProposedRevision/Pages/proposedrevision.aspx?rid=383. Accessed September 30, 2011

15. Lahey BB, Pelham WE, Stein MA, et al. Validity of DSM-IV attention-deficit/hyperactivity disorder for younger children [published correction appears in *J Am Acad Child Adolesc Psychiatry*. 1999;38(2):222]. *J Am Acad Child Adolesc Psychiatry*. 1998;37(7):695–702

16. Pavuluri MN, Luk SL, McGee R. Parent reported preschool attention deficit hyperactivity: measurement and validity. *Eur Child Adolesc Psychiatry*. 1999;8(2): 126–133

17. Harvey EA, Youngwirth SD, Thakar DA, Errazuriz PA. Predicting attention-deficit/hyperactivity disorder and oppositional defiant disorder from preschool diagnostic assessments. *J Consult Clin Psychol*. 2009; 77(2):349–354

18. Keenan K, Wakschlag LS. More than the terrible twos: the nature and severity of behavior problems in clinic-referred preschool children. *J Abnorm Child Psychol*. 2000; 28(1):33–46

19. Gadow KD, Nolan EE, Litcher L, et al. Comparison of attention-deficit/hyperactivity disorder symptoms subtypes in Ukrainian schoolchildren. *J Am Acad Child Adolesc Psychiatry*. 2000;39(12):1520–1527

20. Sprafkin J, Volpe RJ, Gadow KD, Nolan EE, Kelly K. A DSM-IV-referenced screening instrument for preschool children: the Early Childhood Inventory-4. *J Am Acad Child Adolesc Psychiatry*. 2002;41(5): 604–612

21. Poblano A, Romero E. ECI-4 screening of attention deficit-hyperactivity disorder and co-morbidity in Mexican preschool children: preliminary results. *Arq Neuropsiquiatr*. 2006;64(4):932–936

22. McGoey KE, DuPaul GJ, Haley E, Shelton TL. Parent and teacher ratings of attention-deficit/hyperactivity disorder in preschool: the ADHD Rating Scale-IV Preschool Version. *J Psychopathol Behav Assess*. 2007;29(4): 269–276

23. Young J. Common comorbidities seen in adolescents with attention-deficit/hyperactivity disorder. *Adolesc Med State Art Rev*. 2008;19(2): 216–228, vii

24. Freeman R; Tourette Syndrome International Database Consortium. Tic disorders and ADHD: answers from a worldwide clinical dataset on Tourette syndrome [published correction appears in *Eur Child Adolesc Psychiatry*. 2007; 16(8):536]. *Eur Child Adolesc Psychiatry*. 2007;16(1 suppl):15–23

25. Riggs P. Clinical approach to treatment of ADHD in adolescents with substance use disorders and conduct disorder. *J Am Acad Child Adolesc Psychiatry*. 1998;37(3): 331–332

26. Kratochvil CJ, Vaughan BS, Stoner JA, et al. A double-blind, placebo-controlled study of atomoxetine in young children with ADHD. *Pediatrics*. 2011;127(4). Available at: www.pediatrics.org/cgi/content/full/127/4/e862

27. Rowland AS, Lesesne CA, Abramowitz AJ. The epidemiology of attention-deficit/hyperactivity disorder (ADHD): a public health view. *Ment Retard Dev Disabil Res Rev*. 2002;8(3):162–170

28. Cuffe SP, Moore CG, McKeown RE. Prevalence and correlates of ADHD symptoms in the national health interview survey. *J Atten Disord*. 2005;9(2):392–401

29. Pastor PN, Reuben CA. Diagnosed attention deficit hyperactivity disorder and learning disability: United States, 2004–2006. *Vital Health Stat 10*. 2008;(237):1–14

30. Biederman J, Faraone SV, Wozniak J, Mick E, Kwon A, Aleardi M. Further evidence of unique developmental phenotypic correlates of pediatric bipolar disorder: findings from a large sample of clinically referred preadolescent children assessed over the last 7 years. *J Affect Disord*. 2004;82(suppl 1):S45–S58

31. Biederman J, Kwon A, Aleardi M. Absence of gender effects on attention deficit hyperactivity disorder: findings in nonreferred subjects. *Am J Psychiatry*. 2005;162(6): 1083–1089

32. Biederman J, Ball SW, Monuteaux MC, et al. New insights into the comorbidity between ADHD and major depression in adolescent and young adult females. *J Am Acad Child Adolesc Psychiatry*. 2008; 47(4):426–434

33. Biederman J, Melmed RD, Patel A, McBurnett K, Donahue J, Lyne A. Long-term, open-label extension study of guanfacine extended release in children and adolescents with ADHD. *CNS Spectr*. 2008;13(12): 1047–1055

34. Crabtree VM, Ivanenko A, Gozal D. Clinical and parental assessment of sleep in children with attention-deficit/hyperactivity disorder referred to a pediatric sleep medicine center. *Clin Pediatr (Phila)*. 2003;42(9): 807–813

35. LeBourgeois MK, Avis K, Mixon M, Olmi J, Harsh J. Snoring, sleep quality, and sleepiness across attention-deficit/hyperactivity disorder subtypes. *Sleep*. 2004;27(3): 520–525

36. Chan E, Zhan C, Homer CJ. Health care use and costs for children with attention-deficit/hyperactivity disorder: national estimates from the medical expenditure panel survey. *Arch Pediatr Adolesc Med*. 2002; 156(5):504–511

37. Newcorn JH, Miller SR, Ivanova I, et al. Adolescent outcome of ADHD: impact of childhood conduct and anxiety disorders. *CNS Spectr*. 2004;9(9):668–678

38. Sung V, Hiscock H, Sciberras E, Efron D. Sleep problems in children with attention-deficit/hyperactivity disorder: prevalence and the effect on the child and family. *Arch Pediatr Adolesc Med*. 2008; 162(4):336–342

39. American Academy of Pediatrics, Task Force on Mental Health. *Addressing Mental Health Concerns in Primary Care: A Clinician's Toolkit* [CD-ROM]. Elk Grove Village, IL: American Academy of Pediatrics; 2010

40. American Academy of Pediatrics, Committee on Child Health Financing. Scope of health care benefits for children from birth through age 26. *Pediatrics*. 2012; In press

41. Brito A, Grant R, Overholt S, et al. The enhanced medical home: the pediatric standard of care for medically underserved children. *Adv Pediatr*. 2008;55:9–28

42. Homer C, Klatka K, Romm D, et al. A review of the evidence for the medical home for children with special health care needs. *Pediatrics*. 2008;122(4). Available at: www.pediatrics.org/cgi/content/full/122/4/e922

43. Ingram S, Hechtman L, Morgenstern G. Outcome issues in ADHD: adolescent and adult long-term outcome. *Ment Retard Dev Disabil Res Rev.* 1999;5(3):243–250

44. Barbaresi WJ, Katusic SK, Colligan RC, Weaver AL, Jacobsen SJ. Modifiers of long-term school outcomes for children with attention-deficit/hyperactivity disorder: does treatment with stimulant medication make a difference? Results from a population-based study. *J Dev Behav Pediatr.* 2007;28(4):274–287

45. Cheng JY, Cheng RY, Ko JS, Ng EM. Efficacy and safety of atomoxetine for attention-deficit/hyperactivity disorder in children and adolescents-meta-analysis and meta-regression analysis. *Psychopharmacology.* 2007;194(2):197–209

46. Michelson D, Allen AJ, Busner J, Casat C, Dunn D, Kratochvil CJ. Once daily atomoxetine treatment for children and adolescents with ADHD: a randomized, placebo-controlled study. *Am J Psychiatry.* 2002; 159(11):1896–1901

47. Biederman J, Melmed RD, Patel A, et al; SPD503 Study Group. A randomized, double-blind, placebo-controlled study of guanfacine extended release in children and adolescents with attention-deficit/hyperactivity disorder. *Pediatrics.* 2008;121(1). Available at: www.pediatrics.org/cgi/content/full/121/1/e73

48. Sallee FR, Lyne A, Wigal T, McGough JJ. Long-term safety and efficacy of guanfacine extended release in children and adolescents with attention-deficit/hyperactivity disorder. *J Child Adolesc Psychopharmacol.* 2009;19(3):215–226

49. Jain R, Segal S, Kollins SH, Khayrallah M. Clonidine extended-release tablets for pediatric patients with attention-deficit/hyperactivity disorder. *J Am Acad Child Adolesc Psychiatry.* 2011;50(2):171–179

50. Newcorn J, Kratochvil CJ, Allen AJ, et al. Atomoxetine and osmotically released methylphenidate for the treatment of attention deficit hyperactivity disorder: acute comparison and differential response. *Am J Psychiatry.* 2008;165(6):721–730

51. Swanson J, Elliott GR, Greenhill LL, et al. Effects of stimulant medication on growth rates across 3 years in the MTA follow-up. *J Am Acad Child Adolesc Psychiatry.* 2007; 46(8):1015–1027

52. Mosholder AD, Gelperin K, Hammad TA, Phelan K, Johann-Liang R. Hallucinations and other psychotic symptoms associated with the use of attention-deficit/hyperactivity disorder drugs in children. *Pediatrics.* 2009;123(2):611–616

53. Avigan M. *Review of AERS Data From Marketed Safety Experience During Stimulant Therapy: Death, Sudden Death, Cardiovascular SAEs (Including Stroke).* Silver Spring, MD: Food and Drug Administration, Center for Drug Evaluation and Research; 2004. Report No. D030403

54. Perrin JM, Friedman RA, Knilans TK, et al; American Academy of Pediatrics, Black Box Working Group, Section on Cardiology and Cardiac Surgery. Cardiovascular monitoring and stimulant drugs for attention-deficit/hyperactivity disorder. *Pediatrics.* 2008;122(2):451–453

55. McCarthy S, Cranswick N, Potts L, Taylor E, Wong IC. Mortality associated with attention-deficit hyperactivity disorder (ADHD) drug treatment: a retrospective cohort study of children, adolescents and young adults using the general practice research database. *Drug Saf.* 2009;32(11): 1089–1110

56. Gould MS, Walsh BT, Munfakh JL, et al. Sudden death and use of stimulant medications in youths. *Am J Psychiatry.* 2009;166(9):992–1001

57. Greenhill L, Kollins S, Abikoff H, McCracken J, Riddle M, Swanson J. Efficacy and safety of immediate-release methylphenidate treatment for preschoolers with ADHD. *J Am Acad Child Adolesc Psychiatry.* 2006;45(11): 1284–1293

58. Low K, Gendaszek AE. Illicit use of psychostimulants among college students: a preliminary study. *Psychol Health Med.* 2002; 7(3):283–287

59. Cox D, Merkel RL, Moore M, Thorndike F, Muller C, Kovatchev B. Relative benefits of stimulant therapy with OROS methylphenidate versus mixed amphetamine salts extended release in improving the driving performance of adolescent drivers with attention-deficit/hyperactivity disorder. *Pediatrics.* 2006;118(3). Available at:

www.pediatrics.org/cgi/content/full/118/3/e704

60. Pelham W, Wheeler T, Chronis A. Empirically supported psychological treatments for attention deficit hyperactivity disorder. *J Clin Child Psychol.* 1998;27(2):190–205

61. Sonuga-Barke E, Daley D, Thompson M, Laver-Bradbury C, Weeks A. Parent-based therapies for preschool attention-deficit/hyperactivity disorder: a randomized, controlled trial with a community sample. *J Am Acad Child Adolesc Psychiatry.* 2001;40(4):402–408

62. Pelham W, Fabiano GA. Evidence-based psychosocial treatments for attention-deficit/hyperactivity disorder. *J Clin Child Psychol.* 2008;37(1):184–214

63. Van Cleave J, Leslie LK. Approaching ADHD as a chronic condition: implications for long-term adherence. *J Psychosoc Nurs Ment Health Serv.* 2008;46(8):28–36

64. A 14-month randomized clinical trial of treatment strategies for attention-deficit/hyperactivity disorder. The MTA Cooperative Group. Multimodal Treatment Study of Children With ADHD. *Arch Gen Psychiatry.* 1999;56(12):1073–1086

65. Jensen P, Hinshaw SP, Swanson JM, et al. Findings from the NIMH multimodal treatment study of ADHD (MTA): implications and applications for primary care providers. *J Dev Behav Pediatr.* 2001;22(1):60–73

66. Pelham WE, Gnagy EM. Psychosocial and combined treatments for ADHD. *Ment Retard Dev Disabil Res Rev.* 1999;5(3):225–236

67. Davila RR, Williams ML, MacDonald JT. Memorandum on clarification of policy to address the needs of children with attention deficit disorders within general and/or special education. In: Parker HC *The ADD Hyperactivity Handbook for Schools.* Plantation, FL: Impact Publications Inc; 1991:261–268

68. The College Board. Services for Students With Disabilities (SSD). Available at: www.collegeboard.com/ssd/student. Accessed July 8, 2011

69. Bodenheimer T, Wagner EH, Grumbach K. Improving primary care for patients with chronic illness. *JAMA* 2002;288:1775–1779

70. Bodenheimer T, Wagner EH, Grumbach K. Improving primary care for patients with chronic illness: the chronic care model, Part 2. *JAMA* 2002;288:1909–1914

Attention-Deficit/Hyperactivity Disorder Clinical Practice Guideline Quick Reference Tools

- Action Statement Summary
  — ADHD: Clinical Practice Guideline for the Diagnosis, Evaluation, and Treatment of Attention-Deficit/Hyperactivity Disorder in Children and Adolescents
- *ICD-10-CM* Coding Quick Reference for ADHD
- Bonus Features
  — ADHD Coding Fact Sheet for Primary Care Physicians
  — Continuum Model for ADHD
- AAP Patient Education Handouts
  — *Understanding ADHD: Information for Parents About Attention-Deficit/Hyperactivity Disorder*
  — *Medicines for ADHD: Questions From Teens Who Have ADHD*
  — *What Is ADHD? Questions From Teens*

Action Statement Summary

ADHD: Clinical Practice Guideline for the Diagnosis, Evaluation, and Treatment of Attention-Deficit/Hyperactivity Disorder in Children and Adolescents

Key Action Statement 1

The primary care clinician should initiate an evaluation for ADHD for any child 4 through 18 years of age who presents with academic or behavioral problems and symptoms of inattention, hyperactivity, or impulsivity (quality of evidence B/strong recommendation).

Key Action Statement 2

To make a diagnosis of ADHD, the primary care clinician should determine that *Diagnostic and Statistical Manual of Mental Disorders, Fourth Edition* (DSM-IV-TR) criteria have been met (including documentation of impairment in more than 1 major setting), and information should be obtained primarily from reports from parents or guardians, teachers, and other school and mental health clinicians involved in the child's care. The primary care clinician should also rule out any alternative cause (quality of evidence B/strong recommendation).

Key Action Statement 3

In the evaluation of a child for ADHD, the primary care clinician should include assessment for other conditions that might coexist with ADHD, including emotional or behavioral (eg, anxiety, depressive, oppositional defiant, and conduct disorders), developmental (eg, learning and language disorders or other neurodevelopmental disorders), and physical (eg, tics, sleep apnea) conditions (quality of evidence B/strong recommendation).

Key Action Statement 4

The primary care clinician should recognize ADHD as a chronic condition and, therefore, consider children and adolescents with ADHD as children and youth with special health care needs. Management of children and youth with special health care needs should follow the principles of the chronic care model and the medical home (quality of evidence B/strong recommendation).

Key Action Statement 5

Recommendations for treatment of children and youth with ADHD vary depending on the patient's age.

Key Action Statement 5a

For *preschool-aged children (4–5 years of age)*, the primary care clinician should prescribe evidence-based parent and/or teacher-administered behavior therapy as the first line of treatment (quality of evidence A/strong recommendation) and may prescribe methylphenidate if the behavior interventions do not provide significant improvement and there is moderate-to-severe continuing disturbance in the child's function. In areas in which evidence-based behavioral treatments are not available, the clinician needs to weigh the risks of starting medication at an early age against the harm of delaying diagnosis and treatment (quality of evidence B/recommendation).

Key Action Statement 5b

For *elementary school-aged children (6–11 years of age)*, the primary care clinician should prescribe FDA-approved medications for ADHD (quality of evidence A/strong recommendation) and/or evidence based parent- and/or teacher-administered behavior therapy as treatment for ADHD, preferably both (quality of evidence B/strong recommendation). The evidence is particularly strong for stimulant medications and sufficient but less strong for atomoxetine, extended-release guanfacine, and extended-release clonidine (in that order) (quality of evidence A/strong recommendation). The school environment, program, or placement is a part of any treatment plan.

Key Action Statement 5c

For *adolescents (12–18 years of age)*, the primary care clinician should prescribe FDA-approved medications for ADHD with the assent of the adolescent (quality of evidence A/strong recommendation) and may prescribe behavior therapy as treatment for ADHD (quality of evidence C/recommendation), preferably both.

Key Action Statement 6

Primary care clinicians should titrate doses of medication for ADHD to achieve maximum benefit with minimum adverse effects (quality of evidence B/strong recommendation).

Coding Quick Reference for ADHD

ICD-10-CM

F90.0 Attention-deficit hyperactivity disorder, predominantly inattentive type

F90.1 Attention-deficit hyperactivity disorder, predominantly hyperactive type

ADHD Coding Fact Sheet for Primary Care Physicians

Current Procedural Terminology (CPT®) (Procedure) Codes

Initial assessment usually involves a lot of time in determining the differential diagnosis, a diagnostic plan, and potential treatment options. Therefore, most pediatricians will report either an office or an outpatient evaluation and management (E/M) code using time as the key factor or a consultation code for the initial assessment.

Physician E/M Services

*99201	Office or other outpatient visit, *new*[a] patient; self limited or minor problem, 10 min.
*99202	low to moderate severity problem, 20 min.
*99203	moderate severity problem, 30 min.
*99204	moderate to high severity problem, 45 min.
*99205	high severity problem, 60 min.
*99211	Office or other outpatient visit, *established* patient; minimal problem, 5 min.
*99212	self limited or minor problem, 10 min.
*99213	low to moderate severity problem, 15 min.
*99214	moderate severity problem, 25 min.
*99215	moderate to high severity problem, 40 min.
*99241	Office or other outpatient *consultation*,[b–d] new or established patient; self-limited or minor problem, 15 min.
*99242	low severity problem, 30 min.
*99243	moderate severity problem, 45 min.
*99244	moderate to high severity problem, 60 min.
*99245	moderate to high severity problem, 80 min.
*+99354	Prolonged physician services in office or other outpatient setting, with direct patient contact; first hour (*use in conjunction with time-based codes* **99201–99215, 99241–99245, 99301–99350, 90837**)
*+99355	each additional 30 min. (*use in conjunction with* **99354**)

- Used when a physician provides prolonged services beyond the usual service (ie, beyond the typical time).
- Time spent does not have to be continuous.
- Prolonged service of less than 15 minutes beyond the first hour or less than 15 minutes beyond the final 30 minutes is not reported separately.
- If reporting E/M service according to time and not key factors (history, examination, and medical decision-making), the physician must reach the typical time in the highest code in the code set being reported (eg, **99205, 99215, 99245**) before face-to-face prolonged services can be reported.
- Refer to *CPT* for clinical staff prolonged services.

[a] A new patient is one who has not received any professional services (face-to-face services) rendered by physicians and other qualified health care professionals who may report E/M services using 1 or more specific *CPT* codes from the physician/qualified health care professional, or another physician/qualified health care professional of the exact same specialty and subspecialty who belongs to the same group practice, within the past 3 years.
[b] Use of these codes (**99241–99245**) requires the following actions:
 1. Written or verbal request for consultation is documented in the medical record.
 2. Consultant's opinion and any services ordered or performed are documented in the medical record.
 3. Consultant's opinion and any services that are performed are prepared in a written report, which is sent to the requesting physician or other appropriate source.
[c] Patients/parents may not initiate a consultation.
[d] For more information on consultation code changes for 2010, see www.aap.org/en-us/professional-resources/practice-transformation/getting-paid/Coding-at-the-AAP/Pages/ADHD-Coding-Fact-Sheet.aspx.

- New *CPT* code
▲ Revised *CPT* code
+ Codes are *add-on codes*, meaning they are reported separately in addition to the appropriate code for the service provided.
* Indicates a *CPT*-approved telemedicine service.

Reporting E/M Services Using "Time"

- When counseling or coordination of care dominates (>50%) the physician/patient or family encounter (face-to-face time in the office or other outpatient setting or floor/unit time in the hospital or nursing facility), **time shall** be considered the key or controlling factor to qualify for a particular level of E/M services.
- This includes time spent with parties who have assumed responsibility for the care of the patient or decision-making, whether or not they are family members (eg, foster parents, person acting in loco parentis, legal guardian). The extent of counseling or coordination of care must be documented in the medical record.
- For coding purposes, face-to-face time for these services is defined as only that time that the physician spends face-to-face with the patient or family. This includes the time in which the physician performs such tasks as obtaining a history, performing an examination, and counseling the patient.
- When codes are ranked in sequential typical times (eg, office-based E/M services, consultation codes) and the actual time is between 2 typical times, the code with the typical time closest to the actual time is used.
  - **Example:** A physician sees an established patient in the office to discuss the current attention-deficit/hyperactivity disorder (ADHD) medication the patient was placed on. The total face-to-face time was 22 minutes, of which 15 minutes was spent in counseling the mom and patient. Because more than 50% of the total time was spent in counseling, the physician would report the E/M service according to time. The physician would report **99214** instead of **99213** because the total face-to-face time was closer to **99214** (25 minutes) than **99213** (15 minutes).

ADHD Follow-up During a Routine Preventive Medicine Service

- A good time to follow up with a patient regarding his or her ADHD could be during a preventive medicine service.
- If the follow-up requires little additional work on behalf of the physician, it should be reported under the preventive medicine service, rather than as a separate service.
- If the follow-up work requires an additional E/M service in addition to the preventive medicine service, it should be reported as a separate service.
- Chronic conditions should be reported only if they are separately addressed.
- When reporting a preventive medicine service in addition to an office-based E/M service and the services are significant and separately identifiable, modifier **25** will be required on the office-based E/M service.
  - **Example:** A 12-year-old established patient presents for his routine preventive medicine service and, while he and Mom are there, Mom asks about changing his ADHD medication because of some side effects he is experiencing. The physician completes the routine preventive medicine check and then addresses the mom's concerns in a separate service. The additional E/M service takes 15 minutes, of which the physician spends about 10 minutes in counseling and coordinating care; therefore, the E/M service is reported according to time.
    ~ Code **99394** and **99213-25** account for both E/M services and link each to the appropriate *International Classification of Diseases, 10th Revision, Clinical Modification (ICD-10-CM)* code.
    ~ Modifier **25** is required on the problem-oriented office visit code (eg, **99213**) when it is significant and separately identifiable from another service.

Physician Non–face-to-face Services

99339   Care Plan Oversight—Individual physician supervision of a patient (patient not present) in home, domiciliary or rest home (e.g., assisted living facility) requiring complex and multidisciplinary care modalities involving regular physician development and/or revision of care plans, review of subsequent reports of patient status, review of related laboratory and other studies, communication (including telephone calls) for purposes of assessment or care decisions with health care professional(s), family member(s), surrogate decision maker(s) (e.g., legal guardian) and/or key caregiver(s) involved in patient's care, integration of new information into the medical treatment plan and/or adjustment of medical therapy, within a calendar month; 15–29 minutes

99340   30 minutes or more

99358   Prolonged physician services without direct patient contact; first hour

+99359   each additional 30 min. (+ *use in conjunction with* **99358**)

99367   Medical team conference by physician with interdisciplinary team of health care professionals, patient and/or family not present, 30 minutes or more

99441   Telephone evaluation and management to patient, parent or guardian not originating from a related E/M service within the previous 7 days nor leading to an E/M service or procedure within the next 24 hours or soonest available appointment; 5–10 minutes of medical discussion

99442   11–20 minutes of medical discussion

99443   21–30 minutes of medical discussion

99444   Online E/M service provided by a physician or other qualified health care professional to an established patient, guardian or health care provider not originating from a related E/M service provided within the previous 7 days, using the internet or similar electronic communications network

Clinical Staff Care Management Services

Codes are selected according to the amount of time spent by clinical staff/physician providing care coordination activities. *CPT* clearly defines which activities are care coordination activities. To report chronic care management codes, you must

1. Provide 24/7 access to physicians or other qualified health care professionals or clinical staff.
2. Use a standardized methodology to identify patients who require chronic complex care coordination services.
3. Have an internal care coordination process/function whereby a patient identified as meeting the requirements for these services starts receiving them in a timely manner.
4. Use a form and format in the medical record that is standardized within the practice.
5. Be able to engage and educate patients and caregivers, as well as coordinate care among all service professionals, as appropriate for each patient (also applies to code **99490** under NPP services).

• New *CPT* code

▲ Revised *CPT* code

+ Codes are *add-on codes*, meaning they are reported separately in addition to the appropriate code for the service provided.

* Indicates a *CPT*-approved telemedicine service.

•99491   Chronic care management services, provided personally by a physician or other qualified health care professional, at least 30 minutes of physician or other qualified health care professional time, per calendar month, with the following required elements:

- multiple (two or more) chronic conditions expected to last at least 12 months, or until the death of the patient;
- chronic conditions place the patient at significant risk of death, acute exacerbation/decompensation, or functional decline;
- comprehensive care plan established, implemented, revised, or monitored.

Psychiatry

+90785   Interactive complexity (Use in conjunction with codes for diagnostic psychiatric evaluation [**90791**, **90792**], psychotherapy [**90832**, **90834**, **90837**], psychotherapy when performed with an evaluation and management service [**90833**, **90836**, **90838**, **99201–99255**, **99304–99337**, **99341–99350**], and group psychotherapy [**90853**])

Psychiatric Diagnostic or Evaluative Interview Procedures

90791   Psychiatric diagnostic interview examination evaluation

90792   Psychiatric diagnostic evaluation with medical services

Psychotherapy

*90832   Psychotherapy, 30 min with patient;

*+90833   with medical E/M (Use in conjunction with **99201–99255**, **99304–99337**, **99341–99350**)

*90834   Psychotherapy, 45 min with patient;

*+90836   with medical E/M services (Use in conjunction with **99201–99255**, **99304–99337**, **99341–99350**)

*90837   Psychotherapy, 60 min with patient;

*+90838   with medical E/M services (Use in conjunction with **99201–99255**, **99304–99337**, **99341–99350**)

+90785   Interactive complexity (Use in conjunction with codes for diagnostic psychiatric evaluation [**90791**, **90792**], psychotherapy [**90832**, **90834**, **90837**], psychotherapy when performed with an evaluation and management service [**90833**, **90836**, **90838**, **99201–99255**, **99304–99337**, **99341–99350**], and group psychotherapy [**90853**])

- Refers to specific communication factors that complicate the delivery of a psychiatric procedure. Common factors include more difficult communication with discordant or emotional family members and engagement of young and verbally undeveloped or impaired patients. Typical encounters include
  — Patients who have other individuals legally responsible for their care
  — Patients who request others to be present or involved in their care such as translators, interpreters, or additional family members
  — Patients who require the involvement of other third parties such as child welfare agencies, schools, or probation officers

*90846   Family psychotherapy (without patient present), 50 min

*90847   Family psychotherapy (conjoint psychotherapy) (with patient present), 50 min

Other Psychiatric Services/Procedures

90863 Pharmacologic management, including prescription and review of medication, when performed with psychotherapy services (Use in conjunction with **90832**, **90834**, **90837**)
- For pharmacologic management with psychotherapy services performed by a physician or other qualified health care professional who may report E/M codes, use the appropriate E/M codes (**99201–99255**, **99281–99285**, **99304–99337**, **99341–99350**) and the appropriate psychotherapy with E/M service (**90833**, **90836**, **90838**).

90887 Interpretation or explanation of results of psychiatric, other medical exams, or other accumulated data to family or other responsible persons, or advising them how to assist patient

90889 Preparation of reports on patient's psychiatric status, history, treatment, or progress (other than for legal or consultative purposes) for other physicians, agencies, or insurance carriers

97127 Therapeutic interventions that focus on cognitive function (eg, attention, memory, reasoning, executive function, problem solving, and/or pragmatic functioning) and compensatory strategies to manage the performance of an activity (eg, managing time or schedules, initiating, organizing and sequencing tasks), direct (one-on-one) patient contact

Developmental/Psychological Testing

96110 Developmental screening, with scoring and documentation, per standardized instrument (Do not use for ADHD screens or assessments)

•96112 Developmental test administration (including assessment of fine and/or gross motor, language, cognitive level, social, memory and/or executive functions by standardized developmental instruments when performed), by physician or other qualified health care professional, with interpretation and report; first hour

•+96113 each additional 30 minutes (Report with **96112**)

*▲96116 Neurobehavioral status examination (clinical assessment of thinking, reasoning and judgment [eg, acquired knowledge, attention, language, memory, planning and problem solving, and visual spatial abilities]), by physician or other qualified health care professional, both face-to-face time with the patient and time interpreting test results and preparing the report; first hour

*•96121 each additional hour (Report with **96116**)

96127 Brief emotional/behavioral assessment (eg, depression inventory, attention-deficit/hyperactivity disorder [ADHD] scale), with scoring and documentation, per standardized instrument

Nonphysician Provider (NPP) Services

99366 Medical team conference with interdisciplinary team of health care professionals, face-to-face with patient and/or family, 30 minutes or more, participation by a nonphysician qualified health care professional

99368 Medical team conference with interdisciplinary team of health care professionals, patient and/or family not present, 30 minutes or more, participation by a nonphysician qualified health care professional

•96146 Psychological or neuropsychological test administration, with single automated, standardized instrument via electronic platform, with automated result only

*96150 Health and behavior assessment performed by nonphysician provider (health-focused clinical interviews, behavior observations) to identify psychological, behavioral, emotional, cognitive or social factors important to management of physical health problems, 15 min., initial assessment

*96151 re-assessment

*96152 Health and behavior intervention performed by nonphysician provider to improve patient's health and well-being using cognitive, behavioral, social, and/or psychophysiological procedures designed to ameliorate specific disease-related problems, individual, 15 min.

*96153 group (2 or more patients)

*96154 family (with the patient present)

96155 family (without the patient present)

Non–face-to-face Services: NPP

98966 Telephone assessment and management service provided by a qualified nonphysician health care professional to an established patient, parent or guardian not originating from a related assessment and management service provided within the previous seven days nor leading to an assessment and management service or procedure within the next 24 hours or soonest available appointment; 5–10 minutes of medical discussion

98967 11–20 minutes of medical discussion

98968 21–30 minutes of medical discussion

98969 Online assessment and management service provided by a qualified nonphysician health care professional to an established patient or guardian not originating from a related assessment and management service provided within the previous seven days nor using the internet or similar electronic communications network

•99490 Chronic care management services, at least 20 minutes of clinical staff time directed by a physician or other qualified health care professional, per calendar month, with the following required elements:
- multiple (two or more) chronic conditions expected to last at least 12 months, or until the death of the patient;
- chronic conditions place the patient at significant risk of death, acute exacerbation/decompensation, or functional decline;
- comprehensive care plan established, implemented, revised, or monitored.

Chronic care management services are provided when medical needs or psychosocial needs (or both types of needs) of the patient require establishing, implementing, revising, or monitoring the care plan. If 20 minutes is not met within a calendar month, you do not report chronic care management. Refer to code **99491** and *CPT* for more information.

• New *CPT* code
▲ Revised *CPT* code
+ Codes are *add-on codes*, meaning they are reported separately in addition to the appropriate code for the service provided.
* Indicates a *CPT*-approved telemedicine service.

Miscellaneous Services

99071   Educational supplies, such as books, tapes, or pamphlets, provided by the physician for the patient's education at cost to the physician

Clinical Staff

99484   Care management services for *behavioral health conditions*, at least 20 minutes of clinical staff time, directed by a physician or other qualified health care professional, per calendar month, with the following required elements:
- initial assessment or follow-up monitoring, including the use of applicable validated rating scales;
- behavioral health care planning in relation to behavioral/ psychiatric health problems, including revision for patients who are not progressing or whose status changes;
- facilitating and coordinating treatment such as psychotherapy, pharmacotherapy, counseling and/ or psychiatric consultation; and
- continuity of care with a designated member of the care team.
- Do not report in conjunction with psychiatric collaborative care management codes (**99492**, **99493**, **99494**) for the same calendar month.

99492   Initial psychiatric collaborative care management, first 70 minutes in the first calendar month of behavioral health care manager activities, in consultation with a psychiatric consultant, and directed by the treating physician or other qualified health care professional, with the following required elements:
- outreach to and engagement in treatment of a patient directed by the treating physician or other qualified health care professional;
- initial assessment of the patient, including administration of validated rating scales, with the development of an individualized treatment plan;
- review by the psychiatric consultant with modifications of the plan if recommended;
- entering patient in a registry and tracking patient follow-up and progress using the registry, with appropriate documentation, and participation in weekly caseload consultation with the psychiatric consultant; and
- provision of brief interventions using evidence-based techniques such as behavioral activation, motivational interviewing, and other focused treatment strategies.

99493   Subsequent psychiatric collaborative care management, first 60 minutes in a subsequent month of behavioral health care manager activities, in consultation with a psychiatric consultant, and directed by the treating physician or other qualified health care professional, with the following required elements:
- tracking patient follow-up and progress using the registry, with appropriate documentation;
- participation in weekly caseload consultation with the psychiatric consultant;

- ongoing collaboration with and coordination of the patient's mental health care with the treating physician or other qualified health care professional and any other treating mental health providers;
- additional review of progress and recommendations for changes in treatment, as indicated, including medications, based on recommendations provided by the psychiatric consultant;
- provision of brief interventions using evidence-based techniques such as behavioral activation, motivational interviewing, and other focused treatment strategies;
- monitoring of patient outcomes using validated rating scales; and
- relapse prevention planning with patients as they achieve remission of symptoms and/or other treatment goals and are prepared for discharge from active treatment.

+99494   Initial or subsequent psychiatric collaborative care management, each additional 30 minutes in a calendar month of behavioral health care manager activities, in consultation with a psychiatric consultant, and directed by the treating physician or other qualified health care professional (Use **99494** in conjunction with **99492**, **99493**)

ICD-10-CM Codes

- Use as many diagnosis codes that apply to document the patient's complexity and report the patient's symptoms or adverse environmental circumstances (or both).
- Once a definitive diagnosis is established, report any appropriate definitive diagnosis codes as the primary codes, plus any other symptoms that the patient is exhibiting as secondary diagnoses that are not part of the usual disease course or are considered incidental.
- *ICD-10-CM* **codes are only valid on or after October 1, 2015.**

Depressive Disorders

F34.1   Dysthymic disorder (depressive personality disorder, dysthymia neurotic depression)
F39   Mood (affective) disorder, unspecified
F30.8   Other manic episode

Anxiety Disorders

F06.4   Anxiety disorder due to known physiological conditions
F40.10   Social phobia, unspecified
F40.11   Social phobia, generalized
F40.8   Phobic anxiety disorders, other (phobic anxiety disorder of childhood)
F40.9   Phobic anxiety disorder, unspecified
F41.1   Generalized anxiety disorder
F41.9   Anxiety disorder, unspecified

Feeding and Eating Disorders/Elimination Disorders

F50.89   Eating disorders, other
F50.9   Eating disorder, unspecified
F98.0   Enuresis not due to a substance or known physiological condition
F98.1   Encopresis not due to a substance or known physiological condition
F98.3   Pica (infancy or childhood)

- New *CPT* code
▲ Revised *CPT* code
+ Codes are *add-on codes,* meaning they are reported separately in addition to the appropriate code for the service provided.
* Indicates a *CPT*-approved telemedicine service.

Impulse Disorders

F63.9   Impulse disorder, unspecified

Trauma- and Stressor-Related Disorders

F43.20   Adjustment disorder, unspecified
F43.21   Adjustment disorder with depressed mood
F43.22   Adjustment disorder with anxiety
F43.23   Adjustment disorder with mixed anxiety and depressed mood
F43.24   Adjustment disorder with disturbance of conduct

Neurodevelopmental/Other Developmental Disorders

F70   Mild intellectual disabilities
F71   Moderate intellectual disabilities
F72   Severe intellectual disabilities
F73   Profound intellectual disabilities
F79   Unspecified intellectual disabilities
F80.0   Phonological (speech) disorder (speech-sound disorder)
F80.1   Expressive language disorder
F80.2   Mixed receptive-expressive language disorder
F80.4   Speech and language developmental delay due to hearing loss (code also hearing loss)
F80.81   Stuttering
F80.82   Social pragmatic communication disorder
F80.89   Other developmental disorders of speech and language
F80.9   Developmental disorder of speech and language, unspecified
F81.0   Specific reading disorder
F81.2   Mathematics disorder
F81.89   Other developmental disorders of scholastic skills
F82   Developmental coordination disorder
F84.0   Autistic disorder (Autism spectrum disorder)
F88   Specified delays in development; other
F89   Unspecified delay in development
F81.9   Developmental disorder of scholastic skills, unspecified

Behavioral/Emotional Disorders

F90.0   Attention-deficit hyperactivity disorder, predominantly inattentive type
F90.1   Attention-deficit hyperactivity disorder, predominantly hyperactive type
F90.8   Attention-deficit hyperactivity disorder, other type
F90.9   Attention-deficit hyperactivity disorder, unspecified type
F91.1   Conduct disorder, childhood-onset type
F91.2   Conduct disorder, adolescent-onset type
F91.3   Oppositional defiant disorder
F91.9   Conduct disorder, unspecified
F93.0   Separation anxiety disorder
F93.8   Other childhood emotional disorders (relationship problems)
F93.9   Childhood emotional disorder, unspecified
F94.9   Childhood disorder of social functioning, unspecified
F95.0   Transient tic disorder
F95.1   Chronic motor or vocal tic disorder
F95.2   Tourette's disorder
F95.9   Tic disorder, unspecified
F98.8   Other specified behavioral and emotional disorders with onset usually occurring in childhood and adolescence (nail-biting, nose-picking, thumb-sucking)

Other

F07.81   Postconcussional syndrome
F07.89   Personality and behavioral disorders due to known physiological condition, other
F07.9   Personality and behavioral disorder due to known physiological condition, unspecified
F45.41   Pain disorder exclusively related to psychological factors
F48.8   Nonpsychotic mental disorders, other (neurasthenia)
F48.9   Nonpsychotic mental disorders, unspecified
F51.01   Primary insomnia
F51.02   Adjustment insomnia
F51.03   Paradoxical insomnia
F51.04   Psychophysiologic insomnia
F51.05   Insomnia due to other mental disorder (Code also associated mental disorder)
F51.09   Insomnia, other (not due to a substance or known physiological condition)
F51.3   Sleepwalking [somnambulism]
F51.4   Sleep terrors [night terrors]
F51.8   Other sleep disorders
F93.8   Childhood emotional disorders, other
R46.89   Other symptoms and signs involving appearance and behavior

Substance-Related and Addictive Disorders

If a provider documents multiple patterns of use, only 1 should be reported. Use the following hierarchy: use–abuse–dependence (eg, if use and dependence are documented, only code for dependence).

When a minus symbol (-) is included in codes **F10–F17**, a last character is required. Be sure to include the last character from the following list:

0 anxiety disorder

2 sleep disorder

8 other disorder

9 unspecified disorder

Alcohol

F10.10   Alcohol abuse, uncomplicated (alcohol use disorder, mild)
F10.14   Alcohol abuse with alcohol-induced mood disorder
F10.159   Alcohol abuse with alcohol-induced psychotic disorder, unspecified
F10.18-   Alcohol abuse with alcohol-induced
F10.19   Alcohol abuse with unspecified alcohol-induced disorder
F10.20   Alcohol dependence, uncomplicated
F10.21   Alcohol dependence, in remission
F10.24   Alcohol dependence with alcohol-induced mood disorder
F10.259   Alcohol dependence with alcohol-induced psychotic disorder, unspecified
F10.28-   Alcohol dependence with alcohol-induced
F10.29   Alcohol dependence with unspecified alcohol-induced disorder

---

• New *CPT* code
▲ Revised *CPT* code
+ Codes are *add-on codes,* meaning they are reported separately in addition to the appropriate code for the service provided.
* Indicates a *CPT*-approved telemedicine service.

F10.94	Alcohol use, unspecified with alcohol-induced mood disorder
F10.959	Alcohol use, unspecified with alcohol-induced psychotic disorder, unspecified
F10.98-	Alcohol use, unspecified with alcohol-induced
F10.99	Alcohol use, unspecified with unspecified alcohol-induced disorder

Cannabis

F12.10	Cannabis abuse, uncomplicated (cannabis use disorder, mild)
F12.18-	Cannabis abuse with cannabis-induced
F12.19	Cannabis abuse with unspecified cannabis-induced disorder
F12.20	Cannabis dependence, uncomplicated
F12.21	Cannabis dependence, in remission
F12.28-	Cannabis dependence with cannabis-induced
F12.29	Cannabis dependence with unspecified cannabis-induced disorder
F12.90	Cannabis use, unspecified, uncomplicated
F12.98-	Cannabis use, unspecified with
F12.99	Cannabis use, unspecified with unspecified cannabis-induced disorder

Sedatives

F13.10	Sedative, hypnotic or anxiolytic abuse, uncomplicated (sedative, hypnotic, or anxiolytic use disorder, mild)
F13.129	Sedative, hypnotic or anxiolytic abuse with intoxication, unspecified
F13.14	Sedative, hypnotic or anxiolytic abuse with sedative, hypnotic or anxiolytic-induced mood disorder
F13.18-	Sedative, hypnotic or anxiolytic abuse with sedative, hypnotic or anxiolytic-induced
F13.21	Sedative, hypnotic or anxiolytic dependence, in remission
F13.90	Sedative, hypnotic or anxiolytic use, unspecified, uncomplicated
F13.94	Sedative, hypnotic or anxiolytic use, unspecified with sedative, hypnotic or anxiolytic-induced mood disorder
F13.98-	Sedative, hypnotic or anxiolytic use, unspecified with sedative, hypnotic or anxiolytic-induced
F13.99	Sedative, hypnotic or anxiolytic use, unspecified with unspecified sedative, hypnotic or anxiolytic-induced disorder

Stimulants (eg, caffeine, amphetamines)

F15.10	Other stimulant (amphetamine-related disorders or caffeine) abuse, uncomplicated (amphetamine, other or unspecified type substance use disorder, mild)
F15.14	Other stimulant (amphetamine-related disorders or caffeine) abuse with stimulant-induced mood disorder
F15.18-	Other stimulant (amphetamine-related disorders or caffeine) abuse with stimulant-induced
F15.19	Other stimulant (amphetamine-related disorders or caffeine) abuse with unspecified stimulant-induced disorder
F15.20	Other stimulant (amphetamine-related disorders or caffeine) dependence, uncomplicated

F15.21	Other stimulant (amphetamine-related disorders or caffeine) dependence, in remission
F15.24	Other stimulant (amphetamine-related disorders or caffeine) dependence with stimulant-induced mood disorder
F15.28-	Other stimulant (amphetamine-related disorders or caffeine) dependence with stimulant-induced
F15.29	Other stimulant (amphetamine-related disorders or caffeine) dependence with unspecified stimulant-induced disorder
F15.90	Other stimulant (amphetamine-related disorders or caffeine) use, unspecified, uncomplicated
F15.94	Other stimulant (amphetamine-related disorders or caffeine) use, unspecified with stimulant-induced mood disorder
F15.98-	Other stimulant (amphetamine-related disorders or caffeine) use, unspecified with stimulant-induced
F15.99	Other stimulant (amphetamine-related disorders or caffeine) use, unspecified with unspecified stimulant-induced disorder

Nicotine (eg, cigarettes)

F17.200	Nicotine dependence, unspecified, uncomplicated (tobacco use disorder, mild, moderate or severe)
F17.201	Nicotine dependence, unspecified, in remission
F17.203	Nicotine dependence, unspecified, with withdrawal
F17.20-	Nicotine dependence, unspecified, with
F17.210	Nicotine dependence, cigarettes, uncomplicated
F17.211	Nicotine dependence, cigarettes, in remission
F17.213	Nicotine dependence, cigarettes, with withdrawal
F17.218-	Nicotine dependence, cigarettes, with

Symptoms, Signs, and Ill-defined Conditions

Use these codes in absence of a definitive mental diagnosis or when the sign or symptom is not part of the disease course or is considered incidental.

G47.9	Sleep disorder, unspecified
H90.0	Conductive hearing loss, bilateral
H90.11	Conductive hearing loss, unilateral, right ear, with unrestricted hearing on the contralateral side
H90.12	Conductive hearing loss, unilateral, left ear, with unrestricted hearing on the contralateral side
H90.A1-	Conductive hearing loss, unilateral, with restricted hearing on the contralateral side
H90.A2-	Sensorineural hearing loss, unilateral, with restricted hearing on the contralateral side
H90.A3-	Mixed conductive and sensorineural hearing loss, unilateral, with restricted hearing on the contralateral side
	(Codes under category **H90** require a 6th digit: 1– right ear, 2–left ear)
K11.7	Disturbance of salivary secretions
K59.00	Constipation, unspecified
N39.44	Nocturnal enuresis
R10.0	Acute abdomen pain
R11.11	Vomiting without nausea
R11.2	Nausea with vomiting, unspecified
R19.7	Diarrhea, unspecified
R21	Rash, NOS
R25.0	Abnormal head movements
R25.1	Tremor, unspecified
R25.3	Twitching, NOS
R25.8	Other abnormal involuntary movements
R25.9	Unspecified abnormal involuntary movements

R27.8	Other lack of coordination (excludes ataxia)
R27.9	Unspecified lack of coordination
R41.83	Borderline intellectual functioning
R42	Dizziness
R48.0	Alexia/dyslexia, NOS
R51	Headache
R62.0	Delayed milestone in childhood
R62.52	Short stature (child)
R63.3	Feeding difficulties
R63.4	Abnormal weight loss
R63.5	Abnormal weight gain
R68.2	Dry mouth, unspecified
T56.0X1A	Toxic effect of lead and its compounds, accidental (unintentional), initial encounter

Z Codes

Z codes represent reasons for encounters. Categories **Z00–Z99** are provided for occasions when circumstances other than a disease, an injury, or an external cause classifiable to categories **A00–Y89** are recorded as *diagnoses* or *problems*. This can arise in 2 main ways.

1. When a person who may or may not be sick encounters the health services for some specific purpose, such as to receive limited care or service for a current condition, to donate an organ or tissue, to receive prophylactic vaccination (immunization), or to discuss a problem that is, in itself, not a disease or an injury

2. When some circumstance or problem is present that influences the person's health status but is not, in itself, a current illness or injury

Z55.0	Illiteracy and low-level literacy
Z55.2	Failed school examinations
Z55.3	Underachievement in school
Z55.4	Educational maladjustment and discord with teachers and classmates
Z55.8	Other problems related to education and literacy
Z55.9	Problems related to education and literacy, unspecified (**Z55** codes exclude those conditions reported with **F80–F89**)
Z60.4	Social exclusion and rejection
Z60.8	Other problems related to social environment
Z60.9	Problem related to social environment, unspecified
Z62.0	Inadequate parental supervision and control
Z62.21	Foster care status (child welfare)
Z62.6	Inappropriate (excessive) parental pressure
Z62.810	Personal history of physical and sexual abuse in childhood

Z62.811	Personal history of psychological abuse in childhood
Z62.820	Parent-biological child conflict
Z62.821	Parent-adopted child conflict
Z62.822	Parent-foster child conflict
Z63.72	Alcoholism and drug addiction in family
Z63.8	Other specified problems related to primary support group
Z65.3	Problems related to legal circumstances
Z71.89	Counseling, other specified
Z71.9	Counseling, unspecified
Z72.0	Tobacco use
Z77.011	Contact with and (suspected) exposure to lead
Z79.899	Other long term (current) drug therapy
Z81.0	Family history of intellectual disabilities (conditions classifiable to **F70–F79**)
Z81.8	Family history of other mental and behavioral disorders
Z83.2	Family history of diseases of the blood and blood-forming organs (anemia) (conditions classifiable to **D50–D89**)
Z86.2	Personal history of diseases of the blood and blood-forming organs
Z86.39	Personal history of other endocrine, nutritional, and metabolic disease
Z86.59	Personal history of other mental and behavioral disorders
Z86.69	Personal history of other diseases of the nervous system and sense organs
Z87.09	Personal history of other diseases of the respiratory system
Z87.19	Personal history of other diseases of the digestive system
Z87.798	Personal history of other (corrected) congenital malformations
Z87.820	Personal history of traumatic brain injury
Z91.128	Patient's intentional underdosing of medication regimen for other reason (report drug code)
Z91.138	Patient's unintentional underdosing of medication regimen for other reason (report drug code)
Z91.14	Patient's other noncompliance with medication regimen
Z91.19	Patient's noncompliance with other medical treatment and regimen
Z91.411	Personal history of adult psychological abuse

• New *CPT* code
▲ Revised *CPT* code
+ Codes are *add-on codes,* meaning they are reported separately in addition to the appropriate code for the service provided.
* Indicates a *CPT*-approved telemedicine service.

Continuum Model for ADHD

The following continuum model from *Coding for Pediatrics 2019* has been devised to express the various levels of service for ADHD. This model demonstrates the cumulative effect of the key criteria for each level of service using a single diagnosis as the common denominator. It also shows the importance of other variables, such as patient age, duration and severity of illness, social contexts, and comorbid conditions, that often have key roles in pediatric cases.

Quick Reference for Codes Used in Continuum for ADHD—Established Patients[a]					
E/M Code Level	**History**	**Examination**	**MDM**	**Time**	
99211[b]	NA	NA	NA	5 min	
99212	Problem-focused	Problem-focused	Straightforward	10 min	
99213	Expanded problem-focused	Expanded problem-focused	Low	15 min	
99214	Detailed	Detailed	Moderate	25 min	
99215	Comprehensive	Comprehensive	High	40 min	

Abbreviations: ADHD, attention-deficit/hyperactivity disorder; E/M, evaluation and management; MDM, medical decision-making; NA, not applicable.

[a] Use of a code level requires that you meet or exceed 2 of the 3 key components on the basis of medical necessity.

[b] Low level E/M service that may not require the presence of a physician.

Adapted from American Academy of Pediatrics. *Coding for Pediatrics 2019: A Manual for Pediatric Documentation and Payment.* 24th ed. Itasca, IL: American Academy of Pediatrics; 2019.

Continuum Model for Attention-Deficit/Hyperactivity Disorder

Code selection at any level above **99211** may be based on time when documentation states that more than 50% of the total face-to-face time of the encounter is spent in counseling and/or coordination of care. Select the code with the typical time closest to the total face-to-face time.

CPT® Code Vignette	History	Physical Examination (systems)	Medical Decision-making (2 of 3 diagnoses, data, risk)
99211 Nurse visit to check growth or blood pressure prior to renewing prescription for psychoactive drugs	No specific key components required. Must indicate continuation of physician's plan of care, medical necessity, assessment, and/or education provided. CC: Check growth or blood pressure. HPI: Existing medications and desired/undesired effects. Documentation of height, weight, and blood pressure. Assessment: Doing well. Obtained physician approval for prescription refill. Keep appointment with physician in 1 month.		
99212 (Typical time: 10 min) Visit to recheck recent weight loss in patient with established ADHD otherwise stable on stimulant medication	**Problem focused** CC: Weight loss, ADHD HPI: Appetite, signs and symptoms, duration since last weight check	**Problem focused** 1. Constitutional (weight, blood pressure, overall appearance)	**Straightforward** 1. Stable established problem 2. No tests ordered/data reviewed 3. Risk: 1 chronic illness with side effects of treatment and prescription drug management
99213 (Typical time: 15 min) 3- to 6-month visit for child with ADHD who is presently doing well using medication and without other problems	**Expanded problem focused** CC: ADHD HPI: Effect of medication on appetite, mood, sleep, quality of schoolwork (eg, review report cards) ROS: Neurologic (no tics) PFSH: Review of medications	**Expanded problem focused** 1. Constitutional (temperature, weight, blood pressure) 2. Neurologic 3. Psychiatric (alert and oriented, mood and affect)	**Low complexity** 1. Stable established problem 2. Data reviewed: Rating scale results and feedback materials from teacher 3. Risk: Prescription drug management *or* Time: Documented faced-to-face time and >50% spent in counseling and/or coordination and context of discussion of 6-month treatment plan with adjustment of medication
99214 (Typical time: 25 min) Follow-up evaluation of an established patient with ADHD with failure to improve on medication and/or weight loss and new symptoms of depression	**Detailed** CC: ADHD with failure to improve HPI: Signs and symptoms since start of medication; modifying factors; quality of schoolwork (eg, review report cards) ROS: Gastrointestinal and psychiatric PFSH: Current medications; allergies; school attendance; substance use	**Detailed** 1. General multisystem examination with details of affected systems (2–7 systems in all) or detailed single organ system examination of neurologic system	**Moderate complexity** 1. Established problem, not improving with current therapy, and new problem without additional workup planned 2. Data reviewed: Rating scale results and feedback materials from teacher; depression screening score 3. Risk: Prescription drug management *or* Time: Documented face-to-face time with >50% spent in discussion of possible interventions, including, but not limited to a. Educational intervention b. Alteration in medications c. Obtaining drug levels d. Psychiatric intervention e. Behavioral modification program

Continuum Model for Attention-Deficit/Hyperactivity Disorder (*continued*)

Code selection at any level above **99211** may be based on time when documentation states that more than 50% of the total face-to-face time of the encounter is spent in counseling and/or coordination of care. Select the code with the typical time closest to the total face-to-face time.

CPT® Code Vignette	History	Physical Examination (systems)	Medical Decision-making (2 of 3 diagnoses, data, risk)
99215 (Typical time: 40 min) Initial evaluation of an established patient experiencing difficulty in classroom, home, or social situation and suspected of having ADHD	**Comprehensive** CC: Difficulty in school, home, and social situations HPI: Signs and symptoms, duration, modifying factors, severity ROS: Constitutional, eyes, ENMT, cardiovascular, respiratory, musculoskeletal, integumentary, neurological, psychiatric, endocrine	Comprehensive examination of ≥8 systems or comprehensive neurologic/psychiatric examination (1997 guidelines	**High complexity** 1. New problem with additional workup 2. Tests ordered and data reviewed: ADHD assessment instruments; history obtained from parents; and case discussion with another provider (eg, school counselor) 3. Risk: Undiagnosed new problem

Abbreviations: ADHD, attention-deficit/hyperactivity disorder; CC, chief complaint; CPT, Current Procedural Terminology; ENMT, ears, nose, mouth, throat; HPI, history of present illness; PFSH, past, family, and social history; ROS, review of systems.

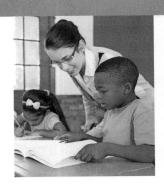

Understanding ADHD:
Information for Parents About Attention-Deficit/Hyperactivity Disorder

Almost all children have times when their behavior veers out of control. However, for some children, these kinds of behaviors are more than an occasional problem.

Children with attention-deficit/hyperactivity disorder (ADHD) have behavioral problems that are so frequent and severe that they interfere with their ability to live normal lives. An impulsive nature may put them in actual physical danger. They may speed about in constant motion, make noise nonstop, refuse to wait their turn, and crash into everything around them. At other times, they may drift as if in a daydream, unable to pay attention or finish what they start. Those who have trouble paying attention usually have trouble learning.

Left untreated, ADHD in some children will continue to cause serious, lifelong problems, such as poor grades in school, run-ins with the law, failed relationships, and the inability to keep a job. Children with ADHD often have trouble getting along with siblings and other children at school, at home, and in other settings. They may be labeled "bad kids" or "space cadets."

If your child has ADHD, effective treatment is available. Your child's doctor can offer a long-term treatment plan to help your child lead a happy and healthy life. As a parent, you have a very important role in this treatment. Here is more information from the American Academy of Pediatrics about ADHD and how you can help your child.

NOTE: To make reading this publication easier, the pronoun he is used to describe a child or teen.

What is ADHD?

ADHD is a condition of the brain that makes it difficult for children to control their behavior. It is one of the most common chronic conditions of childhood. It affects 6% to 12% of school-aged children. ADHD is diagnosed about 3 times more often in boys than in girls. The condition affects behavior in specific ways. See section, *What are the symptoms of ADHD?*

What are the symptoms of ADHD?

ADHD includes 3 groups of behavioral symptoms: inattention, hyperactivity, and impulsivity. See Table 1.

Are there different types of ADHD?

Children with ADHD may have one or more of the symptoms listed in Table 1. The symptoms are usually classified as the following types of ADHD:

- **Inattentive only (formerly known as *attention-deficit disorder* [*ADD*])** — Children with this form of ADHD are not overly active. Because they do not disrupt the classroom or other activities, their symptoms may not be noticed. Among girls with ADHD, this form is more common.
- **Hyperactive/impulsive** — Children with this type of ADHD have both hyperactive and impulsive behavior, but they can pay attention. They are the least common group and are often younger.

Table 1. Symptoms of ADHD

Symptom	How a Child With This Symptom May Behave
Inattention	Often has a hard time paying attention, daydreams
	Often does not seem to listen
	Is easily distracted from work or play
	Often does not seem to care about details, makes careless mistakes
	Frequently does not follow through on instructions or finish tasks
	Is disorganized
	Frequently loses a lot of important things
	Often forgets things
	Frequently avoids doing things that require ongoing mental effort
Hyperactivity	Is in constant motion, as if "driven by a motor"
	Cannot stay seated
	Frequently squirms and fidgets
	Talks too much
	Often runs, jumps, and climbs when this is not permitted
	Cannot play quietly
Impulsivity	Frequently acts and speaks without thinking
	May run into the street without looking for traffic first
	Frequently has trouble taking turns
	Cannot wait for things
	Often calls out answers before the question is complete
	Frequently interrupts others

- **Combined inattentive/hyperactive/impulsive** — Children with this type of ADHD have behaviors from all 3 symptoms. It is the type most people think of when they think of ADHD.

How can I tell if my child has ADHD?

Remember, it is common for all children to show some of these symptoms from time to time. Your child may be reacting to stress at school or at home. He may be bored or going through a difficult stage of life. It does not mean he has ADHD.

Sometimes a teacher is the first to notice inattention, hyperactivity, and/or impulsivity and will inform the parents.

Keep Safety in Mind

If your child shows any symptoms of ADHD, it is very important that you pay close attention to safety. A child with ADHD may not always be aware of dangers and can get hurt easily. Be especially careful around

- Traffic
- Firearms
- Swimming pools
- Tools and equipment, such as lawn mowers
- Poisonous chemicals, cleaning supplies, or medicines

Maybe questions from your child's doctor raised the issue. At well-child visits, your child's doctor may ask

- How is your child doing in school?
- Are there any problems with learning that you or your child's teachers have seen?
- Is your child happy in school?
- Is your child having problems completing class work or homework?
- Are you concerned with any behavioral problems in school, at home, or when your child is playing with friends?

Your answers to these questions may lead to further evaluation for ADHD.

If your child has shown symptoms of ADHD on a regular basis for more than 6 months, discuss this with his doctor.

How is ADHD diagnosed?

Your child's doctor will determine whether he has ADHD by using standard guidelines developed by the American Academy of Pediatrics specifically for children 4 to 18 years of age.

It is difficult to diagnose ADHD in children younger than 4 years. This is because younger children change very rapidly. It is also more difficult to diagnose ADHD once a child becomes a teen.

There is no single test for ADHD. The process requires several steps and involves gathering information from multiple sources. You, your child, your child's school, and other caregivers should be involved in assessing your child's behavior.

Children with ADHD show signs of inattention, hyperactivity, and/or impulsivity in specific ways. (See the behaviors listed in Table 1.) Your child's doctor will look at how your child's behavior compares to that of other children his age, based on the information reported about your child by you, his teacher, and any other caregivers who spend time with your child, such as coaches or child care workers.

Here are guidelines used to confirm a diagnosis of ADHD.

- Some symptoms occur in 2 or more settings, such as home, school, and social situations, and cause some impairment.
- In a child 4 to 17 years of age, 6 or more symptoms must be identified.
- In a teen 17 years and older, 5 or more symptoms must be identified.
- Symptoms significantly impair your child's ability to function in some daily activities, such as doing schoolwork, maintaining relationships

with parents and siblings, building relationships with friends, or having the ability to function in groups such as sports teams.

In addition to looking at your child's behavior, your child's doctor will conduct a physical and neurological examination. A full medical history will be needed to put your child's behavior in context and screen for other conditions that may affect his behavior. Your child's doctor will also talk with your child about how he acts and feels.

Your child's doctor may refer your child to a pediatric subspecialist or mental health clinician if there are concerns in any of the following areas:

- Intellectual disability (previously called *mental retardation*)
- Developmental disorder, such as speech or motor disorders or a learning disability
- Chronic illness being treated with a medication that may interfere with learning
- Trouble seeing and/or hearing
- History of abuse
- Major anxiety or major depression
- Severe aggression
- Possible seizure disorder
- Possible sleep disorder

How can parents help with the diagnosis?

As a parent, you will provide crucial information about your child's behavior and how it affects his life at home, in school, and in other social settings. Your child's doctor will want to know what symptoms your child is experiencing, how long the symptoms have occurred, and how the behavior affects your child and your family. You may need to fill in checklists or rating scales about your child's behavior.

In addition, sharing your family history can offer important clues about your child's condition.

How will my child's school be involved?

For an accurate diagnosis, your child's doctor will need to get information about your child directly from his classroom teacher or another school professional. Children at least 4 years and older spend many of their waking hours at preschool or school. Teachers provide valuable insights. Your child's teacher may write a report or discuss the following topics with your child's doctor:

- Your child's behavior in the classroom
- Your child's learning patterns
- How long the symptoms have been a problem
- How the symptoms are affecting your child's progress at school
- Ways the classroom program is being adapted to help your child
- Whether other conditions may be affecting the symptoms

In addition, your child's doctor may want to see report cards, standardized tests, and samples of your child's schoolwork.

How will others who care for my child be involved?

Other caregivers may also provide important information about your child's behavior. Former teachers, religious and scout leaders, or coaches may have valuable input. If your child is homeschooled, it is especially important to assess his behavior in settings outside of the home.

Your child may not behave the same way at home as he does in other settings. Direct information about the way your child acts in more than one setting is required. It is important to consider other possible causes of your child's symptoms in these settings.

In some cases, other mental health care professionals, such as child psychologists or psychiatrists, may also need to be involved in gathering information for the diagnosis.

What are coexisting conditions?

As part of the diagnosis, your child's doctor will look for other conditions that cause the same types of symptoms as ADHD. Your child may simply have a different condition or ADHD combined with another condition (a *coexisting* condition). Most children with a diagnosis of ADHD have at least one additional condition.

Common coexisting conditions include

- **Learning disabilities** — Learning disabilities are conditions that make it difficult for a child to master specific skills, such as reading or math. ADHD is not a learning disability. However, ADHD can make it hard for a child to do well in school. Diagnosing learning disabilities requires conducting evaluations, such as IQ and academic achievement tests, and it requires educational interventions.

- **Oppositional defiant disorder or conduct disorder** — Up to 35% of children with ADHD also have oppositional defiant disorder or conduct disorder.

  — Children with oppositional defiant disorder tend to lose their temper easily and annoy people on purpose, and they are defiant and hostile toward authority figures.

  — Children with conduct disorder break rules, destroy property, get suspended or expelled from school, violate the rights of other people, or can be cruel to other children or animals.

  — Children with coexisting conduct disorder are at much higher risk for getting into trouble with the law or having substance use problems than children who have only ADHD. Studies show that this type of coexisting condition is more common among children with the primarily hyperactive/impulsive and combination types of ADHD. Your child's doctor may recommend behavioral therapy for your child if he has this condition.

- **Mood disorders/depression** — About 18% of children with ADHD also have mood disorders, such as depression or bipolar disorder (formerly called *manic depressive disorder*). There is often a family history of these conditions. Coexisting mood disorders may put children at higher risk for suicide, especially during the teen years. These disorders are more common among children with inattentive and combined types of ADHD. Children with mood disorders or depression often require additional interventions or a different type of medication than those typically used to treat ADHD.

- **Anxiety disorders** — About 25% of children with ADHD also have anxiety disorders. Children with anxiety disorders have extreme feelings of fear, worry, or panic that make it difficult to function. These disorders can produce physical symptoms, such as racing pulse, sweating, diarrhea, and nausea. Counseling and/or different medication may be needed to treat these coexisting conditions.

- **Language disorders** — Children with ADHD may have difficulty with how they use language. This is referred to as a *pragmatic language disorder*. It may not show up with standard tests of language. A speech-and-language clinician can detect it by observing how a child uses language in his day-to-day activities.

Are there other tests for ADHD?

You may have heard theories about other tests for ADHD. There are no other proven diagnostic tests at this time.

Many theories have been presented, but studies have shown that the following evaluations add little value in diagnosing the disorder:

- Screening for thyroid problems
- Computerized continuous performance tests
- Brain imaging studies, such as computed tomography (CT) scans and magnetic resonance imaging (MRI)
- Electroencephalography (EEG) or brain-wave testing

While these evaluations are not helpful in diagnosing ADHD, your child's doctor may see other signs or symptoms in your child that warrant blood tests, brain imaging studies, or EEG.

What causes ADHD?

ADHD is one of the most studied conditions of childhood, and it may be caused by a number of things.

Research to date has shown

- ADHD is a neurobiological condition in which symptoms are also dependent on the child's environment.
- A lower level of activity in the parts of the brain that control attention and activity level may be associated with ADHD.
- ADHD often runs in families. Sometimes ADHD is diagnosed in a parent at the same time it is diagnosed in the child.
- In very rare cases, toxins in the environment may lead to ADHD. For instance, lead in the body can affect child development and behavior. Lead may be found in many places, including homes built before 1978, when lead was added to paint.
- Significant head injuries may cause ADHD in some cases.
- Preterm birth increases the risk of developing ADHD.
- Prenatal substance exposures, such as alcohol or nicotine from smoking, increase the risk of developing ADHD.

There is little evidence that ADHD is caused by

- Eating too much sugar
- Food additives or food colorings
- Allergies
- Immunizations

How is ADHD treated?

Once the diagnosis is confirmed, the outlook for most children who receive treatment for ADHD is encouraging. There is no specific cure for ADHD, but there are many treatment options available, and some children learn to compensate for the difficulties as they mature.

Each child's treatment must be tailored to meet his individual needs. In most cases, treatment for ADHD should include

- A long-term management plan with
  — Target outcomes for behavior
  — Follow-up activities
  — Monitoring

- Education about ADHD
- Teamwork among doctors, parents, teachers, caregivers, other health care professionals, and the child
- Behavioral therapy, including parent training
- Individual and family counseling
- Medication

Treatment for ADHD is based on the same principles that are used to treat other chronic conditions, like asthma or diabetes. Long-term planning for many children is needed because these conditions are not curable. However, some children learn to compensate once they are adults. Families must manage chronic conditions on an ongoing basis. In the case of ADHD, schools and other caregivers must also be involved in managing the condition.

Educating the people involved with your child is a key part of treatment for ADHD. As a parent, you will need to learn about the condition. Read about it and talk with people who understand it. This will help you manage the ways ADHD affects your child and your family on a day-to-day basis. It will also help your child learn to help himself.

What are target outcomes?

At the beginning of treatment, your child's doctor should help you set around 3 target outcomes (goals) for your child's behavior. These target outcomes will guide the treatment plan. Your child's target outcomes should be chosen to help him function as well as possible at home, at school, and in your community. You need to identify what behaviors are most preventing your child from succeeding.

Here are examples of target outcomes.

- Improved relationships with parents, siblings, teachers, and friends — for example, fewer arguments with brothers or sisters or being invited more often to friends' houses or parties.
- Better schoolwork practices — for example, completing all classwork or homework assignments.
- More independence in self-care or homework — for example, getting ready for school in the morning without supervision.
- Improved self-esteem, such as feeling that he can get his work done.
- Fewer disruptive behaviors — for example, decreasing the number of times he refuses to obey rules.
- Safer behavior in the community — for example, being careful when crossing streets.

The target outcomes should be

- Realistic
- Something your child will be able to do
- Behaviors that you can observe and count (with rating scales)

Your child's treatment plan will be set up to help him achieve these goals.

What is behavioral therapy?

Most experts recommend using both behavioral therapy and medication to treat ADHD. This is known as a *multimodal treatment approach*.

There are many forms of behavioral therapy, but all have a common goal — to change the child's physical and social environments to help the child improve his behavior.

Table 2. Behavioral Therapy Techniques

Technique	Description	Example
Positive reinforcement	Complimenting the child and providing rewards or privileges in response to a desired behavior.	The child completes an assignment and is permitted to play on the computer.
Time-out	Removing access to a desired activity because of unwanted behavior.	The child hits a sibling and, as a result, must sit for 5 minutes in the corner of the room.
Response cost	Withdrawing rewards or privileges because of unwanted behavior.	The child loses free-time privileges for not completing homework.
Token economy	Combining reward and consequence. The child earns rewards and privileges when exhibiting desired behaviors. He loses rewards and privileges for unwanted behaviors.	The child earns stars or points for completing assignments and loses stars for getting out of his seat. He cashes in the sum of his stars or points at the end of the week for a prize.

Behavioral therapy has 3 basic principles.

1. **Set specific, doable goals.** Set clear and reasonable goals for your child, such as staying focused on homework for a certain amount of time or sharing toys with friends.
2. **Provide rewards and consequences.** Give your child a specified reward (positive reinforcement) every time he demonstrates the desired behavior. Give your child a consequence (unwanted result or punishment) consistently when he exhibits inappropriate behaviors.
3. **Keep using the rewards and consequences.** Using the rewards and consequences consistently for a long time will shape your child's behavior in a positive way.

Under this approach, parents, teachers, and other caregivers learn better ways to work with and relate to the child with ADHD. You will learn how to set and enforce rules, help your child understand what he needs to do, use discipline effectively, and encourage good behavior. Your child will learn better ways to control his behavior as a result. You will learn how to be more consistent.

Table 2 shows specific behavioral therapy techniques that can be effective with children who have ADHD.

Behavioral therapy is designed to recognize the limits that having ADHD puts on a child. It focuses on how the important people and places in the child's life can adapt to encourage good behavior and discourage unwanted behavior. It is different from play therapy or other therapies that focus mainly on the child and his emotions.

How can I help my child control his behavior?

As the child's primary caregivers, parents play a major role in behavioral therapy. Parent training is available to help you learn more about ADHD and specific, positive ways to respond to ADHD-type behaviors. This will help your child improve. In many cases, attending parenting classes with other parents will be sufficient, but with more challenging children, individual work with a counselor or coach may be needed.

Taking care of yourself will also help your child. Being the parent of a child with ADHD can be tiring and trying. It can test the limits of even the best parents. Parent training and support groups made up of other families who are dealing with ADHD can be a great source of help. Learn stress-management techniques to help you respond calmly to your child. Seek counseling if you feel overwhelmed or hopeless.

Ask your child's doctor to help you find parent training, counseling, and support groups in your community. See the *Resources* section.

What you can do

- **Keep your child on a daily schedule.** Try to keep the time that your child wakes up, eats, bathes, leaves for school, and goes to sleep the same each day.

- **Cut down on distractions.** Loud music, computer games, and TV can be overstimulating to your child. Make it a rule to keep the TV or music turned off during mealtime and while your child is doing homework. Don't place a TV in your child's bedroom. Whenever possible, avoid taking your child to places that may be too stimulating, such as busy shopping malls.

- **Organize your house.** If your child has specific and logical places to keep his schoolwork, toys, and clothes, he is less likely to lose them. Save a spot near the front door for his school backpack so he can grab it on the way out the door.

- **Reward positive behavior.** Offer kind words, hugs, or small prizes for reaching goals in a timely manner or for good behavior. Praise and reward your child's efforts to pay attention.

- **Set small, reachable goals.** Aim for slow progress rather than instant results. Be sure that your child understands that he can take small steps toward learning to control himself.

- **Help your child stay "on task."** Use charts and checklists to track progress with homework or chores. Keep instructions brief. Offer frequent, friendly reminders.

- **Limit choices.** Help your child learn to make good decisions by giving him only 2 or 3 options at a time.

- **Find activities at which your child can succeed.** All children need to experience success to feel good about themselves.

- **Use calm discipline.** Use consequences such as time-out, removing the child from the situation, or distraction. Sometimes it is best to simply ignore the behavior. Physical punishment, such as spanking or slapping, is not helpful. Discuss your child's behavior with him when both of you are calm.

- **Reach out to teachers.** Develop a good communication system with your child's teachers so that you can coordinate your efforts and monitor your child's progress.

How can my child's school help?

Your child's school is a key partner in providing effective behavioral therapy for your child. In fact, these principles work well in the classroom for most students.

Classroom management techniques may include

- Keeping a set routine and schedule for activities

- Using a system of clear rewards and consequences, such as a point system or token economy (see Table 2)

- Sending daily or weekly report cards or behavioral charts to parents to inform them about the child's progress

- Seating the child near the teacher

- Using small groups for activities

- Encouraging students to pause a moment before answering questions

- Keeping assignments short or breaking them into sections

- Supervising the child closely and giving frequent, positive cues to stay on task

- Changing where and how tests are given so students can succeed — for example, allowing students to take tests in a less distracting environment or allowing more time to complete tests

Your child's school should work with you and your child's doctor to develop strategies to assist your child in the classroom.

When a child has ADHD that is severe enough to interfere with his ability to learn, 2 federal laws offer help. These laws require public schools to provide or cover costs of evaluating the educational needs of the affected child and providing the needed services.

1. **The Individuals With Disabilities Education Act (IDEA), Part B,** requires public schools to provide or cover costs of evaluating the educational needs of the affected child and providing the needed special education services if your child qualifies because his learning is impaired by his ADHD. The diagnosis alone will not necessarily qualify your child for these services.

2. **Section 504 of the Rehabilitation Act of 1973** does not have strict qualification criteria but is limited to changes in the classroom, modifications in homework assignments, and taking tests in a less distracting environment or allowing more time to complete tests. Usually, the diagnosis alone will qualify your child for these services.

If your child has ADHD and a coexisting condition, he may need additional special services, such as a classroom aide, private tutoring, special classroom settings, or, in rare cases, a special school.

It is important to remember that once ADHD is diagnosed and treated, children with the disorder are more likely to achieve their goals in school.

What types of medication relieve ADHD symptoms?

For most children, stimulant medications are a safe and effective way to relieve ADHD symptoms. Just as glasses focus a person's eyesight so they can see better, these medications help children with ADHD focus their thoughts better and ignore distractions. This makes them more able to pay attention and control their behavior.

Stimulants may be used alone or in combination with behavioral therapy. Studies show that about 80% of children with ADHD who are treated with stimulants improve a great deal once the right medication and dose are determined.

Two forms of stimulants are available: immediate release (short acting) and extended release (intermediate acting and long acting). (See Table 3.) Immediate-release medications are usually taken every 4 hours, when needed. They are the cheapest of the medications. Extended-release medications are usually taken once in the morning.

Children who use extended-release forms of stimulants can avoid taking medication at school or after school. It is important not to chew or crush extended-release capsules or tablets. However, extended-release capsules that are made up of beads and lisdexamfetamine can be opened and sprinkled onto food for children who have difficulties swallowing tablets or capsules.

Nonstimulants can be tried when stimulant medications don't work or if they cause bothersome side effects.

Table 3. Common ADHD Medications

Type of Medication	Brand Name	Generic Name	Duration
Short-acting amphetamine stimulants	Adderall	Mixed amphetamine salts	4 to 6 hours
	Dexedrine	Dextroamphetamine	4 to 6 hours
Short-acting methylphenidate stimulants	Focalin	Dexmethylphenidate	3 to 5 hours
	Methylin	Methylphenidate (tablet, liquid, and chewable tablets)	3 to 5 hours
	Ritalin	Methylphenidate	3 to 5 hours
Mildly extended-release methylphenidate stimulants	Metadate ER	Methylphenidate	4 to 6 hours
	Methylin ER	Methylphenidate	4 to 6 hours
Intermediate-acting extended-release methylphenidate stimulants	Focalin XR	Dexmethylphenidate	6 to 8 hours
	Metadate CD	Methylphenidate	6 to 8 hours
	Ritalin LA	Methylphenidate	6 to 8 hours
Long-acting extended-release amphetamine stimulants	Adderall XR	Mixed amphetamine salts	8 to 12 hours
	Adzenys XR-ODT	Amphetamine	8 to 12 hours
	Dyanavel XR	Amphetamine (liquid)	8 to 12 hours
	Vyvanse	Lisdexamfetamine	8 to 12 hours
Long-acting extended-release methylphenidate stimulants	Concerta	Methylphenidate	10 to 12 hours
	Daytrana	Methylphenidate (skin patch)	11 to 12 hours
	Quillivant XR	Methylphenidate (liquid)	10 to 12 hours
α-Adrenergic agents (nonstimulants)	Intuniv	Guanfacine	24 hours
	Kapvay	Clonidine	12 hours
Selective norepinephrine reuptake inhibitors (nonstimulants)	Strattera	Atomoxetine	24 hours

Products are mentioned for informational purposes only and do not imply an endorsement by the American Academy of Pediatrics. Your doctor or pharmacist can provide you with important safety information for the products listed.

Which medication is best for my child?

It may take some time to find the best medication, dosage, and dosing schedule for your child.

Your child may need to try different types of stimulants or other medication. Some children respond to one type of stimulant but not another.

The amount of medication (dosage) that your child needs may also need to be adjusted. The dosage is not based solely on his weight. Your child's doctor will vary the dosage over time to get the best results and control possible side effects.

The medication schedule may also be adjusted, depending on the target outcome. For example, if the goal is to relieve symptoms that mostly occur at school, your child may take the medication only on school days.

It is important for your child to have regular medical checkups to monitor how well the medication is working and check for possible side effects.

What side effects can stimulants cause?

Side effects occur sometimes. These tend to happen early in treatment and are usually mild and short-lived, but in rare cases, they can be prolonged or more severe.

The most common side effects include

• Decreased appetite/weight loss

• Sleep problems

• Social withdrawal

Some less common side effects include

• Rebound effect (increased activity or a bad mood as the medication wears off)

• Transient muscle movements or sounds, called *tics*

• Minor growth delay

Very rare side effects include

• Significant increase in blood pressure or heart rate

• Bizarre behaviors

• Hallucinations

The same sleep problems do not exist for atomoxetine, but initially, this medication may make your child sleepy or upset his stomach. There have been very rare cases of atomoxetine needing to be stopped because it was causing liver damage. Rarely, atomoxetine increased thoughts of suicide. Extended-release guanfacine or clonidine can cause drowsiness, fatigue, or decreased blood pressure.

More than half of children who have tic disorders, such as Tourette syndrome, also have ADHD. Tourette syndrome is a familial condition associated with frequent tics and unusual vocal sounds. The effect of stimulants on tics is not predictable, although most studies indicate that stimulants are safe for children with ADHD and tic disorders in most cases. It is also possible to use atomoxetine or guanfacine for children with ADHD and Tourette syndrome.

Most side effects can be relieved by

- Changing the medication dosage
- Adjusting the schedule of medication
- Using a different stimulant or trying a nonstimulant (see Table 3)

Regular communication with your child's doctor is required until you find the best medication and dose for your child. After that, periodic monitoring by your doctor is important to maintain the best effects. To monitor the effects of the medication, your child's doctor will probably have you and your child's teacher(s) fill out behavior rating scales, observe changes in your child's target goals, notice any side effects, and monitor your child's height, weight, pulse, and blood pressure.

Stimulants, atomoxetine, and extended-release guanfacine or clonidine may not be an option for children who are taking certain other medications or who have some medical conditions, such as congenital heart disease.

How do I know if my child's treatment plan is working?

Ongoing monitoring of your child's behavior and medications is required to find out if the treatment plan is working. Office visits, phone conversations, behavioral checklists, written reports from teachers, and behavioral report cards are common tools for following your child's progress.

Treatment plans for ADHD usually require long-term efforts on the part of families and schools. Medication schedules may be complex. Behavioral therapies require education and patience. Sometimes it can be hard for everyone to stick with it. Your efforts play an important part in building a healthy future for your child.

Ask your child's doctor to help you find ways to keep your child's treatment plan on track.

What if my child does not reach his target outcomes?

Most school-aged children with ADHD respond well when their treatment plan includes both medication and behavioral therapy. If your child is not achieving his goals, your child's doctor will assess the following factors:

- Were the target outcomes realistic?
- Is more information needed about your child's behavior?
- Is the diagnosis correct?
- Is another condition hindering treatment?
- Is the treatment plan being followed?
- Has the treatment failed?

While treatment for ADHD should improve your child's behavior, it may not completely eliminate the symptoms of inattention, hyperactivity, and impulsivity. Children who are being treated successfully may still have trouble with their friends or schoolwork.

However, if your child is clearly not meeting his specific target outcomes, your child's doctor will need to reassess the treatment plan.

How can I help my child during the teen years?

The teen years can be a special challenge. Academic and social demands increase. In some cases, symptoms may be better controlled as your child grows older; however, frequently, the demands for performance also increase, so that in most cases, ADHD symptoms persist and continue to interfere with your child's ability to function

adequately. According to the National Institute of Mental Health, about 80% of those who required medication for ADHD as children still need it during the teen years.

Parents play an important role in helping their teens become independent. Encourage your teen to help himself with strategies such as

- Using a daily planner for assignments and appointments
- Being safety conscious, such as always wearing seat belts and using protective gear for sports
- Getting enough sleep
- Keeping a routine
- Making lists
- Organizing storage for items such as school supplies, clothes, CDs, and sports equipment
- Setting aside a quiet time and place to do homework
- Talking about problems with someone he trusts
- Understanding his increased risk of abusing substances, such as tobacco and alcohol

Activities such as sports, drama, and debate teams can be good places to channel excess energy and develop friendships. Find what your teen does well and support his efforts to "go for it."

Milestones such as learning to drive and dating offer new freedom and risks. Parents must stay involved and set limits for safety. Your teen's ADHD increases his risk of incurring traffic violations and accidents.

It remains important for parents of teens to keep in touch with teachers and make sure that their teen's schoolwork is going well.

Talk with your teen's doctor if your teen shows signs of severe problems, such as depression, drug abuse, or gang-related activities.

What about other types of treatments?

You may have heard media reports or seen advertisements for "miracle cures" for ADHD. Carefully research any such claims. Consider whether the source of the information is valid. At this time, there is no scientifically proven cure for this condition.

The following methods have no scientific evidence to prove that they work:

- Megavitamins and mineral supplements
- Anti-motion-sickness medication (to treat the inner ear)
- Treatment for *Candida* yeast infection
- EEG biofeedback (training to increase brain-wave activity)
- Applied kinesiology (realigning bones in the skull)
- Optometric vision training (which asserts that faulty eye movement and sensitivities cause the behavioral problems)

Always tell your child's doctor about any alternative therapies, supplements, or medications your child is using. These may interact with prescribed medications and harm your child.

Frequently Asked Questions

Q: Will my child outgrow ADHD? What about a cure?

A: ADHD continues into adulthood in most cases. However, by developing their strengths, structuring their environments, and using medication when needed, adults with ADHD can lead very productive lives. In some careers, having a high-energy behavioral pattern can be an asset.

There is no cure for ADHD at this time. However, research is ongoing to learn more about the role of the brain in ADHD, long-term outcomes for people with ADHD, and the best ways to treat the disorder.

Q: Why do so many children have ADHD?

A: The number of children getting treatment for ADHD has risen. It is not clear whether more children have ADHD or more children are receiving a diagnosis of ADHD. Also, more children with ADHD are getting treatment for a longer period. ADHD is one of the most common and most studied conditions of childhood. Because of more awareness and better ways of diagnosing and treating this disorder, more children are being helped. It may also be the case that school performance has become more important because of the higher technical demand of many jobs, and ADHD often interferes with a child's ability to function in school.

Q: Are schools putting children on ADHD medication?

A: Teachers are often the first to notice behavioral signs of possible ADHD. However, only physicians can prescribe medications to treat ADHD. The diagnosis of ADHD should follow a careful process.

Q: Can children get high on stimulant medications?

A: When taken as directed by a doctor, there is no evidence that children are getting high on stimulant drugs such as methylphenidate and amphetamine. At therapeutic doses, these drugs also do not sedate or tranquilize children and do not increase the risk of addiction.

However, stimulants are classified as Schedule II drugs by the US Drug Enforcement Administration because there is potential for abuse of this class of medication. If your child is taking medication, it is always best to supervise the use of the medication closely. Atomoxetine and guanfacine are not Schedule II drugs because they don't have potential for abuse, even in adults.

Q: Will use of stimulant medications lead to illegal drug or alcohol use?

A: People with ADHD are naturally impulsive and tend to take risks. But patients with ADHD who are taking stimulants are not at a greater risk of using other drugs and may actually be at a lower risk. Children and teens who have ADHD combined with coexisting conditions may be at higher risk for drug and alcohol use, regardless of the medication used.

Resources

Here is a list of ADHD support groups and resources. Also, your child's doctor may know about resources in your community.

CHADD–The National Resource Center on ADHD
800/233-4050
www.chadd.org

ADDA (Attention Deficit Disorder Association)
www.add.org

Center for Parent Information and Resources
www.parentcenterhub.org

National Institute of Mental Health
866/615-6464
www.nimh.nih.gov

Tourette Association of America
888/4-TOURET (486-8738)
www.tourette.org

From Your Doctor

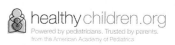

American Academy of Pediatrics
DEDICATED TO THE HEALTH OF ALL CHILDREN®

healthy children.org
Powered by pediatricians. Trusted by parents.
from the American Academy of Pediatrics

The American Academy of Pediatrics (AAP) is an organization of 66,000 primary care pediatricians, pediatric medical subspecialists, and pediatric surgical specialists dedicated to the health, safety, and well-being of infants, children, adolescents, and young adults.

medicines for ADHD questions from teens who have ADHD

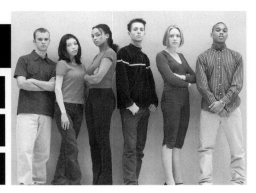

Q: What can I do besides taking medicines?

A: Medicines and behavior therapies are the only treatments that have been shown by scientific studies to work consistently for ADHD symptoms. Medicines are prescribed by a doctor, while behavior therapies usually are done with a trained counselor in behavior treatment. These 2 treatments are probably best used together, but you might be able to do well with one or the other. You can't rely on other treatments such as biofeedback, allergy treatments, special diets, vision training, or chiropractic because there isn't enough evidence that shows they work.

Counseling may help you learn how to cope with some issues you may face. And there are things you can do to help yourself. For example, things that may help you stay focused include using a daily planner for schoolwork and other activities, making to-do lists, and even getting enough sleep. Counseling can help you find an organization system or a checklist.

Q: How can medicines help me?

A: There are several different ADHD medicines. They work by causing the brain to have more *neurotransmitters* in the right places. Neurotransmitters are chemicals in the brain that help us focus our attention, control our impulses, organize and plan, and stick to routines. Medicines for ADHD can help you focus your thoughts and ignore distractions so that you can reach your full potential. They also can help you control your emotions and behavior. Check with your doctor to learn more about this.

Q: Are medicines safe?

A: For most teens with ADHD, stimulant medicines are safe and effective if taken as recommended. However, like most medicines, there could be side effects. Luckily, the side effects tend to happen early on, are usually mild, and don't last too long. If you have any side effects, tell your doctor. Changes may need to be made in your medicines or their dosages.

- **Most common side effects** include decreased appetite or weight loss, problems falling asleep, headaches, jitteriness, and stomachaches.
- **Less common side effects** include a bad mood as medicines wear off (called the rebound effect) and facial twitches or tics.

Q: Will medicines change my personality?

A: Medicines won't change who you are and should not change your personality. If you notice changes in your mood or personality, tell your doctor. Occasionally when medicines wear off, some teens become more irritable for a short time. An adjustment of the medicines by your doctor may be helpful.

Q: Will medicines affect my growth?

A: Medicines will not keep you from growing. Significant growth delay is a very rare side effect of some medicines prescribed for ADHD. Most scientific studies show that taking these medicines has little to no long-term effect on growth in most cases.

Q: Do I need to take medicines at school?

A: There are 3 types of medicines used for teens with ADHD: **short acting** (immediate release), **intermediate acting**, and **long acting.** You can avoid taking medicines at school if you take the intermediate- or long-acting kind. Long-acting medicines usually are taken once in the morning or evening. Short-acting medicines usually are taken every 4 hours.

Q: Does taking medicines make me a drug user?

A: No! Although you may need medicines to help you stay in control of your behavior, medicines used to treat ADHD do not lead to drug abuse. In fact, taking medicines as prescribed by your doctor and doing better in school may help you avoid drug use and abuse. (But never give or share your medicines with anyone else.)

Q: Will I have to take medicines forever?

A: In most cases, ADHD continues later in life. Whether you need to keep taking medicines as an adult depends on your own needs. The need for medicines may change over time. Many adults with ADHD have learned how to succeed in life without medicines by using behavior therapies or finding jobs that suit their strengths and weaknesses.

American Academy
of Pediatrics

DEDICATED TO THE HEALTH OF ALL CHILDREN™

The American Academy of Pediatrics is an organization of 60,000 primary care pediatricians, pediatric medical subspecialists, and pediatric surgical specialists dedicated to the health, safety, and well-being of infants, children, adolescents, and young adults.

American Academy of Pediatrics
Web site—www.HealthyChildren.org

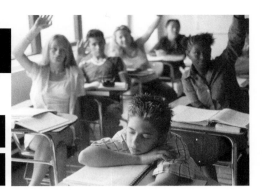

what is ADHD?
questions from teens

Attention-deficit/hyperactivity disorder (ADHD) is a condition of the brain that makes it difficult for people to concentrate or pay attention in certain areas where it is easy for others, like school or homework. The following are quick answers to some common questions:

Q: What causes ADHD?

A: There isn't just one cause. Research shows that

- ADHD is a medical condition caused by small changes in how the brain works. It seems to be related to 2 chemicals in your brain called *dopamine* and *norepinephrine*. These chemicals help send messages between nerve cells in the brain—especially those areas of the brain that control attention and activity level.
- ADHD most often runs in families.
- In a few people with ADHD, being born prematurely or being exposed to alcohol during the pregnancy can contribute to ADHD.
- Immunizations and eating too much sugar do NOT cause ADHD. And there isn't enough evidence that shows allergies and food additives cause ADHD.

Q: How can you tell if someone has ADHD?

A: You can't tell if someone has ADHD just by looks. People with ADHD don't look any different, but how they act may make them stand out from the crowd. Some people with ADHD are very hyperactive (they move around a lot and are not able to sit still) and have behavior problems that are obvious to everyone. Other people with ADHD are quiet and more laid back on the outside, but on the inside struggle with attention to schoolwork and other tasks. They are distracted by people and things around them when they try to study; they may have trouble organizing schoolwork or forget to turn in assignments.

Q: Can ADHD cause someone to act up or get in trouble?

A: Having ADHD can cause you to struggle in school or have problems controlling your behavior. Some people may say or think that your struggles and problems are because you are bad, lazy, or not smart. But they're wrong. It's important that you get help so your impulses don't get you into serious trouble.

Q: Don't little kids who have ADHD outgrow it by the time they are teens?

A: Often kids with the hyperactive kind of ADHD get less hyperactive as they get into their teens, but usually they still have a lot of difficulty paying attention, remembering what they have read, and getting their work done. They may or may not have other behavior problems. Some kids with ADHD have never been hyperactive at all, but usually their attention problems also continue into their teens.

Q: If I have trouble with homework or tests, do I have ADHD?

A: There could be many reasons why a student struggles with schoolwork and tests. ADHD could be one reason. It may or may not be, but your doctor is the best person to say for sure. Kids with ADHD often say it's hard to concentrate, focus on a task (for example, schoolwork, chores, or a job), manage their time, and finish tasks. This could explain why they may have trouble with schoolwork and tests. Whatever the problem, there are many people willing to help you. You need to find the approach that works best for you.

Q: Does having ADHD mean a person is not very smart?

A: Absolutely not! People who have trouble paying attention may have problems in school, but that doesn't mean they're not smart. In fact, some people with ADHD are very smart, but may not be able to reach their potential in school until they get treatment.

ADHD is a common problem. Teens with ADHD have the potential to do well in school and live a normal life with the right treatment.

Q: Is ADHD more common in boys?

A: More boys than girls are diagnosed with ADHD—about 2 or 3 boys to every 1 girl. However, these numbers do not include the number of girls with the inattentive type of ADHD who are not diagnosed. Girls with the inattentive type of ADHD tend to be overlooked entirely or do not attract attention until they are older.

Q: What do I do if I think I have ADHD?

A: Don't be afraid to talk with your parents or other adults that you trust. Together you can meet with your doctor and find out if you really have ADHD. If you do, your doctor will help you learn how to live with ADHD and find ways to deal with your condition.

The persons whose photographs are depicted in this publication are professional models. They have no relation to the issues discussed. Any characters they are portraying are fictional.

The information contained in this publication should not be used as a substitute for the medical care and advice of your pediatrician. There may be variations in treatment that your pediatrician may recommend based on individual facts and circumstances.

From your doctor

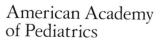

American Academy of Pediatrics

DEDICATED TO THE HEALTH OF ALL CHILDREN™

The American Academy of Pediatrics is an organization of 60,000 primary care pediatricians, pediatric medical subspecialists, and pediatric surgical specialists dedicated to the health, safety, and well-being of infants, children, adolescents, and young adults.

American Academy of Pediatrics
Web site—www.HealthyChildren.org

Brief Resolved Unexplained Events (Formerly Apparent Life-Threatening Events) and Evaluation of Lower-Risk Infants

- *Clinical Practice Guideline*

    - *PPI: AAP Partnership for Policy Implementation
      See Appendix 1 for more information.*

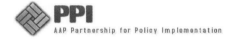

- *Executive Summary*

    - *PPI: AAP Partnership for Policy Implementation
      See Appendix 1 for more information.*

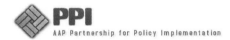

CLINICAL PRACTICE GUIDELINE   Guidance for the Clinician in Rendering Pediatric Care

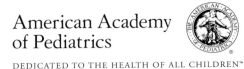

American Academy
of Pediatrics

DEDICATED TO THE HEALTH OF ALL CHILDREN™

Brief Resolved Unexplained Events (Formerly Apparent Life-Threatening Events) and Evaluation of Lower-Risk Infants

Joel S. Tieder, MD, MPH, FAAP, Joshua L. Bonkowsky, MD, PhD, FAAP, Ruth A. Etzel, MD, PhD, FAAP, Wayne H. Franklin, MD, MPH, MMM, FAAP, David A. Gremse, MD, FAAP, Bruce Herman, MD, FAAP, Eliot S. Katz, MD, FAAP, Leonard R. Krilov, MD, FAAP, J. Lawrence Merritt II, MD, FAAP, Chuck Norlin, MD, FAAP, Jack Percelay, MD, MPH, FAAP, Robert E. Sapién, MD, MMM, FAAP, Richard N. Shiffman, MD, MCIS, FAAP, Michael B.H. Smith, MB, FRCPCH, FAAP, for the SUBCOMMITTEE ON APPARENT LIFE THREATENING EVENTS

abstract

This is the first clinical practice guideline from the American Academy of Pediatrics that specifically applies to patients who have experienced an apparent life-threatening event (ALTE). This clinical practice guideline has 3 objectives. First, it recommends the replacement of the term ALTE with a new term, brief resolved unexplained event (BRUE). Second, it provides an approach to patient evaluation that is based on the risk that the infant will have a repeat event or has a serious underlying disorder. Finally, it provides management recommendations, or key action statements, for lower-risk infants. The term BRUE is defined as an event occurring in an infant younger than 1 year when the observer reports a sudden, brief, and now resolved episode of ≥1 of the following: (1) cyanosis or pallor; (2) absent, decreased, or irregular breathing; (3) marked change in tone (hyper- or hypotonia); and (4) altered level of responsiveness. A BRUE is diagnosed only when there is no explanation for a qualifying event after conducting an appropriate history and physical examination. By using this definition and framework, infants younger than 1 year who present with a BRUE are categorized either as (1) a lower-risk patient on the basis of history and physical examination for whom evidence-based recommendations for evaluation and management are offered or (2) a higher-risk patient whose history and physical examination suggest the need for further investigation and treatment but for whom recommendations are not offered. This clinical practice guideline is intended to foster a patient- and family-centered approach to care, reduce unnecessary and costly medical interventions, improve patient outcomes, support implementation, and provide direction for future research. Each key action statement indicates a level of evidence, the benefit-harm relationship, and the strength of recommendation.

DOI: 10.1542/peds.2016-0590

PEDIATRICS (ISSN Numbers: Print, 0031-4005; Online, 1098-4275).

To cite: Tieder JS, Bonkowsky JL, Etzel RA, et al. Brief Resolved Unexplained Events (Formerly Apparent Life-Threatening Events) and Evaluation of Lower-Risk Infants. *Pediatrics.* 2016;137(5):e20160590

INTRODUCTION

This clinical practice guideline applies to infants younger than 1 year and is intended for pediatric clinicians. This guideline has 3 primary objectives. First, it recommends the replacement of the term apparent life-threatening event (ALTE) with a new term, brief resolved unexplained event (BRUE). Second, it provides an approach to patient evaluation that is based on the risk that the infant will have a recurring event or has a serious underlying disorder. Third, it provides evidence-based management recommendations, or key action statements, for lower-risk patients whose history and physical examination are normal. It does not offer recommendations for higher-risk patients whose history and physical examination suggest the need for further investigation and treatment (because of insufficient evidence or the availability of clinical practice guidelines specific to their presentation). This clinical practice guideline also provides implementation support and suggests directions for future research.

The term ALTE originated from a 1986 National Institutes of Health Consensus Conference on Infantile Apnea and was intended to replace the term "near-miss sudden infant death syndrome" (SIDS).[1] An ALTE was defined as "an episode that is frightening to the observer and that is characterized by some combination of apnea (central or occasionally obstructive), color change (usually cyanotic or pallid but occasionally erythematous or plethoric), marked change in muscle tone (usually marked limpness), choking, or gagging. In some cases, the observer fears that the infant has died."[2] Although the definition of ALTE eventually enabled researchers to establish that these events are separate entities from SIDS, the clinical application of this classification, which describes a constellation of observed, subjective, and nonspecific symptoms, has raised significant challenges for clinicians and parents in the evaluation and care of these infants.[3] Although a broad range of disorders can present as an ALTE (eg, child abuse, congenital abnormalities, epilepsy, inborn errors of metabolism, and infections), for a majority of infants who appear well after the event, the risk of a serious underlying disorder or a recurrent event is extremely low.[2]

CHANGE IN TERMINOLOGY AND DIAGNOSIS

The imprecise nature of the original ALTE definition is difficult to apply to clinical care and research.[3] As a result, the clinician is often faced with several dilemmas. First, under the ALTE definition, the infant is often, but not necessarily, asymptomatic on presentation. The evaluation and management of symptomatic infants (eg, those with fever or respiratory distress) need to be distinguished from that of asymptomatic infants. Second, the reported symptoms under the ALTE definition, although often concerning to the caregiver, are not intrinsically life-threatening and frequently are a benign manifestation of normal infant physiology or a self-limited condition. A definition needs enough precision to allow the clinician to base clinical decisions on events that are characterized as abnormal after conducting a thorough history and physical examination. For example, a constellation of symptoms suggesting hemodynamic instability or central apnea needs to be distinguished from more common and less concerning events readily characterized as periodic breathing of the newborn, breath-holding spells, dysphagia, or gastroesophageal reflux (GER). Furthermore, events defined as ALTEs are rarely a manifestation of a more serious illness that, if left undiagnosed, could lead to morbidity or death. Yet, the perceived potential for recurring events or a serious underlying disorder often provokes concern in caregivers and clinicians.[2,4,5] This concern can compel testing or admission to the hospital for observation, which can increase parental anxiety and subject the patient to further risk and does not necessarily lead to a treatable diagnosis or prevention of future events. A more precise definition could prevent the overuse of medical interventions by helping clinicians distinguish infants with lower risk. Finally, the use of ALTE as a diagnosis may reinforce the caregivers' perceptions that the event was indeed "life-threatening," even when it most often was not. For these reasons, a replacement of the term ALTE with a more specific term could improve clinical care and management.

In this clinical practice guideline, a more precise definition is introduced for this group of clinical events: brief resolved unexplained event (BRUE). The term BRUE is intended to better reflect the transient nature and lack of clear cause and removes the "life-threatening" label. The authors of this guideline recommend that the term ALTE no longer be used by clinicians to describe an event or as a diagnosis. Rather, the term BRUE should be used to describe events occurring in infants younger than 1 year of age that are characterized by the observer as "brief" (lasting <1 minute but typically <20–30 seconds) and "resolved" (meaning the patient returned to baseline state of health after the event) and with a reassuring history, physical examination, and vital signs at the time of clinical evaluation by trained medical providers (Table 1). For example, the presence of respiratory symptoms or fever would preclude classification of an event as a BRUE. BRUEs are also "unexplained," meaning that a clinician is unable to explain the cause of the event after an appropriate history and physical examination. Similarly, an event characterized as choking or gagging associated with spitting up is not included in the BRUE definition, because clinicians will want to pursue the cause of vomiting, which may be related to GER, infection, or central nervous system (CNS) disease. However, until BRUE-specific codes are available, for billing and coding purposes, it is reasonable to apply the ALTE International Classification of Diseases, 9th Revision, and International Classification of Diseases, 10th revision, codes to patients determined to have experienced a BRUE (see section entitled "Dissemination and Implementation").

BRUE DEFINITION

Clinicians should use the term BRUE to describe an event occurring in an infant <1 year of age when the observer reports a sudden, brief, and now resolved episode of ≥1 of the following:

- **cyanosis or pallor**
- **absent, decreased, or irregular breathing**
- **marked change in tone (hyper- or hypotonia)**
- **altered level of responsiveness**

Moreover, clinicians should diagnose a BRUE only when there is no explanation for a qualifying event after conducting an appropriate history and physical examination (Tables 2 and 3).

Differences between the terms ALTE and BRUE should be noted. First, the BRUE definition has a strict age limit. Second, an event is only a BRUE if there is no other likely explanation. Clinical symptoms such as fever, nasal congestion, and increased work of breathing may indicate temporary airway obstruction from viral infection. Events characterized as choking after vomiting may indicate

TABLE 1 BRUE Definition and Factors for Inclusion and Exclusion

		Includes	Excludes
Brief		Duration <1 min; typically 20–30 s	Duration ≥1 min
Resolved		Patient returned to his or her baseline state of health after the event	At the time of medical evaluation:
		Normal vital signs	
		Normal appearance	Fever or recent fever
			Tachypnea, bradypnea, apnea
			Tachycardia or bradycardia
			Hypotension, hypertension, or hemodynamic instability
			Mental status changes, somnolence, lethargy
			Hypotonia or hypertonia
			Vomiting
			Bruising, petechiae, or other signs of injury/trauma
			Abnormal weight, growth, or head circumference
			Noisy breathing (stridor, sturgor, wheezing)
			Repeat event(s)
Unexplained		Not explained by an identifiable medical condition	Event consistent with GER, swallow dysfunction, nasal congestion, etc
			History or physical examination concerning for child abuse, congenital airway abnormality, etc
Event Characterization			
Cyanosis or pallor		Central cyanosis: blue or purple coloration of face, gums, trunk	Acrocyanosis or perioral cyanosis
		Central pallor: pale coloration of face or trunk	Rubor
Absent, decreased, or irregular breathing		Central apnea	Periodic breathing of the newborn
		Obstructive apnea	Breath-holding spell
		Mixed obstructive apnea	
Marked change in tone (hyper- or hypotonia)		Hypertonia	Hypertonia associated with crying, choking, or gagging due to GER or feeding problems
		Hypotonia	Tone changes associated with breath-holding spell
			Tonic eye deviation or nystagmus
			Tonic-clonic seizure activity
			Infantile spasms
Altered responsiveness		Loss of consciousness	Loss of consciousness associated with breath-holding spell
		Mental status change	
		Lethargy	
		Somnolence	
		Postictal phase	

a gastrointestinal cause, such as GER. Third, a BRUE diagnosis is based on the clinician's characterization of features of the event and not on a caregiver's perception that the event was life-threatening. Although such perceptions are understandable and important to address, such risk can only be assessed after the event has been objectively characterized by a clinician. Fourth, the clinician should determine whether the infant had episodic cyanosis or pallor, rather

than just determining whether "color change" occurred. Episodes of rubor or redness are not consistent with BRUE, because they are common in healthy infants. Fifth, BRUE expands the respiratory criteria beyond "apnea" to include absent breathing, diminished breathing, and other breathing irregularities. Sixth, instead of the less specific criterion of "change in muscle tone," the clinician should determine whether there was marked change in tone, including hypertonia or hypotonia. Seventh, because choking and gagging usually indicate common diagnoses such as GER or respiratory infection, their presence suggests an event was not a BRUE. Finally, the use of "altered level of responsiveness" is a new criterion, because it can be an important component of an episodic but serious cardiac, respiratory, metabolic, or neurologic event.

For infants who have experienced a BRUE, a careful history and physical examination are necessary to characterize the event, assess the risk of recurrence, and determine the presence of an underlying disorder (Tables 2 and 3). The recommendations provided in this guideline focus on infants with a lower risk of a subsequent event or serious underlying disorder (see section entitled "Risk Assessment: Lower- Versus Higher-Risk BRUE"). In the absence of identifiable risk factors, infants are at lower risk and laboratory studies, imaging studies, and other diagnostic procedures are unlikely to be useful or necessary. However, if the clinical history or physical examination reveals abnormalities, the patient may be at higher risk and further evaluation should focus on the specific areas of concern. For example,

- possible child abuse may be considered when the event history is reported inconsistently or is incompatible with the child's developmental age, or when, on physical examination, there is unexplained bruising or a torn labial or lingual frenulum;

- a cardiac arrhythmia may be considered if there is a family history of sudden, unexplained death in first-degree relatives; and

- infection may be considered if there is fever or persistent respiratory symptoms.

TABLE 2 Historical Features To Be Considered in the Evaluation of a Potential BRUE

Features To Be Considered
Considerations for possible child abuse:
Multiple or changing versions of the history/circumstances
History/circumstances inconsistent with child's developmental stage
History of unexplained bruising
Incongruence between caregiver expectations and child's developmental stage, including assigning negative attributes to the child
History of the event
General description
Who reported the event?
Witness of the event? Parent(s), other children, other adults? Reliability of historian(s)?
State immediately before the event
Where did it occur (home/elsewhere, room, crib/floor, etc)?
Awake or asleep?
Position: supine, prone, upright, sitting, moving?
Feeding? Anything in the mouth? Availability of item to choke on? Vomiting or spitting up?
Objects nearby that could smother or choke?
State during the event
Choking or gagging noise?
Active/moving or quiet/flaccid?
Conscious? Able to see you or respond to voice?
Muscle tone increased or decreased?
Repetitive movements?
Appeared distressed or alarmed?
Breathing: yes/no, struggling to breathe?
Skin color: normal, pale, red, or blue?
Bleeding from nose or mouth?
Color of lips: normal, pale, or blue?
End of event
Approximate duration of the event?
How did it stop: with no intervention, picking up, positioning, rubbing or clapping back, mouth-to-mouth, chest compressions, etc?
End abruptly or gradually?
Treatment provided by parent/caregiver (eg, glucose-containing drink or food)?
911 called by caregiver?
State after event
Back to normal immediately/gradually/still not there?
Before back to normal, was quiet, dazed, fussy, irritable, crying?
Recent history
Illness in preceding day(s)?
If yes, detail signs/symptoms (fussiness, decreased activity, fever, congestion, rhinorrhea, cough, vomiting, diarrhea, decreased intake, poor sleep)
Injuries, falls, previous unexplained bruising?
Past medical history
Pre-/perinatal history
Gestational age
Newborn screen normal (for IEMs, congenital heart disease)?
Previous episodes/BRUE?
Reflux? If yes, obtain details, including management
Breathing problems? Noisy ever? Snoring?
Growth patterns normal?
Development normal? Assess a few major milestones across categories, any concerns about development or behavior?
Illnesses, injuries, emergencies?
Previous hospitalization, surgery?
Recent immunization?
Use of over-the-counter medications?
Family history
Sudden unexplained death (including unexplained car accident or drowning) in first- or second-degree family members before age 35, and particularly as an infant?
Apparent life-threatening event in sibling?
Long QT syndrome?
Arrhythmia?

TABLE 2 Continued

Features To Be Considered
Inborn error of metabolism or genetic disease?
Developmental delay?
Environmental history
Housing: general, water damage, or mold problems?
Exposure to tobacco smoke, toxic substances, drugs?
Social history
Family structure, individuals living in home?
Housing: general, mold?
Recent changes, stressors, or strife?
Exposure to smoke, toxic substances, drugs?
Recent exposure to infectious illness, particularly upper respiratory illness, paroxysmal cough, pertussis?
Support system(s)/access to needed resources?
Current level of concern/anxiety; how family manages adverse situations?
Potential impact of event/admission on work/family?
Previous child protective services or law enforcement involvement (eg, domestic violence, animal abuse), alerts/reports for this child or others in the family (when available)?
Exposure of child to adults with history of mental illness or substance abuse?

The key action statements in this clinical practice guideline do not apply to higher-risk patients but rather apply only to infants who meet the lower-risk criteria by having an otherwise normal history and physical examination.

RISK ASSESSMENT: LOWER- VERSUS HIGHER-RISK BRUE

Patients who have experienced a BRUE may have a recurrent event or an undiagnosed serious condition (eg, child abuse, pertussis, etc) that confers a risk of adverse outcomes. Although this risk has been difficult to quantify historically and no studies have fully evaluated patient-centered outcomes (eg, family experience survey), the systematic review of the ALTE literature identified a subset of BRUE patients who are unlikely to have a recurrent event or undiagnosed serious conditions, are at lower risk of adverse outcomes, and can likely be managed safely without extensive diagnostic evaluation or hospitalization.[3] In the systematic review of ALTE studies in which it was possible to identify BRUE patients, the following characteristics most consistently conferred higher risk: infants <2 months of age, those with a history of prematurity, and those with more

than 1 event. There was generally an increased risk from prematurity in infants born at <32 weeks' gestation, and the risk attenuated once infants born at <32 weeks' gestation reached 45 weeks' postconceptional age. Two ALTE studies evaluated the duration of the event.[6,7] Although duration did not appear to be predictive of hospital admission, it was difficult to discern a BRUE population from the heterogeneous ALTE populations. Nonetheless, most events were less than one minute. By consensus, the subcommittee established <1 minute as the upper limit of a "brief event," understanding that objective, verifiable measurements were rarely, if ever, available. Cariopulmonary resuscitation (CPR) was identified as a risk factor in the older ALTE studies and confirmed in a recent study,[6] but it was unclear how the need for CPR was determined. Therefore, the committee agreed by consensus that the need for CPR should be determined by trained medical providers.

PATIENT FACTORS THAT DETERMINE A LOWER RISK

To be designated lower risk, the following criteria should be met (see Fig 1):

- Age >60 days

- Prematurity: gestational age ≥32 weeks and postconceptional age ≥45 weeks

- First BRUE (no previous BRUE ever and not occurring in clusters)

- Duration of event <1 minute

- No CPR required by trained medical provider

- No concerning historical features (see Table 2)

- No concerning physical examination findings (see Table 3)

Infants who have experienced a BRUE who do not qualify as lower-risk patients are, by definition, at higher risk. Unfortunately, the outcomes data from ALTE studies in the heterogeneous higher-risk population are unclear and preclude the derivation of evidence-based recommendations regarding management. Thus, pending further research, this guideline does not provide recommendations for the management of the higher-risk infant. Nonetheless, it is important for clinicians and researchers to recognize that some studies suggest that higher-risk BRUE patients may be more likely to have a serious underlying cause, recurrent event, or an adverse outcome. For example, infants younger than 2 months who experience a BRUE may be more likely to have a congenital or infectious cause and be at higher risk of an adverse outcome. Infants who have experienced multiple events or a concerning social assessment for child abuse may warrant increased observation to better document the events or contextual factors. A list of differential diagnoses for BRUE patients is provided in Supplemental Table 6.

METHODS

In July 2013, the American Academy of Pediatrics (AAP) convened a multidisciplinary subcommittee composed of primary care clinicians

TABLE 3 Physical Examination Features To Be Considered in the Evaluation of a Potential BRUE

Physical Examination
General appearance
Craniofacial abnormalities (mandible, maxilla, nasal)
Age-appropriate responsiveness to environment
Growth variables
Length, weight, occipitofrontal circumference
Vital signs
Temperature, pulse, respiratory rate, blood pressure, oxygen saturation
Skin
Color, perfusion, evidence of injury (eg, bruising or erythema)
Head
Shape, fontanelles, bruising or other injury
Eyes
General, extraocular movement, pupillary response
Conjunctival hemorrhage
Retinal examination, if indicated by other findings
Ears
Tympanic membranes
Nose and mouth
Congestion/coryza
Blood in nares or oropharynx
Evidence of trauma or obstruction
Torn frenulum
Neck
Mobility
Chest
Auscultation, palpation for rib tenderness, crepitus, irregularities
Heart
Rhythm, rate, auscultation
Abdomen
Organomegaly, masses, distention
Tenderness
Genitalia
Any abnormalities
Extremities
Muscle tone, injuries, limb deformities consistent with fracture
Neurologic
Alertness, responsiveness
Response to sound and visual stimuli
General tone
Pupillary constriction in response to light
Presence of symmetrical reflexes
Symmetry of movement/tone/strength

and experts in the fields of general pediatrics, hospital medicine, emergency medicine, infectious diseases, child abuse, sleep medicine, pulmonary medicine, cardiology, neurology, biochemical genetics, gastroenterology, environmental health, and quality improvement. The subcommittee also included a parent representative, a guideline methodologist/informatician, and an epidemiologist skilled in systematic reviews. All panel members declared potential conflicts on the basis of the AAP policy on Conflict of Interest and Voluntary Disclosure. Subcommittee members repeated this process annually and upon publication of the guideline. All potential conflicts of interest are listed at the end of this document. The project was funded by the AAP.

The subcommittee performed a comprehensive review of the literature related to ALTEs from 1970 through 2014. Articles from 1970 through 2011 were identified and evaluated by using "Management of Apparent Life Threatening Events in Infants: A Systematic Review," authored by the Society of Hospital Medicine's ALTE Expert Panel (which included 4 members of the subcommittee).[3] The subcommittee partnered with the Society of Hospital Medicine Expert Panel and a librarian to update the original systematic review with articles published through December 31, 2014, with the use of the same methodology as the original systematic review. PubMed, Cumulative Index to Nursing and Allied Health Literature, and Cochrane Library databases were searched for studies involving children younger than 24 months by using the stepwise approach specified in the Preferred Reporting Items for Systematic Reviews and Meta-Analyses (PRISMA) statement.[8] Search terms included "ALTE(s)," "apparent life threatening event(s)," "life threatening event(s)," "near miss SIDS" or "near miss sudden infant death syndrome," "aborted crib death" or "aborted sudden infant death syndrome," and "aborted SIDS" or "aborted cot death" or "infant death, sudden." The Medical Subject Heading "infantile apparent life-threatening event," introduced in 2011, was also searched but did not identify additional articles.

In updating the systematic review published in 2012, pairs of 2 subcommittee members used validated methodology to independently score the newly identified abstracts from English-language articles ($n = 120$) for relevance to the clinical questions (Supplemental Fig 3).[9,10] Two independent reviewers then critically appraised the full text of the identified articles ($n = 23$) using a structured data collection form based on published guidelines for evaluating medical literature.[11,12] They recorded each study's relevance to the clinical question, research design, setting, time period covered, sample size, patient eligibility criteria, data source, variables collected, key results, study

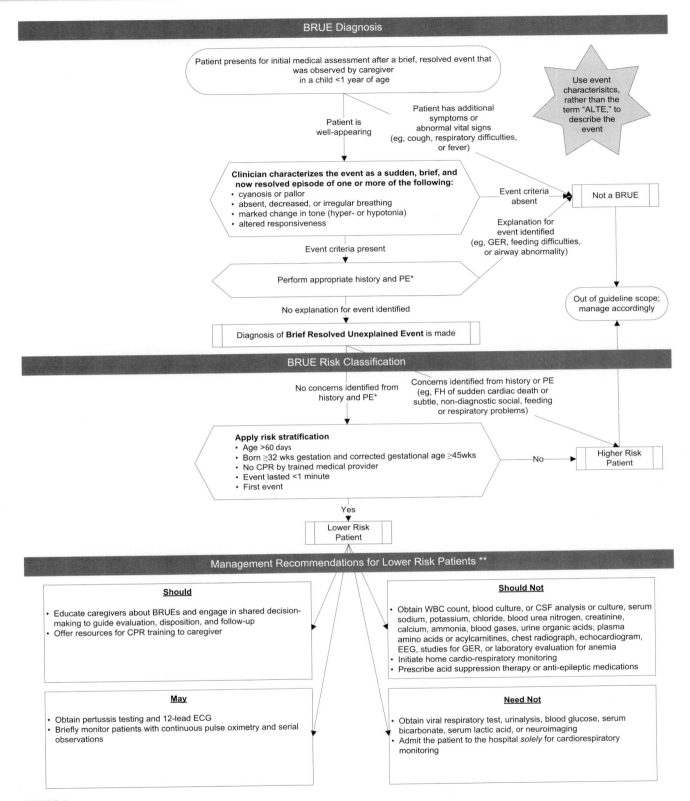

FIGURE 1

Diagnosis, risk classification, and recommended management of a BRUE. *See Tables 3 and 4 for the determination of an appropriate and negative FH and PE. **See Fig 2 for the AAP method for rating of evidence and recommendations. CSF, cerebrospinal fluid; FH, family history; PE, physical examination; WBC, white blood cell.

Figure 1, shown here, has been updated per the erratum at http://pediatrics.aappublications.org/content/138/2/e20161487.

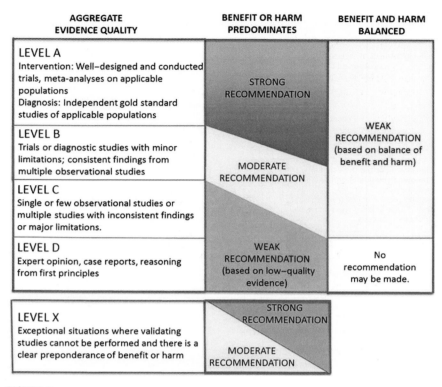

AGGREGATE EVIDENCE QUALITY	BENEFIT OR HARM PREDOMINATES	BENEFIT AND HARM BALANCED
LEVEL A Intervention: Well–designed and conducted trials, meta-analyses on applicable populations Diagnosis: Independent gold standard studies of applicable populations	STRONG RECOMMENDATION	
LEVEL B Trials or diagnostic studies with minor limitations; consistent findings from multiple observational studies		WEAK RECOMMENDATION (based on balance of benefit and harm)
LEVEL C Single or few observational studies or multiple studies with inconsistent findings or major limitations.	MODERATE RECOMMENDATION	
LEVEL D Expert opinion, case reports, reasoning from first principles	WEAK RECOMMENDATION (based on low–quality evidence)	No recommendation may be made.
LEVEL X Exceptional situations where validating studies cannot be performed and there is a clear preponderance of benefit or harm	STRONG RECOMMENDATION MODERATE RECOMMENDATION	

FIGURE 2
AAP rating of evidence and recommendations.

a systematic grading of the quality of evidence from the updated literature review by 2 independent reviewers and incorporation of the previous systematic review. Expert consensus was used when definitive data were not available. If committee members disagreed with the rest of the consensus, they were encouraged to voice their concern until full agreement was reached. If full agreement could not be reached, each committee member reserved the right to state concern or disagreement in the publication (which did not occur). Because the recommendations of this guideline were based on the ALTE literature, we relied on the studies and outcomes that could be attributable to the new definition of lower- or higher-risk BRUE patients.

Key action statements (summarized in Table 5) were generated by using BRIDGE-Wiz (Building Recommendations in a Developers Guideline Editor), an interactive software tool that leads guideline development teams through a series of questions that are intended to create clear, transparent, and actionable key action statements.[30] BRIDGE-Wiz integrates the quality of available evidence and a benefit-harm assessment into the final determination of the strength of each recommendation. Evidence-based guideline recommendations from the AAP may be graded as strong,

limitations, potential sources of bias, and stated conclusions. If at least 1 reviewer judged an article to be relevant on the basis of the full text, subsequently at least 2 reviewers critically appraised the article and determined by consensus what evidence, if any, should be cited in the systematic review. Selected articles used in the earlier review were also reevaluated for their quality. The final recommendations were based on articles identified in the updated ($n = 18$) and original ($n = 37$) systematic review (Supplemental Table 7).[6,7,13–28] The resulting systematic review was used to develop the guideline recommendations by following the policy statement from the AAP Steering Committee on Quality Improvement and Management, "Classifying Recommendations for Clinical Practice Guidelines."[29] Decisions and the strength of recommendations were based on

TABLE 4 Guideline Definitions for Key Action Statements

Statement	Definition	Implication
Strong recommendation	A particular action is favored because anticipated benefits clearly exceed harms (or vice versa) and quality of evidence is excellent or unobtainable.	Clinicians should follow a strong recommendation unless a clear and compelling rationale for an alternative approach is present.
Moderate recommendation	A particular action is favored because anticipated benefits clearly exceed harms (or vice versa) and the quality of evidence is good but not excellent (or is unobtainable).	Clinicians would be prudent to follow a moderate recommendation but should remain alert to new information and sensitive to patient preferences.
Weak recommendation (based on low-quality evidence)	A particular action is favored because anticipated benefits clearly exceed harms (or vice versa), but the quality of evidence is weak.	Clinicians would be prudent follow a weak recommendation but should remain alert to new information and very sensitive to patient preferences.
Weak recommendation (based on balance of benefits and harms)	Weak recommendation is provided when the aggregate database shows evidence of both benefit and harm that appear to be similar in magnitude for any available courses of action.	Clinicians should consider the options in their decision-making, but patient preference may have a substantial role.

TABLE 5 Summary of Key Action Statements for Lower-Risk BRUEs

When managing an infant aged >60 d and <1 y and who, on the basis of a thorough history and physical examination, meets criteria for having experienced a lower-risk BRUE, clinicians:	Evidence Quality; Strength of Recommendation
1. Cardiopulmonary evaluation	
1A. Need not admit infants to the hospital solely for cardiorespiratory monitoring.	B; Weak
1B. May briefly monitor patients with continuous pulse oximetry and serial observations.	D; Weak
1C. Should not obtain a chest radiograph.	B; Moderate
1D. Should not obtain a measurement of venous or arterial blood gas.	B; Moderate
1E. Should not obtain an overnight polysomnograph.	B; Moderate
1F. May obtain a 12-lead electrocardiogram.	C; Weak
1G. Should not obtain an echocardiogram.	C; Moderate
1H. Should not initiate home cardiorespiratory monitoring.	B; Moderate
2. Child abuse evaluation	
2A. Need not obtain neuroimaging (CT, MRI, or ultrasonography) to detect child abuse.	C; Weak
2B. Should obtain an assessment of social risk factors to detect child abuse.	C; Moderate
3. Neurologic evaluation	
3A. Should not obtain neuroimaging (CT, MRI, or ultrasonography) to detect neurologic disorders.	C; Moderate
3B. Should not obtain an EEG to detect neurologic disorders.	C; Moderate
3C. Should not prescribe antiepileptic medications for potential neurologic disorders.	C; Moderate
4. Infectious disease evaluation	
4A. Should not obtain a WBC count, blood culture, or cerebrospinal fluid analysis or culture to detect an occult bacterial infection.	B; Strong
4B. Need not obtain a urinalysis (bag or catheter).	C; Weak
4C. Should not obtain chest radiograph to assess for pulmonary infection.	B; Moderate
4D. Need not obtain respiratory viral testing if rapid testing is available.	C; Weak
4E. May obtain testing for pertussis.	B; Weak
5. Gastrointestinal evaluation	
5A. Should not obtain investigations for GER (eg, upper gastrointestinal tract series, pH probe, endoscopy, barium contrast study, nuclear scintigraphy, and ultrasonography).	C; Moderate
5B. Should not prescribe acid suppression therapy.	C; Moderate
6. IEM evaluation	
6A. Need not obtain measurement of serum lactic acid or serum bicarbonate.	C; Weak
6B. Should not obtain a measurement of serum sodium, potassium, chloride, blood urea nitrogen, creatinine, calcium, or ammonia.	C; Moderate
6C. Should not obtain a measurement of venous or arterial blood gases.	C; Moderate
6D. Need not obtain a measurement of blood glucose.	C; Weak
6E. Should not obtain a measurement of urine organic acids, plasma amino acids, or plasma acylcarnitines.	C; Moderate
7. Anemia evaluation	
7A. Should not obtain laboratory evaluation for anemia.	C; Moderate
8. Patient- and family-centered care	
8A. Should offer resources for CPR training to caregiver.	C; Moderate
8B. Should educate caregivers about BRUEs.	C; Moderate
8C. Should use shared decision-making.	C; Moderate

CPR, cardiopulmonary resuscitation; CT, computed tomography; GER, gastroesophageal reflux; WBC, white blood cell.

moderate, weak based on low-quality evidence, or weak based on balance between benefits and harms. Strong and moderate recommendations are associated with "should" and "should not" recommendation statements, whereas weak recommendation may be recognized by use of "may" or "need not" (Fig 2, Table 4).

A strong recommendation means that the committee's review of the evidence indicates that the benefits of the recommended approach clearly exceed the harms of that approach (or, in the case of a strong negative recommendation, that the

harms clearly exceed the benefits) and that the quality of the evidence supporting this approach is excellent. Clinicians are advised to follow such guidance unless a clear and compelling rationale for acting in a contrary manner is present. A moderate recommendation means that the committee believes that the benefits exceed the harms (or, in the case of a negative recommendation, that the harms exceed the benefits), but the quality of the evidence on which this recommendation is based is not as strong. Clinicians are also encouraged to follow such guidance

but also should be alert to new information and sensitive to patient preferences.

A weak recommendation means either that the evidence quality that exists is suspect or that well-designed, well-conducted studies have shown little clear advantage to one approach versus another. Weak recommendations offer clinicians flexibility in their decision-making regarding appropriate practice, although they may set boundaries on alternatives. Family and patient preference should have a substantial role in influencing clinical

1A. Clinicians Need Not Admit Infants Presenting With a Lower-Risk BRUE to the Hospital Solely for Cardiorespiratory Monitoring (Grade B, Weak Recommendation)

Aggregate Evidence Quality	Grade B
Benefits	Reduce unnecessary testing and caregiver/infant anxiety
	Avoid consequences of false-positive result, health care–associated infections, and other patient safety risks
Risks, harm, cost	May rarely miss a recurrent event or diagnostic opportunity for rare underlying condition
Benefit-harm assessment	The benefits of reducing unnecessary testing, nosocomial infections, and false-positive results, as well as alleviating caregiver and infant anxiety, outweigh the rare missed diagnostic opportunity for an underlying condition
Intentional vagueness	None
Role of patient preferences	Caregiver anxiety and access to quality follow-up care may be important considerations in determining whether a hospitalization for cardiovascular monitoring is indicated
Exclusions	None
Strength	Weak recommendation (because of equilibrium between benefits and harms)
Key references	31, 32

1B. Clinicians May Briefly Monitor Infants Presenting With a Lower-Risk BRUE With Continuous Pulse Oximetry and Serial Observations (Grade D, Weak Recommendation)

Aggregate Evidence Quality	Grade D
Benefits	Identification of hypoxemia
Risks, harm, cost	Increased costs due to monitoring over time and the use of hospital resources
	False-positive results may lead to subsequent testing and hospitalization
	False reassurance from negative test results
Benefit-harm assessment	The potential benefit of detecting hypoxemia outweighs the harm of cost and false results
Intentional vagueness	Duration of time to monitor patients with continuous pulse oximetry and the number and frequency of serial observations may vary
Role of patient preferences	Level of caregiver concern may influence the duration of oximetry monitoring
Exclusions	None
Strength	Weak recommendation (based on low quality of evidence)
Key references	33, 36

decision-making, particularly when recommendations are expressed as weak. Key action statements based on that evidence and expert consensus are provided. A summary is provided in Table 5.

The practice guideline underwent a comprehensive review by stakeholders before formal approval by the AAP, including AAP councils, committees, and sections; selected outside organizations; and individuals identified by the subcommittee as experts in the field.

All comments were reviewed by the subcommittee and incorporated into the final guideline when appropriate.

This guideline is intended for use primarily by clinicians providing care for infants who have experienced a BRUE and their families. This guideline may be of interest to parents and payers, but it is not intended to be used for reimbursement or to determine insurance coverage. This guideline is not intended as the sole source of guidance in the evaluation and

management of BRUEs but rather is intended to assist clinicians by providing a framework for clinical decision-making.

KEY ACTION STATEMENTS FOR LOWER-RISK BRUE

1. Cardiopulmonary

1A. Clinicians Need Not Admit Infants Presenting With a Lower-Risk BRUE to the Hospital Solely for Cardiorespiratory Monitoring (Grade B, Weak Recommendation)

Infants presenting with an ALTE often have been admitted for observation and testing. Observational data indicate that 12% to 14% of infants presenting with a diagnosis of ALTE had a subsequent event or condition that required hospitalization.[7,31] Thus, research has sought to identify risk factors that could be used to identify infants likely to benefit from hospitalization. A long-term follow-up study in infants hospitalized with an ALTE showed that no infants subsequently had SIDS but 11% were victims of child abuse and 4.9% had adverse neurologic outcomes (see 3. Neurology).[32] The ALTE literature supports that infants presenting with a lower-risk BRUE do not have an increased rate of cardiovascular or other events during admission and hospitalization may not be required, but close follow-up is recommended. Careful outpatient follow-up is advised (repeat clinical history and physical examination within 24 hours after the initial evaluation) to identify infants with ongoing medical concerns that would indicate further evaluation and treatment.

Al-Kindy et al[33] used documented monitoring in 54% of infants admitted for an ALTE (338 of 625) and identified 46 of 338 (13.6%) with "extreme" cardiovascular events (central apnea >30 seconds, oxygen saturation <80% for 10 seconds, decrease in heart rate <50–60/minutes for 10 seconds on the basis of postconceptional age). However, no adverse outcomes were noted for any of their cohort (although whether there is a protective effect of observation alone is not known). Some of the infants with extreme events developed symptoms of upper respiratory infection 1 to 2 days after the ALTE presentation. The risk factors for "extreme" events were prematurity, postconceptional age <43 weeks, and (presence of) upper respiratory infection symptoms. Importantly, infants with a postconceptional age >48 weeks were not documented as having an extreme event in this cohort. A previous longitudinal study also identified "extreme" events that occurred with comparable frequency in otherwise normal term infants and that were not statistically increased in term infants with a history of ALTE.[34]

Preterm infants have been shown to have more serious events, although an ALTE does not further increase that risk compared with asymptomatic preterm infants without ALTE.[34] Claudius and Keens[31] performed an observational prospective study in 59 infants presenting with ALTE who had been born at >30 weeks' gestation and had no significant medical illness. They evaluated factors in the clinical history and physical examination that, according to the authors, would warrant hospital admission on the basis of adverse outcomes (including recurrent cardiorespiratory events, infection, child abuse, or any life-threatening condition). Among these otherwise well infants, those with multiple ALTEs or age <1 month experienced adverse outcomes necessitating hospitalization. Prematurity was also a risk factor predictive of subsequent adverse events after an ALTE. Paroxysmal decreases in oxygen saturation in infants immediately before and during viral illnesses have been

well documented.[33,35] However, the significance of these brief hypoxemic events has not been established.

1B. Clinicians May Briefly Monitor Infants Presenting With a Lower-Risk BRUE With Continuous Pulse Oximetry and Serial Observations (Grade D, Weak Recommendation)

A normal physical examination, including vital signs and oximetry, is needed for a patient who has experienced a BRUE to be considered lower-risk. An evaluation at a single point in time may not be as accurate as a longer interval of observation. Unfortunately, there are few data to suggest the optimal duration of this period, the value of repeat examinations, and the effect of false-positive evaluations on family-centered care. Several studies have documented intermittent episodes of hypoxemia after admission for ALTE.[7,31,33] Pulse oximetry identified more infants with concerning paroxysmal events than cardiorespiratory monitoring alone.[33] However, occasional oxygen desaturations are commonly observed in normal infants, especially during sleep.[36] Furthermore, normative oximetry data are dependent on the specific machine, averaging interval, altitude, behavioral state, and postconceptional age. Similarly, there may be considerable variability in the vital signs and the clinical appearance of an infant. Pending further research into this important issue, clinicians may choose to monitor and provide serial examinations of infants in the lower-risk group for a brief period of time, ranging from 1 to 4 hours, to establish that the vital signs, physical examination, and symptomatology remain stable.

1C. Clinicians Should Not Obtain a Chest Radiograph in Infants Presenting With a Lower-Risk BRUE (Grade B, Moderate Recommendation)

Infectious processes can precipitate apnea. In 1 ALTE study, more than 80% of these infections involved the

respiratory tract.[37] Most, but not all, infants with significant lower respiratory tract infections will be symptomatic at the time of ALTE presentation. However, 2 studies have documented pneumonia in infants presenting with ALTE and an otherwise noncontributory history and physical examination.[4,37] These rare exceptions have generally been in infants younger than 2 months and would have placed them in the higher-risk category for a BRUE in this guideline. Similarly, Davies and Gupta[38] reported that 9 of 65 patients (ages unknown) who had ALTEs had abnormalities on chest radiography (not fully specified) despite no suspected respiratory disorder on clinical history or physical examination. Some of the radiographs were performed up to 24 hours after presentation. Davies and Gupta further reported that 33% of infants with ALTEs that were ultimately associated with a respiratory disease had a normal initial respiratory examination.[38] Kant et al[18] reported that 2 of 176 infants discharged after admission for ALTE died within 2 weeks, both of pneumonia. One infant had a normal chest radiograph initially; the other, with a history of prematurity, had a "possible" infiltrate. Thus, most experience has shown that a chest radiograph in otherwise well-appearing infants rarely alters clinical management.[7] Careful follow-up within 24 hours is important in infants with a nonfocal clinical history and physical examination to identify those who will ultimately have a lower respiratory tract infection diagnosed.

1D. Clinicians Should Not Obtain Measurement of Venous or Arterial Blood Gases in Infants Presenting With a Lower-Risk BRUE (Grade B, Moderate Recommendation)

Blood gas measurements have not been shown to add significant clinical information in otherwise well-appearing infants presenting with an ALTE.[4] Although not part of

1C. Clinicians Should Not Obtain Chest Radiograph in Infants Presenting With a Lower-Risk BRUE (Grade B, Moderate Recommendation)

Aggregate Evidence Quality	Grade B
Benefits	Reduce costs, unnecessary testing, radiation exposure, and caregiver/infant anxiety
	Avoid consequences of false-positive results
Risks, harm, cost	May rarely miss diagnostic opportunity for early lower respiratory tract or cardiac disease
Benefit-harm assessment	The benefits of reducing unnecessary testing, radiation exposure, and false-positive results, as well as alleviating caregiver and infant anxiety, outweigh the rare missed diagnostic opportunity for lower respiratory tract or cardiac disease
Intentional vagueness	None
Role of patient preferences	Caregiver may express concern regarding a longstanding breathing pattern in his/her infant or a recent change in breathing that might influence the decision to obtain chest radiography
Exclusions	None
Strength	Moderate recommendation
Key references	4, 37

1D. Clinicians Should Not Obtain Measurement of Venous or Arterial Blood Gases in Infants Presenting With a Lower-Risk BRUE (Grade B, Moderate Recommendation)

Aggregate Evidence Quality	Grade B
Benefits	Reduce costs, unnecessary testing, pain, risk of thrombosis, and caregiver/infant anxiety
	Avoid consequences of false-positive results
Risks, harm, cost	May miss rare instances of hypercapnia and acid-base imbalances
Benefit-harm assessment	The benefits of reducing unnecessary testing and false-positive results, as well as alleviating caregiver and infant anxiety, outweigh the rare missed diagnostic opportunity for hypercapnia and acid-base imbalances
Intentional vagueness	None
Role of patient preferences	None
Exclusions	None
Strength	Moderate recommendation
Key reference	4

this guideline, future research may demonstrate that blood gases are helpful in select infants with a higher risk BRUE to support the diagnosis of pulmonary disease, control-of-breathing disorders, or inborn errors of metabolism (IEMs).

1E. Clinicians Should Not Obtain an Overnight Polysomnograph in Infants Presenting With a Lower-Risk BRUE (Grade B, Moderate Recommendation)

Polysomnography consists of 8 to 12 hours of documented monitoring, including EEG, electro-oculography, electromyography, nasal/oral airflow, electrocardiography, end-tidal carbon dioxide, chest/abdominal excursion, and oximetry. Polysomnography is considered by many to be the gold standard for identifying obstructive sleep apnea (OSA), central sleep apnea, and periodic breathing and may identify seizures. Some data have suggested using polysomnography in infants presenting with ALTEs as a means to predict the likelihood of recurrent significant cardiorespiratory events. A study in which polysomnography was performed in a cohort of infants with ALTEs (including recurrent episodes) reported that polysomnography may reveal respiratory pauses of >20 seconds or brief episodes of bradycardia that are predictive of ensuing events over the next several months.[40] However, without a control population, the clinical significance of these events is uncertain, because respiratory pauses are frequently observed in otherwise normal infants.[35] Similarly, Kahn and Blum[41] reported that 10 of 71 infants with a clinical history of "benign" ALTEs had an abnormal polysomnograph, including periodic breathing (7 of 10) or obstructive apnea (4 of 100), but specific data were not presented. These events were not found in a control group of 181 infants. The severity of the periodic breathing (frequency of arousals and extent of oxygen desaturation) could not be evaluated from these data. Daniëls et al[42] performed polysomnography in 422 infants with ALTEs and identified 11 infants with significant bradycardia, OSA, and/or oxygen desaturation. Home monitoring revealed episodes of bradycardia (<50 per minute) in 7 of 11 infants and concluded that polysomnography is a useful modality. However, the clinical history, physical examination, and laboratory findings were not presented. GER has also been associated with specific episodes of severe bradycardia in monitored infants.[43] Overall, most polysomnography studies have shown minimal or nonspecific findings in infants presenting with ALTEs.[44,45] Polysomnography studies generally have not been predictive of ALTE recurrence and do not identify those infants at risk of SIDS.[46] Thus, the routine use of polysomnography in infants presenting with a lower-risk BRUE is likely to have a low diagnostic yield and is unlikely to lead to changes in therapy.

OSA has been occasionally associated with ALTEs in many series, but not all.[39,47–49] The use of overnight polysomnography to evaluate for OSA should be guided by an assessment of risk on the basis of a

1E. Clinicians Should Not Obtain an Overnight Polysomnograph in Infants Presenting With a Lower-Risk BRUE (Grade B, Moderate Recommendation)

Aggregate Evidence Quality	Grade B
Benefits	Reduce costs, unnecessary testing, and caregiver/infant anxiety Avoid consequences of false-positive results
Risks, harm, cost	May miss rare instances of hypoxemia, hypercapnia, and/or bradycardia that would be detected by polysomnography
Benefit-harm assessment	The benefits of reducing unnecessary testing and false-positive results, as well as alleviating caregiver and infant anxiety, outweigh the rare missed diagnostic opportunity for hypoxemia, hypercapnia, and/or bradycardia
Intentional vagueness	None
Role of patient preferences	Caregivers may report concern regarding some aspects of their infant's sleep pattern that may influence the decision to perform polysomnography
Exclusions	None
Strength	Moderate recommendation
Key reference	39

1F. Clinicians May Obtain a 12-Lead Electrocardiogram for Infants Presenting With Lower-Risk BRUE (Grade C, Weak Recommendation)

Aggregate Evidence Quality	Grade C
Benefits	May identify BRUE patients with channelopathies (long QT syndrome, short QT syndrome, and Brugada syndrome), ventricular pre-excitation (Wolff-Parkinson-White syndrome), cardiomyopathy, or other heart disease
Risks, harm, cost	False-positive results may lead to further workup, expert consultation, anxiety, and cost False reassurance from negative results Cost and availability of electrocardiography testing and interpretation
Benefit-harm assessment	The benefit of identifying patients at risk of sudden cardiac death outweighs the risk of cost and false results
Intentional vagueness	None
Role of patient preferences	Caregiver may decide not to have testing performed
Exclusions	None
Strength	Weak recommendation (because of equilibrium between benefits and harms)
Key references	4, 16

comprehensive clinical history and physical examination.[50] Symptoms of OSA, which may be subtle or absent in infants, include snoring, noisy respirations, labored breathing, mouth breathing, and profuse sweating.[51] Occasionally, infants with OSA will present with failure to thrive, witnessed apnea, and/or developmental delay.[52] Snoring may be absent in younger infants with OSA, including those with micrognathia. In addition, snoring in otherwise normal infants is present at least 2 days per week in 11.8% and at least 3 days per week in 5.3% of infants.[53] Some infants with OSA

may be asymptomatic and have a normal physical examination.[54] However, some studies have reported a high incidence of snoring in infants with (26%–44%) and without (22%–26%) OSA, making the distinction difficult.[55] Additional risk factors for infant OSA include prematurity, maternal smoking, bronchopulmonary dysplasia, obesity, and specific medical conditions including laryngomalacia, craniofacial abnormalities, neuromuscular weakness, Down syndrome, achondroplasia, Chiari malformations, and Prader-Willi syndrome.[34,56-58]

1F. Clinicians May Obtain a 12-Lead Electrocardiogram for Infants Presenting With Lower-Risk BRUE (Grade C, Weak Recommendation)

ALTE studies have examined screening electrocardiograms (ECGs). A study by Brand et al[4] found no positive findings on 24 ECGs performed on 72 patients (33%) without a contributory history or physical examination. Hoki et al[16] reported a 4% incidence of cardiac disease found in 485 ALTE patients; ECGs were performed in 208 of 480 patients (43%) with 3 of 5 abnormal heart rhythms identified by the ECG and the remaining 2 showing structural heart disease. Both studies had low positive-predictive values of ECGs (0% and 1%, respectively). Hoki et al had a negative predictive value of 100% (96%–100%), and given the low prevalence of disease, there is little need for further testing in patients with a negative ECG.

Some cardiac conditions that may present as a BRUE include channelopathies (long QT syndrome, short QT syndrome, Brugada syndrome, and catecholaminergic polymorphic ventricular tachycardia), ventricular pre-excitation (Wolff-Parkinson-White syndrome), and cardiomyopathy/myocarditis (hypertrophic cardiomyopathy, dilated cardiomyopathy). Resting ECGs are ineffective in identifying patients with catecholaminergic polymorphic ventricular tachycardia. Family history is important in identifying individuals with channelopathies.

Severe potential outcomes of any of these conditions, if left undiagnosed or untreated, include sudden death or neurologic injury.[59] However, many patients do not ever experience symptoms in their lifetime and adverse outcomes are uncommon. A genetic autopsy study in infants who died of SIDS in Norway showed an association between 9.5% and 13.0% of infants with abnormal

1G. Clinicians Should Not Obtain an Echocardiogram in Infants Presenting With Lower-Risk BRUE (Grade C, Moderate Recommendation)

Aggregate Evidence Quality	Grade C
Benefits	Reduce costs, unnecessary testing, caregiver/infant anxiety, and sedation risk
	Avoid consequences of false-positive results
Risks, harm, cost	May miss rare diagnosis of cardiac disease
Benefit-harm assessment	The benefits of reducing unnecessary testing and sedation risk, as well as alleviating caregiver and infant anxiety, outweigh the rare missed diagnostic opportunity for cardiac causes
Intentional vagueness	Abnormal cardiac physical examination reflects the clinical judgment of the clinician
Role of patient preferences	Some caregivers may prefer to have echocardiography performed
Exclusions	Patients with an abnormal cardiac physical examination
Strength	Moderate recommendation
Key references	4, 16

1H. Clinicians Should Not Initiate Home Cardiorespiratory Monitoring in Infants Presenting With a Lower-Risk BRUE (Grade B, Moderate Recommendation)

Aggregate Evidence Quality	Grade B
Benefits	Reduce costs, unnecessary testing, and caregiver/infant anxiety
	Avoid consequences of false-positive results
Risks, harm, cost	May rarely miss an infant with recurrent central apnea or cardiac arrhythmias
Benefit-harm assessment	The benefits of reducing unnecessary testing and false-positive results, as well as alleviating caregiver and infant anxiety, outweigh the rare missed diagnostic opportunity for recurrent apnea or cardiac arrhythmias
Intentional vagueness	None
Role of patient preferences	Caregivers will frequently request monitoring be instituted after an ALTE in their infant; a careful explanation of the limitations and disadvantages of this technology should be given
Exclusions	None
Strength	Moderate recommendation
Key reference	34

or novel gene findings at the long QT loci.[60] A syncopal episode, which could present as a BRUE, is strongly associated with subsequent sudden cardiac arrest in patients with long QT syndrome.[61] The incidence and risk in those with other channelopathies have not been adequately studied. The incidence of sudden cardiac arrest in patients with ventricular pre-excitation (Wolff-Parkinson-White syndrome) is 3% to 4% over the lifetime of the individual.[62]

1G. Clinicians Should Not Obtain an Echocardiogram in Infants Presenting With Lower-Risk BRUE (Grade C, Moderate Recommendation)

Cardiomyopathy (hypertrophic and dilated cardiomyopathy) and myocarditis could rarely present as a lower-risk BRUE and can be identified with echocardiography. The cost of an echocardiogram is high and accompanied by sedation risks.

In a study in ALTE patients, Hoki et al[16] did not recommend echocardiography as an initial cardiac test unless there are findings on examination or from an echocardiogram consistent with heart disease. The majority of abnormal echocardiogram findings in their study were not perceived to be life-threatening or related to a cause for the ALTE (eg, septal defects or mild valve abnormalities), and they would have been detected on echocardiogram or physical examination. Brand et al[4] reported 32 echocardiograms in 243 ALTE patients and found only 1 abnormal echocardiogram, which was suspected because of an abnormal history and physical examination (double aortic arch).

1H. Clinicians Should Not Initiate Home Cardiorespiratory Monitoring in Infants Presenting With a Lower-Risk BRUE (Grade B, Moderate Recommendation)

The use of ambulatory cardiorespiratory monitors in infants presenting with ALTEs has been proposed as a modality to identify subsequent events, reduce the risk of SIDS, and alert caregivers of the need for intervention. Monitors can identify respiratory pauses and bradycardia in many infants presenting with ALTE; however, these events are also occasionally observed in otherwise normal infants.[34,40] In addition, infant monitors are prone to artifact and have not been shown to improve outcomes or prevent SIDS or improve neurodevelopmental outcomes.[63] Indeed, caregiver anxiety may be exacerbated with the use of infant monitors and potential false alarms. The overwhelming majority of monitor-identified alarms, including many with reported clinical symptomatology, do not reveal abnormalities on cardiorespiratory recordings.[64–66] Finally, there are several studies showing a lack of correlation between ALTEs and SIDS.[24,32]

Kahn and Blum[41] monitored 50 infants considered at "high risk" of SIDS and reported that 80% had alarms at home. All infants with alarms had at least 1 episode of parental intervention motivated by the alarms, although the authors acknowledged that some cases of parental intervention may have been attributable to parental anxiety. Nevertheless, the stimulated infants did not die of SIDS or require rehospitalization and therefore it was concluded that monitoring resulted in successful resuscitation, but this was not firmly established. Côté et al[40] reported "significant events" involving central apnea and bradycardia with long-term monitoring. However, these events were later shown to be frequently present in otherwise well infants.[34] There are insufficient data to support the use of commercial infant monitoring devices marketed directly to parents for the purposes of SIDS prevention.[63] These monitors may be prone to false alarms, produce anxiety, and disrupt sleep. Furthermore, these machines are frequently used without a medical support system and in the absence of specific training to respond to alarms. Although it is beyond the scope of this clinical practice guideline, future research may show that home monitoring (cardiorespiratory and/or oximetry) is appropriate for some infants with higher-risk BRUE.

2. Child Abuse

2A. Clinicians Need Not Obtain Neuroimaging (Computed Tomography, MRI, or Ultrasonography) To Detect Child Abuse in Infants Presenting With a Lower-Risk BRUE (Grade C, Weak Recommendation)

2B. Clinicians Should Obtain an Assessment of Social Risk Factors To Detect Child Abuse in Infants Presenting With a Lower-Risk BRUE (Grade C, Moderate Recommendation)

Child abuse is a common and serious cause of an ALTE. Previous research has suggested that this occurs in up to 10% of ALTE cohorts.[3,67] Abusive head trauma is the most common form of child maltreatment associated with an ALTE. Other forms of child abuse that can present as an ALTE, but would not be identified by radiologic evaluations, include caregiver-fabricated illness (formally known as Münchausen by proxy), smothering, and poisoning.

Children who have experienced child abuse, most notably abusive head trauma, may present with a

2A. Clinicians Need Not Obtain Neuroimaging (Computed Tomography, MRI, or Ultrasonography) To Detect Child Abuse in Infants Presenting With a Lower-Risk BRUE (Grade C, Weak Recommendation)

Aggregate Evidence Quality	Grade C
Benefits	Decrease cost
	Avoid sedation, radiation exposure, consequences of false-positive results
Risks, harm, cost	May miss cases of child abuse and potential subsequent harm
Benefit-harm assessment	The benefits of reducing unnecessary testing, sedation, radiation exposure, and false-positive results, as well as alleviating caregiver and infant anxiety, outweigh the rare missed diagnostic opportunity for child abuse
Intentional vagueness	None
Role of patient preferences	Caregiver concerns may lead to requests for CNS imaging
Exclusions	None
Strength	Weak recommendation (based on low quality of evidence)
Key references	3, 67

2B. Clinicians Should Obtain an Assessment of Social Risk Factors To Detect Child Abuse in Infants Presenting With a Lower-Risk BRUE (Grade C, Moderate Recommendation)

Aggregate Evidence Quality	Grade C
Benefits	Identification of child abuse
	May benefit the safety of other children in the home
	May identify other social risk factors and needs and help connect caregivers with appropriate resources (eg, financial distress)
Risks, harm, cost	Resource intensive and not always available, particularly for smaller centers
	Some social workers may have inadequate experience in child abuse assessment
	May decrease caregiver's trust in the medical team
Benefit-harm assessment	The benefits of identifying child abuse and identifying and addressing social needs outweigh the cost of attempting to locate the appropriate resources or decreasing the trust in the medical team
Intentional vagueness	None
Role of patient preferences	Caregivers may perceive social services involvement as unnecessary and intrusive
Exclusions	None
Strength	Moderate recommendation
Key reference	68

BRUE. Four studies reported a low incidence (0.54%–2.5%) of abusive head trauma in infants presenting to the emergency department with an ALTE.[22,37,67,69] If only those patients meeting lower-risk BRUE criteria were included, the incidence of abusive head trauma would have been <0.3%. Although missing abusive head trauma can result in significant morbidity and mortality, the yield of performing neuroimaging to screen for abusive head trauma is extremely low and has associated risks of sedation and radiation exposure.[32,70]

Unfortunately, the subtle presentation of child abuse may lead to a delayed diagnosis of abuse and result in significant morbidity and mortality.[70] A thorough history and physical examination is the best way to identify infants at risk of these conditions.[67,71] Significant concerning features for child abuse (especially abusive head trauma) can include a developmentally inconsistent or discrepant history provided by the caregiver(s), a previous ALTE, a recent emergency service telephone call, vomiting, irritability, or bleeding from the nose or mouth.[67,71]

Clinicians and medical team members (eg, nurses and social workers) should obtain an assessment of social risk factors in infants with a BRUE, including negative attributions to and unrealistic expectations of the child, mental health problems, domestic violence/intimate partner violence, social service involvement, law enforcement involvement, and substance abuse.[68] In addition, clinicians and medical team members can help families identify and use resources that may expand and strengthen their network of social support.

In previously described ALTE cohorts, abnormal physical findings were associated with an increased risk of abusive head trauma. These findings include bruising, subconjunctival hemorrhage, bleeding from the nose or mouth, and a history of rapid head enlargement or head circumference >95th percentile.[67,70–74] It is important to perform a careful physical examination to identify subtle findings of child abuse, including a large or full/bulging anterior fontanel, scalp bruising or bogginess, oropharynx or frenula damage, or skin findings such as bruising or petechiae, especially on the trunk, face, or ears. A normal physical examination does not rule out the possibility of abusive head trauma. Although beyond the scope of this guideline, it is important for the clinician to note that according to the available evidence, brain neuroimaging is probably indicated in patients who qualify as higher-risk because of concerns about abuse resulting from abnormal history or physical findings.[67]

A social and environmental assessment should evaluate the risk of intentional poisoning, unintentional poisoning, and environmental exposure (eg, home environment), because these can be associated with the symptoms of ALTEs in infants.[75–78] In 1 study, 8.4% of children presenting to the emergency department after an ALTE were found to have a clinically significant, positive comprehensive toxicology screen.[76] Ethanol or other drugs have also been associated with ALTEs.[79] Pulmonary hemorrhage can be caused by environmental exposure to moldy, water-damaged homes; it would usually present with hemoptysis and thus probably would not qualify as a BRUE.[80]

3. Neurology

3A. Clinicians Should Not Obtain Neuroimaging (Computed Tomography, MRI, or Ultrasonography) To Detect Neurologic Disorders in Infants Presenting With a Lower-Risk BRUE (Grade C, Moderate Recommendation)

Epilepsy or an abnormality of brain structure can present as a lower-risk BRUE. CNS imaging is 1 method for evaluating whether underlying abnormalities of brain development or structure might have led to the BRUE. The long-term risk of a diagnosis of neurologic disorders ranges from 3% to 11% in historical cohorts of ALTE patients.[2,32] One retrospective study in 243 ALTE patients reported that CNS imaging contributed to a neurologic diagnosis in 3% to 7% of patients.[4] However, the study population included all ALTEs, including those with a significant past medical history, non–well-appearing infants, and those with tests ordered as part of the emergency department evaluation.

In a large study of ALTE patients, the utility of CNS imaging studies in potentially classifiable lower-risk BRUE patients was found to be low.[32] The cohort of 471 patients was followed both acutely and long-term

for the development of epilepsy and other neurologic disorders, and the sensitivity and positive-predictive value of abnormal CNS imaging for subsequent development of epilepsy was 6.7% (95% confidence interval [CI]: 0.2%–32%) and 25% (95% CI: 0.6%–81%), respectively.

The available evidence suggests minimal utility of CNS imaging to evaluate for neurologic disorders, including epilepsy, in lower-risk patients. This situation is particularly true for pediatric epilepsy, in which even if a patient is determined ultimately to have seizures/epilepsy, there is no evidence of benefit from starting therapy after the first seizure compared with starting therapy after a second seizure in terms of achieving seizure remission.[81–83] However, our recommendations for BRUEs are not based on any prospective studies and only on a single retrospective study. Future work should track both short- and long-term neurologic outcomes when considering this issue.

3B. Clinicians Should Not Obtain an EEG To Detect Neurologic Disorders in Infants Presenting With a Lower-Risk BRUE (Grade C, Moderate Recommendation)

Epilepsy may first present as a lower-risk BRUE. The long-term risk of epilepsy ranges from 3% to 11% in historical cohorts of ALTE patients.[2,32] EEG is part of the typical evaluation for diagnosis of seizure disorders. However, the utility of obtaining an EEG routinely was found to be low in 1 study.[32] In a cohort of 471 ALTE patients followed both acutely and long-term for the development of epilepsy, the sensitivity and positive-predictive value of an abnormal EEG for subsequent development of epilepsy was 15% (95% CI: 2%–45%) and 33% (95% CI: 4.3%–48%), respectively. In contrast, another retrospective study in 243 ALTE patients reported that EEG contributed to a neurologic diagnosis in 6% of patients.[4] This study

3A. Clinicians Should Not Obtain Neuroimaging (Computed Tomography, MRI, or Ultrasonography) To Detect Neurologic Disorders in Infants Presenting With a Lower-Risk BRUE (Grade C, Moderate Recommendation)

Aggregate Evidence Quality	Grade C
Benefits	Reduce unnecessary testing, radiation exposure, sedation, caregiver/infant anxiety, and costs
	Avoid consequences of false-positive results
Risks, harm, cost	May rarely miss diagnostic opportunity for CNS causes of BRUEs
	May miss unexpected cases of abusive head trauma
Benefit-harm assessment	The benefits of reducing unnecessary testing, radiation exposure, sedation, and false-positive results, as well as alleviating caregiver and infant anxiety, outweigh the rare missed diagnostic opportunity for CNS cause
Intentional vagueness	None
Role of patient preferences	Caregivers may seek reassurance from neuroimaging and may not understand the risks from radiation and sedation
Exclusions	None
Strength	Moderate recommendation
Key references	2, 32, 81

3B. Clinicians Should Not Obtain an EEG To Detect Neurologic Disorders in Infants Presenting With a Lower-Risk BRUE (Grade C, Moderate Recommendation)

Aggregate Evidence Quality	Grade C
Benefits	Reduce unnecessary testing, sedation, caregiver/infant anxiety, and costs
	Avoid consequences of false-positive or nonspecific results
Risks, harm, cost	Could miss early diagnosis of seizure disorder
Benefit-harm assessment	The benefits of reducing unnecessary testing, sedation, and false-positive results, as well as alleviating caregiver and infant anxiety, outweigh the rare missed diagnostic opportunity for epilepsy
Intentional vagueness	None
Role of patient preferences	Caregivers may seek reassurance from an EEG, but they may not appreciate study limitations and the potential of false-positive results
Exclusions	None
Strength	Moderate recommendation
Key references	32, 84, 85

population differed significantly from that of Bonkowsky et al[32] in that all ALTE patients with a significant past medical history and non–well-appearing infants were included in the analysis and that tests ordered in the emergency department evaluation were also included in the measure of EEG yield.

A diagnosis of seizure is difficult to make from presenting symptoms of an ALTE.[30] Although EEG is recommended by the American Academy of Neurology after a first-time nonfebrile seizure, the yield and sensitivity of an EEG after a first-time ALTE in a lower-risk child are low.[86] Thus, the evidence available suggests no utility for routine EEG to evaluate for epilepsy in a lower-risk BRUE. However, our recommendations for BRUEs are based on no prospective studies and on only a single retrospective study. Future work should track both short- and long-term epilepsy when considering this issue.

Finally, even if a patient is determined ultimately to have seizures/epilepsy, the importance of an EEG for a first-time ALTE is low, because there is little evidence that shows a benefit from starting therapy after the first seizure compared with after a second seizure in terms of achieving seizure remission.[81–83,85]

3C. Clinicians Should Not Prescribe Antiepileptic Medications for Potential Neurologic Disorders in Infants Presenting With a Lower-Risk BRUE (Grade C, Moderate Recommendation)

Once epilepsy is diagnosed, treatment can consist of therapy with an antiepileptic medication. In a cohort of 471 ALTE patients followed both acutely and long-term for the development of epilepsy, most patients who developed epilepsy had a second event within 1 month of their initial presentation.[32,87] Even if a patient is determined ultimately to have seizures/epilepsy, there is no evidence of benefit from starting therapy after the first seizure compared with starting therapy after a second seizure in terms of achieving seizure remission.[81–83,85] Sudden unexpected death in epilepsy (SUDEP) has a frequency close to 1 in 1000 patient-years, but the risks of SUDEP are distinct from ALTEs/BRUEs and include adolescent age and presence of epilepsy for more than 5 years. These data do not support prescribing an antiepileptic medicine for a first-time possible seizure because of a concern for SUDEP. Thus, the evidence available for ALTEs suggests lack of benefit for starting an antiepileptic medication for a lower-risk BRUE. However, our recommendations for BRUEs are based on no prospective studies and on only a single retrospective study. Future work should track both short- and long-term epilepsy when considering this issue.

4. Infectious Diseases

4A. Clinicians Should Not Obtain a White Blood Cell Count, Blood Culture, or Cerebrospinal Fluid Analysis or Culture To Detect an Occult Bacterial Infection in Infants Presenting With a Lower-Risk BRUE (Grade B, Strong Recommendation)

Some studies reported that ALTEs are the presenting complaint of an invasive infection, including bacteremia and/or meningitis

3C. Clinicians Should Not Prescribe Antiepileptic Medications for Potential Neurologic Disorders in Infants Presenting With a Lower-Risk BRUE (Grade C, Moderate Recommendation)

Aggregate Evidence Quality	Grade C
Benefits	Reduce medication adverse effects and risks, avoid treatment with unproven efficacy, and reduce cost
Risks, harm, cost	Delay in treatment of epilepsy could lead to subsequent BRUE or seizure
Benefit-harm assessment	The benefits of reducing medication adverse effects, avoiding unnecessary treatment, and reducing cost outweigh the risk of delaying treatment of epilepsy
Intentional vagueness	None
Role of patient preferences	Caregivers may feel reassured by starting a medicine but may not understand the medication risks
Exclusions	None
Strength	Moderate recommendation
Key references	32, 85, 87

4A. Clinicians Should Not Obtain a White Blood Cell Count, Blood Culture, or Cerebrospinal Fluid Analysis or Culture To Detect an Occult Bacterial Infection in Infants Presenting With a Lower-Risk BRUE (Grade B, Strong Recommendation)

Aggregate Evidence Quality	Grade B
Benefits	Reduce unnecessary testing, pain, exposure, caregiver/infant anxiety, and costs
	Avoid unnecessary antibiotic use and hospitalization pending culture results
	Avoid consequences of false-positive results/contaminants
Risks, harm, cost	Could miss serious bacterial infection at presentation
Benefit-harm assessment	The benefits of reducing unnecessary testing, pain, exposure, costs, unnecessary antibiotic use, and false-positive results, as well as alleviating caregiver and infant anxiety, outweigh the rare missed diagnostic opportunity for a bacterial infection
Intentional vagueness	None
Role of patient preferences	Caregiver concerns over possible infectious etiology may lead to requests for antibiotic therapy
Exclusions	None
Strength	Strong recommendation
Key references	4, 37, 88

detected during the initial workup. However, on further review of such cases with serious bacterial infections, these infants did not qualify as lower-risk BRUEs, because they had risk factors (eg, age <2 months) and/or appeared ill and had abnormal findings on physical examination (eg, meningeal signs, nuchal rigidity, hypothermia, shock, respiratory failure) suggesting a possible severe bacterial infection. After eliminating those cases, it appears extremely unlikely that meningitis or sepsis will be the etiology of a lower-risk BRUE.[2-4,37,88,89] Furthermore,

performing these tests for bacterial infection may then lead the clinician to empirically treat with antibiotics with the consequent risks of medication adverse effects, intravenous catheters, and development of resistant organisms. Furthermore, false-positive blood cultures (eg, coagulase negative staphylococci, *Bacillus* species, *Streptococcus viridans*) are likely to occur at times, leading to additional testing, longer hospitalization and antibiotic use, and increased parental anxiety until they are confirmed as contaminants.

Thus, the available evidence suggests that a complete blood cell count,

blood culture, and lumbar puncture are not of benefit in infants with the absence of risk factors or findings from the patient's history, vital signs, and physical examination (ie, a lower-risk BRUE).

4B. Clinicians Need Not Obtain a Urinalysis (Bag or Catheter) in Infants Presenting With a Lower-Risk BRUE (Grade C, Weak Recommendation)

Case series of infants with ALTEs have suggested that a urinary tract infection (UTI) may be detected at the time of first ALTE presentation in up to 8% of cases.[3,4,37,88] Claudius et al[88] provided insight into 17 cases of certain (*n* = 13) or possible (*n* = 4) UTI. However, 14 of these cases would not meet the criteria for a lower-risk BRUE on the basis of age younger than 2 months or being ill-appearing and/or having fever at presentation.

Furthermore, these studies do not always specify the method of urine collection, urinalysis findings, and/or the specific organisms and colony-forming units per milliliter of the isolates associated with the reported UTIs that would confirm the diagnosis. AAP guidelines for the diagnosis and management of UTIs in children 2 to 24 months of age assert that the diagnosis of UTI requires "*both* urinalysis results that suggest infection (pyuria and/or bacteriuria) *and* the presence of at least 50 000 colony-forming units/mL of a uropathogen cultured from a urine specimen obtained through catheterization or suprapubic aspirate."[90] Thus, it seems unlikely for a UTI to present as a lower-risk BRUE.

Pending more detailed studies that apply a rigorous definition of UTI to infants presenting with a lower-risk BRUE, a screening urinalysis need not be obtained routinely. If it is decided to evaluate the infant for a possible UTI, then a urinalysis can be obtained but should only be followed up with a culture if the urinalysis has

4B. Clinicians Need Not Obtain a Urinalysis (Bag or Catheter) in Infants Presenting With a Lower-Risk BRUE (Grade C, Weak Recommendation)

Aggregate Evidence Quality	Grade C
Benefits	Reduce unnecessary testing, pain, iatrogenic infection, caregiver/infant anxiety, and costs
	Avoid consequences of false-positive results
	Avoid delay from time it takes to obtain a bag urine
Risks, harm, cost	May delay diagnosis of infection
Benefit-harm assessment	The benefits of reducing unnecessary testing, iatrogenic infection, pain, costs, and false-positive results, as well as alleviating caregiver and infant anxiety, outweigh the rare missed diagnostic opportunity for a urinary tract infection
Intentional vagueness	None
Role of patient preferences	Caregiver concerns may lead to preference for testing
Exclusions	None
Strength	Weak recommendation (based on low quality of evidence)
Key references	4, 88

4C. Clinicians Should Not Obtain a Chest Radiograph To Assess for Pulmonary Infection in Infants Presenting With a Lower-Risk BRUE (Grade B, Moderate Recommendation)

Aggregate Evidence Quality	Grade B
Benefits	Reduce costs, unnecessary testing, radiation exposure, and caregiver/infant anxiety
	Avoid consequences of false-positive results
Risks, harm, cost	May miss early lower respiratory tract infection
Benefit-harm assessment	The benefits of reducing unnecessary testing, radiation exposure, and false-positive results, as well as alleviating caregiver and infant anxiety, outweigh the rare missed diagnostic opportunity for pulmonary infection
Intentional vagueness	None
Role of patient preferences	Caregiver concerns may lead to requests for a chest radiograph
Exclusions	None
Strength	Moderate recommendation
Key references	4, 18, 37

abnormalities suggestive of possible infection (eg, increased white blood cell count, positive nitrates, and/or leukocyte esterase).

4C. Clinicians Should Not Obtain a Chest Radiograph To Assess for Pulmonary Infection in Infants Presenting With a Lower-Risk BRUE (Grade B, Moderate Recommendation)

Chest radiography is unlikely to yield clinical benefit in a well-appearing infant presenting with a lower-risk BRUE. In the absence of abnormal respiratory findings (eg, cough, tachypnea, decreased oxygen saturation, auscultatory changes), lower respiratory tract infection is unlikely to be present.

Studies in children presenting with an ALTE have described occasional cases with abnormal findings on chest radiography in the absence of respiratory findings on history or physical examination.[4,37] However, the nature of the abnormalities and their role in the ALTE presentation in the absence of further details about the radiography results make it difficult to interpret the significance of these observations. For instance, descriptions of increased interstitial markings or small areas of atelectasis would not have the same implication as a focal consolidation or pleural effusion.

Kant et al,[18] in a follow-up of 176 children admitted for an ALTE, reported that 2 infants died within 2 weeks of discharge and both were found to have pneumonia on postmortem examination. This observation does not support the potential indication for an initial radiograph. In fact, one of the children had a normal radiograph during the initial evaluation. The finding of pneumonia on postmortem examination may reflect an agonal aspiration event. Brand et al[4] reported 14 cases of pneumonia identified at presentation in their analysis of 95 cases of ALTEs. However, in 13 of the patients, findings suggestive of lower respiratory infection, such as tachypnea, stridor, retractions, use of accessory muscles, or adventitious sounds on auscultation, were detected at presentation, leading to the request for chest radiography.

4D. Clinicians Need Not Obtain Respiratory Viral Testing If Rapid Testing Is Available in Infants Presenting With a Lower-Risk BRUE (Grade C, Weak Recommendation)

Respiratory viral infections (especially with respiratory syncytial virus [RSV]) have been reported as presenting with apnea or an ALTE, with anywhere from 9% to 82% of patients tested being positive for RSV.[2,4,37,88] However, this finding was observed predominantly in children younger than 2 months and/or those who were born prematurely. Recent data suggest that apnea or an ALTE presentation is not unique to RSV and may be seen with a spectrum of respiratory viral infections.[90] The data in ALTE cases do not address the potential role of other respiratory viruses in ALTEs or BRUEs.

In older children, respiratory viral infection would be expected to present with symptoms ranging from upper respiratory to lower respiratory tract infection rather than as an isolated BRUE. A history of respiratory symptoms and illness exposure; findings of congestion and/or cough, tachypnea, or lower respiratory tract abnormalities; and local epidemiology regarding currently circulating viruses are

4D. Clinicians Need Not Obtain Respiratory Viral Testing If Rapid Testing Is Available in Infants Presenting With a Lower-Risk BRUE (Grade C, Weak Recommendation)

Aggregate Evidence Quality	Grade C
Benefits	Reduce costs, unnecessary testing, and caregiver/infant discomfort
	Avoid false-negative result leading to missed diagnosis and false reassurance
Risks, harm, cost	Failure to diagnose a viral etiology
	Not providing expectant management for progression and appropriate infection control interventions for viral etiology
Benefit-harm assessment	The benefits of reducing unnecessary testing, pain, costs, false reassurance, and false-positive results, as well as alleviating caregiver and infant anxiety and challenges associated with providing test results in a timely fashion, outweigh the rare missed diagnostic opportunity for a viral infection
Intentional vagueness	"Rapid testing"; time to results may vary
Role of patient preferences	Caregiver may feel reassured by a specific viral diagnosis
Exclusions	None
Strength	Weak recommendation (based on low-quality evidence)
Key references	4, 37, 91

4E. Clinicians May Obtain Testing for Pertussis in Infants Presenting With a Lower-Risk BRUE (Grade B, Weak Recommendation)

Aggregate Evidence Quality	Grade B
Benefits	Identify a potentially treatable infection
	Monitor for progression of symptoms, additional apneic episodes
	Potentially prevent secondary spread and/or identify and treat additional cases
Risks, harm, cost	Cost of test
	Discomfort of nasopharyngeal swab
	False-negative results leading to missed diagnosis and false reassurance
	Rapid testing not always available
	False reassurance from negative results
Benefit-harm assessment	The benefits of identifying and treating pertussis and preventing apnea and secondary spread outweigh the cost, discomfort, and consequences of false test results and false reassurance; the benefits are greatest in at-risk populations (exposed, underimmunized, endemic, and during outbreaks)
Intentional vagueness	None
Role of patient preferences	Caregiver may feel reassured if a diagnosis is obtained and treatment can be implemented
Exclusions	None
Strength	Weak recommendation (based on balance of benefit and harm)
Key reference	93

considerations in deciding whether to order rapid testing for respiratory viruses. Because lower-risk BRUE patients do not have these symptoms, clinicians need not perform such testing.

In addition, until recently and in reports of ALTE patients to date, RSV testing was performed by using antigen detection tests. More recently, automated nucleic acid amplification-based tests have entered clinical practice. These assays are more sensitive than antigen detection tests and can detect multiple viruses from a single nasopharyngeal swab. The use of these tests in future research may allow better elucidation of the role of respiratory viruses in patients presenting with an ALTE in general and whether they play a role in BRUEs.

As a cautionary note, detection of a virus in a viral multiplex assay may not prove causality, because some agents, such as rhinovirus and adenovirus, may persist for periods beyond the acute infection (up to 30 days) and may or may not be related to the present episode.[92] In a lower-risk BRUE without respiratory symptoms testing for viral infection may not be indicated, but in the presence of congestion and/or cough, or recent exposure to a viral respiratory infection, such testing may provide useful information regarding the cause of the child's symptoms and for infection control management. Anticipatory guidance and arranging close follow-up at the initial presentation could be helpful if patients subsequently develop symptoms of a viral infection.

4E. Clinicians May Obtain Testing for Pertussis in Infants Presenting With a Lower-Risk BRUE (Grade B, Weak Recommendation)

Pertussis infection has been reported to cause ALTEs in infants, because it can cause gagging, gasping, and color change followed by respiratory pause. Such infants can be afebrile and may not develop cough or lower respiratory symptoms for several days afterward.

The decision to test a lower-risk BRUE patient for pertussis should consider potential exposures, vaccine history (including intrapartum immunization of the mother as well as the infant's vaccination history), awareness of pertussis activity in the community, and turnaround time for results. Polymerase chain reaction testing for pertussis on a nasopharyngeal specimen, if available, offers the advantage of rapid turnaround time to results.[94] Culture for the organism requires selective media and will take days to yield results but may still be useful in the face of identified risk of exposure. In patients in whom there is a high index of suspicion on the basis of the aforementioned risk factors, clinicians may consider prolonging the observation period and starting empirical antibiotics while awaiting test results (more information is available from the Centers for Disease Control and Prevention).[95]

5. Gastroenterology

5A. Clinicians Should Not Obtain Investigations for GER (eg, Upper Gastrointestinal Series, pH Probe, Endoscopy, Barium Contrast Study, Nuclear Scintigraphy, and Ultrasonography) in Infants Presenting With a Lower-Risk BRUE (Grade C, Moderate Recommendation)

GER occurs in more than two-thirds of infants and is the topic of discussion with pediatricians at one-quarter of all routine 6-month infant visits.[96] GER can lead to airway obstruction, laryngospasm, or aspiration. Although ALTEs that can be attributed to GER symptoms (eg, choking after spitting up) qualify as an ALTE according to the National Institutes of Health definition, importantly, they do not qualify as a BRUE.

GER may still be a contributing factor to a lower-risk BRUE if the patient's GER symptoms were not witnessed or well described by caregivers. However, the available evidence suggests no utility of routine diagnostic testing to evaluate for GER in these patients. The brief period of observation that occurs during an upper gastrointestinal series is inadequate to rule out the occurrence of pathologic reflux at other times, and the high prevalence of nonpathologic reflux that often occurs during the study can encourage false-positive diagnoses. In addition, the observation of the reflux of a barium column into the esophagus during gastrointestinal contrast studies may not correlate with the severity of GER or the degree of esophageal mucosal inflammation in patients with reflux esophagitis. Routine performance

of an upper gastrointestinal series to diagnose GER is not justified and should be reserved to screen for anatomic abnormalities associated with vomiting (which is a symptom that precludes the diagnosis of a lower-risk BRUE).[98] Gastroesophageal scintigraphy scans for reflux of ^{99m}Tc-labeled solids or liquids into the esophagus or lungs after the administration of the test material into the stomach. The lack of standardized techniques and age-specific normal values limits the usefulness of this test. Therefore, gastroesophageal scintigraphy is not recommended in the routine evaluation of pediatric patients with GER symptoms or a lower-risk BRUE.[97] Multiple intraluminal impedance (MII) is useful for detecting both acidic and nonacidic reflux, thereby providing a more detailed picture of esophageal events than pH monitoring. Combined pH/MII testing is evolving into the test of choice to detect temporal relationships between specific symptoms and the reflux of both acid and nonacid gastric contents. In particular, MII has been used in recent years to investigate how GER correlates with respiratory symptoms, such as apnea or

cough. Performing esophageal pH +/- impedance monitoring is not indicated in the routine evaluation of infants presenting with a lower-risk BRUE, although it may be considered in patients with recurrent BRUEs and GER symptoms even if these occur independently.

Problems with the coordination of feedings can lead to ALTEs and BRUEs. In a study in Austrian newborns, infants who experienced an ALTE had a more than twofold increase in feeding difficulties (multivariate relative risk: 2.5; 95% CI: 1.3–4.6).[99] In such patients, it is likely that poor suck-swallow-breathe coordination triggered choking or laryngospasm. A clinical speech therapy evaluation may help to evaluate any concerns for poor coordination swallowing with feeding.

5B. Clinicians Should Not Prescribe Acid Suppression Therapy for Infants Presenting With a Lower-Risk BRUE (Grade C, Moderate Recommendation)

The available evidence suggests no proven efficacy of acid suppression therapy for esophageal reflux in patients presenting with a lower-risk BRUE. Acid suppression therapy with H2-receptor antagonists or proton

5A. Clinicians Should Not Obtain Investigations for GER (eg, Upper Gastrointestinal Series, pH Probe, Endoscopy, Barium Contrast Study, Nuclear Scintigraphy, and Ultrasonography) in Infants Presenting With a Lower-Risk BRUE (Grade C, Moderate Recommendation)

Aggregate Evidence Quality	Grade C
Benefits	Reduce unnecessary testing, procedural complications (sedation, intestinal perforation, bleeding), pain, radiation exposure, caregiver/infant anxiety, and costs Avoid consequences of false-positive results
Risks, harm, cost	Delay diagnosis of rare but serious gastrointestinal abnormalities (eg, tracheoesophageal fistula) Long-term morbidity of repeated events (eg, chronic lung disease)
Benefit-harm assessment	The benefits of reducing unnecessary testing, complications, radiation, pain, costs, and false-positive results, as well as alleviating caregiver and infant anxiety, outweigh the rare missed diagnostic opportunity for a gastrointestinal abnormality or morbidity from repeat events
Intentional vagueness	None
Role of patient preferences	Caregiver may be reassured by diagnostic evaluation of GER
Exclusions	None
Strength	Moderate recommendation
Key references	96, 97

5B. Clinicians Should Not Prescribe Acid Suppression Therapy for Infants Presenting With a Lower-Risk BRUE (Grade C, Moderate Recommendation)

Aggregate Evidence Quality	Grade C
Benefits	Reduce unnecessary medication use, adverse effects, and cost from treatment with unproven efficacy
Risks, harm, cost	Delay treatment of rare but undiagnosed gastrointestinal disease, which could lead to complications (eg, esophagitis)
Benefit-harm assessment	The benefits of reducing medication adverse effects, avoiding unnecessary treatment, and reducing cost outweigh the risk of delaying treatment of gastrointestinal disease
Intentional vagueness	None
Role of patient preferences	Caregiver concerns may lead to requests for treatment
Exclusions	None
Strength	Moderate recommendation
Key reference	98

pump inhibitors may be indicated in selected pediatric patients with GER disease (GERD), which is diagnosed in patients when reflux of gastric contents causes troublesome symptoms or complications.[98] Infants with spitting up or throat-clearing coughs that are not troublesome do not meet diagnostic criteria for GERD. Indeed, the inappropriate administration of acid suppression therapy may have harmful adverse effects because it exposes infants to an increased risk of pneumonia or gastroenteritis.[100]

GER leading to apnea is not always clinically apparent and can be the cause of a BRUE. Acid reflux into the esophagus has been shown to be temporally associated with oxygen desaturation and obstructive apnea, suggesting that esophageal reflux may be one of the underlying conditions in selected infants presenting with BRUEs.[101] Respiratory symptoms are more likely to be associated with GER when gross emesis occurs at the time of a BRUE, when episodes occur while the infant is awake and supine (sometimes referred to as "awake apnea"), and when a pattern of obstructive apnea is observed while the infant is making respiratory efforts without effective air movement.[102]

Wenzl et al[103] reported a temporal association between 30% of the nonpathologic, short episodes of central apnea and GER by analyzing combined data from simultaneous esophageal and cardiorespiratory monitoring. These findings cannot be extrapolated to pathologic infant apnea and may represent a normal protective cessation of breathing during regurgitation. Similarly, Mousa et al[104] analyzed data from 527 apneic events in 25 infants and observed that only 15.2% were temporally associated with GER. Furthermore, there was no difference in the linkage between apneic events and acid reflux (7.0%) and nonacid reflux (8.2%). They concluded that there is little evidence for an association between acid reflux or nonacid reflux and the frequency of apnea. Regression analysis revealed a significant association between apnea and reflux in 4 of 25 infants. Thus, in selected infants, a clear temporal relationship between apnea and ALTE can be shown. However, larger studies have not proven a causal relationship between pathologic apnea and GER.[105]

As outlined in the definition of a BRUE, when an apparent explanation for the event, such as GER, is evident at the time of initial evaluation, the patient should be managed as appropriate for the clinical situation. However, BRUEs can be caused by episodes of reflux-related laryngospasm (sometimes referred to as "silent reflux"), which may not be clinically apparent at the time of initial evaluation. Laryngospasm may also occur during feeding in the absence of GER. Measures that have been shown to be helpful in the nonpharmacologic management of GER in infants include avoiding overfeeding, frequent burping during feeding, upright positioning in the caregiver's arms after feeding, and avoidance of secondhand smoke.[106] Thickening feedings with commercially thickened formula for infants without milk-protein intolerance does not alter esophageal acid exposure detected by esophageal pH study but has been shown to decrease the frequency of regurgitation. Given the temporal association observed between GER and respiratory symptoms in selected infants, approaches that decrease the height of the reflux column, the volume of refluxate, and the frequency of reflux episodes may theoretically be beneficial.[98] Combined pH/MII testing has shown that, although the frequency of reflux events is unchanged with thickened formula, the height of the column of refluxate is decreased. Studies have shown that holding the infant on the caregiver's shoulders for 10 to 20 minutes to allow for adequate burping after a feeding before placing the infant in the "back to sleep position" can decrease the frequency of GER in infants. In contrast, placing an infant in a car seat or in other semisupine positions, such as in an infant carrier, exacerbates esophageal reflux and should be avoided.[98] The frequency of GER has been reported to be decreased in breastfed compared with formula-fed infants. Thus, the benefits of breastfeeding are preferred over the theoretical effect of thickened formula feeding, so exclusive breastfeeding should be encouraged whenever possible.

6. Inborn Errors of Metabolism

6A. Clinicians Need Not Obtain Measurement of Serum Lactic Acid or Serum Bicarbonate To Detect an IEM in Infants Presenting With a Lower-Risk BRUE (Grade C, Weak Recommendation)

6B. Clinicians Should Not Obtain a Measurement of Serum Sodium, Potassium, Chloride, Blood Urea Nitrogen, Creatinine, Calcium, or Ammonia To Detect an IEM on Infants Presenting With a Lower-Risk BRUE (Grade C, Moderate Recommendation)

6C. Clinicians Should Not Obtain a Measurement of Venous or Arterial Blood Gases To Detect an IEM in Infants Presenting With Lower-Risk BRUE (Grade C, Moderate Recommendation)

6D. Clinicians Need Not Obtain a Measurement of Blood Glucose To Detect an IEM in Infants Presenting With a Lower-Risk BRUE (Grade C, Weak Recommendation)

6E. Clinicians Should Not Obtain Measurements of Urine Organic Acids, Plasma Amino Acids, or Plasma Acylcarnitines To Detect an IEM in Infants Presenting With a Lower-Risk BRUE (Grade C, Moderate Recommendation)

IEMs are reported to cause an ALTE in 0% to 5% of cases.[2,27,38,99,107,108] On the basis of the information provided by the authors for these patients, it seems unlikely that events could have been classified as a lower-risk BRUE, either because the patient had a positive history or physical examination or a recurrent event. The most commonly reported disorders include fatty acid oxidation disorders or urea cycle disorders.[107,109] In cases of vague or resolved symptoms, a careful history can help determine whether the infant had not received previous treatment (eg, feeding after listlessness for suspected hypoglycemia). These rare circumstances could include milder or later-onset presentations of IEMs.

Infants may be classified as being at a higher risk of BRUE because

6A. Clinicians Need Not Obtain Measurement of Serum Lactic Acid or Serum Bicarbonate To Detect an IEM in Infants Presenting With a Lower-Risk BRUE (Grade C, Weak Recommendation)

Aggregate Evidence Quality	Grade C
Benefits	Reduce unnecessary testing, caregiver/infant anxiety, and costs
	Avoid consequences of false-positive or nonspecific results
Risks, harm, cost	May miss detection of an IEM
Benefit-harm assessment	The benefits of reducing unnecessary testing, cost, and false-positive results, as well as alleviating caregiver and infant anxiety, outweigh the rare missed diagnostic opportunity for an IEM
Intentional vagueness	Detection of higher lactic acid or lower bicarbonate levels should be considered to have a lower likelihood of being a false-positive result and may warrant additional investigation
Role of patient preferences	Caregiver concerns may lead to requests for diagnostic testing
Exclusions	None
Strength	Weak recommendation (based on low-quality evidence)
Key reference	38

6B. Clinicians Should Not Obtain a Measurement of Serum Sodium, Potassium, Chloride, Blood Urea Nitrogen, Creatinine, Calcium, or Ammonia To Detect an IEM on Infants Presenting With a Lower-Risk BRUE (Grade C, Moderate Recommendation)

Aggregate Evidence Quality	Grade C
Benefits	Reduce costs, unnecessary testing, pain, and caregiver/infant anxiety
	Avoid consequences of false-positive results
Risks, harm, cost	May miss detection of an IEM
Benefit-harm assessment	The benefits of reducing unnecessary testing, cost, and false-positive results, as well as alleviating caregiver and infant anxiety, outweigh the rare missed diagnostic opportunity for an IEM
Intentional vagueness	None
Role of patient preferences	Caregiver concerns may lead to requests for diagnostic testing
Exclusions	None
Strength	Moderate recommendation
Key reference	4

of a family history of an IEM, developmental disabilities, SIDS, or a medical history of abnormal newborn screening results, unexplained infant death, age younger than 2 months, a prolonged event (>1 minute), or multiple events without an explanation. Confirmation that a newborn screen is complete and is negative is an important aspect of the medical history, but the clinician must consider that not all potential disorders are included in current newborn screening panels in the United States.

Lactic Acid

Measurement of lactic acid can result in high false-positive rates if the sample is not collected properly, making the decision to check a lactic

acid problematic. In addition, lactic acid may be elevated because of metabolic abnormalities attributable to other conditions, such as sepsis, and are not specific for IEMs.

Only 2 studies evaluated the specific measurement of lactic acid.[27,38] Davies and Gupta[38] reported 65 infants with consistent laboratory evaluations and found that 54% of infants had a lactic acid >2 mmol/L but only 15% had levels >3 mmol/L. The latter percentage of infants are more likely to be clinically significant and less likely to reflect a false-positive result. Five of 7 infants with a lactic acid >3 mmol/L had a "specific, serious diagnosis," although the specifics of these diagnoses were not included and no IEM was

6C. Clinicians Should Not Obtain a Measurement of Venous or Arterial Blood Gases To Detect an IEM in Infants Presenting With Lower-Risk BRUE (Grade C, Moderate Recommendation)

Aggregate Evidence Quality	Grade C
Benefits	Reduce costs, unnecessary testing, pain, risk of thrombosis, and caregiver/infant anxiety
	Avoid consequences of false-positive results
Risks, harm, cost	May miss detection of an IEM
Benefit-harm assessment	The benefits of reducing unnecessary testing, cost, and false-positive results, as well as alleviating caregiver and infant anxiety, outweigh the rare missed diagnostic opportunity for an IEM
Intentional vagueness	None
Role of patient preferences	Caregiver concerns may lead to requests for diagnostic testing
Exclusions	None
Strength	Moderate recommendation
Key reference	4

6D. Clinicians Need Not Obtain a Measurement of Blood Glucose To Detect an IEM in Infants Presenting With a Lower-Risk BRUE (Grade C, Weak Recommendation)

Aggregate Evidence Quality	Grade C
Benefits	Reduce costs, unnecessary testing, pain, risk of thrombosis, and caregiver/infant anxiety
	Avoid consequences of false-positive results
Risks, harm, cost	May miss rare instances of hypoglycemia attributable to undiagnosed IEM
Benefit-harm assessment	The benefits of reducing unnecessary testing, cost, and false-positive results, as well as alleviating caregiver and infant anxiety, outweigh the rare missed diagnostic opportunity for an IEM
Intentional vagueness	Measurement of glucose is often performed immediately through a simple bedside test; no abnormalities have been reported in asymptomatic infants, although studies often do not distinguish between capillary or venous measurement
Role of patient preferences	Caregiver concerns may lead to requests for diagnostic testing
Exclusions	None
Strength	Weak recommendation (based on low-quality evidence)
Key reference	4

confirmed in this study. This study also reported a 20% positive yield of testing for a bicarbonate <20 mmol/L and commented that there was a trend for lower bicarbonate and higher lactic acid levels in those with a recurrent event or a definitive diagnosis. The second publication[27] found no elevations of lactate in 4 of 49 children who had an initial abnormal venous blood gas, of which all repeat blood gas measurements were normal.

Serum Bicarbonate

Abnormal serum bicarbonate levels have been studied in 11 infants, of whom 7 had a diagnosis of sepsis or seizures.[38] Brand et al[4] studied 215 infants who had bicarbonate measured and found only 9 abnormal results, and only 3 of these contributed to the final diagnosis. Although unknown, it is most likely that the event in those infants would not have been classified as a BRUE under the new classification, because those infants were most likely symptomatic on presentation.

Serum Glucose

Abnormal blood glucose levels were evaluated but not reported in 3 studies.[4,38,110] Although

abnormalities of blood glucose can occur from various IEMs, such as medium-chain acyl–coenzyme A dehydrogenase deficiency or other fatty acid oxidation disorders, their prevalence has not been increased in SIDS and near-miss SIDS but could be considered as a cause of higher-risk BRUEs.[111] It is important to clarify through a careful medical history evaluation that the infant was not potentially hypoglycemic at discovery of the event and improved because of enteral treatment, because these disorders will not typically self-resolve without intervention (ie, feeding).

Serum Electrolytes and Calcium

ALTE studies evaluating the diagnostic value of electrolytes, including sodium, potassium, blood urea nitrogen, and creatinine, reported the rare occurrence of abnormalities, ranging from 0% to 4.3%.[4,38,110] Abnormal calcium levels have been reported in 0% to 1.5% of infants with ALTE, although these reports did not provide specific causes of hypocalcemia. Another study reported profound vitamin D deficiency with hypocalcemia in 5 of 25 infants with a diagnosis of an ALTE over a 2-year period in Saudi Arabia.[4,21,38,110] In lower-risk BRUE infants, clinicians should not obtain a calcium measurement unless the clinical history raises suspicion of hypocalcemia (eg, vitamin D deficiency or hypoparathyroidism).

Ammonia

Elevations of ammonia are typically associated with persistent symptoms and recurring events, and therefore testing would not be indicated in lower-risk BRUEs. Elevations of ammonia were reported in 11 infants (7 whom had an IEM) in a report of infants with recurrent ALTE and SIDS, limiting extrapolation to lower-risk BRUEs.[109] Elevations of ammonia >100 mmol/L were found in 4% of 65 infants, but this publication did not document a confirmed IEM.[38] Weiss et al[27] reported no abnormal elevations of ammonia in 4 infants with abnormal venous blood gas.

Venous or Arterial Blood Gas

Blood gas abnormalities leading to a diagnosis have not been reported in previous ALTE studies. Brand et al[4] reported 53 of 60 with positive findings, with none contributing to the final diagnosis. Weiss et al[27] reported 4 abnormal findings of 49 completed, all of which were normal on repeat measurements (along with normal lactate and ammonia levels). Blood gas detection is a routine test performed in acutely symptomatic patients who are being evaluated for suspected IEMs and may be considered in higher-risk BRUEs.

Urine Organic Acids, Plasma Amino Acids, Plasma Acylcarnitines

The role of advanced screening for IEMs has been reported in only 1 publication. Davies and Gupta[38] reported abnormalities of urine organic acids in 2% of cases and abnormalities of plasma amino acids in 4% of cases. Other reports have described an "unspecified metabolic screen" that was abnormal in 4.5% of cases but did not provide further description of specifics within that "screen."[4] Other reports have frequently included the descriptions of ALTEs with urea cycle disorders, organic acidemias, lactic acidemias, and fatty acid oxidation disorders such as medium chain acyl–coenzyme A dehydrogenase deficiency but did not distinguish between SIDS and near-miss SIDS.[107,109,111] Specific testing of urine organic acids, plasma amino acids, or plasma acylcarnitines may have a role in patients with a higher-risk BRUE.

6E. Clinicians Should Not Obtain Measurements of Urine Organic Acids, Plasma Amino Acids, or Plasma Acylcarnitines To Detect an IEM in Infants Presenting With a Lower-Risk BRUE (Grade C, Moderate Recommendation)

Aggregate Evidence Quality	Grade C
Benefits	Reduce costs, unnecessary testing, pain, risk of thrombosis, and caregiver/infant anxiety
	Avoid consequences of false-positive results
Risks, harm, cost	May miss detection of an IEM
Benefit-harm assessment	The benefits of reducing unnecessary testing, cost, and false-positive results, as well as alleviating caregiver and infant anxiety, outweigh the rare missed diagnostic opportunity for an IEM
Intentional vagueness	Lower-risk BRUEs will have a very low likelihood of disease, but these tests may be indicated in rare cases in which there is no documentation of a newborn screen being performed
Role of patient preferences	Caregiver concerns may lead to requests for diagnostic testing
Exclusions	None
Strength	Moderate recommendation
Key references	4, 38

7A. Clinicians Should Not Obtain Laboratory Evaluation for Anemia in Infants Presenting With a Lower-Risk BRUE (Grade C, Moderate Recommendation)

Aggregate Evidence Quality	Grade C
Benefits	Reduce costs, unnecessary testing, pain, risk of thrombosis, and caregiver/infant anxiety
	Avoid consequences of false-positive results
Risks, harm, cost	May miss diagnosis of anemia
Benefit-harm assessment	The benefits of reducing unnecessary testing, cost, and false-positive results, as well as alleviating caregiver and infant anxiety, outweigh the missed diagnostic opportunity for anemia
Intentional vagueness	None
Role of patient preferences	Caregivers may be reassured by testing
Exclusions	None
Strength	Moderate recommendation
Key reference	22

7. Anemia

7A. Clinicians Should Not Obtain Laboratory Evaluation for Anemia in Infants Presenting With a Lower-Risk BRUE (Grade C, Moderate Recommendation)

Anemia has been associated with ALTEs in infants, but the significance and causal association with the event itself are unclear.[38,112,113] Normal hemoglobin concentrations have also been reported in many other ALTE populations.[69,112,114] Brand et al[4] reported an abnormal hemoglobin in 54 of 223 cases, but in only 2 of 159 was the hemoglobin concentration associated with the final diagnosis (which was abusive head injury in both). Parker and Pitetti[22] also reported that infants who presented with ALTEs and ultimately were determined to be victims of child abuse were more likely to have a lower mean hemoglobin (10.6 vs 12.7 g/dL; *P* = .02).

8. Patient- and Family-Centered Care

8A. Clinicians Should Offer Resources for CPR Training to Caregivers (Grade C, Moderate Recommendation)

The majority of cardiac arrests in children result from a respiratory deterioration. Bystander CPR has been reported to have been conducted in 37% to 48% of pediatric out-of-hospital cardiac arrests and in 34% of respiratory arrests.[116] Bystander CPR results in significant improvement in 1-month survival rates in both cardiac and respiratory arrest.[117–119]

Although lower-risk BRUEs are neither a cardiac nor a respiratory arrest, the AAP policy statement on CPR recommends that pediatricians advocate for life-support training for caregivers and the general public.[115] A technical report that accompanies the AAP policy statement on CPR proposes that this can improve overall community health.[115] CPR training has not been shown to increase caregiver anxiety, and in fact, caregivers have reported a sense of empowerment.[120–122] There are many accessible and effective methods for CPR training (eg, e-learning).

8B. Clinicians Should Educate Caregivers About BRUEs (Grade C, Moderate Recommendation)

Pediatric providers are an important source of this health information and can help guide important conversations around BRUEs. A study by Feudtner et al[123] identified 4 groups of attributes of a "good parent": (1) making sure the child feels loved, (2) focusing on the child's health, (3) advocating for the child and being informed, and (4) ensuring the child's spiritual well-being. Clinicians should be the source of information for caregivers.

Informed caregivers can advocate for their child in all of the attribute areas/domains, and regardless of health literacy levels, prefer being offered choices and being asked for information.[124] A patient- and family-centered care approach results in better health outcomes.[125,126]

8C. Clinicians Should Use Shared Decision-Making for Infants Presenting With a Lower-Risk BRUE (Grade C, Moderate Recommendation)

Shared decision-making is a partnership between the clinician and the patient and family.[125,126] The general principles of shared decision-making are as follows: (1) information sharing, (2) respect and honoring differences, (3) partnership and collaboration, (4) negotiation, and (5) care in the context of family and community.[125] The benefits include improved care and outcomes; improved patient, family, and clinician satisfaction; and better use of health resources.[126] It is advocated for by organizations such as the AAP and the Institute of Medicine.[126,127] The 5 principles can be applied to all aspects of the infant who has experienced a BRUE, through each step (assessment, stabilization, management, disposition, and follow-up). Shared decision-making will empower families and foster a stronger clinician-patient/family alliance as they make decisions together in the face of a seemingly uncertain situation.

DISSEMINATION AND IMPLEMENTATION

Dissemination and implementation efforts are needed to facilitate guideline use across pediatric medicine, family medicine, emergency medicine, research, and patient/family communities.[128] The following general approaches and a Web-based toolkit are proposed for the dissemination and implementation of this guideline.

8A. Clinicians Should Offer Resources for CPR Training to Caregivers (Grade C, Moderate Recommendation)

Aggregate Evidence Quality	Grade C
Benefits	Decrease caregiver anxiety and increase confidence
	Benefit to society
Risks, harm, cost	May increase caregiver anxiety
	Cost and availability of training
Benefit-harm assessment	The benefits of decreased caregiver anxiety and increased confidence, as well as societal benefits, outweigh the increase in caregiver anxiety, cost, and resources
Intentional vagueness	None
Role of patient preferences	Caregiver may decide not to seek out the training
Exclusions	None
Strength	Moderate recommendation
Key reference	115

8B. Clinicians Should Educate Caregivers About BRUEs (Grade C, Moderate Recommendation)

Aggregate Evidence Quality	Grade C
Benefits	Improve caregiver empowerment and health literacy and decrease anxiety
	May reduce unnecessary return visits
	Promotion of the medical home
Risks, harm, cost	Increase caregiver anxiety and potential for caregiver intimidation in voicing concerns
	Increase health care costs and length of stay
Benefit-harm assessment	The benefits of decreased caregiver anxiety and increased empowerment and health literacy outweigh the increase in cost, length of stay, and caregiver anxiety and intimidation
Intentional vagueness	None
Role of patient preferences	Caregiver may decide not to listen to clinician
Exclusions	None
Strength	Moderate recommendation
Key references	None

8C. Clinicians Should Use Shared Decision-Making for Infants Presenting With a Lower-Risk BRUE (Grade C, Moderate Recommendation)

Aggregate Evidence Quality	Grade C
Benefits	Improve caregiver empowerment and health literacy and decrease anxiety
	May reduce unnecessary return visits
	Promotion of the medical home
Risks, harm, cost	Increase cost, length of stay, and caregiver anxiety and intimidation in voicing concerns
Benefit-harm assessment	The benefits of decreased caregiver anxiety and unplanned return visits and increased empowerment, health, literacy, and medical home promotion outweigh the increase in cost, length of stay, and caregiver anxiety and information
Intentional vagueness	None
Role of patient preferences	Caregiver may decide not to listen to clinician
Exclusions	None
Strength	Moderate recommendation
Key references	None

1. Education

Education will be partially achieved through the AAP communication outlets and educational services (*AAP News, Pediatrics,* and PREP). Further support will be sought from stakeholder organizations (American Academy of Family Physicians, American College of Emergency Physicians, American Board of Pediatrics, Society of Hospital Medicine). A Web-based toolkit (to be published online) will include caregiver handouts and a shared decision-making tool to facilitate patient- and family-centered care. Efforts will address appropriate disease classification and diagnosis coding.

2. Integration of Clinical Workflow

An algorithm is provided (Fig 1) for diagnosis and management. Structured history and physical examination templates also are provided to assist in addressing all of the relevant risk factors for BRUEs (Tables 2 and 3). Order sets and modified documents will be hosted on a Web-based learning platform that promotes crowd-sourcing.

3. Administrative and Research

International Classification of Diseases, 9th Revision, and International Classification of Diseases, 10th Revision, diagnostic codes are used for billing, quality improvement, and research; and new codes for lower- and higher-risk BRUEs will need to be developed. In the interim, the current code for an ALTE (799.82) will need to be used for billing purposes. Efforts will be made to better reflect present knowledge and to educate clinicians and payers in appropriate use of codes for this condition.

4. Quality Improvement

Quality improvement initiatives that provide Maintenance of Certification credit, such as the AAP's PREP and EQIPP courses, or collaborative opportunities through the AAP's Quality Improvement Innovation Networks, will engage clinicians in the use and improvement of the guideline. By using proposed quality measures, adherence and outcomes can be assessed and benchmarked with others to inform continual improvement efforts. Proposed measures include process evaluation (use of definition and evaluation), outcome assessment (family experience and diagnostic outcomes), and balancing issues (cost and length of visit). Future research will need to be conducted to validate any measures.

FUTURE RESEARCH

The transition in nomenclature from the term ALTE to BRUE after 30 years reflects the expanded understanding of the etiology and consequences of this entity. Previous research has been largely retrospective or observational in nature, with little long-term follow-up data available. The more-precise definition, the classification of lower- and higher-risk groups, the recommendations for the lower-risk group, and the implementation toolkit will serve as the basis for future research. Important areas for future prospective research include the following.

1. Epidemiology

- Incidence of BRUEs in all infants (in addition to those seeking medical evaluation)

- Influence of race, gender, ethnicity, seasonality, environmental exposures, and socioeconomic status on incidence and outcomes

2. Diagnosis

- Use and effectiveness of the BRUE definition

- Screening tests and risk of UTI

- Quantify and better understand risk in higher- and lower-risk groups

- Risk and benefit of screening tests

- Risk and benefit and optimal duration of observation and monitoring periods

- Effect of prematurity on risk

- Appropriate indications for subspecialty referral

- Early recognition of child maltreatment

- Importance of environmental history taking

- Role of human psychology on accuracy of event characterization

- Type and length of monitoring in the acute setting

3. Pathophysiology

- Role of abnormalities of swallowing, laryngospasm, GER, and autonomic function

4. Outcomes

- Patient- and family-centered outcomes, including caregiver satisfaction, anxiety, and family dynamics (eg, risk of vulnerable child syndrome)

- Long-term health and cognitive consequences

5. Treatment

- Empirical GER treatment on recurrent BRUEs

- Caregiver education strategies, including basic life support, family-centered education, and postpresentation clinical visits

6. Follow-up

- Strategies for timely follow-up and surveillance

SUBCOMMITTEE ON BRIEF RESOLVED UNEXPLAINED EVENTS (FORMERLY REFERRED TO AS APPARENT LIFE THREATENING EVENTS) (OVERSIGHT BY THE COUNCIL ON QUALITY IMPROVEMENT AND PATIENT SAFETY)

Joel S. Tieder, MD, MPH, FAAP, Chair (no financial conflicts, published research related to BRUEs/ALTEs)

Joshua L. Bonkowsky, MD, PhD, FAAP, Pediatric Neurologist

Ruth A. Etzel, MD, PhD, FAAP, Pediatric Epidemiologist

Wayne H. Franklin, MD, MPH, MMM, FAAP, Pediatric Cardiologist

David A. Gremse, MD, FAAP, Pediatric Gastroenterologist

Bruce Herman, MD, FAAP, Child Abuse and Neglect

Eliot Katz, MD, FAAP, Pediatric Pulmonologist

Leonard R. Krilov, MD, FAAP, Pediatric Infectious Diseases

J. Lawrence Merritt II, MD, FAAP, Clinical Genetics and Biochemical Genetics

Chuck Norlin, MD, FAAP, Pediatrician

Robert E. Sapién, MD, MMM, FAAP, Pediatric Emergency Medicine

Richard Shiffman, MD, FAAP, Partnership for Policy Implementation Representative

Michael B.H. Smith, MB, FRCPCH, FAAP, Hospital Medicine

Jack Percelay, MD, MPH, FAAP, Liaison, Society for Hospital Medicine

STAFF

Kymika Okechukwu, MPA

ABBREVIATIONS

AAP: American Academy of Pediatrics

ALTE: apparent life-threatening event

BRUE: brief resolved unexplained event

CI: confidence interval

CNS: central nervous system

CPR: cardiopulmonary resuscitation

ECG: electrocardiogram

GER: gastroesophageal reflux

IEM: inborn error of metabolism

MII: multiple intraluminal impedance

OSA: obstructive sleep apnea

RSV: respiratory syncytial virus

SIDS: sudden infant death syndrome

SUDEP: sudden unexpected death in epilepsy

UTI: urinary tract infection

REFERENCES

1. National Institutes of Health Consensus Development Conference on Infantile Apnea and Home Monitoring, Sept 29 to Oct 1, 1986. *Pediatrics*. 1987;79(2):292–299

2. McGovern MC, Smith MB. Causes of apparent life threatening events in infants: a systematic review. *Arch Dis Child*. 2004;89(11):1043–1048

3. Tieder JS, Altman RL, Bonkowsky JL, et al Management of apparent life-threatening events in infants: a systematic review. *J Pediatr*. 2013;163(1):94–99, e91–e96

4. Brand DA, Altman RL, Purtill K, Edwards KS. Yield of diagnostic testing in infants who have had an apparent

life-threatening event. *Pediatrics*. 2005;115(4):885–893

5. Green M. Vulnerable child syndrome and its variants. *Pediatr Rev*. 1986;8(3):75–80

6. Kaji AH, Claudius I, Santillanes G, et al. Apparent life-threatening event: multicenter prospective cohort study to develop a clinical decision rule for admission to the hospital. *Ann Emerg Med*. 2013;61(4):379–387.e4

7. Mittal MK, Sun G, Baren JM. A clinical decision rule to identify infants with apparent life-threatening event who can be safely discharged from the emergency department. *Pediatr Emerg Care*. 2012;28(7):599–605

8. Moher D, Liberati A, Tetzlaff J, Altman DG; PRISMA Group. Preferred reporting items for systematic reviews and meta-analyses: the PRISMA statement. *Ann Intern Med*. 2009;151(4):264–269, W64

9. Haynes RB, Cotoi C, Holland J, et al; McMaster Premium Literature Service (PLUS) Project. Second-order peer review of the medical literature for clinical practitioners. *JAMA*. 2006;295(15):1801–1808

10. Lokker C, McKibbon KA, McKinlay RJ, Wilczynski NL, Haynes RB. Prediction of citation counts for clinical articles at two years using data available within three weeks of publication: retrospective cohort study. *BMJ*. 2008;336(7645):655–657

11. Laupacis A, Wells G, Richardson WS, Tugwell P; Evidence-Based Medicine Working Group. Users' guides to the medical literature. V. How to use an article about prognosis. *JAMA*. 1994;272(3):234–237

12. Jaeschke R, Guyatt G, Sackett DL. Users' guides to the medical literature. III. How to use an article about a diagnostic test. A. Are the results of the study valid? Evidence-Based Medicine Working Group. *JAMA*. 1994;271(5):389–391

13. Anjos AM, Nunes ML. Prevalence of epilepsy and seizure disorders as causes of apparent life-threatening event (ALTE) in children admitted to a tertiary hospital. *Arq Neuropsiquiatr*. 2009;67(3a 3A):616–620

14. Doshi A, Bernard-Stover L, Kuelbs C, Castillo E, Stucky E. Apparent lifethreatening event admissions and gastroesophageal reflux disease: the value of hospitalization. *Pediatr Emerg Care*. 2012;28(1):17–21

15. Franco P, Montemitro E, Scaillet S, et al. Fewer spontaneous arousals in infants with apparent life-threatening event. *Sleep*. 2011;34(6):733–743

16. Hoki R, Bonkowsky JL, Minich LL, Srivastava R, Pinto NM. Cardiac testing and outcomes in infants after an apparent life-threatening event. *Arch Dis Child*. 2012;97(12):1034–1038

17. Kaji AH, Santillanes G, Claudius I, et al. Do infants less than 12 months of age with an apparent life-threatening event need transport to a pediatric critical care center? *Prehosp Emerg Care*. 2013;17(3):304–311

18. Kant S, Fisher JD, Nelson DG, Khan S. Mortality after discharge in clinically stable infants admitted with a fi rsttime apparent life-threatening event. *Am J Emerg Med*. 2013;31(4):730–733

19. Miano S, Castaldo R, Ferri R, et al. Sleep cyclic alternating pattern analysis in infants with apparent life-threatening events: a daytime polysomnographic study. *Clin Neurophysiol*. 2012;123(7):1346–1352

20. Mittal MK, Donda K, Baren JM. Role of pneumography and esophageal pH monitoring in the evaluation of infants with apparent life-threatening event: a prospective observational study. *Clin Pediatr (Phila)*. 2013;52(4):338–343

21. Mosalli RM, Elsayed YY, Paes BA. Acute life threatening events associated with hypocalcemia and vitamin D defi ciency in early infancy: a single center experience from the Kingdom of Saudi Arabia. *Saudi Med J*. 2011;32(5):528–530

22. Parker K, Pitetti R. Mortality and child abuse in children presenting with apparent life-threatening events. *Pediatr Emerg Care*. 2011;27(7):591–595

23. Poets A, Urschitz MS, Steinfeldt R, Poets CF. Risk factors for early sudden deaths and severe apparent lifethreatening events.

Arch Dis Child Fetal Neonatal Ed. 2012;97(6):F395–F397

24. Semmekrot BA, van Sleuwen BE, Engelberts AC, et al. Surveillance study of apparent life-threatening events (ALTE) in the Netherlands. *Eur J Pediatr*. 2010;169(2):229–236

25. Tieder JS, Altman RL, Bonkowsky JL, et al. Management of apparent life-threatening events in infants: a systematic review. *J Pediatr*. 2013;163(1):94–9.e1, 6

26. Wasilewska J, Sienkiewicz-Szłapka E, Kuźbida E, Jarmołowska B, Kaczmarski M, Kostyra E. The exogenous opioid peptides and DPPIV serum activity in infants with apnoea expressed as apparent life threatening events (ALTE). *Neuropeptides*. 2011;45(3):189–195

27. Weiss K, Fattal-Valevski A, Reif S. How to evaluate the child presenting with an apparent life-threatening event? *Isr Med Assoc J*. 2010;12(3):154–157

28. Zimbric G, Bonkowsky JL, Jackson WD, Maloney CG, Srivastava R. Adverse outcomes associated with gastroesophageal reflux disease are rare following an apparent life-threatening event. *J Hosp Med*. 2012;7(6):476–481

29. American Academy of Pediatrics Steering Committee on Quality Improvement and Management. Classifying recommendations for clinical practice guidelines. *Pediatrics*. 2004;114(3):874–877

30. Shiffman RN, Michel G, Rosenfeld RM, Davidson C. Building better guidelines with BRIDGE-Wiz: development and evaluation of a software assistant to promote clarity, transparency, and implementability. *J Am Med Inform Assoc*. 2012;19(1):94–101

31. Claudius I, Keens T. Do all infants with apparent life-threatening events need to be admitted? *Pediatrics*. 2007;119(4):679–683

32. Bonkowsky JL, Guenther E, Filloux FM, Srivastava R. Death, child abuse, and adverse neurological outcome of infants after an apparent lifethreatening event. *Pediatrics*. 2008;122(1):125–131

33. Al-Kindy HA, Gelinas JF, Hatzakis G, Cote A. Risk factors for extreme events

in infants hospitalized for apparent life-threatening events. *J Pediatr*. 2009;154(3):332–337, 337.e1–337.e2

34. Ramanathan R, Corwin MJ, Hunt CE, et al; Collaborative Home Infant Monitoring Evaluation (CHIME) Study Group. Cardiorespiratory events recorded on home monitors: comparison of healthy infants with those at increased risk for SIDS. *JAMA*. 2001;285(17):2199–2207

35. Poets CF, Stebbens VA, Alexander JR, Arrowsmith WA, Salfield SA, Southall DP. Hypoxaemia in infants with respiratory tract infections. *Acta Paediatr*. 1992;81(6–7):536–541

36. Hunt CE, Corwin MJ, Lister G, et al; Collaborative Home Infant Monitoring Evaluation (CHIME) Study Group. Longitudinal assessment of hemoglobin oxygen saturation in healthy infants during the first 6 months of age. *J Pediatr*. 1999;135(5):580–586

37. Altman RL, Li KI, Brand DA. Infections and apparent life-threatening events. *Clin Pediatr (Phila)*. 2008;47(4):372–378

38. Davies F, Gupta R. Apparent life threatening events in infants presenting to an emergency department. *Emerg Med J*. 2002;19(1):11–16

39. Guilleminault C, Ariagno R, Korobkin R, et al. Mixed and obstructive sleep apnea and near miss for sudden infant death syndrome: 2. Comparison of near miss and normal control infants by age. *Pediatrics*. 1979;64(6):882–891

40. Côté A, Hum C, Brouillette RT, Themens M. Frequency and timing of recurrent events in infants using home cardiorespiratory monitors. *J Pediatr*. 1998;132(5):783–789

41. Kahn A, Blum D. Home monitoring of infants considered at risk for the sudden infant death syndrome: four years' experience (1977-1981). *Eur J Pediatr*. 1982;139(2):94–100

42. Daniëls H, Naulaers G, Deroost F, Devlieger H. Polysomnography and home documented monitoring of cardiorespiratory pattern. *Arch Dis Child*. 1999;81(5):434–436

43. Marcus CL, Hamer A. Significance of isolated bradycardia detected

by home monitoring. *J Pediatr.* 1999;135(3):321–326

44. Rebuffat E, Groswasser J, Kelmanson I, Sottiaux M, Kahn A. Polygraphic evaluation of night-to-night variability in sleep characteristics and apneas in infants. *Sleep.* 1994;17(4):329–332

45. Horemuzova E, Katz-Salamon M, Milerad J. Increased inspiratory effort in infants with a history of apparent life-threatening event. *Acta Paediatr.* 2002;91(3):280–286; discussion: 260–261

46. Schechtman VL, Harper RM, Wilson AJ, Southall DP. Sleep state organization in normal infants and victims of the sudden infant death syndrome. *Pediatrics.* 1992;89(5 Pt 1):865–870

47. Arad-Cohen N, Cohen A, Tirosh E. The relationship between gastroesophageal reflux and apnea in infants. *J Pediatr.* 2000;137(3):321–326

48. Harrington C, Kirjavainen T, Teng A, Sullivan CE. Altered autonomic function and reduced arousability in apparent life-threatening event infants with obstructive sleep apnea. *Am J Respir Crit Care Med.* 2002;165(8):1048–1054

49. Guilleminault C, Pelayo R, Leger D, Philip P. Apparent life-threatening events, facial dysmorphia and sleep-disordered breathing. *Eur J Pediatr.* 2000;159(6):444–449

50. Aurora RN, Zak RS, Karippot A, et al; American Academy of Sleep Medicine. Practice parameters for the respiratory indications for polysomnography in children. *Sleep.* 2011;34(3):379–388

51. Kahn A, Groswasser J, Sottiaux M, Rebuffat E, Franco P. Mechanisms of obstructive sleep apneas in infants. *Biol Neonate.* 1994;65(3–4):235–239

52. Leiberman A, Tal A, Brama I, Sofer S. Obstructive sleep apnea in young infants. *Int J Pediatr Otorhinolaryngol.* 1988;16(1):39–44

53. Montgomery-Downs HE, Gozal D. Sleep habits and risk factors for sleep-disordered breathing in infants and young toddlers in Louisville, Kentucky. *Sleep Med.* 2006;7(3):211–219

54. Brouillette RT, Fernbach SK, Hunt CE. Obstructive sleep apnea in infants and children. *J Pediatr.* 1982;100(1):31–40

55. Kahn A, Groswasser J, Sottiaux M, et al. Clinical symptoms associated with brief obstructive sleep apnea in normal infants. *Sleep.* 1993;16(5):409–413

56. Kahn A, Groswasser J, Sottiaux M, et al. Prenatal exposure to cigarettes in infants with obstructive sleep apneas. *Pediatrics.* 1994;93(5):778–783

57. Kahn A, Mozin MJ, Rebuffat E, et al. Sleep pattern alterations and brief airway obstructions in overweight infants. *Sleep.* 1989;12(5):430–438

58. Fajardo C, Alvarez J, Wong A, Kwiatkowski K, Rigatto H. The incidence of obstructive apneas in preterm infants with and without bronchopulmonary dysplasia. *Early Hum Dev.* 1993;32(2–3):197–206

59. Horigome H, Nagashima M, Sumitomo N, et al. Clinical characteristics and genetic background of congenital long-QT syndrome diagnosed in fetal, neonatal, and infantile life: a nationwide questionnaire survey in Japan. *Circ Arrhythm Electrophysiol.* 2010;3(1):10–17

60. Arnestad M, Crotti L, Rognum TO, et al. Prevalence of long-QT syndrome gene variants in sudden infant death syndrome. *Circulation.* 2007;115(3):361–367

61. Goldenberg I, Moss AJ, Peterson DR, et al. Risk factors for aborted cardiac arrest and sudden cardiac death in children with the congenital long-QT syndrome. *Circulation.* 2008;117(17):2184–2191

62. Munger TM, Packer DL, Hammill SC, et al. A population study of the natural history of Wolff-Parkinson-White syndrome in Olmsted County, Minnesota, 1953-1989. *Circulation.* 1993;87(3):866–873

63. American Academy of Pediatrics, Committee on Fetus and Newborn. Apnea, sudden infant death syndrome, and home monitoring. *Pediatrics.* 2003;111(4 pt 1):914–917

64. Krongrad E, O'Neill L. Near miss sudden infant death syndrome episodes? A clinical and electrocardiographic correlation. *Pediatrics.* 1986;77(6):811–815

65. Nathanson I, O'Donnell J, Commins MF. Cardiorespiratory patterns

during alarms in infants using apnea/bradycardia monitors. *Am J Dis Child.* 1989;143(4):476–480

66. Weese-Mayer DE, Brouillette RT, Morrow AS, Conway LP, Klemka-Walden LM, Hunt CE. Assessing validity of infant monitor alarms with event recording. *J Pediatr.* 1989;115(5 pt 1):702–708

67. Guenther E, Powers A, Srivastava R, Bonkowsky JL. Abusive head trauma in children presenting with an apparent life-threatening event. *J Pediatr.* 2010;157(5):821–825

68. Pierce MC, Kaczor K, Thompson R. Bringing back the social history. *Pediatr Clin North Am.* 2014;61(5):889–905

69. Pitetti RD, Maffei F, Chang K, Hickey R, Berger R, Pierce MC. Prevalence of retinal hemorrhages and child abuse in children who present with an apparent life-threatening event. *Pediatrics.* 2002;110(3):557–562

70. Jenny C, Hymel KP, Ritzen A, Reinert SE, Hay TC. Analysis of missed cases of abusive head trauma. *JAMA.* 1999;281(7):621–626

71. Southall DP, Plunkett MC, Banks MW, Falkov AF, Samuels MP. Covert video recordings of life-threatening child abuse: lessons for child protection. *Pediatrics.* 1997;100(5):735–760

72. Sugar NF, Taylor JA, Feldman KW; Puget Sound Pediatric Research Network. Bruises in infants and toddlers: those who don't cruise rarely bruise. *Arch Pediatr Adolesc Med.* 1999;153(4):399–403

73. Harper NS, Feldman KW, Sugar NF, Anderst JD, Lindberg DM; Examining Siblings To Recognize Abuse Investigators. Additional injuries in young infants with concern for abuse and apparently isolated bruises. *J Pediatr.* 2014;165(2):383–388, e1

74. DeRidder CA, Berkowitz CD, Hicks RA, Laskey AL. Subconjunctival hemorrhages in infants and children: a sign of nonaccidental trauma. *Pediatr Emerg Care.* 2013;29(2):222–226

75. Buck ML, Blumer JL. Phenothiazine-associated apnea in two siblings. *DICP.* 1991;25(3):244–247

76. Hardoin RA, Henslee JA, Christenson CP, Christenson PJ, White M. Colic

medication and apparent life-threatening events. *Clin Pediatr (Phila)*. 1991;30(5):281–285

77. Hickson GB, Altemeier WA, Martin ED, Campbell PW. Parental administration of chemical agents: a cause of apparent life-threatening events. *Pediatrics*. 1989;83(5):772–776

78. Pitetti RD, Whitman E, Zaylor A. Accidental and nonaccidental poisonings as a cause of apparent life-threatening events in infants. *Pediatrics*. 2008;122(2). Available at: www.pediatrics.org/cgi/content/full/122/2/e359

79. McCormick T, Levine M, Knox O, Claudius I. Ethanol ingestion in two infants under 2 months old: a previously unreported cause of ALTE. *Pediatrics*. 2013;131(2). Available at: www.pediatrics.org/cgi/content/full/131/2/e604

80. Dearborn DG, Smith PG, Dahms BB, et al. Clinical profile of 30 infants with acute pulmonary hemorrhage in Cleveland. *Pediatrics*. 2002;110(3):627–637

81. Leone MA, Solari A, Beghi E; First Seizure Trial (FIRST) Group. Treatment of the first tonic-clonic seizure does not affect long-term remission of epilepsy. *Neurology*. 2006;67(12):2227–2229

82. Musicco M, Beghi E, Solari A, Viani F; First Seizure Trial (FIRST) Group. Treatment of first tonic-clonic seizure does not improve the prognosis of epilepsy. *Neurology*. 1997;49(4):991–998

83. Camfield P, Camfield C, Smith S, Dooley J, Smith E. Long-term outcome is unchanged by antiepileptic drug treatment after a first seizure: a 15-year follow-up from a randomized trial in childhood. *Epilepsia*. 2002;43(6):662–663

84. Gilbert DL, Buncher CR. An EEG should not be obtained routinely after first unprovoked seizure in childhood. *Neurology*. 2000;54(3):635–641

85. Arts WF, Geerts AT. When to start drug treatment for childhood epilepsy: the clinical-epidemiological evidence. *Eur J Paediatr Neurol*. 2009;13(2):93–101

86. Hirtz D, Ashwal S, Berg A, et al. Practice parameter: evaluating a first nonfebrile seizure in children: report of the Quality Standards Subcommittee of the American Academy of Neurology, The Child Neurology Society, and The American Epilepsy Society. *Neurology*. 2000;55(5):616–623

87. Bonkowsky JL, Guenther E, Srivastava R, Filloux FM. Seizures in children following an apparent life-threatening event. *J Child Neurol*. 2009;24(6):709–713

88. Claudius I, Mittal MK, Murray R, Condie T, Santillanes G. Should infants presenting with an apparent life-threatening event undergo evaluation for serious bacterial infections and respiratory pathogens? *J Pediatr*. 2014;164(5):1231–1233, e1

89. Mittal MK, Shofer FS, Baren JM. Serious bacterial infections in infants who have experienced an apparent life-threatening event. *Ann Emerg Med*. 2009;54(4):523–527

90. Roberts KB; Subcommittee on Urinary Tract Infection, Steering Committee on Quality Improvement and Management. Urinary tract infection: clinical practice guideline for the diagnosis and management of the initial UTI in febrile infants and children 2 to 24 months. *Pediatrics*. 2011;128(3):595–610

91. Schroeder AR, Mansbach JM, Stevenson M, et al. Apnea in children hospitalized with bronchiolitis. *Pediatrics*. 2013;132(5). Available at: www.pediatrics.org/cgi/content/full/132/5/e1194

92. Loeffelholz MJ, Trujillo R, Pyles RB, et al. Duration of rhinovirus shedding in the upper respiratory tract in the first year of life. *Pediatrics*. 2014;134(6):1144–1150

93. Crowcroft NS, Booy R, Harrison T, et al. Severe and unrecognised: pertussis in UK infants. *Arch Dis Child*. 2003;88(9):802–806

94. Centers for Disease Control and Prevention. Pertussis (whooping cough): diagnostic testing. Available at: www.cdc.gov/pertussis/clinical/diagnostic-testing/index.html. Accessed June 26, 2015

95. Centers for Disease Control and Prevention. Pertussis (whooping cough): treatment. Available at: www.cdc.gov/pertussis/clinical/treatment.html. Accessed June 26, 2015

96. Campanozzi A, Boccia G, Pensabene L, et al. Prevalence and natural history of gastroesophageal reflux: pediatric prospective survey. *Pediatrics*. 2009;123(3):779–783

97. Lightdale JR, Gremse DA; American Academy of Pediatrics, Section on Gastroenterology, Hepatology, and Nutrition. Gastroesophageal reflux: management guidance for the pediatrician. *Pediatrics*. 2013;131(5). Available at: www.pediatrics.org/cgi/content/full/131/5/e1684

98. Vandenplas Y, Rudolph CD, Di Lorenzo C, et al; North American Society for Pediatric Gastroenterology Hepatology and Nutrition; European Society for Pediatric Gastroenterology Hepatology and Nutrition. Pediatric gastroesophageal reflux clinical practice guidelines: joint recommendations of the North American Society for Pediatric Gastroenterology, Hepatology, and Nutrition (NASPGHAN) and the European Society for Pediatric Gastroenterology, Hepatology, and Nutrition (ESPGHAN). *J Pediatr Gastroenterol Nutr*. 2009;49(4):498–547

99. Kiechl-Kohlendorfer U, Hof D, Peglow UP, Traweger-Ravanelli B, Kiechl S. Epidemiology of apparent life threatening events. *Arch Dis Child*. 2005;90(3):297–300

100. Chung EY, Yardley J. Are there risks associated with empiric acid suppression treatment of infants and children suspected of having gastroesophageal reflux disease? *Hosp Pediatr*. 2013;3(1):16–23

101. Herbst JJ, Minton SD, Book LS. Gastroesophageal reflux causing respiratory distress and apnea in newborn infants. *J Pediatr*. 1979;95(5 pt 1):763–768

102. Orenstein SR. An overview of reflux-associated disorders in infants: apnea, laryngospasm, and aspiration. *Am J Med*. 2001;111(suppl 8A):60S–63S

103. Wenzl TG, Schenke S, Peschgens T, Silny J, Heimann G, Skopnik H. Association of

apnea and nonacid gastroesophageal reflux in infants: investigations with the intraluminal impedance technique. *Pediatr Pulmonol.* 2001;31(2):144–149

104. Mousa H, Woodley FW, Metheney M, Hayes J. Testing the association between gastroesophageal reflux and apnea in infants. *J Pediatr Gastroenterol Nutr.* 2005;41(2):169–177

105. Kahn A, Rebuffat E, Sottiaux M, Dufour D, Cadranel S, Reiterer F. Lack of temporal relation between acid reflux in the proximal oesophagus and cardiorespiratory events in sleeping infants. *Eur J Pediatr.* 1992;151(3):208–212

106. Orenstein SR, McGowan JD. Efficacy of conservative therapy as taught in the primary care setting for symptoms suggesting infant gastroesophageal reflux. *J Pediatr.* 2008;152(3): 310–314

107. Kahn A; European Society for the Study and Prevention of Infant Death. Recommended clinical evaluation of infants with an apparent life-threatening event: consensus document of the European Society for the Study and Prevention of Infant Death, 2003. *Eur J Pediatr.* 2004;163(2):108–115

108. Veereman-Wauters G, Bochner A, Van Caillie-Bertrand M. Gastroesophageal reflux in infants with a history of near-miss sudden infant death. *J Pediatr Gastroenterol Nutr.* 1991;12(3): 319–323

109. Arens R, Gozal D, Williams JC, Ward SL, Keens TG. Recurrent apparent life-threatening events during infancy: a manifestation of inborn errors of metabolism. *J Pediatr.* 1993;123(3):415–418

110. See CC, Newman LJ, Berezin S, et al. Gastroesophageal reflux-induced hypoxemia in infants with apparent life-threatening event(s). *Am J Dis Child.* 1989;143(8):951–954

111. Penzien JM, Molz G, Wiesmann UN, Colombo JP, Bühlmann R, Wermuth B. Medium-chain acyl-CoA dehydrogenase deficiency does not correlate with apparent life-threatening events and

the sudden infant death syndrome: results from phenylpropionate loading tests and DNA analysis. *Eur J Pediatr.* 1994;153(5):352–357

112. Pitetti RD, Lovallo A, Hickey R. Prevalence of anemia in children presenting with apparent life-threatening events. *Acad Emerg Med.* 2005;12(10):926–931

113. Gray C, Davies F, Molyneux E. Apparent life-threatening events presenting to a pediatric emergency department. *Pediatr Emerg Care.* 1999;15(3):195–199

114. Poets CF, Samuels MP, Wardrop CA, Picton-Jones E, Southall DP. Reduced haemoglobin levels in infants presenting with apparent life-threatening events—a retrospective investigation. *Acta Paediatr.* 1992;81(4):319–321

115. Pyles LA, Knapp J; American Academy of Pediatrics Committee on Pediatric Emergency Medicine. Role of pediatricians in advocating life support training courses for parents and the public. *Pediatrics.* 2004;114(6). Available at: www.pediatrics.org/cgi/content/full/114/6/e761

116. Tunik MG, Richmond N, Treiber M, et al. Pediatric prehospital evaluation of NYC respiratory arrest survival (PHENYCS). *Pediatr Emerg Care.* 2012;28(9):859–863

117. Foltin GL, Richmond N, Treiber M, et al. Pediatric prehospital evaluation of NYC cardiac arrest survival (PHENYCS). *Pediatr Emerg Care.* 2012;28(9):864–868

118. Akahane M, Tanabe S, Ogawa T, et al. Characteristics and outcomes of pediatric out-of-hospital cardiac arrest by scholastic age category. *Pediatr Crit Care Med.* 2013;14(2): 130–136

119. Atkins DL, Everson-Stewart S, Sears GK, et al; Resuscitation Outcomes Consortium Investigators. Epidemiology and outcomes from out-of-hospital cardiac arrest in children: the Resuscitation Outcomes Consortium Epistry-Cardiac Arrest.

Circulation. 2009;119(11): 1484–1491

120. McLauchlan CA, Ward A, Murphy NM, Griffith MJ, Skinner DV, Camm AJ. Resuscitation training for cardiac patients and their relatives—its effect on anxiety. *Resuscitation.* 1992;24(1):7–11

121. Higgins SS, Hardy CE, Higashino SM. Should parents of children with congenital heart disease and life-threatening dysrhythmias be taught cardiopulmonary resuscitation? *Pediatrics.* 1989;84(6):1102–1104

122. Dracup K, Moser DK, Taylor SE, Guzy PM. The psychological consequences of cardiopulmonary resuscitation training for family members of patients at risk for sudden death. *Am J Public Health.* 1997;87(9):1434–1439

123. Feudtner C, Walter JK, Faerber JA, et al. Good-parent beliefs of parents of seriously ill children. *JAMA Pediatr.* 2015;169(1):39–47

124. Yin HS, Dreyer BP, Vivar KL, MacFarland S, van Schaick L, Mendelsohn AL. Perceived barriers to care and attitudes towards shared decision-making among low socioeconomic status parents: role of health literacy. *Acad Pediatr.* 2012;12(2):117–124

125. Kuo DZ, Houtrow AJ, Arango P, Kuhlthau KA, Simmons JM, Neff JM. Family-centered care: current applications and future directions in pediatric health care. *Matern Child Health J.* 2012;16(2):297–305

126. American Academy of Pediatrics, Committee on Hospital Care; Institute for Patient- and Family-Centered Care. Patient- and family-centered care and the pediatrician's role. *Pediatrics.* 2012;129(2):394–404

127. Institute of Medicine. *Crossing the Quality Chasm: A New Health System for the 21st Century.* Washington, DC: Institute of Medicine, Committee on Quality Healthcare in America National Academies Press; 2001

128. Pronovost PJ. Enhancing physicians' use of clinical guidelines. *JAMA.* 2013;310(23):2501–2502

CLINICAL PRACTICE GUIDELINE Guidance for the Clinician in Rendering Pediatric Care

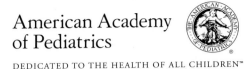

American Academy
of Pediatrics

DEDICATED TO THE HEALTH OF ALL CHILDREN™

Brief Resolved Unexplained Events (Formerly Apparent Life-Threatening Events) and Evaluation of Lower-Risk Infants: Executive Summary

Joel S. Tieder, MD, MPH, FAAP, Joshua L. Bonkowsky, MD, PhD, FAAP, Ruth A. Etzel, MD, PhD, FAAP, Wayne H. Franklin, MD, MPH, MMM, FAAP, David A. Gremse, MD, FAAP, Bruce Herman, MD, FAAP, Eliot S. Katz, MD, FAAP, Leonard R. Krilov, MD, FAAP, J. Lawrence Merritt II, MD, FAAP, Chuck Norlin, MD, FAAP, Jack Percelay, MD, MPH, FAAP, Robert E. Sapién, MD, MMM, FAAP, Richard N. Shiffman, MD, MCIS, FAAP, Michael B.H. Smith, MB, FRCPCH, FAAP, SUBCOMMITTEE ON APPARENT LIFE THREATENING EVENTS

EXECUTIVE SUMMARY

This clinical practice guideline has 2 primary objectives. First, it recommends the replacement of the term "apparent life-threatening event" (ALTE) with a new term, "brief resolved unexplained event" (BRUE). Second, it provides an approach to evaluation and management that is based on the risk that the infant will have a repeat event or has a serious underlying disorder.

Clinicians should use the term BRUE to describe an event occurring in an infant younger than 1 year when the observer reports a sudden, brief, and now resolved episode of ≥1 of the following: (1) cyanosis or pallor; (2) absent, decreased, or irregular breathing; (3) marked change in tone (hyper- or hypotonia); and (4) altered level of responsiveness. Moreover, clinicians should diagnose a BRUE only when there is no explanation for a qualifying event after conducting an appropriate history and physical examination (see Tables 2 and 3 in www.pediatrics.org/cgi/doi/10.1542/peds.2016-0590). Among infants who present for medical attention after a BRUE, the guideline identifies (1) lower-risk patients on the basis of history and physical examination, for whom evidence-based guidelines for evaluation and management are offered, and (2) higher-risk patients, whose history and physical examination suggest the need for further investigation, monitoring, and/or treatment, but for whom recommendations are not offered (because of insufficient evidence or the availability of guidance from other clinical practice guidelines specific to their presentation or diagnosis). Recommendations in this guideline apply only to lower-risk patients,

DOI: 10.1542/peds.2016-0591

PEDIATRICS (ISSN Numbers: Print, 0031-4005; Online, 1098-4275).

To cite: Tieder JS, Bonkowsky JL, Etzel RA, et al. Brief Resolved Unexplained Events (Formerly Apparent Life-Threatening Events) and Evaluation of Lower-Risk Infants: Executive Summary. *Pediatrics.* 2016;137(5):e20160591

who are defined by (1) age >60 days; (2) gestational age ≥32 weeks and postconceptional age ≥45 weeks; (3) occurrence of only 1 BRUE (no prior BRUE ever and not occurring in clusters); (4) duration of BRUE <1 minute; (5) no cardiopulmonary resuscitation by trained medical provider required; (6) no concerning historical features; and (7) no concerning physical examination findings (Fig 1). This clinical practice guideline also provides implementation support and suggests directions for future research.

The term ALTE originated from a 1986 National Institutes of Health Consensus Conference on Infantile Apnea and was intended to replace the term "near-miss sudden infant death syndrome (SIDS)."[1] An ALTE was defined as "[a]n episode that is frightening to the observer and that is characterized by some combination of apnea (central or occasionally obstructive), color change (usually cyanotic or pallid but occasionally erythematous or plethoric), marked change in muscle tone (usually marked limpness), choking, or gagging. In some cases, the observer fears that the infant has died."[2] Although the definition of ALTE enabled researchers to establish over time that these events were a separate entity from SIDS, the clinical application of this classification, which describes a constellation of observed, subjective, and nonspecific symptoms, has raised significant challenges for clinicians and parents in the evaluation and care of these infants.[3] Although a broad range of disorders can present as an ALTE (eg, child abuse, congenital abnormalities, epilepsy, inborn errors of metabolism, and infections), for a majority of well-appearing infants, the risk of a recurrent event or a serious underlying disorder is extremely low.

ALTEs can create a feeling of uncertainty in both the caregiver and the clinician. Clinicians may feel compelled to perform tests and hospitalize the patient even though this may subject the patient to unnecessary risk and is unlikely to lead to a treatable diagnosis or prevent future events.[2,4,5] Understanding the risk of an adverse outcome for an infant who has experienced an ALTE has been difficult because of the nonspecific nature and variable application of the ALTE definition in research. A recent systematic review of nearly 1400 ALTE publications spanning 4 decades concluded that risk of a subsequent or underlying disorder could not be quantified because of the variability in case definitions across studies.[3] Although there are history and physical examination factors that can determine lower or higher risk, it is clear that the term ALTE must be replaced to advance the quality of care and improve research.

This guideline is intended for use primarily by clinicians providing care for infants who have experienced a BRUE, as well as their families. The guideline may be of interest to payers, but it is not intended to be used for reimbursement or to determine insurance coverage. This guideline is not intended as the sole source of guidance in the evaluation and management of BRUEs and specifically does not address higher-risk BRUE patients. Rather, it is intended to assist clinicians by providing a framework for clinical decision making. It is not intended to replace clinical judgment, and these recommendations may not provide the only appropriate approach to the management of this problem.

This guideline is intended to provide a patient- and family-centered approach to

care, reduce unnecessary and costly medical interventions, and improve patient outcomes. It includes recommendations for diagnosis, risk-based stratification, monitoring, disposition planning, effective communication with the patient and family, guideline implementation and evaluation, and future research. In addition, it aims to help clinicians determine the presence of a serious underlying cause and a safe disposition by alerting them to the most significant features of the clinical history and physical examination on which to base an approach for diagnostic testing and hospitalization. Key action statements are summarized in Table 1.

SUBCOMMITTEE ON BRIEF RESOLVED UNEXPLAINED EVENTS (FORMERLY REFERRED TO AS APPARENT LIFE THREATENING EVENTS); OVERSIGHT BY THE COUNCIL ON QUALITY IMPROVEMENT AND PATIENT SAFETY

Joel S. Tieder, MD, MPH, FAAP, Chair
Joshua L. Bonkowsky, MD, PhD, FAAP, Pediatric Neurologist
Ruth A. Etzel, MD, PhD, FAAP, Pediatric Epidemiologist
Wayne H. Franklin, MD, MPH, MMM, FAAP, Pediatric Cardiologist
David A. Gremse, MD, FAAP, Pediatric Gastroenterologist
Bruce Herman, MD, FAAP, Child Abuse and Neglect
Eliot Katz, MD, FAAP, Pediatric Pulmonologist
Leonard R. Krilov, MD, FAAP, Pediatric Infectious Diseases
J. Lawrence Merritt, II, MD, FAAP, Clinical Genetics and Biochemical Genetics
Chuck Norlin, MD, FAAP, Pediatrician
Robert E. Sapién, MD, MMM, FAAP, Pediatric Emergency Medicine
Richard Shiffman, MD, FAAP, Partnership for Policy Implementation Representative
Michael B.H. Smith, MB, FRCPCH, FAAP, Hospital Medicine

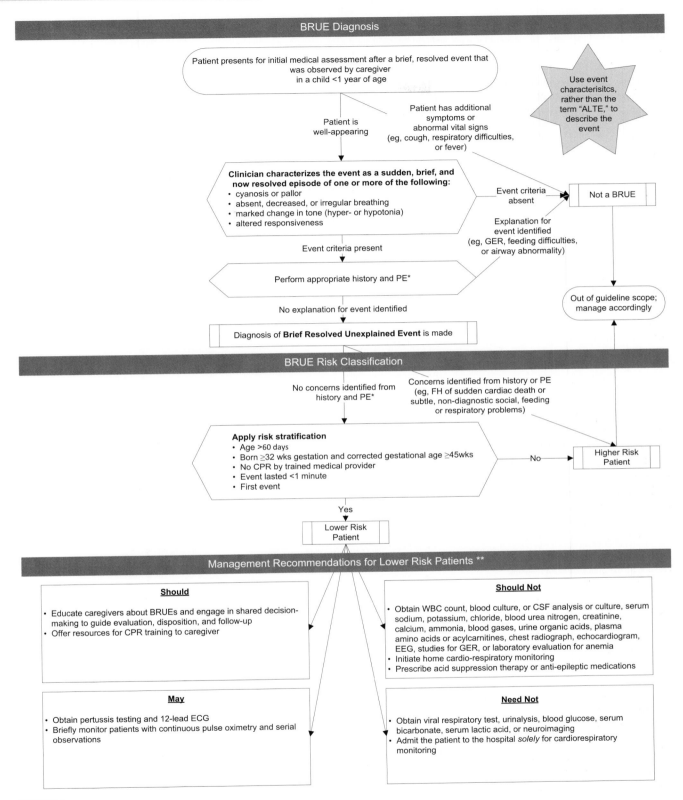

FIGURE 1

Diagnosis, risk classification, and recommended management of a BRUE. *Refer to Tables 3 and 4 in www.pediatrics.org/cgi/doi/10.1542/peds.2016-0591 for the determination of an appropriate and negative history and PE. **Refer to Figure 2 in www.pediatrics.org/cgi/doi/10.1542/peds.2016-0591 for the American Academy of Pediatrics method for rating of evidence and recommendations. CPR, cardiopulmonary resuscitation; CSF, cerebrospinal fluid; ECG, electrocardiogram; FH, family history; GER, gastroesophageal reflux; PE, physical examination; WBC, white blood cell.

Figure 1, shown here, has been updated per the erratum at http://pediatrics.aappublications.org/content/138/2/e20161488.

TABLE 1 Summary of Key Action Statements for Lower-Risk BRUEs

When managing an infant who is >60 d and <1 y of age and who, on the basis of a thorough history and physical examination, meets criteria for having experienced a lower-risk BRUE, clinicians:	Evidence Quality; Strength of Recommendation
1. Cardiopulmonary Evaluation	
1A. Need not admit infants to the hospital solely for cardiorespiratory monitoring.	B; Weak
1B. May briefly monitor patients with continuous pulse oximetry and serial observations.	D; Weak
1C. Should not obtain chest radiograph.	B; Moderate
1D. Should not obtain a measurement of venous or arterial blood gas.	B; Moderate
1E. Should not obtain an overnight polysomnograph.	B; Moderate
1F. May obtain a 12-lead electrocardiogram.	C; Weak
1G. Should not obtain an echocardiogram.	C; Moderate
1H. Should not initiate home cardiorespiratory monitoring.	B; Moderate
2. Child Abuse Evaluation	
2A. Need not obtain neuroimaging (CT, MRI, or ultrasonography) to detect child abuse.	C; Weak
2B. Should obtain an assessment of social risk factors to detect child abuse.	C; Moderate
3. Neurologic Evaluation	
3A. Should not obtain neuroimaging (CT, MRI, or ultrasonography) to detect neurologic disorders.	C; Moderate
3B. Should not obtain an EEG to detect neurologic disorders.	C; Moderate
3C. Should not prescribe antiepileptic medications for potential neurologic disorders.	C; Moderate
4. Infectious Disease Evaluation	
4A. Should not obtain a WBC count, blood culture, or cerebrospinal fluid analysis or culture to detect an occult bacterial infection.	B; Strong
4B. Need not obtain a urinalysis (bag or catheter).	C; Weak
4C. Should not obtain chest radiograph to assess for pulmonary infection.	B; Moderate
4D. Need not obtain respiratory viral testing if rapid testing is available.	C; Weak
4E. May obtain testing for pertussis.	B; Weak
5. Gastrointestinal Evaluation	
5A. Should not obtain investigations for GER (eg, upper gastrointestinal tract series, pH probe, endoscopy, barium contrast study, nuclear scintigraphy, and ultrasonography).	C; Moderate
5B. Should not prescribe acid suppression therapy.	C; Moderate
6. Inborn Error of Metabolism Evaluation	
6A. Need not obtain measurement of serum lactic acid or serum bicarbonate.	C; Weak
6B. Should not obtain a measurement of serum sodium, potassium, chloride, blood urea nitrogen, creatinine, calcium, or ammonia.	C; Moderate
6C. Should not obtain a measurement of venous or arterial blood gases.	C; Moderate
6D. Need not obtain a measurement of blood glucose.	C; Weak
6E. Should not obtain measurements of urine organic acids, plasma amino acids, or plasma acylcarnitines.	C; Moderate
7. Anemia Evaluation	
7A. Should not obtain laboratory evaluation for anemia.	C; Moderate
8. Patient- and Family-Centered Care	
8A. Should offer resources for CPR training to caregiver.	C; Moderate
8B. Should educate caregivers about BRUEs.	C; Moderate
8C. Should use shared decision making.	C; Moderate

CPR, cardiopulmonary resuscitation; CT, computed tomography; GER, gastroesophageal reflux; WBC, white blood cell.

Jack Percelay, MD, MPH, FAAP, Liaison, Society for Hospital Medicine

STAFF

Kymika Okechukwu, MPA

ABBREVIATIONS

ALTE: apparent life-threatening event
BRUE: brief resolved unexplained event
SIDS: sudden infant death syndrome

REFERENCES

1. National Institutes of Health Consensus Development Conference on Infantile Apnea and Home Monitoring, Sept 29 to Oct 1, 1986. *Pediatrics.* 1987;79(2). Available at: www.pediatrics.org/cgi/content/full/79/2/e292

2. McGovern MC, Smith MB. Causes of apparent life threatening events in infants: a systematic review. *Arch Dis Child.* 2004;89(11):1043–1048

3. Tieder JS, Altman RL, Bonkowsky JL, et al Management of apparent life-threatening events in infants: a systematic review. *J Pediatr.* 2013;163(1):94–99, e91–e96

4. Brand DA, Altman RL, Purtill K, Edwards KS. Yield of diagnostic testing in infants who have had an apparent life-threatening event. *Pediatrics.* 2005;115(4). Available at: www.pediatrics.org/cgi/content/full/115/4/e885

5. Green M. Vulnerable child syndrome and its variants. *Pediatr Rev.* 1986; 8(3):75–80

Brief Resolved Unexplained Events Clinical Practice Guideline Quick Reference Tools

• •

- Action Statement Summary
  — Brief Resolved Unexplained Events (Formerly Apparent Life-Threatening Events) and Evaluation of Lower-Risk Infants
- *ICD-10-CM* Coding Quick Reference for Brief Resolved Unexplained Events
- AAP Patient Education Handout
  — *Brief Resolved Unexplained Event: What Parents and Caregivers Need to Know*

Action Statement Summary

Brief Resolved Unexplained Events (Formerly Apparent Life-Threatening Events) and Evaluation of Lower-Risk Infants

Key Action Statement 1
Cardiopulmonary

Key Action Statement 1A
Clinicians need not admit infants presenting with a lower-risk BRUE to the hospital solely for cardiorespiratory monitoring (grade B, weak recommendation)

Key Action Statement 1B
Clinicians may briefly monitor infants presenting with a lower-risk BRUE with continuous pulse oximetry and serial observations (grade D, weak recommendation)

Key Action Statement 1C
Clinicians should not obtain a chest radiograph in infants presenting with a lower-risk BRUE (grade B, moderate recommendation)

Key Action Statement 1D
Clinicians should not obtain measurement of venous or arterial blood gases in infants presenting with a lower-risk BRUE (grade B, moderate recommendation)

Key Action Statement 1E
Clinicians should not obtain an overnight polysomnograph in infants presenting with a lower-risk BRUE (grade B, moderate recommendation)

Key Action Statement 1F
Clinicians may obtain a 12-lead electrocardiogram for infants presenting with lower-risk BRUE (grade C, weak recommendation)

Key Action Statement 1G
Clinicians should not obtain an echocardiogram in infants presenting with lower-risk BRUE (grade C, moderate recommendation)

Key Action Statement 1H
Clinicians should not initiate home cardiorespiratory monitoring in infants presenting with a lower-risk BRUE (grade B, moderate recommendation)

Key Action Statement 2
Child abuse

Key Action Statement 2A
Clinicians need not obtain neuroimaging (computed tomography, MRI, or ultrasonography) to detect child abuse in infants presenting with a lower-risk BRUE (grade C, weak recommendation)

Key Action Statement 2B
Clinicians should obtain an assessment of social risk factors to detect child abuse in infants presenting with a lower-risk BRUE (grade C, moderate recommendation)

Key Action Statement 3
Neurology

Key Action Statement 3A
Clinicians should not obtain neuroimaging (computed tomography, MRI, or ultrasonography) to detect neurologic disorders in infants presenting with a lower-risk BRUE (grade C, moderate recommendation)

Key Action Statement 3B
Clinicians should not obtain an EEG to detect neurologic disorders in infants presenting with a lower-risk BRUE (grade C, moderate recommendation)

Key Action Statement 3C
Clinicians should not prescribe antiepileptic medications for potential neurologic disorders in infants presenting with a lower-risk BRUE (grade C, moderate recommendation)

Key Action Statement 4
Infectious diseases

Key Action Statement 4A
Clinicians should not obtain a white blood cell count, blood culture, or cerebrospinal fluid analysis or culture to detect an occult bacterial infection in infants presenting with a lower-risk BRUE (grade B, strong recommendation)

Key Action Statement 4B
Clinicians need not obtain a urinalysis (bag or catheter) in infants presenting with a lower-risk BRUE (grade C, weak recommendation)

Key Action Statement 4C

Clinicians should not obtain a chest radiograph to assess for pulmonary infection in infants presenting with a lower-risk BRUE (grade B, moderate recommendation)

Key Action Statement 4D

Clinicians need not obtain respiratory viral testing if rapid testing is available in infants presenting with a lower-risk BRUE (grade C, weak recommendation)

Key Action Statement 4E

Clinicians may obtain testing for pertussis in infants presenting with a lower-risk BRUE (grade B, weak recommendation)

Key Action Statement 5

Gastroenterology

Key Action Statement 5A

Clinicians should not obtain investigations for GER (eg, upper gastrointestinal series, pH probe, endoscopy, barium contrast study, nuclear scintigraphy, and ultrasonography) in infants presenting with a lower-risk BRUE (grade C, moderate recommendation)

Key Action Statement 5B

Clinicians should not prescribe acid suppression therapy for infants presenting with a lower-risk BRUE (grade C, moderate recommendation)

Key Action Statement 6

Inborn errors of metabolism

Key Action Statement 6A

Clinicians need not obtain measurement of serum lactic acid or serum bicarbonate to detect an IEM in infants presenting with a lower-risk BRUE (grade C, weak recommendation)

Key Action Statement 6B

Clinicians should not obtain a measurement of serum sodium, potassium, chloride, blood urea nitrogen, creatinine, calcium, or ammonia to detect an IEM in infants presenting with a lower-risk BRUE (grade C, moderate recommendation)

Key Action Statement 6C

Clinicians should not obtain a measurement of venous or arterial blood gases to detect an IEM in infants presenting with lower-risk BRUE (grade C, moderate recommendation)

Key Action Statement 6D

Clinicians need not obtain a measurement of blood glucose to detect an IEM in infants presenting with a lower-risk BRUE (grade C, weak recommendation)

Key Action Statement 6E

Clinicians should not obtain measurements of urine organic acids, plasma amino acids, or plasma acylcarnitines to detect an IEM in infants presenting with a lower-risk BRUE (grade C, moderate recommendation)

Key Action Statement 7

Anemia

Key Action Statement 7A

Clinicians should not obtain laboratory evaluation for anemia in infants presenting with a lower-risk BRUE (grade C, moderate recommendation)

Key Action Statement 8

Patient- and family-centered care

Key Action Statement 8A

Clinicians should offer resources for CPR training to caregivers (grade C, moderate recommendation)

Key Action Statement 8B

Clinicians should educate caregivers about BRUEs (grade C, moderate recommendation)

Key Action Statement 8C

Clinicians should use shared decision-making for infants presenting with a lower-risk BRUE (grade C, moderate recommendation)

Coding Quick Reference for Brief Resolved Unexplained Events
ICD-10-CM
R68.13 Apparent life threatening event (ALTE) in infant (includes brief resolved unexplained events [BRUE])

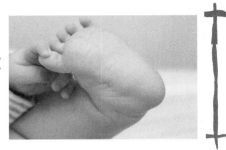

Brief Resolved Unexplained Event:
What Parents and Caregivers Need to Know

What is a brief resolved unexplained event?

A **b**rief **r**esolved **u**nexplained **e**vent (or BRUE for short) occurs suddenly and can be scary for parents and caregivers. A brief resolved unexplained event is a diagnosis made after your baby's doctor or health care professional has examined your baby and determined that there was no known concerning cause for the event.

When a brief resolved unexplained event occurs, babies may seem to stop breathing, their skin color may change to pale or blue, their muscles may relax or tighten, or they may seem to pass out. After a brief period of time, they recover (with or without any medical help) and are soon back to normal.

Though we can never say that a baby who has had a brief resolved unexplained event is at *no* risk for future problems, we can say that babies are at lower risk if

- They are older than 60 days.
- They were born on time (not premature).
- They did not need CPR (cardiopulmonary resuscitation) by a health care professional.
- The brief resolved unexplained event lasted less than 1 minute.
- This was their only such event.

Frequently asked questions after a brief resolved unexplained event

Q: Why did my baby have this event?

A: Your baby's doctor was unable to find a cause based on the results of your baby's examination and cannot tell you why this event happened. If it happens again or your baby develops additional problems, contact your baby's doctor or health care professional. The doctor may decide to have your baby return for another visit.

Q: Should my baby stay in the hospital?

A: Babies who are felt to be at lower risk by their doctors or health care professionals do not need to stay in the hospital. They are safe to go home without doing blood tests or imaging that uses x-rays, and they do not need home monitoring of their heart or lungs.

Q: Does having a brief resolved unexplained event increase my baby's risk for sudden infant death syndrome (SIDS)?

A: No—though the causes of SIDS are not known, events like these do not increase the risk of SIDS. For all babies, it is important to create a safe home and sleeping environment. Your baby should not be exposed to smoky environments. Visit **www.HealthyChildren.org/safesleep** to learn more about how to create a safe sleeping environment for your baby.

Q: What should I do if it happens again?

A: If you are worried that this new event is life threatening, call 911 or your local emergency numbers. If not, call your baby's doctor if you have any questions or worries and to let the doctor know about the event.

Q: Does my baby need extra care after having a brief resolved unexplained event? Is my baby more delicate or weak?

A: No special care is needed. Continue to love and care for your baby as you normally do.

A few important reminders for parents and caregivers of healthy infants

- Remember to take your baby to regular well-child visits to help keep your child healthy and safe.
- Though your baby is not more likely to need it, it is a good idea for everyone who cares for an infant to learn CPR. If you know CPR, you may also use it one day to help someone else in need. For classes near you, contact your child's doctor, the American Red Cross, the American Heart Association, or a national or local organization that offers training.

Listing of resources does not imply an endorsement by the American Academy of Pediatrics (AAP). The AAP is not responsible for the content of external resources. Information was current at the time of publication.

The information contained in this publication should not be used as a substitute for the medical care and advice of your pediatrician. There may be variations in treatment that your pediatrician may recommend based on individual facts and circumstances.

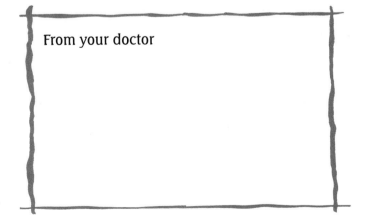

From your doctor

American Academy
of Pediatrics

DEDICATED TO THE HEALTH OF ALL CHILDREN™

The American Academy of Pediatrics (AAP) is an organization of 64,000 primary care pediatricians, pediatric medical subspecialists, and pediatric surgical specialists dedicated to the health, safety, and well-being of all infants, children, adolescents, and young adults.

American Academy of Pediatrics
Web site — www.HealthyChildren.org

The Diagnosis, Management, and Prevention of Bronchiolitis

- *Clinical Practice Guideline*
  - *PPI: AAP Partnership for Policy Implementation*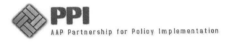
    See Appendix 1 for more information.

CLINICAL PRACTICE GUIDELINE

Clinical Practice Guideline: The Diagnosis, Management, and Prevention of Bronchiolitis

abstract

This guideline is a revision of the clinical practice guideline, "Diagnosis and Management of Bronchiolitis," published by the American Academy of Pediatrics in 2006. The guideline applies to children from 1 through 23 months of age. Other exclusions are noted. Each key action statement indicates level of evidence, benefit-harm relationship, and level of recommendation. Key action statements are as follows: *Pediatrics* 2014;134:e1474–e1502

Shawn L. Ralston, MD, FAAP, Allan S. Lieberthal, MD, FAAP, H. Cody Meissner, MD, FAAP, Brian K. Alverson, MD, FAAP, Jill E. Baley, MD, FAAP, Anne M. Gadomski, MD, MPH, FAAP, David W. Johnson, MD, FAAP, Michael J. Light, MD, FAAP, Nizar F. Maraqa, MD, FAAP, Eneida A. Mendonca, MD, PhD, FAAP, FACMI, Kieran J. Phelan, MD, MSc, Joseph J. Zorc, MD, MSCE, FAAP, Danette Stanko-Lopp, MA, MPH, Mark A. Brown, MD, Ian Nathanson, MD, FAAP, Elizabeth Rosenblum, MD, Stephen Sayles III, MD, FACEP, and Sinsi Hernandez-Cancio, JD

KEY WORDS
bronchiolitis, infants, children, respiratory syncytial virus, evidence-based, guideline

ABBREVIATIONS
AAP—American Academy of Pediatrics
AOM—acute otitis media
CI—confidence interval
ED—emergency department
KAS—Key Action Statement
LOS—length of stay
MD—mean difference
PCR—polymerase chain reaction
RSV—respiratory syncytial virus
SBI—serious bacterial infection

Dedicated to the memory of Dr Caroline Breese Hall.

www.pediatrics.org/cgi/doi/10.1542/peds.2014-2742

doi:10.1542/peds.2014-2742

PEDIATRICS (ISSN Numbers: Print, 0031-4005; Online, 1098-4275).

DIAGNOSIS

1a. Clinicians should diagnose bronchiolitis and assess disease severity on the basis of history and physical examination (Evidence Quality: B; Recommendation Strength: Strong Recommendation).

1b. Clinicians should assess risk factors for severe disease, such as age less than 12 weeks, a history of prematurity, underlying cardiopulmonary disease, or immunodeficiency, when making decisions about evaluation and management of children with bronchiolitis (Evidence Quality: B; Recommendation Strength: Moderate Recommendation).

1c. When clinicians diagnose bronchiolitis on the basis of history and physical examination, radiographic or laboratory studies should not be obtained routinely (Evidence Quality: B; Recommendation Strength: Moderate Recommendation).

TREATMENT

2. Clinicians should not administer albuterol (or salbutamol) to infants and children with a diagnosis of bronchiolitis (Evidence Quality: B; Recommendation Strength: Strong Recommendation).

3. Clinicians should not administer epinephrine to infants and children with a diagnosis of bronchiolitis (Evidence Quality: B; Recommendation Strength: Strong Recommendation).

4a. Nebulized hypertonic saline should not be administered to infants with a diagnosis of bronchiolitis in the emergency department (Evidence Quality: B; Recommendation Strength: Moderate Recommendation).

4b. Clinicians may administer nebulized hypertonic saline to infants and children hospitalized for bronchiolitis (Evidence Quality: B; Recommendation Strength: Weak Recommendation [based on randomized controlled trials with inconsistent findings]).

5. Clinicians should not administer systemic corticosteroids to infants with a diagnosis of bronchiolitis in any setting (Evidence Quality: A; Recommendation Strength: Strong Recommendation).

6a. Clinicians may choose not to administer supplemental oxygen if the oxyhemoglobin saturation exceeds 90% in infants and children with a diagnosis of bronchiolitis (Evidence Quality: D; Recommendation Strength: Weak Recommendation [based on low level evidence and reasoning from first principles]).

6b. Clinicians may choose not to use continuous pulse oximetry for infants and children with a diagnosis of bronchiolitis (Evidence Quality: D; Recommendation Strength: Weak Recommendation [based on low-level evidence and reasoning from first principles]).

7. Clinicians should not use chest physiotherapy for infants and children with a diagnosis of bronchiolitis (Evidence Quality: B; Recommendation Strength: Moderate Recommendation).

8. Clinicians should not administer antibacterial medications to infants and children with a diagnosis of bronchiolitis unless there is a concomitant bacterial infection, or a strong suspicion of one (Evidence Quality: B; Recommendation Strength: Strong Recommendation).

9. Clinicians should administer nasogastric or intravenous fluids for infants with a diagnosis of bronchiolitis who cannot maintain hydration orally (Evidence Quality: X; Recommendation Strength: Strong Recommendation).

PREVENTION

10a. Clinicians should not administer palivizumab to otherwise healthy infants with a gestational age of 29 weeks, 0 days or greater (Evidence Quality: B; Recommendation Strength: Strong Recommendation).

10b. Clinicians should administer palivizumab during the first year of life to infants with hemodynamically significant heart disease or chronic lung disease of prematurity defined as preterm infants <32 weeks 0 days' gestation who require >21% oxygen for at least the first 28 days of life (Evidence Quality: B; Recommendation Strength: Moderate Recommendation).

10c. Clinicians should administer a maximum 5 monthly doses (15 mg/kg/dose) of palivizumab during the respiratory syncytial virus season to infants who qualify for palivizumab in the first year of life (Evidence Quality: B; Recommendation Strength: Moderate Recommendation).

11a. All people should disinfect hands before and after direct contact with patients, after contact with inanimate objects in the direct vicinity of the patient, and after removing gloves (Evidence Quality: B; Recommendation Strength: Strong Recommendation).

11b. All people should use alcohol-based rubs for hand decontamination when caring for children with bronchiolitis. When alcohol-based rubs are not available, individuals should wash their hands with soap and water (Evidence Quality: B; Recommendation Strength: Strong Recommendation).

12a. Clinicians should inquire about the exposure of the infant or child to tobacco smoke when assessing infants and children for bronchiolitis (Evidence Quality: C; Recommendation Strength: Moderate Recommendation).

12b. Clinicians should counsel caregivers about exposing the infant or child to environmental tobacco smoke and smoking cessation when assessing a child for bronchiolitis (Evidence Quality: B; Recommendation Strength: Strong).

13. Clinicians should encourage exclusive breastfeeding for at least 6 months to decrease the morbidity of respiratory infections. (Evidence Quality: B; Recommendation Strength: Moderate Recommendation).

14. Clinicians and nurses should educate personnel and family members on evidence-based diagnosis, treatment, and prevention in bronchiolitis. (Evidence Quality: C; observational studies; Recommendation Strength: Moderate Recommendation).

INTRODUCTION

In October 2006, the American Academy of Pediatrics (AAP) published the clinical practice guideline "Diagnosis and Management of Bronchiolitis."[1] The guideline offered recommendations ranked according to level of evidence and the benefit-harm relationship. Since completion of the original evidence review in July 2004, a significant body of literature on bronchiolitis has been published. This update of the 2006 AAP bronchiolitis guideline evaluates published evidence, including that used in the 2006 guideline as well as evidence published since 2004. Key action statements (KASs) based on that evidence are provided.

The goal of this guideline is to provide an evidence-based approach to the diagnosis, management, and prevention of bronchiolitis in children from 1 month through 23 months of age. The guideline is intended for pediatricians, family physicians, emergency medicine specialists, hospitalists, nurse practitioners, and physician assistants who care for these children. The guideline does not apply to children with immunodeficiencies, including those with HIV infection or recipients of solid organ or hematopoietic stem cell transplants. Children with underlying respiratory illnesses, such as recurrent wheezing, chronic neonatal lung disease (also known as bronchopulmonary dysplasia), neuromuscular disease, or cystic fibrosis and those with hemodynamically significant congenital heart disease are excluded from the sections on management unless otherwise noted but are included in the discussion of prevention. This guideline will not address long-term sequelae of bronchiolitis, such as recurrent wheezing or risk of asthma, which is a field with a large and distinct literature.

Bronchiolitis is a disorder commonly caused by viral lower respiratory tract infection in infants. Bronchiolitis is characterized by acute inflammation, edema, and necrosis of epithelial cells lining small airways, and increased mucus production. Signs and symptoms typically begin with rhinitis and cough, which may progress to tachypnea, wheezing, rales, use of accessory muscles, and/or nasal flaring.[2]

Many viruses that infect the respiratory system cause a similar constellation of signs and symptoms. The most common etiology of bronchiolitis is respiratory syncytial virus (RSV), with the highest incidence of infection occurring between December and March in North America; however, regional variations occur[3] (Fig 1).[4] Ninety percent of children are infected with RSV in the first 2 years of life,[5] and up to 40% will experience lower respiratory tract infection during the initial infection.[6,7] Infection with RSV does not grant permanent or long-term immunity, with reinfections common throughout life.[8] Other viruses that cause bronchiolitis include human rhinovirus, human meta-

pneumovirus, influenza, adenovirus, coronavirus, human, and parainfluenza viruses. In a study of inpatients and outpatients with bronchiolitis,[9] 76% of patients had RSV, 39% had human rhinovirus, 10% had influenza, 2% had coronavirus, 3% had human metapneumovirus, and 1% had parainfluenza viruses (some patients had coinfections, so the total is greater than 100%).

Bronchiolitis is the most common cause of hospitalization among infants during the first 12 months of life. Approximately 100 000 bronchiolitis admissions occur annually in the United States at an estimated cost of $1.73 billion.[10] One prospective, population-based study sponsored by the Centers for Disease Control and Prevention reported the

average RSV hospitalization rate was 5.2 per 1000 children younger than 24 months of age during the 5-year period between 2000 and 2005.[11] The highest age-specific rate of RSV hospitalization occurred among infants between 30 days and 60 days of age (25.9 per 1000 children). For preterm infants (<37 weeks' gestation), the RSV hospitalization rate was 4.6 per 1000 children, a number similar to the RSV hospitalization rate for term infants of 5.2 per 1000. Infants born at <30 weeks' gestation had the highest hospitalization rate at 18.7 children per 1000, although the small number of infants born before 30 weeks' gestation make this number unreliable. Other studies indicate the RSV hospitalization rate in extremely

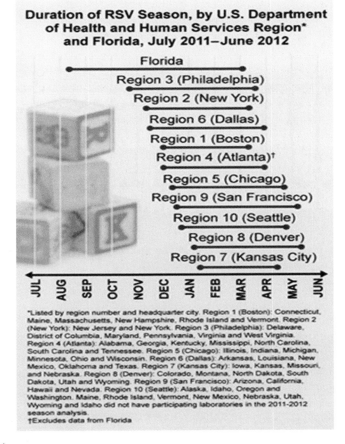

FIGURE 1

RSV season by US regions. Centers for Disease Control and Prevention. RSV activity—United States, July 2011–Jan 2013. *MMWR Morb Mortal Wkly Rep.* 2013;62(8):141–144.

preterm infants is similar to that of term infants.[12,13]

METHODS

In June 2013, the AAP convened a new subcommittee to review and revise the 2006 bronchiolitis guideline. The subcommittee included primary care physicians, including general pediatricians, a family physician, and pediatric subspecialists, including hospitalists, pulmonologists, emergency physicians, a neonatologist, and pediatric infectious disease physicians. The subcommittee also included an epidemiologist trained in systematic reviews, a guideline methodologist/informatician, and a parent representative. All panel members reviewed the AAP Policy on Conflict of Interest and Voluntary Disclosure and were given an opportunity to declare any potential conflicts. Any conflicts can be found in the author listing at the end of this guideline. All funding was provided by the AAP, with travel assistance from the American Academy of Family Physicians, the American College of Chest Physicians, the American Thoracic Society, and the American College of Emergency Physicians for their liaisons.

The evidence search and review included electronic database searches in *The Cochrane Library*, Medline via Ovid, and CINAHL via EBSCO. The search strategy is shown in the Appendix. Related article searches were conducted in PubMed. The bibliographies of articles identified by database searches were also reviewed by 1 of 4 members of the committee, and references identified in this manner were added to the review. Articles included in the 2003 evidence report on bronchiolitis in preparation of the AAP 2006 guideline2 also were reviewed. In addition, the committee reviewed articles published after completion of the systematic review for these updated guidelines. The current literature re-

view encompasses the period from 2004 through May 2014.

The evidence-based approach to guideline development requires that the evidence in support of a policy be identified, appraised, and summarized and that an explicit link between evidence and recommendations be defined. Evidence-based recommendations reflect the quality of evidence and the balance of benefit and harm that is anticipated when the recommendation is followed. The AAP policy statement "Classifying Recommendations for Clinical Practice"[14] was followed in designating levels of recommendation (Fig 2; Table 1).

A draft version of this clinical practice guideline underwent extensive peer review by committees, councils, and sections within AAP; the American Thoracic Society, American College of Chest Physicians, American Academy of Family Physicians, and American College of Emergency Physicians; other outside organizations; and other individuals identified by the subcommittee as experts in the field. The resulting comments were reviewed by the subcommittee and, when appropriate, incorporated into the guideline.

This clinical practice guideline is not intended as a sole source of guidance in the management of children with bronchiolitis. Rather, it is intended to assist clinicians in decision-making. It is not intended to replace clinical judgment or establish a protocol for the care of all children with bronchiolitis. These recommendations may not provide the only appropriate approach to the management of children with bronchiolitis.

All AAP guidelines are reviewed every 5 years.

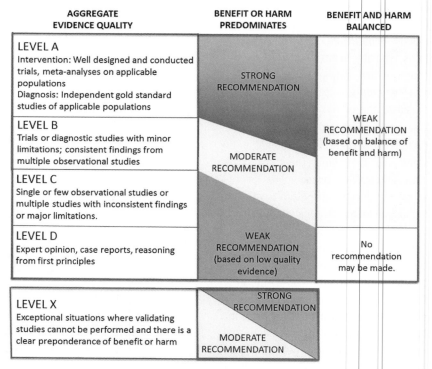

FIGURE 2

Integrating evidence quality appraisal with an assessment of the anticipated balance between benefits and harms leads to designation of a policy as a strong recommendation, moderate recommendation, or weak recommendation.

TABLE 1 Guideline Definitions for Evidence-Based Statements

Statement	Definition	Implication
Strong recommendation	A particular action is favored because anticipated benefits clearly exceed harms (or vice versa), and quality of evidence is excellent or unobtainable.	Clinicians should follow a strong recommendation unless a clear and compelling rationale for an alternative approach is present.
Moderate recommendation	A particular action is favored because anticipated benefits clearly exceed harms (or vice versa), and the quality of evidence is good but not excellent (or is unobtainable).	Clinicians would be prudent to follow a moderate recommendation but should remain alert to new information and sensitive to patient preferences.
Weak recommendation (based on low-quality evidence	A particular action is favored because anticipated benefits clearly exceed harms (or vice versa), but the quality of evidence is weak.	Clinicians would be prudent to follow a weak recommendation but should remain alert to new information and very sensitive to patient preferences.
Weak recommendation (based on balance of benefits and harms)	Weak recommendation is provided when the aggregate database shows evidence of both benefit and harm that appear similar in magnitude for any available courses of action	Clinicians should consider the options in their decision making, but patient preference may have a substantial role.

DIAGNOSIS

Key Action Statement 1a

Clinicians should diagnose bronchiolitis and assess disease severity on the basis of history and physical examination (Evidence Quality: B; Recommendation Strength: Strong Recommendation).

Action Statement Profile KAS 1a

Aggregate evidence quality	B
Benefits	Inexpensive, noninvasive, accurate
Risk, harm, cost	Missing other diagnoses
Benefit-harm assessment	Benefits outweigh harms
Value judgments	None
Intentional vagueness	None
Role of patient preferences	None
Exclusions	None
Strength	Strong recommendation
Differences of opinion	None

Key Action Statement 1b

Clinicians should assess risk factors for severe disease, such as age <12 weeks, a history of prematurity, underlying cardiopulmonary disease, or immunodeficiency, when making decisions about eval-

uation and management of children with bronchiolitis (Evidence Quality: B; Recommendation Strength: Moderate Recommendation).

Action Statement Profile KAS 1b

Aggregate evidence quality	B
Benefits	Improved ability to predict course of illness, appropriate disposition
Risk, harm, cost	Possible unnecessary hospitalization parental anxiety
Benefit-harm assessment	Benefits outweigh harms
Value judgments	None
Intentional vagueness	"Assess" is not defined
Role of patient preferences	None
Exclusions	None
Strength	Moderate recommendation
Differences of opinion	None

Key Action Statement 1c

When clinicians diagnose bronchiolitis on the basis of history and physical examination, radiographic or laboratory studies should not be obtained routinely (Evidence Quality: B; Recommendation Strength: Moderate Recommendation).

Action Statement Profile KAS 1b

Aggregate evidence quality	B
Benefits	Decreased radiation exposure, noninvasive (less procedure-associated discomfort), decreased antibiotic use, cost savings, time saving
Risk, harm, cost	Misdiagnosis, missed diagnosis of comorbid condition
Benefit-harm assessment	Benefits outweigh harms
Value judgments	None
Intentional vagueness	None
Role of patient preferences	None
Exclusions	Infants and children with unexpected worsening disease
Strength	Moderate recommendation
Differences of opinion	None

The main goals in the history and physical examination of infants presenting with wheeze or other lower respiratory tract symptoms, particularly in the winter season, is to differentiate infants with probable viral bronchiolitis from those with other disorders. In addition, an estimate of disease severity (increased respiratory rate, retractions, decreased oxygen saturation) should be made. Most clinicians recognize bronchiolitis as a constellation of clinical signs and symptoms occurring in children younger than 2 years, including a viral upper respiratory tract prodrome followed by increased respiratory effort and wheezing. Clinical signs and symptoms of bronchiolitis consist of rhinorrhea, cough, tachypnea, wheezing, rales, and increased respiratory effort manifested as grunting, nasal flaring, and intercostal and/or subcostal retractions.

The course of bronchiolitis is variable and dynamic, ranging from transient events, such as apnea, to progressive respiratory distress from lower airway obstruction. Important issues to assess in the history include the effects of respiratory symptoms on mental status, feeding, and hydration. The clinician should assess the ability of the family to care for the child and to return for further evaluation if needed. History of underlying conditions, such as prematurity, cardiac disease, chronic pulmonary disease, immunodeficiency, or episodes of previous wheezing, should be identified. Underlying conditions that may be associated with an increased risk of progression to severe disease or mortality include hemodynamically significant congenital heart disease, chronic lung disease (bronchopulmonary dysplasia), congenital anomalies,[15–17] in utero smoke exposure,[18] and the presence of an immunocompromising state.[19,20] In addition, genetic abnormalities have been associated with more severe presentation with bronchiolitis.[21]

Assessment of a child with bronchiolitis, including the physical examination, can be complicated by variability in the disease state and may require serial observations over time to fully assess the child's status. Upper airway obstruction contributes to work of breathing. Suctioning and positioning may decrease the work of breathing and improve the quality of the examination. Respiratory

rate in otherwise healthy children changes considerably over the first year of life.[22–25] In hospitalized children, the 50th percentile for respiratory rate decreased from 41 at 0 to 3 months of age to 31 at 12 to 18 months of age.[26] Counting respiratory rate over the course of 1 minute is more accurate than shorter observations.[27] The presence of a normal respiratory rate suggests that risk of significant viral or bacterial lower respiratory tract infection or pneumonia in an infant is low (negative likelihood ratio approximately 0.5),[27–29] but the presence of tachypnea does not distinguish between viral and bacterial disease.[30,31]

The evidence relating the presence of specific findings in the assessment of bronchiolitis to clinical outcomes is limited. Most studies addressing this issue have enrolled children when presenting to hospital settings, including a large, prospective, multicenter study that assessed a variety of outcomes from the emergency department (ED) and varied inpatient settings.[18,32,33] Severe adverse events, such as ICU admission and need for mechanical ventilation, are uncommon among children with bronchiolitis and limit the power of these studies to detect clinically important risk factors associated with disease progression.[16,34,35] Tachypnea, defined as a respiratory rate $\geq$70 per minute, has been associated with increased risk of severe disease in some studies[35–37] but not others.[38] Many scoring systems have been developed in an attempt to objectively quantify respiratory distress, although none has achieved widespread acceptance and few have demonstrated any predictive validity, likely because of the substantial temporal variability in physical findings in infants with bronchiolitis.[39]

Pulse oximetry has been rapidly adopted into clinical assessment of children with bronchiolitis on the basis of data

suggesting that it reliably detects hypoxemia not suspected on physical examination[36,40]; however, few studies have assessed the effectiveness of pulse oximetry to predict clinical outcomes. Among inpatients, perceived need for supplemental oxygen on the basis of pulse oximetry has been associated with prolonged hospitalization, ICU admission, and mechanical ventilation.[16,34,41] Among outpatients, available evidence differs on whether mild reductions in pulse oximetry (<95% on room air) predict progression of disease or need for a return observational visit.[38]

Apnea has been reported to occur with a wide range of prevalence estimates and viral etiologies.[42,43] Retrospective, hospital-based studies have included a high proportion of infants with risk factors, such as prematurity or neuromuscular disease, that may have biased the prevalence estimates. One large study found no apnea events for infants assessed as low risk by using several risk factors: age >1 month for full-term infants or 48 weeks' postconceptional age for preterm infants, and absence of any previous apneic event at presentation to the hospital.[44] Another large multicenter study found no association between the specific viral agent and risk of apnea in bronchiolitis.[42]

The literature on viral testing for bronchiolitis has expanded in recent years with the availability of sensitive polymerase chain reaction (PCR) assays. Large studies of infants hospitalized for bronchiolitis have consistently found that 60% to 75% have positive test results for RSV, and have noted coinfections in up to one-third of infants.[32,33,45] In the event an infant receiving monthly prophylaxis is hospitalized with bronchiolitis, testing should be performed to determine if RSV is the etiologic agent. If a breakthrough RSV infection is determined to be present based on antigen detection or other assay, monthly palivizumab prophylaxis should be discontinued because of the very low likelihood of a second RSV infection in the same year. Apart from this setting, routine virologic testing is not recommended.

Infants with non-RSV bronchiolitis, in particular human rhinovirus, appear to have a shorter courses and may represent a different phenotype associated with repeated wheezing.[32] PCR assay results should be interpreted cautiously, given that the assay may detect prolonged viral shedding from an unrelated previous illness, particularly with rhinovirus. In contrast, RSV detected by PCR assay almost always is associated with disease. At the individual patient level, the value of identifying a specific viral etiology causing bronchiolitis has not been demonstrated.[33]

Current evidence does not support routine chest radiography in children with bronchiolitis. Although many infants with bronchiolitis have abnormalities on chest radiography, data are insufficient to demonstrate that chest radiography correlates well with disease severity. Atelectasis on chest radiography was associated with increased risk of severe disease in 1 outpatient study.[16] Further studies, including 1 randomized trial, suggest children with suspected lower respiratory tract infection who had radiography performed were more likely to receive antibiotics without any difference in outcomes.[46,47] Initial radiography should be reserved for cases in which respiratory effort is severe enough to warrant ICU admission or where signs of an airway complication (such as pneumothorax) are present.

TREATMENT

ALBUTEROL

Key Action Statement 2

Clinicians should not administer albuterol (or salbutamol) to infants

and children with a diagnosis of bronchiolitis (Evidence Quality: B; Recommendation Strength: Strong Recommendation).

Action Statement Profile KAS 2

Aggregate evidence quality	B
Benefits	Avoid adverse effects, avoid ongoing use of ineffective medication, lower costs
Risk, harm, cost	Missing transient benefit of drug
Benefit-harm assessment	Benefits outweigh harms
Value judgments	Overall ineffectiveness outweighs possible transient benefit
Intentional vagueness	None
Role of patient preferences	None
Exclusions	None
Strength	Strong recommendation
Differences of opinion	None
Notes	This guideline no longer recommends a trial of albuterol, as was considered in the 2006 AAP bronchiolitis guideline

Although several studies and reviews have evaluated the use of bronchodilator medications for viral bronchiolitis, most randomized controlled trials have failed to demonstrate a consistent benefit from α- or β-adrenergic agents. Several meta-analyses and systematic reviews[48–53] have shown that bronchodilators may improve clinical symptom scores, but they do not affect disease resolution, need for hospitalization, or length of stay (LOS). Because clinical scores may vary from one observer to the next[39,54] and do not correlate with more objective measures, such as pulmonary function tests,[55] clinical scores are not validated measures of the efficacy of bronchodilators. Although transient improvements in clinical score have been observed, most infants treated with bronchodilators will not benefit from their use.

A recently updated Cochrane systematic review assessing the impact of bronchodilators on oxygen saturation, the primary outcome measure, reported 30 randomized controlled trials involving 1992 infants in 12 countries.[56] Some studies included in this review evaluated agents other than albuterol/salbutamol (eg, ipratropium and metaproterenol) but did not include epinephrine. Small sample sizes, lack of standardized methods for outcome evaluation (eg, timing of assessments), and lack of standardized intervention (various bronchodilators, drug dosages, routes of administration, and nebulization delivery systems) limit the interpretation of these studies. Because of variable study designs as well as the inclusion of infants who had a history of previous wheezing in some studies, there was considerable heterogeneity in the studies. Sensitivity analysis (ie, including only studies at low risk of bias) significantly reduced heterogeneity measures for oximetry while having little effect on the overall effect size of oximetry (mean difference [MD] −0.38, 95% confidence interval [CI] −0.75 to 0.00). Those studies showing benefit[57–59] are methodologically weaker than other studies and include older children with recurrent wheezing. Results of the Cochrane review indicated no benefit in the clinical course of infants with bronchiolitis who received bronchodilators. The potential adverse effects (tachycardia and tremors) and cost of these agents outweigh any potential benefits.

In the previous iteration of this guideline, a trial of β-agonists was included as an option. However, given the greater strength of the evidence demonstrating no benefit, and that there is no well-established way to determine an "objective method of response" to bronchodilators in bronchiolitis, this option has been removed. Although it is true that a small subset of children with bronchiolitis may have reversible airway obstruction resulting from smooth muscle constriction, attempts to define a subgroup of responders have not been successful to date. If a clinical trial of bronchodilators is undertaken, clinicians should note that the variability of the disease process, the host's airway, and the clinical assessments, particularly scoring, would limit the clinician's ability to observe a clinically relevant response to bronchodilators.

Chavasse et al[60] reviewed the available literature on use of β-agonists for children younger than 2 years with recurrent wheezing. At the time of that review, there were 3 studies in the outpatient setting, 2 in the ED, and 3 in the pulmonary function laboratory setting. This review concluded there were no clear benefits from the use of β-agonists in this population. The authors noted some conflicting evidence, but further study was recommended only if the population could be clearly defined and meaningful outcome measures could be identified.

The population of children with bronchiolitis studied in most trials of bronchodilators limits the ability to make recommendations for all clinical scenarios. Children with severe disease or with respiratory failure were generally excluded from these trials, and this evidence cannot be generalized to these situations. Studies using pulmonary function tests show no effect of albuterol among infants hospitalized with bronchiolitis.[56,61] One study in a critical care setting showed a small decrease in inspiratory resistance after albuterol in one group and levalbuterol in another group, but therapy was accompanied by clinically significant tachycardia.[62] This small clinical change occurring with significant adverse effects does not justify recommending albuterol for routine care.

EPINEPHRINE

Key Action Statement 3

Clinicians should not administer epinephrine to infants and children with a diagnosis of bronchiolitis (Evidence Quality: B; Recommendation Strength: Strong Recommendation).

Action Statement Profile KAS 3

Aggregate evidence quality	B
Benefits	Avoiding adverse effects, lower costs, avoiding ongoing use of ineffective medication
Risk, harm, cost	Missing transient benefit of drug
Benefit-harm assessment	Benefits outweigh harms
Value judgments	The overall ineffectiveness outweighs possible transient benefit
Intentional vagueness	None
Role of patient preferences	None
Exclusions	Rescue treatment of rapidly deteriorating patients
Strength	Strong recommendation
Differences of opinion	None

Epinephrine is an adrenergic agent with both β- and α-receptor agonist activity that has been used to treat upper and lower respiratory tract illnesses both as a systemic agent and directly into the respiratory tract, where it is typically administered as a nebulized solution. Nebulized epinephrine has been administered in the racemic form and as the purified L-enantiomer, which is commercially available in the United States for intravenous use. Studies in other diseases, such as croup, have found no difference in efficacy on the basis of preparation,[63] although the comparison has not been specifically studied for bronchiolitis. Most studies have compared L-epinephrine to placebo or albuterol. A recent Cochrane meta-

analysis by Hartling et al[64] systematically evaluated the evidence on this topic and found no evidence for utility in the inpatient setting. Two large, multicenter randomized trials comparing nebulized epinephrine to placebo[65] or albuterol[66] in the hospital setting found no improvement in LOS or other inpatient outcomes. A recent, large multicenter trial found a similar lack of efficacy compared with placebo and further demonstrated longer LOS when epinephrine was used on a fixed schedule compared with an as-needed schedule.[67] This evidence suggests epinephrine should not be used in children hospitalized for bronchiolitis, except potentially as a rescue agent in severe disease, although formal study is needed before a recommendation for the use of epinephrine in this setting.

The role of epinephrine in the outpatient setting remains controversial. A major addition to the evidence base came from the Canadian Bronchiolitis Epinephrine Steroid Trial.[68] This multicenter randomized trial enrolled 800 patients with bronchiolitis from 8 EDs and compared hospitalization rates over a 7-day period. This study had 4 arms: nebulized epinephrine plus oral dexamethasone, nebulized epinephrine plus oral placebo, nebulized placebo plus oral dexamethasone, and nebulized placebo plus oral placebo. The group of patients who received epinephrine concomitantly with corticosteroids had a lower likelihood of hospitalization by day 7 than the double placebo group, although this effect was no longer statistically significant after adjusting for multiple comparisons.

The systematic review by Hartling et al[64] concluded that epinephrine reduced hospitalizations compared with placebo on the day of the ED visit but not overall. Given that epinephrine has a transient effect and home administration is not routine practice, discharging an infant after observing a response in a monitored setting raises concerns for subsequent progression of illness. Studies have not found a difference in revisit rates, although the numbers of revisits are small and may not be adequately powered for this outcome. In summary, the current state of evidence does not support a routine role for epinephrine for bronchiolitis in outpatients, although further data may help to better define this question.

HYPERTONIC SALINE

Key Action Statement 4a

Nebulized hypertonic saline should not be administered to infants with a diagnosis of bronchiolitis in the emergency department (Evidence Quality: B; Recommendation Strength: Moderate Recommendation).

Action Statement Profile KAS 4a

Aggregate evidence quality	B
Benefits	Avoiding adverse effects, such as wheezing and excess secretions, cost
Risk, harm, cost	None
Benefit-harm assessment	Benefits outweigh harms
Value judgments	None
Intentional vagueness	None
Role of patient preferences	None
Exclusions	None
Strength	Moderate recommendation
Differences of opinion	None

Key Action Statement 4b

Clinicians may administer nebulized hypertonic saline to infants and children hospitalized for bronchiolitis (Evidence Quality: B; Recommendation Strength: Weak

Recommendation [based on randomized controlled trials with inconsistent findings]).

Action Statement Profile KAS 4b

Aggregate evidence quality	B
Benefits	May shorten hospital stay if LOS is >72 h
Risk, harm, cost	Adverse effects such as wheezing and excess secretions; cost
Benefit-harm assessment	Benefits outweigh harms for longer hospital stays
Value judgments	Anticipating an individual child's LOS is difficult. Most US hospitals report an average LOS of <72 h for patients with bronchiolitis. This weak recommendation applies only if the average length of stay is >72 h
Intentional vagueness	This weak recommendation is based on an average LOS and does not address the individual patient.
Role of patient preferences	None
Exclusions	None
Strength	Weak
Differences of opinion	None

Nebulized hypertonic saline is an increasingly studied therapy for acute viral bronchiolitis. Physiologic evidence suggests that hypertonic saline increases mucociliary clearance in both normal and diseased lungs.[69-71] Because the pathology in bronchiolitis involves airway inflammation and resultant mucus plugging, improved mucociliary clearance should be beneficial, although there is only indirect evidence to support such an assertion. A more specific theoretical mechanism of action has been proposed on the basis of the concept of rehydration of the airway surface liquid, although again, evidence remains indirect.[72]

A 2013 Cochrane review[73] included 11 trials involving 1090 infants with mild to moderate disease in both inpatient and emergency settings. There were 6 studies involving 500 inpatients providing data

for the analysis of LOS with an aggregate 1-day decrease reported, a result largely driven by the inclusion of 3 studies with relatively long mean length of stay of 5 to 6 days. The analysis of effect on clinical scores included 7 studies involving 640 patients in both inpatient and outpatient settings and demonstrated incremental positive effect with each day posttreatment from day 1 to day 3 (−0.88 MD on day 1, −1.32 MD on day 2, and −1.51 MD on day 3). Finally, Zhang et al[73] found no effect on hospitalization rates in the pooled analysis of 1 outpatient and 3 ED studies including 380 total patients.

Several randomized trials published after the Cochrane review period further informed the current guideline recommendation. Four trials evaluated admission rates from the ED, 3 using 3% saline and 1 using 7% saline.[74-76] A single trial[76] demonstrated a difference in admission rates from the ED favoring hypertonic saline, although the other 4 studies were concordant with the studies included in the Cochrane review. However, contrary to the studies included in the Cochrane review, none of the more recent trials reported improvement in LOS and, when added to the older studies for an updated meta-analysis, they significantly attenuate the summary estimate of the effect on LOS.[76,77] Most of the trials included in the Cochrane review occurred in settings with typical LOS of more than 3 days in their usual care arms. Hence, the significant decrease in LOS noted by Zhang et al[73] may not be generalizable to the United States where the average LOS is 2.4 days.[10] One other ongoing clinical trial performed in the United States, unpublished except in abstract form, further supports the observation that hypertonic saline does not decrease LOS in settings where expected stays are less than 3 days.[78]

The preponderance of the evidence suggests that 3% saline is safe and effective at improving symptoms of mild to moderate bronchiolitis after 24 hours of use and reducing hospital LOS in settings in which the duration of stay typically exceeds 3 days. It has not been shown to be effective at reducing hospitalization in emergency settings or in areas where the length of usage is brief. It has not been studied in intensive care settings, and most trials have included only patients with mild to moderate disease. Most studies have used a 3% saline concentration, and most have combined it with bronchodilators with each dose; however, there is retrospective evidence that the rate of adverse events is similar without bronchodilators,[79] as well as prospective evidence extrapolated from 2 trials without bronchodilators.[79,80] A single study was performed in the ambulatory outpatient setting[81]; however, future studies in the United States should focus on sustained usage on the basis of pattern of effects discerned in the available literature.

CORTICOSTEROIDS

Key Action Statement 5

Clinicians should not administer systemic corticosteroids to infants with a diagnosis of bronchiolitis in any setting (Evidence Quality: A; Recommendation Strength: Strong Recommendation).

Action Statement Profile KAS 5

Aggregate evidence quality	A
Benefits	No clinical benefit, avoiding adverse effects
Risk, harm, cost	None
Benefit-harm assessment	Benefits outweigh harms
Value judgments	None
Intentional vagueness	None
Role of patient preferences	None
Exclusions	None
Strength	Strong recommendation
Differences of opinion	None

Although there is good evidence of benefit from corticosteroids in other

respiratory diseases, such as asthma and croup,[82–84] the evidence on corticosteroid use in bronchiolitis is negative. The most recent Cochrane systematic review shows that corticosteroids do not significantly reduce outpatient admissions when compared with placebo (pooled risk ratio, 0.92; 95% CI, 0.78 to 1.08; and risk ratio, 0.86; 95% CI, 0.7 to 1.06, respectively) and do not reduce LOS for inpatients (MD −0.18 days; 95% CI −0.39 to 0.04).[85] No other comparisons showed relevant differences for either primary or secondary outcomes. This review contained 17 trials with 2596 participants and included 2 large ED-based randomized trials, neither of which showed reductions in hospital admissions with treatment with corticosteroids as compared with placebo.[69,86]

One of these large trials, the Canadian Bronchiolitis Epinephrine Steroid Trial, however, did show a reduction in hospitalizations 7 days after treatment with combined nebulized epinephrine and oral dexamethasone as compared with placebo.[69] Although an unadjusted analysis showed a relative risk for hospitalization of 0.65 (95% CI 0.45 to 0.95; $P = .02$) for combination therapy as compared with placebo, adjustment for multiple comparison rendered the result insignificant ($P = .07$). These results have generated considerable controversy.[87] Although there is no standard recognized rationale for why combination epinephrine and dexamethasone would be synergistic in infants with bronchiolitis, evidence in adults and children older than 6 years with asthma shows that adding inhaled long-acting β agonists to moderate/high doses of inhaled corticosteroids allows reduction of the corticosteroid dose by, on average, 60%.[88] Basic science studies focused on understanding the interaction between β agonists and corticosteroids have shown potential mechanisms for

why simultaneous administration of these drugs could be synergistic.[89–92] However, other bronchiolitis trials of corticosteroids administered by using fixed simultaneous bronchodilator regimens have not consistently shown benefit[93–97]; hence, a recommendation regarding the benefit of combined dexamethasone and epinephrine therapy is premature.

The systematic review of corticosteroids in children with bronchiolitis cited previously did not find any differences in short-term adverse events as compared with placebo.[86] However, corticosteroid therapy may prolong viral shedding in patients with bronchiolitis.[17]

In summary, a comprehensive systematic review and large multicenter randomized trials provide clear evidence that corticosteroids alone do not provide significant benefit to children with bronchiolitis. Evidence for potential benefit of combined corticosteroid and agents with both α- and β-agonist activity is at best tentative, and additional large trials are needed to clarify whether this therapy is effective.

Further, although there is no evidence of short-term adverse effects from corticosteroid therapy, other than prolonged viral shedding, in infants and children with bronchiolitis, there is inadequate evidence to be certain of safety.

OXYGEN

Key Action Statement 6a

Clinicians may choose not to administer supplemental oxygen if the oxyhemoglobin saturation exceeds 90% in infants and children with a diagnosis of bronchiolitis (Evidence Quality: D; Recommendation Strength: Weak Recommendation [based on low-level evidence and reasoning from first principles]).

Action Statement Profile KAS 6a

Benefits	Decreased hospitalizations, decreased LOS
Risk, harm, cost	Hypoxemia, physiologic stress, prolonged LOS, increased hospitalizations, increased LOS, cost
Benefit-harm assessment	Benefits outweigh harms
Value judgments	Oxyhemoglobin saturation >89% is adequate to oxygenate tissues; the risk of hypoxemia with oxyhemoglobin saturation >89% is minimal
Intentional vagueness	None
Role of patient preferences	Limited
Exclusions	Children with acidosis or fever
Strength	Weak recommendation (based on low-level evidence/ reasoning from first principles)
Differences of opinion	None

Key Action Statement 6b

Clinicians may choose not to use continuous pulse oximetry for infants and children with a diagnosis of bronchiolitis (Evidence Quality: C; Recommendation Strength: Weak Recommendation [based on lower-level evidence]).

Action Statement Profile KAS 6b

Aggregate evidence quality	C
Benefits	Shorter LOS, decreased alarm fatigue, decreased cost
Risk, harm, cost	Delayed detection of hypoxemia, delay in appropriate weaning of oxygen
Benefit-harm assessment	Benefits outweigh harms
Value judgments	None
Intentional vagueness	None
Role of patient preferences	Limited
Exclusions	None
Strength	Weak recommendation (based on lower level of evidence)
Differences of opinion	None

Although oxygen saturation is a poor predictor of respiratory distress, it is associated closely with a perceived need for hospitalization in infants with bronchiolitis.[98,99] Additionally, oxygen saturation has been implicated as a primary determinant of LOS in bronchiolitis.[40,100,101]

Physiologic data based on the oxyhemoglobin dissociation curve (Fig 3) demonstrate that small increases in arterial partial pressure of oxygen are associated with marked improvement in pulse oxygen saturation when the latter is less than 90%; with pulse oxygen saturation readings greater than 90% it takes very large elevations in arterial partial pressure of oxygen to affect further increases. In infants and children with bronchiolitis, no data exist to suggest such increases result in any clinically significant difference in physiologic function, patient symptoms, or clinical outcomes. Although it is well understood that acidosis, temperature, and 2,3-diphosphoglutarate influence the oxyhemoglobin dissociation curve, there has never been research to demonstrate how those influences practically affect infants with hypoxemia. The risk of hypoxemia must be weighed against the risk of hospitalization when making any decisions about site of care. One study of hospitalized children with bronchiolitis, for example, noted a 10% adverse error or near-miss rate for harm-causing interventions.[103] There are no studies on the effect of short-term, brief periods of hypoxemia such as may be seen in bronchiolitis. Transient hypoxemia is common in healthy infants.[104] Travel of healthy children even to moderate altitudes of 1300 m results in transient sleep desaturation to an average of 84% with no known adverse consequences.[105] Although children with chronic hypoxemia do incur developmental and behavioral problems, children who suffer intermittent hypoxemia from diseases such as asthma do not have impaired intellectual abilities or behavioral disturbance.[106–108]

Supplemental oxygen provided for infants not requiring additional respiratory support is best initiated with nasal prongs, although exact measurement of fraction of inspired oxygen is unreliable with this method.[109]

Pulse oximetry is a convenient method to assess the percentage of hemoglobin bound by oxygen in children. Pulse oximetry has been erroneously used in bronchiolitis as a proxy for respiratory distress. Accuracy of pulse oximetry is poor, especially in the 76% to 90% range.[110] Further, it has been well demonstrated that oxygen saturation has much less impact on respiratory drive than carbon dioxide concentrations in the blood.[111] There is very poor correlation between respiratory distress and oxygen saturations among infants with lower respiratory tract infections.[112] Other than cyanosis, no published clinical sign, model, or score accurately identifies hypoxemic children.[113]

Among children admitted for bronchiolitis, continuous pulse oximetry measurement is not well studied and potentially problematic for children who do not require oxygen. Transient desaturation is a normal phenomenon in healthy infants. In 1 study of 64 healthy infants between 2 weeks and 6 months of age, 60% of these infants exhibited a transient oxygen desaturation below 90%, to values as low as 83%.[105] A retrospective study of the role of continuous measurement of oxygenation in infants hospitalized with bronchiolitis found that 1 in 4 patients incur unnecessarily prolonged hospitalization as a result of a perceived need for oxygen outside of other symptoms[40] and no evidence of benefit was found.

Pulse oximetry is prone to errors of measurement. Families of infants hospitalized with continuous pulse oximeters are exposed to frequent alarms that

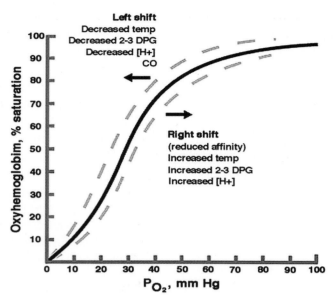

FIGURE 3
Oxyhemoglobin dissociation curve showing percent saturation of hemoglobin at various partial pressures of oxygen (reproduced with permission from the educational Web site www.anaesthesiauk. com).[102]

may negatively affect sleep. Alarm fatigue is recognized by The Joint Commission as a contributor toward in-hospital morbidity and mortality.[114] One adult study demonstrated very poor documentation of hypoxemia alerts by pulse oximetry, an indicator of alarm fatigue.[115] Pulse oximetry probes can fall off easily, leading to inaccurate measurements and alarms.[116] False reliance on pulse oximetry may lead to less careful monitoring of respiratory status. In one study, continuous pulse oximetry was associated with increased risk of minor adverse events in infants admitted to a general ward.[117] The pulse oximetry–monitored patients were found to have less-effective surveillance of their severity of illness when controlling for other variables.

There are a number of new approaches to oxygen delivery in bronchiolitis, 2 of which are home oxygen and high-frequency nasal cannula. There is emerging evidence for the role of home oxygen in reducing LOS or admission rate for infants with bronchiolitis, in-

cluding 2 randomized trials.[118,119] Most of the studies have been performed in areas of higher altitude, where prolonged hypoxemia is a prime determinant of LOS in the hospital.[120,121] Readmission rates may be moderately higher in patients discharged with home oxygen; however, overall hospital use may be reduced,[122] although not in all settings.[123] Concerns have been raised that home pulse oximetry may complicate care or confuse families.[124] Communication with follow-up physicians is important, because primary care physicians may have difficulty determining safe pulse oximetry levels for discontinuation of oxygen.[125] Additionally, there may be an increased demand for follow-up outpatient visits associated with home oxygen use.[124]

Use of humidified, heated, high-flow nasal cannula to deliver air-oxygen mixtures provides assistance to infants with bronchiolitis through multiple proposed mechanisms.[126] There is evidence that high-flow nasal cannula improves physiologic measures of respiratory effort and can generate

continuous positive airway pressure in bronchiolitis.[127–130] Clinical evidence suggests it reduces work of breathing[131,132] and may decrease need for intubation,[133–136] although studies are generally retrospective and small. The therapy has been studied in the ED[136,137] and the general inpatient setting,[134,138] as well as the ICU. The largest and most rigorous retrospective study to date was from Australia,[138] which showed a decline in intubation rate in the subgroup of infants with bronchiolitis (*n* = 330) from 37% to 7% after the introduction of high-flow nasal cannula, while the national registry intubation rate remained at 28%. A single pilot for a randomized trial has been published to date.[139] Although promising, the absence of any completed randomized trial of the efficacy of high-flow nasal cannula in bronchiolitis precludes specific recommendations on it use at present. Pneumothorax is a reported complication.

CHEST PHYSIOTHERAPY

Key Action Statement 7

Clinicians should not use chest physiotherapy for infants and children with a diagnosis of bronchiolitis (Evidence Quality: B; Recommendation Strength: Moderate Recommendation).

Action Statement Profile KAS 7

Aggregate evidence quality	B
Benefits	Decreased stress from therapy, reduced cost
Risk, harm, cost	None
Benefit-harm assessment	Benefits outweigh harms
Value judgments	None
Intentional vagueness	None
Role of patient preferences	None
Exclusions	None
Strength	Moderate recommendation
Differences of opinion	None

Airway edema, sloughing of respiratory epithelium into airways, and generalized hyperinflation of the lungs, coupled with poorly developed collateral ventilation, put infants with bronchiolitis at risk for atelectasis. Although lobar atelectasis is not characteristic of this disease, chest radiographs may show evidence of subsegmental atelectasis, prompting clinicians to consider ordering chest physiotherapy to promote airway clearance. A Cochrane Review[140] found 9 randomized controlled trials that evaluated chest physiotherapy in hospitalized patients with bronchiolitis. No clinical benefit was found by using vibration or percussion (5 trials)[141–144] or passive expiratory techniques (4 trials).[145–148] Since that review, a study[149] of the passive expiratory technique found a small, but significant reduction in duration of oxygen therapy, but no other benefits.

Suctioning of the nasopharynx to remove secretions is a frequent practice in infants with bronchiolitis. Although suctioning the nares may provide temporary relief of nasal congestion or upper airway obstruction, a retrospective study reported that deep suctioning[150] was associated with longer LOS in hospitalized infants 2 to 12 months of age. The same study also noted that lapses of greater than 4 hours in noninvasive, external nasal suctioning were also associated with longer LOS. Currently, there are insufficient data to make a recommendation about suctioning, but it appears that routine use of "deep" suctioning[151,153] may not be beneficial.

ANTIBACTERIALS

Key Action Statement 8

Clinicians should not administer antibacterial medications to infants and children with a diagnosis of bronchiolitis unless there is a concomitant bacterial infection, or a strong suspicion of one. (Evidence

Quality: B; Recommendation Strength: Strong Recommendation).

Action Statement Profile KAS 8

Aggregate evidence quality	B
Benefits	Fewer adverse effects, less resistance to antibacterial agents, lower cost
Risk, harm, cost	None
Benefit-harm assessment	Benefits outweigh harms
Value judgments	None
Intentional vagueness	Strong suspicion is not specifically defined and requires clinician judgment. An evaluation for the source of possible serious bacterial infection should be completed before antibiotic use
Role of patient preferences	None
Exclusions	None
Strength	Strong recommendation
Differences of opinion	None

Infants with bronchiolitis frequently receive antibacterial therapy because of fever,[152] young age,[153] and concern for secondary bacterial infection.[154] Early randomized controlled trials[155,156] showed no benefit from routine antibacterial therapy for children with bronchiolitis. Nonetheless, antibiotic therapy continues to be overused in young infants with bronchiolitis because of concern for an undetected bacterial infection. Studies have shown that febrile infants without an identifiable source of fever have a risk of bacteremia that may be as high as 7%. However, a child with a distinct viral syndrome, such as bronchiolitis, has a lower risk (much less than 1%) of bacterial infection of the cerebrospinal fluid or blood.[157]

Ralston et al[158] conducted a systematic review of serious bacterial infections (SBIs) occurring in hospitalized febrile infants between 30 and 90 days of age with bronchiolitis. Instances of bacteremia or meningitis were extremely rare.

Enteritis was not evaluated. Urinary tract infection occurred at a rate of approximately 1%, but asymptomatic bacteriuria may have explained this finding. The authors concluded routine screening for SBI among hospitalized febrile infants with bronchiolitis between 30 and 90 days of age is not justified. Limited data suggest the risk of bacterial infection in hospitalized infants with bronchiolitis younger than 30 days of age is similar to the risk in older infants. An abnormal white blood cell count is not useful for predicting a concurrent SBI in infants and young children hospitalized with RSV lower respiratory tract infection.[159] Several retrospective studies support this conclusion.[160–166] Four prospective studies of SBI in patients with bronchiolitis and/or RSV infections also demonstrated low rates of SBI.[167–171]

Approximately 25% of hospitalized infants with bronchiolitis have radiographic evidence of atelectasis, and it may be difficult to distinguish between atelectasis and bacterial infiltrate or consolidation.[169] Bacterial pneumonia in infants with bronchiolitis without consolidation is unusual.[170] Antibiotic therapy may be justified in some children with bronchiolitis who require intubation and mechanical ventilation for respiratory failure.[172,173]

Although acute otitis media (AOM) in infants with bronchiolitis may be attributable to viruses, clinical features generally do not permit differentiation of viral AOM from those with a bacterial component.[174] Two studies address the frequency of AOM in patients with bronchiolitis. Andrade et al[175] prospectively identified AOM in 62% of 42 patients who presented with bronchiolitis. AOM was present in 50% on entry to the study and developed in an additional 12% within 10 days. A subsequent report[176] followed 150 children hospitalized for bronchiolitis for the development of AOM. Seventy-nine (53%) developed AOM, two-thirds within the first 2 days of hospitalization. AOM did not influence the clinical course or laboratory findings of bronchiolitis. The current AAP guideline on AOM[177] recommends that a diagnosis of AOM should include bulging of the tympanic membrane. This is based on bulging being the best indicator for the presence of bacteria in multiple tympanocentesis studies and on 2 articles comparing antibiotic to placebo therapy that used a bulging tympanic membrane as a necessary part of the diagnosis.[178,179] New studies are needed to determine the incidence of AOM in bronchiolitis by using the new criterion of bulging of the tympanic membrane. Refer to the AOM guideline[180] for recommendations regarding the management of AOM.

NUTRITION AND HYDRATION

Key Action Statement 9

Clinicians should administer nasogastric or intravenous fluids for infants with a diagnosis of bronchiolitis who cannot maintain hydration orally (Evidence Quality: X; Recommendation Strength: Strong Recommendation).

Action Statement Profile KAS 9

Aggregate evidence quality	X
Benefits	Maintaining hydration
Risk, harm, cost	Risk of infection, risk of aspiration with nasogastric tube, discomfort, hyponatremia, intravenous infiltration, overhydration
Benefit-harm assessment	Benefits outweigh harms
Value judgments	None
Intentional vagueness	None
Role of patient preferences	Shared decision as to which mode is used
Exclusions	None
Strength	Strong recommendation
Differences of opinion	None

The level of respiratory distress attributable to bronchiolitis guides the indications for fluid replacement. Conversely, food intake in the previous 24 hours may be a predictor of oxygen saturation among infants with bron-

chiolitis. One study found that food intake at less than 50% of normal for the previous 24 hours is associated with a pulse oximetry value of <95%.[180] Infants with mild respiratory distress may require only observation, particularly if feeding remains unaffected. When the respiratory rate exceeds 60 to 70 breaths per minute, feeding may be compromised, particularly if nasal secretions are copious. There is limited evidence to suggest coordination of breathing with swallowing may be impaired among infants with bronchiolitis.[181] These infants may develop increased nasal flaring, retractions, and prolonged expiratory wheezing when fed and may be at increased risk of aspiration.[182]

One study estimated that one-third of infants hospitalized for bronchiolitis require fluid replacement.[183] One case series[184] and 2 randomized trials,[185,186] examined the comparative efficacy and safety of the intravenous and nasogastric routes for fluid replacement. A pilot trial in Israel that included 51 infants younger than 6 months demonstrated no significant differences in the duration of oxygen needed or time to full oral feeds between

infants receiving intravenous 5% dextrose in normal saline solution or nasogastric breast milk or formula.[187] Infants in the intravenous group had a shorter LOS (100 vs 120 hours) but it was not statistically

significant. In a larger open randomized trial including infants between 2 and 12 months of age and conducted in Australia and New Zealand, there were no significant differences in rates of admission to ICUs, need for ventilatory support, and adverse events between 381 infants assigned to nasogastric hydration and 378 infants assigned to intravenous hydration.[188] There was a difference of 4 hours in mean LOS between the intravenous group (82.2 hours) and the nasogastric group (86.2 hours) that was not statistically significant. The nasogastric route had a higher success rate of insertion than the intravenous route. Parental satisfaction scores did not differ between the intravenous and nasogastric groups. These studies suggest that infants who have difficulty feeding safely because of respiratory distress can receive either intravenous or nasogastric fluid replacement; however, more evidence is needed to increase the strength of this recommendation.

The possibility of fluid retention related to production of antidiuretic hormone has been raised in patients with bronchiolitis.[187–189] Therefore, receipt of hypotonic fluid replacement and maintenance fluids may increase the risk of iatrogenic hyponatremia in these infants. A recent meta-analysis demonstrated that among hospitalized children requiring maintenance fluids, the use of hypotonic fluids was associated with significant hyponatremia compared with isotonic fluids in older children.[190] Use of isotonic fluids, in general, appears to be safer.

PREVENTION

Key Action Statement 10a

Clinicians should not administer palivizumab to otherwise healthy

infants with a gestational age of 29 weeks, 0 days or greater (Evidence Quality: B; Recommendation Strength: Strong Recommendation).

Action Statement Profile KAS 10a

Aggregate evidence quality	B
Benefits	Reduced pain of injections, reduced use of a medication that has shown minimal benefit, reduced adverse effects, reduced visits to health care provider with less exposure to illness
Risk, harm, cost	Minimal increase in risk of RSV hospitalization
Benefit-harm assessment	Benefits outweigh harms
Value judgments	None
Intentional vagueness	None
Role of patient preferences	Parents may choose to not accept palivizumab
Exclusions	Infants with chronic lung disease of prematurity and hemodynamically significant cardiac disease (as described in KAS 10b)
Strength	Recommendation
Differences of opinion	None
Notes	This KAS is harmonized with the AAP policy statement on palivizumab

Key Action Statement 10b

Clinicians should administer palivizumab during the first year of life to infants with hemodynamically significant heart disease or chronic lung disease of prematurity defined as preterm infants <32 weeks, 0 days' gestation who require >21% oxygen for at least the first 28 days of life (Evidence Quality: B; Recommendation Strength: Moderate Recommendation).

Action Statement Profile KAS 10b

Aggregate evidence quality	B
Benefits	Reduced risk of RSV hospitalization
Risk, harm, cost	Injection pain; increased risk of illness from increased visits to clinician office or clinic; cost; side effects from palivizumab
Benefit-harm assessment	Benefits outweigh harms
Value judgments	None
Intentional vagueness	None
Role of patient preferences	Parents may choose to not accept palivizumab
Exclusions	None
Strength	Moderate recommendation
Differences of opinion	None
Notes	This KAS is harmonized with the AAP policy statement on palivizumab[191,192]

Key Action Statement 10c

Clinicians should administer a maximum 5 monthly doses (15 mg/kg/dose) of palivizumab during the RSV season to infants who qualify for palivizumab in the first year of life (Evidence Quality: B, Recommendation Strength: Moderate Recommendation).

Action Statement Profile KAS 10c

Aggregate evidence quality	B
Benefits	Reduced risk of hospitalization; reduced admission to ICU
Risk, harm, cost	Injection pain; increased risk of illness from increased visits to clinician office or clinic; cost; adverse effects of palivizumab
Benefit-harm assessment	Benefits outweigh harms
Value judgments	None
Intentional vagueness	None
Role of patient preferences	None
Exclusions	Fewer doses should be used if the bronchiolitis season ends before the completion of 5 doses; if the child is hospitalized with a breakthrough RSV, monthly prophylaxis should be discontinued
Strength	Moderate recommendation
Differences of opinion	None
Notes	This KAS is harmonized with the AAP policy statement on palivizumab[191,192]

Detailed evidence to support the policy statement on palivizumab and this palivizumab section can be found in the technical report on palivizumab.[192]

Palivizumab was licensed by the US Food and Drug Administration in June 1998 largely on the basis of results of 1 clinical trial.[193] The results of a second clinical trial among children with congenital heart disease were reported in December 2003.[194] No other prospective, randomized, placebo-controlled trials have been conducted in any subgroup. Since licensure of palivizumab, new peer-reviewed publications provide greater insight into the epidemiology of disease caused by RSV.[195–197] As a result of new data, the Bronchiolitis Guideline Committee and the Committee on Infectious Diseases have updated recommendations for use of prophylaxis.

PREMATURITY

Monthly palivizumab prophylaxis should be restricted to infants born before 29 weeks, 0 days' gestation, except for infants who qualify on the basis of congenital heart disease or chronic lung disease of prematurity. Data show that infants born at or after 29 weeks, 0 days' gestation have an RSV hospitalization rate similar to the rate of full-term infants.[11,198] Infants with a gestational age of 28 weeks, 6 days or less who will be younger than 12 months at the start of the RSV season should receive a maximum of 5 monthly doses of palivizumab or until the end of the RSV season, whichever comes first. Depending on the month of birth, fewer than 5 monthly doses will provide protection for most infants for the duration of the season.

CONGENITAL HEART DISEASE

Despite the large number of subjects enrolled, little benefit from palivizumab prophylaxis was found in the industry-sponsored cardiac study among infants in the cyanotic group (7.9% in control group versus 5.6% in palivizumab group, or 23 fewer hospitalizations per1000 children; P = .285).[197] In the acyanotic group (11.8% vs 5.0%), there were 68 fewer RSV hospitalizations per 1000 prophylaxis recipients (P = .003).[197,199,200]

CHRONIC LUNG DISEASE OF PREMATURITY

Palivizumab prophylaxis should be administered to infants and children younger than 12 months who develop chronic lung disease of prematurity, defined as a requirement for 28 days of more than 21% oxygen beginning at birth. If a child meets these criteria and is in the first 24 months of life and continues to require supplemental oxygen, diuretic therapy, or chronic corticosteroid therapy within 6 months of the start of the RSV season, monthly prophylaxis should be administered for the remainder of the season.

NUMBER OF DOSES

Community outbreaks of RSV disease usually begin in November or December, peak in January or February, and end by late March or, at times, in April.[4] Figure 1 shows the 2011–2012 bronchiolitis season, which is typical of most years. Because 5 monthly doses will provide more than 24 weeks of protective serum palivizumab concentration, administration of more than 5 monthly doses is not recommended within the continental United States. For infants who qualify for 5 monthly doses, initiation of prophylaxis in November and continua-

tion for a total of 5 doses will provide protection into April.[201] If prophylaxis is initiated in October, the fifth and final dose should be administered in February, and protection will last into March for most children.

SECOND YEAR OF LIFE

Because of the low risk of RSV hospitalization in the second year of life, palivizumab prophylaxis is not recommended for children in the second year of life with the following exception. Children who satisfy the definition of chronic lung disease of infancy and continue to require supplemental oxygen, chronic corticosteroid therapy, or diuretic therapy within 6 months of the onset of the second RSV season may be considered for a second season of prophylaxis.

OTHER CONDITIONS

Insufficient data are available to recommend routine use of prophylaxis in children with Down syndrome, cystic fibrosis, pulmonary abnormality, neuromuscular disease, or immune compromise.

Down Syndrome

Routine use of prophylaxis for children in the first year of life with Down syndrome is not recommended unless the child qualifies because of cardiac disease or prematurity.[202]

Cystic Fibrosis

Routine use of palivizumab prophylaxis in patients with cystic fibrosis is not recommended.[203,204] Available studies indicate the incidence of RSV hospitalization in children with cystic fibrosis is low and unlikely to be different from children without cystic fibrosis. No evidence suggests a benefit from palivizumab prophylaxis in patients with cystic fibrosis. A randomized clinical trial involving 186 children with cystic

fibrosis from 40 centers reported 1 subject in each group was hospitalized because of RSV infection. Although this study was not powered for efficacy, no clinically meaningful differences in outcome were reported.[205] A survey of cystic fibrosis center directors published in 2009 noted that palivizumab prophylaxis is not the standard of care for patients with cystic fibrosis.[206] If a neonate is diagnosed with cystic fibrosis by newborn screening, RSV prophylaxis should not be administered if no other indications are present. A patient with cystic fibrosis with clinical evidence of chronic lung disease in the first year of life may be considered for prophylaxis.

Neuromuscular Disease and Pulmonary Abnormality

The risk of RSV hospitalization is not well defined in children with pulmonary abnormalities or neuromuscular disease that impairs ability to clear secretions from the lower airway because of ineffective cough, recurrent gastroesophageal tract reflux, pulmonary malformations, tracheoesophageal fistula, upper airway conditions, or conditions requiring tracheostomy. No data on the relative risk of RSV hospitalization are available for this cohort. Selected infants with disease or congenital anomaly that impairs their ability to clear secretions from the lower airway because of ineffective cough may be considered for prophylaxis during the first year of life.

Immunocompromised Children

Population-based data are not available on the incidence or severity of RSV hospitalization in children who undergo solid organ or hematopoietic stem cell transplantation, receive chemotherapy, or are immunocompromised because of other conditions. Prophylaxis may be considered for hematopoietic stem cell transplant patients who undergo transplantation and are profoundly immunosuppressed during the RSV season.[207]

MISCELLANEOUS ISSUES

Prophylaxis is not recommended for prevention of nosocomial RSV disease in the NICU or hospital setting.[208,209]

No evidence suggests palivizumab is a cost-effective measure to prevent recurrent wheezing in children. Prophylaxis should not be administered to reduce recurrent wheezing in later years.[210,211]

Monthly prophylaxis in Alaska Native children who qualify should be determined by locally generated data regarding season onset and end.

Continuation of monthly prophylaxis for an infant or young child who experiences breakthrough RSV hospitalization is not recommended.

HAND HYGIENE

Key Action Statement 11a

All people should disinfect hands before and after direct contact with patients, after contact with inanimate objects in the direct vicinity of the patient, and after removing gloves (Evidence Quality: B; Recommendation Strength: Strong Recommendation).

Action Statement Profile KAS 11a

Aggregate evidence quality	B
Benefits	Decreased transmission of disease
Risk, harm, cost	Possible hand irritation
Benefit-harm assessment	Benefits outweigh harms
Value judgments	None
Intentional vagueness	None
Role of patient preferences	None
Exclusions	None
Strength	Strong recommendation
Differences of opinion	None

Key Action Statement 11b

All people should use alcohol-based rubs for hand decontamination when caring for children with bronchiolitis. When alcohol-based rubs are not available, individuals should wash their hands with soap and water (Evidence Quality: B; Recommendation Strength: Strong Recommendation).

Action Statement Profile KAS 11b

Aggregate evidence quality	B
Benefits	Less hand irritation
Risk, harm, cost	If there is visible dirt on the hands, hand washing is necessary; alcohol-based rubs are not effective for *Clostridium difficile*, present a fire hazard, and have a slight increased cost
Benefit-harm assessment	Benefits outweigh harms
Value judgments	None
Intentional vagueness	None
Role of patient preferences	None
Exclusions	None
Strength	Strong recommendation
Differences of opinion	None

Efforts should be made to decrease the spread of RSV and other causative agents of bronchiolitis in medical settings, especially in the hospital. Secretions from infected patients can be found on beds, crib railings, tabletops, and toys.[12] RSV, as well as many other viruses, can survive better on hard surfaces than on porous surfaces or hands. It can remain infectious on counter tops for $\geq$6 hours, on gowns or paper tissues for 20 to 30 minutes, and on skin for up to 20 minutes.[212]

It has been shown that RSV can be carried and spread to others on the hands of caregivers.[213] Studies have shown that health care workers have acquired infection by performing activities such as feeding, diaper change, and playing with the RSV-infected infant. Caregivers who had contact only with surfaces contaminated with the infants' secretions or touched inanimate objects in patients' rooms also acquired RSV. In these studies, health care workers contaminated their hands (or gloves) with RSV and inoculated their oral or conjunctival mucosa.[214] Frequent hand washing by health care workers has been shown to reduce the spread of RSV in the health care setting.[215]

The Centers for Disease Control and Prevention published an extensive review of the hand-hygiene literature and made recommendations as to indications for hand washing and hand antisepsis.[216] Among the recommendations are that hands should be disinfected before and after direct contact with every patient, after contact with inanimate objects in the direct vicinity of the patient, and before putting on and after removing gloves. If hands are not visibly soiled, an alcohol-based rub is preferred. In guidelines published in 2009, the World Health Organization also recommended alcohol-based hand-rubs as the standard for hand hygiene in health care.[217] Specifically, systematic reviews show them to remove organisms more effectively, require less time, and irritate skin less often than hand washing with soap or other antiseptic agents and water. The availability of bedside alcohol-based solutions increased compliance with hand hygiene among health care workers.[214]

When caring for hospitalized children with clinically diagnosed bronchiolitis, strict adherence to hand decontamination and use of personal protective equipment (ie, gloves and gowns) can reduce the risk of cross-infection in the health care setting.[215]

Other methods of infection control in viral bronchiolitis include education of personnel and family members, surveillance for the onset of RSV season, and wearing masks when anticipating exposure to aerosolized secretions while performing patient care activities. Programs that implement the aforementioned principles, in conjunction with effective hand decontamination and cohorting of patients, have been shown to reduce the spread of RSV in the health care setting by 39% to 50%.[218,219]

TOBACCO SMOKE

Key Action Statement 12a

Clinicians should inquire about the exposure of the infant or child to tobacco smoke when assessing infants and children for bronchiolitis (Evidence Quality: C; Recommendation Strength: Moderate Recommendation).

Action Statement Profile KAS 12a

Aggregate evidence quality	C
Benefits	Can identify infants and children at risk whose family may benefit from counseling, predicting risk of severe disease
Risk, harm, cost	Time to inquire
Benefit-harm assessment	Benefits outweigh harms
Value judgments	None
Intentional vagueness	None
Role of patient preferences	Parent may choose to deny tobacco use even though they are, in fact, users
Exclusions	None
Strength	Moderate recommendation
Differences of opinion	None

Key Action Statement 12b

Clinicians should counsel caregivers about exposing the infant or child to environmental tobacco smoke and smoking cessation when assessing a child for bronchiolitis (Evidence Quality: B; Recommendation Strength: Strong Recommendation).

Action Statement Profile KAS 12b

Aggregate evidence quality	B
Benefits	Reinforces the detrimental effects of smoking, potential to decrease smoking
Risk, harm, cost	Time to counsel
Benefit-harm assessment	Benefits outweigh harms
Value judgments	None
Intentional vagueness	None
Role of patient preferences	Parents may choose to ignore counseling
Exclusions	None
Strength	Moderate recommendation
Differences of opinion	None
Notes	Counseling for tobacco smoke prevention should begin in the prenatal period and continue in family-centered care and at all well-infant visits

Tobacco smoke exposure increases the risk and severity of bronchiolitis. Strachan and Cook[220] first delineated the effects of environmental tobacco smoke on rates of lower respiratory tract disease in infants in a meta-analysis including 40 studies. In a more recent systematic review, Jones et al[221] found a pooled odds ratio of 2.51 (95% CI 1.96 to 3.21) for tobacco smoke exposure and bronchiolitis hospitalization among the 7 studies specific to the condition. Other investigators have consistently reported tobacco smoke exposure increases both severity of illness and risk of hospitalization for bronchiolitis.[222–225] The AAP issued a technical report on the risks of secondhand smoke in 2009. The report makes recommendations regarding effective ways to eliminate or reduce secondhand smoke exposure, including education of parents.[226]

Despite our knowledge of this important risk factor, there is evidence to suggest health care providers identify fewer than half of children exposed to tobacco smoke in the outpatient, inpatient, or ED settings.[227–229] Furthermore, there is evidence that counseling parents in these settings is well received and has a measurable impact. Rosen et al[230] performed a meta-analysis of the effects of interventions in pediatric settings on parental cessation and found a pooled risk ratio of 1.3 for cessation among the 18 studies reviewed.

In contrast to many of the other recommendations, protecting children from tobacco exposure is a recommendation that is primarily implemented outside of the clinical setting. As such, it is critical that parents are fully educated about the importance of not allowing smoking in the home and that smoke lingers on clothes and in the environment for prolonged periods.[231] It should be provided in plain language and in a respectful, culturally effective manner that is family centered, engages parents as partners in their child's health, and factors in their literacy, health literacy, and primary language needs.

BREASTFEEDING

Key Action Statement 13

Clinicians should encourage exclusive breastfeeding for at least 6 months to decrease the morbidity of respiratory infections (Evidence Quality: Grade B; Recommendation Strength: Moderate Recommendation).

Action Statement Profile KAS 13

Aggregate evidence quality	B
Benefits	May reduce the risk of bronchiolitis and other illnesses; multiple benefits of breastfeeding unrelated to bronchiolitis
Risk, harm, cost	None
Benefit-harm assessment	Benefits outweigh risks
Value judgments	None
Intentional vagueness	None
Role of patient preferences	Parents may choose to feed formula rather than breastfeed
Exclusions	None
Strength	Moderate recommendation
Notes	Education on breastfeeding should begin in the prenatal period

In 2012, the AAP presented a general policy on breastfeeding.[232] The policy statement was based on the proven benefits of breastfeeding for at least 6 months. Respiratory infections were shown to be significantly less common in breastfed children. A primary resource was a meta-analysis from the Agency for Healthcare Research and Quality that showed an overall 72% reduction in the risk of hospitalization secondary to respiratory diseases in infants who were exclusively breastfed for 4 or more months compared with those who were formula fed.[233]

The clinical evidence also supports decreased incidence and severity of illness in breastfed infants with bronchiolitis. Dornelles et al[234] concluded that the duration of exclusive breastfeeding was inversely related to the length of oxygen use and the length of hospital stay in previously healthy infants with acute bronchiolitis. In a large prospective study in Australia, Oddy et al[235] showed that breastfeeding for less than 6 months was associated

with an increased risk for 2 or more medical visits and hospital admission for wheezing lower respiratory illness. In Japan, Nishimura et al[236] looked at 3 groups of RSV-positive infants defined as full, partial, or token breastfeeding. There were no significant differences in the hospitalization rate among the 3 groups; however, there were significant differences in the duration of hospitalization and the rate of requiring oxygen therapy, both favoring breastfeeding.

FAMILY EDUCATION

Key Action Statement 14

Clinicians and nurses should educate personnel and family members on evidence-based diagnosis, treatment, and prevention in bronchiolitis (Evidence Quality: C; observational studies; Recommendation Strength; Moderate Recommendation).

Action Statement Profile KAS 14

Aggregate evidence quality	C
Benefits	Decreased transmission of disease, benefits of breastfeeding, promotion of judicious use of antibiotics, risks of infant lung damage attributable to tobacco smoke
Risk, harm, cost	Time to educate properly
Benefit-harm assessment	Benefits outweigh harms
Value judgments	None
Intentional vagueness	Personnel is not specifically defined but should include all people who enter a patient's room
Role of patient preferences	None
Exclusions	None
Strength	Moderate recommendation
Differences of opinion	None

Shared decision-making with parents about diagnosis and treatment of bronchiolitis is a key tenet of patient-centered care. Despite the absence of effective therapies for viral bronchiolitis, caregiver education by clinicians may have a significant impact on care patterns in the disease. Children with bronchiolitis typically suffer from symptoms for 2 to 3 weeks, and parents often seek care in multiple settings during that time period.[237] Given that children with RSV generally shed virus for 1 to 2 weeks and from 30% to 70% of family members may become ill,[238,239] education about prevention of transmission of disease is key. Restriction of visitors to newborns during the respiratory virus season should be considered. Consistent evidence suggests that parental education is helpful in the promotion of judicious use of antibiotics and that clinicians may misinterpret parental expectations about therapy unless the subject is openly discussed.[240–242]

FUTURE RESEARCH NEEDS

- Better algorithms for predicting the course of illness

- Impact of clinical score on patient outcomes

- Evaluating different ethnic groups and varying response to treatments

- Does epinephrine alone reduce admission in outpatient settings?

- Additional studies on epinephrine in combination with dexamethasone or other corticosteroids

- Hypertonic saline studies in the outpatient setting and in in hospitals with shorter LOS

- More studies on nasogastric hydration

- More studies on tonicity of intravenous fluids

- Incidence of true AOM in bronchiolitis by using 2013 guideline definition
- More studies on deep suctioning and nasopharyngeal suctioning
- Strategies for monitoring oxygen saturation
- Use of home oxygen
- Appropriate cutoff for use of oxygen in high altitude
- Oxygen delivered by high-flow nasal cannula
- RSV vaccine and antiviral agents
- Use of palivizumab in special populations, such as cystic fibrosis, neuromuscular diseases, Down syndrome, immune deficiency
- Emphasis on parent satisfaction/patient-centered outcomes in all research (ie, not LOS as the only measure)

SUBCOMMITTEE ON BRONCHIOLITIS (OVERSIGHT BY THE COUNCIL ON QUALITY IMPROVEMENT AND PATIENT SAFETY, 2013–2014)

Shawn L. Ralston, MD, FAAP: Chair, Pediatric Hospitalist (no financial conflicts; published research related to bronchiolitis)

Allan S. Lieberthal, MD, FAAP: Chair, General Pediatrician with Expertise in Pulmonology (no conflicts)

Brian K. Alverson, MD, FAAP: Pediatric Hospitalist, AAP Section on Hospital Medicine Representative (no conflicts)

Jill E. Baley, MD, FAAP: Neonatal-Perinatal Medicine, AAP Committee on Fetus and Newborn Representative (no conflicts)

Anne M. Gadomski, MD, MPH, FAAP: General Pediatrician and Research Scientist (no financial conflicts; published research related to bronchiolitis including Cochrane review of bronchodilators)

David W. Johnson, MD, FAAP: Pediatric Emergency Medicine Physician (no financial conflicts; published research related to bronchiolitis)

Michael J. Light, MD, FAAP: Pediatric Pulmonologist, AAP Section on Pediatric Pulmonology Representative (no conflicts)

Nizar F. Maraqa, MD, FAAP: Pediatric Infectious Disease Physician, AAP Section on Infectious Diseases Representative (no conflicts)

H. Cody Meissner, MD, FAAP: Pediatric Infectious Disease Physician, AAP Committee on Infectious Diseases Representative (no conflicts)

Eneida A. Mendonca, MD, PhD, FAAP, FACMI: Informatician/Academic Pediatric Intensive Care Physician, Partnership for Policy Implementation Representative (no conflicts)

Kieran J. Phelan, MD, MSc: General Pediatrician (no conflicts)

Joseph J. Zorc, MD, MSCE, FAAP: Pediatric Emergency Physician, AAP Section on Emergency Medicine Representative (no financial conflicts; published research related to bronchiolitis)

Danette Stanko-Lopp, MA, MPH: Methodologist, Epidemiologist (no conflicts)

Mark A. Brown, MD: Pediatric Pulmonologist, American Thoracic Society Liaison (no conflicts)

Ian Nathanson, MD, FAAP: Pediatric Pulmonologist, American College of Chest Physicians Liaison (no conflicts)

Elizabeth Rosenblum, MD: Academic Family Physician, American Academy of Family Physicians liaison (no conflicts).

Stephen Sayles, III, MD, FACEP: Emergency Medicine Physician, American College of Emergency Physicians Liaison (no conflicts)

Sinsi Hernández-Cancio, JD: Parent/Consumer Representative (no conflicts)

STAFF

Caryn Davidson, MA
Linda Walsh, MAB

REFERENCES

1. American Academy of Pediatrics Subcommittee on Diagnosis and Management of Bronchiolitis. Diagnosis and management of bronchiolitis. *Pediatrics.* 2006;118 (4):1774–1793

2. Agency for Healthcare Research and Quality. Management of Bronchiolitis in Infants and Children. Evidence Report/Technology Assessment No. 69. Rockville, MD: Agency for Healthcare Research and Quality; 2003. AHRQ Publication No. 03-E014

3. Mullins JA, Lamonte AC, Bresee JS, Anderson LJ. Substantial variability in community respiratory syncytial virus season timing. *Pediatr Infect Dis J.* 2003; 22(10):857–862

4. Centers for Disease Control and Prevention. Respiratory syncytial virus activity—United States, July 2011-January 2013. *MMWR Morb Mortal Wkly Rep.* 2013; 62(8):141–144

5. Greenough A, Cox S, Alexander J, et al. Health care utilisation of infants with chronic lung disease, related to hospitalisation for RSV infection. *Arch Dis Child.* 2001;85(6):463–468

6. Parrott RH, Kim HW, Arrobio JO, et al. Epidemiology of respiratory syncytial virus infection in Washington, D.C. II. Infection and disease with respect to age, immunologic status, race and sex. *Am J Epidemiol.* 1973;98(4):289–300

7. Meissner HC. Selected populations at increased risk from respiratory syncytial virus infection. *Pediatr Infect Dis J.* 2003; 22(suppl 2):S40–S44, discussion S44–S45

8. Shay DK, Holman RC, Roosevelt GE, Clarke MJ, Anderson LJ. Bronchiolitis-associated mortality and estimates of respiratory syncytial virus-associated deaths among US children, 1979-1997. *J Infect Dis.* 2001; 183(1):16–22

9. Miller EK, Gebretsadik T, Carroll KN, et al. Viral etiologies of infant bronchiolitis, croup and upper respiratory illness during 4 consecutive years. *Pediatr Infect Dis J.* 2013;32(9):950–955

10. Hasegawa K, Tsugawa Y, Brown DF, Mansbach JM, Camargo CA Jr. Trends in bronchiolitis hospitalizations in the United States, 2000-2009. *Pediatrics.* 2013;132(1): 28–36

11. Hall CB, Weinberg GA, Blumkin AK, et al. Respiratory syncytial virus-associated hospitalizations among children less than 24 months of age. *Pediatrics.* 2013; 132(2). Available at: www.pediatrics.org/cgi/content/full/132/2/e341

12. Hall CB. Nosocomial respiratory syncytial virus infections: the "Cold War" has not ended. *Clin Infect Dis.* 2000;31(2): 590–596

13. Stevens TP, Sinkin RA, Hall CB, Maniscalco WM, McConnochie KM. Respiratory syncytial virus and premature infants born at 32 weeks' gestation or earlier: hospitalization and economic implications of prophylaxis. *Arch Pediatr Adolesc Med.* 2000; 154(1):55–61

14. American Academy of Pediatrics Steering Committee on Quality Improvement and Management. Classifying recommendations for clinical practice guidelines. *Pediatrics.* 2004;114(3):874–877

15. Ricart S, Marcos MA, Sarda M, et al. Clinical risk factors are more relevant than respiratory viruses in predicting bronchiolitis severity. *Pediatr Pulmonol.* 2013;48(5):456–463

16. Shaw KN, Bell LM, Sherman NH. Outpatient assessment of infants with bronchiolitis. *Am J Dis Child.* 1991;145(2):151–155

17. Hall CB, Powell KR, MacDonald NE, et al. Respiratory syncytial viral infection in children with compromised immune function. *N Engl J Med.* 1986;315(2):77–81

18. Mansbach JM, Piedra PA, Stevenson MD, et al; MARC-30 Investigators. Prospective multicenter study of children with bronchiolitis requiring mechanical ventilation. *Pediatrics.* 2012;130(3). Available at: www.pediatrics.org/cgi/content/full/130/3/e492

19. Prescott WA Jr, Hutchinson DJ. Respiratory syncytial virus prophylaxis in special populations: is it something worth considering in cystic fibrosis and immunosuppression? *J Pediatr Pharmacol Ther.* 2011;16(2):77–86

20. Armstrong D, Grimwood K, Carlin JB, et al. Severe viral respiratory infections in infants with cystic fibrosis. *Pediatr Pulmonol.* 1998;26(6):371–379

21. Alvarez AE, Marson FA, Bertuzzo CS, Arns CW, Ribeiro JD. Epidemiological and genetic characteristics associated with the severity of acute viral bronchiolitis by respiratory syncytial virus. *J Pediatr (Rio J).* 2013;89(6):531–543

22. Iliff A, Lee VA. Pulse rate, respiratory rate, and body temperature of children between two months and eighteen years of age. *Child Dev.* 1952;23(4):237–245

23. Rogers MC. Respiratory monitoring. In: Rogers MC, Nichols DG, eds. *Textbook of Pediatric Intensive Care.* Baltimore, MD: Williams & Wilkins; 1996:332–333

24. Berman S, Simoes EA, Lanata C. Respiratory rate and pneumonia in infancy. *Arch Dis Child.* 1991;66(1):81–84

25. Fleming S, Thompson M, Stevens R, et al. Normal ranges of heart rate and respiratory rate in children from birth to 18 years of age: a systematic review of observational studies. *Lancet.* 2011;377(9770):1011–1018

26. Bonafide CP, Brady PW, Keren R, Conway PH, Marsolo K, Daymont C. Development of heart and respiratory rate percentile curves for hospitalized children. *Pediatrics.* 2013;131(4). Available at: www.pediatrics.org/cgi/content/full/131/4/e1150

27. Margolis P, Gadomski A. The rational clinical examination. Does this infant have pneumonia? *JAMA.* 1998;279(4):308–313

28. Mahabee-Gittens EM, Grupp-Phelan J, Brody AS, et al. Identifying children with pneumonia in the emergency department. *Clin Pediatr (Phila).* 2005;44(5):427–435

29. Brooks AM, McBride JT, McConnochie KM, Aviram M, Long C, Hall CB. Predicting deterioration in previously healthy infants hospitalized with respiratory syncytial virus infection. *Pediatrics.* 1999;104(3 pt 1):463–467

30. Neuman MI, Monuteaux MC, Scully KJ, Bachur RG. Prediction of pneumonia in a pediatric emergency department. *Pediatrics.* 2011;128(2):246–253

31. Shah S, Bachur R, Kim D, Neuman MI. Lack of predictive value of tachypnea in the diagnosis of pneumonia in children. *Pediatr Infect Dis J.* 2010;29(5):406–409

32. Mansbach JM, McAdam AJ, Clark S, et al. Prospective multicenter study of the viral etiology of bronchiolitis in the emergency department. *Acad Emerg Med.* 2008;15(2):111–118

33. Mansbach JM, Piedra PA, Teach SJ, et al; MARC-30 Investigators. Prospective multicenter study of viral etiology and hospital length of stay in children with severe bronchiolitis. *Arch Pediatr Adolesc Med.* 2012;166(8):700–706

34. Navas L, Wang E, de Carvalho V, Robinson J; Pediatric Investigators Collaborative Network on Infections in Canada. Improved outcome of respiratory syncytial virus infection in a high-risk hospitalized population of Canadian children. *J Pediatr.* 1992;121(3):348–354

35. Wang EE, Law BJ, Stephens D. Pediatric Investigators Collaborative Network on Infections in Canada (PICNIC) prospective study of risk factors and outcomes in patients hospitalized with respiratory syncytial viral lower respiratory tract infection. *J Pediatr.* 1995;126(2):212–219

36. Chan PW, Lok FY, Khatijah SB. Risk factors for hypoxemia and respiratory failure in respiratory syncytial virus bronchiolitis. *Southeast Asian J Trop Med Public Health.* 2002;33(4):806–810

37. Roback MG, Baskin MN. Failure of oxygen saturation and clinical assessment to predict which patients with bronchiolitis discharged from the emergency department will return requiring admission. *Pediatr Emerg Care.* 1997;13(1):9–11

38. Lowell DI, Lister G, Von Koss H, McCarthy P. Wheezing in infants: the response to epinephrine. *Pediatrics.* 1987;79(6):939–945

39. Destino L, Weisgerber MC, Soung P, et al. Validity of respiratory scores in bronchiolitis. *Hosp Pediatr.* 2012;2(4):202–209

40. Schroeder AR, Marmor AK, Pantell RH, Newman TB. Impact of pulse oximetry and oxygen therapy on length of stay in bronchiolitis hospitalizations. *Arch Pediatr Adolesc Med.* 2004;158(6):527–530

41. Dawson KP, Long A, Kennedy J, Mogridge N. The chest radiograph in acute bronchiolitis. *J Paediatr Child Health.* 1990;26(4):209–211

42. Schroeder AR, Mansbach JM, Stevenson M, et al. Apnea in children hospitalized with bronchiolitis. *Pediatrics.* 2013;132(5). Available at: www.pediatrics.org/cgi/content/full/132/5/e1194

43. Ralston S, Hill V. Incidence of apnea in infants hospitalized with respiratory syncytial virus bronchiolitis: a systematic review. *J Pediatr.* 2009;155(5):728–733

44. Willwerth BM, Harper MB, Greenes DS. Identifying hospitalized infants who have bronchiolitis and are at high risk for apnea. *Ann Emerg Med.* 2006;48(4):441–447

45. García CG, Bhore R, Soriano-Fallas A, et al. Risk factors in children hospitalized with RSV bronchiolitis versus non-RSV bronchiolitis. *Pediatrics.* 2010;126(6). Available at: www.pediatrics.org/cgi/content/full/126/6/e1453

46. Swingler GH, Hussey GD, Zwarenstein M. Randomised controlled trial of clinical outcome after chest radiograph in ambulatory acute lower-respiratory infection in children. *Lancet.* 1998;351(9100):404–408

47. Schuh S, Lalani A, Allen U, et al. Evaluation of the utility of radiography in acute bronchiolitis. *J Pediatr.* 2007;150(4):429–433

48. Kellner JD, Ohlsson A, Gadomski AM, Wang EE. Efficacy of bronchodilator therapy in bronchiolitis. A meta-analysis. *Arch Pediatr Adolesc Med.* 1996;150(11):1166–1172

49. Flores G, Horwitz RI. Efficacy of beta2-agonists in bronchiolitis: a reappraisal and meta-analysis. *Pediatrics.* 1997;100(2 pt 1):233–239

50. Hartling L, Wiebe N, Russell K, Patel H, Klassen TP. A meta-analysis of randomized controlled trials evaluating the efficacy of epinephrine for the treatment of acute viral bronchiolitis. *Arch Pediatr Adolesc Med.* 2003;157(10):957–964

51. King VJ, Viswanathan M, Bordley WC, et al. Pharmacologic treatment of bronchiolitis in infants and children: a systematic review. *Arch Pediatr Adolesc Med.* 2004;158(2):127–137

52. Zorc JJ, Hall CB. Bronchiolitis: recent evidence on diagnosis and management. *Pediatrics.* 2010;125(2):342–349

53. Wainwright C. Acute viral bronchiolitis in children—a very common condition with few therapeutic options. *Paediatr Respir Rev.* 2010;11(1):39–45, quiz 45

54. Walsh P, Caldwell J, McQuillan KK, Friese S, Robbins D, Rothenberg SJ. Comparison of nebulized epinephrine to albuterol in bronchiolitis. *Acad Emerg Med.* 2008;15 (4):305–313

55. Scarlett EE, Walker S, Rovitelli A, Ren CL. Tidal breathing responses to albuterol and normal saline in infants with viral bronchiolitis. *Pediatr Allergy Immunol Pulmonol.* 2012;25(4):220–225

56. Gadomski AM, Scribani MB. Bronchodilators for bronchiolitis. *Cochrane Database Syst Rev.* 2014;(6):CD001266

57. Mallol J, Barrueto L, Girardi G, et al. Use of nebulized bronchodilators in infants under 1 year of age: analysis of four forms of therapy. *Pediatr Pulmonol.* 1987;3(5):298–303

58. Lines DR, Kattampallil JS, Liston P. Efficacy of nebulized salbutamol in bronchiolitis. *Pediatr Rev Commun.* 1990;5(2):121–129

59. Alario AJ, Lewander WJ, Dennehy P, Seifer R, Mansell AL. The efficacy of nebulized metaproterenol in wheezing infants and young children. *Am J Dis Child.* 1992;146 (4):412–418

60. Chavasse RJPG, Seddon P, Bara A, McKean MC. Short acting beta2-agonists for recurrent wheeze in children under two years of age. *Cochrane Database Syst Rev.* 2009;(2):CD002873

61. Totapally BR, Demerci C, Zureikat G, Nolan B. Tidal breathing flow-volume loops in bronchiolitis in infancy: the effect of albuterol [ISRCTN47364493]. *Crit Care.* 2002;6(2):160–165

62. Levin DL, Garg A, Hall LJ, Slogic S, Jarvis JD, Leiter JC. A prospective randomized controlled blinded study of three bronchodilators in infants with respiratory syncytial virus bronchiolitis on mechanical ventilation. *Pediatr Crit Care Med.* 2008;9(6):598–604

63. Bjornson C, Russell K, Vandermeer B, Klassen TP, Johnson DW. Nebulized epinephrine for croup in children. *Cochrane Database Syst Rev.* 2013;(10):CD006619

64. Hartling L, Fernandes RM, Bialy L, et al. Steroids and bronchodilators for acute bronchiolitis in the first two years of life: systematic review and meta-analysis. *BMJ.* 2011;342:d1714

65. Wainwright C, Altamirano L, Cheney M, et al. A multicenter, randomized, double-blind, controlled trial of nebulized epinephrine in infants with acute bronchiolitis. *N Engl J Med.* 2003;349(1):27–35

66. Patel H, Gouin S, Platt RW. Randomized, double-blind, placebo-controlled trial of oral albuterol in infants with mild-to-moderate acute viral bronchiolitis. *J Pediatr.* 2003;142(5):509–514

67. Skjerven HO, Hunderi JO, Brügmann-Pieper SK, et al. Racemic adrenaline and inhalation strategies in acute bronchiolitis. *N Engl J Med.* 2013;368(24):2286–2293

68. Plint AC, Johnson DW, Patel H, et al; Pediatric Emergency Research Canada (PERC). Epinephrine and dexamethasone in children with bronchiolitis. *N Engl J Med.* 2009;360(20):2079–2089

69. Wark PA, McDonald V, Jones AP. Nebulised hypertonic saline for cystic fibrosis. *Cochrane Database Syst Rev.* 2005;(3):CD001506

70. Daviskas E, Anderson SD, Gonda I, et al. Inhalation of hypertonic saline aerosol enhances mucociliary clearance in asthmatic and healthy subjects. *Eur Respir J.* 1996;9(4):725–732

71. Sood N, Bennett WD, Zeman K, et al. Increasing concentration of inhaled saline with or without amiloride: effect on mucociliary clearance in normal subjects. *Am J Respir Crit Care Med.* 2003;167(2):158–163

72. Mandelberg A, Amirav I. Hypertonic saline or high volume normal saline for viral bronchiolitis: mechanisms and rationale. *Pediatr Pulmonol.* 2010;45(1):36–40

73. Zhang L, Mendoza-Sassi RA, Wainwright C, Klassen TP. Nebulized hypertonic saline solution for acute bronchiolitis in infants. *Cochrane Database Syst Rev.* 2008;(4):CD006458

74. Jacobs JD, Foster M, Wan J, Pershad J. 7% Hypertonic saline in acute bronchiolitis: a randomized controlled trial. *Pediatrics.* 2014;133(1). Available at: www.pediatrics.org/cgi/content/full/133/1/e8

75. Wu S, Baker C, Lang ME, et al. Nebulized hypertonic saline for bronchiolitis: a randomized clinical trial. *JAMA Pediatr.* 2014;168(7):657–663

76. Florin TA, Shaw KN, Kittick M, Yakscoe S, Zorc JJ. Nebulized hypertonic saline for bronchiolitis in the emergency department: a randomized clinical trial. *JAMA Pediatr.* 2014;168(7):664–670

77. Sharma BS, Gupta MK, Rafik SP. Hypertonic (3%) saline vs 0.93% saline nebulization for acute viral bronchiolitis: a randomized controlled trial. *Indian Pediatr.* 2013;50(8):743–747

78. Silver AH. Randomized controlled trial of the efficacy of nebulized 3% saline without bronchodilators for infants admitted with bronchiolitis: preliminary data [abstr E-PAS2014:2952.685]. Paper presented at: Pediatric Academic Societies Annual Meeting; May 3–6, 2014; Vancouver, British Columbia, Canada

79. Ralston S, Hill V, Martinez M. Nebulized hypertonic saline without adjunctive bronchodilators for children with bronchiolitis. *Pediatrics.* 2010;126(3). Available at: www.pediatrics.org/cgi/content/full/126/3/e520

80. Luo Z, Liu E, Luo J, et al. Nebulized hypertonic saline/salbutamol solution treatment in hospitalized children with mild to moderate bronchiolitis. *Pediatr Int.* 2010;52(2):199–202

81. Sarrell EM, Tal G, Witzling M, et al. Nebulized 3% hypertonic saline solution treatment in ambulatory children with viral bronchiolitis decreases symptoms. *Chest.* 2002;122(6):2015–2020

82. Rowe BH, Spooner C, Ducharme FM, Bretzlaff JA, Bota GW. Early emergency department treatment of acute asthma with systemic corticosteroids. *Cochrane Database Syst Rev.* 2001;(1):CD002178

83. Smith M, Iqbal S, Elliott TM, Everard M, Rowe BH. Corticosteroids for hospitalised children with acute asthma. *Cochrane Database Syst Rev.* 2003;(2):CD002886

84. Russell KF, Liang Y, O'Gorman K, Johnson DW, Klassen TP. Glucocorticoids for croup. *Cochrane Database Syst Rev.* 2011;(1):CD001955

85. Fernandes RM, Bialy LM, Vandermeer B, et al. Glucocorticoids for acute viral bronchiolitis in infants and young children. *Cochrane Database Syst Rev.* 2013;(6):CD004878

86. Corneli HM, Zorc JJ, Mahajan P, et al; Bronchiolitis Study Group of the Pediatric Emergency Care Applied Research Network (PECARN). A multicenter, randomized, controlled trial of dexamethasone for bronchiolitis [published correction appears in *N Engl J Med* 2008;359(18):1972]. *N Engl J Med.* 2007;357(4):331–339

87. Frey U, von Mutius E. The challenge of managing wheezing in infants. *N Engl J Med.* 2009;360(20):2130–2133

88. Gibson PG, Powell H, Ducharme F. Long-acting beta2-agonists as an inhaled corticosteroid-sparing agent for chronic asthma in adults and children. *Cochrane Database Syst Rev.* 2005;(4):CD005076

89. Barnes PJ. Scientific rationale for using a single inhaler for asthma control. *Eur Respir J.* 2007;29(3):587–595

90. Giembycz MA, Kaur M, Leigh R, Newton R. A Holy Grail of asthma management: toward understanding how long-acting beta(2)-adrenoceptor agonists enhance the clinical efficacy of inhaled corticosteroids. *Br J Pharmacol.* 2008;153(6):1090–1104

91. Kaur M, Chivers JE, Giembycz MA, Newton R. Long-acting beta2-adrenoceptor agonists synergistically enhance glucocorticoid-dependent transcription in human airway

epithelial and smooth muscle cells. *Mol Pharmacol.* 2008;73(1):203–214

92. Holden NS, Bell MJ, Rider CF, et al. β2-Adrenoceptor agonist-induced RGS2 expression is a genomic mechanism of bronchoprotection that is enhanced by glucocorticoids. *Proc Natl Acad Sci U S A.* 2011;108(49):19713–19718

93. Schuh S, Coates AL, Binnie R, et al. Efficacy of oral dexamethasone in outpatients with acute bronchiolitis. *J Pediatr.* 2002;140(1):27–32

94. Bentur L, Shoseyov D, Feigenbaum D, Gorichovsky Y, Bibi H. Dexamethasone inhalations in RSV bronchiolitis: a double-blind, placebo-controlled study. *Acta Paediatr.* 2005;94(7):866–871

95. Kuyucu S, Unal S, Kuyucu N, Yilgor E. Additive effects of dexamethasone in nebulized salbutamol or L-epinephrine treated infants with acute bronchiolitis. *Pediatr Int.* 2004;46(5):539–544

96. Mesquita M, Castro-Rodríguez JA, Heinichen L, Fariña E, Iramain R. Single oral dose of dexamethasone in outpatients with bronchiolitis: a placebo controlled trial. *Allergol Immunopathol (Madr).* 2009;37(2):63–67

97. Alansari K, Sakran M, Davidson BL, Ibrahim K, Alrefai M, Zakaria I. Oral dexamethasone for bronchiolitis: a randomized trial. *Pediatrics.* 2013;132(4). Available at: www.pediatrics.org/cgi/content/full/132/4/e810

98. Mallory MD, Shay DK, Garrett J, Bordley WC. Bronchiolitis management preferences and the influence of pulse oximetry and respiratory rate on the decision to admit. *Pediatrics.* 2003;111(1). Available at: www.pediatrics.org/cgi/content/full/111/1/e45

99. Corneli HM, Zorc JJ, Holubkov R, et al; Bronchiolitis Study Group for the Pediatric Emergency Care Applied Research Network. Bronchiolitis: clinical characteristics associated with hospitalization and length of stay. *Pediatr Emerg Care.* 2012;28(2):99–103

100. Unger S, Cunningham S. Effect of oxygen supplementation on length of stay for infants hospitalized with acute viral bronchiolitis. *Pediatrics.* 2008;121(3):470–475

101. Cunningham S, McMurray A. Observational study of two oxygen saturation targets for discharge in bronchiolitis. *Arch Dis Child.* 2012;97(4):361–363

102. Anaesthesia UK. Oxygen dissociation curve. Available at: http://www.anaesthesiauk.com/SearchRender.aspx?DocId=1419&Index=D%3a\dtSearch\UserData\AUK&HitCount=19&hits=4+5+d+e+23+24+37+58+59+a7+a8+14a+14b+17e+180+181+1a9+1aa+1d4 Accessed July 15, 2014

103. McBride SC, Chiang VW, Goldmann DA, Landrigan CP. Preventable adverse events in infants hospitalized with bronchiolitis. *Pediatrics.* 2005;116(3):603–608

104. Hunt CE, Corwin MJ, Lister G, et al; Collaborative Home Infant Monitoring Evaluation (CHIME) Study Group. Longitudinal assessment of hemoglobin oxygen saturation in healthy infants during the first 6 months of age. *J Pediatr.* 1999;135(5):580–586

105. Gavlak JC, Stocks J, Laverty A, et al. The Young Everest Study: preliminary report of changes in sleep and cerebral blood flow velocity during slow ascent to altitude in unacclimatised children. *Arch Dis Child.* 2013;98(5):356–362

106. O'Neil SL, Barysh N, Setear SJ. Determining school programming needs of special population groups: a study of asthmatic children. *J Sch Health.* 1985;55(6):237–239

107. Bender BG, Belleau L, Fukuhara JT, Mrazek DA, Strunk RC. Psychomotor adaptation in children with severe chronic asthma. *Pediatrics.* 1987;79(5):723–727

108. Rietveld S, Colland VT. The impact of severe asthma on schoolchildren. *J Asthma.* 1999;36(5):409–417

109. Sung V, Massie J, Hochmann MA, Carlin JB, Jamsen K, Robertson CF. Estimating inspired oxygen concentration delivered by nasal prongs in children with bronchiolitis. *J Paediatr Child Health.* 2008;44(1-2):14–18

110. Ross PA, Newth CJL, Khemani RG. Accuracy of pulse oximetry in children. *Pediatrics.* 2014;133(1):22–29

111. Hasselbalch KA. Neutralitatsregulation und reizbarkeit des atemzentrums in ihren Wirkungen auf die koklensaurespannung des Blutes. *Biochem Ztschr.* 1912;46:403–439

112. Wang EE, Milner RA, Navas L, Maj H. Observer agreement for respiratory signs and oximetry in infants hospitalized with lower respiratory infections. *Am Rev Respir Dis.* 1992;145(1):106–109

113. Rojas MX, Granados Rugeles C, Charry-Anzola LP. Oxygen therapy for lower respiratory tract infections in children between 3 months and 15 years of age. *Cochrane Database Syst Rev.* 2009;(1):CD005975

114. Mitka M. Joint commission warns of alarm fatigue: multitude of alarms from monitoring devices problematic. *JAMA.* 2013;309(22):2315–2316

115. Bowton DL, Scuderi PE, Harris L, Haponik EF. Pulse oximetry monitoring outside the intensive care unit: progress or problem? *Ann Intern Med.* 1991;115(6):450–454

116. Groothuis JR, Gutierrez KM, Lauer BA. Respiratory syncytial virus infection in children with bronchopulmonary dysplasia. *Pediatrics.* 1988;82(2):199–203

117. Voepel-Lewis T, Pechlavanidis E, Burke C, Talsma AN. Nursing surveillance moderates the relationship between staffing levels and pediatric postoperative serious adverse events: a nested case-control study. *Int J Nurs Stud.* 2013;50(7):905–913

118. Bajaj L, Turner CG, Bothner J. A randomized trial of home oxygen therapy from the emergency department for acute bronchiolitis. *Pediatrics.* 2006;117(3):633–640

119. Tie SW, Hall GL, Peter S, et al. Home oxygen for children with acute bronchiolitis. *Arch Dis Child.* 2009;94(8):641–643

120. Halstead S, Roosevelt G, Deakyne S, Bajaj L. Discharged on supplemental oxygen from an emergency department in patients with bronchiolitis. *Pediatrics.* 2012;129(3). Available at: www.pediatrics.org/cgi/content/full/129/3/e605

121. Sandweiss DR, Mundorff MB, Hill T, et al. Decreasing hospital length of stay for bronchiolitis by using an observation unit and home oxygen therapy. *JAMA Pediatr.* 2013;167(5):422–428

122. Flett KB, Breslin K, Braun PA, Hambidge SJ. Outpatient course and complications associated with home oxygen therapy for mild bronchiolitis. *Pediatrics.* 2014;133(5):769–775

123. Gauthier M, Vincent M, Morneau S, Chevalier I. Impact of home oxygen therapy on hospital stay for infants with acute bronchiolitis. *Eur J Pediatr.* 2012;171(12):1839–1844

124. Bergman AB. Pulse oximetry: good technology misapplied. *Arch Pediatr Adolesc Med.* 2004;158(6):594–595

125. Sandweiss DR, Kadish HA, Campbell KA. Outpatient management of patients with bronchiolitis discharged home on oxygen: a survey of general pediatricians. *Clin Pediatr (Phila).* 2012;51(5):442–446

126. Dysart K, Miller TL, Wolfson MR, Shaffer TH. Research in high flow therapy: mechanisms of action. *Respir Med.* 2009;103(10):1400–1405

127. Milési C, Baleine J, Matecki S, et al. Is treatment with a high flow nasal cannula effective in acute viral bronchiolitis? A physiologic study [published correction appears in *Intensive Care Med.* 2013;39(6):1170]. *Intensive Care Med.* 2013;39(6):1088–1094

128. Arora B, Mahajan P, Zidan MA, Sethuraman U. Nasopharyngeal airway pressures in bronchiolitis patients treated with high-flow nasal cannula oxygen therapy. *Pediatr Emerg Care.* 2012;28(11):1179–1184

129. Spentzas T, Minarik M, Patters AB, Vinson B, Stidham G. Children with respiratory distress treated with high-flow nasal cannula. *J Intensive Care Med.* 2009;24(5):323–328

130. Hegde S, Prodhan P. Serious air leak syndrome complicating high-flow nasal cannula therapy: a report of 3 cases. *Pediatrics.* 2013;131(3). Available at: www.pediatrics.org/cgi/content/full/131/3/e939

131. Pham TM, O'Malley L, Mayfield S, Martin S, Schibler A. The effect of high flow nasal cannula therapy on the work of breathing in infants with bronchiolitis [published online ahead of print May 21, 2014]. *Pediatr Pulmonol.* doi:doi:10.1002/ppul.23060

132. Bressan S, Balzani M, Krauss B, Pettenazzo A, Zanconato S, Baraldi E. High-flow nasal cannula oxygen for bronchiolitis in a pediatric ward: a pilot study. *Eur J Pediatr.* 2013;172(12):1649–1656

133. Ganu SS, Gautam A, Wilkins B, Egan J. Increase in use of non-invasive ventilation for infants with severe bronchiolitis is associated with decline in intubation rates over a decade. *Intensive Care Med.* 2012;38(7):1177–1183

134. Wing R, James C, Maranda LS, Armsby CC. Use of high-flow nasal cannula support in the emergency department reduces the need for intubation in pediatric acute respiratory insufficiency. *Pediatr Emerg Care.* 2012;28(11):1117–1123

135. McKiernan C, Chua LC, Visintainer PF, Allen H. High flow nasal cannulae therapy in infants with bronchiolitis. *J Pediatr.* 2010;156(4):634–638

136. Schibler A, Pham TM, Dunster KR, et al. Reduced intubation rates for infants after introduction of high-flow nasal prong oxygen delivery. *Intensive Care Med.* 2011;37(5):847–852

137. Kelly GS, Simon HK, Sturm JJ. High-flow nasal cannula use in children with respiratory distress in the emergency department: predicting the need for subsequent intubation. *Pediatr Emerg Care.* 2013;29(8):888–892

138. Kallappa C, Hufton M, Millen G, Ninan TK. Use of high flow nasal cannula oxygen (HFNCO) in infants with bronchiolitis on a paediatric ward: a 3-year experience. *Arch Dis Child.* 2014;99(8):790–791

139. Hilliard TN, Archer N, Laura H, et al. Pilot study of vapotherm oxygen delivery in moderately severe bronchiolitis. *Arch Dis Child.* 2012;97(2):182–183

140. Roqué i Figuls M, Giné-Garriga M, Granados Rugeles C, Perrotta C. Chest physiotherapy for acute bronchiolitis in paediatric patients between 0 and 24 months old. *Cochrane Database Syst Rev.* 2012;(2):CD004873

141. Aviram M, Damri A, Yekutielli C, Bearman J, Tal A. Chest physiotherapy in acute bronchiolitis [abstract]. *Eur Respir J.* 1992;5(suppl 15):229–230

142. Webb MS, Martin JA, Cartlidge PH, Ng YK, Wright NA. Chest physiotherapy in acute bronchiolitis. *Arch Dis Child.* 1985;60(11):1078–1079

143. Nicholas KJ, Dhouieb MO, Marshal TG, Edmunds AT, Grant MB. An evaluation of chest physiotherapy in the management of acute bronchiolitis: changing clinical practice. *Physiotherapy.* 1999;85(12):669–674

144. Bohé L, Ferrero ME, Cuestas E, Polliotto L, Genoff M. Indications of conventional chest physiotherapy in acute bronchiolitis [in Spanish]. *Medicina (B Aires).* 2004;64(3):198–200

145. De Córdoba F, Rodrigues M, Luque A, Cadrobbi C, Faria R, Solé D. Fisioterapia respiratória em lactentes com bronquiolite: realizar ou não? *Mundo Saúde.* 2008;32(2):183–188

146. Gajdos V, Katsahian S, Beydon N, et al. Effectiveness of chest physiotherapy in infants hospitalized with acute bronchiolitis: a multicenter, randomized, controlled trial. *PLoS Med.* 2010;7(9):e1000345

147. Rochat I, Leis P, Bouchardy M, et al. Chest physiotherapy using passive expiratory techniques does not reduce bronchiolitis severity: a randomised controlled trial. *Eur J Pediatr.* 2012;171(3):457–462

148. Postiaux G, Louis J, Labasse HC, et al. Evaluation of an alternative chest physiotherapy method in infants with respiratory syncytial virus bronchiolitis. *Respir Care.* 2011;56(7):989–994

149. Sánchez Bayle M, Martín Martín R, Cano Fernández J, et al. Chest physiotherapy and bronchiolitis in the hospitalised infant. Double-blind clinical trial [in Spanish]. *An Pediatr (Barc).* 2012;77(1):5–11

150. Mussman GM, Parker MW, Statile A, Sucharew H, Brady PW. Suctioning and length of stay in infants hospitalized with bronchiolitis. *JAMA Pediatr.* 2013;167(5):414–421

151. Weisgerber MC, Lye PS, Li SH, et al. Factors predicting prolonged hospital stay for infants with bronchiolitis. *J Hosp Med.* 2011;6(5):264–270

152. Nichol KP, Cherry JD. Bacterial-viral interrelations in respiratory infections of children. *N Engl J Med.* 1967;277(13):667–672

153. Field CM, Connolly JH, Murtagh G, Slattery CM, Turkington EE. Antibiotic treatment of epidemic bronchiolitis—a double-blind trial. *BMJ.* 1966;1(5479):83–85

154. Antonow JA, Hansen K, McKinstry CA, Byington CL. Sepsis evaluations in hospitalized infants with bronchiolitis. *Pediatr Infect Dis J.* 1998;17(3):231–236

155. Friis B, Andersen P, Brenøe E, et al. Antibiotic treatment of pneumonia and bronchiolitis. A prospective randomised study. *Arch Dis Child.* 1984;59(11):1038–1045

156. Greenes DS, Harper MB. Low risk of bacteremia in febrile children with recognizable viral syndromes. *Pediatr Infect Dis J.* 1999;18(3):258–261

157. Spurling GK, Doust J, Del Mar CB, Eriksson L. Antibiotics for bronchiolitis in children. *Cochrane Database Syst Rev.* 2011;(6):CD005189

158. Ralston S, Hill V, Waters A. Occult serious bacterial infection in infants younger than 60 to 90 days with bronchiolitis: a systematic review. *Arch Pediatr Adolesc Med.* 2011;165(10):951–956

159. Purcell K, Fergie J. Lack of usefulness of an abnormal white blood cell count for predicting a concurrent serious bacterial infection in infants and young children hospitalized with respiratory syncytial virus lower respiratory tract infection. *Pediatr Infect Dis J.* 2007;26(4):311–315

160. Purcell K, Fergie J. Concurrent serious bacterial infections in 2396 infants and children hospitalized with respiratory syncytial virus lower respiratory tract infections. *Arch Pediatr Adolesc Med.* 2002;156(4):322–324

161. Purcell K, Fergie J. Concurrent serious bacterial infections in 912 infants and children hospitalized for treatment of respiratory syncytial virus lower respiratory tract infection. *Pediatr Infect Dis J.* 2004;23(3):267–269

162. Kuppermann N, Bank DE, Walton EA, Senac MO Jr, McCaslin I. Risks for bacteremia and urinary tract infections in young febrile children with bronchiolitis. *Arch Pediatr Adolesc Med.* 1997;151(12):1207–1214

163. Titus MO, Wright SW. Prevalence of serious bacterial infections in febrile infants with respiratory syncytial virus infection. *Pediatrics.* 2003;112(2):282–284

164. Melendez E, Harper MB. Utility of sepsis evaluation in infants 90 days of age or younger with fever and clinical bronchiolitis. *Pediatr Infect Dis J.* 2003;22(12):1053–1056

165. Hall CB, Powell KR, Schnabel KC, Gala CL, Pincus PH. Risk of secondary bacterial

infection in infants hospitalized with respiratory syncytial viral infection. *J Pediatr.* 1988;113(2):266–271

166. Hall CB. Respiratory syncytial virus: a continuing culprit and conundrum. *J Pediatr.* 1999;135(2 pt 2):2–7

167. Davies HD, Matlow A, Petric M, Glazier R, Wang EE. Prospective comparative study of viral, bacterial and atypical organisms identified in pneumonia and bronchiolitis in hospitalized Canadian infants. *Pediatr Infect Dis J.* 1996;15(4):371–375

168. Levine DA, Platt SL, Dayan PS, et al; Multicenter RSV-SBI Study Group of the Pediatric Emergency Medicine Collaborative Research Committee of the American Academy of Pediatrics. Risk of serious bacterial infection in young febrile infants with respiratory syncytial virus infections. *Pediatrics.* 2004;113(6):1728–1734

169. Kellner JD, Ohlsson A, Gadomski AM, Wang EE. Bronchodilators for bronchiolitis. *Cochrane Database Syst Rev.* 2000;(2):CD001266

170. Pinto LA, Pitrez PM, Luisi F, et al. Azithromycin therapy in hospitalized infants with acute bronchiolitis is not associated with better clinical outcomes: a randomized, double-blinded, and placebo-controlled clinical trial. *J Pediatr.* 2012;161(6):1104–1108

171. McCallum GB, Morris PS, Chang AB. Antibiotics for persistent cough or wheeze following acute bronchiolitis in children. *Cochrane Database Syst Rev.* 2012;(12):CD009834

172. Levin D, Tribuzio M, Green-Wrzesinki T, et al. Empiric antibiotics are justified for infants with RSV presenting with respiratory failure. *Pediatr Crit Care.* 2010;11(3):390–395

173. Thorburn K, Reddy V, Taylor N, van Saene HK. High incidence of pulmonary bacterial co-infection in children with severe respiratory syncytial virus (RSV) bronchiolitis. *Thorax.* 2006;61(7):611–615

174. Gomaa MA, Galal O, Mahmoud MS. Risk of acute otitis media in relation to acute bronchiolitis in children. *Int J Pediatr Otorhinolaryngol.* 2012;76(1):49–51

175. Andrade MA, Hoberman A, Glustein J, Paradise JL, Wald ER. Acute otitis media in children with bronchiolitis. *Pediatrics.* 1998;101(4 pt 1):617–619

176. Shazberg G, Revel-Vilk S, Shoseyov D, Ben-Ami A, Klar A, Hurvitz H. The clinical course of bronchiolitis associated with acute otitis media. *Arch Dis Child.* 2000;83(4):317–319

177. Lieberthal AS, Carroll AE, Chonmaitree T, et al. The diagnosis and management of acute otitis media [published correction appears in *Pediatrics.* 2014;133(2):346]. *Pediatrics.* 2013;131(3). Available at: www.pediatrics.org/cgi/content/full/131/3/e964

178. Hoberman A, Paradise JL, Rockette HE, et al. Treatment of acute otitis media in children under 2 years of age. *N Engl J Med.* 2011;364(2):105–115

179. Tähtinen PA, Laine MK, Huovinen P, Jalava J, Ruuskanen O, Ruohola A. A placebo-controlled trial of antimicrobial treatment for acute otitis media. *N Engl J Med.* 2011;364(2):116–126

180. Corrard F, de La Rocque F, Martin E, et al. Food intake during the previous 24 h as a percentage of usual intake: a marker of hypoxia in infants with bronchiolitis: an observational, prospective, multicenter study. *BMC Pediatr.* 2013;13:6

181. Pinnington LL, Smith CM, Ellis RE, Morton RE. Feeding efficiency and respiratory integration in infants with acute viral bronchiolitis. *J Pediatr.* 2000;137(4):523–526

182. Khoshoo V, Edell D. Previously healthy infants may have increased risk of aspiration during respiratory syncytial viral bronchiolitis. *Pediatrics.* 1999;104(6):1389–1390

183. Kennedy N, Flanagan N. Is nasogastric fluid therapy a safe alternative to the intravenous route in infants with bronchiolitis? *Arch Dis Child.* 2005;90(3):320–321

184. Sammartino L, James D, Goutzamanis J, Lines D. Nasogastric rehydration does have a role in acute paediatric bronchiolitis. *J Paediatr Child Health.* 2002;38(3):321–322

185. Kugelman A, Raibin K, Dabbah H, et al. Intravenous fluids versus gastric-tube feeding in hospitalized infants with viral bronchiolitis: a randomized, prospective pilot study. *J Pediatr.* 2013;162(3):640–642.e1

186. Oakley E, Borland M, Neutze J, et al; Paediatric Research in Emergency Departments International Collaborative (PREDICT). Nasogastric hydration versus intravenous hydration for infants with bronchiolitis: a randomised trial. *Lancet Respir Med.* 2013;1(2):113–120

187. Gozal D, Colin AA, Jaffe M, Hochberg Z. Water, electrolyte, and endocrine homeostasis in infants with bronchiolitis. *Pediatr Res.* 1990;27(2):204–209

188. van Steensel-Moll HA, Hazelzet JA, van der Voort E, Neijens HJ, Hackeng WH. Excessive secretion of antidiuretic hormone in infections with respiratory syncytial virus. *Arch Dis Child.* 1990;65(11):1237–1239

189. Rivers RP, Forsling ML, Olver RP. Inappropriate secretion of antidiuretic hormone in infants with respiratory infections. *Arch Dis Child.* 1981;56(5):358–363

190. Wang J, Xu E, Xiao Y. Isotonic versus hypotonic maintenance IV fluids in hospitalized children: a meta-analysis. *Pediatrics.* 2014;133(1):105–113

191. American Academy of Pediatrics, Committee on Infectious Diseases and Bronchiolitis Guidelines Committee. Policy statement: updated guidance for palivizumab prophylaxis among infants and young children at increased risk of hospitalization for respiratory syncytial virus infection. *Pediatrics.* 2014;134(2):415–420

192. American Academy of Pediatrics; Committee on Infectious Diseases and Bronchiolitis Guidelines Committee. Technical report: updated guidance for palivizumab prophylaxis among infants and young children at increased risk of hospitalization for respiratory syncytial virus infection. *Pediatrics.* 2014;134(2):e620–e638.

193. IMpact-RSV Study Group. Palivizumab, a humanized respiratory syncytial virus monoclonal antibody, reduces hospitalization from respiratory syncytial virus infection in high-risk infants. The IMpact-RSV Study Group. *Pediatrics.* 1998;102(3):531–537

194. Feltes TF, Cabalk AK, Meissner HC, et al. Palivizumab prophylaxis reduces hospitalization due to respiratory syncytial virus in young children with hemodynamically significant congenital heart disease. *J Pediatr.* 2003;143(4):532–540

195. Andabaka T, Nickerson JW, Rojas-Reyes MX, Rueda JD, Bacic VV, Barsic B. Monoclonal antibody for reducing the risk of respiratory syncytial virus infection in children. *Cochrane Database Syst Rev.* 2013;(4):CD006602

196. Wang D, Bayliss S, Meads C. Palivizumab for immunoprophylaxis of respiratory syncytial virus (RSV) bronchiolitis in high-risk infants and young children: a systematic review and additional economic modelling of subgroup analyses. *Health Technol Assess.* 2011;1(5):iii–iv, 1–124

197. Hampp C, Kauf TL, Saidi AS, Winterstein AG. Cost-effectiveness of respiratory syncytial virus prophylaxis in various indications. *Arch Pediatr Adolesc Med.* 2011;165(6):498–505

198. Hall CB, Weinberg GA, Iwane MK, et al. The burden of respiratory syncytial virus infection in young children. *N Engl J Med.* 2009;360(6):588–598

199. Dupenthaler A, Ammann RA, Gorgievski-Hrisoho M, et al. Low incidence of respiratory syncytial virus hospitalisations in haemodynamically significant congenital

heart disease. *Arch Dis Child.* 2004;89:961–965

200. Geskey JM, Thomas NJ, Brummel GL. Palivizumab in congenital heart disease: should international guidelines be revised? *Expert Opin Biol Ther.* 2007;7(11):1615–1620

201. Robbie GJ, Zhao L, Mondick J, Losonsky G, Roskos LK. Population pharmacokinetics of palivizumab, a humanized anti-respiratory syncytial virus monoclonal antibody, in adults and children. *Antimicrob Agents Chemother.* 2012;56(9):4927–4936

202. Megged O, Schlesinger Y. Down syndrome and respiratory syncytial virus infection. *Pediatr Infect Dis J.* 2010;29(7):672–673

203. Robinson KA, Odelola OA, Saldanha IJ, Mckoy NA. Palivizumab for prophylaxis against respiratory syncytial virus infection in children with cystic fibrosis. *Cochrane Database Syst Rev.* 2012;(2):CD007743

204. Winterstein AG, Eworuke E, Xu D, Schuler P. Palivizumab immunoprophylaxis effectiveness in children with cystic fibrosis. *Pediatr Pulmonol.* 2013;48(9):874–884

205. Cohen AH, Boron ML, Dingivan C. A phase IV study of the safety of palivizumab for prophylaxis of RSV disease in children with cystic fibrosis [abstract]. *American Thoracic Society Abstracts,* 2005 International Conference; 2005. p. A178

206. Giusti R. North American synagis prophylaxis survey. *Pediatr Pulmonol.* 2009;44(1):96–98

207. El Saleeby CM, Somes GW, DeVincenzo HP, Gaur AH. Risk factors for severe respiratory syncytial virus disease in children with cancer: the importance of lymphopenia and young age. *Pediatrics.* 2008;121(2):235–243

208. Berger A, Obwegeser E, Aberle SW, Langgartner M, Popow-Kraupp T. Nosocomial transmission of respiratory syncytial virus in neonatal intensive care and intermediate care units. *Pediatr Infect Dis J.* 2010;29(7):669–670

209. Ohler KH, Pham JT. Comparison of the timing of initial prophylactic palivizumab dosing on hospitalization of neonates for respiratory syncytial virus. *Am J Health Syst Pharm.* 2013;70(15):1342–1346

210. Blanken MO, Robers MM, Molenaar JM, et al. Respiratory syncytial virus and recurrent wheeze in healthy preterm infants. *N Engl J Med.* 2013;368(19):1794–1799

211. Yoshihara S, Kusuda S, Mochizuki H, Okada K, Nishima S, Simões EAF; C-CREW Investigators. Effect of palivizumab prophylaxis on subsequent recurrent wheezing in preterm infants. *Pediatrics.* 2013;132(5):811–818

212. Hall CB, Douglas RG Jr, Geiman JM. Possible transmission by fomites of respiratory syncytial virus. *J Infect Dis.* 1980;141(1):98–102

213. Sattar SA, Springthorpe VS, Tetro J, Vashon R, Keswick B. Hygienic hand antiseptics: should they not have activity and label claims against viruses? *Am J Infect Control.* 2002;30(6):355–372

214. Picheansathian W. A systematic review on the effectiveness of alcohol-based solutions for hand hygiene. *Int J Nurs Pract.* 2004;10(1):3–9

215. Hall CB. The spread of influenza and other respiratory viruses: complexities and conjectures. *Clin Infect Dis.* 2007;45(3):353–359

216. Boyce JM, Pittet D; Healthcare Infection Control Practices Advisory Committee; HICPAC/SHEA/APIC/IDSA Hand Hygiene Task Force; Society for Healthcare Epidemiology of America/Association for Professionals in Infection Control/Infectious Diseases Society of America. Guideline for Hand Hygiene in Health-Care Settings. Recommendations of the Healthcare Infection Control Practices Advisory Committee and the HICPAC/SHEA/APIC/IDSA Hand Hygiene Task Force. *MMWR Recomm Rep.* 2002;51(RR-16):1–45, quiz CE1–CE4

217. World Health Organization. Guidelines on hand hygiene in health care. Geneva, Switzerland: World Health Organization; 2009. Available at: http://whqlibdoc.who.int/publications/2009/9789241597906_eng.pdf. Accessed July 15, 2014

218. Karanfil LV, Conlon M, Lykens K, et al. Reducing the rate of nosocomially transmitted respiratory syncytial virus. [published correction appears in Am J Infect Control. 1999;27(3):303] *Am J Infect Control.* 1999;27(2):91–96

219. Macartney KK, Gorelick MH, Manning ML, Hodinka RL, Bell LM. Nosocomial respiratory syncytial virus infections: the cost-effectiveness and cost-benefit of infection control. *Pediatrics.* 2000;106(3):520–526

220. Strachan DP, Cook DG. Health effects of passive smoking. 1. Parental smoking and lower respiratory illness in infancy and early childhood. *Thorax.* 1997;52(10):905–914

221. Jones LL, Hashim A, McKeever T, Cook DG, Britton J, Leonardi-Bee J. Parental and household smoking and the increased risk of bronchitis, bronchiolitis and other lower respiratory infections in infancy: systematic review and meta-analysis. *Respir Res.* 2011;12:5

222. Bradley JP, Bacharier LB, Bonfiglio J, et al. Severity of respiratory syncytial virus bronchiolitis is affected by cigarette smoke exposure and atopy. *Pediatrics.* 2005;115(1). Available at: www.pediatrics.org/cgi/content/full/115/1/e7

223. Al-Shawwa B, Al-Huniti N, Weinberger M, Abu-Hasan M. Clinical and therapeutic variables influencing hospitalisation for bronchiolitis in a community-based paediatric group practice. *Prim Care Respir J.* 2007;16(2):93–97

224. Carroll KN, Gebretsadik T, Griffin MR, et al. Maternal asthma and maternal smoking are associated with increased risk of bronchiolitis during infancy. *Pediatrics.* 2007;119(6):1104–1112

225. Semple MG, Taylor-Robinson DC, Lane S, Smyth RL. Household tobacco smoke and admission weight predict severe bronchiolitis in infants independent of deprivation: prospective cohort study. *PLoS ONE.* 2011;6(7):e22425

226. Best D; Committee on Environmental Health; Committee on Native American Child Health; Committee on Adolescence. From the American Academy of Pediatrics: Technical report—Secondhand and prenatal tobacco smoke exposure. *Pediatrics.* 2009;124(5). Available at: www.pediatrics.org/cgi/content/full/124/5/e1017

227. Wilson KM, Wesgate SC, Best D, Blumkin AK, Klein JD. Admission screening for secondhand tobacco smoke exposure. *Hosp Pediatr.* 2012;2(1):26–33

228. Mahabee-Gittens M. Smoking in parents of children with asthma and bronchiolitis in a pediatric emergency department. *Pediatr Emerg Care.* 2002;18(1):4–7

229. Dempsey DA, Meyers MJ, Oh SS, et al. Determination of tobacco smoke exposure by plasma cotinine levels in infants and children attending urban public hospital clinics. *Arch Pediatr Adolesc Med.* 2012;166(9):851–856

230. Rosen LJ, Noach MB, Winickoff JP, Hovell MF. Parental smoking cessation to protect young children: a systematic review and meta-analysis. *Pediatrics.* 2012;129(1):141–152

231. Matt GE, Quintana PJ, Destaillats H, et al. Thirdhand tobacco smoke: emerging evidence and arguments for a multidisciplinary research agenda. *Environ Health Perspect.* 2011;119(9):1218–1226

232. Section on Breastfeeding. Breastfeeding and the use of human milk. *Pediatrics.* 2012;129(3). Available at: www.pediatrics.org/cgi/content/full/129/3/e827

233. Ip S, Chung M, Raman G, et al. *Breastfeeding and Maternal and Infant Health Outcomes in Developed Countries.* Rockville,

MD: Agency for Healthcare Research and Quality; 2007

234. Dornelles CT, Piva JP, Marostica PJ. Nutritional status, breastfeeding, and evolution of infants with acute viral bronchiolitis. *J Health Popul Nutr.* 2007;25(3):336–343

235. Oddy WH, Sly PD, de Klerk NH, et al. Breast feeding and respiratory morbidity in infancy: a birth cohort study. *Arch Dis Child.* 2003;88(3):224–228

236. Nishimura T, Suzue J, Kaji H. Breastfeeding reduces the severity of respiratory syncytial virus infection among young infants: a multi-center prospective study. *Pediatr Int.* 2009;51(6):812–816

237. Petruzella FD, Gorelick MH. Duration of illness in infants with bronchiolitis evaluated in the emergency department. *Pediatrics.* 2010;126(2):285–290

238. von Linstow ML, Eugen-Olsen J, Koch A, Winther TN, Westh H, Hogh B. Excretion patterns of human metapneumovirus and respiratory syncytial virus among young children. *Eur J Med Res.* 2006;11(8):329–335

239. Sacri AS, De Serres G, Quach C, Boulianne N, Valiquette L, Skowronski DM. Transmission of acute gastroenteritis and respiratory illness from children to parents. *Pediatr Infect Dis J.* 2014;33(6):583–588

240. Taylor JA, Kwan-Gett TS, McMahon EM Jr. Effectiveness of an educational intervention in modifying parental attitudes about antibiotic usage in children. *Pediatrics.* 2003;111 (5 pt 1). Available at: www.pediatrics.org/cgi/content/full/111/5pt1/e548

241. Kuzujanakis M, Kleinman K, Rifas-Shiman S, Finkelstein JA. Correlates of parental antibiotic knowledge, demand, and reported use. *Ambul Pediatr.* 2003;3(4):203–210

242. Mangione-Smith R, McGlynn EA, Elliott MN, Krogstad P, Brook RH. The relationship between perceived parental expectations and pediatrician antimicrobial prescribing behavior. *Pediatrics.* 1999;103(4 pt 1):711–718

APPENDIX 1 SEARCH TERMS BY TOPIC

Introduction

MedLine

(("bronchiolitis"[MeSH]) OR ("respiratory syncytial viruses"[MeSH]) NOT "bronchiolitis obliterans"[All Fields])

1. and exp Natural History/
2. and exp Epidemiology/
3. and (exp economics/ or exp "costs and cost analysis"/ or exp "cost allocation"/ or exp cost-benefit analysis/ or exp "cost control"/ or exp "cost of illness"/ or exp "cost sharing"/ or exp health care costs/ or exp health expenditures/)
4. and exp Risk Factors/

Limit to English Language AND Humans AND ("all infant (birth to 23 months)" or "newborn infant (birth to 1 month)" or "infant (1 to 23 months)")

CINAHL

(MM "Bronchiolitis+") AND ("natural history" OR (MM "Epidemiology") OR (MM "Costs and Cost Analysis") OR (MM "Risk Factors"))

The Cochrane Library

Bronchiolitis AND (epidemiology OR risk factor OR cost)

Diagnosis/Severity

MedLine

exp BRONCHIOLITIS/di [Diagnosis] OR exp Bronchiolitis, Viral/di [Diagnosis]

limit to English Language AND ("all infant (birth to 23 months)" or "newborn infant (birth to 1 month)" or "infant (1 to 23 months)")

CINAHL

(MH "Bronchiolitis/DI")

The Cochrane Library

Bronchiolitis AND Diagnosis

*Upper Respiratory Infection Symptoms

MedLine

(exp Bronchiolitis/ OR exp Bronchiolitis, Viral/) AND exp *Respiratory Tract Infections/

Limit to English Language

Limit to "all infant (birth to 23 months)" OR "newborn infant (birth to 1 month)" OR "infant (1 to 23 months)")

CINAHL

(MM "Bronchiolitis+") AND (MM "Respiratory Tract Infections+")

The Cochrane Library

Bronchiolitis AND Respiratory Infection

Inhalation Therapies

*Bronchodilators & Corticosteroids

MedLine

(("bronchiolitis"[MeSH]) OR ("respiratory syncytial viruses"[MeSH]) NOT "bronchiolitis obliterans"[All Fields])

AND (exp Receptors, Adrenergic, β-2/ OR exp Receptors, Adrenergic, β/ OR exp Receptors, Adrenergic, β-1/ OR β adrenergic*.mp. OR exp ALBUTEROL/ OR levalbuterol.mp. OR exp EPINEPHRINE/ OR exp Cholinergic Antagonists/ OR exp IPRATROPIUM/ OR exp Anti-Inflammatory Agents/ OR ics.mp. OR inhaled corticosteroid*.mp. OR exp Adrenal Cortex Hormones/ OR exp Leukotriene Antagonists/ OR montelukast.mp. OR exp Bronchodilator Agents/)

Limit to English Language AND ("all infant (birth to 23 months)" or "newborn infant (birth to 1 month)" or "infant (1 to 23 months)")

CINAHL

(MM "Bronchiolitis+") AND (MM "Bronchodilator Agents")

The Cochrane Library

Bronchiolitis AND (bronchodilator OR epinephrine OR albuterol OR salbutamol OR corticosteroid OR steroid)

*Hypertonic Saline

MedLine

(("bronchiolitis"[MeSH]) OR ("respiratory syncytial viruses"[MeSH]) NOT "bronchiolitis obliterans"[All Fields])

AND (exp Saline Solution, Hypertonic/ OR (aerosolized saline.mp. OR (exp AEROSOLS/ AND exp Sodium Chloride/)) OR (exp Sodium Chloride/ AND exp "Nebulizers and Vaporizers"/) OR nebulized saline.mp.)

Limit to English Language

Limit to "all infant (birth to 23 months)" OR "newborn infant (birth to 1 month)" OR "infant (1 to 23 months)")

CINAHL

(MM "Bronchiolitis+") AND (MM "Saline Solution, Hypertonic")

The Cochrane Library

Bronchiolitis AND Hypertonic Saline

Oxygen

MedLine

(("bronchiolitis"[MeSH]) OR ("respiratory syncytial viruses"[MeSH]) NOT "bronchiolitis obliterans"[All Fields])

1. AND (exp Oxygen Inhalation Therapy/ OR supplemental oxygen.mp. OR oxygen saturation.mp. OR *Oxygen/ad, st [Administration & Dosage, Standards] OR oxygen treatment.mp.)
2. AND (exp OXIMETRY/ OR oximeters.mp.) AND (exp "Reproducibility of Results"/ OR reliability.mp. OR function.mp. OR technical specifications.mp.) OR (percutaneous measurement*.mp. OR exp Blood Gas Analysis/)

Limit to English Language

Limit to "all infant (birth to 23 months)" OR "newborn infant (birth to 1 month)" OR "infant (1 to 23 months)")

CINAHL

(MM "Bronchiolitis+") AND

((MM "Oxygen Therapy") OR (MM "Oxygen+") OR (MM "Oxygen Saturation") OR (MM "Oximetry+") OR (MM "Pulse Oximetry") OR (MM "Blood Gas Monitoring, Transcutaneous"))

The Cochrane Library

Bronchiolitis AND (oxygen OR oximetry)

Chest Physiotherapy and Suctioning

MedLine

((("bronchiolitis"[MeSH]) OR ("respiratory syncytial viruses"[MeSH]) NOT "bronchiolitis obliterans"[All Fields])

1. AND (Chest physiotherapy.mp. OR (exp Physical Therapy Techniques/ AND exp Thorax/))

2. AND (Nasal Suction.mp. OR (exp Suction/))

Limit to English Language

Limit to "all infant (birth to 23 months)" OR "newborn infant (birth to 1 month)" OR "infant (1 to 23 months)"

CINAHL

(MM "Bronchiolitis+")

1. AND ((MH "Chest Physiotherapy (Saba CCC)") OR (MH "Chest Physical Therapy+") OR (MH "Chest Physiotherapy (Iowa NIC)"))

2. AND (MH "Suctioning, Nasopharyngeal")

The Cochrane Library

Bronchiolitis AND (chest physiotherapy OR suction*)

Hydration

MedLine

((("bronchiolitis"[MeSH]) OR ("respiratory syncytial viruses"[MeSH])

NOT "bronchiolitis obliterans"[All Fields])

AND (exp Fluid Therapy/ AND (exp infusions, intravenous OR exp administration, oral))

Limit to English Language

Limit to ("all infant (birth to 23 months)" or "newborn infant (birth to 1 month)" or "infant (1 to 23 months)")

CINAHL

(MM "Bronchiolitis+") AND

((MM "Fluid Therapy+") OR (MM "Hydration Control (Saba CCC)") OR (MM "Hydration (Iowa NOC)"))

The Cochrane Library

Bronchiolitis AND (hydrat* OR fluid*)

SBI and Antibacterials

MedLine

((("bronchiolitis"[MeSH]) OR ("respiratory syncytial viruses"[MeSH]) NOT "bronchiolitis obliterans"[All Fields])

AND

(exp Bacterial Infections/ OR exp Bacterial Pneumonia/ OR exp Otitis Media/ OR exp Meningitis/ OR exp *Anti-bacterial Agents/ OR exp Sepsis/ OR exp Urinary Tract Infections/ OR exp Bacteremia/ OR exp Tracheitis OR serious bacterial infection.mp.)

Limit to English Language

Limit to ("all infant (birth to 23 months)" or "newborn infant (birth to 1 month)" or "infant (1 to 23 months)")

CINAHL

(MM "Bronchiolitis+") AND

((MM "Pneumonia, Bacterial+") OR (MM "Bacterial Infections+") OR (MM "Otitis Media+") OR (MM "Meningitis, Bacterial+") OR (MM "Antiinfective Agents+") OR (MM "Sepsis+") OR (MM

"Urinary Tract Infections+") OR (MM "Bacteremia"))

The Cochrane Library

Bronchiolitis AND (serious bacterial infection OR sepsis OR otitis media OR meningitis OR urinary tract infection or bacteremia OR pneumonia OR antibacterial OR antimicrobial OR antibiotic)

Hand Hygiene, Tobacco, Breastfeeding, Parent Education

MedLine

((("bronchiolitis"[MeSH]) OR ("respiratory syncytial viruses"[MeSH]) NOT "bronchiolitis obliterans"[All Fields])

1. AND (exp Hand Disinfection/ OR hand decontamination.mp. OR handwashing.mp.)

2. AND exp Tobacco/

3. AND (exp Breast Feeding/ OR exp Milk, Human/ OR exp Bottle Feeding/)

Limit to English Language

Limit to ("all infant (birth to 23 months)" or "newborn infant (birth to 1 month)" or "infant (1 to 23 months)")

CINAHL

(MM "Bronchiolitis+")

1. AND (MH "Handwashing+")

2. AND (MH "Tobacco+")

3. AND (MH "Breast Feeding+" OR MH "Milk, Human+" OR MH "Bottle Feeding+")

The Cochrane Library

Bronchiolitis

1. AND (Breast Feeding OR breastfeeding)

2. AND tobacco

3. AND (hand hygiene OR handwashing OR hand decontamination)

Bronchiolitis Clinical Practice Guideline Quick Reference Tools

- Action Statement Summary
  — The Diagnosis, Management, and Prevention of Bronchiolitis
- *ICD-10-CM* Coding Quick Reference for Bronchiolitis
- AAP Patient Education Handout
  — *Bronchiolitis and Your Young Child*

Action Statement Summary

The Diagnosis, Management, and Prevention of Bronchiolitis

Key Action Statement 1a

Clinicians should diagnose bronchiolitis and assess disease severity on the basis of history and physical examination (Evidence Quality: B; Recommendation Strength: Strong Recommendation).

Key Action Statement 1b

Clinicians should assess risk factors for severe disease, such as age <12 weeks, a history of prematurity, underlying cardiopulmonary disease, or immunodeficiency, when making decisions about evaluation and management of children with bronchiolitis (Evidence Quality: B; Recommendation Strength: Moderate Recommendation).

Key Action Statement 1c

When clinicians diagnose bronchiolitis on the basis of history and physical examination, radiographic or laboratory studies should not be obtained routinely (Evidence Quality: B; Recommendation Strength: Moderate Recommendation).

Key Action Statement 2

Clinicians should not administer albuterol (or salbutamol) to infants and children with a diagnosis of bronchiolitis (Evidence Quality: B; Recommendation Strength: Strong Recommendation).

Key Action Statement 3

Clinicians should not administer epinephrine to infants and children with a diagnosis of bronchiolitis (Evidence Quality: B; Recommendation Strength: Strong Recommendation).

Key Action Statement 4a

Nebulized hypertonic saline should not be administered to infants with a diagnosis of bronchiolitis in the emergency department (Evidence Quality: B; Recommendation Strength: Moderate Recommendation).

Key Action Statement 4b

Clinicians may administer nebulized hypertonic saline to infants and children hospitalized for bronchiolitis (Evidence Quality: B; Recommendation Strength: Weak Recommendation [based on randomized controlled trials with inconsistent findings]).

Key Action Statement 5

Clinicians should not administer systemic corticosteroids to infants with a diagnosis of bronchiolitis in any setting (Evidence Quality: A; Recommendation Strength: Strong Recommendation).

Key Action Statement 6a

Clinicians may choose not to administer supplemental oxygen if the oxyhemoglobin saturation exceeds 90% in infants and children with a diagnosis of bronchiolitis (Evidence Quality: D; Recommendation Strength: Weak Recommendation [based on low-level evidence and reasoning from first principles]).

Key Action Statement 6b

Clinicians may choose not to use continuous pulse oximetry for infants and children with a diagnosis of bronchiolitis (Evidence Quality: C; Recommendation Strength: Weak Recommendation [based on lower-level evidence]).

Key Action Statement 7

Clinicians should not use chest physiotherapy for infants and children with a diagnosis of bronchiolitis (Evidence Quality: B; Recommendation Strength: Moderate Recommendation).

Key Action Statement 8

Clinicians should not administer antibacterial medications to infants and children with a diagnosis of bronchiolitis unless there is a concomitant bacterial infection, or a strong suspicion of one. (Evidence Quality: B; Recommendation Strength: Strong Recommendation).

Key Action Statement 9

Clinicians should administer nasogastric or intravenous fluids for infants with a diagnosis of bronchiolitis who cannot maintain hydration orally (Evidence Quality: X; Recommendation Strength: Strong Recommendation).

Key Action Statement 10a

Clinicians should not administer palivizumab to otherwise healthy infants with a gestational age of 29 weeks, 0 days or greater (Evidence Quality: B; Recommendation Strength: Strong Recommendation).

Key Action Statement 10b

Clinicians should administer palivizumab during the first year of life to infants with hemodynamically significant heart disease or chronic lung disease of prematurity defined as preterm infants <32 weeks, 0 days' gestation who require >21% oxygen for at least the first 28 days of life (Evidence Quality: B; Recommendation Strength: Moderate Recommendation).

Key Action Statement 10c

Clinicians should administer a maximum 5 monthly doses (15 mg/kg/dose) of palivizumab during the RSV season to infants who qualify for palivizumab in the first year of life (Evidence Quality: B, Recommendation Strength: Moderate Recommendation).

Key Action Statement 11a

All people should disinfect hands before and after direct contact with patients, after contact with inanimate objects in the direct vicinity of the patient, and after removing gloves (Evidence Quality: B; Recommendation Strength: Strong Recommendation).

Key Action Statement 11b

All people should use alcohol-based rubs for hand decontamination when caring for children with bronchiolitis. When alcohol-based rubs are not available, individuals should wash their hands with soap and water (Evidence Quality: B; Recommendation Strength: Strong Recommendation).

Key Action Statement 12a

Clinicians should inquire about the exposure of the infant or child to tobacco smoke when assessing infants and children for bronchiolitis (Evidence Quality: C; Recommendation Strength: Moderate Recommendation).

Key Action Statement 12b

Clinicians should counsel caregivers about exposing the infant or child to environmental tobacco smoke and smoking cessation when assessing a child for bronchiolitis (Evidence Quality: B; Recommendation Strength: Strong Recommendation).

Key Action Statement 13

Clinicians should encourage exclusive breastfeeding for at least 6 months to decrease the morbidity of respiratory infections (Evidence Quality: Grade B; Recommendation Strength: Moderate Recommendation).

Key Action Statement 14

Clinicians and nurses should educate personnel and family members on evidence-based diagnosis, treatment, and prevention in bronchiolitis (Evidence Quality: C; observational studies; Recommendation Strength; Moderate Recommendation).

Coding Quick Reference for Bronchiolitis
ICD-10-CM
J21.0 Acute bronchiolitis due to syncytial virus
J21.1 Acute bronchiolitis due to human metapneumovirus
J21.8 Acute bronchiolitis due to other specified organisms
J21.9 Acute bronchiolitis, unspecified

Bronchiolitis and Your Young Child

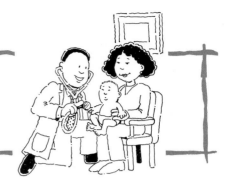

Bronchiolitis is a common respiratory illness among infants. One of its symptoms is trouble breathing, which can be scary for parents and young children. Read on for more information from the American Academy of Pediatrics about bronchiolitis, causes, signs and symptoms, how to treat it, and how to prevent it.

What is bronchiolitis?

Bronchiolitis is an infection that causes the small breathing tubes of the lungs (bronchioles) to swell. This blocks airflow through the lungs, making it hard to breathe. It occurs most often in infants because their airways are smaller and more easily blocked than in older children. Bronchiolitis is not the same as bronchitis, which is an infection of the larger, more central airways that typically causes problems in adults.

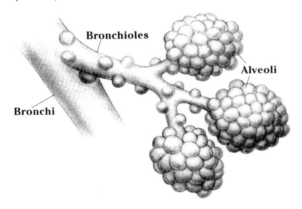

What causes bronchiolitis?

Bronchiolitis is caused by one of several respiratory viruses such as influenza, respiratory syncytial virus (RSV), parainfluenza, and human metapneumovirus. Other viruses can also cause bronchiolitis.

Infants with RSV infection are more likely to get bronchiolitis with wheezing and difficulty breathing. Most adults and many older children with RSV infection only get a cold. RSV is spread by contact with an infected person's mucus or saliva (respiratory droplets produced during coughing or wheezing). It often spreads through families and child care centers. (See "How can you prevent your baby from getting bronchiolitis?").

What are the signs and symptoms of bronchiolitis?

Bronchiolitis often starts with signs of a cold, such as a runny nose, mild cough, and fever. After 1 or 2 days, the cough may get worse and an infant will begin to breathe faster. Your child may become dehydrated if he cannot comfortably drink fluids

If your child shows any signs of troubled breathing or dehydration, call your child's doctor.

Signs of troubled breathing

- He may widen his nostrils and squeeze the muscles under his rib cage to try to get more air into and out of his lungs.
- When he breathes, he may grunt and tighten his stomach muscles.
- He will make a high-pitched whistling sound, called a wheeze, when he breathes out.
- He may have trouble drinking because he may have trouble sucking and swallowing.
- If it gets very hard for him to breathe, you may notice a bluish tint around his lips and fingertips. This tells you his airways are so blocked that there is not enough oxygen getting into his blood.

Signs of dehydration

- Drinking less than normal
- Dry mouth
- Crying without tears
- Urinating less often than normal

Bronchiolitis and children with severe chronic illness

Bronchiolitis may cause more severe illness in children who have a chronic illness. If you think your child has bronchiolitis and she has any of the following conditions, call her doctor:

- Cystic fibrosis
- Congenital heart disease
- Chronic lung disease (seen in some infants who were on breathing machines or respirators as newborns)
- Immune deficiency disease (eg, acquired immunodeficiency syndrome [AIDS])
- Organ or bone marrow transplant
- A cancer for which she is receiving chemotherapy

Can bronchiolitis be treated at home?

There is no specific treatment for RSV or other viruses that cause bronchiolitis. Antibiotics are not helpful because they treat illnesses caused by bacteria, not viruses. However, you can try to ease your child's symptoms.

To relieve a stuffy nose

- Thin the mucus using saline nose drops recommended by your child's doctor. Never use nonprescription nose drops that contain medicine.
- Clear your baby's nose with a suction bulb.

Squeeze the bulb first. Gently put the rubber tip into one nostril, and slowly release the bulb.

This suction will draw the clogged mucus out of the nose. This works best when your baby is younger than 6 months.

To relieve fever

Give your baby acetaminophen. (Follow the recommended dosage for your baby's age.) Do not give your baby aspirin because it has been associated with Reye syndrome, a disease that affects the liver and brain. Check with your child's doctor first before giving any other cold medicines.

To prevent dehydration

Make sure your baby drinks lots of fluid. She may want clear liquids rather than milk or formula. She may feed more slowly or not feel like eating because she is having trouble breathing.

How will your child's doctor treat bronchiolitis?

Your child's doctor will evaluate your child and advise you on nasal suctioning, fever control, and observation, as well as when to call back.

Some children with bronchiolitis need to be treated in a hospital for breathing problems or dehydration. Breathing problems may need to be treated with oxygen and medicine. Dehydration is treated with a special liquid diet or intravenous (IV) fluids.

In very rare cases when these treatments aren't working, an infant might have to be put on a respirator. This is usually only temporary until the infection is gone.

How can you prevent your baby from getting bronchiolitis?

The best steps you can follow to reduce the risk that your baby becomes infected with RSV or other viruses that cause bronchiolitis include
- Make sure everyone washes their hands before touching your baby.
- Keep your baby away from anyone who has a cold, fever, or runny nose.
- Avoid sharing eating utensils and drinking cups with anyone who has a cold, fever, or runny nose.

If you have questions about the treatment of bronchiolitis, call your child's doctor.

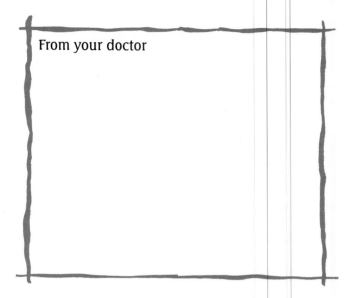

From your doctor

American Academy
of Pediatrics

DEDICATED TO THE HEALTH OF ALL CHILDREN™

The American Academy of Pediatrics (AAP) is an organization of 62,000 primary care pediatricians, pediatric medical subspecialists, and pediatric surgical specialists dedicated to the health, safety, and well-being of all infants, children, adolescents, and young adults.

American Academy of Pediatrics
Web site — www.HealthyChildren.org

Management of Newly Diagnosed Type 2 Diabetes Mellitus (T2DM) in Children and Adolescents

- *Clinical Practice Guideline*

CLINICAL PRACTICE GUIDELINE

Management of Newly Diagnosed Type 2 Diabetes Mellitus (T2DM) in Children and Adolescents

Kenneth C. Copeland, MD, Janet Silverstein, MD, Kelly R. Moore, MD, Greg E. Prazar, MD, Terry Raymer, MD, CDE, Richard N. Shiffman, MD, Shelley C. Springer, MD, MBA, Vidhu V. Thaker, MD, Meaghan Anderson, MS, RD, LD, CDE, Stephen J. Spann, MD, MBA, and Susan K. Flinn, MA

KEY WORDS
diabetes, type 2 diabetes mellitus, childhood, youth, clinical practice guidelines, comanagement, management, treatment

ABBREVIATIONS
AAP—American Academy of Pediatrics
AAFP—American Academy of Family Physicians
BG—blood glucose
FDA—US Food and Drug Administration
HbA1c—hemoglobin A1c
PES—Pediatric Endocrine Society
T1DM—type 1 diabetes mellitus
T2DM—type 2 diabetes mellitus
TODAY—Treatment Options for type 2 Diabetes in Adolescents and Youth

This document is copyrighted and is property of the American Academy of Pediatrics and its Board of Directors. All authors have filed conflict of interest statements with the American Academy of Pediatrics. Any conflicts have been resolved through a process approved by the Board of Directors. The American Academy of Pediatrics has neither solicited nor accepted any commercial involvement in the development of the content of this publication.

The recommendations in this report do not indicate an exclusive course of treatment or serve as a standard of medical care. Variations, taking into account individual circumstances, may be appropriate.

All clinical practice guidelines from the American Academy of Pediatrics automatically expire 5 years after publication unless reaffirmed, revised, or retired at or before that time.

abstract

Over the past 3 decades, the prevalence of childhood obesity has increased dramatically in North America, ushering in a variety of health problems, including type 2 diabetes mellitus (T2DM), which previously was not typically seen until much later in life. The rapid emergence of childhood T2DM poses challenges to many physicians who find themselves generally ill-equipped to treat adult diseases encountered in children. This clinical practice guideline was developed to provide evidence-based recommendations on managing 10- to 18-year-old patients in whom T2DM has been diagnosed. The American Academy of Pediatrics (AAP) convened a Subcommittee on Management of T2DM in Children and Adolescents with the support of the American Diabetes Association, the Pediatric Endocrine Society, the American Academy of Family Physicians, and the Academy of Nutrition and Dietetics (formerly the American Dietetic Association). These groups collaborated to develop an evidence report that served as a major source of information for these practice guideline recommendations. The guideline emphasizes the use of management modalities that have been shown to affect clinical outcomes in this pediatric population. Recommendations are made for situations in which either insulin or metformin is the preferred first-line treatment of children and adolescents with T2DM. The recommendations suggest integrating lifestyle modifications (ie, diet and exercise) in concert with medication rather than as an isolated initial treatment approach. Guidelines for frequency of monitoring hemoglobin A1c (HbA1c) and finger-stick blood glucose (BG) concentrations are presented. Decisions were made on the basis of a systematic grading of the quality of evidence and strength of recommendation. The clinical practice guideline underwent peer review before it was approved by the AAP. This clinical practice guideline is not intended to replace clinical judgment or establish a protocol for the care of all children with T2DM, and its recommendations may not provide the only appropriate approach to the management of children with T2DM. Providers should consult experts trained in the care of children and adolescents with T2DM when treatment goals are not met or when therapy with insulin is initiated. The AAP acknowledges that some primary care clinicians may not be confident of their ability to successfully treat T2DM in a child because of the child's age, coexisting conditions, and/or other concerns. At any point at which a clinician feels he or she is not adequately trained or is uncertain about treatment, a referral to a pediatric medical subspecialist should be made. If a diagnosis of T2DM is made by a pediatric medical subspecialist, the primary care clinician should develop a comanagement strategy with the subspecialist to ensure that the child continues to receive appropriate care consistent with a medical home model in which the pediatrician partners with parents to ensure that all health needs are met. *Pediatrics* 2013;131:364–382

www.pediatrics.org/cgi/doi/10.1542/peds.2012-3494

doi:10.1542/peds.2012-3494

PEDIATRICS (ISSN Numbers: Print, 0031-4005; Online, 1098-4275).

Key action statements are as follows:

1. Clinicians must ensure that insulin therapy is initiated for children and adolescents with T2DM who are ketotic or in diabetic ketoacidosis and in whom the distinction between types 1 and 2 diabetes mellitus is unclear and, in usual cases, should initiate insulin therapy for patients

   a. who have random venous or plasma BG concentrations ≥250 mg/dL; or

   b. whose HbA1c is >9%.

2. In all other instances, clinicians should initiate a lifestyle modification program, including nutrition and physical activity, and start metformin as first-line therapy for children and adolescents at the time of diagnosis of T2DM.

3. The committee suggests that clinicians monitor HbA1c concentrations every 3 months and intensify treatment if treatment goals for finger-stick BG and HbA1c concentrations are not being met (intensification is defined in the Definitions box).

4. The committee suggests that clinicians advise patients to monitor finger-stick BG (see Key Action Statement 4 in the guideline for further details) concentrations in patients who

   a. are taking insulin or other medications with a risk of hypoglycemia; or

   b. are initiating or changing their diabetes treatment regimen; or

   c. have not met treatment goals; or

   d. have intercurrent illnesses.

5. The committee suggests that clinicians incorporate the Academy of Nutrition and Dietetics' *Pediatric Weight Management Evidence-Based Nutrition Practice Guidelines* in their dietary or nutrition counseling of patients with T2DM at the time of diagnosis and as part of ongoing management.

6. The committee suggests that clinicians encourage children and adolescents with T2DM to engage in moderate-to-vigorous exercise for at least 60 minutes daily and to limit nonacademic "screen time" to less than 2 hours a day.

Definitions

Adolescent: an individual in various stages of maturity, generally considered to be between 12 and 18 years of age.

Childhood T2DM: disease in the child who typically

- is overweight or obese (BMI ≥85th–94th and >95th percentile for age and gender, respectively);

- has a strong family history of T2DM;

- has substantial residual insulin secretory capacity at diagnosis (reflected by normal or elevated insulin and C-peptide concentrations);

- has insidious onset of disease;

- demonstrates insulin resistance (including clinical evidence of polycystic ovarian syndrome or acanthosis nigricans);

- lacks evidence for diabetic autoimmunity (negative for autoantibodies typically associated with T1DM). These patients are more likely to have hypertension and dyslipidemia than are those with T1DM.

Clinician: any provider within his or her scope of practice; includes medical practitioners (including physicians and physician extenders), dietitians, psychologists, and nurses.

Diabetes: according to the American Diabetes Association criteria, defined as

1. HbA1c ≥6.5% (test performed in an appropriately certified laboratory); or

2. fasting (defined as no caloric intake for at least 8 hours) plasma glucose ≥126 mg/dL (7.0 mmol/L); or

3. 2-hour plasma glucose ≥200 mg/dL (11.1 mmol/L) during an oral glucose tolerance test performed as described by the World Health Organization by using a glucose load containing the equivalent of 75 g anhydrous glucose dissolved in water; or

4. a random plasma glucose ≥200 mg/dL (11.1 mmol/L) with symptoms of hyperglycemia.

(In the absence of unequivocal hyperglycemia, criteria 1–3 should be confirmed by repeat testing.)

Diabetic ketoacidosis: acidosis resulting from an absolute or relative insulin deficiency, causing fat breakdown and formation of β hydroxybutyrate. Symptoms include nausea, vomiting, dehydration, Kussmaul respirations, and altered mental status.

Fasting blood glucose: blood glucose obtained before the first meal of the day and after a fast of at least 8 hours.

Glucose toxicity: The effect of high blood glucose causing both insulin resistance and impaired β-cell production of insulin.

Intensification: Increase frequency of blood glucose monitoring and adjustment of the dose and type of medication in an attempt to normalize blood glucose concentrations.

Intercurrent illnesses: Febrile illnesses or associated symptoms severe enough to cause the patient to stay home from school and/or seek medical care.

Microalbuminuria: Albumin:creatinine ratio ≥30 mg/g creatinine but <300 mg/g creatinine.

Moderate hyperglycemia: blood glucose = 180–250 mg/dL.

Moderate-to-vigorous exercise: exercise that makes the individual breathe hard and perspire and that raises his or her heart rate. An easy way to define exercise intensity for patients is the "talk test": during moderate physical activity a person can talk, but not sing. During vigorous activity, a person cannot talk without pausing to catch a breath.

Obese: BMI ≥95th percentile for age and gender.

Overweight: BMI between the 85th and 94th percentile for age and gender.

Prediabetes: Fasting plasma glucose ≥100–125 mg/dL or 2-hour glucose concentration during an oral glucose tolerance test ≥126 but <200 mg/dL or an HbA1c of 5.7% to 6.4%.

Severe hyperglycemia: blood glucose >250 mg/dL.

Thiazolidinediones (TZDs): Oral hypoglycemic agents that exert their effect at least in part by activation of the peroxisome proliferator-activated receptor γ.

Type 1 diabetes mellitus (T1DM): Diabetes secondary to autoimmune destruction of β cells resulting in absolute (complete or near complete) insulin deficiency and requiring insulin injections for management.

Type 2 diabetes mellitus (T2DM): The investigators' designation of the diagnosis was used for the purposes of the literature review. The committee acknowledges the distinction between T1DM and T2DM in this population is not always clear cut, and clinical judgment plays an important role. Typically, this diagnosis is made when hyperglycemia is secondary to insulin resistance accompanied by impaired β-cell function resulting in inadequate insulin production to compensate for the degree of insulin resistance.

Youth: used interchangeably with "adolescent" in this document.

INTRODUCTION

Over the past 3 decades, the prevalence of childhood obesity has increased dramatically in North America,[1–5] ushering in a variety of health problems, including type 2 diabetes mellitus (T2DM), which previously was not typically seen until much later in life. Currently, in the United States, up to 1 in 3 new cases of diabetes mellitus diagnosed in youth younger than 18 years is T2DM (depending on the ethnic composition of the patient population),[6,7] with a disproportionate representation in ethnic minorities[8,9] and occurring most commonly among youth between 10 and 19 years of age.[5,10] This trend is not limited to the United States but is occurring internationally[11]; it is projected that by the year 2030, an estimated 366 million people worldwide will have diabetes mellitus.[12]

The rapid emergence of childhood T2DM poses challenges to many physicians who find themselves generally ill-equipped to treat adult diseases encountered in children. Most diabetes education materials designed for pediatric patients are directed primarily to families of children with type 1 diabetes mellitus (T1DM) and emphasize insulin treatment and glucose monitoring, which may or may not be appropriate for children with

T2DM.[13,14] The National Diabetes Education Program TIP sheets (which can be ordered or downloaded from www.yourdiabetesinfo.org or ndep.nih.gov) provide guidance on healthy eating, physical activity, and dealing with T2DM in children and adolescents, but few other resources are available that are directly targeted at youth with this disease.[15] Most medications used for T2DM have been tested for safety and efficacy only in people older than 18 years, and there is scant scientific evidence for optimal management of children with T2DM.[16,17] Recognizing the scarcity of evidence-based data, this report provides a set of guidelines for the management and treatment of children with T2DM that is based on a review of current medical literature covering a period from January 1, 1990, to July 1, 2008.

Despite these limitations, the practicing physician is likely to be faced with the need to provide care for children with T2DM. Thus, the American Academy of Pediatrics (AAP), the Pediatric Endocrine Society (PES), the American Academy of Family Physicians (AAFP), American Diabetes Association, and the Academy of Nutrition and Dietetics (formerly the American Dietetic Association) partnered to develop a set of guidelines that might benefit endocrinologists and generalists, including pediatricians and family physicians alike. This clinical practice guideline may not provide the only appropriate approach to the management of children with T2DM. It is not expected to serve as a sole source of guidance in the management of children and adolescents with T2DM, nor is it intended to replace clinical judgment or establish a protocol for the care of all children with this condition. Rather, it is intended to assist clinicians in decision-making.

Primary care providers should endeavor to obtain the requisite skills to care for children and adolescents with T2DM, and should communicate and work closely with a diabetes team of subspecialists when such consultation is available, practical, and appropriate. The frequency of such consultations will vary, but should usually be obtained at diagnosis and then at least annually if possible. When treatment goals are not met, the committee encourages clinicians to consult with an expert trained in the care of children and adolescents with T2DM.[18,19] When first-line therapy (eg, metformin) fails, recommendations for intensifying therapy should be generally the same for pediatric and adult populations. The picture is constantly changing, however, as new drugs are introduced, and some drugs that initially appeared to be safe demonstrate adverse effects with wider use. Clinicians should, therefore, remain alert to new developments with regard to treatment of T2DM. Seeking the advice of an expert can help ensure that the treatment goals are appropriately set and that clinicians benefit from cutting-edge treatment information in this rapidly changing area.

The Importance of Family-Centered Diabetes Care

Family structure, support, and education help inform clinical decision-making and negotiations with the patient and family about medical preferences that affect medical decisions, independent of existing clinical recommendations. Because adherence is a major issue in any lifestyle intervention, engaging the family is critical not only to maintain needed changes in lifestyle but also to foster medication adherence.[20-22] The family's ideal role in lifestyle interventions varies, however, depending on the child's age. Behavioral interventions in younger children have shown a favorable effect. With adolescents, however, interventions based on target-age behaviors (eg, including phone or Internet-based interventions as well as face-to-face or peer-enhanced activities) appear to foster better results, at least for weight management.[23]

Success in making lifestyle changes to attain therapeutic goals requires the initial and ongoing education of the patient and the entire family about healthy nutrition and exercise. Any behavior change recommendations must establish realistic goals and take into account the families' health beliefs and behaviors. Understanding the patient and family's perception of the disease (and overweight status) before establishing a management plan is important to dispel misconceptions and promote adherence.[24] Because T2DM disproportionately affects minority populations, there is a need to ensure culturally appropriate, family-centered care along with ongoing education.[25-28] Several observational studies cite the importance of addressing cultural issues within the family.[20-22]

Restrictions in Creating This Document

In developing these guidelines, the following restrictions governed the committee's work:

- Although the importance of diabetes detection and screening of at-risk populations is acknowledged and referenced, the guidelines are restricted to patients meeting the diagnostic criteria for diabetes (eg, this document focuses on treatment postdiagnosis). Specifically, this document and its recommendations do not pertain to patients with impaired fasting plasma glucose (100–125 mg/dL) or impaired glucose tolerance (2-hour oral glucose tolerance test plasma glucose: 140–200 mg/dL) or isolated insulin resistance.

- Although it is noted that the distinction between types 1 and 2 diabetes mellitus in children may be difficult,[29,30] these recommendations pertain specifically to patients 10 to less than 18 years of age with T2DM (as defined above).

- Although the importance of high-risk care and glycemic control in pregnancy, including pregravid glycemia, is affirmed, the evidence considered and recommendations contained in this document do not pertain to diabetes in pregnancy, including diabetes in pregnant adolescents.

- Recommended screening schedules and management tools for select comorbid conditions (hypertension, dyslipidemia, nephropathy, microalbuminuria, and depression) are provided as resources in the accompanying technical report.[31] These therapeutic recommendations were adapted from other recommended guideline documents with references, without an independent assessment of their supporting evidence.

METHODS

A systematic review was performed and is described in detail in the accompanying technical report.[31] To develop the clinical practice guideline on the management of T2DM in children and adolescents, the AAP convened the Subcommittee on Management of T2DM in Children and Adolescents with the support of the American Diabetes Association, the PES, the AAFP, and the Academy of Nutrition and Dietetics. The subcommittee was co-chaired by 2 pediatric endocrinologists preeminent in their field and included experts in general pediatrics, family medicine, nutrition, Native American health, epidemiology, and medical informatics/guideline methodology. All panel members reviewed the AAP policy on Conflict of Interest and Voluntary Disclosure and declared all potential conflicts (see conflicts statements in the Task Force member list).

These groups partnered to develop an evidence report that served as a major source of information for these practice guideline recommendations.[31] Specific clinical questions addressed in the evidence review were as follows: (1) the effectiveness of treatment modalities for T2DM in children and adolescents, (2) the efficacy of pharmaceutical therapies for treatment of children and adolescents with T2DM, (3) appropriate recommendations for screening for comorbidities typically associated with T2DM in children and adolescents, and (4) treatment recommendations for comorbidities of T2DM in children and adolescents. The accompanying technical report contains more information on comorbidities.[31]

Epidemiologic project staff searched Medline, the Cochrane Collaboration, and Embase. MESH terms used in various combinations in the search included diabetes, mellitus, type 2, type 1, treatment, prevention, diet, pediatric, T2DM, T1DM, NIDDM, metformin, lifestyle, RCT, meta-analysis, child, adolescent, therapeutics, control, adult, obese, gestational, polycystic ovary syndrome, metabolic syndrome, cardiovascular, dyslipidemia, men, and women. In addition, the Boolean operators NOT, AND, OR were included in various combinations. Articles addressing treatment of diabetes mellitus were prospectively limited to those that were published in English between January 1990 and June 2008, included abstracts, and addressed children between the ages of 120 and 215 months with an established diagnosis of T2DM. Studies in adults were considered for inclusion if >10% of the study population was 45 years of age or younger. The Medline search limits included the following: clinical trial; meta-analysis; randomized controlled trial; review; child: 6–12 years; and adolescent: 13–18 years. Additional articles were identified by review of reference lists of relevant articles and ongoing studies recommended by a technical expert advisory group. All articles were reviewed for compliance with the search limitations and appropriateness for inclusion in this document.

Initially, 199 abstracts were identified for possible inclusion, of which 52 were retained for systematic review. Results of the literature review were presented in evidence tables and published in the final evidence report. An additional literature search of Medline and the Cochrane Database of

Evidence Quality	Preponderance of Benefit or Harm	Balance of Benefit and Harm
A. Well-designed RCTs or diagnostic studies on relevant population	Strong Recommendation	
B. RCTs or diagnostic studies with minor limitations; overwhelmingly consistent evidence from observational studies		Option
C. Observational studies (case-control and cohort design)	Recommendation	
D. Expert opinion, case reports, reasoning from first principles	Option	No Rec
X. Exceptional situations where validating studies cannot be performed and there is a clear preponderance of benefit or harm	Strong Recommendation / Recommendation	

FIGURE 1

Evidence quality. Integrating evidence quality appraisal with an assessment of the anticipated balance between benefits and harms if a policy is carried out leads to designation of a policy as a strong recommendation, recommendation, option, or no recommendation.[32] RCT, randomized controlled trial; Rec, recommendation.

TABLE 1 Definitions and Recommendation Implications

Statement	Definition	Implication
Strong recommendation	A *strong recommendation* in favor of a particular action is made when the anticipated benefits of the recommended intervention clearly exceed the harms (as a strong recommendation against an action is made when the anticipated harms clearly exceed the benefits) and the quality of the supporting evidence is excellent. In some clearly identified circumstances, strong recommendations may be made when high-quality evidence is impossible to obtain and the anticipated benefits strongly outweigh the harms.	Clinicians should follow a strong recommendation unless a clear and compelling rationale for an alternative approach is present.
Recommendation	A *recommendation* in favor of a particular action is made when the anticipated benefits exceed the harms but the quality of evidence is not as strong. Again, in some clearly identified circumstances, recommendations may be made when high-quality evidence is impossible to obtain but the anticipated benefits outweigh the harms.	Clinicians would be prudent to follow a recommendation but should remain alert to new information and sensitive to patient preferences.
Option	*Options* define courses that may be taken when either the quality of evidence is suspect or carefully performed studies have shown little clear advantage to 1 approach over another.	Clinicians should consider the option in their decision-making, and patient preference may have a substantial role.
No recommendation	*No recommendation* indicates that there is a lack of pertinent published evidence and that the anticipated balance of benefits and harms is presently unclear.	Clinicians should be alert to new published evidence that clarifies the balance of benefit versus harm.

It should be noted that, because childhood T2DM is a relatively recent medical phenomenon, there is a paucity of evidence for many or most of the recommendations provided. In some cases, supporting references for a specific recommendation are provided that do not deal specifically with childhood T2DM, such as T1DM, childhood obesity, or childhood "prediabetes," or that were not included in the original comprehensive search. Committee members have made every effort to identify those references that did not affect or alter the level of evidence for specific recommendations.

Systematic Reviews was performed in July 2009 for articles discussing recommendations for screening and treatment of 5 recognized comorbidities of T2DM: cardiovascular disease, dyslipidemia, retinopathy, nephropathy, and peripheral vascular disease. Search criteria were the same as for the search on treatment of T2DM, with the inclusion of the term "type 1 diabetes mellitus." Search terms included, in various combinations, the following: diabetes, mellitus, type 2, type 1, pediatric, T2DM, T1DM, NIDDM, hyperlipidemia, retinopathy, microalbuminuria, comorbidities, screening, RCT, meta-analysis, child, and adolescent. Boolean operators and search limits mirrored those of the primary search.

An additional 336 abstracts were identified for possible inclusion, of which 26 were retained for systematic review. Results of this subsequent literature review were also presented in evidence tables and published in the final evidence report. An epidemiologist appraised the methodologic quality of the research before it was considered by the committee members.

The evidence-based approach to guideline development requires that the evidence in support of each key action statement be identified, appraised, and summarized and that an explicit link between evidence and recommendations be defined. Evidence-based recommendations reflect the quality of evidence and the balance of benefit and harm that is anticipated when the recommendation is followed. The AAP policy statement, "Classifying Recommendations for Clinical Practice Guidelines,"[32] was followed in designating levels of recommendation (see Fig 1 and Table 1).

To ensure that these recommendations can be effectively implemented, the Guidelines Review Group at Yale Center for Medical Informatics provided feedback on a late draft of these recommendations, using the GuideLine Implementability Appraisal.[33] Several potential obstacles to successful implementation were identified and resolved in the final guideline. Evidence was incorporated systematically into 6 key action statements about appropriate management facilitated by BRIDGE-Wiz software (Building Recommendations in a Developer's Guideline Editor; Yale Center for Medical Informatics).

A draft version of this clinical practice guideline underwent extensive peer review by 8 groups within the AAP, the American Diabetes Association, PES, AAFP, and the Academy of Nutrition and Dietetics. Members of the subcommittee were invited to distribute the draft to other representatives and committees within their specialty organizations. The resulting comments were reviewed by the subcommittee and incorporated into the guideline, as appropriate. All AAP guidelines are reviewed every 5 years.

KEY ACTION STATEMENTS

Key Action Statement 1

Clinicians must ensure that insulin therapy is initiated for children and adolescents with T2DM who are ketotic or in diabetic ketoacidosis and in whom the distinction between T1DM and T2DM is unclear; and, in usual cases, should initiate insulin therapy for patients:

a. **who have random venous or plasma BG concentrations ≥250 mg/dL; or**

b. **whose HbA1c is >9%.**

(Strong Recommendation: evidence quality X, validating studies cannot be performed, and C, observational studies and expert opinion; preponderance of benefit over harm.)

process, blood glucose (BG) concentrations may be normal much of the time and the patient likely will be asymptomatic. At this stage, the disease may only be detected by abnormal BG concentrations identified during screening. As insulin secretion declines further, the patient is likely to develop symptoms of hyperglycemia, occasionally with ketosis or frank ketoacidosis. High glucose concentrations can cause a reversible toxicity to islet β cells that contributes further to insulin deficiency. Of adolescents in whom T2DM is subsequently diagnosed, 5% to 25% present with ketoacidosis.[34]

Diabetic ketoacidosis must be treated with insulin and fluid and electrolyte replacement to prevent worsening

T2DM. Patients in whom ketoacidosis is diagnosed require immediate treatment with insulin and fluid replacement in an inpatient setting under the supervision of a physician who is experienced in treating this complication.

Youth and adolescents who present with T2DM with poor glycemic control (BG concentrations ≥250 mg/dL or HbA1c >9%) but who lack evidence of ketosis or ketoacidosis may also benefit from initial treatment with insulin, at least on a short-term basis.[34] This allows for quicker restoration of glycemic control and, theoretically, may allow islet β cells to "rest and recover."[35,36] Furthermore, it has been noted that initiation of insulin may increase long-term adherence to treatment in children and adolescents with T2DM by enhancing the patient's perception of the seriousness of the disease.[7,37–40] Many patients with T2DM can be weaned gradually from insulin therapy and subsequently managed with metformin and lifestyle modification.[34]

As noted previously, in some children and adolescents with newly diagnosed diabetes mellitus, it may be difficult to distinguish between type 1 and type 2 disease (eg, an obese child presenting with ketosis).[39,41] These patients are best managed initially with insulin therapy while appropriate tests are performed to differentiate between T1DM and T2DM. The care of children and adolescents who have either newly diagnosed T2DM or undifferentiated-type diabetes and who require initial insulin treatment should be supervised by a physician experienced in treating diabetic patients with insulin.

Key Action Statement 2

In all other instances, clinicians should initiate a lifestyle modification program, including nutrition

Action Statement Profile KAS 1

Aggregate evidence quality	X (validating studies cannot be performed)
Benefits	Avoidance of progression of diabetic ketoacidosis (DKA) and worsening metabolic acidosis; resolution of acidosis and hyperglycemia; avoidance of coma and/or death. Quicker restoration of glycemic control, potentially allowing islet β cells to "rest and recover," increasing long-term adherence to treatment; avoiding progression to DKA if T1DM. Avoiding hospitalization. Avoidance of potential risks associated with the use of other agents (eg, abdominal discomfort, bloating, loose stools with metformin; possible cardiovascular risks with sulfonylureas).
Harms/risks/cost	Potential for hypoglycemia, insulin-induced weight gain, cost, patient discomfort from injection, necessity for BG testing, more time required by the health care team for patient training.
Benefits-harms assessment	Preponderance of benefit over harm.
Value judgments	Extensive clinical experience of the expert panel was relied on in making this recommendation.
Role of patient preferences	Minimal.
Exclusions	None.
Intentional vagueness	None.
Strength	Strong recommendation.

The presentation of T2DM in children and adolescents varies according to the disease stage. Early in the disease, before diabetes diagnostic criteria are met, insulin resistance predominates with compensatory high insulin secretion, resulting in normoglycemia. Over time, β cells lose their ability to secrete adequate amounts of insulin to overcome insulin resistance, and hyperglycemia results. Early in this

metabolic acidosis, coma, and death. Children and adolescents with symptoms of hyperglycemia (polyuria, polydipsia, and polyphagia) who are diagnosed with diabetes mellitus should be evaluated for ketosis (serum or urine ketones) and, if positive, for ketoacidosis (venous pH), even if their phenotype and risk factor status (obesity, acanthosis nigricans, positive family history of T2DM) suggests

and physical activity, and start metformin as first-line therapy for children and adolescents at the time of diagnosis of T2DM. (Strong recommendation: evidence quality B; 1 RCT showing improved outcomes with metformin versus lifestyle; preponderance of benefits over harms.)

Action Statement Profile KAS 2

Aggregate evidence quality	B (1 randomized controlled trial showing improved outcomes with metformin versus lifestyle combined with expert opinion).
Benefit	Lower HbA1c, target HbA1c sustained longer, less early deterioration of BG, less chance of weight gain, improved insulin sensitivity, improved lipid profile.
Harm (of using metformin)	Gastrointestinal adverse effects or potential for lactic acidosis and vitamin B_{12} deficiency, cost of medications, cost to administer, need for additional instruction about medication, self-monitoring blood glucose (SMBG), perceived difficulty of insulin use, possible metabolic deterioration if T1DM is misdiagnosed and treated as T2DM, potential risk of lactic acidosis in the setting of ketosis or significant dehydration. It should be noted that there have been no cases reported of vitamin B_{12} deficiency or lactic acidosis with the use of metformin in children.
Benefits-harms assessment	Preponderance of benefit over harm.
Value judgments	Committee members valued faster achievement of BG control over not medicating children.
Role of patient preferences	Moderate; precise implementation recommendations likely will be dictated by patient preferences regarding healthy nutrition, potential medication adverse reaction, exercise, and physical activity.
Exclusions	Although the recommendation to start metformin applies to all, certain children and adolescents with T2DM will not be able to tolerate metformin. In addition, certain older or more debilitated patients with T2DM may be restricted in the amount of moderate-to-vigorous exercise they can perform safely. Nevertheless, this recommendation applies to the vast majority of children and adolescents with T2DM.
Intentional vagueness	None.
Policy level	Strong recommendation.

Metformin as First-Line Therapy

Because of the low success rate with diet and exercise alone in pediatric patients diagnosed with T2DM, metformin should be initiated along with the promotion of lifestyle changes, unless insulin is needed to reverse glucose toxicity in the case of significant hyperglycemia or ketoacidosis (see Key Action Statement 1). Because gastrointestinal adverse effects are common with metformin therapy, the committee recommends starting the drug at a low dose of 500 mg daily, increasing by 500 mg every 1 to 2 weeks, up to an ideal and maximum dose of 2000 mg daily in divided doses.[41] It should be noted that the main gastrointestinal adverse effects (abdominal pain, bloating, loose stools) present at initiation of metformin often are transient and often disappear completely if medication is continued. Generally, doses higher than 2000 mg daily do not provide additional therapeutic benefit.[34,42,43] In addition, the use of extended-release metformin, especially with evening dosing, may be considered, although data regarding the frequency of adverse effects with this preparation are scarce. Metformin is generally better tolerated when taken with food. It is important to recognize the paucity of credible RCTs in adolescents with T2DM. The evidence to recommend initiating metformin at diagnosis along with lifestyle changes comes from 1 RCT, several observational studies, and consensus recommendations.

Lifestyle modifications (including nutrition interventions and increased physical activity) have long been the cornerstone of therapy for T2DM. Yet, medical practitioners recognize that effecting these changes is both challenging and often accompanied by regression over time to behaviors not conducive to maintaining the target range of BG concentrations. In pediatric patients, lifestyle change is most likely to be successful when a multidisciplinary approach is used and the entire family is involved. (Encouragement of healthy eating and physical exercise are discussed in Key Action Statements 5 and 6.) Unfortunately, efforts at lifestyle change often fail for a variety of reasons, including high rates of loss to follow-up; a high rate of depression in teenagers, which affects adherence; and peer pressure to participate in activities that often center on unhealthy eating.

Expert consensus is that fewer than 10% of pediatric T2DM patients will attain their BG goals through lifestyle interventions alone.[6,35,44] It is possible that the poor long-term success rates observed from lifestyle interventions stem from patients' perception that the intervention is not important because medications are not being prescribed. One might speculate that prescribing medications, particularly insulin therapy, may convey a greater degree of concern for the patient's health and the seriousness of the diagnosis, relative to that conveyed when medications are not needed, and that improved treatment adherence and follow-up may result from the use of medication. Indeed, 2 prospective observational studies revealed that treatment with lifestyle modification alone is associated with a higher rate of loss to follow-up than that found in patients who receive medication.[45]

Before initiating treatment with metformin, a number of important considerations must be taken into account. First, it is important to determine whether the child with a new diagnosis has T1DM or T2DM, and it is critical to err on the side of caution if there is any uncertainty. The 2009 *Clinical Practice Consensus Guidelines on Type 2 Diabetes in Children and Adolescents* from the International Society for Pediatric and Adolescent Diabetes provides more information on the classification of diabetes in children and adolescents with new diagnoses.[46] If the diagnosis is unclear (as may be the case when an obese child with diabetes presents also with ketosis), the adolescent must be treated with insulin until the T2DM diagnosis is confirmed.[47] Although it is recognized that some children with newly diagnosed T2DM may respond to metformin alone, the committee believes that the presence of either ketosis or ketoacidosis dictates an absolute initial requirement for insulin replacement. (This is addressed in Key Action Statement 1.)

Although there is little debate that a child presenting with significant hyperglycemia and/or ketosis requires insulin, children presenting with more modest levels of hyperglycemia (eg, random BG of 200–249 mg/dL) or asymptomatic T2DM present additional therapeutic challenges to the clinician. In such cases, metformin alone, insulin alone, or metformin with insulin all represent reasonable options. Additional agents are likely to become reasonable options for initial pharmacologic management in the near future. Although metformin and insulin are the only antidiabetic agents currently approved by the US Food and Drug Administration (FDA) for use in children, both thiazolidinediones and incretins are occasionally used in adolescents younger than 18 years.[48]

Metformin is recommended as the initial pharmacologic agent in adolescents presenting with mild hyperglycemia and without ketonuria or severe hyperglycemia. In addition to improving hepatic insulin sensitivity, metformin has a number of practical advantages over insulin:

● Potential weight loss or weight neutrality.[37,48]

● Because of a lower risk of hypoglycemia, less frequent finger-stick BG measurements are required with metformin, compared with insulin therapy or sulfonylureas.[37,42,49–51]

● Improves insulin sensitivity and may normalize menstrual cycles in females with polycystic ovary syndrome. (Because metformin may also improve fertility in patients with polycystic ovary syndrome, contraception is indicated for sexually active patients who wish to avoid pregnancy.)

● Taking pills does not have the discomfort associated with injections.

● Less instruction time is required to start oral medication, making it easier for busy practitioners to prescribe.

● Adolescents do not always accept injections, so oral medication might enhance adherence.[52]

Potential advantages of insulin over metformin for treatment at diabetes onset include the following:

● Metabolic control may be achieved more rapidly with insulin compared with metformin therapy.[37]

● With appropriate education and targeting the regimen to the individual, adolescents are able to accept and use insulin therapy with improved metabolic outcomes.[53]

● Insulin offers theoretical benefits of improved metabolic control while preserving β-cell function or even reversing β-cell damage.[34,35]

● Initial use of insulin therapy may convey to the patient a sense of seriousness of the disease.[7,53]

Throughout the writing of these guidelines, the authors have been following the progress of the National Institute of Diabetes and Digestive and Kidney Diseases–supported Treatment Options for type 2 Diabetes in Adolescents and Youth (TODAY) trial,[54] designed to compare standard (metformin alone) therapy versus more aggressive therapy as the initial treatment of youth with recent-onset T2DM. Since the completion of these guidelines, results of the TODAY trial have become available and reveal that metformin alone is inadequate in effecting sustained glycemic control in the majority of youth with diabetes. The study also revealed that the addition of rosiglitazone to metformin is superior to metformin alone in preserving glycemic control. Direct application of these findings to clinical practice is problematic, however, because rosiglitazone is not FDA-approved for use in children, and its use, even in adults, is now severely restricted by the FDA because of serious adverse effects reported in adults. Thus, the results suggest that therapy that is more aggressive than metformin monotherapy may be required in these adolescents to prevent loss of glycemic control, but they do not provide specific guidance because it is not known whether the effect of the additional agent was specific to rosiglitazone or would be seen with the addition of other agents. Unfortunately, there are limited data for the use of other currently available oral or injected hypoglycemic agents in this age range, except for insulin. Therefore, the writing group for these guidelines continues to recommend metformin as first-line therapy in this age group but with close monitoring for glycemic deterioration and the early addition of insulin or another pharmacologic agent if needed.

Lifestyle Modification, Including Nutrition and Physical Activity

Although lifestyle changes are considered indispensable to reaching treatment goals in diabetes, no significant data from RCTs provide information on success rates with such an approach alone.

A potential downside for initiating lifestyle changes alone at T2DM onset is potential loss of patients to follow-up and worse health outcomes. The value of lifestyle modification in the management of adolescents with T2DM is likely forthcoming after a more detailed analysis of the lifestyle intervention arm of the multicenter TODAY trial becomes available.[54] As noted previously, although it was published after

plus-rosiglitazone intervention in maintaining glycemic control over time.[54]

Summary

As noted previously, metformin is a safe and effective agent for use at the time of diagnosis in conjunction with lifestyle changes. Although observational studies and expert opinion strongly support lifestyle changes as a key component of the regimen in addition to metformin, randomized trials are needed to delineate whether using lifestyle options alone is a reasonable first step in treating any select subgroups of children with T2DM.

Key Action Statement 3

The committee suggests that clinicians monitor HbA1c concentrations every 3 months and intensify treatment if treatment goals for BG and HbA1c concentrations are not being met. (Option: evidence quality D; expert opinion and studies in children with T1DM and in adults with T2DM; preponderance of benefits over harms.)

evaluated the relationship between glycemic control and the risk of developing microvascular and/or macrovascular complications in children and adolescents with T2DM. A number of studies of children with T1DM[55–57] and adults with T2DM have, however, shown a significant relationship between glycemic control (as measured by HbA1c concentration) and the risk of microvascular complications (eg, retinopathy, nephropathy, and neuropathy).[58,59] The relationship between HbA1c concentration and risk of microvascular complications appears to be curvilinear; the lower the HbA1c concentration, the lower the downstream risk of microvascular complications, with the greatest risk reduction seen at the highest HbA1c concentrations.[57]

It is generally recommended that HbA1c concentrations be measured every 3 months.[60] For adults with T1DM, the American Diabetes Association recommends target HbA1c concentrations of less than 7%; the American Association of Clinical Endocrinologists recommends target concentrations of less than 6.5%. Although HbA1c target concentrations for children and adolescents with T1DM are higher,[13] several review articles suggest target HbA1c concentrations of less than 7% for children and adolescents with T2DM.[40,61–63] The committee concurs that, ideally, target HbA1c concentration should be less than 7% but notes that specific goals must be achievable for the individual patient and that this concentration may not be applicable for all patients. For patients in whom a target concentration of less than 7% seems unattainable, individualized goals should be set, with the ultimate goal of reaching guideline target concentrations. In addition, in the absence of hypoglycemia, even lower HbA1c target concentrations can be considered on the basis of an absence of hypoglycemic events and other individual considerations.

Action Statement Profile KAS 3

Aggregate evidence quality	D (expert opinion and studies in children with T1DM and in adults with T2DM; no studies have been performed in children and adolescents with T2DM).
Benefit	Diminishing the risk of progression of disease and deterioration resulting in hospitalization; prevention of microvascular complications of T2DM.
Harm	Potential for hypoglycemia from overintensifying treatment to reach HbA1c target goals; cost of frequent testing and medical consultation; possible patient discomfort.
Benefits-harms assessment	Preponderance of benefits over harms.
Value judgments	Recommendation dictated by widely accepted standards of diabetic care.
Role of patient preferences	Minimal; recommendation dictated by widely accepted standards of diabetic care.
Exclusions	None.
Intentional vagueness	Intentional vagueness in the recommendation as far as setting goals and intensifying treatment attributable to limited evidence.
Policy level	Option.

this guideline was developed, the TODAY trial indicated that results from the metformin-plus-lifestyle intervention were not significantly different from either metformin alone or the metformin-

HbA1c provides a measure of glycemic control in patients with diabetes mellitus and allows an estimation of the individual's average BG over the previous 8 to 12 weeks. No RCTs have

When concentrations are found to be above the target, therapy should be intensified whenever possible, with the goal of bringing the concentration to target. Intensification activities may include, but are not limited to, increasing the frequency of clinic visits, engaging in more frequent BG monitoring, adding 1 or more antidiabetic agents, meeting with a registered dietitian and/or diabetes educator, and increasing attention to diet and exercise regimens. Patients whose HbA1c concentrations remain relatively stable may only need to be tested every 6 months. Ideally, real-time HbA1c concentrations should be available at the time of the patient's visit with the clinician to allow the physician and patient and/or parent to discuss intensification of therapy during the visit, if needed.

Key Action Statement 4

The committee suggests that clinicians advise patients to monitor finger-stick BG concentrations in those who

a. are taking insulin or other medications with a risk of hypoglycemia; or

b. are initiating or changing their diabetes treatment regimen; or

c. have not met treatment goals; or

d. have intercurrent illnesses.

(Option: evidence quality D; expert consensus. Preponderance of benefits over harms.)

Glycemic control correlates closely with the frequency of BG monitoring in adolescents with T1DM.[64,65] Although studies evaluating the efficacy of frequent BG monitoring have not been conducted in children and adolescents with T2DM, benefits have been described in insulin-treated adults with T2DM who tested their BG 4 times per day, compared with adults following a less frequent monitoring regimen.[66] These data support the value of BG monitoring in adults treated with insulin, and likely are relevant to youth with T2DM as well, especially those treated with insulin, at the onset of the disease, when treatment goals are not met, and when the treatment regimen is changed. The committee believes that current (2011) ADA recommendations for finger-stick BG monitoring apply to most youth with T2DM[67]:

- Finger-stick BG monitoring should be performed 3 or more times daily for patients using multiple insulin injections or insulin pump therapy.

- For patients using less-frequent insulin injections, noninsulin therapies, or medical nutrition therapy alone, finger-stick BG monitoring may be useful as a guide to the success of therapy.

- To achieve postprandial glucose targets, postprandial finger-stick BG monitoring may be appropriate.

Recognizing that current practices may not always reflect optimal care, a 2004 survey of practices among members of the PES revealed that 36% of pediatric endocrinologists asked their pediatric patients with T2DM to monitor BG concentrations twice daily; 12% asked patients to do so once daily; 13% asked patients to do so 3 times per day; and 12% asked patients to do so 4 times daily.[61] The questionnaire provided to the pediatric endocrinologists did not ask about the frequency of BG monitoring in relationship to the diabetes regimen, however.

Although normoglycemia may be difficult to achieve in adolescents with T2DM, a fasting BG concentration of 70 to 130 mg/dL is a reasonable target for most. In addition, because postprandial hyperglycemia has been associated with increased risk of cardiovascular events in adults, postprandial BG testing may be valuable in select patients. BG concentrations obtained 2 hours after meals (and paired with pre-meal concentrations) provide an index of glycemic excursion, and may be useful in improving glycemic control, particularly for the patient whose fasting plasma glucose is normal but whose HbA1c is not at target.[68] Recognizing the limited evidence for benefit of FSBG testing in this population, the committee provides suggested guidance for testing frequency, tailored to the medication regimen, as follows:

BG Testing Frequency for Patients With Newly Diagnosed T2DM: Fasting, Premeal, and Bedtime Testing

The committee suggests that all patients with newly diagnosed T2DM, regardless of prescribed treatment plan, should perform finger-stick BG monitoring before meals (including a morning fasting concentration) and

Action Statement Profile KAS 4

Aggregate evidence quality	D (expert consensus).
Benefit	Potential for improved metabolic control, improved potential for prevention of hypoglycemia, decreased long-term complications.
Harm	Patient discomfort, cost of materials.
Benefits-harms assessment	Benefit over harm.
Value judgments	Despite lack of evidence, there were general committee perceptions that patient safety concerns related to insulin use or clinical status outweighed any risks from monitoring.
Role of patient preferences	Moderate to low; recommendation driven primarily by safety concerns.
Exclusions	None.
Intentional vagueness	Intentional vagueness in the recommendation about specific approaches attributable to lack of evidence and the need to individualize treatment.
Policy level	Option.

at bedtime until reasonable metabolic control is achieved.[69] Once BG concentrations are at target levels, the frequency of monitoring can be modified depending on the medication used, the regimen's intensity, and the patient's metabolic control. Patients who are prone to marked hyperglycemia or hypoglycemia or who are on a therapeutic regimen associated with increased risk of hypoglycemia will require continued frequent BG testing. Expectations for frequency and timing of BG monitoring should be clearly defined through shared goal-setting between the patient and clinician. The adolescent and family members should be given a written action plan stating the medication regimen, frequency and timing of expected BG monitoring, as well as follow-up instructions.

BG Testing Frequency for Patients on Single Insulin Daily Injections and Oral Agents

Single bedtime long-acting insulin: The simplest insulin regimen consists of a single injection of long-acting insulin at bedtime (basal insulin only). The appropriateness of the insulin dose for patients using this regimen is best defined by the fasting/prebreakfast BG test. For patients on this insulin regimen, the committee suggests daily fasting BG measurements. This regimen is associated with some risk of hypoglycemia (especially overnight or fasting hypoglycemia) and may not provide adequate insulin coverage for mealtime ingestions throughout the day, as reflected by fasting BG concentrations in target, but daytime readings above target. In such cases, treatment with meglitinide (Prandin [Novo Nordisk Pharmaceuticals] or Starlix [Novartis Pharmaceuticals]) or a short-acting insulin before meals (see below) may be beneficial.

Oral agents: Once treatment goals are met, the frequency of monitoring can be decreased; however, the committee recommends some continued BG testing for all youth with T2DM, at a frequency determined within the clinical context (e.g. medication regimen, HbA1c, willingness of the patient, etc.). For example, an infrequent or intermittent monitoring schedule may be adequate when the patient is using exclusively an oral agent associated with a low risk of hypoglycemia and if HbA1c concentrations are in the ideal or non-diabetic range. A more frequent monitoring schedule should be advised during times of illness or if symptoms of hyperglycemia or hypoglycemia develop.

Oral agent plus a single injection of a long-acting insulin: Some youth with T2DM can be managed successfully with a single injection of long-acting insulin in conjunction with an oral agent. Twice a day BG monitoring (fasting plus a second BG concentration — ideally 2-hour post prandial) often is recommended, as long as HbA1c and BG concentrations remain at goal and the patient remains asymptomatic.

BG Testing Frequency for Patients Receiving Multiple Daily Insulin Injections (eg, Basal Bolus Regimens): Premeal and Bedtime Testing

Basal bolus regimens are commonly used in children and youth with T1DM and may be appropriate for some youth with T2DM as well. They are the most labor intensive, providing both basal insulin plus bolus doses of short-acting insulin at meals. Basal insulin is provided through either the use of long-acting, relatively peak-free insulin (by needle) or via an insulin pump. Bolus insulin doses are given at meal-time, using one of the rapid-acting insulin analogs. The bolus dose is calculated by using a correction algorithm for the premeal BG concentration as well as a "carb ratio," in which 1 unit of

a rapid-acting insulin analog is given for "X" grams of carbohydrates ingested (see box below). When using this method, the patient must be willing and able to count the number of grams of carbohydrates in the meal and divide by the assigned "carb ratio (X)" to know how many units of insulin should be taken. In addition, the patient must always check BG concentrations before the meal to determine how much additional insulin should be given as a correction dose using an algorithm assigned by the care team if the fasting BG is not in target. Insulin pumps are based on this concept of "basal-bolus" insulin administration and have the capability of calculating a suggested bolus dosage, based on inputted grams of carbohydrates and BG concentrations. Because the BG value determines the amount of insulin to be given at each meal, the recommended testing frequency for patients on this regimen is before every meal.

Box 1 Example of Basal Bolus Insulin Regimen

If an adolescent has a BG of 250 mg/dL, is to consume a meal containing 60 g of carbohydrates, with a carbohydrate ratio of 1:10 and an assigned correction dose of 1:25>125 (with 25 being the insulin sensitivity and 125 mg/dL the target blood glucose level), the mealtime bolus dose of insulin would be as follows:

60 g/10 "carb ratio" =

6 units rapid-acting insulin for meal

plus

(250−125)/25 = 125/25 =

5 units rapid-acting insulin for correction

Thus, total bolus insulin coverage at mealtime is: **11 U** (6 + 5) of rapid-acting insulin.

Key Action Statement 5

The committee suggests that clinicians incorporate the Academy of Nutrition and Dietetics' *Pediatric Weight Management Evidence-Based Nutrition Practice Guidelines* **in the nutrition counseling of patients with T2DM both at the time of diagnosis and as part of ongoing management. (Option; evidence quality D; expert opinion; preponderance of benefits over harms. Role of patient preference is dominant.)**

Action Statement Profile KAS 5

Aggregate evidence quality	D (expert opinion).
Benefit	Promotes weight loss; improves insulin sensitivity; contributes to glycemic control; prevents worsening of disease; facilitates a sense of well-being; and improves cardiovascular health.
Harm	Costs of nutrition counseling; inadequate reimbursement of clinicians' time; lost opportunity costs vis-a-vis time and resources spent in other counseling activities.
Benefits-harms assessment	Benefit over harm.
Value judgments	There is a broad societal agreement on the benefits of dietary recommendations.
Role of patient preference	Dominant. Patients may have different preferences for how they wish to receive assistance in managing their weight-loss goals. Some patients may prefer a referral to a nutritionist while others might prefer accessing online sources of help. Patient preference should play a significant role in determining an appropriate weight-loss strategy.
Exclusions	None.
Intentional vagueness	Intentional vagueness in the recommendation about specific approaches attributable to lack of evidence and the need to individualize treatment.
Policy level	Option.

Consuming more calories than one uses results in weight gain and is a major contributor to the increasing incidence of T2DM in children and adolescents. Current literature is inconclusive about a single best meal plan for patients with diabetes mellitus, however, and studies specifically addressing the diet of children and adolescents with T2DM are limited. Challenges to making recommendations stem from the small sample size of these studies, limited specificity for children and adolescents, and difficulties in generalizing the data from dietary research studies to the general population.

Although evidence is lacking in children with T2DM, numerous studies have been conducted in overweight children and adolescents, because the great majority of children with T2DM are obese or overweight at diagnosis.[26] The committee suggests that clinicians encourage children and adolescents with T2DM to follow the Academy of Nutrition and Dietetics' recommendations for maintaining healthy weight to promote health and reduce obesity in this population. The committee recommends that clinicians refer patients to a registered dietitian who has expertise in the nutritional needs of youth with T2DM. Clinicians should incorporate the Academy of Nutrition and Dietetics' *Pediatric Weight Management Evidence-Based Nutrition Practice Guidelines*, which describe effective, evidence-based treatment options for weight management, summarized below (A complete list of these recommendations is accessible to health care professionals at: http://www.andevidencelibrary.com/topic.cfm?cat=4102&auth=1.)

According to the Academy of Nutrition and Dietetics' guidelines, when incorporated with lifestyle changes, balanced macronutrient diets at 900 to 1200 kcal per day are associated with both short- and long-term (eg, ≥ 1 year) improvements in weight status and body composition in children 6 to 12 years of age.[70] These calorie recommendations are to be incorporated with lifestyle changes, including increased activity and possibly medication. Restrictions of no less than 1200 kcal per day in adolescents 13 to 18 years old result in improved weight status and body composition as well.[71] The Diabetes Prevention Program demonstrated that participants assigned to the intensive lifestyle-intervention arm had a reduction in daily energy intake of 450 kcal and a 58% reduction in progression to diabetes at the 2.8-year follow-up.[71] At the study's end, 50% of the lifestyle-arm participants had achieved the goal weight loss of at least 7% after the 24-week curriculum and 38% showed weight loss of at least 7% at the time of their most recent visit.[72] The Academy of Nutrition and Dietetics recommends that protein-sparing, modified-fast (ketogenic) diets be restricted to children who are >120% of their ideal body weight and who have a serious medical complication that would benefit from rapid weight loss.[71] Specific recommendations are for the intervention to be short-term (typically 10 weeks) and to be conducted under the supervision of a multidisciplinary team specializing in pediatric obesity.

Regardless of the meal plan prescribed, some degree of nutrition education must be provided to maximize adherence and positive results. This education should encourage patients to follow healthy eating patterns, such as consuming 3 meals with planned snacks per day, not eating while watching television or using computers, using smaller plates to make portions appear larger, and leaving small amounts of food on the plate.[73] Common dietary recommendations to reduce calorie intake and to promote weight loss in children include the following: (1) eating regular meals and snacks; (2) reducing portion sizes; (3) choosing calorie-free beverages, except for milk; (4) limiting juice to 1 cup per day; (5) increasing consumption of fruits and vegetables; (6) consuming 3 or 4 servings of low-fat dairy products per day; (7) limiting intake of high-fat foods; (8) limiting frequency and size of snacks; and (9) reducing calories consumed in fast-food meals.[74]

Key Action Statement 6

The committee suggests that clinicians encourage children and adolescents with T2DM to engage in moderate-to-vigorous exercise for at least 60 minutes daily and to limit nonacademic screen time to less than 2 hours per day. (Option: evidence quality D, expert opinion and evidence from studies of metabolic syndrome and obesity; preponderance of benefits over harms. Role of patient preference is dominant.)

Action Statement Profile KAS 6

Aggregate evidence quality	D (expert opinion and evidence from studies of metabolic syndrome and obesity).
Benefit	Promotes weight loss; contributes to glycemic control; prevents worsening of disease; facilitates the ability to perform exercise; improves the person's sense of well-being; and fosters cardiovascular health.
Harm	Cost for patient of counseling, food, and time; costs for clinician in taking away time that could be spent on other activities; inadequate reimbursement for clinician's time.
Benefits-harms assessment	Preponderance of benefit over harm.
Value judgments	Broad consensus.
Role of patient preference	Dominant. Patients may seek various forms of exercise. Patient preference should play a significant role in creating an exercise plan.
Exclusions	Although certain older or more debilitated patients with T2DM may be restricted in the amount of moderate-to-vigorous exercise they can perform safely, this recommendation applies to the vast majority of children and adolescents with T2DM.
Intentional vagueness	Intentional vagueness on the sequence of follow-up contact attributable to the lack of evidence and the need to individualize care.
Policy level	Option.

Recommendations From the Academy of Nutrition and Dietetics

Pediatric Weight Management Evidence-Based Nutrition Practice Guidelines

Recommendation	Strength
Interventions to reduce pediatric obesity should be multicomponent and include diet, physical activity, nutritional counseling, and parent or caregiver participation.	Strong
A nutrition prescription should be formulated as part of the dietary intervention in a multicomponent pediatric weight management program.	Strong
Dietary factors that may be associated with an increased risk of overweight are increased total dietary fat intake and increased intake of calorically sweetened beverages.	Strong
Dietary factors that may be associated with a decreased risk of overweight are increased fruit and vegetable intake.	Strong
A balanced macronutrient diet that contains no fewer than 900 kcal per day is recommended to improve weight status in children aged 6–12 y who are medically monitored.	Strong
A balanced macronutrient diet that contains no fewer than 1200 kcal per day is recommended to improve weight status in adolescents aged 13–18 y who are medically monitored.	Strong
Family diet behaviors that are associated with an increased risk of pediatric obesity are parental restriction of highly palatable foods, consumption of food away from home, increased meal portion size, and skipping breakfast.	Fair

Engaging in Physical Activity

Physical activity is an integral part of weight management for prevention and treatment of T2DM. Although there is a paucity of available data from children and adolescents with T2DM, several well-controlled studies performed in obese children and adolescents at risk of metabolic syndrome and T2DM provide guidelines for physical activity. (See the Resources section for tools on this subject.) A summary of the references supporting the evidence for this guideline can be found in the technical report.[31]

At present, moderate-to-vigorous exercise of at least 60 minutes daily is recommended for reduction of BMI and improved glycemic control in patients with T2DM.[75] "Moderate to vigorous exercise" is defined as exercise that makes the individual breathe hard and perspire and that raises his or her heart rate. An easy way to define exercise intensity for patients is the "talk test"; during moderate physical activity a person can talk but not sing. During vigorous activity, a person cannot talk without pausing to catch a breath.[76]

Adherence may be improved if clinicians provide the patient with a written prescription to engage in physical activity, including a "dose" describing ideal duration, intensity, and frequency.[75] When prescribing physical exercise, clinicians are encouraged to be sensitive to the needs of children, adolescents, and their families. Routine, organized exercise may be beyond the family's logistical and/or financial means, and some families may not be able to provide structured exercise programs for their children. It is most helpful to recommend an individualized approach that can be incorporated into the daily routine, is tailored to the patients' physical abilities and preferences, and recognizes the families' circumstances.[77] For example, clinicians might recommend only daily walking, which has been shown to improve weight loss and insulin sensitivity in adults with T2DM[78] and may constitute "moderate to vigorous activity" for some children with T2DM. It is also important to recognize that the recommended 60 minutes of exercise do not have to be accomplished in 1 session but can be completed through several, shorter increments (eg, 10–15 minutes). Patients should be encouraged to identify a variety of forms of activity that can be performed both easily and frequently.[77] In addition, providers should be cognizant of the potential need to adjust the medication dosage, especially if the patient is receiving insulin, when initiating an aggressive physical activity program.

Reducing Screen Time

Screen time contributes to a sedentary lifestyle, especially when the child or adolescent eats while watching television or playing computer games. The US Department of Health and Human Services recommends that individuals limit "screen time" spent watching television and/or using computers and handheld devices to less than 2 hours per day unless the use is related to work or homework.[79] Physical activity may be gained either through structured games and sports or through everyday activities, such as walking, ideally with involvement of the parents as good role models.

Increased screen time and food intake and reduced physical activity are associated with obesity. There is good evidence that modifying these factors can help prevent T2DM by reducing the individual's rate of weight gain. The evidence profile in pediatric patients with T2DM is inadequate at this time, however. Pending new data, the committee suggests that clinicians follow the AAP Committee on Nutrition's guideline, *Prevention of Pediatric Overweight and Obesity.* The guideline recommends restricting nonacademic screen time to a maximum of 2 hours per day and discouraging the presence of video screens and television sets in children's bedrooms.[80–82] The American Medical Association's Expert Panel on Childhood Obesity has endorsed this guideline.

Valuable recommendations for enhancing patient health include the following:

- With patients and their families, jointly determining an individualized plan that includes specific goals to reduce sedentary behaviors and increase physical activity.
- Providing a written prescription for engaging in 60-plus minutes of moderate-to-vigorous physical activities per day that includes

dose, timing, and duration. It is important for clinicians to be sensitive to the needs of children, adolescents, and their families in encouraging daily physical exercise. Graded duration of exercise is recommended for those youth who cannot initially be active for 60 minutes daily, and the exercise may be accomplished through several, shorter increments (eg, 10–15 minutes).

- Incorporating physical activities into children's and adolescents' daily routines. Physical activity may be gained either through structured games and sports or through everyday activities, such as walking.
- Restricting nonacademic screen time to a maximum of 2 hours per day.
- Discouraging the presence of video screens and television sets in children's bedrooms.

Conversations pertaining to the Key Action Statements should be clearly documented in the patient's medical record.

AREAS FOR FUTURE RESEARCH

As noted previously, evidence for medical interventions in children in general is scant and is especially lacking for interventions directed toward children who have developed diseases not previously seen commonly in youth, such as childhood T2DM. Recent studies such as the Search for Diabetes in Youth Study (SEARCH)—an observational multicenter study in 2096 youth with T2DM funded by the Centers for Disease Control and Prevention and the National Institute of Diabetes and Digestive and Kidney Diseases—now provide a detailed description of childhood diabetes. Subsequent trials will describe the short-term and enduring effects of specific interventions on the progression of the disease with time.

Although it is likely that children and adolescents with T2DM have an aggressive form of diabetes, as reflected by the age of onset, future research should determine whether the associated comorbidities and complications of diabetes also are more aggressive in pediatric populations than in adults and if they are more or less responsive to therapeutic interventions. Additional research should explore whether early introduction of insulin or the use of particular oral agents will preserve β-cell function in these children, and whether recent technologic advances (such as continuous glucose monitoring and insulin pumps) will benefit this population. Additional issues that require further study include the following:

- To delineate whether using lifestyle options without medication is a reliable first step in treating selected children with T2DM.

- To determine whether BG monitoring should be recommended to all children and youth with T2DM, regardless of therapy used; what the optimal frequency of BG monitoring is for pediatric patients on the basis of treatment regimen; and which subgroups will be able to successfully maintain glycemic goals with less frequent monitoring.

- To explore the efficacy of school- and clinic-based diet and physical activity interventions to prevent and manage pediatric T2DM.

- To explore the association between increased "screen time" and reduced physical activity with respect to T2DM's risk factors.

RESOURCES

Several tools are available online to assist providers in improving patient adherence to lifestyle modifications, including examples of activities to be recommended for patients:

- The American Academy of Pediatrics:
  - www.healthychildren.org
  - www.letsmove.gov
  - Technical Report: Management of Type 2 Diabetes Mellitus in Children and Adolescents.[31]
    - Includes an overview and screening tools for a variety of comorbidities.

  - Gahagan S, Silverstein J; Committee on Native American Child Health and Section on Endocrinology. Clinical report: prevention and treatment of type 2 diabetes mellitus in children, with special emphasis on American Indian and Alaska Native Children. *Pediatrics*. 2003;112 (4):e328–e347. Available at: http://www.pediatrics.org/cgi/content/full/112/4/e328[63]
    - Fig 3 presents a screening tool for microalbumin.

  - Bright Futures: http://brightfutures.aap.org/

  - Daniels SR, Greer FR; Committee on Nutrition. Lipid screening and cardiovascular health in childhood. *Pediatrics*. 2008;122 (1):198–208. Available at:

- The American Diabetes Association: www.diabetes.org
  - Management of dyslipidemia in children and adolescents with diabetes. *Diabetes Care*. 2003;26(7):2194–2197. Available at: http://care.diabetesjournals.org/content/26/7/2194.full

- Academy of Nutrition and Dietetics:
  - http://www.eatright.org/childhoodobesity/
  - http://www.eatright.org/kids/
  - http://www.eatright.org/cps/rde/xchg/ada/hs.xsl/index.html

- Pediatric Weight Management Evidence-Based Nutrition Practice Guidelines: http://www.adaevidencelibrary.com/topic.cfm?cat=2721

- American Heart Association:
  - American Heart Association *Circulation*. 2006 Dec 12;114(24):2710-2738. Epub 2006 Nov 27. Review.

- Centers for Disease Control and Prevention:
  - http://www.cdc.gov/obesity/childhood/solutions.html
  - BMI and other growth charts can be downloaded and printed from the CDC Web site: http://www.cdc.gov/growthcharts.
  - Center for Epidemiologic Studies Depression Scale (CES-D): http://www.chcr.brown.edu/pcoc/cesdscale.pdf; see attachments

- *Diagnostic and Statistical Manual of Mental Disorders*. 4th ed. Washington, DC: American Psychiatric Association; 1994

- Let's Move Campaign: www.letsmove.gov

- The Reach Institute. *Guidelines for Adolescent Depression in Primary Care (GLAD-PC) Toolkit*, 2007. Contains a listing of the criteria for major depressive disorder as defined by the DSM-IV-TR. Available at: http://www.gladpc.org

- The National Heart, Lung, and Blood Institute (NHLBI) hypertension guidelines: http://www.nhlbi.nih.gov/guidelines/hypertension/child_tbl.htm

- The National Diabetes Education Program and TIP sheets (including tip sheets on youth transitioning to adulthood and adult providers, Staying Active, Eating Healthy, Ups and Downs of Diabetes, etc): www.ndep.nih.gov or www.yourdiabetesinfo.org

- National High Blood Pressure Education Program Working Group on High Blood Pressure in Children and Adolescents, The Fourth Report on the Diagnosis, Evaluation, and Treatment of High Blood Pressure in Children and Adolescents: *Pediatrics*. 2004;114:555–576. Available at: http://pediatrics.aappublications.org/content/114/Supplement_2/555.long

- National Initiative for Children's Healthcare Quality (NICHQ): childhood obesity section: http://www.nichq.org/childhood_obesity/index.html

- The National Institute of Child Health and Human Development (NICHD): www.NICHD.org

- President's Council on Physical Fitness and Sports: http://www.presidentschallenge.org/home_kids.aspx

- US Department of Agriculture's "My Pyramid" Web site:

- http://www.choosemyplate.gov/

- http://fnic.nal.usda.gov/life-cycle-nutrition/child-nutrition-and-health

SUBCOMMITTEE ON TYPE 2 DIABETES (OVERSIGHT BY THE STEERING COMMITTEE ON QUALITY IMPROVEMENT AND MANAGEMENT, 2008–2012)

Kenneth Claud Copeland, MD, FAAP: Co-chair—Endocrinology and Pediatric Endocrine Society Liaison (2009: Novo Nordisk, Genentech, Endo [National Advisory Groups]; 2010: Novo Nordisk [National Advisory Group]); published research related to type 2 diabetes

Janet Silverstein, MD, FAAP: Co-chair—Endocrinology and American Diabetes Association Liaison (small grants with Pfizer, Novo Nordisk, and Lilly; grant review committee for Genentech; was on an advisory committee for Sanofi Aventis, and Abbott Laboratories for a 1-time meeting); published research related to type 2 diabetes

Kelly Roberta Moore, MD, FAAP: General Pediatrics, Indian Health, AAP Committee on Native American Child Health Liaison (board member of the Merck Company Foundation Alliance to Reduce Disparities in Diabetes. Their national program office is the University of Michigan's Center for Managing Chronic Disease.)

Greg Edward Prazar, MD, FAAP: General Pediatrics (no conflicts)

Terry Raymer, MD, CDE: Family Medicine, Indian Health Service (no conflicts)

Richard N. Shiffman, MD, FAAP: Partnership for Policy Implementation Informatician, General Pediatrics (no conflicts)

Shelley C. Springer, MD, MBA, FAAP: Epidemiologist (no conflicts)

Meaghan Anderson, MS, RD, LD, CDE: Academy of Nutrition and Dietetics Liaison (formerly a Certified Pump Trainer for Animas)

Stephen J. Spann, MD, MBA, FAAFP: American Academy of Family Physicians Liaison (no conflicts)

Vidhu V. Thaker, MD, FAAP: QuIIN Liaison, General Pediatrics (no conflicts)

CONSULTANT

Susan K. Flinn, MA: Medical Writer (no conflicts)

STAFF

Caryn Davidson, MA

REFERENCES

1. Centers for Disease Control and Prevention. Data and Statistics. Obesity rates among children in the United States. Available at: www.cdc.gov/obesity/childhood/prevalence.html. Accessed August 13, 2012

2. Copeland KC, Chalmers LJ, Brown RD. Type 2 diabetes in children: oxymoron or medical metamorphosis? *Pediatr Ann*. 2005;34 (9):686–697

3. Narayan KM, Boyle JP, Thompson TJ, Sorensen SW, Williamson DF. Lifetime risk for diabetes mellitus in the United States. *JAMA*. 2003;290(14):1884–1890

4. Chopra M, Galbraith S, Darnton-Hill I. A global response to a global problem: the epidemic of overnutrition. *Bull World Health Organ*. 2002;80(12):952–958

5. Liese AD, D'Agostino RB, Jr, Hamman RF, et al; SEARCH for Diabetes in Youth Study Group. The burden of diabetes mellitus among US youth: prevalence estimates from the SEARCH for Diabetes in Youth Study. *Pediatrics*. 2006;118(4):1510–1518

6. Silverstein JH, Rosenbloom AL. Type 2 diabetes in children. *Curr Diab Rep*. 2001;1 (1):19–27

7. Pinhas-Hamiel O, Zeitler P. Clinical presentation and treatment of type 2 diabetes in children. *Pediatr Diabetes*. 2007;8(suppl 9):16–27

8. Dabelea D, Bell RA, D'Agostino RB Jr, et al; Writing Group for the SEARCH for Diabetes in Youth Study Group. Incidence of diabetes in youth in the United States. *JAMA*. 2007; 297(24):2716–2724

9. Mayer-Davis EJ, Bell RA, Dabelea D, et al; SEARCH for Diabetes in Youth Study Group. The many faces of diabetes in American youth: type 1 and type 2 diabetes in five race and ethnic populations: the SEARCH for Diabetes in Youth Study. *Diabetes Care*. 2009;32(suppl 2):S99–S101

10. Copeland KC, Zeitler P, Geffner M, et al; TODAY Study Group. Characteristics of adolescents and youth with recent-onset type 2 diabetes: the TODAY cohort at baseline. *J Clin Endocrinol Metab*. 2011;96(1):159–167

11. Narayan KM, Williams R. Diabetes—a global problem needing global solutions. *Prim Care Diabetes*. 2009;3(1):3–4

12. Wild S, Roglic G, Green A, Sicree R, King H. Global prevalence of diabetes: estimates for the year 2000 and projections for 2030. *Diabetes Care*. 2004;27(5):1047–1053

13. Silverstein J, Klingensmith G, Copeland K, et al; American Diabetes Association. Care of children and adolescents with type 1 diabetes: a statement of the American Diabetes Association. *Diabetes Care*. 2005;28 (1):186–212

14. Pinhas-Hamiel O, Zeitler P. Barriers to the treatment of adolescent type 2 diabetes—a survey of provider perceptions. *Pediatr Diabetes*. 2003;4(1):24–28

15. Moore KR, McGowan MK, Donato KA, Kollipara S, Roubideaux Y. Community resources for promoting youth nutrition and physical activity. *Am J Health Educ*. 2009;40(5):298–303

16. Zeitler P, Epstein L, Grey M, et al; The TODAY Study Group. Treatment Options for type 2 diabetes mellitus in Adolescents and Youth: a study of the comparative efficacy of metformin alone or in combination with rosiglitazone or lifestyle intervention in adolescents with type 2 diabetes mellitus. *Pediatr Diabetes*. 2007;8(2):74–87

17. Kane MP, Abu-Baker A, Busch RS. The utility of oral diabetes medications in type 2

diabetes of the young. *Curr Diabetes Rev.* 2005;1(1):83–92

18. De Berardis G, Pellegrini F, Franciosi M, et al. Quality of care and outcomes in type 2 diabetes patientes. *Diabetes Care.* 2004;27(2):398–406

19. Ziemer DC, Miller CD, Rhee MK, et al. Clinical inertia contributes to poor diabetes control in a primary care setting. *Diabetes Educ.* 2005;31(4):564–571

20. Bradshaw B. The role of the family in managing therapy in minority children with type 2 diabetes mellitus. *J Pediatr Endocrinol Metab.* 2002;15(suppl 1):547–551

21. Pinhas-Hamiel O, Standiford D, Hamiel D, Dolan LM, Cohen R, Zeitler PS. The type 2 family: a setting for development and treatment of adolescent type 2 diabetes mellitus. *Arch Pediatr Adolesc Med.* 1999; 153(10):1063–1067

22. Mulvaney SA, Schlundt DG, Mudasiru E, et al. Parent perceptions of caring for adolescents with type 2 diabetes. *Diabetes Care.* 2006;29(5):993–997

23. Summerbell CD, Ashton V, Campbell KJ, Edmunds L, Kelly S, Waters E. Interventions for treating obesity in children. *Cochrane Database Syst Rev.* 2003;(3):CD001872

24. Skinner AC, Weinberger M, Mulvaney S, Schlundt D, Rothman RL. Accuracy of perceptions of overweight and relation to self-care behaviors among adolescents with type 2 diabetes and their parents. *Diabetes Care.* 2008;31(2):227–229

25. American Diabetes Association. Type 2 diabetes in children and adolescents. *Diabetes Care.* 2000;23(3):381–389

26. Pinhas-Hamiel O, Zeitler P. Type 2 diabetes in adolescents, no longer rare. *Pediatr Rev.* 1998;19(12):434–435

27. Fagot-Campagna A, Pettitt DJ, Engelgau MM, et al. Type 2 diabetes among North American children and adolescents: an epidemiologic review and a public health perspective. *J Pediatr.* 2000;136(5):664–672

28. Rothman RL, Mulvaney S, Elasy TA, et al. Self-management behaviors, racial disparities, and glycemic control among adolescents with type 2 diabetes. *Pediatrics.* 2008;121(4). Available at: www.pediatrics.org/cgi/content/full/121/4/e912

29. Scott CR, Smith JM, Cradock MM, Pihoker C. Characteristics of youth-onset noninsulin-dependent diabetes mellitus and insulin-dependent diabetes mellitus at diagnosis. *Pediatrics.* 1997;100(1):84–91

30. Libman IM, Pietropaolo M, Arslanian SA, LaPorte RE, Becker DJ. Changing prevalence of overweight children and adolescents at onset of insulin-treated diabetes. *Diabetes Care.* 2003;26(10):2871–2875

31. Springer SC, Copeland KC, Silverstein J, et al. Technical report: management of type 2 diabetes mellitus in children and adolescents. *Pediatrics.* 2012, In press

32. American Academy of Pediatrics Steering Committee on Quality Improvement and Management. Classifying recommendations for clinical practice guidelines. *Pediatrics.* 2004;114(3):874–877

33. Shiffman RN, Dixon J, Brandt C, et al. The GuideLine Implementability Appraisal (GLIA): development of an instrument to identify obstacles to guideline implementation. *BMC Med Inform Decis Mak.* 2005;5:23

34. Gungor N, Hannon T, Libman I, Bacha F, Arslanian S. Type 2 diabetes mellitus in youth: the complete picture to date. *Pediatr Clin North Am.* 2005;52(6):1579–1609

35. Daaboul JJ, Siverstein JH. The management of type 2 diabetes in children and adolescents. *Minerva Pediatr.* 2004;56(3):255–264

36. Kadmon PM, Grupposo PA. Glycemic control with metformin or insulin therapy in adolescents with type 2 diabetes mellitus. *J Pediatr Endocrinol.* 2004;17(9):1185–1193

37. Owada M, Nitadori Y, Kitagawa T. Treatment of NIDDM in youth. *Clin Pediatr (Phila).* 1998;37(2):117–121

38. Pinhas-Hamiel O, Zeitler P. Advances in epidemiology and treatment of type 2 diabetes in children. *Adv Pediatr.* 2005;52:223–259

39. Jones KL, Haghi M. Type 2 diabetes mellitus in children and adolescence: a primer. *Endocrinologist.* 2000;10:389–396

40. Kawahara R, Amemiya T, Yoshino M, et al. Dropout of young non-insulin-dependent diabetics from diabetic care. *Diabetes Res Clin Pract.* 1994;24(3):181–185

41. Kaufman FR. Type 2 diabetes mellitus in children and youth: a new epidemic. *J Pediatr Endocrinol Metab.* 2002;15(suppl 2):737–744

42. Garber AJ, Duncan TG, Goodman AM, Mills DJ, Rohlf JL. Efficacy of metformin in type II diabetes: results of a double-blind, placebo-controlled, dose-response trial. *Am J Med.* 1997;103(6):491–497

43. Dabelea D, Pettitt DJ, Jones KL, Arslanian SA. Type 2 diabetes mellitus in minority children and adolescents: an emerging problem. *Endocrinol Metabo Clin North Am.* 1999;28(4):709–729

44. Miller JL, Silverstein JH. The management of type 2 diabetes mellitus in children and adolescents. *J Pediatr Endocrinol Metab.* 2005;18(2):111–123

45. Reinehr T, Schober E, Roth CL, Wiegand S, Holl R; DPV-Wiss Study Group. Type 2 diabetes in children and adolescents in a 2-year

follow-up: insufficient adherence to diabetes centers. *Horm Res.* 2008;69(2):107–113

46. Rosenbloom AL, Silverstein JH, Amemiya S, Zeitler P, Klingensmith GJ. Type 2 diabetes in children and adolescents. *Pediatr Diabetes.* 2009;10(suppl 12):17–32

47. Zuhri-Yafi MI, Brosnan PG, Hardin DS. Treatment of type 2 diabetes mellitus in children and adolescents. *J Pediatr Endocrinol Metab.* 2002;15(suppl 1):541–546

48. Rapaport R, Silverstein JH, Garzarella L, Rosenbloom AL. Type 1 and type 2 diabetes mellitus in childhood in the United States: practice patterns by pediatric endocrinologists. *J Pediatr Endocrinol Metab.* 2004;17(6):871–877

49. Glaser N, Jones KL. Non-insulin-dependent diabetes mellitus in children and adolescents. *Adv Pediatr.* 1996;43:359–396

50. Miller JL, Silverstein JH. The treatment of type 2 diabetes mellitus in youth: which therapies? *Treat Endocrinol.* 2006;5(4):201–210

51. Silverstein JH, Rosenbloom AL. Treatment of type 2 diabetes mellitus in children and adolescents. *J Pediatr Endocrinol Metab.* 2000;13(suppl 6):1403–1409

52. Dean H. Treatment of type 2 diabetes in youth: an argument for randomized controlled studies. *Paediatr Child Health (Oxford).* 1999;4(4):265–270

53. Sellers EAC, Dean HJ. Short-term insulin therapy in adolescents with type 2 diabetes mellitus. *J Pediatr Endocrinol Metab.* 2004; 17(11):1561–1564

54. Zeitler P, Hirst K, Pyle L, et al; TODAY Study Group. A clinical trial to maintain glycemic control in youth with type 2 diabetes. *N Engl J Med.* 2012;366(24):2247–2256

55. White NH, Cleary PA, Dahms W, Goldstein D, Malone J, Tamborlane WV; Diabetes Control and Complications Trial (DCCT)/Epidemiology of Diabetes Interventions and Complications (EDIC) Research Group. Beneficial effects of intensive therapy of diabetes during adolescence: outcomes after the conclusion of the Diabetes Control and Complications Trial (DCCT). *J Pediatr.* 2001;139(6):804–812

56. The Diabetes Control and Complications Trial Research Group. The effect of intensive treatment of diabetes on the development and progression of long-term complications in insulin-dependent diabetes mellitus. *N Engl J Med.* 1993;329(14):977–986

57. Orchard TJ, Olson JC, Erbey JR, et al. Insulin resistance-related factors, but not glycemia, predict coronary artery disease in type 1 diabetes: 10-year follow-up data from the Pittsburgh Epidemiology of Diabetes Complications Study. *Diabetes Care.* 2003;26(5):1374–1379

58. UK Prospective Diabetes Study Group. U.K. prospective diabetes study 16. Overview of 6 years' therapy of type II diabetes: a progressive disease. *Diabetes.* 1995;44(11): 1249–1258

59. Shichiri M, Kishikawa H, Ohkubo Y, Wake N. Long-term results of the Kumamoto Study on optimal diabetes control in type 2 diabetic patients. *Diabetes Care.* 2000;23 (suppl 2):B21–B29

60. Baynes JW, Bunn HF, Goldstein D, et al; National Diabetes Data Group. National Diabetes Data Group: report of the expert committee on glucosylated hemoglobin. *Diabetes Care.* 1984;7(6):602–606

61. Dabiri G, Jones K, Krebs J, et al. Benefits of rosiglitazone in children with type 2 diabetes mellitus [abstract]. *Diabetes.* 2005; A457

62. Ponder SW, Sullivan S, McBath G. Type 2 diabetes mellitus in teens. *Diabetes Spectrum.* 2000;13(2):95–119

63. Gahagan S, Silverstein J, and the American Academy of Pediatrics Committee on Native American Child Health. Prevention and treatment of type 2 diabetes mellitus in children, with special emphasis on American Indian and Alaska Native children. *Pediatrics.* 2003;112(4). Available at: www.pediatrics.org/cgi/content/full/112/4/e328

64. Levine BS, Anderson BJ, Butler DA, Antisdel JE, Brackett J, Laffel LM. Predictors of glycemic control and short-term adverse outcomes in youth with type 1 diabetes. *J Pediatr.* 2001;139(2):197–203

65. Haller MJ, Stalvey MS, Silverstein JH. Predictors of control of diabetes: monitoring may be the key. *J Pediatr.* 2004;144(5):660–661

66. Murata GH, Shah JH, Hoffman RM, et al; Diabetes Outcomes in Veterans Study (DOVES). Intensified blood glucose monitoring improves glycemic control in stable, insulin-treated veterans with type 2 diabetes: the Diabetes Outcomes in Veterans Study (DOVES). *Diabetes Care.* 2003;26(6): 1759–1763

67. American Diabetes Association. Standards of medical care in diabetes—2011. *Diabetes Care.* 2011;34(suppl 1):S11–S61

68. Hanefeld M, Fischer S, Julius U, et al. Risk factors for myocardial infarction and death in newly detected NIDDM: the Diabetes Intervention Study, 11-year follow-up. *Diabetologia.* 1996;39(12):1577–1583

69. Franciosi M, Pellegrini F, De Berardis G, et al; QuED Study Group. The impact of blood glucose self-monitoring on metabolic control and quality of life in type 2 diabetic patients: an urgent need for better educational strategies. *Diabetes Care.* 2001;24 (11):1870–1877

70. American Dietetic Association. Recommendations summary: pediatric weight management (PWM) using protein sparing modified fast diets for pediatric weight loss. Available at: www.adaevidencelibrary. com/template.cfm?template=guide_-summary&key=416. Accessed August 13, 2012

71. Knowler WC, Barrett-Connor E, Fowler SE, et al; Diabetes Prevention Program Research Group. Reduction in the incidence of type 2 diabetes with lifestyle intervention or metformin. *N Engl J Med.* 2002;346(6): 393–403

72. Willi SM, Martin K, Datko FM, Brant BP. Treatment of type 2 diabetes in childhood using a very-low-calorie diet. *Diabetes Care.* 2004;27(2):348–353

73. Berry D, Urban A, Grey M. Management of type 2 diabetes in youth (part 2). *J Pediatr Health Care.* 2006;20(2):88–97

74. Loghmani ES. Nutrition therapy for overweight children and adolescents with type 2 diabetes. *Curr Diab Rep.* 2005;5(5):385–390

75. McGavock J, Sellers E, Dean H. Physical activity for the prevention and management of youth-onset type 2 diabetes mellitus: focus on cardiovascular complications. *Diab Vasc Dis Res.* 2007;4(4):305–310

76. Centers for Disease Control and Prevention. Physical activity for everyone: how much physical activity do you need? Atlanta, GA: Centers for Disease Control and Prevention; 2008. Available at: www.cdc.gov/physicalactivity/everyone/guidelines/children.html. Accessed August 13, 2012

77. Pinhas-Hamiel O, Zeitler P. A weighty problem: diagnosis and treatment of type 2 diabetes in adolescents. *Diabetes Spectrum.* 1997;10(4):292–298

78. Yamanouchi K, Shinozaki T, Chikada K, et al. Daily walking combined with diet therapy is a useful means for obese NIDDM patients not only to reduce body weight but also to improve insulin sensitivity. *Diabetes Care.* 1995;18(6):775–778

79. National Heart, Lung, and Blood Institute, US Department of Health and Human Services, National Institutes of Health. Reduce screen time. Available at: www.nhlbi. nih.gov/health/public/heart/obesity/wecan/reduce-screen-time/index.htm. Accessed August 13, 2012

80. Krebs NF, Jacobson MS; American Academy of Pediatrics Committee on Nutrition. Prevention of pediatric overweight and obesity. *Pediatrics.* 2003;112(2):424–430

81. American Academy of Pediatrics Committee on Public Education. American Academy of Pediatrics: children, adolescents, and television. *Pediatrics.* 2001;107(2):423–426

82. American Medical Association. Appendix. Expert Committee recommendations on the assessment, prevention, and treatment of child and adolescent overweight and obesity. Chicago, IL: American Medical Association; January 25, 2007. Available at: www.ama-assn.org/ama1/pub/upload/mm/433/ped_obesity_recs.pdf. Accessed August 13, 2012

ERRATA

Several inaccuracies occurred in the American Academy of Pediatrics "Clinical Practice Guideline: Management of Newly Diagnosed Type 2 Diabetes Mellitus (T2DM) in Children and Adolescents" published in the February 2013 issue of *Pediatrics* (2013;131[2]:364–382).

On page 366 in the table of definitions, "Prediabetes" should be defined as "Fasting plasma glucose ≥100–125 mg/dL or 2-hour glucose concentration during an oral glucose tolerance test of ≥140 but <200 mg/dL or an HbA1c of 5.7% to 6.4%."

On page 378, middle column, under "Reducing Screen Time," the second sentence should read as follows: "The US Department of Health and Human Services reflects the American Academy of Pediatrics policies by recommending that individuals limit "screen time" spent watching television and/or using computers and handheld devices to <2 hours per day unless the use is related to work or homework."[79–81,83]

Also on page 378, middle column, in the second paragraph under "Reducing Screen Time," the fourth sentence should read: "Pending new data, the committee suggests that clinicians follow the policy statement 'Children, Adolescents, and Television' from the AAP Council on Communications and Media (formerly the Committee on Public Education)." The references cited in the next sentence should be 80–83.

Reference 82 should be replaced with the following reference: Barlow SE; Expert Committee. Expert committee recommendations regarding the prevention, assessment, and treatment of child and adolescent overweight and obesity: summary report. *Pediatrics*. 2007;120(suppl 4):S164–S192

Finally, a new reference 83 should be added: American Academy of Pediatrics, Council on Communications and Media. Policy statement: children, adolescents, obesity, and the media. *Pediatrics*. 2011;128(1):201–208

doi:10.1542/peds.2013-0666

Diabetes Clinical Practice Guideline Quick Reference Tools

- Action Statement Summary
  — Management of Newly Diagnosed Type 2 Diabetes Mellitus (T2DM) in Children and Adolescents
- *ICD-10-CM* Coding Quick Reference for Type 2 Diabetes Mellitus
- AAP Patient Education Handout
  — *Type 2 Diabetes: Tips for Healthy Living*

Action Statement Summary

Management of Newly Diagnosed Type 2 Diabetes Mellitus (T2DM) in Children and Adolescents

Key Action Statement 1

Clinicians must ensure that insulin therapy is initiated for children and adolescents with T2DM who are ketotic or in diabetic ketoacidosis and in whom the distinction between T1DM and T2DM is unclear; and, in usual cases, should initiate insulin therapy for patients:

- who have random venous or plasma BG concentrations ≥250 mg/dL; or
- whose HbA1c is >9%.

(Strong Recommendation: evidence quality X, validating studies cannot be performed, and C, observational studies and expert opinion; preponderance of benefit over harm.)

Key Action Statement 2

In all other instances, clinicians should initiate a lifestyle modification program, including nutrition and physical activity, and start metformin as first-line therapy for children and adolescents at the time of diagnosis of T2DM. (Strong recommendation: evidence quality B; 1 RCT showing improved outcomes with metformin versus lifestyle; preponderance of benefits over harms.)

Key Action Statement 3

The committee suggests that clinicians monitor HbA1c concentrations every 3 months and intensify treatment if treatment goals for BG and HbA1c concentrations are not being met. (Option: evidence quality D; expert opinion and studies in children with T1DM and in adults with T2DM; preponderance of benefits over harms.)

Key Action Statement 4

The committee suggests that clinicians advise patients to monitor finger-stick BG concentrations in those who

- are taking insulin or other medications with a risk of hypoglycemia; or
- are initiating or changing their diabetes treatment regimen; or
- have not met treatment goals; or
- have intercurrent illnesses.

(Option: evidence quality D; expert consensus. Preponderance of benefits over harms.)

Key Action Statement 5

The committee suggests that clinicians incorporate the Academy of Nutrition and Dietetics' *Pediatric Weight Management Evidence-Based Nutrition Practice Guidelines* in the nutrition counseling of patients with T2DM both at the time of diagnosis and as part of ongoing management. (Option; evidence quality D; expert opinion; preponderance of benefits over harms. Role of patient preference is dominant.)

Key Action Statement 6

The committee suggests that clinicians encourage children and adolescents with T2DM to engage in moderate-to-vigorous exercise for at least 60 minutes daily and to limit nonacademic screen time to less than 2 hours per day. (Option: evidence quality D, expert opinion and evidence from studies of metabolic syndrome and obesity; preponderance of benefits over harms. Role of patient preference is dominant.)

Coding Quick Reference for Type 2 Diabetes Mellitus	
ICD-10-CM	
E11.649	Type 2 diabetes mellitus with hypoglycemia without coma
E11.65	Type 2 diabetes mellitus with hyperglycemia
E11.8	Type 2 diabetes mellitus with unspecified complications
E11.9	Type 2 diabetes mellitus without complications
E13.9	Other specified diabetes mellitus without complications
Use codes above (**E11.8–E13.9**). *ICD-10-CM* does not discern between controlled and uncontrolled.	

Type 2 Diabetes: Tips for Healthy Living

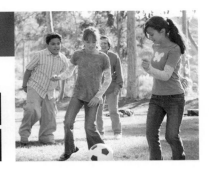

Children with type 2 diabetes can live a healthy life. If your child has been diagnosed with type 2 diabetes, your child's doctor will talk with you about the importance of lifestyle and medication in keeping your child's blood glucose (blood sugar) levels under control.

Read on for information from the American Academy of Pediatrics (AAP) about managing blood glucose and creating plans for healthy living.

What is blood glucose?

Glucose is found in the blood and is the body's main source of energy. The food your child eats is broken down by the body into glucose. Glucose is a type of sugar that gives energy to the cells in the body.

The cells need the help of insulin to take the glucose from the blood to the cells. Insulin is made by an organ called the pancreas.

In children with type 2 diabetes, the pancreas does not make enough insulin and the cells don't use the insulin very well.

Why is it important to manage blood glucose levels?

Glucose will build up in the blood if it cannot be used by the cells. High blood glucose levels can damage many parts of the body, such as the eyes, kidneys, nerves, and heart.

Your child's blood glucose levels may need to be checked on a regular schedule to make sure the levels do not get too high. Your child's doctor will tell you what your child's blood glucose level should be. You and your child will need to learn how to use a glucose meter. Blood glucose levels can be quickly and easily measured using a glucose meter. First, a lancet is used to prick the skin; then a drop of blood from your child's finger is placed on a test strip that is inserted into the meter.

Are there medicines for type 2 diabetes?

Insulin in a shot or another medicine by mouth may be prescribed by your child's doctor if needed to help control your child's blood glucose levels. If your child's doctor has prescribed a medicine, it's important that your child take it as directed. Side effects from certain medicines may include bloating or gassiness. Check with your child's doctor if you have questions.

Along with medicines, your child's doctor will suggest changes to your child's diet and encourage your child to be physically active.

Tips for healthy living

A healthy diet and staying active are especially important for children with type 2 diabetes. Your child's blood glucose levels are easier to manage when you child is at a healthy weight.

Create a plan for eating healthy

Talk with your child's doctor and registered dietitian about a meal plan that meets the needs of your child. The following tips can help you select foods that are healthy and contain a high content of nutrients (protein, vitamins, and minerals):

- Eat at least 5 servings of fruits and vegetables each day.
- Include high-fiber, whole-grain foods such as brown rice, whole-grain pasta, corns, peas, and breads and cereals at meals. Sweet potatoes are also a good choice.
- Choose lower-fat or fat-free toppings like grated low-fat parmesan cheese, salsa, herbed cottage cheese, nonfat/low-fat gravy, low-fat sour cream, low-fat salad dressing, or yogurt.
- Select lean meats such as skinless chicken and turkey, fish, lean beef cuts (round, sirloin, chuck, loin, lean ground beef—no more than 15% fat content), and lean pork cuts (tenderloin, chops, ham). Trim off all visible fat. Remove skin from cooked poultry before eating.
- Include healthy oils such as canola or olive oil in your diet. Choose margarine and vegetable oils without trans fats made from canola, corn, sunflower, soybean, or olive oils.
- Use nonstick vegetable sprays when cooking.
- Use fat-free cooking methods such as baking, broiling, grilling, poaching, or steaming when cooking meat, poultry, or fish.
- Serve vegetable- and broth-based soups, or use nonfat (skim) or low-fat (1%) milk or evaporated skim milk when making cream soups.
- Use the Nutrition Facts label on food packages to find foods with less saturated fat per serving. Pay attention to the serving size as you make choices. Remember that the percent daily values on food labels are based on portion sizes and calorie levels for adults.

Create a plan for physical activity

Physical activity, along with proper nutrition, promotes lifelong health. Following are some ideas on how to get fit:

- **Encourage your child to be active at least 1 hour a day.** Active play is the best exercise for younger children! Parents can join their children and have fun while being active too. School-aged child should participate every day in 1 hour or more of moderate to vigorous physical activity that is right for their age, is enjoyable, and involves a variety of activities.
- **Limit television watching and computer use.** The AAP discourages TV and other media use by children younger than 2 years and encourages interactive play. For older children, total entertainment screen time should be limited to less than 1 to 2 hours per day.
- **Keep an activity log.** The use of activity logs can help children and teens keep track of their exercise programs and physical activity. Online tools can be helpful.

- **Get the whole family involved.** It is a great way to spend time together. Also, children who regularly see their parents enjoying sports and physical activity are more likely to do so themselves.
- **Provide a safe environment.** Make sure your child's equipment and chosen site for the sport or activity are safe. Make sure your child's clothing is comfortable and appropriate.

For more information

National Diabetes Education Program

http://ndep.nih.gov

Listing of resources does not imply an endorsement by the American Academy of Pediatrics (AAP). The AAP is not responsible for the content of the resources mentioned in this publication. Web site addresses are as current as possible, but may change at any time.

The persons whose photographs are depicted in this publication are professional models. They have no relation to the issues discussed. Any characters they are portraying are fictional.

The information contained in this publication should not be used as a substitute for the medical care and advice of your pediatrician. There may be variations in treatment that your pediatrician may recommend based on individual facts and circumstances.

From your doctor

American Academy
of Pediatrics

DEDICATED TO THE HEALTH OF ALL CHILDREN™

The American Academy of Pediatrics is an organization of 60,000 primary care pediatricians, pediatric medical subspecialists, and pediatric surgical specialists dedicated to the health, safety, and well-being of infants, children, adolescents, and young adults.

American Academy of Pediatrics
Web site—www.HealthyChildren.org

Early Detection of Developmental Dysplasia of the Hip

- *Clinical Practice Guideline*

AMERICAN ACADEMY OF PEDIATRICS

Committee on Quality Improvement, Subcommittee on Developmental Dysplasia of the Hip

Clinical Practice Guideline: Early Detection of Developmental Dysplasia of the Hip

ABSTRACT. *Developmental dysplasia of the hip* is the preferred term to describe the condition in which the femoral head has an abnormal relationship to the acetabulum. Developmental dysplasia of the hip includes frank dislocation (luxation), partial dislocation (subluxation), instability wherein the femoral head comes in and out of the socket, and an array of radiographic abnormalities that reflect inadequate formation of the acetabulum. Because many of these findings may not be present at birth, the term *developmental* more accurately reflects the biologic features than does the term *congenital*. The disorder is uncommon. The earlier a dislocated hip is detected, the simpler and more effective is the treatment. Despite newborn screening programs, dislocated hips continue to be diagnosed later in infancy and childhood,[1–11] in some instances delaying appropriate therapy and leading to a substantial number of malpractice claims. The objective of this guideline is to reduce the number of dislocated hips detected later in infancy and childhood. The target audience is the primary care provider. The target patient is the healthy newborn up to 18 months of age, excluding those with neuromuscular disorders, myelodysplasia, or arthrogryposis.

ABBREVIATIONS. DDH, developmental dysplasia of the hip; AVN, avascular necrosis of the hip.

BIOLOGIC FEATURES AND NATURAL HISTORY

Understanding the developmental nature of developmental dysplasia of the hip (DDH) and the subsequent spectrum of hip abnormalities requires a knowledge of the growth and development of the hip joint.[12] Embryologically, the femoral head and acetabulum develop from the same block of primitive mesenchymal cells. A cleft develops to separate them at 7 to 8 weeks' gestation. By 11 weeks' gestation, development of the hip joint is complete. At birth, the femoral head and the acetabulum are primarily cartilaginous. The acetabulum continues to develop postnatally. The growth of the fibrocartilaginous rim (the labrum) that surrounds the bony acetabulum deepens the socket. Development of the femoral head and acetabulum are intimately related, and normal adult hip joints depend on further growth of these structures. Hip dysplasia may occur in utero, perinatally, or during infancy and childhood.

The acronym DDH includes hips that are unstable, subluxated, dislocated (luxated), and/or have malformed acetabula. A hip is *unstable* when the tight fit between the femoral head and the acetabulum is lost and the femoral head is able to move within (subluxated) or outside (dislocated) the confines of the acetabulum. A *dislocation* is a complete loss of contact of the femoral head with the acetabulum. Dislocations are divided into 2 types: teratologic and typical.[12] *Teratologic dislocations* occur early in utero and often are associated with neuromuscular disorders, such as arthrogryposis and myelodysplasia, or with various dysmorphic syndromes. The *typical dislocation* occurs in an otherwise healthy infant and may occur prenatally or postnatally.

During the immediate newborn period, laxity of the hip capsule predominates, and, if clinically significant enough, the femoral head may spontaneously dislocate and relocate. If the hip spontaneously relocates and stabilizes within a few days, subsequent hip development usually is normal. If subluxation or dislocation persists, then structural anatomic changes may develop. A deep concentric position of the femoral head in the acetabulum is necessary for normal development of the hip. When not deeply reduced (subluxated), the labrum may become everted and flattened. Because the femoral head is not reduced into the depth of the socket, the acetabulum does not grow and remodel and, therefore, becomes shallow. If the femoral head moves further out of the socket (dislocation), typically superiorly and laterally, the inferior capsule is pulled upward over the now empty socket. Muscles surrounding the hip, especially the adductors, become contracted, limiting abduction of the hip. The hip capsule constricts; once this capsular constriction narrows to less than the diameter of the femoral head, the hip can no longer be reduced by manual manipulative maneuvers, and operative reduction usually is necessary.

The hip is at risk for dislocation during 4 periods: 1) the 12th gestational week, 2) the 18th gestational week, 3) the final 4 weeks of gestation, and 4) the postnatal period. During the 12th gestational week, the hip is at risk as the fetal lower limb rotates medially. A dislocation at this time is termed teratologic. All elements of the hip joint develop abnor-

The recommendations in this statement do not indicate an exclusive course of treatment or serve as a standard of medical care. Variations, taking into account individual circumstances, may be appropriate.

The Practice Guideline, "Early Detection of Developmental Dysplasia of the Hip," was reviewed by appropriate committees and sections of the American Academy of Pediatrics (AAP) including the Chapter Review Group, a focus group of office-based pediatricians representing each AAP District: Gene R. Adams, MD; Robert M. Corwin, MD; Diane Fuquay, MD; Barbara M. Harley, MD; Thomas J. Herr, MD, Chair; Kenneth E. Matthews, MD; Robert D. Mines, MD; Lawrence C. Pakula, MD; Howard B. Weinblatt, MD; and Delosa A. Young, MD. The Practice Guideline was also reviewed by relevant outside medical organizations as part of the peer review process.

mally. The hip muscles develop around the 18th gestational week. Neuromuscular problems at this time, such as myelodysplasia and arthrogryposis, also lead to teratologic dislocations. During the final 4 weeks of pregnancy, mechanical forces have a role. Conditions such as oligohydramnios or breech position predispose to DDH.[13] Breech position occurs in ~3% of births, and DDH occurs more frequently in breech presentations, reportedly in as many as 23%. The frank breech position of hip flexion and knee extension places a newborn or infant at the highest risk. Postnatally, infant positioning such as swaddling, combined with ligamentous laxity, also has a role.

The true incidence of dislocation of the hip can only be presumed. There is no "gold standard" for diagnosis during the newborn period. Physical examination, plane radiography, and ultrasonography all are fraught with false-positive and false-negative results. Arthrography (insertion of contrast medium into the hip joint) and magnetic resonance imaging, although accurate for determining the precise hip anatomy, are inappropriate methods for screening the newborn and infant.

The reported incidence of DDH is influenced by genetic and racial factors, diagnostic criteria, the experience and training of the examiner, and the age of the child at the time of the examination. Wynne-Davies[14] reported an increased risk to subsequent children in the presence of a diagnosed dislocation (6% risk with healthy parents and an affected child, 12% risk with an affected parent, and 36% risk with an affected parent and 1 affected child). DDH is not always detectable at birth, but some newborn screening surveys suggest an incidence as high as 1 in 100 newborns with evidence of instability, and 1 to 1.5 cases of dislocation per 1000 newborns. The incidence of DDH is higher in girls. Girls are especially susceptible to the maternal hormone relaxin, which may contribute to ligamentous laxity with the resultant instability of the hip. The left hip is involved 3 times as commonly as the right hip, perhaps related to the left occiput anterior positioning of most nonbreech newborns. In this position, the left hip resides posteriorly against the mother's spine, potentially limiting abduction.

PHYSICAL EXAMINATION

DDH is an evolving process, and its physical findings on clinical examination change.[12,15,16] The newborn must be relaxed and preferably examined on a firm surface. Considerable patience and skill are required. The physical examination changes as the child grows older. No signs are pathognomonic for a dislocated hip. The examiner must look for asymmetry. Indeed, bilateral dislocations are more difficult to diagnose than unilateral dislocations because symmetry is retained. Asymmetrical thigh or gluteal folds, better observed when the child is prone, apparent limb length discrepancy, and restricted motion, especially abduction, are significant, albeit not pathognomonic signs. With the infant supine and the pelvis stabilized, abduction to 75° and adduction to 30° should occur readily under normal circumstances.

The 2 maneuvers for assessing hip stability in the newborn are the Ortolani and Barlow tests. The Ortolani elicits the sensation of the dislocated hip reducing, and the Barlow detects the unstable hip dislocating from the acetabulum. The Ortolani is performed with the newborn supine and the examiner's index and middle fingers placed along the greater trochanter with the thumb placed along the inner thigh. The hip is flexed to 90° but not more, and the leg is held in neutral rotation. The hip is gently abducted while lifting the leg anteriorly. With this maneuver, a "clunk" is felt as the dislocated femoral head reduces into the acetabulum. This is a positive Ortolani sign. The Barlow provocative test is performed with the newborn positioned supine and the hips flexed to 90°. The leg is then gently adducted while posteriorly directed pressure is placed on the knee. A palpable clunk or sensation of movement is felt as the femoral head exits the acetabulum posteriorly. This is a positive Barlow sign. The Ortolani and Barlow maneuvers are performed 1 hip at a time. Little force is required for the performance of either of these tests. The goal is not to prove that the hip can be dislocated. Forceful and repeated examinations can break the seal between the labrum and the femoral head. These strongly positive signs of Ortolani and Barlow are distinguished from a large array of soft or equivocal physical findings present during the newborn period. High-pitched clicks are commonly elicited with flexion and extension and are inconsequential. A dislocatable hip has a rather distinctive clunk, whereas a subluxable hip is characterized by a feeling of looseness, a sliding movement, but without the true Ortolani and Barlow clunks. Separating true dislocations (clunks) from a feeling of instability and from benign adventitial sounds (clicks) takes practice and expertise. This guideline recognizes the broad range of physical findings present in newborns and infants and the confusion of terminology generated in the literature. By 8 to 12 weeks of age, the capsule laxity decreases, muscle tightness increases, and the Barlow and Ortolani maneuvers are no longer positive regardless of the status of the femoral head. In the 3-month-old infant, limitation of abduction is the most reliable sign associated with DDH. Other features that arouse suspicion include asymmetry of thigh folds, a positive Allis or Galeazzi sign (relative shortness of the femur with the hips and knees flexed), and discrepancy of leg lengths. These physical findings alert the examiner that abnormal relationships of the femoral head to the acetabulum (dislocation and subluxation) *may* be present.

Maldevelopments of the acetabulum alone (acetabular dysplasia) can be determined only by imaging techniques. Abnormal physical findings may be absent in an infant with acetabular dysplasia but no subluxation or dislocation. Indeed, because of the confusion, inconsistencies, and misuse of language in the literature (eg, an Ortolani sign called a click by some and a clunk by others), this guideline uses the following definitions.

- A *positive examination* result for DDH is the Barlow or Ortolani sign. This is the clunk of dislocation or reduction.
- An *equivocal examination* or *warning signs* include an array of physical findings that may be found in children with DDH, in children with another orthopaedic disorder, or in children who are completely healthy. These physical findings include asymmetric thigh or buttock creases, an apparent or true short leg, and limited abduction. These signs, used singly or in combination, serve to raise the pediatrician's index of suspicion and act as a threshold for referral. Newborn soft tissue hip clicks are not predictive of DDH[17] but may be confused with the Ortolani and Barlow clunks by some screening physicians and thereby be a reason for referral.

IMAGING

Radiographs of the pelvis and hips have historically been used to assess an infant with suspected DDH. During the first few months of life when the femoral heads are composed entirely of cartilage, radiographs have limited value. Displacement and instability may be undetectable, and evaluation of acetabular development is influenced by the infant's position at the time the radiograph is performed. By 4 to 6 months of age, radiographs become more reliable, particularly when the ossification center develops in the femoral head. Radiographs are readily available and relatively low in cost.

Real-time ultrasonography has been established as an accurate method for imaging the hip during the first few months of life.[15,18–25] With ultrasonography, the cartilage can be visualized and the hip can be viewed while assessing the stability of the hip and the morphologic features of the acetabulum. In some clinical settings, ultrasonography can provide information comparable to arthrography (direct injection of contrast into the hip joint), without the need for sedation, invasion, contrast medium, or ionizing radiation. Although the availability of equipment for ultrasonography is widespread, accurate results in hip sonography require training and experience. Although expertise in pediatric hip ultrasonography is increasing, this examination may not always be available or obtained conveniently. Ultrasonographic techniques include *static evaluation* of the morphologic features of the hip, as popularized in Europe by Graf,[26] and a *dynamic evaluation*, as developed by Harcke[20] that assesses the hip for stability of the femoral head in the socket, as well as static anatomy. Dynamic ultrasonography yields more useful information. With both techniques, there is considerable interobserver variability, especially during the first 3 weeks of life.[7,27]

Experience with ultrasonography has documented its ability to detect abnormal position, instability, and dysplasia not evident on clinical examination. Ultrasonography during the first 4 weeks of life often reveals the presence of minor degrees of instability and acetabular immaturity. Studies[7,28,29] indicate that nearly all these mild early findings, which will not be apparent on physical examination, resolve spontaneously without treatment. Newborn screening with ultrasonography has required a high frequency of reexamination and results in a large number of hips being unnecessarily treated. One study[23] demonstrates that a screening process with higher false-positive results also yields increased prevention of late cases. Ultrasonographic screening of all infants at 4 to 6 weeks of age would be expensive, requiring considerable resources. This practice is yet to be validated by clinical trial. *Consequently, the use of ultrasonography is recommended as an adjunct to the clinical evaluation.* It is the technique of choice for clarifying a physical finding, assessing a high-risk infant, and monitoring DDH as it is observed or treated. Used in this selective capacity, it can guide treatment and may prevent overtreatment.

PRETERM INFANTS

DDH may be unrecognized in prematurely born infants. When the infant has cardiorespiratory problems, the diagnosis and management are focused on providing appropriate ventilatory and cardiovascular support, and careful examination of the hips may be deferred until a later date. The most complete examination the infant receives may occur at the time of discharge from the hospital, and this single examination may not detect subluxation or dislocation. Despite the medical urgencies surrounding the preterm infant, it is critical to examine the entire child.

METHODS FOR GUIDELINE DEVELOPMENT

Our goal was to develop a practice parameter by using a process that would be based whenever possible on available evidence. The methods used a combination of expert panel, decision modeling, and evidence synthesis[30] (see the Technical Report available on *Pediatrics electronic pages* at www.pediatrics.org). The predominant methods recommended for such evidence synthesis are generally of 2 types: a *data-driven* method and a *model-driven*[31,32] method. In data-driven methods, the analyst finds the best data available and induces a conclusion from these data. A model-driven method, in contrast, begins with an effort to define the context for evidence and then searches for the data as defined by that context. Data-driven methods are useful when the quality of evidence is high. A careful review of the medical literature revealed that the published evidence about DDH did not meet the criteria for high quality. There was a paucity of randomized clinical trials.[8] We decided, therefore, to use the model-driven method.

A decision model was constructed based on the perspective of practicing clinicians and determining the best strategy for screening and diagnosis. The target child was a full-term newborn with no obvious orthopaedic abnormalities. We focused on the various options available to the pediatrician* for the detection of DDH, including screening by physical examination, screening by ultrasonography, and episodic screening during health supervision. Because

---

*In this guideline, the term *pediatrician* includes the range of pediatric primary care providers, eg, family practitioners and pediatric nurse practitioners.

the detection of a dislocated hip usually results in referral by the pediatrician, and because management of DDH is not in the purview of the pediatrician's care, treatment options are not included. We also included in our model a wide range of options for detecting DDH during the first year of life if the results of the newborn screen are negative.

The outcomes on which we focused were a dislocated hip at 1 year of age as the major morbidity of the disease and avascular necrosis of the hip (AVN) as the primary complication of DDH treatment. AVN is a loss of blood supply to the femoral head resulting in abnormal hip development, distortion of shape, and, in some instances, substantial morbidity. Ideally, a gold standard would be available to define DDH at any point in time. However, as noted, no gold standard exists except, perhaps, arthrography of the hip, which is an inappropriate standard for use in a detection model. Therefore, we defined outcomes in terms of the *process of care*. We reviewed the literature extensively. The purpose of the literature review was to provide the probabilities required by the decision model since there were no randomized clinical trials. The article or chapter title and the abstracts were reviewed by 2 members of the methodology team and members of the subcommittee. Articles not rejected were reviewed, and data were abstracted that would provide evidence for the probabilities required by the decision model. As part of the literature abstraction process, the evidence quality in each article was assessed. A computer-based literature search, hand review of recent publications, or examination of the reference section for other articles ("ancestor articles") identified 623 articles; 241 underwent detailed review, 118 of which provided some data. Of the 100 ancestor articles, only 17 yielded useful articles, suggesting that our accession process was complete. By traditional epidemiologic standards,[33] the quality of the evidence in this set of articles was uniformly low. There were few controlled trials and few studies of the follow-up of infants for whom the results of newborn examinations were negative. When the evidence was poor or lacking entirely, extensive discussions among members of the committee and the expert opinion of outside consultants were used to arrive at a consensus. No votes were taken. Disagreements were discussed, and consensus was achieved.

The available evidence was distilled in 3 ways.

First, estimates were made of DDH at birth in infants without risk factors. These estimates constituted the baseline risk. Second, estimates were made of the rates of DDH in the children with risk factors. These numbers guide clinical actions: rates that are too high might indicate referral or different follow-up despite negative physical findings. Third, each screening strategy (pediatrician-based, orthopaedist-based, and ultrasonography-based) was scored for the estimated number of children given a diagnosis of DDH at birth, at mid-term (4–12 months of age), and at late-term (12 months of age and older) and for the estimated number of cases of AVN incurred, assuming that all children given a diagnosis of DDH would be treated. These numbers suggest the best strategy, balancing DDH detection with incurring adverse effects.

The baseline estimate of DDH based on orthopaedic screening was 11.5/1000 infants. Estimates from pediatric screening were 8.6/1000 and from ultrasonography were 25/1000. The 11.5/1000 rate translates into a rate for not-at-risk boys of 4.1/1000 boys and a rate for not-at-risk girls of 19/1000 girls. These numbers derive from the facts that the relative risk—the rate in girls divided by the rate in boys across several studies—is 4.6 and because infants are split evenly between boys and girls, so $.5 \times 4.1/1000 + .5 \times 19/1000 = 11.5/1000$.[34,35] We used these baseline rates for calculating the rates in other risk groups. Because the relative risk of DDH for children with a positive family history (first-degree relatives) is 1.7, the rate for boys with a positive family history is $1.7 \times 4.1 = 6.4/1000$ boys, and for girls with a positive family history, $1.7 \times 19 = 32/1000$ girls. Finally, the relative risk of DDH for breech presentation (of all kinds) is 6.3, so the risk for breech boys is $7.0 \times 4.1 = 29/1000$ boys and for breech girls, $7.0 \times 19 = 133/1000$ girls. These numbers are summarized in Table 1.

These numbers suggest that boys without risk or those with a family history have the lowest risk; girls without risk and boys born in a breech presentation have an intermediate risk; and girls with a positive family history, and especially girls born in a breech presentation, have the highest risks. Guidelines, considering the risk factors, should follow these risk profiles. Reports of newborn screening for DDH have included various screening techniques. In some, the screening clinician was an orthopaedist, in

TABLE 1.   Relative and Absolute Risks for Finding a Positive Examination Result at Newborn Screening by Using the Ortolani and Barlow Signs

Newborn Characteristics	Relative Risk of a Positive Examination Result	Absolute Risk of a Positive Examination Result per 1000 Newborns With Risk Factors
All newborns	. . .	11.5
Boys	1.0	4.1
Girls	4.6	19
Positive family history	1.7	
Boys	. . .	6.4
Girls	. . .	32
Breech presentation	7.0	
Boys	. . .	29
Girls	. . .	133

TABLE 2.   Newborn Strategy*

Outcome	Orthopaedist PE	Pediatrician PE	Ultrasonography
DDH in newborn	12	8.6	25
DDH at ~6 mo of age	.1	.45	.28
DDH at 12 mo of age or more	.16	.33	.1
AVN at 12 mo of age	.06	.1	.1

* PE indicates physical examination. Outcome per 1000 infants initially screened.

others, a pediatrician, and in still others, a physiotherapist. In addition, screening has been performed by ultrasonography. In assessing the expected effect of each strategy, we estimated the newborn DDH rates, the mid-term DDH rates, and the late-term DDH rates for each of the 3 strategies, as shown in Table 2. We also estimated the rate of AVN for DDH treated before 2 months of age (2.5/1000 treated) and after 2 months of age (109/1000 treated). We could not distinguish the AVN rates for children treated between 2 and 12 months of age from those treated later. Table 2 gives these data. The total cases of AVN per strategy are calculated, assuming that all infants with positive examination results are treated.

Table 2 shows that a strategy using pediatricians to screen newborns would give the lowest newborn rate but the highest mid- and late-term DDH rates. To assess how much better an ultrasonography-only screening strategy would be, we could calculate a cost-effectiveness ratio. In this case, the "cost" of ultrasonographic screening is the number of "extra" newborn cases that probably include children who do not need to be treated. (The cost from AVN is the same in the 2 strategies.) By using these cases as the cost and the number of later cases averted as the effect, a ratio is obtained of 71 children treated neonatally because of a positive ultrasonographic screen for each later case averted. Because this number is high, and because the presumption of better late-term efficacy is based on a single study, we do not recommend ultrasonographic screening at this time.

RECOMMENDATIONS AND NOTES TO ALGORITHM (Fig 1)

1. **All newborns are to be screened by physical examination**. The evidence† for this recommendation is good. The expert consensus‡ is strong. Although initial screening by orthopaedists§ would be optimal (Table 2), it is doubtful that if widely practiced, such a strategy would give the same good results as those published from pediatric orthopaedic research centers. **It is recommended that screening be done by a properly trained health care provider** (eg, physician, pediatric nurse practitioner, physician assistant, or physical therapist). (Evidence for this recommendation is strong.) A number of studies performed by properly trained nonphysicians report results

indistinguishable from those performed by physicians.[36] The examination after discharge from the neonatal intensive care unit should be performed as a newborn examination with appropriate screening. **Ultrasonography of all newborns is not recommended.** (Evidence is fair; consensus is strong.) Although there is indirect evidence to support the use of ultrasonographic screening of all newborns, it is not advocated because it is operator-dependent, availability is questionable, it increases the rate of treatment, and interobserver variability is high. There are probably some increased costs. We considered a strategy of "no newborn screening." This arm is politically indefensible because screening newborns is inherent in pediatrician's care. The technical report details this limb through decision analysis. Regardless of the screening method used for the newborn, DDH is detected in 1 in 5000 infants at 18 months of age.[3] The evidence and consensus for newborn screening remain strong.

Newborn Physical Examination and Treatment

2. **If a positive Ortolani or Barlow sign is found in the newborn examination, the infant should be referred to an orthopaedist**. Orthopaedic referral is recommended when the Ortolani sign is unequivocally positive (a clunk). Orthopaedic referral is not recommended for any softly positive finding in the examination (eg, hip click without dislocation). The precise time frame for the newborn to be evaluated by the orthopaedist cannot be determined from the literature. However, the literature suggests that the majority of "abnormal" physical findings of hip examinations at birth (clicks and clunks) will resolve by 2 weeks; therefore, consultation and possible initiation of treatment are recommended by that time. The data recommending that all those with a positive Ortolani sign be referred to an orthopaedist are limited, but expert panel consensus, nevertheless, was strong, because pediatricians do not have the training to take full responsibility and because true Ortolani clunks are rare and their management is more appropriately performed by the orthopaedist.

If the results of the physical examination at birth are "equivocally" positive (ie, soft click, mild asymmetry, but neither an Ortolani nor a Barlow sign is present), then a follow-up hip examination by the pediatrician in 2 weeks is recommended. (Evidence is good; consensus is strong.) The available data suggest that most clicks resolve by 2 weeks and that these "benign hip clicks" in the newborn period do

---

†In this guideline, evidence is listed as good, fair, or poor based on the methodologist's evaluation of the literature quality. (See the Technical Report.)

‡Opinion or consensus is listed as *strong* if opinion of the expert panel was unanimous or *mixed* if there were dissenting points of view.

§In this guideline, the term *orthopaedist* refers to an orthopaedic surgeon with expertise in pediatric orthopaedic conditions.

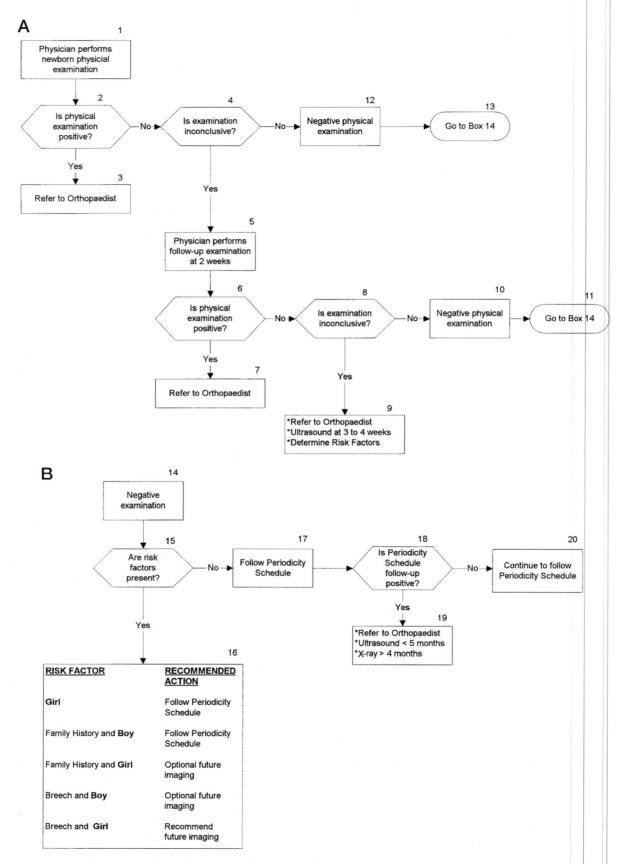

Fig 1. Screening for developmental hip dysplasia—clinical algorithm.

not lead to later hip dysplasia.[9,17,28,37] Thus, for an infant with softly positive signs, the pediatrician should reexamine the hips at 2 weeks before making referrals for orthopaedic care or ultrasonography. We recognize the concern of pediatricians about adherence to follow-up care regimens, but this concern regards all aspects of health maintenance and is not a reason to request ultrasonography or other diagnostic study of the newborn hips.

3. **If the results of the newborn physical examination are positive (ie, presence of an Ortolani or a Barlow sign), ordering an ultrasonographic examination of the newborn is not recommended.** (Evidence is poor; opinion is strong.) Treatment decisions are not influenced by the results of ultrasonography but are based on the results of the physical examination. The treating physician may use a variety of imaging studies during clinical management. **If the results of the newborn physical examination are positive, obtaining a radiograph of the newborn's pelvis and hips is not recommended** (evidence is poor; opinion is strong), because they are of limited value and do not influence treatment decisions.

The use of triple diapers when abnormal physical signs are detected during the newborn period is not recommended. (Evidence is poor; opinion is strong.) Triple diaper use is common practice despite the lack of data on the effectiveness of triple diaper use; and, in instances of frank dislocation, the use of triple diapers may delay the initiation of more appropriate treatment (such as with the Pavlik harness). Often, the primary care pediatrician may not have performed the newborn examination in the hospital. The importance of communication cannot be overemphasized, and triple diapers may aid in follow-up as a reminder that a possible abnormal physical examination finding was present in the newborn.

2-Week Examination

4. **If the results of the physical examination are positive (eg, positive Ortolani or Barlow sign) at 2 weeks, refer to an orthopaedist.** (Evidence is strong; consensus is strong.) Referral is urgent but is not an emergency. Consensus is strong that, as in the newborn, the presence of an Ortolani or Barlow sign at 2 weeks warrants referral to an orthopaedist. An Ortolani sign at 2 weeks may be a new finding or a finding that was not apparent at the time of the newborn examination.

5. **If at the 2-week examination the Ortolani and Barlow signs are absent but physical findings raise suspicions, consider referral to an orthopaedist or request ultrasonography at age 3 to 4 weeks.** Consensus is mixed about the follow-up for softly positive or equivocal findings at 2 weeks of age (eg, adventitial click, thigh asymmetry, and apparent leg length difference). Because it is necessary to confirm the status of the hip joint, the pediatrician can consider referral to an orthopaedist or for ultrasonography if the constellation of physical findings raises a high level of suspicion.

However, if the physical findings are minimal, continuing follow-up by the periodicity schedule with focused hip examinations is also an option, provided risk factors are considered. (See "Recommendations" 7 and 8.)

6. **If the results of the physical examination are negative at 2 weeks, follow-up is recommended at the scheduled well-baby periodic examinations.** (Evidence is good; consensus is strong.)

7. **Risk factors. If the results of the newborn examination are negative (or equivocally positive), risk factors may be considered.**[13,21,38-41] Risk factors are a study of thresholds to act.[42] Table 1 gives the risk of finding a positive Ortolani or Barlow sign at the time of the initial newborn screening. If this examination is negative, the absolute risk of there being a true dislocated hip is greatly reduced. Nevertheless, the data in Table 1 may influence the pediatrician to perform confirmatory evaluations. Action will vary based on the individual clinician. The following recommendations are made (evidence is strong; opinion is strong):

   - **Girl** (newborn risk of 19/1000). When the results of the newborn examination are negative or equivocally positive, hips should be reevaluated at 2 weeks of age. If negative, continue according to the periodicity schedule; if positive, refer to an orthopaedist or for ultrasonography at 3 weeks of age.

   - **Infants with a positive family history of DDH** (newborn risk for boys of 9.4/1000 and for girls, 44/1000). When the results of the newborn examination in boys are negative or equivocally positive, hips should be reevaluated at 2 weeks of age. If negative, continue according to the periodicity schedule; if positive, refer to an orthopaedist or for ultrasonography at 3 weeks of age. In girls, the absolute risk of 44/1000 may exceed the pediatrician's threshold to act, and imaging with an ultrasonographic examination at 6 weeks of age or a radiograph of the pelvis at 4 months of age is recommended.

   - **Breech presentation** (newborn risk for boys of 26/1000 and for girls, 120/1000). **For negative or equivocally positive newborn examinations, the infant should be reevaluated at regular intervals (according to the periodicity schedule) if the examination results remain negative.** Because an absolute risk of 120/1000 (12%) probably exceeds most pediatricians' threshold to act, imaging with an ultrasonographic examination at 6 weeks of age or with a radiograph of the pelvis and hips at 4 months of age is recommended. In addition, because some reports show a high incidence of hip abnormalities detected at an older age in children born breech, this imaging strategy remains an option for all children born breech, not just girls. These hip abnormalities are, for the most part, inadequate development of the acetabulum. Acetabular dysplasia is best found by a radiographic examination at 6 months of age or older. A suggestion of poorly formed acetabula may be observed at 6 weeks of age by ultrasonography, but the best study remains a radiograph performed closer to 6 months of age. Ultrasonographic newborn screening of all breech infants will not eliminate the possibility of later acetabular dysplasia.

8. **Periodicity. The hips must be examined at every well-baby visit according to the recommended periodicity schedule for well-baby examinations (2–4 days for newborns discharged in less than 48 hours after delivery, by 1 month, 2 months, 4 months, 6 months, 9 months, and 12 months of age).** If at any time during the follow-up period DDH is suspected because of an abnormal physical examination or by a parental complaint of difficulty diapering or abnormal appearing legs, the pediatrician must confirm that the hips are stable, in the sockets, and developing normally. Confirmation can be made by a focused physical examination when the infant is calm and relaxed, by consultation with another primary care pediatrician, by consultation with an orthopaedist, by ultrasonography if the infant is younger than 5 months of age, or by radiography if the infant is older than 4 months of age. (Between 4 and 6 months of age, ultrasonography and radiography seem to be equally effective diagnostic imaging studies.)

DISCUSSION

DDH is an important term because it accurately reflects the biologic features of the disorder and the susceptibility of the hip to become dislocated at various times. Dislocated hips always will be diagnosed later in infancy and childhood because not every dislocated hip is detectable at birth, and hips continue to dislocate throughout the first year of life. Thus, this guideline requires that the pediatrician follow *a process of care for the detection of DDH.* The process recommended for early detection of DDH includes the following:

- Screen all newborns' hips by physical examination.
- Examine all infants' hips according to a periodicity schedule and follow-up until the child is an established walker.
- Record and document physical findings.
- Be aware of the changing physical examination for DDH.
- If physical findings raise suspicion of DDH, or if parental concerns suggest hip disease, confirmation is required by expert physical examination, referral to an orthopaedist, or by an age-appropriate imaging study.

When this process of care is followed, the number of dislocated hips diagnosed at 1 year of age should be minimized. However, the problem of late detection of dislocated hips will not be eliminated. The results of screening programs have indicated that 1 in 5000 children have a dislocated hip detected at 18 months of age or older.[3]

TECHNICAL REPORT

The Technical Report is available from the American Academy of Pediatrics from several sources. The Technical Report is published in full-text on *Pediatrics electronic pages.* It is also available in a compendium of practice guidelines that contains guidelines and evidence reports together. The objective was to create a recommendation to pediatricians and other primary care providers about their role as screeners for detecting DDH. The patients are a theoretical cohort of newborns. A model-based method using decision analysis was the foundation. Components of the approach include:

- Perspective: primary care provider
- Outcomes: DDH and AVN
- Preferences: expected rates of outcomes
- Model: influence diagram assessed from the subcommittee and from the methodology team with critical feedback from the subcommittee
- Evidence sources: Medline and EMBase (detailed in "Methods" section)
- Evidence quality: assessed on a custom, subjective scale, based primarily on the fit of the evidence in the decision model

The results are detailed in the "Methods" section. Based on the raw evidence and Bayesian hierarchical meta-analysis,[34,35] estimates for the incidence of DDH based on the type of screener (orthopaedist vs pediatrician); the odds ratio for DDH given risk factors of sex, family history, and breech presentation; and estimates for late detection and AVN were determined and are detailed in the "Methods" section and in Tables 1 and 2.

The decision model (reduced based on available evidence) suggests that orthopaedic screening is optimal, but because orthopaedists in the published studies and in practice would differ in pediatric expertise, the supply of pediatric orthopaedists is relatively limited, and the difference between orthopaedists and pediatricians is statistically insignificant, we conclude that pediatric screening is to be recommended. The place for ultrasonography in the screening process remains to be defined because of the limited data available regarding late diagnosis in ultrasonography screening to permit definitive recommendations.

These data could be used by others to refine the conclusion based on costs, parental preferences, or physician style. Areas for research are well defined by our model-based method. All references are in the Technical Report.

RESEARCH QUESTIONS

The quality of the literature suggests many areas for research, because there is a paucity of randomized clinical trials and case-controlled studies. The following is a list of possibilities:

1. Minimum diagnostic abilities of a screener. Although there are data for pediatricians in general, few, if any, studies evaluated the abilities of an individual examiner. What should the minimum

sensitivity and specificity be, and how should they be assessed?

2. Intercurrent screening. There were few studies on systemic processes for screening after the newborn period.[2,43,44] Although several studies assessed postneonatal DDH, the data did not specify how many examinations were performed on each child before the abnormal result was found.

3. Trade-offs. Screening always results in false-positive results, and these patients suffer the adverse effects of therapy. How many unnecessary AVNs are we—families, physicians, and society—willing to tolerate from a screening program for every appropriately treated infant in whom late DDH was averted? This assessment depends on people's values and preferences and is not strictly an epidemiologic issue.

4. Postneonatal DDH after ultrasonographic screening. Although we concluded that ultrasonographic screening did not result in fewer diagnoses of postneonatal DDH, that conclusion was based on only 1 study.[36] Further study is needed.

5. Cost-effectiveness. If ultrasonographic screening reduces the number of postneonatal DDH diagnoses, then there will be a cost trade-off between the resources spent up front to screen everyone with an expensive technology, as in the case of ultrasonography, and the resources spent later to treat an expensive adverse event, as in the case of physical examination-based screening. The level at which the cost per case of postneonatal DDH averted is no longer acceptable is a matter of social preference, not of epidemiology.

ACKNOWLEDGMENTS

We acknowledge and appreciate the help of our methodology team, Richard Hinton, MD, Paola Morello, MD, and Jeanne Santoli, MD, who diligently participated in the literature review and abstracting the articles into evidence tables, and the subcommittee on evidence analysis.

We would also like to thank Robert Sebring, PhD, for assisting in the management of this process; Bonnie Cosner for managing the workflow; and Chris Kwiat, MLS, from the American Academy of Pediatrics Bakwin Library, who performed the literature searches.

REFERENCES

1. Bjerkreim I, Hagen O, Ikonomou N, Kase T, Kristiansen T, Arseth P. Late diagnosis of developmental dislocation of the hip in Norway during the years 1980–1989. J Pediatr Orthop B. 1993;2:112–114
2. Clarke N, Clegg J, Al-Chalabi A. Ultrasound screening of hips at risk for CDH: failure to reduce the incidence of late cases. J Bone Joint Surg Br. 1989;71:9–12
3. Dezateux C, Godward C. Evaluating the national screening programme for congenital dislocation of the hip. J Med Screen. 1995;2:200–206
4. Hadlow V. Neonatal screening for congenital dislocation of the hip: a prospective 21-year survey. J Bone Joint Surg Br. 1988;70:740–743
5. Krikler S, Dwyer N. Comparison of results of two approaches to hip screening in infants. J Bone Joint Surg Br. 1992;74:701–703
6. Macnicol M. Results of a 25-year screening programme for neonatal hip instability. J Bone Joint Surg Br. 1990;72:1057–1060
7. Marks DS, Clegg J, Al-Chalabi AN. Routine ultrasound screening for neonatal hip instability: can it abolish late-presenting congenital dislocation of the hip? J Bone Joint Surg Br. 1994;76:534–538
8. Rosendahl K, Markestad T, Lie R. Congenital dislocation of the hip: a prospective study comparing ultrasound and clinical examination. Acta Paediatr. 1992;81:177–181
9. Sanfridson J, Redlund-Johnell I, Uden A. Why is congenital dislocation of the hip still missed? Analysis of 96,891 infants screened in Malmo 1956–1987. Acta Orthop Scand. 1991;62:87–91
10. Tredwell S, Bell H. Efficacy of neonatal hip examination. J Pediatr Orthop. 1981;1:61–65
11. Yngve D, Gross R. Late diagnosis of hip dislocation in infants. J Pediatr Orthop. 1990;10:777–779
12. Aronsson DD, Goldberg MJ, Kling TF, Roy DR. Developmental dysplasia of the hip. Pediatrics. 1994;94:201–212
13. Hinderaker T, Daltveit AK, Irgens LM, Uden A, Reikeras O. The impact of intra-uterine factors on neonatal hip instability: an analysis of 1,059,479 children in Norway. Acta Orthop Scand. 1994;65:239–242
14. Wynne-Davies R. Acetabular dysplasia and familial joint laxity: two etiological factors in congenital dislocation of the hip: a review of 589 patients and their families. J Bone Joint Surg Br. 1970;52:704–716
15. De Pellegrin M. Ultrasound screening for congenital dislocation of the hip: results and correlations between clinical and ultrasound findings. Ital J Orthop Traumatol. 1991;17:547–553
16. Stoffelen D, Urlus M, Molenaers G, Fabry G. Ultrasound, radiographs, and clinical symptoms in developmental dislocation of the hip: a study of 170 patients. J Pediatr Orthop B. 1995;4:194–199
17. Bond CD, Hennrikus WL, Della Maggiore E. Prospective evaluation of newborn soft tissue hip clicks with ultrasound. J Pediatr Orthop. 1997;17:199–201
18. Bialik V, Wiener F, Benderly A. Ultrasonography and screening in developmental displacement of the hip. J Pediatr Orthop B. 1992;1:51–54
19. Castelein R, Sauter A. Ultrasound screening for congenital dysplasia of the hip in newborns: its value. J Pediatr Orthop. 1988;8:666–670
20. Clarke NMP, Harcke HT, McHugh P, Lee MS, Borns PF, MacEwen GP. Real-time ultrasound in the diagnosis of congenital dislocation and dysplasia of the hip. J Bone Joint Surg Br. 1985;67:406–412
21. Garvey M, Donoghue V, Gorman W, O'Brien N, Murphy J. Radiographic screening at four months of infants at risk for congenital hip dislocation. J Bone Joint Surg Br. 1992;74:704–707
22. Langer R. Ultrasonic investigation of the hip in newborns in the diagnosis of congenital hip dislocation: classification and results of a screening program. Skeletal Radiol. 1987;16:275–279

23. Rosendahl K, Markestad T, Lie RT. Ultrasound screening for developmental dysplasia of the hip in the neonate: the effect on treatment rate and prevalence of late cases. *Pediatrics*. 1994;94:47–52

24. Terjesen T. Ultrasound as the primary imaging method in the diagnosis of hip dysplasia in children aged <2 years. *J Pediatr Orthop B*. 1996;5: 123–128

25. Vedantam R, Bell M. Dynamic ultrasound assessment for monitoring of treatment of congenital dislocation of the hip. *J Pediatr Orthop*. 1995;15: 725–728

26. Graf R. Classification of hip joint dysplasia by means of sonography. *Arch Orthop Trauma Surg*. 1984;102:248–255

27. Berman L, Klenerman L. Ultrasound screening for hip abnormalities: preliminary findings in 1001 neonates. *Br Med J (Clin Res Ed)*. 1986;293: 719–722

28. Castelein R, Sauter A, de Vlieger M, van Linge B. Natural history of ultrasound hip abnormalities in clinically normal newborns. *J Pediatr Orthop*. 1992;12:423–427

29. Clarke N. Sonographic clarification of the problems of neonatal hip stability. *J Pediatr Orthop*. 1986;6:527–532

30. Eddy DM. The confidence profile method: a Bayesian method for assessing health technologies. *Operations Res*. 1989;37:210–228

31. Howard RA, Matheson JE. Influence diagrams. In: Matheson JE, ed. *Readings on the Principles and Applications of Decision Analysis*. Menlo Park, CA: Strategic Decisions Group; 1981:720–762

32. Nease RF, Owen DK. Use of influence diagrams to structure medical decisions. *Med Decis Making*. 1997;17:265–275

33. Guyatt GH, Sackett DL, Sinclair JC, Hayward R, Cook DJ, Cook RJ. Users' guide to the medical literature, IX: a method for grading health care recommendations. *JAMA*. 1995;274:1800–1804

34. Gelman A, Carlin JB, Stern HS, Rubin DB. *Bayesian Data Analysis*. London, UK: Chapman and Hall; 1997

35. Spiegelhalter D, Thomas A, Best N, Gilks W. *BUGS 0.5: Bayesian Inference Using Gibbs Sampling Manual, II*. Cambridge, MA: MRC Biostatistics Unit, Institute of Public Health; 1996. Available at: http://www.mrc-bsu.cam.ac.uk/bugs/software/software.html

36. Fiddian NJ, Gardiner JC. Screening for congenital dislocation of the hip by physiotherapists: results of a ten-year study. *J Bone Joint Surg Br*. 1994;76:458–459

37. Dunn P, Evans R, Thearle M, Griffiths H, Witherow P. Congenital dislocation of the hip: early and late diagnosis and management compared. *Arch Dis Child*. 1992;60:407–414

38. Holen KJ, Tegnander A, Terjesen T, Johansen OJ, Eik-Nes SH. Ultrasonographic evaluation of breech presentation as a risk factor for hip dysplasia. *Acta Paediatr*. 1996;85:225–229

39. Jones D, Powell N. Ultrasound and neonatal hip screening: a prospective study of "high risk" babies. *J Bone Joint Surg Br*. 1990;72:457–459

40. Teanby DN, Paton RW. Ultrasound screening for congenital dislocation of the hip: a limited targeted programme. *J Pediatr Orthop*. 1997;17: 202–204

41. Tonnis D, Storch K, Ulbrich H. Results of newborn screening for CDH

42. Pauker SG, Kassirer JP. The threshold approach to clinical decision making. *N Engl J Med*. 1980;302:1109–1117

43. Bower C, Stanley F, Morgan B, Slattery H, Stanton C. Screening for congenital dislocation of the hip by child-health nurses in western Australia. *Med J Aust*. 1989;150:61–65

44. Franchin F, Lacalendola G, Molfetta L, Mascolo V, Quagliarella L. Ultrasound for early diagnosis of hip dysplasia. *Ital J Orthop Traumatol*. 1992;18:261–269

with and without sonography and correlation of risk factors. *J Pediatr Orthop*. 1990;10:145–152

ADDENDUM TO REFERENCES FOR THE DDH GUIDELINE

New information is generated constantly. Specific details of this report must be changed over time.

New articles (additional articles 1–7) have been published since the completion of our literature search and construction of this Guideline. These articles taken alone might seem to contradict some of the Guideline's estimates as detailed in the article and in the Technical Report. However, taken in context with the literature synthesis carried out for the construction of this Guideline, our estimates remain intact and no conclusions are obviated.

ADDITIONAL ARTICLES

1. Bialik V, Bialik GM, Blazer S, Sujov P, Wiener F, Berant M. Developmental dysplasia of the hip: a new approach to incidence. *Pediatrics*. 1999;103:93–99

2. Clegg J, Bache CE, Raut VV. Financial justification for routine ultrasound screening of the neonatal hip. *J Bone Joint Surg*. 1999;81-B:852–857

3. Holen KJ, Tegnander A, Eik-Nes SH, Terjesen T. The use of ultrasound in determining the initiation in treatment in instability of the hips in neonates. *J Bone Joint Surg*. 1999;81-B:846–851

4. Lewis K, Jones DA, Powell N. Ultrasound and neonatal hip screening: the five-year results of a prospective study in high risk babies. *J Pediatr Orthop*. 1999;19:760–762

5. Paton RW, Srinivasan MS, Shah B, Hollis S. Ultrasound screening for hips at risk in developmental dysplasia: is it worth it? *J Bone Joint Surg*. 1999;81-B:255–258

6. Sucato DJ, Johnston CE, Birch JG, Herring JA, Mack P. Outcomes of ultrasonographic hip abnormalities in clinically stable hips. *J Pediatr Orthop*. 1999;19:754–759

7. Williams PR, Jones DA, Bishay M. Avascular necrosis and the aberdeen splint in developmental dysplasia of the hip. *J Bone Joint Surg*. 1999;81-B:1023–1028

Dysplasia of the Hip Clinical Practice Guideline
Quick Reference Tools

- Recommendation Summary
  — Early Detection of Developmental Dysplasia of the Hip
- *ICD-10-CM* Coding Quick Reference for Dysplasia of the Hip
- AAP Patient Education Handout
  — *Hip Dysplasia (Developmental Dysplasia of the Hip)*

Recommendation Summary
Early Detection of Developmental Dysplasia of the Hip

Recommendation 1

A. All newborns are to be screened by physical examination. (The evidence for this recommendation is good. The expert consensus is strong.)
B. It is recommended that screening be done by a properly trained health care provider (eg, physician, pediatric nurse practitioner, physician assistant, or physical therapist). (Evidence for this recommendation is strong.)
C. Ultrasonography of all newborns is not recommended. (Evidence is fair; consensus is strong.)

Recommendation 2

A. If a positive Ortolani or Barlow sign is found in the newborn examination, the infant should be referred to an orthopaedist. (The data recommending that all those with a positive Ortolani sign be referred to an orthopaedist are limited, but expert panel consensus, nevertheless, was strong....)
B. If the results of the physical examination at birth are "equivocally" positive (ie, soft click, mild asymmetry, but neither an Ortolani nor a Barlow sign is present), then a follow-up hip examination by the pediatrician in 2 weeks is recommended. (Evidence is good; consensus is strong.)

Recommendation 3

A. If the results of the newborn physical examination are positive (ie, presence of an Ortolani or a Barlow sign), ordering an ultrasonographic examination of the newborn is not recommended. (Evidence is poor; opinion is strong.)
B. If the results of the newborn physical examination are positive, obtaining a radiograph of the newborn's pelvis and hips is not recommended. (Evidence is poor; opinion is strong.)
C. The use of triple diapers when abnormal physical signs are detected during the newborn period is not recommended. (Evidence is poor; opinion is strong.)

Recommendation 4

If the results of the physical examination are positive (eg, positive Ortolani or Barlow sign) at 2 weeks, refer to an orthopaedist. (Evidence is strong; consensus is strong.)

Recommendation 5

If at the 2-week examination the Ortolani and Barlow signs are absent but physical findings raise suspicions, consider referral to an orthopaedist or request ultrasonography at age 3 to 4 weeks.

Recommendation 6

If the results of the physical examination are negative at 2 weeks, follow-up is recommended at the scheduled well-baby periodic examinations. (Evidence is good; consensus is strong.)

Recommendation 7

Risk factors. If the results of the newborn examination are negative (or equivocally positive), risk factors may be considered. The following recommendations are made (evidence is strong; opinion is strong):

A. Girl (newborn risk of 19/1000). When the results of the newborn examination are negative or equivocally positive, hips should be reevaluated at 2 weeks of age. If negative, continue according to the periodicity schedule; if positive, refer to an orthopaedist or for ultrasonography at 3 weeks of age.
B. Infants with a positive family history of DDH (newborn risk for boys of 9.4/1000 and for girls, 44/1000). When the results of the newborn examination in boys are negative or equivocally positive, hips should be reevaluated at 2 weeks of age. If negative, continue according to the periodicity schedule; if positive, refer to an orthopaedist or for ultrasonography at 3 weeks of age. In girls, the absolute risk of 44/1000 may exceed the pediatrician's threshold to act, and imaging with an ultrasonographic examination at 6 weeks of age or a radiograph of the pelvis at 4 months of age is recommended.
C. Breech presentation (newborn risk for boys of 26/1000 and for girls, 120/1000). For negative or equivocally positive newborn examinations, the infant should be reevaluated at regular intervals (according to the periodicity schedule) if the examination results remain negative.

Recommendation 8

Periodicity. The hips must be examined at every well-baby visit according to the recommended periodicity schedule for well-baby examinations (2–4 days for newborns discharged in less than 48 hours after delivery, by 1 month, 2 months, 4 months, 6 months, 9 months, and 12 months of age).

Coding Quick Reference for Dysplasia of the Hip	
ICD-10-CM	
Q65.0-	Congenital dislocation of hip, unilateral
Q65.1	Congenital dislocation of hip, bilateral
Q65.3-	Congenital partial dislocation of hip, unilateral
Q65.4	Congenital partial dislocation of hip, bilateral
Q65.6	Congenital unstable hip (Congenital dislocatable hip)
Q65.89	Other specified congenital deformities of hip

Symbol "-" requires a fifth character; **1** = right; **2** = left.

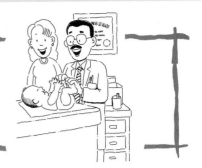

Hip Dysplasia
(Developmental Dysplasia of the Hip)

Hip dysplasia (developmental dysplasia of the hip) is a condition in which a child's upper thighbone is dislocated from the hip socket. It can be present at birth or develop during a child's first year of life.

Hip dysplasia is not always detectable at birth or even during early infancy. In spite of careful screening of children for hip dysplasia during regular well-child exams, a number of children with hip dysplasia are not diagnosed until after they are 1 year old.

Hip dysplasia is rare. However, if your baby is diagnosed with the condition, quick treatment is important.

What causes hip dysplasia?

No one is sure why hip dysplasia occurs (or why the left hip dislocates more often than the right hip). One reason may have to do with the hormones a baby is exposed to before birth. While these hormones serve to relax muscles in the pregnant mother's body, in some cases they also may cause a baby's joints to become too relaxed and prone to dislocation. This condition often corrects itself in several days, and the hip develops normally. In some cases, these dislocations cause changes in the hip anatomy that need treatment.

Who is at risk?

Factors that may increase the risk of hip dysplasia include
- Sex—more frequent in girls
- Family history—more likely when other family members have had hip dysplasia
- Birth position—more common in infants born in the breech position
- Birth order—firstborn children most at risk for hip dysplasia

Detecting hip dysplasia

Your pediatrician will check your newborn for hip dysplasia right after birth and at every well-child exam until your child is walking normally.

During the exam, your child's pediatrician will carefully flex and rotate your child's legs to see if the thighbones are properly positioned in the hip sockets. This does not require a great deal of force and will not hurt your baby.

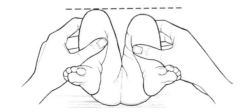

Your child's pediatrician also will look for other signs that may suggest a problem, including
- Limited range of motion in either leg
- One leg is shorter than the other
- Thigh or buttock creases appear uneven or lopsided

If your child's pediatrician suspects a problem with your child's hip, you may be referred to an orthopedic specialist who has experience treating hip dysplasia.

Treating hip dysplasia

Early treatment is important. The sooner treatment begins, the simpler it will be. In the past parents were told to double or triple diaper their babies to keep the legs in a position where dislocation was unlikely. *This practice is not recommended.* The diapering will not prevent hip dysplasia and will only delay effective treatment. Failure to treat this condition can result in permanent disability.

If your child is diagnosed with hip dysplasia before she is 6 months old, she will most likely be treated with a soft brace (such as the Pavlik harness) that holds the legs flexed and apart to allow the thighbones to be secure in the hip sockets.

The orthopedic consultant will tell you how long and when your baby will need to wear the brace. Your child also will be examined frequently during this time to make sure that the hips remain normal and stable.

In resistant cases or in older children, hip dysplasia may need to be treated with a combination of braces, casts, traction, or surgery. Your child will be admitted to the hospital if surgery is necessary. After surgery, your child will be placed in a hip spica cast for about 3 months. A hip spica cast is a hard cast that immobilizes the hips and keeps them in the correct position. When the cast is removed, your child will need to wear a removable hip brace for several more months.

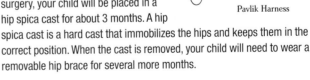

Pavlik Harness

Remember

If you have any concerns about your child's walking, talk with his pediatrician. If the cause is hip dysplasia, prompt treatment is important.

The information contained in this publication should not be used as a substitute for the medical care and advice of your pediatrician. There may be variations in treatment that your pediatrician may recommend based on individual facts and circumstances.

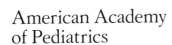
American Academy of Pediatrics
DEDICATED TO THE HEALTH OF ALL CHILDREN™

The American Academy of Pediatrics is an organization of 60,000 primary care pediatricians, pediatric medical subspecialists, and pediatric surgical specialists dedicated to the health, safety, and well-being of infants, children, adolescents, and young adults.

American Academy of Pediatrics
Web site—www.aap.org

Copyright © 2003
American Academy of Pediatrics

Febrile Seizures: Clinical Practice Guideline for the Long-term Management of the Child With Simple Febrile Seizures

- *Clinical Practice Guideline*

Febrile Seizures: Clinical Practice Guideline for the Long-term Management of the Child With Simple Febrile Seizures

Steering Committee on Quality Improvement and Management, Subcommittee on Febrile Seizures

ABSTRACT

Febrile seizures are the most common seizure disorder in childhood, affecting 2% to 5% of children between the ages of 6 and 60 months. Simple febrile seizures are defined as brief (<15-minute) generalized seizures that occur once during a 24-hour period in a febrile child who does not have an intracranial infection, metabolic disturbance, or history of afebrile seizures. This guideline (a revision of the 1999 American Academy of Pediatrics practice parameter [now termed clinical practice guideline] "The Long-term Treatment of the Child With Simple Febrile Seizures") addresses the risks and benefits of both continuous and intermittent anticonvulsant therapy as well as the use of antipyretics in children with simple febrile seizures. It is designed to assist pediatricians by providing an analytic framework for decisions regarding possible therapeutic interventions in this patient population. It is not intended to replace clinical judgment or to establish a protocol for all patients with this disorder. Rarely will these guidelines be the only approach to this problem. *Pediatrics* 2008;121:1281–1286

www.pediatrics.org/cgi/doi/10.1542/peds.2008-0939

doi:10.1542/peds.2008-0939

All clinical reports from the American Academy of Pediatrics automatically expire 5 years after publication unless reaffirmed, revised, or retired at or before that time.

The guidance in this report does not indicate an exclusive course of treatment or serve as a standard of medical care. Variations, taking into account individual circumstances, may be appropriate.

Key Word
fever

Abbreviation
AAP—American Academy of Pediatrics

PEDIATRICS (ISSN Numbers: Print, 0031-4005; Online, 1098-4275). Copyright © 2008 by the American Academy of Pediatrics

The expected outcomes of this practice guideline include:

1. optimizing practitioner understanding of the scientific basis for using or avoiding various proposed treatments for children with simple febrile seizures;

2. improving the health of children with simple febrile seizures by avoiding therapies with high potential for adverse effects and no demonstrated ability to improve children's long-term outcomes;

3. reducing costs by avoiding therapies that will not demonstrably improve children's long-term outcomes; and

4. helping the practitioner educate caregivers about the low risks associated with simple febrile seizures.

The committee determined that with the exception of a high rate of recurrence, no long-term effects of simple febrile seizures have been identified. The risk of developing epilepsy in these patients is extremely low, although slightly higher than that in the general population. No data, however, suggest that prophylactic treatment of children with simple febrile seizures would reduce the risk, because epilepsy likely is the result of genetic predisposition rather than structural damage to the brain caused by recurrent simple febrile seizures. Although antipyretics have been shown to be ineffective in preventing recurrent febrile seizures, there is evidence that continuous anticonvulsant therapy with phenobarbital, primidone, or valproic acid and intermittent therapy with diazepam are effective in reducing febrile-seizure recurrence. The potential toxicities associated with these agents, however, outweigh the relatively minor risks associated with simple febrile seizures. As such, the committee concluded that, on the basis of the risks and benefits of the effective therapies, neither continuous nor intermittent anticonvulsant therapy is recommended for children with 1 or more simple febrile seizures.

INTRODUCTION

Febrile seizures are seizures that occur in febrile children between the ages of 6 and 60 months who do not have an intracranial infection, metabolic disturbance, or history of afebrile seizures. Febrile seizures are subdivided into 2 categories: simple and complex. Simple febrile seizures last for less than 15 minutes, are generalized (without a focal component), and occur once in a 24-hour period, whereas complex febrile seizures are prolonged (>15 minutes), are focal, or occur more than once in 24 hours.[1] Despite the frequency of febrile seizures (2%–5%), there is no unanimity of opinion about management options. This clinical practice guideline addresses potential therapeutic interventions in neurologically normal children with simple febrile seizures. It is not intended for patients with complex febrile seizures and does not pertain to children with previous neurologic insults, known central nervous system abnormalities, or a history of afebrile seizures. This clinical practice guideline is a revision of a 1999 American Academy of Pediatrics (AAP) clinical practice parameter, "The Long-term Treatment of the Child With Simple Febrile Seizures."[2]

For a child who has experienced a simple febrile seizure, there are potentially 4 adverse outcomes that theoretically may be altered by an effective therapeutic agent: (1) decline in IQ; (2) increased risk of epilepsy; (3) risk of recurrent febrile seizures; and (4) death. Neither a decline in IQ, academic performance or neurocognitive inattention nor behavioral abnormalities have been shown to be a consequence of recurrent simple febrile seizures.[3] Ellenberg and Nelson[4] studied 431 children who experienced febrile seizures and observed no significant difference in their learning compared with sibling controls. In a similar study by Verity et al,[5] 303 children with febrile seizures were compared with control children. No difference in learning was identified, except in those children who had neurologic abnormalities before their first seizure.

The second concern, increased risk of epilepsy, is more complex. Children with simple febrile seizures have approximately the same risk of developing epilepsy by the age of 7 years as does the general population (ie, 1%).[6] However, children who have had multiple simple febrile seizures, are younger than 12 months at the time of their first febrile seizure, and have a family history of epilepsy are at higher risk, with generalized afebrile seizures developing by 25 years of age in 2.4%.[7] Despite this fact, no study has demonstrated that successful treatment of simple febrile seizures can prevent this later development of epilepsy, and there currently is no evidence that simple febrile seizures cause structural damage to the brain. Indeed, it is most likely that the increased risk of epilepsy in this population is the result of genetic predisposition.

In contrast to the slightly increased risk of developing epilepsy, children with simple febrile seizures have a high rate of recurrence. The risk varies with age. Children younger than 12 months at the time of their first simple febrile seizure have an approximately 50% probability of having recurrent febrile seizures. Children older than 12 months at the time of their first event have an approximately 30% probability of a second febrile seizure; of those who do have a second febrile seizure, 50% have a chance of having at least 1 additional recurrence.[8]

Finally, there is a theoretical risk of a child dying during a simple febrile seizure as a result of documented injury, aspiration, or cardiac arrhythmia, but to the committee's knowledge, it has never been reported.

In summary, with the exception of a high rate of recurrence, no long-term adverse effects of simple febrile seizures have been identified. Because the risks associated with simple febrile seizures, other than recurrence, are so low and because the number of children who have febrile seizures in the first few years of life is so high, to be commensurate, a proposed therapy would need to be exceedingly low in risks and adverse effects, inexpensive, and highly effective.

METHODS

To update the clinical practice guideline on the treatment of children with simple febrile seizures, the AAP reconvened the Subcommittee on Febrile Seizures. The committee was chaired by a child neurologist and consisted of a neuroepidemiologist, 2 additional child neurologists, and a practicing pediatrician. All panel members reviewed and signed the AAP voluntary disclosure and conflict-of-interest form. The guideline was reviewed by members of the AAP Steering Committee on Quality Improvement and Management; members of the AAP Sections on Neurology, Pediatric Emergency Medicine, Developmental and Behavioral Pediatrics, and Epidemiology; members of the AAP Committees on Pediatric Emergency Medicine and Medical Liability and Risk Management; members of the AAP Councils on Children With Disabilities and Community Pediatrics; and members of outside organizations including the Child Neurology Society and the American Academy of Neurology.

A comprehensive review of the evidence-based literature published since 1998 was conducted with the aim of addressing possible therapeutic interventions in the management of children with simple febrile seizures. The review focused on both the efficacy and potential adverse effects of the proposed treatments. Decisions were made on the basis of a systematic grading of the quality of evidence and strength of recommendations.

The AAP established a partnership with the University of Kentucky (Lexington, KY) to develop an evidence report, which served as a major source of information for these practice-guideline recommendations. The specific issues addressed were (1) effectiveness of continuous anticonvulsant therapy in preventing recurrent febrile seizures, (2) effectiveness of intermittent anticonvulsant therapy in preventing recurrent febrile seizures, (3) effectiveness of antipyretics in preventing recurrent febrile seizures, and (4) adverse effects of either continuous or intermittent anticonvulsant therapy.

In the original practice parameter, more than 300 medical journal articles reporting studies of the natural history of simple febrile seizures or the therapy of these seizures were reviewed and abstracted.[2] An additional 65 articles were reviewed and abstracted for the update. Emphasis was placed on articles that differentiated simple febrile seizures from other types of seizures, that carefully matched treatment and control groups, and that described adherence to the drug regimen. Tables were constructed from the 65 articles that best fit these criteria. A more comprehensive review of the literature on which this report is based can be found in a forthcoming technical report (the initial technical report can be accessed at http://aappolicy.aappublications.org/cgi/content/full/pediatrics;103/6/e86). The technical report also will contain dosing information.

The evidence-based approach to guideline development requires that the evidence in support of a recommendation be identified, appraised, and summarized and that an explicit link between evidence and recommendations be defined. Evidence-based recommendations reflect the quality of evidence and the balance of benefit and harm that is

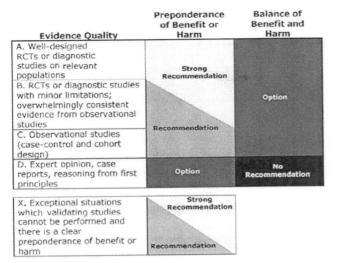

FIGURE 1
Integrating evidence-quality appraisal with an assessment of the anticipated balance between benefits and harms if a policy is conducted leads to designation of a policy as a strong recommendation, recommendation, option, or no recommendation. RCT indicates randomized, controlled trial.

anticipated when the recommendation is followed. The AAP policy statement "Classifying Recommendations for Clinical Practice Guidelines"[9] was followed in designating levels of recommendations (see Fig 1 and Table 1).

RECOMMENDATION

On the basis of the risks and benefits of the effective therapies, neither continuous nor intermittent anticonvulsant therapy is recommended for children with 1 or more simple febrile seizures.

- Aggregate evidence quality: B (randomized, controlled trials and diagnostic studies with minor limitations).

- Benefit: prevention of recurrent febrile seizures, which are not harmful and do not significantly increase the risk for development of future epilepsy.

- Harm: adverse effects including rare fatal hepatotoxicity (especially in children younger than 2 years who are also at greatest risk of febrile seizures), thrombocytopenia, weight loss and gain, gastrointestinal disturbances, and pancreatitis with valproic acid and hyperactivity, irritability, lethargy, sleep disturbances, and hypersensitivity reactions with phenobarbital; lethargy, drowsiness, and ataxia for intermittent diazepam as well as the risk of masking an evolving central nervous system infection.

- Benefits/harms assessment: preponderance of harm over benefit.

- Policy level: recommendation.

BENEFITS AND RISKS OF CONTINUOUS ANTICONVULSANT THERAPY

Phenobarbital

Phenobarbital is effective in preventing the recurrence of simple febrile seizures.[10] In a controlled double-blind study, daily therapy with phenobarbital reduced the rate of subsequent febrile seizures from 25 per 100 subjects per year to 5 per 100 subjects per year.[11] For the agent to be effective, however, it must be given daily and maintained in the therapeutic range. In a study by Farwell et al,[12] for example, children whose phenobarbital levels were in the therapeutic range had a reduction in recurrent seizures, but because noncompliance was so high, an overall benefit with phenobarbital therapy was not identified.

The adverse effects of phenobarbital include hyperactivity, irritability, lethargy, sleep disturbances, and hypersensitivity reactions. The behavioral adverse effects

TABLE 1   Guideline Definitions for Evidence-Based Statements

Statement	Definition	Implication
Strong recommendation	A strong recommendation in favor of a particular action is made when the anticipated benefits of the recommended intervention clearly exceed the harms (as a strong recommendation against an action is made when the anticipated harms clearly exceed the benefits) and the quality of the supporting evidence is excellent. In some clearly identified circumstances, strong recommendations may be made when high-quality evidence is impossible to obtain and the anticipated benefits strongly outweigh the harms.	Clinicians should follow a strong recommendation unless a clear and compelling rationale for an alternative approach is present.
Recommendation	A recommendation in favor of a particular action is made when the anticipated benefits exceed the harms but the quality of evidence is not as strong. Again, in some clearly identified circumstances, recommendations may be made when high-quality evidence is impossible to obtain but the anticipated benefits outweigh the harms.	Clinicians would be prudent to follow a recommendation but should remain alert to new information and sensitive to patient preferences.
Option	Options define courses that may be taken when either the quality of evidence is suspect or carefully performed studies have shown little clear advantage to 1 approach over another.	Clinicians should consider the option in their decision-making, and patient preference may have a substantial role.
No recommendation	No recommendation indicates that there is a lack of pertinent published evidence and that the anticipated balance of benefits and harms is presently unclear.	Clinicians should be alert to new published evidence that clarifies the balance of benefit versus harm.

may occur in up to 20% to 40% of patients and may be severe enough to necessitate discontinuation of the drug.[13-16]

Primidone

Primidone, in doses of 15 to 20 mg/kg per day, has also been shown to reduce the recurrence rate of febrile seizures.[17,18] It is of interest that the derived phenobarbital level in a Minigawa and Miura study[17] was below therapeutic (16 μg/mL) in 29 of the 32 children, suggesting that primidone itself may be active in preventing seizure recurrence. As with phenobarbital, adverse effects include behavioral disturbances, irritability, and sleep disturbances.[18]

Valproic Acid

In randomized, controlled studies, only 4% of children taking valproic acid, as opposed to 35% of control subjects, had a subsequent febrile seizure. Therefore, valproic acid seems to be at least as effective in preventing recurrent simple febrile seizures as phenobarbital and significantly more effective than placebo.[19-21]

Drawbacks to therapy with valproic acid include its rare association with fatal hepatotoxicity (especially in children younger than 2 years, who are also at greatest risk of febrile seizures), thrombocytopenia, weight loss and gain, gastrointestinal disturbances, and pancreatitis. In studies in which children received valproic acid to prevent recurrence of febrile seizures, no cases of fatal hepatotoxicity were reported.[15]

Carbamazepine

Carbamazepine has not been shown to be effective in preventing the recurrence of simple febrile seizures. Antony and Hawke[13] compared children who had been treated with therapeutic levels of either phenobarbital or carbamazepine, and 47% of the children in the carbamazepine-treated group had recurrent seizures compared with only 10% of those in the phenobarbital group. In another study, Camfield et al[22] treated children (whose conditions failed to improve with phenobarbital therapy) with carbamazepine. Despite good compliance, 13 of the 16 children treated with carbamazepine had a recurrent febrile seizure within 18 months. It is theoretically possible that these excessively high rates of recurrences might have been attributable to adverse effects of carbamazepine.

Phenytoin

Phenytoin has not been shown to be effective in preventing the recurrence of simple febrile seizures, even when the agent is in the therapeutic range.[23,24] Other anticonvulsants have not been studied for the continuous treatment of simple febrile seizures.

BENEFITS AND RISKS OF INTERMITTENT ANTICONVULSANT THERAPY

Diazepam

A double-blind controlled study of patients with a history of febrile seizures demonstrated that administration of oral diazepam (given at the time of fever) could reduce the recurrence of febrile seizures. Children with a history of febrile seizures were given either oral diazepam (0.33 mg/kg, every 8 hours for 48 hours) or a placebo at the time of fever. The risk of febrile seizures per person-year was decreased 44% with diazepam.[25] In a more recent study, children with a history of febrile seizures were given oral diazepam at the time of fever and then compared with children in an untreated control group. In the oral diazepam group, there was an 11% recurrence rate compared with a 30% recurrence rate in the control group.[26] It should be noted that all children for whom diazepam was considered a failure had been noncompliant with drug administration, in part because of adverse effects of the medication.

There is also literature that demonstrates the feasibility and safety of interrupting a simple febrile seizure lasting less than 5 minutes with rectal diazepam and with both intranasal and buccal midazolam.[27,28] Although these agents are effective in terminating the seizure, it is questionable whether they have any long-term influence on outcome. In a study by Knudsen et al,[29] children were given either rectal diazepam at the time of fever or only at the onset of seizure. Twelve-year follow-up found that the long-term prognosis of the children in the 2 groups did not differ regardless of whether treatment was aimed at preventing seizures or treating them.

A potential drawback to intermittent medication is that a seizure could occur before a fever is noticed. Indeed, in several of these studies, recurrent seizures were likely attributable to failure of method rather than failure of the agent.

Adverse effects of oral and rectal diazepam[26] and both intranasal and buccal midazolam include lethargy, drowsiness, and ataxia. Respiratory depression is extremely rare, even when given by the rectal route.[28,30] Sedation caused by any of the benzodiazepines, whether administered by the oral, rectal, nasal, or buccal route, have the potential of masking an evolving central nervous system infection. If used, the child's health care professional should be contacted.

BENEFITS AND RISKS OF INTERMITTENT ANTIPYRETICS

No studies have demonstrated that antipyretics, in the absence of anticonvulsants, reduce the recurrence risk of simple febrile seizures. Camfield et al[11] treated 79 children who had had a first febrile seizure with either a placebo plus antipyretic instruction (either aspirin or acetaminophen) versus daily phenobarbital plus antipyretic instruction (either aspirin or acetaminophen). Recurrence risk was significantly lower in the phenobarbital-treated group, suggesting that antipyretic instruction, including the use of antipyretics, is ineffective in preventing febrile-seizure recurrence.

Whether antipyretics are given regularly (every 4 hours) or sporadically (contingent on a specific body-temperature elevation) does not influence outcome. Acetaminophen was either given every 4 hours or only for temperature elevations of more than 37.9°C in 104 children. The incidence of febrile episodes did not differ significantly between the 2 groups, nor did the early recurrence of febrile seizures. The authors determined that administering prophylactic acetaminophen during febrile episodes was ineffective in preventing or reducing fever and in preventing febrile-seizure recurrence.[31]

In a randomized double-blind placebo-controlled trial, acetaminophen was administered along with low-dose oral diazepam.[32] Febrile-seizure recurrence was not reduced, compared with control groups. As with acetaminophen, ibuprofen also has been shown to be ineffective in preventing recurrence of febrile seizures.[33–35]

In general, acetaminophen and ibuprofen are considered to be safe and effective antipyretics for children. However, hepatotoxicity (with acetaminophen) and respiratory failure, metabolic acidosis, renal failure, and coma (with ibuprofen) have been reported in children after overdose or in the presence of risk factors.[36,37]

CONCLUSIONS

The subcommittee has determined that a simple febrile seizure is a benign and common event in children between the ages of 6 and 60 months. Nearly all children have an excellent prognosis. The committee concluded that although there is evidence that both continuous antiepileptic therapy with phenobarbital, primidone, or valproic acid and intermittent therapy with oral diazepam are effective in reducing the risk of recurrence, the potential toxicities associated with antiepileptic drugs outweigh the relatively minor risks associated with simple febrile seizures. As such, long-term therapy is not recommended. In situations in which parental anxiety associated with febrile seizures is severe, intermittent oral diazepam at the onset of febrile illness may be effective in preventing recurrence. Although antipyretics may improve the comfort of the child, they will not prevent febrile seizures.

SUBCOMMITTEE ON FEBRILE SEIZURES, 2002–2008

Patricia K. Duffner, MD, Chairperson
Robert J. Baumann, MD, Methodologist
Peter Berman, MD
John L. Green, MD
Sanford Schneider, MD

STEERING COMMITTEE ON QUALITY IMPROVEMENT AND MANAGEMENT, 2007–2008

Elizabeth S. Hodgson, MD, Chairperson
Gordon B. Glade, MD
Norman "Chip" Harbaugh, Jr, MD
Thomas K. McInerny, MD
Marlene R. Miller, MD, MSc
Virginia A. Moyer, MD, MPH
Xavier D. Sevilla, MD
Lisa Simpson, MB, BCh, MPH
Glenn S. Takata, MD

LIAISONS

Denise Dougherty, PhD
    Agency for Healthcare Research and Quality
Daniel R. Neuspiel, MD
    Section on Epidemiology

Ellen Schwalenstocker, MBA
    National Association of Children's Hospitals and Related Institutions

STAFF

Caryn Davidson, MA

REFERENCES

1. Nelson KB, Ellenberg JH. Prognosis in children with febrile seizures. *Pediatrics*. 1978;61(5):720–727
2. American Academy of Pediatrics, Committee on Quality Improvement, Subcommittee on Febrile Seizures. The long-term treatment of the child with simple febrile seizures. *Pediatrics*. 1999;103(6 pt 1):1307–1309
3. Chang YC, Guo NW, Huang CC, Wang ST, Tsai JJ. Neurocognitive attention and behavior outcome of school age children with a history of febrile convulsions: a population study. *Epilepsia*. 2000;41(4):412–420
4. Ellenberg JH, Nelson KB. Febrile seizures and later intellectual performance. *Arch Neurol*. 1978;35(1):17–21
5. Verity CM, Butler NR, Golding J. Febrile convulsions in a national cohort followed up from birth. II: medical history and intellectual ability at 5 years of age. *BMJ*. 1985;290(6478):1311–1315
6. Nelson KB, Ellenberg JH. Predictors of epilepsy in children who have experienced febrile seizures. *N Engl J Med*. 1976;295(19):1029–1033
7. Annegers JF, Hauser WA, Shirts SB, Kurland LT. Factors prognostic of unprovoked seizures after febrile convulsions. *N Engl J Med*. 1987;316(9):493–498
8. Berg AT, Shinnar S, Darefsky AS, et al. Predictors of recurrent febrile seizures: a prospective cohort study. *Arch Pediatr Adolesc Med*. 1997;151(4):371–378
9. American Academy of Pediatrics, Steering Committee on Quality Improvement and Management. Classifying recommendations for clinical practice guidelines. *Pediatrics*. 2004;114(3):874–877
10. Wolf SM, Carr A, Davis DC, Davidson S, et al. The value of phenobarbital in the child who has had a single febrile seizure: a controlled prospective study. *Pediatrics*. 1977;59(3):378–385
11. Camfield PR, Camfield CS, Shapiro SH, Cummings C. The first febrile seizure: antipyretic instruction plus either phenobarbital or placebo to prevent recurrence. *J Pediatr*. 1980;97(1):16–21
12. Farwell JR, Lee JY, Hirtz DG, Sulzbacher SI, Ellenberg JH, Nelson KB. Phenobarbital for febrile seizures: effects on intelligence and on seizure recurrence [published correction appears in *N Engl J Med*. 1992;326(2):144]. *N Engl J Med*. 1990;322(6):364–369
13. Antony JH, Hawke SHB. Phenobarbital compared with carbamazepine in prevention of recurrent febrile convulsions. *Am J Dis Child*. 1983;137(9):892–895
14. Knudsen Fu, Vestermark S. Prophylactic diazepam or phenobarbitone in febrile convulsions: a prospective, controlled study. *Arch Dis Child*. 1978;53(8):660–663
15. Lee K, Melchior JC. Sodium valproate versus phenobarbital in the prophylactic treatment of febrile convulsions in childhood. *Eur J Pediatr*. 1981;137(2):151–153
16. Camfield CS, Chaplin S, Doyle AB, Shapiro SH, Cummings C, Camfield PR. Side effects of phenobarbital in toddlers: behavioral and cognitive aspects. *J Pediatr*. 1979;95(3):361–365
17. Minagawa K, Miura H. Phenobarbital, primidone and sodium valproate in the prophylaxis of febrile convulsions. *Brain Dev*. 1981;3(4):385–393
18. Herranz JL, Armijo JA, Arteaga R. Effectiveness and toxicity of phenobarbital, primidone, and sodium valproate in the pre-

vention of febrile convulsions, controlled by plasma levels. *Epilepsia.* 1984;25(1):89–95

19. Wallace SJ, Smith JA. Successful prophylaxis against febrile convulsions with valproic acid or phenobarbitone. *BMJ.* 1980; 280(6211):353–354

20. Mamelle N, Mamelle JC, Plasse JC, Revol M, Gilly R. Prevention of recurrent febrile convulsions: a randomized therapeutic assay—sodium valproate, phenobarbitone and placebo. *Neuropediatrics.* 1984;15(1):37–42

21. Ngwane E, Bower B. Continuous sodium valproate or phenobarbitone in the prevention of "simple" febrile convulsions. *Arch Dis Child.* 1980;55(3):171–174

22. Camfield PR, Camfield CS, Tibbles JA. Carbamazepine does not prevent febrile seizures in phenobarbital failures. *Neurology.* 1982;32(3):288–289

23. Bacon CJ, Hierons AM, Mucklow JC, Webb JK, Rawlins MD, Weightman D. Placebo-controlled study of phenobarbitone and phenytoin in the prophylaxis of febrile convulsions. *Lancet.* 1981;2(8247):600–604

24. Melchior JC, Buchthal F, Lennox Buchthal M. The ineffectiveness of diphenylhydantoin in preventing febrile convulsions in the age of greatest risk, under 3 years. *Epilepsia.* 1971;12(1): 55–62

25. Rosman NP, Colton T, Labazzo J, et al. A controlled trial of diazepam administered during febrile illnesses to prevent recurrence of febrile seizures. *N Engl J Med.* 1993;329(2):79–84

26. Verrotti A, Latini G, di Corcia G, et al. Intermittent oral diazepam prophylaxis in febrile convulsions: its effectiveness for febrile seizure recurrence. *Eur J Pediatr Neurol.* 2004;8(3): 131–134

27. Lahat E, Goldman M, Barr J, Bistritzer T, Berkovitch M. Comparison of intranasal midazolam with intravenous diazepam for treating febrile seizures in children: prospective randomized study. *BMJ.* 2000;321(7253):83–86

28. McIntyre J, Robertson S, Norris E, et al. Safety and efficacy of buccal midazolam versus rectal diazepam for emergency treatment of seizures in children: a randomized controlled trial. *Lancet.* 2005;366(9481):205–210

29. Knudsen FU, Paerregaard A, Andersen R, Andresen J. Long term outcome of prophylaxis for febrile convulsions. *Arch Dis Child.* 1996;74(1):13–18

30. Pellock JM, Shinnar S. Respiratory adverse events associated with diazepam rectal gel. *Neurology.* 2005;64(10):1768–1770

31. Schnaiderman D, Lahat E, Sheefer T, Aladjem M. Antipyretic effectiveness of acetaminophen in febrile seizures: ongoing prophylaxis versus sporadic usage. *Eur J Pediatr.* 1993;152(9): 747–749

32. Uhari M, Rantala H, Vainionpaa L, Kurttila R. Effect of acetaminophen and of low dose intermittent doses of diazepam on prevention of recurrences of febrile seizures. *J Pediatr.* 1995; 126(6):991–995

33. van Stuijvenberg M, Derksen-Lubsen G, Steyerberg EW, Habbema JDF, Moll HA. Randomized, controlled trial of ibuprofen syrup administered during febrile illnesses to prevent febrile seizure recurrences. *Pediatrics.* 1998;102(5). Available at: www.pediatrics.org/cgi/content/full/102/5/e51

34. van Esch A, Van Steensel-Moll HA, Steyerberg EW, Offringa M, Habbema JDF, Derksen-Lubsen G. Antipyretic efficacy of ibuprofen and acetaminophen in children with febrile seizures. *Arch Pediatr Adolesc Med.* 1995;149(6):632–637

35. van Esch A, Steyerberg EW, Moll HA, et al. A study of the efficacy of antipyretic drugs in the prevention of febrile seizure recurrence. *Ambul Child Health.* 2000;6(1):19–26

36. Easley RB, Altemeier WA. Central nervous system manifestations of an ibuprofen overdose reversed by naloxone. *Pediatr Emerg Care.* 2000;16(1):39–41

37. American Academy of Pediatrics, Committee on Drugs. Acetaminophen toxicity in children. *Pediatrics.* 2001;108(4): 1020–1024

Febrile Seizures: Guideline for the Neurodiagnostic Evaluation of the Child With a Simple Febrile Seizure

- *Clinical Practice Guideline*

Clinical Practice Guideline—Febrile Seizures: Guideline for the Neurodiagnostic Evaluation of the Child With a Simple Febrile Seizure

SUBCOMMITTEE ON FEBRILE SEIZURES

KEY WORD

seizure

ABBREVIATIONS

AAP—American Academy of Pediatrics
Hib—*Haemophilus influenzae* type b
EEG—electroencephalogram
CT—computed tomography

www.pediatrics.org/cgi/doi/10.1542/peds.2010-3318

doi:10.1542/peds.2010-3318

All clinical practice guidelines from the American Academy of Pediatrics automatically expire 5 years after publication unless reaffirmed, revised, or retired at or before that time.

PEDIATRICS (ISSN Numbers: Print, 0031-4005; Online, 1098-4275).

abstract

OBJECTIVE: To formulate evidence-based recommendations for health care professionals about the diagnosis and evaluation of a simple febrile seizure in infants and young children 6 through 60 months of age and to revise the practice guideline published by the American Academy of Pediatrics (AAP) in 1996.

METHODS: This review included search and analysis of the medical literature published since the last version of the guideline. Physicians with expertise and experience in the fields of neurology and epilepsy, pediatrics, epidemiology, and research methodologies constituted a subcommittee of the AAP Steering Committee on Quality Improvement and Management. The steering committee and other groups within the AAP and organizations outside the AAP reviewed the guideline. The subcommittee member who reviewed the literature for the 1996 AAP practice guidelines searched for articles published since the last guideline through 2009, supplemented by articles submitted by other committee members. Results from the literature search were provided to the subcommittee members for review. Interventions of direct interest included lumbar puncture, electroencephalography, blood studies, and neuroimaging. Multiple issues were raised and discussed iteratively until consensus was reached about recommendations. The strength of evidence supporting each recommendation and the strength of the recommendation were assessed by the committee member most experienced in informatics and epidemiology and graded according to AAP policy.

CONCLUSIONS: Clinicians evaluating infants or young children after a simple febrile seizure should direct their attention toward identifying the cause of the child's fever. Meningitis should be considered in the differential diagnosis for any febrile child, and lumbar puncture should be performed if there are clinical signs or symptoms of concern. For any infant between 6 and 12 months of age who presents with a seizure and fever, a lumbar puncture is an option when the child is considered deficient in *Haemophilus influenzae* type b (Hib) or *Streptococcus pneumoniae* immunizations (ie, has not received scheduled immunizations as recommended), or when immunization status cannot be determined, because of an increased risk of bacterial meningitis. A lumbar puncture is an option for children who are pretreated with antibiotics. In general, a simple febrile seizure does not usually require further evaluation, specifically electroencephalography, blood studies, or neuroimaging. *Pediatrics* 2011;127:389–394

DEFINITION OF THE PROBLEM

This practice guideline provides recommendations for the neurodiagnostic evaluation of neurologically healthy infants and children 6 through 60 months of age who have had a simple febrile seizure and present for evaluation within 12 hours of the event. It replaces the 1996 practice parameter.[1] This practice guideline is not intended for patients who have had complex febrile seizures (prolonged, focal, and/or recurrent), and it does not pertain to children with previous neurologic insults, known central nervous system abnormalities, or history of afebrile seizures.

TARGET AUDIENCE AND PRACTICE SETTING

This practice guideline is intended for use by pediatricians, family physicians, child neurologists, neurologists, emergency physicians, nurse practitioners, and other health care providers who evaluate children for febrile seizures.

BACKGROUND

A febrile seizure is a seizure accompanied by fever (temperature $\geq$ 100.4°F or 38°C[2] by any method), without central nervous system infection, that occurs in infants and children 6 through 60 months of age. Febrile seizures occur in 2% to 5% of all children and, as such, make up the most common convulsive event in children younger than 60 months. In 1976, Nelson and Ellenberg,[3] using data from the National Collaborative Perinatal Project, further defined febrile seizures as being either simple or complex. Simple febrile seizures were defined as primary generalized seizures that lasted for less than 15 minutes and did not recur within 24 hours. Complex febrile seizures were defined as focal, prolonged ($\geq$15 minutes), and/or recurrent within 24 hours. Children who had simple febrile seizures had no evidence of increased mortality, hemiplegia, or mental retardation. During follow-up evaluation, the risk of epilepsy after a simple febrile seizure was shown to be only slightly higher than that of the general population, whereas the chief risk associated with simple febrile seizures was recurrence in one-third of the children. The authors concluded that simple febrile seizures are benign events with excellent prognoses, a conclusion reaffirmed in the 1980 consensus statement from the National Institutes of Health.[3,4]

The expected outcomes of this practice guideline include the following:

1. Optimize clinician understanding of the scientific basis for the neurodiagnostic evaluation of children with simple febrile seizures.

2. Aid the clinician in decision-making by using a structured framework.

3. Optimize evaluation of the child who has had a simple febrile seizure by detecting underlying diseases, minimizing morbidity, and reassuring anxious parents and children.

4. Reduce the costs of physician and emergency department visits, hospitalizations, and unnecessary testing.

5. Educate the clinician to understand that a simple febrile seizure usually does not require further evaluation, specifically electroencephalography, blood studies, or neuroimaging.

METHODOLOGY

To update the clinical practice guideline on the neurodiagnostic evaluation of children with simple febrile seizures,[1] the American Academy of Pediatrics (AAP) reconvened the Subcommittee on Febrile Seizures. The committee was chaired by a child neurologist and consisted of a neuroepidemiologist, 3 additional child neurologists, and a practicing pediatrician. All panel members reviewed and signed the AAP voluntary disclosure and conflict-of-interest form. No conflicts were reported. Participation in the guideline process was voluntary and not paid. The guideline was reviewed by members of the AAP Steering Commit-tee on Quality Improvement and Management; members of the AAP Section on Administration and Practice Management, Section on Developmental and Behavioral Pediatrics, Section on Epidemiology, Section on Infectious Diseases, Section on Neurology, Section on Neurologic Surgery, Section on Pediatric Emergency Medicine, Committee on Pediatric Emergency Medicine, Committee on Practice and Ambulatory Medicine, Committee on Child Health Financing, Committee on Infectious Diseases, Committee on Medical Liability and Risk Management, Council on Children With Disabilities, and Council on Community Pediatrics; and members of outside organizations including the Child Neurology Society, the American Academy of Neurology, the American College of Emergency Physicians, and members of the Pediatric Committee of the Emergency Nurses Association.

A comprehensive review of the evidence-based literature published from 1996 to February 2009 was conducted to discover articles that addressed the diagnosis and evaluation of children with simple febrile seizures. Preference was given to population-based studies, but given the scarcity of such studies, data from hospital-based studies, groups of young children with febrile illness, and comparable groups were reviewed. Decisions were made on the basis of a systematic grading of the quality of evidence and strength of recommendations.

In the original practice parameter,[1] 203 medical journal articles were reviewed and abstracted. An additional 372 articles were reviewed and abstracted for this update. Emphasis was placed on articles that differentiated simple febrile seizures from other types of seizures. Tables were constructed from the 70 articles that best fit these criteria.

The evidence-based approach to guideline development requires that the evidence in support of a recommendation be identified, appraised, and summarized and that an explicit link between

Evidence Quality	Preponderance of Benefit or Harm	Balance of Benefit and Harm
A. Well-designed RCTs or diagnostic studies on relevant population	Strong	
B. RCTs or diagnostic studies with minor limitations; overwhelmingly consistent evidence from observational studies		Option
C. Observational studies (case-control and cohort design)	Rec	
D. Expert opinion, case reports, reasoning from first principles	Option	No Rec
X. Exceptional situations for which validating studies cannot be performed and there is a clear preponderance of benefit or harm	Strong Rec	

FIGURE 1

Integrating evidence quality appraisal with an assessment of the anticipated balance between benefits and harms if a policy is carried out leads to designation of a policy as a strong recommendation, recommendation, option, or no recommendation. RCT indicates randomized controlled trial; Rec, recommendation.

evidence and recommendations be defined. Evidence-based recommendations reflect the quality of evidence and the balance of benefit and harm that is anticipated when the recommendation is followed. The AAP policy statement "Classifying Recommendations for Clinical Practice Guidelines"[5] was followed in designating levels of recommendations (see Fig 1).

KEY ACTION STATEMENTS

Action Statement 1

Action Statement 1a

A lumbar puncture should be performed in any child who presents with a seizure and a fever and has meningeal signs and symptoms (eg, neck stiffness, Kernig and/or Brudzinski signs) or in any child whose history or examination suggests the presence of meningitis or intracranial infection.

- Aggregate evidence level: B (overwhelming evidence from observational studies).
- Benefits: Meningeal signs and symptoms strongly suggest meningitis, which, if bacterial in etiology, will likely be fatal if left untreated.
- Harms/risks/costs: Lumbar puncture is an invasive and often painful procedure and can be costly.

- Benefits/harms assessment: Preponderance of benefit over harm.
- Value judgments: Observational data and clinical principles were used in making this judgment.
- Role of patient preferences: Although parents may not wish to have their child undergo a lumbar puncture, health care providers should explain that if meningitis is not diagnosed and treated, it could be fatal.
- Exclusions: None.
- Intentional vagueness: None.
- Policy level: Strong recommendation.

Action Statement 1b

In any infant between 6 and 12 months of age who presents with a seizure and fever, a lumbar puncture is an option when the child is considered deficient in *Haemophilus influenzae* type b (Hib) or *Streptococcus pneumoniae* immunizations (ie, has not received scheduled immunizations as recommended) or when immunization status cannot be determined because of an increased risk of bacterial meningitis.

- Aggregate evidence level: D (expert opinion, case reports).
- Benefits: Meningeal signs and symptoms strongly suggest meningitis, which, if bacterial in etiology, will

likely be fatal or cause significant long-term disability if left untreated.

- Harms/risks/costs: Lumbar puncture is an invasive and often painful procedure and can be costly.
- Benefits/harms assessment: Preponderance of benefit over harm.
- Value judgments: Data on the incidence of bacterial meningitis from before and after the existence of immunizations against Hib and *S pneumoniae* were used in making this recommendation.
- Role of patient preferences: Although parents may not wish their child to undergo a lumbar puncture, health care providers should explain that in the absence of complete immunizations, their child may be at risk of having fatal bacterial meningitis.
- Exclusions: This recommendation applies only to children 6 to 12 months of age. The subcommittee felt that clinicians would recognize symptoms of meningitis in children older than 12 months.
- Intentional vagueness: None.
- Policy level: Option.

Action Statement 1c

A lumbar puncture is an option in the child who presents with a seizure and fever and is pretreated with antibiotics, because antibiotic treatment can mask the signs and symptoms of meningitis.

- Aggregate evidence level: D (reasoning from clinical experience, case series).
- Benefits: Antibiotics may mask meningeal signs and symptoms but may be insufficient to eradicate meningitis; a diagnosis of meningitis, if bacterial in etiology, will likely be fatal if left untreated.
- Harms/risks/costs: Lumbar puncture is an invasive and often painful procedure and can be costly.

- Benefits/harms assessment: Preponderance of benefit over harm.
- Value judgments: Clinical experience and case series were used in making this judgment while recognizing that extensive data from studies are lacking.
- Role of patient preferences: Although parents may not wish to have their child undergo a lumbar puncture, medical providers should explain that in the presence of pretreatment with antibiotics, the signs and symptoms of meningitis may be masked. Meningitis, if untreated, can be fatal.
- Exclusions: None.
- Intentional vagueness: Data are insufficient to define the specific treatment duration necessary to mask signs and symptoms. The committee determined that the decision to perform a lumbar puncture will depend on the type and duration of antibiotics administered before the seizure and should be left to the individual clinician.
- Policy level: Option.

The committee recognizes the diversity of past and present opinions regarding the need for lumbar punctures in children younger than 12 months with a simple febrile seizure. Since the publication of the previous practice parameter,[1] however, there has been widespread immunization in the United States for 2 of the most common causes of bacterial meningitis in this age range: Hib and *S pneumoniae*. Although compliance with all scheduled immunizations as recommended does not completely eliminate the possibility of bacterial meningitis from the differential diagnosis, current data no longer support routine lumbar puncture in well-appearing, fully immunized children who present with a simple febrile seizure.[6–8] Moreover, although approximately 25% of young children with meningitis have seizures as the presenting sign of the disease, some are ei-

ther obtunded or comatose when evaluated by a physician for the seizure, and the remainder most often have obvious clinical signs of meningitis (focal seizures, recurrent seizures, petechial rash, or nuchal rigidity).[9–11] Once a decision has been made to perform a lumbar puncture, then blood culture and serum glucose testing should be performed concurrently to increase the sensitivity for detecting bacteria and to determine if there is hypoglycorrhachia characteristic of bacterial meningitis, respectively.

Recent studies that evaluated the outcome of children with simple febrile seizures have included populations with a high prevalence of immunization.[7,8] Data for unimmunized or partially immunized children are lacking. Therefore, lumbar puncture is an option for young children who are considered deficient in immunizations or those in whom immunization status cannot be determined. There are also no definitive data on the outcome of children who present with a simple febrile seizure while already on antibiotics. The authors were unable to find a definition of "pretreated" in the literature, so they consulted with the AAP Committee on Infectious Diseases. Although there is no formal definition, pretreatment can be considered to include systemic antibiotic therapy by any route given within the days before the seizure. Whether pretreatment will affect the presentation and course of bacterial meningitis cannot be predicted but will depend, in part, on the antibiotic administered, the dose, the route of administration, the drug's cerebrospinal fluid penetration, and the organism causing the meningitis. Lumbar puncture is an option in any child pretreated with antibiotics before a simple febrile seizure.

Action Statement 2

An electroencephalogram (EEG) should not be performed in the evaluation of a neurologically healthy child with a simple febrile seizure.

- Aggregate evidence level: B (overwhelming evidence from observational studies).
- Benefits: One study showed a possible association with paroxysmal EEGs and a higher rate of afebrile seizures.[12]
- Harms/risks/costs: EEGs are costly and may increase parental anxiety.
- Benefits/harms assessment: Preponderance of harm over benefit.
- Value judgments: Observational data were used for this judgment.
- Role of patient preferences: Although an EEG might have limited prognostic utility in this situation, parents should be educated that the study will not alter outcome.
- Exclusions: None.
- Intentional vagueness: None.
- Policy level: Strong recommendation.

There is no evidence that EEG readings performed either at the time of presentation after a simple febrile seizure or within the following month are predictive of either recurrence of febrile seizures or the development of afebrile seizures/epilepsy within the next 2 years.[13,14] There is a single study that found that a paroxysmal EEG was associated with a higher rate of afebrile seizures.[12] There is no evidence that interventions based on this test would alter outcome.

Action Statement 3

The following tests should not be performed routinely for the sole purpose of identifying the cause of a simple febrile seizure: measurement of serum electrolytes, calcium, phosphorus, magnesium, or blood glucose or complete blood cell count.

- Aggregate evidence level: B (overwhelming evidence from observational studies).
- Benefits: A complete blood cell count may identify children at risk for bacte-

remia; however, the incidence of bacteremia in febrile children younger than 24 months is the same with or without febrile seizures.

- Harms/risks/costs: Laboratory tests may be invasive and costly and provide no real benefit.
- Benefits/harms assessment: Preponderance of harm over benefit.
- Value judgments: Observational data were used for this judgment.
- Role of patient preferences: Although parents may want blood tests performed to explain the seizure, they should be reassured that blood tests should be directed toward identifying the source of their child's fever.
- Exclusions: None.
- Intentional vagueness: None.
- Policy level: Strong recommendation.

There is no evidence to suggest that routine blood studies are of benefit in the evaluation of the child with a simple febrile seizure.[15–18] Although some children with febrile seizures have abnormal serum electrolyte values, their condition should be identifiable by obtaining appropriate histories and performing careful physical examinations. It should be noted that as a group, children with febrile seizures have relatively low serum sodium concentrations. As such, physicians and caregivers should avoid overhydration with hypotonic fluids.[18] Complete blood cell counts may be useful as a means of identifying young children at risk of bacteremia. It should be noted, however, that the incidence of bacteremia in children younger than 24 months with or without febrile seizures is the same. When fever is present, the decision regarding the need for laboratory testing should be directed toward identifying the source of the fever rather than as part of the routine evaluation of the seizure itself.

Action Statement 4

Neuroimaging should not be performed in the routine evaluation of the child with a simple febrile seizure.

- Aggregate evidence level: B (overwhelming evidence from observational studies).
- Benefits: Neuroimaging might provide earlier detection of fixed structural lesions, such as dysplasia, or very rarely, abscess or tumor.
- Harms/risks/costs: Neuroimaging tests are costly, computed tomography (CT) exposes children to radiation, and MRI may require sedation.
- Benefits/harms assessment: Preponderance of harm over benefit.
- Value judgments: Observational data were used for this judgment.
- Role of patient preferences: Although parents may want neuroimaging performed to explain the seizure, they should be reassured that the tests carry risks and will not alter outcome for their child.
- Exclusions: None.
- Intentional vagueness: None.
- Policy level: Strong recommendation.

The literature does not support the use of skull films in evaluation of the child with a febrile seizure.[15,19] No data have been published that either support or negate the need for CT or MRI in the evaluation of children with simple febrile seizures. Data, however, show that CT scanning is associated with radiation exposure that may escalate future cancer risk. MRI is associated with risks from required sedation and high cost.[20,21] Extrapolation of data from the literature on the use of CT in neurologically healthy children who have generalized epilepsy has shown that clinically important intracranial structural abnormalities in this patient population are uncommon.[22,23]

CONCLUSIONS

Clinicians evaluating infants or young children after a simple febrile seizure should direct their attention toward identifying the cause of the child's fever. Meningitis should be considered in the differential diagnosis for any febrile child, and lumbar puncture should be performed if the child is ill-appearing or if there are clinical signs or symptoms of concern. A lumbar puncture is an option in a child 6 to 12 months of age who is deficient in Hib and *S pneumoniae* immunizations or for whom immunization status is unknown. A lumbar puncture is an option in children who have been pretreated with antibiotics. In general, a simple febrile seizure does not usually require further evaluation, specifically EEGs, blood studies, or neuroimaging.

SUBCOMMITTEE ON FEBRILE SEIZURES, 2002–2010

Patricia K. Duffner, MD (neurology, no conflicts)
Peter H. Berman, MD (neurology, no conflicts)
Robert J. Baumann, MD (neuroepidemiology, no conflicts)
Paul Graham Fisher, MD (neurology, no conflicts)
John L. Green, MD (general pediatrics, no conflicts)
Sanford Schneider, MD (neurology, no conflicts)

STAFF
Caryn Davidson, MA

OVERSIGHT BY THE STEERING COMMITTEE ON QUALITY IMPROVEMENT AND MANAGEMENT, 2009–2011

REFERENCES

1. American Academy of Pediatrics, Provisional Committee on Quality Improvement and Subcommittee on Febrile Seizures. Practice parameter: the neurodiagnostic evaluation of a child with a first simple febrile seizure. *Pediatrics.* 1996;97(5): 769–772; discussion 773–775

2. Michael Marcy S, Kohl KS, Dagan R, et al; Brighton Collaboration Fever Working Group. Fever as an adverse event following immunization: case definition and guidelines of data collection, analysis, and presentation. *Vaccine.* 2004;22(5–6):551–556

3. Nelson KB, Ellenberg JH. Predictors of epilepsy in children who have experienced febrile seizures. *N Engl J Med.* 1976;295(19): 1029–1033

4. Consensus statement: febrile seizures—long-term management of children with fever-associated seizures. *Pediatrics.* 1980; 66(6):1009–1012

5. American Academy of Pediatrics, Steering Committee on Quality Improvement and Management. Classifying recommendations for clinical practice guidelines. *Pediatrics.* 2004;114(3):874–877

6. Trainor JL, Hampers LC, Krug SE, Listernick R. Children with first-time simple febrile seizures are at low risk of serious bacterial illness. *Acad Emerg Med.* 2001;8(8):781–787

7. Shaked O, Peña BM, Linares MY, Baker RL. Simple febrile seizures: are the AAP guidelines regarding lumbar puncture being followed? *Pediatr Emerg Care.* 2009;25(1): 8–11

8. Kimia AA, Capraro AJ, Hummel D, Johnston P, Harper MB. Utility of lumbar puncture for first simple febrile seizure among children 6 to 18 months of age. *Pediatrics.* 2009; 123(1):6–12

9. Warden CR, Zibulewsky J, Mace S, Gold C, Gausche-Hill M. Evaluation and management of febrile seizures in the out-of-hospital and emergency department settings. *Ann Emerg Med.* 2003;41(2):215–222

10. Rutter N, Smales OR. Role of routine investigations in children presenting with their first febrile convulsion. *Arch Dis Child.* 1977; 52(3):188–191

11. Green SM, Rothrock SG, Clem KJ, Zurcher RF, Mellick L. Can seizures be the sole manifestation of meningitis in febrile children? *Pediatrics.* 1993;92(4):527–534

12. Kuturec M, Emoto SE, Sofijanov N, et al. Febrile seizures: is the EEG a useful predictor of recurrences? *Clin Pediatr (Phila).* 1997; 36(1):31–36

13. Frantzen E, Lennox-Buchthal M, Nygaard A. Longitudinal EEG and clinical study of children with febrile convulsions. *Electroencephalogr Clin Neurophysiol.* 1968;24(3): 197–212

14. Thorn I. The significance of electroencephalography in febrile convulsions. In: Akimoto H, Kazamatsuri H, Seino M, Ward A, eds. *Advances in Epileptology: XIIIth International Epilepsy Symposium.* New York, NY: Raven Press; 1982:93–95

15. Jaffe M, Bar-Joseph G, Tirosh E. Fever and convulsions: indications for laboratory investigations. *Pediatrics.* 1981;67(5): 729–731

16. Gerber MA, Berliner BC. The child with a "simple" febrile seizure: appropriate diagnostic evaluation. *Am J Dis Child.* 1981; 135(5):431–443

17. Heijbel J, Blom S, Bergfors PG. Simple febrile convulsions: a prospective incidence study and an evaluation of investigations initially needed. *Neuropadiatrie.* 1980;11(1): 45–56

18. Thoman JE, Duffner PK, Shucard JL. Do serum sodium levels predict febrile seizure recurrence within 24 hours? *Pediatr Neurol.* 2004;31(5):342–344

19. Nealis GT, McFadden SW, Ames RA, Ouellette EM. Routine skull roentgenograms in the management of simple febrile seizures. *J Pediatr.* 1977;90(4):595–596

20. Stein SC, Hurst RW, Sonnad SS. Meta-analysis of cranial CT scans in children: a mathematical model to predict radiation-induced tumors associated with radiation exposure that may escalate future cancer risk. *Pediatr Neurosurg.* 2008;44(6): 448–457

21. Brenner DJ, Hall EJ. Computed tomography: an increasing source of radiation exposure. *N Engl J Med.* 2007;357(22):2277–2284

22. Yang PJ, Berger PE, Cohen ME, Duffner PK. Computed tomography and childhood seizure disorders. *Neurology.* 1979;29(8): 1084–1088

23. Bachman DS, Hodges FJ, Freeman JM. Computerized axial tomography in chronic seizure disorders of childhood. *Pediatrics.* 1976;58(6):828–832

Febrile Seizures Clinical Practice Guidelines
Quick Reference Tools

- Recommendation Summaries
  — Febrile Seizures: Clinical Practice Guideline for the Long-term Management of the Child With Simple Febrile Seizures
  — Febrile Seizures: Guideline for the Neurodiagnostic Evaluation of the Child With a Simple Febrile Seizure
- *ICD-10-CM* Coding Quick Reference for Febrile Seizures
- AAP Patient Education Handout
  — *Febrile Seizures*

Recommendation Summaries

Febrile Seizures: Clinical Practice Guideline for the Long-term Management of the Child With Simple Febrile Seizures

On the basis of the risks and benefits of the effective therapies, neither continuous nor intermittent anticonvulsant therapy is recommended for children with 1 or more simple febrile seizures.

- Aggregate evidence quality: B (randomized, controlled trials and diagnostic studies with minor limitations).
- Benefit: prevention of recurrent febrile seizures, which are not harmful and do not significantly increase the risk for development of future epilepsy.
- Harm: adverse effects including rare fatal hepatotoxicity (especially in children younger than 2 years who are also at greatest risk of febrile seizures), thrombocytopenia, weight loss and gain, gastrointestinal disturbances, and pancreatitis with valproic acid and hyperactivity, irritability, lethargy, sleep disturbances, and hypersensitivity reactions with phenobarbital; lethargy, drowsiness, and ataxia for intermittent diazepam as well as the risk of masking an evolving central nervous system infection.
- Benefits/harms assessment: preponderance of harm over benefit.
- Policy level: recommendation.

Febrile Seizures: Guideline for the Neurodiagnostic Evaluation of the Child With a Simple Febrile Seizure

Action Statement 1a

A lumbar puncture should be performed in any child who presents with a seizure and a fever and has meningeal signs and symptoms (eg, neck stiffness, Kernig and/or Brudzinski signs) or in any child whose history or examination suggests the presence of meningitis or intracranial infection.

Action Statement 1b

In any infant between 6 and 12 months of age who presents with a seizure and fever, a lumbar puncture is an option when the child is considered deficient in *Haemophilus influenzae* type b (Hib) or *Streptococcus pneumoniae* immunizations (ie, has not received scheduled immunizations as recommended) or when immunization status cannot be determined because of an increased risk of bacterial meningitis.

Action Statement 1c

A lumbar puncture is an option in the child who presents with a seizure and fever and is pretreated with antibiotics, because antibiotic treatment can mask the signs and symptoms of meningitis.

Action Statement 2

An electroencephalogram (EEG) should not be performed in the evaluation of a neurologically healthy child with a simple febrile seizure.

Action Statement 3

The following tests should not be performed routinely for the sole purpose of identifying the cause of a simple febrile seizure: measurement of serum electrolytes, calcium, phosphorus, magnesium, or blood glucose or complete blood cell count.

Action Statement 4

Neuroimaging should not be performed in the routine evaluation of the child with a simple febrile seizure.

Coding Quick Reference for Febrile Seizures
ICD-10-CM
R56.00 Simple febrile convulsions
R56.01 Complex febrile convulsions

Febrile Seizures

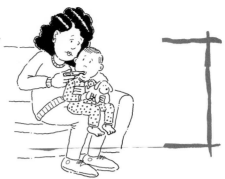

In some children, fevers can trigger seizures. Febrile seizures occur in 2% to 5% of all children between the ages of 6 months and 5 years. Seizures, sometimes called "fits" or "spells," are frightening, but they usually are harmless. Read on for information from the American Academy of Pediatrics that will help you understand febrile seizures and what happens if your child has one.

What is a febrile seizure?

A febrile seizure usually happens during the first few hours of a fever. The child may look strange for a few moments, then stiffen, twitch, and roll his eyes. He will be unresponsive for a short time, his breathing will be disturbed, and his skin may appear a little darker than usual. After the seizure, the child quickly returns to normal. Seizures usually last less than 1 minute but, although uncommon, can last for up to 15 minutes.

Febrile seizures rarely happen more than once within a 24-hour period. Other kinds of seizures (ones that are not caused by fever) last longer, can affect only one part of the body, and may occur repeatedly.

What do I do if my child has a febrile seizure?

If your child has a febrile seizure, act immediately to prevent injury.

- Place her on the floor or bed away from any hard or sharp objects.
- Turn her head to the side so that any saliva or vomit can drain from her mouth.
- Do not put anything into her mouth; she will not swallow her tongue.
- Call your child's doctor.
- If the seizure does not stop after 5 minutes, call 911 or your local emergency number.

Will my child have more seizures?

Febrile seizures tend to run in families. The risk of having seizures with other episodes of fever depends on the age of your child. Children younger than 1 year of age at the time of their first seizure have about a 50% chance of having another febrile seizure. Children older than 1 year of age at the time of their first seizure have only a 30% chance of having a second febrile seizure.

Will my child get epilepsy?

Epilepsy is a term used for multiple and recurrent seizures. Epileptic seizures are not caused by fever. Children with a history of febrile seizures are at only a slightly higher risk of developing epilepsy by age 7 than children who have not had febrile seizures.

Are febrile seizures dangerous?

While febrile seizures may be very scary, they are harmless to the child. Febrile seizures do not cause brain damage, nervous system problems, paralysis, intellectual disability (formerly called mental retardation), or death.

How are febrile seizures treated?

If your child has a febrile seizure, call your child's doctor right away. He or she will want to examine your child in order to determine the cause of your child's fever. It is more important to determine and treat the cause of the fever rather than the seizure. A spinal tap may be done to be sure your child does not have a serious infection like meningitis, especially if your child is younger than 1 year of age.

In general, doctors do not recommend treatment of a simple febrile seizure with preventive medicines. However, this should be discussed with your child's doctor. In cases of prolonged or repeated seizures, the recommendation may be different.

Medicines like acetaminophen and ibuprofen can help lower a fever, but they do not prevent febrile seizures. Your child's doctor will talk with you about the best ways to take care of your child's fever.

If your child has had a febrile seizure, do not fear the worst. These types of seizures are not dangerous to your child and do not cause long-term health problems. If you have concerns about this issue or anything related to your child's health, talk with your child's doctor.

The information contained in this publication should not be used as a substitute for the medical care and advice of your pediatrician. There may be variations in treatment that your pediatrician may recommend based on individual facts and circumstances.

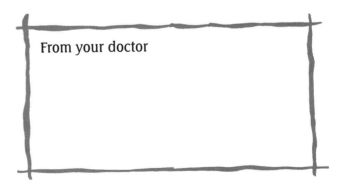

From your doctor

American Academy
of Pediatrics

DEDICATED TO THE HEALTH OF ALL CHILDREN™

The American Academy of Pediatrics is an organization of 60,000 primary care pediatricians, pediatric medical subspecialists, and pediatric surgical specialists dedicated to the health, safety, and well-being of infants, children, adolescents, and young adults.

American Academy of Pediatrics
Web site — www.HealthyChildren.org

Copyright © 1999
American Academy of Pediatrics, Updated 1/12
All rights reserved.

Clinical Practice Guideline for Screening and Management of High Blood Pressure in Children and Adolescents

- *Clinical Practice Guideline*
- *PPI: AAP Partnership for Policy Implementation*
  See Appendix 1 for more information.

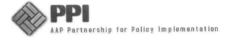

CLINICAL PRACTICE GUIDELINE Guidance for the Clinician in Rendering Pediatric Care

American Academy
of Pediatrics

DEDICATED TO THE HEALTH OF ALL CHILDREN™

Clinical Practice Guideline for Screening and Management of High Blood Pressure in Children and Adolescents

Joseph T. Flynn, MD, MS, FAAP,[a] David C. Kaelber, MD, PhD, MPH, FAAP, FACP, FACMI,[b] Carissa M. Baker-Smith, MD, MS, MPH, FAAP, FAHA,[c] Douglas Blowey, MD,[d] Aaron E. Carroll, MD, MS, FAAP,[e] Stephen R. Daniels, MD, PhD, FAAP,[f] Sarah D. de Ferranti, MD, MPH, FAAP,[g] Janis M. Dionne, MD, FRCPC,[h] Bonita Falkner, MD,[i] Susan K. Flinn, MA,[j] Samuel S. Gidding, MD,[k] Celeste Goodwin,[l] Michael G. Leu, MD, MS, MHS, FAAP,[m] Makia E. Powers, MD, MPH, FAAP,[n] Corinna Rea, MD, MPH, FAAP,[o] Joshua Samuels, MD, MPH, FAAP,[p] Madeline Simasek, MD, MSCP, FAAP,[q] Vidhu V. Thaker, MD, FAAP,[r] Elaine M. Urbina, MD, MS, FAAP,[s] SUBCOMMITTEE ON SCREENING AND MANAGEMENT OF HIGH BLOOD PRESSURE IN CHILDREN

abstract

These pediatric hypertension guidelines are an update to the 2004 "Fourth Report on the Diagnosis, Evaluation, and Treatment of High Blood Pressure in Children and Adolescents." Significant changes in these guidelines include (1) the replacement of the term "prehypertension" with the term "elevated blood pressure," (2) new normative pediatric blood pressure (BP) tables based on normal-weight children, (3) a simplified screening table for identifying BPs needing further evaluation, (4) a simplified BP classification in adolescents ≥13 years of age that aligns with the forthcoming American Heart Association and American College of Cardiology adult BP guidelines, (5) a more limited recommendation to perform screening BP measurements only at preventive care visits, (6) streamlined recommendations on the initial evaluation and management of abnormal BPs, (7) an expanded role for ambulatory BP monitoring in the diagnosis and management of pediatric hypertension, and (8) revised recommendations on when to perform echocardiography in the evaluation of newly diagnosed hypertensive pediatric patients (generally only before medication initiation), along with a revised definition of left ventricular hypertrophy. These guidelines include 30 Key Action Statements and 27 additional recommendations derived from a comprehensive review of almost 15 000 published articles between January 2004 and July 2016. Each Key Action Statement includes level of evidence, benefit-harm relationship, and strength of recommendation. This clinical practice guideline, endorsed by the American Heart Association, is intended to foster a patient- and family-centered approach to care, reduce unnecessary and costly medical interventions, improve patient diagnoses and outcomes, support implementation, and provide direction for future research.

[a]Dr. Robert O. Hickman Endowed Chair in Pediatric Nephrology, Division of Nephrology, Department of Pediatrics, University of Washington and Seattle Children's Hospital, Seattle, Washington; [b]Departments of Pediatrics, Internal Medicine, Population and Quantitative Health Sciences, Center for Clinical Informatics Research and Education, Case Western Reserve University and MetroHealth System, Cleveland, Ohio; [c]Division of Pediatric Cardiology, School of Medicine, University of Maryland, Baltimore, Maryland; [d]Children's Mercy Hospital, University of Missouri-Kansas City and Children's Mercy Integrated Care Solutions, Kansas City, Missouri; [e]Department of Pediatrics, School of Medicine, Indiana University, Bloomington, Indiana; [f]Department of Pediatrics, School of Medicine, University of Colorado-Denver and Pediatrician in Chief, Children's Hospital Colorado, Aurora, Colorado; [g]Director, Preventive Cardiology Clinic, Boston Children's Hospital, Department of Pediatrics, Harvard Medical School, Boston, Massachusetts; [h]Division of Nephrology, Department of Pediatrics, University of British Columbia and British Columbia Children's Hospital, Vancouver, British Columbia, Canada; Departments of [i]Medicine and Pediatrics, Sidney Kimmel Medical College, Thomas Jefferson University, Philadelphia, Pennsylvania; [j]Consultant, American Academy of Pediatrics, Washington, District of Columbia; [k]Cardiology Division Head, Nemours Cardiac Center, Alfred I. duPont Hospital for Children, Wilmington, Delaware; [l]National Pediatric Blood Pressure Awareness Foundation, Prairieville, Louisiana; Departments of [m]Pediatrics and Biomedical Informatics and Medical Education, University of Washington, University of Washington Medicine and Information Technology Services, and Seattle Children's Hospital,

To cite: Flynn JT, Kaelber DC, Baker-Smith CM, et al. Clinical Practice Guideline for Screening and Management of High Blood Pressure in Children and Adolescents. Pediatrics. 2017;140(3):e20171904

1. INTRODUCTION

1. Scope of the Clinical Practice Guideline

Interest in childhood hypertension (HTN) has increased since the 2004 publication of the "Fourth Report on the Diagnosis, Evaluation, and Treatment of High Blood Pressure in Children and Adolescents" (Fourth Report).[1] Recognizing ongoing evidence gaps and the need for an updated, thorough review of the relevant literature, the American Academy of Pediatrics (AAP) and its Council on Quality Improvement and Patient Safety developed this practice guideline to provide an update on topics relevant to the diagnosis, evaluation, and management of pediatric HTN. It is primarily directed at clinicians caring for children and adolescents in the outpatient setting. This guideline is endorsed by the American Heart Association.

When it was not possible to identify sufficient evidence, recommendations are based on the consensus opinion of the expert members of the Screening and Management of High Blood Pressure in Children Clinical Practice Guideline Subcommittee (henceforth, "the subcommittee"). The subcommittee intends to regularly update this guideline as new evidence becomes available. Implementation tools for this guideline are available on the AAP Web site (https://www.aap.org/en-us/about-the-aap/Committees-Councils-Sections/coqips/Pages/Implementation-Guide.aspx).

1.1 Methodology

The subcommittee was co-chaired by a pediatric nephrologist and a general pediatrician and consisted of 17 members, including a parent representative. All subcommittee members were asked to disclose relevant financial or proprietary conflicts of interest for members or their family members at the start of and throughout the guideline preparation process. Potential conflicts of interest were addressed and resolved by the AAP. A detailed list of subcommittee members and affiliations can be found in the Consortium section at the end of this article. A listing of subcommittee members with conflicts of interest will be included in the forthcoming technical report.

The subcommittee epidemiologist created a detailed content outline, which was reviewed and approved by the subcommittee. The outline contained a list of primary and secondary topics generated to guide a thorough literature search and meet the goal of providing an up-to-date systemic review of the literature pertaining to the diagnosis, management, and treatment of pediatric HTN as well as the prevalence of pediatric HTN and its associated comorbidities.

Of the topics covered in the outline, ~80% were researched by using a Patient, Intervention/Indicator, Comparison, Outcome, and Time (PICOT) format to address the following key questions:

1. How should systemic HTN (eg, primary HTN, renovascular HTN, white coat hypertension [WCH], and masked hypertension [MH]) in children be diagnosed, and what is the optimal approach to diagnosing HTN in children and adolescents?

2. What is the recommended workup for pediatric HTN? How do we best identify the underlying etiologies of secondary HTN in children?

3. What is the optimal goal systolic blood pressure (SBP) and/or diastolic blood pressure (DBP) for children and adolescents?

4. In children 0 to 18 years of age, how does treatment with lifestyle versus antihypertensive agents influence indirect measures of cardiovascular disease (CVD) risk, such as carotid intimamedia thickness (cIMT), flow-mediated dilation (FMD), left ventricular hypertrophy (LVH), and other markers of vascular dysfunction?

To address these key questions, a systematic search and review of literature was performed. The initial search included articles published between the publication of the Fourth Report (January 2004) and August 2015. The process used to conduct the systematic review was consistent with the recommendations of the Institute of Medicine for systematic reviews.[2]

For the topics not researched by using the PICOT format, separate searches were conducted. Not all topics (eg, economic aspects of pediatric HTN) were appropriate for the PICOT format. A third and final search was conducted at the time the Key Action Statements (KASs) were generated to identify any additional relevant articles published between August 2015 and July 2016. (See Table 1 for a complete list of KASs.)

A detailed description of the methodology used to conduct the literature search and systematic review for this clinical practice guideline will be included in the forthcoming technical report. In brief, reference selection involved a multistep process. First, 2 subcommittee members reviewed the titles and abstracts of references identified for each key question. The epidemiologist provided a deciding vote when required. Next, 2 subcommittee members and the epidemiologist conducted full-text reviews of the selected articles. Although many subcommittee members have extensively published articles on topics covered in this guideline, articles were not preferentially selected on the basis of authorship.

Articles selected at this stage were mapped back to the relevant main topic in the outline. Subcommittee members were then assigned to

TABLE 1 Summary of KASs for Screening and Management of High BP in Children and Adolescents

KAS	Evidence Quality, Strength of Recommendation
1. BP should be measured annually in children and adolescents ≥3 y of age.	C, moderate
2. BP should be checked in all children and adolescents ≥3 y of age at every health care encounter if they have obesity, are taking medications known to increase BP, have renal disease, a history of aortic arch obstruction or coarctation, or diabetes.	C, moderate
3. Trained health care professionals in the office setting should make a diagnosis of HTN if a child or adolescent has auscultatory-confirmed BP readings ≥95th percentile at 3 different visits.	C, moderate
4. Organizations with EHRs used in an office setting should consider including flags for abnormal BP values, both when the values are being entered and when they are being viewed.	C, weak
5. Oscillometric devices may be used for BP screening in children and adolescents. When doing so, providers should use a device that has been validated in the pediatric age group. If elevated BP is suspected on the basis of oscillometric readings, confirmatory measurements should be obtained by auscultation.	B, strong
6. ABPM should be performed for confirmation of HTN in children and adolescents with office BP measurements in the elevated BP category for 1 year or more or with stage 1 HTN over 3 clinic visits.	C, moderate
7. Routine performance of ABPM should be strongly considered in children and adolescents with high-risk conditions (see Table 12) to assess HTN severity and determine if abnormal circadian BP patterns are present, which may indicate increased risk for target organ damage.	B, moderate
8. ABPM should be performed by using a standardized approach (see Table 13) with monitors that have been validated in a pediatric population, and studies should be interpreted by using pediatric normative data.	C, moderate
9. Children and adolescents with suspected WCH should undergo ABPM. Diagnosis is based on the presence of mean SBP and DBP <95th percentile and SBP and DBP load <25%.	B, strong
10. Home BP monitoring should not be used to diagnose HTN, MH, or WCH but may be a useful adjunct to office and ambulatory BP measurement after HTN has been diagnosed.	C, moderate
11. Children and adolescents ≥6 y of age do not require an extensive evaluation for secondary causes of HTN if they have a positive family history of HTN, are overweight or obese, and/or do not have history or physical examination findings (Table 14) suggestive of a secondary cause of HTN.	C, moderate
12. Children and adolescents who have undergone coarctation repair should undergo ABPM for the detection of HTN (including MH).	B, strong
13. In children and adolescents being evaluated for high BP, the provider should obtain a perinatal history, appropriate nutritional history, physical activity history, psychosocial history, and family history and perform a physical examination to identify findings suggestive of secondary causes of HTN.	B, strong
14. Clinicians should not perform electrocardiography in hypertensive children and adolescents being evaluated for LVH.	B, strong
15-1. It is recommended that echocardiography be performed to assess for cardiac target organ damage (LV mass, geometry, and function) at the time of consideration of pharmacologic treatment of HTN.	C, moderate
15-2. LVH should be defined as LV mass >51 g/m$^{2.7}$ (boys and girls) for children and adolescents older than age 8 y and defined by LV mass >115 g/BSA for boys and LV mass >95 g/BSA for girls.	
15-3. Repeat echocardiography may be performed to monitor improvement or progression of target organ damage at 6- to 12-mo intervals. Indications to repeat echocardiography include persistent HTN despite treatment, concentric LV hypertrophy, or reduced LV ejection fraction.	
15-4. In patients without LV target organ injury at initial echocardiographic assessment, repeat echocardiography at yearly intervals may be considered in those with stage 2 HTN, secondary HTN, or chronic stage 1 HTN incompletely treated (noncompliance or drug resistance) to assess for the development of worsening LV target organ injury.	
16. Doppler renal ultrasonography may be used as a noninvasive screening study for the evaluation of possible RAS in normal-wt children and adolescents ≥8 y of age who are suspected of having renovascular HTN and who will cooperate with the procedure.	C, moderate
17. In children and adolescents suspected of having RAS, either CTA or MRA may be performed as noninvasive imaging studies. Nuclear renography is less useful in pediatrics and should generally be avoided.	D, weak
18. Routine testing for MA is not recommended for children and adolescents with primary HTN.	C, moderate
19. In children and adolescents diagnosed with HTN, the treatment goal with nonpharmacologic and pharmacologic therapy should be a reduction in SBP and DBP to <90th percentile and <130/80 mm Hg in adolescents ≥ 13 years old.	C, moderate
20. At the time of diagnosis of elevated BP or HTN in a child or adolescent, clinicians should provide advice on the DASH diet and recommend moderate to vigorous physical activity at least 3 to 5 d per week (30–60 min per session) to help reduce BP.	C, weak
21. In hypertensive children and adolescents who have failed lifestyle modifications (particularly those who have LV hypertrophy on echocardiography, symptomatic HTN, or stage 2 HTN without a clearly modifiable factor [eg, obesity]), clinicians should initiate pharmacologic treatment with an ACE inhibitor, ARB, long-acting calcium channel blocker, or thiazide diuretic.	B, moderate
22. ABPM may be used to assess treatment effectiveness in children and adolescents with HTN, especially when clinic and/or home BP measurements indicate insufficient BP response to treatment.	B, moderate
23-1. Children and adolescents with CKD should be evaluated for HTN at each medical encounter.	B, strong
23-2. Children or adolescents with both CKD and HTN should be treated to lower 24-hr MAP <50th percentile by ABPM.	
23-3. Regardless of apparent control of BP with office measures, children and adolescents with CKD and a history of HTN should have BP assessed by ABPM at least yearly to screen for MH.	
24. Children and adolescents with CKD and HTN should be evaluated for proteinuria.	B, strong
25. Children and adolescents with CKD, HTN, and proteinuria should be treated with an ACE inhibitor or ARB.	B, strong

TABLE 1 Continued

KAS	Evidence Quality, Strength of Recommendation
26. Children and adolescents with T1DM or T2DM should be evaluated for HTN at each medical encounter and treated if BP ≥95th percentile or >130/80 mm Hg in adolescents ≥13 y of age.	C, moderate
27. In children and adolescents with acute severe HTN and life-threatening symptoms, immediate treatment with short-acting antihypertensive medication should be initiated, and BP should be reduced by no more than 25% of the planned reduction over the first 8 h.	Expert opinion, D, weak
28. Children and adolescents with HTN may participate in competitive sports once hypertensive target organ effects and cardiovascular risk have been assessed.	C, moderate
29. Children and adolescents with HTN should receive treatment to lower BP below stage 2 thresholds before participation in competitive sports.	C, moderate
30. Adolescents with elevated BP or HTN (whether they are receiving antihypertensive treatment) should typically have their care transitioned to an appropriate adult care provider by 22 y of age (recognizing that there may be individual cases in which this upper age limit is exceeded, particularly in the case of youth with special health care needs). There should be a transfer of information regarding HTN etiology and past manifestations and complications of the patient's HTN.	X, strong

writing teams that evaluated the evidence quality for selected topics and generated appropriate KASs in accordance with an AAP grading matrix (see Fig 1 and the detailed discussion in the forthcoming technical report).[3] Special working groups were created to address 2 specific topics for which evidence was lacking and expert opinion was required to generate KASs, "Definition of HTN" and "Definition of LVH." References for any topics not covered by the key questions were selected on the basis of additional literature searches and reviewed by the epidemiologist and subcommittee members assigned to the topic. When applicable, searches were conducted by using the PICOT format .

In addition to the 30 KASs listed above, this guideline also contains 27 additional recommendations that are based on the consensus expert opinion of the subcommittee members. These recommendations, along with their locations in the document, are listed in Table 2.

2. EPIDEMIOLOGY AND CLINICAL SIGNIFICANCE

2.1 Prevalence of HTN in Children

Information on the prevalence of high blood pressure (BP) in children is largely derived from data from the NHANES and typically is based on a single BP measurement session. These surveys, conducted since 1988, indicate that there has been an increase in the prevalence of childhood high BP, including both HTN and elevated BP.[4,5] High BP is consistently greater in boys (15%–19%) than in girls (7%–12%). The prevalence of high BP is higher among Hispanic and non-Hispanic African American children compared with non-Hispanic white children, with higher rates among adolescents than among younger children.[6]

However, in a clinical setting and with repeated BP measurements, the prevalence of confirmed HTN is lower in part because of inherent BP variability as well as an adjustment to the experience of having BP measured (also known as the accommodation effect). Therefore, the actual prevalence of clinical HTN in children and adolescents is ~3.5%.[7,8] The prevalence of persistently elevated BP (formerly termed "prehypertension," including BP values from the 90th to 94th percentiles or between 120/80 and 130/80 mm Hg in adolescents) is also ~2.2% to 3.5%, with higher rates among children and adolescents who have overweight and obesity.[7,9]

Data on BP tracking from childhood to adulthood demonstrate that higher BP in childhood correlates with higher BP in adulthood and the onset of HTN in young adulthood. The strength of the tracking relationship is stronger in older children and adolescents.[10]

Trajectory data on BP (including repeat measurements from early childhood into midadulthood) confirm the association of elevated BP in adolescence with HTN in early adulthood[11] and that normal BP in childhood is associated with a lack of HTN in midadulthood.[11]

2.2 Awareness, Treatment, and Control of HTN in Children

Of the 32.6% of US adults who have HTN, almost half (17.2%) are not aware they have HTN; even among those who are aware of their condition, only approximately half (54.1%) have controlled BP.[12] Unfortunately, there are no large studies in which researchers have systematically studied BP awareness or control in youth, although an analysis of prescribing patterns from a nationwide prescription drug provider found an increase in the number of prescriptions written for high BP in youth from 2004 to 2007.[13]

The SEARCH for Diabetes in Youth study found that only 7.4% of youth with type 1 diabetes mellitus (T1DM) and 31.9% of youth with type 2 diabetes mellitus (T2DM) demonstrated knowledge of their BP status.[14] Even after becoming aware of the diagnosis, only 57.1% of patients with T1DM and 40.6% of patients with T2DM achieved good BP control.[14] The HEALTHY Primary Prevention Trial of Risk Factors for

TABLE 2 Additional Consensus Opinion Recommendations and Text Locations

Recommendation	CPG Section(s)
1. Follow the revised classification scheme in Table 3 for childhood BP levels, including the use of the term "elevated BP," the new definition of stage 2 HTN, and the use of similar BP levels as adults for adolescents ≥13 y of age.	3.1
2. Use simplified BP tables (Table 4) to screen for BP values that may require further evaluation by a clinician.	3.2a
3. Use reference data on neonatal BP from ref 80 to identify elevated BP values in neonates up to 44 wk postmenstrual age and BP curves from the 1987 Second Task Force report to identify elevated BP values in infants 1–12 mo of age.	3.3
4. Use the standardized technique for measuring BP by auscultation described in Table 7 and Fig 2 (including appropriate cuff size, extremity, and patient positioning) to obtain accurate BP values.	4.1
5. If the initial BP at an office visit is elevated, as described in Fig 3, obtain 2 additional BP measurements at the same visit and average them; use the averaged auscultatory BP measurement to determine the patient's BP category.	4.1
6. Oscillometric devices are used to measure BP in infants and toddlers until they are able to cooperate with auscultatory BP. Follow the same rules for BP measurement technique and cuff size as for older children.	4.1a
7. Measure BP at every health care encounter in children <3 y of age if they have an underlying condition listed in Table 9 that increases their risk for HTN.	4.2
8. After a patient's BP has been categorized, follow Table 11 for when to obtain repeat BP readings, institute lifestyle changes, or proceed to a workup for HTN.	4.3
9. When an oscillometric BP reading is elevated, obtain repeat readings, discard the first reading, and average subsequent readings to approximate auscultatory BP.	4.5
10. Wrist and forearm BP measurements should not be used in children and adolescents for the diagnosis or management of HTN.	4.6
11. Use ABPM to evaluate high-risk patients (those with obesity, CKD, or repaired aortic coarctation) for potential MH.	4.7a, 4.8
12. Routine use of BP readings obtained in the school setting is not recommended for diagnosis of HTN in children and adolescents.	4.10
13. Use the history and physical examination to identify possible underlying causes of HTN, such as heart disease, kidney disease, renovascular disease, endocrine HTN (Table 15), drug-induced HTN (Table 8), and OSAS-associated HTN (Table 18).	5.2–5.4, 5.7, 9.2
14. Suspect monogenic HTN in patients with a family history of early-onset HTN, hypokalemia, suppressed plasma renin, or an elevated ARR.	5.8
15. Obtain laboratory studies listed in Table 10 to evaluate for underlying secondary causes of HTN when indicated.	6.4
16. Routine use of vascular imaging, such as carotid intimal-media measurements or PWV measurements, is not recommended in the evaluation of HTN in children and adolescents.	6.7
17. Suspect renovascular HTN in selected children and adolescents with stage 2 HTN, significant diastolic HTN, discrepant kidney sizes on ultrasound, hypokalemia on screening laboratories, or an epigastric and/or upper abdominal bruit on physical examination.	6.8a
18. Routine measurement of serum UA is not recommended for children and adolescents with elevated BP.	6.9
19. Offer intensive weight-loss programs to hypertensive children and adolescents with obesity; consider using MI as an adjunct to the treatment of obesity.	7.2c
20. Follow-up children and adolescents treated with antihypertensive medications every 4–6 wk until BP is controlled, then extend the interval. Follow-up every 3–6 mo is appropriate for patients treated with lifestyle modification only.	7.3c
21. Evaluate and treat children and adolescents with apparent treatment-resistant HTN in a similar manner to that recommended for adults with resistant HTN.	7.4
22. Treat hypertensive children and adolescents with dyslipidemia according to current, existing pediatric lipid guidelines.	9.1
23. Use ABPM to evaluate for potential HTN in children and adolescents with known or suspected OSAS.	9.2
24. Racial, ethnic, and sex differences need not be considered in the evaluation and management of children and adolescents with HTN.	10
25. Use ABPM to evaluate BP in pediatric heart- and kidney-transplant recipients.	11.3

Type 2 Diabetes in Middle-School Youth, which examined a school-based intervention designed to reduce cardiovascular (CV) risk among middle school students, found the prevalence of stage 1 or 2 HTN to be ~9.5%.[15] There was no significant reduction in HTN in the control group after the intervention; the intervention group saw a reduction in the prevalence of HTN of ~1%, leaving 8.5% with BP still above the ideal range.

Researchers in a number of small, single-center studies have evaluated BP control in children and adolescents with HTN. One study found that lifestyle change and medications produced adequate BP control in 46 of 65 youth (70%) with HTN.[16] Another study in which researchers used ambulatory blood pressure monitoring (ABPM) to assess BP control among a group of 38 children (of whom 84% had chronic kidney disease [CKD]) found that only 13 children (34%) achieved adequate BP control even among those who received more than 1 drug.[17] A similar study found that additional drugs did increase rates of BP control in children with CKD, however.[18]

2.3 Prevalence of HTN Among Children With Various Chronic Conditions

It is well recognized that HTN rates are higher in children with certain chronic conditions, including children with obesity, sleep-disordered breathing (SDB), CKD, and those born preterm. These are described below.

2.3a Children With Obesity

HTN prevalence ranges from 3.8% to 24.8% in youth with overweight and obesity. Rates of HTN increase in a graded fashion with increasing adiposity.[19–24] Similar relationships are seen between HTN and increasing waist circumference.[4,25,26] Systematic reviews of 63 studies on BMI[27] and 61 studies on various measures

TABLE 2 Continued

Recommendation	CPG Section(s)
26. Reasonable strategies for HTN prevention include the maintenance of a normal BMI, consuming a DASH-type diet, avoidance of excessive sodium consumption, and regular vigorous physical activity.	13.2
27. Provide education about HTN to patients and their parents to improve patient involvement in their care and better achieve therapeutic goals.	15.2, 15.3

Based on the expert opinion of the subcommittee members (level of evidence = D; strength of recommendations = weak). CPG, clinical practice guideline.

of abdominal adiposity[28] have shown associations between these conditions and HTN. Obesity is also associated with a lack of circadian variability of BP,[29,30] with up to 50% of children who have obesity not experiencing the expected nocturnal BP dip.[31–33]

Studies have shown that childhood obesity is also related to the development of future HTN.[22] Elevated BMI as early as infancy is associated with higher future BP.[34] This risk appears to increase with obesity severity; there is a fourfold increase in BP among those with severe obesity (BMI >99th percentile) versus a twofold increase in those with obesity (BMI 95th–98th percentiles) compared with normal-weight children and adolescents.[35]

Collectively, the results of these cross-sectional and longitudinal studies firmly establish an increasing prevalence of HTN with increasing BMI percentile. The study results also underscore the importance of monitoring BP in all children with overweight and/or obesity at every clinical encounter.

Obesity in children with HTN may be accompanied by additional cardiometabolic risk factors (eg, dyslipidemia and disordered glucose metabolism)[36,37] that may have their own effects on BP or may represent comorbid conditions arising from the same adverse lifestyle behaviors.[25,38] Some argue that the presence of multiple risk factors, including obesity and HTN, leads to far greater increases in CV risk than is explained by the individual risk factors alone. Although this phenomenon has been

hard to demonstrate definitively, the Strong Heart Study did show that American Indian adolescents with multiple cardiometabolic risk factors had a higher prevalence of LVH (43.2% vs 11.7%), left atrial dilation (63.1% vs 21.9%; $P < .001$), and reduced LV systolic and diastolic function compared with those without multiple cardiometabolic risk factors.[39] Notably, both obesity and HTN were drivers of these CV abnormalities, with obesity being a stronger determinant of cardiac abnormalities than HTN (odds ratio, 4.17 vs 1.03).

2.3b Children With SDB

SDB occurs on a spectrum that includes (1) primary snoring, (2) sleep fragmentation, and (3) obstructive sleep apnea syndrome (OSAS). Researchers in numerous studies have identified an association between SDB and HTN in the pediatric population.[40–42] Studies suggest that children who sleep 7 hours or less per night are at increased risk for HTN.[43] Small studies of youth with sleep disorders have found the prevalence of high BP to range between 3.6% and 14%.[40,41] The more severe the OSAS, the more likely a child is to have HTN.[44,45] Even inadequate duration of sleep and poor-quality sleep have been associated with elevated BP.[43]

2.3c Children With CKD

There are well-established pathophysiologic links between childhood HTN and CKD. Certain forms of CKD can lead to HTN, and untreated HTN can lead to CKD in adults, although evidence for the

latter in pediatric patients is lacking. Among children and adolescents with CKD, ~50% are known to be hypertensive.[46–48] In children and adolescents with end-stage renal disease (either those on dialysis or after transplant), ~48% to 79% are hypertensive, with 20% to 70% having uncontrolled HTN.[49–53] Almost 20% of pediatric HTN may be attributable to CKD.[54]

2.3d Children With History of Prematurity

Abnormal birth history—including preterm birth and low birth weight—has been identified as a risk factor for HTN and other CVD in adults[55]; only low birth weight has been associated with elevated BP in the pediatric age range.[56] One retrospective cohort study showed a prevalence of HTN of 7.3% among 3 year olds who were born preterm.[57] Researchers in another retrospective case series noted a high prevalence of HTN in older children with a history of preterm birth.[58] It also appears that preterm birth may result in abnormal circadian BP patterns in childhood.[59] These data are intriguing but limited. Further study is needed to determine how often preterm birth results in childhood HTN.

2.4 Importance of Diagnosing HTN in Children and Adolescents

Numerous studies have shown that elevated BP in childhood increases the risk for adult HTN and metabolic syndrome.[10,60–62] Youth with higher BP levels in childhood are also more likely to have persistent HTN as adults.[60,63] One recent study found that adolescents with elevated BP progressed to HTN at a rate of 7% per year, and elevated BMI predicted sustained BP elevations.[64] In addition, young patients with HTN are likely to experience accelerated vascular aging. Both autopsy[65] and imaging studies[66] have demonstrated BP-related CV damage in youth. These intermediate markers of CVD (eg, increased LV mass,[67] cIMT,[68] and pulse wave velocity [PWV][69]) are known to predict CV events in adults, making it crucial to diagnose and treat HTN early.

Eighty million US adults (1 in 3) have HTN, which is a major contributor to CVD.[12] Key contributors to CV health have been identified by the American Heart Association (AHA) as "Life's Simple 7," including 4 ideal health behaviors (not smoking, normal BMI, physical activity at goal levels, and a healthy diet) and 3 ideal health factors (untreated, normal total cholesterol; normal fasting blood glucose; and normal untreated BP, defined in childhood as ≤90th percentile or <120/80 mm Hg). Notably, elevated BP is the least common abnormal health factor in children and adolescents[70]; 89% of youth (ages 12–19 years) are in the ideal BP category.[6]

Given the prevalence of known key contributors in youth (ie, tobacco exposure, obesity, inactivity, and nonideal diet[12,71]), adult CVD likely has its origins in childhood. One-third of US adolescents report having tried a cigarette in the past 30 days.[72] Almost half (40%–48%) of teenagers have elevated BMI, and the rates of severe obesity (BMI >99th percentile) continue to climb, particularly in girls and adolescents.[73–75] Physical activity measured by accelerometry shows less than half of school-aged boys and only one-third of school-aged girls meet the goal for ideal physical activity levels.[72] More than 80% of youth 12 to 19 years of age have a poor diet (as defined by AHA metrics for ideal CV health); only ~10% eat adequate fruits and vegetables, and only ~15% consume <1500 mg per day of sodium, both of which are key dietary determinants of HTN.[76]

Finally, measuring BP at routine well-child visits enables the early detection of primary HTN as well as the detection of asymptomatic HTN secondary to another underlying

disorder. Early detection of HTN is vital given the greater relative prevalence of secondary causes of HTN in children compared with adults.

3. DEFINITION OF HTN

3.1 Definition of HTN (1–18 Years of Age)

Given the lack of outcome data, the current definition of HTN in children and adolescents is based on the normative distribution of BP in healthy children.[1] Because it is a major determinant of BP in growing children, height has been incorporated into the normative data since the publication of the 1996 Working Group Report.[1] BP levels should be interpreted on the basis of sex, age, and height to avoid misclassification of children who are either extremely tall or extremely short. It should be noted that the normative data were collected by using an auscultatory technique,[1] which may provide different values than measurement obtained by using oscillometric devices or from ABPM.

In the Fourth Report, "normal blood pressure" was defined as SBP and DBP values <90th percentile (on the basis of age, sex, and height percentiles). For the preadolescent, "prehypertension" was defined as SBP and/or DBP ≥90th percentile and <95th percentile (on the basis of age, sex, and height tables). For adolescents, "prehypertension" was defined as BP ≥120/80 mm Hg to <95th percentile, or ≥90th and <95th percentile, whichever was

lower. HTN was defined as average clinic measured SBP and/or DBP ≥95th percentile (on the basis of age, sex, and height percentiles) and was further classified as stage 1 or stage 2 HTN.

There are still no data to identify a specific level of BP in childhood that leads to adverse CV outcomes in adulthood. Therefore, the subcommittee decided to maintain a statistical definition for childhood HTN. The staging criteria have been revised for stage 1 and stage 2 HTN for ease of implementation compared with the Fourth Report. For children ≥13 years of age, this staging scheme will seamlessly interface with the 2017 AHA and American College of Cardiology (ACC) adult HTN guideline.* Additionally, the term "prehypertension" has been replaced by the term "elevated blood pressure," to be consistent with the AHA and ACC guideline and convey the importance of lifestyle measures to prevent the development of HTN (see Table 3).

3.2 New BP Tables

New normative BP tables based on normal-weight children are included with these guidelines (see Tables 4 and 5). Similar to the tables in the

TABLE 3 Updated Definitions of BP Categories and Stages

For Children Aged 1–13 y	For Children Aged ≥13 y
Normal BP: <90th percentile	Normal BP: <120/<80 mm Hg
Elevated BP: ≥90th percentile to <95th percentile or 120/80 mm Hg to <95th percentile (whichever is lower)	Elevated BP: 120/<80 to 129/<80 mm Hg
Stage 1 HTN: ≥95th percentile to <95th percentile + 12 mmHg, or 130/80 to 139/89 mm Hg (whichever is lower)	Stage 1 HTN: 130/80 to 139/89 mm Hg
Stage 2 HTN: ≥95th percentile + 12 mm Hg, or ≥140/90 mm Hg (whichever is lower)	Stage 2 HTN: ≥140/90 mm Hg

*Whelton PK, Carey RM, Aranow WS, et al. ACC/AHA/APPA/ABC/ACPM/AGS/APhA/ASH/ASPC/NMA/PCNA Guideline for the prevention, detection, evaluation and managament of high blood pressure in adults: A report of the American College of Cardiology/American Heart Association Task Force on Clinical Practice Guidelines. *Hypertension.* 2017, In press.

Fourth Report,[1] they include SBP and DBP values arranged by age, sex, and height (and height percentile). These values are based on auscultatory measurements obtained from ~50 000 children and adolescents. A new feature in these tables is that the BP values are categorized according to the scheme presented in Table 3 as normal (50th percentile), elevated BP (>90th percentile), stage 1 HTN (≥95th percentile), and stage 2 HTN (≥95th percentile + 12 mm Hg). Additionally, actual heights in centimeters and inches are provided.

Unlike the tables in the Fourth Report,[1] the BP values in these tables do not include children and adolescents with overweight and obesity (ie, those with a BMI ≥85th percentile); therefore, they represent normative BP values for normal-weight youth. The decision to create these new tables was based on evidence of the strong association of both overweight and obesity with elevated BP and HTN. Including patients with overweight and obesity in normative BP tables was thought to create bias. The practical effect of this change is that the BP values in Tables 4 and 5 are several millimeters of mercury lower than in the similar tables in the Fourth Report.[1] These tables are based on the same population data excluding participants with overweight and obesity, and the same methods used in the Fourth Report.[1] The methods and results have been published elsewhere.[77] For researchers and others interested in the equations used to calculate the tables' BP values, detailed methodology and the Statistical Analysis System (SAS) code can be found at: http://sites. google.com/a/channing.harvard. edu/bernardrosner/pediatric-blood-press/childhood-blood-pressure.

There are slight differences between the actual percentile-based values in these tables and the cut-points in Table 3, particularly for teenagers ≥13 years of age. Clinicians should understand that the scheme in Table 3 was chosen to align with the new adult guideline and facilitate the management of older adolescents with high BP. The percentile-based values in Tables 4 and 5 are provided to aid researchers and others interested in a more precise classification of BP.

3.2a. Simplified BP Table

This guideline includes a new, simplified table for initial BP screening (see Table 6) based on the 90th percentile BP for age and sex for children at the 5th percentile of height, which gives the values in the table a negative predictive value of >99%.[78] This simplified table is designed as a screening tool only for the identification of children and adolescents who need further evaluation of their BP starting with repeat BP measurements. It should not be used to diagnose elevated BP or HTN by itself. To diagnose elevated BP or HTN, it is important to locate the actual cutoffs in the complete BP tables because the SBP and DBP cutoffs may be as much as 9 mm Hg higher depending on a child's age and length or height. A typical-use case for this simplified table is for nursing staff to quickly identify BP that may need further evaluation by a clinician. For adolescents ≥13 years of age, a threshold of 120/80 mm Hg is used in the simplified table regardless of sex to align with adult guidelines for the detection of elevated BP.

3.3 Definition of HTN in the Neonate and Infant (0–1 Year of Age)

Although a reasonably strict definition of HTN has been developed for older children, it is more difficult to define HTN in neonates given the well-known changes in BP that occur during the first few weeks of life.[79] These BP changes can be significant in preterm infants, in whom BP depends on a variety of factors, including postmenstrual age, birth weight, and maternal conditions.[80]

In an attempt to develop a more standardized approach to the HTN definition in preterm and term neonates, Dionne et al[79] compiled available data on neonatal BP and generated a summary table of BP values, including values for the 95th and 99th percentiles for infants from 26 to 44 weeks' postmenstrual age. The authors proposed that by using these values, a similar approach to that used to identify older children with elevated BP can be followed in neonates, even in those who are born preterm.

At present, no alternative data have been developed, and no outcome data are available on the consequences of high BP in this population; thus, it is reasonable to use these compiled BP values in the assessment of elevated BP in newborn infants. Of note, the 1987 "Report of the Second Task Force on Blood Pressure Control in Children" published curves of normative BP values in older infants up to 1 year of age.[81] These normative values should continue to be used given the lack of more contemporary data for this age group.

4. MEASUREMENT OF BP

4.1 BP Measurement Technique

BP in childhood may vary considerably between visits and even during the same visit. There are many potential etiologies for isolated elevated BP in children and adolescents, including such factors as anxiety and recent caffeine intake.[82] BP generally decreases with repeated measurements during a single visit,[83] although the variability may not be large enough to affect BP classification.[84] BP measurements can also vary across visits[64,85]; one study in adolescents found that only 56% of the sample had the same HTN stage on 3 different occasions.[8] Therefore, it is important to obtain multiple measurements over time before diagnosing HTN.

TABLE 4 BP Levels for Boys by Age and Height Percentile

Age (y)	BP Percentile	SBP (mm Hg)							DBP (mm Hg)						
		Height Percentile or Measured Height							Height Percentile or Measured Height						
		5%	10%	25%	50%	75%	90%	95%	5%	10%	25%	50%	75%	90%	95%
1	Height (in)	30.4	30.8	31.6	32.4	33.3	34.1	34.6	30.4	30.8	31.6	32.4	33.3	34.1	34.6
	Height (cm)	77.2	78.3	80.2	82.4	84.6	86.7	87.9	77.2	78.3	80.2	82.4	84.6	86.7	87.9
	50th	85	85	86	86	87	88	88	40	40	40	41	41	42	42
	90th	98	99	99	100	100	101	101	52	52	53	53	54	54	54
	95th	102	102	103	103	104	105	105	54	54	55	55	56	57	57
	95th + 12 mm Hg	114	114	115	115	116	117	117	66	66	67	67	68	69	69
2	Height (in)	33.9	34.4	35.3	36.3	37.3	38.2	38.8	33.9	34.4	35.3	36.3	37.3	38.2	38.8
	Height (cm)	86.1	87.4	89.6	92.1	94.7	97.1	98.5	86.1	87.4	89.6	92.1	94.7	97.1	98.5
	50th	87	87	88	89	89	90	91	43	43	44	44	45	46	46
	90th	100	100	101	102	103	103	104	55	55	56	56	57	58	58
	95th	104	105	105	106	107	107	108	57	58	58	59	60	61	61
	95th + 12 mm Hg	116	117	117	118	119	119	120	69	70	70	71	72	73	73
3	Height (in)	36.4	37	37.9	39	40.1	41.1	41.7	36.4	37	37.9	39	40.1	41.1	41.7
	Height (cm)	92.5	93.9	96.3	99	101.8	104.3	105.8	92.5	93.9	96.3	99	101.8	104.3	105.8
	50th	88	89	89	90	91	92	92	45	46	46	47	48	49	49
	90th	101	102	102	103	104	105	105	58	58	59	59	60	61	61
	95th	106	106	107	107	108	109	109	60	61	61	62	63	64	64
	95th + 12 mm Hg	118	118	119	119	120	121	121	72	73	73	74	75	76	76
4	Height (in)	38.8	39.4	40.5	41.7	42.9	43.9	44.5	38.8	39.4	40.5	41.7	42.9	43.9	44.5
	Height (cm)	98.5	100.2	102.9	105.9	108.9	111.5	113.2	98.5	100.2	102.9	105.9	108.9	111.5	113.2
	50th	90	90	91	92	93	94	94	48	49	49	50	51	52	52
	90th	102	103	104	105	105	106	107	60	61	62	62	63	64	64
	95th	107	107	108	108	109	110	110	63	64	65	66	67	67	68
	95th + 12 mm Hg	119	119	120	120	121	122	122	75	76	77	78	79	79	80
5	Height (in)	41.1	41.8	43.0	44.3	45.5	46.7	47.4	41.1	41.8	43.0	44.3	45.5	46.7	47.4
	Height (cm)	104.4	106.2	109.1	112.4	115.7	118.6	120.3	104.4	106.2	109.1	112.4	115.7	118.6	120.3
	50th	91	92	93	94	95	96	96	51	51	52	53	54	55	55
	90th	103	104	105	106	107	108	108	63	64	65	65	66	67	67
	95th	107	108	109	109	110	111	112	66	67	68	69	70	71	71
	95th + 12 mm Hg	119	120	121	121	122	123	124	78	79	80	81	82	83	83
6	Height (in)	43.4	44.2	45.4	46.8	48.2	49.4	50.2	43.4	44.2	45.4	46.8	48.2	49.4	50.2
	Height (cm)	110.3	112.2	115.3	118.9	122.4	125.6	127.5	110.3	112.2	115.3	118.9	122.4	125.6	127.5
	50th	93	93	94	95	96	97	98	54	54	55	56	57	57	58
	90th	105	105	106	107	109	110	110	66	66	67	68	68	69	69
	95th	108	109	110	111	112	113	114	69	70	70	71	72	72	73
	95th + 12 mm Hg	120	121	122	123	124	125	126	81	82	82	83	84	84	85
7	Height (in)	45.7	46.5	47.8	49.3	50.8	52.1	52.9	45.7	46.5	47.8	49.3	50.8	52.1	52.9
	Height (cm)	116.1	118	121.4	125.1	128.9	132.4	134.5	116.1	118	121.4	125.1	128.9	132.4	134.5
	50th	94	94	95	97	98	98	99	56	56	57	58	58	59	59
	90th	106	107	108	109	110	111	111	68	68	69	70	70	71	71
	95th	110	110	111	112	114	115	116	71	71	72	73	73	74	74
	95th + 12 mm Hg	122	122	123	124	126	127	128	83	83	84	85	85	86	86

TABLE 4 Continued

Age (y)	BP Percentile	SBP (mmHg) Height Percentile or Measured Height							DBP (mmHg) Height Percentile or Measured Height						
		5%	10%	25%	50%	75%	90%	95%	5%	10%	25%	50%	75%	90%	95%
8	Height (in)	47.8	48.6	50	51.6	53.2	54.6	55.5	47.8	48.6	50	51.6	53.2	54.6	55.5
	Height (cm)	121.4	123.5	127	131	135.1	138.8	141	121.4	123.5	127	131	135.1	138.8	141
	50th	95	96	97	98	99	99	100	57	57	58	59	59	60	60
	90th	107	108	109	110	111	112	112	69	70	70	71	72	72	73
	95th	111	112	112	114	115	116	117	72	73	73	74	75	75	75
	95th + 12 mm Hg	123	124	124	126	127	128	129	84	85	85	86	87	87	87
9	Height (in)	49.6	50.5	52	53.7	55.4	56.9	57.9	49.6	50.5	52	53.7	55.4	56.9	57.9
	Height (cm)	126	128.3	132.1	136.3	140.7	144.7	147.1	126	128.3	132.1	136.3	140.7	144.7	147.1
	50th	96	97	98	99	100	101	101	57	58	59	60	61	62	62
	90th	107	108	109	110	112	113	114	70	71	72	73	74	74	74
	95th	112	112	113	115	116	118	119	74	74	75	76	76	77	77
	95th + 12 mm Hg	124	124	125	127	128	130	131	86	86	87	88	88	89	89
10	Height (in)	51.3	52.2	53.8	55.6	57.4	59.1	60.1	51.3	52.2	53.8	55.6	57.4	59.1	60.1
	Height (cm)	130.2	132.7	136.7	141.3	145.9	150.1	152.7	130.2	132.7	136.7	141.3	145.9	150.1	152.7
	50th	97	98	99	100	101	102	103	59	60	61	62	63	63	64
	90th	108	109	111	112	113	115	116	72	73	74	74	75	75	76
	95th	112	113	114	116	118	120	121	76	76	77	77	78	78	78
	95th + 12 mm Hg	124	125	126	128	130	132	133	88	88	89	89	90	90	90
11	Height (in)	53	54	55.7	57.6	59.6	61.3	62.4	53	54	55.7	57.6	59.6	61.3	62.4
	Height (cm)	134.7	137.3	141.5	146.4	151.3	155.8	158.6	134.7	137.3	141.5	146.4	151.3	155.8	158.6
	50th	99	99	101	102	103	104	106	61	61	62	63	63	63	63
	90th	110	111	112	114	116	117	118	74	74	75	75	76	76	76
	95th	114	114	116	118	120	123	124	77	78	78	78	78	78	78
	95th + 12 mm Hg	126	126	128	130	132	135	136	89	90	90	90	90	90	90
12	Height (in)	55.2	56.3	58.1	60.1	62.2	64	65.2	55.2	56.3	58.1	60.1	62.2	64	65.2
	Height (cm)	140.3	143	147.5	152.7	157.9	162.6	165.5	140.3	143	147.5	152.7	157.9	162.6	165.5
	50th	101	101	102	104	106	108	109	61	61	62	62	62	63	63
	90th	113	114	115	117	119	121	122	75	75	75	75	75	76	76
	95th	116	117	118	121	124	126	128	78	78	78	78	78	79	79
	95th + 12 mm Hg	128	129	130	133	136	138	140	90	90	90	90	90	91	91
13	Height (in)	57.9	59.1	61	63.1	65.2	67.1	68.3	57.9	59.1	61	63.1	65.2	67.1	68.3
	Height (cm)	147	150	154.9	160.3	165.7	170.5	173.4	147	150	154.9	160.3	165.7	170.5	173.4
	50th	103	104	105	108	110	111	112	61	60	61	63	64	65	65
	90th	115	116	118	121	124	126	126	74	74	74	75	76	77	77
	95th	119	120	122	125	128	130	131	78	78	78	78	80	81	81
	95th + 12 mm Hg	131	132	134	137	140	142	143	90	90	90	90	92	93	93
14	Height (in)	60.6	61.8	63.8	65.9	68.0	69.8	70.9	60.6	61.8	63.8	65.9	68.0	69.8	70.9
	Height (cm)	153.8	156.9	162	167.5	172.7	177.4	180.1	153.8	156.9	162	167.5	172.7	177.4	180.1
	50th	105	106	109	111	112	113	113	60	60	62	64	65	66	67
	90th	119	120	123	126	127	128	129	74	74	75	77	78	79	80
	95th	123	125	127	130	132	133	134	77	78	79	81	82	83	84
	95th + 12 mm Hg	135	137	139	142	144	145	146	89	90	91	93	94	95	96

TABLE 4 Continued

Age (y)	BP Percentile	SBP (mm Hg)							DBP (mm Hg)						
		Height Percentile or Measured Height							Height Percentile or Measured Height						
		5%	10%	25%	50%	75%	90%	95%	5%	10%	25%	50%	75%	90%	95%
15	Height (in)	62.6	63.8	65.7	67.8	69.8	71.5	72.5	62.6	63.8	65.7	67.8	69.8	71.5	72.5
	Height (cm)	159	162	166.9	172.2	177.2	181.6	184.2	159	162	166.9	172.2	177.2	181.6	184.2
	50th	108	110	112	113	114	114	114	61	62	64	65	66	67	68
	90th	123	124	126	128	129	130	130	75	76	78	79	80	81	81
	95th	127	129	131	132	134	135	135	78	79	81	83	84	85	85
	95th + 12 mm Hg	139	141	143	144	146	147	147	90	91	93	95	96	97	97
16	Height (in)	63.8	64.9	66.8	68.8	70.7	72.4	73.4	63.8	64.9	66.8	68.8	70.7	72.4	73.4
	Height (cm)	162.1	165	169.6	174.6	179.5	183.8	186.4	162.1	165	169.6	174.6	179.5	183.8	186.4
	50th	111	112	114	115	115	116	116	63	64	66	67	68	69	69
	90th	126	127	128	129	131	131	132	77	78	79	80	81	82	82
	95th	130	131	133	134	135	136	137	80	81	83	84	85	86	86
	95th + 12 mm Hg	142	143	145	146	147	148	149	92	93	95	96	97	98	98
17	Height (in)	64.5	65.5	67.3	69.2	71.1	72.8	73.8	64.5	65.5	67.3	69.2	71.1	72.8	73.8
	Height (cm)	163.8	166.5	170.9	175.8	180.7	184.9	187.5	163.8	166.5	170.9	175.8	180.7	184.9	187.5
	50th	114	115	116	117	117	118	118	65	66	67	68	69	70	70
	90th	128	129	130	131	132	133	134	78	79	80	81	82	82	83
	95th	132	133	134	135	137	138	138	81	82	84	85	86	86	87
	95th + 12 mm Hg	144	145	146	147	149	150	150	93	94	96	97	98	98	99

Use percentile values to stage BP readings according to the scheme in Table 3 (elevated BP: ≥90th percentile; stage 1 HTN: ≥95th percentile; and stage 2 HTN: ≥95th percentile + 12 mm Hg). The 50th, 90th, and 95th percentiles were derived by using quantile regression on the basis of normal-weight children (BMI <85th percentile).[77]

TABLE 5 BP Levels for Girls by Age and Height Percentile

Age (y)	BP Percentile	SBP (mm Hg)							DBP (mm Hg)						
		Height Percentile or Measured Height							Height Percentile or Measured Height						
		5%	10%	25%	50%	75%	90%	95%	5%	10%	25%	50%	75%	90%	95%
1	Height (in)	29.7	30.2	30.9	31.8	32.7	33.4	33.9	29.7	30.2	30.9	31.8	32.7	33.4	33.9
	Height (cm)	75.4	76.6	78.6	80.8	83	84.9	86.1	75.4	76.6	78.6	80.8	83	84.9	86.1
	50th	84	85	86	86	87	88	88	41	42	42	43	44	45	46
	90th	98	99	99	100	101	102	102	54	55	56	56	57	58	58
	95th	101	102	102	103	104	105	105	59	59	60	60	61	62	62
	95th + 12 mm Hg	113	114	114	115	116	117	117	71	71	72	72	73	74	74
2	Height (in)	33.4	34	34.9	35.9	36.9	37.8	38.4	33.4	34	34.9	35.9	36.9	37.8	38.4
	Height (cm)	84.9	86.3	88.6	91.1	93.7	96	97.4	84.9	86.3	88.6	91.1	93.7	96	97.4
	50th	87	87	88	89	90	91	91	45	46	47	48	49	50	51
	90th	101	101	102	103	104	105	106	58	58	59	60	61	62	62
	95th	104	105	106	106	107	108	109	62	63	63	64	65	66	66
	95th + 12 mm Hg	116	117	118	118	119	120	121	74	75	75	76	77	78	78
3	Height (in)	35.8	36.4	37.3	38.4	39.6	40.6	41.2	35.8	36.4	37.3	38.4	39.6	40.6	41.2
	Height (cm)	91	92.4	94.9	97.6	100.5	103.1	104.6	91	92.4	94.9	97.6	100.5	103.1	104.6
	50th	88	89	89	90	91	92	93	48	48	49	50	51	53	53
	90th	102	103	104	104	105	106	107	60	61	61	62	63	64	65
	95th	106	106	107	108	109	110	110	64	65	65	66	67	68	69
	95th + 12 mm Hg	118	118	119	120	121	122	122	76	77	77	78	79	80	81
4	Height (in)	38.3	38.9	39.9	41.1	42.4	43.5	44.2	38.3	38.9	39.9	41.1	42.4	43.5	44.2
	Height (cm)	97.2	98.8	101.4	104.5	107.6	110.5	112.2	97.2	98.8	101.4	104.5	107.6	110.5	112.2
	50th	89	90	91	92	93	94	94	50	51	51	53	54	55	55
	90th	103	104	105	106	107	108	108	62	63	64	65	66	67	67
	95th	107	108	109	109	110	111	112	66	67	68	69	70	70	71
	95th + 12 mm Hg	119	120	121	121	122	123	124	78	79	80	81	82	82	83
5	Height (in)	40.8	41.5	42.6	43.9	45.2	46.5	47.3	40.8	41.5	42.6	43.9	45.2	46.5	47.3
	Height (cm)	103.6	105.3	108.2	111.5	114.9	118.1	120	103.6	105.3	108.2	111.5	114.9	118.1	120
	50th	90	91	92	93	94	95	96	52	52	53	55	56	57	57
	90th	104	105	106	107	108	109	110	64	65	66	67	68	69	70
	95th	108	109	109	110	111	112	113	68	69	70	71	72	73	73
	95th + 12 mm Hg	120	121	121	122	123	124	125	80	81	82	83	84	85	85
6	Height (in)	43.3	44	45.2	46.6	48.1	49.4	50.3	43.3	44	45.2	46.6	48.1	49.4	50.3
	Height (cm)	110	111.8	114.9	118.4	122.1	125.6	127.7	110	111.8	114.9	118.4	122.1	125.6	127.7
	50th	92	92	93	94	96	97	97	54	54	55	56	57	58	59
	90th	105	106	107	108	109	110	111	67	67	68	69	70	71	71
	95th	109	109	110	111	112	113	114	70	71	72	72	73	74	74
	95th + 12 mm Hg	121	121	122	123	124	125	126	82	83	84	84	85	86	86
7	Height (in)	45.6	46.4	47.7	49.2	50.7	52.1	53	45.6	46.4	47.7	49.2	50.7	52.1	53
	Height (cm)	115.9	117.8	121.1	124.9	128.8	132.5	134.7	115.9	117.8	121.1	124.9	128.8	132.5	134.7
	50th	92	93	94	95	97	98	99	55	55	56	57	58	59	60
	90th	106	106	107	109	110	111	112	68	68	69	70	71	72	72
	95th	109	110	111	112	113	114	115	72	72	73	73	74	74	75
	95th + 12 mm Hg	121	122	123	124	125	126	127	84	84	85	85	86	86	87

TABLE 5 Continued

Age (y)	BP Percentile	SBP (mm Hg)							DBP (mm Hg)						
		Height Percentile or Measured Height							Height Percentile or Measured Height						
		5%	10%	25%	50%	75%	90%	95%	5%	10%	25%	50%	75%	90%	95%
8	Height (in)	47.6	48.4	49.8	51.4	53	54.5	55.5	47.6	48.4	49.8	51.4	53	54.5	55.5
	Height (cm)	121	123	126.5	130.6	134.7	138.5	140.9	121	123	126.5	130.6	134.7	138.5	140.9
	50th	93	94	95	97	98	99	100	56	56	57	59	60	61	61
	90th	107	107	108	110	111	112	113	69	70	71	72	72	73	73
	95th	110	111	112	113	115	116	117	72	73	74	74	75	75	75
	95th + 12 mm Hg	122	123	124	125	127	128	129	84	85	86	86	87	87	87
9	Height (in)	49.3	50.2	51.7	53.4	55.1	56.7	57.7	49.3	50.2	51.7	53.4	55.1	56.7	57.7
	Height (cm)	125.3	127.6	131.3	135.6	140.1	144.1	146.6	125.3	127.6	131.3	135.6	140.1	144.1	146.6
	50th	95	95	97	98	99	100	101	57	58	59	60	60	61	61
	90th	108	108	109	111	112	113	114	71	71	72	73	73	73	73
	95th	112	112	113	114	116	117	118	74	74	75	75	75	75	75
	95th + 12 mm Hg	124	124	125	126	128	129	130	86	86	87	87	87	87	87
10	Height (in)	51.1	52	53.7	55.5	57.4	59.1	60.2	51.1	52	53.7	55.5	57.4	59.1	60.2
	Height (cm)	129.7	132.2	136.3	141	145.8	150.2	152.8	129.7	132.2	136.3	141	145.8	150.2	152.8
	50th	96	97	98	99	101	102	103	58	59	59	60	61	61	62
	90th	109	110	111	112	113	115	116	72	73	73	73	73	73	73
	95th	113	114	114	116	117	119	120	75	75	76	76	76	76	76
	95th + 12 mm Hg	125	126	126	128	129	131	132	87	87	88	88	88	88	88
11	Height (in)	53.4	54.5	56.2	58.2	60.2	61.9	63	53.4	54.5	56.2	58.2	60.2	61.9	63
	Height (cm)	135.6	138.3	142.8	147.8	152.8	157.3	160	135.6	138.3	142.8	147.8	152.8	157.3	160
	50th	98	99	101	102	104	105	106	60	60	60	61	62	63	64
	90th	111	112	113	114	116	118	120	74	74	74	74	74	75	75
	95th	115	116	117	118	120	123	124	76	77	77	77	77	77	77
	95th + 12 mm Hg	127	128	129	130	132	135	136	88	89	89	89	89	89	89
12	Height (in)	56.2	57.3	59	60.9	62.8	64.5	65.5	56.2	57.3	59	60.9	62.8	64.5	65.5
	Height (cm)	142.8	145.5	149.9	154.8	159.6	163.8	166.4	142.8	145.5	149.9	154.8	159.6	163.8	166.4
	50th	102	102	104	105	107	108	108	61	61	61	62	64	65	65
	90th	114	115	116	118	120	122	123	75	75	75	75	76	76	76
	95th	118	119	120	122	124	125	126	78	78	78	79	79	79	79
	95th + 12 mm Hg	130	131	132	134	136	137	138	90	90	90	91	91	91	91
13	Height (in)	58.3	59.3	60.9	62.7	64.5	66.1	67	58.3	59.3	60.9	62.7	64.5	66.1	67
	Height (cm)	148.1	150.6	154.7	159.2	163.7	167.8	170.2	148.1	150.6	154.7	159.2	163.7	167.8	170.2
	50th	104	105	106	107	108	108	109	62	62	63	64	65	65	66
	90th	116	117	119	121	122	123	123	75	75	75	76	76	76	76
	95th	121	122	123	124	126	126	127	79	79	79	79	80	80	81
	95th + 12 mm Hg	133	134	135	136	138	138	139	91	91	91	91	92	92	93
14	Height (in)	59.3	60.2	61.8	63.5	65.2	66.8	67.7	59.3	60.2	61.8	63.5	65.2	66.8	67.7
	Height (cm)	150.6	153	156.9	161.3	165.7	169.7	172.1	150.6	153	156.9	161.3	165.7	169.7	172.1
	50th	105	106	107	108	109	109	109	63	63	64	64	65	66	66
	90th	118	118	119	122	123	123	123	76	76	76	76	77	77	77
	95th	123	123	124	125	126	127	127	80	80	80	80	81	81	82
	95th + 12 mm Hg	135	135	136	137	138	139	139	92	92	92	92	93	93	94

TABLE 5 Continued

Age (y)	BP Percentile	SBP (mm Hg) Height Percentile or Measured Height							DBP (mm Hg) Height Percentile or Measured Height						
		5%	10%	25%	50%	75%	90%	95%	5%	10%	25%	50%	75%	90%	95%
15	Height (in)	59.7	60.6	62.2	63.9	65.6	67.2	68.1	59.7	60.6	62.2	63.9	65.6	67.2	68.1
	Height (cm)	151.7	154	157.9	162.3	166.7	170.6	173	151.7	154	157.9	162.3	166.7	170.6	173
	50th	105	106	107	108	109	109	109	64	64	64	65	66	67	67
	90th	118	119	121	122	123	123	124	76	76	76	77	77	78	78
	95th	124	124	125	126	127	127	128	80	80	80	81	82	82	82
	95th + 12 mm Hg	136	136	137	138	139	139	140	92	92	92	93	94	94	94
16	Height (in)	59.9	60.8	62.4	64.1	65.8	67.3	68.3	59.9	60.8	62.4	64.1	65.8	67.3	68.3
	Height (cm)	152.1	154.5	158.4	162.8	167.1	171.1	173.4	152.1	154.5	158.4	162.8	167.1	171.1	173.4
	50th	106	107	108	109	109	110	110	64	64	65	66	66	67	67
	90th	119	120	122	123	124	124	124	76	76	76	77	78	78	78
	95th	124	125	125	127	127	128	128	80	80	80	81	82	82	82
	95th + 12 mm Hg	136	137	137	139	139	140	140	92	92	92	93	94	94	94
17	Height (in)	60.0	60.9	62.5	64.2	65.9	67.4	68.4	60.0	60.9	62.5	64.2	65.9	67.4	68.4
	Height (cm)	152.4	154.7	158.7	163.0	167.4	171.3	173.7	152.4	154.7	158.7	163.0	167.4	171.3	173.7
	50th	107	108	109	110	110	110	111	64	64	65	66	66	66	67
	90th	120	121	123	124	124	125	125	76	76	77	77	78	78	78
	95th	125	125	126	127	128	128	128	80	80	80	81	82	82	82
	95th + 12 mm Hg	137	137	138	139	140	140	140	92	92	92	93	94	94	94

Use percentile values to stage BP readings according to the scheme in Table 3 (elevated BP: ≥90th percentile; stage 1 HTN: ≥95th percentile; and stage 2 HTN: ≥95th percentile + 12 mm Hg). The 50th, 90th, and 95th percentiles were derived by using quantile regression on the basis of normal-weight children (BMI <85th percentile).[77]

The initial BP measurement may be oscillometric (on a calibrated machine that has been validated for use in the pediatric population) or auscultatory (by using a mercury or aneroid sphygmomanometer[86,87]). (Validation status for oscillometric BP devices, including whether they are validated in the pediatric age group, can be checked at www.dableducational.org.) BP should be measured in the right arm by using standard measurement practices unless the child has atypical aortic arch anatomy, such as right aortic arch and aortic coarctation or left aortic arch with aberrant right subclavian artery (see Table 7). Other important aspects of proper BP measurement are illustrated in an AAP video available at http://youtu.be/JLzkNBpqwi0. Care should be taken that providers follow an accurate and consistent measurement technique.[88,89]

An appropriately sized cuff should be used for accurate BP measurement.[83] Researchers in 3 studies in the United Kingdom and 1 in Brazil documented the lack of availability of an appropriately sized cuff in both the inpatient and outpatient settings.[91–94] Pediatric offices should have access to a wide range of cuff sizes, including a thigh cuff for use in children and adolescents with severe obesity. For children in whom the appropriate cuff size is difficult to determine, the midarm circumference (measured as the midpoint between the acromion of the scapula and olecranon of the elbow, with the shoulder in a neutral position and the elbow flexed to 90°[86,95,96]) should be obtained for an accurate determination of the correct cuff size (see Fig 2 and Table 7).[95]

If the initial BP is elevated (≥90th percentile), providers should perform 2 additional oscillometric or auscultatory BP measurements at the same visit and average them. If using auscultation, this averaged measurement is used to determine the child's BP category (ie, normal,

TABLE 6 Screening BP Values Requiring Further Evaluation

Age, y	BP, mm Hg			
	Boys		Girls	
	Systolic	DBP	Systolic	DBP
1	98	52	98	54
2	100	55	101	58
3	101	58	102	60
4	102	60	103	62
5	103	63	104	64
6	105	66	105	67
7	106	68	106	68
8	107	69	107	69
9	107	70	108	71
10	108	72	109	72
11	110	74	111	74
12	113	75	114	75
≥13	120	80	120	80

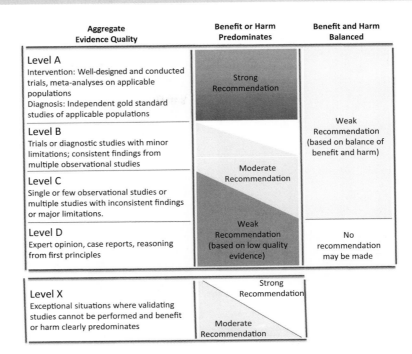

FIGURE 1
AAP grading matrix.

elevated BP, stage 1 HTN, or stage 2 HTN). If the averaged oscillometric reading is ≥90th percentile, 2 auscultatory measurements should be taken and averaged to define the BP category (see Fig 3).

4.1a Measurement of BP in the Neonate

Multiple methods are available for the measurement of BP in hospitalized neonates, including direct intra-arterial measurements using indwelling catheters as well as indirect measurements using the oscillometric technique. In the office, however, the oscillometric technique typically is used at least until the infant is able to cooperate with manual BP determination (which also depends on the ability of the individual measuring the BP to obtain auscultatory BP in infants

and toddlers). Normative values for neonatal and infant BP have generally been determined in the right upper arm with the infant supine, and a similar approach should be followed in the outpatient setting.

As with older children, proper cuff size is important in obtaining accurate BP readings in neonates. The cuff bladder length should encircle 80% to 100% of the arm circumference; a cuff bladder with a width-to-arm circumference ratio of 0.45 to 0.55 is recommended.[79,97,98]

Offices that will be obtaining BP measurements in neonates need to have a variety of cuff sizes available. In addition, the oscillometric device used should be validated in neonates and programmed to have an initial inflation value appropriate for infants (generally ≤120 mm Hg). Auscultation becomes technically feasible once the infant's upper arm is large enough for the smallest cuff available for auscultatory devices. Measurements are best taken when the infant is in a calm state; multiple readings may be needed if the first

TABLE 7 Best BP Measurement Practices

1. The child should be seated in a quiet room for 3–5 min before measurement, with the back supported and feet uncrossed on the floor.
2. BP should be measured in the right arm for consistency, for comparison with standard tables, and to avoid a falsely low reading from the left arm in the case of coarctation of the aorta. The arm should be at heart level,[90] supported, and uncovered above the cuff. The patient and observer should not speak while the measurement is being taken.
3. The correct cuff size should be used. The bladder length should be 80%–100% of the circumference of the arm, and the width should be at least 40%.
4. For an auscultatory BP, the bell of the stethoscope should be placed over the brachial artery in the antecubital fossa, and the lower end of the cuff should be 2–3 cm above the antecubital fossa. The cuff should be inflated to 20–30 mm Hg above the point at which the radial pulse disappears. Overinflation should be avoided. The cuff should be deflated at a rate of 2–3 mm Hg per second. The first (phase I Korotkoff) and last (phase V Korotkoff) audible sounds should be taken as SBP and DBP. If the Korotkoff sounds are heard to 0 mm Hg, the point at which the sound is muffled (phase IV Korotkoff) should be taken as the DBP, or the measurement repeated with less pressure applied over the brachial artery. The measurement should be read to the nearest 2 mm Hg.
5. To measure BP in the legs, the patient should be in the prone position, if possible. An appropriately sized cuff should be placed midthigh and the stethoscope placed over the popliteal artery. The SBP in the legs is usually 10%–20% higher than the brachial artery pressure.

Adapted from Pickering TG, Hall JE, Appel LJ, et al. Recommendations for blood pressure measurement in humans and experimental animals: part 1: blood pressure measurement in humans: a statement for professionals from the Subcommittee of Professional and Public Education of the American Heart Association Council on High Blood Pressure Research. *Circulation*. 2005;111(5):697–716.

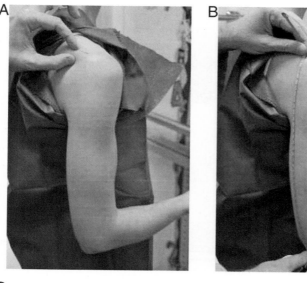

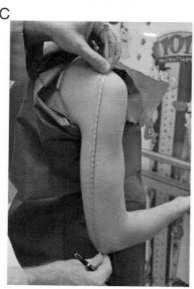

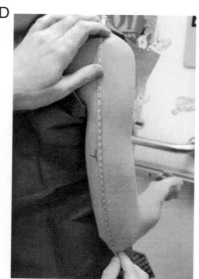

FIGURE 2
Determination of proper BP cuff size.[95] A, Marking spine extending from acromion process. B, Correct tape placement for upper arm length. C, Incorrect tape placement for upper arm length. D, Marking upper arm length midpoint.

reading is elevated, similar to the technique recommended for older children.[99,100]

4.2 BP Measurement Frequency

It remains unclear what age is optimal to begin routine BP measurement in children, although available data suggest that prevention and intervention efforts should begin at a young age.[10,60,101–106] The subcommittee believes that the recommendation to measure BP in the ambulatory setting beginning at 3 years of age should remain unchanged.[1] For otherwise healthy children, however, BP need only be measured annually rather than during every health care encounter.

Some children should have BP measured at every health encounter, specifically those with obesity (BMI ≥95 percentile),[5,27,107–109] renal disease,[46] diabetes,[110,111] aortic arch obstruction or coarctation, or those who are taking medications known

to increase BP (see Table 8 and the "Secondary Causes: Medication-related" section of this guideline).[112,113]

Children younger than 3 years should have BP measurements taken at well-child care visits if they are at increased risk for developing HTN (see Table 9).[1]

Key Action Statement 1

BP should be measured annually in children and adolescents ≥3 years of age (grade C, moderate recommendation).

Key Action Statement 2

BP should be checked in all children and adolescents ≥3 years of age at every health care encounter if they have obesity, are taking medications known to increase BP, have renal disease, a history of aortic arch obstruction or coarctation, or diabetes (see Table 9) (grade C, moderate recommendation).

4.3 Patient Management on the Basis of Office BP

4.3a Normal BP

If BP is normal or normalizes after repeat readings (ie, BP <90th percentile), then no additional action is needed. Practitioners should measure the BP at the next routine well-child care visit.

4.3b Elevated BP

1. If the BP reading is at the elevated BP level (Table 3), lifestyle interventions should be recommended (ie, healthy diet, sleep, and physical activity); the measurement should be repeated in 6 months by auscultation. Nutrition and/or weight management referral should be considered as appropriate;

2. If BP remains at the elevated BP level after 6 months, upper and lower extremity BP should be checked (right arm, left arm, and 1 leg), lifestyle counseling should be repeated, and BP should be

Key Action Statement 1. BP should be measured annually in children and adolescents ≥3 years of age (grade C, moderate recommendation).

Aggregate Evidence Quality	Grade C
Benefits	Early detection of asymptomatic HTN; prevention of short- and long-term HTN-related morbidity
Risks, harm, cost	Overtesting, misclassification, unnecessary treatment, discomfort from BP measurement procedure, time involved in measuring BP
Benefit–harm assessment	Benefit of annual BP measurement exceeds potential harm
Intentional vagueness	None
Role of patient preferences	Increased visit time, discomfort of cuff
Exclusions	None
Strength	Moderate recommendation
Key references	10,60,102,103

Key Action Statement 2. BP should be checked in all children and adolescents ≥3 years of age at every health care encounter if they have obesity, are taking medications known to increase BP, have renal disease, a history of aortic arch obstruction or coarctation, or diabetes (see Table 9) (grade C, moderate recommendation).

Aggregate Evidence Quality	Grade C
Benefits	Early detection of HTN and prevention of CV morbidity in predisposed children and adolescents
Risks, harm, cost	Time for and difficulty of conducting measurements
Benefit–harm assessment	Benefits exceed harm
Intentional vagueness	Frequency of evaluation
Role of patient preferences	Increased visit time, discomfort of cuff
Exclusions	Children and adolescents who are not at increased risk for HTN
Strength	Moderate recommendation
Key references	27,46,107,110–112

rechecked in 6 months (ie, at the next well-child care visit) by auscultation;

3. If BP continues at the elevated BP level after 12 months (eg, after 3 auscultatory measurements), ABPM should be ordered (if available), and diagnostic evaluation should be conducted

(see Table 10 for a list of screening tests and the populations in which they should be performed). Consider subspecialty referral (ie, cardiology or nephrology) (see Table 11); and

4. If BP normalizes at any point, return to annual BP screening at well-child care visits.

4.3c Stage 1 HTN

1. If the BP reading is at the stage 1 HTN level (Table 3) and

the patient is asymptomatic, provide lifestyle counseling and recheck the BP in 1 to 2 weeks by auscultation;

2. If the BP reading is still at the stage 1 level, upper and lower extremity BP should be checked (right arm, left arm, and 1 leg), and BP should be rechecked in 3 months by auscultation. Nutrition and/or weight management referral should be considered as appropriate; and

3. If BP continues to be at the stage 1 HTN level after 3 visits, ABPM should be ordered (if available), diagnostic evaluation should be conducted, and treatment should be initiated. Subspecialty referral should be considered (see Table 11).

4.3d Stage 2 HTN

1. If the BP reading is at the stage 2 HTN level (Table 3), upper and lower extremity BP should be checked (right arm, left arm, and 1 leg), lifestyle recommendations given, and the BP measurement should be repeated within 1 week. Alternatively, the patient could be referred to subspecialty care within 1 week;

2. If the BP reading is still at the stage 2 HTN level when repeated, then diagnostic evaluation, including ABPM, should be conducted and treatment should be initiated, or the patient should

TABLE 8 Common Pharmacologic Agents Associated With Elevated BP in Children

Over-the-counter drugs	Decongestants
	Caffeine
	Nonsteroidal anti-inflammatory drugs
	Alternative therapies, herbal and nutritional supplements
Prescription drugs	Stimulants for attention-deficit/hyperactivity disorder
	Hormonal contraception
	Steroids
	Tricyclic antidepressants
Illicit drugs	Amphetamines
	Cocaine

Adapted from the Fourth Report.[1]

TABLE 9 Conditions Under Which Children Younger Than 3 Years Should Have BP Measured

History of prematurity <32 week's gestation or small for gestational age, very low birth weight, other neonatal complications requiring intensive care, umbilical artery line
Congenital heart disease (repaired or unrepaired)
Recurrent urinary tract infections, hematuria, or proteinuria
Known renal disease or urologic malformations
Family history of congenital renal disease
Solid-organ transplant
Malignancy or bone marrow transplant
Treatment with drugs known to raise BP
Other systemic illnesses associated with HTN (neurofibromatosis, tuberous sclerosis, sickle cell disease,[114] etc)
Evidence of elevated intracranial pressure

Adapted from Table 3 in the Fourth Report.[1]

Key Action Statement 3. Trained health care professionals in the office setting should make a diagnosis of HTN if a child or adolescent has auscultatory-confirmed BP readings ≥95th percentile on 3 different visits (grade C, moderate recommendation).

Aggregate Evidence Quality	Grade C
Benefits	Early detection of HTN; prevention of CV morbidity in predisposed children and adolescents; identification of secondary causes of HTN
Risks, harm, cost	Overtesting, misclassification, unnecessary treatment, discomfort from BP measurement, time involved in taking BP
Benefit–harm assessment	Benefits of repeated BP measurement exceeds potential harm
Intentional vagueness	None
Role of patient preferences	Families may have varying levels of concern about elevated BP readings and may request evaluation on a different time line
Exclusions	None
Strength	Moderate recommendation
Key references	8,84,85

be referred to subspecialty care within 1 week (see Table 11); and

3. If the BP reading is at the stage 2 HTN level and the patient is symptomatic, or the BP is >30 mm Hg above the 95th percentile (or >180/120 mm Hg in an adolescent), refer to an immediate source of care, such as an emergency department (ED).

Key Action Statement 3

Trained health care professionals in the office setting should make a diagnosis of HTN if a child or adolescent has auscultatory-confirmed BP readings ≥95th percentile on 3 different visits (grade C, moderate recommendation).

4.4 Use of Electronic Health Records

Studies have demonstrated that primary care providers frequently fail to measure BP and often underdiagnose HTN.[85,115,116]

One analysis using nationally representative survey data found that providers measured BP at only 67% of preventive visits for children 3 to 18 years of age. Older children and children with overweight or obesity were more likely to be screened.[117] In a large cohort study of 14 187 children, 507 patients met the criteria for HTN, but only 131 (26%) had the diagnosis documented in their electronic health records (EHRs). Elevated BP was only recognized in 11% of cases.[7]

It is likely that the low rates of screening and diagnosis of pediatric HTN are related, at least in part, to the need to use detailed reference tables incorporating age, sex, and height to classify BP levels.[118] Studies have shown that using health information technology can increase adherence to clinical guidelines and improve practitioner performance.[119–121] In fact, applying

decision support in conjunction with an EHR in adult populations has also been associated with improved BP screening, recognition, medication prescribing, and control; pediatric data are limited, however.[122–125] Some studies failed to show improvement in BP screening or control,[122,126] but given the inherent complexity in the interpretation of pediatric BP measurements, EHRs should be designed to flag abnormal values both at the time of measurement and on entry into the EHR.

Key Action Statement 4

Organizations with EHRs used in an office setting should consider including flags for abnormal BP values both when the values are being entered and when they are being viewed (grade C, weak recommendation).

4.5 Oscillometric Versus Auscultatory (Manual) BP Measurement

Although pediatric normative BP data are based on auscultatory measurements, oscillometric BP devices have become commonplace in health care settings.[127] Ease of use, a lack of digit preference, and automation are all perceived benefits of using oscillometric devices. Unlike auscultatory measurement, however, oscillometric devices measure the oscillations transmitted from disrupted arterial flow by using the cuff as a transducer to determine mean arterial pressure (MAP). Rather than directly measuring any pressure that correlates to SBP or DBP, the device uses a proprietary algorithm to calculate these values from the directly measured MAP.[127] Because the algorithms vary for different brands of oscillometric devices, there is no standard oscillometric BP.[128]

Researchers in several studies have evaluated the accuracy of oscillometric devices[127,129–134] and compared auscultatory and

Key Action Statement 4. Organizations with EHRs used in an office setting should consider including flags for abnormal BP values both when the values are being entered and when they are being viewed (grade C, weak recommendation).

Aggregate Evidence Quality	Grade C
Benefits	Improved rate of screening and recognition of elevated BP
Risks, harm, cost	Cost of EHR development, alert fatigue
Benefit–harm assessment	Benefit of EHR flagging of elevated BP outweighs harm from development cost and potential for alert fatigue
Intentional vagueness	None
Role of patient preferences	None
Exclusions	None
Strength	Weak recommendation (because of a lack of pediatric data)
Key references	7,117,120,125

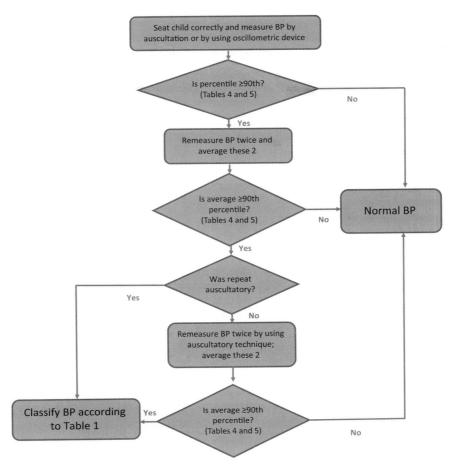

FIGURE 3
Modified BP measurement algorithm.

oscillometric readings' ability to predict target organ damage.[135] These studies demonstrated that oscillometric devices systematically overestimate SBP and DBP compared with values obtained by auscultation.[129,133] BP status potentially can be misclassified because of the different values obtained by these 2 methods, which may be magnified in the office setting.[86,88,129] Target organ damage (such as increased LV mass and elevated PWV) was best predicted by BPs obtained by auscultation.[135]

A major issue with oscillometric devices is that there appears to be great within-visit variation with inaccurately high readings obtained on initial measurement.[136] An elevated initial oscillometric reading should be ignored and

repeat measures averaged to approximate values obtained by auscultation.

TABLE 10 Screening Tests and Relevant Populations

Patient Population	Screening Tests
All patients	Urinalysis
	Chemistry panel, including electrolytes, blood urea nitrogen, and creatinine
	Lipid profile (fasting or nonfasting to include high-density lipoproteina and total cholesterol)
	Renal ultrasonography in those <6 y of age or those with abnormal urinalysis or renal function
In the obese (BMI >95th percentile) child or adolescent, in addition to the above	Hemoglobin A1c (accepted screen for diabetes)
	Aspartate transaminase and alanine transaminase (screen for fatty liver)
	Fasting lipid panel (screen for dyslipidemia)
Optional tests to be obtained on the basis of history, physical examination, and initial studies	Fasting serum glucose for those at high risk for diabetes mellitus
	Thyroid-stimulating hormone
	Drug screen
	Sleep study (if loud snoring, daytime sleepiness, or reported history of apnea)
	Complete blood count, especially in those with growth delay or abnormal renal function

Adapted from Wiesen J, Adkins M, Fortune S, et al. Evaluation of pediatric patients with mild-to-moderate hypertension: yield of diagnostic testing. *Pediatrics.* 2008;122(5). Available at: www.pediatrics.org/cgi/content/full/122/5/e988.

Key Action Statement 5
Oscillometric devices may be used for BP screening in children

TABLE 11 Patient Evaluation and Management According to BP Level

BP Category (See Table 3)	BP Screening Schedule	Lifestyle Counseling (Weight and Nutrition)	Check Upper and Lower Extremity BP	ABPM[a]	Diagnostic Evaluation[b]	Initiate Treatment[c]	Consider Subspecialty Referral
Normal	Annual	X	—	—	—	—	—
Elevated BP	Initial measurement	X	—	—	—	—	—
	Second measurement: repeat in 6 mo	X	X	—	—	—	—
	Third measurement: repeat in 6 mo	X	—	X	X	—	X
Stage 1 HTN	Initial measurement	X	—	—	—	—	—
	Second measurement: repeat in 1–2 wk	X	X	—	—	—	—
	Third measurement: repeat in 3 mo	X	—	X	X	X	X
Stage 2 HTN[d]	Initial measurement	X	X	—	—	—	—
	Second measurement: repeat, refer to specialty care within 1 wk	X	—	X	X	X	X

X, recommended intervention; —, not applicable.

[a] ABPM is done to confirm HTN before initiating a diagnostic evaluation.

[b] See Table 15 for recommended studies.

[c] Treatment may be initiated by a primary care provider or subspecialist.

[d] If the patient is symptomatic or BP is >30 mm Hg above the 95th percentile (or >180/120 mm Hg in an adolescent), send to an ED.

and adolescents. When doing so, providers should use a device that has been validated in the pediatric age group. If elevated BP is suspected on the basis of oscillometric readings, confirmatory measurements should be obtained by auscultation (grade B, strong recommendation).

4.6 Forearm and/or Wrist BP Measurement

Wrist monitors have several potential advantages when compared with arm devices. They are smaller; they can be placed more easily; and, because wrist diameter is less affected by BMI, they do not need to be modified for patients with obesity.[83,137] Several studies in adults have found excellent reproducibility of wrist BP measurements, equivalence to readings obtained by mercury sphygmomanometers or ABPM, and better correlation with left ventricular mass index (LVMI) than systolic office BP.[138,139]

Although many wrist devices have been validated in adults,[140–142] some studies have shown greater variation and decreased accuracy in the resulting measurements.[143–146] These negative outcomes may possibly result from differences in the number of measurements taken,[139] the position of the wrist in relation to the heart,[147] flexion or extension of the wrist during measurement,[148] or differences in pulse pressure.[149] Technologies are being developed to help standardize wrist position.[150,151]

Few studies using wrist monitors have been conducted in children. One study in adolescents compared a wrist digital monitor with a mercury sphygmomanometer and found high agreement between systolic measurements but lower agreement for diastolic measurements, which was clinically relevant.[152] Researchers in 2 small studies conducted in PICUs compared wrist monitors with indwelling arterial lines and found good agreement between the 2 measurement modalities.[153,154] No large comparative studies or formal validation studies of wrist monitors have been conducted in children, however. Because of limited data, the use of wrist and forearm monitors is not recommended in the diagnosis or

Key Action Statement 5. Oscillometric devices may be used for BP screening in children and adolescents. When doing so, providers should use a device that has been validated in the pediatric age group. If elevated BP is suspected on the basis of oscillometric readings, confirmatory measurements should be obtained by auscultation (grade B, strong recommendation).

Aggregate Evidence Quality	Grade B
Benefits	Use of auscultatory readings prevents potential misclassification of patients as hypertensive because of inaccuracy of oscillometric devices
Risks, harm, cost	Auscultation requires more training and experience and has flaws such as digit preference
Benefit–harm assessment	Benefit exceeds harm
Intentional vagueness	None
Role of patient preferences	Patients may prefer the convenience of oscillometric monitors
Exclusions	None
Strength	Strong recommendation
Key references	86,88,128–136

TABLE 12 High-Risk Conditions for Which ABPM May Be Useful

Condition	Rationale
Secondary HTN	Severe ambulatory HTN or nocturnal HTN indicates higher likelihood of secondary HTN[161,167]
CKD or structural renal abnormalities	Evaluate for MH or nocturnal HTN,[168–172] better control delays progression of renal disease[173]
T1DM and T2DM	Evaluate for abnormal ABPM patterns,[174,175] better BP control delays the development of MA[176–178]
Solid-organ transplant	Evaluate for MH or nocturnal HTN, better control BP[179–188]
Obesity	Evaluate for WCH and MH[23,189–192]
OSAS	Evaluate for nondipping and accentuated morning BP surge[43,46,193,194]
Aortic coarctation (repaired)	Evaluate for sustained HTN and MH[58,112,113]
Genetic syndromes associated with HTN (neurofibromatosis, Turner syndrome, Williams syndrome, coarctation of the aorta)	HTN associated with increased arterial stiffness may only be manifest with activity during ABPM[58,195]
Treated hypertensive patients	Confirm 24-h BP control[155]
Patient born prematurely	Evaluate for nondipping[196]
Research, clinical trials	To reduce sample size[197]

TABLE 13 Recommended Procedures for the Application of ABPM

Procedure	Recommendation
Device	Should be validated by the Association for the Advancement of Medical Instrumentation or the British Hypertension Society for use in children
	May be oscillometric or auscultatory
Application	Trained personnel should apply the monitor
	Correct cuff size should be selected
	Right and left arm and a lower extremity BP should be obtained to rule out coarctation of the aorta
	Use nondominant arm unless there is large difference in size between the left arm and right arm, then apply to the arm with the higher BP
	Take readings every 15–20 min during the day and every 20–30 min at night
	Compare (calibrate) the device to resting BP measured by the same technique (oscillometric or auscultatory)
	Record time of medications, activity, and sleep
Assessment	A physician who is familiar with pediatric ABPM should interpret the results
	Interpret only recordings of adequate quality. Minimum of 1 reading per hour, 40–50 for a full day, 65%–75% of all possible recordings
	Edit outliers by inspecting for biologic plausibility, edit out calibration measures
	Calculate mean BP, BP load (% of readings above threshold), and dipping (% decline in BP from wake to sleep)
	Interpret with pediatric ABPM normal data by sex and height
	Use AHA staging schema[155]
	Consider interpretation of 24-h, daytime, and nighttime MAP, especially in patients with CKD[173,198]

Adapted from Flynn JT, Daniels SR, Hayman LL, et al; American Heart Association Atherosclerosis, Hypertension and Obesity in Youth Committee of the Council on Cardiovascular Disease in the Young. Update: ambulatory blood pressure monitoring in children and adolescents: a scientific statement from the American Heart Association. *Hypertension.* 2014;63(5):1116–1135.

management of HTN in children and adolescents at this time.

4.7 ABPM

An ambulatory BP monitor consists of a BP cuff attached to a box slightly larger than a cell phone, which records BP periodically (usually every 20–30 minutes) throughout the day and night; these data are later downloaded to a computer for analysis.[155]

ABPM has been recommended by the US Preventive Services Task Force for the confirmation of HTN in adults before starting treatment.[156] Although a growing number of

pediatric providers have access to ABPM, there are still gaps in access and knowledge regarding the optimal application of ABPM to the evaluation of children's BP.[155,157] For example, there are currently no reference data for children whose height is <120 cm. Because no outcome data exist linking ABPM data from childhood to hard CV events in adulthood, recommendations either rely largely on surrogate outcome markers or are extrapolated from adult studies.

However, sufficient data exist to demonstrate that ABPM is more accurate for the diagnosis of HTN than clinic-measured

BP,[158,159] is more predictive of future BP,[160] and can assist in the detection of secondary HTN.[161] Furthermore, increased LVMI and LVH correlate more strongly with ABPM parameters than casual BP.[162–166] In addition, ABPM is more reproducible than casual or home BP measurements.[159] For these reasons, the routine application of ABPM is recommended, when available, as indicated below (see also Tables 12 and 13). Obtaining ABPM may require referral to a specialist.

Key Action Statement 6

ABPM should be performed for the confirmation of HTN in children and adolescents with office BP measurements in the elevated BP category for 1 year or more or with stage 1 HTN over 3 clinic visits (grade C, moderate recommendation).

For technical reasons, ABPM may need to be limited to children ≥5 years of age who can tolerate the procedure and those for whom reference data are available.

Key Action Statement 7

The routine performance of ABPM should be strongly considered in children and adolescents with high-risk conditions (see Table 12) to assess HTN severity and determine if abnormal circadian BP patterns are present, which may indicate increased risk for target organ damage (grade B, moderate recommendation).

Key Action Statement 8

ABPM should be performed by using a standardized approach (see Table 13) with monitors that have been validated in a pediatric population, and studies should be interpreted by using pediatric normative data (grade C, moderate recommendation).

4.7a Masked Hypertension

MH occurs when patients have normal office BP but elevated BP on ABPM, and it has been found in 5.8% of unselected children studied by ABPM.[199] There is growing evidence

that compared with those with normal 24-hour BP, these patients have significant risk for end organ hypertensive damage.[200,203] Patients who are at risk of MH include patients with obesity and secondary forms of HTN, such as CKD or repaired aortic coarctation. MH is particularly prevalent in patients with CKD[48] and is associated with target organ damage.[203] Children with CKD should be periodically evaluated using ABPM for MH as part of routine CKD management.[201,204–206]

4.7b White Coat Hypertension

WCH is defined as BP ≥95th percentile in the office or clinical setting but <95th percentile outside of the office or clinical setting. WCH is diagnosed by ABPM when the mean SBP and DBP are <95th percentile and SBP and DBP load are <25%; load is defined as the percentage of valid ambulatory BP measurements above a set threshold value (eg, 95th percentile) for age, sex, and height.[155,156,206] It is estimated that up to half of children who are evaluated for elevated office BP have WCH.[207,208]

In adults, compared with normotension, WCH is associated with only a slightly increased risk of adverse outcomes but at a much lower risk compared with those

with established HTN.[209] Most (but not all) studies suggest that WCH is not associated with increased LV mass.[200,207,210] Although the distinction between WCH and true HTN is important, abnormal BP response to exercise and increased LVM has been found to occur in children with WCH.[207] Furthermore, the identification of WCH may reduce costs by reducing the number of additional tests performed and decreasing the number of children who are exposed to antihypertensive medications.[208] Children and adolescents with WCH should have screening BP measured at regular well-child care visits with consideration of a repeat ABPM in 1 to 2 years.

Key Action Statement 9

Children and adolescents with suspected WCH should undergo ABPM. Diagnosis is based on the presence of mean SBP and DBP <95th percentile and SBP and DBP load <25% (grade B, strong recommendation).

4.8 Measurement in Children With Obesity

Accurate BP measurement can be challenging in individuals with obesity.[23,211,212] Elevated BMI in children and adolescents is associated with an increase in the midarm circumference,[96] requiring the use of a larger cuff to obtain accurate BP measurements.[83] During NHANES 2007–2010, among children 9 to 11 years of age with obesity, one-third of boys and one-quarter of girls required an adult BP cuff, and a fraction required a large adult cuff or an adult thigh cuff for an accurate measurement of BP.[213] Researchers in studies of adults have also noted the influence of the conical upper arm shape on BP measurements in people with obesity.[214,215] ABPM is a valuable tool in the diagnosis of HTN in children with obesity because of the discrepancies between casual and

Key Action Statement 6. ABPM should be performed for the confirmation of HTN in children and adolescents with office BP measurements in the elevated BP category for 1 year or more or with stage 1 HTN over 3 clinic visits (grade C, moderate recommendation).

Aggregate Evidence Quality	Grade C
Benefits	Avoids unnecessarily exposing youth with WCH to extensive diagnostic testing or medication
Risks, harm, cost	Risk of discomfort to patient. Some insurance plans may not reimburse for the test
Benefit–harm assessment	The risk of ABPM is lower than the risk of unnecessary treatment. The use of ABPM has also been shown to be more cost-effective than other approaches to diagnosing HTN
Intentional vagueness	None
Role of patient preferences	Some patients may prefer repeat office or home measurements to ABPM
Exclusions	None
Strength	Moderate recommendation
Key references	23,155,158,159

Key Action Statement 7. The routine performance of ABPM should be strongly considered in children and adolescents with high-risk conditions (see Table 12) to assess HTN severity and determine if abnormal circadian BP patterns are present, which may indicate increased risk for target organ damage (grade B, moderate recommendation).

Aggregate Evidence Quality	Grade B
Benefits	Improved 24-h control of BP improves outcomes. Recognition of MH or nocturnal HTN might lead to therapeutic changes that will limit end organ damage
Risks, harm, cost	Risk of discomfort to patient. Some insurance plans may not reimburse for the test. The risk of diagnosing and labeling a patient as having MH or nocturnal HTN might lead to increased anxiety and cost of evaluation
Benefit–harm assessment	The risk of ABPM is much lower than the risk of inadequate treatment
Intentional vagueness	Frequency at which normal or abnormal ABPM should be repeated is not known
Role of patient preferences	Some patients may prefer repeat office or home measurements to ABPM
Exclusions	None
Strength	Moderate recommendation
Key references	47,155,199–202

Key Action Statement 8. ABPM should be performed by using a standardized approach (see Table 13) with monitors that have been validated in a pediatric population, and studies should be interpreted by using pediatric normative data (grade C, moderate recommendation).

Aggregate Evidence Quality	Grade C
Benefits	Validated monitors applied and interpreted correctly will provide the most accurate results
Risks, harm, cost	Risk of discomfort to patient. Some insurance plans may not reimburse for the test. Monitors validated in the pediatric population and expertise in reading pediatric ABPM may not be universally available
Benefit–harm assessment	There is substantial evidence showing incorrect application or interpretation reduces the accuracy of results
Intentional vagueness	None
Role of patient preferences	Some patients may prefer repeat office or home measurements to ABPM
Exclusions	None
Strength	Moderate recommendation
Key references	155

ambulatory BP[23,33] and the higher prevalence of MH.[26,29,155,216,217]

4.9. At-Home Measurement

Home measurement (or self-monitoring) of BP has advantages over both office and ambulatory monitoring, including convenience and the ability to obtain repeated measurements over time.[83,218] Furthermore, automated devices with memory capacity are straightforward to use and avoid potential problems, such as observer bias, inaccurate reporting, and terminal digit preference (ie, overreporting of certain digits, like 0, as the terminal digit in recording BP).[219,220]

Numerous studies have shown that it is feasible for families to conduct repeated measurements at home.[221–223] Home BP measurements appear to be more reproducible than those conducted in the office, likely because of the familiarity of the home environment and greater comfort with repeated measurements.[159,223,224] Inaccuracies occur when measurements obtained at home are either excluded or inappropriately recorded.[219] Inconsistencies in home, office, and ambulatory BP measurements seem to be influenced by both age and HTN status, with ABPM tending to be higher than home BP measurements

in children.[222,225–227] Home BP measurements show no consistent pattern when compared with office measurements.[228–230]

There are several practical concerns with the use of home BP measurement, however. The only normative data available are from the relatively small Arsakeion School study.[231] In addition, only a few automated devices have been validated for use in the pediatric population, and available cuff sizes for them are limited. Furthermore, there is no consensus regarding how many home measurements across what period of time are needed to evaluate BP.

Key Action Statement 10

Home BP monitoring should not be used to diagnose HTN, MH, or WCH but may be a useful adjunct to office and ambulatory BP measurement after HTN has been diagnosed (grade C, moderate recommendation).

4.10 School Measurement and the Role of School-Based Health Professionals

There is limited evidence to support school-based measurement of children's BP.[8,232] Observational studies demonstrate that school measurements can be reliable[233] and that longitudinal follow-up is feasible.[8,232,234] Available data do not distinguish between the efficacy of school-based screening programs in which measurements are obtained by trained clinical personnel (not a school nurse) versus measurements obtained by the school nurse. Because of insufficient evidence and a lack of established protocols, the routine use of school-based measurements to diagnose HTN cannot be recommended. However, school-based BP measurement can be a useful tool to identify children who require formal evaluation as well as a helpful adjunct in the monitoring of diagnosed HTN. Note: School-based health clinics are considered part of

Key Action Statement 9. Children and adolescents with suspected WCH should undergo ABPM. Diagnosis is based on the presence of mean SBP and DBP <95th percentile and SBP and DBP load <25% (grade B, strong recommendation).

Aggregate Evidence Quality	Grade B (Evidence Level A in Adults)
Benefits	Improved diagnosis of WCH and the benefit of fewer additional laboratory tests and/or treatment of primary HTN. Costs might be reduced if the treatment of those misdiagnosed as hypertensive is prevented
Risks, harm, cost	Additional costs; costs may not be covered by insurance companies. The ambulatory BP monitor is uncomfortable for some patients
Benefit–harm assessment	Benefit exceeds risk
Intentional vagueness	None
Role of patient preferences	Important; some patients may not want to undergo ABPM. Benefits of the procedure should be reviewed with families to assist in decision-making
Exclusions	None
Strength	Strong recommendation
Key references	206

Key Action Statement 10. Home BP monitoring should not be used to diagnose HTN, MH, or WCH but may be a useful adjunct to office and ambulatory BP measurement after HTN has been diagnosed (grade C, moderate recommendation).

Aggregate Evidence Quality	Grade C
Benefits	Convenient, cost-effective, widely available, can be used over time
Risks, harm, cost	Risk of inaccurate diagnosis. Unclear what norms or schedule should be used. Few validated devices in children, and cuff sizes are limited
Benefit–harm assessment	Benefits outweigh harm when used as an adjunctive measurement technique
Intentional vagueness	None
Role of patient preferences	Patients may find home BP more convenient and accessible than office or ambulatory BP
Exclusions	None
Strength	Moderate recommendation
Key references	159,221–225,227,230

systems of pediatric primary care, and these comments would not apply to them.

5. PRIMARY AND SECONDARY CAUSES OF HTN

5.1 Primary HTN

Primary HTN is now the predominant diagnosis for hypertensive children and adolescents seen in referral centers in the United States,[235,236] although single-center studies from outside the United States still find primary HTN to be uncommon.[237] Although prospective, multicenter studies are generally lacking, at least one large study in which researchers used insurance claims data confirmed that primary HTN is significantly

more common than secondary HTN among American youth.[238]

General characteristics of children with primary HTN include older age (≥6 years),[239,240] positive family history (in a parent and/or grandparent) of HTN,[236,237,240] and overweight and/or obesity.[16,236,237,239] Severity of BP elevation has not differed significantly between children with primary and secondary HTN in some studies,[235,237] but DBP elevation appears to be more predictive of secondary HTN,[239,240] whereas systolic HTN appears to be more predictive of primary HTN.[236,239]

Key Action Statement 11

Children and adolescents ≥6 years of age do not require an extensive

evaluation for secondary causes of HTN if they have a positive family history of HTN, are overweight or obese, and/or do not have history or physical examination findings (Table 14) suggestive of a secondary cause of HTN (grade C, moderate recommendation).

5.2 Secondary Causes: Renal and/or Renovascular

Renal disease and renovascular disease are among the most common secondary causes of HTN in children. Renal parenchymal disease and renal structural abnormalities accounted for 34% to 79% of patients with secondary HTN in 3 retrospective, single-center case series, and renovascular disease was present in 12% to 13%.[101,240,241] The literature suggests that renal disease is a more common cause of HTN in younger children.[239] Renal disorders (including vascular problems) accounted for 63% to 74% of children <6 years of age who were enrolled in 3 recent clinical trials of angiotensin receptor blockers (ARBs).[239,242–244] No increased frequency was seen in younger patients in a recent single-center case series, however.[101] It is appropriate to have a high index of suspicion for renal and renovascular disease in hypertensive pediatric patients, particularly in those <6 years of age.

5.3 Secondary Causes: Cardiac, Including Aortic Coarctation

Coarctation of the aorta is a congenital abnormality of the aortic arch characterized by discrete narrowing of the aortic arch, generally at the level of the aortic isthmus. It is usually associated with HTN and right arm BP that is 20 mm Hg (or more) greater than the lower extremity BP. Repair in infants is often surgical; adolescents may be treated with angioplasty or stenting. Long-segment narrowing of the abdominal aorta can also cause HTN and should be considered in children with refractory

Key Action Statement 11. Children and adolescents ≥6 years of age do not require an extensive evaluation for secondary causes of HTN if they have a positive family history of HTN, are overweight or obese, and/or do not have history or physical examination findings (Table 14) suggestive of a secondary cause of HTN (grade C, moderate recommendation).

	Grade C
Aggregate Evidence Quality	
Benefits	Avoidance of unnecessary diagnostic evaluation
Risks, harm, cost	Potential to miss some children with secondary HTN
Benefit–harm assessment	Benefit equals harm
Intentional vagueness	Not applicable
Role of patient preferences	Some families may want further testing performed
Exclusions	Hypertensive children <6 y of age
Strength	Moderate recommendation
Key references	16,129,235–240

HTN and a gradient between the upper and lower extremities in which the upper extremity SBP exceeds the lower extremity SBP by 20 mm Hg.[245] Of note, children with abdominal aortic obstruction may have neurofibromatosis, Williams syndrome, Alagille syndrome, or Takayasu arteritis.

Patients with coarctation can remain hypertensive or develop HTN even after early and successful repair, with reported prevalence varying from 17% to 77%.[112] HTN can be a manifestation of recoarctation. Recoarctation in repaired patients should be assessed for by using 4 extremity BP measurements and echocardiography. HTN can also occur without recoarctation.[246] The prevalence of HTN increases over time after successful coarctation repair.[112]

Routine office BP measurement alone is often insufficient for diagnosing HTN after coarctation repair.[113,246] Children who have undergone coarctation repair may have normal in-office BP but high BP out of the office, which is consistent with MH.[58,112] Of children with a history of aortic coarctation, ~45% have MH at ~1 to 14 years after coarctation repair.[58,113] Children with a history of repaired aortic coarctation and normal in-office BP are at risk for LVH,[58] HTN, and MH.[58,112]

ABPM has emerged as the gold standard for diagnosing HTN among individuals who have undergone coarctation repair, and it is likely more useful than casual BP.[58,245–247] Screening is recommended as a part of usual care on an annual basis beginning, at most, 12 years after coarctation repair. Earlier screening may be considered on the basis of risk factors and clinician discretion.

Key Action Statement 12

Children and adolescents who have undergone coarctation repair should undergo ABPM for the detection of HTN (including MH) (grade B, strong recommendation).

5.4 Secondary Causes: Endocrine HTN

HTN resulting from hormonal excess accounts for a relatively small proportion of children with secondary HTN. Although rare (with a prevalence ranging from 0.05% to 6% in children[101,237,239,240]), an accurate diagnosis of endocrine HTN provides the clinician with a unique treatment opportunity to render a surgical cure or achieve a dramatic response with pharmacologic therapy.[248] Known endocrine causes with associated molecular defects (when known) are summarized in Table 15.

5.5 Secondary Causes: Environmental Exposures

Several environmental exposures have been associated with higher childhood BP, although most studies are limited to small case series. Among the most prominent are lead, cadmium, mercury, and phthalates.

- Lead: Long-term exposure to lead in adults has been associated with higher BP in population studies[295,296] and in studies of industrial workers with high lead exposure,[297] although findings have not been consistent.[298] At least 1 cross-sectional study of 122 children demonstrated that children with higher blood lead concentrations had higher BP; lower socioeconomic status was also seen in this group, which may have confounded the BP results.[299] Furthermore, in a randomized study of lead-exposed children, those who received chelation with succimer did not have lower BP than in those who received a placebo.[300]

- Cadmium: Environmental cadmium exposure has been linked to higher BP levels and the development of HTN in adults, particularly among women.[296,301–303] Although cross-sectional studies have

Key Action Statement 12. Children and adolescents who have undergone coarctation repair should undergo ABPM for the detection of HTN (including MH) (grade B, strong recommendation).

Aggregate Evidence Quality	Grade B (Aggregate Level of Evidence Equals B, Given 3 Studies With Similar Findings)
Benefits	Early detection of HTN
Risks, harm, cost	Additional costs related to the placement of ABPM
Benefit–harm assessment	Benefits exceed harms
Intentional vagueness	Frequency of measurement. Because the development of HTN after coarctation repair is influenced by many factors, the ideal onset of screening for HTN (including MH) is unknown
Role of patient preferences	None
Exclusions	Individuals with a history of residual aortic arch obstruction
Strength	Strong recommendation
Key references	58,112,113

TABLE 14 Examples of Physical Examination Findings and History Suggestive of Secondary HTN or Related to End Organ Damage Secondary to HTN

Body System	Finding, History	Possible Etiology
Vital signs	Tachycardia	Hyperthyroidism
		PCC
		Neuroblastoma
	Decreased lower extremity pulses; drop in BP from upper to lower extremities	Coarctation of the aorta
Eyes	Proptosis	Hyperthyroidism
	Retinal changes[a]	Severe HTN, more likely to be associated with secondary HTN
Ear, nose, throat	Adenotonsillar hypertrophy	SDB
	History of snoring	Sleep apnea
Height, weight	Growth retardation	Chronic renal failure
	Obesity (high BMI)	Cushing syndrome
	Truncal obesity	Insulin resistance syndrome
Head, neck	Elfin facies	Williams syndrome
	Moon facies	Cushing syndrome
	Thyromegaly, goiter	Hyperthyroidism
	Webbed neck	Turner syndrome
Skin	Pallor, flushing, diaphoresis	PCC
	Acne, hirsutism, striae	Cushing syndrome
		Anabolic steroid abuse
	Café-au-lait spots	Neurofibromatosis
	Adenoma sebaceum	Tuberous sclerosis
	Malar rash	Systemic lupus
	Acanthosis nigricans	T2DM
Hematologic	Pallor	Renal disease
	Sickle cell anemia	
Chest, cardiac	Chest pain	Heart disease
	Palpitations	
	Exertional dyspnea	
	Widely spaced nipples	Turner syndrome
	Heart murmur	Coarctation of the aorta
	Friction rub	Systemic lupus (pericarditis)
		Collagen vascular disease
	Apical heave[a]	LVH
Abdomen	Abdominal mass	Wilms tumor
		Neuroblastoma
		PCC
	Epigastric, flank bruit	RAS
	Palpable kidneys	Polycystic kidney disease
		Hydronephrosis
		Multicystic dysplastic kidney
Genitourinary	Ambiguous or virilized genitalia	Congenital adrenal hyperplasia
	Urinary tract infection	Renal disease
	Vesicoureteral reflux	
	Hematuria, edema, fatigue	
	Abdominal trauma	
Extremities	Joint swelling	Systemic lupus
		Collagen vascular disease
	Muscle weakness	Hyperaldosteronism
		Liddle syndrome
Neurologic, metabolic	Hypokalemia, headache, dizziness, polyuria, nocturia	Reninoma
	Muscle weakness, hypokalemia	Monogenic HTN (Liddle syndrome, GRA, AME)

AME, apparent mineralocorticoid excess; GRA, glucocorticoid-remediable aldosteronism. Adapted from Flynn JT. Evaluation and management of hypertension in childhood. *Prog Pediatr Cardiol*. 2001;12(2):177–188; National High Blood Pressure Education Program Working Group on Hypertension Control in Children and Adolescents. The fourth report on the diagnosis, evaluation, and treatment of high blood pressure in children and adolescents. *Pediatrics*. 2004;114(2):555–576.
[a] Findings that may be indicative of end organ damage related to HTN.

confirmed potential nephrotoxicity of cadmium in children,[304] no definite effect on BP has been demonstrated.[304,305]

- Mercury: Mercury is a known nephrotoxin, particularly in its elemental form.[306,307] Severe mercury intoxication has been linked to acute HTN in children in several case reports; patients' symptoms may resemble those seen in patients with pheochromocytoma (PCC).[308–310]

- Phthalates: Antenatal and childhood exposure to phthalates has recently been associated with higher childhood BP[311–313] but not with the development of overt HTN. Specific metabolites of these ubiquitous chemicals may have differential effects on BP,[313] indicating that much more detailed study is needed to completely understand the effect of such exposure.

5.6 Secondary Causes: Neurofibromatosis

Neurofibromatosis type 1 (NF-1) (also known as Von Recklinghausen disease) is a rare autosomal dominant disorder characterized by distinct clinical examination findings. These include the following: cafe-au-lait macules, neurofibromas, Lisch nodules of the iris, axillary freckling, optic nerve gliomas, and distinctive bone lesions. Patients with NF-1 have several unique and potential secondary causes of HTN, most commonly renal artery stenosis (RAS); coarctation of the aorta, middle aortic syndrome, and PCC are also well described.[314–319]

Additionally, an increased incidence of idiopathic HTN has been documented in patients with NF-1, as high as 6.1% in a recent pediatric case series, which is a much greater incidence than in the general population.[320] PCC has also been well described in patients with NF-1, although exact incidences are difficult

TABLE 15 Endocrine Causes of HTN

Name of Disorder	Genetic Mutation	Mode of Inheritance	Clinical Feature(s)	Biochemical Mechanism and Notes	Ref No(s).
Catecholamine excess PCC, paraganglioma	VHL (49%) SDHB (15%) SDHD (10%) RET	De novo, AD	HTN Palpitations, headache, sweating Abdominal mass Incidental radiographic finding Family screening	Diagnostic test: fractionated plasma[a] and/or urine metanephrines and normetanephrines	248–254
Mineralocorticoid excess Specific etiologies addressed below Consider if: Early onset HTN Potassium level abnormalities Family history of primary aldosteronism Resistant HTN			Screening test: ARR: PAC, PRA preferably obtained between 8:00 and 10:00 AM		255,256
Congenital adrenal hyperplasia 11β-hydroxylase deficiency	CYP11B1 (loss of function)	AR	HTN Hypokalemia Acne, hirsutism, and virilization in girls Pseudoprecocious puberty in boys 11% of congenital adrenal hyperplasia	Elevated levels of DOC, 11-deoxycortisol, androstenedione, testosterone, and DHEAS Higher prevalence in Moroccan Jews	257–259
17-α hydroxylase deficiency	CYP17 (loss of function)	AR	HTN and hypokalemia Low aldosterone and renin Undervirilized boys, sexual infantilism in girls <1% of congenital adrenal hyperplasia	Elevated DOC and corticosterone Decreased androstenedione, testosterone and DHEAS Prominent in Dutch Mennonites	260–262
Familial hyperaldosteronism Type 1	Hybrid CYP11B1 and CYP11B2 (11β-hydroxylase–aldosterone synthase, gain of function)	AD	Young subjects with PA Family history of young strokes	Excessive, ACTH-regulated aldosterone production Prescription with low-dose dexamethasone May add low-dose spironolactone, calcium channel blocker, or potassium supplementation	263,264
Type 2	Unknown, possibly 7p22	AD (prevalence varies from 1.2% to 6%)	PA in the patient with an affected first-degree relative Unresponsive to dexamethasone May have adrenal adenoma or bilateral adrenal hyperplasia	Excessive autonomous aldosterone production	265–267
Type 3	KCNJ5 G-protein potassium channel (loss of function)	AD	Early onset severe HTN in the first family described Milder phenotypes also seen	Mutation leads to loss of potassium+ sensitivity causing sodium+ influx that activates Ca++ channels, leading to aldosterone synthesis	268–270
Type 4	CACNA1D coding for calcium channel (gain of function)	AD	PA and HTN age <10 y Variable developmental abnormalities	Increased Ca++ channel sensitivity causing increased aldosterone synthesis	271,272
Other genetic causes					

TABLE 15 Continued

Name of Disorder	Genetic Mutation	Mode of Inheritance	Clinical Feature(s)	Biochemical Mechanism and Notes	Ref No(s).
Carney complex	PRKAR1A	AD	Skin pigmentation Pituitary and other tumors	Rare familial cause	273,274
McCune Albright syndrome	GNAS, α-subunit	Somatic	Cutaneous pigmentation Fibrous dysplasia	Tumors in the breast, thyroid, pituitary gland, or testicles may be present	275,276
Primary glucocorticoid resistance (Chrousos syndrome)	NR3C1 (loss of function glucocorticoid receptor)	AD	HTN Ambiguous genitalia Precocious puberty Androgen excess, menstrual abnormalities or infertility in women	Loss of function of glucocorticoid receptor	277–279
Apparent mineralocorticoid excess	HSD11B2 (loss of function)	AR	HTN Hypokalemia Low birth weight Failure to thrive Polyuria, polydipsia	Reduced or absent activity of 11 β-HSD2: cortisol gains access to MR Mimicked by licorice toxicity	280,281
Liddle syndrome	SCNN1B β-subunit—SCNN1G γ-subunit (activating mutation)		Severe HTN Hypokalemia Metabolic alkalosis Muscle weakness	Constitutive activation of the epithelial sodium channel causing salt retention and volume expansion	282,283
Geller syndrome	MCR (mineralocorticoid-d receptor; activating mutation)	AD	Onset of HTN <20 y Exacerbated by pregnancy	Constitutive activation of MR Also activated by progesterone	284
Pseudohypo-aldosteronism type 2 (Gordon syndrome)	WNK1,4; KLHL3; CUL3; SPAK (activating mutation)	AD	Short stature Hyperkalemic and hyperchloremic metabolic acidosis Borderline HTN	Increased activity of sodium chloride cotransporter causing salt retention and volume expansion	285–287
Glucocorticoid excess Cushing syndrome, adrenocortical carcinoma, iatrogenic excess	To be discovered	—	HTN Other signs of Cushing syndrome	Likely attributable to increased DOC, sensitivity to vasoconstriction, cardiac output, activation of RAS	288–290
Other endocrine abnormalities Hyperthyroidism	To be discovered	—	Tachycardia HTN Tremors Other signs of hyperthyroidism	Mechanism increased cardiac output, stroke volume, and decreased peripheral resistance Initial prescription with β blockers	291,292
Hyperparathyroidism	—	—	Hypercalcemia Other signs of hyperparathyroidism	Mechanism unknown, may not remit after treatment of hyperparathyroidism	293,294

ACTH, adrenocorticotropic hormone; AD, autosomal dominant; AR, autosomal recessive; DHEAS, dehydroepiandrosterone sulfate; DOC, deoxycortisol; MR, magnetic resonance; PA, primary hyperaldosteronism; PAC, plasma aldosterone concentration; RAS, renin angiotensin system; —, not applicable.

a Influenced by posture, specialized center preferred.

to determine, and patients may not have classic symptoms of PCC.[321,322]

Vascular causes of HTN and PCC all require specific treatment and follow-up, so maintaining a high index of suspicion for these disorders is important in evaluating hypertensive children and adolescents with NF-1.

5.7 Secondary Causes: Medication Related

Many over-the-counter drugs, prescription medications, alternative therapies (ie, herbal and nutritional supplements), dietary products, and recreational drugs can increase BP. Common prescription medications associated with a rise in BP include oral contraceptives,[323–325] central nervous system stimulants,[326] and corticosteroids.[1,327] When a child has elevated BP measurements, the practitioner should inquire about the intake of pharmacologic agents (see Table 8).

Usually, the BP elevation is mild and reversible on discontinuation of the medication, but a significant increase in BP can occasionally occur with higher doses or as an idiosyncratic response. Over-the-counter cold medications that contain decongestants (eg, pseudoephedrine and phenylpropanolamine) may cause a mild increase in BP with the recommended dosing, but severe HTN has been observed as an idiosyncratic response with appropriate dosing as well as with excessive doses.

Nonsteroidal anti-inflammatory drugs may antagonize the BP-lowering effect of antihypertensive medications (specifically, angiotensin-converting enzyme [ACE] inhibitors) but do not appear to have an impact on BP in those without HTN. The commonly used supplement ephedra (ma haung) likely contains some amount of ephedrine and caffeine that can cause an unpredictable rise in BP. Recreational drugs associated with HTN include stimulants (eg, cocaine and amphetamine derivatives) and anabolic steroids.

5.8 Monogenic HTN

Monogenic forms of HTN are uncommon, although the exact incidence is unknown. In a study of select hypertensive children without a known etiology, genetic testing for familial hyperaldosteronism type I (FH-I), or glucocorticoid-remediable aldosteronism, confirmed responsible genetic mutations in 3% of the population.[263]

Other monogenic forms of HTN in children include Liddle syndrome, pseudohypoaldosteronism type II (Gordon syndrome), apparent mineralocorticoid excess, familial glucocorticoid resistance, mineralocorticoid receptor activating mutation, and congenital adrenal hyperplasia (see "Secondary Causes: Endocrine Causes of Hypertension").[328] All manifest as HTN with suppressed plasma renin activity (PRA) and increased sodium absorption in the distal tubule. Other features may include serum potassium abnormalities, metabolic acid-base disturbances, and abnormal plasma aldosterone concentrations, although the clinical presentations can be highly variable.[263,328,329] In the study of FH-I, all affected children had suppressed PRA and an aldosterone to renin ratio (ARR) (ng/dL and ng/M1 per hour, respectively) of >10; the authors suggest that an ARR >10 is an indication to perform genetic testing in a hypertensive child.[263] Monogenic forms of HTN should be suspected in hypertensive children with a suppressed PRA or elevated ARR, especially if there is a family history of early-onset HTN.

6. DIAGNOSTIC EVALUATION

6.1 Patient Evaluation

As with any medical condition, appropriate diagnostic evaluation is a critical component in the evaluation of a patient with suspected HTN. Evaluation focuses on determining possible causes of and/or comorbidities associated with HTN. Evaluation, as is detailed in the following sections, should include appropriate patient history, family history, physical examination, laboratory evaluation, and imaging.

6.2 History

The first step in the evaluation of the child or adolescent with elevated BP is to obtain a history. The various components of the history include the perinatal history, past medical history, nutritional history, activity history, and psychosocial history. Each is discussed in the following sections.

6.2a Perinatal History

As discussed, perinatal factors such as maternal HTN and low birth weight have been shown to influence later BP, even in childhood.[56,330] Additionally, a high incidence of preterm birth among hypertensive children has recently been reported in 1 large case series.[101] Thus, it is appropriate to obtain a history of pertinent prenatal information, including maternal pregnancy complications; gestational age; birth weight; and, if pertinent, complications occurring in the neonatal nursery and/or ICU. It is also appropriate to document pertinent procedures, such as umbilical catheter placement.

6.2b Nutritional History

High sodium intake has been linked to childhood HTN and increased LVMI and is the focus of several population health campaigns.[4,331] In NHANES 2003–2008, among children 8 to 18 years of age (*n* = 6235), higher sodium intake (as assessed by dietary recall) was associated with a twofold increase in the combined outcome of elevated BP or HTN. The effect was threefold among participants with obesity.[332] Limited data suggest the same effect is seen in younger children.[333] One study found that high intake of total fat and saturated fat, as well as adiposity and central obesity, were also predictors of SBP.[334–336]

Nutrition history is an important part of the patient assessment because it may identify dietary contributors to HTN and detect areas in which lifestyle modification may be appropriate. The important components to discuss include salt intake (including salt added in the kitchen and at the table and sodium hidden in processed and fast food), consumption of high-fat foods, and consumption of sugary beverages.[337,338] Infrequent consumption of fruits, vegetables, and low-fat dairy products should also be identified.

6.2c Physical Activity History

A detailed history of physical activity and inactivity is an integral part of the patient assessment, not only to understand contributors to the development of HTN but also to direct lifestyle modification counseling as an important part of management.[339–344]

6.2d Psychosocial History

Providers should obtain a psychosocial history in children and adolescents with suspected or confirmed HTN. Adverse experiences both prenatally[345] and during childhood (including maltreatment, early onset depression, and anxiety) are associated with adult-onset HTN.[346,347] The identification of stress may suggest a diagnosis of WCH. The psychosocial history should include questions about feelings of depression and anxiety, bullying, and body perceptions. The latter is particularly important for patients with overweight or obesity because ~70% of these children report having bullying and body perception concerns.[348] Starting at 11 years of age, the psychosocial history should include questions about smoking,[349,350] alcohol, and other drug use.[351]

6.2e Family History

Taking and updating the family history is a quick and easy way to risk-stratify pediatric patients with an increased risk for HTN. It is important to update the family history for HTN over the course of the pediatric patient's lifetime in the practice (typically until 18–21 years of age) because first- and second-degree relatives may develop HTN during this time. All too often, the diagnosis of HTN in the pediatric patient stimulates the collection of a detailed family history of HTN, sometimes even years after the pediatric patient has had elevated BP, instead of the other way around.[352]

6.3 Physical Examination

A complete physical examination may provide clues to potential secondary causes of HTN and assess possible hypertensive end organ damage. The child's height, weight, calculated BMI, and percentiles for age should be determined at the start of the physical examination. Poor growth may indicate an underlying chronic illness.

At the second visit with confirmed elevated BP or stage 1 HTN or the first visit with confirmed stage 2 HTN, BP should be measured in both arms and in a leg. Normally, BP is 10 to 20 mm Hg higher in the legs than the arms. If the leg BP is lower than the arm BP, or if femoral pulses are weak or absent, coarctation of the aorta may be present. Obesity alone is an insufficient explanation for diminished femoral pulses in the presence of high BP.

The remainder of the physical examination should pursue clues found in the history and should focus on body systems and findings that may indicate secondary HTN and/ or end organ damage related to HTN. Table 14 lists important physical examination findings in hypertensive children.[353] These are examples of history and physical findings and do not represent all possible history and

physical examination findings. The physical examination in hypertensive children is frequently normal except for the BP elevation.

Key Action Statement 13

In children and adolescents being evaluated for high BP, the provider should obtain a perinatal history, appropriate nutritional history, physical activity history, psychosocial history, and family history and perform a physical examination to identify findings suggestive of secondary causes of HTN (grade B, strong recommendation).

6.4 Laboratory Evaluation

The purpose of the laboratory evaluation is to identify underlying secondary causes of HTN (eg, renal or endocrine disease) that would require specific treatment guided by a subspecialist. In general, such testing includes a basic set of screening tests and additional, specific tests; the latter are selected on the basis of clues obtained from the history and physical examination and/or the results of the initial screening tests.[354] Table 10 provides a list of screening tests and the populations in which they should be performed.

6.5 Electrocardiography

Approximately one-half of adolescents with HTN have undergone electrocardiography at least once as an assessment for LVH.[355] Unlike echocardiography, electrocardiography takes little time and is a relatively low-cost test. Electrocardiography has high specificity but poor sensitivity for identifying children and adolescents with LVH.[356–358] The positive predictive value of electrocardiography to identify LVH is extremely low.[359]

Key Action Statement 14

Clinicians should not perform electrocardiography in hypertensive

Key Action Statement 13. In children and adolescents being evaluated for high BP, the provider should obtain a perinatal history, appropriate nutritional history, physical activity history, psychosocial history, and family history and perform a physical examination to identify findings suggestive of secondary causes of HTN (grade B, strong recommendation).

Aggregate Evidence Quality	Grade B
Benefits	Identify personal risk factors for HTN
Risks, harm, cost	None
Benefit–harm assessment	Identification of personal risk factors is useful in the assessment of childhood HTN
Intentional vagueness	None
Role of patient preferences	None
Exclusions	Children with normal BP
Strength	Strong recommendation
Key references	56,330

children and adolescents being evaluated for LVH (grade B, strong recommendation).

6.6 Imaging Evaluation, Echocardiography: Detection of Target Organ Damage

Echocardiography was identified in the Fourth Report as a tool to measure left ventricular (LV) target organ injury related to HTN in children.[1] The basis for this assessment is as follows: (1) the relationship of LV mass to BP,[361] (2) the independent and strong relationship of LVH to adverse CVD outcomes in adults,[362–364] and (3) that a significant percentage of children and adolescents with HTN demonstrate the degree of LVH associated with adverse outcomes in adults.[365–367] Antihypertensive treatment reduces LVH. Observational data suggest that the regression of LVH independently predicts outcomes in adults.[368]

The best-studied measures of LV target organ injury are measures of LV structure (LV mass and the relationship of LV wall thickness or mass to LV cavity volume) and systolic function (LV ejection fraction). LV structure is usually stratified into 4 groups on the basis of LV mass (normal or hypertrophied) and relative LV wall thickness (normal or increased). These 4 are as follows: (1) normal geometry with normal LV mass and wall thickness, (2) concentric geometry with normal LV mass and increased LV wall thickness, (3) eccentric LVH with increased LV mass and normal LV wall thickness, and (4) concentric LVH with both increased LV mass and increased relative wall thickness.[369,370]

The American Society of Echocardiography recommendations should be followed with regard to image acquisition and LV measurement for calculating LV ejection fraction, mass, and relative wall thickness.[369,371] LV ejection fraction may be significantly decreased in severe or acute onset HTN with associated congestive heart failure.[1] Rarely, LV ejection fraction may be mildly depressed in chronic HTN.

Because the heart increases in size in relation to body size, indexing LV mass is required.[361] Indexing LV mass is particularly important in infants and younger children because of their rapid growth.[372,373] Physical training increases LV mass in a healthful manner. Lean body mass is more strongly associated with LV mass than fat mass.[370] Because body composition is not routinely measured clinically, surrogate formulae for indexing are required. It is unclear whether expected values for LV mass should be derived from reference populations of normal weight and normotensive children or should include normotensive children who have overweight or obesity. The best method for indexing LV mass in children is an area of active investigation.

For this document, the following definitions for LV target organ injury have been chosen regarding hypertrophy, relative wall thickness, and ejection fraction. These definitions are based on published guidelines from the American Society of Echocardiography and associations of thresholds for indexed LV mass with adverse outcomes in adults[362,363,369]:

- LVH is defined as LV mass >51 g/m$^{2.7}$ or LV mass >115 g per body surface area (BSA) for boys and LV mass >95 g/BSA for girls. (Note that the values for LVH are well above the 95th percentile for distributions of LV mass in children and adolescents.[369] The clinical significance of values between the

Key Action Statement 14. Clinicians should not perform electrocardiography in hypertensive children and adolescents being evaluated for LVH (grade B, strong recommendation).

Aggregate Evidence Quality	Grade B (Aggregate of Level of Evidence Equals B Because of Multiple Level of Evidence C References With Similar Findings)
Benefits	Electrocardiography is less expensive than echocardiography or other imaging modalities for identifying LVH
Risks, harm, cost	Electrocardiography has a low sensitivity for detecting LVH
Benefit–harm assessment	The risk of concluding that a child with HTN does not have LVH on the basis of a normal electrocardiogram means that a diagnosis of end organ injury is potentially missed
Intentional vagueness	None
Role of patient preferences	Patients and families may prefer electrocardiography because of cost and convenience, but the sensitivity of the test is poor
Exclusions	None
Strength	Strong recommendation
Key references	1,355–360

95th percentile of a population-based distribution and these thresholds is uncertain[372]);

- An LV relative wall thickness >0.42 cm indicates concentric geometry. LV wall thickness >1.4 cm is abnormal[373]; and

- Decreased LV ejection fraction is a value <53%.

There are a number of additional evidence gaps related to the echocardiographic assessment of LV target organ injury. The value of LV mass assessment in risk reclassification independent of conventional risk assessment has not been established in adults.[364] The costs and benefits of incorporation of echocardiography into HTN care has not been assessed. Quality control regarding reproducibility of measurements across laboratories may be suboptimal.[374] The most accurate method to measure LV mass (M-mode; two-dimensional; or, in the near future, three-dimensional techniques) requires further research.

Key Action Statement 15

1. It is recommended that echocardiography be performed to assess for cardiac target organ damage (LV mass, geometry, and function) at the time of consideration of pharmacologic treatment of HTN;

2. LVH should be defined as LV mass >51 g/m$^{2.7}$ (boys and girls) for children and adolescents older than 8 years and defined by LV mass >115 g/BSA for boys and LV mass >95 g/BSA for girls;

3. Repeat echocardiography may be performed to monitor improvement or progression of target organ damage at 6- to 12-month intervals. Indications to repeat echocardiography include persistent HTN despite treatment, concentric LV hypertrophy, or reduced LV ejection fraction; and

TABLE 16 DASH Diet Recommendations

Food	Servings per Day
Fruits and vegetables	4–5
Low-fat milk products	≥2
Whole grains	6
Fish, poultry, and lean red meats	≤2
Legumes and nuts	1
Oils and fats	2–3
Added sugar and sweets (including sweetened beverages)	≤1
Dietary sodium	<2300 mg per d

Adapted from Barnes TL, Crandell JL, Bell RA, Mayer-Davis EJ, Dabelea D, Liese AD. Change in DASH diet score and cardiovascular risk factors in youth with type 1 and type 2 diabetes mellitus: the SEARCH for Diabetes in Youth study. *Nutr Diabetes*. 2013;3:e91; US Department of Health and Human Services, US Department of Agriculture. Appendix 7. Nutritional goals for age-sex groups based on dietary reference intakes and dietary guidelines recommendations. In: *2015-2020 Dietary Guidelines for Americans*. Washington, DC: US Department of Health and Human Services, US Department of Agriculture; 2015; and Expert Panel on Integrated Guidelines for Cardiovascular Health and Risk Reduction in Children and Adolescents; National Heart, Lung, and Blood Institute. Expert Panel on Integrated Guidelines for Cardiovascular Health and Risk Reduction in Children and Adolescents: Summary Report. *Pediatrics*. 2011;128 (suppl 5): S213–S256.

4. In patients without LV target organ injury at initial echocardiographic assessment, repeat echocardiography at yearly intervals may be considered in those with stage 2 HTN, secondary HTN, or chronic stage 1 HTN incompletely treated (noncompliance or drug resistance) to assess for the development of worsening LV target organ injury (grade C, moderate recommendation).

6.7 Vascular Structure and Function

Emerging data demonstrate an association of higher levels of BP in youth with adverse changes in measures of vascular structure and function, including ultrasonography of the cIMT, PWV, a robust measure of central arterial stiffness[66] that is related to hard CV events in adults

Key Action Statement 15. It is recommended that echocardiography be performed to assess for cardiac target organ damage (LV mass, geometry, and function) at the time of consideration of pharmacologic treatment of HTN;

LVH should be defined as LV mass >51 g/m2.7 (boys and girls) for children and adolescents older than 8 years and defined by LV mass >115 g/BSA for boys and LV mass >95 g/BSA for girls;

Repeat echocardiography may be performed to monitor improvement or progression of target organ damage at 6- to 12-month intervals. Indications to repeat echocardiography include persistent HTN despite treatment, concentric LV hypertrophy, or reduced LV ejection fraction; and

In patients without LV target organ injury at initial echocardiographic assessment, repeat echocardiography at yearly intervals may be considered in those with stage 2 HTN, secondary HTN, or chronic stage 1 HTN incompletely treated (noncompliance or drug resistance) to assess for the development of worsening LV target organ injury (grade C, moderate recommendation).

Aggregate Evidence Quality	Grade C
Benefits	Severe LV target organ damage can only be identified with LV imaging. May improve risk stratification
Risks, harm, cost	Adds cost; improvement in outcomes from incorporating echocardiography into clinical care is not established
Benefit–harm assessment	Benefits exceed harms
Intentional vagueness	None
Role of patient preferences	Patients may elect to not to have the study
Exclusions	None
Strength	Moderate recommendation
Key references	361,363,364,367–369

(eg, stroke, myocardial infarction, etc),[69] and FMD, which assesses endothelial function and describes the ability of the endothelium to release nitric oxide in response to stress.[375]

Although there are multiple large studies of PWV in youth,[376–381] they all suffer from notable limitations, primarily the lack of racial and ethnic diversity and differences in measurement devices and protocols. Researchers in the largest study of PWV in youth to date ($N = 6576$) only evaluated 10 and 11 year olds and measured only carotid-radial PWV across the arm; this measure has not been linked to CV events in adults.[382] Researchers in one large study of FMD performed in youth ($N = 5809$) only included 10- to 11-year-old children in England.[382] The largest set of data for cIMT included 1155 European youth who were 6 to 18 years of age.[383] No racial and ethnic breakdown was provided for this study. The wide heterogeneity in the methods for cIMT measurement hinders the pooling of data. For instance, researchers in the aforementioned article only measured common carotid,[383] although the bulb and internal carotid are the sites of earliest atherosclerotic disease.[384]

Many studies have had significant issues related to methodology. For example, carotid-femoral PWV is not measured identically with different devices and is not equivalent to other measures of PWV, such as brachial-femoral PWV.[385,386] No direct comparisons have been made between carotid-femoral and brachial-ankle PWV, methods in which brachial-ankle PWV provide values considerably higher than carotid-femoral PWV.[378] The brachial-ankle PWV measures stiffness along both a central elastic artery (aorta) and the medium muscular arteries of the leg.

Therefore, insufficient normative data are available to define clinically actionable cut-points between normal and abnormal for these vascular parameters. The routine measurement of vascular structure and function to stratify risk in hypertensive youth cannot be recommended at this time.

6.8 Imaging for Renovascular Disease

There are no evidence-based criteria for the identification of children and adolescents who may be more likely to have RAS. Some experts will do a more extensive evaluation for RAS in children and adolescents with stage 2 HTN, those with significant diastolic HTN (especially on ABPM), those with HTN and hypokalemia on screening laboratories, and those with a notable size discrepancy between the kidneys on standard ultrasound imaging. Bruits over the renal arteries are also suggestive of RAS but are not always present. Consultation with a subspecialist is recommended to help decide which patients warrant further investigation and to aid in the selection of the appropriate imaging modality.

6.8a Renal Ultrasonography

The utility of Doppler renal ultrasonography as a noninvasive screening study for the identification of RAS in children and adolescents has been examined in at least 2 recent case series; sensitivity has been reported to be 64% to 90%, with a specificity of 68% to 70%.[387,388] In another study that included both children and adults, sensitivity and specificity for the detection of renal artery stenoses was 75% and 89%, respectively.[389] Factors that may affect the accuracy of Doppler ultrasonography include patient cooperation, the technician's experience, the age of the child, and the child's BMI. Best results are obtained in older (≥8 years),[388] nonobese (BMI ≤85th percentile), cooperative children and adolescents who are examined in a facility with extensive pediatric vascular imaging experience. Doppler ultrasonography should probably not be obtained in patients who do not meet these criteria or in facilities that lack appropriate pediatric experience.

Key Action Statement 16

Doppler renal ultrasonography may be used as a noninvasive screening study for the evaluation of possible RAS in normal-weight children and adolescents ≥8 years of age who are suspected of having renovascular HTN and who will cooperate with the procedure (grade C, moderate recommendation).

6.8b Computed Tomographic Angiography, Magnetic Resonance Angiography, and Renography

Other noninvasive imaging studies that have been assessed for their ability to identify RAS include computed tomographic angiography (CTA), magnetic resonance angiography (MRA), and nuclear medicine studies. Each of these

Key Action Statement 16. Doppler renal ultrasonography may be used as a noninvasive screening study for the evaluation of possible RAS in normal-weight children and adolescents ≥8 years of age who are suspected of having renovascular HTN and who will cooperate with the procedure (grade C, moderate recommendation).

Aggregate Evidence Quality	Grade C
Benefits	Avoidance of complications of invasive procedure (angiography) or radiation from traditional or computed tomography angiography
Risks, harm, cost	Potential false-positive or false-negative results
Benefit–harm assessment	Potential for avoidance of an invasive procedure outweighs risk of false-negative or false-positive results
Intentional vagueness	None
Role of patient preferences	None
Exclusions	Children and adolescents without suspected renovascular HTN
Strength	Moderate recommendation
Key references	387–390

TABLE 17 Dosing Recommendations for the Initial Prescription of Antihypertensive Drugs for Outpatient Management of Chronic HTN

Drug	Age	Initial Dose	Maximal Dose	Dosing Interval	Formulations
ACE inhibitors					
Contraindications: pregnancy, angioedema					
Common adverse effects: cough, headache, dizziness, asthenia					
Severe adverse effects: hyperkalemia, acute kidney injury, angioedema, fetal toxicity					
Benazepril	≥6 y[a]	0.2 mg/kg per d (up to 10 mg per d)	0.6 mg/kg per d (up to 40 mg per d)	Daily	Tablet: 5, 10, 20, 40 mg (generic)
					Extemporaneous liquid: 2 mg/mL
Captopril	Infants	0.05 mg/kg per dose	6 mg/kg per d	Daily to 4 times a day	Tablet: 12.5, 25, 50, 100 mg (generic)
	Children	0.5 mg/kg per dose	6 mg/kg per d	Three times a day	Extemporaneous liquid: 1 mg/mL
Enalapril	≥1 mo[a]	0.08 mg/kg per d (up to 5 mg per d)	0.6 mg/kg per d (up to 40 mg per d)	Daily to twice a day	Tablet: 2.5, 5, 10, 20 mg (generic)
					Solution: 1 mg/mL
Fosinopril	≥6 y	0.1 mg/kg per d (up to 5 mg per d)	40 mg per d	Daily	Tablet: 10, 20, 40 mg (generic)
	<50 kg				
	≥50 kg[a]	5 mg per d	40 mg per d		
Lisinopril	≥6 y[a]	0.07 mg/kg per d (up to 5 mg per d)	0.6 mg/kg per d (up to 40 mg per d)	Daily	Tablet: 2.5, 5, 10, 20, 30, 40 mg (generic)
					Solution: 1 mg/mL
Ramipril	—	1.6 mg/m² per d	6 mg/m² per d	Daily	Capsule: 1.25, 2.5, 5 10 mg (generic)
Quinapril	—	5 mg per d	80 mg per d	Daily	Tablet: 5, 10, 20, 40 mg (generic)
ARBs					
Contraindications: pregnancy					
Common adverse effects: headache, dizziness					
Severe adverse effects: hyperkalemia, acute kidney injury, fetal toxicity					
Candesartan	1–5 y[a]	0.02 mg/kg per d (up to 4 mg per d)	0.4 mg/kg per d (up to 16 mg per d)	Daily to twice a day	Tablet: 4, 8, 16, 32 mg
	≥6 y[a]				Extemporaneous liquid: 1 mg/mL
	<50 kg	4 mg per d	16 mg per d		
	≥50 kg	8 mg per d	32 mg per d		
Irbesartan	6–12 y	75 mg per d	150 mg per d	Daily	Tablet: 75, 150, 300 mg (generic)
	≥13	150 mg per d	300 mg per d		
Losartan	≥6 y[a]	0.7 mg/kg (up to 50 mg)	1.4 mg/kg (up to 100 mg)	Daily	Tablet: 25, 50 100 (generic)
					Extemporaneous liquid: 2.5 mg/mL
Olmesartan	≥6 y[a]	—	—	Daily	Tablet: 5, 20, 40 mg
	<35 kg	10 mg	20 mg		Extemporaneous liquid: 2 mg/mL
	≥35 kg	20 mg	40 mg		
Valsartan	≥6 y[a]	1.3 mg/kg (up to 40 mg)	2.7 mg/kg (up to 160 mg)	Daily	Tablet: 40, 80, 160, 320 mg (generic)
					Extemporaneous liquid: 4 mg/mL
Thiazide diuretics					
Contraindications: anuria					
Common adverse effects: dizziness, hypokalemia					
Severe adverse effects: cardiac dysrhythmias, cholestatic jaundice, new onset diabetes mellitus, pancreatitis					
Chlorthalidone	Child	0.3 mg/kg	2 mg/k per d (50 mg)	Daily	Tablet: 25, 50, 100 mg (generic)
Chlorothiazide	Child[a]	10 mg/kg per d	20 mg/kg per d (up to 375 mg per d)	Daily to twice a day	Tablet: 250, 500 mg (generic)
					Suspension: 250/5 mL
					Extemporaneous liquid: 1 mg/mL
Hydrochlorothiazide	Child[a]	1 mg/kg per d	2 mg/kg per d (up to 37.5 mg per d)	Daily to twice a day	Tablet: 12.5, 25, 50 mg

TABLE 17 Continued

Drug	Age	Initial Dose	Maximal Dose	Dosing Interval	Formulations
Calcium channel blockers					
Contraindications: hypersensitivity to CCBs					
Common adverse effects: flushing, peripheral edema, dizziness					
Severe adverse effects: angioedema					
Amlodipine	1–5 y	0.1 mg/kg	0.6 mg/kg (up to 5 mg per d)	Daily	Tablet: 2.5, 5,10 mg; Extemporaneous liquid: 1 mg/mL
	≥6 y[a]	2.5 mg	10 mg		
Felodipine	≥6 y	2.5 mg	10 mg	Daily	Tablet (extended release): 2.5,5,10 mg (generic)
Isradipine	Child	0.05–0.1 mg/kg	0.6 mg/kg (up to 10 mg per d)	Capsule: twice daily to 3 times a day; extended-release tablet: daily	Capsule: 2.5, 5 mg; Extended-release tablet: 5, 10 mg
Nifedipine extended release	Child	0.2–0.5 mg/kg per d	3 mg/kg/d (up to 120 mg per d)	Daily to twice a day	Tablet (extended-release): 30, 60, 90 mg (generic)

—, not applicable.
[a] FDA pediatric labeling.

has been compared with the gold standard, renal arteriography. CTA and MRA have generally been found to be acceptable as noninvasive imaging modalities for the identification of hemodynamically significant vascular stenosis. One study that included both pediatric and adult patients showed that the sensitivity and specificity for the detection of RAS was 94% and 93% for CTA and 90% and 94% for MRA, respectively.[389]

Unfortunately, studies of either technique that include only pediatric patients are limited at best for CTA and are nonexistent for MRA. Despite this, expert opinion holds that either modality may be used for noninvasive screening for suspected RAS, but neither is a substitute for angiography.[390] CTA typically involves significant radiation exposure, and MRA generally requires sedation or anesthesia in young children, which are factors that must be considered when deciding to use one of these modalities.

Nuclear renography is based on the principle that after the administration of an agent affecting the renin-angiotensin-aldosterone system (RAAS), there will be reduced blood flow to a kidney or kidney segment affected by hemodynamically significant RAS. Such reduced blood flow can be detected by a comparison of perfusion before and after the administration of the RAAS agent. Limited pediatric nuclear renography studies exist that show variable sensitivity and specificity, ranging from 48% to 85.7% and 73% to 92.3%, respectively.[391–393] The utility of nuclear renography may be less in children then adults because children with RAS often have more complicated vascular abnormalities than adults.[394] Given these issues, nuclear renography has generally been abandoned as a screening test for RAS in children and adolescents.[390]

Key Action Statement 17

In children and adolescents suspected of having RAS, either CTA or MRA may be performed as a noninvasive imaging study. Nuclear renography is less useful in pediatrics and should generally be avoided (grade D, weak recommendation).

6.9 Uric Acid

Cross-sectional data have suggested a relationship between elevated serum uric acid (UA) levels and HTN. Two recent studies of adolescents included in NHANES 1999–2000 and a small study conducted in Italy found that elevated UA levels were associated with higher BP.[395–397] In the Italian study and in another US study of youth with obesity and HTN,[397,398] elevated UA was also associated with other markers of CV risk. These findings suggest that the measurement of UA levels may best be viewed as 1 component of CV risk assessment, especially in those with obesity.

A causative role for elevated UA in the development of childhood HTN has not been definitively established, although recent studies suggest that it may be on the causal pathway. A longitudinal study in which researchers followed a group of children for an average of 12 years demonstrated that childhood UA levels were associated with adult BP levels even after controlling for baseline BP.[399] A few small, single-center clinical trials have

also shown that lowering UA can decrease BP levels, and increased UA levels blunt the efficacy of lifestyle modifications on BP control.[400–404] No large-scale, multicenter study has yet been conducted to confirm these preliminary findings. Hence, there is currently not sufficient evidence to support the routine measurement of serum UA in the evaluation and management of children with elevated BP.

6.10 Microalbuminuria

Microalbuminuria (MA), which should be differentiated from proteinuria in CKD, has been shown to be a marker of HTN-related kidney injury and a predictor of CVD in adults.[405–408] MA has been shown to be effectively reduced via the use of ARBs and ACE inhibitors in adults. Lowering the degree of MA in adults has been associated with decreased CVD risk.

In contrast, data to support a clear relationship between HTN and MA in pediatric patients with primary HTN are limited.[408–410] A single, retrospective study of children with primary HTN and WCH found that 20% of the former had MA versus 0% of the latter.[411] MA appears to be a nonspecific finding in children that can occur in the absence of HTN; it can occur in children who have obesity, insulin resistance, diabetes, dyslipidemia, and even in those who have recently participated in vigorous physical activity.[412] The previously mentioned study by

Seeman et al[411] did not control for these potential confounders.

Limited, single-center data suggest that a reduction in the degree of MA, more than a reduction in BMI or SBP, is associated with a decrease in LVMI. In particular, researchers in this single-center, nonrandomized, prospective study of 64 hypertensive children without kidney disease who were 11 to 19 years of age evaluated the children at baseline and after 12 months of combination ACE and hydrochlorothiazide ($N = 59$) or ACE, hydrochlorothiazide, and ARB therapy ($N = 5$). Results found that lowering MA in children is associated with a regression of LVH.[413] Given the single-center design and lack of a control group, however, the applicability of these findings to the general population of children with primary HTN is unknown.

Key Action Statement 18

Routine testing for MA is not recommended for children and adolescents with primary HTN (grade C, moderate recommendation).

7. TREATMENT

7.1 Overall Goals

The overall goals for the treatment of HTN in children and adolescents, including both primary and secondary HTN, include achieving a BP level that not only reduces the risk for target organ damage in childhood but also reduces the risk for HTN and related CVD in adulthood. Several studies have shown that currently available treatment options can even reverse target organ damage in hypertensive youth.[105,414,415]

The previous recommendations for HTN treatment target in children without CKD or diabetes were SBP and DBP <95th percentile. Since that recommendation was made, evidence has emerged that markers of target organ damage, such as increased LVMI, can be detected among some

Key Action Statement 17. In children and adolescents suspected of having RAS, either CTA or MRA may be performed as a noninvasive imaging study. Nuclear renography is less useful in pediatrics and should generally be avoided (grade D, weak recommendation).

Aggregate Evidence Quality	Grade D
Benefits	Avoidance of complications of an invasive procedure (angiography)
Risks, harm, cost	Potential false-positive or false-negative results
Benefit–harm assessment	Potential for avoidance of an invasive procedure outweighs risk of false-negative or false-positive results
Intentional vagueness	None
Role of patient preferences	None
Exclusions	Children and adolescents without suspected RAS
Strength	Weak recommendation; pediatric data are limited
Key references	389,390

Key Action Statement 18. Routine testing for MA is not recommended for children and adolescents with primary HTN (grade C, moderate recommendation).

Aggregate Evidence Quality	Grade C
Benefits	Avoid improper detection of MA in children with HTN. Detection of MA is strongly influenced by other factors, such as recent participation in rigorous physical activity, obesity, insulin resistance and diabetes. Hence, there is no clear benefit for testing for MA in the absence of other known comorbidities
Risks, harm, cost	No known risks given a lack of clear association between MA and primary HTN in children
Benefit–harm assessment	Limited data to support any real benefit for screening children for MA
Intentional vagueness	Screening of children with primary HTN versus screening of children with single kidney or CKD and HTN
Role of patient preferences	Unknown
Exclusions	None
Strength	Moderate recommendation
Key references	408,410,411,413

children with BP >90th percentile (or >120/80 mm Hg) but <95th percentile.[66,416,417] Longitudinal studies on BP from childhood to adulthood that include indirect measures of CV injury indicate that the risk for subsequent CVD in early adulthood increases as the BP level in adolescence exceeds 120/80 mm Hg.[11,103,418] In addition, there is some evidence that targeting a BP <90th percentile results in reductions in LVMI and prevalence of LVH.[104] Therefore, an optimal BP level to be achieved with treatment of childhood HTN is <90th percentile or <130/80 mm Hg, whichever is lower.

Treatment and management options are discussed below, including lifestyle modifications and pharmacologic therapy to achieve optimal BP levels in children and adolescents with HTN.

Key Action Statement 19

In children and adolescents diagnosed with HTN, the treatment goal with nonpharmacologic and pharmacologic therapy should be a reduction in SBP and DBP to <90th percentile and <130/80 mm Hg in adolescents ≥ 13 years old (grade C, moderate recommendation).

7.2 Lifestyle and Nonpharmacologic Interventions

Lifestyle interventions are recommended to lower BP. There is good evidence from studies in adults showing that nutritional interventions lower BP,[419] including clinical trials demonstrating that reducing dietary sodium results in lower BP and CV mortality,[338] and a diet high in olive oil polyphenols lowers BP.[420] Studies of hypertensive youth suggest

that the relationship between diet, physical activity, and BP in childhood is similar to that observed in adults.

7.2a Diet

The Dietary Approaches to Stop Hypertension (DASH) approach and specific elements of that diet have been the primary dietary strategy tested in the literature. These elements include a diet that is high in fruits, vegetables, low-fat milk products, whole grains, fish, poultry, nuts, and lean red meats; it also includes a limited intake of sugar and sweets along with lower sodium intake (see Table 16). Cross-sectional studies demonstrate associations between elements of the DASH diet and BP. For example, population-based data from NHANES show correlations between dietary sodium and BP in childhood and elevated BP and HTN, particularly in people with excess weight.[332]

A high intake of fruits, vegetables, and legumes (ie, a plant-strong diet) is associated with lower BP.[421] A lack of fruit consumption in childhood has been linked to increases in cIMT in young adulthood in the Young Finns study.[422] Higher intake of low-fat dairy products has been associated with lower BP in childhood.[423]

Longitudinal, observational, and interventional data also support relationships between diet and BP in youth. The National Heart Lung and Blood Institute's Growth and Health Study, which followed 2185 girls over 10 years, demonstrated that consuming ≥2 servings of dairy and ≥3 servings of fruits and vegetables daily was associated with lower BP in childhood and a 36% lower risk of high BP by young adulthood.[424] Similar associations have been demonstrated in children and adolescents with diabetes.[425] Moreover, an improvement in diet

Key Action Statement 19. In children and adolescents diagnosed with HTN, the treatment goal with nonpharmacologic and pharmacologic therapy should be a reduction in SBP and DBP to <90th percentile and <130/80 mm Hg in adolescents ≥ 13 years old (grade C, moderate recommendation).

Aggregate Evidence Quality	Grade C
Benefits	Lower risk of childhood target organ damage, lower risk of adulthood HTN and CVD
Risk, harm, cost	Risk of drug adverse effects and polypharmacy
Benefit–harm assessment	Preponderance of benefit
Intentional vagueness	None
Role of patient preferences	Patient may have preference for nonpharmacologic or pharmacologic treatment
Exclusions	None
Strength	Moderate recommendation
Key references	11,66,103,104,416–418

led to lower BP in some studies of adolescents with elevated BP,[426] youth with overweight,[427] girls with metabolic syndrome,[428] and youth with T2DM.[429] However, consuming a healthier diet may increase costs.[430]

7.2b Physical Activity

Observational data support a relationship between physical activity and lower BP, although the data are scant.[339] Interventional data demonstrate increasing physical activity leads to lower BP. A review of 9 studies of physical activity interventions in children and adolescents with obesity suggested that 40 minutes of moderate to vigorous, aerobic physical activity at least 3 to 5 days per week improved SBP by an average of 6.6 mm Hg and prevented vascular dysfunction.[340] A number of subsequent, additional studies with small sample sizes support a benefit of physical activity on BP.[341] A more recent analysis of 12 randomized controlled trials including 1266 subjects found reductions of 1% and 3% for resting SBP and DBP, respectively. These results did not reach statistical significance, however, and the authors suggested that longer studies with larger sample sizes are needed.[344] Any type of exercise, whether it's aerobic training, resistance training, or combined training, appears to be beneficial[342] (see "HTN and the Athlete").

Programs that combine diet and physical activity can have a beneficial effect on SBP, as is shown in several studies designed to prevent childhood obesity and address cardiometabolic risk.[431]

Key Action Statement 20

At the time of diagnosis of elevated BP or HTN in a child or adolescent, clinicians should provide advice on the DASH diet and recommend moderate to vigorous physical activity at least 3 to 5 days per week (30–60 minutes per session) to help reduce BP (grade C, weak recommendation).

7.2c Weight Loss and Related CV Risk Factors

As is true for children and adolescents with isolated HTN, a DASH diet[426,432] and vigorous physical activity[431] are recommended in pediatric patients with multiple obesity-related risk factors as part of intensive weight-loss therapy.[433,434] Motivational interviewing (MI) is a tool recommended for pediatricians' use by the AAP Expert Committee Statement on Obesity.[435] MI may be a useful counseling tool to use in combination with other behavioral techniques to address overweight and obesity in children.[436] Studies in hypertensive adults support the use of MI to improve adherence to antihypertensive medications[437] and decrease SBP.[436] Although there are no trials investigating the use of MI in the care of hypertensive youth, a number of studies have shown that MI can be used successfully to address or prevent childhood obesity by promoting physical activity and dietary changes.[438–441] However, other studies have been less promising.[442,443] In addition to the standard lifestyle approaches, intensive weight-loss therapy

TABLE 18 OSAS Symptoms and Signs

History of frequent snoring (≥3 nights per week)
Labored breathing during sleep
Gasps, snorting noises, observed episodes of apnea
Sleep enuresis (especially secondary enuresis)
Sleeping in a seated position or with the neck hyperextended
Cyanosis
Headaches on awakening
Daytime sleepiness
Attention-deficit/hyperactivity disorder
Learning problems
Physical examination
Underweight or overweight
Tonsillar hypertrophy
Adenoidal facies
Micrognathia, retrognathia
High-arched palate
Failure to thrive
HTN

Adapted from Marcus CL, Brooks LJ, Draper KA, et al; American Academy of Pediatrics. Diagnosis and management of childhood obstructive sleep apnea syndrome. *Pediatrics.* 2012;130(3). Available at: www.pediatrics.org/cgi/content/full/130/3/e714.

Key Action Statement 20. At the time of diagnosis of elevated BP or HTN in a child or adolescent, clinicians should provide advice on the DASH diet and recommend moderate to vigorous physical activity at least 3 to 5 days per week (30–60 minutes per session) to help reduce BP (grade C, weak recommendation).

Aggregate Evidence Quality	Grade C
Benefits	Potential to reduce BP
Risk, harm, cost	No or low potential for harm. Following a healthier diet may increase costs to patients and families
Benefit–harm assessment	Potential benefit outweighs lack of harm and minimal cost
Intentional vagueness	None
Role of patient preferences	Level of caregiver and patient concern may influence adoption of the DASH diet and physical activity. Patients may also have preferences around the use of a medication. These factors may influence the efficacy of lifestyle change
Exclusions	None
Strength	Weak recommendation
Key references	332,339–342,424–431

involving regular patient and/or family contact and at least 1 hour of moderate to vigorous physical activity on a daily basis should be offered to children and adolescents with obesity and HTN.[444]

7.2d Stress Reduction

Complimentary medicine interventions have shown some promise in studies in normotensive children and adolescents and in those with elevated BP. Breathing-awareness meditation, a component of the Mindfulness-Based Stress Reduction Program at the University of Massachusetts Memorial Medical Center,[445] led to a reduction in daytime, nighttime, and 24-hour SBP (3–4 mm Hg) and DPB (1 mm Hg) in normotensive African American adolescents and African American adolescents with elevated BP.[446] Another study of transcendental meditation showed no significant BP effect but did lead to a decrease in LVM in African American adolescents with elevated BP.[447] Scant data suggest yoga may also be helpful.[448]

7.3 Pharmacologic Treatment

Children who remain hypertensive despite a trial of lifestyle modifications or who have symptomatic HTN, stage 2 HTN without a clearly modifiable factor (eg, obesity), or any stage of HTN associated with CKD or diabetes mellitus therapy should be initiated with a single medication at the low end of the dosing range (see Table 17). Depending on repeated BP measurements, the dose of the initial medication can be increased every 2 to 4 weeks until BP is controlled (eg, <90th percentile), the maximal dose is reached, or adverse effects occur. Although the dose can be titrated every 2 to 4 weeks using home BP measurements, the patient should be seen every 4 to 6 weeks until BP has normalized. If BP is not controlled with a single agent, a second agent can be added to the regimen and titrated as with the

initial drug. Because of the salt and water retention that occurs with many antihypertensive medications, a thiazide diuretic is often the preferred second agent.

Lifestyle modifications should be continued in children requiring pharmacologic therapy. An ongoing emphasis on a healthy, plant-strong diet rich in fruits and vegetables; reduced sodium intake; and increased exercise can improve the effectiveness of antihypertensive medications. The use of a combination product as initial treatment has been studied only for bisoprolol and hydrochlorothiazide,[449] so the routine use of combination products to initiate treatment in children cannot be recommended. Once BP control has been achieved, a combination product can be considered as a means to improve adherence and reduce cost if the dose and formulation are appropriate.

7.3a Pharmacologic Treatment and Pediatric Exclusivity Studies

Studies completed in hypertensive children show that antihypertensive drugs decrease BP with few adverse effects.[173,202,242–244,450–467] There are few studies in children in which researchers compare different antihypertensive agents.[453] These studies do not show clinically significant differences in the degree of BP lowering between agents. There are no clinical trials in children that have CV end points as outcomes. Long-term studies on the safety of antihypertensive medications in children and their impact on future CVD are limited.[455]

Because of legislative acts that provide incentives and mandates for drug manufacturers to complete pediatric assessments,[468] most of the newer antihypertensive medications have undergone some degree of efficacy and safety evaluation. Antihypertensive drugs without patent protection have not been, and are unlikely to be, studied in children

despite their continued widespread use.[238]

7.3b Pharmacologic Treatment: Choice of Agent

Pharmacologic treatment of HTN in children and adolescents should be initiated with an ACE inhibitor, ARB,[469] long-acting calcium channel blocker, or a thiazide diuretic. Because African American children may not have as robust a response to ACE inhibitors,[470,471] a higher initial dose for the ACE inhibitor may be considered; alternatively, therapy may be initiated with a thiazide diuretic or long-acting calcium channel blocker. In view of the expanded adverse effect profile and lack of association in adults with improved outcomes compared with other agents, β-blockers are not recommended as initial treatment in children. ACE inhibitors and ARBs are contraindicated in pregnancy because these agents can cause injury and death to the developing fetus. Adolescents of childbearing potential should be informed of the potential risks of these agents on the developing fetus; alternative medications (eg, calcium channel blocker, β-blocker) can be considered when appropriate.

In children with HTN and CKD, proteinuria, or diabetes mellitus, an ACE inhibitor or ARB is recommended as the initial antihypertensive agent unless there is an absolute contraindication. Other antihypertensive medications (eg, α-blockers, β-blockers, combination α- and β-blockers, centrally acting agents, potassium-sparing diuretics, and direct vasodilators) should be reserved for children who are not responsive to 2 or more of the preferred agents (see "Treatment in CKD").

Key Action Statement 21

In hypertensive children and adolescents who have failed lifestyle modifications (particularly those

TABLE 19 Oral and Intravenous Antihypertensive Medications for Acute Severe HTN

Drug	Class	Route	Dose	Comments
Useful for Severely Hypertensive Patients With Life-Threatening Symptoms				
Esmolol	β-adrenergic blocker	Intravenous infusion	100–500 mcg/kg per min	Short acting; constant infusion preferred. May cause profound bradycardia
Hydralazine	Direct vasodilator	Intravenous, intramuscular	0.1–0.2 mg/kg per dose up to 0.4 mg/kg per dose	Causes tachycardia
Labetalol	α- and β-adrenergic blocker	Intravenous bolus or infusion	Bolus: 0.20–1.0 mg/kg per dose up to 40 mg per dose; Infusion: 0.25–3.0 mg/kg per h	Give every 4 h when given intravenous bolus. Asthma and overt heart failure are relative contraindications
Nicardipine	Calcium channel blocker	Intravenous bolus or infusion	Bolus: 30 mcg/kg up to 2 mg per dose; Infusion: 0.5–4 mcg/kg per min	May cause reflex tachycardia. Increases cyclosporine and tacrolimus levels
Sodium nitroprusside	Direct vasodilator	Intravenous infusion	Starting: 0–3 mcg/kg per min; Maximum: 10 mcg/kg per min	Monitor cyanide levels with prolonged (>72 h) use or in renal failure; or coadminister with sodium thiosulfate
Useful for Severely Hypertensive Patients With Less Significant Symptoms				
Clonidine	Central α-agonist	Oral	2–5 mcg/kg per dose up to 10 mcg/kg per dose given every 6–8 h	Adverse effects include dry mouth and drowsiness
Fenoldopam	Dopamine receptor agonist	Intravenous infusion	0.2–0.5 mcg/kg per min up to 0.8 mcg/kg per min	Higher doses worsen tachycardia without further reducing BP
Hydralazine	Direct vasodilator	Oral	0.25 mg/kg per dose up to 25 mg per dose given every 6–8 h	Half-life varies with genetically determined acetylation rates
Isradipine	Calcium channel blocker	Oral	0.05–0.1 mg/kg per dose up to 5 mg per dose given every 6–8 h	Exaggerated decrease in BP can be seen in patients receiving azole antifungal agents
Minoxidil	Direct vasodilator	Oral	0.1–0.2 mg/kg per dose up to 10 mg per dose given Q 8–12 h	Most potent oral vasodilator; long acting

who have LV hypertrophy on echocardiography, symptomatic HTN, or stage 2 HTN without a clearly modifiable factor [eg, obesity]), clinicians should initiate pharmacologic treatment with an ACE inhibitor, ARB, long-acting calcium channel blocker, or thiazide diuretic (grade B, moderate recommendation).

7.3c Treatment: Follow-Up and Monitoring

Treatment of a child or adolescent with HTN requires ongoing monitoring because goal BP can be difficult to achieve.[472] If the decision has been made to initiate treatment with medication, the patient should be seen frequently (every 4–6 weeks) for dose adjustments and/or addition of a second or third agent until goal BP has been achieved (see the preceding section). After that, the frequency of visits can be extended to every 3 to 4 months.

If the decision has been made to proceed with lifestyle changes only, then follow-up visits can occur at longer intervals (every 3–6 months) so that adherence to lifestyle change can be reinforced and the need for initiation of medication can be reassessed.

In patients treated with antihypertensive medications, home BP measurement is frequently used to get a better assessment of BP control (see "At-Home Measurement"). Repeat ABPM may also be used to assess BP control and is especially important in patients with CKD (see "Treatment: Use of ABPM and Assessment").

At each follow-up visit, the patient should be assessed for adherence to prescribed therapy and for any adverse effects of the prescribed medication; such assessment may include laboratory testing depending on the medication (for example, electrolyte monitoring if the patient is on a diuretic). It is also important to continually reinforce adherence

Key Action Statement 21. In hypertensive children and adolescents who have failed lifestyle modifications (particularly those who have LV hypertrophy on echocardiography, symptomatic HTN, or stage 2 HTN without a clearly modifiable factor [eg, obesity]), clinicians should initiate pharmacologic treatment with an ACE inhibitor, ARB, long-acting calcium channel blocker, or thiazide diuretic (grade B, moderate recommendation).

Aggregate Evidence Quality	Grade B
Benefits	Potential prevention of progressive CVD; regression or avoidance of target organ damage; resolution of hypertensive symptoms; improved cognition; avoidance of worsening HTN; potential avoidance of stroke, heart failure, coronary artery disease, kidney failure
Risks, harm, cost	Potential for hypotension, financial cost, chronic medication treatment, adverse medication effects, impact on insurability (health and life)
Benefit–harm assessment	Preponderance of benefits over harms
Intentional vagueness	None
Role of patient preferences	The choice of which antihypertensive medication to use should be made in close discussion with the patient and parent regarding risk, benefits, and adverse effects
Exclusions	None
Strength	Moderate recommendation
Key references	452,455,467

to lifestyle changes because effective treatment will depend on the combination of effects from both medication and lifestyle measures. Finally, known hypertensive target organ damage (such as LVH) should be reassessed according to the recommendations in "Imaging Evaluation, Echocardiography: Coarctation of the Aorta and Detection of Target Organ Damage."

7.3d Treatment: Use of ABPM to Assess Treatment

ABPM can be an objective method to evaluate treatment effect during antihypertensive drug therapy. Data obtained in a multicenter, single-blind, crossover study in which hypertensive children received a placebo or no treatment demonstrated no change in ABPM after receiving the placebo.[473] A report from a single center found that among hypertensive children receiving antihypertensive drugs, BP data from ABPM resulted in medication changes in 63% of patients.[474] Another study of 38 hypertensive children used ABPM to evaluate the effectiveness of antihypertensive therapy (nonpharmacologic and pharmacologic). After 1 year of

treatment, ABPM results indicated that treatment-goal BP was achieved in only one-third of children with HTN.[17]

Key Action Statement 22

ABPM may be used to assess treatment effectiveness in children and adolescents with HTN, especially when clinic and/or home BP measurements indicate insufficient BP response to treatment (grade B, moderate recommendation).

7.4 Treatment-Resistant HTN

Resistant HTN in adults is defined as persistently elevated BP

despite treatment with 3 or more antihypertensive agents of different classes. All of these drugs should be prescribed at maximally effective doses, and at least 1 should be a diuretic. Key to the identification of patients with true resistant HTN is correct office BP measurement, confirmation of adherence to current therapy, and confirmation of treatment resistance by ABPM.

The treatment of patients with resistant HTN includes dietary sodium restriction, the elimination of substances known to elevate BP, the identification of previously undiagnosed secondary causes of HTN, the optimization of current therapy, and the addition of additional agents as needed.[475] Recent clinical trial data suggest that an aldosterone receptor antagonist (such as spironolactone) is the optimal additional agent in adults with resistant HTN; it helps address volume excess as well as untreated hyperaldosteronism, which is common in adult patients with true resistant HTN.[476,477]

At present, there are no data on whether true treatment-resistant HTN exists in pediatric patients. Evaluation and management strategies similar to those proven effective in adults with resistant HTN would be reasonable in children and adolescents who present with apparent treatment resistance.

Key Action Statement 22. ABPM may be used to assess treatment effectiveness in children and adolescents with HTN, especially when clinic and/or home BP measurements indicate insufficient BP response to treatment (grade B, moderate recommendation).

Aggregate Evidence Quality	Grade B
Benefits	ABPM results can guide adjustment in medication. ABPM can facilitate achieving treatment-goal BP levels
Risks, harm, cost	Inconvenience and patient annoyance in wearing an ABPM monitor. Cost of ABPM monitors
Benefit–harm assessment	Overall benefit
Intentional vagueness	None
Role of patient preferences	Patients may choose not to wear the ambulatory BP monitor repeatedly, which may necessitate alternative approaches to evaluate treatment efficacy
Exclusions	Uncomplicated HTN with satisfactory BP control
Strength	Moderate recommendation
Key references	17,474,475

8. TREATMENT IN SPECIAL POPULATIONS

8.1 Treatment in Patients With CKD and Proteinuria

8.1a CKD

Children and adolescents with CKD often present with or develop HTN.[478] HTN is a known risk factor for the progression of kidney disease in adults and children.[173,479,480] Evidence suggests that the treatment of HTN in children with CKD might slow the progression of or reverse end organ damage.[173,415] When evaluated by 24-hour ABPM, children and adolescents with CKD often have poor BP control even if BP measured in the clinic appears to be normal.[48] MH is associated with end organ damage, such as LVH.[203,481] Threshold values that define HTN are not different in children with CKD, although there is some evidence that lower treatment goals might improve outcomes.

In the European Effect of Strict Blood Pressure Control and ACE-Inhibition on Progression of Chronic Renal Failure in Pediatric Patients study, researchers randomly assigned children with CKD to standard antihypertensive therapy (with a treatment goal of 24-hour MAP <90th percentile by ABPM) or

to intensive BP control (24-hour MAP <50th percentile by ABPM). The study demonstrated fewer composite CKD outcomes in children with the lower BP target.[173] Recent adult data from the Systolic Blood Pressure Intervention Trial suggest lower BP targets may be beneficial in preventing other, adverse CV outcomes as well.[482]

Key Action Statement 23

1. Children and adolescents with CKD should be evaluated for HTN at each medical encounter;

2. Children or adolescents with both CKD and HTN should be treated to lower 24-hour MAP to <50th percentile by ABPM; and

3. Regardless of apparent control of BP with office measures, children and adolescents with CKD and a history of HTN should have BP assessed by ABPM at least yearly to screen for MH (grade B; strong recommendation).

8.1b Proteinuria

Proteinuric renal disease is often associated with HTN and a rapid decline in glomerular filtration.[483] Studies in both adults and children have indicated that both BP control and a reduction in proteinuria are

beneficial for preserving renal function. Researchers in multiple studies have evaluated the utility of RAAS blockade therapy in patients with CKD and HTN.[452,464,465,484–487] These medications have been shown to benefit both BP and proteinuria.

The benefit of such therapies may not be sustained, however.[173,488] The Effect of Strict Blood Pressure Control and ACE-Inhibition on Progression of Chronic Renal Failure in Pediatric Patients study demonstrated an initial 50% reduction in proteinuria in children with CKD after treatment with ramipril but with a rebound effect after 36 months.[450,464,488] This study also showed that BP reduction with a ramipril-based antihypertensive regimen improved renal outcomes. In children with HTN related to underlying CKD, the assessment of proteinuria and institution of RAAS blockade therapy appears to have important prognostic implications.

Key Action Statement 24

Children and adolescents with CKD and HTN should be evaluated for proteinuria (grade B, strong recommendation).

Key Action Statement 25

Children and adolescents with CKD, HTN, and proteinuria should be treated with an ACE inhibitor or ARB (grade B, strong recommendation).

8.2. Treatment in Patients With Diabetes

Based on the Fourth Report criteria for the diagnosis of HTN,[1] between 4% and 16% of children and adolescents with T1DM are found to have HTN.[14,489–491] In the SEARCH study of 3691 youth between the ages of 3 and 17 years, elevated BP was documented in 6% of children with T1DM, with the highest prevalence in Asian Pacific Islander and American Indian children followed by African American and Hispanic children and those with

---

Key Action Statement 23. Children and adolescents with CKD should be evaluated for HTN at each medical encounter;

Children or adolescents with both CKD and HTN should be treated to lower 24-hour MAP to <50th percentile by ABPM; and

Regardless of apparent control of BP with office measures, children and adolescents with CKD and a history of HTN should have BP assessed by ABPM at least yearly to screen for MH (grade B; strong recommendation).

Aggregate Evidence Quality	Grade B
Benefits	Control of BP in children and adolescents with CKD has been shown to decrease CKD progression and lead to resolution of LVH
Risks, harm, cost	Cost of ABPM and BP control, both financial and nonfinancial
Benefit–harm assessment	Benefits of BP control in patients with CKD outweigh treatment risks
Intentional vagueness	Threshold
Role of patient preferences	Patients may not want to wear the ambulatory BP monitor repeatedly, which should lead to detailed counseling regarding the benefits of this procedure in CKD
Exclusions	None
Strength	Strong recommendation
Key references	47,173,203,415,480–483

higher glycosylated hemoglobin A1c levels.[14] An office-based study in Australia found much higher rates (16%) and a positive correlation with BMI.[490] BP >130/90 mm Hg has been associated with a more-than-fourfold increase in the relative risk of coronary artery disease and mortality at 10-year follow-up of individuals with T1DM.[492]

The prevalence of HTN is higher in youth with T2DM compared with T1DM, ranging from 12% at baseline (N = 699) in the Treatment Options for Type 2 Diabetes in Adolescents and Youth study[493] to 31% (N = 598) in the Pediatric Diabetes Consortium Type 2 Diabetes Clinic Registry.[494] BP and arterial stiffness in cohort studies have correlated with BMI, male sex, African American race, and age of onset of diabetes.[14,494,495] Unlike T1DM, HTN in T2DM is not correlated with glycosylated hemoglobin A1c levels or glycemic failure, and it develops early in the course of the disease.[496] It is also associated with rapid onset of adverse cardiac changes[111,497] and may not respond to diet changes.[425] The concurrence of obesity and T2DM compounds the risks for target end organ damage.[111,498]

Empirical evidence shows a poor awareness of HTN in youth with T1DM and T2DM.[14] Additionally, only a fraction of children with HTN and diabetes were found to be on pharmacologic therapy[14,490,498,499] despite treatment recommendations from the American Diabetes Association,[499] the International Society for Pediatric and Adolescent Diabetes,[500] AHA,[110] and the National Heart, Lung, and Blood Institute.[501]

Key Action Statement 26

Children and adolescents with T1DM or T2DM should be evaluated for HTN at each medical encounter and treated if BP is ≥95th percentile or >130/80 mm Hg in adolescents ≥13 years of age (grade C, moderate recommendation).

9. COMORBIDITIES

9.1 Comorbidities: Dyslipidemia

Children and adolescents with HTN are at increased risk for lipid disorders attributable to the "common soil" phenomenon,[502] in which poor diet, inactivity, and obesity contribute to both disorders. Some observational pediatric data confirm this association.[503–506] Furthermore, both HTN and dyslipidemias are associated with subclinical atherosclerosis[206] and are risk factors for future CVD.[503] Screening is recommended to identify those at increased risk for early atherosclerosis.[503] Treatment of lipid disorders identified in the setting of HTN should follow existing pediatric lipid guidelines with lifestyle advice, including weight loss and pharmacotherapy, as necessary.[503]

9.2 Comorbidities: OSAS

Children with snoring, daytime sleepiness (in adolescents), or hyperactivity (in younger children) may have OSAS and consequent HTN.[507] The more severe the OSAS, the more likely a child is to have elevated BP[44,45] (see Table 18). Children with moderate to severe OSAS are at increased risk for HTN. However, it is not known whether OSAS treatment with continuous positive airway pressure results in improved BP in all children.[44] Furthermore, adenotonsillectomy may not result in BP improvement in all children with OSAS. In particular, children who have obesity and OSAS may be less likely to experience a lowering of BP after an adenotonsillectomy.[508]

Therefore, children with signs of OSAS (eg, daytime fatigue, snoring, hyperactivity, etc) should undergo evaluation for elevated BP regardless of treatment status. Given that both nighttime and daytime BP is affected by OSAS, the use of ABPM is the recommended method for assessing the BP of children with suspected OSAS.

9.3 Comorbidities: Cognitive Impairment

Data from studies conducted in adults suggest that the central nervous system is a target organ that can be affected by HTN.[419] Preliminary studies suggest that this is true in children as well. Hypertensive children score lower on tests of neurocognition and on parental reports of executive function compared with normotensive controls.[509,510] Adams et al[511] found an increased prevalence of learning disabilities in children with primary HTN compared with normotensive controls. The postulated mechanism for these findings is impaired cerebrovascular reactivity.[512–515] At the present time, these findings do not have specific clinical implications with respect to the diagnostic evaluation of childhood HTN, although they underscore the importance of early detection and treatment.

Key Action Statement 24. Children and adolescents with CKD and HTN should be evaluated for proteinuria (grade B, strong recommendation).

Aggregate Evidence Quality	Grade B
Benefits	Detection of proteinuria among children with CKD and HTN may foster early detection and treatment of children at risk for more advanced renal disease
Risks, harm, cost	Additional testing
Benefit–harm assessment	Benefit of detection of a higher-risk group exceeds the risk of testing
Intentional vagueness	Whether to screen children with HTN without CKD for proteinuria
Role of patient preferences	None
Exclusions	Children without CKD
Strength	Strong recommendation
Key references	47,484

Key Action Statement 25. Children and adolescents with CKD, HTN, and proteinuria should be treated with an ACE inhibitor or ARB (grade B, strong recommendation).

Aggregate Evidence Quality	Grade B
Benefits	ACE inhibitor and ARB therapy has been shown in the short-term to be effective in reducing urine proteinuria
Risks, harm, cost	Positive effect on urine protein concentrations after the receipt of an ACE inhibitor may not be sustained over time
Benefit–harm assessment	Treatment with an ACE inhibitor or ARB may lower the rate of progression of renal disease even if the effect is not sustained in the long-term
Intentional vagueness	Whether to aggressively treat the BP so that it is <90th percentile
Role of patient preferences	Patients may have concerns about the choice of medication, which should be addressed
Exclusions	Children without CKD
Strength	Strong recommendation
Key references	173,464,465,485,487,488

Key Action Statement 26. Children and adolescents with T1DM or T2DM should be evaluated for HTN at each medical encounter and treated if BP is ≥95th percentile or >130/80 mm Hg in adolescents ≥13 years of age (grade C, moderate recommendation).

Aggregate Evidence Quality	Grade C
Benefits	Early detection and treatment of HTN in children with T1DM and T2DM may reduce future CV and kidney disease
Risks, harm, cost	Risk of drug adverse effects and polypharmacy
Benefit–harm assessment	Preponderance of benefit
Intentional vagueness	None
Role of patient preferences	Family concerns about additional testing and/or medication may need to be addressed
Exclusions	None
Strength	Weak to moderate recommendation
Key references	14,110,111,494

10. SEX, RACIAL, AND ETHNIC DIFFERENCES IN BP AND MEDICATION CHOICE

BP differences between various ethnic groups are well described in the adult population.[216,516] Large, cross-sectional studies have demonstrated that, per capita, minority ethnic groups have both a higher prevalence of HTN and more significant end organ damage and outcomes.[517,518] Although a growing body of evidence indicates that racial and ethnic differences in BP appear during adolescence,[519–521] the cause of these differences and when they develop in childhood are yet to be fully determined. The risk of HTN correlates more with obesity status than with ethnicity or race, although there may be some interaction.[216] At this time, although limited data suggest that there may be a racial difference in response to ACE inhibitors in the pediatric age group,[471] the strength of available evidence is insufficient to recommend using racial, sex, or ethnic factors to inform the evaluation or management of HTN in children.

11. SPECIAL POPULATIONS AND SITUATIONS

11.1 Acute Severe HTN

There is a lack of robust evidence to guide the evaluation and management of children and adolescents with acute presentations of severe HTN. Thus, much of what is known is derived from studies conducted in adults, including medication choice.[522] The evidence base has been enhanced somewhat over the past decade by the publication of several pediatric clinical trials and case series of antihypertensive agents that can be used to treat such patients.[465,523–530]

Although children and adolescents can become symptomatic from HTN at lesser degrees of BP elevation, in general, patients who present with acute severe HTN will have BP elevation well above the stage 2 HTN threshold. In a study of 55 children presenting to a pediatric ED in Taiwan with hypertensive crisis, 96% had SBP greater than that of stage 2 HTN, and 76% had DBP greater than that of stage 2 HTN.[531] The major clinical issue in such children is that this level of BP elevation may produce acute target organ effects, including encephalopathy, acute kidney injury, and congestive heart failure. Clinicians should be concerned about the development of these complications when a child's BP increases 30 mm Hg or more above the 95th percentile.

Although a few children with primary HTN may present with features of acute severe HTN,[532] the vast majority will have an underlying secondary cause of HTN.[532,533] Thus, for patients who present with acute severe HTN, an evaluation for secondary causes is appropriate and should be conducted expediently. Additionally, target organ effects should be assessed with renal function, echocardiography, and central nervous system imaging, among others.

Given the potential for the development of potentially life-threatening complications, expert opinion holds that children and adolescents who present with acute severe HTN require immediate treatment with short-acting antihypertensive medications that may abort such sequelae.[533,534] Treatment may be initiated with oral agents if the patient is able to tolerate oral therapy and if

TABLE 20 Comparison of HTN Screening Strategies

Dimension	Option A (Clinic BP Alone)	Option B (Clinic BP Confirmed by ABPM)	Option C (ABPM Only)	Preferred Option	Assumptions Made
Population: 170 cardiology, nephrology referred patients; analyzed at single-patient level	Auscultatory or oscillatory BP >95%	Auscultatory or oscillatory BP >90% then ABPM	Patients referred to provider who only used ABPM	—	—
Operational factors					
Percent adherence to care (goal of 80%)	Assumes 100%	Assumes 100%	Assumes 100%	—	—
Care delivery team effects	Baseline	Additional work to arrange or interpret confirmatory ABPM	Additional work to arrange and interpret ABPM for all patients	—	Assumes ABPM can be arranged and interpreted correctly
Patient, family effects	Baseline	Less desirable to have more visits; more desirable to have better accuracy		Family opinion depends on family's values	—
Benefits					
Clinical significance	Baseline	If HTN, treatment improves long-term outcome	If HTN, treatment improves long-term outcome	C	WCH estimated at 35%, ABPM results in fewer false-positive screening results
Cost of options				B	
Visit, diagnosis costs (annual estimated cost for 1 patient)	$1880 for visits and laboratory tests	$1330 for visits, ABPM, and laboratory tests	$1880 for visits, ABPM, and laboratory tests		
Costs from complications, adverse events, nonoptimal treatment					
Likelihood of nonoptimal treatment	60% undiagnosed patients; 35% of those diagnosed with WCH	30% undiagnosed patients	All patients correctly diagnosed; fewer complications	C	Assumes treatment benefit for correctly diagnosed HTN has no complications
Costs of nonoptimal treatment	Increased mortality for not treating undiagnosed HTN; inconvenience of treatment of patients with WCH	Increased mortality for not treating undiagnosed HTN	All patients correctly diagnosed who are treated	C	—

—, none.

life-threatening complications have not yet developed. Intravenous agents are indicated when oral therapy is not possible because of the patient's clinical status or when a severe complication has developed (such as congestive heart failure) that warrants a more controlled BP reduction. In such situations, the BP should be reduced by no more than 25% of the planned reduction over the first 8 hours, with the remainder of the planned reduction over the next 12 to 24 hours.[533,534] The ultimate short-term BP goal in such patients should generally be around the 95th percentile. Table 19 lists suggested doses for oral and intravenous antihypertensive medications that may be used to treat patients with acute severe HTN.

Key Action Statement 27

In children and adolescents with acute severe HTN and life-threatening symptoms, immediate treatment with short-acting antihypertensive medication should be initiated, and BP should be reduced by no more than 25% of the planned reduction over the first 8 hours (grade expert opinion D, weak recommendation).

11.2 HTN and the Athlete

Sports participation and increased physical activity should be encouraged in children with HTN. In adults, physical fitness is associated with lower all-cause mortality.[536] Although meta-analyses and randomized controlled trials consistently show lower BP after exercise training in adults,[535] the results are less robust in children.[340] On the basis of this evidence, sports participation should improve BP over time. Additionally, there is evidence that exercise itself has a beneficial effect on cardiac structure in adolescents.[537]

The athlete interested in participating in competitive sports and/or intense training presents a special circumstance. Existing guidelines present conflicting recommendations.[1,538] Although increased LV wall dimension may be a consequence of athletic training,[360] recommendations from AHA and ACC include the following: (1) limiting competitive athletic participation among athletes with LVH beyond that seen with athlete's heart until BP is normalized by appropriate antihypertensive drug therapy, and (2) restricting athletes with stage 2 HTN (even among those without evidence of target organ injury) from participating in high-static sports (eg, weight lifting, boxing, and wrestling) until HTN is controlled with either lifestyle modification or drug therapy.[539]

The AAP policy statement "Athletic Participation by Children and Adolescents Who Have Systemic Hypertension" recommends that children with stage 2 HTN be restricted from high-static sports (classes IIIA to IIIC) in the absence of end organ damage, including LVH or concomitant heart disease, until their BP is in the normal range after lifestyle modification and/or drug therapy.[538] It is further recommended that athletes be promptly referred and evaluated by a qualified pediatric medical subspecialist within 1 week if they are asymptomatic or immediately if they are symptomatic. The subcommittee agrees with these recommendations.

It should be acknowledged that there are no data linking the presence of HTN to sudden death related to sports participation in children, although many cases of sudden death are of unknown etiology. That said, athletes identified as hypertensive (eg, during preparticipation sports screening) should undergo appropriate evaluation as outlined above. For athletes with more severe HTN (stage 2 or greater), treatment should be initiated before sports participation.

Key Action Statement 28

Children and adolescents with HTN may participate in competitive sports once hypertensive target organ effects and risk have been assessed (grade C, moderate recommendation).

Key Action Statement 29

Children and adolescents with HTN should receive treatment to lower BP below stage 2 thresholds before participating in competitive sports (grade C, weak recommendation).

11.3 HTN and the Posttransplant Patient

HTN is common in children after solid-organ transplants, with prevalence rates ranging from 50% to 90%.[179,180,540,541] Contributing factors include the use of steroids, calcineurin inhibitors, and mTOR (mammalian target of rapamycin) inhibitors. In patients with renal

transplants, the presence of native kidneys, CKD, and transplant glomerulopathy are additional risk factors for HTN. HTN rates are higher by 24-hour ABPM compared with clinic BP measurements because these populations commonly have MH and nocturnal HTN.[179–183,542] Control of HTN in renal-transplant patients has been improved with the use of annual ABPM.[184,185] Therefore, ABPM should be used to identify and monitor nocturnal BP abnormalities and MH in pediatric kidney and heart-transplant recipients. The use of home BP assessment may provide a comparable alternative to ABPM for BP assessment after transplant as well.[186]

The management of identified HTN in the pediatric transplant patient can be challenging. Rates of control of HTN in renal-transplant patients generally range from 33% to 55%.[180,187] In studies by Seeman et al,[188] intensified antihypertensive treatment in pediatric renal-transplant recipients improved nocturnal SBP and significantly reduced proteinuria.[543] Children in these studies who achieved normotension had stable graft function, whereas those who remained hypertensive at 2 years had a progression of renal disease.[544]

Antihypertensive medications have rarely been systematically studied in this population. There is limited evidence that ACE inhibitors and ARBs may be superior to other agents in achieving BP control and improving long-term graft survival in renal-transplant patients.[185,543,544] However, the combination of ACE inhibitors and ARBs in renal-transplant patients has been associated with acidosis and hyperkalemia and is not recommended.[545]

12. LIFETIME HTN TREATMENT AND TRANSITION TO ADULTHOOD

For adolescents with HTN requiring ongoing treatment, the

Key Action Statement 27. In children and adolescents with acute severe HTN and life-threatening symptoms, immediate treatment with short-acting antihypertensive medication should be initiated, and BP should be reduced by no more than 25% of the planned reduction over the first 8 hours (grade expert opinion D, weak recommendation).

Aggregate Evidence Quality	Expert Opinion, D
Benefits	Avoidance of complications caused by rapid BP reduction
Risks, harm, cost	Severe BP elevation may persist
Benefit–harm assessment	Benefit outweighs harm
Intentional vagueness	None
Role of patient preferences	None
Exclusions	Patients without acute severe HTN and life-threatening symptoms
Strength	Weak recommendation because of expert opinion
Key references	240,533,535

Key Action Statement 28. Children and adolescents with HTN may participate in competitive sports once hypertensive target organ effects and risk have been assessed (grade C, moderate recommendation).

Aggregate Evidence Quality	Grade C
Benefits	Aerobic exercise improves CVD risk factors in children and adolescents with HTN
Risks, harm, cost	Unknown, but theoretical risk related to a rise in BP with strenuous exercise may exist
Benefit–harm assessment	The benefits of exercise likely outweigh the potential risk in the vast majority of children and adolescents with HTN
Intentional vagueness	None
Role of patient preferences	Families may have different opinions about sports participation in children with HTN
Exclusions	None
Strength	Moderate recommendation
Key references	341,360,538,540,541

Key Action Statement 29. Children and adolescents with HTN should receive treatment to lower BP below stage 2 thresholds before participating in competitive sports (grade C, weak recommendation).

Aggregate Evidence Quality	Grade C
Benefits	Aerobic exercise improves CVD risk factors in children and adolescents with HTN
Risks, harm, cost	Unknown, but theoretical risk related to a rise in BP with strenuous exercise may exist
Benefit–harm assessment	The benefits of exercise likely outweigh the potential risk in the vast majority of children and adolescents with HTN
Intentional vagueness	None
Role of patient preferences	None
Exclusions	None
Strength	Weak recommendation
Key references	341,360,538,540,541

transition from pediatric care to an adult provider is essential.[546] HTN definition and treatment recommendations in this guideline are generally consistent with the forthcoming adult HTN treatment guideline, so diagnosis and treatment should not typically change with transition.

Key Action Statement 30

Adolescents with elevated BP or HTN (whether they are receiving antihypertensive treatment) should typically have their care transitioned to an appropriate adult care provider by 22 years of age (recognizing that there may be individual cases in which this upper age limit is exceeded, particularly in the case of youth with special health care needs). There should be a transfer

of information regarding HTN etiology and past manifestations and complications of the patient's HTN (grade X, strong recommendation).

13. PREVENTION OF HTN

13.1 Importance of Preventing HTN

BP levels tend to increase with time even after adult height is reached. The rate of progression to frank HTN in a study of more than 12 000 Japanese adults (20–35 years of age at baseline, followed for 9 years) was 36.5% and was greater with higher baseline BP category.[548] The rate of progression may also be accelerated in African American individuals. Similarly, both the Bogalusa Heart[63] and Fels Longitudinal[60] studies have clearly

demonstrated that the risk of HTN in early adulthood is dependent on childhood BP, with greater numbers of elevated BP measurements in childhood conferring an increased risk of adult HTN.

Because the tracking of BP levels in children has also been well documented,[10] it is not surprising that analyses of the National Childhood BP database found 7% of adolescents with elevated BP per year progressed to true hypertensive BP levels. Of note, initial BMI and change in BMI were major determinants of the development of HTN.[22] Therefore, in both children and adults, efforts (discussed below) should be made to prevent progression to sustained HTN and to avoid the development of hypertensive CV diseases.

13.2 Strategies for Prevention

One of the largest trials of preventing progression to HTN in adults, the Trial of Preventing Hypertension study, proved that 2 years of treatment with candesartan reduced the number of subjects with elevated BP from developing stage 1 HTN even after the drug was withdrawn.[547] However, no similar study has been conducted in youth; for this reason, prevention efforts to date have focused on lifestyle modification, especially dietary intervention,[426] exercise,[549] and treatment of obesity.[550] The best evidence for the potential of such prevention strategies comes from epidemiologic evidence for risk factors for the development of HTN or from studies focused on the treatment of established HTN. These risk factors include positive family history, obesity, a high-sodium diet, the absence of a DASH-type diet, larger amounts of

Key Action Statement 30. Adolescents with elevated BP or HTN (whether they are receiving antihypertensive treatment) should typically have their care transitioned to an appropriate adult care provider by 22 years of age (recognizing that there may be individual cases in which this upper age limit is exceeded, particularly in the case of youth with special health care needs). There should be a transfer of information regarding HTN etiology and past manifestations and complications of the patient's HTN (grade X, strong recommendation).

Aggregate Evidence Quality	Grade X
Benefits	Provides continuity of care for patients
Risks, harm, cost	None
Benefit–harm assessment	No risk
Intentional vagueness	None
Role of patient preferences	Patient can pick adult care provider
Exclusions	None
Strength	Strong recommendation
Key references	547

sedentary time, and possibly other dietary factors.[551–553]

Because family history is immutable, it is difficult to build a preventive strategy around it. However, a positive family history of HTN should suggest the need for closer BP monitoring to detect HTN if it occurs.

Appropriate energy balance with calories eaten balanced by calories expended in physical activity is important. This is the best strategy to maintain an appropriate BMI percentile for age and sex and to avoid the development of obesity.[554] From a broader dietary perspective, a DASH-type diet (ie, high in fruits, vegetables, whole grains, and low-fat dairy, with decreased intake of foods high in saturated fat or sugar) may be beneficial (see Table 16).[423,427] Avoiding high-sodium foods may prove helpful in preventing HTN, particularly for individuals who are more sensitive to dietary sodium intake.[555]

Adhering to recommendations for 60 minutes a day of moderate to vigorous physical activity can be important to maintaining an appropriate weight and may be independently helpful to maintaining a lower BP.[344] The achievement of normal sleep habits

and avoidance of tobacco products are also reasonable strategies to reduce CV risk.

These preventive strategies can be implemented as part of routine primary health care for children and adolescents.

14. CHALLENGES IN THE IMPLEMENTATION OF PEDIATRIC HTN GUIDELINES

Many studies have shown that physicians fail to meet benchmarks with respect to screening, especially universal screening for high BP in children.[7,115] Although the reasons for this failure likely vary from practice to practice, a number of common challenges can be identified.

The first challenge is determining how to identify every child in a clinic who merits a BP measurement. This could be accomplished through flags in an EHR, documentation rules for specific patients, and/or clinic protocols.

The second challenge is establishing a local clinic protocol for measuring BP correctly on the basis of the algorithms in this guideline. It is important to determine the optimal approach on the basis of the available equipment, the skills of clinic personnel, and the clinic's throughput needs.

The third challenge is for clinic personnel to be aware of what to do with high BP measurements when they occur. Knowing when to counsel patients, order tests or laboratory work, and reach out for help is essential. Making this part of standard practice so every child follows the prescribed pathway may be challenging.

The final diagnosis of HTN also relies on a number of sequential visits. Ensuring that patients return for all of these visits and are not lost to follow-up may require new clinic processes or mechanisms. Information technology may help remind providers to schedule these visits and remind patients to attend these visits; even with that assistance, however, completing all the visits may be difficult for some patients.

In addition, family medicine physicians and general pediatricians may face challenges in having normative pediatric BP values available for use at all times. Although adult BP cutoffs are easy to memorize, pediatric BP percentile cutoffs are greatly dependent on age and height. The BP tables in this guideline provide cutoffs to use for the proper diagnosis of HTN; their availability will simplify the recognition of abnormal BP values.

The AAP Education in Quality Improvement for Pediatric Practice module on HTN identification and management[556] and its accompanying implementation guide[557] should be of assistance to practitioners who wish to improve their approach to identifying and managing childhood HTN. This module is currently being updated to incorporate the new recommendations in this guideline.

15. OTHER TOPICS

15.1 Economic Impact of BP Management

Researchers in a small number of studies have examined the potential economic impacts related to pediatric BP management.[208,558,559] Wang et al[558] estimated both the effectiveness and cost-effectiveness of 3 screening strategies and interventions to normalize pediatric BP based on the literature and through a simulation of children (n = 4 017 821). The 3 screening strategies included the following: (1) no screening; (2) selected screening and treatment, as well as "treating everyone" (ie, with population-wide interventions, such as targeted programs for overweight adolescents [eg, weight-loss programs, exercise programs, and salt-reduction programs]); and (3) nontargeted programs for exercise and salt reduction.

The simulation suggested that these various strategies could reduce mortality, with a modest expected survival benefit of 0.5 to 8.6 days. The researchers also examined quality-adjusted life-years (QALYs) and the cost per QALY. Only 1 intervention, a nontargeted salt-reduction campaign, had a negative cost per QALY. This intervention and the other 2 described in that article support the concept that population-wide interventions may be the most cost-effective way to improve CV health. The article has serious limitations, however, including the fact that population-wide interventions for exercise and the reduction of sodium intake have not, thus far, been effective.

The accurate determination of those who actually have HTN (as opposed to WCH) is fundamental to providing sound care to patients. Researchers in two studies examined the effects of using ABPM in the diagnosis of HTN.[208,559] Davis et al[559] compared 3 HTN

screening strategies; these options are summarized in the following value-analysis framework (see Table 20).[560] It appears that the implementation of ABPM for all patients is not ensured. The next best option, screening clinic BP with ABPM, is most likely to be implementable and has significant clinical benefit given the high prevalence of WCH.

Swartz et al[208] conducted a retrospective review of 267 children with elevated clinic BP measurements referred for ABPM. Of the 126 patients who received ABPM, 46% had WCH, 49% had stage 1 HTN, and 5% had stage 2 HTN. This is consistent with the concept that screening with clinic BP alone results in high numbers of false-positive results for HTN. The diagnosis of HTN in this study resulted in an additional $3420 for evaluation (includes clinic visit, facility fee, laboratory testing, renal ultrasound, and echocardiography) vs $1265 (includes clinic visit, facility fee, and ABPM). This suggests that ABPM is cost-effective because of the reduction of unnecessary testing in patients with WCH.

When examining these costs, the availability of ABPM, and the availability of practitioners who are skilled in pediatric interpretation, the most cost-effective and implementable screening solution is to measure clinic BP and confirm elevated readings by ABPM.

15.2 Patient Perspective and Pediatric HTN

Children and adolescents are not just patients; they are active participants in their health management. If children and adolescents lack a clear understanding of what is happening inside their bodies, they will not be able to make informed choices in their daily activities. Better

choices lead to better decisions executed in self-care. For clear judgments to be made, there needs to be open communication between physicians and families, a provision of appropriate education on optimal HTN management, and a strong partnership assembled within a multidisciplinary health care team including physicians, advanced practice providers, dietitians, nurses, and medical and clinical assistants.

It is important for physicians to be mindful that children and adolescents want, and need, to be involved in their medical care. Pediatric HTN patients are likely to feel excluded when clinicians or other providers speak to their parents instead of including them in the conversation. When patients are neither included in the discussion nor encouraged to ask questions, their anxiety can increase, thus worsening their HTN. Keeping an open line of communication is important and is best done by using a team approach consisting of the patient, the family, health care support staff, and physicians. With practical education on HTN management provided in easily understandable terms, the patients will be more likely to apply the concepts presented to them. Education is important and should be given in a way that is appropriate for young children and their families to understand. Education should consist of suitable medication dosing, a proper diet and level of activity, the identification of symptoms, and appropriate BP monitoring (including cuff size).

15.3 Parental Perspective and Pediatric HTN

Parents play a key role in the management and care of their children's health. Parents and physicians should act as a cohesive unit to foster the best results. It is vital for physicians to provide concise information in plain language and do so using a team approach. This will facilitate parents having a clear understanding of the required tests, medications, follow-ups, and outcomes.

Patient Perspective, by Matthew Goodwin

"I am not just a 13 year old, I am a teenager who has lived with hypertension, renal disease, and midaortic syndrome since I was 4 years old. I have experienced surgeries, extended hospitalizations, daily medications, procedures, tests, continued blood pressure monitoring, lifestyle changes, and dietary restrictions. Hypertension is a part of my everyday life. It will always be a component of me. I had to learn the effects of hypertension at a young age. I knew what would happen to me if I ate too much salt or did not fully hydrate, thus I became watchful. I did this so I could efficiently communicate with my physicians any changes I physically felt or any symptoms that were new or different regarding my illness. This has allowed me, my family, and my doctors to work effectively as one unit. I am grateful for my doctors listening to me as a person and not as a kid."

Parents of children with hypertensive issues can encounter 1 or more specialists in addition to their pediatric clinician. This can prove to be overwhelming, frightening, and may fill the parent with anxiety. Taking these things into account and creating unified partners, built with the physician and family, will encourage the family to be more involved in the patient's health management. Plain language in a team approach will yield the most positive outcomes for the patient.

Understanding the family and patient's perception of HTN and any underlying disease that may be contributing to it is important to resolve any misconceptions and encourage adherence to the physician's recommendations. To attain therapeutic goals, proper education must be provided to the family as a whole. This education should include proper medication dosages, recommended sodium intake, any dietary changes, exercise expectations, and any other behavioral changes. It is equally important to stress to the family the short- and long-term effects of HTN if it is not properly managed. Parents with younger children will carry the ultimate burden of daily decisions as it applies to medications, food choices, and activity. Parents of older adolescents will partner with the children to encourage the right choices. Education as a family unit is important for everyone involved to understand the consequences.

A family-based approach is important for all pediatric diseases but plays a particular role in conditions that are substantially influenced by lifestyle behaviors. This has been shown in several pediatric populations, including those with T2DM and obesity.[561–565]

16. EVIDENCE GAPS AND PROPOSED FUTURE DIRECTIONS

In general, the pediatric HTN literature is not as robust as the adult HTN literature. The reasons for this are many, but the 2 most important are as follows: (1) the lower prevalence of HTN in childhood compared with adults, and (2) the lack of adverse CV events (myocardial infarction, stroke, and death) attributable to HTN in young patients. These factors make it difficult to conduct

the types of clinical trials that are needed to produce high-quality evidence. For example, no large pediatric cohort has ever been assembled to answer the question of whether routine BP measurement in childhood is useful to prevent adult CVD.[566] Given this, other types of evidence, such as from cross-sectional and observational cohort studies, must be examined to guide practice.[567]

From the standpoint of the primary care provider, the most significant evidence gaps relate to whether diagnosing elevated BP and HTN in children and adolescents truly has long-term health consequences, whether antihypertensive medications should be used in a child or adolescent with elevated BP, and what medications should be preferentially used. These evidence gaps have been alluded to previously in this document.

Other important evidence gaps should be highlighted, including the following:

- Is there a specific BP level in childhood that predicts adverse outcomes, and can a single number (or numbers) be used to define HTN, as in adults?

- Can and should ABPM ever replace auscultation in the diagnosis of childhood HTN?

- Are the currently used, normative standards for ABPM appropriate, or are new normative data needed?[568]

- What is the best diagnostic evaluation to confidently exclude secondary causes of HTN?

- Are other assessments of hypertensive target organ damage (such as urine MA or vascular studies) better than echocardiography?

- How confident can we be that a child or teenager with elevated BP will have HTN and/or CVD disease as an adult?

Some of these questions may eventually be answered by research that is currently in progress, such as further analysis of the International Childhood Cardiovascular Cohort Consortium[569] and the promising Adult Hypertension Onset in Youth study, which seeks to better define the level of BP in childhood that predicts the development of hypertensive target organ damage.[570] Other studies will need to be performed in children and adolescents to fill in the remaining gaps, including more rigorous validation studies of automated BP devices in the pediatric population, expanded trials of lifestyle interventions, further comparative trials of antihypertensive medications, and studies of the clinical applicability of hypertensive target organ assessments.

Furthermore, and perhaps more crucially, there needs to be prospective assessment of the recommendations made in this document with regular updates based on new evidence as it is generated (generally, per AAP policy, these occur approximately every 5 years). With such ongoing reassessment and revision, it is hoped that this document and its future revisions will come to be viewed as an effective guide to practice and will improve the care of the young patients who are entrusted to us.

Implementation tools for this guideline are available on the AAP Web site (https://www.aap.org/en-us/about-the-aap/Committees-Councils-Sections/coqips/Pages/Implementation-Guide.aspx).

AUTHORS

Joseph T. Flynn, MD, MS, FAAP
David C. Kaelber, MD, PhD, MPH, FAAP, FACP, FACMI
Carissa M. Baker-Smith, MD, MS, MPH, FAAP, FAHA
Douglas Blowey, MD
Aaron E. Carroll, MD, MS, FAAP
Stephen R. Daniels, MD, PhD, FAAP
Sarah D. de Ferranti, MD, MPH, FAAP
Janis M. Dionne, MD, FRCPC

Susan K. Flinn, MA
Bonita Falkner, MD
Samuel S. Gidding, MD
Celeste Goodwin
Michael G. Leu, MD, MS, MHS, FAAP
Makia E. Powers, MD, MPH, FAAP
Corinna Rea, MD, MPH, FAAP
Joshua Samuels, MD, MPH, FAAP
Madeline Simasek, MD, MSCP, FAAP
Vidhu V. Thaker, MD, FAAP
Elaine M. Urbina, MD, MS, FAAP

SUBCOMMITTEE ON SCREENING AND MANAGEMENT OF HIGH BLOOD PRESSURE IN CHILDREN (OVERSIGHT BY THE COUNCIL ON QUALITY IMPROVEMENT AND PATIENT SAFETY)†

Joseph T. Flynn, MD, MS, FAAP, Co-chair, Section on Nephrology
David Kaelber, MD, MPH, PhD, FAAP, Co-chair, Section on Medicine-Pediatrcs, Council on Clinical Information Technology
Carissa M. Baker-Smith, MD, MS, MPH, Epidemiologist and Methodologist
Aaron Carroll, MD, MS, FAAP, Partnership for Policy Implementation
Stephen R. Daniels, MD, PhD, FAAP, Committee on Nutrition
Sarah D. de Ferranti, MD, MPH, FAAP, Committee on Cardiology and Cardiac Surgery
Michael G. Leu, MD, MS, MHS, FAAP, Council on Quality Improvement and Patient Safety
Makia Powers, MD, MPH, FAAP, Committee on Adolescence
Corinna Rea, MD, MPH, FAAP, Section on Early Career Physicians
Joshua Samuels, MD, MPH, FAAP, Section on Nephrology
Madeline Simasek, MD, FAAP, Quality Improvement Innovation Networks
Vidhu Thaker, MD, FAAP, Section on Obesity

LIAISONS

Douglas Blowey, MD, *American Society of Pediatric Nephrology*
Janis Dionne, MD, FRCPC, *Canadian Association of Paediatric Nephrologists*
Bonita Falkner, MD, *International Pediatric Hypertension Association*
Samuel Gidding, MD, *American College of Cardiology, American Heart Association*
Celeste Goodwin, *National Pediatric Blood Pressure Awareness Foundation*
Elaine Urbina, MD, FAAP, *American Heart Association AHOY Committee*

MEDICAL WRITER

Susan K. Flinn, MA

STAFF

Kymika Okechukwu, MPA, Manager, Evidence-Based Practice Initiatives

ABBREVIATIONS

AAP: American Academy of Pediatrics
ABPM: ambulatory blood pressure monitoring
ACC: American College of Cardiology
ACE: angiotensin-converting enzyme
AHA: American Heart Association
ARB: angiotensin receptor blocker
ARR: aldosterone to renin ratio
BP: blood pressure
BSA: body surface area
cIMT: carotid intimamedia thickness
CKD: chronic kidney disease
CTA: computed tomographic angiography
CV: cardiovascular
CVD: cardiovascular disease
DASH: Dietary Approaches to Stop Hypertension
DBP: diastolic blood pressure
ED: emergency department
EHR: electronic health record
FMD: flow-mediated dilation
HTN: hypertension
LVH: left ventricular hypertrophy
LVMI: left ventricular mass index
MA: microalbuminuria
MAP: mean arterial pressure
MH: masked hypertension
MI: motivational interviewing
MRA: magnetic resonance angiography
NF-1: neurofibromatosis type 1
OSAS: obstructive sleep apnea syndrome
PCC: pheochromocytoma
PICOT: Patient, Intervention/Indicator, Comparison, Outcome, and Time
PRA: plasma renin activity
PWV: pulse wave velocity
QALY: quality-adjusted life-year
RAAS: renin-angiotensin-aldosterone system
RAS: renal artery stenosis
SBP: systolic blood pressure
SDB: sleep-disordered breathing
T1DM: type 1 diabetes mellitus
T2DM: type 2 diabetes mellitus
UA: uric acid
WCH: white coat hypertension

Seattle, Washington; [n]Department of Pediatrics, School of Medicine, Morehouse College, Atlanta, Georgia; [o]Associate Director, General Academic Pediatric Fellowship, Staff Physician, Boston's Children's Hospital Primary Care at Longwood, Instructor, Harvard Medical School, Boston, Massachusetts; Departments of [p]Pediatrics and Internal Medicine, McGovern Medical School, University of Texas, Houston, Texas; [q]Pediatric Education, University of Pittsburgh Medical Center Shadyside Family Medicine Residency, Clinical Associate Professor of Pediatrics, Children's Hospital of Pittsburgh of University of Pittsburgh Medical Center, and School of Medicine, University of Pittsburgh, Pittsburgh, Pennsylvania; [r]Division of Molecular Genetics, Department of Pediatrics, Columbia University Medical Center, New York, New York; and [s]Preventive Cardiology, Cincinnati Children's Hospital Medical Center, Department of Pediatrics, University of Cincinnati, Cincinnati, Ohio

Drs Flynn and Kaelber served as the specialty and primary care chairs of the Subcommittee and had lead roles in developing the framework for the guidelines and coordinating the overall guideline development; Dr Baker-Smith served as the epidemiologist and led the evidence review and synthesis; Ms. Flinn compiled the first draft of the manuscript and coordinated manuscript revisions; All other authors were significantly involved in all aspects of the guideline creation including initial scoping, literature review and synthesis, draft manuscript creation and manuscript review; and all authors approved the final manuscript as submitted.

Endorsed by the American Heart Association.

DOI: https://doi.org/10.1542/peds.2017-1904

Address correspondence to Joseph T Flynn. Email: joseph.flynn@seattlechildrens.org

PEDIATRICS (ISSN Numbers: Print, 0031-4005; Online, 1098-4275).

FUNDING: The American Academy of Pediatrics provided funding to cover travel costs for subcommittee members to attend subcommittee meetings, to pay for the epidemiologist (Dr Baker-Smith) and consultant (Susan Flynn), and to produce the revised normative blood pressure tables.

REFERENCES

1. National High Blood Pressure Education Program Working Group on High Blood Pressure in Children and Adolescents. The fourth report on the diagnosis, evaluation, and treatment of high blood pressure in children and adolescents. *Pediatrics*. 2004;114(2, suppl 4th Report):555–576

2. Institute of Medicine, Committee on Standards for Systematic Reviews of Comparative Effectiveness Research. In: Eden J, Levit L, Berg A, Morton S, eds. *Finding What Works in Health Care: Standards for Systematic Reviews*. Washington, DC: National Academies Press; 2011

3. American Academy of Pediatrics Steering Committee on Quality Improvement and Management. Classifying recommendations for clinical practice guidelines. *Pediatrics*. 2004;114(3):874–877

4. Rosner B, Cook NR, Daniels S, Falkner B. Childhood blood pressure trends and risk factors for high blood pressure: the NHANES experience 1988-2008. *Hypertension*. 2013;62(2):247–254

5. Din-Dzietham R, Liu Y, Bielo MV, Shamsa F. High blood pressure trends in children and adolescents in national surveys, 1963 to 2002. *Circulation*. 2007;116(13):1488–1496

6. Kit BK, Kuklina E, Carroll MD, Ostchega Y, Freedman DS, Ogden CL. Prevalence of and trends in dyslipidemia and blood pressure among US children and adolescents, 1999-2012. *JAMA Pediatr*. 2015;169(3):272–279

7. Hansen ML, Gunn PW, Kaelber DC. Underdiagnosis of hypertension in children and adolescents. *JAMA*. 2007;298(8):874–879

8. McNiece KL, Poffenbarger TS, Turner JL, Franco KD, Sorof JM, Portman RJ. Prevalence of hypertension and pre-hypertension among adolescents. *J Pediatr*. 2007;150(6):640–644, 644.e1

9. Chiolero A, Cachat F, Burnier M, Paccaud F, Bovet P. Prevalence of hypertension in schoolchildren based on repeated measurements and association with overweight. *J Hypertens*. 2007;25(11):2209–2217

10. Chen X, Wang Y. Tracking of blood pressure from childhood to adulthood: a systematic review and meta-regression analysis. *Circulation*. 2008;117(25):3171–3180

11. Theodore RF, Broadbent J, Nagin D, et al. Childhood to early-midlife systolic blood pressure trajectories: early-life predictors, effect modifiers, and adult cardiovascular outcomes. *Hypertension*. 2015;66(6):1108–1115

12. Mozaffarian D, Benjamin EJ, Go AS, et al; Writing Group Members; American Heart Association Statistics Committee; Stroke Statistics Subcommittee. Executive summary: heart disease and stroke statistics—2016 update: a report from the American Heart Association. *Circulation*. 2016;133(4):447–454

13. Liberman JN, Berger JE, Lewis M. Prevalence of antihypertensive, antidiabetic, and dyslipidemic prescription medication use among children and adolescents. *Arch Pediatr Adolesc Med*. 2009;163(4):357–364

14. Rodriguez BL, Dabelea D, Liese AD, et al; SEARCH Study Group. Prevalence and correlates of elevated blood pressure in youth with diabetes mellitus: the

SEARCH for diabetes in youth study. *J Pediatr.* 2010;157(2):245–251.e1

15. Willi SM, Hirst K, Jago R, et al; HEALTHY Study Group. Cardiovascular risk factors in multi-ethnic middle school students: the HEALTHY primary prevention trial. *Pediatr Obes.* 2012;7(3):230–239

16. DiPietro A, Kees-Folts D, DesHarnais S, Camacho F, Wassner SJ. Primary hypertension at a single center: treatment, time to control, and extended follow-up. *Pediatr Nephrol.* 2009;24(12):2421–2428

17. Seeman T, Gilík J. Long-term control of ambulatory hypertension in children: improving with time but still not achieving new blood pressure goals. *Am J Hypertens.* 2013;26(7):939–945

18. Foglia CF, von Vigier RO, Fossali E, et al. A simplified antihypertensive drug regimen does not ameliorate control of childhood hypertension. *J Hum Hypertens.* 2005;19(8):653–654

19. Sorof J, Daniels S. Obesity hypertension in children: a problem of epidemic proportions. *Hypertension.* 2002;40(4):441–447

20. Sorof JM, Lai D, Turner J, Poffenbarger T, Portman RJ. Overweight, ethnicity, and the prevalence of hypertension in school-aged children. *Pediatrics.* 2004;113(3, pt 1):475–482

21. Koebnick C, Black MH, Wu J, et al. High blood pressure in overweight and obese youth: implications for screening. *J Clin Hypertens (Greenwich).* 2013;15(11):793–805

22. Falkner B, Gidding SS, Ramirez-Garnica G, Wiltrout SA, West D, Rappaport EB. The relationship of body mass index and blood pressure in primary care pediatric patients. *J Pediatr.* 2006;148(2):195–200

23. Lurbe E, Invitti C, Torro I, et al. The impact of the degree of obesity on the discrepancies between office and ambulatory blood pressure values in youth [published correction appears in *J Hypertens.* 2007;25(1):258]. *J Hypertens.* 2006;24(8):1557–1564

24. Skinner AC, Perrin EM, Moss LA, Skelton JA. Cardiometabolic risks and severity of obesity in children

and young adults. *N Engl J Med.* 2015;373(14):1307–1317

25. Zhang T, Zhang H, Li S, et al. Impact of adiposity on incident hypertension is modified by insulin resistance in adults: longitudinal observation from the Bogalusa Heart Study. *Hypertension.* 2016;67(1):56–62

26. So H-K, Yip GW-K, Choi K-C, et al; Hong Kong ABP Working Group. Association between waist circumference and childhood-masked hypertension: a community-based study. *J Paediatr Child Health.* 2016;52(4):385–390

27. Friedemann C, Heneghan C, Mahtani K, Thompson M, Perera R, Ward AM. Cardiovascular disease risk in healthy children and its association with body mass index: systematic review and meta-analysis. *BMJ.* 2012;345:e4759

28. Kelishadi R, Mirmoghtadaee P, Najafi H, Keikha M. Systematic review on the association of abdominal obesity in children and adolescents with cardio-metabolic risk factors. *J Res Med Sci.* 2015;20(3):294–307

29. Török K, Pálfi A, Szelényi Z, Molnár D. Circadian variability of blood pressure in obese children. *Nutr Metab Cardiovasc Dis.* 2008;18(6):429–435

30. Framme J, Dangardt F, Mårild S, Osika W, Währborg P, Friberg P. 24-h systolic blood pressure and heart rate recordings in lean and obese adolescents. *Clin Physiol Funct Imaging.* 2006;26(4):235–239

31. Westerståhl M, Marcus C. Association between nocturnal blood pressure dipping and insulin metabolism in obese adolescents. *Int J Obes.* 2010;34(3):472–477

32. Westerståhl M, Hedvall Kallerman P, Hagman E, Ek AE, Rössner SM, Marcus C. Nocturnal blood pressure non-dipping is prevalent in severely obese, prepubertal and early pubertal children. *Acta Paediatr.* 2014;103(2):225–230

33. Macumber IR, Weiss NS, Halbach SM, Hanevold CD, Flynn JT. The association of pediatric obesity with nocturnal non-dipping on 24-hour ambulatory blood pressure monitoring. *Am J Hypertens.* 2016;29(5):647–652

34. Perng W, Rifas-Shiman SL, Kramer MS, et al. Early weight gain, linear growth,

and mid-childhood blood pressure: a prospective study in project viva. *Hypertension.* 2016;67(2):301–308

35. Parker ED, Sinaiko AR, Kharbanda EO, et al. Change in weight status and development of hypertension. *Pediatrics.* 2016;137(3):e20151662

36. Yip J, Facchini FS, Reaven GM. Resistance to insulin-mediated glucose disposal as a predictor of cardiovascular disease. *J Clin Endocrinol Metab.* 1998;83(8):2773–2776

37. Kashyap SR, Defronzo RA. The insulin resistance syndrome: physiological considerations. *Diab Vasc Dis Res.* 2007;4(1):13–19

38. Lurbe E, Torro I, Aguilar F, et al. Added impact of obesity and insulin resistance in nocturnal blood pressure elevation in children and adolescents. *Hypertension.* 2008;51(3):635–641

39. Chinali M, de Simone G, Roman MJ, et al. Cardiac markers of pre-clinical disease in adolescents with the metabolic syndrome: the strong heart study. *J Am Coll Cardiol.* 2008;52(11):932–938

40. Archbold KH, Vasquez MM, Goodwin JL, Quan SF. Effects of sleep patterns and obesity on increases in blood pressure in a 5-year period: report from the Tucson Children's Assessment of Sleep Apnea Study. *J Pediatr.* 2012;161(1):26–30

41. Javaheri S, Storfer-Isser A, Rosen CL, Redline S. Sleep quality and elevated blood pressure in adolescents. *Circulation.* 2008;118(10):1034–1040

42. Hartzell K, Avis K, Lozano D, Feig D. Obstructive sleep apnea and periodic limb movement disorder in a population of children with hypertension and/or nocturnal nondipping blood pressures. *J Am Soc Hypertens.* 2016;10(2):101–107

43. Au CT, Ho CK, Wing YK, Lam HS, Li AM. Acute and chronic effects of sleep duration on blood pressure. *Pediatrics.* 2014;133(1). Available at: www.pediatrics.org/cgi/content/full/133/1/e64

44. Li AM, Au CT, Ng C, Lam HS, Ho CKW, Wing YK. A 4-year prospective follow-up study of childhood OSA

and its association with BP. *Chest.* 2014;145(6):1255–1263

45. Li AM, Au CT, Sung RY, et al. Ambulatory blood pressure in children with obstructive sleep apnoea: a community based study. *Thorax.* 2008;63(9):803–809

46. Flynn JT, Mitsnefes M, Pierce C, et al; Chronic Kidney Disease in Children Study Group. Blood pressure in children with chronic kidney disease: a report from the Chronic Kidney Disease in Children study. *Hypertension.* 2008;52(4):631–637

47. Samuels J, Ng D, Flynn JT, et al; Chronic Kidney Disease in Children Study Group. Ambulatory blood pressure patterns in children with chronic kidney disease. *Hypertension.* 2012;60(1):43–50

48. Shatat IF, Flynn JT. Hypertension in children with chronic kidney disease. *Adv Chronic Kidney Dis.* 2005;12(4):378–384

49. Chavers BM, Solid CA, Daniels FX, et al. Hypertension in pediatric long-term hemodialysis patients in the United States. *Clin J Am Soc Nephrol.* 2009;4(8):1363–1369

50. Seeman T. Hypertension after renal transplantation. *Pediatr Nephrol.* 2009;24(5):959–972

51. Tkaczyk M, Nowicki M, Bałasz-Chmielewska I, et al. Hypertension in dialysed children: the prevalence and therapeutic approach in Poland—a nationwide survey. *Nephrol Dial Transplant.* 2006;21(3):736–742

52. Kramer AM, van Stralen KJ, Jager KJ, et al. Demographics of blood pressure and hypertension in children on renal replacement therapy in Europe. *Kidney Int.* 2011;80(10):1092–1098

53. Halbach SM, Martz K, Mattoo T, Flynn J. Predictors of blood pressure and its control in pediatric patients receiving dialysis. *J Pediatr.* 2012;160(4):621–625.e1

54. Kaelber DC. IBM explorys cohort discovery tool. Available at: www.ibm.com/watson/health/explorys. Accessed February 3, 2017

55. Barker DJ. The fetal and infant origins of adult disease. *BMJ.* 1990;301(6761):1111

56. Edvardsson VO, Steinthorsdottir SD, Eliasdottir SB, Indridason OS, Palsson R. Birth weight and childhood blood pressure. *Curr Hypertens Rep.* 2012;14(6):596–602

57. Mhanna MJ, Iqbal AM, Kaelber DC. Weight gain and hypertension at three years of age and older in extremely low birth weight infants. *J Neonatal Perinatal Med.* 2015;8(4):363–369

58. Di Salvo G, Castaldi B, Baldini L, et al. Masked hypertension in young patients after successful aortic coarctation repair: impact on left ventricular geometry and function. *J Hum Hypertens.* 2011;25(12):739–745

59. Bayrakci US, Schaefer F, Duzova A, Yigit S, Bakkaloglu A. Abnormal circadian blood pressure regulation in children born preterm. *J Pediatr.* 2007;151(4):399–403

60. Sun SS, Grave GD, Siervogel RM, Pickoff AA, Arslanian SS, Daniels SR. Systolic blood pressure in childhood predicts hypertension and metabolic syndrome later in life. *Pediatrics.* 2007;119(2):237–246

61. Juhola J, Oikonen M, Magnussen CG, et al. Childhood physical, environmental, and genetic predictors of adult hypertension: the cardiovascular risk in young Finns study. *Circulation.* 2012;126(4):402–409

62. Juhola J, Magnussen CG, Viikari JS, et al. Tracking of serum lipid levels, blood pressure, and body mass index from childhood to adulthood: the Cardiovascular Risk in Young Finns Study. *J Pediatr.* 2011;159(4):584–590

63. Bao W, Threefoot SA, Srinivasan SR, Berenson GS. Essential hypertension predicted by tracking of elevated blood pressure from childhood to adulthood: the Bogalusa Heart Study. *Am J Hypertens.* 1995;8(7):657–665

64. Falkner B, Gidding SS, Portman R, Rosner B. Blood pressure variability and classification of prehypertension and hypertension in adolescence. *Pediatrics.* 2008;122(2):238–242

65. Tracy RE, Newman WP III, Wattigney WA, Srinivasan SR, Strong JP, Berenson GS. Histologic features of atherosclerosis and hypertension from autopsies of young individuals in a defined geographic population: the

Bogalusa Heart Study. *Atherosclerosis.* 1995;116(2):163–179

66. Urbina EM, Khoury PR, McCoy C, Daniels SR, Kimball TR, Dolan LM. Cardiac and vascular consequences of pre-hypertension in youth. *J Clin Hypertens (Greenwich).* 2011;13(5):332–342

67. de Simone G, Devereux RB, Daniels SR, Koren MJ, Meyer RA, Laragh JH. Effect of growth on variability of left ventricular mass: assessment of allometric signals in adults and children and their capacity to predict cardiovascular risk. *J Am Coll Cardiol.* 1995;25(5):1056–1062

68. O'Leary DH, Polak JF, Kronmal RA, Manolio TA, Burke GL, Wolfson SK Jr; Cardiovascular Health Study Collaborative Research Group. Carotid-artery intima and media thickness as a risk factor for myocardial infarction and stroke in older adults. *N Engl J Med.* 1999;340(1):14–22

69. Mitchell GF, Hwang SJ, Vasan RS, et al. Arterial stiffness and cardiovascular events: the Framingham Heart Study. *Circulation.* 2010;121(4):505–511

70. Lloyd-Jones DM, Hong Y, Labarthe D, et al; American Heart Association Strategic Planning Task Force and Statistics Committee. Defining and setting national goals for cardiovascular health promotion and disease reduction: the American Heart Association's strategic impact goal through 2020 and beyond. *Circulation.* 2010;121(4):586–613

71. Ning H, Labarthe DR, Shay CM, et al. Status of cardiovascular health in US children up to 11 years of age: the National Health and Nutrition Examination Surveys 2003-2010. *Circ Cardiovasc Qual Outcomes.* 2015;8(2):164–171

72. Steinberger J, Daniels SR, Hagberg N, et al; American Heart Association Atherosclerosis, Hypertension, and Obesity in the Young Committee of the Council on Cardiovascular Disease in the Young; Council on Cardiovascular and Stroke Nursing; Council on Epidemiology and Prevention; Council on Functional Genomics and Translational Biology; Stroke Council. Cardiovascular health promotion in children: challenges and opportunities for 2020 and beyond: a

scientific statement from the American Heart Association. *Circulation*. 2016;134(12):e236–e255

73. Ogden CL, Carroll MD, Lawman HG, et al. Trends in obesity prevalence among children and adolescents in the United States, 1988-1994 through 2013-2014. *JAMA*. 2016;315(21):2292–2299

74. Skinner AC, Perrin EM, Skelton JA. Prevalence of obesity and severe obesity in US children, 1999-2014. *Obesity (Silver Spring)*. 2016;24(5):1116–1123

75. Skinner AC, Skelton JA. Prevalence and trends in obesity and severe obesity among children in the United States, 1999-2012. *JAMA Pediatr*. 2014;168(6):561–566

76. Shay CM, Ning H, Daniels SR, Rooks CR, Gidding SS, Lloyd-Jones DM. Status of cardiovascular health in US adolescents: prevalence estimates from the National Health and Nutrition Examination Surveys (NHANES) 2005-2010. *Circulation*. 2013;127(13):1369–1376

77. Rosner B, Cook N, Portman R, Daniels S, Falkner B. Determination of blood pressure percentiles in normal-weight children: some methodological issues. *Am J Epidemiol*. 2008;167(6):653–666

78. Kaelber DC, Pickett F. Simple table to identify children and adolescents needing further evaluation of blood pressure. *Pediatrics*. 2009;123(6). Available at: www.pediatrics.org/cgi/content/full/123/6/e972

79. Dionne JM, Abitbol CL, Flynn JT. Hypertension in infancy: diagnosis, management and outcome [published correction appears in *Pediatr Nephrol*. 2012;27(1):159-60]. *Pediatr Nephrol*. 2012;27(1):17–32

80. Kent AL, Chaudhari T. Determinants of neonatal blood pressure. *Curr Hypertens Rep*. 2013;15(5):426–432

81. Report of the second task force on blood pressure control in children–1987. Task force on blood pressure control in children. National Heart, Lung, and Blood Institute, Bethesda, Maryland. *Pediatrics*. 1987;79(1):1–25

82. Savoca MR, MacKey ML, Evans CD, Wilson M, Ludwig DA, Harshfield GA.

Association of ambulatory blood pressure and dietary caffeine in adolescents. *Am J Hypertens*. 2005;18(1):116–120

83. Pickering TG, Hall JE, Appel LJ, et al. Recommendations for blood pressure measurement in humans and experimental animals: part 1: blood pressure measurement in humans: a statement for professionals from the Subcommittee of Professional and Public Education of the American Heart Association Council on High Blood Pressure Research. *Circulation*. 2005;111(5):697–716

84. Becton LJ, Egan BM, Hailpern SM, Shatat IF. Blood pressure reclassification in adolescents based on repeat clinic blood pressure measurements. *J Clin Hypertens (Greenwich)*. 2013;15(10):717–722

85. Daley MF, Sinaiko AR, Reifler LM, et al. Patterns of care and persistence after incident elevated blood pressure. *Pediatrics*. 2013;132(2). Available at: www.pediatrics.org/cgi/content/full/132/2/e349

86. Ostchega Y, Prineas RJ, Nwankwo T, Zipf G. Assessing blood pressure accuracy of an aneroid sphygmomanometer in a national survey environment. *Am J Hypertens*. 2011;24(3):322–327

87. Ma Y, Temprosa M, Fowler S, et al; Diabetes Prevention Program Research Group. Evaluating the accuracy of an aneroid sphygmomanometer in a clinical trial setting. *Am J Hypertens*. 2009;22(3):263–266

88. Podoll A, Grenier M, Croix B, Feig DI. Inaccuracy in pediatric outpatient blood pressure measurement. *Pediatrics*. 2007;119(3). Available at: www.pediatrics.org/cgi/content/full/119/3/e538

89. Mourad A, Carney S. Arm position and blood pressure: an audit. *Intern Med J*. 2004;34(5):290–291

90. Mourad A, Carney S, Gillies A, Jones B, Nanra R, Trevillian P. Arm position and blood pressure: a risk factor for hypertension? *J Hum Hypertens*. 2003;17(6):389–395

91. Zaheer S, Watson L, Webb NJ. Unmet needs in the measurement of blood pressure in primary care. *Arch Dis Child*. 2014;99(5):463–464

92. Veiga EV, Arcuri EAM, Cloutier L, Santos JL. Blood pressure measurement: arm circumference and cuff size availability. *Rev Lat Am Enfermagem*. 2009;17(4):455–461

93. Thomas M, Radford T, Dasgupta I. Unvalidated blood pressure devices with small cuffs are being used in hospitals. *BMJ*. 2001;323(7309):398

94. Burke MJ, Towers HM, O'Malley K, Fitzgerald DJ, O'Brien ET. Sphygmomanometers in hospital and family practice: problems and recommendations. *Br Med J (Clin Res Ed)*. 1982;285(6340):469–471

95. Centers for Disease Control and Prevention. National Health and Nutrition Examination Survey (NHANES) Anthropometry Procedures Manual. Available at: https://www.cdc.gov/nchs/data/nhanes/nhanes_07_08/manual_an.pdf. Published January 2013. Accessed May 9, 2016

96. Prineas RJ, Ostchega Y, Carroll M, Dillon C, McDowell M. US demographic trends in mid-arm circumference and recommended blood pressure cuffs for children and adolescents: data from the National Health and Nutrition Examination Survey 1988-2004. *Blood Press Monit*. 2007;12(2):75–80

97. Kimble KJ, Darnall RA Jr, Yelderman M, Ariagno RL, Ream AK. An automated oscillometric technique for estimating mean arterial pressure in critically ill newborns. *Anesthesiology*. 1981;54(5):423–425

98. Sonesson SE, Broberger U. Arterial blood pressure in the very low birthweight neonate. Evaluation of an automatic oscillometric technique. *Acta Paediatr Scand*. 1987;76(2):338–341

99. Duncan AF, Rosenfeld CR, Morgan JS, Ahmad N, Heyne RJ. Interrater reliability and effect of state on blood pressure measurements in infants 1 to 3 years of age. *Pediatrics*. 2008;122(3). Available at: www.pediatrics.org/cgi/content/full/122/3/e590

100. Nwankwo MU, Lorenz JM, Gardiner JC. A standard protocol for blood pressure measurement in the newborn. *Pediatrics*. 1997;99(6). Available at: www.pediatrics.org/cgi/content/full/99/6/e10

101. Gupta-Malhotra M, Banker A, Shete S, et al. Essential hypertension vs. secondary hypertension among children. *Am J Hypertens.* 2015;28(1):73–80

102. Kelly RK, Thomson R, Smith KJ, Dwyer T, Venn A, Magnussen CG. Factors affecting tracking of blood pressure from childhood to adulthood: the Childhood Determinants of Adult Health Study. *J Pediatr.* 2015;167(6):1422–1428.e2

103. Juhola J, Magnussen CG, Berenson GS, et al. Combined effects of child and adult elevated blood pressure on subclinical atherosclerosis: the International Childhood Cardiovascular Cohort Consortium. *Circulation.* 2013;128(3):217–224

104. Sladowska-Kozłowska J, Litwin M, Niemirska A, Wierzbicka A, Wawer ZT, Janas R. Change in left ventricular geometry during antihypertensive treatment in children with primary hypertension. *Pediatr Nephrol.* 2011;26(12):2201–2209

105. Litwin M, Niemirska A, Sladowska-Kozlowska J, et al. Regression of target organ damage in children and adolescents with primary hypertension. *Pediatr Nephrol.* 2010;25(12):2489–2499

106. Meyer AA, Kundt G, Lenschow U, Schuff-Werner P, Kienast W. Improvement of early vascular changes and cardiovascular risk factors in obese children after a six-month exercise program. *J Am Coll Cardiol.* 2006;48(9):1865–1870

107. Juonala M, Magnussen CG, Berenson GS, et al. Childhood adiposity, adult adiposity, and cardiovascular risk factors. *N Engl J Med.* 2011;365(20):1876–1885

108. Lo JC, Chandra M, Sinaiko A, et al. Severe obesity in children: prevalence, persistence and relation to hypertension. *Int J Pediatr Endocrinol.* 2014;2014(1):3

109. Rademacher ER, Jacobs DR Jr, Moran A, Steinberger J, Prineas RJ, Sinaiko A. Relation of blood pressure and body mass index during childhood to cardiovascular risk factor levels in young adults. *J Hypertens.* 2009;27(9):1766–1774

110. Maahs DM, Daniels SR, de Ferranti SD, et al; American Heart Association Atherosclerosis, Hypertension and Obesity in Youth Committee of the Council on Cardiovascular Disease in the Young; Council on Clinical Cardiology; Council on Cardiovascular and Stroke Nursing; Council for High Blood Pressure Research; Council on Lifestyle and Cardiometabolic Health. Cardiovascular disease risk factors in youth with diabetes mellitus: a scientific statement from the American Heart Association. *Circulation.* 2014;130(17):1532–1558

111. Levitt Katz L, Gidding SS, Bacha F, et al; TODAY Study Group. Alterations in left ventricular, left atrial, and right ventricular structure and function to cardiovascular risk factors in adolescents with type 2 diabetes participating in the TODAY clinical trial. *Pediatr Diabetes.* 2015;16(1):39–47

112. Hager A, Kanz S, Kaemmerer H, Schreiber C, Hess J. Coarctation Long-term Assessment (COALA): significance of arterial hypertension in a cohort of 404 patients up to 27 years after surgical repair of isolated coarctation of the aorta, even in the absence of restenosis and prosthetic material. *J Thorac Cardiovasc Surg.* 2007;134(3):738–745

113. O'Sullivan JJ, Derrick G, Darnell R. Prevalence of hypertension in children after early repair of coarctation of the aorta: a cohort study using casual and 24 hour blood pressure measurement. *Heart.* 2002;88(2):163–166

114. Becker AM, Goldberg JH, Henson M, et al. Blood pressure abnormalities in children with sickle cell anemia. *Pediatr Blood Cancer.* 2014;61(3):518–522

115. Brady TM, Solomon BS, Neu AM, Siberry GK, Parekh RS. Patient-, provider-, and clinic-level predictors of unrecognized elevated blood pressure in children. *Pediatrics.* 2010;125(6). Available at: www.pediatrics.org/cgi/content/full/125/6/e1286

116. Stabouli S, Sideras L, Vareta G, et al. Hypertension screening during healthcare pediatric visits. *J Hypertens.* 2015;33(5):1064–1068

117. Shapiro DJ, Hersh AL, Cabana MD, Sutherland SM, Patel AI. Hypertension screening during ambulatory pediatric visits in the United States, 2000-2009. *Pediatrics.* 2012;130(4):604–610

118. Bijlsma MW, Blufpand HN, Key Action Statementpers GJ, Bökenkamp A. Why pediatricians fail to diagnose hypertension: a multicenter survey. *J Pediatr.* 2014;164(1):173–177.e7

119. Chaudhry B, Wang J, Wu S, et al. Systematic review: impact of health information technology on quality, efficiency, and costs of medical care. *Ann Intern Med.* 2006;144(10):742–752

120. Shojania KG, Jennings A, Mayhew A, Ramsay CR, Eccles MP, Grimshaw J. The effects of on-screen, point of care computer reminders on processes and outcomes of care. *Cochrane Database Syst Rev.* 2009;(3):CD001096

121. Garg AX, Adhikari NKJ, McDonald H, et al. Effects of computerized clinical decision support systems on practitioner performance and patient outcomes: a systematic review. *JAMA.* 2005;293(10):1223–1238

122. Hicks LS, Sequist TD, Ayanian JZ, et al. Impact of computerized decision support on blood pressure management and control: a randomized controlled trial. *J Gen Intern Med.* 2008;23(4):429–441

123. Samal L, Linder JA, Lipsitz SR, Hicks LS. Electronic health records, clinical decision support, and blood pressure control. *Am J Manag Care.* 2011;17(9):626–632

124. Heymann AD, Hoch I, Valinsky L, Shalev V, Silber H, Kokia E. Mandatory computer field for blood pressure measurement improves screening. *Fam Pract.* 2005;22(2):168–169

125. Brady TM, Neu AM, Miller ER III, Appel LJ, Siberry GK, Solomon BS. Real-time electronic medical record alerts increase high blood pressure recognition in children. *Clin Pediatr (Phila).* 2015;54(7):667–675

126. Romano MJ, Stafford RS. Electronic health records and clinical decision support systems: impact on national ambulatory care quality. *Arch Intern Med.* 2011;171(10):897–903

127. Alpert BS, Quinn D, Gallick D. Oscillometric blood pressure: a review for clinicians. *J Am Soc Hypertens.* 2014;8(12):930–938

128. Alpert BS. Oscillometric blood pressure values are algorithm-specific. *Am J Cardiol.* 2010;106(10):1524–1525, author reply 1524–1525

129. Flynn JT, Pierce CB, Miller ER III, et al; Chronic Kidney Disease in Children Study Group. Reliability of resting blood pressure measurement and classification using an oscillometric device in children with chronic kidney disease. *J Pediatr.* 2012;160(3):434–440.e1

130. Kamath N, Goud BR, Phadke KD, Iyengar A. Use of oscillometric devices for the measurement of blood pressure-comparison with the gold standard. *Indian J Pediatr.* 2012;79(9):1230–1232

131. Chiolero A, Bovet P, Stergiou GS. Automated oscillometric blood pressure measurement in children. *J Clin Hypertens (Greenwich).* 2014;16(6):468

132. Chiolero A, Paradis G, Lambert M. Accuracy of oscillometric devices in children and adults. *Blood Press.* 2010;19(4):254–259

133. Chio SS, Urbina EM, Lapointe J, Tsai J, Berenson GS. Korotkoff sound versus oscillometric cuff sphygmomanometers: comparison between auscultatory and DynaPulse blood pressure measurements. *J Am Soc Hypertens.* 2011;5(1):12–20

134. Eliasdottir SB, Steinthorsdottir SD, Indridason OS, Palsson R, Edvardsson VO. Comparison of aneroid and oscillometric blood pressure measurements in children. *J Clin Hypertens (Greenwich).* 2013;15(11):776–783

135. Urbina EM, Khoury PR, McCoy CE, Daniels SR, Dolan LM, Kimball TR. Comparison of mercury sphygmomanometry blood pressure readings with oscillometric and central blood pressure in predicting target organ damage in youth. *Blood Press Monit.* 2015;20(3):150–156

136. Negroni-Balasquide X, Bell CS, Samuel J, Samuels JA. Is one measurement enough to evaluate blood pressure among adolescents? A blood pressure screening experience in more than 9000 children with a subset comparison of auscultatory to mercury measurements. *J Am Soc Hypertens.* 2016;10(2):95–100

137. Leblanc M-É, Croteau S, Ferland A, et al. Blood pressure assessment in severe obesity: validation of a forearm approach. *Obesity (Silver Spring).* 2013;21(12):E533–E541

138. Altunkan S, Genç Y, Altunkan E. A comparative study of an ambulatory blood pressure measuring device and a wrist blood pressure monitor with a position sensor versus a mercury sphygmomanometer. *Eur J Intern Med.* 2007;18(2):118–123

139. Uen S, Fimmers R, Brieger M, Nickenig G, Mengden T. Reproducibility of wrist home blood pressure measurement with position sensor and automatic data storage. *BMC Cardiovasc Disord.* 2009;9:20

140. Fania C, Benetti E, Palatini P. Validation of the A&D BP UB-543 wrist device for home blood pressure measurement according to the European Society of Hypertension International Protocol revision 2010. *Blood Press Monit.* 2015;20(4):237–240

141. Kang Y-Y, Chen Q, Li Y, Wang JG. Validation of the SCIAN LD-735 wrist blood pressure monitor for home blood pressure monitoring according to the European Society of Hypertension International Protocol revision 2010. *Blood Press Monit.* 2016;21(4):255–258

142. Xie P, Wang Y, Xu X, Huang F, Pan J. Validation of the Pangao PG-800A11 wrist device assessed according to the European Society of Hypertension and the British Hypertension Society protocols. *Blood Press Monit.* 2015;20(2):108–111

143. Zweiker R, Schumacher M, Fruhwald FM, Watzinger N, Klein W. Comparison of wrist blood pressure measurement with conventional sphygmomanometry at a cardiology outpatient clinic. *J Hypertens.* 2000;18(8):1013–1018

144. Altunkan S, Yildiz S, Azer S. Wrist blood pressure-measuring devices: a comparative study of accuracy with a standard auscultatory method using a mercury manometer. *Blood Press Monit.* 2002;7(5):281–284

145. Palatini P, Longo D, Toffanin G, Bertolo O, Zaetta V, Pessina AC. Wrist blood pressure overestimates blood pressure measured at the upper arm. *Blood Press Monit.* 2004;9(2):77–81

146. Stergiou GS, Christodoulakis GR, Nasothimiou EG, Giovas PP, Kalogeropoulos PG. Can validated wrist devices with position sensors replace arm devices for self-home blood pressure monitoring? A randomized crossover trial using ambulatory monitoring as reference. *Am J Hypertens.* 2008;21(7):753–758

147. Khoshdel AR, Carney S, Gillies A. The impact of arm position and pulse pressure on the validation of a wrist-cuff blood pressure measurement device in a high risk population. *Int J Gen Med.* 2010;3:119–125

148. Kikuya M, Chonan K, Imai Y, Goto E, Ishii M; Research Group to Assess the Validity of Automated Blood Pressure Measurement Devices in Japan. Accuracy and reliability of wrist-cuff devices for self-measurement of blood pressure. *J Hypertens.* 2002;20(4):629–638

149. Westhoff TH, Schmidt S, Meissner R, Zidek W, van der Giet M. The impact of pulse pressure on the accuracy of wrist blood pressure measurement. *J Hum Hypertens.* 2009;23(6):391–395

150. Deutsch C, Krüger R, Saito K, et al. Comparison of the Omron RS6 wrist blood pressure monitor with the positioning sensor on or off with a standard mercury sphygmomanometer. *Blood Press Monit.* 2014;19(5):306–313

151. Yarows SA. Comparison of the Omron HEM-637 wrist monitor to the auscultation method with the wrist position sensor on or disabled. *Am J Hypertens.* 2004;17(1):54–58

152. Menezes AMB, Dumith SC, Noal RB, et al. Validity of a wrist digital monitor for blood pressure measurement in comparison to a mercury sphygmomanometer. *Arq Bras Cardiol.* 2010;94(3):345–349, 365–370

153. Wankum PC, Thurman TL, Holt SJ, Hall RA, Simpson PM, Heulitt MJ. Validation of a noninvasive blood pressure

monitoring device in normotensive and hypertensive pediatric intensive care patients. *J Clin Monit Comput.* 2004;18(4):253–263

154. Cua CL, Thomas K, Zurakowski D, Laussen PC. A comparison of the Vasotrac with invasive arterial blood pressure monitoring in children after pediatric cardiac surgery. *Anesth Analg.* 2005;100(5): 1289–1294

155. Flynn JT, Daniels SR, Hayman LL, et al; American Heart Association Atherosclerosis, Hypertension and Obesity in Youth Committee of the Council on Cardiovascular Disease in the Young. Update: ambulatory blood pressure monitoring in children and adolescents: a scientific statement from the American Heart Association. *Hypertension.* 2014;63(5): 1116–1135

156. Siu AL; U.S. Preventive Services Task Force. Screening for high blood pressure in adults: U.S. Preventive Services Task Force recommendation statement. *Ann Intern Med.* 2015;163(10):778–786

157. Díaz LN, Garin EH. Comparison of ambulatory blood pressure and Task Force criteria to identify pediatric hypertension. *Pediatr Nephrol.* 2007;22(4):554–558

158. Salice P, Ardissino G, Zanchetti A, et al. Age-dependent differences in office (OBP) vs ambulatory blood pressure monitoring (ABPM) in hypertensive children and adolescents: 8C.03. *J Hypertens.* 2010;28:e423–e424

159. Stergiou GS, Alamara CV, Salgami EV, Vaindirlis IN, Dacou-Voutetakis C, Mountokalakis TD. Reproducibility of home and ambulatory blood pressure in children and adolescents. *Blood Press Monit.* 2005;10(3):143–147

160. Li Z, Snieder H, Harshfield GA, Treiber FA, Wang X. A 15-year longitudinal study on ambulatory blood pressure tracking from childhood to early adulthood. *Hypertens Res.* 2009;32(5):404–410

161. Seeman T, Palyzová D, Dusek J, Janda J. Reduced nocturnal blood pressure dip and sustained nighttime hypertension are specific markers of secondary hypertension. *J Pediatr.* 2005;147(3):366–371

162. Bjelakovic B, Jaddoe VW, Vukomanovic V, et al. The relationship between currently recommended ambulatory systolic blood pressure measures and left ventricular mass index in pediatric hypertension. *Curr Hypertens Rep.* 2015;17(4):534

163. Brady TM, Fivush B, Flynn JT, Parekh R. Ability of blood pressure to predict left ventricular hypertrophy in children with primary hypertension. *J Pediatr.* 2008;152(1):73–78, 78.e1

164. McNiece KL, Gupta-Malhotra M, Samuels J, et al; National High Blood Pressure Education Program Working Group. Left ventricular hypertrophy in hypertensive adolescents: analysis of risk by 2004 National High Blood Pressure Education Program Working Group staging criteria. *Hypertension.* 2007;50(2):392–395

165. Richey PA, Disessa TG, Hastings MC, Somes GW, Alpert BS, Jones DP. Ambulatory blood pressure and increased left ventricular mass in children at risk for hypertension. *J Pediatr.* 2008;152(3):343–348

166. Conkar S, Yılmaz E, Hacıkara Ş, Bozabalı S, Mir S. Is daytime systolic load an important risk factor for target organ damage in pediatric hypertension? *J Clin Hypertens (Greenwich).* 2015;17(10):760–766

167. Flynn JT. Differentiation between primary and secondary hypertension in children using ambulatory blood pressure monitoring. *Pediatrics.* 2002;110(1, pt 1):89–93

168. Dursun H, Bayazit AK, Cengiz N, et al. Ambulatory blood pressure monitoring and renal functions in children with a solitary kidney. *Pediatr Nephrol.* 2007;22(4):559–564

169. Patzer L, Seeman T, Luck C, Wühl E, Janda J, Misselwitz J. Day- and night-time blood pressure elevation in children with higher grades of renal scarring. *J Pediatr.* 2003;142(2):117–122

170. Fidan K, Kandur Y, Buyukkaragoz B, Akdemir UO, Soylemezoglu O. Hypertension in pediatric patients with renal scarring in association with vesicoureteral reflux. *Urology.* 2013;81(1):173–177

171. Basiratnia M, Esteghamati M, Ajami GH, et al. Blood pressure profile in renal transplant recipients and its relation to diastolic function: tissue Doppler echocardiographic study. *Pediatr Nephrol.* 2011;26(3):449–457

172. Chaudhuri A, Sutherland SM, Begin B, et al. Role of twenty-four-hour ambulatory blood pressure monitoring in children on dialysis. *Clin J Am Soc Nephrol.* 2011;6(4):870–876

173. Wühl E, Trivelli A, Picca S, et al; ESCAPE Trial Group. Strict blood-pressure control and progression of renal failure in children. *N Engl J Med.* 2009;361(17):1639–1650

174. Chatterjee M, Speiser PW, Pellizzarri M, et al. Poor glycemic control is associated with abnormal changes in 24-hour ambulatory blood pressure in children and adolescents with type 1 diabetes mellitus. *J Pediatr Endocrinol Metab.* 2009;22(11):1061–1067

175. Darcan S, Goksen D, Mir S, et al. Alterations of blood pressure in type 1 diabetic children and adolescents. *Pediatr Nephrol.* 2006;21(5):672–676

176. Dost A, Klinkert C, Kapellen T, et al; DPV Science Initiative. Arterial hypertension determined by ambulatory blood pressure profiles: contribution to microalbuminuria risk in a multicenter investigation in 2,105 children and adolescents with type 1 diabetes. *Diabetes Care.* 2008;31(4):720–725

177. Ettinger LM, Freeman K, DiMartino-Nardi JR, Flynn JT. Microalbuminuria and abnormal ambulatory blood pressure in adolescents with type 2 diabetes mellitus. *J Pediatr.* 2005;147(1):67–73

178. Lurbe E, Redon J, Kesani A, et al. Increase in nocturnal blood pressure and progression to microalbuminuria in type 1 diabetes. *N Engl J Med.* 2002;347(11):797–805

179. Nagasako SS, Nogueira PC, Machado PG, Pestana JO. Risk factors for hypertension 3 years after renal transplantation in children. *Pediatr Nephrol.* 2007;22(9):1363–1368

180. Roche SL, Kaufmann J, Dipchand AI, Kantor PF. Hypertension after pediatric heart transplantation is primarily associated with immunosuppressive

regimen. *J Heart Lung Transplant.* 2008;27(5):501–507

181. Paripovic D, Kostic M, Spasojevic B, Kruscic D, Peco-Antic A. Masked hypertension and hidden uncontrolled hypertension after renal transplantation. *Pediatr Nephrol.* 2010;25(9):1719–1724

182. Ferraris JR, Ghezzi L, Waisman G, Krmar RT. ABPM vs office blood pressure to define blood pressure control in treated hypertensive paediatric renal transplant recipients. *Pediatr Transplant.* 2007;11(1):24–30

183. McGlothan KR, Wyatt RJ, Ault BH, et al. Predominance of nocturnal hypertension in pediatric renal allograft recipients. *Pediatr Transplant.* 2006;10(5):558–564

184. Balzano R, Lindblad YT, Vavilis G, Jogestrand T, Berg UB, Krmar RT. Use of annual ABPM, and repeated carotid scan and echocardiography to monitor cardiovascular health over nine yr in pediatric and young adult renal transplant recipients. *Pediatr Transplant.* 2011;15(6):635–641

185. Krmar RT, Berg UB. Blood pressure control in hypertensive pediatric renal transplants: role of repeated ABPM following transplantation. *Am J Hypertens.* 2008;21(10):1093–1099

186. Ambrosi P, Kreitmann B, Habib G. Home blood pressure monitoring in heart transplant recipients: comparison with ambulatory blood pressure monitoring. *Transplantation.* 2014;97(3):363–367

187. Seeman T, Simková E, Kreisinger J, et al. Reduction of proteinuria during intensified antihypertensive therapy in children after renal transplantation. *Transplant Proc.* 2007;39(10):3150–3152

188. Seeman T, Simková E, Kreisinger J, et al. Improved control of hypertension in children after renal transplantation: results of a two-yr interventional trial. *Pediatr Transplant.* 2007;11(5):491–497

189. Lurbe E, Alvarez V, Liao Y, et al. The impact of obesity and body fat distribution on ambulatory blood pressure in children and adolescents. *Am J Hypertens.* 1998;11(4, pt 1):418–424

190. Lurbe E, Alvarez V, Redon J. Obesity, body fat distribution, and ambulatory blood pressure in children and adolescents. *J Clin Hypertens (Greenwich).* 2001;3(6):362–367

191. Marcovecchio ML, Patricelli L, Zito M, et al. Ambulatory blood pressure monitoring in obese children: role of insulin resistance. *J Hypertens.* 2006;24(12):2431–2436

192. Shatat IF, Freeman KD, Vuguin PM, Dimartino-Nardi JR, Flynn JT. Relationship between adiponectin and ambulatory blood pressure in obese adolescents. *Pediatr Res.* 2009;65(6):691–695

193. Amin RS, Carroll JL, Jeffries JL, et al. Twenty-four-hour ambulatory blood pressure in children with sleep-disordered breathing. *Am J Respir Crit Care Med.* 2004;169(8):950–956

194. Leung LC, Ng DK, Lau MW, et al. Twenty-four-hour ambulatory BP in snoring children with obstructive sleep apnea syndrome. *Chest.* 2006;130(4):1009–1017

195. Akyürek N, Atabek ME, Eklioglu BS, Alp H. Ambulatory blood pressure and subclinical cardiovascular disease in children with turner syndrome. *Pediatr Cardiol.* 2014;35(1):57–62

196. Salgado CM, Jardim PC, Teles FB, Nunes MC. Low birth weight as a marker of changes in ambulatory blood pressure monitoring. *Arq Bras Cardiol.* 2009;92(2):107–121

197. Gimpel C, Wühl E, Arbeiter K, et al; ESCAPE Trial Group. Superior consistency of ambulatory blood pressure monitoring in children: implications for clinical trials. *J Hypertens.* 2009;27(8):1568–1574

198. Suláková T, Feber J. Should mean arterial pressure be included in the definition of ambulatory hypertension in children? *Pediatr Nephrol.* 2013;28(7):1105–1112

199. Lurbe E, Torro I, Alvarez V, et al. Prevalence, persistence, and clinical significance of masked hypertension in youth. *Hypertension.* 2005;45(4):493–498

200. Stabouli S, Kotsis V, Toumanidis S, Papamichael C, Constantopoulos A, Zakopoulos N. White-coat and masked hypertension in children: association with target-organ damage. *Pediatr Nephrol.* 2005;20(8):1151–1155

201. Furusawa ÉA, Filho UD, Junior DM, Koch VH. Home and ambulatory blood pressure to identify white coat and masked hypertension in the pediatric patient. *Am J Hypertens.* 2011;24(8):893–897

202. Wells TG, Portman R, Norman P, Haertter S, Davidai G, Fei Wang. Safety, efficacy, and pharmacokinetics of telmisartan in pediatric patients with hypertension. *Clin Pediatr (Phila).* 2010;49(10):938–946

203. Mitsnefes M, Flynn J, Cohn S, et al; CKiD Study Group. Masked hypertension associates with left ventricular hypertrophy in children with CKD. *J Am Soc Nephrol.* 2010;21(1):137–144

204. Lurbe E, Redon J. Discrepancies in office and ambulatory blood pressure in adolescents: help or hindrance? *Pediatr Nephrol.* 2008;23(3):341–345

205. Pogue V, Rahman M, Lipkowitz M, et al; African American Study of Kidney Disease and Hypertension Collaborative Research Group. Disparate estimates of hypertension control from ambulatory and clinic blood pressure measurements in hypertensive kidney disease. *Hypertension.* 2009;53(1):20–27

206. Urbina EM, Williams RV, Alpert BS, et al; American Heart Association Atherosclerosis, Hypertension, and Obesity in Youth Committee of the Council on Cardiovascular Disease in the Young. Noninvasive assessment of subclinical atherosclerosis in children and adolescents: recommendations for standard assessment for clinical research: a scientific statement from the American Heart Association. *Hypertension.* 2009;54(5):919–950

207. Kavey RE, Kveselis DA, Atallah N, Smith FC. White coat hypertension in childhood: evidence for end-organ effect. *J Pediatr.* 2007;150(5):491–497

208. Swartz SJ, Srivaths PR, Croix B, Feig DI. Cost-effectiveness of ambulatory blood pressure monitoring in the initial evaluation of hypertension in children. *Pediatrics.* 2008;122(6):1177–1181

209. Briasoulis A, Androulakis E, Palla M, Papageorgiou N, Tousoulis D. White-coat hypertension and cardiovascular events: a meta-analysis. *J Hypertens.* 2016;34(4):593–599

210. Valent-Morić B, Zigman T, Zaja-Franulović O, Malenica M, Cuk M. The importance of ambulatory blood pressure monitoring in children and adolescents. *Acta Clin Croat.* 2012;51(1):59–64

211. Palatini P, Parati G. Blood pressure measurement in very obese patients: a challenging problem. *J Hypertens.* 2011;29(3):425–429

212. Halm MA. Arm circumference, shape, and length: how interplaying variables affect blood pressure measurement in obese persons. *Am J Crit Care.* 2014;23(2):166–170

213. Ostchega Y, Hughes JP, Prineas RJ, Zhang G, Nwankwo T, Chiappa MM. Mid-arm circumference and recommended blood pressure cuffs for children and adolescents aged between 3 and 19 years: data from the National Health and Nutrition Examination Survey, 1999-2010. *Blood Press Monit.* 2014;19(1):26–31

214. Bonso E, Saladini F, Zanier A, Benetti E, Dorigatti F, Palatini P. Accuracy of a single rigid conical cuff with standard-size bladder coupled to an automatic oscillometric device over a wide range of arm circumferences. *Hypertens Res.* 2010;33(11):1186–1191

215. Palatini P, Benetti E, Fania C, Malipiero G, Saladini F. Rectangular cuffs may overestimate blood pressure in individuals with large conical arms. *J Hypertens.* 2012;30(3):530–536

216. Aguilar A, Ostrow V, De Luca F, Suarez E. Elevated ambulatory blood pressure in a multi-ethnic population of obese children and adolescents. *J Pediatr.* 2010;156(6):930–935

217. Ostrow V, Wu S, Aguilar A, Bonner R Jr, Suarez E, De Luca F. Association between oxidative stress and masked hypertension in a multi-ethnic population of obese children and adolescents. *J Pediatr.* 2011;158(4):628–633.e1

218. Woroniecki RP, Flynn JT. How are hypertensive children evaluated and managed? A survey of North American pediatric nephrologists. *Pediatr Nephrol.* 2005;20(6):791–797

219. Mengden T, Hernandez Medina RM, Beltran B, Alvarez E, Kraft K, Vetter H. Reliability of reporting self-measured blood pressure values by hypertensive patients. *Am J Hypertens.* 1998;11(12):1413–1417

220. Palatini P, Frick GN. Techniques for self-measurement of blood pressure: limitations and needs for future research. *J Clin Hypertens (Greenwich).* 2012;14(3):139–143

221. Stergiou GS, Karpettas N, Kapoyiannis A, Stefanidis CJ, Vazeou A. Home blood pressure monitoring in children and adolescents: a systematic review. *J Hypertens.* 2009;27(10):1941–1947

222. Stergiou GS, Nasothimiou E, Giovas P, Kapoyiannis A, Vazeou A. Diagnosis of hypertension in children and adolescents based on home versus ambulatory blood pressure monitoring. *J Hypertens.* 2008;26(8):1556–1562

223. Furusawa EA, Filho UD, Koch VH. Home blood pressure monitoring in paediatric chronic hypertension. *J Hum Hypertens.* 2009;23(7):464–469

224. Stergiou GS, Nasothimiou EG, Giovas PP, Rarra VC. Long-term reproducibility of home vs. office blood pressure in children and adolescents: the Arsakeion school study. *Hypertens Res.* 2009;32(4):311–315

225. Wühl E, Hadtstein C, Mehls O, Schaefer F; Escape Trial Group. Home, clinic, and ambulatory blood pressure monitoring in children with chronic renal failure. *Pediatr Res.* 2004;55(3):492–497

226. Stergiou GS, Karpettas N, Panagiotakos DB, Vazeou A. Comparison of office, ambulatory and home blood pressure in children and adolescents on the basis of normalcy tables. *J Hum Hypertens.* 2011;25(4):218–223

227. Stergiou GS, Alamara CV, Kalkana CB, et al. Out-of-office blood pressure in children and adolescents: disparate findings by using home or ambulatory monitoring. *Am J Hypertens.* 2004;17(10):869–875

228. Stergiou GS, Rarra VC, Yiannes NG. Changing relationship between home and office blood pressure with increasing age in children: the Arsakeion School study. *Am J Hypertens.* 2008;21(1):41–46

229. Salgado CM, Jardim PC, Viana JK, Jardim TS, Velasquez PP. Home blood pressure in children and adolescents: a comparison with office and ambulatory blood pressure measurements. *Acta Paediatr.* 2011;100(10):e163–e168

230. Stergiou GS, Ntineri A, Kollias A, Destounis A, Nasothimiou E, Roussias L. Changing relationship among clinic, home, and ambulatory blood pressure with increasing age. *J Am Soc Hypertens.* 2015;9(7):544–552

231. Stergiou GS, Yiannes NG, Rarra VC, Panagiotakos DB. Home blood pressure normalcy in children and adolescents: the Arsakeion School study. *J Hypertens.* 2007;25(7):1375–1379

232. Sorof JM, Turner J, Franco K, Portman RJ. Characteristics of hypertensive children identified by primary care referral compared with school-based screening. *J Pediatr.* 2004;144(4):485–489

233. King CA, Meadows BB, Engelke MK, Swanson M. Prevalence of elevated body mass index and blood pressure in a rural school-aged population: implications for school nurses. *J Sch Health.* 2006;76(4):145–149

234. Underwood SM, Averhart L, Dean A, et al. Clinical evaluation and follow-up of body mass and blood pressure in pre-elementary school children: program review. *J Natl Black Nurses Assoc.* 2012;23(1):8–15

235. Kapur G, Ahmed M, Pan C, Mitsnefes M, Chiang M, Mattoo TK. Secondary hypertension in overweight and stage 1 hypertensive children: a Midwest Pediatric Nephrology Consortium report. *J Clin Hypertens (Greenwich).* 2010;12(1):34–39

236. Flynn JT, Alderman MH. Characteristics of children with primary hypertension seen at a referral center. *Pediatr Nephrol.* 2005;20(7):961–966

237. Gomes RS, Quirino IG, Pereira RM, et al. Primary versus secondary

hypertension in children followed up at an outpatient tertiary unit. *Pediatr Nephrol.* 2011;26(3):441–447

238. Welch WP, Yang W, Taylor-Zapata P, Flynn JT. Antihypertensive drug use by children: are the drugs labeled and indicated? *J Clin Hypertens (Greenwich).* 2012;14(6):388–395

239. Flynn J, Zhang Y, Solar-Yohay S, Shi V. Clinical and demographic characteristics of children with hypertension. *Hypertension.* 2012;60(4):1047–1054

240. Baracco R, Kapur G, Mattoo T, et al. Prediction of primary vs secondary hypertension in children. *J Clin Hypertens (Greenwich).* 2012;14(5):316–321

241. Silverstein DM, Champoux E, Aviles DH, Vehaskari VM. Treatment of primary and secondary hypertension in children. *Pediatr Nephrol.* 2006;21(6):820–827

242. Flynn JT, Meyers KEC, Neto JP, et al; Pediatric Valsartan Study Group. Efficacy and safety of the angiotensin receptor blocker valsartan in children with hypertension aged 1 to 5 years. *Hypertension.* 2008;52(2):222–228

243. Schaefer F, van de Walle J, Zurowska A, et al; Candesartan in Children with Hypertension Investigators. Efficacy, safety and pharmacokinetics of candesartan cilexetil in hypertensive children from 1 to less than 6 years of age. *J Hypertens.* 2010;28(5):1083–1090

244. Webb NJ, Wells TG, Shahinfar S, et al. A randomized, open-label, dose-response study of losartan in hypertensive children. *Clin J Am Soc Nephrol.* 2014;9(8):1441–1448

245. Coleman DM, Eliason JL, Ohye RG, Stanley JC. Long-segment thoracoabdominal aortic occlusions in childhood. *J Vasc Surg.* 2012;56(2):482–485

246. Lee MG, Kowalski R, Galati JC, et al. Twenty-four-hour ambulatory blood pressure monitoring detects a high prevalence of hypertension late after coarctation repair in patients with hypoplastic arches. *J Thorac Cardiovasc Surg.* 2012;144(5):1110–1116

247. Agnoletti G, Bonnet C, Bonnet D, Sidi D, Aggoun Y. Mid-term effects of implanting stents for relief of aortic recoarctation on systemic hypertension, carotid mechanical properties, intimal medial thickness and reflection of the pulse wave. *Cardiol Young.* 2005;15(3):245–250

248. Young WF. Endocrine hypertension. In: Melmed S, Polonsky KS, Larsen R, Kronenberg HM, eds. *Williams Textbook of Endocrinology.* 13th ed. Philadelphia, PA: Elsevier Inc; 2016:556–588

249. Bausch B, Wellner U, Bausch D, et al. Long-term prognosis of patients with pediatric pheochromocytoma. *Endocr Relat Cancer.* 2013;21(1):17–25

250. Waguespack SG, Rich T, Grubbs E, et al. A current review of the etiology, diagnosis, and treatment of pediatric pheochromocytoma and paraganglioma. *J Clin Endocrinol Metab.* 2010;95(5):2023–2037

251. Fishbein L, Merrill S, Fraker DL, Cohen DL, Nathanson KL. Inherited mutations in pheochromocytoma and paraganglioma: why all patients should be offered genetic testing. *Ann Surg Oncol.* 2013;20(5):1444–1450

252. Barontini M, Levin G, Sanso G. Characteristics of pheochromocytoma in a 4- to 20-year-old population. *Ann N Y Acad Sci.* 2006;1073:30–37

253. Welander J, Söderkvist P, Gimm O. Genetics and clinical characteristics of hereditary pheochromocytomas and paragangliomas. *Endocr Relat Cancer.* 2011;18(6):R253–R276

254. Eisenhofer G, Peitzsch M. Laboratory evaluation of pheochromocytoma and paraganglioma. *Clin Chem.* 2014;60(12):1486–1499

255. Funder JW, Carey RM, Mantero F, et al. The management of primary aldosteronism: case detection, diagnosis, and treatment: an Endocrine Society clinical practice guideline. *J Clin Endocrinol Metab.* 2016;101(5):1889–1916

256. Stowasser M, Gordon RD. Monogenic mineralocorticoid hypertension. *Best Pract Res Clin Endocrinol Metab.* 2006;20(3):401–420

257. White PC, Dupont J, New MI, Leiberman E, Hochberg Z, Rösler A. A mutation in CYP11B1 (Arg-448---His) associated with steroid 11 beta-hydroxylase deficiency in Jews of Moroccan origin. *J Clin Invest.* 1991;87(5):1664–1667

258. Parsa AA, New MI. Low-renin hypertension of childhood. *Endocrinol Metab Clin North Am.* 2011;40(2):369–377, viii

259. Parajes S, Loidi L, Reisch N, et al. Functional consequences of seven novel mutations in the CYP11B1 gene: four mutations associated with nonclassic and three mutations causing classic 11beta-hydroxylase deficiency. *J Clin Endocrinol Metab.* 2010;95(2):779–788

260. New MI, Geller DS, Fallo F, Wilson RC. Monogenic low renin hypertension. *Trends Endocrinol Metab.* 2005;16(3):92–97

261. Imai T, Yanase T, Waterman MR, Simpson ER, Pratt JJ. Canadian Mennonites and individuals residing in the Friesland region of The Netherlands share the same molecular basis of 17 alpha-hydroxylase deficiency. *Hum Genet.* 1992;89(1):95–96

262. Dhir V, Reisch N, Bleicken CM, et al. Steroid 17alpha-hydroxylase deficiency: functional characterization of four mutations (A174E, V178D, R440C, L465P) in the CYP17A1 gene. *J Clin Endocrinol Metab.* 2009;94(8):3058–3064

263. Aglony M, Martínez-Aguayo A, Carvajal CA, et al. Frequency of familial hyperaldosteronism type 1 in a hypertensive pediatric population: clinical and biochemical presentation. *Hypertension.* 2011;57(6):1117–1121

264. Speiser PW, White PC. Congenital adrenal hyperplasia. *N Engl J Med.* 2003;349(8):776–788

265. Funder JW. Genetic disorders in primary aldosteronism — familial and somatic. *J Steroid Biochem Mol Biol.* 2017;165(pt A):154–157

266. Carss KJ, Stowasser M, Gordon RD, O'Shaughnessy KM. Further study of chromosome 7p22 to identify the molecular basis of familial hyperaldosteronism type II. *J Hum Hypertens.* 2011;25(9):560–564

267. So A, Duffy DL, Gordon RD, et al. Familial hyperaldosteronism type II is linked to the chromosome 7p22 region but also shows predicted heterogeneity. *J Hypertens.* 2005;23(8):1477–1484

268. Geller DS, Zhang J, Wisgerhof MV, Shackleton C, Key Action Statementhgarian M, Lifton RP. A novel form of human mendelian hypertension featuring nonglucocorticoid-remediable aldosteronism. *J Clin Endocrinol Metab.* 2008;93(8):3117–3123

269. Boulkroun S, Beuschlein F, Rossi GP, et al. Prevalence, clinical, and molecular correlates of KCNJ5 mutations in primary aldosteronism. *Hypertension.* 2012;59(3):592–598

270. Scholl UI, Nelson-Williams C, Yue P, et al. Hypertension with or without adrenal hyperplasia due to different inherited mutations in the potassium channel KCNJ5. *Proc Natl Acad Sci USA.* 2012;109(7):2533–2538

271. Scholl UI, Goh G, Stölting G, et al. Somatic and germline CACNA1D calcium channel mutations in aldosterone-producing adenomas and primary aldosteronism. *Nat Genet.* 2013;45(9):1050–1054

272. Scholl UI, Stölting G, Nelson-Williams C, et al. Recurrent gain of function mutation in calcium channel CACNA1H causes early-onset hypertension with primary aldosteronism. *Elife.* 2015;4:e06315

273. Rothenbuhler A, Stratakis CA. Clinical and molecular genetics of Carney complex. *Best Pract Res Clin Endocrinol Metab.* 2010;24(3):389–399

274. Stratakis CA, Salpea P, Raygada M. *Carney Complex.* Seattle, WA: University of Washington; 2015

275. Lietman SA, Schwindinger WF, Levine MA. Genetic and molecular aspects of McCune-Albright syndrome. *Pediatr Endocrinol Rev.* 2007;4(suppl 4):380–385

276. Lumbroso S, Paris F, Sultan C. McCune-Albright syndrome: molecular genetics. *J Pediatr Endocrinol Metab.* 2002;15(suppl 3):875–882

277. Malchoff CD, Javier EC, Malchoff DM, et al. Primary cortisol resistance presenting as isosexual precocity. *J Clin Endocrinol Metab.* 1990;70(2):503–507

278. Nicolaides NC, Charmandari E. Chrousos syndrome: from molecular pathogenesis to therapeutic management. *Eur J Clin Invest.* 2015;45(5):504–514

279. Malchoff DM, Brufsky A, Reardon G, et al. A mutation of the glucocorticoid receptor in primary cortisol resistance. *J Clin Invest.* 1993;91(5):1918–1925

280. Ferrari P. The role of 11β-hydroxysteroid dehydrogenase type 2 in human hypertension. *Biochim Biophys Acta.* 2010;1802(12):1178–1187

281. Morineau G, Sulmont V, Salomon R, et al. Apparent mineralocorticoid excess: report of six new cases and extensive personal experience. *J Am Soc Nephrol.* 2006;17(11):3176–3184

282. Nesterov V, Krueger B, Bertog M, Dahlmann A, Palmisano R, Korbmacher C. In Liddle syndrome, epithelial sodium channel is hyperactive mainly in the early part of the aldosterone-sensitive distal nephron. *Hypertension.* 2016;67(6):1256–1262

283. Hanukoglu I, Hanukoglu A. Epithelial sodium channel (ENaC) family: Phylogeny, structure-function, tissue distribution, and associated inherited diseases. *Gene.* 2016;579(2):95–132

284. Geller DS, Farhi A, Pinkerton N, et al. Activating mineralocorticoid receptor mutation in hypertension exacerbated by pregnancy. *Science.* 2000;289(5476):119–123

285. Wilson FH, Disse-Nicodème S, Choate KA, et al. Human hypertension caused by mutations in WNK kinases. *Science.* 2001;293(5532):1107–1112

286. Boyden LM, Choi M, Choate KA, et al. Mutations in kelch-like 3 and cullin 3 cause hypertension and electrolyte abnormalities. *Nature.* 2012;482(7383):98–102

287. Stowasser M, Pimenta E, Gordon RD. Familial or genetic primary aldosteronism and Gordon syndrome. *Endocrinol Metab Clin North Am.* 2011;40(2):343–368, viii

288. Sacerdote A, Weiss K, Tran T, Rokeya Noor B, McFarlane SI. Hypertension in patients with Cushing's disease: pathophysiology, diagnosis, and management. *Curr Hypertens Rep.* 2005;7(3):212–218

289. Baid S, Nieman LK. Glucocorticoid excess and hypertension. *Curr Hypertens Rep.* 2004;6(6):493–499

290. Michalkiewicz E, Sandrini R, Figueiredo B, et al. Clinical and outcome characteristics of children with adrenocortical tumors: a report from the International Pediatric Adrenocortical Tumor Registry. *J Clin Oncol.* 2004;22(5):838–845

291. Danzi S, Klein I. Thyroid hormone and blood pressure regulation. *Curr Hypertens Rep.* 2003;5(6):513–520

292. Bahn RS, Burch HB, Cooper DS, et al; American Thyroid Association; American Association of Clinical Endocrinologists. Hyperthyroidism and other causes of thyrotoxicosis: management guidelines of the American Thyroid Association and American Association of Clinical Endocrinologists. *Endocr Pract.* 2011;17(3):456–520

293. Heyliger A, Tangpricha V, Weber C, Sharma J. Parathyroidectomy decreases systolic and diastolic blood pressure in hypertensive patients with primary hyperparathyroidism. *Surgery.* 2009;146(6):1042–1047

294. Rydberg E, Birgander M, Bondeson AG, Bondeson L, Willenheimer R. Effect of successful parathyroidectomy on 24-hour ambulatory blood pressure in patients with primary hyperparathyroidism. *Int J Cardiol.* 2010;142(1):15–21

295. Gambelunghe A, Sallsten G, Borné Y, et al. Low-level exposure to lead, blood pressure, and hypertension in a population-based cohort. *Environ Res.* 2016;149:157–163

296. Lee BK, Ahn J, Kim NS, Lee CB, Park J, Kim Y. Association of blood pressure with exposure to lead and cadmium: analysis of data from the 2008-2013 Korean National Health and Nutrition Examination Survey. *Biol Trace Elem Res.* 2016;174(1):40–51

297. Rapisarda V, Ledda C, Ferrante M, et al. Blood pressure and occupational

exposure to noise and lead (Pb): a cross-sectional study. *Toxicol Ind Health*. 2016;32(10):1729–1736

298. Hara A, Thijs L, Asayama K, et al. Blood pressure in relation to environmental lead exposure in the national health and nutrition examination survey 2003 to 2010. *Hypertension*. 2015;65(1):62–69

299. Gump BB, Reihman J, Stewart P, Lonky E, Darvill T, Matthews KA. Blood lead (Pb) levels: a potential environmental mechanism explaining the relation between socioeconomic status and cardiovascular reactivity in children. *Health Psychol*. 2007;26(3):296–304

300. Chen A, Rhoads GG, Cai B, Salganik M, Rogan WJ. The effect of chelation on blood pressure in lead-exposed children: a randomized study. *Environ Health Perspect*. 2006;114(4):579–583

301. Chen X, Zhu G, Lei L, Jin T. The association between blood pressure and blood cadmium in a Chinese population living in cadmium polluted area. *Environ Toxicol Pharmacol*. 2013;36(2):595–599

302. Tellez-Plaza M, Navas-Acien A, Crainiceanu CM, Guallar E. Cadmium exposure and hypertension in the 1999-2004 National Health and Nutrition Examination Survey (NHANES). *Environ Health Perspect*. 2008;116(1):51–56

303. Gallagher CM, Meliker JR. Blood and urine cadmium, blood pressure, and hypertension: a systematic review and meta-analysis. *Environ Health Perspect*. 2010;118(12):1676–1684

304. Swaddiwudhipong W, Mahasakpan P, Jeekeeree W, et al. Renal and blood pressure effects from environmental cadmium exposure in Thai children. *Environ Res*. 2015;136:82–87

305. Cao Y, Chen A, Radcliffe J, et al. Postnatal cadmium exposure, neurodevelopment, and blood pressure in children at 2, 5, and 7 years of age. *Environ Health Perspect*. 2009;117(10):1580–1586

306. Park JD, Zheng W. Human exposure and health effects of inorganic and elemental mercury. *J Prev Med Public Health*. 2012;45(6):344–352

307. Weidemann DK, Weaver VM, Fadrowski JJ. Toxic environmental exposures and kidney health in children. *Pediatr Nephrol*. 2016;31(11):2043–2054

308. Torres AD, Rai AN, Hardiek ML. Mercury intoxication and arterial hypertension: report of two patients and review of the literature. *Pediatrics*. 2000;105(3). Available at: www.pediatrics.org/cgi/content/full/105/3/e34

309. Brannan EH, Su S, Alverson BK. Elemental mercury poisoning presenting as hypertension in a young child. *Pediatr Emerg Care*. 2012;28(8):812–814

310. Mercer JJ, Bercovitch L, Muglia JJ. Acrodynia and hypertension in a young girl secondary to elemental mercury toxicity acquired in the home. *Pediatr Dermatol*. 2012;29(2):199–201

311. Valvi D, Casas M, Romaguera D, et al. Prenatal phthalate exposure and childhood growth and blood pressure: evidence from the Spanish INMA-Sabadell Birth Cohort Study. *Environ Health Perspect*. 2015;123(10):1022–1029

312. Trasande L, Sathyanarayana S, Spanier AJ, Trachtman H, Attina TM, Urbina EM. Urinary phthalates are associated with higher blood pressure in childhood. *J Pediatr*. 2013;163(3):747–753.e1

313. Trasande L, Attina TM. Association of exposure to di-2-ethylhexylphthalate replacements with increased blood pressure in children and adolescents. *Hypertension*. 2015;66(2):301–308

314. Saif I, Seriki D, Moore R, Woywodt A. Midaortic syndrome in neurofibromatosis type 1 resulting in bilateral renal artery stenosis. *Am J Kidney Dis*. 2010;56(6):1197–1201

315. Kimura M, Kakizaki S, Kawano K, Sato S, Kure S. Neurofibromatosis type 1 complicated by atypical coarctation of the thoracic aorta. *Case Rep Pediatr*. 2013;2013:458543

316. Malav IC, Kothari SS. Renal artery stenosis due to neurofibromatosis. *Ann Pediatr Cardiol*. 2009;2(2):167–169

317. Mavani G, Kesar V, Devita MV, Rosenstock JL, Michelis MF, Schwimmer JA. Neurofibromatosis type 1-associated hypertension secondary to coarctation of the thoracic aorta. *Clin Kidney J*. 2014;7(4):394–395

318. Duan L, Feng K, Tong A, Liang Z. Renal artery stenosis due to neurofibromatosis type 1: case report and literature review. *Eur J Med Res*. 2014;19:17

319. Srinivasan A, Krishnamurthy G, Fontalvo-Herazo L, et al. Spectrum of renal findings in pediatric fibromuscular dysplasia and neurofibromatosis type 1. *Pediatr Radiol*. 2011;41(3):308–316

320. Dubov T, Toledano-Alhadef H, Chernin G, Constantini S, Cleper R, Ben-Shachar S. High prevalence of elevated blood pressure among children with neurofibromatosis type 1. *Pediatr Nephrol*. 2016;31(1):131–136

321. Erem C, Onder Ersöz H, Ukinç K, et al. Neurofibromatosis type 1 associated with pheochromocytoma: a case report and a review of the literature. *J Endocrinol Invest*. 2007;30(1):59–64

322. Zinnamosca L, Petramala L, Cotesta D, et al. Neurofibromatosis type 1 (NF1) and pheochromocytoma: prevalence, clinical and cardiovascular aspects. *Arch Dermatol Res*. 2011;303(5):317–325

323. Nawrot TS, Den Hond E, Fagard RH, Hoppenbrouwers K, Staessen JA. Blood pressure, serum total cholesterol and contraceptive pill use in 17-year-old girls. *Eur J Cardiovasc Prev Rehabil*. 2003;10(6):438–442

324. Le-Ha C, Beilin LJ, Burrows S, et al. Oral contraceptive use in girls and alcohol consumption in boys are associated with increased blood pressure in late adolescence. *Eur J Prev Cardiol*. 2013;20(6):947–955

325. Du Y, Rosner BM, Knopf H, Schwarz S, Dören M, Scheidt-Nave C. Hormonal contraceptive use among adolescent girls in Germany in relation to health behavior and biological cardiovascular risk factors. *J Adolesc Health*. 2011;48(4):331–337

326. Samuels JA, Franco K, Wan F, Sorof JM. Effect of stimulants on 24-h ambulatory blood pressure in children with ADHD: a double-blind, randomized, cross-over trial. *Pediatr Nephrol*. 2006;21(1):92–95

327. Covar RA, Leung DY, McCormick D, Steelman J, Zeitler P, Spahn JD. Risk

factors associated with glucocorticoid-induced adverse effects in children with severe asthma. *J Allergy Clin Immunol.* 2000;106(4):651–659

328. Vehaskari VM. Heritable forms of hypertension. *Pediatr Nephrol.* 2009;24(10):1929–1937

329. Halperin F, Dluhy RG. Glucocorticoid-remediable aldosteronism. *Endocrinol Metab Clin North Am.* 2011;40(2):333–341, viii

330. Staley JR, Bradley J, Silverwood RJ, et al. Associations of blood pressure in pregnancy with offspring blood pressure trajectories during childhood and adolescence: findings from a prospective study. *J Am Heart Assoc.* 2015;4(5):e001422

331. Daniels SD, Meyer RA, Loggie JM. Determinants of cardiac involvement in children and adolescents with essential hypertension. *Circulation.* 1990;82(4):1243–1248

332. Yang Q, Zhang Z, Kuklina EV, et al. Sodium intake and blood pressure among US children and adolescents. *Pediatrics.* 2012;130(4):611–619

333. He FJ, MacGregor GA. Importance of salt in determining blood pressure in children: meta-analysis of controlled trials. *Hypertension.* 2006;48(5):861–869

334. Aeberli I, Spinas GA, Lehmann R, l'Allemand D, Molinari L, Zimmermann MB. Diet determines features of the metabolic syndrome in 6- to 14-year-old children. *Int J Vitam Nutr Res.* 2009;79(1):14–23

335. Colín-Ramírez E, Castillo-Martínez L, Orea-Tejeda A, Villa Romero AR, Vergara Castañeda A, Asensio Lafuente E. Waist circumference and fat intake are associated with high blood pressure in Mexican children aged 8 to 10 years. *J Am Diet Assoc.* 2009;109(6):996–1003

336. Niinikoski H, Jula A, Viikari J, et al. Blood pressure is lower in children and adolescents with a low-saturated-fat diet since infancy: the special turku coronary risk factor intervention project. *Hypertension.* 2009;53(6):918–924

337. Institute of Medicine. *Strategies to Reduce Sodium Intake in the United States.* Washington, DC: National Academies Press; 2010

338. Adler AJ, Taylor F, Martin N, Gottlieb S, Taylor RS, Ebrahim S. Reduced dietary salt for the prevention of cardiovascular disease. *Cochrane Database Syst Rev.* 2014;(12):CD009217

339. Rebholz CM, Gu D, Chen J, et al; GenSalt Collaborative Research Group. Physical activity reduces salt sensitivity of blood pressure: the Genetic Epidemiology Network of Salt Sensitivity study. *Am J Epidemiol.* 2012;176(suppl 7):S106–S113

340. Torrance B, McGuire KA, Lewanczuk R, McGavock J. Overweight, physical activity and high blood pressure in children: a review of the literature. *Vasc Health Risk Manag.* 2007;3(1):139–149

341. Chen HH, Chen YL, Huang CY, Lee SD, Chen SC, Kuo CH. Effects of one-year swimming training on blood pressure and insulin sensitivity in mild hypertensive young patients. *Chin J Physiol.* 2010;53(3):185–189

342. Farpour-Lambert NJ, Aggoun Y, Marchand LM, Martin XE, Herrmann FR, Beghetti M. Physical activity reduces systemic blood pressure and improves early markers of atherosclerosis in pre-pubertal obese children. *J Am Coll Cardiol.* 2009;54(25):2396–2406

343. Cai L, Wu Y, Cheskin LJ, Wilson RF, Wang Y. Effect of childhood obesity prevention programmes on blood lipids: a systematic review and meta-analysis. *Obes Rev.* 2014;15(12):933–944

344. Kelley GA, Kelley KS, Tran ZV. The effects of exercise on resting blood pressure in children and adolescents: a meta-analysis of randomized controlled trials. *Prev Cardiol.* 2003;6(1):8–16

345. van Dijk AE, van Eijsden M, Stronks K, Gemke RJ, Vrijkotte TG. The association between prenatal psychosocial stress and blood pressure in the child at age 5-7 years. *PLoS One.* 2012;7(8):e43548

346. Stein DJ, Scott K, Haro Abad JM, et al. Early childhood adversity and later hypertension: data from the World Mental Health Survey. *Ann Clin Psychiatry.* 2010;22(1):19–28

347. Halonen JI, Stenholm S, Pentti J, et al. Childhood psychosocial adversity and adult neighborhood disadvantage as predictors of cardiovascular disease: a cohort study. *Circulation.* 2015;132(5):371–379

348. Maggio AB, Martin XE, Saunders Gasser C, et al. Medical and non-medical complications among children and adolescents with excessive body weight. *BMC Pediatr.* 2014;14:232

349. Yun M, Li S, Sun D, et al. Tobacco smoking strengthens the association of elevated blood pressure with arterial stiffness: the Bogalusa Heart Study. *J Hypertens.* 2015;33(2):266–274

350. Priest JR, Nead KT, Wehner MR, Cooke JP, Leeper NJ. Self-reported history of childhood smoking is associated with an increased risk for peripheral arterial disease independent of lifetime smoking burden. *PLoS One.* 2014;9(2):e88972

351. Hagan JFSJ, Duncan PM. *Bright Futures: Guidelines for Health Supervision of Infants, Children, and Adolescents.* 3rd ed. Elk Grove Village, IL: American Academy of Pediatrics; 2008

352. Benson L, Baer HJ, Greco PJ, Kaelber DC. When is family history obtained? - Lack of timely documentation of family history among overweight and hypertensive paediatric patients. *J Paediatr Child Health.* 2010;46(10):600–605

353. Flynn JT. Evaluation and management of hypertension in childhood. *Prog Pediatr Cardiol.* 2001;12(2):177–188

354. Wiesen J, Adkins M, Fortune S, et al. Evaluation of pediatric patients with mild-to-moderate hypertension: yield of diagnostic testing. *Pediatrics.* 2008;122(5). Available at: www.pediatrics.org/cgi/content/full/122/5/e988

355. Yoon EY, Cohn L, Rocchini A, et al. Use of diagnostic tests in adolescents with essential hypertension. *Arch Pediatr Adolesc Med.* 2012;166(9):857–862

356. Killian L, Simpson JM, Savis A, Rawlins D, Sinha MD. Electrocardiography is a poor screening test to detect left ventricular hypertrophy in children. *Arch Dis Child.* 2010;95(10):832–836

357. Ramaswamy P, Patel E, Fahey M, Mahgerefteh J, Lytrivi ID, Kupferman JC. Electrocardiographic predictors of left ventricular hypertrophy in pediatric hypertension. *J Pediatr.* 2009;154(1):106–110

358. Rijnbeek PR, van Herpen G, Kapusta L, Ten Harkel AD, Witsenburg M, Kors JA. Electrocardiographic criteria for left ventricular hypertrophy in children. *Pediatr Cardiol.* 2008;29(5):923–928

359. Grossman A, Prokupetz A, Koren-Morag N, Grossman E, Shamiss A. Comparison of usefulness of Sokolow and Cornell criteria for left ventricular hypertrophy in subjects aged <20 years versus >30 years. *Am J Cardiol.* 2012;110(3):440–444

360. Caselli S, Maron MS, Urbano-Moral JA, Pandian NG, Maron BJ, Pelliccia A. Differentiating left ventricular hypertrophy in athletes from that in patients with hypertrophic cardiomyopathy. *Am J Cardiol.* 2014;114(9):1383–1389

361. Urbina EM, Gidding SS, Bao W, Pickoff AS, Berdusis K, Berenson GS. Effect of body size, ponderosity, and blood pressure on left ventricular growth in children and young adults in the Bogalusa Heart Study. *Circulation.* 1995;91(9):2400–2406

362. Kuznetsova T, Haddad F, Tikhonoff V, et al; European Project On Genes in Hypertension (EPOGH) Investigators. Impact and pitfalls of scaling of left ventricular and atrial structure in population-based studies. *J Hypertens.* 2016;34(6):1186–1194

363. Armstrong AC, Gidding S, Gjesdal O, Wu C, Bluemke DA, Lima JA. LV mass assessed by echocardiography and CMR, cardiovascular outcomes, and medical practice. *JACC Cardiovasc Imaging.* 2012;5(8):837–848

364. Armstrong AC, Jacobs DR Jr, Gidding SS, et al. Framingham score and LV mass predict events in young adults: CARDIA study. *Int J Cardiol.* 2014;172(2):350–355

365. Gidding SS, Palermo RA, DeLoach SS, Keith SW, Falkner B. Associations of cardiac structure with obesity, blood pressure, inflammation, and insulin resistance in African-American adolescents. *Pediatr Cardiol.* 2014;35(2):307–314

366. Hanevold C, Waller J, Daniels S, Portman R, Sorof J; International Pediatric Hypertension Association. The effects of obesity, gender, and ethnic group on left ventricular hypertrophy and geometry in hypertensive children: a collaborative study of the International Pediatric Hypertension Association. *Pediatrics.* 2004;113(2):328–333

367. Daniels SR, Loggie JM, Khoury P, Kimball TR. Left ventricular geometry and severe left ventricular hypertrophy in children and adolescents with essential hypertension. *Circulation.* 1998;97(19):1907–1911

368. Devereux RB, Wachtell K, Gerdts E, et al. Prognostic significance of left ventricular mass change during treatment of hypertension. *JAMA.* 2004;292(19):2350–2356

369. Lang RM, Badano LP, Mor-Avi V, et al. Recommendations for cardiac chamber quantification by echocardiography in adults: an update from the American Society of Echocardiography and the European Association of Cardiovascular Imaging. *J Am Soc Echocardiogr.* 2015;28(1):1–39.e14

370. Daniels SR, Kimball TR, Morrison JA, Khoury P, Witt S, Meyer RA. Effect of lean body mass, fat mass, blood pressure, and sexual maturation on left ventricular mass in children and adolescents. Statistical, biological, and clinical significance. *Circulation.* 1995;92(11):3249–3254

371. Lopez L, Colan SD, Frommelt PC, et al. Recommendations for quantification methods during the performance of a pediatric echocardiogram: a report from the Pediatric Measurements Writing Group of the American Society of Echocardiography Pediatric and Congenital Heart Disease Council. *J Am Soc Echocardiogr.* 2010;23(5):465–495, quiz 576–577

372. Foster BJ, Khoury PR, Kimball TR, Mackie AS, Mitsnefes M. New reference centiles for left ventricular mass relative to lean body mass in children. *J Am Soc Echocardiogr.* 2016;29(5):441–447.e2

373. Khoury PR, Mitsnefes M, Daniels SR, Kimball TR. Age-specific reference intervals for indexed left ventricular mass in children. *J Am Soc Echocardiogr.* 2009;22(6):709–714

374. Lipshultz SE, Easley KA, Orav EJ, et al. Reliability of multicenter pediatric echocardiographic measurements of left ventricular structure and function: the prospective P(2)C(2) HIV study. *Circulation.* 2001;104(3):310–316

375. Urbina EM. Abnormalities of vascular structure and function in pediatric hypertension. *Pediatr Nephrol.* 2016;31(7):1061–1070

376. Elmenhorst J, Hulpke-Wette M, Barta C, Dalla Pozza R, Springer S, Oberhoffer R. Percentiles for central blood pressure and pulse wave velocity in children and adolescents recorded with an oscillometric device. *Atherosclerosis.* 2015;238(1):9–16

377. Hidvégi EV, Illyés M, Benczúr B, et al. Reference values of aortic pulse wave velocity in a large healthy population aged between 3 and 18 years. *J Hypertens.* 2012;30(12):2314–2321

378. Miyai N, Utsumi M, Gowa Y, et al. Age-specific nomogram of brachial-ankle pulse wave velocity in Japanese adolescents. *Clin Exp Hypertens.* 2013;35(2):95–101

379. Urbina EM, Khoury PR, McCoy CE, Dolan LM, Daniels SR, Kimball TR. Triglyceride to HDL-C ratio and increased arterial stiffness in children, adolescents, and young adults [published correction appears in *Pediatrics.* 2013;132(4):780]. *Pediatrics.* 2013;131(4). Available at: www.pediatrics.org/cgi/content/full/131/4/e1082

380. Lurbe E, Torro I, Garcia-Vicent C, Alvarez J, Fernández-Fornoso JA, Redon J. Blood pressure and obesity exert independent influences on pulse wave velocity in youth. *Hypertension.* 2012;60(2):550–555

381. Zhu H, Yan W, Ge D, et al. Relationships of cardiovascular phenotypes with healthy weight, at risk of overweight, and overweight in US youths. *Pediatrics.* 2008;121(1):115–122

382. Charakida M, Jones A, Falaschetti E, et al. Childhood obesity and vascular

phenotypes: a population study. *J Am Coll Cardiol.* 2012;60(25):2643–2650

383. Doyon A, Kracht D, Bayazit AK, et al; 4C Study Consortium. Carotid artery intima-media thickness and distensibility in children and adolescents: reference values and role of body dimensions. *Hypertension.* 2013;62(3):550–556

384. Urbina EM, Kimball TR, McCoy CE, Khoury PR, Daniels SR, Dolan LM. Youth with obesity and obesity-related type 2 diabetes mellitus demonstrate abnormalities in carotid structure and function. *Circulation.* 2009;119(22):2913–2919

385. Keehn L, Milne L, McNeill K, Chowienczyk P, Sinha MD. Measurement of pulse wave velocity in children: comparison of volumetric and tonometric sensors, brachial-femoral and carotid-femoral pathways. *J Hypertens.* 2014;32(7):1464–1469, discussion 1469

386. Kis E, Cseprekál O, Kerti A, et al. Measurement of pulse wave velocity in children and young adults: a comparative study using three different devices. *Hypertens Res.* 2011;34(11):1197–1202

387. Chhadia S, Cohn RA, Vural G, Donaldson JS. Renal Doppler evaluation in the child with hypertension: a reasonable screening discriminator? *Pediatr Radiol.* 2013;43(12):1549–1556

388. Castelli PK, Dillman JR, Kershaw DB, Khalatbari S, Stanley JC, Smith EA. Renal sonography with Doppler for detecting suspected pediatric renin-mediated hypertension - is it adequate? *Pediatr Radiol.* 2014;44(1):42–49

389. Rountas C, Vlychou M, Vassiou K, et al. Imaging modalities for renal artery stenosis in suspected renovascular hypertension: prospective intraindividual comparison of color Doppler US, CT angiography, GD-enhanced MR angiography, and digital substraction angiography. *Ren Fail.* 2007;29(3):295–302

390. Marks SD, Tullus K. Update on imaging for suspected renovascular hypertension in children and adolescents. *Curr Hypertens Rep.* 2012;14(6):591–595

391. Lagomarsino E, Orellana P, Muñoz J, Velásquez C, Cavagnaro F, Valdés F. Captopril scintigraphy in the study of arterial hypertension in pediatrics. *Pediatr Nephrol.* 2004;19(1):66–70

392. Abdulsamea S, Anderson P, Biassoni L, et al. Pre- and postcaptopril renal scintigraphy as a screening test for renovascular hypertension in children. *Pediatr Nephrol.* 2010;25(2):317–322

393. Günay EC, Oztürk MH, Ergün EL, et al. Losartan renography for the detection of renal artery stenosis: comparison with captopril renography and evaluation of dose and timing. *Eur J Nucl Med Mol Imaging.* 2005;32(9):1064–1074

394. Reusz GS, Kis E, Cseprekál O, Szabó AJ, Kis E. Captopril-enhanced renal scintigraphy in the diagnosis of pediatric hypertension. *Pediatr Nephrol.* 2010;25(2):185–189

395. Loeffler LF, Navas-Acien A, Brady TM, Miller ER III, Fadrowski JJ. Uric acid level and elevated blood pressure in US adolescents: National Health and Nutrition Examination Survey, 1999-2006. *Hypertension.* 2012;59(4):811–817

396. Shatat IF, Abdallah RT, Sas DJ, Hailpern SM. Serum uric acid in U.S. adolescents: distribution and relationship to demographic characteristics and cardiovascular risk factors. *Pediatr Res.* 2012;72(1):95–100

397. Viazzi F, Antolini L, Giussani M, et al. Serum uric acid and blood pressure in children at cardiovascular risk. *Pediatrics.* 2013;132(1). Available at: www.pediatrics.org/cgi/content/full/132/1/e93

398. Reschke LD, Miller ER III, Fadrowski JJ, et al. Elevated uric acid and obesity-related cardiovascular disease risk factors among hypertensive youth. *Pediatr Nephrol.* 2015;30(12):2169–2176

399. Alper AB Jr, Chen W, Yau L, Srinivasan SR, Berenson GS, Hamm LL. Childhood uric acid predicts adult blood pressure: the Bogalusa Heart Study. *Hypertension.* 2005;45(1):34–38

400. Soletsky B, Feig DI. Uric acid reduction rectifies prehypertension

in obese adolescents. *Hypertension.* 2012;60(5):1148–1156

401. Feig DI, Soletsky B, Johnson RJ. Effect of allopurinol on blood pressure of adolescents with newly diagnosed essential hypertension: a randomized trial. *JAMA.* 2008;300(8):924–932

402. Assadi F. Allopurinol enhances the blood pressure lowering effect of enalapril in children with hyperuricemic essential hypertension. *J Nephrol.* 2014;27(1):51–56

403. Feig DI, Nakagawa T, Karumanchi SA, et al. Hypothesis: uric acid, nephron number, and the pathogenesis of essential hypertension. *Kidney Int.* 2004;66(1):281–287

404. Viazzi F, Rebora P, Giussani M, et al. Increased serum uric acid levels blunt the antihypertensive efficacy of lifestyle modifications in children at cardiovascular risk. *Hypertension.* 2016;67(5):934–940

405. Klausen K, Borch-Johnsen K, Feldt-Rasmussen B, et al. Very low levels of microalbuminuria are associated with increased risk of coronary heart disease and death independently of renal function, hypertension, and diabetes. *Circulation.* 2004;110(1):32–35

406. Bigazzi R, Bianchi S, Baldari D, Campese VM. Microalbuminuria predicts cardiovascular events and renal insufficiency in patients with essential hypertension. *J Hypertens.* 1998;16(9):1325–1333

407. Chugh A, Bakris GL. Microalbuminuria: what is it? Why is it important? What should be done about it? An update. *J Clin Hypertens (Greenwich).* 2007;9(3):196–200

408. Flynn JT. Microalbuminuria in children with primary hypertension. *J Clin Hypertens (Greenwich).* 2016;18(10):962–965

409. Radhakishun NN, van Vliet M, von Rosenstiel IA, Beijnen JH, Diamant M. Limited value of routine microalbuminuria assessment in multi-ethnic obese children. *Pediatr Nephrol.* 2013;28(7):1145–1149

410. Tsioufis C, Mazaraki A, Dimitriadis K, Stefanidis CJ, Stefanadis C. Microalbuminuria in the paediatric age: current knowledge and

emerging questions. *Acta Paediatr.* 2011;100(9):1180–1184

411. Seeman T, Pohl M, Palyzova D, John U. Microalbuminuria in children with primary and white-coat hypertension. *Pediatr Nephrol.* 2012;27(3):461–467

412. Sanad M, Gharib A. Evaluation of microalbuminuria in obese children and its relation to metabolic syndrome. *Pediatr Nephrol.* 2011;26(12):2193–2199

413. Assadi F. Effect of microalbuminuria lowering on regression of left ventricular hypertrophy in children and adolescents with essential hypertension. *Pediatr Cardiol.* 2007;28(1):27–33

414. Niemirska A, Litwin M, Feber J, Jurkiewicz E. Blood pressure rhythmicity and visceral fat in children with hypertension. *Hypertension.* 2013;62(4):782–788

415. Kupferman JC, Paterno K, Mahgerefteh J, et al. Improvement of left ventricular mass with antihypertensive therapy in children with hypertension. *Pediatr Nephrol.* 2010;25(8):1513–1518

416. Falkner B, DeLoach S, Keith SW, Gidding SS. High risk blood pressure and obesity increase the risk for left ventricular hypertrophy in African-American adolescents. *J Pediatr.* 2013;162(1):94–100

417. Stabouli S, Kotsis V, Rizos Z, et al. Left ventricular mass in normotensive, prehypertensive and hypertensive children and adolescents. *Pediatr Nephrol.* 2009;24(8):1545–1551

418. Tirosh A, Afek A, Rudich A, et al. Progression of normotensive adolescents to hypertensive adults: a study of 26,980 teenagers. *Hypertension.* 2010;56(2):203–209

419. Chobanian AV, Bakris GL, Black HR; National Heart, Lung, and Blood Institute Joint National Committee on Prevention, Detection, Evaluation, and Treatment of High Blood Pressure; National High Blood Pressure Education Program Coordinating Committee. The seventh report of the Joint National Committee on prevention, detection, evaluation, and treatment of high blood pressure: the JNC 7 report [published correction appears in *JAMA.* 2003;290(2):197]. *JAMA.* 2003;289(19):2560–2571

420. Moreno-Luna R, Muñoz-Hernandez R, Miranda ML, et al. Olive oil polyphenols decrease blood pressure and improve endothelial function in young women with mild hypertension. *Am J Hypertens.* 2012;25(12):1299–1304

421. Damasceno MM, de Araújo MF, de Freitas RW, de Almeida PC, Zanetti ML. The association between blood pressure in adolescents and the consumption of fruits, vegetables and fruit juice--an exploratory study. *J Clin Nurs.* 2011;20(11–12):1553–1560

422. Juonala M, Viikari JS, Kähönen M, et al. Life-time risk factors and progression of carotid atherosclerosis in young adults: the Cardiovascular Risk in Young Finns study. *Eur Heart J.* 2010;31(14):1745–1751

423. Yuan WL, Kakinami L, Gray-Donald K, Czernichow S, Lambert M, Paradis G. Influence of dairy product consumption on children's blood pressure: results from the QUALITY cohort. *J Acad Nutr Diet.* 2013;113(7):936–941

424. Moore LL, Bradlee ML, Singer MR, Qureshi MM, Buendia JR, Daniels SR. Dietary approaches to stop hypertension (DASH) eating pattern and risk of elevated blood pressure in adolescent girls. *Br J Nutr.* 2012;108(9):1678–1685

425. Günther AL, Liese AD, Bell RA, et al. Association between the dietary approaches to hypertension diet and hypertension in youth with diabetes mellitus. *Hypertension.* 2009;53(1):6–12

426. Couch SC, Saelens BE, Levin L, Dart K, Falciglia G, Daniels SR. The efficacy of a clinic-based behavioral nutrition intervention emphasizing a DASH-type diet for adolescents with elevated blood pressure. *J Pediatr.* 2008;152(4):494–501

427. Davis JN, Ventura EE, Cook LT, Gyllenhammer LE, Gatto NMLA. LA Sprouts: a gardening, nutrition, and cooking intervention for Latino youth improves diet and reduces obesity. *J Am Diet Assoc.* 2011;111(8):1224–1230

428. Saneei P, Hashemipour M, Kelishadi R, Rajaei S, Esmaillzadeh A.
Effects of recommendations to follow the dietary approaches to stop hypertension (DASH) diet v. usual dietary advice on childhood metabolic syndrome: a randomised cross-over clinical trial. *Br J Nutr.* 2013;110(12):2250–2259

429. Barnes TL, Crandell JL, Bell RA, Mayer-Davis EJ, Dabelea D, Liese AD. Change in DASH diet score and cardiovascular risk factors in youth with type 1 and type 2 diabetes mellitus: the SEARCH for Diabetes in Youth study. *Nutr Diabetes.* 2013;3:e91

430. Rao M, Afshin A, Singh G, Mozaffarian D. Do healthier foods and diet patterns cost more than less healthy options? A systematic review and meta-analysis. *BMJ Open.* 2013;3(12):e004277

431. Monzavi R, Dreimane D, Geffner ME, et al. Improvement in risk factors for metabolic syndrome and insulin resistance in overweight youth who are treated with lifestyle intervention. *Pediatrics.* 2006;117(6). Available at: www.pediatrics.org/cgi/content/full/117/6/e1111

432. Asghari G, Yuzbashian E, Mirmiran P, Hooshmand F, Najafi R, Azizi F. Dietary approaches to stop hypertension (DASH) dietary pattern is associated with reduced incidence of metabolic syndrome in children and adolescents. *J Pediatr.* 2016;174:178–184.e1

433. Pacifico L, Anania C, Martino F, et al. Management of metabolic syndrome in children and adolescents. *Nutr Metab Cardiovasc Dis.* 2011;21(6):455–466

434. Puri M, Flynn JT. Management of hypertension in children and adolescents with the metabolic syndrome. *J Cardiometab Syndr.* 2006;1(4):259–268

435. Davis MM, Gance-Cleveland B, Hassink S, Johnson R, Paradis G, Resnicow K. Recommendations for prevention of childhood obesity. *Pediatrics.* 2007;120(suppl 4):S229–S253

436. Ogedegbe G, Chaplin W, Schoenthaler A, et al. A practice-based trial of motivational interviewing and adherence in hypertensive African Americans. *Am J Hypertens.* 2008;21(10):1137–1143

437. Bosworth HB, Olsen MK, Neary A, et al. Take Control of Your Blood Pressure (TCYB) study: a multifactorial tailored behavioral and educational intervention for achieving blood pressure control. *Patient Educ Couns.* 2008;70(3):338–347

438. Resnicow K, McMaster F, Bocian A, et al. Motivational interviewing and dietary counseling for obesity in primary care: an RCT. *Pediatrics.* 2015;135(4):649–657

439. Davoli AM, Broccoli S, Bonvicini L, et al. Pediatrician-led motivational interviewing to treat overweight children: an RCT. *Pediatrics.* 2013;132(5). Available at: www.pediatrics.org/cgi/content/full/132/5/e1236

440. Broccoli S, Davoli AM, Bonvicini L, et al. Motivational interviewing to treat overweight children: 24-month follow-up of a randomized controlled trial. *Pediatrics.* 2016;137(1):e20151979

441. Flattum C, Friend S, Neumark-Sztainer D, Story M. Motivational interviewing as a component of a school-based obesity prevention program for adolescent girls. *J Am Diet Assoc.* 2009;109(1):91–94

442. Schwartz RP, Hamre R, Dietz WH, et al. Office-based motivational interviewing to prevent childhood obesity: a feasibility study. *Arch Pediatr Adolesc Med.* 2007;161(5):495–501

443. Döring N, Ghaderi A, Bohman B, et al. Motivational interviewing to prevent childhood obesity: a cluster RCT. *Pediatrics.* 2016;137(5):1–10

444. Spear BA, Barlow SE, Ervin C, et al. Recommendations for treatment of child and adolescent overweight and obesity. *Pediatrics.* 2007;120(4, suppl 4):S254–S288

445. Kabat-Zinn J, Hanh TN. *Full Catastrophe Living: Using the Wisdom of Your Body and Mind to Face Stress, Pain, and Illness.* New York, NY: Delta; 1990

446. Gregoski MJ, Barnes VA, Tingen MS, Harshfield GA, Treiber FA. Breathing awareness meditation and LifeSkills Training programs influence upon ambulatory blood pressure and sodium excretion among African American adolescents. *J Adolesc Health.* 2011;48(1):59–64

447. Barnes VA, Kapuku GK, Treiber FA. Impact of transcendental meditation on left ventricular mass in African American adolescents. *Evid Based Complement Alternat Med.* 2012;2012:923153

448. Sieverdes JC, Mueller M, Gregoski MJ, et al. Effects of Hatha yoga on blood pressure, salivary α-amylase, and cortisol function among normotensive and prehypertensive youth. *J Altern Complement Med.* 2014;20(4):241–250

449. Sorof JM, Cargo P, Graepel J, et al. β-blocker/thiazide combination for treatment of hypertensive children: a randomized double-blind, placebo-controlled trial. *Pediatr Nephrol.* 2002;17(5):345–350

450. Trachtman H, Hainer JW, Sugg J, Teng R, Sorof JM, Radcliffe J; Candesartan in Children with Hypertension (CINCH) Investigators. Efficacy, safety, and pharmacokinetics of candesartan cilexetil in hypertensive children aged 6 to 17 years. *J Clin Hypertens (Greenwich).* 2008;10(10):743–750

451. Herder SD, Weber E, Winkemann A, Herder C, Morck H. Efficacy and safety of angiotensin II receptor type 1 antagonists in children and adolescents. *Pediatr Nephrol.* 2010;25(5):801–811

452. Schaefer F, Litwin M, Zachwieja J, et al. Efficacy and safety of valsartan compared to enalapril in hypertensive children: a 12-week, randomized, double-blind, parallel-group study. *J Hypertens.* 2011;29(12):2484–2490

453. Gartenmann AC, Fossali E, von Vigier RO, et al. Better renoprotective effect of angiotensin II antagonist compared to dihydropyridine calcium channel blocker in childhood. *Kidney Int.* 2003;64(4):1450–1454

454. Chaturvedi S, Lipszyc DH, Licht C, Craig JC, Parekh R. Pharmacological interventions for hypertension in children. *Evid Based Child Health.* 2014;9(3):498–580

455. Flynn JT. Efficacy and safety of prolonged amlodipine treatment in hypertensive children. *Pediatr Nephrol.* 2005;20(5):631–635

456. Schaefer F, Coppo R, Bagga A, et al. Efficacy and safety of valsartan in hypertensive children 6 months to 5 years of age. *J Hypertens.* 2013;31(5):993–1000

457. Batisky DL, Sorof JM, Sugg J, et al; Toprol-XL Pediatric Hypertension Investigators. Efficacy and safety of extended release metoprolol succinate in hypertensive children 6 to 16 years of age: a clinical trial experience. *J Pediatr.* 2007;150(2):134–139, 139.e1

458. Wells T, Blumer J, Meyers KE, et al; Valsartan Pediatric Hypertension Study Group. Effectiveness and safety of valsartan in children aged 6 to 16 years with hypertension. *J Clin Hypertens (Greenwich).* 2011;13(5):357–365

459. Trachtman H, Frank R, Mahan JD, et al. Clinical trial of extended-release felodipine in pediatric essential hypertension. *Pediatr Nephrol.* 2003;18(6):548–553

460. Shahinfar S, Cano F, Soffer BA, et al. A double-blind, dose-response study of losartan in hypertensive children. *Am J Hypertens.* 2005;18(2, pt 1):183–190

461. Hazan L, Hernández Rodriguez OA, Bhorat AE, Miyazaki K, Tao B, Heyrman R; Assessment of Efficacy and Safety of Olmesartan in Pediatric Hypertension Study Group. A double-blind, dose-response study of the efficacy and safety of olmesartan medoxomil in children and adolescents with hypertension. *Hypertension.* 2010;55(6):1323–1330

462. Flynn JT, Newburger JW, Daniels SR, et al; PATH-1 Investigators. A randomized, placebo-controlled trial of amlodipine in children with hypertension. *J Pediatr.* 2004;145(3):353–359

463. Simonetti GD, Rizzi M, Donadini R, Bianchetti MG. Effects of antihypertensive drugs on blood pressure and proteinuria in childhood. *J Hypertens.* 2007;25(12):2370–2376

464. Seeman T, Dusek J, Vondrák K, Flögelová H, Geier P, Janda J. Ramipril in the treatment of hypertension and proteinuria in children with chronic kidney diseases. *Am J Hypertens.* 2004;17(5, pt 1):415–420

465. Hammer GB, Verghese ST, Drover DR, Yaster M, Tobin JR. Pharmacokinetics and pharmacodynamics of fenoldopam mesylate for blood pressure control

in pediatric patients. *BMC Anesthesiol.* 2008;8:6

466. Blowey DL. Update on the pharmacologic treatment of hypertension in pediatrics. *J Clin Hypertens (Greenwich).* 2012;14(6):383–387

467. Li JS, Flynn JT, Portman R, et al. The efficacy and safety of the novel aldosterone antagonist eplerenone in children with hypertension: a randomized, double-blind, dose-response study. *J Pediatr.* 2010;157(2):282–287

468. U.S. Food and Drug Administration. Pediatric product development. Available at: www.fda.gov/Drugs/ DevelopmentApprovalProcess/ DevelopmentResources/ucm049867. htm. Accessed February 6, 2017

469. Croxall JD. Valsartan: in children and adolescents with hypertension. *Paediatr Drugs.* 2012;14(3):201–207

470. Menon S, Berezny KY, Kilaru R, et al. Racial differences are seen in blood pressure response to fosinopril in hypertensive children. *Am Heart J.* 2006;152(2):394–399

471. Li JS, Baker-Smith CM, Smith PB, et al. Racial differences in blood pressure response to angiotensin-converting enzyme inhibitors in children: a meta-analysis. *Clin Pharmacol Ther.* 2008;84(3):315–319

472. Seeman T, Dostálek L, Gilík J. Control of hypertension in treated children and its association with target organ damage. *Am J Hypertens.* 2012;25(3):389–395

473. Redwine K, Howard L, Simpson P, et al; Network of Pediatric Pharmacology Research Units. Effect of placebo on ambulatory blood pressure monitoring in children. *Pediatr Nephrol.* 2012;27(10):1937–1942

474. Halbach SM, Hamman R, Yonekawa K, Hanevold C. Utility of ambulatory blood pressure monitoring in the evaluation of elevated clinic blood pressures in children. *J Am Soc Hypertens.* 2016;10(5):406–412

475. White WB, Turner JR, Sica DA, et al. Detection, evaluation, and treatment of severe and resistant hypertension: proceedings from an American Society of Hypertension Interactive forum held in Bethesda, MD, U.S.A., October 10th, 2013. *J Am Soc Hypertens.* 2014;8(10):743–757

476. Narayan H, Webb DJ. New evidence supporting the use of mineralocorticoid receptor blockers in drug-resistant hypertension. *Curr Hypertens Rep.* 2016;18(5):34

477. Williams B, MacDonald TM, Morant S, et al; British Hypertension Society's PATHWAY Studies Group. Spironolactone versus placebo, bisoprolol, and doxazosin to determine the optimal treatment for drug-resistant hypertension (PATHWAY-2): a randomised, double-blind, crossover trial. *Lancet.* 2015;386(10008):2059–2068

478. Mitsnefes M, Ho PL, McEnery PT. Hypertension and progression of chronic renal insufficiency in children: a report of the North American Pediatric Renal Transplant Cooperative Study (NAPRTCS). *J Am Soc Nephrol.* 2003;14(10):2618–2622

479. Dionne JM. Evidence-based guidelines for the management of hypertension in children with chronic kidney disease. *Pediatr Nephrol.* 2015;30(11):1919–1927

480. VanDeVoorde RG, Mitsnefes MM. Hypertension and CKD. *Adv Chronic Kidney Dis.* 2011;18(5):355–361

481. Mitsnefes MM, Kimball TR, Kartal J, et al. Progression of left ventricular hypertrophy in children with early chronic kidney disease: 2-year follow-up study. *J Pediatr.* 2006;149(5):671–675

482. Wright JT Jr, Williamson JD, Whelton PK, et al; SPRINT Research Group. A randomized trial of intensive versus standard blood-pressure control. *N Engl J Med.* 2015;373(22):2103–2116

483. Wong H, Mylrea K, Feber J, Drukker A, Filler G. Prevalence of complications in children with chronic kidney disease according to KDOQI. *Kidney Int.* 2006;70(3):585–590

484. Simonetti GD, von Vigier RO, Konrad M, Rizzi M, Fossali E, Bianchetti MG. Candesartan cilexetil in children with hypertension or proteinuria: preliminary data. *Pediatr Nephrol.* 2006;21(10):1480–1482

485. White CT, Macpherson CF, Hurley RM, Matsell DG. Antiproteinuric effects of enalapril and losartan: a pilot study. *Pediatr Nephrol.* 2003;18(10):1038–1043

486. Webb NJ, Lam C, Loeys T, et al. Randomized, double-blind, controlled study of losartan in children with proteinuria. *Clin J Am Soc Nephrol.* 2010;5(3):417–424

487. Webb NJ, Shahinfar S, Wells TG, et al. Losartan and enalapril are comparable in reducing proteinuria in children. *Kidney Int.* 2012;82(7):819–826

488. Wühl E, Mehls O, Schaefer F; ESCAPE Trial Group. Antihypertensive and antiproteinuric efficacy of ramipril in children with chronic renal failure. *Kidney Int.* 2004;66(2):768–776

489. Eppens MC, Craig ME, Cusumano J, et al. Prevalence of diabetes complications in adolescents with type 2 compared with type 1 diabetes. *Diabetes Care.* 2006;29(6):1300–1306

490. Mayer-Davis EJ, Ma B, Lawson A, et al; SEARCH for Diabetes in Youth Study Group. Cardiovascular disease risk factors in youth with type 1 and type 2 diabetes: implications of a factor analysis of clustering. *Metab Syndr Relat Disord.* 2009;7(2):89–95

491. Margeirsdottir HD, Larsen JR, Brunborg C, Overby NC, Dahl-Jørgensen K; Norwegian Study Group for Childhood Diabetes. High prevalence of cardiovascular risk factors in children and adolescents with type 1 diabetes: a population-based study. *Diabetologia.* 2008;51(4):554–561

492. Orchard TJ, Forrest KY, Kuller LH, Becker DJ; Pittsburgh Epidemiology of Diabetes Complications Study. Lipid and blood pressure treatment goals for type 1 diabetes: 10-year incidence data from the Pittsburgh Epidemiology of Diabetes Complications Study. *Diabetes Care.* 2001;24(6):1053–1059

493. Copeland KC, Zeitler P, Geffner M, et al; TODAY Study Group. Characteristics of adolescents and youth with recent-onset type 2 diabetes: the TODAY cohort at baseline. *J Clin Endocrinol Metab.* 2011;96(1):159–167

494. Klingensmith GJ, Connor CG, Ruedy KJ, et al; Pediatric Diabetes Consortium. Presentation of youth with type 2

diabetes in the Pediatric Diabetes Consortium. *Pediatr Diabetes*. 2016;17(4):266–273

495. Shah AS, Dolan LM, Gao Z, Kimball TR, Urbina EM. Racial differences in arterial stiffness among adolescents and young adults with type 2 diabetes. *Pediatr Diabetes*. 2012;13(2):170–175

496. TODAY Study Group. Rapid rise in hypertension and nephropathy in youth with type 2 diabetes: the TODAY clinical trial. *Diabetes Care*. 2013;36(6):1735–1741

497. Shah AS, Khoury PR, Dolan LM, et al. The effects of obesity and type 2 diabetes mellitus on cardiac structure and function in adolescents and young adults. *Diabetologia*. 2011;54(4):722–730

498. Nambam B, DuBose SN, Nathan BM, et al; T1D Exchange Clinic Network. Therapeutic inertia: underdiagnosed and undertreated hypertension in children participating in the T1D Exchange Clinic Registry. *Pediatr Diabetes*. 2016;17(1):15–20

499. American Diabetes Association. Supplemental issue: standards of medical care in diabetes - 2016. *Diabetes Care*. 2016;39(suppl 1):S1–S2

500. Donaghue KC, Chiarelli F, Trotta D, Allgrove J, Dahl-Jorgensen K. Microvascular and macrovascular complications associated with diabetes in children and adolescents. *Pediatr Diabetes*. 2009;10(suppl 12): 195–203

501. Expert Panel on Integrated Guidelines for Cardiovascular Health and Risk Reduction in Children and Adolescents; National Heart, Lung, and Blood Institute. Expert panel on integrated guidelines for cardiovascular health and risk reduction in children and adolescents: summary report. *Pediatrics*. 2011;128(suppl 5):S213–S256

502. Stern MP. Diabetes and cardiovascular disease. The "common soil" hypothesis. *Diabetes*. 1995;44(4):369–374

503. Martino F, Puddu PE, Pannarale G, et al. Hypertension in children and adolescents attending a lipid clinic. *Eur J Pediatr*. 2013;172(12):1573–1579

504. Rodríguez-Morán M, Guerrero-Romero F, Aradillas-García C, et al. Atherogenic indices and prehypertension in obese and non-obese children. *Diab Vasc Dis Res*. 2013;10(1):17–24

505. Li J, Motsko SP, Goehring EL Jr, Vendiola R, Maneno M, Jones JK. Longitudinal study on pediatric dyslipidemia in population-based claims database. *Pharmacoepidemiol Drug Saf*. 2010;19(1):90–98

506. Liao CC, Su TC, Chien KL, et al. Elevated blood pressure, obesity, and hyperlipidemia. *J Pediatr*. 2009;155(1):79–83, 83.e1

507. Marcus CL, Brooks LJ, Draper KA, et al; American Academy of Pediatrics. Diagnosis and management of childhood obstructive sleep apnea syndrome. *Pediatrics*. 2012;130(3). Available at: www.pediatrics.org/cgi/content/full/130/3/e714

508. Kuo YL, Kang KT, Chiu SN, Weng WC, Lee PL, Hsu WC. Blood pressure after surgery among obese and nonobese children with obstructive sleep apnea. *Otolaryngol Head Neck Surg*. 2015;152(5):931–940

509. Lande MB, Adams HR, Kupferman JC, Hooper SR, Szilagyi PG, Batisky DL. A multicenter study of neurocognition in children with hypertension: methods, challenges, and solutions. *J Am Soc Hypertens*. 2013;7(5):353–362

510. Lande MB, Adams H, Falkner B, et al. Parental assessments of internalizing and externalizing behavior and executive function in children with primary hypertension. *J Pediatr*. 2009;154(2):207–212

511. Adams HR, Szilagyi PG, Gebhardt L, Lande MB. Learning and attention problems among children with pediatric primary hypertension. *Pediatrics*. 2010;126(6). Available at: www.pediatrics.org/cgi/content/full/126/6/e1425

512. Settakis G, Páll D, Molnár C, Katona E, Bereczki D, Fülesdi B. Hyperventilation-induced cerebrovascular reactivity among hypertensive and healthy adolescents. *Kidney Blood Press Res*. 2006;29(5):306–311

513. Wong LJ, Kupferman JC, Prohovnik I, et al. Hypertension impairs vascular

reactivity in the pediatric brain. *Stroke*. 2011;42(7):1834–1838

514. Lande MB, Kupferman JC, Adams HR. Neurocognitive alterations in hypertensive children and adolescents. *J Clin Hypertens (Greenwich)*. 2012;14(6):353–359

515. Ostrovskaya MA, Rojas M, Kupferman JC, et al. Executive function and cerebrovascular reactivity in pediatric hypertension. *J Child Neurol*. 2015;30(5):543–546

516. Ong KL, Cheung BM, Man YB, Lau CP, Lam KS. Prevalence, awareness, treatment, and control of hypertension among United States adults 1999-2004. *Hypertension*. 2007;49(1):69–75

517. Guo F, He D, Zhang W, Walton RG. Trends in prevalence, awareness, management, and control of hypertension among United States adults, 1999 to 2010. *J Am Coll Cardiol*. 2012;60(7):599–606

518. Hajjar I, Kotchen TA. Trends in prevalence, awareness, treatment, and control of hypertension in the United States, 1988-2000. *JAMA*. 2003;290(2):199–206

519. Daniels SR, McMahon RP, Obarzanek E, et al. Longitudinal correlates of change in blood pressure in adolescent girls. *Hypertension*. 1998;31(1):97–103

520. Wang X, Poole JC, Treiber FA, Harshfield GA, Hanevold CD, Snieder H. Ethnic and gender differences in ambulatory blood pressure trajectories: results from a 15-year longitudinal study in youth and young adults. *Circulation*. 2006;114(25):2780–2787

521. Rosner B, Cook N, Portman R, Daniels S, Falkner B. Blood pressure differences by ethnic group among United States children and adolescents. *Hypertension*. 2009;54(3):502–508

522. Peacock WF IV, Hilleman DE, Levy PD, Rhoney DH, Varon J. A systematic review of nicardipine vs labetalol for the management of hypertensive crises. *Am J Emerg Med*. 2012;30(6):981–993

523. Wiest DB, Garner SS, Uber WE, Sade RM. Esmolol for the management of pediatric hypertension after cardiac operations. *J Thorac Cardiovasc Surg*. 1998;115(4):890–897

524. Flynn JT, Mottes TA, Brophy PD, Kershaw DB, Smoyer WE, Bunchman TE. Intravenous nicardipine for treatment of severe hypertension in children. *J Pediatr.* 2001;139(1):38–43

525. Tabbutt S, Nicolson SC, Adamson PC, et al. The safety, efficacy, and pharmacokinetics of esmolol for blood pressure control immediately after repair of coarctation of the aorta in infants and children: a multicenter, double-blind, randomized trial. *J Thorac Cardiovasc Surg.* 2008;136(2):321–328

526. Miyashita Y, Peterson D, Rees JM, Flynn JT. Isradipine for treatment of acute hypertension in hospitalized children and adolescents. *J Clin Hypertens (Greenwich).* 2010;12(11):850–855

527. Thomas CA, Moffett BS, Wagner JL, Mott AR, Feig DI. Safety and efficacy of intravenous labetalol for hypertensive crisis in infants and small children. *Pediatr Crit Care Med.* 2011;12(1):28–32

528. Kako H, Gable A, Martin D, et al. A prospective, open-label trial of clevidipine for controlled hypotension during posterior spinal fusion. *J Pediatr Pharmacol Ther.* 2015;20(1):54–60

529. Hammer GB, Lewandowski A, Drover DR, et al. Safety and efficacy of sodium nitroprusside during prolonged infusion in pediatric patients. *Pediatr Crit Care Med.* 2015;16(5):397–403

530. Flynn JT, Bradford MC, Harvey EM. Intravenous hydralazine in hospitalized children and adolescents with hypertension. *J Pediatr.* 2016;168:88–92

531. Yang WC, Zhao LL, Chen CY, Wu YK, Chang YJ, Wu HP. First-attack pediatric hypertensive crisis presenting to the pediatric emergency department. *BMC Pediatr.* 2012;12:200

532. Baracco R, Mattoo TK. Pediatric hypertensive emergencies. *Curr Hypertens Rep.* 2014;16(8):456

533. Flynn JT, Tullus K. Severe hypertension in children and adolescents: pathophysiology and treatment [published correction appears in *Pediatr Nephrol.* 2012;27(3):503–504]. *Pediatr Nephrol.* 2009;24(6):1101–1112

534. Patel NH, Romero SK, Kaelber DC. Evaluation and management of pediatric hypertensive crises: hypertensive urgency and hypertensive emergencies. *Open Access Emerg Med.* 2012;4:85–92

535. Chen YL, Liu YF, Huang CY, et al. Normalization effect of sports training on blood pressure in hypertensives. *J Sports Sci.* 2010;28(4):361–367

536. Hupin D, Roche F, Gremeaux V, et al. Even a low-dose of moderate-to-vigorous physical activity reduces mortality by 22% in adults aged ≥60 years: a systematic review and meta-analysis. *Br J Sports Med.* 2015;49(19):1262–1267

537. Di Paolo FM, Schmied C, Zerguini YA, et al. The athlete's heart in adolescent Africans: an electrocardiographic and echocardiographic study. *J Am Coll Cardiol.* 2012;59(11):1029–1036

538. McCambridge TM, Benjamin HJ, Brenner JS, et al; Council on Sports Medicine and Fitness. Athletic participation by children and adolescents who have systemic hypertension. *Pediatrics.* 2010;125(6):1287–1294

539. Black HR, Sica D, Ferdinand K, White WB. Eligibility and disqualification recommendations for competitive athletes with cardiovascular abnormalities: Task Force 6: hypertension: a scientific statement from the American Heart Association and the American College of Cardiology. *J Am Coll Cardiol.* 2015;66(21):2393–2397

540. Tainio J, Qvist E, Miettinen J, et al. Blood pressure profiles 5 to 10 years after transplant in pediatric solid organ recipients. *J Clin Hypertens (Greenwich).* 2015;17(2):154–161

541. Seeman T, Simková E, Kreisinger J, et al. Control of hypertension in children after renal transplantation. *Pediatr Transplant.* 2006;10(3):316–322

542. Gülhan B, Topaloğlu R, Karabulut E, et al. Post-transplant hypertension in pediatric kidney transplant recipients. *Pediatr Nephrol.* 2014;29(6):1075–1080

543. Arbeiter K, Pichler A, Stemberger R, et al. ACE inhibition in the treatment of children after renal transplantation. *Pediatr Nephrol.* 2004;19(2):222–226

544. Suszynski TM, Rizzari MD, Gillingham KJ, et al. Antihypertensive pharmacotherapy and long-term outcomes in pediatric kidney transplantation. *Clin Transplant.* 2013;27(3):472–480

545. Sakallı H, Baskın E, Bayrakçı US, Moray G, Haberal M. Acidosis and hyperkalemia caused by losartan and enalapril in pediatric kidney transplant recipients. *Exp Clin Transplant.* 2014;12(4):310–313

546. Cooley WC, Sagerman PJ; American Academy of Pediatrics; American Academy of Family Physicians; American College of Physicians; Transitions Clinical Report Authoring Group. Supporting the health care transition from adolescence to adulthood in the medical home. *Pediatrics.* 2011;128(1):182–200

547. Julius S, Nesbitt SD, Egan BM, et al; Trial of Preventing Hypertension (TROPHY) Study Investigators. Feasibility of treating prehypertension with an angiotensin-receptor blocker. *N Engl J Med.* 2006;354(16):1685–1697

548. Kurioka S, Horie S, Inoue A, Mafune K, Tsuda Y, Otsuji Y. Risk of progression to hypertension in nonhypertensive Japanese workers aged 20-64 years. *J Hypertens.* 2014;32(2):236–244

549. Stabouli S, Papakatsika S, Kotsis V. The role of obesity, salt and exercise on blood pressure in children and adolescents. *Expert Rev Cardiovasc Ther.* 2011;9(6):753–761

550. Holm JC, Gamborg M, Neland M, et al. Longitudinal changes in blood pressure during weight loss and regain of weight in obese boys and girls. *J Hypertens.* 2012;30(2):368–374

551. Gillman MW, Ellison RC. Childhood prevention of essential hypertension. *Pediatr Clin North Am.* 1993;40(1):179–194

552. Krousel-Wood MA, Muntner P, He J, Whelton PK. Primary prevention of essential hypertension. *Med Clin North Am.* 2004;88(1):223–238

553. Whelton PK, He J, Appel LJ, et al; National High Blood Pressure Education Program Coordinating Committee. Primary prevention of

hypertension: clinical and public health advisory from the National High Blood Pressure Education Program. *JAMA*. 2002;288(15):1882–1888

554. Kim N, Seo DC, King MH, Lederer AM, Sovinski D. Long-term predictors of blood pressure among adolescents during an 18-month school-based obesity prevention intervention. *J Adolesc Health*. 2014;55(4):521–527

555. Aburto NJ, Ziolkovska A, Hooper L, Elliott P, Cappuccio FP, Meerpohl JJ. Effect of lower sodium intake on health: systematic review and meta-analyses. *BMJ*. 2013;346:f1326

556. American Academy of Pediatrics. EQIPP: hypertension recognition and management. Available at: http://shop.aap.org/eqipp-hypertension-identification-and-management. Accessed February 6, 2017

557. American Academy of Pediatrics, Council on Quality Improvement and Patient Safety. Implementation guide. Available at: https://www.aap.org/en-us/about-the-aap/Committees-Councils-Sections/coqips/Pages/Implementation-Guide.aspx. Accessed July 28, 2017

558. Wang YC, Cheung AM, Bibbins-Domingo K, et al. Effectiveness and cost-effectiveness of blood pressure screening in adolescents in the United States. *J Pediatr*. 2011;158(2):257–264. e1–e7

559. Davis ML, Ferguson MA, Zachariah JP. Clinical predictors and impact of ambulatory blood pressure monitoring in pediatric hypertension referrals. *J Am Soc Hypertens*. 2014;8(9):660–667

560. Leu MG, Austin E, Foti JL, et al. A framework for evaluating value of new clinical recommendations. *Hosp Pediatr*. 2016;6(10):578–586

561. Bradshaw B. The role of the family in managing therapy in minority children with type 2 diabetes mellitus. *J Pediatr Endocrinol Metab*. 2002;15(suppl 1):547–551

562. Pinhas-Hamiel O, Standiford D, Hamiel D, Dolan LM, Cohen R, Zeitler PS. The type 2 family: a setting for development and treatment of adolescent type 2 diabetes mellitus. *Arch Pediatr Adolesc Med*. 1999;153(10):1063–1067

563. Mulvaney SA, Schlundt DG, Mudasiru E, et al. Parent perceptions of caring for adolescents with type 2 diabetes. *Diabetes Care*. 2006;29(5):993–997

564. Summerbell CD, Ashton V, Campbell KJ, Edmunds L, Kelly S, Waters E. Interventions for treating obesity in children. *Cochrane Database Syst Rev*. 2003;(3):CD001872

565. Skinner AC, Weinberger M, Mulvaney S, Schlundt D, Rothman RL. Accuracy of perceptions of overweight and relation to self-care behaviors among adolescents with type 2 diabetes and their parents. *Diabetes Care*. 2008;31(2):227–229

566. Thompson M, Dana T, Bougatsos C, Blazina I, Norris SL. Screening for hypertension in children and adolescents to prevent cardiovascular disease. *Pediatrics*. 2013;131(3):490–525

567. Urbina EM, de Ferranti S, Steinberger J. Observational studies may be more important than randomized clinical trials: weaknesses in US Preventive Services Task Force recommendation on blood pressure screening in youth. *Hypertension*. 2014;63(4):638–640

568. Flynn JT. Ambulatory blood pressure monitoring in children: imperfect yet essential. *Pediatr Nephrol*. 2011;26(12):2089–2094

569. Juonala M, Magnussen CG, Venn A, et al. Influence of age on associations between childhood risk factors and carotid intima-media thickness in adulthood: the Cardiovascular Risk in Young Finns Study, the Childhood Determinants of Adult Health Study, the Bogalusa Heart Study, and the Muscatine Study for the International Childhood Cardiovascular Cohort (i3C) Consortium. *Circulation*. 2010;122(24):2514–2520

570. Muntner P, Becker RC, Calhoun D, et al. Introduction to the American Heart Association's hypertension strategically focused research network. *Hypertension*. 2016;67(4):674–680

High Blood Pressure Clinical Practice Guideline
Quick Reference Tools

- Action Statement Summary
  — Clinical Practice Guideline for Screening and Management of High Blood Pressure in Children and Adolescents
- *ICD-10-CM* Coding Quick Reference for High Blood Pressure

Action Statement Summary

Clinical Practice Guideline for Screening and Management of High Blood Pressure in Children and Adolescents

Key Action Statement 1

BP should be measured annually in children and adolescents ≥3 years of age (grade C, moderate recommendation).

Key Action Statement 2

BP should be checked in all children and adolescents ≥3 years of age at every health care encounter if they have obesity, are taking medications known to increase BP, have renal disease, a history of aortic arch obstruction or coarctation, or diabetes (grade C, moderate recommendation).

Key Action Statement 3

Trained health care professionals in the office setting should make a diagnosis of HTN if a child or adolescent has auscultatory-confirmed BP readings ≥95th percentile on 3 different visits (grade C, moderate recommendation).

Key Action Statement 4

Organizations with EHRs used in an office setting should consider including flags for abnormal BP values both when the values are being entered and when they are being viewed (grade C, weak recommendation).

Key Action Statement 5

Oscillometric devices may be used for BP screening in children and adolescents. When doing so, providers should use a device that has been validated in the pediatric age group. If elevated BP is suspected on the basis of oscillometric readings, confirmatory measurements should be obtained by auscultation (grade B, strong recommendation).

Key Action Statement 6

ABPM should be performed for the confirmation of HTN in children and adolescents with office BP measurements in the elevated BP category for 1 year or more or with stage 1 HTN over 3 clinic visits (grade C, moderate recommendation).

Key Action Statement 7

The routine performance of ABPM should be strongly considered in children and adolescents with high-risk conditions to assess HTN severity and determine if abnormal circadian BP patterns are present, which may indicate increased risk for target organ damage (grade B, moderate recommendation).

Key Action Statement 8

ABPM should be performed by using a standardized approach with monitors that have been validated in a pediatric population, and studies should be interpreted by using pediatric normative data (grade C, moderate recommendation).

Key Action Statement 9

Children and adolescents with suspected WCH should undergo ABPM. Diagnosis is based on the presence of mean SBP and DBP <95th percentile and SBP and DBP load <25% (grade B, strong recommendation).

Key Action Statement 10

Home BP monitoring should not be used to diagnose HTN, MH, or WCH but may be a useful adjunct to office and ambulatory BP measurement after HTN has been diagnosed (grade C, moderate recommendation).

Key Action Statement 11

Children and adolescents ≥6 years of age do not require an extensive evaluation for secondary causes of HTN if they have a positive family history of HTN, are overweight or obese, and/or do not have history or physical examination findings suggestive of a secondary cause of HTN (grade C, moderate recommendation).

Key Action Statement 12

Children and adolescents who have undergone coarctation repair should undergo ABPM for the detection of HTN (including MH) (grade B, strong recommendation).

Key Action Statement 13

In children and adolescents being evaluated for high BP, the provider should obtain a perinatal history, appropriate nutritional history, physical activity history, psychosocial history, and family history and perform a physical examination to identify findings suggestive of secondary causes of HTN (grade B, strong recommendation).

Key Action Statement 14

Clinicians should not perform electrocardiography in hypertensive children and adolescents being evaluated for LVH (grade B, strong recommendation).

Key Action Statement 15

1. It is recommended that echocardiography be performed to assess for cardiac target organ damage (LV mass, geometry, and function) at the time of consideration of pharmacologic treatment of HTN;
2. LVH should be defined as LV mass >51 g/m$^{2.7}$ (boys and girls) for children and adolescents older than 8 years and defined by LV mass >115 g/BSA for boys and LV mass >95 g/BSA for girls;
3. Repeat echocardiography may be performed to monitor improvement or progression of target organ damage at 6- to 12-month intervals. Indications to repeat echocardiography include persistent HTN despite treatment, concentric LV hypertrophy, or reduced LV ejection fraction; and
4. In patients without LV target organ injury at initial echocardiographic assessment, repeat echocardiography at yearly intervals may be considered in those with stage 2 HTN, secondary HTN, or chronic stage 1 HTN incompletely treated (noncompliance or drug resistance) to assess for the development of worsening LV target organ injury (grade C, moderate recommendation).

Key Action Statement 16

Doppler renal ultrasonography may be used as a noninvasive screening study for the evaluation of possible RAS in normal-weight children and adolescents ≥8 years of age who are suspected of having renovascular HTN and who will cooperate with the procedure (grade C, moderate recommendation).

Key Action Statement 17

In children and adolescents suspected of having RAS, either CTA or MRA may be performed as a noninvasive imaging study. Nuclear renography is less useful in pediatrics and should generally be avoided (grade D, weak recommendation).

Key Action Statement 18

Routine testing for MA is not recommended for children and adolescents with primary HTN (grade C, moderate recommendation).

Key Action Statement 19

In children and adolescents diagnosed with HTN, the treatment goal with nonpharmacologic and pharmacologic therapy should be a reduction in SBP and DBP to <90th percentile and <130/80 mm Hg in adolescents ≥13 years of age (grade C, moderate recommendation).

Key Action Statement 20

At the time of diagnosis of elevated BP or HTN in a child or adolescent, clinicians should provide advice on the DASH diet and recommend moderate to vigorous physical activity at least 3 to 5 days per week (30–60 minutes per session) to help reduce BP (grade C, weak recommendation).

Key Action Statement 21

In hypertensive children and adolescents who have failed lifestyle modifications (particularly those who have LV hypertrophy on echocardiography, symptomatic HTN, or stage 2 HTN without a clearly modifiable factor [eg, obesity]), clinicians should initiate pharmacologic treatment with an ACE inhibitor, ARB, long-acting calcium channel blocker, or thiazide diuretic (grade B, moderate recommendation).

Key Action Statement 22

ABPM may be used to assess treatment effectiveness in children and adolescents with HTN, especially when clinic and/or home BP measurements indicate insufficient BP response to treatment (grade B, moderate recommendation).

Key Action Statement 23

1. Children and adolescents with CKD should be evaluated for HTN at each medical encounter;
2. Children or adolescents with both CKD and HTN should be treated to lower 24-hour MAP to <50th percentile by ABPM; and
3. Regardless of apparent control of BP with office measures, children and adolescents with CKD and a history of HTN should have BP assessed by ABPM at least yearly to screen for MH (grade B, strong recommendation).

Key Action Statement 24

Children and adolescents with CKD and HTN should be evaluated for proteinuria (grade B, strong recommendation).

Key Action Statement 25

Children and adolescents with CKD, HTN, and proteinuria should be treated with an ACE inhibitor or ARB (grade B, strong recommendation).

Key Action Statement 26

Children and adolescents with T1DM or T2DM should be evaluated for HTN at each medical encounter and treated if BP is ≥95th percentile or >130/80 mm Hg in adolescents ≥13 years of age (grade C, moderate recommendation).

Key Action Statement 27

In children and adolescents with acute severe HTN and life-threatening symptoms, immediate treatment with short-acting antihypertensive medication should be initiated, and BP should be reduced by no more than 25% of the planned reduction over the first 8 hours (grade expert opinion D, weak recommendation).

Key Action Statement 28

Children and adolescents with HTN may participate in competitive sports once hypertensive target organ effects and risk have been assessed (grade C, moderate recommendation).

Key Action Statement 29

Children and adolescents with HTN should receive treatment to lower BP below stage 2 thresholds before participating in competitive sports (grade C, weak recommendation).

Key Action Statement 30

Adolescents with elevated BP or HTN (whether they are receiving antihypertensive treatment) should typically have their care transitioned to an appropriate adult care provider by 22 years of age (recognizing that there may be individual cases in which this upper age limit is exceeded, particularly in the case of youth with special health care needs). There should be a transfer of information regarding HTN etiology and past manifestations and complications of the patient's HTN (grade X, strong recommendation).

Coding Quick Reference for High Blood Pressure

ICD-10-CM	
I10	**Essential (primary) hypertension**
I11.9	Hypertensive heart disease without heart failure
I12.0	Hypertensive chronic kidney disease with stage 5 chronic kidney disease or end stage renal disease*
I12.9	Hypertensive chronic kidney disease with stage 1 through stage 4 chronic kidney disease, or unspecified chronic kidney disease*
I15.0 Renovascular hypertension [secondary] **I15.1** Hypertension secondary to other renal disorders **I15.2** Hypertension secondary to endocrine disorders **I15.8** Other secondary hypertension **I15.9** Secondary hypertension, unspecified	Underlying cause coded in addition*
R03.0	Elevated blood-pressure reading, without diagnosis of hypertension
P29.2	Neonatal hypertension
***Underlying Causes**	
E25.0	Congenital adrenogenital disorders associated with enzyme deficiency
E26.02	Glucocorticoid-remediable aldosteronism
N18.1	Chronic kidney disease, stage 1
N18.2	Chronic kidney disease, stage 2 (mild)
N18.3	Chronic kidney disease, stage 3 (moderate)
N18.4	Chronic kidney disease, stage 4 (severe)
N18.5	Chronic kidney disease, stage 5
N18.9	Chronic kidney disease, unspecified
Q25.1	Coarctation of aorta
Q25.71	Coarctation of pulmonary artery
Q27.1	Congenital renal artery stenosis
Q85.00	Neurofibromatosis, unspecified
Q85.01	Neurofibromatosis, type 1
Z83.49	Family history of other endocrine, nutritional and metabolic diseases [hyperaldosteronism]
Z87.74	Personal history of (corrected) congenital malformations of heart and circulatory system [coarctation repair]

Coding Quick Reference for High Blood Pressure, continued

Z77.011	Contact with and (suspected) exposure to lead
Z77.018	Contact with and (suspected) exposure to other hazardous metals
Z79.3	Long term (current) use of hormonal contraceptives
Z79.51	Long term (current) use of inhaled steroids
Z79.52	Long term (current) use of systemic steroids
Z79.899	Other long term (current) drug therapy [CNS stimulant]

Management of Hyperbilirubinemia in the Newborn Infant 35 or More Weeks of Gestation

• •

- *Clinical Practice Guideline*

AMERICAN ACADEMY OF PEDIATRICS

CLINICAL PRACTICE GUIDELINE

Subcommittee on Hyperbilirubinemia

Management of Hyperbilirubinemia in the Newborn Infant 35 or More Weeks of Gestation

ABSTRACT. Jaundice occurs in most newborn infants. Most jaundice is benign, but because of the potential toxicity of bilirubin, newborn infants must be monitored to identify those who might develop severe hyperbilirubinemia and, in rare cases, acute bilirubin encephalopathy or kernicterus. The focus of this guideline is to reduce the incidence of severe hyperbilirubinemia and bilirubin encephalopathy while minimizing the risks of unintended harm such as maternal anxiety, decreased breastfeeding, and unnecessary costs or treatment. Although kernicterus should almost always be preventable, cases continue to occur. These guidelines provide a framework for the prevention and management of hyperbilirubinemia in newborn infants of 35 or more weeks of gestation. In every infant, we recommend that clinicians 1) promote and support successful breastfeeding; 2) perform a systematic assessment before discharge for the risk of severe hyperbilirubinemia; 3) provide early and focused follow-up based on the risk assessment; and 4) when indicated, treat newborns with phototherapy or exchange transfusion to prevent the development of severe hyperbilirubinemia and, possibly, bilirubin encephalopathy (kernicterus). *Pediatrics* 2004; 114:297–316; *hyperbilirubinemia, newborn, kernicterus, bilirubin encephalopathy, phototherapy.*

ABBREVIATIONS. AAP, American Academy of Pediatrics; TSB, total serum bilirubin; TcB, transcutaneous bilirubin; G6PD, glucose-6-phosphate dehydrogenase; ETCO$_c$, end-tidal carbon monoxide corrected for ambient carbon monoxide; B/A, bilirubin/albumin; UB, unbound bilirubin.

BACKGROUND

In October 1994, the Provisional Committee for Quality Improvement and Subcommittee on Hyperbilirubinemia of the American Academy of Pediatrics (AAP) produced a practice parameter dealing with the management of hyperbilirubinemia in the healthy term newborn.[1] The current guideline represents a consensus of the committee charged by the AAP with reviewing and updating the existing guideline and is based on a careful review of the evidence, including a comprehensive literature review by the New England Medical Center Evidence-Based Practice Center.[2] (See "An Evidence-Based Review of Important Issues Concerning Neonatal Hyperbilirubinemia"[3] for a description of the methodology, questions addressed, and conclusions of this report.) This guideline is intended for use by hospitals and pediatricians, neonatologists, family physicians, physician assistants, and advanced practice nurses who treat newborn infants in the hospital and as outpatients. A list of frequently asked questions and answers for parents is available in English and Spanish at www.aap.org/family/jaundicefaq.htm.

DEFINITION OF RECOMMENDATIONS

The evidence-based approach to guideline development requires that the evidence in support of a policy be identified, appraised, and summarized and that an explicit link between evidence and recommendations be defined. Evidence-based recommendations are based on the quality of evidence and the balance of benefits and harms that is anticipated when the recommendation is followed. This guideline uses the definitions for quality of evidence and balance of benefits and harms established by the AAP Steering Committee on Quality Improvement Management.[4] See Appendix 1 for these definitions.

The draft practice guideline underwent extensive peer review by committees and sections within the AAP, outside organizations, and other individuals identified by the subcommittee as experts in the field. Liaison representatives to the subcommittee were invited to distribute the draft to other representatives and committees within their specialty organizations. The resulting comments were reviewed by the subcommittee and, when appropriate, incorporated into the guideline.

BILIRUBIN ENCEPHALOPATHY AND KERNICTERUS

Although originally a pathologic diagnosis characterized by bilirubin staining of the brainstem nuclei and cerebellum, the term "kernicterus" has come to be used interchangeably with both the acute and chronic findings of bilirubin encephalopathy. Bilirubin encephalopathy describes the clinical central nervous system findings caused by bilirubin toxicity to the basal ganglia and various brainstem nuclei. To avoid confusion and encourage greater consistency in the literature, the committee recommends that in infants the term "acute bilirubin encephalopathy" be used to describe the acute manifestations of bilirubin

PEDIATRICS (ISSN 0031 4005). Copyright © 2004 by the American Academy of Pediatrics.

toxicity seen in the first weeks after birth and that the term "kernicterus" be reserved for the chronic and permanent clinical sequelae of bilirubin toxicity.

See Appendix 1 for the clinical manifestations of acute bilirubin encephalopathy and kernicterus.

FOCUS OF GUIDELINE

The overall aim of this guideline is to promote an approach that will reduce the frequency of severe neonatal hyperbilirubinemia and bilirubin encephalopathy and minimize the risk of unintended harm such as increased anxiety, decreased breastfeeding, or unnecessary treatment for the general population and excessive cost and waste. Recent reports of kernicterus indicate that this condition, although rare, is still occurring.[2,5–10]

Analysis of these reported cases of kernicterus suggests that if health care personnel follow the recommendations listed in this guideline, kernicterus would be largely preventable.

These guidelines emphasize the importance of universal systematic assessment for the risk of severe hyperbilirubinemia, close follow-up, and prompt intervention when indicated. The recommendations apply to the care of infants at 35 or more weeks of gestation. These recommendations seek to further the aims defined by the Institute of Medicine as appropriate for health care:[11] safety, effectiveness, efficiency, timeliness, patient-centeredness, and equity. They specifically emphasize the principles of patient safety and the key role of timeliness of interventions to prevent adverse outcomes resulting from neonatal hyperbilirubinemia.

The following are the key elements of the recommendations provided by this guideline. Clinicians should:

1. Promote and support successful breastfeeding.
2. Establish nursery protocols for the identification and evaluation of hyperbilirubinemia.
3. Measure the total serum bilirubin (TSB) or transcutaneous bilirubin (TcB) level on infants jaundiced in the first 24 hours.
4. Recognize that visual estimation of the degree of jaundice can lead to errors, particularly in darkly pigmented infants.
5. Interpret all bilirubin levels according to the infant's age in hours.
6. Recognize that infants at less than 38 weeks' gestation, particularly those who are breastfed, are at higher risk of developing hyperbilirubinemia and require closer surveillance and monitoring.
7. Perform a systematic assessment on all infants before discharge for the risk of severe hyperbilirubinemia.
8. Provide parents with written and verbal information about newborn jaundice.
9. Provide appropriate follow-up based on the time of discharge and the risk assessment.
10. Treat newborns, when indicated, with phototherapy or exchange transfusion.

PRIMARY PREVENTION

In numerous policy statements, the AAP recommends breastfeeding for all healthy term and near-term newborns. This guideline strongly supports this general recommendation.

RECOMMENDATION 1.0: Clinicians should advise mothers to nurse their infants at least 8 to 12 times per day for the first several days[12] (evidence quality C: benefits exceed harms).

Poor caloric intake and/or dehydration associated with inadequate breastfeeding may contribute to the development of hyperbilirubinemia.[6,13,14] Increasing the frequency of nursing decreases the likelihood of subsequent significant hyperbilirubinemia in breastfed infants.[15–17] Providing appropriate support and advice to breastfeeding mothers increases the likelihood that breastfeeding will be successful.

Additional information on how to assess the adequacy of intake in a breastfed newborn is provided in Appendix 1.

RECOMMENDATION 1.1: The AAP recommends against routine supplementation of nondehydrated breast-fed infants with water or dextrose water (evidence quality B and C: harms exceed benefits).

Supplementation with water or dextrose water will not prevent hyperbilirubinemia or decrease TSB levels.[18,19]

SECONDARY PREVENTION

RECOMMENDATION 2.0: Clinicians should perform ongoing systematic assessments during the neonatal period for the risk of an infant developing severe hyperbilirubinemia.

Blood Typing

RECOMMENDATION 2.1: All pregnant women should be tested for ABO and Rh (D) blood types and have a serum screen for unusual isoimmune antibodies (evidence quality B: benefits exceed harms).
RECOMMENDATION 2.1.1: If a mother has not had prenatal blood grouping or is Rh-negative, a direct antibody test (or Coombs' test), blood type, and an Rh (D) type on the infant's (cord) blood are strongly recommended (evidence quality B: benefits exceed harms).
RECOMMENDATION 2.1.2: If the maternal blood is group O, Rh-positive, it is an option to test the cord blood for the infant's blood type and direct antibody test, but it is not required provided that there is appropriate surveillance, risk assessment before discharge, and follow-up[20] (evidence quality C: benefits exceed harms).

Clinical Assessment

RECOMMENDATION 2.2: Clinicians should ensure that all infants are routinely monitored for the development of jaundice, and nurseries should have established protocols for the assessment of jaundice. Jaundice should be assessed whenever the infant's vital signs are measured but no less than every 8 to 12 hours (evidence quality D: benefits versus harms exceptional).

In newborn infants, jaundice can be detected by blanching the skin with digital pressure, revealing the underlying color of the skin and subcutaneous tissue. The assessment of jaundice must be per-

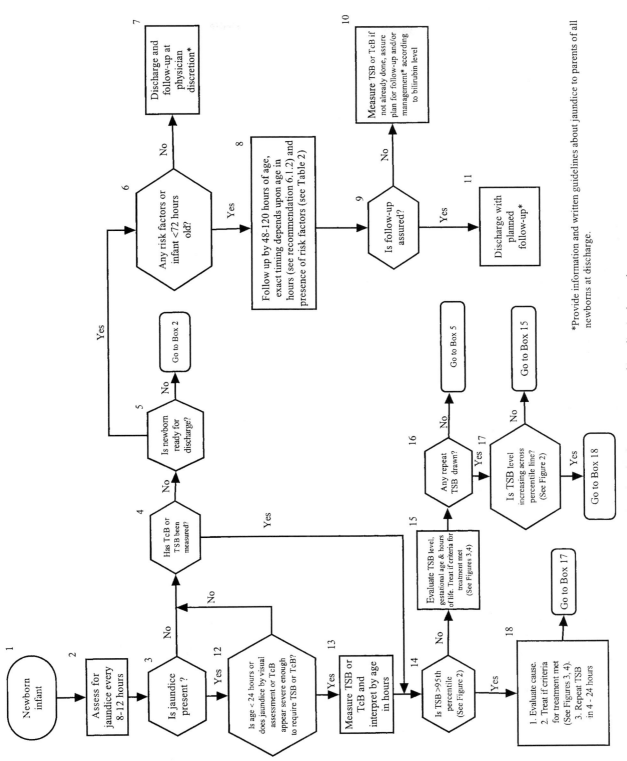

Fig 1. Algorithm for the management of jaundice in the newborn nursery.

formed in a well-lit room or, preferably, in daylight at a window. Jaundice is usually seen first in the face and progresses caudally to the trunk and extremities,[21] but visual estimation of bilirubin levels from the degree of jaundice can lead to errors.[22–24] In most infants with TSB levels of less than 15 mg/dL (257 μmol/L), noninvasive TcB-measurement devices can provide a valid estimate of the TSB level.[2,25–29] See Appendix 1 for additional information on the clinical evaluation of jaundice and the use of TcB measurements.

RECOMMENDATION 2.2.1: Protocols for the assessment of jaundice should include the circumstances in which nursing staff can obtain a TcB level or order a TSB measurement (evidence quality D: benefits versus harms exceptional).

Laboratory Evaluation

RECOMMENDATION 3.0: A TcB and/or TSB measurement should be performed on every infant who is jaundiced in the first 24 hours after birth (Fig 1 and Table 1)[30] (evidence quality C: benefits exceed harms). The need for and timing of a repeat TcB or TSB measurement will depend on the zone in which the TSB falls (Fig 2),[25,31] the age of the infant, and the evolution of the hyperbilirubinemia. Recommendations for TSB measurements after the age of 24 hours are provided in Fig 1 and Table 1.

See Appendix 1 for capillary versus venous bilirubin levels.

RECOMMENDATION 3.1: A TcB and/or TSB measurement should be performed if the jaundice appears excessive for the infant's age (evidence quality D: benefits versus harms exceptional). If there is any doubt about the degree of jaundice, the TSB or TcB should be measured. Visual estimation of bilirubin levels from the degree of jaundice can lead to errors, particularly in darkly pigmented infants (evidence quality C: benefits exceed harms).

RECOMMENDATION 3.2: All bilirubin levels should be interpreted according to the infant's age in hours (Fig 2) (evidence quality C: benefits exceed harms).

Cause of Jaundice

RECOMMENDATION 4.1: The possible cause of jaundice should be sought in an infant receiving phototherapy or whose TSB level is rising rapidly (ie, crossing percentiles [Fig 2]) and is not explained by the history and physical examination (evidence quality D: benefits versus harms exceptional).

RECOMMENDATION 4.1.1: Infants who have an elevation of direct-reacting or conjugated bilirubin should have a urinalysis and urine culture.[32] Additional laboratory evaluation for sepsis should be performed if indicated by history and physical examination (evidence quality C: benefits exceed harms).

See Appendix 1 for definitions of abnormal levels of direct-reacting and conjugated bilirubin.

RECOMMENDATION 4.1.2: Sick infants and those who are jaundiced at or beyond 3 weeks should have a measurement of total and direct or conjugated bilirubin to identify cholestasis (Table 1) (evidence quality D: benefit versus harms exceptional). The results of the newborn thyroid and galactosemia screen should also be checked in these infants (evidence quality D: benefits versus harms exceptional).

RECOMMENDATION 4.1.3: If the direct-reacting or conjugated bilirubin level is elevated, additional evaluation for the causes of cholestasis is recommended (evidence quality C: benefits exceed harms).

RECOMMENDATION 4.1.4: Measurement of the glucose-6-phosphate dehydrogenase (G6PD) level is recommended for a jaundiced infant who is receiving phototherapy and whose family history or ethnic or geographic origin suggest the likelihood of G6PD deficiency or for an infant in whom the response to phototherapy is poor (Fig 3) (evidence quality C: benefits exceed harms).

G6PD deficiency is widespread and frequently unrecognized, and although it is more common in the populations around the Mediterranean and in the Middle East, Arabian peninsula, Southeast Asia, and Africa, immigration and intermarriage have transformed G6PD deficiency into a global problem.[33,34]

TABLE 1. Laboratory Evaluation of the Jaundiced Infant of 35 or More Weeks' Gestation

Indications	Assessments
Jaundice in first 24 h	Measure TcB and/or TSB
Jaundice appears excessive for infant's age	Measure TcB and/or TSB
Infant receiving phototherapy or TSB rising rapidly (ie, crossing percentiles [Fig 2]) and unexplained by history and physical examination	Blood type and Coombs' test, if not obtained with cord blood
	Complete blood count and smear
	Measure direct or conjugated bilirubin
	It is an option to perform reticulocyte count, G6PD, and ETCO$_c$, if available
	Repeat TSB in 4–24 h depending on infant's age and TSB level
TSB concentration approaching exchange levels or not responding to phototherapy	Perform reticulocyte count, G6PD, albumin, ETCO$_c$, if available
Elevated direct (or conjugated) bilirubin level	Do urinalysis and urine culture. Evaluate for sepsis if indicated by history and physical examination
Jaundice present at or beyond age 3 wk, or sick infant	Total and direct (or conjugated) bilirubin level
	If direct bilirubin elevated, evaluate for causes of cholestasis
	Check results of newborn thyroid and galactosemia screen, and evaluate infant for signs or symptoms of hypothyroidism

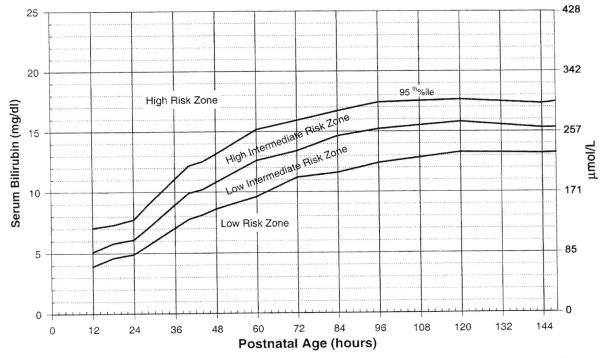

Fig 2. Nomogram for designation of risk in 2840 well newborns at 36 or more weeks' gestational age with birth weight of 2000 g or more or 35 or more weeks' gestational age and birth weight of 2500 g or more based on the hour-specific serum bilirubin values. The serum bilirubin level was obtained before discharge, and the zone in which the value fell predicted the likelihood of a subsequent bilirubin level exceeding the 95th percentile (high-risk zone) as shown in Appendix 1, Table 4. Used with permission from Bhutani et al.[31] See Appendix 1 for additional information about this nomogram, which should not be used to represent the natural history of neonatal hyperbilirubinemia.

Furthermore, G6PD deficiency occurs in 11% to 13% of African Americans, and kernicterus has occurred in some of these infants.[5,33] In a recent report, G6PD deficiency was considered to be the cause of hyperbilirubinemia in 19 of 61 (31.5%) infants who developed kernicterus.[5] (See Appendix 1 for additional information on G6PD deficiency.)

Risk Assessment Before Discharge

RECOMMENDATION 5.1: Before discharge, every newborn should be assessed for the risk of developing severe hyperbilirubinemia, and all nurseries should establish protocols for assessing this risk. Such assessment is particularly important in infants who are discharged before the age of 72 hours (evidence quality C: benefits exceed harms).

RECOMMENDATION 5.1.1: The AAP recommends 2 clinical options used individually or in combination for the systematic assessment of risk: predischarge measurement of the bilirubin level using TSB or TcB and/or assessment of clinical risk factors. Whether either or both options are used, appropriate follow-up after discharge is essential (evidence quality C: benefits exceed harms).

The best documented method for assessing the risk of subsequent hyperbilirubinemia is to measure the TSB or TcB level[25,31,35–38] and plot the results on a nomogram (Fig 2). A TSB level can be obtained at the time of the routine metabolic screen, thus obviating the need for an additional blood sample. Some authors have suggested that a TSB measurement should be part of the routine screening of all newborns.[5,31] An infant whose predischarge TSB is in the low-risk zone (Fig 2) is at very low risk of developing severe hyperbilirubinemia.[5,38]

Table 2 lists those factors that are clinically signif-

TABLE 2. Risk Factors for Development of Severe Hyperbilirubinemia in Infants of 35 or More Weeks' Gestation (in Approximate Order of Importance)

Major risk factors
  Predischarge TSB or TcB level in the high-risk zone (Fig 2)[25,31]
  Jaundice observed in the first 24 h[30]
  Blood group incompatibility with positive direct antiglobulin test, other known hemolytic disease (eg, G6PD deficiency), elevated ETCO$_c$
  Gestational age 35–36 wk[39,40]
  Previous sibling received phototherapy[40,41]
  Cephalohematoma or significant bruising[39]
  Exclusive breastfeeding, particularly if nursing is not going well and weight loss is excessive[39,40]
  East Asian race[39]*
Minor risk factors
  Predischarge TSB or TcB level in the high intermediate-risk zone[25,31]
  Gestational age 37–38 wk[39,40]
  Jaundice observed before discharge[40]
  Previous sibling with jaundice[40,41]
  Macrosomic infant of a diabetic mother[42,43]
  Maternal age ≥25 y[39]
  Male gender[39,40]
Decreased risk (these factors are associated with decreased risk of significant jaundice, listed in order of decreasing importance)
  TSB or TcB level in the low-risk zone (Fig 2)[25,31]
  Gestational age ≥41 wk[39]
  Exclusive bottle feeding[39,40]
  Black race[38]*
  Discharge from hospital after 72 h[40,44]

* Race as defined by mother's description.

icant and most frequently associated with an increase in the risk of severe hyperbilirubinemia. But, because these risk factors are common and the risk of hyperbilirubinemia is small, individually the factors are of limited use as predictors of significant hyperbilirubinemia.[39] Nevertheless, if no risk factors are present, the risk of severe hyperbilirubinemia is extremely low, and the more risk factors present, the greater the risk of severe hyperbilirubinemia.[39] The important risk factors most frequently associated with severe hyperbilirubinemia are breastfeeding, gestation below 38 weeks, significant jaundice in a previous sibling, and jaundice noted before discharge.[39,40] A formula-fed infant of 40 or more weeks' gestation is at very low risk of developing severe hyperbilirubinemia.[39]

Hospital Policies and Procedures

RECOMMENDATION 6.1: All hospitals should provide written and verbal information for parents at the time of discharge, which should include an explanation of jaundice, the need to monitor infants for jaundice, and advice on how monitoring should be done (evidence quality D: benefits versus harms exceptional).

An example of a parent-information handout is available in English and Spanish at www.aap.org/family/jaundicefaq.htm.

Follow-up

RECOMMENDATION 6.1.1: All infants should be examined by a qualified health care professional in the first few days after discharge to assess infant well-being and the presence or absence of jaundice. The timing and location of this assessment will be determined by the length of stay in the nursery, presence or absence of risk factors for hyperbilirubinemia (Table 2 and Fig 2), and risk of other neonatal problems (evidence quality C: benefits exceed harms).

Timing of Follow-up

RECOMMENDATION 6.1.2: Follow-up should be provided as follows:

Infant Discharged	Should Be Seen by Age
Before age 24 h	72 h
Between 24 and 47.9 h	96 h
Between 48 and 72 h	120 h

For some newborns discharged before 48 hours, 2 follow-up visits may be required, the first visit between 24 and 72 hours and the second between 72 and 120 hours. Clinical judgment should be used in determining follow-up. Earlier or more frequent follow-up should be provided for those who have risk factors for hyperbilirubinemia (Table 2), whereas those discharged with few or no risk factors can be seen after longer intervals (evidence quality C: benefits exceed harms).

RECOMMENDATION 6.1.3: If appropriate follow-up cannot be ensured in the presence of elevated risk for developing severe hyperbilirubinemia, it may be necessary to delay discharge either until appropriate follow-up can be ensured or the period of greatest risk has passed (72-96 hours) (evidence quality D: benefits versus harms exceptional).

Follow-up Assessment

RECOMMENDATION 6.1.4: The follow-up assessment should include the infant's weight and percent change from birth weight, adequacy of intake, the pattern of voiding and stooling, and the presence or absence of jaundice (evidence quality C: benefits exceed harms). Clinical judgment should be used to determine the need for a bilirubin measurement. If there is any doubt about the degree of jaundice, the TSB or TcB level should be measured. Visual estimation of bilirubin levels can lead to errors, particularly in darkly pigmented infants (evidence quality C: benefits exceed harms).

See Appendix 1 for assessment of the adequacy of intake in breastfeeding infants.

TREATMENT

Phototherapy and Exchange Transfusion

RECOMMENDATION 7.1: Recommendations for treatment are given in Table 3 and Figs 3 and 4 (evidence quality C: benefits exceed harms). If the TSB does not fall or continues to rise despite intensive phototherapy, it is very likely that hemolysis is occurring. The committee's recommendations for discontinuing phototherapy can be found in Appendix 2.

RECOMMENDATION 7.1.1: In using the guidelines for phototherapy and exchange transfusion (Figs 3 and 4), the direct-reacting (or conjugated) bilirubin level should not be subtracted from the total (evidence quality D: benefits versus harms exceptional).

In unusual situations in which the direct bilirubin level is 50% or more of the total bilirubin, there are no good data to provide guidance for therapy, and consultation with an expert in the field is recommended.

RECOMMENDATION 7.1.2: If the TSB is at a level at which exchange transfusion is recommended (Fig 4) or if the TSB level is 25 mg/dL (428 μmol/L) or higher at any time, it is a medical emergency and the infant should be admitted immediately and directly to a hospital pediatric service for intensive phototherapy. These infants should not be referred to the emergency department, because it delays the initiation of treatment[54] (evidence quality C: benefits exceed harms).

RECOMMENDATION 7.1.3: Exchange transfusions should be performed only by trained personnel in a neonatal intensive care unit with full monitoring and resuscitation capabilities (evidence quality D: benefits versus harms exceptional).

RECOMMENDATION 7.1.4: In isoimmune hemolytic disease, administration of intravenous γ-globulin (0.5-1 g/kg over 2 hours) is recommended if the TSB is rising despite intensive phototherapy or the TSB level is within 2 to 3 mg/dL (34-51 μmol/L) of the exchange level (Fig 4).[55] If necessary, this dose can be repeated in 12 hours (evidence quality B: benefits exceed harms).

Intravenous γ-globulin has been shown to reduce the need for exchange transfusions in Rh and ABO hemolytic disease.[55–58] Although data are limited, it is reasonable to assume that intravenous γ-globulin will also be helpful in the other types of Rh hemolytic disease such as anti-C and anti-E.

TABLE 3. Example of a Clinical Pathway for Management of the Newborn Infant Readmitted for Phototherapy or Exchange Transfusion

Treatment
  Use intensive phototherapy and/or exchange transfusion as indicated in Figs 3 and 4 (see Appendix 2 for details of phototherapy use)
Laboratory tests
  TSB and direct bilirubin levels
  Blood type (ABO, Rh)
  Direct antibody test (Coombs')
  Serum albumin
  Complete blood cell count with differential and smear for red cell morphology
  Reticulocyte count
  $ETCO_c$ (if available)
  G6PD if suggested by ethnic or geographic origin or if poor response to phototherapy
  Urine for reducing substances
  If history and/or presentation suggest sepsis, perform blood culture, urine culture, and cerebrospinal fluid for protein, glucose, cell count, and culture
Interventions
  If TSB ≥25 mg/dL (428 μmol/L) or ≥20 mg/dL (342 μmol/L) in a sick infant or infant <38 wk gestation, obtain a type and crossmatch, and request blood in case an exchange transfusion is necessary
  In infants with isoimmune hemolytic disease and TSB level rising in spite of intensive phototherapy or within 2–3 mg/dL (34–51 μmol/L) of exchange level (Fig 4), administer intravenous immunoglobulin 0.5–1 g/kg over 2 h and repeat in 12 h if necessary
  If infant's weight loss from birth is >12% or there is clinical or biochemical evidence of dehydration, recommend formula or expressed breast milk. If oral intake is in question, give intravenous fluids.
For infants receiving intensive phototherapy
  Breastfeed or bottle-feed (formula or expressed breast milk) every 2–3 h
  If TSB ≥25 mg/dL (428 μmol/L), repeat TSB within 2–3 h
  If TSB 20–25 mg/dL (342–428 μmol/L), repeat within 3–4 h. If TSB <20 mg/dL (342 μmol/L), repeat in 4–6 h. If TSB continues to fall, repeat in 8–12 h
  If TSB is not decreasing or is moving closer to level for exchange transfusion or the TSB/albumin ratio exceeds levels shown in Fig 4, consider exchange transfusion (see Fig 4 for exchange transfusion recommendations)
  When TSB is <13–14 mg/dL (239 μmol/L), discontinue phototherapy
  Depending on the cause of the hyperbilirubinemia, it is an option to measure TSB 24 h after discharge to check for rebound

Serum Albumin Levels and the Bilirubin/Albumin Ratio

RECOMMENDATION 7.1.5: It is an option to measure the serum albumin level and consider an albumin level of less than 3.0 g/dL as one risk factor for lowering the threshold for phototherapy use (see Fig 3) (evidence quality D: benefits versus risks exceptional.).

RECOMMENDATION 7.1.6: If an exchange transfusion is being considered, the serum albumin level should be measured and the bilirubin/albumin (B/A) ratio used in conjunction with the TSB level and other factors in determining the need for exchange transfusion (see Fig 4) (evidence quality D: benefits versus harms exceptional).

The recommendations shown above for treating hyperbilirubinemia are based primarily on TSB levels and other factors that affect the risk of bilirubin encephalopathy. This risk might be increased by a prolonged (rather than a brief) exposure to a certain TSB level.[59,60] Because the published data that address this issue are limited, however, it is not possible to provide specific recommendations for intervention based on the duration of hyperbilirubinemia.

See Appendix 1 for the basis for recommendations 7.1 through 7.1.6 and for the recommendations provided in Figs 3 and 4. Appendix 1 also contains a discussion of the risks of exchange transfusion and the use of B/A binding.

Acute Bilirubin Encephalopathy

RECOMMENDATION 7.1.7: Immediate exchange transfusion is recommended in any infant who is jaun-diced and manifests the signs of the intermediate to advanced stages of acute bilirubin encephalopathy[61,62] (hypertonia, arching, retrocollis, opisthotonos, fever, high-pitched cry) even if the TSB is falling (evidence quality D: benefits versus risks exceptional).

Phototherapy

RECOMMENDATION 7.2: All nurseries and services treating infants should have the necessary equipment to provide intensive phototherapy (see Appendix 2) (evidence quality D: benefits exceed risks).

Outpatient Management of the Jaundiced Breastfed Infant

RECOMMENDATION 7.3: In breastfed infants who require phototherapy (Fig 3), the AAP recommends that, if possible, breastfeeding should be continued (evidence quality C: benefits exceed harms). It is also an option to interrupt temporarily breastfeeding and substitute formula. This can reduce bilirubin levels and/or enhance the efficacy of phototherapy[63–65] (evidence quality B: benefits exceed harms). In breastfed infants receiving phototherapy, supplementation with expressed breast milk or formula is appropriate if the infant's intake seems inadequate, weight loss is excessive, or the infant seems dehydrated.

IMPLEMENTATION STRATEGIES

The Institute of Medicine[11] recommends a dramatic change in the way the US health care system

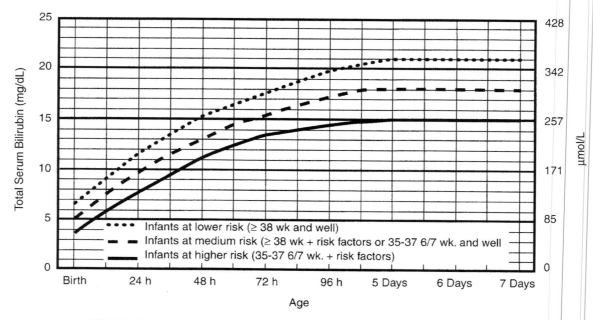

- Use total bilirubin. Do not subtract direct reacting or conjugated bilirubin.
- Risk factors = isoimmune hemolytic disease, G6PD deficiency, asphyxia, significant lethargy, temperature instability, sepsis, acidosis, or albumin < 3.0g/dL (if measured)
- For well infants 35-37 6/7 wk can adjust TSB levels for intervention around the medium risk line. It is an option to intervene at lower TSB levels for infants closer to 35 wks and at higher TSB levels for those closer to 37 6/7 wk.
- It is an option to provide conventional phototherapy in hospital or at home at TSB levels 2-3 mg/dL (35-50mmol/L) below those shown but home phototherapy should not be used in any infant with risk factors.

Fig 3. Guidelines for phototherapy in hospitalized infants of 35 or more weeks' gestation.

Note: These guidelines are based on limited evidence and the levels shown are approximations. The guidelines refer to the use of intensive phototherapy which should be used when the TSB exceeds the line indicated for each category. Infants are designated as "higher risk" because of the potential negative effects of the conditions listed on albumin binding of bilirubin,[45–47] the blood-brain barrier,[48] and the susceptibility of the brain cells to damage by bilirubin.[48]

"Intensive phototherapy" implies irradiance in the blue-green spectrum (wavelengths of approximately 430–490 nm) of at least 30 μW/cm^2 per nm (measured at the infant's skin directly below the center of the phototherapy unit) and delivered to as much of the infant's surface area as possible. Note that irradiance measured below the center of the light source is much greater than that measured at the periphery. Measurements should be made with a radiometer specified by the manufacturer of the phototherapy system.

See Appendix 2 for additional information on measuring the dose of phototherapy, a description of intensive phototherapy, and of light sources used. If total serum bilirubin levels approach or exceed the exchange transfusion line (Fig 4), the sides of the bassinet, incubator, or warmer should be lined with aluminum foil or white material.[50] This will increase the surface area of the infant exposed and increase the efficacy of phototherapy.[51]

If the total serum bilirubin does not decrease or continues to rise in an infant who is receiving intensive phototherapy, this strongly suggests the presence of hemolysis.

Infants who receive phototherapy and have an elevated direct-reacting or conjugated bilirubin level (cholestatic jaundice) may develop the bronze-baby syndrome. See Appendix 2 for the use of phototherapy in these infants.

ensures the safety of patients. The perspective of safety as a purely individual responsibility must be replaced by the concept of safety as a property of systems. Safe systems are characterized by a shared knowledge of the goal, a culture emphasizing safety, the ability of each person within the system to act in a manner that promotes safety, minimizing the use of memory, and emphasizing the use of standard procedures (such as checklists), and the involvement of patients/families as partners in the process of care.

These principles can be applied to the challenge of preventing severe hyperbilirubinemia and kernicterus. A systematic approach to the implementation of these guidelines should result in greater safety. Such approaches might include

- The establishment of standing protocols for nursing assessment of jaundice, including testing TcB and TSB levels, without requiring physician orders.

- Checklists or reminders associated with risk factors, age at discharge, and laboratory test results that provide guidance for appropriate follow-up.
- Explicit educational materials for parents (a key component of all AAP guidelines) concerning the identification of newborns with jaundice.

FUTURE RESEARCH

Epidemiology of Bilirubin-Induced Central Nervous System Damage

There is a need for appropriate epidemiologic data to document the incidence of kernicterus in the newborn population, the incidence of other adverse effects attributable to hyperbilirubinemia and its management, and the number of infants whose TSB levels exceed 25 or 30 mg/dL (428-513 μmol/L). Organizations such as the Centers for Disease Control and Prevention should implement strategies for appropriate data gathering to identify the number of

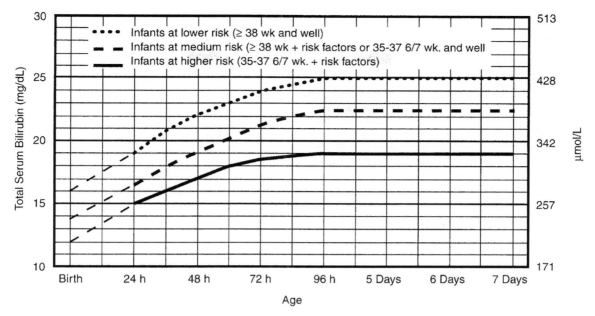

- The dashed lines for the first 24 hours indicate uncertainty due to a wide range of clinical circumstances and a range of responses to phototherapy.
- Immediate exchange transfusion is recommended if infant shows signs of acute bilirubin encephalopathy (hypertonia, arching, retrocollis, opisthotonos, fever, high pitched cry) or if TSB is ≥5 mg/dL (85 μmol/L) above these lines.
- Risk factors - isoimmune hemolytic disease, G6PD deficiency, asphyxia, significant lethargy, temperature instability, sepsis, acidosis.
- Measure serum albumin and calculate B/A ratio (See legend)
- Use total bilirubin. Do not subtract direct reacting or conjugated bilirubin
- If infant is well and 35-37 6/7 wk (median risk) can individualize TSB levels for exchange based on actual gestational age.

Fig 4. Guidelines for exchange transfusion in infants 35 or more weeks' gestation.

Note that these suggested levels represent a consensus of most of the committee but are based on limited evidence, and the levels shown are approximations. See ref. 3 for risks and complications of exchange transfusion. During birth hospitalization, exchange transfusion is recommended if the TSB rises to these levels despite intensive phototherapy. For readmitted infants, if the TSB level is above the exchange level, repeat TSB measurement every 2 to 3 hours and consider exchange if the TSB remains above the levels indicated after intensive phototherapy for 6 hours.

The following B/A ratios can be used together with but in not in lieu of the TSB level as an additional factor in determining the need for exchange transfusion[52]:

Risk Category	B/A Ratio at Which Exchange Transfusion Should be Considered	
	TSB mg/dL/Alb, g/dL	TSB μmol/L/Alb, μmol/L
Infants ≥38 0/7 wk	8.0	0.94
Infants 35 0/7–36 6/7 wk and well or ≥38 0/7 wk if higher risk or isoimmune hemolytic disease or G6PD deficiency	7.2	0.84
Infants 35 0/7–37 6/7 wk if higher risk or isoimmune hemolytic disease or G6PD deficiency	6.8	0.80

If the TSB is at or approaching the exchange level, send blood for immediate type and crossmatch. Blood for exchange transfusion is modified whole blood (red cells and plasma) crossmatched against the mother and compatible with the infant.[53]

infants who develop serum bilirubin levels above 25 or 30 mg/dL (428-513 μmol/L) and those who develop acute and chronic bilirubin encephalopathy. This information will help to identify the magnitude of the problem; the number of infants who need to be screened and treated to prevent 1 case of kernicterus; and the risks, costs, and benefits of different strategies for prevention and treatment of hyperbilirubinemia. In the absence of these data, recommendations for intervention cannot be considered definitive.

Effect of Bilirubin on the Central Nervous System

The serum bilirubin level by itself, except when it is extremely high and associated with bilirubin encephalopathy, is an imprecise indicator of long-term neurodevelopmental outcome.[2] Additional studies are needed on the relationship between central nervous system damage and the duration of hyperbilirubinemia, the binding of bilirubin to albumin, and changes seen in the brainstem auditory evoked response. These studies could help to better identify risk, clarify the effect of bilirubin on the central nervous system, and guide intervention.

Identification of Hemolysis

Because of their poor specificity and sensitivity, the standard laboratory tests for hemolysis (Table 1) are frequently unhelpful.[66,67] However, end-tidal carbon monoxide, corrected for ambient carbon monoxide ($ETCO_c$), levels can confirm the presence or absence of hemolysis, and measurement of $ETCO_c$ is the only clinical test that provides a direct measurement of the rate of heme catabolism and the rate of bilirubin production.[68,69] Thus, $ETCO_c$ may be helpful in determining the degree of surveillance needed and the timing of intervention. It is not yet known, however, how $ETCO_c$ measurements will affect management.

Nomograms and the Measurement of Serum and TcB

It would be useful to develop an age-specific (by hour) nomogram for TSB in populations of newborns that differ with regard to risk factors for hyperbilirubinemia. There is also an urgent need to improve the precision and accuracy of the measurement of TSB in the clinical laboratory.[70,71] Additional studies are also needed to develop and validate noninvasive (transcutaneous) measurements of serum bilirubin and to understand the factors that affect these measurements. These studies should also assess the cost-effectiveness and reproducibility of TcB measurements in clinical practice.[2]

Pharmacologic Therapy

There is now evidence that hyperbilirubinemia can be effectively prevented or treated with tin-mesoporphyrin,[72-75] a drug that inhibits the production of heme oxygenase. Tin-mesoporphyrin is not approved by the US Food and Drug Administration. If approved, tin-mesoporphyrin could find immediate application in preventing the need for exchange transfusion in infants who are not responding to phototherapy.[75]

Dissemination and Monitoring

Research should be directed toward methods for disseminating the information contained in this guideline to increase awareness on the part of physicians, residents, nurses, and parents concerning the issues of neonatal hyperbilirubinemia and strategies for its management. In addition, monitoring systems should be established to identify the impact of these guidelines on the incidence of acute bilirubin encephalopathy and kernicterus and the use of phototherapy and exchange transfusions.

CONCLUSIONS

Kernicterus is still occurring but should be largely preventable if health care personnel follow the recommendations listed in this guideline. These recommendations emphasize the importance of universal, systematic assessment for the risk of severe hyperbilirubinemia, close follow-up, and prompt intervention, when necessary.

SUBCOMMITTEE ON HYPERBILIRUBINEMIA
M. Jeffrey Maisels, MB, BCh, Chairperson
Richard D. Baltz, MD
Vinod K. Bhutani, MD
Thomas B. Newman, MD, MPH
Heather Palmer, MB, BCh
Warren Rosenfeld, MD
David K. Stevenson, MD
Howard B. Weinblatt, MD

CONSULTANT
Charles J. Homer, MD, MPH, Chairperson
American Academy of Pediatrics Steering
Committee on Quality Improvement and
Management

STAFF
Carla T. Herrerias, MPH

ACKNOWLEDGMENTS

M.J.M. received grant support from Natus Medical, Inc, for multinational study of ambient carbon monoxide; WellSpring Pharmaceutical Corporation for study of Stannsoporfin (tin-mesoporphyrin); and Minolta, Inc, for study of the Minolta/Hill-Rom Air-Shields transcutaneous jaundice meter model JM-103. V.K.B. received grant support from WellSpring Pharmaceutical Corporation for study of Stannsoporfin (tin-mesoporphyrin) and Natus Medical, Inc, for multinational study of ambient carbon monoxide and is a consultant (volunteer) to SpectrX (BiliChek transcutaneous bilirubinometer). D.K.S. is a consultant to and holds stock options through Natus Medical, Inc.

The American Academy of Pediatrics Subcommittee on Hyperbilirubinemia gratefully acknowledges the help of the following organizations, committees, and individuals who reviewed drafts of this guideline and provided valuable criticisms and commentary: American Academy of Pediatrics Committee on Nutrition; American Academy of Pediatrics Committee on Practice and Ambulatory Medicine; American Academy of Pediatrics Committee on Child Health Financing; American Academy of Pediatrics Committee on Medical Liability; American Academy of Pediatrics Committee on Fetus and Newborn; American Academy of Pediatrics Section on Perinatal Pediatrics; Centers for Disease Control and Prevention; Parents of Infants and Children With Kernicterus (PICK); Charles Ahlfors, MD; Daniel Batton, MD; Thomas Bojko, MD; Sarah Clune, MD; Sudhakar Ezhuthachan, MD; Lawrence Gartner, MD; Cathy Hammerman, MD; Thor Hansen, MD; Lois Johnson, MD; Michael Kaplan, MB, ChB; Tony McDonagh, PhD; Gerald Merenstein, MD; Mary O'Shea, MD; Max Perlman, MD; Ronald Poland, MD; Alex Robertson, MD; Firmino Rubaltelli, MD; Steven Shapiro, MD; Stanford Singer, MD; Ann Stark, MD; Gautham Suresh, MD; Margot VandeBor, MD; Hank Vreman, PhD; Philip Walson, MD; Jon Watchko, MD; Richard Wennberg, MD; and Chap-Yung Yeung, MD.

REFERENCES

1. American Academy of Pediatrics, Provisional Committee for Quality Improvement and Subcommittee on Hyperbilirubinemia. Practice parameter: management of hyperbilirubinemia in the healthy term newborn. *Pediatrics*. 1994;94:558–562

2. Ip S, Glicken S, Kulig J, Obrien R, Sege R, Lau J. *Management of Neonatal Hyperbilirubinemia*. Rockville, MD: US Department of Health and Human Services, Agency for Healthcare Research and Quality; 2003. AHRQ Publication 03-E011

3. Ip S, Chung M, Kulig J. et al. An evidence-based review of important issues concerning neonatal hyperbilirubinemia. *Pediatrics*. 2004;113(6). Available at: www.pediatrics.org/cgi/content/full/113/6/e644

4. American Academy of Pediatrics, Steering Committee on Quality Improvement and Management. A taxonomy of recommendations. *Pediatrics*. 2004; In press

5. Johnson LH, Bhutani VK, Brown AK. System-based approach to management of neonatal jaundice and prevention of kernicterus. *J Pediatr*. 2002;140:396–403

6. Maisels MJ, Newman TB. Kernicterus in otherwise healthy, breast-fed term newborns. *Pediatrics*. 1995;96:730–733

7. MacDonald M. Hidden risks: early discharge and bilirubin toxicity due to glucose-6-phosphate dehydrogenase deficiency. *Pediatrics*. 1995;96:734–738

8. Penn AA, Enzman DR, Hahn JS, Stevenson DK. Kernicterus in a full term infant. *Pediatrics*. 1994;93:1003–1006

9. Washington EC, Ector W, Abboud M, Ohning B, Holden K. Hemolytic jaundice due to G6PD deficiency causing kernicterus in a female newborn. *South Med J*. 1995;88:776–779

10. Ebbesen F. Recurrence of kernicterus in term and near-term infants in Denmark. *Acta Paediatr*. 2000;89:1213–1217

11. Institue of Medicine. *Crossing the Quality Chasm: A New Health System for the 21st Century*. Washington, DC: National Academy Press; 2001

12. American Academy of Pediatrics, American College of Obstetricians and Gynecologists. *Guidelines for Perinatal Care*. 5th ed. Elk Grove Village, IL: American Academy of Pediatrics; 2002:220–224

13. Bertini G, Dani C, Trochin M, Rubaltelli F. Is breastfeeding really favoring early neonatal jaundice? *Pediatrics*. 2001;107(3). Available at: www.pediatrics.org/cgi/content/full/107/3/e41

14. Maisels MJ, Gifford K. Normal serum bilirubin levels in the newborn and the effect of breast-feeding. *Pediatrics*. 1986;78:837–843

15. Yamauchi Y, Yamanouchi I. Breast-feeding frequency during the first 24 hours after birth in full-term neonates. *Pediatrics*. 1990;86:171–175

16. De Carvalho M, Klaus MH, Merkatz RB. Frequency of breastfeeding and serum bilirubin concentration. *Am J Dis Child*. 1982;136:737–738

17. Varimo P, Similä S, Wendt L, Kolvisto M. Frequency of breast feeding and hyperbilirubinemia [letter]. *Clin Pediatr (Phila)*. 1986;25:112

18. De Carvalho M, Holl M, Harvey D. Effects of water supplementation on physiological jaundice in breast-fed babies. *Arch Dis Child*. 1981;56:568–569

19. Nicoll A, Ginsburg R, Tripp JH. Supplementary feeding and jaundice in newborns. *Acta Paediatr Scand*. 1982;71:759–761

20. Madlon-Kay DJ. Identifying ABO incompatibility in newborns: selective vs automatic testing. *J Fam Pract*. 1992;35:278–280

21. Kramer LI. Advancement of dermal icterus in the jaundiced newborn. *Am J Dis Child*. 1969;118:454–458

22. Moyer VA, Ahn C, Sneed S. Accuracy of clinical judgment in neonatal jaundice. *Arch Pediatr Adolesc Med*. 2000;154:391–394

23. Davidson LT, Merritt KK, Weech AA. Hyperbilirubinemia in the newborn. *Am J Dis Child*. 1941;61:958–980

24. Tayaba R, Gribetz D, Gribetz I, Holzman IR. Noninvasive estimation of serum bilirubin. *Pediatrics*. 1998;102(3). Available at: www.pediatrics.org/cgi/content/full/102/3/e28

25. Bhutani V, Gourley GR, Adler S, Kreamer B, Dalman C, Johnson LH. Noninvasive measurement of total serum bilirubin in a multiracial predischarge newborn population to assess the risk of severe hyperbilirubinemia. *Pediatrics*. 2000;106(2). Available at: www.pediatrics.org/cgi/content/full/106/2/e17

26. Yasuda S, Itoh S, Isobe K, et al. New transcutaneous jaundice device with two optical paths. *J Perinat Med*. 2003;31:81–88

27. Maisels MJ, Ostrea EJ Jr, Touch S, et al. Evaluation of a new transcutaneous bilirubinometer. *Pediatrics*. 2004;113:1638–1645

28. Ebbesen F, Rasmussen LM, Wimberley PD. A new transcutaneous bilirubinometer, bilicheck, used in the neonatal intensive care unit and the maternity ward. *Acta Paediatr*. 2002;91:203–211

29. Rubaltelli FF, Gourley GR, Loskamp N, et al. Transcutaneous bilirubin measurement: a multicenter evaluation of a new device. *Pediatrics*. 2001;107:1264–1271

30. Newman TB, Liljestrand P, Escobar GJ. Jaundice noted in the first 24 hours after birth in a managed care organization. *Arch Pediatr Adolesc Med*. 2002;156:1244–1250

31. Bhutani VK, Johnson L, Sivieri EM. Predictive ability of a predischarge hour-specific serum bilirubin for subsequent significant hyperbilirubinemia in healthy term and near-term newborns. *Pediatrics*. 1999;103:6–14

32. Garcia FJ, Nager AL. Jaundice as an early diagnostic sign of urinary tract infection in infancy. *Pediatrics*. 2002;109:846–851

33. Kaplan M, Hammerman C. Severe neonatal hyperbilirubinemia: a potential complication of glucose-6-phosphate dehydrogenase deficiency. *Clin Perinatol*. 1998;25:575–590

34. Valaes T. Severe neonatal jaundice associated with glucose-6-phosphate dehydrogenase deficiency: pathogenesis and global epidemiology. *Acta Paediatr Suppl*. 1994;394:58–76

35. Alpay F, Sarici S, Tosuncuk HD, Serdar MA, Inanç N, Gökçay E. The value of first-day bilirubin measurement in predicting the development of significant hyperbilirubinemia in healthy term newborns. *Pediatrics*. 2000;106(2). Available at: www.pediatrics.org/cgi/content/full/106/2/e16

36. Carbonell X, Botet F, Figueras J, Riu-Godo A. Prediction of hyperbilirubinaemia in the healthy term newborn. *Acta Paediatr*. 2001;90:166–170

37. Kaplan M, Hammerman C, Feldman R, Brisk R. Predischarge bilirubin screening in glucose-6-phosphate dehydrogenase-deficient neonates. *Pediatrics*. 2000;105:533–537

38. Stevenson DK, Fanaroff AA, Maisels MJ, et al. Prediction of hyperbilirubinemia in near-term and term infants. *Pediatrics*. 2001;108:31–39

39. Newman TB, Xiong B, Gonzales VM, Escobar GJ. Prediction and prevention of extreme neonatal hyperbilirubinemia in a mature health maintenance organization. *Arch Pediatr Adolesc Med*. 2000;154:1140–1147

40. Maisels MJ, Kring EA. Length of stay, jaundice, and hospital readmission. *Pediatrics*. 1998;101:995–998

41. Gale R, Seidman DS, Dollberg S, Stevenson DK. Epidemiology of neonatal jaundice in the Jerusalem population. *J Pediatr Gastroenterol Nutr*. 1990;10:82–86

42. Berk MA, Mimouni F, Miodovnik M, Hertzberg V, Valuck J. Macrosomia in infants of insulin-dependent diabetic mothers. *Pediatrics*. 1989;83:1029–1034

43. Peevy KJ, Landaw SA, Gross SJ. Hyperbilirubinemia in infants of diabetic mothers. *Pediatrics*. 1980;66:417–419

44. Soskolne El, Schumacher R, Fyock C, Young ML, Schork A. The effect of early discharge and other factors on readmission rates of newborns. *Arch Pediatr Adolesc Med*. 1996;150:373–379

45. Ebbesen F, Brodersen R. Risk of bilirubin acid precipitation in preterm infants with respiratory distress syndrome: considerations of blood/brain bilirubin transfer equilibrium. *Early Hum Dev*. 1982;6:341–355

46. Cashore WJ, Oh W, Brodersen R. Reserve albumin and bilirubin toxicity index in infant serum. *Acta Paediatr Scand*. 1983;72:415–419

47. Cashore WJ. Free bilirubin concentrations and bilirubin-binding affinity in term and preterm infants. *J Pediatr*. 1980;96:521–527

48. Bratlid D. How bilirubin gets into the brain. *Clin Perinatol*. 1990;17:449–465

49. Wennberg RP. Cellular basis of bilirubin toxicity. *N Y State J Med*. 1991;91:493–496

50. Eggert P, Stick C, Schroder H. On the distribution of irradiation intensity in phototherapy. Measurements of effective irradiance in an incubator. *Eur J Pediatr*. 1984;142:58–61

51. Maisels MJ. Why use homeopathic doses of phototherapy? *Pediatrics*. 1996;98:283–287

52. Ahlfors CE. Criteria for exchange transfusion in jaundiced newborns. *Pediatrics*. 1994;93:488–494

53. American Association of Blood Banks Technical Manual Committee. Perinatal issues in transfusion practice. In: Brecher M, ed. *Technical Manual*. Bethesda, MD: American Association of Blood Banks; 2002:497–515

54. Garland JS, Alex C, Deacon JS, Raab K. Treatment of infants with indirect hyperbilirubinemia. Readmission to birth hospital vs nonbirth hospital. *Arch Pediatr Adolesc Med*. 1994;148:1317–1321

55. Gottstein R, Cooke R. Systematic review of intravenous immunoglobulin in haemolytic disease of the newborn. *Arch Dis Child Fetal Neonatal Ed*. 2003;88:F6–F10

56. Sato K, Hara T, Kondo T, Iwao H, Honda S, Ueda K. High-dose intravenous gammaglobulin therapy for neonatal immune haemolytic jaundice due to blood group incompatibility. *Acta Paediatr Scand*. 1991;80:163–166

57. Rubo J, Albrecht K, Lasch P, et al. High-dose intravenous immune globulin therapy for hyperbilirubinemia caused by Rh hemolytic disease. *J Pediatr*. 1992;121:93–97

58. Hammerman C, Kaplan M, Vreman HJ, Stevenson DK. Intravenous immune globulin in neonatal ABO isoimmunization: factors associated with clinical efficacy. *Biol Neonate*. 1996;70:69–74

59. Johnson L, Boggs TR. Bilirubin-dependent brain damage: incidence and indications for treatment. In: Odell GB, Schaffer R, Simopoulos AP, eds. *Phototherapy in the Newborn: An Overview*. Washington, DC: National Academy of Sciences; 1974:122–149

60. Ozmert E, Erdem G, Topcu M. Long-term follow-up of indirect hyperbilirubinemia in full-term Turkish infants. *Acta Paediatr*. 1996;85:1440–1444

61. Volpe JJ. *Neurology of the Newborn*. 4th ed. Philadelphia, PA: W. B. Saunders; 2001

62. Harris M, Bernbaum J, Polin J, Zimmerman R, Polin RA. Developmental follow-up of breastfed term and near-term infants with marked hyperbilirubinemia. *Pediatrics*. 2001;107:1075–1080

63. Osborn LM, Bolus R. Breast feeding and jaundice in the first week of life. *J Fam Pract*. 1985;20:475–480

64. Martinez JC, Maisels MJ, Otheguy L, et al. Hyperbilirubinemia in the breast-fed newborn: a controlled trial of four interventions. *Pediatrics.* 1993;91:470–473

65. Amato M, Howald H, von Muralt G. Interruption of breast-feeding versus phototherapy as treatment of hyperbilirubinemia in full-term infants. *Helv Paediatr Acta.* 1985;40:127–131

66. Maisels MJ, Gifford K, Antle CE, Leib GR. Jaundice in the healthy newborn infant: a new approach to an old problem. *Pediatrics.* 1988;81:505–511

67. Newman TB, Easterling MJ. Yield of reticulocyte counts and blood smears in term infants. *Clin Pediatr (Phila).* 1994;33:71–76

68. Herschel M, Karrison T, Wen M, Caldarelli L, Baron B. Evaluation of the direct antiglobulin (Coombs') test for identifying newborns at risk for hemolysis as determined by end-tidal carbon monoxide concentration (ETCOc); and comparison of the Coombs' test with ETCOc for detecting significant jaundice. *J Perinatol.* 2002;22:341–347

69. Stevenson DK, Vreman HJ. Carbon monoxide and bilirubin production in neonates. *Pediatrics.* 1997;100:252–254

70. Vreman HJ, Verter J, Oh W, et al. Interlaboratory variability of bilirubin measurements. *Clin Chem.* 1996;42:869–873

71. Lo S, Doumas BT, Ashwood E. Performance of bilirubin determinations in US laboratories—revisited. *Clin Chem.* 2004;50:190–194

72. Kappas A, Drummond GS, Henschke C, Valaes T. Direct comparison of Sn-mesoporphyrin, an inhibitor of bilirubin production, and phototherapy in controlling hyperbilirubinemia in term and near-term newborns. *Pediatrics.* 1995;95:468–474

73. Martinez JC, Garcia HO, Otheguy L, Drummond GS, Kappas A. Control of severe hyperbilirubinemia in full-term newborns with the inhibitor of bilirubin production Sn-mesoporphyrin. *Pediatrics.* 1999;103:1–5

74. Suresh G, Martin CL, Soll R. Metalloporphyrins for treatment of unconjugated hyperbilirubinemia in neonates. *Cochrane Database Syst Rev.* 2003;2:CD004207

75. Kappas A, Drummond GS, Munson DP, Marshall JR. Sn-mesoporphyrin interdiction of severe hyperbilirubinemia in Jehovah's Witness newborns as an alternative to exchange transfusion. *Pediatrics.* 2001;108:1374–1377

APPENDIX 1: Additional Notes

Definitions of Quality of Evidence and Balance of Benefits and Harms

The Steering Committee on Quality Improvement and Management categorizes evidence quality in 4 levels:

1. Well-designed, randomized, controlled trials or diagnostic studies on relevant populations
2. Randomized, controlled trials or diagnostic studies with minor limitations; overwhelming, consistent evidence from observational studies
3. Observational studies (case-control and cohort design)
4. Expert opinion, case reports, reasoning from first principles

The AAP defines evidence-based recommendations as follows:[1]

- Strong recommendation: the committee believes that the benefits of the recommended approach clearly exceed the harms of that approach and that the quality of the supporting evidence is either excellent or impossible to obtain. Clinicians should follow these recommendations unless a clear and compelling rationale for an alternative approach is present.
- Recommendation: the committee believes that the benefits exceed the harms, but the quality of evidence on which this recommendation is based is not as strong. Clinicians should also generally follow these recommendations but should be alert to new information and sensitive to patient prefer-

ences. In this guideline, the term "should" implies a recommendation by the committee.

- Option: either the quality of the evidence that exists is suspect or well-performed studies have shown little clear advantage to one approach over another. Patient preference should have a substantial role in influencing clinical decision-making when a policy is described as an option.
- No recommendation: there is a lack of pertinent evidence and the anticipated balance of benefits and harms is unclear.

Anticipated Balance Between Benefits and Harms

The presence of clear benefits or harms supports stronger statements for or against a course of action. In some cases, however, recommendations are made when analysis of the balance of benefits and harms provides an exceptional dysequilibrium and it would be unethical or impossible to perform clinical trials to "prove" the point. In these cases the balance of benefit and harm is termed "exceptional."

Clinical Manifestations of Acute Bilirubin Encephalopathy and Kernicterus

Acute Bilirubin Encephalopathy

In the early phase of acute bilirubin encephalopathy, severely jaundiced infants become lethargic and hypotonic and suck poorly.[2,3] The intermediate phase is characterized by moderate stupor, irritability, and hypertonia. The infant may develop a fever and high-pitched cry, which may alternate with drowsiness and hypotonia. The hypertonia is manifested by backward arching of the neck (retrocollis) and trunk (opisthotonos). There is anecdotal evidence that an emergent exchange transfusion at this stage, in some cases, might reverse the central nervous system changes.[4] The advanced phase, in which central nervous system damage is probably irreversible, is characterized by pronounced retrocollis-opisthotonos, shrill cry, no feeding, apnea, fever, deep stupor to coma, sometimes seizures, and death.[2,3,5]

Kernicterus

In the chronic form of bilirubin encephalopathy, surviving infants may develop a severe form of athetoid cerebral palsy, auditory dysfunction, dental-enamel dysplasia, paralysis of upward gaze, and, less often, intellectual and other handicaps. Most infants who develop kernicterus have manifested some or all of the signs listed above in the acute phase of bilirubin encephalopathy. However, occasionally there are infants who have developed very high bilirubin levels and, subsequently, the signs of kernicterus but have exhibited few, if any, antecedent clinical signs of acute bilirubin encephalopathy.[3,5,6]

Clinical Evaluation of Jaundice and TcB Measurements

Jaundice is usually seen in the face first and progresses caudally to the trunk and extremities,[7] but because visual estimation of bilirubin levels from the degree of jaundice can lead to errors,[8–10] a low threshold should be used for measuring the TSB.

Devices that provide a noninvasive TcB measurement have proven very useful as screening tools,[11] and newer instruments give measurements that provide a valid estimate of the TSB level.[12–17] Studies using the new TcB-measurement instruments are limited, but the data published thus far suggest that in most newborn populations, these instruments generally provide measurements within 2 to 3 mg/dL (34–51 μmol/L) of the TSB and can replace a measurement of serum bilirubin in many circumstances, particularly for TSB levels less than 15 mg/dL (257 μmol/L).[12–17] Because phototherapy "bleaches" the skin, both visual assessment of jaundice and TcB measurements in infants undergoing phototherapy are not reliable. In addition, the ability of transcutaneous instruments to provide accurate measurements in different racial groups requires additional study.[18,19] The limitations of the accuracy and reproducibility of TSB measurements in the clinical laboratory[20–22] must also be recognized and are discussed in the technical report.[23]

Capillary Versus Venous Serum Bilirubin Measurement

Almost all published data regarding the relationship of TSB levels to kernicterus or developmental outcome are based on capillary blood TSB levels. Data regarding the differences between capillary and venous TSB levels are conflicting.[24,25] In 1 study the capillary TSB levels were higher, but in another they were lower than venous TSB levels.[24,25] Thus, obtaining a venous sample to "confirm" an elevated capillary TSB level is not recommended, because it will delay the initiation of treatment.

Direct-Reacting and Conjugated Bilirubin

Although commonly used interchangeably, direct-reacting bilirubin is not the same as conjugated bilirubin. Direct-reacting bilirubin is the bilirubin that reacts directly (without the addition of an accelerating agent) with diazotized sulfanilic acid. Conjugated bilirubin is bilirubin made water soluble by binding with glucuronic acid in the liver. Depending on the technique used, the clinical laboratory will report total and direct-reacting or unconjugated and conjugated bilirubin levels. In this guideline and for clinical purposes, the terms may be used interchangeably.

Abnormal Direct and Conjugated Bilirubin Levels

Laboratory measurement of direct bilirubin is not precise,[26] and values between laboratories can vary widely. If the TSB is at or below 5 mg/dL (85 μmol/L), a direct or conjugated bilirubin of more than 1.0 mg/dL (17.1 μmol/L) is generally considered abnormal. For TSB values higher than 5 mg/dL (85 μmol/L), a direct bilirubin of more than 20% of the TSB is considered abnormal. If the hospital laboratory measures conjugated bilirubin using the Vitros (formerly Ektachem) system (Ortho-Clinical Diagnostics, Raritan, NJ), any value higher than 1 mg/dL is considered abnormal.

Assessment of Adequacy of Intake in Breastfeeding Infants

The data from a number of studies[27–34] indicate that unsupplemented, breastfed infants experience their maximum weight loss by day 3 and, on average, lose 6.1% $\pm$ 2.5% (SD) of their birth weight. Thus, ~5% to 10% of fully breastfed infants lose 10% or more of their birth weight by day 3, suggesting that adequacy of intake should be evaluated and the infant monitored if weight loss is more than 10%.[35] Evidence of adequate intake in breastfed infants also includes 4 to 6 thoroughly wet diapers in 24 hours and the passage of 3 to 4 stools per day by the fourth day. By the third to fourth day, the stools in adequately breastfed infants should have changed from meconium to a mustard yellow, mushy stool.[36] The above assessment will also help to identify breastfed infants who are at risk for dehydration because of inadequate intake.

Nomogram for Designation of Risk

Note that this nomogram (Fig 2) does not describe the natural history of neonatal hyperbilirubinemia, particularly after 48 to 72 hours, for which, because of sampling bias, the lower zones are spuriously elevated.[37] This bias, however, will have much less effect on the high-risk zone (95th percentile in the study).[38]

G6PD Dehydrogenase Deficiency

It is important to look for G6PD deficiency in infants with significant hyperbilirubinemia, because some may develop a sudden increase in the TSB. In addition, G6PD-deficient infants require intervention at lower TSB levels (Figs 3 and 4). It should be noted also that in the presence of hemolysis, G6PD levels can be elevated, which may obscure the diagnosis in the newborn period so that a normal level in a hemolyzing neonate does not rule out G6PD deficiency.[39] If G6PD deficiency is strongly suspected, a repeat level should be measured when the infant is 3 months old. It is also recognized that immediate laboratory determination of G6PD is generally not available in most US hospitals, and thus translating the above information into clinical practice is cur-

TABLE 4. Risk Zone as a Predictor of Hyperbilirubinemia[39]

TSB Before Discharge	Newborns (Total = 2840), n (%)	Newborns Who Subsequently Developed a TSB Level >95th Percentile, n (%)
High-risk zone (>95th percentile)	172 (6.0)	68 (39.5)
High intermediate-risk zone	356 (12.5)	46 (12.9)
Low intermediate-risk zone	556 (19.6)	12 (2.26)
Low-risk zone	1756 (61.8)	0

rently difficult. Nevertheless, practitioners are reminded to consider the diagnosis of G6PD deficiency in infants with severe hyperbilirubinemia, particularly if they belong to the population groups in which this condition is prevalent. This is important in the African American population, because these infants, as a group, have much lower TSB levels than white or Asian infants.[40,41] Thus, severe hyperbilirubinemia in an African American infant should always raise the possibility of G6PD deficiency.

Basis for the Recommendations 7.1.1 Through 7.1.6 and Provided in Figs 3 and 4

Ideally, recommendations for when to implement phototherapy and exchange transfusions should be based on estimates of when the benefits of these interventions exceed their risks and cost. The evidence for these estimates should come from randomized trials or systematic observational studies. Unfortunately, there is little such evidence on which to base these recommendations. As a result, treatment guidelines must necessarily rely on more uncertain estimates and extrapolations. For a detailed discussion of this question, please see "An Evidence-Based Review of Important Issues Concerning Neonatal Hyperbilirubinemia."[23]

The recommendations for phototherapy and exchange transfusion are based on the following principles:

- The main demonstrated value of phototherapy is that it reduces the risk that TSB levels will reach a level at which exchange transfusion is recommended.[42–44] Approximately 5 to 10 infants with TSB levels between 15 and 20 mg/dL (257–342 μmol/L) will receive phototherapy to prevent the TSB in 1 infant from reaching 20 mg/dL (the number needed to treat).[12] Thus, 8 to 9 of every 10 infants with these TSB levels will not reach 20 mg/dL (342 μmol/L) even if they are not treated. Phototherapy has proven to be a generally safe procedure, although rare complications can occur (see Appendix 2).
- Recommended TSB levels for exchange transfusion (Fig 4) are based largely on the goal of keeping TSB levels below those at which kernicterus has been reported.[12,45–48] In almost all cases, exchange transfusion is recommended only after phototherapy has failed to keep the TSB level below the exchange transfusion level (Fig 4).
- The recommendations to use phototherapy and exchange transfusion at lower TSB levels for infants of lower gestation and those who are sick are based on limited observations suggesting that sick infants (particularly those with the risk factors listed in Figs 3 and 4)[49–51] and those of lower gestation[51–54] are at greater risk for developing kernicterus at lower bilirubin levels than are well infants of more than 38 6/7 weeks' gestation. Nevertheless, other studies have not confirmed all of these associations.[52,55,56] There is no doubt, however, that infants at 35 to 37 6/7 weeks' gestation are at a much greater risk of developing very high

TSB levels.[57,58] Intervention for these infants is based on this risk as well as extrapolations from more premature, lower birth-weight infants who do have a higher risk of bilirubin toxicity.[52,53]
- For all newborns, treatment is recommended at lower TSB levels at younger ages because one of the primary goals of treatment is to prevent additional increases in the TSB level.

Subtle Neurologic Abnormalities Associated With Hyperbilirubinemia

There are several studies demonstrating measurable transient changes in brainstem-evoked potentials, behavioral patterns, and the infant's cry[59–63] associated with TSB levels of 15 to 25 mg/dL (257–428 μmol/L). In these studies, the abnormalities identified were transient and disappeared when the serum bilirubin levels returned to normal with or without treatment.[59,60,62,63]

A few cohort studies have found an association between hyperbilirubinemia and long-term adverse neurodevelopmental effects that are more subtle than kernicterus.[64–67] Current studies, however, suggest that although phototherapy lowers the TSB levels, it has no effect on these long-term neurodevelopmental outcomes.[68–70]

Risks of Exchange Transfusion

Because exchange transfusions are now rarely performed, the risks of morbidity and mortality associated with the procedure are difficult to quantify. In addition, the complication rates listed below may not be generalizable to the current era if, like most procedures, frequency of performance is an important determinant of risk. Death associated with exchange transfusion has been reported in approximately 3 in 1000 procedures,[71,72] although in otherwise well infants of 35 or more weeks' gestation, the risk is probably much lower.[71–73] Significant morbidity (apnea, bradycardia, cyanosis, vasospasm, thrombosis, necrotizing enterocolitis) occurs in as many as 5% of exchange transfusions,[71] and the risks associated with the use of blood products must always be considered.[74] Hypoxic-ischemic encephalopathy and acquired immunodeficiency syndrome have occurred in otherwise healthy infants receiving exchange transfusions.[73,75]

Serum Albumin Levels and the B/A Ratio

The legends to Figs 3 and 4 and recommendations 7.1.5 and 7.1.6 contain references to the serum albumin level and the B/A ratio as factors that can be considered in the decision to initiate phototherapy (Fig 3) or perform an exchange transfusion (Fig 4). Bilirubin is transported in the plasma tightly bound to albumin, and the portion that is unbound or loosely bound can more readily leave the intravascular space and cross the intact blood-brain barrier.[76] Elevations of unbound bilirubin (UB) have been associated with kernicterus in sick preterm newborns.[77,78] In addition, elevated UB concentrations are more closely associated than TSB levels with transient abnormalities in the audiometric brainstem response in term[79] and preterm[80] infants. Long-term studies relating B/A binding in infants to developmental outcome are limited and conflicting.[69,81,82] In addition, clinical laboratory measurement of UB is not currently available in the United States.

The ratio of bilirubin (mg/dL) to albumin (g/dL) does correlate with measured UB in newborns[83] and can be used as an approximate surrogate for the measurement of UB. It must be recognized, however, that both albumin levels and the ability of albumin to bind bilirubin vary significantly between newborns.[83,84] Albumin binding of bilirubin is impaired in sick infants,[84–86] and some studies show an increase in binding with increasing gestational[86,87] and postnatal[87,88] age, but others have not found a significant effect of gestational age on binding.[89] Furthermore, the risk of bilirubin encephalopathy is unlikely to be a simple function of the TSB level or the concentration of UB but is more likely a combination of both (ie, the total amount of bilirubin available [the miscible pool of bilirubin] as well as the tendency of bilirubin to enter the tissues [the UB concentration]).[83] An additional factor is the possible susceptibility of the cells of the central nervous system to damage by bilirubin.[90] It is therefore a clinical option to use the B/A ratio together with, but not in lieu of, the TSB level as an additional factor in determining the need for exchange transfusion[83] (Fig 4).

REFERENCES

1. American Academy of Pediatrics, Steering Committee on Quality Improvement and Management. Classification of recommendations for clinical practice guidelines. *Pediatrics.* 2004; In press

2. Johnson LH, Bhutani VK, Brown AK. System-based approach to management of neonatal jaundice and prevention of kernicterus. *J Pediatr.* 2002;140:396–403

3. Volpe JJ. *Neurology of the Newborn.* 4th ed. Philadelphia, PA: W. B. Saunders; 2001

4. Harris M, Bernbaum J, Polin J, Zimmerman R, Polin RA. Developmental follow-up of breastfed term and near-term infants with marked hyperbilirubinemia. *Pediatrics.* 2001;107:1075–1080

5. Van Praagh R. Diagnosis of kernicterus in the neonatal period. *Pediatrics.* 1961;28:870–876

6. Jones MH, Sands R, Hyman CB, Sturgeon P, Koch FP. Longitudinal study of incidence of central nervous system damage following erythroblastosis fetalis. *Pediatrics.* 1954;14:346–350

7. Kramer LI. Advancement of dermal icterus in the jaundiced newborn. *Am J Dis Child.* 1969;118:454–458

8. Moyer VA, Ahn C, Sneed S. Accuracy of clinical judgment in neonatal jaundice. *Arch Pediatr Adolesc Med.* 2000;154:391–394

9. Davidson LT, Merritt KK, Weech AA. Hyperbilirubinemia in the newborn. *Am J Dis Child.* 1941;61:958–980

10. Tayaba R, Gribetz D, Gribetz I, Holzman IR. Noninvasive estimation of serum bilirubin. *Pediatrics.* 1998;102(3). Available at: www.pediatrics.org/cgi/content/full/102/3/e28

11. Maisels MJ, Kring E. Transcutaneous bilirubinometry decreases the need for serum bilirubin measurements and saves money. *Pediatrics.* 1997;99:599–601

12. Ip S, Glicken S, Kulig J, Obrien R, Sege R, Lau J. *Management of Neonatal Hyperbilirubinemia.* Rockville, MD: US Department of Health and Human Services, Agency for Healthcare Research and Quality; 2003. AHRQ Publication 03-E011

13. Bhutani V, Gourley GR, Adler S, Kreamer B, Dalman C, Johnson LH. Noninvasive measurement of total serum bilirubin in a multiracial predischarge newborn population to assess the risk of severe hyperbilirubinemia. *Pediatrics.* 2000;106(2). Available at: www.pediatrics.org/cgi/content/full/106/2/e17

14. Yasuda S, Itoh S, Isobe K, et al. New transcutaneous jaundice device with two optical paths. *J Perinat Med.* 2003;31:81–88

15. Maisels MJ, Ostrea EJ Jr, Touch S, et al. Evaluation of a new transcutaneous bilirubinometer. *Pediatrics.* 2004;113:1638–1645

16. Ebbesen F, Rasmussen LM, Wimberley PD. A new transcutaneous bilirubinometer, bilicheck, used in the neonatal intensive care unit and the maternity ward. *Acta Paediatr.* 2002;91:203–211

17. Rubaltelli FF, Gourley GR, Loskamp N, et al. Transcutaneous bilirubin measurement: a multicenter evaluation of a new device. *Pediatrics.* 2001;107:1264–1271

18. Engle WD, Jackson GL, Sendelbach D, Manning D, Frawley W. Assessment of a transcutaneous device in the evaluation of neonatal hyperbilirubinemia in a primarily Hispanic population. *Pediatrics.* 2002;110:61–67

19. Schumacher R. Transcutaneous bilirubinometry and diagnostic tests: "the right job for the tool." *Pediatrics.* 2002;110:407–408

20. Vreman HJ, Verter J, Oh W, et al. Interlaboratory variability of bilirubin measurements. *Clin Chem.* 1996;42:869–873

21. Doumas BT, Eckfeldt JH. Errors in measurement of total bilirubin: a perennial problem. *Clin Chem.* 1996;42:845–848

22. Lo S, Doumas BT, Ashwood E. Performance of bilirubin determinations in US laboratories—revisited. *Clin Chem.* 2004;50:190–194

23. Ip S, Chung M, Kulig J. et al. An evidence-based review of important issues concerning neonatal hyperbilirubinemia. *Pediatrics.* 2004;113(6). Available at: www.pediatrics.org/cgi/content/full/113/6/e644

24. Leslie GI, Philips JB, Cassady G. Capillary and venous bilirubin values: are they really different? *Am J Dis Child.* 1987;141:1199–1200

25. Eidelman AI, Schimmel MS, Algur N, Eylath U. Capillary and venous bilirubin values: they are different—and how [letter]! *Am J Dis Child.* 1989;143:642

26. Watkinson LR, St John A, Penberthy LA. Investigation into paediatric bilirubin analyses in Australia and New Zealand. *J Clin Pathol.* 1982;35:52–58

27. Bertini G, Dani C, Trochin M, Rubaltelli F. Is breastfeeding really favoring early neonatal jaundice? *Pediatrics.* 2001;107(3). Available at: www.pediatrics.org/cgi/content/full/107/3/e41

28. De Carvalho M, Klaus MH, Merkatz RB. Frequency of breastfeeding and serum bilirubin concentration. *Am J Dis Child.* 1982;136:737–738

29. De Carvalho M, Holl M, Harvey D. Effects of water supplementation on physiological jaundice in breast-fed babies. *Arch Dis Child.* 1981;56:568–569

30. Nicoll A, Ginsburg R, Tripp JH. Supplementary feeding and jaundice in newborns. *Acta Paediatr Scand.* 1982;71:759–761

31. Butler DA, MacMillan JP. Relationship of breast feeding and weight loss to jaundice in the newborn period: review of the literature and results of a study. *Cleve Clin Q.* 1983;50:263–268

32. De Carvalho M, Robertson S, Klaus M. Fecal bilirubin excretion and serum bilirubin concentration in breast-fed and bottle-fed infants. *J Pediatr.* 1985;107:786–790

33. Gourley GR, Kreamer B, Arend R. The effect of diet on feces and jaundice during the first three weeks of life. *Gastroenterology.* 1992;103:660–667

34. Maisels MJ, Gifford K. Breast-feeding, weight loss, and jaundice. *J Pediatr.* 1983;102:117–118

35. Laing IA, Wong CM. Hypernatraemia in the first few days: is the incidence rising? *Arch Dis Child Fetal Neonatal Ed.* 2002;87:F158–F162

36. Lawrence RA. Management of the mother-infant nursing couple. In: *A Breastfeeding Guide for the Medical Profession.* 4th ed. St Louis, MO: Mosby-Year Book, Inc; 1994:215–277

37. Maisels MJ, Newman TB. Predicting hyperbilirubinemia in newborns: the importance of timing. *Pediatrics.* 1999;103:493–495

38. Bhutani VK, Johnson L, Sivieri EM. Predictive ability of a predischarge hour-specific serum bilirubin for subsequent significant hyperbilirubinemia in healthy term and near-term newborns. *Pediatrics.* 1999;103:6–14

39. Beutler E. Glucose-6-phosphate dehydrogenase deficiency. *Blood.* 1994;84:3613–3636

40. Linn S, Schoenbaum SC, Monson RR, Rosner B, Stubblefield PG, Ryan KJ. Epidemiology of neonatal hyperbilirubinemia. *Pediatrics.* 1985;75:770–774

41. Newman TB, Easterling MJ, Goldman ES, Stevenson DK. Laboratory evaluation of jaundiced newborns: frequency, cost and yield. *Am J Dis Child.* 1990;144:364–368

42. Martinez JC, Maisels MJ, Otheguy L, et al. Hyperbilirubinemia in the breast-fed newborn: a controlled trial of four interventions. *Pediatrics.* 1993;91:470–473

43. Maisels MJ. Phototherapy—traditional and nontraditional. *J Perinatol.* 2001;21(suppl 1):S93–S97

44. Brown AK, Kim MH, Wu PY, Bryla DA. Efficacy of phototherapy in prevention and management of neonatal hyperbilirubinemia. *Pediatrics.* 1985;75:393–400

45. Armitage P, Mollison PL. Further analysis of controlled trials of treatment of hemolytic disease of the newborn. *J Obstet Gynaecol Br Emp.* 1953;60:602–605

46. Mollison PL, Walker W. Controlled trials of the treatment of haemolytic disease of the newborn. *Lancet.* 1952;1:429–433

47. Hsia DYY, Allen FH, Gellis SS, Diamond LK. Erythroblastosis fetalis. VIII. Studies of serum bilirubin in relation to kernicterus. *N Engl J Med.* 1952;247:668–671

48. Newman TB, Maisels MJ. Does hyperbilirubinemia damage the brain of healthy full-term infants? *Clin Perinatol.* 1990;17:331–358

49. Ozmert E, Erdem G, Topcu M. Long-term follow-up of indirect hyperbilirubinemia in full-term Turkish infants. *Acta Paediatr.* 1996;85:1440–1444

50. Perlman JM, Rogers B, Burns D. Kernicterus findings at autopsy in 2 sick near-term infants. *Pediatrics.* 1997;99:612–615

51. Gartner LM, Snyder RN, Chabon RS, Bernstein J. Kernicterus: high incidence in premature infants with low serum bilirubin concentration. *Pediatrics.* 1970;45:906–917

52. Watchko JF, Oski FA. Kernicterus in preterm newborns: past, present, and future. *Pediatrics.* 1992;90:707–715

53. Watchko J, Claassen D. Kernicterus in premature infants: current prevalence and relationship to NICHD Phototherapy Study exchange criteria. *Pediatrics.* 1994;93(6 Pt 1):996–999

54. Stern L, Denton RL. Kernicterus in small, premature infants. *Pediatrics.* 1965;35:486–485

55. Turkel SB, Guttenberg ME, Moynes DR, Hodgman JE. Lack of identifiable risk factors for kernicterus. *Pediatrics.* 1980;66:502–506

56. Kim MH, Yoon JJ, Sher J, Brown AK. Lack of predictive indices in kernicterus. A comparison of clinical and pathologic factors in infants with or without kernicterus. *Pediatrics.* 1980;66:852–858

57. Newman TB, Xiong B, Gonzales VM, Escobar GJ. Prediction and prevention of extreme neonatal hyperbilirubinemia in a mature health maintenance organization. *Arch Pediatr Adolesc Med.* 2000;154:1140–1147

58. Newman TB, Escobar GJ, Gonzales VM, Armstrong MA, Gardner MN, Folck BF. Frequency of neonatal bilirubin testing and hyperbilirubinemia in a large health maintenance organization. *Pediatrics.* 1999;104:1198–1203

59. Vohr BR. New approaches to assessing the risks of hyperbilirubinemia. *Clin Perinatol.* 1990;17:293–306

60. Perlman M, Fainmesser P, Sohmer H, Tamari H, Wax Y, Pevsmer B. Auditory nerve-brainstem evoked responses in hyperbilirubinemic neonates. *Pediatrics.* 1983;72:658–664

61. Nakamura H, Takada S, Shimabuku R, Matsuo M, Matsuo T, Negishi H. Auditory and brainstem responses in newborn infants with hyperbilirubinemia. *Pediatrics.* 1985;75:703–708

62. Nwaesei CG, Van Aerde J, Boyden M, Perlman M. Changes in auditory brainstem responses in hyperbilirubinemic infants before and after exchange transfusion. *Pediatrics.* 1984;74:800–803

63. Wennberg RP, Ahlfors CE, Bickers R, McMurtry CA, Shetter JL. Abnormal auditory brainstem response in a newborn infant with hyperbilirubinemia: improvement with exchange transfusion. *J Pediatr.* 1982;100:624–626

64. Soorani-Lunsing I, Woltil H, Hadders-Algra M. Are moderate degrees of hyperbilirubinemia in healthy term neonates really safe for the brain? *Pediatr Res.* 2001;50:701–705

65. Grimmer I, Berger-Jones K, Buhrer C, Brandl U, Obladen M. Late neurological sequelae of non-hemolytic hyperbilirubinemia of healthy term neonates. *Acta Paediatr.* 1999;88:661–663

66. Seidman DS, Paz I, Stevenson DK, Laor A, Danon YL, Gale R. Neonatal hyperbilirubinemia and physical and cognitive performance at 17 years of age. *Pediatrics.* 1991;88:828–833

67. Newman TB, Klebanoff MA. Neonatal hyperbilirubinemia and long-term outcome: another look at the collaborative perinatal project. *Pediatrics.* 1993;92:651–657

68. Scheidt PC, Bryla DA, Nelson KB, Hirtz DG, Hoffman HJ. Phototherapy for neonatal hyperbilirubinemia: six-year follow-up of the National Institute of Child Health and Human Development clinical trial. *Pediatrics.* 1990;85:455–463

69. Scheidt PC, Graubard BI, Nelson KB, et al. Intelligence at six years in relation to neonatal bilirubin levels: follow-up of the National Institute of Child Health and Human Development Clinical Trial of Phototherapy. *Pediatrics.* 1991;87:797–805

70. Seidman DS, Paz I, Stevenson DK, Laor A, Danon YL, Gale R. Effect of phototherapy for neonatal jaundice on cognitive performance. *J Perinatol.* 1994;14:23–28

71. Keenan WJ, Novak KK, Sutherland JM, Bryla DA, Fetterly KL. Morbidity and mortality associated with exchange transfusion. *Pediatrics.* 1985;75:417–421

72. Hovi L, Siimes MA. Exchange transfusion with fresh heparinized blood is a safe procedure: Experiences from 1069 newborns. *Acta Paediatr Scand.* 1985;74:360–365

73. Jackson JC. Adverse events associated with exchange transfusion in healthy and ill newborns. *Pediatrics.* 1997;99(5):e7. Available at: www.pediatrics.org/cgi/content/full/99/5/e7

74. Schreiber GB, Busch MP, Kleinman SH, Korelitz JJ. The risk of transfusion-transmitted viral infections. *N Engl J Med.* 1996;334:1685–1690

75. Maisels MJ, Newman TB. Kernicterus in otherwise healthy, breast-fed term newborns. *Pediatrics.* 1995;96:730–733

76. Bratlid D. How bilirubin gets into the brain. *Clin Perinatol.* 1990;17:449–465

77. Cashore WJ, Oh W. Unbound bilirubin and kernicterus in low-birth-weight infants. *Pediatrics.* 1982;69:481–485

78. Nakamura H, Yonetani M, Uetani Y, Funato M, Lee Y. Determination of serum unbound bilirubin for prediction of kernicterus in low birth-weight infants. *Acta Paediatr Jpn.* 1992;34:642–647

79. Funato M, Tamai H, Shimada S, Nakamura H. Vigintiphobia, unbound bilirubin, and auditory brainstem responses. *Pediatrics.* 1994;93:50–53

80. Amin SB, Ahlfors CE, Orlando MS, Dalzell LE, Merle KS, Guillet R. Bilirubin and serial auditory brainstem responses in premature infants. *Pediatrics.* 2001;107:664–670

81. Johnson L, Boggs TR. Bilirubin-dependent brain damage: incidence and indications for treatment. In: Odell GB, Schaffer R, Simopoulos AP, eds. *Phototherapy in the Newborn: An Overview.* Washington, DC: National Academy of Sciences; 1974:122–149

82. Odell GB, Storey GNB, Rosenberg LA. Studies in kernicterus. 3. The saturation of serum proteins with bilirubin during neonatal life and its relationship to brain damage at five years. *J Pediatr.* 1970;76:12–21

83. Ahlfors CE. Criteria for exchange transfusion in jaundiced newborns. *Pediatrics.* 1994;93:488–494

84. Cashore WJ. Free bilirubin concentrations and bilirubin-binding affinity in term and preterm infants. *J Pediatr.* 1980;96:521–527

85. Ebbesen F, Brodersen R. Risk of bilirubin acid precipitation in preterm infants with respiratory distress syndrome: considerations of blood/brain bilirubin transfer equilibrium. *Early Hum Dev.* 1982;6:341–355

86. Cashore WJ, Oh W, Brodersen R. Reserve albumin and bilirubin toxicity index in infant serum. *Acta Paediatr Scand.* 1983;72:415–419

87. Ebbesen F, Nyboe J. Postnatal changes in the ability of plasma albumin to bind bilirubin. *Acta Paediatr Scand.* 1983;72:665–670

88. Esbjorner E. Albumin binding properties in relation to bilirubin and albumin concentrations during the first week of life. *Acta Paediatr Scand.* 1991;80:400–405

89. Robertson A, Sharp C, Karp W. The relationship of gestational age to reserve albumin concentration for binding of bilirubin. *J Perinatol.* 1988;8:17–18

90. Wennberg RP. Cellular basis of bilirubin toxicity. *N Y State J Med.* 1991;91:493–496

APPENDIX 2: Phototherapy

There is no standardized method for delivering phototherapy. Phototherapy units vary widely, as do the types of lamps used in the units. The efficacy of phototherapy depends on the dose of phototherapy administered as well as a number of clinical factors (Table 5).[1]

Measuring the Dose of Phototherapy

Table 5 shows the radiometric quantities used in measuring the phototherapy dose. The quantity most commonly reported in the literature is the spectral irradiance. In the nursery, spectral irradiance can be measured by using commercially available radiometers. These instruments take a single measurement across a band of wavelengths, typically 425 to 475 or 400 to 480 nm. Unfortunately, there is no standardized method for reporting phototherapy dosages in the clinical literature, so it is difficult to compare published studies on the efficacy of phototherapy and manufacturers' data for the irradiance produced by different systems.[2] Measurements of irradiance from the same system, using different radiometers,

TABLE 5. Factors That Affect the Dose and Efficacy of Phototherapy

Factor	Mechanism/Clinical Relevance	Implementation and Rationale	Clinical Application
Spectrum of light emitted	Blue-green spectrum is most effective. At these wavelengths, light penetrates skin well and is absorbed maximally by bilirubin.	Special blue fluorescent tubes or other light sources that have most output in the blue-green spectrum and are most effective in lowering TSB.	Use special blue tubes or LED light source with output in blue-green spectrum for intensive PT.
Spectral irradiance (irradiance in certain wavelength band) delivered to surface of infant	↑ irradiance → ↑ rate of decline in TSB	Irradiance is measured with a radiometer as $\mu W/cm^2$ per nm. Standard PT units deliver 8–10 $\mu W/cm^2$ per nm (Fig 6). Intensive PT requires >30 $\mu W/cm^2$ per nm.	If special blue fluorescent tubes are used, bring tubes as close to infant as possible to increase irradiance (Fig 6). Note: This cannot be done with halogen lamps because of the danger of burn. Special blue tubes 10–15 cm above the infant will produce an irradiance of at least 35 $\mu W/cm^2$ per nm.
Spectral power (average spectral irradiance across surface area)	↑ surface area exposed → ↑ rate of decline in TSB	For intensive PT, expose maximum surface area of infant to PT.	Place lights above and fiber-optic pad or special blue fluorescent tubes* below the infant. For maximum exposure, line sides of bassinet, warmer bed, or incubator with aluminum foil.
Cause of jaundice	PT is likely to be less effective if jaundice is due to hemolysis or if cholestasis is present. (↑ direct bilirubin)		When hemolysis is present, start PT at lower TSB levels. Use intensive PT. Failure of PT suggests that hemolysis is the cause of jaundice. If ↑ direct bilirubin, watch for bronze baby syndrome or blistering.
TSB level at start of PT	The higher the TSB, the more rapid the decline in TSB with PT.		Use intensive PT for higher TSB levels. Anticipate a more rapid decrease in TSB when TSB >20 mg/dL (342 $\mu mol/L$).

PT indicates phototherapy; LED, light-emitting diode.
* Available in the Olympic BiliBassinet (Olympic Medical, Seattle, WA).

can also produce significantly different results. The width of the phototherapy lamp's emissions spectrum (narrow versus broad) will affect the measured irradiance. Measurements under lights with a very focused emission spectrum (eg, blue light-emitting diode) will vary significantly from one radiometer to another, because the response spectra of the radiometers vary from manufacturer to manufacturer. Broader-spectrum lights (fluorescent and halogen) have fewer variations among radiometers. Manufacturers of phototherapy systems generally recommend the specific radiometer to be used in measuring the dose of phototherapy when their system is used.

It is important also to recognize that the measured irradiance will vary widely depending on where the measurement is taken. Irradiance measured below the center of the light source can be more than double that measured at the periphery, and this dropoff at the periphery will vary with different phototherapy units. Ideally, irradiance should be measured at multiple sites under the area illuminated by the unit and the measurements averaged. The International Electrotechnical Commission[3] defines the "effective surface area" as the intended treatment surface that is illuminated by the phototherapy light. The commission uses 60 × 30 cm as the standard-sized surface.

Is It Necessary to Measure Phototherapy Doses Routinely?

Although it is not necessary to measure spectral irradiance before each use of phototherapy, it is important to perform periodic checks of phototherapy units to make sure that an adequate irradiance is being delivered.

The Dose-Response Relationship of Phototherapy

Figure 5 shows that there is a direct relationship between the irradiance used and the rate at which the serum bilirubin declines under phototherapy.[4] The data in Fig 5 suggest that there is a saturation point beyond which an increase in the irradiance produces no added efficacy. We do not know, however, that a saturation point exists. Because the conversion of bilirubin to excretable photoproducts is partly irreversible and follows first-order kinetics, there may not be a saturation point, so we do not know the maximum effective dose of phototherapy.

Effect on Irradiance of the Light Spectrum and the Distance Between the Infant and the Light Source

Figure 6 shows that as the distance between the light source and the infant decreases, there is a corresponding increase in the spectral irradiance.[5] Fig 6 also demonstrates the dramatic difference in irradi-

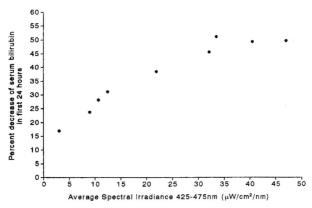

Fig 5. Relationship between average spectral irradiance and decrease in serum bilirubin concentration. Term infants with nonhemolytic hyperbilirubinemia were exposed to special blue lights (Phillips TL 52/20W) of different intensities. Spectral irradiance was measured as the average of readings at the head, trunk, and knees. Drawn from the data of Tan.[4] Source: *Pediatrics*. 1996;98: 283-287.

ance produced within the important 425- to 475-nm band by different types of fluorescent tubes.

What is Intensive Phototherapy?

Intensive phototherapy implies the use of high levels of irradiance in the 430- to 490-nm band (usually 30 μW/cm^2 per nm or higher) delivered to as much of the infant's surface area as possible. How this can be achieved is described below.

Using Phototherapy Effectively

Light Source

The spectrum of light delivered by a phototherapy unit is determined by the type of light source and

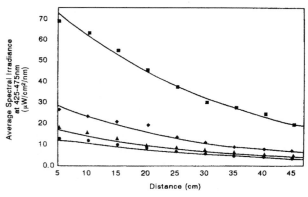

Fig 6. Effect of light source and distance from the light source to the infant on average spectral irradiance. Measurements were made across the 425- to 475-nm band by using a commercial radiometer (Olympic Bilimeter Mark II) and are the average of measurements taken at different locations at each distance (irradiance at the center of the light is much higher than at the periphery). The phototherapy unit was fitted with eight 24-in fluorescent tubes. ■ indicates special blue, General Electric 20-W F20T12/BB tube; ◆, blue, General Electric 20-W F20T12/B tube; ▲, daylight blue, 4 General Electric 20-W F20T12/B blue tubes and 4 Sylvania 20-W F20T12/D daylight tubes; •, daylight, Sylvania 20-W F20T12/D daylight tube. Curves were plotted by using linear curve fitting (True Epistat, Epistat Services, Richardson, TX). The best fit is described by the equation $y = Ae^{Bx}$. Source: *Pediatrics*. 1996;98:283-287.

any filters used. Commonly used phototherapy units contain daylight, cool white, blue, or "special blue" fluorescent tubes. Other units use tungsten-halogen lamps in different configurations, either free-standing or as part of a radiant warming device. Recently, a system using high-intensity gallium nitride light-emitting diodes has been introduced.[6] Fiber-optic systems deliver light from a high-intensity lamp to a fiber-optic blanket. Most of these devices deliver enough output in the blue-green region of the visible spectrum to be effective for standard phototherapy use. However, when bilirubin levels approach the range at which intensive phototherapy is recommended, maximal efficiency must be sought. The most effective light sources currently commercially available for phototherapy are those that use special blue fluorescent tubes[7] or a specially designed light-emitting diode light (Natus Inc, San Carlos, CA).[6] The special blue fluorescent tubes are labeled F20T12/BB (General Electric, Westinghouse, Sylvania) or TL52/20W (Phillips, Eindhoven, The Netherlands). It is important to note that special blue tubes provide much greater irradiance than regular blue tubes (labeled F20T12/B) (Fig 6). Special blue tubes are most effective because they provide light predominantly in the blue-green spectrum. At these wavelengths, light penetrates skin well and is absorbed maximally by bilirubin.[7]

There is a common misconception that ultraviolet light is used for phototherapy. The light systems used do not emit significant ultraviolet radiation, and the small amount of ultraviolet light that is emitted by fluorescent tubes and halogen bulbs is in longer wavelengths than those that cause erythema. In addition, almost all ultraviolet light is absorbed by the glass wall of the fluorescent tube and the Plexiglas cover of the phototherapy unit.

Distance From the Light

As can be seen in Fig 6, the distance of the light source from the infant has a dramatic effect on the spectral irradiance, and this effect is most significant when special blue tubes are used. To take advantage of this effect, the fluorescent tubes should be placed as close to the infant as possible. To do this, the infant should be in a bassinet, not an incubator, because the top of the incubator prevents the light from being brought sufficiently close to the infant. In a bassinet, it is possible to bring the fluorescent tubes within approximately 10 cm of the infant. Naked term infants do not become overheated under these lights. It is important to note, however, that the halogen spot phototherapy lamps cannot be positioned closer to the infant than recommended by the manufacturers without incurring the risk of a burn. When halogen lamps are used, manufacturers recommendations should be followed. The reflectors, light source, and transparent light filters (if any) should be kept clean.

Surface Area

A number of systems have been developed to provide phototherapy above and below the infant.[8,9] One commercially available system that does this is the BiliBassinet (Olympic Medical, Seattle, WA). This unit provides special blue fluorescent tubes above and below the infant. An alternative is to place fiber-optic pads below an infant with phototherapy lamps above. One disadvantage of fiber-optic pads is that they cover a relatively small surface area so that 2 or 3 pads may be needed.[5] When bilirubin levels are extremely high and must be lowered as rapidly as possible, it is essential to expose as much of the infant's surface area to phototherapy as possible. In these situations, additional surface-area exposure can be achieved by lining the sides of the bassinet with aluminum foil or a white cloth.[10]

In most circumstances, it is not necessary to remove the infant's diaper, but when bilirubin levels approach the exchange transfusion range, the diaper should be removed until there is clear evidence of a significant decline in the bilirubin level.

What Decline in the Serum Bilirubin Can You Expect?

The rate at which the bilirubin declines depends on the factors listed in Table 5, and different responses can be expected depending on the clinical circumstances. When bilirubin levels are extremely high (more than 30 mg/dL [513 μmol/L]), and intensive phototherapy is used, a decline of as much as 10 mg/dL (171 μmol/L) can occur within a few hours,[11] and a decrease of at least 0.5 to 1 mg/dL per hour can be expected in the first 4 to 8 hours.[12] On average, for infants of more than 35 weeks' gestation readmitted for phototherapy, intensive phototherapy can produce a decrement of 30% to 40% in the initial bilirubin level by 24 hours after initiation of phototherapy.[13] The most significant decline will occur in the first 4 to 6 hours. With standard phototherapy systems, a decrease of 6% to 20% of the initial bilirubin level can be expected in the first 24 hours.[8,14]

Intermittent Versus Continuous Phototherapy

Clinical studies comparing intermittent with continuous phototherapy have produced conflicting results.[15–17] Because all light exposure increases bilirubin excretion (compared with darkness), no plausible scientific rationale exists for using intermittent phototherapy. In most circumstances, however, phototherapy does not need to be continuous. Phototherapy may be interrupted during feeding or brief parental visits. Individual judgment should be exercised. If the infant's bilirubin level is approaching the exchange transfusion zone (Fig 4), phototherapy should be administered continuously until a satisfactory decline in the serum bilirubin level occurs or exchange transfusion is initiated.

Hydration

There is no evidence that excessive fluid administration affects the serum bilirubin concentration. Some infants who are admitted with high bilirubin levels are also mildly dehydrated and may need supplemental fluid intake to correct their dehydration. Because these infants are almost always breast-fed, the best fluid to use in these circumstances is a milk-based formula, because it inhibits the enterohepatic circulation of bilirubin and should help to lower the serum bilirubin level. Because the photo-products responsible for the decline in serum bilirubin are excreted in urine and bile,[18] maintaining adequate hydration and good urine output should help to improve the efficacy of phototherapy. Unless there is evidence of dehydration, however, routine intravenous fluid or other supplementation (eg, with dextrose water) of term and near-term infants receiving phototherapy is not necessary.

When Should Phototherapy Be Stopped?

There is no standard for discontinuing phototherapy. The TSB level for discontinuing phototherapy depends on the age at which phototherapy is initiated and the cause of the hyperbilirubinemia.[13] For infants who are readmitted after their birth hospitalization (usually for TSB levels of 18 mg/dL [308 μmol/L] or higher), phototherapy may be discontinued when the serum bilirubin level falls below 13 to 14 mg/dL (239-239 μmol/L). Discharge from the hospital need not be delayed to observe the infant for rebound.[13,19,20] If phototherapy is used for infants with hemolytic diseases or is initiated early and discontinued before the infant is 3 to 4 days old, a follow-up bilirubin measurement within 24 hours after discharge is recommended.[13] For infants who are readmitted with hyperbilirubinemia and then discharged, significant rebound is rare, but a repeat TSB measurement or clinical follow-up 24 hours after discharge is a clinical option.[13]

Home Phototherapy

Because the devices available for home phototherapy may not provide the same degree of irradiance or surface-area exposure as those available in the hospital, home phototherapy should be used only in infants whose bilirubin levels are in the "optional phototherapy" range (Fig 3); it is not appropriate for infants with higher bilirubin concentrations. As with hospitalized infants, it is essential that serum bilirubin levels be monitored regularly.

Sunlight Exposure

In their original description of phototherapy, Cremer et al[21] demonstrated that exposure of newborns to sunlight would lower the serum bilirubin level. Although sunlight provides sufficient irradiance in the 425- to 475-nm band to provide phototherapy, the practical difficulties involved in safely exposing a naked newborn to the sun either inside or outside (and avoiding sunburn) preclude the use of sunlight as a reliable therapeutic tool, and it therefore is not recommended.

Complications

Phototherapy has been used in millions of infants for more than 30 years, and reports of significant toxicity are exceptionally rare. Nevertheless, phototherapy in hospital separates mother and infant, and eye patching is disturbing to parents. The most important, but uncommon, clinical complication occurs in infants with cholestatic jaundice. When these infants are exposed to phototherapy, they may develop a dark, grayish-brown discoloration of the skin, serum, and urine (the bronze infant syndrome).[22] The pathogenesis of this syndrome is unknown, but it may be related to an accumulation of porphyrins and other metabolites in the plasma of infants who develop cholestasis.[22,23] Although it occurs exclusively in infants with cholestasis, not all infants with cholestatic jaundice develop the syndrome.

This syndrome generally has had few deleterious consequences, and if there is a need for phototherapy, the presence of direct hyperbilirubinemia should not be considered a contraindication to its use. This is particularly important in sick neonates. Because the products of phototherapy are excreted in the bile, the presence of cholestasis will decrease the efficacy of phototherapy. Nevertheless, infants with direct hyperbilirubinemia often show some response to phototherapy. In infants receiving phototherapy who develop the bronze infant syndrome, exchange transfusion should be considered if the TSB is in the intensive phototherapy range and phototherapy does not promptly lower the TSB. Because of the paucity of data, firm recommendations cannot be made. Note, however, that the direct serum bilirubin should not be subtracted from the TSB concentration in making decisions about exchange transfusions (see Fig 4).

Rarely, purpura and bullous eruptions have been described in infants with severe cholestatic jaundice receiving phototherapy,[24,25] and severe blistering and photosensitivity during phototherapy have occurred in infants with congenital erythropoietic porphyria.[26,27] Congenital porphyria or a family history of porphyria is an absolute contraindication to the use of phototherapy, as is the concomitant use of drugs or agents that are photosensitizers.[28]

REFERENCES

1. Maisels MJ. Phototherapy—traditional and nontraditional. J Perinatol. 2001;21(suppl 1):S93–S97
2. Fiberoptic phototherapy systems. Health Devices. 1995;24:132–153
3. International Electrotechnical Commission. Medical electrical equipment—part 2-50: particular requirements for the safety of infant phototherapy equipment. 2000. IEC 60601-2-50. Available at www.iec.ch. Accessed June 7, 2004
4. Tan KL. The pattern of bilirubin response to phototherapy for neonatal hyperbilirubinemia. Pediatr Res. 1982;16:670–674
5. Maisels MJ. Why use homeopathic doses of phototherapy? Pediatrics. 1996;98:283–287
6. Seidman DS, Moise J, Ergaz Z, et al. A new blue light-emitting phototherapy device: a prospective randomized controlled study. J Pediatr. 2000;136:771–774
7. Ennever JF. Blue light, green light, white light, more light: treatment of neonatal jaundice. Clin Perinatol. 1990;17:467–481
8. Garg AK, Prasad RS, Hifzi IA. A controlled trial of high-intensity double-surface phototherapy on a fluid bed versus conventional phototherapy in neonatal jaundice. Pediatrics. 1995;95:914–916
9. Tan KL. Phototherapy for neonatal jaundice. Clin Perinatol. 1991;18:423–439
10. Eggert P, Stick C, Schroder H. On the distribution of irradiation intensity in phototherapy. Measurements of effective irradiance in an incubator. Eur J Pediatr. 1984;142:58–61
11. Hansen TW. Acute management of extreme neonatal jaundice—the potential benefits of intensified phototherapy and interruption of enterohepatic bilirubin circulation. Acta Paediatr. 1997;86:843–846
12. Newman TB, Liljestrand P, Escobar GJ. Infants with bilirubin levels of 30 mg/dL or more in a large managed care organization. Pediatrics. 2003;111(6 Pt 1):1303–1311
13. Maisels MJ, Kring E. Bilirubin rebound following intensive phototherapy. Arch Pediatr Adolesc Med. 2002;156:669–672
14. Tan KL. Comparison of the efficacy of fiberoptic and conventional phototherapy for neonatal hyperbilirubinemia. J Pediatr. 1994;125:607–612
15. Rubaltelli FF, Zanardo V, Granati B. Effect of various phototherapy regimens on bilirubin decrement. Pediatrics. 1978;61:838–841
16. Maurer HM, Shumway CN, Draper DA, Hossaini AA. Controlled trial comparing agar, intermittent phototherapy, and continuous phototherapy for reducing neonatal hyperbilirubinemia. J Pediatr. 1973;82:73–76
17. Lau SP, Fung KP. Serum bilirubin kinetics in intermittent phototherapy of physiological jaundice. Arch Dis Child. 1984;59:892–894
18. McDonagh AF, Lightner DA. 'Like a shrivelled blood orange'—bilirubin, jaundice, and phototherapy. Pediatrics. 1985;75:443–455
19. Yetman RJ, Parks DK, Huseby V, Mistry K, Garcia J. Rebound bilirubin levels in infants receiving phototherapy. J Pediatr. 1998;133:705–707
20. Lazar L, Litwin A, Merlob P. Phototherapy for neonatal nonhemolytic hyperbilirubinemia. Analysis of rebound and indications for discontinuing therapy. Clin Pediatr (Phila). 1993;32:264–267
21. Cremer RJ, Perryman PW, Richards DH. Influence of light on the hyperbilirubinemia of infants. Lancet. 1958;1(7030):1094–1097
22. Rubaltelli FF, Jori G, Reddi E. Bronze baby syndrome: a new porphyrin-related disorder. Pediatr Res. 1983;17:327–330
23. Meisel P, Jahrig D, Theel L, Ordt A, Jahrig K. The bronze baby syndrome: consequence of impaired excretion of photobilirubin? Photobiochem Photobiophys. 1982;3:345–352
24. Mallon E, Wojnarowska F, Hope P, Elder G. Neonatal bullous eruption as a result of transient porphyrinemia in a premature infant with hemolytic disease of the newborn. J Am Acad Dermatol. 1995;33:333–336
25. Paller AS, Eramo LR, Farrell EE, Millard DD, Honig PJ, Cunningham BB. Purpuric phototherapy-induced eruption in transfused neonates: relation to transient porphyrinemia. Pediatrics. 1997;100:360–364
26. Tonz O, Vogt J, Filippini L, Simmler F, Wachsmuth ED, Winterhalter KH. Severe light dermatosis following phototherapy in a newborn infant with congenital erythropoietic urophyria [in German]. Helv Paediatr Acta. 1975;30:47–56
27. Soylu A, Kavukcu S, Turkmen M. Phototherapy sequela in a child with congenital erythropoietic porphyria. Eur J Pediatr. 1999;158:526–527
28. Kearns GL, Williams BJ, Timmons OD. Fluorescein phototoxicity in a premature infant. J Pediatr. 1985;107:796–798

ERRATUM

Two errors appeared in the American Academy of Pediatrics clinical practice guideline, titled "Management of Hyperbilirubinemia in the Newborn Infant 35 or More Weeks of Gestation," that was published in the July 2004 issue of *Pediatrics* (2004;114:297–316). On page 107, Background section, first paragraph, the second sentence should read: "The current guideline represents a consensus of the committee charged by the AAP with reviewing and updating the existing guideline and is based on a careful review of the evidence, including a comprehensive literature review by the Agency for Healthcare Research and Quality and the New England Medical Center Evidence-Based Practice Center."[2] On page 118, Appendix 1, first paragraph, the 4 levels of evidence quality should have been labeled A, B, C, and D rather than 1, 2, 3, and 4, respectively. The American Academy of Pediatrics regrets these errors.

Hyperbilirubinemia Clinical Practice Guideline
Quick Reference Tools

• •

- Recommendation Summary
  — Management of Hyperbilirubinemia in the Newborn Infant 35 or More Weeks of Gestation
- *ICD-10-CM* Coding Quick Reference for Hyperbilirubinemia
- AAP Patient Education Handout
  — *Jaundice and Your Newborn*

Recommendation Summary

Management of Hyperbilirubinemia in the Newborn Infant 35 or More Weeks of Gestation

The following are the key elements of the recommendations provided by this guideline. Clinicians should:

1. Promote and support successful breastfeeding.
2. Establish nursery protocols for the identification and evaluation of hyperbilirubinemia.
3. Measure the total serum bilirubin (TSB) or transcutaneous bilirubin (TcB) level on infants jaundiced in the first 24 hours.
4. Recognize that visual estimation of the degree of jaundice can lead to errors, particularly in darkly pigmented infants.
5. Interpret all bilirubin levels according to the infant's age in hours.
6. Recognize that infants at less than 38 weeks' gestation, particularly those who are breastfed, are at higher risk of developing hyperbilirubinemia and require closer surveillance and monitoring.
7. Perform a systematic assessment on all infants before discharge for the risk of severe hyperbilirubinemia.
8. Provide parents with written and verbal information about newborn jaundice.
9. Provide appropriate follow-up based on the time of discharge and the risk assessment.
10. Treat newborns, when indicated, with phototherapy or exchange transfusion.

Coding Quick Reference for Hyperbilirubinemia	
ICD-10-CM	
P59.0	Neonatal jaundice associated with preterm delivery
P59.3	Neonatal jaundice from breast milk inhibitor
P59.9	Neonatal jaundice, unspecified
R17	Unspecified jaundice

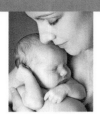

Jaundice and Your Newborn

Congratulations on the birth of your new baby!

To make sure your baby's first week is safe and healthy, it is important that

1. **You find a primary care provider, such as a pediatrician you are comfortable with, for your baby's ongoing care.**

2. **Your baby is checked for jaundice in the hospital.**

3. **If you are breastfeeding, you get the help you need to make sure it is going well.**

4. **You make sure your baby is seen by a doctor or nurse at 3 to 5 days of age.**

5. **If your baby is discharged before age 72 hours, your baby should be seen by a doctor or nurse within 2 days of discharge from the hospital.**

Q: What is jaundice?

A: Jaundice is the yellow color seen in the skin of many newborns. It happens when a chemical called *bilirubin* builds up in the baby's blood. Jaundice can occur in babies of any race or color.

Q: Why is jaundice common in newborns?

A: Everyone's blood contains bilirubin, which comes from red blood cells and is removed by the liver. Before birth, the mother's liver does this for the baby. Most babies develop jaundice in the first few days after birth because it takes a few days for the baby's liver to get better at removing bilirubin.

Q: How can I tell if my baby is jaundiced?

A: The skin of a baby with jaundice usually appears yellow. The best way to see jaundice is in good light, such as daylight or under fluorescent lights. Jaundice usually appears first in the face and then moves to the chest, abdomen, arms, and legs as the bilirubin level increases. The whites of the eyes may also be yellow. Jaundice may be harder to see in babies with darker skin color.

Q: Can jaundice hurt my baby?

A: Most babies have mild jaundice that is harmless, but in unusual situations the bilirubin level can get very high and might cause brain damage. This is why newborns should be checked carefully for jaundice and treated to prevent a high bilirubin level.

Q: How should my baby be checked for jaundice?

A: If your baby looks jaundiced in the first few days after birth, your baby's doctor or nurse may use a skin or blood test to check your baby's bilirubin level. However, because estimating the bilirubin level based on the baby's appearance can be difficult, most experts recommend that a skin or blood test be done in the first 2 days even if your baby does not appear jaundiced. A bilirubin level is always needed if jaundice develops before the baby is 24 hours old. Whether a test is needed after that depends on the baby's age, the amount of jaundice, and whether the baby has other factors that make jaundice more likely or harder to see.

Q: Does breastfeeding affect jaundice?

A: Breast milk (human milk) is the ideal food for your baby. Jaundice is more common in babies who are breastfed than babies who are formula-fed. However, this occurs more often in newborns who are not getting enough breast milk because their mothers are not producing enough milk (especially if the milk comes in late) or if breastfeeding is not going well, such as babies not latching on properly.

For the first 24 hours after birth, normal breastfed newborns receive only about 1 teaspoon of milk with each feeding. The amount of breast milk provided increases with each day. If you are breastfeeding, you should breastfeed your baby at least 8 to 12 times a day for the first few days. This will help you produce enough milk and will help keep the baby's bilirubin level down. If you are having trouble breastfeeding, ask your baby's doctor or nurse or a lactation specialist for help.

Q: When should my baby get checked after leaving the hospital?

A: It is important for your baby to be seen by a nurse or doctor when the baby is between 3 and 5 days old, because this is usually when a baby's bilirubin level is highest. This is why, if your baby is discharged before age 72 hours, your baby should be seen within 2 days of discharge. The timing of this visit may vary depending on your baby's age when released from the hospital and other factors.

Q: Why do some babies need an earlier follow-up visit after leaving the hospital?

A: Some babies have a greater risk for high levels of bilirubin and may need to be seen sooner after discharge from the hospital. Ask your doctor about an early follow-up visit if your baby has any of the following symptoms:

- A high bilirubin level before leaving the hospital
- Early birth (more than 2 weeks before the due date)
- Jaundice in the first 24 hours after birth
- Breastfeeding that is not going well
- A lot of bruising or bleeding under the scalp related to labor and delivery
- A parent, brother, or sister who had a high bilirubin level and received light therapy

Q: When should I call my baby's doctor?

A: Call your baby's doctor if

- Your baby's skin turns more yellow.
- Your baby's abdomen, arms, or legs are yellow.
- The whites of your baby's eyes are yellow.
- Your baby is jaundiced and is hard to wake, fussy, or not nursing or taking formula well.

Q: How is harmful jaundice prevented?

A: Most jaundice requires no treatment. When treatment is necessary, placing your baby under special lights while he or she is undressed will lower the bilirubin level. Depending on your baby's bilirubin level, this can be done in the hospital or at home. Jaundice is treated at levels that are much lower than those at which brain damage is a concern. In some babies, supplementing breast milk with formula can also help to lower the bilirubin level and prevent the need for phototherapy. Treatment can prevent the harmful effects of jaundice.

> **Note:** Exposing your baby to sunlight through a window might help lower the bilirubin level, but this will only work if the baby is undressed. Make sure the temperature in your home is comfortable and not too cold for your baby. Newborns should never be put in direct sunlight outside because they might get sunburned.

Q: When does jaundice go away?

A: In breastfed babies, it is common for jaundice to last 1 month or occasionally longer. In formula-fed babies, most jaundice goes away by 2 weeks. However, if your baby is jaundiced for more than 3 weeks, see your baby's doctor.

From Your Doctor 🖉

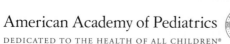

American Academy of Pediatrics

DEDICATED TO THE HEALTH OF ALL CHILDREN®

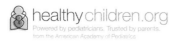

healthy children.org
Powered by pediatricians. Trusted by parents.
from the American Academy of Pediatrics

The American Academy of Pediatrics (AAP) is an organization of 66,000 primary care pediatricians, pediatric medical subspecialists, and pediatric surgical specialists dedicated to the health, safety, and well-being of infants, children, adolescents, and young adults.

The information contained in this publication should not be used as a substitute for the medical care and advice of your pediatrician. There may be variations in treatment that your pediatrician may recommend based on individual facts and circumstances. The persons whose photographs are depicted in this publication are professional models. They have no relation to the issues discussed. Any characters they are portraying are fictional.

Clinical Practice Guideline for the Management of Infantile Hemangiomas

• *Clinical Practice Guideline*

CLINICAL PRACTICE GUIDELINE Guidance for the Clinician in Rendering Pediatric Care

American Academy
of Pediatrics

DEDICATED TO THE HEALTH OF ALL CHILDREN™

Clinical Practice Guideline for the Management of Infantile Hemangiomas

Daniel P. Krowchuk, MD, FAAP,[a] Ilona J. Frieden, MD, FAAP,[b] Anthony J. Mancini, MD, FAAP,[c] David H. Darrow, MD, DDS, FAAP,[d] Francine Blei, MD, MBA, FAAP,[e] Arin K. Greene, MD, FAAP,[f] Aparna Annam, DO, FAAP, [g] Cynthia N. Baker, MD, FAAP,[h] Peter C. Frommelt, MD, FAAP,[i] Amy Hodak, CPMSM,[j] Brian M. Pate, MD, FHM, FAAP,[k] Janice L. Pelletier, MD, FAAP,[l] Deborah Sandrock, MD, FAAP,[m] Stuart T. Weinberg, MD, FAAP,[n] Mary Anne Whelan, MD, PhD, FAAP,[o] SUBCOMMITTEE ON THE MANAGEMENT OF INFANTILE HEMANGIOMAS

abstract

Infantile hemangiomas (IHs) occur in as many as 5% of infants, making them the most common benign tumor of infancy. Most IHs are small, innocuous, self-resolving, and require no treatment. However, because of their size or location, a significant minority of IHs are potentially problematic. These include IHs that may cause permanent scarring and disfigurement (eg, facial IHs), hepatic or airway IHs, and IHs with the potential for functional impairment (eg, periorbital IHs), ulceration (that may cause pain or scarring), and associated underlying abnormalities (eg, intracranial and aortic arch vascular abnormalities accompanying a large facial IH). This clinical practice guideline for the management of IHs emphasizes several key concepts. It defines those IHs that are potentially higher risk and should prompt concern, and emphasizes increased vigilance, consideration of active treatment and, when appropriate, specialty consultation. It discusses the specific growth characteristics of IHs, that is, that the most rapid and significant growth occurs between 1 and 3 months of age and that growth is completed by 5 months of age in most cases. Because many IHs leave behind permanent skin changes, there is a window of opportunity to treat higher-risk IHs and optimize outcomes. Early intervention and/or referral (ideally by 1 month of age) is recommended for infants who have potentially problematic IHs. When systemic treatment is indicated, propranolol is the drug of choice at a dose of 2 to 3 mg/kg per day. Treatment typically is continued for at least 6 months and often is maintained until 12 months of age (occasionally longer). Topical timolol may be used to treat select small, thin, superficial IHs. Surgery and/or laser treatment are most useful for the treatment of residual skin changes after involution and, less commonly, may be considered earlier to treat some IHs.

Departments of [a]Pediatrics and Dermatology, Wake Forest School of Medicine, Winston-Salem, North Carolina; Departments of [b]Dermatology and Pediatrics, School of Medicine, University of California, San Francisco, San Francisco, California; Departments of [c]Pediatrics and Dermatology, Feinberg School of Medicine, Northwestern University and Ann and Robert H. Lurie Children's Hospital of Chicago, Chicago, Illinois; Departments of [d]Otolaryngology and Pediatrics, Eastern Virginia Medical School and Children's Hospital of the King's Daughters, Norfolk, Virginia; [e]Donald and Barbara Zucker School of Medicine, Northwell Health, New York City, New York; [f]Department of Plastic and Oral Surgery, Boston Children's Hospital and Harvard Medical School, Harvard University, Boston, Massachusetts; [g]Department of Radiology, University of Colorado School of Medicine, Children's Hospital Colorado, Aurora, Colorado; [h]Department of Pediatrics, Kaiser Permanente Medical Center, Los Angeles, California; [i]Department of Pediatrics, Cardiology, Medical College of Wisconsin and Children's Hospital of Wisconsin, Milwaukee, Wisconsin; [j]American Board of Pediatrics, Chapel Hill, North Carolina; [k]Department of Pediatrics, University of Kansas School of Medicine-Wichita, Wichita, Kansas; [l]Department of Pediatrics, Northern Light Health, Bangor, Maine; [m]St Christopher's Hospital for Children and College of Medicine, Drexel University, Philadelphia, Pennsylvania; Departments of [n]Biomedical Informatics and Pediatrics, School of Medicine, Vanderbilt University, Nashville, Tennessee; and [o]College of Physicians and Surgeons, Columbia University, New York City, New York

To cite: Krowchuk DP, Frieden IJ, Mancini AJ, et al. Clinical Practice Guideline for the Management of Infantile Hemangiomas. Pediatrics. 2019;143(1):e20183475

INTRODUCTION

This is the first clinical practice guideline (CPG) from the American Academy of Pediatrics (AAP) regarding the management of infantile hemangiomas (IHs). Similar consensus statements have been published by European[1] and Australasian expert groups.[2] In addition, a recent AAP clinical report provided a comprehensive review of the pathogenesis, clinical features, and treatment of IH; it is available at http://pediatrics.aappublications.org/content/136/4/e1060.[3]

IHs occur in approximately 4% to 5% of infants, making them the most common benign tumor of childhood. They are more common in girls, twins, infants born preterm or with low birth weight (up to 30% of infants born weighing <1 kg are affected), and white neonates. The pathogenesis of IHs has yet to be fully defined. A leading hypothesis is that circulating endothelial progenitor cells migrate to locations in which conditions (eg, hypoxia and developmental field disturbances) are favorable for growth.[3]

Knowledge about IHs has advanced dramatically in the past decade, particularly regarding the unique timing and nature of proliferation and involution, risks of sequelae, and newer treatment options. As a result, pediatric providers have an opportunity to improve care and reduce morbidity in infants with IHs by promptly recognizing which

IHs are potentially high risk and when intervention is needed.

In the broadest sense, the goal of this CPG from the AAP is to enhance primary care providers' ability to confidently evaluate, triage, and manage IHs, employing an evidence-based approach. Specifically, the CPG will:

- provide an approach to risk stratification and recognition of potentially problematic IHs;

- emphasize that early and frequent monitoring in the first few weeks and months of life is crucial in identifying those IHs that require intervention because IHs may change rapidly during this time period;

- review the role of imaging in patients who have IHs; and

- offer evidence-based guidance for the management of IHs, including indications for consultation, referral and possible intervention, pharmacologic options for therapy, the role of surgical modalities, and ongoing management and monitoring (including parent education).

This CPG is intended for pediatricians and other primary care providers who (1) manage IHs collaboratively with a hemangioma specialist (defined below), (2) care for children with IHs being managed primarily by a hemangioma specialist, or (3) manage

IHs independently on the basis of their knowledge and expertise. It does not address the management of vascular malformations, congenital hemangiomas, or other vascular tumors. The CPG encourages enhanced communication between primary care clinicians and hemangioma specialists to ensure early assessment and treatment of infants in whom active intervention is indicated, to improve patient outcomes, and to enhance anticipatory guidance. It is not intended to be a sole source of guidance in the management of children with IHs, to replace clinical judgment, or to establish a protocol for all infants with IHs. Rather, it provides a framework for clinical decision-making.

METHODS

The methods of this CPG are discussed in detail in the Methods section of the Supplemental Information. Briefly, a comparative effectiveness review of potential benefits and harms of diagnostic modalities and pharmacologic and surgical treatments was conducted on behalf of the Agency for Healthcare Research and Quality (AHRQ). The literature search strategy employed Medline via the PubMed interface, the Cumulative Index to Nursing and Allied Health Literature (CINAHL), and Excerpta Medica Database (Embase). Searches were limited to the English language and to studies published from 1982 to June

---

TABLE 1 Highlights of This CPG

- IH growth characteristics are different than once taught.
  - Most rapid IH growth occurs between 1 and 3 months of age.
  - Although IHs involute, this process may be incomplete, leaving permanent skin changes that may be life altering. This is especially true for IHs that are thick.
  - There is a window of opportunity to treat problematic IHs. Consult early (by 1 month of age) for lesions that are potentially high risk because of the following associations (Table 3):
    - potential for disfigurement (the most common reason treatment is needed);
    - life-threatening complications;
    - functional impairment;
    - ulceration; and
    - underlying abnormalities.
- Oral propranolol is the treatment of choice for problematic IHs that require systemic therapy.
- Topical timolol may be used to treat some thin and/or superficial IHs.
- Surgery and/or laser treatment are most useful for the treatment of residual skin changes after involution. They may be used earlier to treat selected IHs.

TABLE 2 Definitions

Hemangioma specialist:	Unlike many diseases, management of IHs is not limited to 1 medical or surgical specialty. A hemangioma specialist may have expertise in dermatology, hematologyoncology, pediatrics, facial plastic and reconstructive surgery, ophthalmology, otolaryngology, pediatric surgery, and/or plastic surgery, and his or her practice is often focused primarily or exclusively on the pediatric age group.

Hemangioma specialists should:	• understand the time-sensitive nature of IHs during the growth phase and be able to accommodate requests for urgent evaluation;
	• have experience with accurate risk stratification and potential complications associated with IHs;
	• be able to provide recommendations for various management options, including observation, medical therapies, and surgical or laser procedures, and provide counseling regarding the potential risks and benefits of these interventions for specific patients; and
	• have a thorough knowledge of past and emerging medical literature regarding IHs.
	• Such specialists often have 1 or more of the following characteristics:
	  o participated in a vascular anomalies program during previous medical training;
	  o devotes a significant part of his or her clinical practice to IHs;
	  o is a member of or collaborates with a multidisciplinary vascular anomalies center;
	  o maintains membership in professional organizations or groups with a special interest in IHs;
	  o participates in research studies in the field of IHs; or
	  o publishes medical literature in the field of IHs.

IHs: infantile hemangiomas	Benign vascular tumors of infancy and childhood with unique clinical and histopathologic characteristics that distinguish them from other vascular tumors (eg, congenital hemangiomas) or malformations. These characteristics include development during the first weeks or months of life, a typical natural history of rapid growth followed by gradual involution, and immunohistochemical staining of biopsy specimens with erythrocyte-type glucose transporter protein and other unique markers not present on other benign vascular tumors. Many other entities are also called hemangiomas. Some are true vascular tumors, and others are vascular malformations. Therefore, it is important to use the adjective "infantile" when referring to true IHs. IHs are classified on the basis of soft-tissue depth and the pattern of anatomic involvement (see Supplemental Figs 5–10 for photographic examples).
Soft-tissue depth:	• Superficial: red with little or no evidence of a subcutaneous component (formerly called strawberry" hemangiomas); • Deep: blue and located below the skin surface (formerly called "cavernous" hemangiomas); and • Combined (mixed): both superficial and deep components are present.
Anatomic appearance:	• Localized: well-defined focal lesions (appearing to arise from a central point); • Segmental: IH involving an anatomic region that is often plaque-like and often measuring at >5 cm in diameter; • Indeterminate (undetermined): neither clearly localized or segmental (often called partial segmental); and • Multifocal: multiple discrete IHs at disparate sites.

2015. Because the therapy of IHs has been evolving rapidly, the CPG subcommittee performed an updated literature review for the period of July 2015 to January 2017 to augment the original search. This most recent search employed only Medline because previously, virtually all relevant articles had been accessed via this database. The search was concentrated on pharmacologic interventions, including topical timolol (an emerging therapeutic alternative for which limited data were available at the time of the original search). The original methodology and report, including the evidence search and review, are available in their entirety and as an executive summary at www.effectivehealthcare.ahrq.gov/reports/final.cfm.[4]

DEVELOPMENT OF THE CLINICAL PRACTICE GUIDELINE

In December 2016, the AAP convened a multidisciplinary subcommittee composed of IH experts in the fields of dermatology, cardiology, hematology-oncology, otolaryngology(head and neck surgery), plastic surgery, and radiology. The subcommittee also included general pediatricians, a parent representative, an implementation scientist, a representative from the Partnership for Policy Implementation (https://www.aap.org/en-us/professional-resources/quality-improvement/Pages/Partnership-for-Policy-Implementation.aspx), and an epidemiologist and methodologist. All panel members declared potential conflicts on the basis of the AAP policy on Conflict of Interest and Voluntary Disclosure. Subcommittee members repeated this process at the time of the publication of the guideline. All potential conflicts of interest are listed at the end of this document. The project was funded by the AAP.

The final recommendations were based on articles identified in the AHRQ and updated systematic reviews. Decisions and the strength of recommendations were based on a systematic grading of the quality of evidence by independent reviewers. Expert consensus was used when definitive data were not available. Key action statements (KASs), summarized in Table 4, were generated by subcommittee members authoring individual components of the CPG using

TABLE 3 High-Risk IHs

IH Clinical Findings	IH Risk
Life-threatening	
"Beard-area" IH	Obstructive airway hemangiomas
≥5 cutaneous IHs	Liver hemangiomas, cardiac failure, hypothyroidism
Functional impairment	
Periocular IH (>1 cm)	Astigmatism, anisometropia, proptosis, amblyopia
IH involving lip or oral cavity	Feeding impairment
Ulceration	
Segmental IH: IH of any size involving any of the following sites: lips, columella, superior helix of ear, gluteal cleft and/or perineum, perianal skin, and other intertriginous areas (eg, neck, axillae, inguinal region)	Increased risk of ulceration
Associated structural anomalies	
Segmental IH of face or scalp	PHACE syndrome
Segmental IH of lumbosacral and/or perineal area	LUMBAR syndrome
Disfigurement	
Segmental IH, especially of face and scalp	High risk of scarring and/or permanent disfigurement
Facial IH (measurements refer to size during infancy): nasal tip or lip (any size) or any facial location ≥2 cm (>1 cm if ≤3 mo of age)	Risk of disfigurement via distortion of anatomic landmarks and/or scarring and/or permanent skin changes
Scalp IH >2 cm	Permanent alopecia (especially if the hemangioma becomes thick or bulky); profuse bleeding if ulceration develops (typically more bleeding than at other anatomic sites)
Neck, trunk, or extremity IH >2 cm, especially in growth phase or if abrupt transition from normal to affected skin (ie, ledge effect); thick superficial IH (eg, ≥2 mm thickness)	Greater risk of leaving permanent scarring and/or permanent skin changes depending on anatomic location
Breast IH (female infants)	Permanent changes in breast development (eg, breast asymmetry) or nipple contour

Categorization of IH as high risk is based on published literature (including the AHRQ review and hemangioma severity scores) and consensus of CPG subcommittee members. Given the wide variation in IH location, size, and age at presentation, the subcommittee acknowledges that there may be situations in which an IH meets high-risk criteria and, therefore, merits consultation or referral, but the practitioner and parents do not believe this is necessary or practical. Clinical judgment is always involved in such decisions, and any plan of action needs to be individualized on the basis of a number of factors, including location of the lesion, age of child, family preferences, and geographic access to care.

the results of the literature review. These sections were reviewed and refined by the subcommittee chairperson and co-chairperson and ultimately by all subcommittee members.

Evidence-based guideline recommendations from the AAP may be graded as strong, moderate, weak on the basis of low-quality evidence, or weak on the basis of balance between benefits and harms. Strong and moderate recommendations usually are associated with "should" and "should not" recommendation statements, whereas some moderate and all weak recommendations may be recognized by use of "may" or "need not," signifying that moderate recommendations are based on a range of evidence strengths within the boundaries of the definition (Table 5, Fig 1).

The CPG underwent a comprehensive review by stakeholders (including AAP councils, committees, and sections), selected outside organizations, and individuals identified by the subcommittee as experts in the field before formal approval by the AAP. All comments were reviewed by the subcommittee and incorporated into the final guideline when appropriate.

RISK STRATIFICATION, TRIAGE, AND REFERRAL

Key Action Statement 1A (Table 6)

Clinicians should classify an IH as high risk if there is evidence of or potential for the following: (1) life-threatening complications, (2) functional impairment or ulceration, (3) structural anomalies (eg, in PHACE syndrome or LUMBAR syndrome), or (4) permanent disfigurement (grade X, strong recommendation).

The purpose of this statement is to ensure timely identification of IHs that may require early intervention. Clinicians in the primary care setting caring for infants with IH face 2 major challenges: disease heterogeneity and the unique growth characteristics of IHs.[24] For example, because IHs involute spontaneously, many that are small, are superficial, occur in areas covered by clothing, and/or are unlikely to cause disfigurement do not require hemangioma specialist evaluation or treatment. However, some IHs may be considered high risk, and depending on the clinician's comfort level and local access to specialty care, require a higher level of experience and expertise to determine if additional intervention is indicated. These high-risk IHs and their associated clinical findings are summarized in Table 3 and illustrated in Figs 2–4, Supplemental Table 22, and Supplemental Fig 11. Of particular note and as discussed later, segmental hemangiomas, those that cover an anatomic territory arising from 1 or more developmental units, confer a higher risk of morbidity and life-threatening complications than those that are localized, that is, seeming to arise from a central focal point.[5] At the same time, smaller IHs in particular anatomic locations, such as the cheek, tip of the

TABLE 4 Summary of Key Action Statements (KASs) for the Management of IHs

In Managing IH, Recommendations for Clinicians	Evidence Quality; Strength of Recommendation
1. Risk stratification	
1A. Classify an IH as high risk if there is evidence of or potential for the following: (1) life-threatening complications, (2) functional impairment or ulceration, (3) structural anomalies (eg, in PHACE syndrome or LUMBAR syndrome), or (4) permanent disfigurement	X; strong
1B. After identifying an IH as high risk, facilitate evaluation by a hemangioma specialist as soon possible	X; strong
2. Imaging	
2A. Do not perform imaging unless the diagnosis of IH is uncertain, there are $\geq$5 cutaneous IHs, or associated anatomic abnormalities are suspected	B; moderate
2B. Perform ultrasonography as the initial imaging modality when the diagnosis of IH is uncertain	C; weak
2C. Perform MRI when concerned about associated structural abnormalities (eg, PHACE syndrome or LUMBAR syndrome)	B; moderate
3. Pharmacotherapy	
3A. Use oral propranolol as the first-line agent for IHs requiring systemic treatment	A; strong
3B. Dose propranolol between 2 and 3 mg/kg per d unless there are comorbidities (eg, PHACE syndrome) or adverse effects (eg, sleep disturbance) that necessitate a lower dose	A; moderate
3C. Counsel that propranolol be administered with or after feeding and that doses be held at times of diminished oral intake or vomiting to reduce the risk of hypoglycemia	X; strong
3D. Evaluate patients for and educate caregivers about potential adverse effects of propranolol, including sleep disturbances, bronchial irritation, and clinically symptomatic bradycardia and hypotension	X; strong
3E. May prescribe oral prednisolone or prednisone to treat IHs if there are contraindications or an inadequate response to oral propranolol	B; moderate
3F. May recommend intralesional injection of triamcinolone and/or betamethasone to treat focal, bulky IHs during proliferation or in certain critical anatomic locations (eg, the lip)	B; moderate
3G. May prescribe topical timolol maleate as a therapy for thin and/or superficial IHs	B; moderate
4. Surgical management	
4. May recommend surgery and laser therapy as treatment options in managing selected IHs	C; moderate
5. Parent education	
5. Educate caregivers of infants with an IH about the condition, including the expected natural history and its potential for causing complications or disfigurement	X; strong

TABLE 5 Guideline Definitions for Key Action Statements

Statement	Definition	Implication
Strong recommendation	A particular action is favored because anticipated benefits clearly exceed harms (or vice versa), and quality of evidence is excellent or unobtainable.	Clinicians should follow a strong recommendation unless a clear and compelling rationale for an alternative approach is present.
Moderate recommendation	A particular action is favored because anticipated benefits clearly exceed harms (or vice versa), and the quality of evidence is good but not excellent (or is unobtainable).	Clinicians would be prudent to follow a moderate recommendation but should remain alert to new information and sensitive to patient preferences.
Weak recommendation (based on low-quality evidence)	A particular action is favored because anticipated benefits clearly exceed harms (or vice versa), but the quality of evidence is weak.	Clinicians would be prudent to follow a weak recommendation but should remain alert to new information and sensitive to patient preferences.
Weak recommendation (based on balance of benefits and harms)	A weak recommendation is provided when the aggregate database shows evidence of both benefit and harm that appears to be similar in magnitude for any available courses of action.	Clinicians should consider the options in their decision-making, but patient preference may have a substantial role.

PHACE indicates posterior fossa defects, hemangiomas, cerebrovascular arterial anomalies, cardiovascular anomalies including coarctation of the aorta, and eye anomalies; LUMBAR, lower body IH and other cutaneous defects, urogenital anomalies and ulceration, myelopathy, bony deformities, anorectal malformations, and arterial anomalies and renal anomalies.

nose, and perioral and periocular skin, can confer a high risk of complications as well (see discussion below).

There are 5 major indications for consideration of early treatment or need for further evaluation of IHs:

1. life-threatening complications;

2. functional impairment or risk thereof;

3. ulceration or risk thereof;

4. evaluation to identify important associated structural anomalies; and

5. risk of leaving permanent scarring or distortion of anatomic landmarks

Life-threatening Complications

Life-threatening lesions include obstructing IHs of the airway, liver IHs associated with high-output congestive heart failure and severe hypothyroidism, and, rarely, profuse bleeding from an ulcerated IH. Obstructing IHs of the airway typically involve the subglottis,

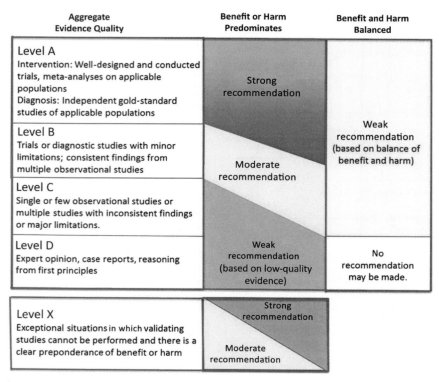

	Aggregate Evidence Quality	Benefit or Harm Predominates	Benefit and Harm Balanced

Level A
Intervention: Well-designed and conducted trials, meta-analyses on applicable populations
Diagnosis: Independent gold-standard studies of applicable populations

Level B
Trials or diagnostic studies with minor limitations; consistent findings from multiple observational studies

Level C
Single or few observational studies or multiple studies with inconsistent findings or major limitations.

Level D
Expert opinion, case reports, reasoning from first principles

Strong recommendation

Moderate recommendation

Weak recommendation (based on low-quality evidence)

Weak recommendation (based on balance of benefit and harm)

No recommendation may be made.

Level X
Exceptional situations in which validating studies cannot be performed and there is a clear preponderance of benefit or harm

Strong recommendation

Moderate recommendation

FIGURE 1
AAP rating of evidence and recommendations.

TABLE 6 Key Action Statement 1A: Clinicians should classify an IH as high risk if there is evidence of or potential for the following: (1) life-threatening complications, (2) functional impairment or ulceration, (3) structural anomalies (eg, in PHACE syndrome or LUMBAR syndrome), or (4) permanent disfigurement (grade X, strong recommendation).

Aggregate Evidence Quality	Grade X
Benefits	Early recognition of high-risk, potentially problematic IHs facilitates early specialist evaluation and management and potential avoidance of complications
Risks, harm, cost	Unnecessary parental concern regarding lesions inappropriately characterized as high-risk IHs
Benefit-harm assessment	The benefits of identifying high-risk IHs outweigh the harm
Intentional vagueness	None
Role of patient preference	None
Exclusions	Vascular lesions that are not true IHs
Strength	Strong recommendation
Key references	5–23

further compromising the narrowest portion of the pediatric airway. Although the mean age at the time of diagnosis is about 4 months, symptoms usually present much earlier but are often mistaken as infectious or inflammatory croup or reactive airway disease.[25–27] Most children who are affected develop biphasic stridor and barky cough as the IH enlarges. Approximately half of infants in whom an airway IH is diagnosed also will have a cutaneous IH. Segmental IH of the lower face ("beard distribution") or anterior neck and oral and/or pharyngeal mucosal IHs are the greatest risk factors for an airway IH.[6,27–29]

Hepatic hemangiomas have been characterized as occurring in 3 patterns: focal, multifocal, and diffuse; the latter 2 are attributable to IHs, whereas focal lesions more often represent congenital hemangiomas.[7,8] Most multifocal hepatic IHs are asymptomatic and do not require treatment. However, a minority of these lesions are associated with macrovascular shunting, causing high flow that can, in rare cases, result in high-output cardiac failure. So-called "diffuse" hepatic IHs are another rare subset that confers an even greater risk for morbidity and mortality. Infants who are affected typically present before 4 months of age with severe hepatomegaly, which can lead to potentially lethal abdominal compartment syndrome attributable to compromised ventilation, renal failure attributable to renal vein compression, or compromised inferior vena cava blood flow to the heart.[7,8] A consumptive form of hypothyroidism caused by the inactivation of thyroid hormones by type 3 iodothyronine deiodinase present in IH tissue can also be a complication of multifocal or diffuse hepatic IHs.[9] Although liver IHs can occasionally be seen in infants with 1 or no IH of the skin, the greatest risk for liver IHs is in infants who have 5 or more cutaneous IHs,[10] for whom screening ultrasonography is recommended (see KAS 2A).[11,30] Other sites of extracutaneous hemangiomas can occur, including the gastrointestinal tract, brain, and other organs. However, such involvement is rare and occurs mostly in association with large segmental IHs, and screening for these extracutaneous hemangiomas is not recommended unless signs or symptoms are present.[31,32] Severe bleeding, although often feared by parents, is an extremely rare complication of ulcerated IHs (see discussion of ulceration). Another potentially life-threatening complication is severe coarctation of the aorta not attributable to IHs but rather to structural anomalies seen in association with IHs in PHACE syndrome.

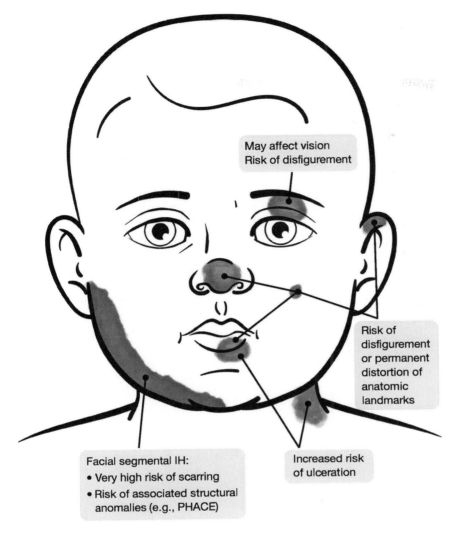

**May affect vision
Risk of disfigurement**

Risk of disfigurement or permanent distortion of anatomic landmarks

Facial segmental IH:
• Very high risk of scarring
• Risk of associated structural anomalies (e.g., PHACE)

Increased risk of ulceration

FIGURE 2
High-risk IHs involving the face and neck.

Functional Impairment

Examples of functional impairment include visual disturbance and interference with feeding because of IH involvement of the lips or mouth. IHs occurring in the periocular region have the potential to cause mechanical ptosis, strabismus, anisometropia, or astigmatism, which can quickly lead to the development of amblyopia.[12,13,33] Specific characteristics that place an infant at a higher risk for amblyopia include an IH size of >1 cm, upper eyelid involvement, associated ptosis, eyelid margin changes, medial location, and segmental morphology or displacement of the globe.[13,34,35] Feeding impairment can occur in infants with IHs involving

either the perioral region or the airway. Infants with ulcerated lip IHs may have feeding difficulties secondary to severe pain.[36] Airway IHs may complicate breathing and swallowing, leading also to impaired feeding.[37]

Ulceration

Skin or mucosal ulceration of the IH surface occurs with an estimated incidence of 5% to 21% in referral populations.[14,38] Ulceration can lead to significant pain, bleeding, and secondary infection and virtually always results in scarring. Depending on the anatomic site of involvement, it can result in disfigurement. Ulceration occurs most frequently in infants

younger than 4 months, during the period of active IH proliferation. Certain types of IHs are at higher risk, including superficial and mixed types, segmental IHs, and those involving the scalp, neck, and perioral, perineal, perianal, and intertriginous sites, the latter likely caused by maceration and friction. In addition, protuberant IHs can ulcerate as a result of trauma. Although concern for potential bleeding in IHs is common among caregivers and providers, most IH bleeding is minor and easily controllable with pressure. In rare cases, particularly IHs involving the scalp or with deep ulceration, bleeding can be more profuse, even life-threatening.[14,15]

Associated Structural Anomalies

A small subset of children with IHs have associated congenital anomalies. The best known phenomenon is PHACE syndrome (OMIM 606519).[39] The acronym "PHACES" is sometimes used instead to include potential ventral midline defects, specifically sternal cleft and/or supraumbilical raphe. Cerebrovascular anomalies, present in more than 90% of patients with PHACE syndrome, are the most common extracutaneous feature of the syndrome, followed by cardiac anomalies (67%) and structural brain anomalies (52%). The hallmark of PHACE syndrome is a large (often >5 cm in diameter) segmental IH that typically involves the face, scalp, and/or neck, although in rare cases, the face or scalp are spared, with a segmental IH located on the torso and upper extremity instead.[5,16] The risk of PHACE syndrome in an infant presenting with a large segmental IH of the head or neck is approximately 30%.[5] Revised consensus criteria for the diagnosis of PHACE syndrome and the care of infants who are affected have recently been published.[16]

LUMBAR syndrome may best be viewed as the "lower half of the body" equivalent of PHACE syndrome.[17] IHs in LUMBAR syndrome are almost invariably segmental, involving the

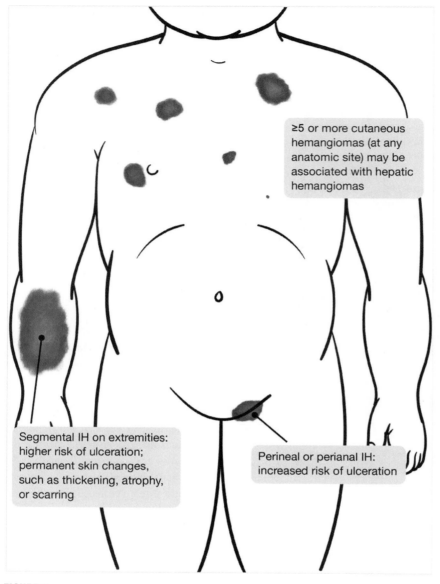

≥5 or more cutaneous hemangiomas (at any anatomic site) may be associated with hepatic hemangiomas

Segmental IH on extremities: higher risk of ulceration; permanent skin changes, such as thickening, atrophy, or scarring

Perineal or perianal IH: increased risk of ulceration

FIGURE 3
High-risk IHs involving the trunk, extremities, and perineum.

This indication for treatment represents a paradigm shift from the hands-off approach of the late 1950s through 1980s, when many experts recommended treatment only for those IHs causing functional impairment.[41] One reason for this change is an increased recognition that although IHs involute, they often leave behind permanent skin changes that, although not life or function threatening, are potentially life altering.[19,20] Moreover, with the advent of β-blocker therapies for IHs, there are now better treatment options with greater efficacy and lower potential toxicity than oral corticosteroids, the previous gold standard. There is also increased recognition that parental and patient quality of life can be adversely affected by visible birthmarks and resultant scarring, particularly in areas that cannot be easily covered with clothing, such as the face, neck, arms, and hands, as well as other emotionally sensitive areas, such as the breasts and genitalia.[42–44]

The precise risk of a patient in a primary care setting having permanent skin changes from an IH is not known, but in a referral setting, such changes are seen in 55% to 69% of those with untreated IHs.[19,20] This risk is greatest in IHs with a prominent and thick superficial (strawberry) component, especially when there is a steep step-off (ie, ledge effect) from affected to surrounding normal skin. However, the degree of superficial thickening may be difficult to predict in early infancy. Thus, even in IHs that do not initially appear to be high risk, it is prudent to serially follow lesion growth and establish a means for prompt evaluation if ongoing or rapid growth is observed because this could alter management.

Key Action Statement 1B (Table 7)

After identifying an IH as high risk, clinicians should facilitate an evaluation by a hemangioma specialist as soon as possible (grade X, strong recommendation).

The purpose of this statement is to ensure timely evaluation by a

lumbosacral or perineal skin and often extending onto 1 leg. Many IHs in LUMBAR syndrome are minimally proliferative morphologically, with telangiectatic vascular stains predominating over bulkier superficial hemangiomas. In such cases, ulceration can be an early clue to the diagnosis.[17] Rarely, undergrowth or overgrowth of an affected limb may be present. Like PHACE syndrome, the cutaneous IH and underlying anomalies in LUMBAR syndrome reveal regional correlation. Myelopathy, particularly

spinal dysraphism, is the most common extracutaneous anomaly.[17]

Disfigurement

IHs can lead to permanent disfigurement either via scarring of the skin or distortion of anatomic landmarks (see Table 3 for specific information). The risk of disfigurement is much higher than the risk of functional or life-threatening consequences. The majority of infants who receive treatment of IHs do so to prevent uncontrolled growth leading to permanent disfigurement.[1,18,40]

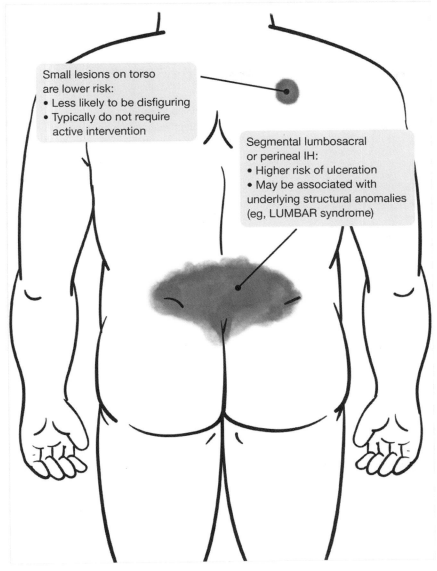

Small lesions on torso are lower risk:
• Less likely to be disfiguring
• Typically do not require active intervention

Segmental lumbosacral or perineal IH:
• Higher risk of ulceration
• May be associated with underlying structural anomalies (eg, LUMBAR syndrome)

FIGURE 4
IHs involving the posterior trunk.

have completed growth by 5 months of age.[22] In a study in which parents' photographs were used, early IH growth was found to be nonlinear, with an accelerated period of rapid growth between 5 and 7 weeks of age, and the optimal time for referral or initiation of treatment was 1 month of age, a time far earlier than the time most infants with IHs are typically referred to (or seen by) hemangioma specialists.[21,22]

These observations regarding growth are helpful, but their impact in individual case management is limited by the tremendous degree of disease heterogeneity of IHs. Even for the most experienced clinicians, it can be difficult to predict the degree of IH growth until several weeks to months after the lesion is first noticed. By that time, damage to the dermis and subcutaneous tissues as well as permanent distortion of important anatomic landmarks, such as the nose or lips, may already have occurred.[19,20,44] Hence, decisions regarding intervention must be based on risk stratification, including the age of the child (in anticipation of possible IH growth), health considerations (like prematurity), anatomic site, the size of the IH, any actual or potential complications, and parental preferences. In high-risk IHs, a wait-and-see approach can result in a missed window of opportunity to prevent adverse outcomes.

The rate of growth and ultimate size of an IH can vary dramatically from patient to patient. Predicting the growth of a particular IH is, therefore, difficult and made even more challenging by the minority of lesions that do not exhibit the typical pattern of proliferation followed by slow involution.[23,45] Differences in growth can even be evident when comparing 1 IH to another on the same patient. For example, in patients who have 2 or more IHs, 1 lesion may become large and problematic, and others may barely grow. A subset of IHs known as infantile hemangiomas with minimal or arrested growth (IH-MAGs) typically present as a patch of fine or coarsely reticulated

hemangioma specialist of an IH identified as high risk. IH is a disease with a window of opportunity in which to intervene and prevent poorer outcomes, and this critical time frame for optimizing outcomes can be missed if there are delays in referral or treatment. Recent literature suggests that the presence and growth of IHs is apparent much earlier than originally thought.[21,22] Premonitory findings appear in the skin during early infancy, including localized blanching or macular telangiectatic erythema.[21] As endothelial

cell proliferation continues, the IH enlarges, becomes more elevated, and develops a rubbery consistency. IHs typically have their clinical onset before 4 weeks of age.[21,22]

Several studies have helped to better characterize the proliferative phase of IHs. Although IHs proliferate for variable periods of time and to varying degrees, the most rapid growth of superficial IHs typically occurs between 1 and 3 months' chronological age.[21] IHs reach 80% of their ultimate size by 3 months of age, and the large majority of IHs

TABLE 7 Key Action Statement 1B: After identifying an IH as high risk, clinicians should facilitate an evaluation by a hemangioma specialist as soon as possible (grade X, strong recommendation).

Aggregate Evidence Quality	Grade X
Benefits	Potential for early intervention for IH at a high risk of causing complications
Risks, harm, cost	Potential for delay in intervention if specialist evaluation cannot be arranged promptly or is unavailable in the geographic region; costs associated with specialist evaluation for IH incorrectly identified as high risk
Benefit-harm assessment	The benefits of specialist evaluation outweigh harms and costs
Intentional vagueness	The subcommittee recognizes the multidisciplinary nature of IH management and the diverse level of expertise among individuals in this field. As a result, the definition of a specialist with expertise in vascular birthmarks is vague. The subcommittee also recognizes that the time frame "as soon as possible" is vague.
Role of patient preference	Parental preference should be considered in the decision to see a specialist and in the choice of specialist
Exclusions	IHs not considered high risk
Strength	Strong recommendation
Key references	19–23

telangiectasias, often within a zone of vasoconstriction.[23] They may be mistaken for a port-wine stain or other vascular birthmark. Although they lack the robust proliferative phase characteristic of many IHs, IH-MAGs may be associated with complications, such as ulceration or, if segmental, structural anomalies. The growth trajectory of deeper IHs or those with deeper soft-tissue components also differs from that of localized superficial IHs, often presenting at a later age (eg, 1–2 months and, occasionally, even later).[22]

On the basis of this information, the consensus recommendation of the subcommittee is that patients with IHs identified as high risk have expedited consultation and/or referral to a hemangioma specialist (Supplemental Table 22, Supplemental Fig 11). The type of hemangioma specialist may depend on the specific concern (eg, a hemangioma specialist experienced in airway management will be needed if concern exists for a subglottic hemangioma). Because the time to appointment with a hemangioma specialist may exceed the window of opportunity during which evaluation and possible treatment would be of maximum benefit, those who care for infants with IHs should have mechanisms in place to expedite such

appointments, including the education of office staff to give young infants with high-risk IHs priority appointments. In-person consultation may not always be possible or mandatory. Clinicians may also use telemedicine (either live interactive or store and forward of photographs taken in the office) to assist with triage, evaluation, and management.

Key Action Statement 2A (Table 8)

Clinicians should not perform imaging unless the diagnosis of IH is uncertain, there are 5 or more cutaneous IHs, or associated anatomic abnormalities are suspected (grade B, moderate recommendation).

The purpose of this statement is to provide guidance to clinicians regarding the indications for imaging of IHs. Most IHs can be diagnosed clinically. Therefore, imaging of IHs is not indicated for diagnostic purposes unless the lesion has an atypical appearance (ie, the diagnosis is uncertain) or it behaves in a manner that is inconsistent with the expected proliferative growth and involution phases within the expected time frame.[46,47] Noninvasive imaging may be used to monitor response to treatment but typically is not required.[47] Occasionally, differentiating an IH from a highly vascularized malignant tumor

may be difficult. Clinical history, response to therapy, and imaging characteristics considered together are extremely important in this differentiation. In rare cases, a tissue biopsy may be needed to confirm the diagnosis.

Clinicians should use imaging, specifically abdominal ultrasonography, if 5 or more cutaneous IHs are present to screen for hepatic IH.[30] Ultrasonography has a sensitivity of 95% for detection of hepatic hemangiomas and avoids the need for sedation and exposure to ionizing radiation.[46] Early detection of these lesions may lead to improved monitoring and initiation of appropriate treatment, resulting in decreased morbidity and mortality.[8,46,49]

Imaging also is indicated if concern exists for structural anomalies, as would be the case in infants at risk for PHACE syndrome or LUMBAR syndrome. These infants would typically have large (eg, >5 cm in diameter) segmental facial or scalp IHs or segmental IHs of the perineum, gluteal cleft, or lumbosacral area, with or without lower extremity IHs (see KAS 2C for further discussion).[16,17,47,48]

Key Action Statement 2B (Table 9)

Clinicians should perform ultrasonography as the initial imaging modality when the diagnosis of IH is uncertain (grade C, weak recommendation).

Ultrasonography (with Doppler imaging) is the initial imaging modality of choice when the diagnosis of IH is uncertain. The study can be performed without sedation and does not necessitate exposure to ionizing radiation, which can be risky, particularly in young infants. On ultrasonography, most IHs appear as a well-defined mass with high-flow vascular characteristics and no arteriovenous shunting (an exception to the latter is that hepatic IHs may exhibit arteriovenous shunting). This may change as the IH involutes and has a more fatty appearance with decreased vascularity.[47,50] Doppler ultrasonography is also the modality of choice when screening for hepatic IHs and can be used to monitor

TABLE 8 Key Action Statement 2A: Clinicians should not perform imaging unless the diagnosis of IH is uncertain, there are 5 or more cutaneous IHs, or associated anatomic abnormalities are suspected (grade B, moderate recommendation).

Aggregate Evidence Quality	Grade B
Benefits	Avoid the cost, risk of sedation, and radiation associated with unnecessary imaging
Risks, harm, cost	Potential misdiagnosis if imaging is not performed
Benefit-harm assessment	Benefits outweigh harm
Intentional vagueness	None
Role of patient preference	Minimal; when parental anxiety is significant, ultrasonography is a low-cost and low-risk means of confirming the diagnosis
Exclusions	None
Strength	Moderate recommendation
Key references	8,46–48

TABLE 9 Key Action Statement 2B: Clinicians should perform ultrasonography as the initial imaging modality when the diagnosis of IH is uncertain (grade C, weak recommendation).

Aggregate Evidence Quality	Grade C
Benefits	Select the appropriate imaging study to aid in diagnosis and identify associated abnormalities; avoid ionizing radiation and sedation
Risks, harm, cost	Risk that ultrasonography may not be sufficiently diagnostic or may result in the misdiagnosis of a lesion believed to represent an IH
Benefit-harm assessment	Benefits outweigh harms
Intentional vagueness	None
Role of patient preference	Minimal
Exclusions	None
Strength	Weak recommendation
Key references	47,50

progression of disease and response to treatment.[47]

Key Action Statement 2C (Table 10)

Clinicians should perform MRI when concerned about associated structural abnormalities (eg, PHACE syndrome or LUMBAR syndrome) (grade B, moderate recommendation).

Imaging for associated structural anomalies is indicated in infants at risk for PHACE syndrome or LUMBAR syndrome. For example, an infant with a large (eg, >5 cm in diameter) segmental facial or scalp IH is at risk for PHACE syndrome, and further evaluation with MRI and/or magnetic resonance angiography (MRA) of the head and neck (including the aortic arch and brachiocephalic origins) and echocardiography is advisable.[16,47]

For patients with segmental IHs of the perineum, gluteal cleft, or lumbosacral area (with or without lower extremity IHs), imaging for LUMBAR syndrome should be considered.[17,48] If there is uncertainty about whether there is a risk of associated structural anomalies, consultation with a hemangioma specialist or other appropriate expert (eg, pediatric neurologist, neurosurgeon, or radiologist) can be helpful to determine if imaging is required and which studies should be performed.

MRI is the optimal imaging modality to define underlying structural abnormalities, and contrast is needed to assess vascular components.[46] MRA can illustrate the vascular anatomy. Thus, MRI and MRA, with and without contrast of the head and neck, are the best studies to detect PHACE syndrome. MRI does not use ionizing radiation but may require sedation given the duration of the examination.[51,52] The duration of imaging is important because it has been theorized that prolonged (>3 hours) or repeated exposures to general anesthetic and sedative drugs in children younger than 3 years may negatively affect brain development.[53,54] Single, brief exposures are unlikely to have similar effects. As more rapid MRI scanning protocols are developed, the need for sedation may diminish. As an alternative to sedation, young infants fed immediately before an MRI and swaddled may sleep through the procedure. Discussion between the radiologist, ordering clinician, and sedation team is critical to determine the optimal imaging and sedation protocols.[55]

In patients in whom there is a risk of LUMBAR syndrome, spinal ultrasonography (for those with a corrected age of less than 6 months) and Doppler ultrasonography of the abdomen and pelvis can be used as an initial screen for abnormalities.[56–58] Ultimately, however, MRI likely will be required to provide greater definition. For example, if a high suspicion for spinal abnormalities remains despite normal ultrasonography (ie, there are associated markers of dysraphism [eg, sacral dimple, skin appendage, tuft of hair, and lipoma]), MRI is a more sensitive diagnostic modality.[47]

Computed tomography is not the modality of choice for imaging IHs because it involves ionizing radiation, which should be avoided in children, particularly young infants, unless absolutely necessary. Advantages of computed tomography are that it can be rapidly performed and may not require sedation.

MANAGEMENT: PHARMACOTHERAPY

Key Action Statement 3A (Table 11)

Clinicians should use oral propranolol as the first-line agent for IHs requiring

TABLE 10 Key Action Statement 2C: Clinicians should perform MRI when concerned about associated structural abnormalities (eg, PHACE syndrome or LUMBAR syndrome) (grade B, moderate recommendation).

Aggregate Evidence Quality	Grade B
Benefits	Select the appropriate imaging study to aid in diagnosis and identify associated abnormalities; avoid ionizing radiation and sedation
Risks, harm, cost	Risk of sedation or general anesthesia
	Cost of MRI (but offers greater diagnostic sensitivity)
Benefit-harm assessment	Benefits outweigh harms
Intentional vagueness	None
Role of patient preference	Minimal
Exclusions	None
Strength	Moderate recommendation
Key references	46,51–55

TABLE 11 Key Action Statement 3A: Clinicians should use oral propranolol as the first-line agent for IHs requiring systemic treatment (grade A, strong recommendation).

Aggregate Evidence Quality	Grade A
Benefits	Improve IH treatment; avoid adverse effects associated with oral steroid therapy
Risks, harm, cost	Occurrence of adverse effects associated with propranolol use (see KAS 3D); medication cost and cost of hospitalization if drug is initiated while infant is an inpatient
Benefit-harm assessment	Benefits outweigh harms
Intentional vagueness	None
Role of patient preference	Parents should be involved in shared decision-making regarding treatment.
Exclusions	Caution (but not exclusion) in infants <5 wk of age, postconceptional age of <48 wk; potential exclusions that require appropriate subspecialty evaluation and/or clearance; evidence of cardiogenic shock or heart failure; sinus bradycardia; heart block greater than first degree; known or suspected PHACE syndrome, including presence or risk of coarctation of the aorta and cerebrovascular anomalies; known asthma and/or reactive airway disease; known hypersensitivity to propranolol
Strength	Strong recommendation
Key references	3,46,59–61

systemic treatment (grade A, strong recommendation).

The purpose of this statement is to advise clinicians that oral propranolol is the current treatment of choice for IHs requiring systemic therapy. After the serendipitous observation of its utility in treating IHs,[59] propranolol, a nonselective antagonist of both β-1 and β-2 adrenergic receptors, has evolved to become the treatment of choice for IHs.[1,3,60] The precise mechanisms of action of propranolol on IHs are unclear but have been hypothesized to be attributable to vasoconstriction, angiogenesis inhibition,

induction of apoptosis, inhibition of nitric oxide production, and regulation of the renin-angiotensin system.[61–69] Oral propranolol hydrochloride (Hemangeol) was approved by the US Food and Drug Administration (FDA) in March 2014 for use in proliferating IHs requiring systemic therapy. This therapy has now replaced the previous gold standard therapy for threatening IHs, systemic or intralesional corticosteroids.[70]

In the AHRQ review, 18 studies were included in a network meta-analysis of the effectiveness and harms of corticosteroids and β-blockers. The

mean estimate of expected clearance for oral propranolol was 95%, which was superior to other interventions.[46] Ten studies compared propranolol versus another modality, including steroids, pulsed-dye laser (PDL), bleomycin, or other treatments (Table 12). Propranolol was more effective in 3 studies, effectiveness did not differ significantly in 2 other studies, and studies comparing propranolol versus steroids to reduce IH size had conflicting results. Harms are discussed in subsequent KASs, but in the AHRQ analysis, propranolol's superior safety profile is confirmed.

The subcommittee's additional review yielded another 19 studies, 4 of which met inclusion criteria for benefits of interventions (and 9 of which met inclusion criteria for harms of interventions). These 4 studies evaluated propranolol versus placebo or observation. Propranolol was associated with significantly greater clearance of IH compared with the control group in all studies. The strength of evidence (SOE) was considered high for greater effectiveness of propranolol versus placebo or observation. The review also confirmed the superiority of oral propranolol over a variety of comparators. Propranolol was superior to ibuprofen and paracetamol in treating ulcerated hemangiomas[71] and to oral captopril in patients with problematic IHs.[72] In a randomized controlled trial (RCT) of oral propranolol compared with observation for IHs, the overall efficacy of propranolol (defined as excellent, good, or medium response) was 98.97%, compared with 31.25% in the observation group ($P < .05$).[73] Last, Aly et al[74] compared oral propranolol alone versus oral propranolol combined with 2 weeks of "priming" with oral prednisolone. Those in the prednisolone-primed propranolol group showed a statistically superior reduction in IH size at weeks 2, 4, and 8 compared with the propranolol group, but the 6-month response was equivocal for both groups regarding all assessed variables.[74]

TABLE 12 AHRQ Summary of Comparative Efficacy of Various Treatments for IHs

Drug	Mean Estimate of Expected Clearance, %	95% Bayesian Credible Interval, %
Propranolol	95	88–99
Topical timolol	62	39–83
Intralesional triamcinolone	58	21–93
Oral steroid	43	21–66
Control	6	1–11

Limited data exist on the utility of β-blockers other than propranolol or different delivery mechanisms for propranolol. The AHRQ review included 3 small studies comparing propranolol versus nadolol or atenolol and 1 study comparing oral, intralesional, and topical propranolol. Atenolol and nadolol each demonstrated effectiveness on lesion size, with little difference in efficacy between propranolol and atenolol and greater efficacy of nadolol in 1 small study. The review did not find differences in response with propranolol, nadolol, or atenolol, but the SOE in comparing these was low.[46] The subcommittee's additional review yielded 1 article on oral atenolol for IH, which did not meet the AHRQ inclusion criteria for comparative effectiveness but revealed an excellent treatment response in 56.5% of patients.[75]

Key Action Statement 3B (Table 13)

Clinicians should dose propranolol between 2 and 3 mg/kg per day unless there are comorbidities (eg, PHACE syndrome) or adverse effects (eg, sleep disturbance) that necessitate a lower dose (grade A, moderate recommendation).

The purpose of this statement is to provide clinicians guidance in dosing oral propranolol for IHs. To date, authors of most studies favor dosing at 2 to 3 mg/kg per day. An RCT of 456 infants compared a placebo versus 1 of 4 propranolol regimens (1 mg/kg per day or 3 mg/kg per day for 3 or 6 months duration). The regimen of 3 mg/kg per day for 6 months was superior, with complete or nearly complete resolution in 60% of patients, compared with 4% of patients in the placebo arm ($P < .0001$).[76] The FDA approval of propranolol hydrochloride oral solution (4.28 mg/mL) recommends a starting dose of 0.6 mg/kg twice daily, with a gradual increase over 2 weeks to a maintenance dose of 1.7 mg/kg twice daily (3.4 mg/kg per day based on expression as the hydrochloride salt of propranolol). As noted in the AHRQ review, other studies typically reported dosing of 2 to 2.5 mg/kg per day,[46] and a multidisciplinary, multiinstitutional expert panel and a European expert consensus group[1,61] support a starting dose of 1 mg/kg per day and a target dose of 2 to 3 mg/kg per day. Data comparing 2 and 3 mg/kg per day are lacking.

Similarly, available data do not permit evidence-based recommendations on dosing frequency (twice daily versus 3 times daily), but both the FDA and the European Medicine Evaluation Agency labeling is for twice-daily dosing. The site for initiation of propranolol (outpatient versus inpatient) is evolving as more evidence accumulates that cardiovascular and other acute toxicities occur rarely. Although in both the aforementioned consensus articles, initiation in an inpatient setting is favored for infants younger than 8 weeks, those with cardiovascular or respiratory comorbidities, and those with poor social support, FDA labeling sanctions initiation in an outpatient setting for infants >5 weeks' corrected gestational age.

A duration of 6 months of therapy was shown to be superior to 3 months in the large RCT conducted by Léauté-Labrèze et al.[76] In the AHRQ review, the duration of propranolol treatment ranged from 3 to 13 months.[46] Rebound growth during tapering or after stopping the medication may occur in 10% to 25% of patients and can occur even after 6 months of therapy.[18,76] A large multicenter retrospective cohort study found the greatest risk of rebound occurred in those in whom therapy was discontinued at <12 months of age (and especially before 9 months), and the lowest risk was in those in whom treatment was discontinued between 12 and 15 months of age.[18] Risk factors for rebound growth noted in this study were the presence of mixed or deep morphology and female sex. These observations have led many experts to recommend continuing therapy until at least 1 year of age.

Dosing may need to be modified in certain situations. Patients with PHACE syndrome may have an increased risk of stroke, and this risk may be greater if certain neurovascular anomalies are present.[16] In patients who merit systemic IH therapy, the benefits and risks must be carefully weighed. Evaluation with MRI and/or MRA of the head and neck and echocardiography should be performed before or shortly after the initiation of therapy.[61] If patients who are at high risk require treatment with propranolol, it is advisable to use the lowest effective dose, slowly titrate the dose, and administer the drug 3 times daily (to minimize abrupt changes in blood pressure); comanagement with a pediatric neurologist is recommended.[1,16,61,77] Other patients who may require lower propranolol doses include those with progressive IH ulceration while receiving therapy and those who experience adverse effects (such as sleep disturbances).

Key Action Statement 3C (Table 14)

Clinicians should counsel that propranolol be administered with or after feeding and that doses be held at times of diminished oral intake or vomiting to reduce the risk of hypoglycemia (grade X, strong recommendation).

TABLE 13 Key Action Statement 3B: Clinicians should dose propranolol between 2 and 3 mg/kg per day unless there are comorbidities (eg, PHACE syndrome) or adverse effects (eg, sleep disturbance) that necessitate a lower dose (grade A, moderate recommendation).

Aggregate Evidence Quality	Grade A
Benefits	The recommended doses have been associated with high clearance rates of IH
Risks, harm, cost	Response rates for higher or lower doses have not been well studied
Benefit-harm assessment	Benefits outweigh harms
Intentional vagueness	None
Role of patient preference	Parents will be involved in the decision about dosing in the setting of PHACE syndrome or the occurrence of adverse effects
Exclusions	See KAS 3A; dosing may be modified if comorbidities exist
Strength	Moderate recommendation
Key references	1,46,61,76

TABLE 14 Key Action Statement 3C: Clinicians should counsel that propranolol be administered with or after feeding and that doses be held at times of diminished oral intake or vomiting to reduce the risk of hypoglycemia (grade X, strong recommendation).

Aggregate Evidence Quality	Grade X
Benefits	Reduce the likelihood of adverse reactions
Risks, harm, cost	Risk that parents will decline therapy because of concerns about potential medication adverse effects
Benefit-harm assessment	Benefits outweigh harms
Intentional vagueness	None
Role of patient preference	None
Exclusions	None
Strength	Strong recommendation
Key references	46,60,61,76,78–80

The purpose of this statement is to reinforce the importance of administering oral propranolol with feeds and of holding therapy at times of restricted oral intake to prevent hypoglycemia and hypoglycemia-induced seizures. The association between hypoglycemia and propranolol in infants and children is well established and is related to effects on glycogenolysis and gluconeogenesis.[78] β-blockade by propranolol can affect these processes, and infants and children may be particularly susceptible to this effect.[78,79] Early clinical features of hypoglycemia in infants, which may be masqueraded by β-adrenergic blockade, include sweating, tachycardia, shakiness, and anxious appearance, whereas later manifestations (signs of neuroglycopenia) may include lethargy, poor feeding, apnea, seizures, stupor, and loss of consciousness.[79]

The AHRQ review identified 24 comparative studies (4 good quality) and 56 case series (4 good quality) that reported harms data of β-blockers for IHs. Rates of clinically important harms (hypoglycemia, hypotension, bradycardia, and bronchospasm) varied widely, and the authors assigned a moderate SOE for the association of propranolol with both clinically important and minor harms (with high study limitations).[46] Harms overall did not cause treatment discontinuation.

The subcommittee's additional review yielded 8 reports that met inclusion criteria for harms regarding oral propranolol for treatment of IHs. These reports provided more detailed information about the occurrence of hypoglycemia. Three of the 8 articles reported hypoglycemia; these articles included 1021 patients, 10 of whom

experienced hypoglycemia (3 of these suffered hypoglycemic seizures in the setting of viral gastroenteritis and poor oral intake).[80–82]

In a large meta-analysis of oral propranolol for IHs not included in the AHRQ review, adverse events were reported for 1945 of 5862 patients who were treated.[60] The investigators identified 24 cases of hypoglycemia and 2 cases of hypoglycemic seizures among 3766 patients who were treated with propranolol from their literature review (some of whom are included in aforementioned studies). Of the 14 events with resolution details, 9 led to dose adjustment or temporary discontinuation of propranolol, and 1 led to permanent discontinuation of treatment. The authors mention that 1 case of hypoglycemic seizure was related to overdose, and the other was associated with diminished oral intake because of infection.[60]

Although the risk of hypoglycemia must be considered when prescribing oral propranolol for IHs, routine glucose screening is not indicated.[1,61] Hypoglycemia occurs infrequently and can be minimized with appropriate education of caregivers on the importance of administering propranolol during or immediately after a feeding and of temporarily withdrawing therapy during periods of fasting (including poor oral intake because of illness or before general anesthesia) or vomiting.[60] Prolonged fasting should be avoided, and parents should be advised that hypoglycemia becomes more likely after ≥8 hours of fasting in infants and young children.[83,84]

Key Action Statement 3D (Table 15)

Clinicians should evaluate patients for and educate caregivers about potential adverse effects of propranolol, including sleep disturbances, bronchial irritation, and clinically symptomatic bradycardia and hypotension (grade X, strong recommendation).

The purpose of this statement is to increase awareness of potential propranolol-associated adverse effects other than hypoglycemia for clinicians and caregivers of patients receiving this medical therapy for IHs. Propranolol has been used in pediatric patients for decades, primarily in an off-label fashion. In young infants, is has been used primarily for cardiac disorders and for the treatment of thyrotoxicosis at doses up to 6 to 8 mg/kg per day. Despite this use, many pediatricians will be unfamiliar with the drug, and reviewing its possible adverse effects is warranted.

As noted in the discussion of KAS 3C, the AHRQ review identified a number of adverse effects during propranolol treatment. Adverse effects most frequently reported included sleep disturbances, cold extremities, gastrointestinal symptoms, bronchial irritation (classified as hyperreactivity, bronchospasm, bronchiolitis, and cold-induced wheezing), and a decrease in heart rate or blood pressure. Rates of clinically important harms (hypoglycemia, hypotension, bradycardia, and bronchospasm) varied widely across the studies, and the authors assigned a moderate SOE for the association of propranolol with both clinically important and minor harms (with high study limitations).[46] Overall, harms did not cause treatment discontinuation.

Our additional review yielded 8 reports that met inclusion criteria for harms of interventions. Sleep disturbance, sleeping disorders, agitation during the night, and nightmares or night terrors were mentioned in 6 of 8 reports and occurred in 2% to 18.5% of patients who were treated.[80,82,85,86,89,90] In 3 of these 6 reports, propranolol treatment was modified (reduction in dosage, earlier-evening dosing, and early discontinuation of therapy) in response to these effects.[80,82,85]

In 4 reports, possible respiratory adverse effects were mentioned, including labored breathing in 0.9%,[86] breathing-related problems in 11.5%,[89] respiratory disorders in 3.4%,[80] and wheezing or bronchiolitis in 12.9%.[82] In 3 of these series treatment modifications in response to the

TABLE 15 Key Action Statement 3D: Clinicians should evaluate patients for and educate caregivers about potential adverse effects of propranolol, including sleep disturbances, bronchial irritation, and clinically symptomatic bradycardia and hypotension (grade X, strong recommendation).

Aggregate Evidence Quality	Grade X
Benefits	Recognition of adverse effects of propranolol treatment
Risks, harm, cost	Risk of caregivers declining medical therapy because of concern about potential adverse effects
Benefit-harm assessment	Benefits outweigh harms
Intentional vagueness	None
Role of patient preference	None
Exclusions	None
Strength	Strong recommendation
Key references	3,46,61,76,80,85–88

respiratory events were mentioned, including temporary discontinuation of therapy[80,82] and decreased dosage of propranolol.[89]

Although bradycardia and hypotension are known to accompany propranolol-associated β-receptor blockade, both tend to be mild and asymptomatic in children treated for IHs who have no preexisting cardiac comorbidities.[3,84,87,88,91–93] In the subcommittee's review, only 1 of the 8 reports mentioned hypotension or bradycardia as an adverse event, with 1 of 906 patients (0.1%) exhibiting bradycardia and 2 of 906 exhibiting asymptomatic hypotension.[80] The use of pretreatment electrocardiography (ECG) is controversial. Although this initially was advocated by some, several studies have revealed no actionable findings with continuous ECG monitoring, and researchers have questioned its value.[61,91] FDA guidelines for patient monitoring do not include routine ECG.[61] In their consensus recommendations, Drolet et al[61] suggest ECG screening only (1) in infants with a baseline heart rate below normal for age, (2) in infants with a family history of congenital heart conditions or arrhythmias or with a maternal history of connective tissue disease, or (3) when there is a history of arrhythmia or one is auscultated during examination. Currently, the FDA-approved administration guidelines mirror those used in the pivotal clinical

trial, with a recommendation for in-office intermittent heart rate and blood pressure monitoring for 2 hours after the first dose of propranolol or for increasing the dose for infants 5 weeks' adjusted gestational age or older.[76] Monitoring for those who are younger or for those with other comorbidities should be individualized and may require brief hospitalization for medication initiation. These recommendations may change over time as more information becomes available now that the medication is in widespread use.

Theoretical concerns about adverse effects of propranolol on brain development have been raised. As a highly lipophilic β-blocker, propranolol has the ability to cross the blood brain barrier.[94] Adult studies have revealed impairments in short- and long-term memory, psychomotor function, and mood, and prenatal β-blockade has been associated with long-term cognitive impairment,[95,96] leading some to question the potential central nervous system effects of this agent when used to treat young children with IHs.[97,98] In the large prospective randomized propranolol trial conducted by Léauté-Labrèze et al,[76] no appreciable neurodevelopmental differences were noted between the propranolol-treated groups and the placebo group at week 96. Four other studies addressing development in infants treated with propranolol for

IHs have yielded conflicting results. In 2 case series (with a total of 272 patients), gross motor delay was reported in 4.8% to 6.9%.[99,100] In contrast, a case series of 141 patients found psychomotor delay in only 1 child, and a controlled trial of 82 children found no increase in the rate of developmental concerns as assessed by the Ages and Stages Questionnaire.[101,102] Although these latter studies are reassuring, further prospective psychometric studies of children treated with oral propranolol for IHs may be warranted.

Key Action Statement 3E (Table 16)

Clinicians may prescribe oral prednisolone or prednisone to treat IHs if there are contraindications or an inadequate response to oral propranolol (grade B, moderate recommendation).

The purpose of this statement is to highlight the utility of systemic corticosteroid therapy for IHs in certain settings, such as for patients in whom β-blocker therapy is contraindicated, poorly tolerated, or ineffective. Systemic therapy with corticosteroids was considered the standard of care for several decades before being supplanted by oral propranolol.

In the AHRQ review, oral steroids had a mean estimate of expected clearance of 43% (Table 12).[46,103] The AHRQ report identified 24 studies (3 RCTs, 1 cohort study, and 20 case series) reporting outcomes and/or harms after corticosteroid use in children with IHs. One RCT was judged as good, 1 as fair, and 1 as poor quality, and the cohort study was judged as fair quality (all case series were judged as poor quality for harms reporting). The steroids studied varied in terms of dose, type, route of administration, and patient ages. Children in steroid treatment arms typically had modest improvement in lesion size, but outcomes were difficult to compare given differences in scales. The optimal dosing of systemic corticosteroids for IHs remains unclear. Dose ranges of prednisone or prednisolone reported

most frequently in the literature are between 2 and 5 mg/kg per day,[3,70,104–106] and most consider optimal dosing to be 2 to 3 mg/kg per day. Typical protocols include treating at full dose for 4 to 12 weeks followed by a gradual taper and completion of therapy by 9 to 12 months of age.[3,70,105,106] Some have advocated for shorter treatment durations (1–6 weeks), with multiple intermittent courses as needed.[107]

In the AHRQ review, steroids were consistently associated with clinically important harms, including Cushingoid appearance, infection, growth retardation, hypertension, and mood changes. The authors considered the SOE to be moderate for the association of steroids with clinically important harms.[46]

Key Action Statement 3F (Table 17)

Clinicians may recommend intralesional injection of triamcinolone and/or betamethasone to treat focal, bulky IHs during proliferation or in certain critical anatomic locations (eg, the lip) (grade B, moderate recommendation).

The purpose of this statement is to highlight the utility of intralesional corticosteroid injection for certain IH subsets. Numerous studies have reported success in the use of steroid injections for IHs, demonstrating it to be safe and effective.[108–114] This modality is most often reserved for IHs that are relatively small and well localized where proliferation is resulting in increased bulk and threatening anatomic landmarks (eg, the lip or nose). Larger or more extensive lesions are poorer candidates for this treatment modality given the larger volume of steroids necessary (and the inherent systemic risks), the difficulty of obtaining even distribution throughout the tumor, and the potential for local complications in lesions that are mostly flat or superficial.[3] Most studies have used triamcinolone either alone or in conjunction with betamethasone, with injections given on average every 4 to 6 weeks (but with wide variability). Repeat

injections are often administered, with the number used ranging in most reports from 1 to 7.[109–112]

The AHRQ review found that intralesional triamcinolone had a mean estimate of expected clearance of 58% (Table 12).[46,103] Overall, the SOE was low for intralesional steroids having a modest effect relative to control, with wide confidence bounds.[46] The subcommittee's additional search yielded 1 report that met inclusion criteria for benefits of interventions as a comparative study. This was a retrospective review of patients with periocular IHs treated with oral propranolol, who were compared with a cohort treated with intralesional corticosteroid injection. Both groups showed a reduction in astigmatism over 12 months, and neither experienced significant adverse effects necessitating dose reduction or treatment cessation.[115] The authors concluded that oral propranolol (given its efficacy and safety profiles) has emerged as the treatment of choice for periocular IHs requiring therapy.[115]

Steroids (oral and intralesional forms were grouped together in the AHRQ harms analysis) were consistently associated with clinically important harms, including Cushingoid appearance, infection, growth retardation, hypertension, and mood changes. The authors considered the SOE to be moderate for the association of steroids with clinically important harms. The most commonly reported complications associated with intralesional steroid injection for IHs are transient Cushingoid features, failure to thrive, and local skin complications.[109–112] Local complications may include fat and/or dermal atrophy and pigmentary changes.[108–110] Adrenal suppression is infrequently reported in association with intralesional steroid injections but has been observed when large doses (eg, >4 mg/kg) have been administered.[116,117] There have been rare reports of central retinal artery embolization, usually after injection into IHs of the upper eyelid, likely related to high injection pressures and/or volumes.[118–121]

TABLE 16 Key Action Statement 3E: Clinicians may prescribe oral prednisolone or prednisone to treat IHs if there are contraindications or an inadequate response to oral propranolol (grade B, moderate recommendation).

Aggregate Evidence Quality	Grade B
Benefits	Modest benefit in IH clearance; medication cost is low
Risks, harm, cost	Clinically important harms; cost associated with the evaluation and treatment of adverse effects
Intentional vagueness	None
Benefit-harm assessment	Benefits outweigh harms
Role of patient preference	Shared decision-making regarding treatment
Exclusions	None
Strength	Moderate recommendation
Key references	46,70,103

TABLE 17 Key Action Statement 3F: Clinicians may recommend intralesional injection of triamcinolone and/or betamethasone to treat focal, bulky IHs during proliferation or in certain critical anatomic locations (eg, the lip) (grade B, moderate recommendation).

Aggregate Evidence Quality	Grade B
Benefits	Modest benefit in IH clearance
Risks, harm, cost	Clinically important harms; cost of medication, visits for injection; risk of anesthesia if used
Benefit-harm assessment	Benefits outweigh harms in selected clinical situations
Intentional vagueness	None
Role of patient preference	Shared decision-making regarding route of drug delivery
Exclusions	None
Strength	Moderate recommendation
Key references	3,46,103,108–112

Key Action Statement 3G (Table 18)

Clinicians may prescribe topical timolol maleate as a therapy for thin and/or superficial IHs (grade B, moderate recommendation).

The purpose of this statement is to highlight the potential utility of topical timolol in treating thin and/or superficial IHs. Topical timolol maleate, a nonselective β-adrenergic receptor inhibitor, has been used in the treatment of pediatric glaucoma as a first-line agent for several decades.[122,127,128] Treatment of IHs with ophthalmic timolol maleate was initially reported in 2010, and since that time, there have been many reports (including some with hundreds of patients), as well as an RCT, with positive findings.[40,122–125,129–134] On the basis of these reports showing efficacy with minimal adverse effects, timolol is increasingly being used for thin and superficial IHs, and many centers report

that their use of timolol exceeds that of oral β-blockers.[135]

In the AHRQ review, 2 RCTs and 4 cohort studies were included. Topical timolol had a mean estimate of expected clearance of 62% (Table 12).[46,103] Timolol was significantly more effective than observation or a placebo in 3 studies; 1 study comparing topical imiquimod with timolol did not demonstrate superiority of either agent but was found to have insufficient SOE.[46] Our subsequent review found 3 further reports meeting criteria for efficacy, including 1 study comparing timolol to an ultrapotent corticosteroid and 2 other studies of timolol alone.[40,133,134] In the largest of these, a multicenter retrospective cohort study of 731 patients, most infants were treated with the 0.5% gel-forming solution. The study reveal improvement in nearly 70% of patients treated for 1 to 3 months and in 92.3% of patients who received

6 to 9 months of therapy. The greatest improvement was in color; however, with a longer duration of treatment, improvement in size, extent, and volume were also observed. Best responses were observed in thinner superficial IHs (ie, <1 mm thick) versus mixed or deep IHs. The large majority of infants studied were 6 months or younger at time of initiation of treatment, and 41% were ≤3 months of age. This suggests that early topical timolol treatment may also inhibit IH growth. Only 7% of infants required subsequent treatment with a systemic β-blocker.[40]

Although pharmacokinetic data are limited, evidence suggests that timolol maleate can be detected in the blood or urine of at least some infants treated topically.[126,136] Additional pharmacokinetic studies are needed given occasional reports of systemic toxicity.[137–139] It should be noted that timolol is significantly more potent than propranolol, and topical application avoids first-pass liver metabolism, as would occur with an oral β-blocker.[127] Pending the results of ongoing studies, these factors should lead to caution when using timolol, especially if prescribing more than 1 drop twice daily or when treating preterm or young infants.

The AHRQ report emphasized that there were far more reports of harms with oral β-blockers than with timolol but did note 1 report of shortness of breath and insomnia.[46] Subsequent to that report, tolerability data have been reassuring overall, but some adverse events have been reported.[40,122,124,125,131–134,140] In the large cohort study of 731 patients conducted by Püttgen et al,[40] adverse events were noted in 3.4% of patients and included local irritation (nearly half of the adverse events) and bronchospasm (in 3 patients); no cardiovascular events were reported. No adverse events were significant enough to necessitate drug discontinuation.[40] In a retrospective case series of 30 children with ulcerated IHs treated with topical timolol maleate 0.5% gel-forming solution and evaluating for

TABLE 18 Key Action Statement 3G: Clinicians may prescribe topical timolol maleate as a therapy for thin and/or superficial IHs (grade B, moderate recommendation).

Aggregate Evidence Quality	Grade B
Benefit	Modest benefit in IH clearance
Harm	Low but possible risk of local irritation, sleep disturbance, cold extremities, bronchospasm, and bradycardia, with more caution needed in preterm infants and those without intact skin (ie, ulceration)
Cost	Cost of medication
Benefits-harm assessment	Benefits outweigh harms
Value judgments	None
Role of patient preference	Parents have a significant role in decision-making regarding the desire to treat small superficial lesions for which timolol may be effective
Intentional vagueness	None
Exclusions	Lesions that are large size, significantly elevated, or life-threatening
Strength	Moderate recommendation
Key references	40,46,85,122–126

adverse events, sleep disturbance was observed in 1 infant (who was treated simultaneously with oral propranolol and topical timolol) and a single episode of cold extremities was reported in another. The remainder had no reported adverse events.[141] Bradycardia, both symptomatic and asymptomatic, was reported in 4 of 22 young and preterm infants given timolol for IHs. Two infants had bradycardia that was mild and asymptomatic, but in 2 (both of whom were born preterm and weighed less than 2500 g at initiation of therapy) there were associated symptoms.[126] To address concerns regarding potential percutaneous absorption and toxicity, many authors have advocated using limited amounts of medication (eg, 1 drop 2–3 times per day),[40] and some have cautioned against application to ulcerated lesions.[127]

SURGICAL MANAGEMENT

Key Action Statement 4 (Table 19)

Clinicians may recommend surgery and laser therapy as treatment options in managing selected IHs (grade C, moderate recommendation).

The purpose of this statement is to support surgery and laser therapy as treatment options for selected IHs, although it is recommended that decisions regarding their use should be made in consultation with a hemangioma specialist, especially in young infants. With the advent of β-blocker therapy, surgical and laser approaches are used less frequently.

In general, surgical interventions are not performed in infancy. During this time, anesthetic risks are of greater concern, and the tumor is highly vascular, posing a higher risk of blood loss, iatrogenic injury, and an inferior outcome.[142,143,145] In certain locations, such as the lip and nasal tip, the final cosmetic result is superior when growth of the lesion has ceased and the number of surgical interventions can be kept to a minimum. Furthermore, there is no psychosocial urgency to improve a deformity caused by IHs in this age group because long-term memory and self-esteem are not established until later in childhood.[143,146–148] There are certain clinical situations, however, in which early surgery can be an important treatment option. These include IHs that ulcerate, obstruct or deform vital structures (such as the airway or orbit), or involve aesthetically sensitive areas. In these circumstances, surgery may be indicated when (1) the lesion has failed to improve with local wound care and/or pharmacotherapy; (2) the lesion is well localized, and early surgery will simplify later reconstruction (eg, a prominent IH involving the ear or eyelid [causing ptosis]); (3) the lesion is well localized in an anatomically favorable area; or (4) resection is likely to be necessary in the future, and the resultant scar would be the same.[142,143,145] The decision to undertake surgery during infancy should take into consideration current knowledge of the risks of general anesthesia in this age group.[53–55]

Surgery also is an important treatment option for IHs that, despite involution, have left residual skin changes (eg, thinned skin, scar, fibrofatty tissue, telangiectasias, and/or anatomic deformities in areas such as the nose, ear, or lip).[19,20,143] In most cases, deferring surgery until the child is 3 to 5 years of age is reasonable because: (1) the lesion may resolve significantly without leaving a deformity that necessitates intervention; (2) the tumor is smaller than it was during infancy, and thus, the operation is often easier, and the resultant scar may be smaller; and (3) the IH primarily is adipose tissue instead of blood vessels, and thus, the operation is safer.[142,143,145] However, it is usually unnecessary to wait longer than 3 to 5 years of age because the previously accepted adage that 50% of IHs complete involution by 5 years of age, 70% by 7 years of age, and 90% by 9 years of age has proven to be incorrect.[19,143,149] In fact, most IHs do not improve significantly after 3 to 4 years of age.[20,143] Moreover, performing surgery at this earlier age can be beneficial in minimizing stigma and impact on a child's self-esteem.[143] There is less urgency to correct a residual deformity in an area that is concealed by clothing (eg, a lesion on the trunk). Some parents may elect to wait until the child is older and able to help in decision-making, especially if the reason for surgery is the management of less disfiguring skin changes.[143]

Laser Management

PDL has been used for several decades to treat IHs. The AHRQ review noted that most studies that were reviewed

TABLE 19 Key Action Statement 4: Clinicians may recommend surgery and laser therapy as treatment options in managing selected IHs (grade C, moderate recommendation).

Aggregate Evidence Quality	Grade C
Benefits	Early surgical intervention after infancy corrects residual deformities before the child's self-esteem develops
Risks, harm, cost	Risk of surgical complications and general anesthesia; costs associated with operative intervention, anesthesia, and postoperative care
Benefits-harm assessment	Preponderance of benefit
Intentional vagueness	None
Role of patient preference	Significant
Exclusions	Children with a nonproblematic IH
Strength	Moderate recommendation
Key references	20,142–144

evaluated PDL (as opposed to other lasers) and examined heterogeneous end points (the latter factor limiting the ability to draw conclusions). However, there is low SOE that PDL is more effective in reducing IH size when compared with observation.[46] There is evidence that PDL is superior to other lasers. In contrast, there is wide recognition that PDL is effective and safe in removing residual macular erythema and superficial telangiectasias in involuting or involuted IHs, but it often requires several treatments to achieve optimal results.[1, 142] Other lasers, such as erbium-yttrium-aluminum-garnet, have been reportedly effective in ameliorating textural changes in small case series.[150] Harms associated with laser therapy that were identified in the AHRQ review included skin atrophy, bleeding, scarring, ulceration, purpura, and pigmentation changes.[46] The AHRQ review also noted that most studies of lasers reviewed evaluated lasers as a first-line treatment, a practice that is less common since the advent of β-blocker treatment.

There is controversy regarding whether PDL should be used to treat IHs early in infancy (ie, during the proliferative phase). Several case reports and case series have revealed an increased risk of ulceration, scarring, and hypopigmentation when PDL is used during this period.[1,144,151] Moreover, PDL penetrates only into the superficial dermis, and thus, although

redness may be diminished, deeper elements of the IH (that increase the risk of residual skin changes) are not affected.[144,152,153]

Some authors advocate for using PDL as a treatment of ulceration. However, evidence supporting the use of PDL for this indication comes from case reports and small case series. Propranolol has been associated with faster healing of ulceration when compared with laser therapy and antibiotics.[46]

PARENT EDUCATION

Key Action Statement 5 (Table 20)

Clinicians should educate parents of infants with an IH about the condition, including the expected natural history, and its potential for causing complications or disfigurement (grade X, strong recommendation).

The purpose of this statement is to ensure that parents are knowledgeable about their child's IH and to provide clinicians with a framework for educating those parents about IHs. The information provided by clinicians should be as specific to the patient's IH as possible (eg, indicating whether and why an IH is low risk and, thus, likely to cause no problems or sequelae or is potentially high risk and requires urgent evaluation or treatment; Table 3, illustrated in

Figs 2–4, Supplemental Table 22, and Supplemental Fig 11).

IHs That Do Not Raise Concern

In a primary care setting, the majority of IHs are not problematic and require no active intervention (ie, are low risk; Supplemental Table 22, Supplemental Fig 11). However, given their appearance, even nonproblematic (that is, low-risk) IHs may cause significant parental anxiety and concern. These emotions may be amplified by information gleaned from Internet searches that show photographs emphasizing the more severe end of the disease spectrum as well as public reactions to the child's IH if the lesion is located at a site not easily covered by clothing.[42,155,156] Formal educational efforts can reduce parental anxiety and enhance comfort with a plan to observe the IH for any unexpected or worrisome changes.[154]

Parents should be educated about the natural history of IHs. Specifically, they may be advised that, although growth characteristics vary from case to case, most superficial IHs have a maximum growth potential between 1 and 3 months of age[3,21,157] and that the majority of growth is complete by 5 months of age.[22] Deeper IHs may have a slightly later onset and a more prolonged duration of growth. During the period of growth, clinicians should encourage parents to call, schedule an office visit, or share photographs of the IH with them to reassess if concerns exist about the lesion's appearance, unexpectedly rapid growth, ulceration, bleeding, or pain, all findings that indicate that a lesion is no longer low risk.

Parents should be advised that by age 5 to 12 months, most IHs have stopped growing and are beginning to involute. For IHs with a superficial component, this appears as a gradual change in color from red to milky-white or gray. Lesions gradually flatten and shrink from the center outward. Involution proceeds more slowly than growth. Newer studies have demonstrated that 90% of IH involution is complete by 4 years of age.[20,143] This is in contrast to traditional teaching that involution proceeds at 10% per year (ie, 50% of IHs resolve by 5 years of age and 90% by 9 years of age). Parents should be advised that even after involution, residual changes, such as telangiectasias, redundant skin, or a scar,[3,19] may be left. It is usually possible to tell whether such changes are going to persist by 4 years of age, and if concerning, consultation for management of these skin changes, particularly laser or surgical treatment, may be pursued.

A collection of serial photographs can be useful to demonstrate to parents the natural history of IHs and the process of spontaneous involution.[154] Such photos are available on the Hemangioma Investigator Group (https://hemangiomaeducation. org/) and Yale Dermatology (http:// medicine.yale.edu/dermatology/patient/ conditions/hemangioma.aspx) Web sites. Information sheets (ie, handouts) are available from the Society for Pediatric Dermatology Web site (http://pedsderm.net/) under the "For Patients and Families" tab, and adapted versions of their hemangioma patient information and propranolol sheets are included in the What Are Hemangiomas? Propranolol for Hemangiomas, and Medication Information sections of the Supplemental Information. A video for parents is also available on the Society for Pediatric Dermatology Web site (https://pedsderm.net/for-patients-families/patient-education-videos/ #InfantileHemangiomas). Information also is available from the AHRQ (https:// effectivehealthcare.ahrq.gov/topics/ infantile-hemangioma/consumer/),[158] and answers to frequently asked questions are available on the Hemangioma Investigator Group and Yale Dermatology Web sites.

IHs That May Be Problematic

When confronted with a potentially problematic IH (ie, high risk; Table 3; illustrated in Figs 2–4, Supplemental Table 22, and Supplemental Fig 11), primary care clinicians are encouraged

TABLE 20 Key Action Statement 5: Clinicians should educate parents of infants with an IH about the condition, including the expected natural history, and its potential for causing complications or disfigurement (grade X, strong recommendation).

Aggregate Evidence Quality	Grade X
Benefits	Promotes parent satisfaction and understanding, may reduce medication errors, may improve clinical outcomes
Risks, harm, cost	May increase parental anxiety because of the need to administer medication; time spent in education, may increase health care costs because of the need for follow-up visits
Benefit-harm assessment	Benefits outweigh harms
Intentional vagueness	None
Role of parental preferences	Essential; shared decision-making regarding the need for treatment is vital
Exclusions	None
Strength	Strong recommendation
Key references	21,22,154

to consult promptly with a hemangioma specialist unless they have the experience and knowledge to manage such patients independently. Because IH proliferation may occur early and be unpredictable and because there is a window of opportunity for optimal treatment, caregivers can be advised that consultation should take place in a timely manner. Unfortunately, this does not always occur. Although caregivers first notice lesions by 1 month of age (on average, at 2 weeks) and the ideal time for consultation may be 4 weeks of age, 1 study found that the mean age at presentation to a dermatologist was 5 months, by which time most growth is complete.[21,22]

Recognizing that it may be difficult to obtain an appointment with a hemangioma specialist in a timely manner, caregivers and clinicians may need to advocate on behalf of the infant. In settings where a hemangioma specialist is not readily available, telemedicine triage or consultation, using photographs taken by caregivers or the clinician, can be helpful. In 1 academic center in Spain, teledermatology triage reduced the age at first evaluation of an infant with an IH from 5.9 to 3.5 months.[159]

Once the hemangioma specialist has an opportunity to meet with parents and evaluate the infant, a

discussion about management can take place. If medical treatment is recommended, the specialist will educate parents about the medication and its dosing, its possible adverse effects, and the expected duration of treatment. If the medication selected is propranolol, as often is the case, a patient information sheet (such as that developed by the Society for Pediatric Dermatology or that provided in the What Are Hemangiomas? and Propranolol for Hemangiomas sections of the Supplemental Information) or information from the article by Martin et al[160] may be provided. For families unable to travel to see a hemangioma specialist, collaborative care may be considered. The hemangioma specialist can evaluate serial photographs and provide the primary care clinician with guidance on treatment. In this case, the primary care clinician will assume a more active role in parent education.

CHALLENGES TO IMPLEMENTING THIS CPG

Several potential challenges exist to implementing this CPG. The first is the dynamic nature of individual IHs with a period of rapid growth, the degree of which can be difficult to predict, particularly in young infants. There are no surrogate markers or imaging studies that have been shown to reliably predict growth. Hence, frequent in-person visits or a review of parental photos may be needed, especially in infants younger than 3 to 4 months. However, this may be complicated by the frequency and timing of well-child visits during this period. After the first-week visit, an infant who is well, has regained birth weight, and has parents who are experienced caregivers may not be seen again until 2 months of age. As noted by Tollefson and Frieden,[21] most superficial IHs have accelerated growth between 5 and 7 weeks of age, and 4 weeks of age may be the ideal time for referral if high-risk features are present. Thus, the most dramatic IH growth (and potentially permanent skin changes) may occur during a time when an infant is not scheduled to see a health care provider. Although awareness of this issue does not justify altering the interval of well-child visits for all infants, it heightens the need for more frequent monitoring in those with possible or definite IHs. Prompt evaluation, either in-person or via photographs, is warranted for any infant reported by parents to have a changing birthmark during the first 2 months of life.

A second challenge is the wide heterogeneity of IHs in terms of size, location, patterns of distribution (ie, segmental versus localized), and depth (ie, superficial, mixed, or deep). This heterogeneity, particularly when combined with the unpredictable growth of any given IH, may lead to uncertainty in management (ie, whether to treat or observe). Although this CPG provides guidance regarding risk stratification and growth characteristics, there is no one-size-fits-all approach. If uncertainty exists, consultation with a hemangioma specialist (whether by an in-person visit or photographic triage) can be helpful.

A third challenge is the long-held tenet that IHs are benign and go away. Because of this myth, parents and caregivers are often reassured that the lesion will disappear, and this is accurate in the vast majority of cases. However, there is ample evidence that

false reassurance can be given even in high-risk cases; indeed, all hemangioma specialists have seen examples of lost opportunities to intervene and prevent poor outcomes because of lack of or delayed referral. The availability of highly effective treatments for IHs makes it critical that this myth is debunked and that practitioners become more comfortable with the concept of identifying high-risk IHs that require close observation or prompt intervention.

Last, some geographical locations lack access to prompt specialty care from hemangioma specialists. Lack of access can also result in delays in referrals or prompt appointments. Possible solutions could include establishing resources for the photographic triage of cases in which risk stratification is uncertain or in which triage to hasten referral can be augmented by this methodology.

EVIDENCE GAPS AND PROPOSED FUTURE DIRECTIONS

The proportion of IHs in primary care settings that are truly high risk is not known. Even in a referral setting, the proportions needing active intervention vary depending on referral patterns.[3,161] This information would be useful to pediatricians and other primary care providers and should be the subject of future research.

Scoring systems for IH severity have been proposed, and one in particular, the Hemangioma Severity Score, has gained some favor as a triage tool.[162–164] However, more research is needed to ensure that it can accurately be interpreted by primary care physicians and to find scores that capture the vast majority of high-risk IHs requiring specialty care without overreferring.

Other important evidence gaps should be highlighted, including the following:

- How safe is topical timolol as a treatment during early infancy, and which patients being treated with the

drug need referral versus which can be observed without referral by the pediatrician?

- Is outpatient in-office cardiovascular monitoring for propranolol truly needed in healthy infants 5 weeks or older? Is blood pressure monitoring necessary, or is measuring heart rate sufficient?

- What is the role of the pediatrician in managing infants placed on β-blocker therapies (both topical and systemic), and are there specific time frames for specialty reevaluation?

- How accurate are primary care physicians in identifying high-risk IHs using parameters such as those outlined in this CPG?

- Are pediatric trainees receiving adequate training in risk stratification and management of IHs?

Some of these questions may be answered by research that is currently underway. Other studies will be needed to identify and remedy remaining gaps. Moreover, because there has been a tremendous accrual of information about IH management, there will need to be periodic updates as new information becomes available (and possibly sooner than the 5 years typical for CPGs). With such ongoing reassessment and revision, the subcommittee hopes this CPG will be viewed as an effective guide to IH triage and management and to minimize poor outcomes from higher-risk IHs. One barrier to a better understanding of IHs and to answering the questions posed here is the imprecision of current diagnostic codes. For example, the *International Classification of Diseases, 10th Revision* code for "hemangioma of the skin and subcutaneous tissues" is not specific to IHs and can include other entities (eg, congenital hemangioma and verrucous hemangioma) that are not IHs. In addition, current diagnostic codes do not contain sufficient detail to permit appreciation of higher-risk features, such as location or multifocality. Advocacy for the creation of a unique and exclusive *International*

Classification of Diseases, 10th Revision code (and appropriate modifiers) for IHs would be an appropriate step in addressing this issue.

Implementation tools for this guideline are available on the AAP Web site at https://www.aap.org/en-us/professional-resources/quality-improvement/Pages/default.aspx (this may leave or stay depending on the Digital Transformation Initiative). A useful resource for clinicians is the AAP Web page, "Diagnosis and Management of Infantile Hemangiomas" (https://www.aap.org/en-us/advocacy-and-policy/aap-health-initiatives/Infantile-Hemangiomas/Pages/default.aspx).

LEAD AUTHORS

Daniel P. Krowchuk, MD, FAAP
Ilona J. Frieden, MD, FAAP
Anthony J. Mancini MD, FAAP
David H. Darrow, MD, DDS, FAAP
Francine Blei, MD, MBA, FAAP
Arin K. Greene, MD, FAAP
Aparna Annam, DO, FAAP
Cynthia N. Baker, MD, FAAP
Peter C. Frommelt, MD
Amy Hodak, CPMSM
Brian M. Pate, MD, FHM, FAAP
Janice L. Pelletier, MD, FAAP
Deborah Sandrock, MD, FAAP
Stuart T. Weinberg, MD, FAAP
Mary Anne Whelan, MD, PhD, FAAP

SUBCOMMITTEE ON THE MANAGEMENT OF INFANTILE HEMANGIOMAS (OVERSIGHT BY THE COUNCIL ON QUALITY IMPROVEMENT AND PATIENT SAFETY)

Daniel P. Krowchuk, MD, FAAP, Chairperson, General Pediatrics and Adolescent Medicine
Ilona Frieden, MD, FAAP, Vice Chairperson, Pediatric Dermatology
Aparna Annam, DO, FAAP, Pediatric Radiology
Cynthia N. Baker, MD, FAAP, General Pediatrics
Francine Blei, MD, MBA, FAAP, Pediatric Hematology-Oncology
David H. Darrow, MD, DDS, FAAP, Otolaryngology Head and Neck Surgery
Peter C. Frommelt, MD, Pediatric Cardiology
Arin K. Greene, MD, FAAP, Plastic Surgery
Amy Hodak, CPMSM, Family Representative
Anthony J. Mancini, MD, FAAP, Pediatric Dermatology
Brian M. Pate, MD, FHM, FAAP, Implementation Scientist
Janice L. Pelletier, MD, FAAP, General Pediatrics
Deborah Sandrock, MD, FAAP, General Pediatrics
Stuart T. Weinberg, MD, FAAP, Partnership for Policy Implementation Representative
Mary Anne Whelan, MD, PhD, FAAP, Epidemiologist and Methodologist

STAFF

Kymika Okechukwu, MPA, Senior Manager, Evidence-Based Medicine Initiatives

ABBREVIATIONS

AAP: American Academy of Pediatrics
AHRQ: Agency for Healthcare Research and Quality
CPG: clinical practice guideline
ECG: electrocardiography
FDA: Food and Drug Administration
IH: infantile hemangioma
IH-MAG: infantile hemangioma with minimal or arrested growth
KAS: key action statement
LUMBAR: lower body infantile hemangiomas and other cutaneous defects, urogenital anomalies and ulceration, myelopathy, bony deformities, anorectal malformations, and arterial anomalies and renal anomalies
MRA: magnetic resonance angiography
PDL: pulsed-dye laser
PHACE: posterior fossa defects, hemangiomas, cerebrovascular arterial anomalies, cardiovascular anomalies (including coarctation of the aorta), and eye anomalies
RCT: randomized controlled trial
SOE: strength of evidence

The guidance in this report does not indicate an exclusive course of treatment or serve as a standard of medical care. Variations, taking into account individual circumstances, may be appropriate.

All clinical practice guidelines from the American Academy of Pediatrics automatically expire 5 years after publication unless reaffirmed, revised, or retired at or before that time.

DOI: https://doi.org/10.1542/peds.2018-3475

Address correspondence to Daniel P. Krowchuk, MD, FAAP. E-mail: krowchuk@wakehealth.edu

PEDIATRICS (ISSN Numbers: Print, 0031-4005; Online, 1098-4275).

FINANCIAL DISCLOSURE: Dr Frieden is a member of the Data Monitoring Safety Board for Pfizer and the Scientific Advisory Board for Venthera/Bridge Bio; Dr Mancini has indicated that he has advisory board relationships with Verrica, Valeant, and Pfizer; the other authors have indicated they have no financial relationships relevant to this article to disclose.

FUNDING: No external funding.

POTENTIAL CONFLICT OF INTEREST: The authors have indicated they have no potential conflicts of interest to disclose.

REFERENCES

1. Hoeger PH, Harper JI, Baselga E, et al. Treatment of infantile haemangiomas: recommendations of a European expert group. *Eur J Pediatr.* 2015;174(7):855–865

2. Smithson SL, Rademaker M, Adams S, et al. Consensus statement for the treatment of infantile haemangiomas with propranolol. *Australas J Dermatol.* 2017;58(2):155–159

3. Darrow DH, Greene AK, Mancini AJ, Nopper AJ; Section on Dermatology; Section on Otolaryngology–Head and Neck Surgery; Section on Plastic Surgery. Diagnosis and management of infantile hemangioma. *Pediatrics.* 2015;136(4). Available at: www.pediatrics.org/cgi/content/full/136/4/e1060

4. Agency for Healthcare Research and Quality. Effective health care program.

Available at: www.effectivehealthcare. ahrq.gov/reports/final.cfm. Accessed February 6, 2018

5. Haggstrom AN, Garzon MC, Baselga E, et al. Risk for PHACE syndrome in infants with large facial hemangiomas. *Pediatrics*. 2010;126(2). Available at: www.pediatrics.org/cgi/content/full/126/2/e418

6. Orlow SJ, Isakoff MS, Blei F. Increased risk of symptomatic hemangiomas of the airway in association with cutaneous hemangiomas in a "beard" distribution. *J Pediatr*. 1997;131(4):643–646

7. Kulungowski AM, Alomari AI, Chawla A, Christison-Lagay ER, Fishman SJ. Lessons from a liver hemangioma registry: subtype classification. *J Pediatr Surg*. 2012;47(1):165–170

8. Rialon KL, Murillo R, Fevurly RD, et al. Risk factors for mortality in patients with multifocal and diffuse hepatic hemangiomas. *J Pediatr Surg*. 2015;50(5):837–841

9. Huang SA, Tu HM, Harney JW, et al. Severe hypothyroidism caused by type 3 iodothyronine deiodinase in infantile hemangiomas. *N Engl J Med*. 2000;343(3):185–189

10. Horii KA, Drolet BA, Frieden IJ, et al; Hemangioma Investigator Group. Prospective study of the frequency of hepatic hemangiomas in infants with multiple cutaneous infantile hemangiomas. *Pediatr Dermatol*. 2011;28(3):245–253

11. Rialon KL, Murillo R, Fevurly RD, et al. Impact of screening for hepatic hemangiomas in patients with multiple cutaneous infantile hemangiomas. *Pediatr Dermatol*. 2015;32(6):808–812

12. Jockin YM, Friedlander SF. Periocular infantile hemangioma. *Int Ophthalmol Clin*. 2010;50(4):15–25

13. Schwartz SR, Blei F, Ceisler E, Steele M, Furlan L, Kodsi S. Risk factors for amblyopia in children with capillary hemangiomas of the eyelids and orbit. *J AAPOS*. 2006;10(3):262–268

14. Chamlin SL, Haggstrom AN, Drolet BA, et al. Multicenter prospective study of ulcerated hemangiomas [published correction appears in *J Pediatr*. 2008;152(4):597]. *J Pediatr*. 2007;151(6):684–689, 689.e1

15. Connelly EA, Viera M, Price C, Waner M. Segmental hemangioma of infancy complicated by life-threatening arterial bleed. *Pediatr Dermatol*. 2009;26(4):469–472

16. Garzon MC, Epstein LG, Heyer GL, et al. PHACE syndrome: consensus-derived diagnosis and care recommendations. *J Pediatr*. 2016;178:24–33.e2

17. Iacobas I, Burrows PE, Frieden IJ, et al. LUMBAR: association between cutaneous infantile hemangiomas of the lower body and regional congenital anomalies. *J Pediatr*. 2010;157(5):795–801.e1–e7

18. Shah SD, Baselga E, McCuaig C, et al. Rebound growth of infantile hemangiomas after propranolol therapy. *Pediatrics*. 2016;137(4):e20151754

19. Bauland CG, Lüning TH, Smit JM, Zeebregts CJ, Spauwen PH. Untreated hemangiomas: growth pattern and residual lesions. *Plast Reconstr Surg*. 2011;127(4):1643–1648

20. Baselga E, Roe E, Coulie J, et al. Risk factors for degree and type of sequelae after involution of untreated hemangiomas of infancy. *JAMA Dermatol*. 2016;152(11):1239–1243

21. Tollefson MM, Frieden IJ. Early growth of infantile hemangiomas: what parents' photographs tell us. *Pediatrics*. 2012;130(2). Available at: www.pediatrics.org/cgi/content/full/130/2/e314

22. Chang LC, Haggstrom AN, Drolet BA, et al; Hemangioma Investigator Group. Growth characteristics of infantile hemangiomas: implications for management. *Pediatrics*. 2008;122(2):360–367

23. Suh KY, Frieden IJ. Infantile hemangiomas with minimal or arrested growth: a retrospective case series. *Arch Dermatol*. 2010;146(9):971–976

24. Luu M, Frieden IJ. Haemangioma: clinical course, complications and management. *Br J Dermatol*. 2013;169(1):20–30

25. Shikhani AH, Jones MM, Marsh BR, Holliday MJ. Infantile subglottic hemangiomas. An update. *Ann Otol Rhinol Laryngol*. 1986;95(4, pt 1):336–347

26. Bitar MA, Moukarbel RV, Zalzal GH. Management of congenital subglottic hemangioma: trends and success over the past 17 years. *Otolaryngol Head Neck Surg*. 2005;132(2):226–231

27. Uthurriague C, Boccara O, Catteau B, et al. Skin patterns associated with upper airway infantile haemangiomas: a retrospective multicentre study. *Acta Derm Venereol*. 2016;96(7):963–966

28. Sherrington CA, Sim DK, Freezer NJ, Robertson CF. Subglottic haemangioma. *Arch Dis Child*. 1997;76(5):458–459

29. Sie KC, McGill T, Healy GB. Subglottic hemangioma: ten years' experience with the carbon dioxide laser. *Ann Otol Rhinol Laryngol*. 1994;103(3):167–172

30. Horii KA, Drolet BA, Baselga E, et al; Hemangioma Investigator Group. Risk of hepatic hemangiomas in infants with large hemangiomas. *Arch Dermatol*. 2010;146(2):201–203

31. Drolet BA, Pope E, Juern AM, et al. Gastrointestinal bleeding in infantile hemangioma: a complication of segmental, rather than multifocal, infantile hemangiomas. *J Pediatr*. 2012;160(6):1021–1026.e3

32. Viswanathan V, Smith ER, Mulliken JB, et al. Infantile hemangiomas involving the neuraxis: clinical and imaging findings. *AJNR Am J Neuroradiol*. 2009;30(5):1005–1013

33. von Noorden GK. Application of basic research data to clinical amblyopia. *Ophthalmology*. 1978;85(5):496–504

34. Dubois J, Milot J, Jaeger BI, McCuaig C, Rousseau E, Powell J. Orbit and eyelid hemangiomas: is there a relationship between location and ocular problems? *J Am Acad Dermatol*. 2006;55(4):614–619

35. Frank RC, Cowan BJ, Harrop AR, Astle WF, McPhalen DF. Visual development in infants: visual complications of periocular haemangiomas. *J Plast Reconstr Aesthet Surg*. 2010;63(1):1–8

36. Yan AC. Pain management for ulcerated hemangiomas. *Pediatr Dermatol*. 2008;25(6):586–589

37. Thomas MW, Burkhart CN, Vaghani SP, Morrell DS, Wagner AM. Failure to thrive in infants with complicated facial hemangiomas. *Pediatr Dermatol*. 2012;29(1):49–52

38. Shin HT, Orlow SJ, Chang MW. Ulcerated haemangioma of infancy: a retrospective review of 47 patients. *Br J Dermatol*. 2007;156(5):1050–1052

39. Frieden IJ, Reese V, Cohen D. PHACE syndrome. The association of posterior fossa brain malformations, hemangiomas, arterial anomalies, coarctation of the aorta and cardiac defects, and eye abnormalities. *Arch Dermatol*. 1996;132(3):307–311

40. Püttgen K, Lucky A, Adams D, et al; Hemangioma Investigator Group. Topical timolol maleate treatment of infantile hemangiomas. *Pediatrics*. 2016;138(3):e20160355

41. Jacobs AH. Strawberry hemangiomas; the natural history of the untreated lesion. *Calif Med*. 1957;86(1):8–10

42. Tanner JL, Dechert MP, Frieden IJ. Growing up with a facial hemangioma: parent and child coping and adaptation. *Pediatrics*. 1998;101 (3, pt 1):446–452

43. Fay A, Nguyen J, Waner M. Conceptual approach to the management of infantile hemangiomas. *J Pediatr*. 2010;157(6):881–888.e1–e5

44. O TM, Scheuermann-Poley C, Tan M, Waner M. Distribution, clinical characteristics, and surgical treatment of lip infantile hemangiomas. *JAMA Facial Plast Surg*. 2013;15(4):292–304

45. Ma EH, Robertson SJ, Chow CW, Bekhor PS. Infantile hemangioma with minimal or arrested growth: further observations on clinical and histopathologic findings of this unique but underrecognized entity. *Pediatr Dermatol*. 2017;34(1):64–71

46. Chinnadurai S, Snyder K, Sathe N, et al. *Diagnosis and Management of Infantile Hemangioma*. Rockville, MD: Agency for Healthcare Research and Quality; 2016

47. Menapace D, Mitkov M, Towbin R, Hogeling M. The changing face of complicated infantile hemangioma treatment. *Pediatr Radiol*. 2016;46(11):1494–1506

48. Bessis D, Bigorre M, Labrèze C. Reticular infantile hemangiomas with minimal or arrested growth associated with lipoatrophy. *J Am Acad Dermatol*. 2015;72(5):828–833

49. Dickie B, Dasgupta R, Nair R, et al. Spectrum of hepatic hemangiomas: management and outcome. *J Pediatr Surg*. 2009;44(1):125–133

50. Rotter A, Samorano LP, de Oliveira Labinas GH, et al. Ultrasonography as an objective tool for assessment of infantile hemangioma treatment with propranolol. *Int J Dermatol*. 2017;56(2):190–194

51. Mamlouk MD, Hess CP. Arterial spin-labeled perfusion for vascular anomalies in the pediatric head and neck. *Clin Imaging*. 2016;40(5):1040–1046

52. Aggarwal N, Tekes A, Bosemani T. Infantile hepatic hemangioma: role of dynamic contrast-enhanced magnetic resonance angiography. *J Pediatr*. 2015;167(4):940–940.e1

53. US Food and Drug Administration. FDA drug safety communications: FDA review results in new warnings about using general anesthetics and sedation drugs in young children and pregnant women. 2016. Available at: www.fda.gov/downloads/Drugs/DrugSafety/UCM533197.pdf. Accessed September 10, 2018

54. American Society of Anesthesiologists. ASA response to the FDA med watch warning - December 16, 2016. 2016. Available at: https://www.asahq.org/advocacy-and-asapac/fda-and-washington-alerts/washington-alerts/2016/12/asa-response-to-the-fda-med-watch. Accessed September 10, 2018

55. Practice advisory on anesthetic care for magnetic resonance imaging: an updated report by the American Society of Anesthesiologists Task Force on Anesthetic Care for Magnetic Resonance Imaging. *Anesthesiology*. 2015;122(3):495–520

56. Drolet BA, Chamlin SL, Garzon MC, et al. Prospective study of spinal anomalies in children with infantile hemangiomas of the lumbosacral skin. *J Pediatr*. 2010;157(5):789–794

57. Schumacher WE, Drolet BA, Maheshwari M, et al. Spinal dysraphism associated with the cutaneous lumbosacral infantile hemangioma: a neuroradiological review. *Pediatr Radiol*. 2012;42(3):315–320

58. Yu J, Maheshwari M, Foy AB, Calkins CM, Drolet BA. Neonatal lumbosacral ulceration masking lumbosacral and intraspinal hemangiomas associated with occult spinal dysraphism. *J Pediatr*. 2016;175:211–215

59. Léauté-Labrèze C, Dumas de la Roque E, Hubiche T, Boralevi F, Thambo JB, Taïeb A. Propranolol for severe hemangiomas of infancy. *N Engl J Med*. 2008;358(24):2649–2651

60. Léaute-Labrèze C, Boccara O, Degrugillier-Chopinet C, et al. Safety of oral propranolol for the treatment of infantile hemangioma: a systematic review. *Pediatrics*. 2016;138(4):e20160353

61. Drolet BA, Frommelt PC, Chamlin SL, et al. Initiation and use of propranolol for infantile hemangioma: report of a consensus conference. *Pediatrics*. 2013;131(1):128–140

62. Itinteang T, Withers AH, Davis PF, Tan ST. Biology of infantile hemangioma. *Front Surg*. 2014;1:38

63. Dai Y, Hou F, Buckmiller L, et al. Decreased eNOS protein expression in involuting and propranolol-treated hemangiomas. *Arch Otolaryngol Head Neck Surg*. 2012;138(2):177–182

64. Greenberger S, Bischoff J. Infantile hemangioma-mechanism(s) of drug action on a vascular tumor. *Cold Spring Harb Perspect Med*. 2011;1(1):a006460

65. Storch CH, Hoeger PH. Propranolol for infantile haemangiomas: insights into the molecular mechanisms of action. *Br J Dermatol*. 2010;163(2):269–274

66. Sans V, de la Roque ED, Berge J, et al. Propranolol for severe infantile hemangiomas: follow-up report. *Pediatrics*. 2009;124(3). Available at: www.pediatrics.org/cgi/content/full/124/3/e423

67. Pan WK, Li P, Guo ZT, Huang Q, Gao Y. Propranolol induces regression of hemangioma cells via the down-regulation of the PI3K/Akt/eNOS/VEGF pathway. *Pediatr Blood Cancer*. 2015;62(8):1414–1420

68. Sharifpanah F, Saliu F, Bekhite MM, Wartenberg M, Sauer H. β-adrenergic receptor antagonists inhibit vasculogenesis of embryonic stem cells by downregulation of nitric oxide generation and interference

with VEGF signalling. *Cell Tissue Res.* 2014;358(2):443–452

69. Ji Y, Chen S, Xu C, Li L, Xiang B. The use of propranolol in the treatment of infantile haemangiomas: an update on potential mechanisms of action. *Br J Dermatol.* 2015;172(1):24–32

70. Greene AK, Couto RA. Oral prednisolone for infantile hemangioma: efficacy and safety using a standardized treatment protocol. *Plast Reconstr Surg.* 2011;128(3):743–752

71. Tiwari P, Pandey V, Gangopadhyay AN, Sharma SP, Gupta DK. Role of propranolol in ulcerated haemangioma of head and neck: a prospective comparative study. *Oral Maxillofac Surg.* 2016;20(1):73–77

72. Zaher H, Rasheed H, El-Komy MM, et al. Propranolol versus captopril in the treatment of infantile hemangioma (IH): a randomized controlled trial. *J Am Acad Dermatol.* 2016;74(3):499–505

73. Wu S, Wang B, Chen L, et al. Clinical efficacy of propranolol in the treatment of hemangioma and changes in serum VEGF, bFGF and MMP-9. *Exp Ther Med.* 2015;10(3):1079–1083

74. Aly MM, Hamza AF, Abdel Kader HM, Saafan HA, Ghazy MS, Ragab IA. Therapeutic superiority of combined propranolol with short steroids course over propranolol monotherapy in infantile hemangioma. *Eur J Pediatr.* 2015;174(11):1503–1509

75. Ji Y, Wang Q, Chen S, et al. Oral atenolol therapy for proliferating infantile hemangioma: a prospective study. *Medicine (Baltimore).* 2016;95(24):e3908

76. Léauté-Labrèze C, Hoeger P, Mazereeuw-Hautier J, et al. A randomized, controlled trial of oral propranolol in infantile hemangioma. *N Engl J Med.* 2015;372(8):735–746

77. Siegel DH, Tefft KA, Kelly T, et al. Stroke in children with posterior fossa brain malformations, hemangiomas, arterial anomalies, coarctation of the aorta and cardiac defects, and eye abnormalities (PHACE) syndrome: a systematic review of the literature. *Stroke.* 2012;43(6):1672–1674

78. Breur JM, de Graaf M, Breugem CC, Pasmans SG. Hypoglycemia as a result of propranolol during treatment of infantile hemangioma: a case report. *Pediatr Dermatol.* 2011;28(2):169–171

79. Holland KE, Frieden IJ, Frommelt PC, Mancini AJ, Wyatt D, Drolet BA. Hypoglycemia in children taking propranolol for the treatment of infantile hemangioma. *Arch Dermatol.* 2010;146(7):775–778

80. Prey S, Voisard JJ, Delarue A, et al. Safety of propranolol therapy for severe infantile hemangioma. *JAMA.* 2016;315(4):413–415

81. Techasatian L, Komwilaisak P, Panombualert S, Uppala R, Jetsrisuparb C. Propranolol was effective in treating cutaneous infantile haemangiomas in Thai children. *Acta Paediatr.* 2016;105(6):e257–e262

82. Stringari G, Barbato G, Zanzucchi M, et al. Propranolol treatment for infantile hemangioma: a case series of sixty-two patients. *Pediatr Med Chir.* 2016;38(2):113

83. Sreekantam S, Preece MA, Vijay S, Raiman J, Santra S. How to use a controlled fast to investigate hypoglycaemia. *Arch Dis Child Educ Pract Ed.* 2017;102(1):28–36

84. Cushing SL, Boucek RJ, Manning SC, Sidbury R, Perkins JA. Initial experience with a multidisciplinary strategy for initiation of propranolol therapy for infantile hemangiomas. *Otolaryngol Head Neck Surg.* 2011;144(1):78–84

85. Ng M, Knuth C, Weisbrod C, Murthy A. Propranolol therapy for problematic infantile hemangioma. *Ann Plast Surg.* 2016;76(3):306–310

86. Chang L, Ye X, Qiu Y, et al. Is propranolol safe and effective for outpatient use for infantile hemangioma? A prospective study of 679 cases from one center in China. *Ann Plast Surg.* 2016;76(5):559–563

87. Liu LS, Sokoloff D, Antaya RJ. Twenty-four-hour hospitalization for patients initiating systemic propranolol therapy for infantile hemangiomas—is it indicated? *Pediatr Dermatol.* 2013;30(5):554–560

88. El Ezzi O, Hohlfeld J, de Buys Roessingh A. Propranolol in infantile haemangioma: simplifying pretreatment monitoring. *Swiss Med Wkly.* 2014;144:w13943

89. Tang LY, Hing JW, Tang JY, et al. Predicting complications with pretreatment testing in infantile haemangioma treated with oral propranolol. *Br J Ophthalmol.* 2016;100(7):902–906

90. Ge J, Zheng J, Zhang L, Yuan W, Zhao H. Oral propranolol combined with topical timolol for compound infantile hemangiomas: a retrospective study. *Sci Rep.* 2016;6:19765

91. Raphael MF, Breugem CC, Vlasveld FA, et al. Is cardiovascular evaluation necessary prior to and during beta-blocker therapy for infantile hemangiomas?: a cohort study. *J Am Acad Dermatol.* 2015;72(3):465–472

92. de Graaf M, Breur JMPJ, Raphaël MF, Vos M, Breugem CC, Pasmans SGMA. Adverse effects of propranolol when used in the treatment of hemangiomas: a case series of 28 infants. *J Am Acad Dermatol.* 2011;65(2):320–327

93. Xu DP, Cao RY, Xue L, Sun NN, Tong S, Wang XK. Treatment of severe infantile hemangiomas with propranolol: an evaluation of the efficacy and effects of cardiovascular parameters in 25 consecutive patients. *J Oral Maxillofac Surg.* 2015;73(3):430–436

94. Street JA, Hemsworth BA, Roach AG, Day MD. Tissue levels of several radiolabelled beta-adrenoceptor antagonists after intravenous administration in rats. *Arch Int Pharmacodyn Ther.* 1979;237(2):180–190

95. Feenstra MG. Functional neuroteratology of drugs acting on adrenergic receptors. *Neurotoxicology.* 1992;13(1):55–63

96. Pitzer M, Schmidt MH, Esser G, Laucht M. Child development after maternal tocolysis with beta-sympathomimetic drugs. *Child Psychiatry Hum Dev.* 2001;31(3):165–182

97. Langley A, Pope E. Propranolol and central nervous system function: potential implications for paediatric patients with infantile haemangiomas. *Br J Dermatol.* 2015;172(1):13–23

98. Bryan BA. Reconsidering the use of propranolol in the treatment of cosmetic infantile hemangiomas. *Angiology: Open Access.* 2013;1:e101

99. Phillips RJ, Penington AJ, Bekhor PS, Crock CM. Use of propranolol for treatment of infantile haemangiomas in an outpatient setting. *J Paediatr Child Health.* 2012;48(10):902–906

100. Gonski K, Wargon O. Retrospective follow up of gross motor development in children using propranolol for treatment of infantile haemangioma at Sydney Children's Hospital. *Australas J Dermatol.* 2014;55(3):209–211

101. Moyakine AV, Hermans DJ, Fuijkschot J, van der Vleuten CJ. Propranolol treatment of infantile hemangiomas does not negatively affect psychomotor development. *J Am Acad Dermatol.* 2015;73(2):341–342

102. Moyakine AV, Kerstjens JM, Spillekom-van Koulil S, van der Vleuten CJ. Propranolol treatment of infantile hemangioma (IH) is not associated with developmental risk or growth impairment at age 4 years. *J Am Acad Dermatol.* 2016;75(1):59–63.e1

103. Chinnadurai S, Fonnesbeck C, Snyder KM, et al. Pharmacologic interventions for infantile hemangioma: a meta-analysis. *Pediatrics.* 2016;137(2):e20153896

104. Frieden IJ, Eichenfield LF, Esterly NB, Geronemus R, Mallory SB; American Academy of Dermatology Guidelines Outcomes Committee. Guidelines of care for hemangiomas of infancy. *J Am Acad Dermatol.* 1997;37(4):631–637

105. Sadan N, Wolach B. Treatment of hemangiomas of infants with high doses of prednisone. *J Pediatr.* 1996;128(1):141–146

106. Bennett ML, Fleischer AB Jr, Chamlin SL, Frieden IJ. Oral corticosteroid use is effective for cutaneous hemangiomas: an evidence-based evaluation. *Arch Dermatol.* 2001;137(9):1208–1213

107. Nieuwenhuis K, de Laat PC, Janmohamed SR, Madern GC, Oranje AP. Infantile hemangioma: treatment with short course systemic corticosteroid therapy as an alternative for propranolol. *Pediatr Dermatol.* 2013;30(1):64–70

108. Sloan GM, Reinisch JF, Nichter LS, Saber WL, Lew K, Morwood DT. Intralesional corticosteroid therapy for infantile hemangiomas. *Plast Reconstr Surg.* 1989;83(3):459–467

109. Chowdri NA, Darzi MA, Fazili Z, Iqbal S. Intralesional corticosteroid therapy for childhood cutaneous hemangiomas. *Ann Plast Surg.* 1994;33(1):46–51

110. Chen MT, Yeong EK, Horng SY. Intralesional corticosteroid therapy in proliferating head and neck hemangiomas: a review of 155 cases. *J Pediatr Surg.* 2000;35(3):420–423

111. Buckmiller LM, Francis CL, Glade RS. Intralesional steroid injection for proliferative parotid hemangiomas. *Int J Pediatr Otorhinolaryngol.* 2008;72(1):81–87

112. Prasetyono TO, Djoenaedi I. Efficacy of intralesional steroid injection in head and neck hemangioma: a systematic review. *Ann Plast Surg.* 2011;66(1):98–106

113. Zarem HA, Edgerton MT. Induced resolution of cavernous hemangiomas following prednisolone therapy. *Plast Reconstr Surg.* 1967;39(1):76–83

114. Kushner BJ. The treatment of periorbital infantile hemangioma with intralesional corticosteroid. *Plast Reconstr Surg.* 1985;76(4):517–526

115. Herlihy EP, Kelly JP, Sidbury R, Perkins JA, Weiss AH. Visual acuity and astigmatism in periocular infantile hemangiomas treated with oral beta-blocker versus intralesional corticosteroid injection. *J AAPOS.* 2016;20(1):30–33

116. Goyal R, Watts P, Lane CM, Beck L, Gregory JW. Adrenal suppression and failure to thrive after steroid injections for periocular hemangioma. *Ophthalmology.* 2004;111(2):389–395

117. Weiss AH. Adrenal suppression after corticosteroid injection of periocular hemangiomas. *Am J Ophthalmol.* 1989;107(5):518–522

118. Shorr N, Seiff SR. Central retinal artery occlusion associated with periocular corticosteroid injection for juvenile hemangioma. *Ophthalmic Surg.* 1986;17(4):229–231

119. Ruttum MS, Abrams GW, Harris GJ, Ellis MK. Bilateral retinal embolization associated with intralesional corticosteroid injection for capillary hemangioma of infancy. *J Pediatr Ophthalmol Strabismus.* 1993;30(1):4–7

120. Egbert JE, Schwartz GS, Walsh AW. Diagnosis and treatment of an ophthalmic artery occlusion during an intralesional injection of corticosteroid into an eyelid capillary hemangioma. *Am J Ophthalmol.* 1996;121(6):638–642

121. Egbert JE, Paul S, Engel WK, Summers CG. High injection pressure during intralesional injection of corticosteroids into capillary hemangiomas. *Arch Ophthalmol.* 2001;119(5):677–683

122. Chan H, McKay C, Adams S, Wargon O. RCT of timolol maleate gel for superficial infantile hemangiomas in 5- to 24-week-olds. *Pediatrics.* 2013;131(6). Available at: www.pediatrics.org/cgi/content/full/131/6/e1739

123. Pope E, Chakkittakandiyil A. Topical timolol gel for infantile hemangiomas: a pilot study. *Arch Dermatol.* 2010;146(5):564–565

124. Chakkittakandiyil A, Phillips R, Frieden IJ, et al. Timolol maleate 0.5% or 0.1% gel-forming solution for infantile hemangiomas: a retrospective, multicenter, cohort study. *Pediatr Dermatol.* 2012;29(1):28–31

125. Chambers CB, Katowitz WR, Katowitz JA, Binenbaum G. A controlled study of topical 0.25% timolol maleate gel for the treatment of cutaneous infantile capillary hemangiomas. *Ophthal Plast Reconstr Surg.* 2012;28(2):103–106

126. Frommelt P, Juern A, Siegel D, et al. Adverse events in young and preterm infants receiving topical timolol for infantile hemangioma. *Pediatr Dermatol.* 2016;33(4):405–414

127. McMahon P, Oza V, Frieden IJ. Topical timolol for infantile hemangiomas: putting a note of caution in "cautiously optimistic". *Pediatr Dermatol.* 2012;29(1):127–130

128. Coppens G, Stalmans I, Zeyen T, Casteels I. The safety and efficacy of glaucoma medication in the pediatric

population. *J Pediatr Ophthalmol Strabismus*. 2009;46(1):12–18

129. Guo S, Ni N. Topical treatment for capillary hemangioma of the eyelid using beta-blocker solution. *Arch Ophthalmol*. 2010;128(2):255–256

130. Ni N, Langer P, Wagner R, Guo S. Topical timolol for periocular hemangioma: report of further study. *Arch Ophthalmol*. 2011;129(3):377–379

131. Moehrle M, Léauté-Labrèze C, Schmidt V, Röcken M, Poets CF, Goelz R. Topical timolol for small hemangiomas of infancy. *Pediatr Dermatol*. 2013;30(2):245–249

132. Yu L, Li S, Su B, et al. Treatment of superficial infantile hemangiomas with timolol: evaluation of short-term efficacy and safety in infants. *Exp Ther Med*. 2013;6(2):388–390

133. Danarti R, Ariwibowo L, Radiono S, Budiyanto A. Topical timolol maleate 0.5% for infantile hemangioma: its effectiveness compared to ultrapotent topical corticosteroids - a single-center experience of 278 cases. *Dermatology*. 2016;232(5):566–571

134. Oranje AP, Janmohamed SR, Madern GC, de Laat PC. Treatment of small superficial haemangioma with timolol 0.5% ophthalmic solution: a series of 20 cases. *Dermatology*. 2011;223(4):330–334

135. Gomulka J, Siegel DH, Drolet BA. Dramatic shift in the infantile hemangioma treatment paradigm at a single institution. *Pediatr Dermatol*. 2013;30(6):751–752

136. Weibel L, Barysch MJ, Scheer HS, et al. Topical timolol for infantile hemangiomas: evidence for efficacy and degree of systemic absorption. *Pediatr Dermatol*. 2016;33(2):184–190

137. Olson RJ, Bromberg BB, Zimmerman TJ. Apneic spells associated with timolol therapy in a neonate. *Am J Ophthalmol*. 1979;88(1):120–122

138. Burnstine RA, Felton JL, Ginther WH. Cardiorespiratory reaction to timolol maleate in a pediatric patient: a case report. *Ann Ophthalmol*. 1982;14(10):905–906

139. Kiryazov K, Stefova M, Iotova V. Can ophthalmic drops cause central nervous system depression and cardiogenic shock in infants? *Pediatr Emerg Care*. 2013; 29(11):1207–1209

140. Semkova K, Kazandjieva J. Topical timolol maleate for treatment of infantile haemangiomas: preliminary results of a prospective study. *Clin Exp Dermatol*. 2013;38(2):143–146

141. Boos MD, Castelo-Soccio L. Experience with topical timolol maleate for the treatment of ulcerated infantile hemangiomas (IH). *J Am Acad Dermatol*. 2016;74(3):567–570

142. Greene AK. Management of hemangiomas and other vascular tumors. *Clin Plast Surg*. 2011;38(1):45–63

143. Couto RA, Maclellan RA, Zurakowski D, Greene AK. Infantile hemangioma: clinical assessment of the involuting phase and implications for management. *Plast Reconstr Surg*. 2012;130(3):619–624

144. Batta K, Goodyear HM, Moss C, Williams HC, Hiller L, Waters R. Randomised controlled study of early pulsed dye laser treatment of uncomplicated childhood haemangiomas: results of a 1-year analysis. *Lancet*. 2002;360(9332):521–527

145. Mulliken JB, Fishman SJ, Burrows PE. Vascular anomalies. *Curr Probl Surg*. 2000;37(8):517–584

146. Charlesworth R. The toddler: affective development. In: *Understanding Child Development*. 6th ed. Delmar Learning; 1994:304

147. Santrock JW. The self and identity. In: *Child Development*. 7th ed. McGraw-Hill; 1996:378–385

148. Neisser U. Memory development: new questions and old. *Dev Rev*. 2004;24(1):154–158

149. Bowers RE, Graham EA, Tomlinson KM. The natural history of the strawberry nevus. *Arch Dermatol*. 1960;82(5):667–680

150. Laubach HJ, Anderson RR, Luger T, Manstein D. Fractional photothermolysis for involuted infantile hemangioma. *Arch Dermatol*. 2009;145(7):748–750

151. Witman PM, Wagner AM, Scherer K, Waner M, Frieden IJ. Complications following pulsed dye laser treatment of superficial hemangiomas. *Lasers Surg Med*. 2006;38(2):116–123

152. Scheepers JH, Quaba AA. Does the pulsed tunable dye laser have a role in the management of infantile hemangiomas? Observations based on 3 years' experience. *Plast Reconstr Surg*. 1995;95(2):305–312

153. Kessels JP, Hamers ET, Ostertag JU. Superficial hemangioma: pulsed dye laser versus wait-and-see. *Dermatol Surg*. 2013;39(3, pt 1):414–421

154. Liu LS, Sowa A, Antaya RJ. Educating caregivers about the natural history of infantile hemangiomas. *Acta Paediatr*. 2015;104(1):9–11

155. Zweegers J, van der Vleuten CJ. The psychosocial impact of an infantile haemangioma on children and their parents. *Arch Dis Child*. 2012;97(10):922–926

156. Minzer-Conzetti K, Garzon MC, Haggstrom AN, et al. Information about infantile hemangiomas on the Internet: how accurate is it? *J Am Acad Dermatol*. 2007;57(6):998–1004

157. Takahashi K, Mulliken JB, Kozakewich HP, Rogers RA, Folkman J, Ezekowitz RA. Cellular markers that distinguish the phases of hemangioma during infancy and childhood. *J Clin Invest*. 1994;93(6):2357–2364

158. Agency for Healthcare Research and Quality. Treating infantile hemangiomas in children. Available at: https://effectivehealthcare.ahrq. gov/topics/infantile-hemangioma/ consumer. Accessed November 27, 2018

159. Bernabeu-Wittel J, Pereyra J, Corb R, Ruiz-Canela J, Tarilonte A M, Conejo-Mir J. Teledermatology for infantile hemangiomas. Comment on: Chang LC, Haggstrom AN, Drolet BA, et al for the Hemangioma Investigator Group. Growth characteristics of infantile hemangiomas: implications for management. Pediatrics. 2008;122:360-367. Available at: http://pediatrics. aappublications.org/content/122/2/ 360.comments

160. Martin K, Blei F, Chamlin SL, et al. Propranolol treatment of infantile hemangiomas: anticipatory guidance for parents and caretakers [published correction appears in *Pediatr*

Dermatol. 2013;30(2):280]. *Pediatr Dermatol.* 2013;30(1):155–159

161. Munden A, Butschek R, Tom WL, et al. Prospective study of infantile haemangiomas: incidence, clinical characteristics and association with placental anomalies. *Br J Dermatol.* 2014;170(4):907–913

162. Moyakine AV, Herwegen B, van der Vleuten CJM. Use of the Hemangioma Severity Scale to facilitate treatment decisions for infantile hemangiomas. *J Am Acad Dermatol.* 2017;77(5): 868–873

163. Mull JL, Chamlin SL, Lai JS, et al. Utility of the Hemangioma Severity Scale as

a triage tool and predictor of need for treatment. *Pediatr Dermatol.* 2017;34(1):78–83

164. Haggstrom AN, Beaumont JL, Lai JS, et al. Measuring the severity of infantile hemangiomas: instrument development and reliability. *Arch Dermatol.* 2012;148(2):197–202

Infantile Hemangiomas Clinical Practice Guideline Quick Reference Tools

- Action Statement Summary
  — Clinical Practice Guideline for the Management of Infantile Hemangiomas
- *ICD-10-CM* Coding Quick Reference for Infantile Hemangiomas

Action Statement Summary

Key Action Statement 1

Risk stratification

Key Action Statement 1A

Clinicians should classify an IH as high risk if there is evidence of or potential for the following: (1) life-threatening complications, (2) functional impairment or ulceration, (3) structural anomalies (eg, in PHACE syndrome or LUMBAR syndrome), or (4) permanent disfigurement (grade X, strong recommendation).

Key Action Statement 1B

After identifying an IH as high risk, clinicians should facilitate an evaluation by a hemangioma specialist as soon as possible (grade X, strong recommendation).

Key Action Statement 2

Imaging

Key Action Statement 2A

Clinicians should not perform imaging unless the diagnosis of IH is uncertain, there are 5 or more cutaneous IHs, or associated anatomic abnormalities are suspected (grade B, moderate recommendation).

Key Action Statement 2B

Clinicians should perform ultrasonography as the initial imaging modality when the diagnosis of IH is uncertain (grade C, weak recommendation).

Key Action Statement 2C

Clinicians should perform MRI when concerned about associated structural abnormalities (eg, PHACE syndrome or LUMBAR syndrome) (grade B, moderate recommendation).

Key Action Statement 3

Pharmacotherapy

Key Action Statement 3A

Clinicians should use oral propranolol as the first-line agent for IHs requiring systemic treatment (grade A, strong recommendation).

Key Action Statement 3B

Clinicians should dose propranolol between 2 and 3 mg/kg per day unless there are comorbidities (eg, PHACE syndrome) or adverse effects (eg, sleep disturbance) that necessitate a lower dose (grade A, moderate recommendation).

Key Action Statement 3C

Clinicians should counsel that propranolol be administered with or after feeding and that doses be held at times of diminished oral intake or vomiting to reduce the risk of hypoglycemia (grade X, strong recommendation).

Key Action Statement 3D

Clinicians should evaluate patients for and educate caregivers about potential adverse effects of propranolol, including sleep disturbances, bronchial irritation, and clinically symptomatic bradycardia and hypotension (grade X, strong recommendation).

Key Action Statement 3E

Clinicians may prescribe oral prednisolone or prednisone to treat IHs if there are contraindications or an inadequate response to oral propranolol (grade B, moderate recommendation).

Key Action Statement 3F

Clinicians may recommend intralesional injection of triamcinolone and/or betamethasone to treat focal, bulky IHs during proliferation or in certain critical anatomic locations (eg, the lip) (grade B, moderate recommendation).

Key Action Statement 3G

Clinicians may prescribe topical timolol maleate as a therapy for thin and/or superficial IHs (grade B, moderate recommendation).

Key Action Statement 4

Clinicians may recommend surgery and laser therapy as treatment options in managing selected IHs (grade C, moderate recommendation).

Key Action Statement 5

Clinicians should educate parents of infants with an IH about the condition, including the expected natural history, and its potential for causing complications or disfigurement (grade X, strong recommendation).

Coding Quick Reference for Infantile Hemangiomas
ICD-10-CM
D18.00 Hemangioma unspecified site
D18.01 Hemangioma of skin and subcutaneous tissue
D18.02 Hemangioma of intracranial structures
D18.03 Hemangioma of intra-abdominal structures
D18.09 Hemangioma of other sites

Clinical Practice Guideline: Maintenance Intravenous Fluids in Children

- *Clinical Practice Guideline*

CLINICAL PRACTICE GUIDELINE Guidance for the Clinician in Rendering Pediatric Care

American Academy
of Pediatrics

DEDICATED TO THE HEALTH OF ALL CHILDREN™

Clinical Practice Guideline: Maintenance Intravenous Fluids in Children

Leonard G. Feld, MD, PhD, MMM, FAAP,[a] Daniel R. Neuspiel, MD, MPH, FAAP,[b] Byron A. Foster, MD, MPH, FAAP,[c] Michael G. Leu, MD, MS, MHS, FAAP,[d] Matthew D. Garber, MD, FHM, FAAP,[e] Kelly Austin, MD, MS, FAAP, FACS,[f] Rajit K. Basu, MD, MS, FCCM,[g,h] Edward E. Conway Jr, MD, MS, FAAP,[i] James J. Fehr, MD, FAAP,[j] Clare Hawkins, MD,[k] Ron L. Kaplan, MD, FAAP,[l] Echo V. Rowe, MD, FAAP,[m] Muhammad Waseem, MD, MS, FAAP, FACEP,[n] Michael L. Moritz, MD, FAAP,[o] SUBCOMMITTEE ON FLUID AND ELECTROLYTE THERAPY

abstract

Maintenance intravenous fluids (IVFs) are used to provide critical supportive care for children who are acutely ill. IVFs are required if sufficient fluids cannot be provided by using enteral administration for reasons such as gastrointestinal illness, respiratory compromise, neurologic impairment, a perioperative state, or being moribund from an acute or chronic illness. Despite the common use of maintenance IVFs, there is high variability in fluid prescribing practices and a lack of guidelines for fluid composition administration and electrolyte monitoring. The administration of hypotonic IVFs has been the standard in pediatrics. Concerns have been raised that this approach results in a high incidence of hyponatremia and that isotonic IVFs could prevent the development of hyponatremia. Our goal in this guideline is to provide an evidence-based approach for choosing the tonicity of maintenance IVFs in most patients from 28 days to 18 years of age who require maintenance IVFs. This guideline applies to children in surgical (postoperative) and medical acute-care settings, including critical care and the general inpatient ward. Patients with neurosurgical disorders, congenital or acquired cardiac disease, hepatic disease, cancer, renal dysfunction, diabetes insipidus, voluminous watery diarrhea, or severe burns; neonates who are younger than 28 days old or in the NICU; and adolescents older than 18 years old are excluded. We specifically address the tonicity of maintenance IVFs in children.

The Key Action Statement of the subcommittee is as follows:

1A: The American Academy of Pediatrics recommends that patients 28 days to 18 years of age requiring maintenance IVFs should receive isotonic solutions with appropriate potassium chloride and dextrose because they significantly decrease the risk of developing hyponatremia (evidence quality: A; recommendation strength: strong)

[a]Retired, Nicklaus Children's Health System, Miami, Florida; [b]Retired, Levine Children's Hospital, Charlotte, North Carolina; [c]Oregon Health and Science University, Portland, Oregon; [d]Department of Pediatric Emergency Medicine, [d]School of Medicine, University of Washington and Seattle Children's Hospital, Seattle, Washington; [e]Department of Pediatrics, College of Medicine – Jacksonville, University of Florida, Jacksonville, Florida; Departments of [f]Surgery and [o]Pediatrics, University of Pittsburgh School of Medicine, Children's Hospital of Pittsburgh, Pittsburgh, Pennsylvania; [g]Division of Critical Care Medicine, Children's Healthcare of Atlanta, Atlanta, Georgia; [h]Department of Pediatrics, School of Medicine, Emory University, Atlanta, Georgia; [i]Division of Pediatric Critical Care Medicine, Department of Pediatrics, Jacobi Medical Center, Bronx, New York; Departments of [j]Anesthesiology and Pediatrics, Washington University in St Louis, St Louis, Missouri; [k]Department of Family Medicine, Houston Methodist Hospital, Houston, Texas; [m]Department of Anesthesia, Stanford University School of Medicine, Stanford, California; and [n]Lincoln Medical Center, Bronx, New York

This document is copyrighted and is property of the American Academy of Pediatrics and its Board of Directors. All authors have filed conflict of interest statements with the American Academy of Pediatrics. Any conflicts have been resolved through a process approved by the Board of Directors. The American Academy of Pediatrics has neither solicited nor accepted any commercial involvement in the development of the content of this publication.

The guidance in this report does not indicate an exclusive course of treatment or serve as a standard of medical care. Variations, taking into account individual circumstances, may be appropriate.

To cite: Feld LG, Neuspiel DR, Foster BA, et al. Clinical Practice Guideline: Maintenance Intravenous Fluids in Children. *Pediatrics.* 2018;142(6):e20183083

INTRODUCTION

Maintenance intravenous fluids (IVFs) are used to provide critical supportive care for children who are acutely ill. IVFs are required if sufficient fluids cannot be provided by using enteral administration for reasons such as gastrointestinal illness, respiratory compromise, neurologic impairment, a perioperative state, or being moribund from an acute or chronic illness. For the purposes of this document, specifying appropriate maintenance IVFs includes the composition of IVF needed to preserve a child's extracellular volume while simultaneously minimizing the risk of developing volume depletion, fluid overload, or electrolyte disturbances, such as hyponatremia or hypernatremia. Because maintenance IVFs may have both potential benefits and harms, they should only be administered when clinically indicated. The administration of hypotonic IVF has been the standard in pediatrics. Concerns have been raised that this approach results in a high incidence of hyponatremia and that isotonic IVF could prevent the development of hyponatremia. Guidelines for maintenance IVF therapy in children have primarily been opinion based, and evidence-based consensus guidelines are lacking.

OBJECTIVE

Despite the common use of maintenance IVFs, there is high variability in fluid prescribing practices and a lack of guidelines for fluid composition and electrolyte monitoring.[1–4] Our goal in this guideline is to provide an evidence-based approach for choosing the tonicity of maintenance IVFs in most patients from 28 days to 18 years of age who require maintenance IVFs. These recommendations do not apply to patients with neurosurgical disorders, congenital or acquired cardiac disease, hepatic disease, cancer, renal dysfunction, diabetes insipidus, voluminous watery diarrhea, or severe burns; neonates who are younger than 28 days old or in the NICU; or adolescents older than 18 years old.

BACKGROUND

Phases of Fluid Therapy

Recent literature has emerged in which researchers describe the context-dependent use of IVFs, which should be prescribed, ordered, dosed, and delivered like any other drug.[5–7] Four distinct physiology-driven time periods exist for children requiring IVFs. The resuscitative phase is the acute presentation window, when IVFs are needed to restore adequate tissue perfusion and prevent or mitigate end-organ injury. The titration phase is the time when IVFs are transitioned from boluses to maintenance; this is a critical window to determine what intravascular repletion has been achieved and the trajectory of fluid gains versus losses in children who are acutely ill. The maintenance phase accounts for fluids administered during the previous 2 stabilization phases and is a time when fluids should be supplied to achieve a precise homeostatic balance between needs and losses. Finally, the convalescent phase reflects the period when exogenous fluid administration is stopped, and the patient returns to intrinsic fluid regulation. The dose of fluid during these 4 phases of fluid therapy needs to be adjusted on the basis of the unique physiologic needs of each patient, and a specific protocoled dose is not able to be applied to all patients.[8,9]

A variety of IVFs are commercially available for use in infants and children. These solutions principally vary by their specific electrolyte composition, the addition of a buffer, and whether they contain glucose (Table 1).[10]

The buffer in plasma is bicarbonate, but buffers in commercially available solutions include various concentrations of lactate, acetate, and gluconate. Multiple balanced salt solutions can be compared with normal saline (0.9% saline), which has the same sodium concentration as plasma but has a supraphysiologic chloride concentration.

Effect of Dextrose on Tonicity

Tonicity is used to describe the net vector of force on cells relative to a semipermeable membrane when in solution. Physiologic relevance occurs with tonicity studied in vivo (eg, as IVF is infused intravascularly). Infused isotonic fluids do not result in osmotic shifts; the cells stay the same size. Cellular expansion occurs during immersion in hypotonic fluids as free water, in higher relative abundance in the extracellular environment, and crosses the semipermeable membrane. The converse happens in hypertonic fluid immersion: free water shifts out of the cells, leading to cellular contraction. A distinct but related concept is the concept of osmolality. Osmolality is measured as osmoles of solute per kilogram of solvent. Serum osmolality can be estimated by the following formula:

$$2 \times Na(mEq/L) + BUN(mg/dL)/2.8 + glucose(mg/dL)/18$$

Osmolality is distinct from tonicity (effective osmolality) in that tonicity relates to both the effect on a cell of a fluid (dependent on the selective permeability of the membrane) and the osmolality of the fluid. In the plasma, urea affects osmolality but not tonicity because urea moves freely across cell membranes with no effect on tonicity. The tonicity of IVF is primarily affected by the sodium and potassium concentration.

Dextrose (D-glucose) can be added to IVFs (Table 1). Although dextrose affects the osmolarity of IVFs, it is not a significant contributor to the plasma osmotic pressure or tonicity

TABLE 1 Composition of Commonly Used Maintenance IVFs

Fluid	Glucose, g/dL	Sodium	Chloride	Potassium, mEq/L	Calcium	Magnesium	Buffer	Osmolarity,[a] mOsm/L
Human plasma	0.07–0.11	135–145	95–105	3.5–5.3	4.4–5.2	1.6–2.4	23–30 bicarbonate	308[b]
Hypotonic solutions								
D_5 0.2% NaCl	5	34	34	0	0	0	0	78
D_5 0.45% NaCl	5	77	77	0	0	0	0	154
Isotonic and/or near-isotonic solutions								
D_5 0.9% NaCl	5	154	154	0	0	0	0	308
D_5 lactated Ringer	5	130	109	4	3	0	28 lactate	273
PlasmaLyte[c,d]	0	140	98	5	0	3	27 acetate and 23 gluconate	294

[a] The osmolarity calculation excludes the dextrose in the solution because dextrose is rapidly metabolized on infusion.

[b] The osmolality for plasma is 275–295 mOsm/kg.

[c] Multiple electrolytes injection, type 1 *United States Pharmacopeia*, is the generic name for PlasmaLyte.

[d] PlasmaLyte with 5% dextrose is not available in the United States from Baxter Healthcare Corporation in Deerfield, Illinois.

in the absence of uncontrolled diabetes because it is rapidly metabolized after entering the blood stream. Thus, although dextrose will affect the osmolarity of solutions, for patients in whom maintenance IVFs are needed, the dextrose component generally is not believed to affect the tonicity of solutions.

Historical Maintenance IVF Practice and Hyponatremia

Hyponatremia (serum sodium concentration <135 mEq/L) is the most common electrolyte abnormality in patients who are hospitalized, affecting approximately 15% to 30% of children and adults.[11, 12] Patients who are acutely ill frequently have disease states associated with arginine vasopressin (AVP) excess that can impair free-water excretion and place the patient at risk for developing hyponatremia when a source of electrolyte-free water is supplied, as in hypotonic fluids.[10] Nonosmotic stimuli of AVP release include pain, nausea, stress, a postoperative state, hypovolemia, medications, and pulmonary and central nervous system (CNS) disorders, including common childhood conditions such as pneumonia and meningitis.[13–15] These conditions can lead to the syndrome of inappropriate antidiuresis (SIAD) or SIAD-like

states, which lead to water retention followed by a physiologic natriuresis in which fluid balance is maintained at the expense of plasma sodium.

Children have historically been administered hypotonic maintenance IVFs.[3,4] This practice is based on theoretical calculations from the 1950s.[16] The water requirement was based on the energy expenditure of healthy children, with 1 mL of fluid provided for each kilocalorie (kcal) expended, or 1500 mL/m² per day. The resting energy expenditure in healthy children is vastly different in those with an acute disease and/or illness or after surgery. When using calorimetric methods, energy expenditure in these patients is closer to the basal metabolic rate proposed by Talbot,[17] which averages 50 to 60 kcal/kg per day.[18] The electrolyte concentration of IVFs was estimated to reflect the composition of human and cow milk. The final composition consisted of 3 mEq of sodium and 2 mEq of potassium per 100 kcal metabolized.[16]

Most hyponatremia in patients who are hospitalized is hospital acquired and related to the administration of hypotonic IVFs in the setting of elevated AVP concentrations.[10,11] Studies in which researchers evaluated hospital-acquired hyponatremia have revealed a

relationship with the administration of hypotonic IVFs.[11,19,20] The most serious complication of hospital-acquired hyponatremia is hyponatremic encephalopathy, which is a medical emergency that can be fatal or lead to irreversible brain injury if inadequately treated.[21–24] The reports of hospital-acquired hyponatremic encephalopathy have occurred primarily in otherwise healthy children who were receiving hypotonic IVFs, in many cases after minor surgical procedures.[21,23] Patients with hospital-acquired hyponatremia are at particular risk for hyponatremic encephalopathy, which usually develops acutely in less than 48 hours, leaving little time for the brain to adapt. Children are at particularly high risk of developing symptomatic hyponatremia because of their larger brain/skull size ratio.[24] Symptoms of hyponatremia can be nonspecific, including fussiness, headache, nausea, vomiting, confusion, lethargy, and muscle cramps, making prompt diagnosis difficult.

After reports of severe hyponatremia and associated neurologic injury were reported in 1992, a significant debate emerged regarding the appropriateness of administering hypotonic maintenance IVFs to children.[21] In 2003, it was recommended that isotonic fluids be administered to children who are acutely ill and require maintenance IVFs to prevent the development of hyponatremia.[24] Since then, the Institute for Safe Medical Practices of both the United States[25] and Canada[26] released reports on deaths from severe hyponatremia in patients who were hospitalized and received hypotonic IVFs. The United Kingdom released a national safety alert reporting 4 deaths and 1 near miss from hospital-acquired hyponatremia,[27] and 50 cases of serious injury or child death from hypotonic IVFs were reported in the international literature.[22]

After the recognition of hospital-acquired hyponatremia in patients receiving hypotonic IVFs and recommendations for avoiding them,[24] the use of 0.2% saline has declined with an increase in the use of 0.45% and 0.9% saline.[3,28] There have been concerns raised about the safety of the proposed use of isotonic maintenance IVFs in children who are acutely ill for the prevention of hospital-acquired hyponatremia.[18] Some believe that this approach could lead to complications such as hypernatremia, fluid overload with edema and hypertension, and hyperchloremic acidosis.[29] In the past 15 years, there have been a multitude of clinical trials and systematic reviews in which researchers have attempted to address this debate.[30–35] Authors of textbooks and review articles in the United States continue to recommend hypotonic fluids.[36–38] Conversely, the National Clinical Guideline Centre in the United Kingdom published evidence-based guidelines for IVF therapy in children younger than 16 years old and recommended isotonic IVFs.[34]

METHODS

In April 2016, the American Academy of Pediatrics (AAP) convened a multidisciplinary subcommittee composed of primary care clinicians and experts in the fields of general pediatrics, hospital medicine, emergency medicine, critical care medicine, nephrology, anesthesiology, surgery, and quality improvement. The subcommittee also included a guideline methodologist and/or informatician and an epidemiologist who were skilled in systematic reviews. All panel members declared potential conflicts on the basis of the AAP policy on conflicts of interest and voluntary disclosure. Subcommittee members repeated this process annually and on publication of the guideline. All potential conflicts of interest are listed at the end of this document. The project was funded by the AAP.

The subcommittee initiated its literature review by combining the search strategies in 7 recent systematic reviews of clinical trials of maintenance IVFs in children and adolescents, which consisted of 11 clinical trials involving 1139 patients.[9,33,34,39–42] The subcommittee then used this combined search strategy to discover 7 additional clinical trials of maintenance IVFs involving 1316 children and adolescents (ages 28 days to 18 years) published since 2013 (the last year included in the previous 6 systematic reviews) in the PubMed, Cumulative Index to Nursing and Allied Health Literature, and Cochrane Library databases. All articles that were initially identified were back searched for other relevant publications. Studies published as of March 15, 2016, were included. Three independent reviewers from the subcommittee then critically appraised the full text of each identified article ($n = 17$) using a structured data collection form that was based on published guidelines for evaluating medical literature.[43,44] These reviews were integrated into an evidence table by the subcommittee epidemiologist (Supplemental Table 3). Forest plots for all included randomized controlled trials (RCTs) in which researchers used random-effects models and Mantel-Haenzel (M-H) statistics with the outcome of hyponatremia are shown in Supplemental Figs 2–4.

To appraise the methodology of the included studies, a risk-of-bias assessment was completed by using the *Cochrane Handbook* risk of bias assessment framework.[45] Using this framework, raters placed a value of low, high, or unclear risk of bias for each article in the areas of selection bias (both random-sequence generation and allocation concealment), performance bias, detection bias, attrition bias, and reporting bias. Two authors independently reviewed each study identified in the systematic review and made an independent judgment. Differences in assessment were resolved via discussion.

The resulting systematic review was used to develop the guideline recommendations by following the Policy Statement from the AAP Steering Committee on Quality Improvement and Management, "Classifying Recommendations for Clinical Practice Guidelines."[46] Decisions and the strength of recommendations were based on a systematic grading of the quality of evidence from the updated literature review by the subcommittee with guidance by the epidemiologist. Expert consensus was used when definitive data were not available. If committee members disagreed with the consensus, they were encouraged to voice their concerns until full agreement was reached. Full agreement was reached on the clinical recommendations below.

Clinical recommendations were entered into Bridge-Wiz 2.1 for AAP software (Building Recommendations in a Developers Guideline Editor), an interactive software tool that is used to lead guideline development

TABLE 2 Key Action Statement 1A

Aggregate Evidence Quality	Grade A
Benefits	More physiologic fluid, less hyponatremia
Risks, harm, cost	Potential harms of hypernatremia, fluid overload, hypertension, hyperchloremic metabolic acidosis, and acute kidney injury have not been found to be of increased risk with isotonic maintenance fluids.
Benefit-harm assessment	Decreased risk of hyponatremia
Intentional vagueness	None
Role of patient preferences	None
Exclusions	Patients with neurosurgical disorders, congenital or acquired cardiac disease, hepatic disease, cancer, renal dysfunction, diabetes insipidus, voluminous watery diarrhea, or severe burns; neonates who are <28 d old or in the NICU; or adolescents >18 y old
Strength	Strong recommendation
Key references	9,33,39–42

teams through a series of questions that are intended to create clear, transparent, and actionable Key Action Statements.[47] The committee was actively involved while the software was used and solicited the inputs of this program, which included strength of evidence and balance of benefits versus harms, and chose which sentences recommended by the program to use as part of the guideline. Bridge-Wiz also integrates the quality of available evidence and a benefit-harm assessment into the final determination of the strength of each recommendation per the guidance in Fig 1.

Before formal approval by the AAP, this guideline underwent a comprehensive review by stakeholders, including AAP councils, committees, and sections; selected outside stakeholder organizations; and individuals who were identified by the subcommittee as experts in the field. All comments were reviewed by the subcommittee and incorporated into the final guideline when appropriate.

On the basis of the reviewed literature, this guideline applies to children 28 days to 18 years of age in surgical (postoperative) and medical acute-care settings, including critical care and the general inpatient ward. This guideline DOES NOT apply to children with neurosurgical disorders, congenital or acquired cardiac disease, hepatic disease, cancer, renal dysfunction, diabetes insipidus, voluminous watery diarrhea, or severe burns; neonates who are younger than 28 days old or in the NICU; or adolescents older than 18 years old because the majority of the researchers in the prospective studies reviewed in this guideline excluded these subsets of patients or did not include patients with these specific high-risk diagnoses.

RESULTS

Key Action Statement

The Key Action Statement is as follows:

1. Composition of Maintenance IVFs

1A: The AAP recommends that patients 28 days to 18 years of age requiring maintenance IVFs should receive isotonic solutions with appropriate potassium chloride (KCl) and dextrose because they significantly decrease the risk of developing hyponatremia (evidence quality: A; recommendation strength: strong; Table 2).

FIGURE 1
AAP rating of evidence and recommendations.

Aggregate Evidence Quality | Benefit or Harm Predominates | Benefit and Harm Balanced

Level A
Intervention: well designed and conducted trials, meta-analyses on applicable populations
Diagnosis: independent gold standard studies of applicable populations

Level B
Trials or diagnostic studies within minor limitations; consistent findings in from multiple observational studies

Level C
Single or few observational studies or multiple studies with inconsistent findings or major limitations

Level D
Expert opinion, case reports, reasoning from first principles

Strong recommendation
Moderate recommendation
Weak recommendation (based on low quality evidence)
Weak recommendation (based on balance of benefit and harm)
No recommendation may be made

Level X
Exceptional situations in which validating studies cannot be performed, and there is a clear preponderance of benefit or harm

Strong recommendation
Moderate recommendation

Isotonic Solutions Versus Hypotonic Solutions

Isotonic fluid has a sodium concentration similar to plasma (135–144 mEq/L). Plasma is approximately 93% aqueous and 7% anhydrous with a sodium concentration in the aqueous phase of plasma of 154 mEq/L and osmolarity of 308 mOsm/L, similar to that of 0.9% sodium chloride (NaCl). Conversely, hypotonic fluid has a sodium concentration lower than that of the aqueous phase of plasma. In the studies evaluated in the formulation of these guidelines, there is some heterogeneity in both the isotonic and hypotonic fluids used. The sodium concentration of isotonic fluids ranged from 131 to 154 mEq/L. Hartmann solution (sodium concentration 131 mEq/L; osmolality 279 mOsm/L) was used in only 46 patients.[48,49] PlasmaLyte (sodium concentration 140 mEq/L; osmolarity 294 mOsm/L) was used in 346 patients.[35] Researchers in the majority of the studies used either 0.9% NaCl (sodium concentration 154 mEq/L; osmolarity 308 mOsm/L) or a fluid of equivalent tonicity. Hypotonic fluids ranged from 30 to 100 mEq/L.[33] Lactated Ringer solution (sodium concentration 130 mEq/L; osmolarity 273 mOsm/L), a slightly hypotonic solution, was not involved in any of the clinical trials. For the purposes of this guideline, isotonic solutions have a sodium concentration similar to PlasmaLyte, or 0.9% NaCl. Recommendations are not made regarding the safety of lactated Ringer solution. Researchers in the majority of studies added dextrose (2.5%–5%) to the intravenous (IV) solution.

The search revealed 17 randomized clinical trials[20,31,32,35,48–60] that met the search criteria, including a total 2455 patients (2313 patients had primary outcome data for analysis in Supplemental Figs 2–4), to help evaluate the question of whether isotonic or hypotonic fluids should be used in children who are hospitalized. Sixteen of the studies revealed that isotonic fluids were superior to hypotonic fluids in preventing hyponatremia. There have also been 7 systematic reviews over the past 11 years in which researchers have synthesized various combinations of the above RCTs.[9,33,34,39–42] The number needed to treat with isotonic fluids to prevent hyponatremia (sodium <135 mEq/L) was 7.5 across all included studies and 27.8 for moderate hyponatremia (sodium <130 mEq/L).

Study appraisal for risk of bias (Supplemental Table 4) revealed the reviewed studies in total to be methodologically sound. Most types of bias were found to be of low risk in all but 2 studies. There was 1 study with 2 bias types of potentially high risk and 11 studies with 1 or more unclear bias areas.

Inclusion and Exclusion Criteria: Rationale for Specific Subgroups

Age

The specific age groups from which data are available from randomized clinical trials range from 1 day (1 trial) to 18 years. Given this broad age range, we specifically evaluated whether there was variability in the outcomes by age, particularly for the lower age range. McNab et al[33] examined this question in their systematic review and found 100 children studied at younger than 1 year of age, 243 children studied between the ages of 1 and 5 years, and 465 children studied at older than 5 years of age. They showed a significant benefit of isotonic IVFs in each age group stratum. There have been 7 additional studies in which researchers have also included children younger than 1 year old, although there are not specific outcome data reported for this age group.[31,32,35,50,51,55,58]

Surgical (Postoperative Patients)

Surgical or postoperative patients have been specifically studied in 7 studies[20,48,49,51,54,56,57] that included 529 patients. McNab[30] showed a pooled risk ratio of 0.48 (95% confidence interval [CI], 0.38–0.60) for the outcome of hyponatremia in favor of isotonic fluids.

Medical (Nonsurgical Patients)

Medical patients are defined here as children who are hospitalized in an acute-care setting with no indication for a surgical operation and no immediate history of a surgical operation. For these patients, there are 4 randomized clinical trials[32,52,55,58] in which researchers enrolled only medical patients and 6 randomized clinical trials[50,51,53,56,57,59] in which researchers enrolled both medical and surgical patients. Some of the mixed studies in which researchers looked at both medical and surgical patients include outcomes for only medical patients, whereas most include combined outcomes for both groups.

Varying Acuity (ICU Versus General Ward)

There are 6 randomized clinical trials[31,49,50,53,56,59] in which researchers enrolled only ICU patients, and all but one[50] revealed a significant difference favoring isotonic IVFs for the prevention of hyponatremia. Researchers in 8 randomized clinical trials enrolled exclusively patients in a general ward setting,[32,51,52,54,55,57,58,60] and those in all but 2[32,57] found a significant reduction in hyponatremia among those receiving isotonic IVFs. McNab et al[35] enrolled patients in both the ICU and general surgical ward, and they were at similar risk for developing hyponatremia.

Exclusion of Specific Populations Not Studied

Patients with neurosurgical disorders, congenital or acquired cardiac disease, hepatic disease, cancer, renal dysfunction, diabetes insipidus, voluminous watery diarrhea, or severe burns; neonates who were younger than 28 days old or in the NICU (researchers in the majority of prospective studies reviewed in this guideline excluded this subset of patients); and adolescents older than 18 years old were excluded. Patients with congenital or acquired heart disease have been either explicitly excluded from every study listed previously or were not described, so no conclusions may be drawn related to this specific population. Similarly, patients with known liver or renal disease or adrenal insufficiency have also been excluded from most of the studies listed, limiting any conclusions for these patients as well. Neurosurgical patients and those with traumatic brain injury were excluded from most studies. Oncology patients have been included in some of the randomized trials, but no specific subanalysis for them has been completed, and data are not available separately to conduct one. Many patients receiving chemotherapy receive high volumes of fluids to prevent renal injury, and there are reports of clinically significant hyponatremia, which is possibly associated with the fluid type.[61] Further study is needed to evaluate the fluid type, rate, and risk of renal injury and hyponatremia for this population. The committee did not specifically review literature for those with the following care needs: patients with significant renal concentrating defects, such as nephrogenic diabetes insipidus, and patients with voluminous diarrhea or severe burns who may have significant ongoing free-water losses.

Complications

Hyponatremia

The reviewed studies revealed the relative risk of developing mild and moderate hyponatremia (defined as a serum sodium concentration

<135 mEq/L and <130 mEq/L, respectively) to be >2 and >5, respectively. The risk related to hyponatremia persisted regardless of age, medical versus surgical status, and intensive care versus general pediatric ward setting. These data strongly reveal an increased risk of hyponatremia when children receive hypotonic versus isotonic IVFs. This association is reinforced by the observations that increased hyponatremia occurs in (1) children with normal sodium at baseline (hospital-acquired hyponatremia) and (2) children who have a low sodium concentration at baseline (hospital-aggravated hyponatremia). This association has been found when using both 0.2% saline (sodium 34 mEq/L) and 0.45% saline (sodium 77 mEq/L). The risk for hyponatremia with hypotonic fluids persisted in the subgroup of patients who received fluids at a restricted rate.[49,54,58,59] A sensitivity analysis in which the Shamim et al[58] study was excluded given the anomalous number of events in both arms revealed no change in the overall estimated relative risk (0.43; 95% CI, 0.35–0.53) compared with that of all the studies included (0.46; 95% CI, 0.37–0.57; Supplemental Fig 2). In the clinical trials in which researchers assessed the possible mechanism for this finding, elevated antidiuretic hormone (ADH) concentration was found to play a putative role.[54]

There is heterogeneity in the design of the above studies in the types of patients enrolled, IVF rate and type, frequency of plasma sodium monitoring, and study duration. Despite this heterogeneity, the increased risk of hyponatremia with hypotonic IVFs is consistent. Some may argue that mild hyponatremia (plasma sodium 130–134 mEq/L) and moderate hyponatremia (plasma sodium 125–129 mEq/L) may not be clinically significant or constitute harm. However, the studies in which

researchers evaluated moderate hyponatremia revealed benefits of isotonic versus hypotonic IVFs (Supplemental Figs 2 and 4). Furthermore, hypotonic solutions have been associated with a larger decrease in serum sodium. Also, the true effects of hypotonic IVFs may have been underestimated because many of the studies also included rigorous monitoring of sodium, during which patients were removed from the study if mild hyponatremia developed. Numerous studies of adults have revealed that mild and asymptomatic hyponatremia is associated with deleterious consequences, is an independent risk factor for mortality,[62,63] and leads to increased length of hospitalization and increases in costs of hospitalization.[64,65] Thus, the subcommittee believes that hyponatremia is an appropriate indicator of potential harm.

Hypernatremia

One of the concerns when providing a higher level of sodium in IVFs is the development of hypernatremia (serum sodium >145 mEq/L). This was evaluated in the most recently published systematic review.[33] Those authors identified that there was no evidence of an increased risk of hypernatremia associated with the administration of isotonic fluids, although the quality of evidence was judged to be low, primarily given the low incidence of hypernatremia in the studies included. To be clear, there was not evidence of no risk; the risk is unclear from the meta-analysis results. The estimated risk ratio from that meta-analysis was 1.24 (95% CI, 0.65–2.38), drawn from 9 studies with 937 patients, although 3 studies had no events and did not contribute to the estimate. Researchers in 2 large studies published since the meta-analysis did not find evidence of an increased risk of hypernatremia with isotonic IVFs. In the study by Friedman et al,[32] there was 1 patient in each randomized group (N = 110) who developed hypernatremia, and in the study by McNab et al,[35] the incidence of hypernatremia was 4% in the isotonic IVF group and 6% in the hypotonic IVF group, with no significant difference noted between the 2 groups ($N = 641$ with data for analysis). The available data among the meta-analysis discussed above and subsequent large RCTs were unable to be used to demonstrate an increased risk of hypernatremia associated with the use of isotonic IVFs.

Acidosis

A hyperchloremic metabolic acidosis has been associated with 0.9% NaCl when it is used as a resuscitation fluid. Researchers in the majority of studies reviewed in this series did not specifically evaluate the development of acidosis or report on it as a complication. Researchers in 4 studies involving 496 patients evaluated the effect of IVF composition on acid and/or base status,[31,49,54,58] and the majority were not able to demonstrate that 0.9% NaCl resulted in acidosis. Two studies in which researchers compared 0.9% NaCl to 0.45% NaCl involving 357 children found no effect on the development of acidosis based on the change in total carbon dioxide (Tco_2), a measure of plasma bicarbonate, with a low Tco_2 being a surrogate marker for acidosis rather than a low pH.[31,54] Researchers in 1 study compared Hartman solution, which has a base equivalent to 0.45% NaCl, involving 79 patients and found no effect on the development of acidosis based on a change in Tco_2.[49] Researchers in 1 study involving 60 patients compared 0.9% NaCl to 0.18% NaCl and demonstrated a decrease in pH from 7.36 to 7.32 in the 0.9% NaCl group compared with an increase in pH from 7.36 to 7.38 in the 0.18% NaCl group ($P = .01$), but the effect on Tco_2 was not reported.[58]

Fluid Overload

Children receiving IVFs are at risk for fluid accumulation leading to a positive fluid balance or volume overload. A combination of excessive fluid and sodium can synergistically increase retained volume, a condition that is exacerbated in children with chronic comorbidities (such as systolic cardiac dysfunction [congestive heart failure (CHF)], cirrhotic hepatic failure, chronic kidney disease, and hepatorenal syndrome) and metabolic disturbances (such as hyperaldosteronism and long-term steroid use). Researchers in recent literature, most notably in the critically ill population (adults and children), have attempted to delineate the causative and outcome associations with significant positive fluid accumulation, termed "fluid overload."[66] In the non-ICU population, researchers in only a handful of studies mention an association between fluid tonicity and volume overload (or "weight gain").[20,59,60] Choong et al[20] reported on "overhydration" as estimated by using total weight gain, finding no significant difference between isotonic and hypotonic IVF administration. In the meta-analyses that encompass 12 different RCTs and more than 750 children, neither weight nor net fluid balance is discussed. Increasing scrutiny is being given to fluid management in the critically ill population.[33] To determine any association in patients who are noncritically ill, more evidence is required.

Specific Groups That May Be at Higher Risk for Developing Hyponatremia

Researchers in the RCTs reviewed for this statement excluded many groups of patients who are at particularly high risk for hyponatremia, such as those with congenital or acquired heart disease, liver disease, renal failure or dysfunction, or adrenal

insufficiency; neurosurgical patients; and patients taking medication known to impair free-water excretion, such as desmopressin. Data on the efficacy of isotonic fluids to prevent hyponatremia and the potential complications related to isotonic fluids in these patients are lacking. Further studies in which researchers evaluate optimal fluid management in these groups of patients are necessary. Patients with edematous states, such as CHF, cirrhosis, and nephrotic syndrome, have an impaired ability to excrete both free water and sodium and are at risk for both volume overload and hyponatremia. Administering isotonic saline at typical maintenance rates will likely be excessive and risk volume overload, and IVFs should be restricted with close monitoring. Renal diseases can have multiple effects on sodium and water homeostasis; patients with glomerulonephritis may avidly reabsorb sodium, whereas those with tubulopathies may have obligatory urinary sodium losses. Patients with renal failure have a relative inability to excrete free water because of the reduced glomerular filtration rate and simultaneously are unable to produce maximally concentrated urine. Patients with adrenal insufficiency can have renal salt wasting and an impaired ability to excrete free water. Patients with CNS disorders can have multiple conditions that impair water excretion, including SIAD and cerebral salt wasting. Patients receiving certain medications are at particularly high risk for developing hyponatremia, such as desmopressin administered perioperatively for Von Willebrand disease, antiepileptic medications (such as carbamazepine), and chemotherapeutic agents (such as IV cyclophosphamide and vincristine). Isotonic IVFs may be the preferred fluid composition for these disease states, but care is needed in dosing the quantity of fluids, and close monitoring of both the volume status and electrolytes is required.

Limitations

The subcommittee's recommendation to use isotonic fluids when maintenance IVFs are required does not mean that there are no indications for administering hypotonic fluids or that isotonic fluids will be safe in all patients. Patients with significant renal concentrating defects, such as nephrogenic diabetes insipidus, could develop hypernatremia if they are administered isotonic fluids. Patients with voluminous diarrhea or severe burns may require a hypotonic fluid to keep up with ongoing free-water losses. Hypotonic fluids may also be required to correct hypernatremia. However, for the vast majority of patients, isotonic fluids are the most appropriate maintenance IVF and are the least likely to result in a disorder in serum sodium.

CONCLUSIONS

For the past 60 years, the prescription for maintenance IVFs for infants and children has been a hypotonic fluid. These recommendations were made on theoretical grounds and were not based on clinical trials. Despite this accepted dogma, over the past decade and longer, there have been increasing reports of the deleterious effect of hyponatremia in the acute care setting with the use of the prevailing hypotonic maintenance solutions. Using an evidence-based approach, recommendations for optimal sodium composition of maintenance IVFs are provided to prevent hyponatremia and acute or permanent neurologic impairment related to it. Recommendations are not made regarding the use of an isotonic buffered crystalloid solution versus saline, the optimal rate of fluid therapy, or the need for providing potassium in maintenance fluids. The

use of this guideline differentiates the applicability to 2 subgroups of children: (1) The guideline applies to surgical (postoperative) medical patients in a critical care setting and the general inpatient ward. (2) The guideline does not apply to patients with neurosurgical disorders, congenital or acquired cardiac disease, hepatic disease, cancer, renal dysfunction, diabetes insipidus, voluminous watery diarrhea, or severe burns; neonates who are younger than 28 days old or in the NICU; or adolescents older than 18 years of age (Supplemental Fig 5).

This guideline is intended for use primarily by clinicians providing acute care for children and adolescents who require maintenance IVFs. It may be of interest to parents and payers, but it is not intended to be used for reimbursement or to determine insurance coverage. This guideline is not intended to be the sole source of guidance in the use of maintenance IVFs but rather is intended to assist clinicians by providing a framework for clinical decision-making.

The Key Action Statement is as follows:

1A: The AAP recommends that patients 28 days to 18 years of age requiring maintenance IVFs should receive isotonic solutions with appropriate KCl and dextrose because they significantly decrease the risk of developing hyponatremia (evidence quality: A; recommendation strength: strong).

BIOCHEMICAL LABORATORY MONITORING

Although the frequency for biochemical laboratory monitoring was not specifically addressed in the 17 RCTs included in the meta-analysis, researchers in most of the studies obtained serial plasma sodium values, with the first plasma

sodium being measured between 6 hours and 12 hours. The incidence of hyponatremia in patients receiving isotonic fluids ranged from 0% to 23%, whereas that of hypotonic fluids ranged from 5% to 100%. This large variability was likely related to the different study designs. Many patients who were hospitalized and received isotonic IVFs will be at risk for hyponatremia if they are receiving IV medications containing free water or are consuming additional free water via the enteral route. For these reasons, clinicians should be aware that even patients receiving isotonic maintenance IVFs are at sufficient risk for developing hyponatremia. If an electrolyte abnormality is discovered, this could provide useful information to adjust maintenance fluid therapy. If patients receiving isotonic maintenance IVFs develop hyponatremia, they should be evaluated to determine if they are receiving other sources of free water or if they may have SIAD and/or an adrenal insufficiency. If hypernatremia develops (plasma sodium >144 mEq/L), patients should be evaluated for renal dysfunction or extrarenal free-water losses.

In patients at high risk for developing electrolyte abnormalities, such as those who have undergone major surgery, those in the ICU, or those with large gastrointestinal losses or receiving diuretics, frequent laboratory monitoring may be necessary. If neurologic symptoms that could be consistent with hyponatremic encephalopathy are present, such as unexplained nausea, vomiting, headache, confusion, or lethargy, electrolytes should be measured.

FUTURE QUALITY-IMPROVEMENT QUESTIONS

Future questions are as follows:

1. How frequently is plasma sodium concentration abnormal, and

is this abnormality clinically significant?

2. Will the widespread use of isotonic maintenance IVFs in the acute-care setting significantly reduce or eliminate hyponatremia- and hyponatremia-related neurologic events?

3. Will the widespread use of 0.9% saline for maintenance IVFs in the acute care setting increase clinically significant metabolic acidosis?

4. Are isotonic-balanced solutions superior to 0.9% saline for the maintenance IVF in the acute-care setting?

5. How frequently should clinicians monitor the serum sodium concentrations when a patient is receiving maintenance IVFs and for patients who are at high risk of sodium abnormalities?

SUBCOMMITTEE ON FLUID AND ELECTROLYTE THERAPY

Leonard G. Feld, MD, PhD, MMM, FAAP – *Chair, Pediatric Nephrology*
Daniel R. Neuspiel, MD, MPH, FAAP – *Pediatric Epidemiologist*
Byron Alexander Foster, MD, MPH, FAAP – *Pediatric Hospitalist*
Matthew D. Garber, MD, FHM, FAAP – *Pediatric Hospitalist; Implementation Scientist*
Michael G. Leu, MD, MS, MHS, FAAP – *Partnership for Policy Implementation*
Rajit K. Basu, MD, MS, FCCM – *Society of Critical Care Medicine, Pediatric Section*
Kelly Austin, MD, MS, FAAP, FACS – *American Pediatric Surgical Association*
Edward E. Conway, Jr, MD, MS, FAAP – *Pediatric Critical Care*
James J. Fehr, MD, FAAP – *Society for Pediatric Anesthesia*
Clare Hawkins, MD – *American Academy of Family Physicians*
Ron L. Kaplan, MD, FAAP – *Pediatric Emergency Medicine*
Echo V. Rowe, MD, FAAP – *Pediatric Anesthesiology and Pain Medicine*
Muhammad Waseem, MD, MS, FAAP, FACEP – *American College of Emergency Physicians*
Michael L. Moritz, MD, FAAP – *Pediatric Nephrology*

STAFF

Kymika Okechukwu, MPA – *Senior Manager, Evidence-Based Medicine Initiatives*

ABBREVIATIONS

AAP: American Academy of Pediatrics
ADH: antidiuretic hormone
AVP: arginine vasopressin
CHF: congestive heart failure
CI: confidence interval
CNS: central nervous system
IV: intravenous
IVF: intravenous fluid
kcal: kilocalorie
KCl: potassium chloride
M-H: Mantel-Haenzel
NaCl: sodium chloride
RCT: randomized controlled trial
SIAD: syndrome of inappropriate antidiuresis
Tco_2: total carbon dioxide

All clinical practice guidelines from the American Academy of Pediatrics automatically expire 5 years after publication unless reaffirmed, revised, or retired at or before that time.

DOI: https://doi.org/10.1542/peds.2018-3083

Address correspondence to Leonard G. Feld, MD, PhD, MMM, FAAP. E-mail: feldllc@gmail.com

PEDIATRICS (ISSN Numbers: Print, 0031-4005; Online, 1098-4275).

Copyright © 2018 by the American Academy of Pediatrics

FINANCIAL DISCLOSURE: The authors have indicated they have no financial relationships relevant to this article to disclose.

FUNDING: No external funding.

POTENTIAL CONFLICT OF INTEREST: The authors have indicated they have no potential conflicts of interest to disclose.

REFERENCES

1. Chawla G, Drummond GB. Textbook coverage of a common topic: fluid management of patients after surgery. *Med Educ.* 2008;42(6):613–618

2. Davies P, Hall T, Ali T, Lakhoo K. Intravenous postoperative fluid prescriptions for children: a survey of practice. *BMC Surg.* 2008;8:10

3. Freeman MA, Ayus JC, Moritz ML. Maintenance intravenous fluid prescribing practices among paediatric residents. *Acta Paediatr.* 2012;101(10):e465–e468

4. Lee JM, Jung Y, Lee SE, et al. Intravenous fluid prescription practices among pediatric residents in Korea. *Korean J Pediatr.* 2013;56(7):282–285

5. Goldstein SL. Fluid management in acute kidney injury. *J Intensive Care Med.* 2014;29(4):183–189

6. Hoste EA, Maitland K, Brudney CS, et al; ADQI XII Investigators Group. Four phases of intravenous fluid therapy: a conceptual model. *Br J Anaesth.* 2014;113(5): 740–747

7. McDermid RC, Raghunathan K, Romanovsky A, Shaw AD, Bagshaw SM. Controversies in fluid therapy: type, dose and toxicity. *World J Crit Care Med.* 2014;3(1):24–33

8. Jackson J, Bolte RG. Risks of intravenous administration of hypotonic fluids for pediatric patients in ED and prehospital settings: let's remove the handle from the pump. *Am J Emerg Med.* 2000;18(3):269–270

9. Wang J, Xu E, Xiao Y. Isotonic versus hypotonic maintenance IV fluids in hospitalized children: a meta-analysis. *Pediatrics.* 2014;133(1):105–113

10. Moritz ML, Ayus JC. Maintenance intravenous fluids in acutely ill patients. *N Engl J Med.* 2015;373(14):1350–1360

11. Carandang F, Anglemyer A, Longhurst CA, et al. Association between

maintenance fluid tonicity and hospital-acquired hyponatremia. *J Pediatr.* 2013;163(6):1646–1651

12. Upadhyay A, Jaber BL, Madias NE. Incidence and prevalence of hyponatremia. *Am J Med.* 2006;119 (7, suppl 1):S30–S35

13. Moritz ML, Ayus JC. Disorders of water metabolism in children: hyponatremia and hypernatremia. *Pediatr Rev.* 2002;23(11):371–380

14. Gerigk M, Gnehm HE, Rascher W. Arginine vasopressin and renin in acutely ill children: implication for fluid therapy. *Acta Paediatr.* 1996;85(5):550–553

15. Judd BA, Haycock GB, Dalton RN, Chantler C. Antidiuretic hormone following surgery in children. *Acta Paediatr Scand.* 1990;79(4):461–466

16. Holliday MA, Segar WE. The maintenance need for water in parenteral fluid therapy. *Pediatrics.* 1957;19(5):823–832

17. Talbot FB. Basal metabolism standards for children. *Am J Dis Child.* 1938;55(3):455–459

18. Hatherill M. Rubbing salt in the wound. *Arch Dis Child.* 2004;89(5):414–418

19. Hoorn EJ, Geary D, Robb M, Halperin ML, Bohn D. Acute hyponatremia related to intravenous fluid administration in hospitalized children: an observational study. *Pediatrics.* 2004;113(5):1279–1284

20. Choong K, Arora S, Cheng J, et al. Hypotonic versus isotonic maintenance fluids after surgery for children: a randomized controlled trial. *Pediatrics.* 2011;128(5):857–866

21. Arieff AI, Ayus JC, Fraser CL. Hyponatraemia and death or permanent brain damage in healthy children. *BMJ.* 1992;304(6836):1218–1222

22. Moritz ML, Ayus JC. Preventing neurological complications from dysnatremias in children. *Pediatr Nephrol.* 2005;20(12):1687–1700

23. Halberthal M, Halperin ML, Bohn D. Lesson of the week: acute hyponatraemia in children admitted to hospital: retrospective analysis of factors contributing to its development and resolution. *BMJ.* 2001;322(7289):780–782

24. Moritz ML, Ayus JC. Prevention of hospital-acquired hyponatremia: a case for using isotonic saline. *Pediatrics.* 2003;111(2):227–230

25. ISMP. Medication safety alert. Plain D5W or hypotonic saline solutions post-op could result in acute hyponatremia and death in healthy children. Available at: ismp.org. Accessed August 14, 2009

26. ISMP Canada. Hospital-acquired acute hyponatremia: two reports of pediatric deaths. *ISMP Canada Saf Bul.* 2009;9(7). Available at: http://www.ismp-canada. org/download/safetyBulletins/ ISMPCSB2009-7-HospitalAcquiredA cuteHyponatremia.pdf. Accessed July 26, 2018

27. National Patient Safety Agency. Reducing the risk of hyponatraemia when administering intravenous infusions to children. 2007. Available at: www.npsa.nhs.uk/health/alerts. Accessed July 6, 2018

28. Drysdale SB, Coulson T, Cronin N, et al. The impact of the National Patient Safety Agency intravenous fluid alert on iatrogenic hyponatraemia in children. *Eur J Pediatr.* 2010;169(7):813–817

29. Holliday MA, Ray PE, Friedman AL. Fluid therapy for children: facts, fashions and questions. *Arch Dis Child.* 2007;92(6):546–550

30. McNab S. Isotonic vs hypotonic intravenous fluids for hospitalized children. *JAMA.* 2015;314(7):720–721

31. Almeida HI, Mascarenhas MI, Loureiro HC, et al. The effect of NaCl 0.9% and NaCl 0.45% on sodium, chloride, and acid-base balance in a PICU population. *J Pediatr (Rio J).* 2015;91(5):499–505

32. Friedman JN, Beck CE, DeGroot J, Geary DF, Sklansky DJ, Freedman SB. Comparison of isotonic and hypotonic intravenous maintenance fluids: a randomized clinical trial. *JAMA Pediatr.* 2015;169(5):445–451

33. McNab S, Ware RS, Neville KA, et al. Isotonic versus hypotonic solutions for maintenance intravenous fluid administration in children. *Cochrane Database Syst Rev.* 2014;(12):CD009457

34. National Clinical Guideline Centre (UK). *IV Fluids in Children: Intravenous Fluid Therapy in Children and Young People*

in Hospital. London, United Kingdom: National Clinical Guideline Centre; 2015. Available at: www.ncbi.nlm.nih. gov/pubmed/26741016. Accessed July 6, 2018

35. McNab S, Duke T, South M, et al. 140 mmol/L of sodium versus 77 mmol/L of sodium in maintenance intravenous fluid therapy for children in hospital (PIMS): a randomised controlled double-blind trial. *Lancet.* 2015;385(9974):1190–1197. Published online December 1, 2014

36. Siegel NJ, ed. Fluids, electrolytes and acid-base. In: *Rudolph's Pediatrics.* 21st ed. New York, NY: McGraw Hill; 2003:1653–1655

37. Greenbaum LA, ed. Pathophysiology of body fluids and fluid therapy. In: *Nelson's Textbook of Pediatrics.* 17th ed. Philadelphia, PA: WB Saunders; 2004:242–245

38. Powers KS. Dehydration: isonatremic, hyponatremic, and hypernatremic recognition and management. *Pediatr Rev.* 2015;36(7):274–283; quiz 284–285

39. Foster BA, Tom D, Hill V. Hypotonic versus isotonic fluids in hospitalized children: a systematic review and meta-analysis. *J Pediatr.* 2014;165(1):163–169.e2

40. Padua AP, Macaraya JR, Dans LF, Anacleto FE Jr. Isotonic versus hypotonic saline solution for maintenance intravenous fluid therapy in children: a systematic review. *Pediatr Nephrol.* 2015;30(7):1163–1172

41. Yang G, Jiang W, Wang X, Liu W. The efficacy of isotonic and hypotonic intravenous maintenance fluid for pediatric patients: a meta-analysis of randomized controlled trials. *Pediatr Emerg Care.* 2015;31(2):122–126

42. Choong K, Kho ME, Menon K, Bohn D. Hypotonic versus isotonic saline in hospitalised children: a systematic review. *Arch Dis Child.* 2006;91(10):828–835

43. Guyatt GH, Sackett DL, Cook DJ. Users' guides to the medical literature. II. How to use an article about therapy or prevention. A. Are the results of the study valid? Evidence-Based Medicine Working Group. *JAMA.* 1993;270(21):2598–2601

44. Guyatt GH, Sackett DL, Cook DJ. Users' guides to the medical literature. II.

How to use an article about therapy or prevention. B. What were the results and will they help me in caring for my patients? Evidence-Based Medicine Working Group. *JAMA.* 1994;271(1):59–63

45. Higgins JP, Green S, eds. *Cochrane Handbook for Systematic Reviews of Interventions. Version 5.1.0. Updated March 2011.* London, United Kingdom: The Cochrane Collaboration; 2011. Available at: http://handbook-5-1.cochrane.org/. Accessed July 6, 2018

46. American Academy of Pediatrics Steering Committee on Quality Improvement and Management. Classifying recommendations for clinical practice guidelines. *Pediatrics.* 2004;114(3):874–877

47. Bridge-Wiz. Guideline quality appraisal. Available at: http://gem.med.yale.edu/BRIDGE-Wiz/BridgeWiz_2.1_AAP.zip. Accessed April 12, 2016

48. Brazel PW, McPhee IB. Inappropriate secretion of antidiuretic hormone in postoperative scoliosis patients: the role of fluid management. *Spine.* 1996;21(6):724–727

49. Coulthard MG, Long DA, Ullman AJ, Ware RS. A randomised controlled trial of Hartmann's solution versus half normal saline in postoperative paediatric spinal instrumentation and craniotomy patients. *Arch Dis Child.* 2012;97(6):491–496

50. Jorro Barón FA, Meregalli CN, Rombola VA, et al. Hypotonic versus isotonic maintenance fluids in critically ill pediatric patients: a randomized controlled trial [in English and Spanish]. *Arch Argent Pediatr.* 2013;111(4):281–287

51. Flores Robles CM, Cuello García CA. A prospective trial comparing isotonic with hypotonic maintenance fluids for prevention of hospital-acquired hyponatraemia. *Paediatr Int Child Health.* 2016;36(3):168–174

52. Kannan L, Lodha R, Vivekanandhan S, Bagga A, Kabra SK, Kabra M. Intravenous fluid regimen and hyponatraemia among children: a randomized controlled trial. *Pediatr Nephrol.* 2010;25(11):2303–2309

53. Montañana PA, Modesto i Alapont V, Ocón AP, López PO, López Prats JL, Toledo Parreño JD. The use of isotonic fluid as maintenance therapy prevents iatrogenic hyponatremia in pediatrics: a randomized, controlled open study. *Pediatr Crit Care Med.* 2008;9(6):589–597

54. Neville KA, Sandeman DJ, Rubinstein A, et al. Prevention of hyponatremia during maintenance intravenous fluid administration: a prospective randomized study of fluid type versus fluid rate. *J Pediatr.* 2010;156(2):313–319.e1–e2

55. Ramanathan S, Kumar P, Mishra K, Dutta AK. Isotonic versus hypotonic parenteral maintenance fluids in very severe pneumonia. *Indian J Pediatr.* 2016;83(1):27–32

56. Rey C, Los-Arcos M, Hernández A, Sánchez A, Díaz JJ, López-Herce J. Hypotonic versus isotonic maintenance fluids in critically ill children: a multicenter prospective randomized study. *Acta Paediatr.* 2011;100(8):1138–1143

57. Saba TG, Fairbairn J, Houghton F, Laforte D, Foster BJ. A randomized controlled trial of isotonic versus hypotonic maintenance intravenous fluids in hospitalized children. *BMC Pediatr.* 2011;11:82

58. Shamim A, Afzal K, Ali SM. Safety and efficacy of isotonic (0.9%) vs. hypotonic (0.18%) saline as maintenance intravenous fluids in children: a randomized controlled trial. *Indian Pediatr.* 2014;51(12):969–974

59. Yung M, Keeley S. Randomised controlled trial of intravenous

maintenance fluids. *J Paediatr Child Health.* 2009;45(1–2):9–14

60. Valadão MC S, Piva JP, Santana JC, Garcia PC. Comparison of two maintenance electrolyte solutions in children in the postoperative appendectomy period: a randomized, controlled trial. *J Pediatr (Rio J).* 2015;91(5):428–434

61. Duke T, Kinney S, Waters K. Hyponatraemia and seizures in oncology patients associated with hypotonic intravenous fluids. *J Paediatr Child Health.* 2005;41(12):685–686

62. Gankam-Kengne F, Ayers C, Khera A, de Lemos J, Maalouf NM. Mild hyponatremia is associated with an increased risk of death in an ambulatory setting. *Kidney Int.* 2013;83(4):700–706

63. Holland-Bill L, Christiansen CF, Heide-Jørgensen U, et al. Hyponatremia and mortality risk: a Danish cohort study of 279508 acutely hospitalized patients. *Eur J Endocrinol.* 2015;173(1):71–81

64. Amin A, Deitelzweig S, Christian R, et al. Evaluation of incremental healthcare resource burden and readmission rates associated with hospitalized hyponatremic patients in the US. *J Hosp Med.* 2012;7(8):634–639

65. Corona G, Giuliani C, Parenti G, et al. The economic burden of hyponatremia: systematic review and meta-analysis. *Am J Med.* 2016;129(8):823–835.e4

66. Alobaidi R, Morgan C, Basu RK, et al. Associations between fluid balance and outcomes in critically ill children: a protocol for a systematic review and meta-analysis. *Can J Kidney Health Dis.* 2017;4:2054358117692560

67. Pemde HK, Dutta AK, Sodani R, Mishra K. Isotonic intravenous maintenance fluid reduces hospital acquired hyponatremia in young children with central nervous system infections. *Indian J Pediatr.* 2015;82(1):13–18

Intravenous Fluids Clinical Practice Guideline Quick Reference Tools

- Action Statement Summary
  — Clinical Practice Guideline: Maintenance Intravenous Fluids in Children
- *ICD-10-CM* Coding Quick Reference for Maintenance Intravenous Fluids

Action Statement Summary
Clinical Practice Guideline: Maintenance Intravenous Fluids in Children

Key Action Statement 1
Composition of Maintenance IVFs

Key Action Statement 1A
The AAP recommends that patients 28 days to 18 years of age requiring maintenance IVFs should receive isotonic solutions with appropriate potassium chloride (KCl) and dextrose because they significantly decrease the risk of developing hyponatremia (evidence quality: A; recommendation strength: strong).

Coding Quick Reference for Maintenance Intravenous Fluids
ICD-10-CM
E86.0 Dehydration

The Diagnosis and Management of Acute Otitis Media

- *Clinical Practice Guideline*

CLINICAL PRACTICE GUIDELINE

The Diagnosis and Management of Acute Otitis Media

abstract

This evidence-based clinical practice guideline is a revision of the 2004 acute otitis media (AOM) guideline from the American Academy of Pediatrics (AAP) and American Academy of Family Physicians. It provides recommendations to primary care clinicians for the management of children from 6 months through 12 years of age with uncomplicated AOM.

In 2009, the AAP convened a committee composed of primary care physicians and experts in the fields of pediatrics, family practice, otolaryngology, epidemiology, infectious disease, emergency medicine, and guideline methodology. The subcommittee partnered with the Agency for Healthcare Research and Quality and the Southern California Evidence-Based Practice Center to develop a comprehensive review of the new literature related to AOM since the initial evidence report of 2000. The resulting evidence report and other sources of data were used to formulate the practice guideline recommendations.

The focus of this practice guideline is the appropriate diagnosis and initial treatment of a child presenting with AOM. The guideline provides a specific, stringent definition of AOM. It addresses pain management, initial observation versus antibiotic treatment, appropriate choices of antibiotic agents, and preventive measures. It also addresses recurrent AOM, which was not included in the 2004 guideline. Decisions were made on the basis of a systematic grading of the quality of evidence and benefit-harm relationships.

The practice guideline underwent comprehensive peer review before formal approval by the AAP.

This clinical practice guideline is not intended as a sole source of guidance in the management of children with AOM. Rather, it is intended to assist primary care clinicians by providing a framework for clinical decision-making. It is not intended to replace clinical judgment or establish a protocol for all children with this condition. These recommendations may not provide the only appropriate approach to the management of this problem. *Pediatrics* 2013;131:e964–e999

Allan S. Lieberthal, MD, FAAP, Aaron E. Carroll, MD, MS, FAAP, Tasnee Chonmaitree, MD, FAAP, Theodore G. Ganiats, MD, Alejandro Hoberman, MD, FAAP, Mary Anne Jackson, MD, FAAP, Mark D. Joffe, MD, FAAP, Donald T. Miller, MD, MPH, FAAP, Richard M. Rosenfeld, MD, MPH, FAAP, Xavier D. Sevilla, MD, FAAP, Richard H. Schwartz, MD, FAAP, Pauline A. Thomas, MD, FAAP, and David E. Tunkel, MD, FAAP, FACS

KEY WORDS
acute otitis media, otitis media, otoscopy, otitis media with effusion, watchful waiting, antibiotics, antibiotic prophylaxis, tympanostomy tube insertion, immunization, breastfeeding

ABBREVIATIONS
AAFP—American Academy of Family Physicians
AAP—American Academy of Pediatrics
AHRQ—Agency for Healthcare Research and Quality
AOM—acute otitis media
CI—confidence interval
FDA—US Food and Drug Administration
LAIV—live-attenuated intranasal influenza vaccine
MEE—middle ear effusion
MIC—minimum inhibitory concentration
NNT—number needed to treat
OM—otitis media
OME—otitis media with effusion
OR—odds ratio
PCV7—heptavalent pneumococcal conjugate vaccine
PCV13—13-valent pneumococcal conjugate vaccine
RD—rate difference
SNAP—safety-net antibiotic prescription
TIV—trivalent inactivated influenza vaccine
TM—tympanic membrane
WASP—wait-and-see prescription

This document is copyrighted and is property of the American Academy of Pediatrics and its Board of Directors. All authors have filed conflict of interest statements with the American Academy of Pediatrics. Any conflicts have been resolved through a process approved by the Board of Directors. The American Academy of Pediatrics has neither solicited nor accepted any commercial involvement in the development of the content of this publication.

The recommendations in this report do not indicate an exclusive course of treatment or serve as a standard of medical care. Variations, taking into account individual circumstances, may be appropriate.

(Continued on last page)

Key Action Statement 1A: Clinicians should diagnose acute otitis media (AOM) in children who present with moderate to severe bulging of the tympanic membrane (TM) *or* new onset of otorrhea not due to acute otitis externa. Evidence Quality: Grade B. Strength: Recommendation.

Key Action Statement 1B: Clinicians should diagnose AOM in children who present with mild bulging of the TM *and* recent (less than 48 hours) onset of ear pain (holding, tugging, rubbing of the ear in a nonverbal child) *or* intense erythema of the TM. Evidence Quality: Grade C. Strength: Recommendation.

Key Action Statement 1C: Clinicians should not diagnose AOM in children who do not have middle ear effusion (MEE) (based on pneumatic otoscopy and/or tympanometry). Evidence Quality: Grade B. Strength: Recommendation.

Key Action Statement 2: The management of AOM should include an assessment of pain. If pain is present, the clinician should recommend treatment to reduce pain. Evidence Quality: Grade B. Strength: Strong Recommendation.

Key Action Statement 3A: Severe AOM: The clinician should prescribe antibiotic therapy for AOM (bilateral or unilateral) in children 6 months and older with severe signs or symptoms (ie, moderate or severe otalgia or otalgia for at least 48 hours or temperature 39°C [102.2°F] or higher). Evidence Quality: Grade B. Strength: Strong Recommendation.

Key Action Statement 3B: Nonsevere bilateral AOM in young children: The clinician should prescribe antibiotic therapy for bilateral AOM in children 6 months through 23 months of age without severe signs or symptoms (ie, mild otalgia for less than 48 hours and temperature less than 39°C [102.2°F]). Evidence Quality: Grade B. Strength: Recommendation.

Key Action Statement 3C: Nonsevere unilateral AOM in young children: The clinician should either prescribe antibiotic therapy *or* offer observation with close follow-up based on joint decision-making with the parent(s)/caregiver for unilateral AOM in children 6 months to 23 months of age without severe signs or symptoms (ie, mild otalgia for less than 48 hours and temperature less than 39°C [102.2°F]). When observation is used, a mechanism must be in place to ensure follow-up and begin antibiotic therapy if the child worsens or fails to improve within 48 to 72 hours of onset of symptoms. Evidence Quality: Grade B. Strength: Recommendation.

Key Action Statement 3D: Nonsevere AOM in older children: The clinician should either prescribe antibiotic therapy *or* offer observation with close follow-up based on joint decision-making with the parent(s)/caregiver for AOM (bilateral or unilateral) in children 24 months or older without severe signs or symptoms (ie, mild otalgia for less than 48 hours and temperature less than 39°C [102.2°F]). When observation is used, a mechanism must be in place to ensure follow-up and begin antibiotic therapy if the child worsens or fails to improve within 48 to 72 hours of onset of symptoms. Evidence Quality: Grade B. Strength: Recommendation.

Key Action Statement 4A: Clinicians should prescribe amoxicillin for AOM when a decision to treat with antibiotics has been made *and* the child has not received amoxicillin in the past 30 days *or* the child does not have concurrent purulent conjunctivitis *or* the child is not allergic to penicillin. Evidence Quality: Grade B. Strength: Recommendation.

Key Action Statement 4B: Clinicians should prescribe an antibiotic with additional β-lactamase coverage for AOM when a decision to treat with antibiotics has been made, *and* the child has received amoxicillin in the last 30 days *or* has concurrent purulent conjunctivitis, *or* has a history of recurrent AOM unresponsive to amoxicillin. Evidence Quality: Grade C. Strength: Recommendation.

Key Action Statement 4C: Clinicians should reassess the patient if the caregiver reports that the child's symptoms have worsened or failed to respond to the initial antibiotic treatment within 48 to 72 hours and determine whether a change in therapy is needed. Evidence Quality: Grade B. Strength: Recommendation.

Key Action Statement 5A: Clinicians should not prescribe prophylactic antibiotics to reduce the frequency of episodes of AOM in children with recurrent AOM. Evidence Quality: Grade B. Strength: Recommendation.

Key Action Statement 5B: Clinicians may offer tympanostomy tubes for recurrent AOM (3 episodes in 6 months or 4 episodes in 1 year with 1 episode in the preceding 6 months). Evidence Quality: Grade B. Strength: Option.

Key Action Statement 6A: Clinicians should recommend pneumococcal conjugate vaccine to all children according to the schedule of the Advisory Committee on Immunization Practices of the Centers for Disease Control and Prevention, American Academy of Pediatrics (AAP), and American Academy of Family Physicians (AAFP). Evidence Quality: Grade B. Strength: Strong Recommendation.

Key Action Statement 6B: Clinicians should recommend annual influenza vaccine to all children according to the schedule of the Advisory Committee on Immunization Practices, AAP, and AAFP. Evidence Quality: Grade B. Strength: Recommendation.

2Key Action Statement 6C: Clinicians should encourage exclusive breastfeeding for at least 6 months. Evidence Quality: Grade B. Strength: Recommendation.

Key Action Statement 6D: Clinicians should encourage avoidance of tobacco smoke exposure. Evidence Quality: Grade C. Strength: Recommendation.

INTRODUCTION

In May 2004, the AAP and AAFP published the "Clinical Practice Guideline: Diagnosis and Management of Acute Otitis Media".[1] The guideline offered 8 recommendations ranked according to level of evidence and benefit-harm relationship. Three of the recommendations—diagnostic criteria, observation, and choice of antibiotics—led to significant discussion, especially among experts in the field of otitis media (OM). Also, at the time the guideline was written, information regarding the heptavalent pneumococcal conjugate vaccine (PCV7) was not yet published. Since completion of the guideline in November 2003 and its publication in May 2004, there has been a significant body of additional literature on AOM.

Although OM remains the most common condition for which antibacterial agents are prescribed for children in the United States[2,3] clinician visits for OM decreased from 950 per 1000 children in 1995–1996 to 634 per 1000 children in 2005–2006. There has been a proportional decrease in antibiotic prescriptions for OM from 760 per 1000 in 1995–1996 to 484 per 1000 in 2005–2006. The percentage of OM visits

resulting in antibiotic prescriptions remained relatively stable (80% in 1995–1996; 76% in 2005–2006).[2] Many factors may have contributed to the decrease in visits for OM, including financial issues relating to insurance, such as copayments, that may limit doctor visits, public education campaigns regarding the viral nature of most infectious diseases, use of the PCV7 pneumococcal vaccine, and increased use of the influenza vaccine. Clinicians may also be more attentive to differentiating AOM from OM with effusion (OME), resulting in fewer visits coded for AOM and fewer antibiotic prescriptions written.

Despite significant publicity and awareness of the 2004 AOM guideline, evidence shows that clinicians are hesitant to follow the guideline recommendations. Vernacchio et al[4] surveyed 489 primary care physicians as to their management of 4 AOM scenarios addressed in the 2004 guideline. No significant changes in practice were noted on this survey, compared with a survey administered before the 2004 AOM guideline. Coco[5] used the National Ambulatory Medical Care Survey from 2002 through 2006 to determine the frequency of AOM visits without antibiotics before and after publication of the 2004 guideline. There was no difference in prescribing rates. A similar response to otitis guidelines was found in Italy as in the United States.[6,7] These findings parallel results of other investigations regarding clinician awareness and adherence to guideline recommendations in all specialties, including pediatrics.[8] Clearly, for clinical practice guidelines to be effective, more must be done to improve their dissemination and implementation.

This revision and update of the AAP/AAFP 2004 AOM guideline[1] will evaluate published evidence on the diagnosis and management of uncomplicated AOM and make recommendations based on that evidence. The guideline is intended

for primary care clinicians including pediatricians and family physicians, emergency department physicians, otolaryngologists, physician assistants, and nurse practitioners. The scope of the guideline is the diagnosis and management of AOM, including recurrent AOM, in children 6 months through 12 years of age. It applies only to an otherwise healthy child without underlying conditions that may alter the natural course of AOM, including but not limited to the presence of tympanostomy tubes; anatomic abnormalities, including cleft palate; genetic conditions with craniofacial abnormalities, such as Down syndrome; immune deficiencies; and the presence of cochlear implants. Children with OME without AOM are also excluded.

Glossary of Terms

AOM—the rapid onset of signs and symptoms of inflammation in the middle ear[9,10]

Uncomplicated AOM—AOM without otorrhea[1]

Severe AOM—AOM with the presence of moderate to severe otalgia or fever equal to or higher than 39°C[9,10]

Nonsevere AOM—AOM with the presence of mild otalgia and a temperature below 39°C[9,10]

Recurrent AOM—3 or more well-documented and separate AOM episodes in the preceding 6 months or 4 or more episodes in the preceding 12 months with at least 1 episode in the past 6 months[11,12]

OME—inflammation of the middle ear with liquid collected in the middle ear; the signs and symptoms of acute infection are absent[9]

MEE—liquid in the middle ear without reference to etiology, pathogenesis, pathology, or duration[9]

Otorrhea—discharge from the ear, originating at 1 or more of the following sites: the external auditory canal, middle ear, mastoid, inner ear, or intracranial cavity

Otitis externa—an infection of the external auditory canal

Tympanometry—measuring acoustic immittance (transfer of acoustic energy) of the ear as a function of ear canal air pressure[13,14]

Number needed to treat (NNT)—the number of patients who need to be treated to prevent 1 additional bad outcome[15]

Initial antibiotic therapy—treatment of AOM with antibiotics that are prescribed at the time of diagnosis with the intent of starting antibiotic therapy as soon as possible after the encounter

Initial observation—initial management of AOM limited to symptomatic relief, with commencement of antibiotic therapy only if the child's condition worsens at any time or does not show clinical improvement within 48 to 72 hours of diagnosis; a mechanism must be in place to ensure follow-up and initiation of antibiotics if the child fails observation

METHODS

Guideline development using an evidence-based approach requires that all evidence related to the guideline is gathered in a systematic fashion, objectively assessed, and then described so readers can easily see the links between the evidence and recommendations made. An evidence-based approach leads to recommendations that are guided by both the quality of the available evidence and the benefit-to-harm ratio that results from following the recommendation. Figure 1 shows the relationship of evidence quality and benefit-harm balance in determining the level of recommendation. Table 1 presents the AAP definitions and implications of different levels of evidence-based recommendations.[16]

In preparing for the 2004 AAP guidelines, the Agency for Healthcare Research and Quality (AHRQ) funded and conducted an exhaustive review of the literature on diagnosis and management of AOM.[17–19] In 2008, the AHRQ and the Southern California Evidence-Based Practice Center began a similar process of reviewing the literature published since the 2001 AHRQ report. The AAP again partnered with AHRQ and the Southern California Evidence-Based Practice Center to develop the evidence report, which served as a major source of data for these practice guideline recommendations.[20,21] New key questions were determined by a technical expert panel. The scope of the new report went beyond the 2001 AHRQ report to include recurrent AOM.

The key questions addressed by AHRQ in the 2010 report were as follows:

1. Diagnosis of AOM: What are the operating characteristics (sensitivity, specificity, and likelihood ratios) of clinical symptoms and otoscopic findings (such as bulging TM) to diagnose uncomplicated AOM and to distinguish it from OME?

2. What has been the effect of the use of heptavalent PCV7 on AOM microbial epidemiology, what organisms (bacterial and viral) are associated with AOM since the introduction of PCV7, and what are the patterns

of antimicrobial resistance in AOM since the introduction of PCV7?

3. What is the comparative effectiveness of various treatment options for treating uncomplicated AOM in average risk children?

4. What is the comparative effectiveness of different management options for recurrent OM (uncomplicated) and persistent OM or relapse of AOM?

5. Do treatment outcomes in Questions 3 and 4 differ by characteristics of the condition (AOM), patient, environment, and/or health care delivery system?

6. What adverse effects have been observed for treatments for which outcomes are addressed in Questions 3 and 4?

For the 2010 review, searches of PubMed and the Cochrane Database of Systematic Reviews, Cochrane Central Register of Controlled Trials, and Education Resources Information Center were conducted by using the same search strategies used for the 2001 report for publications from 1998 through June 2010. Additional terms or conditions not considered in the 2001 review (recurrent OM, new drugs, and heptavalent pneumococcal vaccine) were also included. The Web of Science was also used to search for citations of the 2001 report and its peer-reviewed publications. Titles were screened independently by 2

Evidence Quality	Preponderance of Benefit or Harm	Balance of Benefit and Harm
A. Well designed RCTs or diagnostic studies on relevant population	Strong Recommendation	Option
B. RCTs or diagnostic studies with minor limitations; overwhelmingly consistent evidence from observational studies		
C. Observational studies (case-control and cohort design)	Recommendation	
D. Expert opinion, case reports, reasoning from first principles	Option	No Rec
X. Exceptional situations in which validating studies cannot be performed and there is a clear preponderance of benefit or harm	Strong Recommendation / Recommendation	

FIGURE 1

Relationship of evidence quality and benefit-harm balance in determining the level of recommendation. RCT, randomized controlled trial.

TABLE 1 Guideline Definitions for Evidence-Based Statements

Statement	Definition	Implication
Strong Recommendation	A strong recommendation in favor of a particular action is made when the anticipated benefits of the recommended intervention clearly exceed the harms (as a strong recommendation against an action is made when the anticipated harms clearly exceed the benefits) and the quality of the supporting evidence is excellent. In some clearly identified circumstances, strong recommendations may be made when high-quality evidence is impossible to obtain and the anticipated benefits strongly outweigh the harms.	Clinicians should follow a strong recommendation unless a clear and compelling rationale for an alternative approach is present.
Recommendation	A recommendation in favor of a particular action is made when the anticipated benefits exceed the harms, but the quality of evidence is not as strong. Again, in some clearly identified circumstances, recommendations may be made when high-quality evidence is impossible to obtain but the anticipated benefits outweigh the harms.	Clinicians would be prudent to follow a recommendation but should remain alert to new information and sensitive to patient preferences.
Option	Options define courses that may be taken when either the quality of evidence is suspect or carefully performed studies have shown little clear advantage to 1 approach over another.	Clinicians should consider the option in their decision-making, and patient preference may have a substantial role.
No Recommendation	No recommendation indicates that there is a lack of pertinent published evidence and that the anticipated balance of benefits and harms is presently unclear.	Clinicians should be alert to new published evidence that clarifies the balance of benefit versus harm.

pediatricians with experience in conducting systematic reviews.

For the question pertaining to diagnosis, efficacy, and safety, the search was primarily for clinical trials. For the question pertaining to the effect of PCV7 on epidemiology and microbiology, the group searched for trials that compared microbiology in the same populations before and after introduction of the vaccine or observational studies that compared microbiology across vaccinated and unvaccinated populations.

In total, the reviewers examined 7646 titles, of which 686 titles were identified for further review. Of those, 72 articles that met the predetermined inclusion and exclusion criteria were reviewed in detail. Investigators abstracted data into standard evidence tables, with accuracy checked by a second investigator. Studies were quality-rated by 2 investigators by using established criteria. For randomized controlled trials, the Jadad criteria were used.[22] QUADAS criteria[23] were used to evaluate the studies that pertained to diagnosis. GRADE criteria were applied to pooled analyses.[24] Data abstracted

included parameters necessary to define study groups, inclusion/exclusion criteria, influencing factors, and outcome measures. Some of the data for analysis were abstracted by a biostatistician and checked by a physician reviewer. A sequential resolution strategy was used to match and resolve the screening and review results of the 2 pediatrician reviewers.

For the assessment of treatment efficacy, pooled analyses were performed for comparisons for which 3 or more trials could be identified. Studies eligible for analyses of questions pertaining to treatment efficacy were grouped for comparisons by treatment options. Each comparison consisted of studies that were considered homogeneous across clinical practice. Because some of the key questions were addressed in the 2001 evidence report,[17] studies identified in that report were included with newly identified articles in the 2010 evidence report.[20]

Decisions were made on the basis of a systematic grading of the quality of evidence and strength of recommendations as well as expert consensus when

definitive data were not available. Results of the literature review were presented in evidence tables and published in the final evidence report.[20]

In June 2009, the AAP convened a new subcommittee to review and revise the May 2004 AOM guideline.[1] The subcommittee comprised primary care physicians and experts in the fields of pediatrics, family practice, otolaryngology, epidemiology, infectious disease, emergency medicine, and guideline methodology. All panel members reviewed the AAP policy on conflict of interest and voluntary disclosure and were given an opportunity to present any potential conflicts with the subcommittee's work. All potential conflicts of interest are listed at the end of this document. The project was funded by the AAP. New literature on OM is continually being published. Although the systematic review performed by AHRQ could not be replicated with new literature, members of the Subcommittee on Diagnosis and Management of Acute Otitis Media reviewed additional articles. PubMed was searched by using the single search term "acute otitis media," approximately every 6 months from June 2009 through October 2011 to obtain new articles. Subcommittee members evaluated pertinent articles for quality of methodology and importance of results. Selected articles used in the AHRQ review were also reevaluated for their quality. Conclusions were based on the consensus of the subcommittee after the review of newer literature and reevaluation of the AHRQ evidence. Key action statements were generated using BRIDGE-Wiz (Building Recommendations in a Developers Guideline Editor), an interactive software tool that leads guideline development through a series of questions that are intended to create a more actionable set of key action statements.[25] BRIDGE-Wiz also incorporates the quality of available evidence into the final determination of the strength of each recommendation.

After thorough review by the subcommittee for this guideline, a draft was reviewed by other AAP committees and sections, selected outside organizations, and individuals identified by the subcommittee as experts in the field. Additionally, members of the subcommittee were encouraged to distribute the draft to interested parties in their respective specialties. All comments were reviewed by the writing group and incorporated into the final guideline when appropriate.

This clinical practice guideline is not intended as a sole source of guidance in the management of children with AOM. Rather, it is intended to assist clinicians in decision-making. It is not intended to replace clinical judgment or establish a protocol for the care of all children with this condition. These recommendations may not provide the only appropriate approach to the management of children with AOM.

It is AAP policy to review and update evidence-based guidelines every 5 years.

KEY ACTION STATEMENTS
Key Action Statement 1A

Clinicians should diagnose AOM in children who present with moderate to severe bulging of the TM *or* new onset of otorrhea not due to acute otitis externa. (Evidence Quality: Grade B, Rec. Strength: Recommendation)

Key Action Statement Profile: KAS 1A

Aggregate evidence quality	Grade B
Benefits	• Identify a population of children most likely to benefit from intervention. • Avoid unnecessary treatment of those without highly certain AOM. • Promote consistency in diagnosis.
Risks, harms, cost	May miss AOM that presents with a combination of mild bulging, intense erythema, or otalgia that may not necessarily represent less severe disease and may also benefit from intervention.
Benefits-harms assessment	Preponderance of benefit.
Value judgments	Identification of a population of children with highly certain AOM is beneficial. Accurate, specific diagnosis is helpful to the individual patient. Modification of current behavior of overdiagnosis is a goal. Increased specificity is preferred even as sensitivity is lowered.
Intentional vagueness	By using stringent diagnostic criteria, the TM appearance of less severe illness that might be early AOM has not been addressed.
Role of patient preferences	None
Exclusions	None
Strength	**Recommendation**
Notes	Tympanocentesis studies confirm that using these diagnostic findings leads to high levels of isolation of pathogenic bacteria. Evidence is extrapolated from treatment studies that included tympanocentesis.

Key Action Statement 1B

Clinicians should diagnose AOM in children who present with mild bulging of the TM *and* recent (less than 48 hours) onset of ear pain (holding, tugging, rubbing of the ear in a nonverbal child) or intense erythema of the TM. (Evidence Quality: Grade C, Rec. Strength: Recommendation)

Key Action Statement Profile: KAS 1B

Aggregate evidence quality	Grade C
Benefits	Identify AOM in children when the diagnosis is not highly certain.
Risks, harms, cost	Overdiagnosis of AOM. Reduced precision in diagnosis.
Benefits-harms assessment	Benefits greater than harms.
Value judgments	None.
Intentional vagueness	Criteria may be more subjective.
Role of patient preferences	None
Exclusions	None
Strength	**Recommendation**
Notes	Recent onset of ear pain means within the past 48 hours.

Key Action Statement 1C

Clinicians should not diagnose AOM in children who do not have MEE (based on pneumatic otoscopy and/or tympanometry). (Evidence Quality: Grade B, Rec. Strength: Recommendation)

Key Action Statement Profile: KAS 1C

Aggregate evidence quality	Grade B
Benefits	Reduces overdiagnosis and unnecessary treatment. Increases correct diagnosis of other conditions with symptoms that otherwise might be attributed to AOM. Promotes the use of pneumatic otoscopy and tympanometry to improve diagnostic accuracy.
Risks, harms, cost	Cost of tympanometry. Need to acquire or reacquire skills in pneumatic otoscopy and tympanometry for some clinicians.
Benefits-harms assessment	Preponderance of benefit.
Value judgments	AOM is overdiagnosed, often without adequate visualization of the TM. Early AOM without effusion occurs, but the risk of overdiagnosis supersedes that concern.
Intentional vagueness	None
Role of patient preferences	None
Exclusions	Early AOM evidenced by intense erythema of the TM.
Strength	**Recommendation**

Purpose of This Section

There is no gold standard for the diagnosis of AOM. In fact, AOM has a spectrum of signs as the disease develops.[26] Therefore, the purpose of this section is to provide clinicians and researchers with a working clinical definition of AOM and to differentiate AOM from OME. The criteria were chosen to achieve high specificity recognizing that the resulting decreased sensitivity may exclude less severe presentations of AOM.

Changes From AAP/AAFP 2004 AOM Guideline

Accurate diagnosis of AOM is critical to sound clinical decision-making and high-quality research. The 2004 "Clinical Practice Guideline: Diagnosis and Management of AOM"[1] used a 3-part definition for AOM: (1) acute onset of symptoms, (2) presence of MEE, and (3) signs of acute middle ear inflammation. This definition generated extensive discussion and reanalysis of the AOM diagnostic evidence. The 2004 definition lacked precision to exclude cases of OME, and diagnoses of AOM

could be made in children with acute onset of symptoms, including severe otalgia and MEE, without other otoscopic findings of inflammation.[27] Furthermore, the use of "uncertain diagnosis" in the 2004 AOM guideline may have permitted diagnoses of AOM without clear visualization of the TM. Earlier studies may have enrolled children who had OME rather than AOM, resulting in the possible classification of such children as improved because their nonspecific symptoms would have abated regardless of therapy.[28–30] Two studies, published in 2011, used stringent diagnostic criteria for diagnosing AOM with much less risk of conclusions based on data from mixed patients.[31,32]

Since publication of the 2004 AOM guideline, a number of studies have been conducted evaluating scales for the presence of symptoms. These studies did not show a consistent correlation of symptoms with the initial diagnosis of AOM, especially in preverbal children.[33–35]

Recent research has used precisely stated stringent criteria of AOM for

purposes of the studies.[31,32] The current guideline endorses stringent otoscopic diagnostic criteria as a basis for management decisions (described later). As clinicians use the proposed stringent criteria to diagnose AOM, they should be aware that children with AOM may also present with recent onset of ear pain and intense erythema of the TM as the only otoscopic finding.

Symptoms

Older children with AOM usually present with a history of rapid onset of ear pain. However, in young preverbal children, otalgia as suggested by tugging/rubbing/holding of the ear, excessive crying, fever, or changes in the child's sleep or behavior pattern as noted by the parent are often relatively nonspecific symptoms. A number of studies have attempted to correlate symptom scores with diagnoses of AOM.

A systematic review[36] identified 4 articles that evaluated the accuracy of symptoms.[37–40] Ear pain appeared useful in diagnosing AOM (combined positive likelihood ratio 3.0–7.3, negative likelihood ratio 0.4–0.6); however, it was only present in 50% to 60% of children with AOM. Conclusions from these studies may be limited, because they (1) enrolled children seen by specialists, not likely to represent the whole spectrum of severity of illness; (2) used a clinical diagnosis of AOM based more on symptomatology rather than on tympanocentesis; and (3) included relatively older children.[37,40]

Laine et al[34] used a questionnaire administered to 469 parents who suspected their children, aged 6 to 35 months, had AOM. Of the children, 237 had AOM using strict otoscopic criteria, and 232 had upper respiratory tract infection without AOM. Restless sleep, ear rubbing, fever, and nonspecific respiratory or gastrointestinal tract symptoms did not differentiate children with or without AOM.

McCormick et al[30] used 2 symptom scores—a 3-item score (OM-3), consisting of symptoms of physical suffering such as ear pain or fever, emotional distress (irritability, poor appetite), and limitation in activity; and a 5-item score (Ear Treatment Group Symptom Questionnaire, 5 Items [ETG-5]), including fever, earache, irritability, decreased appetite, and sleep disturbance—to assess AOM symptoms at the time of diagnosis and daily during the 10-day treatment or observation period. They found both to be a responsive measure of changes in clinical symptoms. The same group[35] also tested a visual scale, Acute Otitis Media-Faces Scale (AOM-FS), with faces similar to the Wong-Baker pain scale.[41] None of the scales were adequately sensitive for making the diagnosis of AOM based on symptoms. The AOM-FS combined with an otoscopy score, OS-8,[30] were presented as a double-sided pocket card. The combination of AOM-FS and OS-8 was more responsive to change than either instrument alone.

Shaikh et al[33,42] validated a 7-item parent-reported symptom score (Acute Otitis Media Severity of Symptom Scale [AOM-SOS]) for children with AOM, following stringent guidance of the US Food and Drug Administration (FDA) on the development of patient-reported outcome scales. Symptoms included ear tugging/rubbing/holding, excessive crying, irritability, difficulty sleeping, decreased activity or appetite, and fever. AOM-SOS was correlated with otoscopic diagnoses (AOM, OME, and normal middle ear status). AOM-SOS changed appropriately in response to clinical change. Its day-to-day responsiveness supports its usefulness in following AOM symptoms over time.

Signs of AOM

Few studies have evaluated the relationship of otoscopic findings in AOM

and tympanocentesis. A study by Karma et al[43] is often cited as the best single study of otoscopic findings in AOM. However, the study uses only a symptom-based diagnosis of AOM plus the presence of MEE. Thus, children with acute upper respiratory tract infection symptoms and OME would have been considered to have AOM. There also were significant differences in findings at the 2 centers that participated in the study.

The investigators correlated TM color, mobility, and position with the presence of middle ear fluid obtained by tympanocentesis. At 2 sites in Finland (Tampere and Oulu), 2911 children were followed from 6 months to 2.5 years of age. A single otolaryngologist at Tampere and a single pediatrician at Oulu examined subjects. Color, position, and mobility were recorded. Myringotomy and aspiration were performed if MEE was suspected. AOM was diagnosed if MEE was found and the child had fever, earache, irritability, ear rubbing or tugging, simultaneous other acute respiratory tract symptoms, vomiting, or diarrhea. The presence or absence of MEE was noted, but no analyses of the fluid, including culture, were performed. Pneumatic otoscopic findings were classified as follows: color—hemorrhagic, strongly red, moderately red, cloudy or dull, slightly red, or normal; position—bulging, retracted, or normal; and mobility—distinctly impaired, slightly impaired, or normal.

For this analysis, 11 804 visits were available. For visits with acute symptoms, MEE was found in 84.9% and 81.8% at the 2 sites at which the study was performed. There were significant differences among the results at the 2 centers involved in the study. Table 2 shows specific data for each finding.

The combination of a "cloudy," bulging TM with impaired mobility was the

TABLE 2 Otoscopic Findings in Children With Acute Symptoms and MEE[a]

TM Finding in Acute Visits With MEE	Group I (Tampere, Finland), %	Group II (Oulu, Finland), %
Color		
Distinctly red	69.8	65.6
Hemorrhagic	81.3	62.9
Strongly red	87.7	68.1
Moderately red	59.8	66.0
Slightly red	39.4	16.7
Cloudy	95.7	80.0
Normal	1.7	4.9
Position		
Bulging	96.0	89
Retracted	46.8	48.6
Normal	32.1	22.2
Mobility		
Distinctly impaired	94.0	78.5
Slightly impaired	59.7	32.8
Normal	2.7	4.8

[a] Totals are greater than 100%, because each ear may have had different findings.[43]

best predictor of AOM using the symptom-based diagnosis in this study. Impaired mobility had the highest sensitivity and specificity (approximately 95% and 85%, respectively). Cloudiness had the next best combination of high sensitivity (~74%) and high specificity (~93%) in this study. Bulging had high specificity (~97%) but lower sensitivity (~51%). A TM that was hemorrhagic, strongly red, or moderately red also correlated with the presence of AOM, and a TM that was only "slightly red" was not helpful diagnostically.

McCormick et al reported that a bulging TM was highly associated with the presence of a bacterial pathogen, with or without a concomitant viral pathogen.[44] In a small study, 31 children (40 ears) underwent myringotomy.[45] Bulging TMs had positive bacterial cultures 75% of the time. The percentage of positive cultures for a pathogen increased to 80% if the color of the TM was yellow. The conclusion is that moderate to severe bulging of the TM represents the most important characteristic in the diagnosis of AOM—a finding that has implications for clinical care, research, and education.

The committee recognized that there is a progression from the presence of MEE to the bulging of the TM, and it is often difficult to differentiate this equivocal appearance from the highly certain AOM criteria advocated in this guideline.[26] As such, there is a role for individualized diagnosis and management decisions. Examples of normal, mild bulging, moderate bulging, and severe bulging can be seen in Fig 2.

Distinguishing AOM From OME

OME may occur either as the aftermath of an episode of AOM or as a consequence of eustachian tube dysfunction attributable to an upper respiratory tract infection.[46] However, OME may also precede and predispose to the development of AOM. These 2 forms of OM may be considered segments of a disease continuum.[47] However, because OME does not represent an acute infectious process that benefits from antibiotics, it is of utmost importance for clinicians to become proficient in distinguishing normal middle ear status from OME or AOM. Doing so will avoid unnecessary use of antibiotics, which leads to increased adverse effects of medication and facilitates the development of antimicrobial resistance.

Examination of the TM

Accurate diagnosis of AOM in infants and young children may be difficult.

Symptoms may be mild or overlap with those of an upper respiratory tract illness. The TM may be obscured by cerumen, and subtle changes in the TM may be difficult to discern. Additional factors complicating diagnosis may include lack of cooperation from the child; less than optimal diagnostic equipment, including lack of a pneumatic bulb; inadequate instruments for clearing cerumen from the external auditory canal; inadequate assistance for restraining the child; and lack of experience in removing cerumen and performing pneumatic otoscopy.

The pneumatic otoscope is the standard tool used in diagnosing OM. Valuable also is a surgical head, which greatly facilitates cleaning cerumen from an infant's external auditory canal. Cerumen may be removed by using a curette, gentle suction, or irrigation.[48] The pneumatic otoscope should have a light source of sufficient brightness and an air-tight seal that permits application of positive and negative pressure. In general, nondisposable specula achieve a better seal with less pain because of a thicker, smoother edge and better light transmission properties. The speculum size should be chosen to gently seal at the outer portion of the external auditory canal.

Pneumatic otoscopy permits assessment of the contour of the TM (normal, retracted, full, bulging), its color (gray, yellow, pink, amber, white, red, blue), its translucency (translucent, semiopaque, opaque), and its mobility (normal, increased, decreased, absent). The normal TM is translucent, pearly gray, and has a ground-glass appearance (Fig 2A). Specific landmarks can be visualized. They include the short process and the manubrium of the malleus and the pars flaccida, located superiorly. These are easily observed and help to identify the position of the TM. Inward movement of the TM on positive pressure in the external canal and outward movement on negative pressure should occur, especially in the superior posterior quadrant. When the TM is retracted, the short process of the malleus becomes more prominent, and the manubrium appears shortened because of its change in position within the middle ear. Inward motion occurring with positive pressure is restricted or absent, because the TM is frequently as far inward as its range of motion allows. However, outward mobility can be visualized when negative pressure is applied. If the TM does not move perceptibly with applications of gentle positive or negative pressure, MEE is likely. Sometimes, the application of pressure will make an air-fluid interface behind the TM (which is diagnostic of MEE) more evident.[49]

Instruction in the proper evaluation of the child's middle ear status should begin with the first pediatric rotation in medical school and continue throughout postgraduate training.[50]

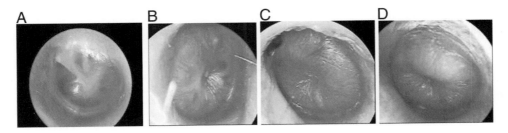

FIGURE 2
A, Normal TM. B, TM with mild bulging. C, TM with moderate bulging. D, TM with severe bulging. Courtesy of Alejandro Hoberman, MD.

Continuing medical education should reinforce the importance of, and retrain the clinician in, the use of pneumatic otoscopy.[51] Training tools include the use of a video-otoscope in residency programs, the use of Web-based educational resources,[49,52] as well as simultaneous or sequential examination of TMs with an expert otoscopist to validate findings by using a double headed or video otoscope. Tools for learning the ear examination can be found in a CD distributed by the Johns Hopkins University School of Medicine and the Institute for Johns

Hopkins Nursing,[53] also available at http://www2.aap.org/sections/infectdis/video.cfm,[54] and through a Web-based program, ePROM: Enhancing Proficiency in Otitis Media.[52]

Key Action Statement 2

The management of AOM should include an assessment of pain. If pain is present, the clinician should recommend treatment to reduce pain. (Evidence Quality: Grade B, Rec. Strength: Strong Recommendation)

with AOM can be substantial in the first few days of illness and often persists longer in young children.[57] Antibiotic therapy of AOM does not provide symptomatic relief in the first 24 hours[58–61] and even after 3 to 7 days, there may be persistent pain, fever, or both in 30% of children younger than 2 years.[62] In contrast, analgesics do relieve pain associated with AOM within 24 hours[63] and should be used whether antibiotic therapy is or is not prescribed; they should be continued as long as needed. The AAP published the policy statement "The Assessment and Management of Acute Pain in Infants, Children, and Adolescents"[64] to assist the clinician in addressing pain in the context of illness. The management of pain, especially during the first 24 hours of an episode of AOM, should be addressed regardless of the use of antibiotics.

Various treatments of otalgia have been used, but none has been well studied. The clinician should select a treatment on the basis of a consideration of benefits and risks and, wherever possible, incorporate parent/caregiver and patient preference (Table 3).

Key Action Statement Profile: KAS 2

Aggregate evidence quality	Grade B
Benefits	Relieves the major symptom of AOM.
Risks, harms, cost	Potential medication adverse effects. Variable efficacy of some modes of treatment.
Benefits-harms assessment	Preponderance of benefit.
Value judgments	Treating pain is essential whether or not antibiotics are prescribed.
Intentional vagueness	Choice of analgesic is not specified.
Role of patient preferences	Parents may assist in the decision as to what means of pain relief they prefer.
Exclusions	Topical analgesics in the presence of a perforated TM.
Strength	**Strong Recommendation**

Purpose of This Section

Pain is the major symptom of AOM. This section addresses and updates the literature on treating otalgia.

Changes From AAP/AAFP 2004 AOM Guideline

Only 2 new articles directly address the treatment of otalgia. Both address topical treatment. The 2 new articles are consistent with the 2004 guideline statement. The text of the 2004 guideline is, therefore, reproduced here, with the addition of discussion of the 2 new articles. Table 3 has been updated to include the new references.

Treatment of Otalgia

Many episodes of AOM are associated with pain.[55] Some children with OME also have ear pain. Although pain is

a common symptom in these illnesses, clinicians often see otalgia as a peripheral concern not requiring direct attention.[56] Pain associated

TABLE 3 Treatments for Otalgia in AOM

Treatment Modality	Comments
Acetaminophen, ibuprofen[63]	Effective analgesia for mild to moderate pain. Readily available. Mainstay of pain management for AOM.
Home remedies (no controlled studies that directly address effectiveness) Distraction External application of heat or cold Oil drops in external auditory canal	May have limited effectiveness.
Topical agents	
Benzocaine, procaine, lidocaine[65,67,70]	Additional, but brief, benefit over acetaminophen in patients older than 5 y.
Naturopathic agents[68]	Comparable to amethocaine/phenazone drops in patients older than 6 y.
Homeopathic agents[71,72]	No controlled studies that directly address pain.
Narcotic analgesia with codeine or analogs	Effective for moderate or severe pain. Requires prescription; risk of respiratory depression, altered mental status, gastrointestinal tract upset, and constipation.
Tympanostomy/myringotomy[73]	Requires skill and entails potential risk.

Since the 2004 guideline was published, there have been only 2 significant new articles.

Bolt et al reported in 2008 on a double-blind placebo-controlled trial at the Australia Children's Hospital emergency department conducted in 2003–2004.[65] They used a convenience sample of children 3 to 17 years of age diagnosed with AOM in the ED. They excluded children with perforation of the TM, pressure-equalizing tube, allergy to local anesthetic or paracetamol, epilepsy, or liver, renal, or cardiac disease. Sixty-three eligible children were randomized to receive aqueous lidocaine or normal saline ear drops up to 3 times in 24 hours. They demonstrated a statistically significant 50% reduction in reported pain at 10 and 30 minutes but not at 20 minutes after application of topical lidocaine, compared with normal saline. Complications were minimal: 3 children reported some dizziness the next day, and none reported tinnitus. A limitation was that some children had received oral acetaminophen before administration of ear drops.

A Cochrane review of topical analgesia for AOM[66] searched the Cochrane register of controlled trials, randomized controlled trials, or quasi-randomized controlled trials that compared otic preparations to placebo or that compared 2 otic preparations. It included studies of adults and children, without TM perforation.

It identified 5 trials in children 3 to 18 years of age. Two (including Bolt et al,[65] discussed above) compared anesthetic drops and placebo at diagnosis of AOM. In both studies, some children also received oral analgesics. Three studies compared anesthetic ear drops with naturopathic herbal drops. Naturopathic drops were favored 15 to 30 minutes after installation, and 1 to 3 days after diagnosis, but the difference was not statistically significant. The Cochrane group concluded that there is limited evidence that ear drops are effective at 30 minutes and unclear if results from these studies are a result of the natural course of illness, placebo effect of receiving treatment, soothing effect of any liquid in the ear, or the drops themselves. Three of the studies included in this review were cited in the 2004 AAP guideline[67–69] and the 1 new paper by Bolt et al.[65]

Key Action Statement 3A

Severe AOM

The clinician should prescribe antibiotic therapy for AOM (bilateral or unilateral) in children 6 months and older with severe signs or symptoms (ie, moderate or severe otalgia or otalgia for at least 48 hours, or temperature 39°C [102.2°F] or higher). (Evidence Quality: Grade B, Rec. Strength: Strong Recommendation)

Key Action Statement Profile: KAS 3A

Aggregate evidence quality	Grade B
Benefits	Increased likelihood of more rapid resolution of symptoms. Increased likelihood of resolution of AOM.
Risks, harms, cost	Adverse events attributable to antibiotics, such as diarrhea, diaper dermatitis, and allergic reactions. Overuse of antibiotics leads to increased bacterial resistance. Cost of antibiotics.
Benefits-harms assessment	Preponderance of benefit over harm.
Value judgments	None
Role of patient preference	None
Intentional vagueness	None
Exclusions	None
Strength	**Strong Recommendation**

Key Action Statement 3B

Nonsevere Bilateral AOM in Young Children

The clinician should prescribe antibiotic therapy for bilateral AOM in children younger than 24 months without severe signs or symptoms (ie, mild otalgia for less than 48 hours, temperature less than 39°C [102.2°F]). (Evidence Quality: Grade B, Rec. Strength: Recommendation)

Key Action Statement Profile: KAS 3B

Aggregate evidence quality	Grade B
Benefits	Increased likelihood of more rapid resolution of symptoms. Increased likelihood of resolution of AOM.
Risks, harms, cost	Adverse events attributable to antibiotics, such as diarrhea, diaper dermatitis, and allergic reactions. Overuse of antibiotics leads to increased bacterial resistance. Cost of antibiotics.
Benefits-harms assessment	Preponderance of benefit over harm.
Value judgments	None
Role of patient preference	None
Intentional vagueness	None
Exclusions	None
Strength	**Recommendation**

Key Action Statement 3C

Nonsevere Unilateral AOM in Young Children

The clinician should either prescribe antibiotic therapy or offer observation with close follow-up based on joint decision-making with the parent(s)/caregiver for unilateral AOM in children 6 months to 23 months of age without severe signs or symptoms (ie, mild otalgia for less than 48 hours, temperature less than 39°C [102.2°F]). When observation is used, a mechanism must be in place to ensure

follow-up and begin antibiotic therapy if the child worsens or fails to improve within 48 to 72 hours of onset of symptoms. (Evidence Quality: Grade B, Rec. Strength: Recommendation)

Key Action Statement Profile: KAS 3C

Aggregate evidence quality	Grade B
Benefits	Moderately increased likelihood of more rapid resolution of symptoms with initial antibiotics. Moderately increased likelihood of resolution of AOM with initial antibiotics.
Risks, harms, cost	Adverse events attributable to antibiotics, such as diarrhea, diaper dermatitis, and allergic reactions. Overuse of antibiotics leads to increased bacterial resistance. Cost of antibiotics.
Benefits-harms assessment	Moderate degree of benefit over harm.
Value judgments	Observation becomes an alternative as the benefits and harms approach balance.
Role of patient preference	Joint decision-making with the family is essential before choosing observation.
Intentional vagueness	Joint decision-making is highly variable from family to family
Exclusions	None
Strength	**Recommendation**
Note	In the judgment of 1 Subcommittee member (AH), antimicrobial treatment of these children is preferred because of a preponderance of benefit over harm. AH did not endorse Key Action Statement 3C

Key Action Statement 3D

Nonsevere AOM in Older Children

The clinician should either prescribe antibiotic therapy *or* offer observation with close follow-up based on joint decision-making with the parent(s)/caregiver for AOM (bilateral or unilateral) in children 24 months or older without severe signs or symptoms (ie, mild otalgia for less than 48 hours, temperature less than 39°C [102.2°F]). When observation is used, a mechanism must be in place to ensure follow-up and begin antibiotic therapy if the child worsens or fails to improve within 48 to 72 hours of onset of symptoms. (Evidence Quality: Grade B, Rec Strength: Recommendation)

Key Action Statement Profile: KAS 3D

Aggregate evidence quality	Grade B
Benefits	*Initial antibiotic treatment*: Slightly increased likelihood of more rapid resolution of symptoms; slightly increased likelihood of resolution of AOM. *Initial observation*: Decreased use of antibiotics; decreased adverse effects of antibiotics; decreased potential for development of bacterial resistance.
Risks, harms, cost	*Initial antibiotic treatment*: Adverse events attributable to antibiotics such as diarrhea, rashes, and allergic reactions. Overuse of antibiotics leads to increased bacterial resistance. *Initial observation*: Possibility of needing to start antibiotics in 48 to 72 h if the patient continues to have symptoms. Minimal risk of adverse consequences of delayed antibiotic treatment. Potential increased phone calls and doctor visits.
Benefits-harms assessment	Slight degree of benefit of initial antibiotics over harm.
Value judgments	Observation is an option as the benefits and harms approach balance.
Role of patient preference	Joint decision-making with the family is essential before choosing observation.
Intentional vagueness	Joint decision-making is highly variable from family to family.
Exclusions	None
Strength	**Recommendation.**

Purpose of This Section

The purpose of this section is to offer guidance on the initial management of AOM by helping clinicians choose between the following 2 strategies:

1. *Initial antibiotic therapy*, defined as treatment of AOM with antibiotics that are prescribed at the time of diagnosis with the intent of starting antibiotic therapy as soon as possible after the encounter.

2. *Initial observation*, defined as initial management of AOM limited to symptomatic relief, with commencement of antibiotic therapy only if the child's condition worsens at any time or does not show clinical improvement within 48 to 72 hours of diagnosis. A mechanism must be in place to ensure follow-up and initiation of antibiotics if the child fails observation.

This section assumes that the clinician has made an accurate diagnosis of AOM by using the criteria and strategies outlined earlier in this guideline. Another assumption is that a clear distinction is made between the role of analgesics and antibiotics in providing symptomatic relief for children with AOM.

Changes From Previous AOM Guideline

The AOM guideline published by the AAP and AAFP in 2004 proposed, for the first time in North America, an "observation option" for selected children with AOM, building on successful implementation of a similar policy in the state of New York[74] and the use of a similar paradigm in many countries in Europe. A common feature of both approaches was to prioritize initial antibiotic therapy according to diagnostic certainty, with greater reliance on observation when the diagnosis was uncertain. In response to criticism that allowing an "uncertain diagnosis" might condone incomplete visualization of the TM or allow inappropriate antibiotic use, this category has been eliminated with greater emphasis now placed on maximizing diagnostic accuracy for AOM.

Since the earlier AOM guideline was published, there has been substantial new research on initial management of AOM, including randomized controlled trials of antibiotic therapy versus placebo or no therapy,[31,32,75] immediate versus delayed antibiotic therapy,[30,76,77] or delayed antibiotic with or without a concurrent prescription.[78] The Hoberman and Tähtinen articles are especially important as they used stringent criteria for diagnosing AOM.[31,32] Systematic reviews have been published on delayed antibiotic therapy,[79] the natural history of AOM in untreated children,[57] predictive factors for antibiotic benefits,[62] and the effect of antibiotics on asymptomatic MEE after therapy.[80] Observational studies provide additional data on outcomes of initial observation with delayed antibiotic therapy, if needed,[81] and on the relationship of previous antibiotic therapy for AOM to subsequent acute mastoiditis.[82,83]

In contrast to the earlier AOM guideline,[1] which recommended antibiotic therapy for all children 6 months to 2 years of age with a certain diagnosis,

the current guideline indicates a choice between initial antibiotic therapy or initial observation in this age group for children with unilateral AOM and mild symptoms but only after joint decision-making with the parent(s)/caregiver (Table 4). This change is supported by evidence on the safety of observation or delayed prescribing in young children.[30,31,32,75,76,81] A mechanism must be in place to ensure follow-up and begin antibiotics if the child fails observation.

Importance of Accurate Diagnosis

The recommendations for management of AOM assume an accurate diagnosis on the basis of criteria outlined in the diagnosis section of this guideline. Many of the studies since the 2004 AAP/AAFP AOM guideline[1] used more stringent and well-defined AOM diagnostic definitions than were previously used. Bulging of the TM was required for diagnosis of AOM for most of the children enrolled in the most recent studies.[31,32] By using the criteria in this guideline, clinicians will more accurately distinguish AOM from OME. The management of OME can be found in guidelines written by the AAP, AAFP, and American Academy of Otolaryngology–Head and Neck Surgery.[84,85]

Age, Severity of Symptoms, Otorrhea, and Laterality

Rovers et al[62] performed a systematic search for AOM trials that (1) used random allocation of children, (2) included children 0 to 12 years of age with AOM, (3) compared antibiotics with placebo or no treatment, and (4) had pain or fever as an outcome. The original investigators were asked for their original data.

Primary outcome was pain and/or fever (>38°C) at 3 to 7 days. The adverse effects of antibiotics were also analyzed. Baseline predictors were age <2 years versus ≥2 years, bilateral AOM versus unilateral AOM, and the presence versus absence of otorrhea. Statistical methods were used to assess heterogeneity and to analyze the data.

Of the 10 eligible studies, the investigators of 6 studies[30,75,86–89] provided the original data requested, and 4 did not. A total of 1642 patients were included in the 6 studies from which data were obtained. Of the cases submitted, the average age was 3 to 4 years, with 35% of children younger than 2 years. Bilateral AOM was present in 34% of children, and 42% of children had a bulging TM. Otorrhea was present in 21% of children. The antibiotic and control groups were comparable for all characteristics.

The rate difference (RD) for pain, fever, or both between antibiotic and control groups was 13% (NNT = 8). For children younger than 2 years, the RD was 15% (NNT = 7); for those ≥2 years, RD was 11% (NNT = 10). For unilateral AOM, the RD was 6% (NNT = 17); for bilateral AOM, the RD was 20% (NNT = 5). When unilateral AOM was broken into age groups, among those younger than 2 years, the RD was 5% (NNT = 20), and among those ≥2 years, the RD was 7% (NNT = 15). For bilateral AOM in children younger than 2 years, the RD was 25% (NNT = 4); for

TABLE 4 Recommendations for Initial Management for Uncomplicated AOM[a]

Age	Otorrhea With AOM[a]	Unilateral or Bilateral AOM[a] With Severe Symptoms[b]	Bilateral AOM[a] Without Otorrhea	Unilateral AOM[a] Without Otorrhea
6 mo to 2 y	Antibiotic therapy	Antibiotic therapy	Antibiotic therapy	Antibiotic therapy or additional observation
≥2 y	Antibiotic therapy	Antibiotic therapy	Antibiotic therapy or additional observation	Antibiotic therapy or additional observation[c]

[a] Applies only to children with well-documented AOM with high certainty of diagnosis (see Diagnosis section).

[b] A toxic-appearing child, persistent otalgia more than 48 h, temperature ≥39°C (102.2°F) in the past 48 h, or if there is uncertain access to follow-up after the visit.

[c] This plan of initial management provides an opportunity for shared decision-making with the child's family for those categories appropriate for additional observation. If observation is offered, a mechanism must be in place to ensure follow-up and begin antibiotics if the child worsens or fails to improve within 48 to 72 h of AOM onset.

bilateral AOM in children ≥2 years, the RD was 12% (NNT = 9). For otorrhea, the RD was 36% (NNT = 3). One child in the control group who developed meningitis had received antibiotics beginning on day 2 because of worsening status. There were no cases of mastoiditis.

In a Cochrane Review, Sanders et al[59] identified 10 studies that met the following criteria: (1) randomized controlled trial, (2) compared antibiotic versus placebo or antibiotic versus observation, (3) age 1 month to 15 years, (4) reported severity and duration of pain, (5) reported adverse events, and (6) reported serious complications of AOM, recurrent attacks, and hearing problems. Studies were analyzed for risk of bias and assessment of heterogeneity. The studies were the same as analyzed by Rovers et al[62] but included the 4 studies for which primary data were not available to Rovers.[60,61,90,91]

The authors' conclusions were that antibiotics produced a small reduction in the number of children with pain 2 to 7 days after diagnosis. They also concluded that most cases spontaneously remitted with no complications (NNT = 16). Antibiotics were most beneficial in children younger than 2 years with bilateral AOM and in children with otorrhea.

Two recent studies only included children younger than 3 years[32] or younger than 2 years.[31] Both included only subjects in whom the diagnosis of AOM was certain. Both studies used improvement of symptoms and improvement in the appearance of the TM in their definitions of clinical success or failure.

Hoberman et al[31] conducted a randomized, double-blind, placebo-controlled study of the efficacy of antimicrobial treatment on AOM. The criteria for AOM were acute symptoms with a score of at least 3 on the AOM-SOS,

a validated symptom scale[33,92]; MEE; and moderate or marked bulging of the TM or slight bulging accompanied by either otalgia or marked erythema of the TM. They chose to use high-dose amoxicillin-clavulanate (90 mg/kg/day) as active treatment, because it has the best oral antibiotic coverage for organisms causing AOM. Included in the study were 291 patients 6 to 23 months of age: 144 in the antibiotic group and 147 in the placebo group. The primary outcome measures were the time to resolution of symptoms and the symptom burden over time. The initial resolution of symptoms (ie, the first recording of an AOM-SOS score of 0 or 1) was recorded among the children who received amoxicillin-clavulanate in 35% by day 2, 61% by day 4, and 80% by day 7. Among children who received placebo, an AOM-SOS score of 0 or 1 was recorded in 28% by day 2, 54% by day 4, and 74% by day 7 (P = .14 for the overall comparison). For sustained resolution of symptoms (ie, the time to the second of 2 successive recordings of an AOM-SOS score of 0 or 1), the corresponding values were 20% at day 2, 41% at day 4, and 67% at day 7 with amoxicillin-clavulanate, compared with 14%, 36%, and 53% with placebo (P = .04 for the overall comparison). The symptom burden (ie, mean AOM-SOS scores) over the first 7 days were lower for the children treated with amoxicillin-clavulanate than for those who received placebo (P = .02). Clinical failure at or before the 4- to 5-day visit was defined as "either a lack of substantial improvement in symptoms, a worsening of signs on otoscopic examination, or both," and clinical failure at the 10- to 12-day visit was defined as "the failure to achieve complete or nearly complete resolution of symptoms and of otoscopic signs, without regard to the persistence or resolution of middle ear

effusion." Treatment failure occurred by day 4 to 5 in 4% of the antimicrobial treatment group versus 23% in the placebo group (P < .001) and at day 10 to 12 in 16% of the antimicrobial treatment group versus 51% in the placebo group (NNT = 2.9, P < .001). In a comparison of outcome in unilateral versus bilateral AOM, clinical failure rates by day 10 to 12 in children with unilateral AOM were 9% in those treated with amoxicillin-clavulanate versus 41% in those treated with placebo (RD, 32%; NNT = 3) and 23% vs 60% (RD, 37%; NNT = 3) in those with bilateral AOM. Most common adverse events were diarrhea (25% vs 15% in the treatment versus placebo groups, respectively; P = .05) and diaper dermatitis (51% vs 35% in the treatment versus placebo groups, respectively; P = .008). One placebo recipient developed mastoiditis. According to these results, antimicrobial treatment of AOM was more beneficial than in previous studies that used less stringent diagnostic criteria.

Tähtinen et al[32] conducted a randomized, double-blind, placebo-controlled, intention-to-treat study of amoxicillin-clavulanate (40 mg/kg/day) versus placebo. Three hundred nineteen patients from 6 to 35 months of age were studied: 161 in the antibiotic group and 158 in the placebo group. AOM definition was the presence of MEE, distinct erythema over a bulging or yellow TM, and acute symptoms such as ear pain, fever, or respiratory symptoms. Compliance was measured by using daily patient diaries and number of capsules remaining at the end of the study. Primary outcome was time to treatment failure defined as a composite of 6 independent components: no improvement in overall condition by day 3, worsening of the child's condition at any time, no improvement in otoscopic signs by day 8, perforation of the TM, development of severe infection (eg, pneumonia, mastoiditis), and any other reason for stopping the study drug/ placebo.

Groups were comparable on multiple parameters. In the treatment group, 135 of 161 patients (84%) were younger than 24 months, and in the placebo group, 124 of 158 patients (78%) were younger than 24 months. Treatment failure occurred in 18.6% of the treatment group and 44.9% in the placebo group (NNT = 3.8, $P < .001$). Rescue treatment was needed in 6.8% of the treatment group and 33.5% of placebo patients ($P < .001$). Contralateral AOM developed in 8.2% and 18.6% of treatment and placebo groups, respectively ($P = .007$). There was no significant difference in use of analgesic or antipyretic medicine, which was used in 84.2% of the amoxicillin-clavulanate group and 85.9% of the placebo group.

Parents of child care attendees on placebo missed more days of work ($P = .005$). Clinical failure rates in children with unilateral AOM were 17.2% in those treated with amoxicillin-clavulanate versus 42.7% in those treated with placebo; for bilateral AOM, clinical failure rates were 21.7% for those treated with amoxicillin-clavulanate versus 46.3% in the placebo group. Reported rates of treatment failure by day 8 were 17.2% in the amoxicillin-clavulanate group versus 42.7% in the placebo group in children with unilateral AOM and 21.7% vs 46.3% among those with bilateral disease.

Adverse events, primarily diarrhea and/or rash, occurred in 52.8% of the treatment group and 36.1% of the placebo group ($P = .003$). Overall condition as evaluated by the parents and otoscopic appearance of the TM showed a benefit of antibiotics over placebo at the end of treatment visit ($P < .001$). Two placebo recipients developed a severe infection; 1 developed pneumococcal bacteremia, and 1 developed radiographically confirmed pneumonia.

Most studies have excluded children with severe illness and all exclude those with bacterial disease other than AOM (pneumonia, mastoiditis, meningitis, streptococcal pharyngitis). Kaleida et al[91] compared myringotomy alone with myringotomy plus antibiotics. Severe AOM was defined as temperature >39°C (102.2°F) or the presence of severe otalgia. Patients with severe AOM in the group that received only myringotomy (without initial antibiotics) had much worse outcomes.

Initial Antibiotic Therapy

The rationale for antibiotic therapy in children with AOM is based on a high prevalence of bacteria in the accompanying MEE.[93] Bacterial and viral cultures of middle ear fluid collected by tympanocentesis from children with AOM showed 55% with bacteria only and 15% with bacteria and viruses. A beneficial effect of antibiotics on AOM was first demonstrated in 1968,[94] followed by additional randomized trials and a meta-analysis[95] showing a 14% increase in absolute rates of clinical improvement. Systematic reviews of the literature published before 2011[21,59,62] revealed increases of clinical improvement with initial antibiotics of 6% to 12%.

Randomized clinical trials using stringent diagnostic criteria for AOM in young children[31,32] show differences in clinical improvement of 26% to 35% favoring initial antibiotic treatment as compared with placebo. Greater benefit of immediate antibiotic therapy was observed for bilateral AOM[62,96] or AOM associated with otorrhea.[62] In most randomized trials,[30,75,77,88,89] antibiotic therapy also decreased the duration of pain, analgesic use, or school absence and parent days missed from work.

Children younger than 2 years with AOM may take longer to improve clinically than older children,[57] and although they are more likely to benefit from antibiotics,[31,32] AOM in many children will resolve without antibiotics.[62] A clinically significant benefit of immediate antibiotic therapy is observed for bilateral AOM,[62,96] *Streptococcus pneumoniae* infection, or AOM associated with otorrhea.[62]

Initial Observation for AOM

In systematic reviews of studies that compare antibiotic therapy for AOM with placebo, a consistent finding has been the overall favorable natural history in control groups (NNT = 8–16).[12,59,62,95] However, randomized trials in these reviews had varying diagnostic criteria that would have permitted inclusion of some children with OME, viral upper respiratory infections, or myringitis, thereby limiting the ability to apply these findings to children with a highly certain AOM diagnosis. In more recent AOM studies[31,32] using stringent diagnostic criteria, approximately half of young children (younger than 2–3 years) experienced clinical success when given placebo, but the effect of antibiotic therapy was substantially greater than suggested by studies without precise diagnosis (NNT = 3–4).

Observation as initial management for AOM in properly selected children does not increase suppurative complications, provided that follow-up is ensured and a rescue antibiotic is given for persistent or worsening symptoms.[17] In contrast, withholding of antibiotics in all children with AOM, regardless of clinical course, would risk a return to the suppurative complications observed in the preantibiotic era. At the population level, antibiotics halve the risk of mastoiditis after AOM, but the high NNT of approximately 4800 patients to prevent 1 case of mastoiditis precludes a strategy of universal antibiotic therapy as a means to prevent mastoiditis.[83]

The favorable natural history of AOM makes it difficult to demonstrate significant differences in efficacy between antibiotic and placebo when a successful outcome is defined by relief or improvement of presenting signs and symptoms. In contrast, when otoscopic improvement (resolution of TM bulging, intense erythema, or both) is also required for a positive outcome,[31,32] the NNT is 3 to 4, compared with 8 to 16 for symptom improvement alone in older studies that used less precise diagnostic criteria. MEE, however, may persist for weeks or months after an AOM episode and is not a criterion for otoscopic failure.

National guidelines for initial observation of AOM in select children were first implemented in the Netherlands[97] and subsequently in Sweden,[98] Scotland,[99] the United States,[1] the United Kingdom,[100] and Italy.[101] All included observation as an initial treatment option under specified circumstances.

In numerous studies, only approximately one-third of children initially observed received a rescue antibiotic for persistent or worsening AOM,[30,32,76,81,89,102] suggesting that antibiotic use could potentially be reduced by 65% in eligible children. Given the high incidence of AOM, this reduction could help substantially in curtailing antibiotic-related adverse events.

McCormick et al[30] reported on 233 patients randomly assigned to receive immediate antibiotics (amoxicillin, 90 mg/kg/day) or to undergo watchful waiting. Criteria for inclusion were symptoms of ear infection, otoscopic evidence of AOM, and nonsevere AOM

based on a 3-item symptom score (OM-3) and TM appearance based on an 8-item scale (OS-8). Primary outcomes were parent satisfaction with AOM care, resolution of AOM symptoms after initial treatment, AOM failure and recurrence, and nasopharyngeal carriage of S pneumoniae strains resistant to antibiotics after treatment. The study was confounded by including patients who had received antibiotics in the previous 30 days.

In the watchful waiting group, 66% of children completed the study without antibiotics. There was no difference in parent satisfaction scores at day 12. A 5-item symptom score (ETG-5) was assessed at days 0 to 10 by using patient diaries. Subjects receiving immediate antibiotics resolved their symptoms faster than did subjects who underwent watchful waiting ($P = .004$). For children younger than 2 years, the difference was greater ($P = .008$). Otoscopic and tympanogram scores were also lower in the antibiotic group as opposed to the watchful waiting group ($P = .02$ for otoscopic score, $P = .004$ for tympanogram). Combining all ages, failure and recurrence rates were lower for the antibiotic group (5%) than for the watchful waiting group (21%) at 12 days. By day 30, there was no difference in failure or recurrence for the antibiotic and watchful waiting groups (23% and 24%, respectively). The association between clinical outcome and intervention group was not significantly different between age groups. Immediate antibiotics resulted in eradication of S pneumoniae carriage in the majority of children, but S pneumoniae strains cultured from children in the antibiotic group at day 12 were more likely to be multidrug resistant than were strains cultured from children in the watchful waiting group.

The decision not to give initial antibiotic treatment and observe should be

a joint decision of the clinician and the parents. In such cases, a system for close follow-up and a means of beginning antibiotics must be in place if symptoms worsen or no improvement is seen in 48 to 72 hours.

Initial observation of AOM should be part of a larger management strategy that includes analgesics, parent information, and provisions for a rescue antibiotic. Education of parents should include an explanation about the self-limited nature of most episodes of AOM, especially in children 2 years and older; the importance of pain management early in the course; and the potential adverse effects of antibiotics. Such an approach can substantially reduce prescription fill rates for rescue antibiotics.[103]

A critical component of any strategy involving initial observation for AOM is the ability to provide a rescue antibiotic if needed. This is often done by using a "safety net" or a "wait-and-see prescription,"[76,102] in which the parent/caregiver is given an antibiotic prescription during the clinical encounter but is instructed to fill the prescription only if the child fails to improve within 2 to 3 days or if symptoms worsen at any time. An alternative approach is not to provide a written prescription but to instruct the parent/caregiver to call or return if the child fails to improve within 2 to 3 days or if symptoms worsen.

In one of the first major studies of observation with a safety-net antibiotic prescription (SNAP), Siegel et al[102] enrolled 194 patients with protocol defined AOM, of whom 175 completed the study. Eligible patients were given a SNAP with instructions to fill the prescription only if symptoms worsened or did not improve in 48 hours. The SNAP was valid for 5 days. Pain medicine was recommended to be taken as needed. A phone interview was conducted 5 to 10 days after diagnosis.

One hundred twenty of 175 families did not fill the prescription. Reasons for filling the prescription (more than 1 reason per patient was acceptable) were as follows: continued pain, 23%; continued fever, 11%; sleep disruption, 6%; missed days of work, 3%; missed days of child care, 3%; and no reason given, 5%. One 16-month-old boy completed observation successfully but 6 weeks later developed AOM in the opposite ear, was treated with antibiotics, and developed postauricular cellulitis.

In a similar study of a "wait-and-see prescription" (WASP) in the emergency department, Spiro et al[76] randomly assigned 283 patients to either a WASP or standard prescription. Clinicians were educated on the 2004 AAP diagnostic criteria and initial treatment options for AOM; however, diagnosis was made at the discretion of the clinician. Patients were excluded if they did not qualify for observation per the 2004 guidelines. The primary outcome was whether the prescription was filled within 3 days of diagnosis. Prescriptions were not filled for 62% and 13% of the WASP and standard prescription patients, respectively ($P < .001$). Reasons for filling the prescription in the WASP group were fever (60%), ear pain (34%), or fussy behavior (6%). No serious adverse events were reported.

Strategies to observe children with AOM who are likely to improve on their own without initial antibiotic therapy reduces common adverse effects of antibiotics, such as diarrhea and diaper dermatitis. In 2 trials, antibiotic therapy significantly increased the absolute rates of diarrhea by 10% to 20% and of diaper rash or dermatitis by 6% to 16%.[31,32] Reduced antibiotic use may also reduce the prevalence of resistant bacterial pathogens. Multidrug-resistant S pneumoniae continues to be a significant concern for AOM, despite universal immunization of

children in the United States with heptavalent pneumococcal conjugate vaccine.[104,105] In contrast, countries with low antibiotic use for AOM have a low prevalence of resistant nasopharyngeal pathogens in children.[106]

Key Action Statement 4A

Clinicians should prescribe amoxicillin for AOM when a decision to treat with antibiotics has been made *and* the child has not received amoxicillin in the past 30 days *or* the child does not have concurrent purulent conjunctivitis *or* the child is not allergic to penicillin. (Evidence Quality: Grade B, Rec. Strength: Recommendation)

Key Action Statement Profile: KAS 4A

Aggregate evidence quality	Grade B
Benefits	Effective antibiotic for most children with AOM. Inexpensive, safe, acceptable taste, narrow antimicrobial spectrum.
Risks, harms, cost	Ineffective against β-lactamase–producing organisms. Adverse effects of amoxicillin.
Benefits-harms assessment	Preponderance of benefit.
Value judgments	Better to use a drug that has reasonable cost, has an acceptable taste, and has a narrow antibacterial spectrum.
Intentional vagueness	The clinician must determine whether the patient is truly penicillin allergic.
Role of patient preferences	Should be considered if previous bad experience with amoxicillin.
Exclusions	Patients with known penicillin allergy.
Strength	**Recommendation.**

Key Action Statement 4B

Clinicians should prescribe an antibiotic with additional β-lactamase coverage for AOM when a decision to treat with antibiotics has been made *and* the child has received amoxicillin in the past 30 days *or* has concurrent purulent conjunctivitis *or* has a history of recurrent AOM unresponsive to amoxicillin. (Evidence Quality: Grade C, Rec. Strength: Recommendation)

Key Action Statement Profile: KAS 4B

Aggregate evidence quality	Grade C
Benefits	Successful treatment of β-lactamase–producing organisms.
Risks, harms, cost	Cost of antibiotic. Increased adverse effects.
Benefits-harms assessment	Preponderance of benefit.
Value judgments	Efficacy is more important than taste.
Intentional vagueness	None.
Role of patient preferences	Concern regarding side effects and taste.
Exclusions	Patients with known penicillin allergy.
Strength	**Recommendation**

Key Action Statement 4C

Clinicians should reassess the patient if the caregiver reports that the child's symptoms have worsened or failed to respond to the initial antibiotic treatment within 48 to 72 hours and determine whether a change in therapy is needed. (Evidence Quality: Grade B, Rec. Strength: Recommendation)

Key Action Statement Profile: KAS 4C

Aggregate evidence quality	Grade B
Benefits	Identify children who may have AOM caused by pathogens resistant to previous antibiotics.
Risks, harms, cost	Cost. Time for patient and clinician to make change. Potential need for parenteral medication.
Benefit-harm assessment	Preponderance of benefit.
Value judgments	None.
Intentional vagueness	"Reassess" is not defined. The clinician may determine the method of assessment.
Role of patient preferences	Limited.
Exclusions	Appearance of TM improved.
Strength	**Recommendation**

Purpose of This Section

If an antibiotic will be used for treatment of a child with AOM, whether as initial management or after a period of observation, the clinician must choose an antibiotic that will have a high likelihood of being effective against the most likely etiologic bacterial pathogens with considerations of cost, taste, convenience, and adverse effects. This section proposes first- and second-line antibiotics that best meet these criteria while balancing potential benefits and harms.

Changes From AAP/AAFP 2004 AOM Guideline

Despite new data on the effect of PCV7 and updated data on the in vitro susceptibility of bacterial pathogens most likely to cause AOM, the recommendations for the first-line antibiotic remains unchanged from 2004. The current guideline contains revised recommendations regarding penicillin allergy based on new data. The increase of multidrug-resistant strains of pneumococci is noted.

Microbiology

Microorganisms detected in the middle ear during AOM include pathogenic bacteria, as well as respiratory viruses.[107–110] AOM occurs most frequently as a consequence of viral upper respiratory tract infection,[111–113] which leads to eustachian tube inflammation/

dysfunction, negative middle ear pressure, and movement of secretions containing the upper respiratory tract infection causative virus and pathogenic bacteria in the nasopharynx into the middle ear cleft. By using comprehensive and sensitive microbiologic testing, bacteria and/or viruses can be detected in the middle ear fluid in up to 96% of AOM cases (eg, 66% bacteria and viruses together, 27% bacteria alone, and 4% virus alone).[114] Studies using less sensitive or less comprehensive microbiologic assays have yielded less positive results for bacteria and much less positive results for viruses.[115–117] The 3 most common bacterial pathogens in AOM are *S pneumoniae*, nontypeable *Haemophilus influenzae*, and *Moraxella catarrhalis*.[111] *Streptococcus pyogenes* (group A β-hemolytic streptococci) accounts for less than 5% of AOM cases. The proportion of AOM cases with pathogenic bacteria isolated from the middle ear fluids varies depending on bacteriologic techniques, transport issues, and stringency of AOM definition. In series of reports from the United States and Europe from 1952–1981 and 1985–1992, the mean percentage of cases with bacterial pathogens isolated from the middle ear fluids was 69% and 72%, respectively.[118] A large series from the University of Pittsburgh Otitis Media Study Group reported bacterial pathogens in 84% of the middle ear fluids

from 2807 cases of AOM.[118] Studies that applied more stringent otoscopic criteria and/or use of bedside specimen plating on solid agar in addition to liquid transport media have a reported rate of recovery of pathogenic bacteria from middle ear exudates ranging from 85% to 90%.[119–121] When using appropriate stringent diagnostic criteria, careful specimen handling, and sensitive microbiologic techniques, the vast majority of cases of AOM will involve pathogenic bacteria either alone or in concert with viral pathogens.

Among AOM bacterial pathogens, *S pneumoniae* was the most frequently cultured in earlier reports. Since the debut and routine use of PCV7 in 2000, the ordinal frequency of these 3 major middle ear pathogens has evolved.[105] In the first few years after PCV7 introduction, *H influenzae* became the most frequently isolated middle ear pathogen, replacing *S pneumoniae*.[122,123] Shortly thereafter, a shift to non-PCV7 serotypes of *S pneumoniae* was described.[124] Pichichero et al[104] later reported that 44% of 212 AOM cases seen in 2003–2006 were caused by *H influenzae*, and 28% were caused by *S pneumoniae*, with a high proportion of highly resistant *S pneumoniae*. In that study, a majority (77%) of cases involved recurrent disease or initial treatment failure. A later report[125] with data from 2007 to 2009, 6 to 8 years after the introduction of PCV7 in the United States, showed that PCV7 strains of *S pneumoniae* virtually disappeared from the middle ear fluid of children with AOM who had been vaccinated. However, the frequency of isolation of non-PCV7 serotypes of *S pneumoniae* from the middle ear fluid overall was increased; this has made isolation of *S pneumoniae* and *H influenzae* of children with AOM nearly equal.

In a study of tympanocentesis over 4 respiratory tract illness seasons in a private practice, the percentage of

S pneumoniae initially decreased relative to *H influenzae*. In 2005–2006 (*N* = 33), 48% of bacteria were *S pneumoniae*, and 42% were *H influenzae*. For 2006–2007 (*N* = 37), the percentages were equal at 41%. In 2007–2008 (*N* = 34), 35% were *S pneumoniae*, and 59% were *H influenzae*. In 2008–2009 (*N* = 24), the percentages were 54% and 38%, respectively, with an increase in intermediate and nonsusceptible *S pneumoniae*.[126] Data on nasopharyngeal colonization from PCV7-immunized children with AOM have shown continued presence of *S pneumoniae* colonization. Revai et al[127] showed no difference in *S pneumoniae* colonization rate among children with AOM who have been unimmunized, underimmunized, or fully immunized with PCV7. In a study during a viral upper respiratory tract infection, including mostly PCV7-immunized children (6 months to 3 years of age), *S pneumoniae* was detected in 45.5% of 968 nasopharyngeal swabs, *H influenzae* was detected in 32.4%, and *M catarrhalis* was detected in 63.1%.[128] Data show that nasopharyngeal colonization of children vaccinated with PCV7 increasingly is caused by *S pneumoniae* serotypes not contained in the vaccine.[129–132] With the use of the recently licensed 13-valent pneumococcal conjugate vaccine (PCV13),[133] the patterns of nasopharyngeal colonization and infection with these common AOM bacterial pathogens will continue to evolve.

Investigators have attempted to predict the type of AOM pathogenic bacteria on the basis of clinical severity, but results have not been promising. *S pyogenes* has been shown to occur more commonly in older children[134] and to cause a greater degree of inflammation of the middle ear and TM, a greater frequency of spontaneous rupture of the TM, and more frequent progression to acute mastoiditis

compared with other bacterial pathogens.[134–136] As for clinical findings in cases with *S pneumoniae* and nontypeable *H influenzae*, some studies suggest that signs and symptoms of AOM caused by *S pneumoniae* may be more severe (fever, severe earache, bulging TM) than those caused by other pathogens.[44,121,137] These findings were refuted by results of the studies that found AOM caused by nontypeable *H influenzae* to be associated with bilateral AOM and more severe inflammation of the TM.[96,138] Leibovitz et al[139] concluded, in a study of 372 children with AOM caused by *H influenzae* (*N* = 138), *S pneumoniae* (*N* = 64), and mixed *H influenzae* and *S pneumoniae* (*N* = 64), that clinical/otologic scores could not discriminate among various bacterial etiologies of AOM. However, there were significantly different clinical/otologic scores between bacterial culture negative and culture positive cases. A study of middle ear exudates of 82 cases of bullous myringitis has shown a 97% bacteria positive rate, primarily *S pneumoniae*. In contrast to the previous belief, mycoplasma is rarely the causative agent in this condition.[140] Accurate prediction of the bacterial cause of AOM on the basis of clinical presentation, without bacterial culture of the middle ear exudates, is not possible, but specific etiologies may be predicted in some situations. Published evidence has suggested that AOM associated with conjunctivitis (otitis-conjunctivitis syndrome) is more likely caused by nontypeable *H influenzae* than by other bacteria.[141–143]

Bacterial Susceptibility to Antibiotics

Selection of antibiotic to treat AOM is based on the suspected type of bacteria and antibiotic susceptibility pattern, although clinical pharmacology

and clinical and microbiologic results and predicted compliance with the drug are also taken into account. Early studies of AOM patients show that 19% of children with *S pneumoniae* and 48% with *H influenzae* cultured on initial tympanocentesis who were not treated with antibiotic cleared the bacteria at the time of a second tympanocentesis 2 to 7 days later.[144] Approximately 75% of children infected with *M catarrhalis* experienced bacteriologic cure even after treatment with amoxicillin, an antibiotic to which it is not susceptible.[145,146]

Antibiotic susceptibility of major AOM bacterial pathogens continues to change, but data on middle ear pathogens have become scanty because tympanocentesis is not generally performed in studies of children with uncomplicated AOM. Most available data come from cases of persistent or recurrent AOM. Current US data from a number of centers indicates that approximately 83% and 87% of isolates of *S pneumoniae* from all age groups are susceptible to regular (40 mg/kg/day) and high-dose amoxicillin (80–90 mg/kg/day divided twice daily), respectively.[130,147–150] Pediatric isolates are smaller in number and include mostly ear isolates collected from recurrent and persistent AOM cases with a high percentage of multidrug-resistant *S pneumoniae*, most frequently nonvaccine serotypes that have recently increased in frequency and importance.[104]

High-dose amoxicillin will yield middle ear fluid levels that exceed the minimum inhibitory concentration (MIC) of all *S pneumoniae* serotypes that are intermediately resistant to penicillin (penicillin MICs, 0.12–1.0 µg/mL), and many but not all highly resistant serotypes (penicillin MICs, ≥2 µg/mL) for a longer period of the dosing interval and has been shown to improve bacteriologic and clinical efficacy compared with the regular dose.[151–153] Hoberman et al[154] reported superior efficacy of high-dose amoxicillin-clavulanate in eradication of S pneumoniae (96%) from the middle ear at days 4 to 6 of therapy compared with azithromycin.

The antibiotic susceptibility pattern for S pneumoniae is expected to continue to evolve with the use of PCV13, a conjugate vaccine containing 13 serotypes of S pneumoniae.[133,155,156] Widespread use of PCV13 could potentially reduce diseases caused by multidrug-resistant pneumococcal serotypes and diminish the need for the use of higher dose of amoxicillin or amoxicillin-clavulanate for AOM.

Some H influenzae isolates produce β-lactamase enzyme, causing the isolate to become resistant to penicillins. Current data from different studies with non-AOM sources and geographic locations that may not be comparable show that 58% to 82% of H influenzae isolates are susceptible to regular- and high-dose amoxicillin.[130,147,148,157,158] These data represented a significant decrease in β-lactamase–producing H influenzae, compared with data reported in the 2004 AOM guideline.

Nationwide data suggest that 100% of M catarrhalis derived from the upper respiratory tract are β-lactamase–positive but remain susceptible to amoxicillin-clavulanate.[159] However, the high rate of spontaneous clinical resolution occurring in children with AOM attributable to M catarrhalis treated with amoxicillin reduces the concern for the first-line coverage for this microorganism.[145,146] AOM attributable to M catarrhalis rarely progresses to acute mastoiditis or intracranial infections.[102,160,161]

Antibiotic Therapy

High-dose amoxicillin is recommended as the first-line treatment in most patients, although there are a number of medications that are clinically effective (Table 5). The justification for the use of amoxicillin relates to its effectiveness against common AOM bacterial pathogens as well as its safety, low cost, acceptable taste, and narrow microbiologic spectrum.[145,151] In children who have taken amoxicillin in the previous 30 days, those with concurrent conjunctivitis, or those for whom coverage for β-lactamase–positive H influenzae and M catarrhalis is desired, therapy should be initiated with high-dose amoxicillin-clavulanate (90 mg/kg/day of amoxicillin, with 6.4 mg/kg/day of clavulanate, a ratio of amoxicillin to clavulanate of 14:1, given in 2 divided doses, which is less likely to cause diarrhea than other amoxicillin-clavulanate preparations).[162]

Alternative initial antibiotics include cefdinir (14 mg/kg per day in 1 or 2 doses), cefuroxime (30 mg/kg per day in 2 divided doses), cefpodoxime (10 mg/kg per day in 2 divided doses), or ceftriaxone (50 mg/kg, administered intramuscularly). It is important to note that alternative antibiotics vary in their efficacy against AOM pathogens. For example, recent US data on in vitro susceptibility of S pneumoniae to cefdinir and cefuroxime are 70% to 80%, compared with 84% to 92% amoxicillin efficacy.[130,147–149] In vitro efficacy of cefdinir and cefuroxime against H influenzae is approximately 98%, compared with 58% efficacy of amoxicillin and nearly 100% efficacy of amoxicillin-clavulanate.[158] A multicenter double tympanocentesis open-label study of

TABLE 5 Recommended Antibiotics for (Initial or Delayed) Treatment and for Patients Who Have Failed Initial Antibiotic Treatment

Initial Immediate or Delayed Antibiotic Treatment		Antibiotic Treatment After 48–72 h of Failure of Initial Antibiotic Treatment	
Recommended First-line Treatment	Alternative Treatment (if Penicillin Allergy)	Recommended First-line Treatment	Alternative Treatment
Amoxicillin (80–90 mg/kg per day in 2 divided doses)	Cefdinir (14 mg/kg per day in 1 or 2 doses)	Amoxicillin-clavulanate[a] (90 mg/kg per day of amoxicillin, with 6.4 mg/kg per day of clavulanate in 2 divided doses)	Ceftriaxone, 3 d Clindamycin (30–40 mg/kg per day in 3 divided doses), with or without third-generation cephalosporin
or	Cefuroxime (30 mg/kg per day in 2 divided doses)	or	Failure of second antibiotic
Amoxicillin-clavulanate[a] (90 mg/kg per day of amoxicillin, with 6.4 mg/kg per day of clavulanate [amoxicillin to clavulanate ratio, 14:1] in 2 divided doses)	Cefpodoxime (10 mg/kg per day in 2 divided doses)	Ceftriaxone (50 mg IM or IV for 3 d)	Clindamycin (30–40 mg/kg per day in 3 divided doses) plus third-generation cephalosporin
	Ceftriaxone (50 mg IM or IV per day for 1 or 3 d)		Tympanocentesis[b] Consult specialist[b]

IM, intramuscular; IV, intravenous.

[a] May be considered in patients who have received amoxicillin in the previous 30 d or who have the otitis-conjunctivitis syndrome.

[b] Perform tympanocentesis/drainage if skilled in the procedure, or seek a consultation from an otolaryngologist for tympanocentesis/drainage. If the tympanocentesis reveals multidrug-resistant bacteria, seek an infectious disease specialist consultation.

[c] Cefdinir, cefuroxime, cefpodoxime, and ceftriaxone are highly unlikely to be associated with cross-reactivity with penicillin allergy on the basis of their distinct chemical structures. See text for more information.

cefdinir in recurrent AOM attributable to H influenzae showed eradication of the organism in 72% of patients.[163]

For penicillin-allergic children, recent data suggest that cross-reactivity among penicillins and cephalosporins is lower than historically reported.[164–167] The previously cited rate of cross-sensitivity to cephalosporins among penicillin-allergic patients (approximately 10%) is likely an overestimate. The rate was based on data collected and reviewed during the 1960s and 1970s. A study analyzing pooled data of 23 studies, including 2400 patients with reported history of penicillin allergy and 39 000 with no penicillin allergic history concluded that many patients who present with a history of penicillin allergy do not have an immunologic reaction to penicillin.[166] The chemical structure of the cephalosporin determines the risk of cross-reactivity between specific agents.[165,168] The degree of cross-reactivity is higher between penicillins and first-generation cephalosporins but is negligible with the second- and third-generation cephalosporins. Because of the differences in the chemical structures, cefdinir, cefuroxime, cefpodoxime, and ceftriaxone are highly unlikely to be associated with cross-reactivity with penicillin.[165] Despite this, the Joint Task Force on Practice Parameters; American Academy of Allergy, Asthma and Immunology; American College of Allergy, Asthma and Immunology; and Joint Council of Allergy, Asthma and Immunology[169] stated that "cephalosporin treatment of patients with a history of penicillin allergy, selecting out those with severe reaction histories, show a reaction rate of 0.1%." They recommend a cephalosporin in cases without severe and/or recent penicillin allergy reaction history when skin test is not available.

Macrolides, such as erythromycin and azithromycin, have limited efficacy against both H influenzae and S pneumoniae.[130,147–149] Clindamycin lacks efficacy against H influenzae. Clindamycin alone (30–40 mg/kg per day in 3 divided doses) may be used for suspected penicillin-resistant S pneumoniae; however, the drug will likely not be effective for the multidrug-resistant serotypes.[130,158,166]

Several of these choices of antibiotic suspensions are barely palatable or frankly offensive and may lead to avoidance behaviors or active rejection by spitting out the suspension. Palatability of antibiotic suspensions has been compared in many studies.[170–172] Specific antibiotic suspensions such as cefuroxime, cefpodoxime, and clindamycin may benefit from adding taste-masking products, such as chocolate or strawberry flavoring agents, to obscure the initial bitter taste and the unpleasant aftertaste.[172,173] In the patient who is persistently vomiting or cannot otherwise tolerate oral medication, even when the taste is masked, ceftriaxone (50 mg/kg, administered intramuscularly in 1 or 2 sites in the anterior thigh, or intravenously) has been demonstrated to be effective for the initial or repeat antibiotic treatment of AOM.[174,175] Although a single injection of ceftriaxone is approved by the US FDA for the treatment of AOM, results of a double tympanocentesis study (before and 3 days after single dose ceftriaxone) by Leibovitz et al[175] suggest that more than 1 ceftriaxone dose may be required to prevent recurrence of the middle ear infection within 5 to 7 days after the initial dose.

Initial Antibiotic Treatment Failure

When antibiotics are prescribed for AOM, clinical improvement should be noted within 48 to 72 hours. During the 24 hours after the diagnosis of AOM,

the child's symptoms may worsen slightly. In the next 24 hours, the patient's symptoms should begin to improve. If initially febrile, the temperature should decline within 48 to 72 hours. Irritability and fussiness should lessen or disappear, and sleeping and drinking patterns should normalize.[176,177] If the patient is not improved by 48 to 72 hours, another disease or concomitant viral infection may be present, or the causative bacteria may be resistant to the chosen therapy.

Some children with AOM and persistent symptoms after 48 to 72 hours of initial antibacterial treatment may have combined bacterial and viral infection, which would explain the persistence of ongoing symptoms despite appropriate antibiotic therapy.[109,178,179] Literature is conflicting on the correlation between clinical and bacteriologic outcomes. Some studies report good correlation ranging from 86% to 91%,[180,181] suggesting continued presence of bacteria in the middle ear in a high proportion of cases with persistent symptoms. Others report that middle ear fluid from children with AOM in whom symptoms are persistent is sterile in 42% to 49% of cases.[123,182] A change in antibiotic may not be required in some children with mild persistent symptoms.

In children with persistent, severe symptoms of AOM and unimproved otologic findings after initial treatment, the clinician may consider changing the antibiotic (Table 5). If the child was initially treated with amoxicillin and failed to improve, amoxicillin-clavulanate should be used. Patients who were given amoxicillin-clavulanate or oral third-generation cephalosporins may receive intramuscular ceftriaxone (50 mg/kg). In the treatment of AOM unresponsive to initial antibiotics, a 3-day course of ceftriaxone has been shown to be better than a 1-day regimen.[175]

Although trimethoprim-sulfamethoxazole and erythromycin-sulfisoxazole had been useful as therapy for patients with AOM, pneumococcal surveillance studies have indicated that resistance to these 2 combination agents is substantial.[130,149,183] Therefore, when patients fail to improve while receiving amoxicillin, neither trimethoprim-sulfamethoxazole[184] nor erythromycin-sulfisoxazole is appropriate therapy.

Tympanocentesis should be considered, and culture of middle ear fluid should be performed for bacteriologic diagnosis and susceptibility testing when a series of antibiotic drugs have failed to improve the clinical condition. If tympanocentesis is not available, a course of clindamycin may be used, with or without an antibiotic that covers nontypeable H influenzae and M catarrhalis, such as cefdinir, cefixime, or cefuroxime.

Because S pneumoniae serotype 19A is usually multidrug-resistant and may not be responsive to clindamycin,[104,149] newer antibiotics that are not approved by the FDA for treatment of AOM, such as levofloxacin or linezolid, may be indicated.[185–187] Levofloxacin is a quinolone antibiotic that is not approved by the FDA for use in children. Linezolid is effective against resistant Gram-positive bacteria. It is not approved by the FDA for AOM treatment and is expensive. In children with repeated treatment failures, every effort should be made for bacteriologic diagnosis by tympanocentesis with Gram stain, culture, and antibiotic susceptibility testing of the organism(s) present. The clinician may consider consulting with pediatric medical subspecialists, such as an otolaryngologist for possible tympanocentesis, drainage, and culture and an infectious disease expert, before use of unconventional drugs such as levofloxacin or linezolid.

When tympanocentesis is not available, 1 possible way to obtain information on the middle ear pathogens and their antimicrobial susceptibility is to obtain a nasopharyngeal specimen for bacterial culture. Almost all middle ear pathogens derive from the pathogens colonizing the nasopharynx, but not all nasopharyngeal pathogens enter the middle ear to cause AOM. The positive predictive value of nasopharyngeal culture during AOM (likelihood that bacteria cultured from the nasopharynx is the middle ear pathogen) ranges from 22% to 44% for S pneumoniae, 50% to 71% for nontypeable H influenzae, and 17% to 19% for M catarrhalis. The negative predictive value (likelihood that bacteria not found in the nasopharynx are not AOM pathogens) ranges from 95% to 99% for all 3 bacteria.[188,189] Therefore, if nasopharyngeal culture is negative for specific bacteria, that organism is likely not the AOM pathogen. A negative culture for S pneumoniae, for example, will help eliminate the concern for multidrug-resistant bacteria and the need for unconventional therapies, such as levofloxacin or linezolid. On the other hand, if S pneumoniae is cultured from the nasopharynx, the antimicrobial susceptibility pattern can help guide treatment.

Duration of Therapy

The optimal duration of therapy for patients with AOM is uncertain; the usual 10-day course of therapy was derived from the duration of treatment of streptococcal pharyngotonsillitis. Several studies favor standard 10-day therapy over shorter courses for children younger than 2 years.[162,190–194] Thus, for children younger than 2 years and children with severe symptoms, a standard 10-day course is recommended. A 7-day course of oral antibiotic appears to be equally effective in children 2 to 5 years of age with mild or moderate AOM. For children 6 years and older with mild to moderate symptoms, a 5- to 7-day course is adequate treatment.

Follow-up of the Patient With AOM

Once the child has shown clinical improvement, follow-up is based on the usual clinical course of AOM. There is little scientific evidence for a routine 10- to 14-day reevaluation visit for all children with an episode of AOM. The physician may choose to reassess some children, such as young children with severe symptoms or recurrent AOM or when specifically requested by the child's parent.

Persistent MEE is common and can be detected by pneumatic otoscopy (with or without verification by tympanometry) after resolution of acute symptoms. Two weeks after successful antibiotic treatment of AOM, 60% to 70% of children have MEE, decreasing to 40% at 1 month and 10% to 25% at 3 months after successful antibiotic treatment.[177,195] The presence of MEE without clinical symptoms is defined as OME. OME must be differentiated clinically from AOM and requires infrequent additional monitoring but not antibiotic therapy. Assurance that OME resolves is particularly important for parents of children with cognitive or developmental delays that may be affected adversely by transient hearing loss associated with MEE. Detailed recommendations for the management of the child with OME can be found in the evidence-based guideline from the AAP/AAFP/American Academy of Otolaryngology-Head and Neck Surgery published in 2004.[84,85]

Key Action Statement 5A

Clinicians should *NOT* prescribe prophylactic antibiotics to reduce the frequency of episodes of AOM in children with recurrent AOM. (Evidence Quality: Grade B, Rec. Strength: Recommendation)

Key Action Statement Profile: KAS 5A

Aggregate evidence quality	Grade B
Benefits	No adverse effects from antibiotic. Reduces potential for development of bacterial resistance. Reduced costs.
Risks, harms, cost	Small increase in episodes of AOM.
Benefit-harm assessment	Preponderance of benefit.
Value judgments	Potential harm outweighs the potential benefit.
Intentional vagueness	None.
Role of patient preferences	Limited.
Exclusions	Young children whose only alternative would be tympanostomy tubes.
Strength	**Recommendation**

Key Action Statement 5B

Clinicians may offer tympanostomy tubes for recurrent AOM (3 episodes in 6 months or 4 episodes in 1 year, with 1 episode in the preceding 6 months). (Evidence Quality: Grade B, Rec. Strength: Option)

Key Action Statement Profile: KAS 5B

Aggregate evidence quality	**Grade B**
Benefits	Decreased frequency of AOM. Ability to treat AOM with topical antibiotic therapy.
Risks, harms, cost	Risks of anesthesia or surgery. Cost. Scarring of TM, chronic perforation, cholesteatoma. Otorrhea.
Benefits-harms assessment	Equilibrium of benefit and harm.
Value judgments	None.
Intentional vagueness	Option based on limited evidence.
Role of patient preferences	Joint decision of parent and clinician.
Exclusions	Any contraindication to anesthesia and surgery.
Strength	**Option**

Purpose of This Section

Recurrent AOM has been defined as the occurrence of 3 or more episodes of AOM in a 6-month period or the occurrence of 4 or more episodes of AOM in a 12-month period that includes at least 1 episode in the preceding 6 months.[20] These episodes should be well documented and separate acute infections.[11]

Winter season, male gender, and passive exposure to smoking have been associated with an increased likelihood of recurrence. Half of children younger than 2 years treated for AOM will experience a recurrence within 6 months. Symptoms that last more than 10 days may also predict recurrence.[196]

Changes From AAP/AAFP 2004 AOM Guideline

Recurrent AOM was not addressed in the 2004 AOM guideline. This section addresses the literature on recurrent AOM.

Antibiotic Prophylaxis

Long-term, low-dose antibiotic use, referred to as antibiotic prophylaxis or chemoprophylaxis, has been used to treat children with recurrent AOM to prevent subsequent episodes.[85] A 2006 Cochrane review analyzed 16 studies of long-term antibiotic use for AOM and found such use prevented 1.5 episodes of AOM per year, reducing in half the number of AOM episodes during the period of treatment.[197] Randomized placebo-controlled trials of prophylaxis reported a decrease of 0.09 episodes per month in the frequency of AOM attributable to therapy (approximately 0.5 to 1.5 AOM episodes per year for 95% of children). An estimated 5 children would need to be treated for 1 year to prevent 1 episode of OM. The effect may be more substantial for children with 6 or more AOM episodes in the preceding year.[12]

This decrease in episodes of AOM occurred only while the prophylactic antibiotic was being given. The modest benefit afforded by a 6-month course of antibiotic prophylaxis does not have longer-lasting benefit after cessation of therapy. Teele showed no differences between children who received prophylactic antibiotics compared with those who received placebo in AOM recurrences or persistence of OME.[198]

Antibiotic prophylaxis is not appropriate for children with long-term MEE or for children with infrequent episodes of AOM. The small reduction in frequency of AOM with long-term antibiotic prophylaxis must be weighed against the cost of such therapy; the potential adverse effects of antibiotics, principally allergic reaction and gastrointestinal tract consequences, such as diarrhea; and their contribution to the emergence of bacterial resistance.

Surgery for Recurrent AOM

The use of tympanostomy tubes for treatment of ear disease in general, and for AOM in particular, has been controversial.[199] Most published studies of surgical intervention for OM focus on children with persistent MEE with or without AOM. The literature on surgery for recurrent AOM as defined here is scant. A lack of consensus among otolaryngologists regarding the role of surgery for recurrent AOM was reported in a survey of Canadian otolaryngologists in which 40% reported they would "never," 30% reported they would "sometimes," and 30% reported they would "often or always" place tympanostomy tubes for a hypothetical 2-year-old child with frequent OM without persistent MEE or hearing loss.[200]

Tympanostomy tubes, however, remain widely used in clinical practice for both OME and recurrent OM.[201] Recurrent

AOM remains a common indication for referral to an otolaryngologist.

Three randomized controlled trials have compared the number of episodes of AOM after tympanostomy tube placement or no surgery.[202] Two found significant improvement in mean number of AOM episodes after tympanostomy tubes during a 6-month follow-up period.[203,204] One study randomly assigned children with recurrent AOM to groups receiving placebo, amoxicillin prophylaxis, or tympanostomy tubes and followed them for 2 years.[205] Although prophylactic antibiotics reduced the rate of AOM, no difference in number of episodes of AOM was noted between the tympanostomy tube group and the placebo group over 2 years. A Cochrane review of studies of tympanostomy tubes for recurrent AOM analyzed 2 studies[204,206] that met inclusion criteria and found that tympanostomy tubes reduced the number of episodes of AOM by 1.5 episodes in the 6 months after surgery.[207] Tympanostomy tube insertion has been shown to improve disease-specific quality-of-life measures in children with OM.[208] One multicenter, nonrandomized observational study showed large improvements in a disease-specific quality-of-life instrument that measured psychosocial domains of physical suffering, hearing loss, speech impairment, emotional distress, activity limitations, and caregiver concerns that are associated with ear infections.[209] These benefits of tympanostomy tubes have been demonstrated in mixed populations of children that include children with OME as well as recurrent AOM.

Beyond the cost, insertion of tympanostomy tubes is associated with a small but finite surgical and anesthetic risk. A recent review looking at protocols to minimize operative risk reported no major complications, such as sensorineural hearing loss, vascular injury,

or ossicular chain disruption, in 10 000 tube insertions performed primarily by residents, although minor complications such as TM tears or displaced tubes in the middle ear were seen in 0.016% of ears.[210] Long-term sequelae of tympanostomy tubes include TM structural changes including focal atrophy, tympanosclerosis, retraction pockets, and chronic perforation. One meta-analysis found tympanosclerosis in 32% of patients after placement of tympanostomy tubes and chronic perforations in 2.2% of patients who had short-term tubes and 16.6% of patients with long-term tubes.[211]

Adenoidectomy, without myringotomy and/or tympanostomy tubes, did not reduce the number of episodes of AOM when compared with chemoprophylaxis or placebo.[212] Adenoidectomy alone should not be used for prevention of AOM but may have benefit when performed with placement of tympanostomy tubes or in children with previous tympanostomy tube placement in OME.[213]

Prevention of AOM: Key Action Statement 6A

Pneumococcal Vaccine

Clinicians should recommend pneumococcal conjugate vaccine to all children according to the schedule of the Advisory Committee on Immunization Practices, AAP, and AAFP. (Evidence Quality: Grade B, Rec. Strength: Strong Recommendation)

Key Action Statement Profile: KAS 6A

Aggregate evidence quality	Grade B
Benefits	Reduced frequency of AOM attributable to vaccine serotypes. Reduced risk of serious pneumococcal systemic disease.
Risks, harms, cost	Potential vaccine side effects. Cost of vaccine.
Benefits-harms assessment	Preponderance of benefit.
Value judgments	Potential vaccine adverse effects are minimal.
Intentional vagueness	None.
Role of patient preferences	Some parents may choose to refuse the vaccine.
Exclusions	Severe allergic reaction (eg, anaphylaxis) to any component of pneumococcal vaccine or any diphtheria toxoid-containing vaccine.
Strength	**Strong Recommendation**

Key Action Statement 6B

Influenza Vaccine: Clinicians should recommend annual influenza vaccine to all children according to the schedule of the Advisory Committee on Immunization Practices, AAP, and AAFP. (Evidence Quality: Grade B, Rec. Strength: Recommendation)

Key Action Statement Profile: KAS 6B

Aggregate evidence quality	Grade B
Benefits	Reduced risk of influenza infection. Reduction in frequency of AOM associated with influenza.
Risks, harms, cost	Potential vaccine adverse effects. Cost of vaccine. Requires annual immunization.
Benefits-harms assessment	Preponderance of benefit.
Value judgments	Potential vaccine adverse effects are minimal.
Intentional vagueness	None
Role of patient preferences	Some parents may choose to refuse the vaccine.
Exclusions	See CDC guideline on contraindications (http://www.cdc.gov/flu/professionals/acip/shouldnot.htm).
Strength	**Recommendation**

Key Action Statement 6C

Breastfeeding: Clinicians should encourage exclusive breastfeeding for at least 6 months. (Evidence Quality: Grade B, Rec. Strength: Recommendation)

Key Action Statement Profile: KAS 6C

Aggregate evidence quality	Grade B
Benefits	May reduce the risk of early AOM. Multiple benefits of breastfeeding unrelated to AOM.
Risk, harm, cost	None
Benefit-harm assessment	Preponderance of benefit.
Value judgments	The intervention has value unrelated to AOM prevention.
Intentional vagueness	None
Role of patient preferences	Some parents choose to feed formula.
Exclusions	None
Strength	**Recommendation**

Key Action Statement 6D

Clinicians should encourage avoidance of tobacco smoke exposure. (Evidence Quality: Grade C, Rec. Strength: Recommendation)

Key Action Statement Profile: KAS 6D

Aggregate evidence quality	Grade C
Benefits	May reduce the risk of AOM.
Risks, harms, cost	None
Benefits-harms assessment	Preponderance of benefit.
Value judgments	Avoidance of tobacco exposure has inherent value unrelated to AOM.
Intentional vagueness	None
Role of patient preferences	Many parents/caregivers choose not to stop smoking. Some also remain addicted, and are unable to quit smoking.
Exclusions	None
Strength	**Recommendation**

Purpose of This Section

The 2004 AOM guideline noted data on immunizations, breastfeeding, and lifestyle changes that would reduce the risk of acquiring AOM. This section addresses new data published since 2004.

Changes From AAP/AAFP 2004 AOM Guideline

PCV7 has been in use in the United States since 2000. PCV13 was introduced in the United States in 2010. The 10-valent pneumococcal nontypeable *H influenzae* protein D-conjugate vaccine was recently licensed in Europe for prevention of diseases attributable to *S pneumoniae* and nontypeable *H influenzae*. Annual influenza immunization is now recommended for all children 6 months of age and older in the United States.[214,215] Updated information regarding these vaccines and their effect on the incidence of AOM is reviewed.

The AAP issued a new breastfeeding policy statement in February 2012.[216] This guideline also includes a recommendation regarding tobacco smoke exposure. Bottle propping, pacifier use, and child care are discussed, but no recommendations are made because of limited evidence. The use of xylitol, a possible adjunct to AOM prevention, is discussed; however, no recommendations are made.

Pneumococcal Vaccine

Pneumococcal conjugate vaccines have proven effective in preventing OM caused by pneumococcal serotypes contained in the vaccines. A meta-analysis of 5 studies with AOM as an outcome determined that there is a 29% reduction in AOM caused by all pneumococcal serotypes among children who received PCV7 before 24 months of age.[217] Although the overall benefit seen in clinical trials for all causes of AOM is small (6%–7%),[218–221] observational studies have shown that medical office visits for otitis were reduced by up to 40% comparing years before and after introduction of PCV7.[222–224] Grijvala[223] reported no effect, however, among children first vaccinated at older ages. Poehling et al[225] reported reductions of frequent AOM and PE tube use after introduction of PCV7. The observations by some of greater benefit observed in the community than in clinical trials is not fully understood but may be related to effects of herd immunity or may be attributed to secular trends or changes in AOM diagnosis patterns over time.[223,226–229] In a 2009 Cochrane review,[221] Jansen et al found that the overall reduction in AOM incidence may only be 6% to 7% but noted that even that small rate may have public health relevance. O'Brien et al concurred and noted in addition the potential for cost savings.[230] There is evidence that serotype replacement may reduce the long-term efficacy of pneumococcal conjugate vaccines against AOM,[231] but it is possible that new pneumococcal conjugate vaccines may demonstrate an increased effect on reduction in AOM.[232–234] Data on AOM reduction secondary to the PCV13 licensed in the United States in 2010 are not yet available.

The *H influenzae* protein D-conjugate vaccine recently licensed in Europe has potential benefit of protection against 10 serotypes of *S pneumoniae* and nontypeable *H influenzae*.[221,234]

Influenza Vaccine

Most cases of AOM follow upper respiratory tract infections caused by viruses, including influenza viruses. As many as two-thirds of young children with influenza may have AOM.[235] Investigators have studied the efficacy of trivalent inactivated influenza vaccine (TIV) and live-attenuated intranasal influenza vaccine (LAIV) in preventing AOM. Many studies have demonstrated 30% to 55% efficacy of influenza vaccine in prevention of AOM during the respiratory illness season.[6,235–239] One study reported no benefit of TIV in reducing AOM burden; however, 1 of the 2 respiratory illness seasons during which this study was conducted had a relatively low influenza activity. A pooled analysis[240] of 8 studies comparing LAIV versus TIV or placebo[241–248] showed a higher efficacy of LAIV compared with both placebo and with TIV. Influenza vaccination is now recommended for all children 6 months of age and older in the United States.[214,215]

Breastfeeding

Multiple studies provide evidence that breastfeeding for at least 4 to 6 months reduces episodes of AOM and recurrent AOM.[249–253] Two cohort studies, 1 retrospective study[250] and 1 prospective study,[253] suggest a dose response, with some protection from partial breastfeeding and the greatest protection from exclusive breastfeeding through 6 months of age. In multivariate analysis controlling for exposure to child care settings, the risk of nonrecurrent otitis is 0.61 (95% confidence interval [CI]: 0.4–0.92) comparing exclusive breastfeeding

through 6 months of age with no breastfeeding or breastfeeding less than 4 months. In a prospective cohort, Scariatti[253] found a significant dose-response effect. In this study, OM was self-reported by parents. In a systematic review, McNiel et al[254] found that when exclusive breastfeeding was set as the normative standard, the recalculated odds ratios (ORs) revealed the risks of any formula use. For example, any formula use in the first 6 months of age was significantly associated with increased incidence of OM (OR: 1.78; 95% CI: 1.19–2.70; OR: 4.55; 95% CI: 1.64–12.50 in the available studies; pooled OR for any formula in the first 3 months of age, 2.00; 95% CI: 1.40–2.78). A number of studies[255–259] addressed the association of AOM and other infectious illness in infants with duration and exclusivity of breastfeeding, but all had limitations and none had a randomized controlled design. However, taken together, they continue to show a protective effect of exclusive breastfeeding. In all studies, there has been a predominance of white subjects, and child care attendance and smoking exposure may not have been completely controlled. Also, feeding methods were self-reported.

The consistent finding of a lower incidence of AOM and recurrent AOM with increased breastfeeding supports the AAP recommendation to encourage exclusive breastfeeding for the first 6 months of life and to continue for at least the first year and beyond for as long as mutually desired by mother and child.[216]

Lifestyle Changes

In addition to its many other benefits,[260] eliminating exposure to passive tobacco smoke has been postulated to reduce the incidence of AOM in infancy.[252,261–264] Bottles and pacifiers have been associated with AOM.

Avoiding supine bottle feeding ("bottle propping") and reducing or eliminating pacifier use in the second 6 months of life may reduce AOM incidence.[265–267] In a recent cohort study, pacifier use was associated with AOM recurrence.[268]

During infancy and early childhood, reducing the incidence of upper respiratory tract infections by altering child care-center attendance patterns can reduce the incidence of recurrent AOM significantly.[249,269]

Xylitol

Xylitol, or birch sugar, is chemically a pentitol or 5-carbon polyol sugar alcohol. It is available as chewing gum, syrup, or lozenges. A 2011 Cochrane review[270] examined the evidence for the use of xylitol in preventing recurrent AOM. A statistically significant 25% reduction in the risk of occurrence of AOM among healthy children at child care centers in the xylitol group compared with the control group (relative risk: 0.75; 95% CI: 0.65 to 0.88; RD: −0.07; 95% CI: −0.12 to −0.03) in the 4 studies met criteria for analysis.[271–274] Chewing gum and lozenges containing xylitol appeared to be more effective than syrup. Children younger than 2 years, those at the greatest risk of having AOM, cannot safely use lozenges or chewing gum. Also, xylitol needs to be given 3 to 5 times a day to be effective. It is not effective for treating AOM and it must be taken daily throughout the respiratory illness season to have an effect. Sporadic or as-needed use is not effective.

Future Research

Despite advances in research partially stimulated by the 2004 AOM guideline, there are still many unanswered clinical questions in the field. Following are possible clinical research questions that still need to be resolved.

Diagnosis

There will probably never be a gold standard for diagnosis of AOM because of the continuum from OME to AOM. Conceivably, new techniques that could be used on the small amount of fluid obtained during tympanocentesis could identify inflammatory markers in addition to the presence of bacteria or viruses. However, performing tympanocentesis studies on children with uncomplicated otitis is likely not feasible because of ethical and other considerations.

Devices that more accurately identify the presence of MEE and bulging that are easier to use than tympanometry during office visits would be welcome, especially in the difficult-to-examine infant. Additional development of inexpensive, easy-to-use video pneumatic otoscopes is still a goal.

Initial Treatment

The recent studies of Hoberman[31] and Tähtinen[32] have addressed clinical and TM appearance by using stringent diagnostic criteria of AOM. However, the outcomes for less stringent diagnostic criteria, a combination of symptoms, MEE, and TM appearance not completely consistent with OME can only be inferred from earlier studies that used less stringent criteria but did not specify outcomes for various grades of findings. Randomized controlled trials on these less certain TM appearances using scales similar to the OS-8 scale[35] could clarify the benefit of initial antibiotics and initial observation for these less certain diagnoses. Such studies must also specify severity of illness, laterality, and otorrhea.

Appropriate end points must be established. Specifically is the appearance of the TM in patients without clinical symptoms at the end of a study significant for relapse, recurrence, or persistent MEE. Such a study would require randomization of patients with unimproved TM appearance to continued observation and antibiotic groups.

The most efficient and acceptable methods of initial observation should continue to be studied balancing the convenience and benefits with the potential risks to the patient.

Antibiotics

Amoxicillin-clavulanate has a broader spectrum than amoxicillin and may be a better initial antibiotic. However, because of cost and adverse effects, the subcommittee has chosen amoxicillin as first-line AOM treatment. Randomized controlled trials comparing the 2 with adequate power to differentiate clinical efficacy would clarify this choice. Stringent diagnostic criteria should be the standard for these studies. Antibiotic comparisons for AOM should now include an observation arm for patients with nonsevere illness to ensure a clinical benefit over placebo. Studies should also have enough patients to show small but meaningful differences.

Although there have been studies on the likelihood of resistant S pneumoniae or H influenzae in children in child care settings and with siblings younger than 5 years, studies are still needed to determine whether these and other risk factors would indicate a need for different initial treatment than noted in the guideline.

New antibiotics that are safe and effective are needed for use in AOM because of the development of multidrug-resistant organisms. Such new antibiotics must be tested against the currently available medications.

Randomized controlled trials using different durations of antibiotic therapy in different age groups are needed to optimize therapy with the possibility of decreasing duration of antibiotic use. These would need to be performed initially with amoxicillin and amoxicillin-clavulanate but should also be performed for any antibiotic used in AOM. Again, an observation arm should be included in nonsevere illness.

Recurrent AOM

There have been adequate studies regarding prophylactic antibiotic use in recurrent AOM. More and better controlled studies of tympanostomy tube placement would help determine its benefit versus harm.

Prevention

There should be additional development of vaccines targeted at common organisms associated with AOM.[275] Focused epidemiologic studies on the benefit of breastfeeding, specifically addressing AOM prevention, including duration of breastfeeding and partial versus exclusive breastfeeding, would clarify what is now a more general database. Likewise, more focused studies of the effects of lifestyle changes would help clarify their effect on AOM.

Complementary and Alternative Medicine

There are no well-designed randomized controlled trials of the usefulness of complementary and alternative medicine in AOM, yet a large number of families turn to these methods. Although most alternative therapies are relatively inexpensive, some may be costly. Such studies should compare the alternative therapy to observation rather than antibiotics and only use an antibiotic arm if the alternative therapy is shown to be better than observation. Such studies should focus on children with less stringent criteria of AOM but using the same descriptive criteria for the patients as noted above.

DISSEMINATION OF GUIDELINES

An Institute of Medicine Report notes that "Effective multifaceted implementation strategies targeting both individuals and healthcare systems should be employed by implementers to promote adherence to trustworthy [clinical practice guidelines]."[230]

Many studies of the effect of clinical practice guidelines have been performed. In general, the studies show little overt change in practice after a guideline is published. However, as was seen after the 2004 AOM guideline, the number of visits for AOM and the number of prescriptions for antibiotics for AOM had decreased publication. Studies of educational and dissemination methods both at the practicing physician level and especially at the resident level need to be examined.

SUBCOMMITTEE ON DIAGNOSIS AND MANAGEMENT OF ACUTE OTITIS MEDIA

Allan S. Lieberthal, MD, FAAP (Chair, general pediatrician, no conflicts)

Aaron E. Carroll, MD, MS, FAAP (Partnership for Policy Implementation [PPI] Informatician, general academic pediatrician, no conflicts)

Tasnee Chonmaitree, MD, FAAP (pediatric infectious disease physician, no financial conflicts; published research related to AOM)

Theodore G. Ganiats, MD (family physician, American Academy of Family Physicians, no conflicts)

Alejandro Hoberman, MD, FAAP (general academic pediatrician, no financial conflicts; published research related to AOM)

Mary Anne Jackson, MD, FAAP (pediatric infectious disease physician, AAP Committee on Infectious Disease, no conflicts)

Mark D. Joffe, MD, FAAP (pediatric emergency medicine physician, AAP Committee/Section on Pediatric Emergency Medicine, no conflicts)

Donald T. Miller, MD, MPH, FAAP (general pediatrician, no conflicts)

Richard M. Rosenfeld, MD, MPH, FAAP (otolaryngologist, AAP Section on Otolaryngology, Head and Neck Surgery, American Academy of Otolaryngology-Head and Neck Surgery, no financial conflicts; published research related to AOM)

Xavier D. Sevilla, MD, FAAP (general pediatrics, Quality Improvement Innovation Network, no conflicts)

Richard H. Schwartz, MD, FAAP (general pediatrician, no financial conflicts; published research related to AOM)

Pauline A. Thomas, MD, FAAP (epidemiologist, general pediatrician, no conflicts)

David E. Tunkel, MD, FAAP, FACS (otolaryngologist, AAP Section on Otolaryngology, Head and Neck Surgery, periodic consultant to Medtronic ENT)

CONSULTANT

Richard N. Shiffman, MD, FAAP, FACMI (informatician, guideline methodologist, general academic pediatrician, no conflicts)

STAFF

Caryn Davidson, MA
Oversight by the Steering Committee on Quality Improvement and Management, 2009–2012

REFERENCES

1. American Academy of Pediatrics Subcommittee on Management of Acute Otitis Media. Diagnosis and management of acute otitis media. *Pediatrics.* 2004;113(5): 1451–1465

2. Grijalva CG, Nuorti JP, Griffin MR. Antibiotic prescription rates for acute respiratory tract infections in US ambulatory settings. *JAMA.* 2009;302(7): 758–766

3. McCaig LF, Besser RE, Hughes JM. Trends in antimicrobial prescribing rates for children and adolescents. *JAMA.* 2002;287 (23):3096–3102

4. Vernacchio L, Vezina RM, Mitchell AA. Management of acute otitis media by primary care physicians: trends since the release of the 2004 American Academy of Pediatrics/American Academy of Family Physicians clinical practice guideline. *Pediatrics.* 2007;120(2):281–287

5. Coco A, Vernacchio L, Horst M, Anderson A. Management of acute otitis media after publication of the 2004 AAP and AAFP clinical practice guideline. *Pediatrics.* 2010;125(2):214–220

6. Marchisio P, Mira E, Klersy C, et al. Medical education and attitudes about acute otitis media guidelines: a survey of Italian pediatricians and otolaryngologists. *Pediatr Infect Dis J.* 2009;28(1): 1–4

7. Arkins ER, Koehler JM. Use of the observation option and compliance with guidelines in treatment of acute otitis media. *Ann Pharmacother.* 2008;42(5): 726–727

8. Flores G, Lee M, Bauchner H, Kastner B. Pediatricians' attitudes, beliefs, and practices regarding clinical practice guidelines: a national survey. *Pediatrics.* 2000;105(3 pt 1):496–501

9. Bluestone CD. Definitions, terminology, and classification. In: Rosenfeld RM, Bluestone CD, eds. *Evidence-Based Otitis Media.* Hamilton, Canada: BC Decker; 2003:120–135

10. Bluestone CD, Klein JO. Definitions, terminology, and classification. In: Bluestone CD, Klein JO, eds. *Otitis Media in Infants and Children.* 4th ed. Hamilton, Canada: BC Decker; 2007:1–19

11. Dowell SF, Marcy MS, Phillips WR, et al. Otitis media: principles of judicious use of antimicrobial agents. *Pediatrics.* 1998;101 (suppl):165–171

12. Rosenfeld RM. Clinical pathway for acute otitis media. In: Rosenfeld RM, Bluestone CD, eds. *Evidence-Based Otitis Media.* 2nd ed. Hamilton, Canada: BC Decker; 2003: 280–302

13. Carlson LH, Carlson RD. Diagnosis. In: Rosenfeld RM, Bluestone CD, eds. *Evidence-Based Otitis Media.* Hamilton, Canada: BC Decker; 2003: 136–146

14. Bluestone CD, Klein JO. Diagnosis. In: *Otitis Media in Infants and Children.* 4th ed. Hamilton, Canada: BC Decker; 2007:147–212

15. University of Oxford, Centre for Evidence Based Medicine. Available at: www.cebm.net/index.aspx?o=1044. Accessed July 17, 2012

16. American Academy of Pediatrics Steering Committee on Quality Improvement and Management. Classifying recommendations for clinical practice guidelines. *Pediatrics.* 2004;114(3):874–877

17. Marcy M, Takata G, Shekelle P, et al. *Management of Acute Otitis Media.* Evidence Report/Technology Assessment No. 15. Rockville, MD: Agency for Healthcare Research and Quality; 2000

18. Chan LS, Takata GS, Shekelle P, Morton SC, Mason W, Marcy SM. Evidence assessment of management of acute otitis media: II. Research gaps and priorities for future research. *Pediatrics.* 2001;108(2): 248–254

19. Takata GS, Chan LS, Shekelle P, Morton SC, Mason W, Marcy SM. Evidence assessment of management of acute otitis media: I. The role of antibiotics in treatment of uncomplicated acute otitis media. *Pediatrics.* 2001;108(2):239–247

20. Shekelle PG, Takata G, Newberry SJ, et al. *Management of Acute Otitis Media: Update.* Evidence Report/Technology Assessment No. 198. Rockville, MD: Agency for Healthcare Research and Quality; 2010

21. Coker TR, Chan LS, Newberry SJ, et al. Diagnosis, microbial epidemiology, and antibiotic treatment of acute otitis media in children: a systematic review. *JAMA.* 2010;304(19):2161–2169

22. Jadad AR, Moore RA, Carroll D, et al. Assessing the quality of reports of randomized clinical trials: is blinding necessary? *Control Clin Trials.* 1996;17(1):1–12

23. Whiting P, Rutjes AW, Reitsma JB, Bossuyt PM, Kleijnen J. The development of QUADAS: a tool for the quality assessment of studies of diagnostic accuracy included in systematic reviews. *BMC Med Res Methodol.* 2003;3:25

24. Guyatt GH, Oxman AD, Vist GE, et al; GRADE Working Group. GRADE: an emerging consensus on rating quality of evidence and strength of recommendations. *BMJ.* 2008; 336(7650):924–926

25. Hoffman RN, Michel G, Rosenfeld RM, Davidson C. Building better guidelines with BRIDGE-Wiz: development and evaluation of a software assistant to promote clarity, transparency, and implementability. *J Am Med Inform Assoc.* 2012;19 (1):94–101

26. Kalu SU, Ataya RS, McCormick DP, Patel JA, Revai K, Chonmaitree T. Clinical spectrum of acute otitis media complicating upper respiratory tract viral infection. *Pediatr Infect Dis J.* 2011;30(2):95–99

27. Block SL, Harrison CJ. *Diagnosis and Management of Acute Otitis Media.* 3rd ed. Caddo, OK: Professional Communications; 2005:48–50

28. Wald ER. Acute otitis media: more trouble with the evidence. *Pediatr Infect Dis J.* 2003;22(2):103–104

29. Paradise JL, Rockette HE, Colborn DK, et al. Otitis media in 2253 Pittsburgh-area infants: prevalence and risk factors during the first two years of life. *Pediatrics.* 1997;99(3):318–333

30. McCormick DP, Chonmaitree T, Pittman C, et al. Nonsevere acute otitis media: a clinical trial comparing outcomes of watchful waiting versus immediate antibiotic treatment. *Pediatrics.* 2005;115(6): 1455–1465

31. Hoberman A, Paradise JL, Rockette HE, et al. Treatment of acute otitis media in children under 2 years of age. *N Engl J Med.* 2011;364(2):105–115

32. Tähtinen PA, Laine MK, Huovinen P, Jalava J, Ruuskanen O, Ruohola A. A placebo-controlled trial of antimicrobial treatment for acute otitis media. *N Engl J Med.* 2011;364(2):116–126

33. Shaikh N, Hoberman A, Paradise JL, et al. Development and preliminary evaluation of a parent-reported outcome instrument for clinical trials in acute otitis media. *Pediatr Infect Dis J.* 2009;28(1):5–8

34. Laine MK, Tähtinen PA, Ruuskanen O, Huovinen P, Ruohola A. Symptoms or symptom-based scores cannot predict acute otitis media at otitis-prone age. *Pediatrics.* 2010;125(5). Available at: www.pediatrics.org/cgi/content/full/125/5/e1154

35. Friedman NR, McCormick DP, Pittman C, et al. Development of a practical tool for assessing the severity of acute otitis media. *Pediatr Infect Dis J.* 2006;25(2):101–107

36. Rothman R, Owens T, Simel DL. Does this child have acute otitis media? *JAMA.* 2003; 290(12):1633–1640

37. Niemela M, Uhari M, Jounio-Ervasti K, Luotonen J, Alho OP, Vierimaa E. Lack of specific symptomatology in children with acute otitis media. *Pediatr Infect Dis J.* 1994;13(9):765–768

38. Heikkinen T, Ruuskanen O. Signs and symptoms predicting acute otitis media. *Arch Pediatr Adolesc Med.* 1995;149(1): 26–29

39. Ingvarsson L. Acute otalgia in children—findings and diagnosis. *Acta Paediatr Scand.* 1982;71(5):705–710

40. Kontiokari T, Koivunen P, Niemelä M, Pokka T, Uhari M. Symptoms of acute otitis media. *Pediatr Infect Dis J.* 1998;17(8):676–679

41. Wong DL, Baker CM. Pain in children: comparison of assessment scales. *Pediatr Nurs.* 1988;14(1):9–17

42. Shaikh N, Hoberman A, Paradise JL, et al. Responsiveness and construct validity of a symptom scale for acute otitis media. *Pediatr Infect Dis J.* 2009;28(1):9–12

43. Karma PH, Penttilä MA, Sipilä MM, Kataja MJ. Otoscopic diagnosis of middle ear effusion in acute and non-acute otitis media. I. The value of different otoscopic findings. *Int J Pediatr Otorhinolaryngol.* 1989;17(1):37–49

44. McCormick DP, Lim-Melia E, Saeed K, Baldwin CD, Chonmaitree T. Otitis media: can clinical findings predict bacterial or viral etiology? *Pediatr Infect Dis J.* 2000; 19(3):256–258

45. Schwartz RH, Stool SE, Rodriguez WJ, Grundfast KM. Acute otitis media: toward a more precise definition. *Clin Pediatr (Phila).* 1981;20(9):549–554

46. Rosenfeld RM. Antibiotic prophylaxis for recurrent acute otitis media. In: Alper CM, Bluestone CD, eds. *Advanced Therapy of Otitis Media.* Hamilton, Canada: BC Decker; 2004

47. Paradise J, Bernard B, Colborn D, Smith C, Rockette H; Pittsburgh-area Child Development/Otitis Media Study Group. Otitis media with effusion: highly prevalent and often the forerunner of acute otitis media during the first year of life [abstract]. *Pediatr Res.* 1993;33:121A

48. Roland PS, Smith TL, Schwartz SR, et al. Clinical practice guideline: cerumen impaction. *Otolaryngol Head Neck Surg.* 2008;139(3 suppl 2):S1–S21

49. Shaikh N, Hoberman A, Kaleida PH, Ploof DL, Paradise JL. Videos in clinical medicine. Diagnosing otitis media—otoscopy and cerumen removal. *N Engl J Med.* 2010; 362(20):e62

50. Pichichero ME. Diagnostic accuracy, tympanocentesis training performance, and antibiotic selection by pediatric residents in management of otitis media. *Pediatrics.* 2002;110(6):1064–1070

51. Kaleida PH, Ploof DL, Kurs-Lasky M, et al. Mastering diagnostic skills: Enhancing Proficiency in Otitis Media, a model for diagnostic skills training. *Pediatrics.* 2009; 124(4). Available at: www.pediatrics.org/cgi/content/full/124/4/e714

52. Kaleida PH, Ploof D. ePROM: Enhancing Proficiency in Otitis Media. Pittsburgh, PA: University of Pittsburgh School of Medicine. Available at: http://pedsed.pitt.edu. Accessed December 31, 2011

53. Innovative Medical Education. *A View Through the Otoscope: Distinguishing Acute Otitis Media from Otitis Media with Effusion.* Paramus, NJ: Innovative Medical Education; 2000

54. American Academy of Pediatrics. Section on Infectious Diseases. A view through the otoscope: distinguishing acute otitis media from otitis media with effusion [video]. Available at: http://www2.aap.org/sections/infectdis/video.cfm. Accessed January 20, 2012

55. Hayden GF, Schwartz RH. Characteristics of earache among children with acute

otitis media. *Am J Dis Child.* 1985;139(7): 721–723

56. Schechter NL. Management of pain associated with acute medical illness. In: Schechter NL, Berde CB, Yaster M, eds. *Pain in Infants, Children, and Adolescents.* Baltimore, MD: Williams & Wilkins; 1993: 537–538

57. Rovers MM, Glasziou P, Appelman CL, et al. Predictors of pain and/or fever at 3 to 7 days for children with acute otitis media not treated initially with antibiotics: a meta-analysis of individual patient data. *Pediatrics.* 2007;119(3):579–585

58. Burke P, Bain J, Robinson D, Dunleavey J. Acute red ear in children: controlled trial of nonantibiotic treatment in children: controlled trial of nonantibiotic treatment in general practice. *BMJ.* 1991;303(6802): 558–562

59. Sanders S, Glasziou PP, DelMar C, Rovers M. Antibiotics for acute otitis media in children [review]. *Cochrane Database Syst Rev.* 2009;(2):1–43

60. van Buchem FL, Dunk JH, van't Hof MA. Therapy of acute otitis media: myringotomy, antibiotics, or neither? A double-blind study in children. *Lancet.* 1981;2(8252): 883–887

61. Thalin A, Densert O, Larsson A, et al. Is penicillin necessary in the treatment of acute otitis media? In: *Proceedings of the International Conference on Acute and Secretory Otitis Media. Part 1.* Amsterdam, Netherlands: Kugler Publications; 1986:441–446

62. Rovers MM, Glasziou P, Appelman CL, et al. Antibiotics for acute otitis media: an individual patient data meta-analysis. *Lancet.* 2006;368(9545):1429–1435

63. Bertin L, Pons G, d'Athis P, et al. A randomized, double-blind, multicentre controlled trial of ibuprofen versus acetaminophen and placebo for symptoms of acute otitis media in children. *Fundam Clin Pharmacol.* 1996;10(4):387–392

64. American Academy of Pediatrics. Committee on Psychosocial Aspects of Child and Family Health; Task Force on Pain in Infants, Children, and Adolescents. The assessment and management of acute pain in infants, children, and adolescents. *Pediatrics.* 2001;108(3): 793–797

65. Bolt P, Barnett P, Babl FE, Sharwood LN. Topical lignocaine for pain relief in acute otitis media: results of a double-blind placebo-controlled randomised trial. *Arch Dis Child.* 2008;93(1):40–44

66. Foxlee R, Johansson AC, Wejfalk J, Dawkins J, Dooley L, Del Mar C. Topical analgesia for

acute otitis media. *Cochrane Database Syst Rev.* 2006;(3):CD005657

67. Hoberman A, Paradise JL, Reynolds EA, Urkin J. Efficacy of Auralgan for treating ear pain in children with acute otitis media. *Arch Pediatr Adolesc Med.* 1997; 151(7):675–678

68. Sarrell EM, Mandelberg A, Cohen HA. Efficacy of naturopathic extracts in the management of ear pain associated with acute otitis media. *Arch Pediatr Adolesc Med.* 2001;155(7):796–799

69. Sarrell EM, Cohen HA, Kahan E. Naturopathic treatment for ear pain in children. *Pediatrics.* 2003;111(5 pt 1):e574–e579

70. Adam D, Federspil P, Lukes M, Petrowicz O. Therapeutic properties and tolerance of procaine and phenazone containing ear drops in infants and very young children. *Arzneimittelforschung.* 2009;59(10):504–512

71. Barnett ED, Levatin JL, Chapman EH, et al. Challenges of evaluating homeopathic treatment of acute otitis media. *Pediatr Infect Dis J.* 2000;19(4):273–275

72. Jacobs J, Springer DA, Crothers D. Homeopathic treatment of acute otitis media in children: a preliminary randomized placebo-controlled trial. *Pediatr Infect Dis J.* 2001;20(2):177–183

73. Rosenfeld RM, Bluestone CD. Clinical efficacy of surgical therapy. In: Rosenfeld RM, Bluestone CD, eds. *Evidence-Based Otitis Media. 2003.* Hamilton, Canada: BC Decker; 2003:227–240

74. Rosenfeld RM. Observation option toolkit for acute otitis media. *Int J Pediatr Otorhinolaryngol.* 2001;58(1):1–8

75. Le Saux N, Gaboury I, Baird M, et al. A randomized, double-blind, placebo-controlled noninferiority trial of amoxicillin for clinically diagnosed acute otitis media in children 6 months to 5 years of age. *CMAJ.* 2005;172(3):335–341

76. Spiro DM, Tay KY, Arnold DH, Dziura JD, Baker MD, Shapiro ED. Wait-and-see prescription for the treatment of acute otitis media: a randomized controlled trial. *JAMA.* 2006;296(10):1235–1241

77. Neumark T, Mölstad S, Rosén C, et al. Evaluation of phenoxymethylpenicillin treatment of acute otitis media in children aged 2–16. *Scand J Prim Health Care.* 2007;25(3):166–171

78. Chao JH, Kunkov S, Reyes LB, Lichten S, Crain EF. Comparison of two approaches to observation therapy for acute otitis media in the emergency department. *Pediatrics.* 2008;121(5). Available at: www.pediatrics.org/cgi/content/full/121/5/e1352

79. Spurling GK, Del Mar CB, Dooley L, Foxlee R. Delayed antibiotics for respiratory infections. *Cochrane Database Syst Rev.* 2007;(3):CD004417

80. Koopman L, Hoes AW, Glasziou PP, et al. Antibiotic therapy to prevent the development of asymptomatic middle ear effusion in children with acute otitis media: a meta-analysis of individual patient data. *Arch Otolaryngol Head Neck Surg.* 2008;134(2):128–132

81. Marchetti F, Ronfani L, Nibali SC, Tamburlini G; Italian Study Group on Acute Otitis Media. Delayed prescription may reduce the use of antibiotics for acute otitis media: a prospective observational study in primary care. *Arch Pediatr Adolesc Med.* 2005; 159(7):679–684

82. Ho D, Rotenberg BW, Berkowitz RG. The relationship between acute mastoiditis and antibiotic use for acute otitis media in children. *Arch Otolaryngol Head Neck Surg.* 2008;34(1):45–48

83. Thompson PL, Gilbert RE, Long PF, Saxena S, Sharland M, Wong IC. Effect of antibiotics for otitis media on mastoiditis in children: a retrospective cohort study using the United Kingdom general practice research database. *Pediatrics.* 2009; 123(2):424–430

84. American Academy of Family Physicians; American Academy of Otolaryngology-Head and Neck Surgery; American Academy of Pediatrics Subcommittee on Otitis Media With Effusion. Otitis media with effusion. *Pediatrics.* 2004;113(5):1412–1429

85. Rosenfeld RM, Culpepper L, Doyle KJ, et al; American Academy of Pediatrics Subcommittee on Otitis Media with Effusion; American Academy of Family Physicians; American Academy of Otolaryngology—Head and Neck Surgery. Clinical practice guideline: otitis media with effusion. *Otolaryngol Head Neck Surg.* 2004;130(suppl 5): S95–S118

86. Appelman CL, Claessen JQ, Touw-Otten FW, Hordijk GJ, de Melker RA. Co-amoxiclav in recurrent acute otitis media: placebo controlled study. *BMJ.* 1991;303(6815): 1450–1452

87. Burke P, Bain J, Robinson D, Dunleavey J. Acute red ear in children: controlled trial of nonantibiotic treatment in children: controlled trial of nonantibiotic treatment in general practice. *BMJ.* 1991;303(6802): 558–562

88. van Balen FA, Hoes AW, Verheij TJ, de Melker RA. Primary care based randomized, double blind trial of amoxicillin versus placebo in children aged under 2 years. *BMJ.* 2000;320(7231):350–354

89. Little P, Gould C, Williamson I, Moore M, Warner G, Dunleavey J. Pragmatic randomised controlled trial of two prescribing strategies for childhood acute otitis media. BMJ. 2001;322(7282):336–342

90. Mygind N, Meistrup-Larsen K-I, Thomsen J, Thomsen VF, Josefsson K, Sørensen H. Penicillin in acute otitis media: a double-blind placebo-controlled trial. Clin Otolaryngol Allied Sci. 1981;6(1):5–13

91. Kaleida PH, Casselbrant ML, Rockette HE, et al. Amoxicillin or myringotomy or both for acute otitis media: results of a randomized clinical trial. Pediatrics. 1991;87 (4):466–474

92. Shaikh N, Hoberman A, Paradise JL, et al. Responsiveness and construct validity of a symptom scale for acute otitis media. Pediatr Infect Dis J. 2009;28(1):9–12

93. Heikkinen T, Chonmaitree T. Importance of respiratory viruses in acute otitis media. Clin Microbiol Rev. 2003;16(2):230–241

94. Halsted C, Lepow ML, Balassanian N, Emmerich J, Wolinsky E. Otitis media. Clinical observations, microbiology, and evaluation of therapy. Am J Dis Child. 1968;115(5):542–551

95. Rosenfeld RM, Vertrees J, Carr J, et al. Clinical efficacy of antimicrobials for acute otitis media: meta-analysis of 5,400 children from 33 randomized trials. J Pediatr. 1994;124(3):355–367

96. McCormick DP, Chandler SM, Chonmaitree T. Laterality of acute otitis media: different clinical and microbiologic characteristics. Pediatr Infect Dis J. 2007;26(7):583–588

97. Appelman CLM, Bossen PC, Dunk JHM, Lisdonk EH, de Melker RA, van Weert HCPM. NHG Standard Otitis Media Acuta (Guideline on acute otitis media of the Dutch College of General Practitioners). Huisarts Wet. 1990;33:242–245

98. Swedish Medical Research Council. Treatment for acute inflammation of the middle ear: consensus statement. Stockholm, Sweden: Swedish Medical Research Council; 2000. Available at: http://soapimg. icecube.snowfall.se/strama/Konsensut_ora_eng.pdf. Accessed July 18, 2012

99. Scottish Intercollegiate Guideline Network. Diagnosis and management of childhood otitis media in primary care. Edinburgh, Scotland: Scottish Intercollegiate Guideline Network; 2000. Available at: www.sign.ac.uk/guidelines/fulltext/66/index.html. Accessed July 18, 2012

100. National Institute for Health and Clinical Excellence, Centre for Clinical Practice. Respiratory tract infections—antibiotic prescribing: prescribing of antibiotics for self-limiting respiratory tract infections in adults and children in primary care. NICE Clinical Guideline 69. London, United Kingdom: National Institute for Health and Clinical Excellence; July 2008. Available at: www.nice.org.uk/CG069. Accessed July 18, 2012

101. Marchisio P, Bellussi L, Di Mauro G, et al. Acute otitis media: from diagnosis to prevention. Summary of the Italian guideline. Int J Pediatr Otorhinolaryngol. 2010;74(11):1209–1216

102. Siegel RM, Kiely M, Bien JP, et al. Treatment of otitis media with observation and a safety-net antibiotic prescription. Pediatrics. 2003;112(3 pt 1):527–531

103. Pshetizky Y, Naimer S, Shvartzman P. Acute otitis media—a brief explanation to parents and antibiotic use. Fam Pract. 2003;20(4):417–419

104. Pichichero ME, Casey JR. Emergence of a multiresistant serotype 19A pneumococcal strain not included in the 7-valent conjugate vaccine as an otopathogen in children. JAMA. 2007;298(15):1772–1778

105. Pichichero ME, Casey JR. Evolving microbiology and molecular epidemiology of acute otitis media in the pneumococcal conjugate vaccine era. Pediatr Infect Dis J. 2007;26(suppl 10):S12–S16

106. Nielsen HUK, Konradsen HB, Lous J, Frimodt-Møller N. Nasopharyngeal pathogens in children with acute otitis media in a low-antibiotic use country. Int J Pediatr Otorhinolaryngol. 2004;68(9):1149–1155

107. Pitkäranta A, Virolainen A, Jero J, Arruda E, Hayden FG. Detection of rhinovirus, respiratory syncytial virus, and coronavirus infections in acute otitis media by reverse transcriptase polymerase chain reaction. Pediatrics. 1998;102(2 pt 1):291–295

108. Heikkinen T, Thint M, Chonmaitree T. Prevalence of various respiratory viruses in the middle ear during acute otitis media. N Engl J Med. 1999;340(4):260–264

109. Chonmaitree T. Acute otitis media is not a pure bacterial disease. Clin Infect Dis. 2006;43(11):1423–1425

110. Williams JV, Tollefson SJ, Nair S, Chonmaitree T. Association of human metapneumovirus with acute otitis media. Int J Pediatr Otorhinolaryngol. 2006;70(7):1189–1193

111. Chonmaitree T, Heikkinen T. Role of viruses in middle-ear disease. Ann N Y Acad Sci. 1997;830:143–157

112. Klein JO, Bluestone CD. Otitis media. In: Feigin RD, Cherry JD, Demmler-Harrison GJ, Kaplan SL, eds. Textbook of Pediatric Infectious Diseases. 6th ed. Philadelphia, PA: Saunders; 2009:216–237

113. Chonmaitree T, Revai K, Grady JJ, et al. Viral upper respiratory tract infection and otitis media complication in young children. Clin Infect Dis. 2008;46(6):815–823

114. Ruohola A, Meurman O, Nikkari S, et al. Microbiology of acute otitis media in children with tympanostomy tubes: prevalences of bacteria and viruses. Clin Infect Dis. 2006; 43(11):1417–1422

115. Ruuskanen O, Arola M, Heikkinen T, Ziegler T. Viruses in acute otitis media: increasing evidence for clinical significance. Pediatr Infect Dis J. 1991;10(6):425–427

116. Chonmaitree T. Viral and bacterial interaction in acute otitis media. Pediatr Infect Dis J. 2000;19(suppl 5):S24–S30

117. Nokso-Koivisto J, Räty R, Blomqvist S, et al. Presence of specific viruses in the middle ear fluids and respiratory secretions of young children with acute otitis media. J Med Virol. 2004;72(2):241–248

118. Bluestone CD, Klein JO. Microbiology. In: Bluestone CD, Klein JO, eds. Otitis Media in Infants and Children. 4th ed. Hamilton, Canada: BC Decker; 2007:101–126

119. Del Beccaro MA, Mendelman PM, Inglis AF, et al. Bacteriology of acute otitis media: a new perspective. J Pediatr. 1992;120(1): 81–84

120. Block SL, Harrison CJ, Hedrick JA, et al. Penicillin-resistant Streptococcus pneumoniae in acute otitis media: risk factors, susceptibility patterns and antimicrobial management. Pediatr Infect Dis J. 1995;14 (9):751–759

121. Rodriguez WJ, Schwartz RH. Streptococcus pneumoniae causes otitis media with higher fever and more redness of tympanic membranes than Haemophilus influenzae or Moraxella catarrhalis. Pediatr Infect Dis J. 1999;18(10):942–944

122. Block SL, Hedrick J, Harrison CJ, et al. Community-wide vaccination with the heptavalent pneumococcal conjugate significantly alters the microbiology of acute otitis media. Pediatr Infect Dis J. 2004;23 (9):829–833

123. Casey JR, Pichichero ME. Changes in frequency and pathogens causing acute otitis media in 1995–2003. Pediatr Infect Dis J. 2004;23(9):824–828

124. McEllistrem MC, Adams JM, Patel K, et al. Acute otitis media due to penicillin-nonsusceptible Streptococcus pneumoniae before and after the introduction of the pneumococcal conjugate vaccine. Clin Infect Dis. 2005;40(12):1738–1744

125. Casey JR, Adlowitz DG, Pichichero ME. New patterns in the otopathogens causing acute otitis media six to eight years after introduction of pneumococcal conjugate vaccine. Pediatr Infect Dis J. 2010;29(4): 304–309

126. Grubb MS, Spaugh DC. Microbiology of acute otitis media, Puget Sound region, 2005–2009. *Clin Pediatr (Phila)*. 2010;49(8): 727–730

127. Revai K, McCormick DP, Patel J, Grady JJ, Saeed K, Chonmaitree T. Effect of pneumococcal conjugate vaccine on nasopharyngeal bacterial colonization during acute otitis media. *Pediatrics*. 2006;117(5): 1823–1829

128. Pettigrew MM, Gent JF, Revai K, Patel JA, Chonmaitree T. Microbial interactions during upper respiratory tract infections. *Emerg Infect Dis*. 2008;14(10):1584–1591

129. O'Brien KL, Millar EV, Zell ER, et al. Effect of pneumococcal conjugate vaccine on nasopharyngeal colonization among immunized and unimmunized children in a community-randomized trial. *J Infect Dis*. 2007;196(8):1211–1220

130. Jacobs MR, Bajaksouzian S, Windau A, Good C. Continued emergence of nonvaccine serotypes of *Streptococcus pneumoniae* in Cleveland. *Proceedings of the 49th Interscience Conference on Antimicrobial Agents and Chemotherapy*, 2009:G1-G1556

131. Hoberman A, Paradise JL, Shaikh N, et al. Pneumococcal resistance and serotype 19A in Pittsburgh-area children with acute otitis media before and after introduction of 7-valent pneumococcal polysaccharide vaccine. *Clin Pediatr (Phila)*. 2011;50(2): 114–120

132. Huang SS, Hinrichsen VL, Stevenson AE, et al. Continued impact of pneumococcal conjugate vaccine on carriage in young children. *Pediatrics*. 2009;124(1). Available at: www.pediatrics.org/cgi/content/full/124/1/e1

133. Centers for Disease Control and Prevention (CDC). Licensure of a 13-valent pneumococcal conjugate vaccine (PCV13) and recommendations for use among children—Advisory Committee on Immunization Practices (ACIP), 2010. *MMWR Morb Mortal Wkly Rep*. 2010;59(9):258–261

134. Segal N, Givon-Lavi N, Leibovitz E, Yagupsky P, Leiberman A, Dagan R. Acute otitis media caused by *Streptococcus pyogenes* in children. *Clin Infect Dis*. 2005;41(1):35–41

135. Luntz M, Brodsky A, Nusem S, et al. Acute mastoiditis—the antibiotic era: a multicenter study. *Int J Pediatr Otorhinolaryngol*. 2001;57(1):1–9

136. Nielsen JC. *Studies on the Aetiology of Acute Otitis Media*. Copenhagen, Denmark: Ejnar Mundsgaard Forlag; 1945

137. Palmu AA, Herva E, Savolainen H, Karma P, Mäkelä PH, Kilpi TM. Association of clinical signs and symptoms with bacterial findings in acute otitis media. *Clin Infect Dis*. 2004;38(2):234–242

138. Leibovitz E, Asher E, Piglansky L, et al. Is bilateral acute otitis media clinically different than unilateral acute otitis media? *Pediatr Infect Dis J*. 2007;26(7):589–592

139. Leibovitz E, Satran R, Piglansky L, et al. Can acute otitis media caused by *Haemophilus influenzae* be distinguished from that caused by *Streptococcus pneumoniae*? *Pediatr Infect Dis J*. 2003;22(6): 509–515

140. Palmu AA, Kotikoski MJ, Kaijalainen TH, Puhakka HJ. Bacterial etiology of acute myringitis in children less than two years of age. *Pediatr Infect Dis J*. 2001;20(6): 607–611

141. Bodor FF. Systemic antibiotics for treatment of the conjunctivitis-otitis media syndrome. *Pediatr Infect Dis J*. 1989;8(5): 287–290

142. Bingen E, Cohen R, Jourenkova N, Gehanno P. Epidemiologic study of conjunctivitis-otitis syndrome. *Pediatr Infect Dis J*. 2005;24(8):731–732

143. Barkai G, Leibovitz E, Givon-Lavi N, Dagan R. Potential contribution by nontypable *Haemophilus influenzae* in protracted and recurrent acute otitis media. *Pediatr Infect Dis J*. 2009;28(6):466–471

144. Howie VM, Ploussard JH. Efficacy of fixed combination antibiotics versus separate components in otitis media. Effectiveness of erythromycin estrolate, triple sulfonamide, ampicillin, erythromycin estolate-triple sulfonamide, and placebo in 280 patients with acute otitis media under two and one-half years of age. *Clin Pediatr (Phila)*. 1972;11(4):205–214

145. Klein JO. Microbiologic efficacy of antibacterial drugs for acute otitis media. *Pediatr Infect Dis J*. 1993;12(12): 973–975

146. Barnett ED, Klein JO. The problem of resistant bacteria for the management of acute otitis media. *Pediatr Clin North Am*. 1995;42(3):509–517

147. Tristram S, Jacobs MR, Appelbaum PC. Antimicrobial resistance in *Haemophilus influenzae*. *Clin Microbiol Rev*. 2007;20(2): 368–389

148. Critchley IA, Jacobs MR, Brown SD, Traczewski MM, Tillotson GS, Janjic N. Prevalence of serotype 19A *Streptococcus pneumoniae* among isolates from U.S. children in 2005≠2006 and activity of faropenem. *Antimicrob Agents Chemother*. 2008;52(7): 2639–2643

149. Jacobs MR, Good CE, Windau AR, et al. Activity of ceftaroline against emerging serotypes of Streptococcus pneumoniae. *Antimicrob Agents Chemother*. 2010;54(6): 2716–2719

150. Jacobs MR. Antimicrobial-resistant *Streptococcus pneumoniae:* trends and management. *Expert Rev Anti Infect Ther*. 2008;6(5):619–635

151. Piglansky L, Leibovitz E, Raiz S, et al. Bacteriologic and clinical efficacy of high dose amoxicillin for therapy of acute otitis media in children. *Pediatr Infect Dis J*. 2003;22(5):405–413

152. Dagan R, Johnson CE, McLinn S, et al. Bacteriologic and clinical efficacy of amoxicillin/clavulanate vs. azithromycin in acute otitis media. *Pediatr Infect Dis J*. 2000;19(2):95–104

153. Dagan R, Hoberman A, Johnson C, et al. Bacteriologic and clinical efficacy of high dose amoxicillin/clavulanate in children with acute otitis media. *Pediatr Infect Dis J*. 2001;20(9):829–837

154. Hoberman A, Dagan R, Leibovitz E, et al. Large dosage amoxicillin/clavulanate, compared with azithromycin, for the treatment of bacterial acute otitis media in children. *Pediatr Infect Dis J*. 2005;24 (6):525–532

155. De Wals P, Erickson L, Poirier B, Pépin J, Pichichero ME. How to compare the efficacy of conjugate vaccines to prevent acute otitis media? *Vaccine*. 2009;27(21): 2877–2883

156. Shouval DS, Greenberg D, Givon-Lavi N, Porat N, Dagan R. Serotype coverage of invasive and mucosal pneumococcal disease in Israeli children younger than 3 years by various pneumococcal conjugate vaccines. *Pediatr Infect Dis J*. 2009;28(4): 277–282

157. Jones RN, Farrell DJ, Mendes RE, Sader HS. Comparative ceftaroline activity tested against pathogens associated with community-acquired pneumonia: results from an international surveillance study. *J Antimicrob Chemother*. 2011;66(suppl 3): iii69–iii80

158. Harrison CJ, Woods C, Stout G, Martin B, Selvarangan R. Susceptibilities of Haemophilus influenzae, Streptococcus pneumoniae, including serotype 19A, and Moraxella catarrhalis paediatric isolates from 2005 to 2007 to commonly used antibiotics. *J Antimicrob Chemother*. 2009;63(3):511–519

159. Doern GV, Jones RN, Pfaller MA, Kugler K. *Haemophilus influenzae* and *Moraxella catarrhalis* from patients with community-acquired respiratory tract infections: antimicrobial susceptibility patterns from the SENTRY antimicrobial Surveillance Program (United States and Canada, 1997).

Antimicrob Agents Chemother. 1999;43(2): 385–389

160. Nussinovitch M, Yoeli R, Elishkevitz K, Varsano I. Acute mastoiditis in children: epidemiologic, clinical, microbiologic, and therapeutic aspects over past years. *Clin Pediatr (Phila).* 2004;43(3):261–267

161. Roddy MG, Glazier SS, Agrawal D. Pediatric mastoiditis in the pneumococcal conjugate vaccine era: symptom duration guides empiric antimicrobial therapy. *Pediatr Emerg Care.* 2007;23(11):779–784

162. Hoberman A, Paradise JL, Burch DJ, et al. Equivalent efficacy and reduced occurrence of diarrhea from a new formulation of amoxicillin/clavulanate potassium (Augmentin) for treatment of acute otitis media in children. *Pediatr Infect Dis J.* 1997;16(5):463–470

163. Arguedas A, Dagan R, Leibovitz E, Hoberman A, Pichichero M, Paris M. A multicenter, open label, double tympanocentesis study of high dose cefdinir in children with acute otitis media at high risk of persistent or recurrent infection. *Pediatr Infect Dis J.* 2006;25(3):211–218

164. Atanasković-Marković M, Velickovic TC, Gavrović-Jankulović M, Vucković O, Nestorović B. Immediate allergic reactions to cephalosporins and penicillins and their cross-reactivity in children. *Pediatr Allergy Immunol.* 2005;16(4):341–347

165. Pichichero ME. Use of selected cephalosporins in penicillin-allergic patients: a paradigm shift. *Diagn Microbiol Infect Dis.* 2007;57(suppl 3):13S–18S

166. Pichichero ME, Casey JR. Safe use of selected cephalosporins in penicillin-allergic patients: a meta-analysis. *Otolaryngol Head Neck Surg.* 2007;136(3):340–347

167. DePestel DD, Benninger MS, Danziger L, et al. Cephalosporin use in treatment of patients with penicillin allergies. *J Am Pharm Assoc (2003).* 2008;48(4):530–540

168. Fonacier L, Hirschberg R, Gerson S. Adverse drug reactions to a cephalosporins in hospitalized patients with a history of penicillin allergy. *Allergy Asthma Proc.* 2005;26(2):135–141

169. Joint Task Force on Practice Parameters; American Academy of Allergy, Asthma and Immunology; American College of Allergy, Asthma and Immunology; Joint Council of Allergy, Asthma and Immunology. Drug allergy: an updated practice parameter. *Ann Allergy Asthma Immunol.* 2010;105(4): 259–273

170. Powers JL, Gooch WM, III, Oddo LP. Comparison of the palatability of the oral suspension of cefdinir vs. amoxicillin/clavulanate potassium, cefprozil and azithromycin in pediatric patients. *Pediatr Infect Dis J.* 2000; 19(suppl 12):S174–S180

171. Steele RW, Thomas MP, Bégué RE. Compliance issues related to the selection of antibiotic suspensions for children. *Pediatr Infect Dis J.* 2001;20(1):1–5

172. Steele RW, Russo TM, Thomas MP. Adherence issues related to the selection of antistaphylococcal or antifungal antibiotic suspensions for children. *Clin Pediatr (Phila).* 2006;45(3):245–250

173. Schwartz RH. Enhancing children's satisfaction with antibiotic therapy: a taste study of several antibiotic suspensions. *Curr Ther Res.* 2000;61(8):570–581

174. Green SM, Rothrock SG. Single-dose intramuscular ceftriaxone for acute otitis media in children. *Pediatrics.* 1993;91(1): 23–30

175. Leibovitz E, Piglansky L, Raiz S, Press J, Leiberman A, Dagan R. Bacteriologic and clinical efficacy of one day vs. three day intramuscular ceftriaxone for treatment of nonresponsive acute otitis media in children. *Pediatr Infect Dis J.* 2000;19(11): 1040–1045

176. Rosenfeld RM, Kay D. Natural history of untreated otitis media. *Laryngoscope.* 2003;113(10):1645–1657

177. Rosenfeld RM, Kay D. Natural history of untreated otitis media. In: Rosenfeld RM, Bluestone CD, eds. *Evidence-Based Otitis Media.* 2nd ed. Hamilton, Canada: BC Decker; 2003:180–198

178. Arola M, Ziegler T, Ruuskanen O. Respiratory virus infection as a cause of prolonged symptoms in acute otitis media. *J Pediatr.* 1990;116(5):697–701

179. Chonmaitree T, Owen MJ, Howie VM. Respiratory viruses interfere with bacteriologic response to antibiotic in children with acute otitis media. *J Infect Dis.* 1990; 162(2):546–549

180. Dagan R, Leibovitz E, Greenberg D, Yagupsky P, Fliss DM, Leiberman A. Early eradication of pathogens from middle ear fluid during antibiotic treatment of acute otitis media is associated with improved clinical outcome. *Pediatr Infect Dis J.* 1998;17(9):776–782

181. Carlin SA, Marchant CD, Shurin PA, Johnson CE, Super DM, Rehmus JM. Host factors and early therapeutic response in acute otitis media. *J Pediatr.* 1991;118(2):178–183

182. Teele DW, Pelton SI, Klein JO. Bacteriology of acute otitis media unresponsive to initial antimicrobial therapy. *J Pediatr.* 1981; 98(4):537–539

183. Doern GV, Pfaller MA, Kugler K, Freeman J, Jones RN. Prevalence of antimicrobial resistance among respiratory tract isolates of *Streptococcus pneumoniae* in North America: 1997 results from the SENTRY antimicrobial surveillance program. *Clin Infect Dis.* 1998;27(4):764–770

184. Leiberman A, Leibovitz E, Piglansky L, et al. Bacteriologic and clinical efficacy of trimethoprim-sulfamethoxazole for treatment of acute otitis media. *Pediatr Infect Dis J.* 2001;20(3):260–264

185. Humphrey WR, Shattuck MH, Zielinski RJ, et al. Pharmacokinetics and efficacy of linezolid in a gerbil model of *Streptococcus pneumoniae*-induced acute otitis media. *Antimicrob Agents Chemother.* 2003; 47(4):1355–1363

186. Arguedas A, Dagan R, Pichichero M, et al. An open-label, double tympanocentesis study of levofloxacin therapy in children with, or at high risk for, recurrent or persistent acute otitis media. *Pediatr Infect Dis J.* 2006;25(12):1102–1109

187. Noel GJ, Blumer JL, Pichichero ME, et al. A randomized comparative study of levofloxacin versus amoxicillin/clavulanate for treatment of infants and young children with recurrent or persistent acute otitis media. *Pediatr Infect Dis J.* 2008;27(6): 483–489

188. Howie VM, Ploussard JH. Simultaneous nasopharyngeal and middle ear exudate culture in otitis media. *Pediatr Digest.* 1971;13:31–35

189. Gehanno P, Lenoir G, Barry B, Bons J, Boucot I, Berche P. Evaluation of nasopharyngeal cultures for bacteriologic assessment of acute otitis media in children. *Pediatr Infect Dis J.* 1996;15(4): 329–332

190. Cohen R, Levy C, Boucherat M, Langue J, de La Rocque F. A multicenter, randomized, double-blind trial of 5 versus 10 days of antibiotic therapy for acute otitis media in young children. *J Pediatr.* 1998;133(5): 634–639

191. Pessey JJ, Gehanno P, Thoroddsen E, et al. Short course therapy with cefuroxime axetil for acute otitis media: results of a randomized multicenter comparison with amoxicillin/clavulanate. *Pediatr Infect Dis J.* 1999;18(10):854–859

192. Cohen R, Levy C, Boucherat M, et al. Five vs. ten days of antibiotic therapy for acute otitis media in young children. *Pediatr Infect Dis J.* 2000;19(5):458–463

193. Pichichero ME, Marsocci SM, Murphy ML, Hoeger W, Francis AB, Green JL. A prospective observational study of 5-, 7-, and 10-day antibiotic treatment for acute otitis media. *Otolaryngol Head Neck Surg.* 2001; 124(4):381–387

194. Kozyrskyj AL, Klassen TP, Moffatt M, Harvey K. Short-course antibiotics for acute otitis media. *Cochrane Database Syst Rev.* 2010; (9):CD001095

195. Shurin PA, Pelton SI, Donner A, Klein JO. Persistence of middle-ear effusion after acute otitis media in children. *N Engl J Med.* 1979;300(20):1121–1123

196. Damoiseaux RA, Rovers MM, Van Balen FA, Hoes AW, de Melker RA. Long-term prognosis of acute otitis media in infancy: determinants of recurrent acute otitis media and persistent middle ear effusion. *Fam Pract.* 2006;23(1):40–45

197. Leach AJ, Morris PS. Antibiotics for the prevention of acute and chronic suppurative otitis media in children. *Cochrane Database Syst Rev.* 2006;(4):CD004401

198. Teele DW, Klein JO, Word BM, et al; Greater Boston Otitis Media Study Group. Antimicrobial prophylaxis for infants at risk for recurrent acute otitis media. *Vaccine.* 2000;19(suppl 1):S140–S143

199. Paradise JL. On tympanostomy tubes: rationale, results, reservations, and recommendations. *Pediatrics.* 1977;60(1):86–90

200. McIsaac WJ, Coyte PC, Croxford R, Asche CV, Friedberg J, Feldman W. Otolaryngologists' perceptions of the indications for tympanostomy tube insertion in children. *CMAJ.* 2000;162(9):1285–1288

201. Casselbrandt ML. Ventilation tubes for recurrent acute otitis media. In: Alper CM, Bluestone CD, eds. *Advanced Therapy of Otitis Media.* Hamilton, Canada: BC Decker; 2004:113–115

202. Shin JJ, Stinnett SS, Hartnick CJ. Pediatric recurrent acute otitis media. In: Shin JJ, Hartnick CJ, Randolph GW, eds. *Evidence-Based Otolaryngology.* New York, NY: Springer; 2008:91–95

203. Gonzalez C, Arnold JE, Woody EA, et al. Prevention of recurrent acute otitis media: chemoprophylaxis versus tympanostomy tubes. *Laryngoscope.* 1986;96(12): 1330–1334

204. Gebhart DE. Tympanostomy tubes in the otitis media prone child. *Laryngoscope.* 1981;91(6):849–866

205. Casselbrant ML, Kaleida PH, Rockette HE, et al. Efficacy of antimicrobial prophylaxis and of tympanostomy tube insertion for prevention of recurrent acute otitis media: results of a randomized clinical trial. *Pediatr Infect Dis J.* 1992;11(4):278–286

206. El-Sayed Y. Treatment of recurrent acute otitis media chemoprophylaxis versus ventilation tubes. *Aust J Otolaryngol.* 1996; 2(4):352–355

207. McDonald S, Langton Hewer CD, Nunez DA. Grommets (ventilation tubes) for re-

current acute otitis media in children. *Cochrane Database Syst Rev.* 2008;(4): CD004741

208. Rosenfeld RM, Bhaya MH, Bower CM, et al. Impact of tympanostomy tubes on child quality of life. *Arch Otolaryngol Head Neck Surg.* 2000;126(5):585–592

209. Witsell DL, Stewart MG, Monsell EM, et al. The Cooperative Outcomes Group for ENT: a multicenter prospective cohort study on the outcomes of tympanostomy tubes for children with otitis media. *Otolaryngol Head Neck Surg.* 2005;132(2):180–188

210. Isaacson G. Six Sigma tympanostomy tube insertion: achieving the highest safety levels during residency training. *Otolaryngol Head Neck Surg.* 2008;139(3):353–357

211. Kay DJ, Nelson M, Rosenfeld RM. Meta-analysis of tympanostomy tube sequelae. *Otolaryngol Head Neck Surg.* 2001;124(4): 374–380

212. Koivunen P, Uhari M, Luotonen J, et al. Adenoidectomy versus chemoprophylaxis and placebo for recurrent acute otitis media in children aged under 2 years: randomised controlled trial. *BMJ.* 2004; 328(7438):487

213. Rosenfeld RM. Surgical prevention of otitis media. *Vaccine.* 2000;19(suppl 1):S134–S139

214. Centers for Disease Control and Prevention (CDC). Prevention and control of influenza with vaccines: recommendations of the Advisory Committee on Immunization Practices (ACIP), 2011. *MMWR Morb Mortal Wkly Rep.* 2011;60(33):1128–1132

215. American Academy of Pediatrics Committee on Infectious Diseases. Recommendations for prevention and control of influenza in children, 2011–2012. *Pediatrics.* 2011;128(4):813–825

216. Section on Breastfeeding. Breastfeeding and the use of human milk. *Pediatrics.* 2012;129(3). Available at: www.pediatrics. org/cgi/content/full/129/3/e827

217. Pavia M, Bianco A, Nobile CG, Marinelli P, Angelillo IF. Efficacy of pneumococcal vaccination in children younger than 24 months: a meta-analysis. *Pediatrics.* 2009; 123(6). Available at: www.pediatrics.org/ cgi/content/full/123/6/e1103

218. Eskola J, Kilpi T, Palmu A, et al; Finnish Otitis Media Study Group. Efficacy of a pneumococcal conjugate vaccine against acute otitis media. *N Engl J Med.* 2001;344(6):403–409

219. Black S, Shinefield H, Fireman B, et al; Northern California Kaiser Permanente Vaccine Study Center Group. Efficacy, safety and immunogenicity of heptavalent

pneumococcal conjugate vaccine in children. *Pediatr Infect Dis J.* 2000;19(3): 187–195

220. Jacobs MR. Prevention of otitis media: role of pneumococcal conjugate vaccines in reducing incidence and antibiotic resistance. *J Pediatr.* 2002;141(2):287–293

221. Jansen AG, Hak E, Veenhoven RH, Damoiseaux RA, Schilder AG, Sanders EA. Pneumococcal conjugate vaccines for preventing otitis media. *Cochrane Database Syst Rev.* 2009;(2):CD001480

222. Fireman B, Black SB, Shinefield HR, Lee J, Lewis E, Ray P. Impact of the pneumococcal conjugate vaccine on otitis media. *Pediatr Infect Dis J.* 2003;22(1):10–16

223. Grijalva CG, Poehling KA, Nuorti JP, et al. National impact of universal childhood immunization with pneumococcal conjugate vaccine on otitis media. *Pediatr Infect Dis J.* 2006;118(3):865–873

224. Zhou F, Shefer A, Kong Y, Nuorti JP. Trends in acute otitis media-related health care utilization by privately insured young children in the United States, 1997–2004. *Pediatrics.* 2008;121(2):253–260

225. Poehling KA, Szilagyi PG, Grijalva CG, et al. Reduction of frequent otitis media and pressure-equalizing tube insertions in children after introduction of pneumococcal conjugate vaccine. *Pediatrics.* 2007; 119(4):707–715

226. Pelton SI. Prospects for prevention of otitis media. *Pediatr Infect Dis J.* 2007;26 (suppl 10):S20–S22

227. Pelton SI, Leibovitz E. Recent advances in otitis media. *Pediatr Infect Dis J.* 2009;28 (suppl 10):S133–S137

228. De Wals P, Erickson L, Poirier B, Pépin J, Pichichero ME. How to compare the efficacy of conjugate vaccines to prevent acute otitis media? *Vaccine.* 2009;27(21): 2877–2883

229. Plasschaert AI, Rovers MM, Schilder AG, Verheij TJ, Hak E. Trends in doctor consultations, antibiotic prescription, and specialist referrals for otitis media in children: 1995–2003. *Pediatrics.* 2006;117(6): 1879–1886

230. O'Brien MA, Prosser LA, Paradise JL, et al. New vaccines against otitis media: projected benefits and cost-effectiveness. *Pediatrics.* 2009;123(6):1452–1463

231. Hanage WP, Auranen K, Syrjänen R, et al. Ability of pneumococcal serotypes and clones to cause acute otitis media: implications for the prevention of otitis media by conjugate vaccines. *Infect Immun.* 2004; 72(1):76–81

232. Prymula R, Peeters P, Chrobok V, et al. Pneumococcal capsular polysaccharides

conjugated to protein D for prevention of acute otitis media caused by both Streptococcus pneumoniae and non-typable *Haemophilus influenzae*: a randomised double-blind efficacy study. *Lancet*. 2006; 367(9512):740–748

233. Prymula R, Schuerman L. 10-valent pneumococcal nontypeable *Haemophilus influenzae* PD conjugate vaccine: Synflorix. *Expert Rev Vaccines*. 2009;8(11):1479–1500

234. Schuerman L, Borys D, Hoet B, Forsgren A, Prymula R. Prevention of otitis media: now a reality? *Vaccine*. 2009;27(42):5748–5754

235. Heikkinen T, Ruuskanen O, Waris M, Ziegler T, Arola M, Halonen P. Influenza vaccination in the prevention of acute otitis media in children. *Am J Dis Child*. 1991;145(4):445–448

236. Clements DA, Langdon L, Bland C, Walter E. Influenza A vaccine decreases the incidence of otitis media in 6- to 30-month-old children in day care. *Arch Pediatr Adolesc Med*. 1995;149(10):1113–1117

237. Belshe RB, Gruber WC. Prevention of otitis media in children with live attenuated influenza vaccine given intranasally. *Pediatr Infect Dis J*. 2000;19(suppl 5):S66–S71

238. Marchisio P, Cavagna R, Maspes B, et al. Efficacy of intranasal virosomal influenza vaccine in the prevention of recurrent acute otitis media in children. *Clin Infect Dis*. 2002;35(2):168–174

239. Ozgur SK, Beyazova U, Kemaloglu YK, et al. Effectiveness of inactivated influenza vaccine for prevention of otitis media in children. *Pediatr Infect Dis J*. 2006;25(5):401–404

240. Block SL, Heikkinen T, Toback SL, Zheng W, Ambrose CS. The efficacy of live attenuated influenza vaccine against influenza-associated acute otitis media in children. *Pediatr Infect Dis J*. 2011;30(3):203–207

241. Ashkenazi S, Vertruyen A, Arístegui J, et al; CAIV-T Study Group. Superior relative efficacy of live attenuated influenza vaccine compared with inactivated influenza vaccine in young children with recurrent respiratory tract infections. *Pediatr Infect Dis J*. 2006;25(10):870–879

242. Belshe RB, Edwards KM, Vesikari T, et al; CAIV-T Comparative Efficacy Study Group. Live attenuated versus inactivated influenza vaccine in infants and young children [published correction appears in *N Engl J Med*. 2007;356(12):1283]. *N Engl J Med*. 2007;356(7):685–696

243. Bracco Neto H, Farhat CK, Tregnaghi MW, et al; D153-P504 LAIV Study Group. Efficacy and safety of 1 and 2 doses of live attenuated influenza vaccine in vaccine-naive children. *Pediatr Infect Dis J*. 2009;28(5): 365–371

244. Tam JS, Capeding MR, Lum LC, et al; Pan-Asian CAIV-T Pediatric Efficacy Trial Network. Efficacy and safety of a live attenuated, cold-adapted influenza vaccine, trivalent against culture-confirmed influenza in young children in Asia. *Pediatr Infect Dis J*. 2007;26(7):619–628

245. Vesikari T, Fleming DM, Aristegui JF, et al; CAIV-T Pediatric Day Care Clinical Trial Network. Safety, efficacy, and effectiveness of cold-adapted influenza vaccine-trivalent against community-acquired, culture-confirmed influenza in young children attending day care. *Pediatrics*. 2006;118(6):2298–2312

246. Forrest BD, Pride MW, Dunning AJ, et al. Correlation of cellular immune responses with protection against culture-confirmed influenza virus in young children. *Clin Vaccine Immunol*. 2008;15(7): 1042–1053

247. Lum LC, Borja-Tabora CF, Breiman RF, et al. Influenza vaccine concurrently administered with a combination measles, mumps, and rubella vaccine to young children. *Vaccine*. 2010;28(6):1566–1574

248. Belshe RB, Mendelman PM, Treanor J, et al. The efficacy of live attenuated, cold-adapted, trivalent, intranasal influenzavirus vaccine in children. *N Engl J Med*. 1998;338(20): 1405–1412

249. Daly KA, Giebink GS. Clinical epidemiology of otitis media. *Pediatr Infect Dis J*. 2000; 19(suppl 5):S31–S36

250. Duncan B, Ey J, Holberg CJ, Wright AL, Martinez FD, Taussig LM. Exclusive breastfeeding for at least 4 months protects against otitis media. *Pediatrics*. 1993;91(5): 867–872

251. Duffy LC, Faden H, Wasielewski R, Wolf J, Krystofik D. Exclusive breastfeeding protects against bacterial colonization and day care exposure to otitis media. *Pediatrics*. 1997;100(4). Available at: www.pediatrics.org/cgi/content/full/100/4/e7

252. Paradise JL. Short-course antimicrobial treatment for acute otitis media: not best for infants and young children. *JAMA*. 1997;278(20):1640–1642

253. Scariati PD, Grummer-Strawn LM, Fein SB. A longitudinal analysis of infant morbidity and the extent of breastfeeding in the United States. *Pediatrics*. 1997;99(6). Available at: www.pediatrics.org/cgi/content/full/99/6/e5

254. McNiel ME, Labbok MH, Abrahams SW. What are the risks associated with formula feeding? A re-analysis and review. *Breastfeed Rev*. 2010;18(2):25–32

255. Chantry CJ, Howard CR, Auinger P. Full breastfeeding duration and associated decrease in respiratory tract infection in US children. *Pediatrics*. 2006;117(2):425–432

256. Hatakka K, Piirainen L, Pohjavuori S, Poussa T, Savilahti E, Korpela R. Factors associated with acute respiratory illness in day care children. *Scand J Infect Dis*. 2010;42(9):704–711

257. Ladomenou F, Kafatos A, Tselentis Y, Galanakis E. Predisposing factors for acute otitis media in infancy. *J Infect*. 2010;61(1):49–53

258. Ladomenou F, Moschandreas J, Kafatos A, Tselentis Y, Galanakis E. Protective effect of exclusive breastfeeding against infections during infancy: a prospective study. *Arch Dis Child*. 2010;95(12):1004–1008

259. Duijts L, Jaddoe VW, Hofman A, Moll HA. Prolonged and exclusive breastfeeding reduces the risk of infectious diseases in infancy. *Pediatrics*. 2010;126(1). Available at: www.pediatrics.org/cgi/content/full/126/1/e18

260. Best D; Committee on Environmental Health; Committee on Native American Child Health; Committee on Adolescence. From the American Academy of Pediatrics: technical report—secondhand and prenatal tobacco smoke exposure. *Pediatrics*. 2009;124(5). Available at: www.pediatrics.org/cgi/content/full/124/5/e1017

261. Etzel RA, Pattishall EN, Haley NJ, Fletcher RH, Henderson FW. Passive smoking and middle ear effusion among children in day care. *Pediatrics*. 1992;90(2 pt 1): 228–232

262. Ilicali OC, Keleş N, Değer K, Savaş I. Relationship of passive cigarette smoking to otitis media. *Arch Otolaryngol Head Neck Surg*. 1999;125(7):758–762

263. Wellington M, Hall CB. Pacifier as a risk factor for acute otitis media [letter]. *Pediatrics*. 2002;109(2):351–352, author reply 353

264. Kerstein R. Otitis media: prevention instead of prescription. *Br J Gen Pract*. 2008;58(550):364–365

265. Brown CE, Magnuson B. On the physics of the infant feeding bottle and middle ear sequela: ear disease in infants can be associated with bottle feeding. *Int J Pediatr Otorhinolaryngol*. 2000;54(1):13–20

266. Niemelä M, Pihakari O, Pokka T, Uhari M. Pacifier as a risk factor for acute otitis media: a randomized, controlled trial of parental counseling. *Pediatrics*. 2000;106(3): 483–488

267. Tully SB, Bar-Haim Y, Bradley RL. Abnormal tympanography after supine bottle feeding. *J Pediatr.* 1995;126(6):S105–S111

268. Rovers MM, Numans ME, Langenbach E, Grobbee DE, Verheij TJ, Schilder AG. Is pacifier use a risk factor for acute otitis media? A dynamic cohort study. *Fam Pract.* 2008;25(4):233–236

269. Adderson EE. Preventing otitis media: medical approaches. *Pediatr Ann.* 1998;27(2):101–107

270. Azarpazhooh A, Limeback H, Lawrence HP, Shah PS. Xylitol for preventing acute otitis media in children up to 12 years of age. *Cochrane Database Syst Rev.* 2011;(11): CD007095

271. Hautalahti O, Renko M, Tapiainen T, Kontiokari T, Pokka T, Uhari M. Failure of xylitol given three times a day for preventing acute otitis media. *Pediatr Infect Dis J.* 2007;26(5):423–427

272. Tapiainen T, Luotonen L, Kontiokari T, Renko M, Uhari M. Xylitol administered only during respiratory infections failed to prevent acute otitis media. *Pediatrics.* 2002;109(2). Available at: www.pediatrics.org/cgi/content/full/109/2/e19

273. Uhari M, Kontiokari T, Koskela M, Niemelä M. Xylitol chewing gum in prevention of acute otitis media: double blind randomised trial. *BMJ.* 1996;313(7066):1180–1184

274. Uhari M, Kontiokari T, Niemelä M. A novel use of xylitol sugar in preventing acute otitis media. *Pediatrics.* 1998;102(4 pt 1):879–884

275. O'Brien MA, Prosser LA, Paradise JL, et al. New vaccines against otitis media: projected benefits and cost-effectiveness. *Pediatrics.* 2009;123(6):1452–1463

(Continued from first page)

All clinical practice guidelines from the American Academy of Pediatrics automatically expire 5 years after publication unless reaffirmed, revised, or retired at or before that time.

www.pediatrics.org/cgi/doi/10.1542/peds.2012-3488

doi:10.1542/peds.2012-3488

PEDIATRICS (ISSN Numbers: Print, 0031-4005; Online, 1098-4275).

Otitis Media With Effusion

- *Clinical Practice Guideline*

AMERICAN ACADEMY OF PEDIATRICS

CLINICAL PRACTICE GUIDELINE

American Academy of Family Physicians, American Academy of Otolaryngology-Head and Neck Surgery, and American Academy of Pediatrics Subcommittee on Otitis Media With Effusion

Otitis Media With Effusion

ABSTRACT. The clinical practice guideline on otitis media with effusion (OME) provides evidence-based recommendations on diagnosing and managing OME in children. This is an update of the 1994 clinical practice guideline "Otitis Media With Effusion in Young Children," which was developed by the Agency for Healthcare Policy and Research (now the Agency for Healthcare Research and Quality). In contrast to the earlier guideline, which was limited to children 1 to 3 years old with no craniofacial or neurologic abnormalities or sensory deficits, the updated guideline applies to children aged 2 months through 12 years with or without developmental disabilities or underlying conditions that predispose to OME and its sequelae. The American Academy of Pediatrics, American Academy of Family Physicians, and American Academy of Otolaryngology-Head and Neck Surgery selected a subcommittee composed of experts in the fields of primary care, otolaryngology, infectious diseases, epidemiology, hearing, speech and language, and advanced-practice nursing to revise the OME guideline.

The subcommittee made a strong recommendation that clinicians use pneumatic otoscopy as the primary diagnostic method and distinguish OME from acute otitis media.

The subcommittee made recommendations that clinicians should 1) document the laterality, duration of effusion, and presence and severity of associated symptoms at each assessment of the child with OME, 2) distinguish the child with OME who is at risk for speech, language, or learning problems from other children with OME and more promptly evaluate hearing, speech, language, and need for intervention in children at risk, and 3) manage the child with OME who is not at risk with watchful waiting for 3 months from the date of effusion onset (if known) or diagnosis (if onset is unknown).

The subcommittee also made recommendations that 4) hearing testing be conducted when OME persists for 3 months or longer or at any time that language delay, learning problems, or a significant hearing loss is suspected in a child with OME, 5) children with persistent OME who are not at risk should be reexamined at 3- to 6-month intervals until the effusion is no longer present, significant hearing loss is identified, or structural abnormalities of the eardrum or middle ear are suspected, and 6) when a child becomes a surgical candidate (tympanostomy tube insertion is the preferred initial procedure). Adenoidectomy should not be performed unless a distinct indication exists (nasal obstruction, chronic adenoiditis); repeat surgery consists of adenoidectomy plus myringotomy with or without tubeinsertion. Tonsillectomy alone or myringotomy alone should not be used to treat OME.

The subcommittee made negative recommendations that 1) population-based screening programs for OME not be performed in healthy, asymptomatic children, and 2) because antihistamines and decongestants are ineffective for OME, they should not be used for treatment; antimicrobials and corticosteroids do not have long-term efficacy and should not be used for routine management.

The subcommittee gave as options that 1) tympanometry can be used to confirm the diagnosis of OME and 2) when children with OME are referred by the primary clinician for evaluation by an otolaryngologist, audiologist, or speech-language pathologist, the referring clinician should document the effusion duration and specific reason for referral (evaluation, surgery) and provide additional relevant information such as history of acute otitis media and developmental status of the child. The subcommittee made no recommendations for 1) complementary and alternative medicine as a treatment for OME, based on a lack of scientific evidence documenting efficacy, or 2) allergy management as a treatment for OME, based on insufficient evidence of therapeutic efficacy or a causal relationship between allergy and OME. Last, the panel compiled a list of research needs based on limitations of the evidence reviewed.

The purpose of this guideline is to inform clinicians of evidence-based methods to identify, monitor, and manage OME in children aged 2 months through 12 years. The guideline may not apply to children more than 12 years old, because OME is uncommon and the natural history is likely to differ from younger children who experience rapid developmental change. The target population includes children with or without developmental disabilities or underlying conditions that predispose to OME and its sequelae. The guideline is intended for use by providers of health care to children, including primary care and specialist physicians, nurses and nurse practitioners, physician assistants, audiologists, speech-language pathologists, and child-development specialists. The guideline is applicable to any setting in which children with OME would be identified, monitored, or managed.

This guideline is not intended as a sole source of guidance in evaluating children with OME. Rather, it is designed to assist primary care and other clinicians by providing an evidence-based framework for decision-making strategies. It is not intended to replace clinical judgment or establish a protocol for all children with this condition and may not provide the only appropriate approach to diagnosing and managing this problem. *Pediatrics* 2004;113:1412–1429; *acute otitis media, antibacterial, antibiotic.*

This document was approved by the American Academy of Otolaryngology–Head and Neck Surgery Foundation, Inc and the American Academy of Pediatrics, and is published in the May 2004 issue of *Otolaryngology-Head and Neck Surgery* and the May 2004 issue of *Pediatrics*.
PEDIATRICS (ISSN 0031 4005). Copyright © 2004 by the American Academy of Otolaryngology–Head and Neck Surgery Foundation, Inc and the American Academy of Pediatrics.

ABBREVIATIONS. OME, otitis media with effusion; AOM, acute otitis media; AAP, American Academy of Pediatrics; AHRQ, Agency for Healthcare Research and Quality; EPC, Southern California Evidence-Based Practice Center; CAM, complementary and alternative medicine; HL, hearing level.

Otitis media with effusion (OME) as discussed in this guideline is defined as the presence of fluid in the middle ear without signs or symptoms of acute ear infection.[1,2] OME is considered distinct from acute otitis media (AOM), which is defined as a history of acute onset of signs and symptoms, the presence of middle-ear effusion, and signs and symptoms of middle-ear inflammation. Persistent middle-ear fluid from OME results in decreased mobility of the tympanic membrane and serves as a barrier to sound conduction.[3] Approximately 2.2 million diagnosed episodes of OME occur annually in the United States, yielding a combined direct and indirect annual cost estimate of $4.0 billion.[2]

OME may occur spontaneously because of poor eustachian tube function or as an inflammatory response following AOM. Approximately 90% of children (80% of individual ears) have OME at some time before school age,[4] most often between ages 6 months and 4 years.[5] In the first year of life, >50% of children will experience OME, increasing to >60% by 2 years.[6] Many episodes resolve spontaneously within 3 months, but ~30% to 40% of children have recurrent OME, and 5% to 10% of episodes last 1 year or longer.[1,4,7]

The primary outcomes considered in the guideline include hearing loss; effects on speech, language, and learning; physiologic sequelae; health care utilization (medical, surgical); and quality of life.[1,2] The high prevalence of OME, difficulties in diagnosis and assessing duration, increased risk of conductive hearing loss, potential impact on language and cognition, and significant practice variations in management[8] make OME an important condition for the use of up-to-date evidence-based practice guidelines.

METHODS

General Methods and Literature Search

In developing an evidence-based clinical practice guideline on managing OME, the American Academy of Pediatrics (AAP), American Academy of Family Physicians, and American Academy of Otolaryngology-Head and Neck Surgery worked with the Agency for Healthcare Research and Quality (AHRQ) and other organizations. This effort included representatives from each partnering organization along with liaisons from audiology, speech-language pathology, informatics, and advanced-practice nursing. The most current literature on managing children with OME was reviewed, and research questions were developed to guide the evidence-review process.

The AHRQ report on OME from the Southern California Evidence-Based Practice Center (EPC) focused on key questions of natural history, diagnostic methods, and long-term speech, language, and hearing outcomes.[2] Searches were conducted through January 2000 in Medline, Embase, and the Cochrane Library. Additional articles were identified by review of reference listings in proceedings, reports, and other guidelines. The EPC accepted 970 articles for full review after screening 3200 abstracts. The EPC reviewed articles by using established quality criteria[9,10] and included randomized trials, prospective cohorts, and validations of diagnostic tests (validating cohort studies).

The AAP subcommittee on OME updated the AHRQ review with articles identified by an electronic Medline search through April 2003 and with additional material identified manually by subcommittee members. Copies of relevant articles were distributed to the subcommittee for consideration. A specific search for articles relevant to complementary and alternative medicine (CAM) was performed by using Medline and the Allied and Complementary Medicine Database through April 2003. Articles relevant to allergy and OME were identified by using Medline through April 2003. The subcommittee met 3 times over a 1-year period, ending in May 2003, with interval electronic review and feedback on each guideline draft to ensure accuracy of content and consistency with standardized criteria for reporting clinical practice guidelines.[11]

In May 2003, the Guidelines Review Group of the Yale Center for Medical Informatics used the Guideline Elements Model[12] to categorize content of the present draft guideline. Policy statements were parsed into component decision variables and actions and then assessed for decidability and executability. Quality appraisal using established criteria[13] was performed with Guideline Elements Model-Q Online.[14,15] Implementation issues were predicted by using the Implementability Rating Profile, an instrument under development by the Yale Guidelines Review Group (R. Shiffman, MD, written communication, May 2003). OME subcommittee members received summary results and modified an advanced draft of the guideline.

The final draft practice guideline underwent extensive peer review by numerous entities identified by the subcommittee. Comments were compiled and reviewed by the subcommittee cochairpersons. The recommendations contained in the practice guideline are based on the best available published data through April 2003. Where data are lacking, a combination of clinical experience and expert consensus was used. A scheduled review process will occur 5 years from publication or sooner if new compelling evidence warrants earlier consideration.

Classification of Evidence-Based Statements

Guidelines are intended to reduce inappropriate variations in clinical care, produce optimal health outcomes for patients, and minimize harm. The evidence-based approach to guideline development requires that the evidence supporting a policy be identified, appraised, and summarized and that an explicit link between evidence and statements be defined. Evidence-based statements reflect the quality of evidence and the balance of benefit and harm that is anticipated when the statement is followed. The AAP definitions for evidence-based statements[16] are listed in Tables 1 and 2.

Guidelines are never intended to overrule professional judgment; rather, they may be viewed as a relative constraint on individual clinician discretion in a particular clinical circumstance. Less frequent variation in practice is expected for a strong recommendation than might be expected with a recommendation. Options offer the opportunity for practice variability.[17] All clinicians should always act and decide in a way that they believe will best serve their patients' interests and needs regardless of guideline recommendations. Guidelines represent the best judgment of a team of experienced clinicians and methodologists addressing the scientific evidence for a particular topic.[16]

Making recommendations about health practices involves value judgments on the desirability of various outcomes associated with management options. Value judgments applied by the OME subcommittee were made in an effort to minimize harm and diminish unnecessary therapy. Emphasis was placed on promptly identifying and managing children at risk for speech, language, or learning problems to maximize opportunities for beneficial outcomes. Direct costs also were considered in the statements concerning diagnosis and screening and to a lesser extent in other statements.

1A. PNEUMATIC OTOSCOPY: CLINICIANS SHOULD USE PNEUMATIC OTOSCOPY AS THE PRIMARY DIAGNOSTIC METHOD FOR OME, AND OME SHOULD BE DISTINGUISHED FROM AOM

This is a strong recommendation based on systematic review of cohort studies and the preponderance of benefit over harm.

TABLE 1. Guideline Definitions for Evidence-Based Statements

Statement	Definition	Implication
Strong Recommendation	A strong recommendation means that the subcommittee believes that the benefits of the recommended approach clearly exceed the harms (or that the harms clearly exceed the benefits in the case of a strong negative recommendation) and that the quality of the supporting evidence is excellent (grade A or B).* In some clearly identified circumstances, strong recommendations may be made based on lesser evidence when high-quality evidence is impossible to obtain and the anticipated benefits strongly outweigh the harms.	Clinicians should follow a strong recommendation unless a clear and compelling rationale for an alternative approach is present.
Recommendation	A recommendation means that the subcommittee believes that the benefits exceed the harms (or that the harms exceed the benefits in the case of a negative recommendation), but the quality of evidence is not as strong (grade B or C).* In some clearly identified circumstances, recommendations may be made based on lesser evidence when high-quality evidence is impossible to obtain and the anticipated benefits outweigh the harms.	Clinicians also should generally follow a recommendation but should remain alert to new information and sensitive to patient preferences.
Option	An option means that either the quality of evidence that exists is suspect (grade D)* or that well-done studies (grade A, B, or C)* show little clear advantage to one approach versus another.	Clinicians should be flexible in their decision-making regarding appropriate practice, although they may set boundaries on alternatives; patient preference should have a substantial influencing role.
No Recommendation	No recommendation means that there is both a lack of pertinent evidence (grade D)* and an unclear balance between benefits and harms.	Clinicians should feel little constraint in their decision-making and be alert to new published evidence that clarifies the balance of benefit versus harm; patient preference should have a substantial influencing role.

* See Table 2 for the definitions of evidence grades.

TABLE 2. Evidence Quality for Grades of Evidence

Grade	Evidence Quality
A	Well-designed, randomized, controlled trials or diagnostic studies performed on a population similar to the guideline's target population
B	Randomized, controlled trials or diagnostic studies with minor limitations; overwhelmingly consistent evidence from observational studies
C	Observational studies (case-control and cohort design)
D	Expert opinion, case reports, or reasoning from first principles (bench research or animal studies)

1B. TYMPANOMETRY: TYMPANOMETRY CAN BE USED TO CONFIRM THE DIAGNOSIS OF OME

This option is based on cohort studies and a balance of benefit and harm.

Diagnosing OME correctly is fundamental to proper management. Moreover, OME must be differentiated from AOM to avoid unnecessary antimicrobial use.[18,19]

OME is defined as fluid in the middle ear without signs or symptoms of acute ear infection.[2] The tympanic membrane is often cloudy with distinctly impaired mobility,[20] and an air-fluid level or bubble may be visible in the middle ear. Conversely, diagnosing AOM requires a history of acute onset of signs and symptoms, the presence of middle-ear effusion, and signs and symptoms of middle-ear inflammation. The critical distinguishing feature is that only AOM has acute signs and symptoms. Distinct redness of the tympanic membrane should not be a criterion for prescribing antibiotics, because it has poor predictive value for AOM and is present in ~5% of ears with OME.[20]

The AHRQ evidence report[2] systematically reviewed the sensitivity, specificity, and predictive values of 9 diagnostic methods for OME. Pneumatic otoscopy had the best balance of sensitivity and specificity, consistent with the 1994 guideline.[1] Meta-analysis revealed a pooled sensitivity of 94% (95% confidence interval: 91%–96%) and specificity of 80% (95% confidence interval: 75%–86%) for validated observers using pneumatic otoscopy versus myringotomy as the gold standard. Pneumatic otoscopy therefore should remain the primary method of OME diagnosis, because the instrument is readily available in practice settings, cost-effective, and accurate in experienced hands. Non–pneumatic otoscopy is not advised for primary diagnosis.

The accuracy of pneumatic otoscopy in routine clinical practice may be less than that shown in published results, because clinicians have varying training and experience.[21,22] When the diagnosis of OME is uncertain, tympanometry or acoustic reflectometry should be considered as an adjunct to pneumatic otoscopy. Tympanometry with a standard 226-Hz probe tone is reliable for infants 4 months old or older and has good interobserver agreement of curve patterns in routine clinical practice.[23,24] Younger infants require specialized equipment with a higher probe tone frequency. Tympanometry generates costs related to instrument purchase, annual calibration, and test administration. Acoustic reflectometry with spectral gradient analysis is a low-cost alternative to tympanometry that does not require an airtight seal in the ear canal; however, validation studies primarily have used children 2 years old or older with a high prevalence of OME.[25–27]

Although no research studies have examined whether pneumatic otoscopy causes discomfort, expert consensus suggests that the procedure does not have to be painful, especially when symptoms of acute infection (AOM) are absent. A nontraumatic examination is facilitated by using a gentle touch, restraining the child properly when necessary, and inserting the speculum only into the outer one third (cartilaginous portion) of the ear canal.[28] The pneumatic bulb should be compressed slightly before insertion, because OME often is associated with a negative middle-ear pressure, which can be assessed more accurately by releasing the already compressed bulb. The otoscope must be fully charged, the bulb (halogen or xenon) bright and luminescent,[29] and the insufflator bulb attached tightly to the head to avoid the loss of an air seal. The window must also be sealed.

Evidence Profile: Pneumatic Otoscopy

- Aggregate evidence quality: A, diagnostic studies in relevant populations.
- Benefit: improved diagnostic accuracy; inexpensive equipment.
- Harm: cost of training clinicians in pneumatic otoscopy.
- Benefits-harms assessment: preponderance of benefit over harm.
- Policy level: strong recommendation.

Evidence Profile: Tympanometry

- Aggregate evidence quality: B, diagnostic studies with minor limitations.
- Benefit: increased diagnostic accuracy beyond pneumatic otoscopy; documentation.
- Harm: acquisition cost, administrative burden, and recalibration.
- Benefits-harms assessment: balance of benefit and harm.
- Policy level: option.

1C. SCREENING: POPULATION-BASED SCREENING PROGRAMS FOR OME ARE NOT RECOMMENDED IN HEALTHY, ASYMPTOMATIC CHILDREN

This recommendation is based on randomized, controlled trials and cohort studies, with a preponderance of harm over benefit.

This recommendation concerns population-based screening programs of all children in a community or a school without regard to any preexisting symptoms or history of disease. This recommendation does not address hearing screening or monitoring of specific children with previous or recurrent OME.

OME is highly prevalent in young children. Screening surveys of healthy children ranging in age from infancy to 5 years old show a 15% to 40% point prevalence of middle-ear effusion.[5,7,30–36] Among children examined at regular intervals for a year, ~50% to 60% of child care center attendees[32] and 25% of school-aged children[37] were found to have a middle-ear effusion at some time during the examination period, with peak incidence during the winter months.

Population-based screening has not been found to influence short-term language outcomes,[33] and its long-term effects have not been evaluated in a randomized, clinical trial. Therefore, the recommendation against screening is based not only on the ability to identify OME but more importantly on a lack of demonstrable benefits from treating children so identified that exceed the favorable natural history of the disease. The New Zealand Health Technology Assessment[38] could not determine whether preschool screening for OME was effective. More recently, the Canadian Task Force on Preventive Health Care[39] reported that insufficient evidence was available to recommend including or excluding routine early screening for OME. Although screening for OME is not inherently harmful, potential risks include inaccurate diagnoses, overtreating self-limited disease, parental anxiety, and the costs of screening and unnecessary treatment.

Population-based screening is appropriate for conditions that are common, can be detected by a sensitive and specific test, and benefit from early detection and treatment.[40] The first 2 requirements are fulfilled by OME, which affects up to 80% of children by school entry[2,5,7] and can be screened easily with tympanometry (see recommendation 1B). Early detection and treatment of OME identified by screening, however, have not been shown to improve intelligence, receptive language, or expressive language.[2,39,41,42] Therefore, population-based screening for early detection of OME in asymptomatic children has not been shown to improve outcomes and is not recommended.

Evidence Profile: Screening

- Aggregate evidence quality: B, randomized, controlled trials with minor limitations and consistent evidence from observational studies.
- Benefit: potentially improved developmental outcomes, which have not been demonstrated in the best current evidence.

- Harm: inaccurate diagnosis (false-positive or false-negative), overtreating self-limited disease, parental anxiety, cost of screening, and/or unnecessary treatment.
- Benefits-harms assessment: preponderance of harm over benefit.
- Policy level: recommendation against.

2. DOCUMENTATION: CLINICIANS SHOULD DOCUMENT THE LATERALITY, DURATION OF EFFUSION, AND PRESENCE AND SEVERITY OF ASSOCIATED SYMPTOMS AT EACH ASSESSMENT OF THE CHILD WITH OME

This recommendation is based on observational studies and strong preponderance of benefit over harm.

Documentation in the medical record facilitates diagnosis and treatment and communicates pertinent information to other clinicians to ensure patient safety and reduce medical errors.[43] Management decisions in children with OME depend on effusion duration and laterality plus the nature and severity of associated symptoms. Therefore, these features should be documented at every medical encounter for OME. Although no studies have addressed documentation for OME specifically, there is room for improvement in documentation of ambulatory care medical records.[44]

Ideally, the time of onset and laterality of OME can be defined through diagnosis of an antecedent AOM, a history of acute onset of signs or symptoms directly referable to fluid in the middle ear, or the presence of an abnormal audiogram or tympanogram closely after a previously normal test. Unfortunately, these conditions are often lacking, and the clinician is forced to speculate on the onset and duration of fluid in the middle ear(s) in a child found to have OME at a routine office visit or school screening audiometry.

In ~40% to 50% of cases of OME, neither the affected children nor their parents or caregivers describe significant complaints referable to a middle-ear effusion.[45,46] In some children, however, OME may have associated signs and symptoms caused by inflammation or the presence of effusion (not acute infection) that should be documented, such as

- Mild intermittent ear pain, fullness, or "popping"
- Secondary manifestations of ear pain in infants, which may include ear rubbing, excessive irritability, and sleep disturbances
- Failure of infants to respond appropriately to voices or environmental sounds, such as not turning accurately toward the sound source
- Hearing loss, even when not specifically described by the child, suggested by seeming lack of attentiveness, behavioral changes, failure to respond to normal conversational-level speech, or the need for excessively high sound levels when using audio equipment or viewing television
- Recurrent episodes of AOM with persistent OME between episodes
- Problems with school performance
- Balance problems, unexplained clumsiness, or delayed gross motor development[47–50]
- Delayed speech or language development

The laterality (unilateral versus bilateral), duration of effusion, and presence and severity of associated symptoms should be documented in the medical record at each assessment of the child with OME. When OME duration is uncertain, the clinician must take whatever evidence is at hand and make a reasonable estimate.

Evidence Profile: Documentation

- Aggregate evidence quality: C, observational studies.
- Benefits: defines severity, duration has prognostic value, facilitates future communication with other clinicians, supports appropriate timing of intervention, and, if consistently unilateral, may identify a problem with specific ear other than OME (eg, retraction pocket or cholesteatoma).
- Harm: administrative burden.
- Benefits-harms assessment: preponderance of benefit over harm.
- Policy level: recommendation.

3. CHILD AT RISK: CLINICIANS SHOULD DISTINGUISH THE CHILD WITH OME WHO IS AT RISK FOR SPEECH, LANGUAGE, OR LEARNING PROBLEMS FROM OTHER CHILDREN WITH OME AND SHOULD EVALUATE HEARING, SPEECH, LANGUAGE, AND NEED FOR INTERVENTION MORE PROMPTLY

This recommendation is based on case series, the preponderance of benefit over harm, and ethical limitations in studying children with OME who are at risk.

The panel defines the child at risk as one who is at increased risk for developmental difficulties (delay or disorder) because of sensory, physical, cognitive, or behavioral factors listed in Table 3. These factors are not caused by OME but can make the child less tolerant of hearing loss or vestibular problems secondary to middle-ear effusion. In contrast the child with OME who is not at risk is otherwise healthy and does not have any of the factors shown in Table 3.

Earlier guidelines for managing OME have applied only to young children who are healthy and exhibit no developmental delays.[1] Studies of the relationship between OME and hearing loss or speech/language development typically exclude children with craniofacial anomalies, genetic syndromes, and other developmental disorders. Therefore, the available literature mainly applies to otherwise healthy children who meet inclusion criteria for randomized,

TABLE 3.   Risk Factors for Developmental Difficulties*

Permanent hearing loss independent of OME
Suspected or diagnosed speech and language delay or disorder
Autism-spectrum disorder and other pervasive developmental disorders
Syndromes (eg, Down) or craniofacial disorders that include cognitive, speech, and language delays
Blindness or uncorrectable visual impairment
Cleft palate with or without associated syndrome
Developmental delay

* Sensory, physical, cognitive, or behavioral factors that place children who have OME at an increased risk for developmental difficulties (delay or disorder).

controlled trials. Few, if any, existing studies dealing with developmental sequelae caused by hearing loss from OME can be generalized to children who are at risk.

Children who are at risk for speech or language delay would likely be affected additionally by hearing problems from OME,[51] although definitive studies are lacking. For example, small comparative studies of children or adolescents with Down syndrome[52] or cerebral palsy[53] show poorer articulation and receptive language associated with a history of early otitis media. Large studies are unlikely to be forthcoming because of methodologic and ethical difficulties inherent in studying children who are delayed or at risk for further delays. Therefore, clinicians who manage children with OME should determine whether other conditions coexist that put a child at risk for developmental delay (Table 3) and then take these conditions into consideration when planning assessment and management.

Children with craniofacial anomalies (eg, cleft palate; Down syndrome; Robin sequence; coloboma, heart defect, choanal atresia, retarded growth and development, genital anomaly, and ear defect with deafness [CHARGE] association) have a higher prevalence of chronic OME, hearing loss (conductive and sensorineural), and speech or language delay than do children without these anomalies.[54–57] Other children may not be more prone to OME but are likely to have speech and language disorders, such as those children with permanent hearing loss independent of OME,[58,59] specific language impairment,[60] autism-spectrum disorders,[61] or syndromes that adversely affect cognitive and linguistic development. Some retrospective studies[52,62,63] have found that hearing loss caused by OME in children with cognitive delays, such as Down syndrome, has been associated with lower language levels. Children with language delays or disorders with OME histories perform more poorly on speech-perception tasks than do children with OME histories alone.[64,65]

Children with severe visual impairments may be more susceptible to the effects of OME, because they depend on hearing more than children with normal vision.[51] Any decrease in their most important remaining sensory input for language (hearing) may significantly compromise language development and their ability to interact and communicate with others. All children with severe visual impairments should be considered more vulnerable to OME sequelae, especially in the areas of balance, sound localization, and communication.

Management of the child with OME who is at increased risk for developmental delays should include hearing testing and speech and language evaluation and may include speech and language therapy concurrent with managing OME, hearing aids or other amplification devices for hearing loss independent of OME, tympanostomy tube insertion,[54,63,66,67] and hearing testing after OME resolves to document improvement, because OME can mask a permanent underlying hearing loss and delay detection.[59,68,69]

Evidence Profile: Child at Risk

- Aggregate evidence quality: C, observational studies of children at risk; D, expert opinion on the ability of prompt assessment and management to alter outcomes.
- Benefits: optimizing conditions for hearing, speech, and language; enabling children with special needs to reach their potential; avoiding limitations on the benefits of educational interventions because of hearing problems from OME.
- Harm: cost, time, and specific risks of medications or surgery.
- Benefits-harms assessment: exceptional preponderance of benefits over harm based on subcommittee consensus because of circumstances to date precluding randomized trials.
- Policy level: recommendation.

4. WATCHFUL WAITING: CLINICIANS SHOULD MANAGE THE CHILD WITH OME WHO IS NOT AT RISK WITH WATCHFUL WAITING FOR 3 MONTHS FROM THE DATE OF EFFUSION ONSET (IF KNOWN) OR DIAGNOSIS (IF ONSET IS UNKNOWN)

This recommendation is based on systematic review of cohort studies and the preponderance of benefit over harm.

This recommendation is based on the self-limited nature of most OME, which has been well documented in cohort studies and in control groups of randomized trials.[2,70]

The likelihood of spontaneous resolution of OME is determined by the cause and duration of effusion.[70] For example, ~75% to 90% of residual OME after an AOM episode resolves spontaneously by 3 months.[71–73] Similar outcomes of defined onset during a period of surveillance in a cohort study are observed for OME.[32,37] Another favorable situation involves improvement (not resolution) of newly detected OME defined as change in tympanogram from type B (flat curve) to non-B (anything other than a flat curve). Approximately 55% of children so defined improve by 3 months,[70] but one third will have OME relapse within the next 3 months.[4] Although a type B tympanogram is an imperfect measure of OME (81% sensitivity and 74% specificity versus myringotomy), it is the most widely reported measure suitable for deriving pooled resolution rates.[2,70]

Approximately 25% of newly detected OME of unknown prior duration in children 2 to 4 years old resolves by 3 months when resolution is defined as a change in tympanogram from type B to type A/C1 (peak pressure >200 daPa).[2,70,74–77] Resolution rates may be higher for infants and young children in whom the preexisting duration of effusion is generally shorter, and particularly for those observed prospectively in studies or in the course of well-child care. Documented bilateral OME of 3 months' duration or longer resolves spontaneously after 6 to 12 months in ~30% of children primarily 2 years old or older, with only marginal benefits if observed longer.[70]

Any intervention for OME (medical or surgical) other than observation carries some inherent harm. There is little harm associated with a specified period of observation in the child who is not at risk for speech, language, or learning problems. When observing children with OME, clinicians should inform the parent or caregiver that the child may experience reduced hearing until the effusion resolves, especially if it is bilateral. Clinicians may discuss strategies for optimizing the listening and learning environment until the effusion resolves. These strategies include speaking in close proximity to the child, facing the child and speaking clearly, repeating phrases when misunderstood, and providing preferential classroom seating.[78,79]

The recommendation for a 3-month period of observation is based on a clear preponderance of benefit over harm and is consistent with the original OME guideline intent of avoiding unnecessary surgery.[1] At the discretion of the clinician, this 3-month period of watchful waiting may include interval visits at which OME is monitored by using pneumatic otoscopy, tympanometry, or both. Factors to consider in determining the optimal interval(s) for follow-up include clinical judgment, parental comfort level, unique characteristics of the child and/or his environment, access to a health care system, and hearing levels (HLs) if known.

After documented resolution of OME in all affected ears, additional follow-up is unnecessary.

Evidence Profile: Watchful Waiting

- Aggregate evidence quality: B, systematic review of cohort studies.
- Benefit: avoid unnecessary interventions, take advantage of favorable natural history, and avoid unnecessary referrals and evaluations.
- Harm: delays in therapy for OME that will not resolve with observation; prolongation of hearing loss.
- Benefits-harms assessment: preponderance of benefit over harm.
- Policy level: recommendation.

5. MEDICATION: ANTIHISTAMINES AND DECONGESTANTS ARE INEFFECTIVE FOR OME AND ARE NOT RECOMMENDED FOR TREATMENT; ANTIMICROBIALS AND CORTICOSTEROIDS DO NOT HAVE LONG-TERM EFFICACY AND ARE NOT RECOMMENDED FOR ROUTINE MANAGEMENT

This recommendation is based on systematic review of randomized, controlled trials and the preponderance of harm over benefit.

Therapy for OME is appropriate only if persistent and clinically significant benefits can be achieved beyond spontaneous resolution. Although statistically significant benefits have been demonstrated for some medications, they are short-term and relatively small in magnitude. Moreover, significant adverse events may occur with all medical therapies.

The prior OME guideline[1] found no data supporting antihistamine-decongestant combinations in treating OME. Meta-analysis of 4 randomized trials showed no significant benefit for antihistamines or decongestants versus placebo. No additional studies have been published since 1994 to change this recommendation. Adverse effects of antihistamines and decongestants include insomnia, hyperactivity, drowsiness, behavioral change, and blood-pressure variability.

Long-term benefits of antimicrobial therapy for OME are unproved despite a modest short-term benefit for 2 to 8 weeks in randomized trials.[1,80,81] Initial benefits, however, can become nonsignificant within 2 weeks of stopping the medication.[82] Moreover, ~7 children would need to be treated with antimicrobials to achieve one short-term response.[1] Adverse effects of antimicrobials are significant and may include rashes, vomiting, diarrhea, allergic reactions, alteration of the child's nasopharyngeal flora, development of bacterial resistance,[83] and cost. Societal consequences include direct transmission of resistant bacterial pathogens in homes and child care centers.[84]

The prior OME guideline[1] did not recommend oral steroids for treating OME in children. A later meta-analysis[85] showed no benefit for oral steroid versus placebo within 2 weeks but did show a short-term benefit for oral steroid plus antimicrobial versus antimicrobial alone in 1 of 3 children treated. This benefit became nonsignificant after several weeks in a prior meta-analysis[1] and in a large, randomized trial.[86] Oral steroids can produce behavioral changes, increased appetite, and weight gain.[1] Additional adverse effects may include adrenal suppression, fatal varicella infection, and avascular necrosis of the femoral head.[3] Although intranasal steroids have fewer adverse effects, one randomized trial[87] showed statistically equivalent outcomes at 12 weeks for intranasal beclomethasone plus antimicrobials versus antimicrobials alone for OME.

Antimicrobial therapy with or without steroids has not been demonstrated to be effective in long-term resolution of OME, but in some cases this therapy can be considered an option because of short-term benefit in randomized trials, when the parent or caregiver expresses a strong aversion to impending surgery. In this circumstance, a single course of therapy for 10 to 14 days may be used. The likelihood that the OME will resolve long-term with these regimens is small, and prolonged or repetitive courses of antimicrobials or steroids are strongly not recommended.

Other nonsurgical therapies that are discussed in the OME literature include autoinflation of the eustachian tube, oral or intratympanic use of mucolytics, and systemic use of pharmacologic agents other than antimicrobials, steroids, and antihistamine-decongestants. Insufficient data exist for any of these therapies to be recommended in treating OME.[3]

Evidence Profile: Medication

- Aggregate evidence quality: A, systematic review of well-designed, randomized, controlled trials.

- Benefit: avoid side effects and reduce cost by not administering medications; avoid delays in definitive therapy caused by short-term improvement then relapse.
- Harm: adverse effects of specific medications as listed previously; societal impact of antimicrobial therapy on bacterial resistance and transmission of resistant pathogens.
- Benefits-harms assessment: preponderance of harm over benefit.
- Policy level: recommendation against.

6. HEARING AND LANGUAGE: HEARING TESTING IS RECOMMENDED WHEN OME PERSISTS FOR 3 MONTHS OR LONGER OR AT ANY TIME THAT LANGUAGE DELAY, LEARNING PROBLEMS, OR A SIGNIFICANT HEARING LOSS IS SUSPECTED IN A CHILD WITH OME; LANGUAGE TESTING SHOULD BE CONDUCTED FOR CHILDREN WITH HEARING LOSS

This recommendation is based on cohort studies and the preponderance of benefit over risk.

Hearing Testing

Hearing testing is recommended when OME persists for 3 months or longer or at any time that language delay, learning problems, or a significant hearing loss is suspected. Conductive hearing loss often accompanies OME[1,88] and may adversely affect binaural processing,[89] sound localization,[90] and speech perception in noise.[91–94] Hearing loss caused by OME may impair early language acquisition,[95–97] but the child's home environment has a greater impact on outcomes[98]; recent randomized trials[41,99,100] suggest no impact on children with OME who are not at risk as identified by screening or surveillance.

Studies examining hearing sensitivity in children with OME report that average pure-tone hearing loss at 4 frequencies (500, 1000, 2000, and 4000 Hz) ranges from normal hearing to moderate hearing loss (0–55 dB). The 50th percentile is an ~25-dB HL, and ~20% of ears exceed 35-dB HL.[101,102] Unilateral OME with hearing loss results in overall poorer binaural hearing than in infants with normal middle-ear function bilaterally.[103,104] However, based on limited research, there is evidence that children experiencing the greatest conductive hearing loss for the longest periods may be more likely to exhibit developmental and academic sequelae.[1,95,105]

Initial hearing testing for children 4 years old or older can be done in the primary care setting.[106] Testing should be performed in a quiet environment, preferably in a separate closed or sound-proofed area set aside specifically for that purpose. Conventional audiometry with earphones is performed with a fail criterion of more than 20-dB HL at 1 or more frequencies (500, 1000, 2000, and 4000 Hz) in either ear.[106,107] Methods not recommended as substitutes for primary care hearing testing include tympanometry and pneumatic otoscopy,[102] caregiver judgment regarding hearing loss,[108,109] speech audiometry, and tuning forks, acoustic reflectometry, and behavioral observation.[1]

Comprehensive audiologic evaluation is recommended for children who fail primary care testing, are less than 4 years old, or cannot be tested in the primary care setting. Audiologic assessment includes evaluating air-conduction and bone-conduction thresholds for pure tones, speech-detection or speech-recognition thresholds,[102] and measuring speech understanding if possible.[94] The method of assessment depends on the developmental age of the child and might include visual reinforcement or conditioned orienting-response audiometry for infants 6 to 24 months old, play audiometry for children 24 to 48 months old, or conventional screening audiometry for children 4 years old and older.[106] The auditory brainstem response and otoacoustic emission are tests of auditory pathway structural integrity, not hearing, and should not substitute for behavioral pure-tone audiometry.[106]

Language Testing

Language testing should be conducted for children with hearing loss (pure-tone average more than 20-dB HL on comprehensive audiometric evaluation). Testing for language delays is important, because communication is integral to all aspects of human functioning. Young children with speech and language delays during the preschool years are at risk for continued communication problems and later delays in reading and writing.[110–112] In one study, 6% to 8% of children 3 years old and 2% to 13% of kindergartners had language impairment.[113] Language intervention can improve communication and other functional outcomes for children with histories of OME.[114]

Children who experience repeated and persistent episodes of OME and associated hearing loss during early childhood may be at a disadvantage for learning speech and language.[79,115] Although Shekelle et al[2] concluded that there was no evidence to support the concern that OME during the first 3 years of life was related to later receptive or expressive language, this meta-analysis should be interpreted cautiously, because it did not examine specific language domains such as vocabulary and the independent variable was OME and not hearing loss. Other meta-analyses[79,115] have suggested at most a small negative association of OME and hearing loss on children's receptive and expressive language through the elementary school years. The clinical significance of these effects for language and learning is unclear for the child not at risk. For example, in one randomized trial,[100] prompt insertion of tympanostomy tubes for OME did not improve developmental outcomes at 3 years old regardless of baseline hearing. In another randomized trial,[116] however, prompt tube insertion achieved small benefits for children with bilateral OME and hearing loss.

Clinicians should ask the parent or caregiver about specific concerns regarding their child's language development. Children's speech and language can be tested at ages 6 to 36 months by direct engagement of a child and interviewing the parent using the Early Language Milestone Scale.[117] Other approaches require interviewing only the child's parent or caregiver, such as the MacArthur Communicative Development Inventory[118] and the Language Development Survey.[119] For older children, the Denver Developmental Screening Test II[120] can be used to screen general development including speech and language. Comprehensive speech and language evaluation is recommended for children who fail testing or whenever the child's parent or caregiver expresses concern.[121]

Evidence Profile: Hearing and Language

- Aggregate evidence quality: B, diagnostic studies with minor limitations; C, observational studies.
- Benefit: to detect hearing loss and language delay and identify strategies or interventions to improve developmental outcomes.
- Harm: parental anxiety, direct and indirect costs of assessment, and/or false-positive results.
- Balance of benefit and harm: preponderance of benefit over harm.
- Policy level: recommendation.

7. SURVEILLANCE: CHILDREN WITH PERSISTENT OME WHO ARE NOT AT RISK SHOULD BE REEXAMINED AT 3- TO 6-MONTH INTERVALS UNTIL THE EFFUSION IS NO LONGER PRESENT, SIGNIFICANT HEARING LOSS IS IDENTIFIED, OR STRUCTURAL ABNORMALITIES OF THE EARDRUM OR MIDDLE EAR ARE SUSPECTED

This recommendation is based on randomized, controlled trials and observational studies with a preponderance of benefit over harm.

If OME is asymptomatic and is likely to resolve spontaneously, intervention is unnecessary even if OME persists for more than 3 months. The clinician should determine whether risk factors exist that would predispose the child to undesirable sequelae or predict nonresolution of the effusion. As long as OME persists, the child is at risk for sequelae and must be reevaluated periodically for factors that would prompt intervention.

The 1994 OME guideline[1] recommended surgery for OME persisting 4 to 6 months with hearing loss but requires reconsideration because of later data on tubes and developmental sequelae.[122] For example, selecting surgical candidates using duration-based criteria (eg, OME >3 months or exceeding a cumulative threshold) does not improve developmental outcomes in infants and toddlers who are not at risk.[41,42,99,100] Additionally, the 1994 OME guideline did not specifically address managing effusion without significant hearing loss persisting more than 6 months.

Asymptomatic OME usually resolves spontaneously, but resolution rates decrease the longer the effusion has been present,[36,76,77] and relapse is common.[123] Risk factors that make spontaneous resolution less likely include[124,125]:

- Onset of OME in the summer or fall season
- Hearing loss more than 30-dB HL in the better-hearing ear

- History of prior tympanostomy tubes
- Not having had an adenoidectomy

Children with chronic OME are at risk for structural damage of the tympanic membrane[126] because the effusion contains leukotrienes, prostaglandins, and arachidonic acid metabolites that invoke a local inflammatory response.[127] Reactive changes may occur in the adjacent tympanic membrane and mucosal linings. A relative underventilation of the middle ear produces a negative pressure that predisposes to focal retraction pockets, generalized atelectasis of the tympanic membrane, and cholesteatoma.

Structural integrity is assessed by carefully examining the entire tympanic membrane, which, in many cases, can be accomplished by the primary care clinician using a handheld pneumatic otoscope. A search should be made for retraction pockets, ossicular erosion, and areas of atelectasis or atrophy. If there is any uncertainty that all observed structures are normal, the patient should be examined by using an otomicroscope. All children with these tympanic membrane conditions, regardless of OME duration, should have a comprehensive audiologic evaluation.

Conditions of the tympanic membrane that generally mandate inserting a tympanostomy tube are posterosuperior retraction pockets, ossicular erosion, adhesive atelectasis, and retraction pockets that accumulate keratin debris. Ongoing surveillance is mandatory, because the incidence of structural damage increases with effusion duration.[128]

As noted in recommendation 6, children with persistent OME for 3 months or longer should have their hearing tested. Based on these results, clinicians can identify 3 levels of action based on HLs obtained for the better-hearing ear using earphones or in sound field using speakers if the child is too young for ear-specific testing.

1. HLs of ≥40 dB (at least a moderate hearing loss): A comprehensive audiologic evaluation is indicated if not previously performed. If moderate hearing loss is documented and persists at this level, surgery is recommended, because persistent hearing loss of this magnitude that is permanent in nature has been shown to impact speech, language, and academic performance.[129–131]
2. HLs of 21 to 39 dB (mild hearing loss): A comprehensive audiologic evaluation is indicated if not previously performed. Mild sensorineural hearing loss has been associated with difficulties in speech, language, and academic performance in school,[129,132] and persistent mild conductive hearing loss from OME may have a similar impact. Further management should be individualized based on effusion duration, severity of hearing loss, and parent or caregiver preference and may include strategies to optimize the listening and learning environment (Table 4) or surgery. Repeat hearing testing should be performed in 3 to 6 months if OME persists at follow-up evaluation or tympanostomy tubes have not been placed.
3. HLs of ≤20 dB (normal hearing): A repeat hearing test should be performed in 3 to 6 months if OME persists at follow-up evaluation.

TABLE 4. Strategies for Optimizing the Listening-Learning Environment for Children With OME and Hearing Loss*

Get within 3 feet of the child before speaking.
Turn off competing audio signals such as unnecessary music and television in the background.
Face the child and speak clearly, using visual clues (hands, pictures) in addition to speech.
Slow the rate, raise the level, and enunciate speech directed at the child.
Read to or with the child, explaining pictures and asking questions.
Repeat words, phrases, and questions when misunderstood.
Assign preferential seating in the classroom near the teacher.
Use a frequency-modulated personal- or sound-field-amplification system in the classroom.

* Modified with permission from Roberts et al.[78,79]

In addition to hearing loss and speech or language delay, other factors may influence the decision to intervene for persistent OME. Roberts et al[98,133] showed that the caregiving environment is more strongly related to school outcome than was OME or hearing loss. Risk factors for delays in speech and language development caused by a poor caregiving environment included low maternal educational level, unfavorable child care environment, and low socioeconomic status. In such cases, these factors may be additive to the hearing loss in affecting lower school performance and classroom behavior problems.

Persistent OME may be associated with physical or behavioral symptoms including hyperactivity, poor attention, and behavioral problems in some studies[134–136] and reduced child quality of life.[46] Conversely, young children randomized to early versus late tube insertion for persistent OME showed no behavioral benefits from early surgery.[41,100] Children with chronic OME also have significantly poorer vestibular function and gross motor proficiency when compared with non-OME controls.[48–50] Moreover, vestibular function, behavior, and quality of life can improve after tympanostomy tube insertion.[47,137,138] Other physical symptoms of OME that, if present and persistent, may warrant surgery include otalgia, unexplained sleep disturbance, and coexisting recurrent AOM. Tubes reduce the absolute incidence of recurrent AOM by ~1 episode per child per year, but the relative risk reduction is 56%.[139]

The risks of continued observation of children with OME must be balanced against the risks of surgery. Children with persistent OME examined regularly at 3- to 6-month intervals, or sooner if OME-related symptoms develop, are most likely at low risk for physical, behavioral, or developmental sequelae of OME. Conversely, prolonged watchful waiting of OME is not appropriate when regular surveillance is impossible or when the child is at risk for developmental sequelae of OME because of co-morbidities (Table 3). For these children, the risks of anesthesia and surgery (see recommendation 9) may be less than those of continued observation.

Evidence Profile: Surveillance

- Aggregate evidence quality: C, observational studies and some randomized trials.

- Benefit: avoiding interventions that do not improve outcomes.
- Harm: allowing structural abnormalities to develop in the tympanic membrane, underestimating the impact of hearing loss on a child, and/or failing to detect significant signs or symptoms that require intervention.
- Balance of benefit and harm: preponderance of benefit over harm.
- Policy level: recommendation.

8. REFERRAL: WHEN CHILDREN WITH OME ARE REFERRED BY THE PRIMARY CARE CLINICIAN FOR EVALUATION BY AN OTOLARYNGOLOGIST, AUDIOLOGIST, OR SPEECH-LANGUAGE PATHOLOGIST, THE REFERRING CLINICIAN SHOULD DOCUMENT THE EFFUSION DURATION AND SPECIFIC REASON FOR REFERRAL (EVALUATION, SURGERY) AND PROVIDE ADDITIONAL RELEVANT INFORMATION SUCH AS HISTORY OF AOM AND DEVELOPMENTAL STATUS OF THE CHILD

This option is based on panel consensus and a preponderance of benefit over harm.

This recommendation emphasizes the importance of communication between the referring primary care clinician and the otolaryngologist, audiologist, and speech-language pathologist. Parents and caregivers may be confused and frustrated when a recommendation for surgery is made for their child because of conflicting information about alternative management strategies. Choosing among management options is facilitated when primary care physicians and advanced-practice nurses who best know the patient's history of ear problems and general medical status provide the specialist with accurate information. Although there are no studies showing improved outcomes from better documentation of OME histories, there is a clear need for better mechanisms to convey information and expectations from primary care clinicians to consultants and subspecialists.[140–142]

When referring a child for evaluation to an otolaryngologist, the primary care physician should explain the following to the parent or caregiver of the patient:

- Reason for referral: Explain that the child is seeing an otolaryngologist for evaluation, which is likely to include ear examination and audiologic testing, and not necessarily simply to be scheduled for surgery.
- What to expect: Explain that surgery may be recommended, and let the parent know that the otolaryngologist will explain the options, benefits, and risks further.
- Decision-making process: Explain that there are many alternatives for management and that surgical decisions are elective; the parent or caregiver should be encouraged to express to the surgeon any concerns he or she may have about the recommendations made.

When referring a child to an otolaryngologist, audiologist, or speech-language pathologist, the minimum information that should be conveyed in writing includes:

- Duration of OME: State how long fluid has been present.
- Laterality of OME: State whether one or both ears have been affected.
- Results of prior hearing testing or tympanometry.
- Suspected speech or language problems: State whether there had been a delay in speech and language development or whether the parent or a caregiver has expressed concerns about the child's communication abilities, school achievement, or attentiveness.
- Conditions that might exacerbate the deleterious effects of OME: State whether the child has conditions such as permanent hearing loss, impaired cognition, developmental delays, cleft lip or palate, or an unstable or nonsupportive family or home environment.
- AOM history: State whether the child has a history of recurrent AOM.

Additional medical information that should be provided to the otolaryngologist by the primary care clinician includes:

- Parental attitude toward surgery: State whether the parents have expressed a strong preference for or against surgery as a management option.
- Related conditions that might require concomitant surgery: State whether there have been other conditions that might warrant surgery if the child is going to have general anesthesia (eg, nasal obstruction and snoring that might be an indication for adenoidectomy or obstructive breathing during sleep that might mean tonsillectomy is indicated).
- General health status: State whether there are any conditions that might present problems for surgery or administering general anesthesia, such as congenital heart abnormality, bleeding disorder, asthma or reactive airway disease, or family history of malignant hyperthermia.

After evaluating the child, the otolaryngologist, audiologist, or speech-language pathologist should inform the referring physician regarding his or her diagnostic impression, plans for additional assessment, and recommendations for ongoing monitoring and management.

Evidence Profile: Referral

- Aggregate evidence quality: C, observational studies.
- Benefit: better communication and improved decision-making.
- Harm: confidentiality concerns, administrative burden, and/or increased parent or caregiver anxiety.
- Benefits-harms assessment: balance of benefit and harm.
- Policy level: option.

9. SURGERY: WHEN A CHILD BECOMES A SURGICAL CANDIDATE, TYMPANOSTOMY TUBE INSERTION IS THE PREFERRED INITIAL PROCEDURE; ADENOIDECTOMY SHOULD NOT BE PERFORMED UNLESS A DISTINCT INDICATION EXISTS (NASAL OBSTRUCTION, CHRONIC ADENOIDITIS). REPEAT SURGERY CONSISTS OF ADENOIDECTOMY PLUS MYRINGOTOMY, WITH OR WITHOUT TUBE INSERTION. TONSILLECTOMY ALONE OR MYRINGOTOMY ALONE SHOULD NOT BE USED TO TREAT OME

This recommendation is based on randomized, controlled trials with a preponderance of benefit over harm.

Surgical candidacy for OME largely depends on hearing status, associated symptoms, the child's developmental risk (Table 3), and the anticipated chance of timely spontaneous resolution of the effusion. Candidates for surgery include children with OME lasting 4 months or longer with persistent hearing loss or other signs and symptoms, recurrent or persistent OME in children at risk regardless of hearing status, and OME and structural damage to the tympanic membrane or middle ear. Ultimately, the recommendation for surgery must be individualized based on consensus between the primary care physician, otolaryngologist, and parent or caregiver that a particular child would benefit from intervention. Children with OME of any duration who are at risk are candidates for earlier surgery.

Tympanostomy tubes are recommended for initial surgery because randomized trials show a mean 62% relative decrease in effusion prevalence and an absolute decrease of 128 effusion days per child during the next year.[139,143–145] HLs improve by a mean of 6 to 12 dB while the tubes remain patent.[146,147] Adenoidectomy plus myringotomy (without tube insertion) has comparable efficacy in children 4 years old or older[143] but is more invasive, with additional surgical and anesthetic risks. Similarly, the added risk of adenoidectomy outweighs the limited, short-term benefit for children 3 years old or older without prior tubes.[148] Consequently, adenoidectomy is not recommended for initial OME surgery unless a distinct indication exists, such as adenoiditis, postnasal obstruction, or chronic sinusitis.

Approximately 20% to 50% of children who have had tympanostomy tubes have OME relapse after tube extrusion that may require additional surgery.[144,145,149] When a child needs repeat surgery for OME, adenoidectomy is recommended (unless the child has an overt or submucous cleft palate), because it confers a 50% reduction in the need for future operations.[143,150,151] The benefit of adenoidectomy is apparent at 2 years old,[150] greatest for children 3 years old or older, and independent of adenoid size.[143,151,152] Myringotomy is performed concurrent with adenoidectomy. Myringotomy plus adenoidectomy is effective for children 4 years old or older,[143] but tube insertion is advised for younger children, when potential relapse of effusion must be minimized (eg, children at risk) or pronounced inflammation of the tympanic membrane and middle-ear mucosa is present.

Tonsillectomy or myringotomy alone (without adenoidectomy) is not recommended to treat OME. Although tonsillectomy is either ineffective[152] or of limited efficacy,[148,150] the risks of hemorrhage (~2%) and additional hospitalization outweigh any potential benefits unless a distinct indication for tonsillectomy exists. Myringotomy alone, without tube placement or adenoidectomy, is ineffective for chronic OME,[144,145] because the incision closes within several days. Laser-assisted myringotomy extends the ventilation period several weeks,[153] but randomized trials with concurrent controls have not been conducted to establish efficacy. In contrast, tympanostomy tubes ventilate the middle ear for an average of 12 to 14 months.[144,145]

Anesthesia mortality has been reported to be ~1: 50 000 for ambulatory surgery,[154] but the current fatality rate may be lower.[155] Laryngospasm and bronchospasm occur more often in children receiving anesthesia than adults. Tympanostomy tube sequelae are common[156] but are generally transient (otorrhea) or do not affect function (tympanosclerosis, focal atrophy, or shallow retraction pocket). Tympanic membrane perforations, which may require repair, are seen in 2% of children after placement of short-term (grommet-type) tubes and 17% after long-term tubes.[156] Adenoidectomy has a 0.2% to 0.5% incidence of hemorrhage[150,157] and 2% incidence of transient velopharyngeal insufficiency.[148] Other potential risks of adenoidectomy, such as nasopharyngeal stenosis and persistent velopharyngeal insufficiency, can be minimized with appropriate patient selection and surgical technique.

There is a clear preponderance of benefit over harm when considering the impact of surgery for OME on effusion prevalence, HLs, subsequent incidence of AOM, and the need for reoperation after adenoidectomy. Information about adenoidectomy in children less than 4 years old, however, remains limited. Although the cost of surgery and anesthesia is nontrivial, it is offset by reduced OME and AOM after tube placement and by reduced need for reoperation after adenoidectomy. Approximately 8 adenoidectomies are needed to avoid a single instance of tube reinsertion; however, each avoided surgery probably represents a larger reduction in the number of AOM and OME episodes, including those in children who did not require additional surgery.[150]

Evidence Profile: Surgery

- Aggregate evidence quality: B, randomized, controlled trials with minor limitations.
- Benefit: improved hearing, reduced prevalence of OME, reduced incidence of AOM, and less need for additional tube insertion (after adenoidectomy).
- Harm: risks of anesthesia and specific surgical procedures; sequelae of tympanostomy tubes.
- Benefits-harms assessment: preponderance of benefit over harm.
- Policy level: recommendation.

10. CAM: NO RECOMMENDATION IS MADE REGARDING CAM AS A TREATMENT FOR OME

There is no recommendation based on lack of scientific evidence documenting efficacy and an uncertain balance of harm and benefit.

The 1994 OME guideline[1] made no recommendation regarding CAM as a treatment for OME, and no subsequent controlled studies have been published to change this conclusion. The current statement of "no recommendation" is based on the lack of scientific evidence documenting efficacy plus the balance of benefit and harm.

Evidence concerning CAM is insufficient to determine whether the outcomes achieved for OME differ from those achieved by watchful waiting and spontaneous resolution. There are no randomized, controlled trials with adequate sample sizes on the efficacy of CAM for OME. Although many case reports and subjective reviews on CAM treatment of AOM were found, little is published on OME treatment or prevention. Homeopathy[158] and chiropractic treatments[159] were assessed in pilot studies with small numbers of patients that failed to show clinically or statistically significant benefits. Consequently, there is no research base on which to develop a recommendation concerning CAM for OME.

The natural history of OME in childhood (discussed previously) is such that almost any intervention can be "shown" to have helped in an anecdotal, uncontrolled report or case series. The efficacy of CAM or any other intervention for OME can only be shown with parallel-group, randomized, controlled trials with valid diagnostic methods and adequate sample sizes. Unproved modalities that have been claimed to provide benefit in middle-ear disease include osteopathic and chiropractic manipulation, dietary exclusions (such as dairy), herbal and other dietary supplements, acupuncture, traditional Chinese medicine, and homeopathy. None of these modalities, however, have been subjected yet to a published, peer-reviewed, clinical trial.

The absence of any published clinical trials also means that all reports of CAM adverse effects are anecdotal. A systematic review of recent evidence[160] found significant serious adverse effects of unconventional therapies for children, most of which were associated with inadequately regulated herbal medicines. One report on malpractice liability associated with CAM therapies[161] did not address childhood issues specifically. Allergic reactions to echinacea occur but seem to be rare in children.[162] A general concern about herbal products is the lack of any governmental oversight into product quality or purity.[160,163,164] Additionally, herbal products may alter blood levels of allopathic medications, including anticoagulants. A possible concern with homeopathy is the worsening of symptoms, which is viewed as a positive, early sign of homeopathic efficacy. The adverse effects of manipulative therapies (such as chiropractic treatments and osteopathy) in children are difficult to assess because of scant evidence, but a case series of 332 children treated for AOM or OME with chiropractic manipulation did not mention any side effects.[165] Quadriplegia has been reported, however, after spinal manipulation in an infant with torticollis.[166]

Evidence Profile: CAM

- Aggregate evidence quality: D, case series without controls.
- Benefit: not established.
- Harm: potentially significant depending on the intervention.
- Benefits-harms assessment: uncertain balance of benefit and harm.
- Policy level: no recommendation.

11. ALLERGY MANAGEMENT: NO RECOMMENDATION IS MADE REGARDING ALLERGY MANAGEMENT AS A TREATMENT FOR OME

There is no recommendation based on insufficient evidence of therapeutic efficacy or a causal relationship between allergy and OME.

The 1994 OME guideline[1] made no recommendation regarding allergy management as a treatment for OME, and no subsequent controlled studies have been published to change this conclusion. The current statement of "no recommendation" is based on insufficient evidence of therapeutic efficacy or a causal relationship between allergy and OME plus the balance of benefit and harm.

A linkage between allergy and OME has long been speculated but to date remains unquantified. The prevalence of allergy among OME patients has been reported to range from less than 10% to more than 80%.[167] Allergy has long been postulated to cause OME through its contribution to eustachian tube dysfunction.[168] The cellular response of respiratory mucosa to allergens has been well studied. Therefore, similar to other parts of respiratory mucosa, the mucosa lining the middle-ear cleft is capable of an allergic response.[169,170] Sensitivity to allergens varies among individuals, and atopy may involve neutrophils in type I allergic reactions that enhance the inflammatory response.[171]

The correlation between OME and allergy has been widely reported, but no prospective studies have examined the effects of immunotherapy compared with observation alone or other management options. Reports of OME cure after immunotherapy or food-elimination diets[172] are impossible to interpret without concurrent control groups because of the favorable natural history of most untreated OME. The documentation of allergy in published reports has been defined inconsistently (medical history, physical examination, skin-prick testing, nasal smears, serum immunoglobulin E and eosinophil counts, inflammatory mediators in effusions). Study groups have been drawn primarily from specialist offices, likely lack heterogeneity, and are not representative of general medical practice.

Evidence Profile: Allergy Management

- Aggregate evidence quality: D, case series without controls.

- Benefit: not established.
- Harm: adverse effects and cost of medication, physician evaluation, elimination diets, and desensitization.
- Benefits-harms assessment: balance of benefit and harm.
- Policy level: no recommendation.

RESEARCH NEEDS

Diagnosis

- Further standardize the definition of OME.
- Assess the performance characteristics of pneumatic otoscopy as a diagnostic test for OME when performed by primary care physicians and advanced-practice nurses in the routine office setting.
- Determine the optimal methods for teaching pneumatic otoscopy to residents and clinicians.
- Develop a brief, reliable, objective method for diagnosing OME.
- Develop a classification method for identifying the presence of OME for practical use by clinicians that is based on quantifiable tympanometric characteristics.
- Assess the usefulness of algorithms combining pneumatic otoscopy and tympanometry for detecting OME in clinical practice.
- Conduct additional validating cohort studies of acoustic reflectometry as a diagnostic method for OME, particularly in children less than 2 years old.

Child At Risk

- Better define the child with OME who is at risk for speech, language, and learning problems.
- Conduct large, multicenter, observational cohort studies to identify the child at risk who is most susceptible to potential adverse sequelae of OME.
- Conduct large, multicenter, observational cohort studies to analyze outcomes achieved with alternative management strategies for OME in children at risk.

Watchful Waiting

- Define the spontaneous resolution of OME in infants and young children (existing data are limited primarily to children 2 years old or older).
- Conduct large-scale, prospective cohort studies to obtain current data on the spontaneous resolution of newly diagnosed OME of unknown prior duration (existing data are primarily from the late 1970s and early 1980s).
- Develop prognostic indicators to identify the best candidates for watchful waiting.
- Determine whether the lack of impact from prompt insertion of tympanostomy tubes on speech and language outcomes seen in asymptomatic young children with OME identified by screening or intense surveillance can be generalized to older children with OME or to symptomatic children with OME referred for evaluation.

Medication

- Clarify which children, if any, should receive antimicrobials, steroids, or both for OME.
- Conduct a randomized, placebo-controlled trial on the efficacy of antimicrobial therapy, with or without concurrent oral steroid, in avoiding surgery in children with OME who are surgical candidates and have not received recent antimicrobials.
- Investigate the role of mucosal surface biofilms in refractory or recurrent OME and develop targeted interventions.

Hearing and Language

- Conduct longitudinal studies on the natural history of hearing loss accompanying OME.
- Develop improved methods for describing and quantifying the fluctuations in hearing of children with OME over time.
- Conduct prospective controlled studies on the relation of hearing loss associated with OME to later auditory, speech, language, behavioral, and academic sequelae.
- Develop reliable, brief, objective methods for estimating hearing loss associated with OME.
- Develop reliable, brief, objective methods for estimating speech or language delay associated with OME.
- Evaluate the benefits and administrative burden of language testing by primary care clinicians.
- Agree on the aspects of language that are vulnerable to or affected by hearing loss caused by OME, and reach a consensus on the best tools for measurement.
- Determine whether OME and associated hearing loss place children from special populations at greater risk for speech and language delays.

Surveillance

- Develop better tools for monitoring children with OME that are suitable for routine clinical care.
- Assess the value of new strategies for monitoring OME, such as acoustic reflectometry performed at home by the parent or caregiver, in optimizing surveillance.
- Improve our ability to identify children who would benefit from early surgery instead of prolonged surveillance.
- Promote early detection of structural abnormalities in the tympanic membrane associated with OME that may require surgery to prevent complications.
- Clarify and quantify the role of parent or caregiver education, socioeconomic status, and quality of the caregiving environment as modifiers of OME developmental outcomes.
- Develop methods for minimizing loss to follow-up during OME surveillance.

Surgery

- Define the role of adenoidectomy in children 3 years old or younger as a specific OME therapy.
- Conduct controlled trials on the efficacy of tympanostomy tubes for developmental outcomes in children with hearing loss, other symptoms, or speech and language delay.
- Conduct randomized, controlled trials of surgery versus no surgery that emphasize patient-based outcome measures (quality of life, functional health status) in addition to objective measures (effusion prevalence, HLs, AOM incidence, reoperation).
- Identify the optimal ways to incorporate parent or caregiver preference into surgical decision-making.

CAM

- Conduct randomized, controlled trials on the efficacy of CAM modalities for OME.
- Develop strategies to identify parents or caregivers who use CAM therapies for their child's OME, and encourage surveillance by the primary care clinician.

Allergy Management

- Evaluate the causal role of atopy in OME.
- Conduct randomized, controlled trials on the efficacy of allergy therapy for OME that are generalizable to the primary care setting.

CONCLUSIONS

This evidence-based practice guideline offers recommendations for identifying, monitoring, and managing the child with OME. The guideline emphasizes appropriate diagnosis and provides options for various management strategies including observation, medical intervention, and referral for surgical intervention. These recommendations should provide primary care physicians and other health care providers with assistance in managing children with OME.

SUBCOMMITTEE ON OTITIS MEDIA WITH EFFUSION
Richard M. Rosenfeld, MD, MPH, Cochairperson
     American Academy of Pediatrics
     American Academy of Otolaryngology-Head and Neck Surgery
Larry Culpepper, MD, MPH, Cochairperson
     American Academy of Family Physicians
Karen J. Doyle, MD, PhD
     American Academy of Otolaryngology-Head and Neck Surgery
Kenneth M. Grundfast, MD
     American Academy of Otolaryngology-Head and Neck Surgery
Alejandro Hoberman, MD
     American Academy of Pediatrics
Margaret A. Kenna, MD
     American Academy of Otolaryngology-Head and Neck Surgery
Allan S. Lieberthal, MD
     American Academy of Pediatrics
Martin Mahoney, MD, PhD
     American Academy of Family Physicians
Richard A. Wahl, MD
     American Academy of Pediatrics
Charles R. Woods, Jr, MD, MS
     American Academy of Pediatrics

Barbara Yawn, MD, MSc
American Academy of Family Physicians

CONSULTANTS
S. Michael Marcy, MD
Richard N. Shiffman, MD

LIAISONS
Linda Carlson, MS, CPNP
National Association of Pediatric Nurse
Practitioners
Judith Gravel, PhD
American Academy of Audiology
Joanne Roberts, PhD
American Speech-Language-Hearing Association
STAFF
Maureen Hannley, PhD
American Academy of Otolaryngology-Head and
Neck Surgery
Carla T. Herrerias, MPH
American Academy of Pediatrics
Bellinda K. Schoof, MHA, CPHQ
American Academy of Family Physicians

ACKNOWLEDGMENTS

Dr Marcy serves as a consultant to Abbott Laboratories Glaxo-SmithKline (vaccines).

REFERENCES

1. Stool SE, Berg AO, Berman S, et al. *Otitis Media With Effusion in Young Children. Clinical Practice Guideline, Number 12.* AHCPR Publication No. 94-0622. Rockville, MD: Agency for Health Care Policy and Research, Public Health Service, US Department of Health and Human Services; 1994

2. Shekelle P, Takata G, Chan LS, et al. *Diagnosis, Natural History, and Late Effects of Otitis Media With Effusion. Evidence Report/Technology Assessment No. 55.* AHRQ Publication No. 03-E023. Rockville, MD: Agency for Healthcare Research and Quality; 2003

3. Williamson I. Otitis media with effusion. *Clin Evid.* 2002;7:469–476

4. Tos M. Epidemiology and natural history of secretory otitis. *Am J Otol.* 1984;5:459–462

5. Paradise JL, Rockette HE, Colborn DK, et al. Otitis media in 2253 Pittsburgh area infants: prevalence and risk factors during the first two years of life. *Pediatrics.* 1997;99:318–333

6. Casselbrant ML, Mandel EM. Epidemiology. In: Rosenfeld RM, Bluestone CD, eds. *Evidence-Based Otitis Media.* 2nd ed. Hamilton, Ontario: BC Decker; 2003:147–162

7. Williamson IG, Dunleavy J, Baine J, Robinson D. The natural history of otitis media with effusion—a three-year study of the incidence and prevalence of abnormal tympanograms in four South West Hampshire infant and first schools. *J Laryngol Otol.* 1994;108:930–934

8. Coyte PC, Croxford R, Asche CV, To T, Feldman W, Friedberg J. Physician and population determinants of rates of middle-ear surgery in Ontario. *JAMA.* 2001;286:2128–2135

9. Tugwell P. How to read clinical journals: III. To learn the clinical course and prognosis of disease. *Can Med Assoc J.* 1981;124:869–872

10. Jaeschke R, Guyatt G, Sackett DL. Users' guides to the medical literature. III. How to use an article about a diagnostic test. A. Are the results of the study valid? Evidence-Based Medicine Working Group. *JAMA.* 1994;271:389–391

11. Shiffman RN, Shekelle P, Overhage JM, Slutsky J, Grimshaw J, Deshpande AM. Standardized reporting of clinical practice guidelines: a proposal from the Conference on Guideline Standardization. *Ann Intern Med.* 2003;139:493–498

12. Shiffman RN, Karras BT, Agrawal A, Chen R, Marenco L, Nath S. GEM: a proposal for a more comprehensive guideline document model using XML. *J Am Med Inform Assoc.* 2000;7:488–498

13. Shaneyfelt TM, Mayo-Smith MF, Rothwangl J. Are guidelines following guidelines? The methodological quality of clinical practice guidelines in the peer-reviewed medical literature. *JAMA.* 1999;281: 1900–1905

14. Agrawal A, Shiffman RN. Evaluation of guideline quality using GEM-Q. *Medinfo.* 2001;10:1097–1101

15. Yale Center for Medical Informatics. GEM: The Guideline Elements Model. Available at: http://ycmi.med.yale.edu/GEM/. Accessed December 8, 2003

16. American Academy of Pediatrics, Steering Committee on Quality Improvement and Management. A taxonomy of recommendations for clinical practice guidelines. *Pediatrics.* 2004; In press

17. Eddy DM. *A Manual for Assessing Health Practices and Designing Practice Policies: The Explicit Approach.* Philadelphia, PA: American College of Physicians; 1992

18. Dowell SF, Marcy MS, Phillips WR, Gerber MA, Schwartz B. Otitis media—principles of judicious use of antimicrobial agents. *Pediatrics.* 1998;101:165–171

19. Dowell SF, Butler JC, Giebink GS, et al. Acute otitis media: management and surveillance in an era of pneumococcal resistance—a report from the Drug-Resistant *Streptococcus pneumoniae* Therapeutic Working Group. *Pediatr Infect Dis J.* 1999;18:1–9

20. Karma PH, Penttila MA, Sipila MM, Kataja MJ. Otoscopic diagnosis of middle ear effusion in acute and non-acute otitis media. I. The value of different otoscopic findings. *Int J Pediatr Otorhinolaryngol.* 1989;17: 37–49

21. Pichichero ME, Poole MD. Assessing diagnostic accuracy and tympanocentesis skills in the management of otitis media. *Arch Pediatr Adolesc Med.* 2001;155:1137–1142

22. Steinbach WJ, Sectish TC. Pediatric resident training in the diagnosis and treatment of acute otitis media. *Pediatrics.* 2002;109:404–408

23. Palmu A, Puhakka H, Rahko T, Takala AK. Diagnostic value of tympanometry in infants in clinical practice. *Int J Pediatr Otorhinolaryngol.* 1999;49:207–213

24. van Balen FA, Aarts AM, De Melker RA. Tympanometry by general practitioners: reliable? *Int J Pediatr Otorhinolaryngol.* 1999;48:117–123

25. Block SL, Mandel E, McLinn S, et al. Spectral gradient acoustic reflectometry for the detection of middle ear effusion by pediatricians and parents. *Pediatr Infect Dis J.* 1998;17:560–564, 580

26. Barnett ED, Klein JO, Hawkins KA, Cabral HJ, Kenna M, Healy G. Comparison of spectral gradient acoustic reflectometry and other diagnostic techniques for detection of middle ear effusion in children with middle ear disease. *Pediatr Infect Dis J.* 1998;17:556–559, 580

27. Block SL, Pichichero ME, McLinn S, Aronovitz G, Kimball S. Spectral gradient acoustic reflectometry: detection of middle ear effusion by pediatricians in suppurative acute otitis media. *Pediatr Infect Dis J.* 1999;18:741–744

28. Schwartz RH. A practical approach to the otitis prone child. *Contemp Pediatr.* 1987;4:30–54

29. Barriga F, Schwartz RH, Hayden GF. Adequate illumination for otoscopy. Variations due to power source, bulb, and head and speculum design. *Am J Dis Child.* 1986;140:1237–1240

30. Sorenson CH, Jensen SH, Tos M. The post-winter prevalence of middle-ear effusion in four-year-old children, judged by tympanometry. *Int J Pediatr Otorhinolaryngol.* 1981;3:119–128

31. Fiellau-Nikolajsen M. Epidemiology of secretory otitis media. A descriptive cohort study. *Ann Otol Rhinol Laryngol.* 1983;92:172–177

32. Casselbrant ML, Brostoff LM, Cantekin EI, et al. Otitis media with effusion in preschool children. *Laryngoscope.* 1985;95:428–436

33. Zielhuis GA, Rach GH, van den Broek P. Screening for otitis media with effusion in preschool children. *Lancet.* 1989;1:311–314

34. Poulsen G, Tos M. Repetitive tympanometric screenings of two-year-old children. *Scand Audiol.* 1980;9:21–28

35. Tos M, Holm-Jensen S, Sorensen CH. Changes in prevalence of secretory otitis from summer to winter in four-year-old children. *Am J Otol.* 1981;2:324–327

36. Thomsen J, Tos M. Spontaneous improvement of secretory otitis. A long-term study. *Acta Otolaryngol.* 1981;92:493–499

37. Lous J, Fiellau-Nikolajsen M. Epidemiology of middle ear effusion and tubal dysfunction. A one-year prospective study comprising monthly tympanometry in 387 non-selected seven-year-old children. *Int J Pediatr Otorhinolaryngol.* 1981;3:303–317

38. New Zealand Health Technology Assessment. *Screening Programmes for the Detection of Otitis Media With Effusion and Conductive Hearing Loss in Pre-School and New Entrant School Children: A Critical Appraisal of the Literature.* Christchurch, New Zealand: New Zealand Health Technology Assessment; 1998:61

39. Canadian Task Force on Preventive Health Care. Screening for otitis media with effusion: recommendation statement from the Canadian Task Force on Preventive Health Care. *CMAJ.* 2001;165:1092–1093

40. US Preventive Services Task Force. *Guide to Clinical Preventive Services.* 2nd ed. Baltimore, MD: Williams & Wilkins; 1995

41. Paradise JL, Feldman HM, Campbell TF, et al. Effect of early or delayed insertion of tympanostomy tubes for persistent otitis media on

developmental outcomes at the age of three years. *N Engl J Med.* 2001;344:1179–1187

42. Rovers MM, Krabble PF, Straatman H, Ingels K, van der Wilt GJ, Zielhuis GA. Randomized controlled trial of the effect of ventilation tubes (grommets) on quality of life at age 1–2 years. *Arch Dis Child.* 2001;84:45–49

43. Wood DL. Documentation guidelines: evolution, future direction, and compliance. *Am J Med.* 2001;110:332–334

44. Soto CM, Kleinman KP, Simon SR. Quality and correlates of medical record documentation in the ambulatory care setting. *BMC Health Serv Res.* 2002;2:22–35

45. Marchant CD, Shurin PA, Turczyk VA, Wasikowski DE, Tutihasi MA, Kinney SE. Course and outcome of otitis media in early infancy: a prospective study. *J Pediatr.* 1984;104:826–831

46. Rosenfeld RM, Goldsmith AJ, Tetlus L, Balzano A. Quality of life for children with otitis media. *Arch Otolaryngol Head Neck Surg.* 1997;123:1049–1054

47. Casselbrant ML, Furman JM, Rubenstein E, Mandel EM. Effect of otitis media on the vestibular system in children. *Ann Otol Rhinol Laryngol.* 1995;104:620–624

48. Orlin MN, Effgen SK, Handler SD. Effect of otitis media with effusion on gross motor ability in preschool-aged children: preliminary findings. *Pediatrics.* 1997;99:334–337

49. Golz A, Angel-Yeger B, Parush S. Evaluation of balance disturbances in children with middle ear effusion. *Int J Pediatr Otorhinolaryngol.* 1998;43:21–26

50. Casselbrant ML, Redfern MS, Furman JM, Fall PA, Mandel EM. Visual-induced postural sway in children with and without otitis media. *Ann Otol Rhinol Laryngol.* 1998;107:401–405

51. Ruben R. Host susceptibility to otitis media sequelae. In: Rosenfeld RM, Bluestone CD, eds. *Evidence-Based Otitis Media.* 2nd ed. Hamilton, ON, Canada: BC Decker; 2003:505–514

52. Whiteman BC, Simpson GB, Compton WC. Relationship of otitis media and language impairment on adolescents with Down syndrome. *Ment Retard.* 1986;24:353–356

53. van der Vyver M, van der Merwe A, Tesner HE. The effects of otitis media on articulation in children with cerebral palsy. *Int J Rehabil Res.* 1988;11:386–389

54. Paradise JL, Bluestone CD. Early treatment of the universal otitis media of infants with cleft palate. *Pediatrics.* 1974;53:48–54

55. Schwartz DM, Schwartz RH. Acoustic impedance and otoscopic findings in young children with Down's syndrome. *Arch Otolaryngol.* 1978;104:652–656

56. Corey JP, Caldarelli DD, Gould HJ. Otopathology in cranial facial dysostosis. *Am J Otol.* 1987;8:14–17

57. Schonweiler R, Schonweiler B, Schmelzeisen R. Hearing capacity and speech production in 417 children with facial cleft abnormalities [in German]. *HNO.* 1994;42:691–696

58. Ruben RJ, Math R. Serous otitis media associated with sensorineural hearing loss in children. *Laryngoscope.* 1978;88:1139–1154

59. Brookhouser PE, Worthington DW, Kelly WJ. Middle ear disease in young children with sensorineural hearing loss. *Laryngoscope.* 1993;103:371–378

60. Rice ML. Specific language impairments: in search of diagnostic markers and genetic contributions. *Ment Retard Dev Disabil Res Rev.* 1997;3:350–357

61. Rosenhall U, Nordin V, Sandstrom M, Ahlsen G, Gillberg C. Autism and hearing loss. *J Autism Dev Disord.* 1999;29:349–357

62. Cunningham C, McArthur K. Hearing loss and treatment in young Down's syndrome children. *Child Care Health Dev.* 1981;7:357–374

63. Shott SR, Joseph A, Heithaus D. Hearing loss in children with Down syndrome. *Int J Pediatr Otorhinolaryngol.* 2001;61:199–205

64. Clarkson RL, Eimas PD, Marean GC. Speech perception in children with histories of recurrent otitis media. *J Acoust Soc Am.* 1989;85:926–933

65. Groenen P, Crul T, Maassen B, van Bon W. Perception of voicing cues by children with early otitis media with and without language impairment. *J Speech Hear Res.* 1996;39:43–54

66. Hubbard TW, Paradise JL, McWilliams BJ, Elster BA, Taylor FH. Consequences of unremitting middle-ear disease in early life. Otologic, audiologic, and developmental findings in children with cleft palate. *N Engl J Med.* 1985;312:1529–1534

67. Nunn DR, Derkay CS, Darrow DH, Magee W, Strasnick B. The effect of very early cleft palate closure on the need for ventilation tubes in the first years of life. *Laryngoscope.* 1995;105:905–908

68. Pappas DG, Flexer C, Shackelford L. Otological and habilitative management of children with Down syndrome. *Laryngoscope.* 1994;104:1065–1070

69. Vartiainen E. Otitis media with effusion in children with congenital or early-onset hearing impairment. *J Otolaryngol.* 2000;29:221–223

70. Rosenfeld RM, Kay D. Natural history of untreated otitis media. *Laryngoscope.* 2003;113:1645–1657

71. Teele DW, Klein JO, Rosner BA. Epidemiology of otitis media in children. *Ann Otol Rhinol Laryngol Suppl.* 1980;89:5–6

72. Mygind N, Meistrup-Larsen KI, Thomsen J, Thomsen VF, Josefsson K, Sorensen H. Penicillin in acute otitis media: a double-blind, placebo-controlled trial. *Clin Otolaryngol.* 1981;6:5–13

73. Burke P, Bain J, Robinson D, Dunleavey J. Acute red ear in children: controlled trial of nonantibiotic treatment in general practice. *BMJ.* 1991;303:558–562

74. Fiellau-Nikolajsen M, Lous J. Prospective tympanometry in 3-year-old children. A study of the spontaneous course of tympanometry types in a nonselected population. *Arch Otolaryngol.* 1979;105:461–466

75. Fiellau-Nikolajsen M. Tympanometry in 3-year-old children. Type of care as an epidemiological factor in secretory otitis media and tubal dysfunction in unselected populations of 3-year-old children. *ORL J Otorhinolaryngol Relat Spec.* 1979;41:193–205

76. Tos M. Spontaneous improvement of secretory otitis and impedance screening. *Arch Otolaryngol.* 1980;106:345–349

77. Tos M, Holm-Jensen S, Sorensen CH, Mogensen C. Spontaneous course and frequency of secretory otitis in 4-year-old children. *Arch Otolaryngol.* 1982;108:4–10

78. Roberts JE, Zeisel SA. *Ear Infections and Language Development.* Rockville, MD: American Speech-Language-Hearing Association and the National Center for Early Development and Learning; 2000

79. Roberts JE, Rosenfeld RM, Zeisel SA. Otitis media and speech and language: a meta-analysis of prospective studies. *Pediatrics.* 2004;113(3). Available at: www.pediatrics.org/cgi/content/full/113/3/e238

80. Williams RL, Chalmers TC, Stange KC, Chalmers FT, Bowlin SJ. Use of antibiotics in preventing recurrent otitis media and in treating otitis media with effusion. A meta-analytic attempt to resolve the brouhaha. *JAMA.* 1993;270:1344–1351

81. Rosenfeld RM, Post JC. Meta-analysis of antibiotics for the treatment of otitis media with effusion. *Otolaryngol Head Neck Surg.* 1992;106:378–386

82. Mandel EM, Rockette HE, Bluestone CD, Paradise JL, Nozza RJ. Efficacy of amoxicillin with and without decongestant-antihistamine for otitis media with effusion in children. Results of a double-blind, randomized trial. *N Engl J Med.* 1987;316:432–437

83. McCormick AW, Whitney CG, Farley MM, et al. Geographic diversity and temporal trends of antimicrobial resistance in *Streptococcus pneumoniae* in the United States. *Nat Med.* 2003;9:424–430

84. Levy SB. *The Antibiotic Paradox. How the Misuse of Antibiotic Destroys Their Curative Powers.* Cambridge, MA: Perseus Publishing; 2002

85. Butler CC, van der Voort JH. Oral or topical nasal steroids for hearing loss associated with otitis media with effusion in children. *Cochrane Database Syst Rev.* 2002;4:CD001935

86. Mandel EM, Casselbrant ML, Rockette HE, Fireman P, Kurs-Lasky M, Bluestone CD. Systemic steroid for chronic otitis media with effusion in children. *Pediatrics.* 2002;110:1071–1080

87. Tracy JM, Demain JG, Hoffman KM, Goetz DW. Intranasal beclomethasone as an adjunct to treatment of chronic middle ear effusion. *Ann Allergy Asthma Immunol.* 1998;80:198–206

88. Joint Committee on Infant Hearing. Year 2000 position statement: principles and guidelines for early hearing detection and intervention programs. *Am J Audiol.* 2000;9:9–29

89. Pillsbury HC, Grose JH, Hall JW III. Otitis media with effusion in children. Binaural hearing before and after corrective surgery. *Arch Otolaryngol Head Neck Surg.* 1991;117:718–723

90. Besing J, Koehnke J A test of virtual auditory localization. *Ear Hear.* 1995;16:220–229

91. Jerger S, Jerger J, Alford BR, Abrams S. Development of speech intelligibility in children with recurrent otitis media. *Ear Hear.* 1983;4:138–145

92. Gravel JS, Wallace IF. Listening and language at 4 years of age: effects of early otitis media. *J Speech Hear Res.* 1992;35:588–595

93. Schilder AG, Snik AF, Straatman H, van den Broek P. The effect of otitis media with effusion at preschool age on some aspects of auditory perception at school age. *Ear Hear.* 1994;15:224–231

94. Rosenfeld RM, Madell JR, McMahon A. Auditory function in normal-hearing children with middle ear effusion. In: Lim DJ, Bluestone CD, Casselbrant M, Klein JO, Ogra PL, eds. *Recent Advances in Otitis Media: Proceedings of the 6th International Symposium.* Hamilton, ON, Canada: BC Decker; 1996:354–356

95. Friel-Patti S, Finitzo T. Language learning in a prospective study of otitis media with effusion in the first two years of life. *J Speech Hear Res.* 1990;33:188–194

96. Wallace IF, Gravel JS, McCarton CM, Stapells DR, Bernstein RS, Ruben RJ. Otitis media, auditory sensitivity, and language outcomes at one year. *Laryngoscope.* 1988;98:64–70

97. Roberts JE, Burchinal MR, Medley LP, et al. Otitis media, hearing sensitivity, and maternal responsiveness in relation to language during infancy. *J Pediatr.* 1995;126:481–489

98. Roberts JE, Burchinal MR, Zeisel SA. Otitis media in early childhood in relation to children's school-age language and academic skills. *Pediatrics.* 2002;110:696–706

99. Rovers MM, Straatman H, Ingels K, van der Wilt GJ, van den Broek P, Zielhuis GA. The effect of ventilation tubes on language development in infants with otitis media with effusion: a randomized trial. *Pediatrics.* 2000;106(3). Available at: www.pediatrics.org/cgi/content/full/106/3/e42

100. Paradise JL, Feldman HM, Campbell TF, et al. Early versus delayed insertion of tympanostomy tubes for persistent otitis media: developmental outcomes at the age of three years in relation to prerandomization illness patterns and hearing levels. *Pediatr Infect Dis J.* 2003;22:309–314

101. Kokko E. Chronic secretory otitis media in children. A clinical study. *Acta Otolaryngol Suppl.* 1974;327:1–44

102. Fria TJ, Cantekin EI, Eichler JA. Hearing acuity of children with otitis media with effusion. *Arch Otolaryngol.* 1985;111:10–16

103. Gravel JS, Wallace IF. Effects of otitis media with effusion on hearing in the first three years of life. *J Speech Lang Hear Res.* 2000;43:631–644

104. Roberts JE, Burchinal MR, Zeisel S, et al. Otitis media, the caregiving environment, and language and cognitive outcomes at 2 years. *Pediatrics.* 1998;102:346–354

105. Gravel JS, Wallace IF, Ruben RJ. Early otitis media and later educational risk. *Acta Otolaryngol.* 1995;115:279–281

106. Cunningham M, Cox EO; American Academy of Pediatrics, Committee on Practice and Ambulatory Medicine, Section on Otolaryngology and Bronchoesophagology. Hearing assessment in infants and children: recommendations beyond neonatal screening. *Pediatrics.* 2003;111:436–440

107. American Speech-Language-Hearing Association Panel on Audiologic Assessment. *Guidelines for Audiologic Screening.* Rockville, MD: American Speech-Language-Hearing Association; 1996

108. Rosenfeld RM, Goldsmith AJ, Madell JR. How accurate is parent rating of hearing for children with otitis media? *Arch Otolaryngol Head Neck Surg.* 1998;124:989–992

109. Brody R, Rosenfeld RM, Goldsmith AJ, Madell JR. Parents cannot detect mild hearing loss in children. *Otolaryngol Head Neck Surg.* 1999;121:681–686

110. Catts HW, Fey ME, Zhang X, Tomblin JB. Language basis of reading and reading disabilities: evidence from a longitudinal investigation. *Sci Stud Read.* 1999;3:331–362

111. Johnson CJ, Beitchman JH, Young A, et al. Fourteen-year follow-up of children with and without speech/language impairments: speech/language stability and outcomes. *J Speech Lang Hear Res.* 1999;42:744–760

112. Scarborough H, Dobrich W. Development of children with early language delay. *J Speech Hear Res.* 1990;33:70–83

113. Tomblin JB, Records NL, Buckwalter P, Zhang X, Smith E, O'Brien M. Prevalence of specific language impairment in kindergarten children. *J Speech Lang Hear Res.* 1997;40:1245–1260

114. Glade MJ. *Diagnostic and Therapeutic Technology Assessment: Speech Therapy in Patients With a Prior History of Recurrent Acute or Chronic Otitis Media With Effusion.* Chicago, IL: American Medical Association; 1996:1–14

115. Casby MW. Otitis media and language development: a meta-analysis. *Am J Speech Lang Pathol.* 2001;10:65–80

116. Maw R, Wilks J, Harvey I, Peters TJ, Golding J. Early surgery compared with watchful waiting for glue ear and effect on language development in preschool children: a randomised trial. *Lancet.* 1999;353:960–963

117. Coplan J. *Early Language Milestone Scale.* 2nd ed. Austin, TX: PRO-ED; 1983

118. Fenson L, Dale PS, Reznick JS, et al. *MacArthur Communicative Development Inventories. User's Guide and Technical Manual.* San Diego, CA: Singular Publishing Group; 1993

119. Rescoria L. The Language Development Survey: a screening tool for delayed language in toddlers. *J Speech Hear Dis.* 1989;54:587–599

120. Frankenburg WK, Dodds JA, Faucal A, et al. *Denver Developmental Screening Test II.* Denver, CO: University of Colorado Press; 1990

121. Klee T, Pearce K, Carson DK. Improving the positive predictive value of screening for developmental language disorder. *J Speech Lang Hear Res.* 2000;43:821–833

122. Shekelle PG, Ortiz E, Rhodes S, et al. Validity of the Agency for Healthcare Research and Quality clinical practice guidelines: how quickly do guidelines become outdated? *JAMA.* 2001;286:1461–1467

123. Zielhuis GA, Straatman H, Rach GH, van den Broek P. Analysis and presentation of data on the natural course of otitis media with effusion in children. *Int J Epidemiol.* 1990;19:1037–1044

124. MRC Multi-centre Otitis Media Study Group. Risk factors for persistence of bilateral otitis media with effusion. *Clin Otolaryngol.* 2001;26:147–156

125. van Balen FA, De Melker RA. Persistent otitis media with effusion: can it be predicted? A family practice follow-up study in children aged 6 months to 6 years. *J Fam Pract.* 2000;49:605–611

126. Sano S, Kamide Y, Schachern PA, Paparella MM. Micropathologic changes of pars tensa in children with otitis media with effusion. *Arch Otolaryngol Head Neck Surg.* 1994;120:815–819

127. Yellon RF, Doyle WJ, Whiteside TL, Diven WF, March AR, Fireman P. Cytokines, immunoglobulins, and bacterial pathogens in middle ear effusions. *Arch Otolaryngol Head Neck Surg.* 1995;121:865–869

128. Maw RA, Bawden R. Tympanic membrane atrophy, scarring, atelectasis and attic retraction in persistent, untreated otitis media with effusion and following ventilation tube insertion. *Int J Pediatr Otorhinolaryngol.* 1994;30:189–204

129. Davis JM, Elfenbein J, Schum R, Bentler RA. Effects of mild and moderate hearing impairment on language, educational, and psychosocial behavior of children. *J Speech Hear Disord.* 1986;51:53–62

130. Carney AE, Moeller MP. Treatment efficacy: hearing loss in children. *J Speech Lang Hear Res.* 1998;41:S61–S84

131. Karchmer MA, Allen TE. The functional assessment of deaf and hard of hearing students. *Am Ann Deaf.* 1999;144:68–77

132. Bess FH, Dodd-Murphy J, Parker RA. Children with minimal sensorineural hearing loss: prevalence, educational performance, and functional status. *Ear Hear.* 1998;19:339–354

133. Roberts JE, Burchinal MR, Jackson SC, et al. Otitis media in early childhood in relation to preschool language and school readiness skills among black children. *Pediatrics.* 2000;106:725–735

134. Haggard MP, Birkin JA, Browning GG, Gatehouse S, Lewis S. Behavior problems in otitis media. *Pediatr Infect Dis J.* 1994;13:S43–S50

135. Bennett KE, Haggard MP. Behaviour and cognitive outcomes from middle ear disease. *Arch Dis Child.* 1999;80:28–35

136. Bennett KE, Haggard MP, Silva PA, Stewart IA. Behaviour and developmental effects of otitis media with effusion into the teens. *Arch Dis Child.* 2001;85:91–95

137. Wilks J, Maw R, Peters TJ, Harvey I, Golding J. Randomised controlled trial of early surgery versus watchful waiting for glue ear: the effect on behavioural problems in pre-school children. *Clin Otolaryngol.* 2000;25:209–214

138. Rosenfeld RM, Bhaya MH, Bower CM, et al. Impact of tympanostomy tubes on child quality of life. *Arch Otolaryngol Head Neck Surg.* 2000;126:585–592

139. Rosenfeld RM, Bluestone CD. Clinical efficacy of surgical therapy. In: Rosenfeld RM, Bluestone CD, eds. *Evidence-Based Otitis Media.* 2nd ed. Hamilton, ON, Canada: BC Decker; 2003:227–240

140. Kuyvenhoven MM, De Melker RA. Referrals to specialists. An exploratory investigation of referrals by 13 general practitioners to medical and surgical departments. *Scand J Prim Health Care.* 1990;8:53–57

141. Haldis TA, Blankenship JC. Telephone reporting in the consultant-generalist relationship. *J Eval Clin Pract.* 2002;8:31–35

142. Reichman S. The generalist's patient and the subspecialist. *Am J Manag Care.* 2002;8:79–82

143. Gates GA, Avery CA, Prihoda TJ, Cooper JC Jr. Effectiveness of adenoidectomy and tympanostomy tubes in the treatment of chronic otitis media with effusion. *N Engl J Med.* 1987;317:1444–1451

144. Mandel EM, Rockette HE, Bluestone CD, Paradise JL, Nozza RJ. Myringotomy with and without tympanostomy tubes for chronic otitis media with effusion. *Arch Otolaryngol Head Neck Surg.* 1989;115:1217–1224

145. Mandel EM, Rockette HE, Bluestone CD, Paradise JL, Nozza RJ. Efficacy of myringotomy with and without tympanostomy tubes for chronic otitis media with effusion. *Pediatr Infect Dis J.* 1992;11:270–277

146. University of York Centre for Reviews and Dissemination. The treatment of persistent glue ear in children. *Eff Health Care.* 1992;4:1–16

147. Rovers MM, Straatman H, Ingels K, van der Wilt GJ, van den Broek P, Zielhuis GA. The effect of short-term ventilation tubes versus watchful waiting on hearing in young children with persistent otitis media with effusion: a randomized trial. *Ear Hear.* 2001;22:191–199

148. Paradise JL, Bluestone CD, Colborn DK, et al. Adenoidectomy and adenotonsillectomy for recurrent acute otitis media: parallel randomized clinical trials in children not previously treated with tympanostomy tubes. *JAMA.* 1999;282:945–953

149. Boston M, McCook J, Burke B, Derkay C. Incidence of and risk factors for additional tympanostomy tube insertion in children. *Arch Otolaryngol Head Neck Surg.* 2003;129:293–296

150. Coyte PC, Croxford R, McIsaac W, Feldman W, Friedberg J. The role of adjuvant adenoidectomy and tonsillectomy in the outcome of insertion of tympanostomy tubes. *N Engl J Med.* 2001;344:1188–1195

151. Paradise JL, Bluestone CD, Rogers KD, et al. Efficacy of adenoidectomy for recurrent otitis media in children previously treated with tympanostomy-tube placement. Results of parallel randomized and nonrandomized trials. *JAMA.* 1990;263:2066–2073

152. Maw AR. Chronic otitis media with effusion (glue ear) and adenotonsillectomy: prospective randomised controlled study. *Br Med J (Clin Res Ed).* 1983;287:1586–1588

153. Cohen D, Schechter Y, Slatkine M, Gatt N, Perez R. Laser myringotomy in different age groups. *Arch Otolaryngol Head Neck Surg.* 2001;127:260–264

154. Holzman RS. Morbidity and mortality in pediatric anesthesia. *Pediatr Clin North Am.* 1994;41:239–256

155. Cottrell JE, Golden S. *Under the Mask: A Guide to Feeling Secure and Comfortable During Anesthesia and Surgery.* New Brunswick, NJ: Rutgers University Press; 2001

156. Kay DJ, Nelson M, Rosenfeld RM. Meta-analysis of tympanostomy tube sequelae. *Otolaryngol Head Neck Surg.* 2001;124:374–380

157. Crysdale WS, Russel D. Complications of tonsillectomy and adenoidectomy in 9409 children observed overnight. *CMAJ.* 1986;135:1139–1142

158. Harrison H, Fixsen A, Vickers A. A randomized comparison of homeopathic and standard care for the treatment of glue ear in children. *Complement Ther Med.* 1999;7:132–135

159. Sawyer CE, Evans RL, Boline PD, Branson R, Spicer A. A feasibility study of chiropractic spinal manipulation versus sham spinal manipulation for chronic otitis media with effusion in children. *J Manipulative Physiol Ther.* 1999;22:292–298

160. Ernst E. Serious adverse effects of unconventional therapies for children and adolescents: a systematic review of recent evidence. *Eur J Pediatr.* 2003;162:72–80

161. Cohen MH, Eisenberg DM. Potential physician malpractice liability associated with complementary and integrative medical therapies. *Ann Intern Med.* 2002;136:596–603

162. Mullins RJ, Heddle R. Adverse reactions associated with echinacea: the Australian experience. *Ann Allergy Asthma Immunol.* 2002;88:42–51

163. Miller LG, Hume A, Harris IM, et al. White paper on herbal products. American College of Clinical Pharmacy. *Pharmacotherapy.* 2000;20:877–891

164. Angell M, Kassirer JP. Alternative medicine—the risks of untested and unregulated remedies. *N Engl J Med.* 1998;339:839–841

165. Fallon JM. The role of chiropractic adjustment in the care and treatment of 332 children with otitis media. *J Clin Chiropractic Pediatr.* 1997;2:167–183

166. Shafrir Y, Kaufman BA. Quadriplegia after chiropractic manipulation in an infant with congenital torticollis caused by a spinal cord astrocytoma. *J Pediatr.* 1992;120:266–269

167. Corey JP, Adham RE, Abbass AH, Seligman I. The role of IgE-mediated hypersensitivity in otitis media with effusion. *Am J Otolaryngol.* 1994;15:138–144

168. Bernstein JM. Role of allergy in eustachian tube blockage and otitis media with effusion: a review. *Otolaryngol Head Neck Surg.* 1996;114:562–568

169. Ishii TM, Toriyama M, Suzuki JI. Histopathological study of otitis media with effusion. *Ann Otol Rhinol Laryngol.* 1980;89(suppl):83–86

170. Hurst DS, Venge P. Evidence of eosinophil, neutrophil, and mast-cell mediators in the effusion of OME patients with and without atopy. *Allergy.* 2000;55:435–441

171. Hurst DS, Venge P. The impact of atopy on neutrophil activity in middle ear effusion from children and adults with chronic otitis media. *Arch Otolaryngol Head Neck Surg.* 2002;128:561–566

172. Hurst DS. Allergy management of refractory serous otitis media. *Otolaryngol Head Neck Surg.* 1990;102:664–669

Otitis Media Clinical Practice Guidelines
Quick Reference Tools

• •

- Action Statement Summary
  — The Diagnosis and Management of Acute Otitis Media
  — Otitis Media With Effusion
- *ICD-10-CM* Coding Quick Reference for Otitis Media
- Bonus Feature
  — Continuum Model for Otitis Media
- AAP Patient Education Handouts
  — *Acute Ear Infections and Your Child*
  — *Middle Ear Fluid and Your Child*

Action Statement Summary

The Diagnosis and Management of Acute Otitis Media

Key Action Statement 1A
Clinicians should diagnose acute otitis media (AOM) in children who present with moderate to severe bulging of the tympanic membrane (TM) *or* new onset of otorrhea not due to acute otitis externa. Evidence Quality: Grade B. Strength: Recommendation.

Key Action Statement 1B
Clinicians should diagnose AOM in children who present with mild bulging of the TM *and* recent (less than 48 hours) onset of ear pain (holding, tugging, rubbing of the ear in a nonverbal child) or intense erythema of the TM. Evidence Quality: Grade C. Strength: Recommendation.

Key Action Statement 1C
Clinicians should not diagnose AOM in children who do not have middle ear effusion (MEE) (based on pneumatic otoscopy and/or tympanometry). Evidence Quality: Grade B. Strength: Recommendation.

Key Action Statement 2
The management of AOM should include an assessment of pain. If pain is present, the clinician should recommend treatment to reduce pain. Evidence Quality: Grade B. Strength: Strong Recommendation.

Key Action Statement 3A
Severe AOM: The clinician should prescribe antibiotic therapy for AOM (bilateral or unilateral) in children 6 months and older with severe signs or symptoms (ie, moderate or severe otalgia or otalgia for at least 48 hours or temperature 39°C [102.2°F] or higher). Evidence Quality: Grade B. Strength: Strong Recommendation.

Key Action Statement 3B
Nonsevere bilateral AOM in young children: The clinician should prescribe antibiotic therapy for bilateral AOM in children 6 months through 23 months of age without severe signs or symptoms (ie, mild otalgia for less than 48 hours and temperature less than 39°C [102.2°F]). Evidence Quality: Grade B. Strength: Recommendation.

Key Action Statement 3C
Nonsevere unilateral AOM in young children: The clinician should either prescribe antibiotic therapy *or* offer observation with close follow-up based on joint decision-making with the parent(s)/caregiver for unilateral AOM in children 6 months to 23 months of age without severe signs or symptoms (ie, mild otalgia for less than 48 hours and temperature less than 39°C [102.2°F]). When observation is used, a mechanism must be in place to ensure follow-up and begin antibiotic therapy if the child worsens or fails to improve within 48 to 72 hours of onset of symptoms. Evidence Quality: Grade B. Strength: Recommendation.

Key Action Statement 3D
Nonsevere AOM in older children: The clinician should either prescribe antibiotic therapy *or* offer observation with close follow-up based on joint decision-making with the parent(s)/caregiver for AOM (bilateral or unilateral) in children 24 months or older without severe signs or symptoms (ie, mild otalgia for less than 48 hours and temperature less than 39°C [102.2°F]). When observation is used, a mechanism must be in place to ensure follow-up and begin antibiotic therapy if the child worsens or fails to improve within 48 to 72 hours of onset of symptoms. Evidence Quality: Grade B. Strength: Recommendation.

Key Action Statement 4A
Clinicians should prescribe amoxicillin for AOM when a decision to treat with antibiotics has been made *and* the child has not received amoxicillin in the past 30 days *or* the child does not have concurrent purulent conjunctivitis *or* the child is not allergic to penicillin. Evidence Quality: Grade B. Strength: Recommendation.

Key Action Statement 4B
Clinicians should prescribe an antibiotic with additional β-lactamase coverage for AOM when a decision to treat with antibiotics has been made, *and* the child has received amoxicillin in the last 30 days *or* has concurrent purulent conjunctivitis, *or* has a history of recurrent AOM unresponsive to amoxicillin. Evidence Quality: Grade C. Strength: Recommendation.

Key Action Statement 4C
Clinicians should reassess the patient if the caregiver reports that the child's symptoms have worsened or failed to respond to the initial antibiotic treatment within 48 to 72 hours and determine whether a change in therapy is needed. Evidence Quality: Grade B. Strength: Recommendation.

Key Action Statement 5A

Clinicians should not prescribe prophylactic antibiotics to reduce the frequency of episodes of AOM in children with recurrent AOM. Evidence Quality: Grade B. Strength: Recommendation.

Key Action Statement 5B

Clinicians may offer tympanostomy tubes for recurrent AOM (3 episodes in 6 months or 4 episodes in 1 year with 1 episode in the preceding 6 months). Evidence Quality: Grade B. Strength: Option.

Key Action Statement 6A

Clinicians should recommend pneumococcal conjugate vaccine to all children according to the schedule of the Advisory Committee on Immunization Practices of the Centers for Disease Control and prevention, American Academy of Pediatrics (AAP), and American Academy of Family Physicians (AAFP). Evidence Quality: Grade B. Strength: Strong Recommendation.

Otitis Media With Effusion

1A. Pneumatic Otoscopy

Clinicians should use pneumatic otoscopy as the primary diagnostic method for OME, and OME should be distinguished from AOM.

This is a strong recommendation based on systematic review of cohort studies and the preponderance of benefit over harm.

1B. Tympanometry

Tympanometry can be used to confirm the diagnosis a of OME.

This option is based on cohort studies and a balance of benefit and harm.

1C. Screening

Population-based screening programs for OME are not recommended in healthy, asymptomatic children.

This recommendation is based on randomized, controlled trials and cohort studies, with a preponderance of harm over benefit.

2. Documentation

Clinicians should document the laterality, duration of effusion, and presence and severity of associated symptoms at each assessment of the child with OME.

This recommendation is based on observational studies and strong preponderance of benefit over harm.

3. Child at Risk

Clinicians should distinguish the child with OME who is at risk for speech, language, or learning problems from other children with OME and should evaluate hearing, speech, language, and need for intervention more promptly.

This recommendation is based on case series, the preponderance of benefit over harm, and ethical limitations in studying children with OME who are at risk.

4. Watchful Waiting

Clinicians should manage the child with OME who is not at risk with watchful waiting for 3 months from the date of effusion onset (if known) or diagnosis (if onset is unknown).

This recommendation is based on systematic review of cohort studies and the preponderance of benefit over harm.

5. Medication

Antihistamines and decongestants are ineffective for OME and are not recommended for treatment; antimicrobials and corticosteroids do not have long-term efficacy and are not recommended for routine management.

This recommendation is based on systematic review of randomized, controlled trials and the preponderance of harm over benefit.

6. Hearing and Language

Hearing testing is recommended when OME persists for 3 months or longer or at any time that language delay, learning problems, or a significant hearing loss is suspected in a child with OME; language testing should be conducted for children with hearing loss.

This recommendation is based on cohort studies and the preponderance of benefit over risk.

7. Surveillance

Children with persistent OME who are not at risk should be reexamined at 3- to 6-month intervals until the effusion is no longer present, significant hearing loss is identified, or structural abnormalities of the eardrum or middle ear are suspected.

This recommendation is based on randomized, controlled trials and observational studies with a preponderance of benefit over harm.

8. Referral

When children with OME are referred by the primary care clinician for evaluation by an otolaryngologist, audiologist, or speech-language pathologist, the referring clinician should document the effusion duration and specific reason for referral (evaluation, surgery) and provide additional relevant information such as history of AOM and developmental status of the child.

This option is based on panel consensus and a preponderance of benefit over harm.

9. Surgery

When a child becomes a surgical candidate, tympanostomy tube insertion is the preferred initial procedure; adenoidectomy should not be performed unless a distinct indication exists (nasal obstruction, chronic adenoiditis). Repeat surgery consists of adenoidectomy plus myringotomy, with or without tube insertion. tonsillectomy alone or myringotomy alone should not be used to treat OME.

This recommendation is based on randomized, controlled trials with a preponderance of benefit over harm.

10. CAM

No recommendation is made regarding CAM as a treatment for OME.

There is no recommendation based on lack of scientific evidence documenting efficacy and an uncertain balance of harm and benefit.

11. Allergy Management

No recommendation is made regarding allergy management as a treatment for OME.

There is no recommendation based on insufficient evidence of therapeutic efficacy or a causal relationship between allergy and OME.

Coding Quick Reference for Otitis Media

ICD-10-CM

H65.01	Acute serous otitis media, right ear
H65.02	Left ear
H65.03	Bilateral
H65.04	Recurrent, right ear
H65.05	Recurrent, left ear
H65.06	Recurrent, bilateral

H65.21	Chronic serous otitis media, right ear
H65.22	Left ear
H65.23	Bilateral

H65.91	Unspecified nonsuppurative otitis media, right ear
H65.92	Left ear
H65.93	Bilateral

H66.001	Acute suppurative otitis media without spontaneous rupture of ear drum, right ear
H66.002	Left ear
H66.003	Bilateral
H66.004	Recurrent, right ear
H66.005	Recurrent, left ear
H66.006	Recurrent, bilateral

H66.011	Acute suppurative otitis media with spontaneous rupture of ear drum, right ear
H66.012	Left ear
H66.013	Bilateral
H66.014	Recurrent, right ear
H66.015	Recurrent, left ear
H66.016	Recurrent, bilateral

H67.1	Otitis media in diseases classified elsewhere, right ear
H67.2	Left ear
H67.3	Bilateral

H66.3X1	Other chronic suppurative otitis media, right ear
H66.3X2	Left ear
H66.3X3	Bilateral

Continuum Model for Otitis Media

The following continuum model from *Coding for Pediatrics 2019* has been devised to express the various levels of service for otitis media. This model demonstrates the cumulative effect of the key criteria for each level of service using a single diagnosis as the common denominator. It also shows the importance of other variables, such as patient age, duration and severity of illness, social contexts, and comorbid conditions, that often have key roles in pediatric cases.

Quick Reference for Codes Used in Continuum for Otitis Media—Established Patients				
E/M Code Level	**History**	**Examination**	**MDM**	**Time**
99211[a]	NA	NA	NA	5 min
99212	Problem-focused	Problem-focused	Straightforward	10 min
99213	Problem-focused	Expanded problem-focused	Low	15 min
99214	Detailed	Detailed	Moderate	25 min
99215	Detailed	Detailed	High	40 min

Abbreviations: E/M, evaluation and management; MDM; medical decision-making; NA, not applicable.

[a] Low level E/M service that may not require the presence of a physician.

Adapted from American Academy of Pediatrics. *Coding for Pediatrics 2019: A Manual for Pediatric Documentation and Payment.* 24th ed. Itasca, IL: American Academy of Pediatrics; 2019.

Continuum Model for Otitis Media

Code selection at any level above 99211 may be based on time when documentation states that more than 50% of the total face-to-face time of the encounter is spent in counseling and/or coordination of care. Select the code with the typical time closest to the total face-to-face time.

CPT® Code Vignette	History	Physical Examination (systems)	Medical Decision-making (diagnoses, data, risk)
99211 Clinical staff evaluations Follow-up on serous fluid or hearing loss with tympanogram (Be sure to code tympanogram [92567] and/or audiogram [92551 series] in addition to 99211.)	No specific key components required. Must indicate continuation of physician's plan of care, medical necessity, assessment, and/or education provided. CC: Follow-up on serous fluid OR on hearing loss. HPI: Mom reports medication completed and previous symptoms resolved. Assessment: Problem resolved. Follow-up with physician for recommended preventive service.		
99212 Follow-up otitis media, uncomplicated	**Problem focused** CC: Follow-up otitis media HPI: History of treatment, difficulties with medication, hearing status	**Problem focused** 1. ENMT	**Straightforward** 1. One established problem, improved 2. No tests ordered/data reviewed 3. Risk: No need for further follow-up
99213 2-year-old presents with tugging at her right ear. Afebrile. Mild otitis media.	**Problem focused** CC: Tugging at right ear HPI: Duration, associated signs/symptoms, and home management, including over-the-counter medications, and response ROS: Constitutional, eyes, ENMT, gastrointestinal, genitourinary	**Expanded problem focused** 1. ENMT 2. Conjunctiva 3. Overall appearance	**Low complexity** 1. Minor problem 2. No tests ordered/data reviewed 3. Risk: Observation and nonprescription analgesics
99214 Infant presents for suspected third episode of otitis media within 3 months. Infant presents with fever and cough.	**Detailed** CC: Fever and cough, suspected otitis media HPI: Duration, severity of fever, other symptoms, modifying factor (medication) ROS: Constitutional, eyes, ENMT, respiratory, gastrointestinal, urinary PSFH: Allergies, frequency of similar infection in past and response to treatment, environmental factors (eg, tobacco exposure, child care), immunization status	**Detailed** 1. Constitutional 2. Eyes 3. ENMT 4. Lungs 5. Skin	**Moderate complexity** 1. Established problem, not responding to management 2. Hearing evaluation planned 3. Risk: Prescription drug management
99215 3-month-old presents with high fever, vomiting, irritability.	**Detailed** CC: Fever, vomiting, irritability HPI: Severity of fever, quality of irritability, duration of symptoms, and modifying factors ROS: Constitutional, eyes, ENMT, respiratory, gastrointestinal, genitourinary PFSH: Medications, allergies, frequency of similar infection in past and response to treatment, environmental factors (eg, tobacco exposure, child care)	**Comprehensive** 1. Overall appearance, hydration status 2. Head 3. Eyes 4. ENMT 5. Neck 6. Cardiovascular 7. Respiratory 8. Skin	**High complexity** 1. New problem with additional work-up planned. 2. Tests ordered: Complete blood cell count with differential, blood culture, blood urea nitrogen, creatinine, electrolytes, urinalysis with culture, chest radiograph, and possible lumbar puncture. 3. Risk: Consider admission to NICU.

Continuum Model for Otitis Media (*continued*)

Code selection at any level above **99211** may be based on time when documentation states that more than 50% of the total face-to-face time of the encounter is spent in counseling and/or coordination of care. Select the code with the typical time closest to the total face-to-face time.

CPT® Code Vignette	History	Physical Examination (systems)	Medical Decision-making (diagnoses, data, risk)
99214 or **99215** **NOTE:** Depending on the variables (ie, time), this example could be reported as **99214** or **99215**. Extended evaluation of child with chronic or recurrent otitis media	Documentation of total face-to-face time and >50% of time spent in extensive discussion of treatment options, including, but not limited to 1. Continued episodic treatment with antibiotics 2. Myringotomy and tube placement 3. Adenoidectomy 4. Allergy evaluation 5. Steroid therapy with weighing of risk to benefit ratio of various therapies **NOTE:** Time is the key factor when counseling and/or coordination of care are more than 50% of the face-to-face time with the patient. For **99214**, the total visit time would be 25 minutes; for **99215**, the total time is 40 minutes. You must document time spent on counseling and/or coordination of care and include the areas discussed.		

Abbreviations: CC, chief complaint; CPT, Current Procedural Terminology; ENMT, ears, nose, throat, mouth; HPI, history of present illness; PFSH, past, family, and social history; ROS, review of systems.

Acute Ear Infections and Your Child

Next to the common cold, an ear infection is the most common childhood illness. In fact, most children have at least one ear infection by the time they are 3 years old. Many ear infections clear up without causing any lasting problems.

The following is information from the American Academy of Pediatrics about the symptoms, treatments, and possible complications of acute *otitis media*, a common infection of the middle ear.

How do ear infections develop?

The ear has 3 parts—the outer ear, middle ear, and inner ear. A narrow channel (eustachian tube) connects the middle ear to the back of the nose. When a child has a cold, nose or throat infection, or allergy, the mucus and fluid can enter the eustachian tube causing a buildup of fluid in the middle ear. If bacteria or a virus infects this fluid, it can cause swelling and pain in the ear. This type of ear infection is called *acute otitis media* (*middle ear inflammation*).

Often after the symptoms of acute otitis media clear up, fluid remains in the ear, creating another kind of ear problem called *otitis media with effusion* (*middle ear fluid*). This condition is harder to detect than acute otitis media because except for the fluid and usually some mild hearing loss, there is often no pain or other symptoms present. This fluid may last several months and, in most cases, disappears on its own. The child's hearing then returns to normal.

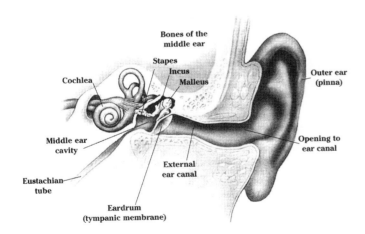

Cross-Section of the Ear

Is my child at risk for developing an ear infection?

Risk factors for developing childhood ear infections include

- **Age.** Infants and young children are more likely to get ear infections than older children. The size and shape of an infant's eustachian tube makes it easier for an infection to develop. Ear infections occur most often in children between 6 months and 3 years of age. Also, the younger a child is at the time of the first ear infection, the greater the chance he will have repeated infections.
- **Family history.** Ear infections can run in families. Children are more likely to have repeated middle ear infections if a parent or sibling also had repeated ear infections.
- **Colds.** Colds often lead to ear infections. Children in group child care settings have a higher chance of passing their colds to each other because they are exposed to more viruses from the other children.
- **Tobacco smoke.** Children who breathe in someone else's tobacco smoke have a higher risk of developing health problems, including ear infections.

How can I reduce the risk of an ear infection?

Some things you can do to help reduce your child's risk of getting an ear infection are

- Breastfeed instead of bottle-feed. Breastfeeding may decrease the risk of frequent colds and ear infections.
- Keep your child away from tobacco smoke, especially in your home or car.
- Throw away pacifiers or limit to daytime use, *if your child is older than 1 year*.
- Keep vaccinations up to date. Vaccines against bacteria (such as pneumococcal vaccine) and viruses (such as influenza vaccine) reduce the number of ear infections in children with frequent infections.

What are the symptoms of an ear infection?

Your child may have many symptoms during an ear infection. Talk with your pediatrician about the best way to treat your child's symptoms.

- **Pain.** The most common symptom of an ear infection is pain. Older children can tell you that their ears hurt. Younger children may only seem irritable and cry. You may notice this more during feedings because sucking and swallowing may cause painful pressure changes in the middle ear.
- **Loss of appetite.** Your child may have less of an appetite because of the ear pain.
- **Trouble sleeping.** Your child may have trouble sleeping because of the ear pain.
- **Fever.** Your child may have a temperature ranging from 100°F (normal) to 104°F.

- **Ear drainage.** You might notice yellow or white fluid, possibly blood-tinged, draining from your child's ear. The fluid may have a foul odor and will look different from normal earwax (which is orange-yellow or reddish-brown). Pain and pressure often decrease after this drainage begins, but this doesn't always mean that the infection is going away. If this happens it's not an emergency, but your child will need to see your pediatrician.
- **Trouble hearing.** During and after an ear infection, your child may have trouble hearing for several weeks. This occurs because the fluid behind the eardrum gets in the way of sound transmission. This is usually temporary and clears up after the fluid from the middle ear drains away.

Important: Your doctor *cannot* diagnose an ear infection over the phone; your child's eardrum must be examined by your doctor to confirm fluid buildup and signs of inflammation.

What causes ear pain?

There are other reasons why your child's ears may hurt besides an ear infection. The following can cause ear pain:

- An infection of the skin of the ear canal, often called "swimmer's ear"
- Reduced pressure in the middle ear from colds or allergies
- A sore throat
- Teething or sore gums
- Inflammation of the eardrum alone during a cold (without fluid buildup)

How are ear infections treated?

Because pain is often the first and most uncomfortable symptom of an ear infection, it's important to help comfort your child by giving her pain medicine. Acetaminophen and ibuprofen are over-the-counter (OTC) pain medicines that may help decrease much of the pain. Be sure to use the right dosage for your child's age and size. *Don't give aspirin to your child.* It has been associated with Reye syndrome, a disease that affects the liver and brain. There are also ear drops that may relieve ear pain for a short time. Ask your pediatrician whether these drops should be used. There is no need to use OTC cold medicines (decongestants and antihistamines), because they don't help clear up ear infections.

Not all ear infections require antibiotics. Some children who don't have a high fever and aren't severely ill may be observed without antibiotics. In most cases, pain and fever will improve in the first 1 to 2 days.

If your child is younger than 2 years, has drainage from the ear, has a fever higher than 102.5°F, seems to be in a lot of pain, is unable to sleep, isn't eating, or is acting ill, it's important to call your pediatrician. If your child is older than 2 years and your child's symptoms are mild, you may wait a couple of days to see if she improves.

Your child's ear pain and fever should improve or go away within 3 days of their onset. If your child's condition doesn't improve within 3 days, or worsens at any time, call your pediatrician. Your pediatrician may wish to see your child and may prescribe an antibiotic to take by mouth, if one wasn't given initially. If an antibiotic was already started, your child may need a different antibiotic. Be sure to follow your pediatrician's instructions closely.

If an antibiotic was prescribed, make sure your child finishes the entire prescription. If you stop the medicine too soon, some of the bacteria that caused the ear infection may still be present and cause an infection to start all over again.

As the infection starts to clear up, your child might feel a "popping" in the ears. This is a normal sign of healing. Children with ear infections don't need to stay home if they are feeling well, as long as a child care provider or someone at school can give them their medicine properly, if needed. If your child needs to travel in an airplane, or wants to swim, contact your pediatrician for specific instructions.

What are signs of hearing problems?

Because your child can have trouble hearing without other symptoms of an ear infection, watch for the following changes in behavior (especially during or after a cold):

- Talking more loudly or softly than usual
- Saying "huh?" or "what?" more than usual
- Not responding to sounds
- Having trouble understanding speech in noisy rooms
- Listening with the TV or radio turned up louder than usual

If you think your child may have difficulty hearing, call your pediatrician. Being able to hear and listen to others talk helps a child learn speech and language. This is especially important during the first few years of life.

Are there complications from ear infections?

Although it's very rare, complications from ear infections can develop, including the following:

- An infection of the inner ear that causes dizziness and imbalance (labyrinthitis)
- An infection of the skull behind the ear (mastoiditis)
- Scarring or thickening of the eardrum
- Loss of feeling or movement in the face (facial paralysis)
- Permanent hearing loss

It's normal for children to have several ear infections when they are young—even as many as 2 separate infections within a few months. Most ear infections that develop in children are minor. Recurring ear infections may be a nuisance, but they usually clear up without any lasting problems. With proper care and treatment, ear infections can usually be managed successfully. But, if your child has one ear infection after another for several months, you may want to talk about other treatment options with your pediatrician.

From your doctor

American Academy of Pediatrics

DEDICATED TO THE HEALTH OF ALL CHILDREN™

The American Academy of Pediatrics is an organization of 66,000 primary care pediatricians, pediatric medical subspecialists, and pediatric surgical specialists dedicated to the health, safety, and well-being of infants, children, adolescents, and young adults.

American Academy of Pediatrics
Web site—www.HealthyChildren.org

Middle Ear Fluid and Your Child

The *middle* ear is the space behind the eardrum that is usually filled with air. When a child has middle ear fluid (otitis media with effusion), it means that a watery or mucus-like fluid has collected in the middle ear. *Otitis media* means *middle ear inflammation*, and *effusion* means *fluid*.

Middle ear fluid is **not** the same as an ear infection. An ear infection occurs when middle ear fluid is infected with viruses, bacteria, or both, often during a cold. Children with middle ear fluid have no signs or symptoms of infection. Most children don't have fever or severe pain, but may have mild discomfort or trouble hearing. About 90% of children get middle ear fluid at some time before age 5.

The following is information from the American Academy of Pediatrics about the causes, symptoms, risk reduction, testing, and treatments for middle ear fluid, as well as how middle ear fluid may affect your child's learning.

What causes middle ear fluid?

There is no one cause for middle ear fluid. Often your child's doctor may not know the cause. Middle ear fluid could be caused by

- A past ear infection
- A cold or flu
- Blockage of the eustachian tube (a narrow channel that connects the middle ear to the back of the nose)

What are the symptoms of middle ear fluid?

Many healthy children with middle ear fluid have little or no problems. They usually get better on their own. Often middle ear fluid is found at a regular checkup. Ear discomfort, if present, is usually mild. Your child may be irritable, rub his ears, or have trouble sleeping. Other symptoms include hearing loss, irritability, sleep problems, clumsiness, speech or language problems, and poor school performance. You may notice your child sitting closer to the TV or turning the sound up louder than usual. Sometimes it may seem like your child isn't paying attention to you, especially when at the playground or in a noisy environment.

Talk with your child's doctor if you are concerned about your child's hearing. Keep a record of your child's ear problems. Write down your child's name, child's doctor's name and number, date and type of ear problem or infection, treatment, and results. This may help your child's doctor find the cause of the middle ear fluid.

Can middle ear fluid affect my child's learning?

Some children with middle ear fluid are at risk for delays in speaking or may have problems with learning or schoolwork, especially children with

- Permanent hearing loss not caused by middle ear fluid
- Speech and language delays or disorders
- Developmental delay of social and communication skills disorders (for example, autism spectrum disorders)
- Syndromes that affect cognitive, speech, and language delays (for example, Down syndrome)
- Craniofacial disorders that affect cognitive, speech, and language delays (for example, cleft palate)
- Blindness or visual loss that can't be corrected

If your child is at risk and has ongoing middle ear fluid, her hearing, speech, and language should be checked.

How can I reduce the risk of middle ear fluid?

Children who live with smokers, attend group child care, or use pacifiers have more ear infections. Because some children who have middle ear infections later get middle ear fluid, you may want to

- Keep your child away from tobacco smoke.
- Keep your child away from children who are sick.
- Throw away pacifiers or limit to daytime use, *if your child is older than 1 year*.

Are there special tests to check for middle ear fluid?

Two tests that can check for middle ear fluid are *pneumatic otoscopy* and *tympanometry*. A pneumatic otoscope is the recommended test for middle ear fluid. With this tool, the doctor looks at the eardrum and uses air to see how well the eardrum moves. Tympanometry is another test for middle ear fluid that uses sound to see how well the eardrum moves. An eardrum with fluid behind it doesn't move as well as a normal eardrum. Your child must sit still for both tests; the tests are painless.

Because these tests don't check hearing level, a hearing test may be given, if needed. Hearing tests measure how well your child hears. Although hearing tests don't test for middle ear fluid, they can measure if the fluid is affecting your child's hearing level. The type of hearing test given depends on your child's age and ability to participate.

How can middle ear fluid be treated?

Middle ear fluid can be treated in several ways. Treatment options include observation and tube surgery or adenoid surgery. Because a treatment that works for one child may not work for another, your child's doctor can help you decide which treatment is best for your child and when you should see an ear, nose, and throat (ENT) specialist. If one treatment doesn't work, another treatment can be tried. Ask your child's doctor or ENT specialist about the costs, advantages, and disadvantages of each treatment.

When should middle ear fluid be treated?

Your child is more likely to need treatment for middle ear fluid if she has any of the following:

- Conditions placing her at risk for developmental delays (see "Can middle ear fluid affect my child's learning?")
- Fluid in both ears, especially if present more than 3 months
- Hearing loss or other significant symptoms (see "What are the symptoms of middle ear fluid?")

What treatments are not recommended?

A number of treatments are **not** recommended for young children with middle ear fluid.

- **Medicines** not recommended include antibiotics, decongestants, antihistamines, and steroids (by mouth or in nasal sprays). All of these have side effects and do not cure middle ear fluid.
- **Surgical treatments** not recommended include myringotomy (draining of fluid without placing a tube) and tonsillectomy (removal of the tonsils). If your child's doctor or ENT specialist suggests one of these surgeries, it may be for another medical reason. Ask your doctor why your child needs the surgery.

What about other treatment options?

There is no evidence that complementary and alternative medicine treatments or that treatment for allergies works to decrease middle ear fluid. Some of these treatments may be harmful and many are expensive.

The information contained in this publication should not be used as a substitute for the medical care and advice of your pediatrician. There may be variations in treatment that your pediatrician may recommend based on individual facts and circumstances.

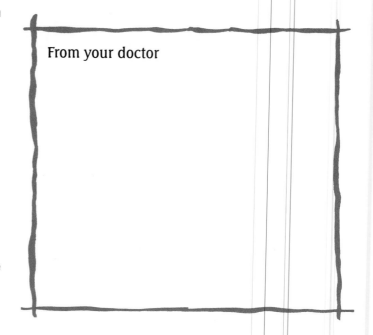

From your doctor

American Academy
of Pediatrics

DEDICATED TO THE HEALTH OF ALL CHILDREN™

The American Academy of Pediatrics is an organization of 66,000 primary care pediatricians, pediatric medical subspecialists, and pediatric surgical specialists dedicated to the health, safety, and well-being of infants, children, adolescents, and young adults.
American Academy of Pediatrics
Web site— www.HealthyChildren.org

Clinical Practice Guideline for the Diagnosis and Management of Acute Bacterial Sinusitis in Children Aged 1 to 18 Years

- *Clinical Practice Guideline*
  - *PPI: AAP Partnership for Policy Implementation*
    See Appendix 1 for more information.

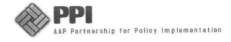

CLINICAL PRACTICE GUIDELINE

Clinical Practice Guideline for the Diagnosis and Management of Acute Bacterial Sinusitis in Children Aged 1 to 18 Years

abstract

OBJECTIVE: To update the American Academy of Pediatrics clinical practice guideline regarding the diagnosis and management of acute bacterial sinusitis in children and adolescents.

METHODS: Analysis of the medical literature published since the last version of the guideline (2001).

RESULTS: The diagnosis of acute bacterial sinusitis is made when a child with an acute upper respiratory tract infection (URI) presents with (1) persistent illness (nasal discharge [of any quality] or daytime cough or both lasting more than 10 days without improvement), (2) a worsening course (worsening or new onset of nasal discharge, daytime cough, or fever after initial improvement), or (3) severe onset (concurrent fever [temperature ≥39°C/102.2°F] and purulent nasal discharge for at least 3 consecutive days). Clinicians should not obtain imaging studies of any kind to distinguish acute bacterial sinusitis from viral URI, because they do not contribute to the diagnosis; however, a contrast-enhanced computed tomography scan of the paranasal sinuses should be obtained whenever a child is suspected of having orbital or central nervous system complications. The clinician should prescribe antibiotic therapy for acute bacterial sinusitis in children with severe onset or worsening course. The clinician should either prescribe antibiotic therapy or offer additional observation for 3 days to children with persistent illness. Amoxicillin with or without clavulanate is the first-line treatment of acute bacterial sinusitis. Clinicians should reassess initial management if there is either a caregiver report of worsening (progression of initial signs/symptoms or appearance of new signs/symptoms) or failure to improve within 72 hours of initial management. If the diagnosis of acute bacterial sinusitis is confirmed in a child with worsening symptoms or failure to improve, then clinicians may change the antibiotic therapy for the child initially managed with antibiotic or initiate antibiotic treatment of the child initially managed with observation.

CONCLUSIONS: Changes in this revision include the addition of a clinical presentation designated as "worsening course," an option to treat immediately or observe children with persistent symptoms for 3 days before treating, and a review of evidence indicating that imaging is not necessary in children with uncomplicated acute bacterial sinusitis. *Pediatrics* 2013;132:e262–e280

Ellen R. Wald, MD, FAAP, Kimberly E. Applegate, MD, MS, FAAP, Clay Bordley, MD, FAAP, David H. Darrow, MD, DDS, FAAP, Mary P. Glode, MD, FAAP, S. Michael Marcy, MD, FAAP, Carrie E. Nelson, MD, MS, Richard M. Rosenfeld, MD, FAAP, Nader Shaikh, MD, MPH, FAAP, Michael J. Smith, MD, MSCE, FAAP, Paul V. Williams, MD, FAAP, and Stuart T. Weinberg, MD, FAAP

KEY WORDS
acute bacterial sinusitis, sinusitis, antibiotics, imaging, sinus aspiration

ABBREVIATIONS
AAP—American Academy of Pediatrics
AOM—acute otitis media
CT—computed tomography
PCV-13—13-valent pneumococcal conjugate vaccine
RABS—recurrent acute bacterial sinusitis
RCT—randomized controlled trial
URI—upper respiratory tract infection

www.pediatrics.org/cgi/doi/10.1542/peds.2013-1071

doi:10.1542/peds.2013-1071

PEDIATRICS (ISSN Numbers: Print, 0031-4005; Online, 1098-4275).

INTRODUCTION

Acute bacterial sinusitis is a common complication of viral upper respiratory infection (URI) or allergic inflammation. Using stringent criteria to define acute sinusitis, it has been observed that between 6% and 7% of children seeking care for respiratory symptoms has an illness consistent with this definition.[1–4]

This clinical practice guideline is a revision of the clinical practice guideline published by the American Academy of Pediatrics (AAP) in 2001.[5] It has been developed by a subcommittee of the Steering Committee on Quality Improvement and Management that included physicians with expertise in the fields of primary care pediatrics, academic general pediatrics, family practice, allergy, epidemiology and informatics, pediatric infectious diseases, pediatric otolaryngology, radiology, and pediatric emergency medicine. None of the participants had financial conflicts of interest, and only money from the AAP was used to fund the development of the guideline. The guideline will be reviewed in 5 years unless new evidence emerges that warrants revision sooner.

The guideline is intended for use in a variety of clinical settings (eg, office, emergency department, hospital) by clinicians who treat pediatric patients. The data on which the recommendations are based are included in a companion technical report, published in the electronic pages.[6] The Partnership for Policy Implementation has developed a series of definitions using accepted health information technology standards to assist in the implementation of this guideline in computer systems and quality measurement efforts. This document is available at: http://www2.aap.org/informatics/PPI.html.

This revision focuses on the diagnosis and management of acute sinusitis in children between 1 and 18 years of age. It does not apply to children with subacute or chronic sinusitis. Similar to the previous guideline, this document does not consider neonates and children younger than 1 year or children with anatomic abnormalities of the sinuses, immunodeficiencies, cystic fibrosis, or primary ciliary dyskinesia. The most significant areas of change from the 2001 guideline are in the addition of a clinical presentation designated as "worsening course," inclusion of new data on the effectiveness of antibiotics in children with acute sinusitis,[4] and a review of evidence indicating that imaging is not necessary to identify those children who will benefit from antimicrobial therapy.

METHODS

The Subcommittee on Management of Sinusitis met in June 2009 to identify research questions relevant to guideline revision. The primary goal was to update the 2001 report by identifying and reviewing additional studies of pediatric acute sinusitis that have been performed over the past decade.

Searches of PubMed were performed by using the same search term as in the 2001 report. All searches were limited to English-language and human studies. Three separate searches were performed to maximize retrieval of the most recent and highest-quality evidence for pediatric sinusitis. The first limited results to all randomized controlled trials (RCTs) from 1966 to 2009, the second to all meta-analyses from 1966 to 2009, and the third to all pediatric studies (limited to ages <18 years) published since the last technical report (1999–2009). Additionally, the Web of Science was queried to identify studies that cited the original AAP guidelines. This literature search was replicated in July 2010

Evidence Quality	Preponderance of Benefit or Harm	Balance of Benefit and Harm
A. Well-designed RCTs or diagnostic studies on relevant population	Strong Recommendation	Option
B. RCTs or diagnostic studies with minor limitations; overwhelmingly consistent evidence from observational studies		
C. Observational studies (case-control and cohort design)	Recommendation	
D. Expert opinion, case reports, reasoning from first principles	Option	No Rec
X. Exceptional situations where validating studies cannot be performed and there is a clear preponderance of benefit or harm	Strong Recommendation / Recommendation	

FIGURE 1
Levels of recommendations. Rec, recommendation.

and November 2012 to capture recently published studies. The complete results of the literature review are published separately in the technical report.[6] In summary, 17 randomized studies of sinusitis in children were identified and reviewed. Only 3 trials met inclusion criteria. Because of significant heterogeneity among these studies, formal meta-analyses were not pursued.

The results from the literature review were used to guide development of the key action statements included in this document. These action statements were generated by using BRIDGE-Wiz (Building Recommendations in a Developers Guideline Editor, Yale School of Medicine, New Haven, CT), an interactive software tool that leads guideline development through a series of questions that are intended to create a more actionable set of key action statements.[7] BRIDGE-Wiz also incorporates the quality of available evidence into the final determination of the strength of each recommendation.

The AAP policy statement "Classifying Recommendations for Clinical Practice Guidelines" was followed in designating levels of recommendations (Fig 1).[8] Definitions of evidence-based statements are provided in Table 1. This guideline was reviewed by multiple groups in the AAP and 2 external organizations. Comments were compiled and reviewed by the subcommittee, and relevant changes were incorporated into the guideline.

KEY ACTION STATEMENTS

Key Action Statement 1

Clinicians should make a presumptive diagnosis of acute bacterial sinusitis when a child with an acute URI presents with the following:

- **Persistent illness, ie, nasal discharge (of any quality) or daytime cough or both lasting more than 10 days without improvement;**

OR

- **Worsening course, ie, worsening or new onset of nasal discharge, daytime cough, or fever after initial improvement;**

OR

- **Severe onset, ie, concurrent fever (temperature ≥39°C/102.2°F) and purulent nasal discharge for at least 3 consecutive days (Evidence Quality: B; Recommendation).**

KAS Profile 1

Aggregate evidence quality: B	
Benefit	Diagnosis allows decisions regarding management to be made. Children likely to benefit from antimicrobial therapy will be identified.
Harm	Inappropriate diagnosis may lead to unnecessary treatment. A missed diagnosis may lead to persistent infection or complications
Cost	Inappropriate diagnosis may lead to unnecessary cost of antibiotics. A missed diagnosis leads to cost of persistent illness (loss of time from school and work) or cost of caring for complications.
Benefits-harm assessment	Preponderance of benefit.
Value judgments	None.
Role of patient preference	Limited.
Intentional vagueness	None.
Exclusions	Children aged <1 year or older than 18 years and with underlying conditions.
Strength	Recommendation.

TABLE 1 Guideline Definitions for Evidence-Based Statements

Statement	Definition	Implication
Strong recommendation	A strong recommendation in favor of a particular action is made when the anticipated benefits of the recommended intervention clearly exceed the harms (as a strong recommendation against an action is made when the anticipated harms clearly exceed the benefits) and the quality of the supporting evidence is excellent. In some clearly identified circumstances, strong recommendations may be made when high-quality evidence is impossible to obtain and the anticipated benefits strongly outweigh the harms.	Clinicians should follow a strong recommendation unless a clear and compelling rationale for an alternative approach is present.
Recommendation	A recommendation in favor of a particular action is made when the anticipated benefits exceed the harms but the quality of evidence is not as strong. Again, in some clearly identified circumstances, recommendations may be made when high-quality evidence is impossible to obtain but the anticipated benefits outweigh the harms.	Clinicians would be prudent to follow a recommendation, but should remain alert to new information and sensitive to patient preferences.
Option	Options define courses that may be taken when either the quality of evidence is suspect or carefully performed studies have shown little clear advantage to one approach over another.	Clinicians should consider the option in their decision-making, and patient preference may have a substantial role.
No recommendation	No recommendation indicates that there is a lack of pertinent published evidence and that the anticipated balance of benefits and harms is presently unclear.	Clinicians should be alert to new published evidence that clarifies the balance of benefit versus harm.

The purpose of this action statement is to guide the practitioner in making a diagnosis of acute bacterial sinusitis on the basis of stringent clinical criteria. To develop criteria to be used in distinguishing episodes of acute bacterial sinusitis from other common respiratory infections, it is helpful to describe the features of an uncomplicated viral URI. Viral URIs are usually characterized by nasal symptoms (discharge and congestion/obstruction) or cough or both. Most often, the nasal discharge begins as clear and watery. Often, however, the quality of nasal discharge changes during the course of the illness. Typically, the nasal discharge becomes thicker and more mucoid and may become purulent (thick, colored, and opaque) for several days. Then the situation reverses, with the purulent discharge becoming mucoid and then clear again or simply resolving. The transition from clear to purulent to clear again occurs in uncomplicated viral URIs without the use of antimicrobial therapy.

Fever, when present in uncomplicated viral URI, tends to occur early in the illness, often in concert with other constitutional symptoms such as headache and myalgias. Typically, the fever and constitutional symptoms disappear in the first 24 to 48 hours, and the respiratory symptoms become more prominent (Fig 2).

The course of most uncomplicated viral URIs is 5 to 7 days.[9–12] As shown in Fig 2, respiratory symptoms usually peak in severity by days 3 to 6 and then begin to improve; however, resolving symptoms and signs may persist in some patients after day 10.[9,10]

Symptoms of acute bacterial sinusitis and uncomplicated viral URI overlap considerably, and therefore it is their persistence without improvement that suggests a diagnosis of acute sinusitis.[9,10,13] Such symptoms include

nasal discharge (of any quality: thick or thin, serous, mucoid, or purulent) or daytime cough (which may be worse at night) or both. Bad breath, fatigue, headache, and decreased appetite, although common, are not specific indicators of acute sinusitis.[14] Physical examination findings are also not particularly helpful in distinguishing sinusitis from uncomplicated URIs. Erythema and swelling of the nasal turbinates are nonspecific findings.[14] Percussion of the sinuses is not useful. Transillumination of the sinuses is difficult to perform correctly in children and has been shown to be unreliable.[15,16] Nasopharyngeal cultures do not reliably predict the etiology of acute bacterial sinusitis.[14,16]

Only a minority (~6%–7%) of children presenting with symptoms of URI will meet criteria for persistence.[3,4,11] As a result, before diagnosing acute bacterial sinusitis, it is important for the practitioner to attempt to (1) differentiate between sequential episodes of uncomplicated viral URI (which may seem to coalesce in the mind of the patient or parent) from the onset of acute bacterial sinusitis with persistent symptoms and (2) establish whether the symptoms are clearly not improving.

A worsening course of signs and symptoms, termed "double sickening," in the context of a viral URI is another presentation of acute bacterial sinusitis.[13,17] Affected children experience substantial and acute worsening of

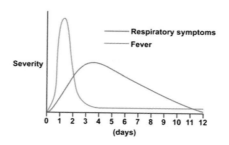

FIGURE 2
Uncomplicated viral URI.

respiratory symptoms (nasal discharge or nasal congestion or daytime cough) or a new fever, often on the sixth or seventh day of illness, after initial signs of recovery from an uncomplicated viral URI. Support for this definition comes from studies in children and adults, for whom antibiotic treatment of worsening symptoms after a period of apparent improvement was associated with better outcomes.[4]

Finally, some children with acute bacterial sinusitis may present with severe onset, ie, concurrent high fever (temperature >39°C) and purulent nasal discharge. These children usually are ill appearing and need to be distinguished from children with uncomplicated viral infections that are unusually severe. If fever is present in uncomplicated viral URIs, it tends to be present early in the illness, usually accompanied by other constitutional symptoms, such as headache and myalgia.[9,13,18] Generally, the constitutional symptoms resolve in the first 48 hours and then the respiratory symptoms become prominent. In most uncomplicated viral infections, including influenza, purulent nasal discharge does not appear for several days. Accordingly, it is the concurrent presentation of high fever and purulent nasal discharge for the first 3 to 4 days of an acute URI that helps to define the severe onset of acute bacterial sinusitis.[13,16,18] This presentation in children is the corollary to acute onset of headache, fever, and facial pain in adults with acute sinusitis.

Allergic and nonallergic rhinitis are predisposing causes of some cases of acute bacterial sinusitis in childhood. In addition, at their onset, these conditions may be mistaken for acute bacterial sinusitis. A family history of atopic conditions, seasonal occurrences, or occurrences with exposure to common allergens and other allergic diatheses in the index patient (eczema, atopic dermatitis, asthma) may suggest the presence of non-infectious rhinitis. The patient may have complaints of pruritic eyes and nasal mucosa, which will provide a clue to the likely etiology of the condition. On physical examination, there may be a prominent nasal crease, allergic shiners, cobblestoning of the conjunctiva or pharyngeal wall, or pale nasal mucosa as other indicators of the diagnosis.

Key Action Statement 2A

Clinicians should not obtain imaging studies (plain films, contrast-enhanced computed tomography [CT], MRI, or ultrasonography) to distinguish acute bacterial sinusitis from viral URI (Evidence Quality: B; Strong Recommendation).

KAS Profile 2A

Aggregate evidence quality: B; overwhelmingly consistent evidence from observational studies.	
Benefit	Avoids exposure to radiation and costs of studies. Avoids unnecessary therapy for false-positive diagnoses.
Harm	None.
Cost	Avoids cost of imaging.
Benefits-harm assessment	Exclusive benefit.
Value judgments	Concern for unnecessary radiation and costs.
Role of patient preference	Limited. Parents may value a negative study and avoidance of antibiotics as worthy of radiation but panel disagrees.
Intentional vagueness	None.
Exclusions	Patients with complications of sinusitis.
Strength	Strong recommendation.

The purpose of this key action statement is to discourage the practitioner from obtaining imaging studies in children with uncomplicated acute bacterial sinusitis. As emphasized in Key Action Statement 1, acute bacterial sinusitis in children is a diagnosis that is made on the basis of stringent clinical criteria that describe signs, symptoms, and temporal patterns of a URI. Although historically imaging has been used as a confirmatory or diagnostic modality in children

suspected to have acute bacterial sinusitis, it is no longer recommended. The membranes that line the nose are continuous with the membranes (mucosa) that line the sinus cavities, the middle ear, the nasopharynx, and the oropharynx. When an individual experiences a viral URI, there is inflammation of the nasal mucosa and, often, the mucosa of the middle ear and paranasal sinuses as well. The continuity of the mucosa of the upper respiratory tract is responsible for the controversy regarding the usefulness of images of the paranasal sinuses in contributing to a diagnosis of acute bacterial sinusitis.

As early as the 1940s, observations were made regarding the frequency of abnormal sinus radiographs in healthy children without signs or symptoms of current respiratory disease.[19] In addition, several investigators in the 1970s and 1980s observed that children with uncomplicated viral URI had frequent abnormalities of the paranasal sinuses on plain radiographs.[20–22] These abnormalities were the same as those considered to be diagnostic of acute bacterial sinusitis (diffuse opacification, mucosal swelling of at least 4 mm, or an air-fluid level).[16]

As technology advanced and CT scanning of the central nervous system and

skull became prevalent, several studies reported on incidental abnormalities of the paranasal sinuses that were observed in children.[23,24] Gwaltney et al[25] showed striking abnormalities (including air-fluid levels) in sinus CT scans of young adults with uncomplicated colds. Manning et al[26] evaluated children undergoing either CT or MRI of the head for indications other than respiratory complaints or suspected sinusitis. Each patient underwent rhinoscopy and otoscopy before imaging and each patient's parent was asked to fill out a questionnaire regarding recent symptoms of URI. Sixty-two percent of patients overall had physical findings or history consistent with an upper respiratory inflammatory process, and 55% of the total group showed some abnormalities on sinus imaging; 33% showed pronounced mucosal thickening or an air-fluid level. Gordts et al[27] made similar observations in children undergoing MRI. Finally, Kristo et al[28] performed MRI in children with URIs and confirmed the high frequency (68%) of major abnormalities seen in the paranasal sinuses.

In summary, when the paranasal sinuses are imaged, either with plain radiographs, contrast-enhanced CT, or MRI in children with uncomplicated URI, the majority of studies will be significantly abnormal with the same kind of findings that are associated with bacterial infection of the sinuses. Accordingly, although normal radiographs or CT or MRI results can ensure that a patient with respiratory symptoms does not have acute bacterial sinusitis, an abnormal image cannot confirm the diagnosis. Therefore, it is not necessary to perform imaging in children with uncomplicated episodes of clinical sinusitis. Similarly, the high likelihood of an abnormal imaging result in a child with an uncomplicated URI indicates that radiographic studies not be performed in an attempt to eliminate the diagnosis of sinusitis.

Key Action Statement 2B

Clinicians should obtain a contrast-enhanced CT scan of the paranasal sinuses and/or an MRI with contrast whenever a child is suspected of having orbital or central nervous system complications of acute bacterial sinusitis (Evidence Quality: B; Strong Recommendation).

KAS Profile 2B

Aggregate evidence quality: B; overwhelmingly consistent evidence from observational studies.	
Benefit	Determine presence of abscesses, which may require surgical intervention; avoid sequelae because of appropriate aggressive management.
Harm	Exposure to ionizing radiation for CT scans; need for sedation for MRI.
Cost	Direct cost of studies.
Benefits-harm assessment	Preponderance of benefit.
Value judgments	Concern for significant complication that may be unrecognized and, therefore, not treated appropriately.
Role of patient preference	Limited.
Intentional vagueness	None.
Exclusions	None.
Strength	Strong recommendation.

The purpose of this key action statement is to have the clinician obtain contrast-enhanced CT images when children are suspected of having serious complications of acute bacterial sinusitis. The most common complication of acute sinusitis involves the orbit in children with ethmoid sinusitis who are younger than 5 years.[29-31] Orbital complications should be suspected when the child presents with a swollen eye, especially if accompanied by proptosis or impaired function of the extraocular muscles. Orbital complications of acute sinusitis have been divided into 5 categories: sympathetic effusion, subperiosteal abscess, orbital cellulitis, orbital abscess, and cavernous sinus thrombosis.[32] Although sympathetic effusion (inflammatory edema) is categorized as an

orbital complication, the site of infection remains confined to the sinus cavities; eye swelling is attributable to the impedance of venous drainage secondary to congestion within the ethmoid sinuses. Alternative terms for sympathetic effusion (inflammatory edema) are preseptal or periorbital cellulitis. The remaining "true" orbital complications are best visualized by contrast-enhanced CT scanning.

Intracranial complications of acute sinusitis, which are substantially less common than orbital complications, are more serious, with higher morbidity and mortality than those involving the orbit. Intracranial complications should be suspected in the patient who presents with a very severe headache, photophobia, seizures, or other focal neurologic findings. Intracranial complications include subdural empyema, epidural empyema, venous thrombosis, brain abscess, and meningitis.[29] Typically, patients with intracranial complications of acute bacterial sinusitis are previously healthy adolescent males with frontal sinusitis.[33,34]

There have been no head-to-head comparisons of the diagnostic accuracy of contrast-enhanced CT scanning to MRI with contrast in the evaluation

of orbital and intracranial complications of sinusitis in children. In general, the contrast-enhanced CT scan has been the preferred imaging study when complications of sinusitis are suspected.[35,36] However, there are documented cases in which a contrast-enhanced CT scan has not revealed the abnormality responsible for the clinical presentation and the MRI with contrast has, especially for intracranial complications and rarely for orbital complications.[37,38] Accordingly, the most recent appropriateness criteria from the American College of Radiology endorse both MRI with contrast and contrast-enhanced CT as complementary examinations when evaluating potential complications of sinusitis.[35] The availability and speed of obtaining the contrast-enhanced CT are desirable; however, there is increasing concern regarding exposure to radiation. The MRI, although very sensitive, takes longer than the contrast-enhanced CT and often requires sedation in young children (which carries its own risks). In older children and adolescents who may not require sedation, MRI with contrast, if available, may be preferred when intracranial complications are likely. Furthermore, MRI with contrast should be performed when there is persistent clinical concern or incomplete information has been provided by the contrast-enhanced CT scan.

Key Action Statement 3

Initial Management of Acute Bacterial Sinusitis

3A: "Severe onset and worsening course" acute bacterial sinusitis. The clinician should prescribe antibiotic therapy for acute bacterial sinusitis in children with severe onset or worsening course (signs, symptoms, or both) (Evidence Quality: B; Strong Recommendation).

KAS Profile 3A

KAS Profile 3A

Aggregate evidence quality: B; randomized controlled trials with limitations.	
Benefit	Increase clinical cures, shorten illness duration, and may prevent suppurative complications in a high-risk patient population.
Harm	Adverse effects of antibiotics.
Cost	Direct cost of therapy.
Benefits-harm assessment	Preponderance of benefit.
Value judgments	Concern for morbidity and possible complications if untreated.
Role of patient preference	Limited.
Intentional vagueness	None.
Exclusions	None.
Strength	Strong recommendation.

3B: "Persistent illness." The clinician should either prescribe antibiotic therapy OR offer additional outpatient observation for 3 days to children with persistent illness (nasal discharge of any quality or cough or both for at least 10 days without evidence of improvement) (Evidence Quality: B; Recommendation).

The purpose of this section is to offer guidance on initial management of persistent illness sinusitis by helping clinicians choose between the following 2 strategies:

1. Antibiotic therapy, defined as initial treatment of acute bacterial sinusitis with antibiotics, with the intent of starting antibiotic therapy as soon as possible after the encounter.

2. Additional outpatient observation, defined as initial management of acute bacterial sinusitis limited to continued observation for 3 days, with commencement of antibiotic therapy if either the child does not improve clinically within several days of diagnosis or if there is clinical worsening of the child's condition at any time.

In contrast to the 2001 AAP guideline,[5] which recommended antibiotic therapy for all children diagnosed with acute bacterial sinusitis, this guideline allows for additional observation of children presenting with persistent illness (nasal discharge of any quality or daytime cough or both for at least 10 days without evidence of improvement). In both guidelines, however, children presenting with severe or worsening illness (which was not defined explicitly in the 2001 guideline[5]) are to receive antibiotic therapy. The rationale for this approach (Table 2) is discussed below.

Antibiotic Therapy for Acute Bacterial Sinusitis

In the United States, antibiotics are prescribed for 82% of children with acute sinusitis.[39] The rationale for antibiotic therapy of acute bacterial sinusitis is based on the recovery of bacteria in high density ($\geq 10^4$ colony-forming units/mL) in 70% of maxillary sinus aspirates obtained from children with a clinical syndrome characterized by persistent nasal discharge, daytime cough, or both.[16,40] Children who present with severe-onset acute bacterial sinusitis are presumed to have bacterial infection, because a temperature of at least 39°C/102.2°F coexisting for at least 3 consecutive days with purulent nasal discharge is not consistent with the well-documented pattern of acute viral URI. Similarly, children with worsening-course acute bacterial sinusitis have a clinical course that is also not consistent with the steady improvement that characterizes an uncomplicated viral URI.[9,10]

KAS Profile 3B

Aggregate evidence quality: B; randomized controlled trials with limitations.	
Benefit	Antibiotics increase the chance of improvement or cure at 10 to 14 days (number needed to treat, 3–5); additional observation may avoid the use of antibiotics with attendant cost and adverse effects.
Harm	Antibiotics have adverse effects (number needed to harm, 3) and may increase bacterial resistance. Observation may prolong illness and delay start of needed antibiotic therapy.
Cost	Direct cost of antibiotics as well as cost of adverse reactions; indirect costs of delayed recovery when observation is used.
Benefits-harm assessment	Preponderance of benefit (because both antibiotic therapy and additional observation with rescue antibiotic, if needed, are appropriate management).
Value judgments	Role for additional brief observation period for selected children with persistent illness sinusitis, similar to what is recommended for acute otitis media, despite the lack of randomized trials specifically comparing additional observation with immediate antibiotic therapy and longer duration of illness before presentation.
Role of patient preference	Substantial role in shared decision-making that should incorporate illness severity, child's quality of life, and caregiver values and concerns.
Intentional vagueness	None.
Exclusions	Children who are excluded from randomized clinical trials of acute bacterial sinusitis, as defined in the text.
Strength	Recommendation.

Three RCTs have compared antibiotic therapy with placebo for the initial management of acute bacterial sinusitis in children. Two trials by Wald et al[4,41] found an increase in cure or improvement after antibiotic therapy compared with placebo with a number needed to treat of 3 to 5 children. Most children in these studies had persistent acute bacterial sinusitis, but children with severe or worsening illness were also included. Conversely, Garbutt et al,[42] who studied only children with persistent acute bacterial sinusitis, found no difference in outcomes for antibiotic versus placebo. Another RCT by Kristo et al,[43] often cited as showing no benefit from antibiotics for acute bacterial sinusitis, will not be considered further because of methodologic flaws, including weak entry criteria and inadequate dosing of antibiotic treatment.

The guideline recommends antibiotic therapy for severe or worsening acute bacterial sinusitis because of the benefits revealed in RCTs[4,41] and a theoretically higher risk of suppurative complications than for children who present with persistent symptoms. Orbital and intracranial complications of acute bacterial sinusitis have not been observed in RCTs, even when placebo was administered; however, sample sizes have inadequate power to preclude an increased risk. This risk, however, has caused some investigators to exclude children with severe acute bacterial sinusitis from trial entry.[42]

Additional Observation for Persistent Onset Acute Bacterial Sinusitis

The guideline recommends either antibiotic therapy or an additional brief period of observation as initial management strategies for children with persistent acute bacterial sinusitis because, although there are benefits to antibiotic therapy (number needed to treat, 3–5), some children improve on their own, and the risk of suppurative

complications is low.[4,41] Symptoms of persistent acute bacterial sinusitis may be mild and have varying effects on a given child's quality of life, ranging from slight (mild cough, nasal discharge) to significant (sleep disturbance, behavioral changes, school or child care absenteeism). The benefits of antibiotic therapy in some trials[4,41] must also be balanced against an increased risk of adverse events (number need to harm, 3), most often self-limited diarrhea, but also including occasional rash.[4]

Choosing between antibiotic therapy or additional observation for initial management of persistent illness sinusitis presents an opportunity for shared decision-making with families (Table 2). Factors that might influence this decision include symptom severity, the child's quality of life, recent antibiotic use, previous experience or outcomes with acute bacterial sinusitis, cost of antibiotics, ease of administration, caregiver concerns about potential adverse effects of antibiotics, persistence of respiratory symptoms, or development of complications. Values and preferences expressed by the caregiver should be taken into consideration (Table 3).

Children with persistent acute bacterial sinusitis who received antibiotic therapy in the previous 4 weeks, those with concurrent bacterial infection (eg, pneumonia, suppurative cervical adenitis, group A streptococcal pharyngitis, or acute otitis media), those with actual or

suspected complications of acute bacterial sinusitis, or those with underlying conditions should generally be managed with antibiotic therapy. The latter group includes children with asthma, cystic fibrosis, immunodeficiency, previous sinus surgery, or anatomic abnormalities of the upper respiratory tract.

Limiting antibiotic use in children with persistent acute bacterial sinusitis who may improve on their own reduces common antibiotic-related adverse events, such as diarrhea, diaper dermatitis, and skin rash. The most recent RCT of acute bacterial sinusitis in children[4] found adverse events of 44% with antibiotic and 14% with placebo.

Limiting antibiotics may also reduce the prevalence of resistant bacterial pathogens. Although this is always a desirable goal, no increase in resistant bacterial species was observed within the group of children treated with a single course of antimicrobial agents (compared with those receiving placebo) in 2 recent large studies of antibiotic versus placebo for children with acute otitis media.[44,45]

Key Action Statement 4

Clinicians should prescribe amoxicillin with or without clavulanate as first-line treatment when a decision has been made to initiate antibiotic treatment of acute bacterial sinusitis (Evidence Quality: B; Recommendation).

KAS Profile 4

Aggregate evidence quality: B; randomized controlled trials with limitations.	
Benefit	Increase clinical cures with narrowest spectrum drug; stepwise increase in broadening spectrum as risk factors for resistance increase.
Harm	Adverse effects of antibiotics including development of hypersensitivity.
Cost	Direct cost of antibiotic therapy.
Benefits-harm assessment	Preponderance of benefit.
Value judgments	Concerns for not encouraging resistance if possible.
Role of patient preference	Potential for shared decision-making that should incorporate the caregiver's experiences and values.
Intentional vagueness	None.
Exclusions	May include allergy or intolerance.
Strength	Recommendation.

TABLE 2 Recommendations for Initial Use of Antibiotics for Acute Bacterial Sinusitis

Clinical Presentation	Severe Acute Bacterial Sinusitis[a]	Worsening Acute Bacterial Sinusitis[b]	Persistent Acute Bacterial Sinusitis[c]
Uncomplicated acute bacterial sinusitis without coexisting illness	Antibiotic therapy	Antibiotic therapy	Antibiotic therapy or additional observation for 3 days[d]
Acute bacterial sinusitis with orbital or intracranial complications	Antibiotic therapy	Antibiotic therapy	Antibiotic therapy
Acute bacterial sinusitis with coexisting acute otitis media, pneumonia, adenitis, or streptococcal pharyngitis	Antibiotic therapy	Antibiotic therapy	Antibiotic therapy

[a] Defined as temperature ≥39°C and purulent (thick, colored, and opaque) nasal discharge present concurrently for at least 3 consecutive days.

[b] Defined as nasal discharge or daytime cough with sudden worsening of symptoms (manifested by new-onset fever ≥38° C/100.4°F or substantial increase in nasal discharge or cough) after having experienced transient improvement of symptoms.

[c] Defined as nasal discharge (of any quality), daytime cough (which may be worse at night), or both, persisting for >10 days without improvement.

[d] Opportunity for shared decision-making with the child's family; if observation is offered, a mechanism must be in place to ensure follow-up and begin antibiotics if the child worsens at any time or fails to improve within 3 days of observation.

The purpose of this key action statement is to guide the selection of antimicrobial therapy once the diagnosis of acute bacterial sinusitis has been made. The microbiology of acute bacterial sinusitis was determined nearly 30 years ago through direct maxillary sinus aspiration in children with compatible signs and symptoms. The major bacterial pathogens recovered at that time were Streptococcus pneumoniae in approximately 30% of children and nontypeable Haemophilus influenzae and Moraxella catarrhalis in approximately 20% each.[16,40] Aspirates from the remaining 25% to 30% of children were sterile.

Maxillary sinus aspiration is rarely performed at the present time unless the course of the infection is unusually prolonged or severe. Although some authorities have recommended obtaining cultures from the middle meatus to determine the cause of a maxillary sinus infection, there are no data in children with acute bacterial sinusitis that have compared such cultures with cultures of a maxillary sinus aspirate. Furthermore, there are data indicating that the middle meatus in healthy children is commonly colonized with S pneumoniae, H influenzae, and M catarrhalis.[46]

Recent estimates of the microbiology of acute sinusitis have, of necessity, been based primarily on that of acute otitis media (AOM), a condition with relatively easy access to infective fluid through performance of tympanocentesis and one with a similar pathogenesis to acute bacterial sinusitis.[47,48] The 3 most common bacterial pathogens recovered from the middle ear fluid of children with AOM are the same as those that have been associated with acute bacterial sinusitis: S pneumoniae, nontypeable H influenzae, and M catarrhalis.[49] The proportion of each has varied from study to study depending on criteria used for diagnosis of AOM, patient characteristics, and bacteriologic techniques. Recommendations since the year 2000 for the routine use in infants of 7-valent and, more recently, 13-valent pneumococcal conjugate vaccine (PCV-13) have been associated with a decrease in recovery of S pneumoniae from ear fluid of children with AOM and a relative increase in the incidence of infections attributable to H influenzae.[50] Thus, on the basis of the proportions of bacteria

found in middle ear infections, it is estimated that S pneumoniae and H influenzae are currently each responsible for approximately 30% of cases of acute bacterial sinusitis in children, and M catarrhalis is responsible for approximately 10%. These percentages are contingent on the assumption that approximately one-quarter of aspirates of maxillary sinusitis would still be sterile, as reported in earlier studies. Staphylococcus aureus is rarely isolated from sinus aspirates in children with acute bacterial sinusitis, and with the exception of acute maxillary sinusitis associated with infections of dental origin,[51] respiratory anaerobes are also rarely recovered.[40,52] Although S aureus is a very infrequent cause of acute bacterial sinusitis in children, it is a significant pathogen in the orbital and intracranial complications of sinusitis. The reasons for this discrepancy are unknown.

Antimicrobial susceptibility patterns for S pneumoniae vary considerably from community to community. Isolates obtained from surveillance centers nationwide indicate that, at the present time, 10% to 15% of upper respiratory tract isolates of S pneumoniae are nonsusceptible to penicillin[53,54]; however, values for penicillin nonsusceptibility as high as 50% to 60% have been reported in some areas.[55,56] Of the organisms that are resistant, approximately half are highly resistant to penicillin and the remaining half are intermediate in resistance.[53,54,56–59] Between 10% and 42% of H influenzae[56–59] and close to 100% of M catarrhalis are likely to be β-lactamase positive and nonsusceptible to amoxicillin. Because of dramatic geographic variability in the prevalence of β-lactamase–positive H influenzae, it is extremely desirable for the practitioner to be familiar with local patterns of susceptibility. Risk factors for the presence of organisms likely to be resistant to amoxicillin include attendance at child care, receipt of antimicrobial treatment within the previous 30 days, and age younger than 2 years.[50,55,60]

Amoxicillin remains the antimicrobial agent of choice for first-line treatment of uncomplicated acute bacterial sinusitis in situations in which antimicrobial resistance is not suspected. This recommendation is based on amoxicillin's effectiveness, safety, acceptable taste, low cost, and relatively narrow microbiologic spectrum. For children aged 2 years or older with uncomplicated acute bacterial sinusitis that is mild to moderate in degree of severity who do not attend child care and who have not been treated with an antimicrobial agent within the last 4 weeks, amoxicillin is recommended at a standard dose of 45 mg/kg per day in 2 divided doses. In communities with a high prevalence of nonsusceptible S pneumoniae (>10%, including intermediate- and high-level resistance), treatment may be initiated at 80 to 90 mg/kg per day in 2 divided doses, with a maximum of 2 g per dose.[55] This high-dose amoxicillin therapy is likely to achieve sinus fluid concentrations that are adequate to overcome the resistance of S pneumoniae, which is attributable to alteration in penicillin-binding proteins on the basis of data derived from patients with AOM.[61] If, within the next several years after licensure of PCV-13, a continuing decrease in isolates of S pneumoniae (including a decrease in isolates of nonsusceptible S pneumoniae) and an increase in β-lactamase–producing H influenzae are observed, standard-dose amoxicillin-clavulanate (45 mg/kg per day) may be most appropriate.

Patients presenting with moderate to severe illness as well as those younger than 2 years, attending child care, or who have recently been treated with an antimicrobial may receive high-dose amoxicillin-clavulanate (80–90 mg/kg per day of the amoxicillin component with 6.4 mg/kg per day of clavulanate in 2 divided doses with a maximum of 2 g per dose). The potassium clavulanate levels are adequate to inhibit all β-lactamase–producing H influenzae and M catarrhalis.[56,59]

A single 50-mg/kg dose of ceftriaxone, given either intravenously or intramuscularly, can be used for children who are vomiting, unable to tolerate oral medication, or unlikely to be adherent to the initial doses of antibiotic.[62–64] The 3 major bacterial pathogens involved in acute bacterial sinusitis are susceptible to ceftriaxone in 95% to 100% of cases.[56,58,59] If clinical improvement is observed at 24 hours, an oral antibiotic can be substituted to complete the course of therapy. Children who are still significantly febrile or symptomatic at 24 hours may require additional parenteral doses before switching to oral therapy.

The treatment of patients with presumed allergy to penicillin has been controversial. However, recent publications indicate that the risk of a serious allergic reaction to second- and third-generation cephalosporins in patients with penicillin or amoxicillin allergy appears to be almost nil and no greater than the risk among patients without such allergy.[65–67] Thus, patients allergic to amoxicillin with a non–type 1 (late or delayed, >72 hours) hypersensitivity reaction can safely be treated with cefdinir, cefuroxime, or cefpodoxime.[66–68] Patients with a history of a serious type 1 immediate or accelerated (anaphylactoid) reaction to amoxicillin can also safely be treated with cefdinir, cefuroxime, or cefpodoxime. In both circumstances, clinicians may wish to determine individual tolerance by referral to an allergist for penicillin and/or cephalosporin skin-testing before initiation of therapy.[66–68] The susceptibility of S pneumoniae to cefdinir, cefpodoxime, and cefuroxime varies from 60% to 75%,[56–59] and the susceptibility of H influenzae to these agents varies from 85% to 100%.[56,58] In young children (<2 years) with a serious type 1 hypersensitivity to penicillin and moderate or more severe sinusitis, it may be prudent to use a combination of clindamycin (or linezolid) and cefixime to achieve the most comprehensive coverage against both resistant S pneumoniae and H influenzae. Linezolid has excellent activity against all S pneumoniae, including penicillin-resistant strains, but lacks activity against H influenzae and M catarrhalis. Alternatively, a quinolone, such as levofloxacin, which has a high level of activity against both S pneumoniae and H influenzae, may be prescribed.[57,58] Although the use of quinolones is usually restricted because of concerns for toxicity, cost, and emerging resistance, their use in this circumstance can be justified.

Pneumococcal and H influenzae surveillance studies have indicated that resistance of these organisms to trimethoprim-sulfamethoxazole and azithromycin is sufficient to preclude their use for treatment of acute bacterial sinusitis in patients with penicillin hypersensitivity.[56,58,59,69]

The optimal duration of antimicrobial therapy for patients with acute bacterial sinusitis has not received systematic study. Recommendations based on clinical observations have varied widely, from 10 to 28 days of treatment. An alternative suggestion has been made that antibiotic therapy be continued for 7 days after the patient becomes free of signs and symptoms.[5] This strategy has the advantage of individualizing the treatment of each patient, results in a minimum course of 10 days, and avoids prolonged antimicrobial therapy in patients who are asymptomatic and therefore unlikely to adhere to the full course of treatment.[5]

Patients who are acutely ill and appear toxic when first seen (see below) can be managed with 1 of 2 options. Consultation can be requested from an otolaryngologist for consideration of maxillary sinus aspiration (with appropriate analgesia/anesthesia) to obtain a sample of sinus secretions for Gram stain, culture, and susceptibility testing so that antimicrobial therapy can be adjusted precisely. Alternatively, inpatient therapy can be initiated with intravenous cefotaxime or ceftriaxone, with referral to an otolaryngologist if the patient's condition worsens or fails to show improvement within 48 hours. If a complication is suspected, management will differ depending on the site and severity.

A recent guideline was published by the Infectious Diseases Society of America for acute bacterial rhinosinusitis in children and adults.[70] Their recommendation for initial empirical antimicrobial therapy for acute bacterial sinusitis in children was amoxicillin-clavulanate based on the concern that there is an increasing prevalence of *H influenzae* as a cause of sinusitis since introduction of the pneumococcal conjugate vaccines and an increasing prevalence of β-lactamase production among these strains. In contrast, this guideline from the AAP allows either amoxicillin or amoxicillin-clavulanate as first-line empirical therapy and is therefore inclusive of the Infectious Diseases Society of America's recommendation. Unfortunately, there are scant data available regarding the precise microbiology of acute bacterial sinusitis in the post–PCV-13 era. Prospective surveillance of nasopharyngeal cultures may be helpful in completely

aligning these recommendations in the future.

Key Action Statement 5A

Clinicians should reassess initial management if there is either a caregiver report of worsening (progression of initial signs/symptoms or appearance of new signs/symptoms) OR failure to improve (lack of reduction in all presenting signs/symptoms) within 72 hours of initial management (Evidence Quality: C; Recommendation).

KAS Profile 5A

Aggregate evidence quality: C; observational studies	
Benefits	Identification of patients who may have been misdiagnosed, those at risk of complications, and those who require a change in management.
Harm	Delay of up to 72 hours in changing therapy if patient fails to improve.
Cost	Additional provider and caregiver time and resources.
Benefits-harm assessment	Preponderance of benefit.
Value judgments	Use of 72 hours to assess progress may result in excessive classification as treatment failures if premature; emphasis on importance of worsening illness in defining treatment failures.
Role of patient preferences	Caregivers determine whether the severity of the patient's illness justifies the report to clinician of the patient's worsening or failure to improve.
Intentional vagueness	None.
Exclusions	Patients with severe illness, poor general health, complicated sinusitis, immune deficiency, previous sinus surgery, or coexisting bacterial illness.
Strength	Recommendation.

The purpose of this key action statement is to ensure that patients with acute bacterial sinusitis who fail to improve symptomatically after initial management are reassessed to be certain that they have been correctly diagnosed and to consider initiation of alternate therapy to hasten resolution of symptoms and avoid complications. "Worsening" is defined as progression of presenting signs or symptoms of acute bacterial sinusitis or onset of new signs or symptoms. "Failure to improve" is lack of reduction in presenting signs or symptoms of acute

bacterial sinusitis by 72 hours after diagnosis and initial management; patients with persistent but improving symptoms do not meet this definition.

The rationale for using 72 hours as the time to assess treatment failure for acute bacterial sinusitis is based on clinical outcomes in RCTs. Wald et al[41] found that 18 of 35 patients (51%) receiving placebo demonstrated symptomatic improvement within 3 days of initiation of treatment; only an additional 3 patients receiving placebo (9%) improved between days 3 and 10. In the same study, 48 of 58 patients (83%) receiving antibiotics were cured or improved within 3 days; at 10 days, the overall rate of improvement was 79%, suggesting that no additional patients improved between days 3 and 10. In a more recent study, 17 of 19 children who ultimately failed initial therapy with either antibiotic or placebo demonstrated failure to improve within 72 hours.[4] Although Garbutt et al[42] did not report the percentage of patients who improved by day 3, they did demonstrate that the majority of improvement in symptoms occurred within the first 3 days of study entry whether they received active treatment or placebo.

Reporting of either worsening or failure to improve implies a shared responsibility between clinician and caregiver. Although the clinician should educate the caregiver regarding the anticipated reduction in symptoms within 3 days, it is incumbent on the caregiver to appropriately notify the clinician of concerns regarding worsening or failure to improve. Clinicians should emphasize the importance of reassessing those children whose symptoms are worsening whether or not antibiotic therapy was prescribed. Reassessment may be indicated before the 72-hour

process by which such reporting occurs should be discussed at the time the initial management strategy is determined.

Key Action Statement 5B

If the diagnosis of acute bacterial sinusitis is confirmed in a child with worsening symptoms or failure to improve in 72 hours, then clinicians may change the antibiotic therapy for the child initially managed with antibiotic OR initiate antibiotic treatment of the child initially managed with observation (Evidence Quality: D; Option based on expert opinion, case reports, and reasoning from first principles).

corresponds to the patient's pattern of illness, as defined in Key Action Statement 1. If caregivers report worsening of symptoms at any time in a patient for whom observation was the initial intervention, the clinician should begin treatment as discussed in Key Action Statement 4. For patients whose symptoms are mild and who have failed to improve but have not worsened, initiation of antimicrobial agents or continued observation (for up to 3 days) is reasonable.

If caregivers report worsening of symptoms after 3 days in a patient initially treated with antimicrobial agents, current signs and symptoms should be reviewed to determine whether acute bacterial sinusitis is still the best diagnosis. If sinusitis is still the best diagnosis, infection with drug-resistant bacteria is probable, and an alternate antimicrobial agent may be administered. Face-to-face reevaluation of the patient is desirable. Once the decision is made to change medications, the clinician should consider the limitations of the initial antibiotic coverage, the anticipated susceptibility of residual bacterial pathogens, and the ability of antibiotics to adequately penetrate the site of infection. Cultures of sinus or nasopharyngeal secretions in patients with initial antibiotic failure have identified a large percentage of bacteria with resistance to the original antibiotic.[71,72] Furthermore, multidrug-resistant *S pneumoniae* and β-lactamase–positive *H influenzae* and *M catarrhalis* are more commonly isolated after previous antibiotic exposure.[73–78] Unfortunately, there are no studies in children that have investigated the microbiology of treatment failure in acute bacterial sinusitis or cure rates using second-line antimicrobial agents. As a result, the likelihood of adequate antibiotic coverage for resistant organisms must be

KAS Profile 5B

Aggregate evidence quality: D; expert opinion and reasoning from first principles.	
Benefit	Prevention of complications, administration of effective therapy.
Harm	Adverse effects of secondary antibiotic therapy.
Cost	Direct cost of medications, often substantial for second-line agents.
Benefits-harm assessment	Preponderance of benefit.
Value judgments	Clinician must determine whether cost and adverse effects associated with change in antibiotic is justified given the severity of illness.
Role of patient preferences	Limited in patients whose symptoms are severe or worsening, but caregivers of mildly affected children who are failing to improve may reasonably defer change in antibiotic.
Intentional vagueness	None.
Exclusions	None.
Strength	Option.

mark if the patient is substantially worse, because it may indicate the development of complications or a need for parenteral therapy. Conversely, in some cases, caregivers may think that symptoms are not severe enough to justify a change to an antibiotic with a less desirable safety profile or even the time, effort, and resources required for reassessment. Accordingly, the circumstances under which caregivers report back to the clinician and the

The purpose of this key action statement is to ensure optimal antimicrobial treatment of children with acute bacterial sinusitis whose symptoms worsen or fail to respond to the initial intervention to prevent complications and reduce symptom severity and duration (see Table 4).

Clinicians who are notified by a caregiver that a child's symptoms are worsening or failing to improve should confirm that the clinical diagnosis of acute bacterial sinusitis

addressed by extrapolations from studies of acute otitis media in children and sinusitis in adults and by using the results of data generated in vitro. A general guide to management of the child who worsens in 72 hours is shown in Table 4.

NO RECOMMENDATION

Adjuvant Therapy

Potential adjuvant therapy for acute sinusitis might include intranasal corticosteroids, saline nasal irrigation or lavage, topical or oral decongestants, mucolytics, and topical or oral antihistamines. A recent Cochrane review on decongestants, antihistamines, and nasal irrigation for acute sinusitis in children found no appropriately designed studies to determine the effectiveness of these interventions.[79]

Intranasal Steroids

The rationale for the use of intranasal corticosteroids in acute bacterial sinusitis is that an antiinflammatory agent may reduce the swelling around the sinus ostia and encourage drainage, thereby hastening recovery. However, there are limited data on how much inflammation is present, whether the inflammation is responsive to steroids, and whether there are differences in responsivity according to age. Nonetheless, there are several RCTs in adolescents and adults, most of which do show significant differences compared with placebo or active comparator that favor intranasal steroids in the reduction of symptoms and the patient's global assessment of overall improvement.[80–85] Several studies in adults with acute bacterial sinusitis provide data supporting the use of intranasal steroids as either monotherapy or adjuvant therapy to antibiotics.[81,86] Only one study did not show efficacy.[85]

There have been 2 trials of intranasal steroids performed exclusively in children: one comparing intranasal corticosteroids versus an oral decongestant[87] and the other comparing intranasal corticosteroids with placebo.[88] These studies showed a greater rate of complete resolution[87] or greater reduction in symptoms in patients receiving the steroid preparation, although the effects were modest.[88] It is important to note that nearly all of these studies (both those reported in children and adults) suffered from substantial methodologic problems. Examples of these methodologic problems are as follows: (1) variable inclusion criteria for sinusitis, (2) mixed populations of allergic and nonallergic subjects, and (3) different outcome criteria. All of these factors make deriving a clear conclusion difficult. Furthermore, the lack of stringent criteria in selecting the subject population increases the chance that the subjects had viral URIs or even persistent allergies rather than acute bacterial sinusitis.

The intranasal steroids studied to date include budesonide, flunisolide, fluticasone, and mometasone. There is no reason to believe that one steroid would be more effective than another, provided equivalent doses are used.

Potential harm in using nasal steroids in children with acute sinusitis includes the increased cost of therapy, difficulty in effectively administering nasal sprays in young children, nasal irritation and epistaxis, and potential systemic adverse effects of steroid use. Fortunately, no clinically significant steroid adverse effects have been discovered in studies in children.[89–96]

Saline Irrigation

Saline nasal irrigation or lavage (not saline nasal spray) has been used to remove debris from the nasal cavity and temporarily reduce tissue edema (hypertonic saline) to promote drainage from the sinuses. There have been very few RCTs using saline nasal irrigation or lavage in acute sinusitis, and these have had mixed results.[97,98] The 1 study in children showed greater improvement in nasal airflow and quality of life as well as a better rate of improvement in total symptom score when compared with placebo in patients treated with antibiotics and decongestants.[98] There are 2 Cochrane reviews published on the use of saline nasal irrigation in acute sinusitis in adults that showed variable results. One review published in 2007[99] concluded that it is a beneficial adjunct, but the other, published in 2010,[100] concluded that most trials were too small or contained too high a risk of bias to be confident about benefits.

Nasal Decongestants, Mucolytics, and Antihistamines

Data are insufficient to make any recommendations about the use of oral or topical nasal decongestants, mucolytics, or oral or nasal spray antihistamines as adjuvant therapy for acute bacterial sinusitis in children.[79] It is the opinion of the expert panel that antihistamines should not be used for the primary indication of acute bacterial sinusitis in any child, although such therapy might be helpful in reducing typical allergic symptoms in patients with atopy who also have acute sinusitis.

OTHER RELATED CONDITIONS

Recurrence of Acute Bacterial Sinusitis

Recurrent acute bacterial sinusitis (RABS) is an uncommon occurrence in healthy children and must be distinguished from recurrent URIs, exacerbations of allergic rhinitis, and chronic sinusitis. The former is defined by episodes of bacterial infection of the paranasal sinuses lasting fewer than 30 days and separated by intervals of

TABLE 3 Parent Information Regarding Initial Management of Acute Bacterial Sinusitis

How common are sinus infections in children?	Thick, colored, or cloudy mucus from your child's nose frequently occurs with a common cold or viral infection and does not by itself mean your child has sinusitis. In fact, fewer than 1 in 15 children get a true bacterial sinus infection during or after a common cold.
How can I tell if my child has bacterial sinusitis or simply a common cold?	Most colds have a runny nose with mucus that typically starts out clear, becomes cloudy or colored, and improves by about 10 d. Some colds will also include fever (temperature >38°C [100.4°F]) for 1 to 2 days. In contrast, acute bacterial sinusitis is likely when the pattern of illness is persistent, severe, or worsening. 1. *Persistent* sinusitis is the most common type, defined as runny nose (of any quality), daytime cough (which may be worse at night), or both for at least 10 days without improvement. 2. *Severe* sinusitis is present when fever (temperature ≥39°C [102.2°F]) lasts for at least 3 days in a row and is accompanied by nasal mucus that is thick, colored, or cloudy. 3. *Worsening* sinusitis starts with a viral cold, which begins to improve but then worsens when bacteria take over and cause new-onset fever (temperature ≥38°C [100.4°F]) or a substantial increase in daytime cough or runny nose.
If my child has sinusitis, should he or she take an antibiotic?	Children with *persistent* sinusitis may be managed with either an antibiotic or with an additional brief period of observation, allowing the child up to another 3 days to fight the infection and improve on his or her own. The choice to treat or observe should be discussed with your doctor and may be based on your child's quality of life and how much of a problem the sinusitis is causing. In contrast, all children diagnosed with *severe* or *worsening* sinusitis should start antibiotic treatment to help them recover faster and more often.
Why not give all children with acute bacterial sinusitis an immediate antibiotic?	Some episodes of *persistent* sinusitis include relatively mild symptoms that may improve on their own in a few days. In addition, antibiotics can have adverse effects, which may include vomiting, diarrhea, upset stomach, skin rash, allergic reactions, yeast infections, and development of resistant bacteria (that make future infections more difficult to treat).

at least 10 days during which the patient is asymptomatic. Some experts require at least 4 episodes in a calendar year to fulfill the criteria for this condition. Chronic sinusitis is manifest as 90 or more uninterrupted days of respiratory symptoms, such as cough, nasal discharge, or nasal obstruction.

Children with RABS should be evaluated for underlying allergies, particularly allergic rhinitis; quantitative and functional immunologic defect(s), chiefly immunoglobulin A and immunoglobulin G deficiency; cystic fibrosis; gastroesophageal reflux disease; or dysmotile cilia syndrome.[101] Anatomic abnormalities obstructing one or more sinus ostia may be present. These include septal deviation, nasal polyps, or concha bullosa (pneumatization of the middle turbinate); atypical ethmoid cells with compromised drainage; a lateralized middle turbinate; and intrinsic ostiomeatal anomalies.[102]

Contrast-enhanced CT, MRI, or endoscopy or all 3 should be performed for detection of obstructive conditions, particularly in children with genetic or acquired craniofacial abnormalities.

The microbiology of RABS is similar to that of isolated episodes of acute bacterial sinusitis and warrants the same treatment.[72] It should be recognized that closely spaced sequential courses of antimicrobial therapy may foster the emergence of antibiotic-resistant bacterial species as the causative agent in recurrent episodes. There are no systematically evaluated options for prevention of RABS in children. In general, the use of prolonged prophylactic antimicrobial therapy should be avoided and is not usually recommended for children with recurrent acute otitis media. However, when there are no recognizable predisposing conditions to remedy in children with RABS, prophylactic antimicrobial agents may be used for several months during the respiratory season. Enthusiasm for this strategy is tempered by concerns regarding the encouragement of bacterial resistance. Accordingly, prophylaxis should only be considered in carefully selected children whose infections have been thoroughly documented.

Influenza vaccine should be administered annually, and PCV-13 should be administered at the recommended ages for all children, including those with RABS. Intranasal steroids and nonsedating antihistamines can be helpful for children with allergic rhinitis, as can antireflux medications for those with gastroesophageal reflux disease. Children with anatomic abnormalities may require endoscopic surgery for removal of or reduction in ostiomeatal obstruction.

The pathogenesis of chronic sinusitis is poorly understood and appears to be multifactorial; however, many of the conditions associated with RABS

TABLE 4 Management of Worsening or Lack of Improvement at 72 Hours

Initial Management	Worse in 72 Hours	Lack of Improvement in 72 Hours
Observation	Initiate amoxicillin with or without clavulanate	Additional observation or initiate antibiotic based on shared decision-making
Amoxicillin	High-dose amoxicillin-clavulanate	Additional observation or high-dose amoxicillin-clavulanate based on shared decision-making
High-dose amoxicillin-clavulanate	Clindamycin[a] and cefixime OR linezolid and cefixime OR levofloxacin	Continued high-dose amoxicillin-clavulanate OR clindamycin[a] and cefixime OR linezolid and cefixime OR levofloxacin

[a] Clindamycin is recommended to cover penicillin-resistant *S pneumoniae*. Some communities have high levels of clindamycin-resistant *S pneumoniae*. In these communities, linezolid is preferred.

have also been implicated in chronic sinusitis, and it is clear that there is an overlap between the 2 syndromes.[101,102] In some cases, there may be episodes of acute bacterial sinusitis superimposed on a chronic sinusitis, warranting antimicrobial therapy to hasten resolution of the acute infection.

Complications of Acute Bacterial Sinusitis

Complications of acute bacterial sinusitis should be diagnosed when the patient develops signs or symptoms of orbital and/or central nervous system (intracranial) involvement. Rarely, complicated acute bacterial sinusitis can result in permanent blindness, other neurologic sequelae, or death if not treated promptly and appropriately. Orbital complications have been classified by Chandler et al.[32] Intracranial complications include epidural or subdural abscess, brain abscess, venous thrombosis, and meningitis.

Periorbital and intraorbital inflammation and infection are the most common complications of acute sinusitis and most often are secondary to acute ethmoiditis in otherwise healthy young children. These disorders are commonly classified in relation to the orbital septum; periorbital or preseptal inflammation involves only the eyelid, whereas postseptal (intraorbital) inflammation involves structures of the orbit. Mild cases of preseptal cellulitis (eyelid <50% closed) may be treated on an outpatient basis with appropriate

oral antibiotic therapy (high-dose amoxicillin-clavulanate for comprehensive coverage) for acute bacterial sinusitis and daily follow-up until definite improvement is noted. If the patient does not improve within 24 to 48 hours or if the infection is progressive, it is appropriate to admit the patient to the hospital for antimicrobial therapy. Similarly, if proptosis, impaired visual acuity, or impaired and/or painful extraocular mobility is present on examination, the patient should be hospitalized, and a contrast-enhanced CT should be performed. Consultation with an otolaryngologist, an ophthalmologist, and an infectious disease expert is appropriate for guidance regarding the need for surgical intervention and the selection of antimicrobial agents.

Intracranial complications are most frequently encountered in previously healthy adolescent males with frontal sinusitis.[33,34] In patients with altered mental status, severe headache, or Pott's puffy tumor (osteomyelitis of the frontal bone), neurosurgical consultation should be obtained. A contrast-enhanced CT scan (preferably coronal thin cut) of the head, orbits, and sinuses is essential to confirm intracranial or intraorbital suppurative complications; in such cases, intravenous antibiotics should be started immediately. Alternatively, an MRI may also be desirable in some cases of intracranial abnormality. Appropriate antimicrobial therapy for intraorbital complications include vancomycin (to cover possible methicillin-resistant

S aureus or penicillin-resistant *S pneumoniae*) and either ceftriaxone, ampicillin-sulbactam, or piperacillin-tazobactam.[103] Given the polymicrobial nature of sinogenic abscesses, coverage for anaerobes (ie, metronidazole) should also be considered for intraorbital complications and should be started in all cases of intracranial complications if ceftriaxone is prescribed.

Patients with small orbital, subperiosteal, or epidural abscesses and minimal ocular and neurologic abnormalities may be managed with intravenous antibiotic treatment for 24 to 48 hours while performing frequent visual and mental status checks.[104] In patients who develop progressive signs and symptoms, such as impaired visual acuity, ophthalmoplegia, elevated intraocular pressure (>20 mm), severe proptosis (>5 mm), altered mental status, headache, or vomiting, as well as those who fail to improve within 24 to 48 hours while receiving antibiotics, prompt surgical intervention and drainage of the abscess should be undertaken.[104] Antibiotics can be tailored to the results of culture and sensitivity studies when they become available.

AREAS FOR FUTURE RESEARCH

Since the publication of the original guideline in 2001, only a small number of high-quality studies of the diagnosis and treatment of acute bacterial sinusitis in children have been published.[5] Ironically, the number of published guidelines on the topic (5) exceeds the number of prospective, placebo-controlled clinical trials of either antibiotics or ancillary treatments of acute bacterial sinusitis. Thus, as was the case in 2001, there are scant data on which to base recommendations. Accordingly, areas for future research include the following:

Etiology

1. Reexamine the microbiology of acute sinusitis in children in the postpneumococcal conjugate vaccine era and determine the value of using newer polymerase chain reaction–based respiratory testing to document viral, bacterial, and polymicrobial disease.

2. Correlate cultures obtained from the middle meatus of the maxillary sinus of infected children with cultures obtained from the maxillary sinus by puncture of the antrum.

3. Conduct more and larger studies to more clearly define and correlate the clinical findings with the various available diagnostic criteria of acute bacterial sinusitis (eg, sinus aspiration and treatment outcome).

4. Develop noninvasive strategies to accurately diagnose acute bacterial sinusitis in children.

5. Develop imaging technology that differentiates bacterial infection from viral infection or allergic inflammation, preferably without radiation.

Treatment

1. Determine the optimal duration of antimicrobial therapy for children with acute bacterial sinusitis.

2. Evaluate a "wait-and-see prescription" strategy for children with persistent symptom presentation of acute sinusitis.

3. Determine the optimal antimicrobial agent for children with acute bacterial sinusitis, balancing the incentives of choosing narrow-spectrum agents against the known microbiology of the disease and resistance patterns of likely pathogens.

4. Determine the causes and treatment of subacute, recurrent acute, and chronic bacterial sinusitis.

5. Determine the efficacy of prophylaxis with antimicrobial agents to prevent RABS.

6. Determine the effects of bacterial resistance among *S pneumoniae*, *H influenzae*, and *M catarrhalis* on outcome of treatment with antibiotics by the performance of randomized, double-blind, placebo-controlled studies in well-defined populations of patients.

7. Determine the role of adjuvant therapies (antihistamines, nasal corticosteroids, mucolytics, decongestants, nasal irrigation, etc) in patients with acute bacterial sinusitis by the performance of prospective, randomized clinical trials.

8. Determine whether early treatment of acute bacterial sinusitis prevents orbital or central nervous system complications.

9. Determine the role of complementary and alternative medicine strategies in patients with acute bacterial sinusitis by performing systematic, prospective, randomized clinical trials.

10. Develop new bacterial and viral vaccines to reduce the incidence of acute bacterial sinusitis.

SUBCOMMITTEE ON ACUTE SINUSITIS

Ellen R. Wald, MD, FAAP (Chair, Pediatric Infectious Disease Physician: no financial conflicts; published research related to sinusitis)

Kimberly E. Applegate, MD, MS, FAAP (Radiologist, AAP Section on Radiology: no conflicts)

Clay Bordley, MD, MPH, FAAP (Pediatric Emergency and Hospitalist Medicine physician: no conflicts)

David H. Darrow, MD, FAAP (Otolaryngologist, AAP Section on Otolaryngology–Head and Neck Surgery: no conflicts)

Mary P. Glode, MD, FAAP (Pediatric Infectious Disease Physician, AAP Committee on Infectious Disease: no conflicts)

S. Michael Marcy, MD, FAAP (General Pediatrician with Infectious Disease Expertise, AAP Section on Infectious Diseases: no conflicts)

Nader Shaikh, MD, FAAP (General Academic Pediatrician: no financial conflicts; published research related to sinusitis)

Michael J. Smith, MD, MSCE, FAAP (Epidemiologist, Pediatric Infectious Disease Physician: research funding for vaccine clinical trials from Sanofi Pasteur and Novartis)

Paul V. Williams, MD, FAAP (Allergist, AAP Section on Allergy, Asthma, and Immunology: no conflicts)

Stuart T. Weinberg, MD, FAAP (PPI Informatician, General Academic Pediatrician: no conflicts)

Carrie E. Nelson, MD, MS (Family Physician, American Academy of Family Physicians: employed by McKesson Health Solutions)

Richard M. Rosenfeld, MD, MPH, FAAP (Otolaryngologist, AAP Section on Otolaryngology–Head and Neck Surgery, American Academy of Otolaryngology–Head and Neck Surgery: no financial conflicts; published research related to sinusitis)

CONSULTANT

Richard N. Shiffman, MD, FAAP (Informatician, Guideline Methodologist, General Academic Pediatrician: no conflicts)

STAFF

Caryn Davidson, MA

REFERENCES

1. Aitken M, Taylor JA. Prevalence of clinical sinusitis in young children followed up by primary care pediatricians. *Arch Pediatr Adolesc Med.* 1998;152(3):244–248

2. Kakish KS, Mahafza T, Batieha A, Ekteish F, Daoud A. Clinical sinusitis in children attending primary care centers. *Pediatr Infect Dis J.* 2000;19(11):1071–1074

3. Ueda D, Yoto Y. The ten-day mark as a practical diagnostic approach for acute paranasal sinusitis in children. *Pediatr Infect Dis J.* 1996;15(7):576–579

4. Wald ER, Nash D, Eickhoff J. Effectiveness of amoxicillin/clavulanate potassium in the treatment of acute bacterial sinusitis in children. Pediatrics. 2009;124(1):9–15

5. American Academy of Pediatrics, Subcommittee on Management of Sinusitis and Committee on Quality Improvement. Clinical practice guideline: management of sinusitis. Pediatrics. 2001;108(3):798–808

6. Smith MJ. AAP technical report: evidence for the diagnosis and treatment of acute uncomplicated sinusitis in children: a systematic review. 2013, In press.

7. Shiffman RN, Michel G, Rosenfeld RM, Davidson C. Building better guidelines with BRIDGE-Wiz: development and evaluation of a software assistant to promote clarity, transparency, and implementability. J Am Med Inform Assoc. 2012;19(1):94–101

8. American Academy of Pediatrics, Steering Committee on Quality Improvement and Management. Classifying recommendations for clinical practice guidelines. Pediatrics. 2004;114(3):874–877

9. Gwaltney JM, Jr, Hendley JO, Simon G, Jordan WS Jr. Rhinovirus infections in an industrial population. II. Characteristics of illness and antibody response. JAMA. 1967;202(6):494–500

10. Pappas DE, Hendley JO, Hayden FG, Winther B. Symptom profile of common colds in school-aged children. Pediatr Infect Dis J. 2008;27(1):8–11

11. Wald ER, Guerra N, Byers C. Frequency and severity of infections in day care: three-year follow-up. J Pediatr. 1991;118(4 pt 1):509–514

12. Wald ER, Guerra N, Byers C. Upper respiratory tract infections in young children: duration of and frequency of complications. Pediatrics. 1991;87(2):129–133

13. Meltzer EO, Hamilos DL, Hadley JA, et al. Rhinosinusitis: establishing definitions for clinical research and patient care. J Allergy Clin Immunol. 2004;114(6 suppl):155–212

14. Shaikh N, Wald ER. Signs and symptoms of acute sinusitis in children. Pediatr Infect Dis J. 2013; in press

15. Wald ER. The diagnosis and management of sinusitis in children: diagnostic considerations. Pediatr Infect Dis. 1985;4(6 suppl):S61–S64

16. Wald ER, Milmoe GJ, Bowen A, Ledesma-Medina J, Salamon N, Bluestone CD. Acute maxillary sinusitis in children. N Engl J Med. 1981;304(13):749–754

17. Lindbaek M, Hjortdahl P, Johnsen UL. Use of symptoms, signs, and blood tests to diagnose acute sinus infections in primary care: comparison with computed tomography. Fam Med. 1996;28(3):183–188

18. Wald ER. Beginning antibiotics for acute rhinosinusitis and choosing the right treatment. Clin Rev Allergy Immunol. 2006;30(3):143–152

19. Maresh MM, Washburn AH. Paranasal sinuses from birth to late adolescence. II. Clinical and roentgenographic evidence of infection. Am J Dis Child. 1940;60:841–861

20. Glasier CM, Mallory GB, Jr, Steele RW. Significance of opacification of the maxillary and ethmoid sinuses in infants. J Pediatr. 1989;114(1):45–50

21. Kovatch AL, Wald ER, Ledesma-Medina J, Chiponis DM, Bedingfield B. Maxillary sinus radiographs in children with non-respiratory complaints. Pediatrics. 1984;73(3):306–308

22. Shopfner CE, Rossi JO. Roentgen evaluation of the paranasal sinuses in children. Am J Roentgenol Radium Ther Nucl Med. 1973;118(1):176–186

23. Diament MJ, Senac MO, Jr, Gilsanz V, Baker S, Gillespie T, Larsson S. Prevalence of incidental paranasal sinuses opacification in pediatric patients: a CT study. J Comput Assist Tomogr. 1987;11(3):426–431

24. Glasier CM, Ascher DP, Williams KD. Incidental paranasal sinus abnormalities on CT of children: clinical correlation. AJNR Am J Neuroradiol. 1986;7(5):861–864

25. Gwaltney JM, Jr, Phillips CD, Miller RD, Riker DK. Computed tomographic study of the common cold. N Engl J Med. 1994;330(1):25–30

26. Manning SC, Biavati MJ, Phillips DL. Correlation of clinical sinusitis signs and symptoms to imaging findings in pediatric patients. Int J Pediatr Otorhinolaryngol. 1996;37(1):65–74

27. Gordts F, Clement PA, Destryker A, Desprechins B, Kaufman L. Prevalence of sinusitis signs on MRI in a non-ENT paediatric population. Rhinology. 1997;35(4):154–157

28. Kristo A, Uhari M, Luotonen J, et al. Paranasal sinus findings in children during respiratory infection evaluated with magnetic resonance imaging. Pediatrics. 2003;111(5 pt 1):e586–e589

29. Brook I. Microbiology and antimicrobial treatment of orbital and intracranial complications of sinusitis in children and their management. Int J Pediatr Otorhinolaryngol. 2009;73(9):1183–1186

30. Sultesz M, Csakanyi Z, Majoros T, Farkas Z, Katona G. Acute bacterial rhinosinusitis and its complications in our pediatric otorhinolaryngological department between 1997 and 2006. Int J Pediatr Otorhinolaryngol. 2009;73(11):1507–1512

31. Wald ER. Periorbital and orbital infections. Infect Dis Clin North Am. 2007;21(2):393–408

32. Chandler JR, Langenbrunner DJ, Stevens ER. The pathogenesis of orbital complications in acute sinusitis. Laryngoscope. 1970;80(9):1414–1428

33. Kombogiorgas D, Seth R, Modha J, Singh J. Suppurative intracranial complications of sinusitis in adolescence. Single institute experience and review of the literature. Br J Neurosurg. 2007;21(6):603–609

34. Rosenfeld EA, Rowley AH. Infectious intracranial complications of sinusitis, other than meningitis in children: 12 year review. Clin Infect Dis. 1994;18(5):750–754

35. American College of Radiology. Appropriateness criteria for sinonasal disease. 2009. Available at: www.acr.org/~/media/8172B4DE503149248E64856857674BB5.pdf. Accessed November 6, 2012

36. Triulzi F, Zirpoli S. Imaging techniques in the diagnosis and management of rhinosinusitis in children. Pediatr Allergy Immunol. 2007;18(suppl 18):46–49

37. McIntosh D, Mahadevan M. Failure of contrast enhanced computed tomography scans to identify an orbital abscess. The benefit of magnetic resonance imaging. J Laryngol Otol. 2008;122(6):639–640

38. Younis RT, Anand VK, Davidson B. The role of computed tomography and magnetic resonance imaging in patients with sinusitis with complications. Laryngoscope. 2002;112(2):224–229

39. Shapiro DJ, Gonzales R, Cabana MD, Hersh AL. National trends in visit rates and antibiotic prescribing for children with acute sinusitis. Pediatrics. 2011;127(1):28–34

40. Wald ER, Reilly JS, Casselbrant M, et al. Treatment of acute maxillary sinusitis in childhood: a comparative study of amoxicillin and cefaclor. J Pediatr. 1984;104(2):297–302

41. Wald ER, Chiponis D, Ledesma-Medina J. Comparative effectiveness of amoxicillin and amoxicillin-clavulanate potassium in acute paranasal sinus infections in children: a double-blind, placebo-controlled trial. Pediatrics. 1986;77(6):795–800

42. Garbutt JM, Goldstein M, Gellman E, Shannon W, Littenberg B. A randomized, placebo-controlled trial of antimicrobial treatment for children with clinically diagnosed acute sinusitis. Pediatrics. 2001;107(4):619–625

43. Kristo A, Uhari M, Luotonen J, Ilkko E, Koivunen P, Alho OP. Cefuroxime axetil versus placebo for children with acute respiratory infection and imaging evidence of sinusitis: a randomized, controlled trial. *Acta Paediatr.* 2005;94(9): 1208–1213

44. Hoberman A, Paradise JL, Rockette HE, et al. Treatment of acute otitis media in children under 2 years of age. *N Engl J Med.* 2011;364(2):105–115

45. Tahtinen PA, Laine MK, Huovinen P, Jalava J, Ruuskanen O, Ruohola A. A placebo-controlled trial of antimicrobial treatment for acute otitis media. *N Engl J Med.* 2011;364(2):116–126

46. Gordts F, Abu Nasser I, Clement PA, Pierard D, Kaufman L. Bacteriology of the middle meatus in children. *Int J Pediatr Otorhinolaryngol.* 1999;48(2):163–167

47. Parsons DS, Wald ER. Otitis media and sinusitis: similar diseases. *Otolaryngol Clin North Am.* 1996;29(1):11–25

48. Revai K, Dobbs LA, Nair S, Patel JA, Grady JJ, Chonmaitree T. Incidence of acute otitis media and sinusitis complicating upper respiratory tract infection: the effect of age. *Pediatrics.* 2007;119(6). Available at: www.pediatrics.org/cgi/content/full/119/6/e1408

49. Klein JO, Bluestone CD. *Textbook of Pediatric Infectious Diseases.* 6th ed. Philadelphia, PA: Saunders; 2009

50. Casey JR, Adlowitz DG, Pichichero ME. New patterns in the otopathogens causing acute otitis media six to eight years after introduction of pneumococcal conjugate vaccine. *Pediatr Infect Dis J.* 2010;29(4): 304–309

51. Brook I, Gober AE. Frequency of recovery of pathogens from the nasopharynx of children with acute maxillary sinusitis before and after the introduction of vaccination with the 7-valent pneumococcal vaccine. *Int J Pediatr Otorhinolaryngol.* 2007;71(4):575–579

52. Wald ER. Microbiology of acute and chronic sinusitis in children. *J Allergy Clin Immunol.* 1992;90(3 pt 2):452–456

53. Centers for Disease Control and Prevention. Effects of new penicillin susceptibility breakpoints for *Streptococcus pneumoniae*—United States, 2006-2007. *MMWR Morb Mortal Wkly Rep.* 2008;57 (50):1353–1355

54. Centers for Disease Control and Prevention. Active Bacterial Core Surveillance (ABCs): Emerging Infections Program Network. 2011. Available at: www.cdc.gov/abcs/reports-findings/survreports/spneu09.html. Accessed November 6, 2012

55. Garbutt J, St Geme JW, III, May A, Storch GA, Shackelford PG. Developing community-specific recommendations for first-line treatment of acute otitis media: is high-dose amoxicillin necessary? *Pediatrics.* 2004;114(2):342–347

56. Harrison CJ, Woods C, Stout G, Martin B, Selvarangan R. Susceptibilities of *Haemophilus influenzae, Streptococcus pneumoniae,* including serotype 19A, and *Moraxella catarrhalis* paediatric isolates from 2005 to 2007 to commonly used antibiotics. *J Antimicrob Chemother.* 2009; 63(3):511–519

57. Critchley IA, Jacobs MR, Brown SD, Traczewski MM, Tillotson GS, Janjic N. Prevalence of serotype 19A *Streptococcus pneumoniae* among isolates from U.S. children in 2005-2006 and activity of faropenem. *Antimicrob Agents Chemother.* 2008;52(7):2639–2643

58. Jacobs MR, Good CE, Windau AR, et al. Activity of ceftaroline against recent emerging serotypes of *Streptococcus pneumoniae* in the United States. *Antimicrob Agents Chemother.* 2010;54(6):2716–2719

59. Tristram S, Jacobs MR, Appelbaum PC. Antimicrobial resistance in *Haemophilus influenzae. Clin Microbiol Rev.* 2007;20(2): 368–389

60. Levine OS, Farley M, Harrison LH, Lefkowitz L, McGeer A, Schwartz B. Risk factors for invasive pneumococcal disease in children: a population-based case-control study in North America. *Pediatrics.* 1999; 103(3). Available at: www.pediatrics.org/cgi/content/full/103/3/e28

61. Seikel K, Shelton S, McCracken GH Jr. Middle ear fluid concentrations of amoxicillin after large dosages in children with acute otitis media. *Pediatr Infect Dis J.* 1997;16(7):710–711

62. Cohen R, Navel M, Grunberg J, et al. One dose ceftriaxone vs. ten days of amoxicillin/clavulanate therapy for acute otitis media: clinical efficacy and change in nasopharyngeal flora. *Pediatr Infect Dis J.* 1999;18(5):403–409

63. Green SM, Rothrock SG. Single-dose intramuscular ceftriaxone for acute otitis media in children. *Pediatrics.* 1993;91(1): 23–30

64. Leibovitz E, Piglansky L, Raiz S, Press J, Leiberman A, Dagan R. Bacteriologic and clinical efficacy of one day vs. three day intramuscular ceftriaxone for treatment of nonresponsive acute otitis media in children. *Pediatr Infect Dis J.* 2000;19(11): 1040–1045

65. DePestel DD, Benninger MS, Danziger L, et al. Cephalosporin use in treatment of patients with penicillin allergies. *J Am Pharm Assoc.* 2008;48(4):530–540

66. Pichichero ME. A review of evidence supporting the American Academy of Pediatrics recommendation for prescribing cephalosporin antibiotics for penicillin-allergic patients. *Pediatrics.* 2005;115(4): 1048–1057

67. Pichichero ME, Casey JR. Safe use of selected cephalosporins in penicillin-allergic patients: a meta-analysis. *Otolaryngol Head Neck Surg.* 2007;136(3): 340–347

68. Park MA, Koch CA, Klemawesch P, Joshi A, Li JT. Increased adverse drug reactions to cephalosporins in penicillin allergy patients with positive penicillin skin test. *Int Arch Allergy Immunol.* 2010;153(3): 268–273

69. Jacobs MR. Antimicrobial-resistant Streptococcus pneumoniae: trends and management. *Expert Rev Anti Infect Ther.* 2008; 6(5):619–635

70. Chow AW, Benninger MS, Brook I, et al; Infectious Diseases Society of America. IDSA clinical practice guideline for acute bacterial rhinosinusitis in children and adults. *Clin Infect Dis.* 2012;54(8):e72–e112

71. Brook I, Gober AE. Resistance to antimicrobials used for therapy of otitis media and sinusitis: effect of previous antimicrobial therapy and smoking. *Ann Otol Rhinol Laryngol.* 1999;108(7 pt 1):645–647

72. Brook I, Gober AE. Antimicrobial resistance in the nasopharyngeal flora of children with acute maxillary sinusitis and maxillary sinusitis recurring after amoxicillin therapy. *J Antimicrob Chemother.* 2004;53(2):399–402

73. Dohar J, Canton R, Cohen R, Farrell DJ, Felmingham D. Activity of telithromycin and comparators against bacterial pathogens isolated from 1,336 patients with clinically diagnosed acute sinusitis. *Ann Clin Microbiol Antimicrob.* 2004;3(3): 15–21

74. Jacobs MR, Bajaksouzian S, Zilles A, Lin G, Pankuch GA, Appelbaum PC. Susceptibilities of *Streptococcus pneumoniae* and *Haemophilus influenzae* to 10 oral antimicrobial agents based on pharmacodynamic parameters: 1997 U.S. surveillance study. *Antimicrob Agents Chemother.* 1999;43(8):1901–1908

75. Jacobs MR, Felmingham D, Appelbaum PC, Gruneberg RN. The Alexander Project 1998-2000: susceptibility of pathogens isolated from community-acquired respiratory tract infection to commonly used antimicrobial agents. *J Antimicrob Chemother.* 2003;52(2):229–246

76. Lynch JP, III, Zhanel GG. *Streptococcus pneumoniae*: epidemiology and risk factors, evolution of antimicrobial resistance, and impact of vaccines. *Curr Opin Pulm Med*. 2010;16(3):217–225

77. Sahm DF, Jones ME, Hickey ML, Diakun DR, Mani SV, Thornsberry C. Resistance surveillance of *Streptococcus pneumoniae*, *Haemophilus influenzae* and *Moraxella catarrhalis* isolated in Asia and Europe, 1997-1998. *J Antimicrob Chemother*. 2000; 45(4):457–466

78. Sokol W. Epidemiology of sinusitis in the primary care setting: results from the 1999-2000 respiratory surveillance program. *Am J Med*. 2001;111(suppl 9A):19S–24S

79. Shaikh N, Wald ER, Pi M. Decongestants, antihistamines and nasal irrigation for acute sinusitis in children. *Cochrane Database Syst Rev*. 2010;(12):CD007909

80. Dolor RJ, Witsell DL, Hellkamp AS, Williams JW, Jr, Califf RM, Simel DL. Comparison of cefuroxime with or without intranasal fluticasone for the treatment of rhinosinusitis. The CAFFS Trial: a randomized controlled trial. *JAMA*. 2001;286(24):3097–3105

81. Meltzer EO, Bachert C, Staudinger H. Treating acute rhinosinusitis: comparing efficacy and safety of mometasone furoate nasal spray, amoxicillin, and placebo. *J Allergy Clin Immunol*. 2005;116(6):1289–1295

82. Meltzer EO, Charous BL, Busse WW, Zinreich SJ, Lorber RR, Danzig MR. Added relief in the treatment of acute recurrent sinusitis with adjunctive mometasone furoate nasal spray. The Nasonex Sinusitis Group. *J Allergy Clin Immunol*. 2000;106 (4):630–637

83. Meltzer EO, Orgel HA, Backhaus JW, et al. Intranasal flunisolide spray as an adjunct to oral antibiotic therapy for sinusitis. *J Allergy Clin Immunol*. 1993;92(6):812–823

84. Nayak AS, Settipane GA, Pedinoff A, et al. Effective dose range of mometasone furoate nasal spray in the treatment of acute rhinosinusitis. *Ann Allergy Asthma Immunol*. 2002;89(3):271–278

85. Williamson IG, Rumsby K, Benge S, et al. Antibiotics and topical nasal steroid for treatment of acute maxillary sinusitis: a randomized controlled trial. *JAMA*. 2007; 298(21):2487–2496

86. Zalmanovici A, Yaphe J. Intranasal steroids for acute sinusitis. *Cochrane Database Syst Rev*. 2009;(4):CD005149

87. Yilmaz G, Varan B, Yilmaz T, Gurakan B. Intranasal budesonide spray as an adjunct to oral antibiotic therapy for acute sinusitis in children. *Eur Arch Otorhinolaryngol*. 2000;257(5):256–259

88. Barlan IB, Erkan E, Bakir M, Berrak S, Basaran MM. Intranasal budesonide spray as an adjunct to oral antibiotic therapy for acute sinusitis in children. *Ann Allergy Asthma Immunol*. 1997;78(6):598–601

89. Bruni FM, De Luca G, Venturoli V, Boner AL. Intranasal corticosteroids and adrenal suppression. *Neuroimmunomodulation*. 2009;16 (5):353–362

90. Kim KT, Rabinovitch N, Uryniak T, Simpson B, O'Dowd L, Casty F. Effect of budesonide aqueous nasal spray on hypothalamic-pituitary-adrenal axis function in children with allergic rhinitis. *Ann Allergy Asthma Immunol*. 2004;93(1):61–67

91. Meltzer EO, Tripathy I, Maspero JF, Wu W, Philpot E. Safety and tolerability of fluticasone furoate nasal spray once daily in paediatric patients aged 6-11 years with allergic rhinitis: subanalysis of three randomized, double-blind, placebo-controlled, multicentre studies. *Clin Drug Investig*. 2009;29(2):79–86

92. Murphy K, Uryniak T, Simpson B, O'Dowd L. Growth velocity in children with perennial allergic rhinitis treated with budesonide aqueous nasal spray. *Ann Allergy Asthma Immunol*. 2006;96(5):723–730

93. Ratner PH, Meltzer EO, Teper A. Mometasone furoate nasal spray is safe and effective for 1-year treatment of children with perennial allergic rhinitis. *Int J Pediatr Otorhinolaryngol*. 2009;73(5):651–657

94. Skoner DP, Gentile DA, Doyle WJ. Effect on growth of long-term treatment with intranasal triamcinolone acetonide aqueous in children with allergic rhinitis. *Ann*

Allergy Asthma Immunol. 2008;101(4): 431–436

95. Weinstein S, Qaqundah P, Georges G, Nayak A. Efficacy and safety of triamcinolone acetonide aqueous nasal spray in children aged 2 to 5 years with perennial allergic rhinitis: a randomized, double-blind, placebo-controlled study with an open-label extension. *Ann Allergy Asthma Immunol*. 2009;102(4):339–347

96. Zitt M, Kosoglou T, Hubbell J. Mometasone furoate nasal spray: a review of safety and systemic effects. *Drug Saf*. 2007;30(4): 317–326

97. Adam P, Stiffman M, Blake RL Jr. A clinical trial of hypertonic saline nasal spray in subjects with the common cold or rhinosinusitis. *Arch Fam Med*. 1998;7(1):39–43

98. Wang YH, Yang CP, Ku MS, Sun HL, Lue KH. Efficacy of nasal irrigation in the treatment of acute sinusitis in children. *Int J Pediatr Otorhinolaryngol*. 2009;73(12): 1696–1701

99. Harvey R, Hannan SA, Badia L, Scadding G. Nasal saline irrigations for the symptoms of chronic rhinosinusitis. *Cochrane Database Syst Rev*. 2007;(3):CD006394

100. Kassel JC, King D, Spurling GK. Saline nasal irrigation for acute upper respiratory tract infections. *Cochrane Database Syst Rev*. 2010;(3):CD006821

101. Shapiro GG, Virant FS, Furukawa CT, Pierson WE, Bierman CW. Immunologic defects in patients with refractory sinusitis. *Pediatrics*. 1991;87(3):311–316

102. Wood AJ, Douglas RG. Pathogenesis and treatment of chronic rhinosinusitis. *Postgrad Med J*. 2010;86(1016):359–364

103. Liao S, Durand ML, Cunningham MJ. Sinogenic orbital and subperiosteal abscesses: microbiology and methicillin-resistant Staphylococcus aureus incidence. *Otolaryngol Head Neck Surg*. 2010;143(3):392–396

104. Oxford LE, McClay J. Medical and surgical management of subperiosteal orbital abscess secondary to acute sinusitis in children. *Int J Pediatr Otorhinolaryngol*. 2006;70(11):1853–1861

Sinusitis Clinical Practice Guideline Quick Reference Tools

- Action Statement Summary
  — Clinical Practice Guideline for the Diagnosis and Management of Acute Bacterial
  Sinusitis in Children Aged 1 to 18 Years
- *ICD-10-CM* Coding Quick Reference for Sinusitis
- AAP Patient Education Handout
  — *Sinusitis and Your Child*

Action Statement Summary

Clinical Practice Guideline for the Diagnosis and Management of Acute Bacterial Sinusitis in Children Aged 1 to 18 Years

Key Action Statement 1

Clinicians should make a presumptive diagnosis of acute bacterial sinusitis when a child with an acute URI presents with the following:

- Persistent illness, ie, nasal discharge (of any quality) or daytime cough or both lasting more than 10 days without improvement;

OR

- Worsening course, ie, worsening or new onset of nasal discharge, daytime cough, or fever after initial improvement;

OR

- Severe onset, ie, concurrent fever (temperature ≥39°C/102.2°F) and purulent nasal discharge for at least 3 consecutive days (Evidence Quality: B; Recommendation).

Key Action Statement 2A

Clinicians should not obtain imaging studies (plain films, contrast-enhanced computed tomography [CT], MRI, or ultrasonography) to distinguish acute bacterial sinusitis from viral URI (Evidence Quality: B; Strong Recommendation).

Key Action Statement 2B

Clinicians should obtain a contrast-enhanced CT scan of the paranasal sinuses and/or an MRI with contrast whenever a child is suspected of having orbital or central nervous system complications of acute bacterial sinusitis (Evidence Quality: B; Strong Recommendation).

Key Action Statement 3

Initial Management of Acute Bacterial Sinusitis

3A: "Severe onset and worsening course" acute bacterial sinusitis. The clinician should prescribe antibiotic therapy for acute bacterial sinusitis in children with severe onset or worsening course (signs, symptoms, or both) (Evidence Quality: B; Strong Recommendation).

3B: "Persistent illness." The clinician should either prescribe antibiotic therapy OR offer additional outpatient observation for 3 days to children with persistent illness (nasal discharge of any quality or cough or both for at least 10 days without evidence of improvement) (Evidence Quality: B; Recommendation).

Key Action Statement 4

Clinicians should prescribe amoxicillin with or without clavulanate as first-line treatment when a decision has been made to initiate antibiotic treatment of acute bacterial sinusitis (Evidence Quality: B; Recommendation).

Key Action Statement 5A

Clinicians should reassess initial management if there is either a caregiver report of worsening (progression of initial signs/symptoms or appearance of new signs/symptoms) OR failure to improve (lack of reduction in all presenting signs/symptoms) within 72 hours of initial management (Evidence Quality: C; Recommendation).

Key Action Statement 5B

If the diagnosis of acute bacterial sinusitis is confirmed in a child with worsening symptoms or failure to improve in 72 hours, then clinicians may change the antibiotic therapy for the child initially managed with antibiotic OR initiate antibiotic treatment of the child initially managed with observation (Evidence Quality: D; Option based on expert opinion, case reports, and reasoning from first principles).

Coding Quick Reference for Sinusitis

ICD-10-CM

J01.00	Acute maxillary sinusitis, unspecified
J01.01	Acute recurrent maxillary sinusitis
J01.10	Acute frontal sinusitis, unspecified
J01.11	Acute recurrent frontal sinusitis
J01.21	Acute recurrent ethmoidal sinusitis
J01.30	Acute sphenoidal sinusitis, unspecified
J01.31	Acute recurrent sphenoidal sinusitis
J01.40	Acute pansinusitis, unspecified
J01.41	Acute recurrent pansinusitis
J01.80	Other acute sinusitis
J01.81	Other acute recurrent sinusitis
J01.90	Acute sinusitis, unspecified
J01.91	Acute recurrent sinusitis, unspecified
J32.9	Sinusitis NOS

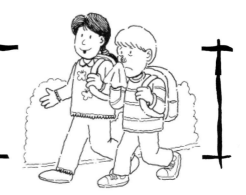

Sinusitis and Your Child

Sinusitis is an inflammation of the lining of the nose and sinuses. It is a very common infection in children.

Viral sinusitis usually accompanies a cold. Allergic sinusitis may accompany allergies such as hay fever. Bacterial sinusitis is a secondary infection caused by the trapping of bacteria in the sinuses during the course of a cold or allergy.

Fluid inside the sinuses

When your child has a viral cold or hay fever, the linings of the nose and sinus cavities swell up and produce more fluid than usual. This is why the nose gets congested and is "runny" during a cold.

Most of the time the swelling disappears by itself as the cold or allergy goes away. However, if the swelling does not go away, the openings that normally allow the sinuses to drain into the back of the nose get blocked and the sinuses fill with fluid. Because the sinuses are blocked and cannot drain properly, bacteria are trapped inside and grow there, causing a secondary infection. Although nose blowing and sniffing may be natural responses to this blockage, when excessive they can make the situation worse by pushing bacteria from the back of the nose into the sinuses.

Is it a cold or bacterial sinusitis?

It is often difficult to tell if an illness is just a viral cold or if it is complicated by a bacterial infection of the sinuses.

Generally viral colds have the following characteristics:

- Colds usually last only 5 to 10 days.
- Colds typically start with clear, watery nasal discharge. After a day or 2, it is normal for the nasal discharge to become thicker and white, yellow, or green. After several days, the discharge becomes clear again and dries.
- Colds include a daytime cough that often gets worse at night.
- If a fever is present, it is usually at the beginning of the cold and is generally low grade, lasting for 1 or 2 days.
- Cold symptoms usually peak in severity at 3 or 5 days, then improve and disappear over the next 7 to 10 days.

Signs and symptoms that your child may have bacterial sinusitis include:

- Cold symptoms (nasal discharge, daytime cough, or both) lasting more than 10 days *without improving*
- Thick yellow nasal discharge *and* a fever for at least 3 or 4 days in a row
- A severe headache behind or around the eyes that gets worse when bending over
- Swelling and dark circles around the eyes, especially in the morning
- Persistent bad breath along with cold symptoms (However, this also could be from a sore throat or a sign that your child is not brushing his teeth!)

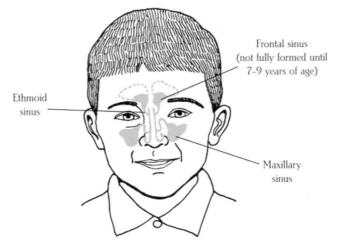

The linings of the sinuses and the nose always produce some fluid (secretions). This fluid keeps the nose and sinus cavities from becoming too dry and adds moisture to the air that you breathe.

In very rare cases, a bacterial sinus infection may spread to the eye or the central nervous system (the brain). If your child has the following symptoms, call your pediatrician immediately:

- Swelling and/or redness around the eyes, not just in the morning but all day
- Severe headache and/or pain in the back of the neck
- Persistent vomiting
- Sensitivity to light
- Increasing irritability

Diagnosing bacterial sinusitis

It may be difficult to tell a sinus infection from an uncomplicated cold, especially in the first few days of the illness. Your pediatrician will most likely be able to tell if your child has bacterial sinusitis after examining your child and hearing about the progression of symptoms. In older children, when the diagnosis is uncertain, your pediatrician may order computed tomographic (CT) scans to confirm the diagnosis.

Treating bacterial sinusitis

If your child has bacterial sinusitis, your pediatrician may prescribe an antibiotic for at least 10 days. Once your child is on the medication, symptoms should start to go away over the next 2 to 3 days—the nasal discharge will clear and the cough will improve. *Even though your child may seem better, continue to give the antibiotics for the prescribed length of time. Ending the medications too early could cause the infection to return.*

When a diagnosis of sinusitis is made in children with cold symptoms lasting more than 10 days without improving, some doctors may choose to continue observation for another few days. If your child's symptoms worsen during this time or do not improve after 3 days, antibiotics should be started.

If your child's symptoms show no improvement 2 to 3 days after starting the antibiotics, talk with your pediatrician. Your child might need a different medication or need to be re-examined.

Treating related symptoms of bacterial sinusitis

Headache or sinus pain. To treat headache or sinus pain, try placing a warm washcloth on your child's face for a few minutes at a time. Pain medications such as acetaminophen or ibuprofen may also help. (However, do not give your child aspirin. It has been associated with a rare but potentially fatal disease called Reye syndrome.)

Nasal congestion. If the secretions in your child's nose are especially thick, your pediatrician may recommend that you help drain them with saline nose drops. These are available without a prescription or can be made at home by adding 1/4 teaspoon of table salt to an 8-ounce cup of water. Unless advised by your pediatrician, do not use nose drops that contain medications because they can be absorbed in amounts that can cause side effects.

Placing a cool-mist humidifier in your child's room may help keep your child more comfortable. Clean and dry the humidifier daily to prevent bacteria or mold from growing in it (follow the instructions that came with the humidifier). Hot water vaporizers are not recommended because they can cause scalds or burns.

Remember

If your child has symptoms of a bacterial sinus infection, see your pediatrician. Your pediatrician can properly diagnose and treat the infection and recommend ways to help alleviate the discomfort from some of the symptoms.

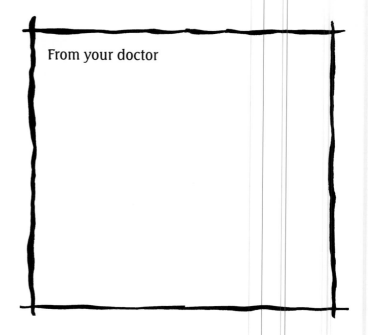

From your doctor

American Academy of Pediatrics

DEDICATED TO THE HEALTH OF ALL CHILDREN™

The American Academy of Pediatrics is an organization of 60,000 primary care pediatricians, pediatric medical subspecialists, and pediatric surgical specialists dedicated to the health, safety, and well-being of infants, children, adolescents, and young adults.

American Academy of Pediatrics
Web site — www.HealthyChildren.org

Diagnosis and Management of
Childhood Obstructive Sleep Apnea Syndrome

· ·

• *Clinical Practice Guideline*

CLINICAL PRACTICE GUIDELINE

Diagnosis and Management of Childhood Obstructive Sleep Apnea Syndrome

abstract

OBJECTIVES: This revised clinical practice guideline, intended for use by primary care clinicians, provides recommendations for the diagnosis and management of the obstructive sleep apnea syndrome (OSAS) in children and adolescents. This practice guideline focuses on uncomplicated childhood OSAS, that is, OSAS associated with adenotonsillar hypertrophy and/or obesity in an otherwise healthy child who is being treated in the primary care setting.

METHODS: Of 3166 articles from 1999–2010, 350 provided relevant data. Most articles were level II–IV. The resulting evidence report was used to formulate recommendations.

RESULTS AND CONCLUSIONS: The following recommendations are made. (1) All children/adolescents should be screened for snoring. (2) Polysomnography should be performed in children/adolescents with snoring and symptoms/signs of OSAS; if polysomnography is not available, then alternative diagnostic tests or referral to a specialist for more extensive evaluation may be considered. (3) Adenotonsillectomy is recommended as the first-line treatment of patients with adenotonsillar hypertrophy. (4) High-risk patients should be monitored as inpatients postoperatively. (5) Patients should be reevaluated postoperatively to determine whether further treatment is required. Objective testing should be performed in patients who are high risk or have persistent symptoms/signs of OSAS after therapy. (6) Continuous positive airway pressure is recommended as treatment if adenotonsillectomy is not performed or if OSAS persists postoperatively. (7) Weight loss is recommended in addition to other therapy in patients who are overweight or obese. (8) Intranasal corticosteroids are an option for children with mild OSAS in whom adenotonsillectomy is contraindicated or for mild postoperative OSAS. *Pediatrics* 2012;130:576–584

Carole L. Marcus, MBBCh, Lee Jay Brooks, MD, Kari A. Draper, MD, David Gozal, MD, Ann Carol Halbower, MD, Jacqueline Jones, MD, Michael S. Schechter, MD, MPH, Stephen Howard Sheldon, DO, Karen Spruyt, PhD, Sally Davidson Ward, MD, Christopher Lehmann, MD, Richard N. Shiffman, MD

KEY WORDS
snoring, sleep-disordered breathing, adenotonsillectomy, continuous positive airway pressure

ABBREVIATIONS
AAP—American Academy of Pediatrics
AHI—apnea hypopnea index
CPAP—continuous positive airway pressure
OSAS—obstructive sleep apnea syndrome

www.pediatrics.org/cgi/doi/10.1542/peds.2012-1671

doi:10.1542/peds.2012-1671

PEDIATRICS (ISSN Numbers: Print, 0031-4005; Online, 1098-4275).

INTRODUCTION

Obstructive sleep apnea syndrome (OSAS) is a common condition in childhood and can result in severe complications if left untreated. In 2002, the American Academy of Pediatrics (AAP) published a practice guideline for the diagnosis and management of childhood OSAS.[1] Since that time, there has been a considerable increase in publications and research on the topic; thus, the guidelines have been revised.

The purposes of this revised clinical practice guideline are to (1) increase the recognition of OSAS by primary care clinicians to minimize delay in diagnosis and avoid serious sequelae of OSAS; (2) evaluate diagnostic techniques; (3) describe treatment options; (4) provide guidelines for follow-up; and (5) discuss areas requiring further research. The recommendations in this statement do not indicate an exclusive course of treatment. Variations, taking into account individual circumstances, may be appropriate.

This practice guideline focuses on uncomplicated childhood OSAS—that is, the OSAS associated with adenotonsillar hypertrophy and/or obesity in an otherwise healthy child who is being treated in the primary care setting. This guideline specifically excludes infants younger than 1 year of age, patients with central apnea or hypoventilation syndromes, and patients with OSAS associated with other medical disorders, including but not limited to Down syndrome, craniofacial anomalies, neuromuscular disease (including cerebral palsy), chronic lung disease, sickle cell disease, metabolic disease, or laryngomalacia. These important patient populations are too complex to discuss within the scope of this article and require consultation with a pediatric subspecialist.

Additional information providing justification for the key action statements and a detailed review of the literature are provided in the accompanying technical report available online.[2]

METHODS OF GUIDELINE DEVELOPMENT

Details of the methods of guideline development are included in the accompanying technical report.[2] The AAP selected a subcommittee composed of pediatricians and other experts in the fields of sleep medicine, pulmonology, and otolaryngology, as well as experts from epidemiology and pediatric practice to develop an evidence base of literature on this topic. The committee included liaison members from the AAP Section on Otolaryngology-Head and Neck Surgery, American Thoracic Society, American Academy of Sleep Medicine, American College of Chest Physicians, and the National Sleep Foundation. Committee members signed forms disclosing conflicts of interest.

An automated search of the literature on childhood OSAS from 1999 to 2008 was performed by using 5 scientific literature search engines.[2] The medical subject heading terms that were used in all fields were snoring, apnea, sleep-disordered breathing, sleep-related breathing disorders, upper airway resistance, polysomnography, sleep study, adenoidectomy, tonsillectomy, continuous positive airway pressure, obesity, adiposity, hypopnea, hypoventilation, cognition, behavior, and neuropsychology. Reviews, case reports, letters to the editor, and abstracts were not included. Non–English-language articles, animal studies, and studies relating to infants younger than 1 year and to special populations (eg, children with craniofacial anomalies or sickle cell disease) were excluded. In several steps, a total of 3166 hits was reduced to 350 articles, which underwent detailed review.[2] Committee members selectively updated this literature search for articles published from 2008 to 2011 specific to guideline categories. Details of the literature grading system are available in the accompanying technical report.

Since publication of the previous guidelines, there has been an improvement in the quality of OSAS studies in the literature; however, there remain few randomized, blinded, controlled studies. Most studies were questionnaire or polysomnography based. Many studies used standard definitions for pediatric polysomnography scoring, but the interpretation of polysomnography (eg, the apnea hypopnea index [AHI] criterion used for diagnosis or to determine treatment) varied widely. The guideline notes the quality of evidence for each key action statement. Additional details are available in the technical report.

The evidence-based approach to guideline development requires that the evidence in support of each key action statement be identified, appraised, and summarized and that an explicit link between evidence and recommendations be defined. Evidence-based recommendations reflect the quality of evidence and the balance of benefit and harm that is anticipated when the recommendation is followed. The AAP policy statement, "Classifying Recommendations for Clinical Practice Guidelines,"[3] was followed in designating levels of recommendation (see Fig 1 and Table 1).

DEFINITION

This guideline defines OSAS in children as a "disorder of breathing during sleep characterized by prolonged partial upper airway obstruction and/or intermittent complete obstruction (obstructive apnea) that disrupts normal ventilation during sleep and normal sleep patterns,"[4] accompanied by symptoms or signs, as listed in Table 2. Prevalence rates based on level I and II studies range from 1.2% to 5.7%.[5–7] Symptoms include habitual snoring (often with intermittent pauses, snorts, or gasps), disturbed sleep, and daytime neurobehavioral problems. Daytime sleepiness may occur, but is uncommon in young children. OSAS is associated with neurocognitive impairment, behavioral problems, failure to thrive, hypertension, cardiac dysfunction, and systemic inflammation. Risk factors include adenotonsillar hypertrophy, obesity, craniofacial anomalies, and neuromuscular disorders. Only the first 2 risk factors are

Evidence Quality	Preponderance of Benefit or Harm	Balance of Benefit and Harm
A. Well designed RCTs or diagnostic studies on relevant population	Strong Recommendation	
B. RCTs or diagnostic studies with minor limitations;overwhelmingly consistent evidence from observational studies		Option
C. Observational studies (case-control and cohort design)	Recommendation	
D. Expert opinion, case reports, reasoning from first principles	Option	No Rec
X. Exceptional situations where validating studies cannot be performed and there is a clear preponderance of benefit or harm	Strong Recommendation / Recommendation	

FIGURE 1

Evidence quality. Integrating evidence quality appraisal with an assessment of the anticipated balance between benefits and harms if a policy is carried out leads to designation of a policy as a strong recommendation, recommendation, option, or no recommendation. RCT, randomized controlled trial; Rec, recommendation.

discussed in this guideline. In this guideline, obesity is defined as a BMI >95th percentile for age and gender.[8]

KEY ACTION STATEMENTS

Key Action Statement 1: Screening for OSAS

As part of routine health maintenance visits, clinicians should inquire whether the child or adolescent snores. If the answer is affirmative or if a child or adolescent presents with signs or symptoms of OSAS (Table 2), clinicians should perform a more focused evaluation. (Evidence Quality: Grade B, Recommendation Strength: Recommendation.)

Evidence Profile KAS 1

- Aggregate evidence quality: B
- Benefit: Early identification of OSAS is desirable, because it is a high-prevalence condition, and identification and treatment can result in alleviation of current symptoms, improved quality of life, prevention of sequelae, education of parents, and decreased health care utilization.
- Harm: Provider time, patient and parent time.
- Benefits-harms assessment: Preponderance of benefit over harm.
- Value judgments: Panelists believe that identification of a serious medical condition outweighs the time expenditure necessary for screening.
- Role of patient preferences: None.
- Exclusions: None.
- Intentional vagueness: None.
- Strength: Recommendation.

Almost all children with OSAS snore,[9–11] although caregivers frequently do not volunteer this information at medical visits.[12] Thus, asking about snoring at each health maintenance visit (as well as at other appropriate times, such as when evaluating for tonsillitis) is a sensitive, albeit nonspecific, screening measure that is quick and easy to perform. Snoring is common in children and adolescents; however, OSAS is less common. Therefore, an affirmative answer should be followed by a detailed history and examination to determine whether further evaluation for OSAS is needed (Table 2); this clinical evaluation alone

TABLE 1 Definitions and Recommendation Implications

Statement	Definition	Implication
Strong recommendation	A strong recommendation in favor of a particular action is made when the anticipated benefits of the recommended intervention clearly exceed the harms (as a strong recommendation against an action is made when the anticipated harms clearly exceed the benefits) and the quality of the supporting evidence is excellent. In some clearly identified circumstances, strong recommendations may be made when high-quality evidence is impossible to obtain and the anticipated benefits strongly outweigh the harms.	Clinicians should follow a strong recommendation unless a clear and compelling rationale for an alternative approach is present.
Recommendation	A recommendation in favor of a particular action is made when the anticipated benefits exceed the harms but the quality of evidence is not as strong. Again, in some clearly identified circumstances, recommendations may be made when high-quality evidence is impossible to obtain but the anticipated benefits outweigh the harms.	It would be prudent for clinicians to follow a recommendation, but they should remain alert to new information and sensitive to patient preferences.
Option	Options define courses that may be taken when either the quality of evidence is suspect or carefully performed studies have shown little clear advantage to one approach over another.	Clinicians should consider the option in their decision-making, and patient preference may have a substantial role.
No recommendation	No recommendation indicates that there is a lack of pertinent published evidence and that the anticipated balance of benefits and harms is presently unclear.	Clinicians should be alert to new published evidence that clarifies the balance of benefit versus harm.

TABLE 2 Symptoms and Signs of OSAS

History
    Frequent snoring ($\geq$3 nights/wk)
    Labored breathing during sleep
    Gasps/snorting noises/observed
       episodes of apnea
    Sleep enuresis (especially secondary enuresis)[a]
    Sleeping in a seated position or with the neck
       hyperextended
    Cyanosis
    Headaches on awakening
    Daytime sleepiness
    Attention-deficit/hyperactivity disorder
    Learning problems
Physical examination
    Underweight or overweight
    Tonsillar hypertrophy
    Adenoidal facies
    Micrognathia/retrognathia
    High-arched palate
    Failure to thrive
    Hypertension

[a] Enuresis after at least 6 mo of continence.

does not establish the diagnosis (see technical report). Occasional snoring, for example, with an upper respiratory tract infection, is less of a concern than snoring that occurs at least 3 times a week and is associated with any of the symptoms or signs listed in Table 2.

Key Action Statement 2A: Polysomnography

If a child or adolescent snores on a regular basis and has any of the complaints or findings shown in Table 2, clinicians should either (1) obtain a polysomnogram (Evidence Quality A, Key Action strength: Recommendation) OR (2) refer the patient to a sleep specialist or otolaryngologist for a more extensive evaluation (Evidence quality D, Key Action strength: Option). (Evidence Quality: Grade A for polysomnography; Grade D for specialist referral, Recommendation Strength: Recommendation.)

Evidence Profile KAS 2A: Polysomnography

- Aggregate evidence quality: A
- Benefits: Establish diagnosis and determine severity of OSAS.

- Harm: Expense, time, anxiety/discomfort.

- Benefits-harms assessment: Preponderance of benefit over harm.

- Value judgments: Panelists weighed the value of establishing a diagnosis as more important than the minor potential harms listed.

- Role of patient preferences: Small because of preponderance of evidence that polysomnography is the most accurate way to make a diagnosis.

- Exclusions: See Key Action Statement 2B regarding lack of availability.

- Intentional vagueness: None.

- Strength: Recommendation.

Evidence Profile KAS 2A: Referral

- Aggregate evidence quality: D

- Benefits: Subspecialist may be better able to establish diagnosis and determine severity of OSAS.

- Harm: Expense, time, anxiety/discomfort.

- Benefits-harms assessment: Preponderance of benefit over harm.

- Value judgments: Panelists weighed the value of establishing a diagnosis as more important than the minor potential harms listed.

- Role of patient preferences: Large.

- Exclusions: None.

- Intentional vagueness: None.

- Strength: Option.

Although history and physical examination are useful to screen patients and determine which patients need further investigation for OSAS, the sensitivity and specificity of the history and physical examination are poor (see accompanying technical report). Physical examination when the child is awake may be normal, and the size of the tonsils cannot be used to predict the presence of OSAS in an individual child. Thus, objective testing is required. The gold standard test

is overnight, attended, in-laboratory polysomnography (sleep study). This is a noninvasive test involving the measurement of a number of physiologic functions overnight, typically including EEG; pulse oximetry; oronasal airflow, abdominal and chest wall movements, partial pressure of carbon dioxide (P_{CO_2}); and video recording.[13] Specific pediatric measuring and scoring criteria should be used.[13] Polysomnography will demonstrate the presence or absence of OSAS. Polysomnography also demonstrates the severity of OSAS, which is helpful in planning treatment and in postoperative short- and long-term management.

Key Action Statement 2B: Alternative Testing

If polysomnography is not available, then clinicians may order alternative diagnostic tests, such as nocturnal video recording, nocturnal oximetry, daytime nap polysomnography, or ambulatory polysomnography. (Evidence Quality: Grade C, Recommendation Strength: Option.)

Evidence Profile KAS 2B

- Aggregate evidence quality: C

- Benefit: Varying positive and negative predictive values for establishing diagnosis.

- Harm: False-negative and false-positive results may underestimate or overestimate severity, expense, time, anxiety/discomfort.

- Benefits-harms assessment: Equilibrium of benefits and harms.

- Value judgments: Opinion of the panel that some objective testing is better than none. Pragmatic decision based on current shortage of pediatric polysomnography facilities (this may change over time).

- Role of patient preferences: Small, if choices are limited by availability;

families may choose to travel to centers where more extensive facilities are available.

- Exclusions: None.
- Intentional vagueness: None.
- Strength: Option.

Although polysomnography is the gold standard for diagnosis of OSAS, there is a shortage of sleep laboratories with pediatric expertise. Hence, polysomnography may not be readily available in certain regions of the country. Alternative diagnostic tests have been shown to have weaker positive and negative predictive values than polysomnography, but nevertheless, objective testing is preferable to clinical evaluation alone. If an alternative test fails to demonstrate OSAS in a patient with a high pretest probability, full polysomnography should be sought.

Key Action Statement 3: Adenotonsillectomy

If a child is determined to have OSAS, has a clinical examination consistent with adenotonsillar hypertrophy, and does not have a contraindication to surgery (see Table 3), the clinician should recommend adenotonsillectomy as the first line of treatment. If the child has OSAS but does not have adenotonsillar hypertrophy, other treatment should be considered (see Key Action Statement 6). Clinical judgment is required to determine the benefits of adenotonsillectomy compared with other treatments in obese children with varying degrees of adenotonsillar hypertrophy. (Evidence Quality: Grade B, Recommendation Strength: Recommendation.)

Evidence Profile KAS 3

- Aggregate evidence quality: B
- Benefit: Improve OSAS and accompanying symptoms and sequelae.

- Harm: Pain, anxiety, dehydration, anesthetic complications, hemorrhage, infection, postoperative respiratory difficulties, velopharyngeal incompetence, nasopharyngeal stenosis, death.
- Benefits-harms assessment: Preponderance of benefit over harm.
- Value judgments: The panel sees the benefits of treating OSAS as more beneficial than the low risk of serious consequences.
- Role of patient preferences: Low; continuous positive airway pressure (CPAP) is an option but involves prolonged, long-term treatment as compared with a single, relatively low-risk surgical procedure.
- Exclusions: See Table 3.
- Intentional vagueness: None.
- Strength: Recommendation.

Adenotonsillectomy is very effective in treating OSAS. Adenoidectomy or tonsillectomy alone may not be sufficient, because residual lymphoid tissue may contribute to persistent obstruction. In otherwise healthy children with adenotonsillar hypertrophy, adenotonsillectomy is associated with improvements in symptoms and sequelae of OSAS. Postoperative polysomnography typically shows a major decrease in the number of obstructive events, although some obstructions may still be present. Although obese children may have less satisfactory results, many will be adequately treated with

TABLE 3 Contraindications for Adenotonsillectomy

Absolute contraindications
  No adenotonsillar tissue (tissue has been surgically removed)
Relative contraindications
  Very small tonsils/adenoid
  Morbid obesity and small tonsils/adenoid
  Bleeding disorder refractory to treatment
  Submucus cleft palate
  Other medical conditions making patient medically unstable for surgery

adenotonsillectomy; however, further research is needed to determine which obese children are most likely to benefit from surgery. In this population, the benefits of a 1-time surgical procedure, with a small but real risk of complications, need to be weighed against long-term treatment with CPAP, which is associated with discomfort, disruption of family lifestyle, and risks of poor adherence. Potential complications of adenotonsillectomy are shown in Table 4. Although serious complications (including death) may occur, the rate of these complications is low, and the risks of complications need to be weighed against the consequences of untreated OSAS. In general, a 1-time only procedure with a relatively low morbidity is preferable to lifelong treatment with CPAP; furthermore, the efficacy of CPAP is limited by generally suboptimal adherence. Other treatment options, such as anti-inflammatory medications, weight loss, or tracheostomy, are less effective, are difficult to achieve, or have higher morbidity, respectively.

Key Action Statement 4: High-Risk Patients Undergoing Adenotonsillectomy

Clinicians should monitor high-risk patients (Table 5) undergoing adenotonsillectomy as inpatients postoperatively. (Evidence Quality: Grade B, Recommendation Strength: Recommendation.)

TABLE 4 Risks of Adenotonsillectomy

Minor
  Pain
  Dehydration attributable to postoperative nausea/vomiting and poor oral intake
Major
  Anesthetic complications
  Acute upper airway obstruction during induction or emergence from anesthesia
  Postoperative respiratory compromise
  Hemorrhage
  Velopharyngeal incompetence
  Nasopharyngeal stenosis
  Death

TABLE 5 Risk Factors for Postoperative Respiratory Complications in Children With OSAS Undergoing Adenotonsillectomy

Younger than 3 y of age
Severe OSAS on polysomnography[a]
Cardiac complications of OSAS
Failure to thrive
Obesity
Craniofacial anomalies[b]
Neuromuscular disorders[b]
Current respiratory infection

[a] It is difficult to provide exact polysomnographic criteria for severity, because these criteria will vary depending on the age of the child; additional comorbidities, such as obesity, asthma, or cardiac complications of OSAS; and other polysomnographic criteria that have not been evaluated in the literature, such as the level of hypercapnia and the frequency of desaturation (as compared with lowest oxygen saturation). Nevertheless, on the basis of published studies (primarily Level III, see Technical Report), it is recommended that all patients with a lowest oxygen saturation <80% (either on preoperative polysomnography or during observation in the recovery room postoperatively) or an AHI $\geq$24/h be observed as inpatients postoperatively as they are at increased risk for postoperative respiratory compromise. Additionally, on the basis of expert consensus, it is recommended that patients with significant hypercapnia on polysomnography (peak P_{CO_2} $\geq$60 mm Hg) be admitted postoperatively. The committee noted that that most published studies were retrospective and not comprehensive, and therefore these recommendations may change if higher-level studies are published. Clinicians may decide to admit patients with less severe polysomnographic abnormalities based on a constellation of risk factors (age, comorbidities, and additional polysomnographic factors) for a particular individual.
[b] Not discussed in these guidelines.

Evidence Profile KAS 4

- Aggregate evidence quality: B
- Benefit: Effectively manage severe respiratory compromise and avoid death.
- Harm: Expense, time, anxiety.
- Benefits-harms assessment: Preponderance of benefit over harm.
- Value judgments: The panel believes that early recognition of any serious adverse events is critically important.
- Role of patient preferences: Minimal; this is an important safety issue.
- Exclusions: None.
- Intentional vagueness: None.
- Strength: Recommendation.

Patients with OSAS may develop respiratory complications, such as worsening of OSAS or pulmonary edema, in the immediate postoperative period. Death attributable to respiratory complications in the immediate postoperative period has been reported in patients with severe OSAS. Identified risk factors are shown in Table 5. High-risk patients should undergo surgery in a center capable of treating complex pediatric patients. They should be hospitalized overnight for close monitoring postoperatively. Children with an acute respiratory infection on the day of surgery, as documented by fever, cough, and/or wheezing, are at increased risk of postoperative complications and, therefore, should be rescheduled or monitored closely postoperatively. Clinicians should decide on an individual basis whether these patients should be rescheduled, taking into consideration the severity of OSAS in the particular patient and keeping in mind that many children with adenotonsillar hypertrophy have chronic rhinorrhea and nasal congestion, even in the absence of viral infections.

Key Action Statement 5: Reevaluation

Clinicians should clinically reassess all patients with OSAS for persisting signs and symptoms after therapy to determine whether further treatment is required. (Evidence Quality: Grade B, Recommendation Strength: Recommendation.)

Evidence Profile KAS 5A

- Aggregate evidence quality: B
- Benefit: Determine effects of treatment.
- Harm: Expense, time.
- Benefits-harms assessment: Preponderance of benefit over harm.
- Value judgments: Data show that a significant proportion of children continue to have abnormalities postoperatively; therefore, the panel determined that the benefits of follow-up outweigh the minor inconveniences.
- Role of patient preferences: Minimal; follow-up is good clinical practice.
- Exclusions: None.
- Intentional vagueness: None.
- Strength: Recommendation.

Clinicians should reassess OSAS-related symptoms and signs (Table 2) after 6 to 8 weeks of therapy to determine whether further evaluation and treatment are indicated. Objective data regarding the timing of the postoperative evaluation are not available. Most clinicians recommend reevaluation 6 to 8 weeks after treatment to allow for healing of the operative site and to allow time for upper airway, cardiac, and central nervous system recovery. Patients who remain symptomatic should undergo objective testing (see Key Action Statement 2) or be referred to a sleep specialist for further evaluation.

Key Action Statement 5B: Reevaluation of High-Risk Patients

Clinicians should reevaluate high-risk patients for persistent OSAS after adenotonsillectomy, including those who had a significantly abnormal baseline polysomnogram, have sequelae of OSAS, are obese, or remain symptomatic after treatment, with an objective test (see Key Action Statement 2) or refer such patients to a sleep specialist. (Evidence Quality: Grade B, Recommendation Strength: Recommendation.)

Evidence Profile KAS 5B

- Aggregate evidence quality: B
- Benefit: Determine effects of treatment.
- Harm: Expense, time, anxiety/discomfort.
- Benefits-harms assessment: Preponderance of benefit over harm.

- Value judgments: Given the panel's concerns about the consequences of OSAS and the frequency of postoperative persistence in high-risk groups, the panel believes that the follow-up costs are outweighed by benefits of recognition of persistent OSAS. A minority of panelists believed that all children with OSAS should have follow-up polysomnography because of the high prevalence of persistent postoperative abnormalities on polysomnography, but most panelists believed that persistent polysomnographic abnormalities in uncomplicated children with mild OSAS were usually mild in patients who were asymptomatic after surgery.

- Role of patient preferences: Minimal. Further evaluation is needed to determine the need for further treatment.

- Exclusions: None.

- Intentional vagueness: None.

- Strength: Recommendation.

Numerous studies have shown that a large proportion of children at high risk continue to have some degree of OSAS postoperatively[10,13,14]; thus, objective evidence is required to determine whether further treatment is necessary.

Key Action Statement 6: CPAP

Clinicians should refer patients for CPAP management if symptoms/signs (Table 2) or objective evidence of OSAS persists after adenotonsillectomy or if adenotonsillectomy is not performed. (Evidence Quality: Grade B, Recommendation Strength: Recommendation.)

Evidence Profile KAS 6

- Aggregate evidence quality: B
- Benefit: Improve OSAS and accompanying symptoms and sequelae.

- Harm: Expense, time, anxiety; parental sleep disruption; nasal and skin adverse effects; possible midface remodeling; extremely rare serious pressure-related complications, such as pneumothorax; poor adherence.

- Benefits-harms assessment: Preponderance of benefit over harm.

- Value judgments: Panelists believe that CPAP is the most effective treatment of OSAS that persists postoperatively and that the benefits of treatment outweigh the adverse effects. Other treatments (eg, rapid maxillary expansion) may be effective in specially selected patients.

- Role of patient preferences: Other treatments may be effective in specially selected patients.

- Exclusions: Rare patients at increased risk of severe pressure complications.

- Intentional vagueness: None.

- Policy level: Recommendation.

CPAP therapy is delivered by using an electronic device that delivers air at positive pressure via a nasal mask, leading to mechanical stenting of the airway and improved functional residual capacity in the lungs. There is no clear advantage of using bilevel pressure over CPAP.[15] CPAP should be managed by an experienced and skilled clinician with expertise in its use in children. CPAP pressure requirements vary among individuals and change over time; thus, CPAP must be titrated in the sleep laboratory before prescribing the device and periodically readjusted thereafter. Behavioral modification therapy may be required, especially for young children or those with developmental delays. Objective monitoring of adherence, by using the equipment software, is important. If adherence is suboptimal, the clinician should institute measures to improve adherence (such as behavioral modification, or treating side effects of

CPAP) and institute alternative treatments if these measures are ineffective.

Key Action Statement 7: Weight Loss

Clinicians should recommend weight loss in addition to other therapy if a child/adolescent with OSAS is overweight or obese. (Evidence Quality: Grade C, Recommendation Strength: Recommendation.)

Evidence Profile KAS 7

- Aggregate evidence quality: C

- Benefit: Improve OSAS and accompanying symptoms and sequelae; non–OSAS-related benefits of weight loss.

- Harm: Hard to achieve and maintain weight loss.

- Benefits-harms assessment: Preponderance of benefit over harm.

- Value judgments: The panel agreed that weight loss is beneficial for both OSAS and other health issues, but clinical experience suggests that weight loss is difficult to achieve and maintain, and even effective weight loss regimens take time; therefore, additional treatment is required in the interim.

- Role of patient preferences: Strong role for patient and family preference regarding nutrition and exercise.

- Exclusions: None.

- Intentional vagueness: None.

- Strength: Recommendation.

Weight loss has been shown to improve OSAS,[16,17] although the degree of weight loss required has not been determined. Because weight loss is a slow and unreliable process, other treatment modalities (such as adenotonsillectomy or CPAP therapy) should be instituted until sufficient weight loss has been achieved and maintained.

Key Action Statement 8: Intranasal Corticosteroids

Clinicians may prescribe topical intranasal corticosteroids for children with mild OSAS in whom adenotonsillectomy is contraindicated or for children with mild postoperative OSAS. (Evidence Quality: Grade B, Recommendation Strength: Option.)

Evidence Profile KAS 8

- Aggregate evidence quality: B
- Benefit: Improves mild OSAS and accompanying symptoms and sequelae.
- Harm: Some subjects may not have an adequate response. It is not known whether therapeutic effect persists long-term; therefore, long-term observation is required. Low risk of steroid-related adverse effects.
- Benefits-harms assessment: Preponderance of benefit over harm.
- Value judgments: The panel agreed that intranasal steroids provide a less invasive treatment than surgery or CPAP and, therefore, may be preferred in some cases despite lower efficacy and lack of data on long-term efficacy.
- Role of patient preferences: Moderate role for patient and family preference if OSAS is mild.
- Exclusions: None.
- Intentional vagueness: None.
- Strength: Option.

Mild OSAS is defined, for this indication, as an AHI <5 per hour, on the basis of studies on intranasal corticosteroids described in the accompanying technical report.[2] Several studies have shown that the use of intranasal steroids decreases the degree of OSAS; however, although

OSAS improves, residual OSAS may remain. Furthermore, there is individual variability in response to treatment, and long-term studies have not been performed to determine the duration of improvement. Therefore, nasal steroids are not recommended as a first-line therapy. The response to treatment should be measured objectively after a course of treatment of approximately 6 weeks. Because the long-term effect of this treatment is unknown, the clinician should continue to observe the patient for symptoms of recurrence and adverse effects of corticosteroids.

AREAS FOR FUTURE RESEARCH

A detailed list of research recommendations is provided in the accompanying technical report.[2] There is a great need for further research into the prevalence of OSAS, sequelae of OSAS, best treatment methods, and the role of obesity. In particular, well-controlled, blinded studies, including randomized controlled trials of treatment, are needed to determine the best care for children and adolescents with OSAS.

SUBCOMMITTEE ON OBSTRUCTIVE SLEEP APNEA SYNDROME*

Carole L. Marcus, MBBCh, Chairperson (Sleep Medicine, Pediatric Pulmonologist; Liaison, American Academy of Sleep Medicine; Research Support from Philips Respironics; Affiliated with an academic sleep center; Published research related to OSAS)

Lee J. Brooks, MD (Sleep Medicine, Pediatric Pulmonologist; Liaison, American College of Chest Physicians; No financial conflicts; Affiliated with an academic sleep center; Published research related to OSAS)

Sally Davidson Ward, MD (Sleep Medicine, Pediatric Pulmonologist; No financial conflicts; Affiliated with an academic sleep center; Published research related to OSAS)

Kari A. Draper, MD (General Pediatrician; No conflicts)

David Gozal, MD (Sleep Medicine, Pediatric Pulmonologist; Research support from AstraZeneca; Speaker for Merck Company; Affiliated with an academic sleep center; Published research related to OSAS)

Ann C. Halbower, MD (Sleep Medicine, Pediatric Pulmonologist; Liaison, American Thoracic Society; Research Funding from Resmed; Affiliated with an academic sleep center; Published research related to OSAS)

Jacqueline Jones, MD (Pediatric Otolaryngologist; AAP Section on Otolaryngology-Head and Neck Surgery; Liaison, American Academy of Otolaryngology-Head and Neck Surgery; No financial conflicts; Affiliated with an academic otolaryngologic practice)

Christopher Lehman, MD (Neonatologist, Informatician; No conflicts)

Michael S. Schechter, MD, MPH (Pediatric Pulmonologist; AAP Section on Pediatric Pulmonology; Consultant to Genentech, Inc and Gilead, Inc, not related to Obstructive Sleep Apnea; Research Support from Mpex Pharmaceuticals, Inc, Vertex Pharmaceuticals Incorporated, PTC Therapeutics, Bayer Healthcare, not related to Obstructive Sleep Apnea)

Stephen Sheldon, MD (Sleep Medicine, General Pediatrician; Liaison, National Sleep Foundation; No financial conflicts; Affiliated with an academic sleep center; Published research related to OSAS)

Richard N. Shiffman, MD, MCIS (General pediatrics, Informatician; No conflicts)

Karen Spruyt, PhD (Clinical Psychologist, Child Neuropsychologist, and Biostatistician/Epidemiologist; No financial conflicts; Affiliated with an academic sleep center)

Oversight from the Steering Committee on Quality Improvement and Management, 2009–2012

STAFF

Caryn Davidson, MA

*Areas of expertise are shown in parentheses after each name.

ACKNOWLEDGMENTS

The committee thanks Jason Caboot, June Chan, Mary Currie, Fiona Healy, Maureen Josephson, Sofia Konstantinopoulou, H. Madan Kumar, Roberta Leu, Darius Loghmanee, Rajeev Bhatia, Argyri Petrocheilou, Harsha Vardhan, and Colleen Walsh for assisting with evidence extraction.

REFERENCES

1. Section on Pediatric Pulmonology, Subcommittee on Obstructive Sleep Apnea Syndrome. American Academy of Pediatrics. Clinical practice guideline: diagnosis and management of childhood obstructive sleep apnea syndrome. *Pediatrics.* 2002;109(4):704–712

2. Marcus CL, Brooks LJ, Davidson C, et al; American Academy of Pediatrics, Subcommittee on Obstructive Sleep Apnea

Syndrome. Technical report: diagnosis and management of childhood obstructive sleep apnea syndrome. *Pediatrics*. 2012; 130(3):In press

3. American Academy of Pediatrics Steering Committee on Quality Improvement and Management. Classifying recommendations for clinical practice guidelines. *Pediatrics*. 2004;114(3):874–877

4. American Thoracic Society. Standards and indications for cardiopulmonary sleep studies in children. *Am J Respir Crit Care Med*. 1996;153(2):866–878

5. Bixler EO, Vgontzas AN, Lin HM, et al. Sleep disordered breathing in children in a general population sample: prevalence and risk factors. *Sleep*. 2009;32(6):731–736

6. Li AM, So HK, Au CT, et al. Epidemiology of obstructive sleep apnoea syndrome in Chinese children: a two-phase community study. *Thorax*. 2010;65(11):991–997

7. O'Brien LM, Holbrook CR, Mervis CB, et al. Sleep and neurobehavioral characteristics of 5- to 7-year-old children with parentally reported symptoms of attention-deficit/hyperactivity disorder. *Pediatrics*. 2003; 111(3):554–563

8. Himes JH, Dietz WH; The Expert Committee on Clinical Guidelines for Overweight in Adolescent Preventive Services. Guidelines for overweight in adolescent preventive services: recommendations from an expert committee. *Am J Clin Nutr*. 1994;59(2):307–316

9. Mitchell RB. Adenotonsillectomy for obstructive sleep apnea in children: outcome evaluated by pre- and postoperative polysomnography. *Laryngoscope*. 2007;117(10):1844–1854

10. Suen JS, Arnold JE, Brooks LJ. Adenotonsillectomy for treatment of obstructive sleep apnea in children. *Arch Otolaryngol Head Neck Surg*. 1995;121(5):525–530

11. Nieminen P, Tolonen U, Löppönen H. Snoring and obstructive sleep apnea in children: a 6-month follow-up study. *Arch Otolaryngol Head Neck Surg*. 2000;126(4):481–486

12. Blunden S, Lushington K, Lorenzen B, Wong J, Balendran R, Kennedy D. Symptoms of sleep breathing disorders in children are underreported by parents at general practice visits. *Sleep Breath*. 2003;7(4):167–176

13. Apostolidou MT, Alexopoulos EI, Chaidas K, et al. Obesity and persisting sleep apnea after adenotonsillectomy in Greek children. *Chest*. 2008;134(6):1149–1155

14. Mitchell RB, Kelly J. Outcome of adenotonsillectomy for severe obstructive sleep apnea in children. *Int J Pediatr Otorhinolaryngol*. 2004;68(11):1375–1379

15. Marcus CL, Rosen G, Ward SL, et al. Adherence to and effectiveness of positive airway pressure therapy in children with obstructive sleep apnea. *Pediatrics*. 2006; 117(3). Available at: www.pediatrics.org/cgi/content/full/117/3/e442

16. Verhulst SL, Franckx H, Van Gaal L, De Backer W, Desager K. The effect of weight loss on sleep-disordered breathing in obese teenagers. *Obesity (Silver Spring)*. 2009;17(6):1178–1183

17. Kalra M, Inge T. Effect of bariatric surgery on obstructive sleep apnoea in adolescents. *Paediatr Respir Rev*. 2006;7(4):260–267

Sleep Apnea Clinical Practice Guideline
Quick Reference Tools

- Action Statement Summary
  — Diagnosis and Management of Childhood Obstructive Sleep Apnea Syndrome
- *ICD-10-CM* Coding Quick Reference for Sleep Apnea
- AAP Patient Education Handout
  — *Sleep Apnea and Your Child*

Action Statement Summary

Diagnosis and Management of Childhood Obstructive Sleep Apnea Syndrome

Key Action Statement 1: Screening for OSAS

As part of routine health maintenance visits, clinicians should inquire whether the child or adolescent snores. If the answer is affirmative or if a child or adolescent presents with signs or symptoms of OSAS (Table 2), clinicians should perform a more focused evaluation. (Evidence Quality: Grade B, Recommendation Strength: Recommendation.)

Key Action Statement 2A: Polysomnography

If a child or adolescent snores on a regular basis and has any of the complaints or findings shown in Table 2, clinicians should either (1) obtain a polysomnogram (Evidence Quality A, Key Action strength: Recommendation) OR (2) refer the patient to a sleep specialist or otolaryngologist for a more extensive evaluation (Evidence quality D, Key Action strength: Option). (Evidence Quality: Grade A for polysomnography; Grade D for specialist referral, Recommendation Strength: Recommendation.)

Key Action Statement 2B: Alternative Testing

If polysomnography is not available, then clinicians may order alternative diagnostic tests, such as nocturnal video recording, nocturnal oximetry, daytime nap polysomnography, or ambulatory polysomnography. (Evidence Quality: Grade C, Recommendation Strength: Option.)

Key Action Statement 3: Adenotonsillectomy

If a child is determined to have OSAS, has a clinical examination consistent with adenotonsillar hypertrophy, and does not have a contraindication to surgery (see Table 3), the clinician should recommend adenotonsillectomy as the first line of treatment. If the child has OSAS but does not have adenotonsillar hypertrophy, other treatment should be considered (see Key Action Statement 6). Clinical judgment is required to determine the benefits of adenotonsillectomy compared with other treatments in obese children with varying degrees of adenotonsillar hypertrophy. (Evidence Quality: Grade B, Recommendation Strength: Recommendation.)

Key Action Statement 4: High-Risk Patients Undergoing Adenotonsillectomy

Clinicians should monitor high-risk patients (Table 5) undergoing adenotonsillectomy as inpatients postoperatively. (Evidence Quality: Grade B, Recommendation Strength: Recommendation.)

Key Action Statement 5: Reevaluation

Clinicians should clinically reassess all patients with OSAS for persisting signs and symptoms after therapy to determine whether further treatment is required. (Evidence Quality: Grade B, Recommendation Strength: Recommendation.)

Key Action Statement 5B: Reevaluation of High-Risk Patients

Clinicians should reevaluate high-risk patients for persistent OSAS after adenotonsillectomy, including those who had a significantly abnormal baseline polysomnogram, have sequelae of OSAS, are obese, or remain symptomatic after treatment, with an objective test (see Key Action Statement 2) or refer such patients to a sleep specialist. (Evidence Quality: Grade B, Recommendation Strength: Recommendation.)

Key Action Statement 6: CPAP

Clinicians should refer patients for CPAP management if symptoms/signs (Table 2) or objective evidence of OSAS persists after adenotonsillectomy or if adenotonsillectomy is not performed. (Evidence Quality: Grade B, Recommendation Strength: Recommendation.)

Key Action Statement 7: Weight Loss

Clinicians should recommend weight loss in addition to other therapy if a child/adolescent with OSAS is overweight or obese. (Evidence Quality: Grade C, Recommendation Strength: Recommendation.)

Key Action Statement 8: Intranasal Corticosteroids

Clinicians may prescribe topical intranasal corticosteroids for children with mild OSAS in whom adenotonsillectomy is contraindicated or for children with mild postoperative OSAS. (Evidence Quality: Grade B, Recommendation Strength: Option.)

Coding Quick Reference for Sleep Apnea
ICD-10-CM
G47.30 Sleep apnea, unspecified
G47.31 Primary central sleep apnea
G47.33 Obstructive sleep apnea (adult) (pediatric) _____ (Code additional underlying conditions.)
J35.3   Hypertrophy of tonsils with hypertrophy of adenoids
E66.01 Morbid (severe) obesity due to excess calories
E66.09 Other obesity due to excess calories
E66.3   Overweight
E66.8   Other obesity
E66.9   Obesity, unspecified

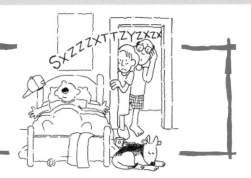

Sleep Apnea and Your Child

Does your child snore a lot? Does he sleep restlessly? Does he have difficulty breathing, or does he gasp or choke, while he sleeps?

If your child has these symptoms, he may have a condition known as sleep apnea.

Sleep apnea is a common problem that affects an estimated 2% of all children, including many who are undiagnosed.

If not treated, sleep apnea can lead to a variety of problems. These include heart, behavior, learning, and growth problems.

How do I know if my child has sleep apnea?

Symptoms of sleep apnea include

- Frequent snoring
- Problems breathing during the night
- Sleepiness during the day
- Difficulty paying attention
- Behavior problems

If you notice any of these symptoms, let your pediatrician know as soon as possible. Your pediatrician may recommend an overnight sleep study called a *polysomnogram.* Overnight polysomnograms are conducted at hospitals and major medical centers. During the study, medical staff will watch your child sleep. Several sensors will be attached to your child to monitor breathing, oxygenation, and brain waves. An electroencephalogram (EEG) is a test that measures brain waves.

The results of the study will show whether your child suffers from sleep apnea. Other specialists, such as pediatric pulmonologists, otolaryngologists, neurologists, and pediatricians with specialty training in sleep disorders, may help your pediatrician make the diagnosis.

What causes sleep apnea?

Many children with sleep apnea have larger tonsils and adenoids.

Tonsils are the round, reddish masses on each side of your child's throat. They help fight infections in the body. You can only see the adenoid with an x-ray or special mirror. It lies in the space between the nose and throat.

Large tonsils and adenoid may block a child's airway while she sleeps. This causes her to snore and wake up often during the night. However, not every child with large tonsils and adenoid has sleep

apnea. A sleep study can tell your doctor whether your child has sleep apnea or if she is simply snoring.

Children born with other medical conditions, such as Down syndrome, cerebral palsy, or craniofacial (skull and face) abnormalities, are at higher risk for sleep apnea. Overweight children are also more likely to suffer from sleep apnea.

How is sleep apnea treated?

The most common way to treat sleep apnea is to remove your child's tonsils and adenoid. This surgery is called a tonsillectomy and adenoidectomy. It is highly effective in treating sleep apnea.

Another effective treatment is nasal continuous positive airway pressure (CPAP), which requires the child to wear a mask while he sleeps. The mask delivers steady air pressure through the child's nose, allowing him to breathe comfortably. Continuous positive airway pressure is usually used in children who do not improve after tonsillectomy and adenoidectomy, or who are not candidates for tonsillectomy and adenoidectomy.

Children who may need additional treatment include children who are overweight or suffering from another complicating condition. Overweight children will improve if they lose weight, but may need to use CPAP until the weight is lost.

Remember

A good night's sleep is important to good health. If your child suffers from the symptoms of sleep apnea, talk with your pediatrician. A proper diagnosis and treatment can mean restful nights and restful days for your child and your family.

The information contained in this publication should not be used as a substitute for the medical care and advice of your pediatrician. There may be variations in treatment that your pediatrician may recommend based on individual facts and circumstances.

From your doctor

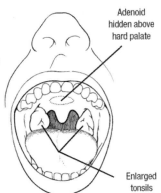

Adenoid hidden above hard palate

Enlarged tonsils

Reaffirmation of AAP Clinical Practice Guideline: The Diagnosis and Management of the Initial Urinary Tract Infection in Febrile Infants and Young Children 2–24 Months of Age

- *Reaffirmation of AAP Clinical Practice Guideline*

- *Clinical Practice Guideline*
  - *PPI: AAP Partnership for Policy Implementation See Appendix 1 for more information.*

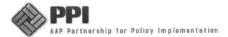

CLINICAL PRACTICE GUIDELINE   Guidance for the Clinician in Rendering Pediatric Care

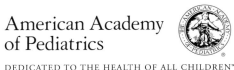

American Academy
of Pediatrics

DEDICATED TO THE HEALTH OF ALL CHILDREN™

Reaffirmation of AAP Clinical Practice Guideline: The Diagnosis and Management of the Initial Urinary Tract Infection in Febrile Infants and Young Children 2–24 Months of Age

SUBCOMMITTEE ON URINARY TRACT INFECTION

It is the policy of the American Academy of Pediatrics to reassess clinical practice guidelines (CPGs) every 5 years and retire, revise, or reaffirm them. The members of the urinary tract infection (UTI) subcommittee who developed the 2011 UTI CPG[1] have reviewed the literature published since 2011 along with unpublished manuscripts and the status of some clinical trials still in progress. With this article, we reaffirm the 2011 UTI CPG and provide an updated review of the supporting evidence. For the convenience of the reader, we reiterate the 7 Key Action Statements here to obviate the need to consult the 2011 UTI CPG, although interested readers may want to review the text of the guideline[1] and/or its accompanying technical report.[2]

ACTION STATEMENT 1

If a clinician decides that a febrile infant with no apparent source for the fever requires antimicrobial therapy to be administered because of ill appearance or another pressing reason, the clinician should ensure that a urine specimen is obtained for both culture and urinalysis before an antimicrobial is administered; the specimen needs to be obtained through catheterization or suprapubic aspiration (SPA), because the diagnosis of UTI cannot be established reliably through culture of urine collected in a bag (evidence quality: A; strong recommendation).

Comment

A key to an accurate diagnosis of UTI is obtaining a sample of urine for culture with minimal contamination before starting antimicrobial

DOI: 10.1542/peds.2016-3026

PEDIATRICS (ISSN Numbers: Print, 0031-4005; Online, 1098-4275).

Copyright © 2016 by the American Academy of Pediatrics

FINANCIAL DISCLOSURE: The authors have indicated they do not have a financial relationship relevant to this article to disclose.

FUNDING: No external funding.

POTENTIAL CONFLICT OF INTEREST: The authors have indicated they have no potential conflicts of interest to disclose.

To cite: AAP SUBCOMMITTEE ON URINARY TRACT INFECTION. Reaffirmation of AAP Clinical Practice Guideline: The Diagnosis and Management of the Initial Urinary Tract Infection in Febrile Infants and Young Children 2–24 Months of Age. *Pediatrics.* 2016;138(6):e20163026

agents. Urine collected in a bag or via a clean catch method is suitable for urinalysis (see Action Statement 2, Option 2), but such specimens (especially urine collected in a bag) are less appropriate for culture. If a culture obtained by bag is positive, the likelihood of a false positive is extremely high, so the result must be confirmed by culturing urine obtained by a more reliable method; if an antimicrobial agent is present in the urine, the opportunity for confirmation is likely to be lost.

Although samples of urine obtained by transurethral catheterization may be contaminated by urethral flora, meticulous technique can reduce this possibility. To avoid contamination, 2 practical steps should be implemented: (1) the first few milliliters obtained by catheter should be discarded (allowed to fall outside of the sterile collecting vessel) and only the subsequent urine cultured; and (2) if the attempt at catheterization is unsuccessful, a new, clean catheter should be used (aided, in girls, by leaving the initial catheter in place as a marker).

ACTION STATEMENT 2

If a clinician assesses a febrile infant with no apparent source for the fever as not being so ill as to require immediate antimicrobial therapy, then the clinician should assess the likelihood of UTI.

Action Statement 2a. If the clinician determines the febrile infant to have a low likelihood of UTI (see text), then clinical follow-up monitoring without testing is sufficient (evidence quality: A; strong recommendation).

Action Statement 2b. If the clinician determines that the febrile infant is not in a low-risk group (see below), then there are 2 choices (evidence quality: A; strong recommendation).

Option 1 is to obtain a urine specimen through catheterization or SPA for culture and urinalysis.

Option 2 is to obtain a urine specimen through the most convenient means and to perform a urinalysis. If the urinalysis results suggest a UTI (positive leukocyte esterase test results or nitrite test or microscopic analysis results for leukocytes or bacteria), then a urine specimen should be obtained through catheterization or SPA and cultured; if urinalysis of fresh (less than 1 hour since void) urine yields negative leukocyte esterase and nitrite results, then it is reasonable to monitor the clinical course without initiating antimicrobial therapy, recognizing that a negative urinalysis does not rule out a UTI with certainty.

Comment

When the patient's degree of illness does not warrant immediate antimicrobial treatment and the risk of UTI is extremely low, the patient may be observed without assessing the urine. (The risk assessment tables in the 2011 UTI CPG have been simplified into algorithm form.[3]) If there is a low but real risk of infection, then either the best possible specimen should be obtained for urinalysis and culture, or a sample of urine obtained by a convenient method and a judgment made about culturing the urine dependent on the findings of the urinalysis or dipstick. A positive urinalysis provides sufficient concern to mandate a properly obtained urine specimen. This 2-step process (Option 2) is not only suitable for office practice but has been demonstrated to be feasible and beneficial in a busy pediatric emergency department, with the catheterization rate decreasing from

63% to fewer than 30% without increasing length of stay or missing UTIs.[4]

ACTION STATEMENT 3

To establish the diagnosis of UTI, clinicians should require both urinalysis results that suggest infection (pyuria and/or bacteriuria) and the presence of at least 50 000 colony-forming units (cfu) per milliliter of a uropathogen cultured from a urine specimen obtained through transurethral catheterization or SPA (evidence quality: C; recommendation).

Comment

The thrust of this key action statement is that the diagnosis of UTI in febrile infants is signaled by the presence of both bacteriuria and pyuria. In general, pyuria without bacteriuria is insufficient to make a diagnosis of UTI because it is nonspecific and occurs in the absence of infection (eg, Kawasaki disease, chemical urethritis, streptococcal infections). Likewise, bacteriuria, without pyuria is attributable to external contamination, asymptomatic bacteriuria, or, rarely, very early infection (before the onset of inflammation). Non–*Escherichia coli* isolates are less frequently associated with pyuria than *E coli*,[5] but the significance of this association is not clear at present. Non–*E coli* uropathogens are of concern because they are more likely to result in scarring than *E coli*,[6] but animal studies demonstrate the host inflammatory response to be what causes scarring rather than the presence of organisms.[7] Moreover, the rate of asymptomatic bacteriuria is sufficient to account for the lack of association with pyuria.

The remaining question is what constitutes "significant" bacteriuria and "significant" pyuria. In 1994, by using single versus multiple organisms to distinguish true UTI from contamination, 50 000 cfu/mL was proposed as the appropriate threshold for specimens obtained by catheterization,[8] recommended in the 2011 UTI CPG and implemented in the Randomized Intervention for Children with Vesicoureteral Reflux (RIVUR) trial.[9] Lower colony counts are sufficient if the urine specimen is obtained by SPA and, thus, less likely to be contaminated, but most (80%) cases of UTI documented with urine obtained by SPA have 10^5 cfu/mL or more. Colony counts lower than 50 000 cfu/mL are currently being considered for the diagnosis of UTI.[10] If 10 000 cfu/mL coupled with symptoms (eg, fever) and evidence of inflammation (pyuria) proves both sensitive and specific, this threshold would be of particular assistance to clinicians who use laboratories that do not specify colony counts between 10 000 and 100 000 cfu/mL and, thereby, make the criterion of 50 000 cfu/mL difficult to use.

Significant pyuria is ≥10 white blood cells/mm^3 on an "enhanced urinalysis" or ≥5 white blood cells per high power field on a centrifuged specimen of urine or any leukocyte esterase on a dipstick.

ACTION STATEMENT 4

Action Statement 4a. When initiating treatment, the clinician should base the choice of route of administration on practical considerations: initiating treatment orally or parenterally is equally efficacious. The clinician should base the choice of agent on local antimicrobial sensitivity patterns (if available) and should adjust the choice according to sensitivity testing of the isolated uropathogen (evidence quality: A; strong recommendation).

Action Statement 4b. The clinician should choose 7 to 14 days as

the duration of antimicrobial therapy (evidence quality B; recommendation).

Comment

Basing the choice of an initial antimicrobial agent on local sensitivity patterns can be difficult because applicable information may not be available. Whether the child has received antimicrobial therapy in the recent past should be considered. This exposure constitutes a risk factor for resistance to the recently prescribed antimicrobial. Further delineation of treatment duration has not been forthcoming, but a randomized controlled trial is currently under way comparing the effectiveness of 5 days versus 10 days of treatment.[11]

Note: The dose of ceftriaxone in Table 2 should be 50 mg/kg, every 24 h.

ACTION STATEMENT 5

Febrile infants with UTIs should undergo renal and bladder ultrasonography (RBUS) (evidence quality: C; recommendation).

Comment

As noted in the 2011 CPG, it is important that the study be a renal and bladder ultrasonogram, not a limited renal ultrasonogram. Ideally, the patient should be well-hydrated for the examination and the bladder should be evaluated while distended. Concern has been raised that RBUS is not effective to detect vesicoureteral reflux (VUR), as it is frequently normal in infants with low-grade VUR and even in some who have high-grade VUR. Moreover, nonspecific RBUS findings, such as mild renal pelvic or ureteral distention, are common and are not necessarily associated with reflux. However, low-grade VUR is generally not considered of concern for renal damage, and most studies (other than the RIVUR trial[9]) have demonstrated continuous antimicrobial prophylaxis

(CAP) to lack benefit in this group.[1,2] Although RBUS is not invariably abnormal in infants with grades IV and V VUR, it does identify most, and, of particular importance, an abnormal RBUS is a major risk factor for scarring.[6]

ACTION STATEMENT 6

Action Statement 6a. Voiding cystourethrography (VCUG) should not be performed routinely after the first febrile UTI; VCUG is indicated if RBUS reveals hydronephrosis, scarring, or other findings that would suggest either high-grade VUR or obstructive uropathy, as well as in other atypical or complex clinical circumstances (evidence quality B; recommendation).

Action Statement 6b. Further evaluation should be conducted if there is a recurrence of febrile UTI (evidence quality: X; recommendation).

Comment

For decades, UTIs in infants were considered harbingers of underlying anatomic and/or physiologic abnormalities, so RBUS and VCUG were recommended to be performed routinely. VUR was a particular concern; CAP was assumed to be effective in preventing UTI and became standard practice when VUR was discovered. In the years leading up to the 2011 guideline, randomized controlled trials of CAP were performed. Authors of the 6 studies published in 2006-2010 graciously provided data to the guideline committee, permitting a meta-analysis of data specifically targeting febrile infants 2 to 24 months of age. CAP was not demonstrated to be effective, so the need to identify VUR by routine voiding cystourethrography was discouraged.[1,2] A recent large trial in the United States, the RIVUR trial, concluded that CAP was of benefit, but, to prevent 1 UTI recurrence required 5840 doses of antimicrobial and did not reduce the rate of renal scarring.[9]

Since the publication of the 2011 guideline, multiple studies have demonstrated that abnormalities are missed by the selective imaging recommended in the guideline; however, there is no evidence that identifying these missed abnormalities is of sufficient clinical benefit to offset the cost, discomfort, and radiation.[12] Compared with performing the full array of imaging tests, the radiation burden incurred with the application of the guideline has been calculated to be reduced by 93%.[13] Moreover, in population studies, the significance of VUR and the value of treating VUR have been questioned.[14,15]

The authors of the RIVUR trial and its companion study, Careful Urinary Tract Infection Evaluation, have called attention to bowel/bladder dysfunction (BBD) as a major risk factor for UTI recurrences and recognize that, in children who have a UTI recurrence, evaluation for BBD (ie, constipation), rather than for VUR, can be performed by nonspecialists and does not incur high cost, cause discomfort, or require radiation.[16] BBD has long been underappreciated and deserves greater consideration.

ACTION STATEMENT 7

After confirmation of UTI, the clinician should instruct parents or guardians to seek prompt medical evaluation (ideally within 48 hours) for future febrile illnesses to ensure that recurrent infections can be detected and treated promptly (evidence quality: C; recommendation).

Comment

Prompt treatment is of clinical benefit to the child with the acute infection. What has been controversial is the definition of "prompt" and the relationship to renal scarring. A recent study identified that the median time to treatment was shorter in infants who did not incur a scar than in those who did (48 vs 72 hours). The study also noted that the rate of scarring increased minimally between days 1 and 2 and between days 2 and 3 but was much higher thereafter.[17]

SUBCOMMITTEE ON URINARY TRACT INFECTION, 2009-2011

Kenneth B. Roberts, MD, FAAP Chair
Stephen M. Downs, MD, MS, FAAP
S. Maria E. Finnell, MD, MS, FAAP
*Stanley Hellerstein, MD (deceased)
Linda D. Shortliffe, MD
Ellen R. Wald, MD, FAAP, Vice-Chair
J. Michael Zerin, MD

STAFF

Kymika Okechukwu, MPA, Manager, Evidence-Based Practice Initiatives

---

ABBREVIATIONS

BBD: bowel/bladder dysfunction
CAP: continuous antimicrobial
     prophylaxis
cfu: colony-forming units
CPG: clinical practice guideline
RBUS: renal and bladder
     ultrasonography
RIVUR: Randomized Intervention
     for Children with
     Vesicoureteral Reflux
SPA: suprapubic aspiration
UTI: urinary tract infection
VCUG: voiding
     cystourethrography
VUR: vesicoureteral reflux

REFERENCES

1. Roberts KB; Subcommittee on Urinary Tract Infection, Steering Committee on Quality Improvement and Management. Urinary tract infection: clinical practice guideline for the diagnosis and management of the initial UTI in febrile infants and children 2 to 24 months. *Pediatrics*. 2011;128(3):595–610

2. Finnell SM, Carroll AE, Downs SM; Subcommittee on Urinary Tract Infection. Technical report—Diagnosis and management of an initial UTI in febrile infants and young children. *Pediatrics*. 2011;128(3). Available at: www.pediatrics.org/cgi/content/full/128/3/e749 PubMed

3. Roberts KB. Revised AAP Guideline on UTI in Febrile Infants and Young Children. *Am Fam Physician*. 2012;86(10):940–946

4. Lavelle JM, Blackstone MM, Funari MK, et al. Two-step process for ED UTI screening in febrile young children: reducing catheterization rates. *Pediatrics*. 2016;138(1):e20153023

5. Shaikh N, Shope TR, Hoberman A, Vigliotti A, Kurs-Lasky M, Martin JM. Association between uropathogen and pyuria. *Pediatrics*. 2016;138(1):e20160087

6. Shaikh N, Craig JC, Rovers MM, et al. Identification of children and adolescents at risk for renal scarring after a first urinary tract infection: a meta-analysis with individual patient data. *JAMA Pediatr*. 2014;168(10):893–900

7. Glauser MP, Meylan P, Bille J. The inflammatory response and tissue damage. The example of renal scars following acute renal infection. *Pediatr Nephrol*. 1987;1(4):615–622

8. Hoberman A, Wald ER, Reynolds EA, Penchansky L, Charron M. Pyuria and bacteriuria in urine specimens obtained by catheter from young children with fever. *J Pediatr*. 1994;124(4):513–519

9. Hoberman A, Greenfield SP, Mattoo TK, et al; RIVUR Trial Investigators. Antimicrobial prophylaxis for children with vesicoureteral reflux. *N Engl J Med*. 2014;370(25):2367–2376

10. Tullus K. Low urinary bacterial counts: do they count? *Pediatr Nephrol*. 2016;31(2):171–174

11. Hoberman A. The SCOUT study: short course therapy for urinary tract infections in children. Available at: https://clinicaltrials.gov/ct2/show/

NCT01595529. Accessed October 14, 2016

12. Narchi H, Marah M, Khan AA, et al Renal tract abnormalities missed in a historical cohort of your children with UTI if the NICE and AAP imaging guidelines were applied. *J Pediatr Urol.* 2015;11(5):252.e1–7

13. La Scola C, De Mutiis C, Hewitt IK, et al. Different guidelines for imaging after first UTI in febrile infants: yield, cost, and radiation. *Pediatrics.* 2013;131(3).

Available at: www.pediatrics.org/cgi/content/full/131/3/e665 PubMed

14. Salo J, Ikäheimo R, Tapiainen T, Uhari M. Childhood urinary tract infections as a cause of chronic kidney disease. *Pediatrics.* 2011;128(5):840–847

15. Craig JC, Williams GJ. Denominators do matter: it's a myth—urinary tract infection does not cause chronic kidney disease. *Pediatrics.* 2011;128(5):984–985

16. Shaikh N, Hoberman A, Keren R, et al. Recurrent urinary tract infections in children with bladder and bowel dysfunction. *Pediatrics.* 2016;137(1):e20152982

17. Shaikh N, Mattoo TK, Keren R, et al. Early antibiotic treatment for pediatric febrile urinary tract infection and renal scarring. *JAMA Pediatr.* 2016;170(9):848–854

459

CLINICAL PRACTICE GUIDELINE

Urinary Tract Infection: Clinical Practice Guideline for the Diagnosis and Management of the Initial UTI in Febrile Infants and Children 2 to 24 Months

SUBCOMMITTEE ON URINARY TRACT INFECTION, STEERING COMMITTEE ON QUALITY IMPROVEMENT AND MANAGEMENT

KEY WORDS
urinary tract infection, infants, children, vesicoureteral reflux, voiding cystourethrography

ABBREVIATIONS
SPA—suprapubic aspiration
AAP—American Academy of Pediatrics
UTI—urinary tract infection
RCT—randomized controlled trial
CFU—colony-forming unit
VUR—vesicoureteral reflux
WBC—white blood cell
RBUS—renal and bladder ultrasonography
VCUG—voiding cystourethrography

www.pediatrics.org/cgi/doi/10.1542/peds.2011-1330

doi:10.1542/peds.2011-1330

PEDIATRICS (ISSN Numbers: Print, 0031-4005; Online, 1098-4275).

Copyright © 2011 by the American Academy of Pediatrics

COMPANION PAPERS: Companions to this article can be found on pages 572 and e749, and online at www.pediatrics.org/cgi/doi/10.1542/peds.2011-1818 and www.pediatrics.org/cgi/doi/10.1542/peds.2011-1332.

abstract

OBJECTIVE: To revise the American Academy of Pediatrics practice parameter regarding the diagnosis and management of initial urinary tract infections (UTIs) in febrile infants and young children.

METHODS: Analysis of the medical literature published since the last version of the guideline was supplemented by analysis of data provided by authors of recent publications. The strength of evidence supporting each recommendation and the strength of the recommendation were assessed and graded.

RESULTS: Diagnosis is made on the basis of the presence of both pyuria and at least 50 000 colonies per mL of a single uropathogenic organism in an appropriately collected specimen of urine. After 7 to 14 days of antimicrobial treatment, close clinical follow-up monitoring should be maintained to permit prompt diagnosis and treatment of recurrent infections. Ultrasonography of the kidneys and bladder should be performed to detect anatomic abnormalities. Data from the most recent 6 studies do not support the use of antimicrobial prophylaxis to prevent febrile recurrent UTI in infants without vesicoureteral reflux (VUR) or with grade I to IV VUR. Therefore, a voiding cystourethrography (VCUG) is not recommended routinely after the first UTI; VCUG is indicated if renal and bladder ultrasonography reveals hydronephrosis, scarring, or other findings that would suggest either high-grade VUR or obstructive uropathy and in other atypical or complex clinical circumstances. VCUG should also be performed if there is a recurrence of a febrile UTI. The recommendations in this guideline do not indicate an exclusive course of treatment or serve as a standard of care; variations may be appropriate. Recommendations about antimicrobial prophylaxis and implications for performance of VCUG are based on currently available evidence. As with all American Academy of Pediatrics clinical guidelines, the recommendations will be reviewed routinely and incorporate new evidence, such as data from the Randomized Intervention for Children With Vesicoureteral Reflux (RIVUR) study.

CONCLUSIONS: Changes in this revision include criteria for the diagnosis of UTI and recommendations for imaging. *Pediatrics* 2011;128:595–610

INTRODUCTION

Since the early 1970s, occult bacteremia has been the major focus of concern for clinicians evaluating febrile infants who have no recognizable source of infection. With the introduction of effective conjugate vaccines against *Haemophilus influenzae* type b and *Streptococcus pneumoniae* (which have resulted in dramatic decreases in bacteremia and meningitis), there has been increasing appreciation of the urinary tract as the most frequent site of occult and serious bacterial infections. Because the clinical presentation tends to be nonspecific in infants and reliable urine specimens for culture cannot be obtained without invasive methods (urethral catheterization or suprapubic aspiration [SPA]), diagnosis and treatment may be delayed. Most experimental and clinical data support the concept that delays in the institution of appropriate treatment of pyelonephritis increase the risk of renal damage.[1,2]

This clinical practice guideline is a revision of the practice parameter published by the American Academy of Pediatrics (AAP) in 1999.[3] It was developed by a subcommittee of the Steering Committee on Quality Improvement and Management that included physicians with expertise in the fields of academic general pediatrics, epidemiology and informatics, pediatric infectious diseases, pediatric nephrology, pediatric practice, pediatric radiology, and pediatric urology. The AAP funded the development of this guideline; none of the participants had any financial conflicts of interest. The guideline was reviewed by multiple groups within the AAP (7 committees, 1 council, and 9 sections) and 5 external organizations in the United States and Canada. The guideline will be reviewed and/or revised in 5 years, unless new evidence emerges that warrants revision sooner. The guideline is intended

for use in a variety of clinical settings (eg, office, emergency department, or hospital) by clinicians who treat infants and young children. This text is a summary of the analysis. The data on which the recommendations are based are included in a companion technical report.[4]

Like the 1999 practice parameter, this revision focuses on the diagnosis and management of initial urinary tract infections (UTIs) in febrile infants and young children (2–24 months of age) who have no obvious neurologic or anatomic abnormalities known to be associated with recurrent UTI or renal damage. (For simplicity, in the remainder of this guideline the phrase "febrile infants" is used to indicate febrile infants and young children 2–24 months of age.) The lower and upper age limits were selected because studies on infants with unexplained fever generally have used these age limits and have documented that the prevalence of UTI is high (~5%) in this age group. In those studies, fever was defined as temperature of at least 38.0°C (≥100.4°F); accordingly, this definition of fever is used in this guideline. Neonates and infants less than 2 months of age are excluded, because there are special considerations in this age group that may limit the application of evidence derived from the studies of 2- to 24-month-old children. Data are insufficient to determine whether the evidence generated from studies of infants 2 to 24 months of age applies to children more than 24 months of age.

METHODS

To provide evidence for the guideline, 2 literature searches were conducted, that is, a surveillance of Medline-listed literature over the past 10 years for significant changes since the guideline was published and a systematic review of the literature on the effective-

ness of prophylactic antimicrobial therapy to prevent recurrence of febrile UTI/pyelonephritis in children with vesicoureteral reflux (VUR). The latter was based on the new and growing body of evidence questioning the effectiveness of antimicrobial prophylaxis to prevent recurrent febrile UTI in children with VUR. To explore this particular issue, the literature search was expanded to include trials published since 1993 in which antimicrobial prophylaxis was compared with no treatment or placebo treatment for children with VUR. Because all except 1 of the recent randomized controlled trials (RCTs) of the effectiveness of prophylaxis included children more than 24 months of age and some did not provide specific data according to grade of VUR, the authors of the 6 RCTs were contacted; all provided raw data from their studies specifically addressing infants 2 to 24 months of age, according to grade of VUR. Meta-analysis of these data was performed.

Results from the literature searches and meta-analyses were provided to committee members. Issues were raised and discussed until consensus was reached regarding recommendations. The quality of evidence supporting each recommendation and the strength of the recommendation were assessed by the committee member most experienced in informatics and epidemiology and were graded according to AAP policy[5] (Fig 1).

The subcommittee formulated 7 recommendations, which are presented in the text in the order in which a clinician would use them when evaluating and treating a febrile infant, as well as in algorithm form in the Appendix. This clinical practice guideline is not intended to be a sole source of guidance for the treatment of febrile infants with UTIs. Rather, it is intended to assist clinicians in decision-making. It is not intended to replace clinical judgment or to

Evidence Quality	Preponderance of Benefit or Harm	Balance of Benefit and Harm
A. Well designed RCTs or diagnostic studies on relevant population	Strong Recommendation	
B. RCTs or diagnostic studies with minor limitations;overwhelmingly consistent evidence from observational studies		Option
C. Observational studies (case-control and cohort design)	Recommendation	
D. Expert opinion, case reports, reasoning from first principles	Option	No Rec
X. Exceptional situations where validating studies cannot be performed and there is a clear preponderance of benefit or harm	Strong Recommendation Recommendation	

FIGURE 1
AAP evidence strengths.

establish an exclusive protocol for the care of all children with this condition.

DIAGNOSIS

Action Statement 1

If a clinician decides that a febrile infant with no apparent source for the fever requires antimicrobial therapy to be administered because of ill appearance or another pressing reason, the clinician should ensure that a urine specimen is obtained for both culture and urinalysis before an antimicrobial agent is administered; the specimen needs to be obtained through catheterization or SPA, because the diagnosis of UTI cannot be established reliably through culture of urine collected in a bag (evidence quality: A; strong recommendation).

When evaluating febrile infants, clinicians make a subjective assessment of the degree of illness or toxicity, in addition to seeking an explanation for the fever. This clinical assessment determines whether antimicrobial therapy should be initiated promptly and affects the diagnostic process regarding UTI. If the clinician determines that the degree of illness warrants immediate antimicrobial therapy, then a urine specimen suitable for culture should be obtained through catheterization or SPA before antimicrobial agents are

administered, because the antimicrobial agents commonly prescribed in such situations would almost certainly obscure the diagnosis of UTI.

SPA has been considered the standard method for obtaining urine that is uncontaminated by perineal flora. Variable success rates for obtaining urine have been reported (23%–90%).[6–8] When ultrasonographic guidance is used, success rates improve.[9,10] The technique has limited risks, but technical expertise and experience are required, and many parents and physicians perceive the procedure as unacceptably invasive, compared with catheterization. However, there may be no acceptable alternative to SPA for boys with moderate or severe phimosis or girls with tight labial adhesions.

Urine obtained through catheterization for culture has a sensitivity of 95% and a specificity of 99%, compared with that obtained through SPA.[7,11,12] The techniques required for catheterization and SPA are well described.[13] When catheterization or SPA is being attempted, the clinician should have a sterile container ready to collect a urine specimen, because the preparation for the procedure may stimulate the child to void. Whether the urine is obtained through catheterization or is voided, the first few drops should be allowed to fall outside the sterile con-

tainer, because they may be contaminated by bacteria in the distal urethra.

Cultures of urine specimens collected in a bag applied to the perineum have an unacceptably high false-positive rate and are valid only when they yield negative results.[6,14–16] With a prevalence of UTI of 5% and a high rate of false-positive results (specificity: ~63%), a "positive" culture result for urine collected in a bag would be a false-positive result 88% of the time. For febrile boys, with a prevalence of UTI of 2%, the rate of false-positive results is 95%; for circumcised boys, with a prevalence of UTI of 0.2%, the rate of false-positive results is 99%. Therefore, in cases in which antimicrobial therapy will be initiated, catheterization or SPA is required to establish the diagnosis of UTI.

- Aggregate quality of evidence: A (diagnostic studies on relevant populations).

- Benefits: A missed diagnosis of UTI can lead to renal scarring if left untreated; overdiagnosis of UTI can lead to overtreatment and unnecessary and expensive imaging. Once antimicrobial therapy is initiated, the opportunity to make a definitive diagnosis is lost; multiple studies of antimicrobial therapy have shown that the urine may be rapidly sterilized.

- Harms/risks/costs: Catheterization is invasive.

- Benefit-harms assessment: Preponderance of benefit over harm.

- Value judgments: Once antimicrobial therapy has begun, the opportunity to make a definitive diagnosis is lost. Therefore, it is important to have the most-accurate test for UTI performed initially.

- Role of patient preferences: There is no evidence regarding patient preferences for bag versus catheterized urine. However, bladder tap has been shown to be more painful than urethral catheterization.

- Exclusions: None.
- Intentional vagueness: The basis of the determination that antimicrobial therapy is needed urgently is not specified, because variability in clinical judgment is expected; considerations for individual patients, such as availability of follow-up care, may enter into the decision, and the literature provides only general guidance.
- Policy level: Strong recommendation.

Individual Risk Factors: Girls
White race Age < 12 mo Temperature ≥ 39°C Fever ≥ 2 d Absence of another source of infection

Probability of UTI	No. of Factors Present
≤1%	No more than 1
≤2%	No more than 2

Individual Risk Factors: Boys
Nonblack race Temperature ≥ 39°C Fever > 24 h Absence of another source of infection

Probability of UTI	No. of Factors Present	
	Uncircumcised	Circumcised
≤1%	a	No more than 2
≤2%	None	No more than 3

FIGURE 2

Probability of UTI Among Febrile Infant Girls[28] and Infant Boys[30] According to Number of Findings Present. [a]Probability of UTI exceeds 1% even with no risk factors other than being uncircumcised.

Action Statement 2

If a clinician assesses a febrile infant with no apparent source for the fever as not being so ill as to require immediate antimicrobial therapy, then the clinician should assess the likelihood of UTI (see below for how to assess likelihood).

Action Statement 2a

If the clinician determines the febrile infant to have a low likelihood of UTI (see text), then clinical follow-up monitoring without testing is sufficient (evidence quality: A; strong recommendation).

Action Statement 2b

If the clinician determines that the febrile infant is not in a low-risk group (see below), then there are 2 choices (evidence quality: A; strong recommendation). Option 1 is to obtain a urine specimen through catheterization or SPA for culture and urinalysis. Option 2 is to obtain a urine specimen through the most convenient means and to perform a urinalysis. If the urinalysis results suggest a UTI (positive leukocyte esterase test results or nitrite test or microscopic analysis results positive for leukocytes or bacteria), then a urine specimen should be obtained through catheterization or SPA and cultured; if urinalysis of fresh (<1 hour since void) urine yields negative leukocyte esterase and nitrite test results, then it is reasonable to monitor the clinical course without initiating antimicrobial therapy, recognizing that negative urinalysis results do not rule out a UTI with certainty.

If the clinician determines that the degree of illness does not require immediate antimicrobial therapy, then the likelihood of UTI should be assessed. As noted previously, the overall prevalence of UTI in febrile infants who have no source for their fever evident on the basis of history or physical examination results is approximately 5%,[17,18] but it is possible to identify groups with higher-than-average likelihood and some with lower-than-average likelihood. The prevalence of UTI among febrile infant girls is more than twice that among febrile infant boys (relative risk: 2.27). The rate for uncircumcised boys is 4 to 20 times higher than that for circumcised boys, whose rate of UTI is only 0.2% to 0.4%.[19–24] The presence of another, clinically obvious source of infection reduces the likelihood of UTI by one-half.[25]

In a survey asking, "What yield is required to warrant urine culture in febrile infants?," the threshold was less than 1% for 10.4% of academicians and 11.7% for practitioners[26]; when the threshold was increased to 1% to 3%, 67.5% of academicians and 45.7% of practitioners considered the yield sufficiently high to warrant urine culture. Therefore, attempting to operationalize "low likelihood" (ie, below a threshold that warrants a urine culture) does not produce an absolute percentage; clinicians will choose a threshold depending on factors such as their confidence that contact will be maintained through the illness (so that a specimen can be obtained at a later time) and comfort with diagnostic uncertainty. Fig 2 indicates the number of risk factors associated with threshold probabilities of UTI of at least 1% and at least 2%.

In a series of studies, Gorelick, Shaw, and colleagues[27–29] derived and validated a prediction rule for febrile infant girls on the basis of 5 risk factors, namely, white race, age less than 12 months, temperature of at least 39°C, fever for at least 2 days, and absence of another source of infection. This prediction rule, with sensitivity of 88% and specificity of 30%, permits some infant girls to be considered in a low-likelihood group (Fig 2). For example, of girls with no identifiable source of infection, those who are nonwhite and more than 12 months of age with a recent onset (<2 days) of low-grade fever (<39°C) have less than a 1% probability of UTI; each additional risk factor increases the probability. It should be noted, however, that some of the factors (eg, duration of fever) may change during the course of the illness, excluding the infant from a low-likelihood designation and prompting testing as described in action statement 2a.

As demonstrated in Fig 2, the major risk factor for febrile infant boys is whether they are circumcised. The probability of UTI can be estimated on the basis of 4 risk factors, namely, nonblack race, temperature of at least 39°C, fever for more than 24 hours, and absence of another source of infection.[4,30]

If the clinician determines that the infant does not require immediate antimicrobial therapy and a urine specimen is desired, then often a urine collection bag affixed to the perineum is used. Many clinicians think that this collection technique has a low contamination rate under the following circumstances: the patient's perineum is properly cleansed and rinsed before application of the collection bag, the urine bag is removed promptly after urine is voided into the bag, and the specimen is refrigerated or processed immediately. Even if contamination from the perineal skin is minimized, however, there may be significant contamination from the vagina in girls or the prepuce in uncircumcised boys, the 2 groups at highest risk of UTI. A "positive" culture result from a specimen collected in a bag cannot be used to document a UTI; confirmation requires culture of a specimen collected through catheterization or SPA. Because there may be substantial delay waiting for the infant to void and a second specimen, obtained through catheterization, may be necessary if the urinalysis suggests the possibility of UTI, many clinicians prefer to obtain a

TABLE 1 Sensitivity and Specificity of Components of Urinalysis, Alone and in Combination

Test	Sensitivity (Range), %	Specificity (Range), %
Leukocyte esterase test	83 (67–94)	78 (64–92)
Nitrite test	53 (15–82)	98 (90–100)
Leukocyte esterase or nitrite test positive	93 (90–100)	72 (58–91)
Microscopy, WBCs	73 (32–100)	81 (45–98)
Microscopy, bacteria	81 (16–99)	83 (11–100)
Leukocyte esterase test, nitrite test, or microscopy positive	99.8 (99–100)	70 (60–92)

definitive urine specimen through catheterization initially.

- Aggregate quality of evidence: A (diagnostic studies on relevant populations).

- Benefits: Accurate diagnosis of UTI can prevent the spread of infection and renal scarring; avoiding overdiagnosis of UTI can prevent overtreatment and unnecessary and expensive imaging.

- Harms/risks/costs: A small proportion of febrile infants, considered at low likelihood of UTI, will not receive timely identification and treatment of their UTIs.

- Benefit-harms assessment: Preponderance of benefit over harm.

- Value judgments: There is a risk of UTI sufficiently low to forestall further evaluation.

- Role of patient preferences: The choice of option 1 or option 2 and the threshold risk of UTI warranting obtaining a urine specimen may be influenced by parents' preference to avoid urethral catheterization (if a bag urine sample yields negative urinalysis results) versus timely evaluation (obtaining a definitive specimen through catheterization).

- Exclusions: Because it depends on a range of patient- and physician-specific considerations, the precise threshold risk of UTI warranting obtaining a urine specimen is left to the clinician but is below 3%.

- Intentional vagueness: None.

- Policy level: Strong recommendation.

Action Statement 3

To establish the diagnosis of UTI, clinicians should require *both* urinalysis results that suggest infection (pyuria and/or bacteriuria) *and* the presence of at least 50 000 colony-forming units (CFUs) per mL of a uropathogen cultured from a urine specimen obtained through catheterization or SPA (evidence quality: C; recommendation).

Urinalysis

General Considerations

Urinalysis cannot substitute for urine culture to document the presence of UTI but needs to be used in conjunction with culture. Because urine culture results are not available for at least 24 hours, there is considerable interest in tests that may predict the results of the urine culture and enable presumptive therapy to be initiated at the first encounter. Urinalysis can be performed on any specimen, including one collected from a bag applied to the perineum. However, the specimen must be fresh (<1 hour after voiding with maintenance at room temperature or <4 hours after voiding with refrigeration), to ensure sensitivity and specificity of the urinalysis. The tests that have received the most attention are biochemical analyses of leukocyte esterase and nitrite through a rapid dipstick method and urine microscopic examination for white blood cells (WBCs) and bacteria (Table 1).

Urine dipsticks are appealing, because they provide rapid results, do not require microscopy, and are eligible for a waiver under the Clinical Laboratory Improvement Amendments. They indicate the presence of leukocyte esterase (as a surrogate marker for pyuria) and urinary nitrite (which is converted from dietary nitrates in the presence of most Gram-negative enteric bacteria in the urine). The conversion of dietary nitrates to nitrites by bacteria requires approximately 4 hours in the bladder.[31] The performance characteristics of both leukocyte esterase and nitrite tests vary according to the definition used for positive urine culture results, the age and symptoms of the population being studied, and the method of urine collection.

Nitrite Test

A nitrite test is not a sensitive marker for children, particularly infants, who empty their bladders frequently. Therefore, negative nitrite test results have little value in ruling out UTI. Moreover, not all urinary pathogens reduce nitrate to nitrite. The test is helpful when the result is positive, however, because it is highly specific (ie, there are few false-positive results).[32]

Leukocyte Esterase Test

The sensitivity of the leukocyte esterase test is 94% when it used in the context of clinically suspected UTI. Overall, the reported sensitivity in various studies is lower (83%), because the results of leukocyte esterase tests were related to culture results without exclusion of individuals with asymptomatic bacteriuria. The absence of leukocyte esterase in the urine of individuals with asymptomatic bacteriuria is an advantage of the test, rather than a limitation, because it distinguishes individuals with asymptomatic bacteriuria from those with true UTI.

The specificity of the leukocyte esterase test (average: 72% [range:

64%–92%]) generally is not as good as the sensitivity, which reflects the nonspecificity of pyuria in general. Accordingly, positive leukocyte esterase test results should be interpreted with caution, because false-positive results are common. With numerous conditions other than UTI, including fever resulting from other conditions (eg, streptococcal infections or Kawasaki disease), and after vigorous exercise, WBCs may be found in the urine. Therefore, a finding of pyuria by no means confirms that an infection of the urinary tract is present.

The absence of pyuria in children with true UTIs is rare, however. It is theoretically possible if a febrile child is assessed before the inflammatory response has developed, but the inflammatory response to a UTI produces both fever and pyuria; therefore, children who are being evaluated because of fever should already have WBCs in their urine. More likely explanations for significant bacteriuria in culture in the absence of pyuria include contaminated specimens, insensitive criteria for pyuria, and asymptomatic bacteriuria. In most cases, when true UTI has been reported to occur in the absence of pyuria, the definition of pyuria has been at fault. The standard method of assessing pyuria has been centrifugation of the urine and microscopic analysis, with a threshold of 5 WBCs per high-power field ($\sim$25 WBCs per μL). If a counting chamber is used, however, the finding of at least 10 WBCs per μL in uncentrifuged urine has been demonstrated to be more sensitive[33] and performs well in clinical situations in which the standard method does not, such as with very young infants.[34]

An important cause of bacteriuria in the absence of pyuria is asymptomatic bacteriuria. Asymptomatic bacteriuria often is associated with school-aged and older girls,[35] but it can be present

during infancy. In a study of infants 2 to 24 months of age, 0.7% of afebrile girls had 3 successive urine cultures with 10^5 CFUs per mL of a single uropathogen.[26] Asymptomatic bacteriuria can be easily confused with true UTI in a febrile infant but needs to be distinguished, because studies suggest that antimicrobial treatment may do more harm than good.[36] The key to distinguishing true UTI from asymptomatic bacteriuria is the presence of pyuria.

Microscopic Analysis for Bacteriuria

The presence of bacteria in a fresh, Gram-stained specimen of uncentrifuged urine correlates with 10^5 CFUs per mL in culture.[37] An "enhanced urinalysis," combining the counting chamber assessment of pyuria noted previously with Gram staining of drops of uncentrifuged urine, with a threshold of at least 1 Gram-negative rod in 10 oil immersion fields, has greater sensitivity, specificity, and positive predictive value than does the standard urinalysis[33] and is the preferred method of urinalysis when appropriate equipment and personnel are available.

Automated Urinalysis

Automated methods to perform urinalysis are now being used in many hospitals and laboratories. Image-based systems use flow imaging analysis technology and software to classify particles in uncentrifuged urine specimens rapidly.[38] Results correlate well with manual methods, especially for red blood cells, WBCs, and squamous epithelial cells. In the future, this may be the most common method by which urinalysis is performed in laboratories.

Culture

The diagnosis of UTI is made on the basis of quantitative urine culture results in addition to evidence of pyuria and/or bacteriuria. Urine specimens should be processed as expediently as possible. If the specimen is not processed promptly, then it should be refrigerated to prevent the growth of organisms that can occur in urine at room temperature; for the same reason, specimens that require transportation to another site for processing should be transported on ice. A properly collected urine specimen should be inoculated on culture medium that will allow identification of urinary tract pathogens.

Urine culture results are considered positive or negative on the basis of the number of CFUs that grow on the culture medium.[36] Definition of significant colony counts with regard to the method of collection considers that the distal urethra and periurethral area are commonly colonized by the same bacteria that may cause UTI; therefore, a low colony count may be present in a specimen obtained through voiding or catheterization when bacteria are not present in bladder urine. Definitions of positive and negative culture results are operational and not absolute. The time the urine resides in the bladder (bladder incubation time) is an important determinant of the magnitude of the colony count. The concept that more than 100 000 CFUs per mL indicates a UTI was based on morning collections of urine from adult women, with comparison of specimens from women without symptoms and women considered clinically to have pyelonephritis; the transition range, in which the proportion of women with pyelonephritis exceeded the proportion of women without symptoms, was 10 000 to 100 000 CFUs per mL.[39] In most instances, an appropriate threshold to consider bacteriuria "significant" in infants and children is the presence of at least 50 000 CFUs per mL of a single urinary pathogen.[40] (Organisms such as *Lactobacillus* spp, coagulase-negative staphylococci, and *Corynebacterium*

spp are not considered clinically relevant urine isolates for otherwise healthy, 2- to 24-month-old children.) Reducing the threshold from 100 000 CFUs per mL to 50 000 CFUs per mL would seem to increase the sensitivity of culture at the expense of decreased specificity; however, because the proposed criteria for UTI now include evidence of pyuria in addition to positive culture results, infants with "positive" culture results alone will be recognized as having asymptomatic bacteriuria rather than a true UTI. Some laboratories report growth only in the following categories: 0 to 1000, 1000 to 10 000, 10 000 to 100 000, and more than 100 000 CFUs per mL. In such cases, results in the 10 000 to 100 000 CFUs per mL range need to be evaluated in context, such as whether the urinalysis findings support the diagnosis of UTI and whether the organism is a recognized uropathogen.

Alternative culture methods, such as dipslides, may have a place in the office setting; sensitivity is reported to be in the range of 87% to 100%, and specificity is reported to be 92% to 98%, but dipslides cannot specify the organism or antimicrobial sensitivities.[41] Practices that use dipslides should do so in collaboration with a certified laboratory for identification and sensitivity testing or, in the absence of such results, may need to perform "test of cure" cultures after 24 hours of treatment.

- Aggregate quality of evidence: C (observational studies).
- Benefits: Accurate diagnosis of UTI can prevent the spread of infection and renal scarring; avoiding overdiagnosis of UTI can prevent overtreatment and unnecessary and expensive imaging. These criteria reduce the likelihood of overdiagnosis of UTI in infants with asymptomatic bacteriuria or contaminated specimens.

- Harms/risks/costs: Stringent diagnostic criteria may miss a small number of UTIs.
- Benefit-harms assessment: Preponderance of benefit over harm.
- Value judgments: Treatment of asymptomatic bacteriuria may be harmful.
- Role of patient preferences: We assume that parents prefer no action in the absence of a UTI (avoiding false-positive results) over a very small chance of missing a UTI.
- Exclusions: None.
- Intentional vagueness: None.
- Policy level: Recommendation.

MANAGEMENT

Action Statement 4

Action Statement 4a

When initiating treatment, the clinician should base the choice of route of administration on practical considerations. Initiating treatment orally or parenterally is equally efficacious. The clinician should base the choice of agent on local antimicrobial sensitivity patterns (if available) and should adjust the choice according to sensitivity testing of the isolated uropathogen (evidence quality: A; strong recommendation).

Action Statement 4b

The clinician should choose 7 to 14 days as the duration of antimicrobial therapy (evidence quality: B; recommendation).

The goals of treatment of acute UTI are to eliminate the acute infection, to prevent complications, and to reduce the likelihood of renal damage. Most children can be treated orally.[42–44] Patients whom clinicians judge to be "toxic" or who are unable to retain oral intake (including medications) should receive an antimicrobial agent parenter-

TABLE 2 Some Empiric Antimicrobial Agents for Parenteral Treatment of UTI

Antimicrobial Agent	Dosage
Ceftriaxone	75 mg/kg, every 24 h
Cefotaxime	150 mg/kg per d, divided every 6–8 h
Ceftazidime	100–150 mg/kg per d, divided every 8 h
Gentamicin	7.5 mg/kg per d, divided every 8 h
Tobramycin	5 mg/kg per d, divided every 8 h
Piperacillin	300 mg/kg per d, divided every 6–8 h

TABLE 3 Some Empiric Antimicrobial Agents for Oral Treatment of UTI

Antimicrobial Agent	Dosage
Amoxicillin-clavulanate	20–40 mg/kg per d in 3 doses
Sulfonamide	
Trimethoprim-sulfamethoxazole	6–12 mg/kg trimethoprim and 30-60 mg/kg sulfamethoxazole per d in 2 doses
Sulfisoxazole	120–150 mg/kg per d in 4 doses
Cephalosporin	
Cefixime	8 mg/kg per d in 1 dose
Cefpodoxime	10 mg/kg per d in 2 doses
Cefprozil	30 mg/kg per d in 2 doses
Cefuroxime axetil	20–30 mg/kg per d in 2 doses
Cephalexin	50–100 mg/kg per d in 4 doses

ally (Table 2) until they exhibit clinical improvement, generally within 24 to 48 hours, and are able to retain orally administered fluids and medications. In a study of 309 febrile infants with UTIs, only 3 (1%) were deemed too ill to be assigned randomly to either parenteral or oral treatment.[42] Parenteral administration of an antimicrobial agent also should be considered when compliance with obtaining an antimicrobial agent and/or administering it orally is uncertain. The usual choices for oral treatment of UTIs include a cephalosporin, amoxicillin plus clavulanic acid, or trimethoprim-sulfamethoxazole (Table 3). It is essential to know local patterns of susceptibility of coliforms to antimicrobial agents, particularly trimethoprim-sulfamethoxazole and cephalexin, because there is substantial geographic variability that needs to be taken into account during selection of an antimicrobial agent before sensitivity results are available. Agents that are excreted in the urine but do not achieve therapeutic concentrations in the bloodstream, such as nitrofurantoin, should not be used to treat febrile infants with UTIs, because parenchymal and serum antimicrobial concentrations may be insufficient to treat pyelonephritis or urosepsis.

Whether the initial route of administration of the antimicrobial agent is oral or parenteral (then changed to oral),

the total course of therapy should be 7 to 14 days. The committee attempted to identify a single, preferred, evidence-based duration, rather than a range, but data comparing 7, 10, and 14 days directly were not found. There is evidence that 1- to 3-day courses for febrile UTIs are inferior to courses in the recommended range; therefore, the minimal duration selected should be 7 days.

- Aggregate quality of evidence: A/B (RCTs).

- Benefits: Adequate treatment of UTI can prevent the spread of infection and renal scarring. Outcomes of short courses (1–3 d) are inferior to those of 7- to 14-d courses.

- Harms/risks/costs: There are minimal harm and minor cost effects of antimicrobial choice and duration of therapy.

- Benefit-harms assessment: Preponderance of benefit over harm.

- Value judgments: Adjusting antimicrobial choice on the basis of available data and treating according to best evidence will minimize cost and consequences of failed or unnecessary treatment.

- Role of patient preferences: It is assumed that parents prefer the most-effective treatment and the least amount of medication that ensures effective treatment.

- Exclusions: None.

- Intentional vagueness: No evidence

distinguishes the benefit of treating 7 vs 10 vs 14 days, and the range is allowable.

- Policy level: Strong recommendation/ recommendation.

Action Statement 5

Febrile infants with UTIs should undergo renal and bladder ultrasonography (RBUS) (evidence quality: C; recommendation).

The purpose of RBUS is to detect anatomic abnormalities that require further evaluation, such as additional imaging or urologic consultation. RBUS also provides an evaluation of the renal parenchyma and an assessment of renal size that can be used to monitor renal growth. The yield of actionable findings is relatively low.[45,46] Widespread application of prenatal ultrasonography clearly has reduced the prevalence of previously unsuspected obstructive uropathy in infants, but the consequences of prenatal screening with respect to the risk of renal abnormalities in infants with UTIs have not yet been well defined. There is considerable variability in the timing and quality of prenatal ultrasonograms, and the report of "normal" ultrasonographic results cannot necessarily be relied on to dismiss completely the possibility of a structural abnormality unless the study was a detailed anatomic survey (with measurements), was performed during the third trimester, and was performed and interpreted by qualified individuals.[47]

The timing of RBUS depends on the clinical situation. RBUS is recommended during the first 2 days of treatment to identify serious complications, such as renal or perirenal abscesses or pyonephrosis associated with obstructive uropathy when the clinical illness is unusually severe or substantial clinical improvement is not occurring. For febrile infants with UTIs who demonstrate substantial clinical improvement, however, imaging does not need to occur early during the acute infection and can even be misleading; animal studies demonstrate that *Escherichia coli* endotoxin can produce dilation during acute infection, which could be confused with hydronephrosis, pyonephrosis, or obstruction.[48] Changes in the size and shape of the kidneys and the echogenicity of renal parenchyma attributable to edema also are common during acute infection. The presence of these abnormalities makes it inappropriate to consider RBUS performed early during acute infection to be a true baseline study for later comparisons in the assessment of renal growth.

Nuclear scanning with technetium-labeled dimercaptosuccinic acid has greater sensitivity for detection of acute pyelonephritis and later scarring than does either RBUS or voiding cystourethrography (VCUG). The scanning is useful in research, because it ensures that all subjects in a study have pyelonephritis to start with and it permits assessment of later renal scarring as an outcome measure. The findings on nuclear scans rarely affect acute clinical management, however, and are not recommended as part of routine evaluation of infants with their first febrile UTI. The radiation dose to the patient during dimercaptosuccinic acid scanning is generally low (~1 mSv),[49] although it may be increased in

children with reduced renal function. The radiation dose from dimercaptosuccinic acid is additive with that of VCUG when both studies are performed.[50] The radiation dose from VCUG depends on the equipment that is used (conventional versus pulsed digital fluoroscopy) and is related directly to the total fluoroscopy time. Moreover, the total exposure for the child will be increased when both acute and follow-up studies are obtained. The lack of exposure to radiation is a major advantage of RBUS, even with recognition of the limitations of this modality that were described previously.

- Aggregate quality of evidence: C (observational studies).

- Benefits: RBUS in this population will yield abnormal results in ~15% of cases, and 1% to 2% will have abnormalities that would lead to action (eg, additional evaluation, referral, or surgery).

- Harms/risks/costs: Between 2% and 3% will be false-positive results, leading to unnecessary and invasive evaluations.

- Benefit-harms assessment: Preponderance of benefit over harm.

- Value judgments: The seriousness of the potentially correctable abnormalities in 1% to 2%, coupled with the absence of physical harm, was judged sufficiently important to tip the scales in favor of testing.

- Role of patient preferences: Because ultrasonography is noninvasive and poses minimal risk, we assume that parents will prefer RBUS over taking even a small risk of missing a serious and correctable condition.

- Exclusions: None.

- Intentional vagueness: None.

- Policy level: Recommendation.

Action Statement 6

Action Statement 6a

VCUG should not be performed routinely after the first febrile UTI; VCUG is indicated if RBUS reveals hydronephrosis, scarring, or other findings that would suggest either high-grade VUR or obstructive uropathy, as well as in other atypical or complex clinical circumstances (evidence quality B; recommendation).

Action Statement 6b

Further evaluation should be conducted if there is a recurrence of febrile UTI (evidence quality: X; recommendation).

For the past 4 decades, the strategy to protect the kidneys from further damage after an initial UTI has been to detect childhood genitourinary abnormalities in which recurrent UTI could increase renal damage. The most common of these is VUR, and VCUG is used to detect this. Management included continuous antimicrobial administration as prophylaxis and surgical intervention if VUR was persistent or recurrences of infection were not prevented with an antimicrobial prophylaxis regimen; some have advocated surgical intervention to correct high-grade reflux even when infection has not recurred. However, it is clear that there are a significant number of infants who develop pyelonephritis in whom VUR cannot be demonstrated, and the effectiveness of antimicrobial prophylaxis for patients who have VUR has been challenged in the past decade. Several studies have suggested that prophylaxis does not confer the desired benefit of preventing recurrent febrile UTI.[51–55] If prophylaxis is, in fact, not beneficial and VUR is not required for development of pyelonephritis, then the rationale for performing VCUG routinely after an initial febrile UTI must be questioned.

RCTs of the effectiveness of prophylaxis performed to date generally included children more than 24 months of age, and some did not provide complete data according to grade of VUR. These 2 factors have compromised meta-analyses. To ensure direct comparisons, the committee contacted the 6 researchers who had conducted the most recent RCTs and requested raw data from their studies.[51–56] All complied, which permitted the creation of a data set with data for 1091 infants 2 to 24 months of age according to grade of VUR. A χ^2 analysis (2-tailed) and a formal meta-analysis did not detect a statistically significant benefit of prophylaxis in preventing recurrence of febrile UTI/pyelonephritis in infants without reflux or those with grades I, II, III, or IV VUR (Table 4 and Fig 3). Only 5 infants with grade V VUR were included in the RCTs; therefore, data for those infants are not included in Table 4 or Fig 3.

The proportion of infants with high-grade VUR among all infants with febrile UTIs is small. Data adapted from current studies (Table 5) indicate that, of a hypothetical cohort of 100 infants with febrile UTIs, only 1 has grade V VUR; 99 do not. With a practice of waiting for a second UTI to perform VCUG, only 10 of the 100 would need to undergo the procedure and the 1 with grade V VUR would be identified. (It also is possible that the 1 infant with grade V VUR might have been identified after the first UTI on the basis of abnormal RBUS results that prompted VCUG to be performed.) Data to quantify additional potential harm to an infant who is not revealed to have high-grade VUR until a second UTI are not precise but suggest that the increment is insufficient to justify routinely subjecting all infants with an initial febrile UTI to VCUG (Fig 4). To minimize any harm incurred by that infant, attempts have been made to identify, at the time of

TABLE 4 Recurrences of Febrile UTI/Pyelonephritis in Infants 2 to 24 Months of Age With and Without Antimicrobial Prophylaxis, According to Grade of VUR

Reflux Grade	Prophylaxis		No Prophylaxis		P
	No. of Recurrences	Total N	No. of Recurrences	Total N	
None	7	210	11	163	.15
I	2	37	2	35	1.00
II	11	133	10	124	.95
III	31	140	40	145	.29
IV	16	55	21	49	.14

the initial UTI, those who have the greatest likelihood of having high-grade VUR. Unfortunately, there are no clinical or laboratory indicators that have been demonstrated to identify infants with high-grade VUR. Indications for VCUG have been proposed on the basis of consensus in the absence of data[57]; the predictive value of any of the indications for VCUG proposed in this manner is not known.

The level of evidence supporting routine imaging with VCUG was deemed insufficient at the time of the 1999 practice parameter to receive a recommendation, but the consensus of the subcommittee was to "strongly encourage" imaging studies. The position of the current subcommittee reflects the new evidence demonstrating antimicrobial prophylaxis not to be effective as presumed previously. Moreover, prompt diagnosis and effective treatment of a febrile UTI recurrence may be of greater importance regardless of whether VUR is present or the child is receiving antimicrobial prophylaxis. A national study (the Randomized Intervention for Children With Vesicoureteral Reflux study) is currently in progress to identify the effects of a prophylactic antimicrobial regimen for children 2 months to 6 years of age who have experienced a UTI, and it is anticipated to provide additional important data[58] (see Areas for Research).

Action Statement 6a

- Aggregate quality of evidence: B (RCTs).

- Benefits: This avoids, for the vast majority of febrile infants with UTIs, radiation exposure (of particular concern near the ovaries in girls), expense, and discomfort.

- Harms/risks/costs: Detection of a small number of cases of high-grade reflux and correctable abnormalities is delayed.

- Benefit-harms assessment: Preponderance of benefit over harm.

- Value judgments: The risks associated with radiation (plus the expense and discomfort of the procedure) for the vast majority of infants outweigh the risk of delaying the detection of the few with correctable abnormalities until their second UTI.

- Role of patient preferences: The judgment of parents may come into play, because VCUG is an uncomfortable procedure involving radiation exposure. In some cases, parents may prefer to subject their children to the procedure even when the chance of benefit is both small and uncertain. Antimicrobial prophylaxis seems to be ineffective in preventing recurrence of febrile UTI/pyelonephritis for the vast majority of infants. Some parents may want to avoid VCUG even after the second UTI. Because the benefit of identifying high-grade reflux is still in some doubt, these preferences should be considered. It is the judgment of the committee that VCUG is indicated after the second UTI.

- Exclusions: None.

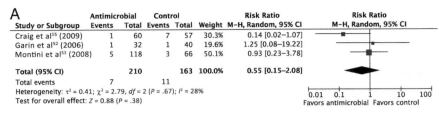

A

Study or Subgroup	Antimicrobial Events	Total	Control Events	Total	Weight	Risk Ratio M–H, Random, 95% CI
Craig et al⁵⁵ (2009)	1	60	7	57	30.3%	0.14 [0.02–1.07]
Garin et al⁵² (2006)	1	32	1	40	19.6%	1.25 [0.08–19.22]
Montini et al⁵³ (2008)	5	118	3	66	50.1%	0.93 [0.23–3.78]
Total (95% CI)		**210**		**163**	**100.0%**	**0.55 [0.15–2.08]**
Total events	7		11			

Heterogeneity: τ² = 0.41; χ² = 2.79, df = 2 (P = .67); I² = 28%
Test for overall effect: Z = 0.88 (P = .38)

Risk Ratio M–H, Random, 95% CI — 0.01 0.1 1 10 100 — Favors antimicrobial Favors control

B

Study or Subgroup	Antimicrobial Events	Total	Control Events	Total	Weight	Risk Ratio M–H, Random, 95% CI
Craig et al⁵⁵ (2009)	1	10	1	12	49.9%	1.20 [0.09–16.84]
Garin et al⁵² (2006)	0	5	0	3		Not estimable
Montini et al⁵³ (2008)	1	15	1	8	50.1%	0.53 [0.04–7.44]
Roussey-Kesler et al⁵⁴ (2008)	0	7	0	12		Not estimable
Total (95% CI)		**37**		**35**	**100.0%**	**0.80 [0.12–5.16]**
Total events	2		2			

Heterogeneity: τ² = 0.00; χ² = 0.18, df = 1 (P = .67); I² = 0%
Test for overall effect: z = 0.24 (P = .81)

Risk Ratio M–H, Random, 95% CI — 0.01 0.1 1 10 100 — Favors antimicrobial Favors control

C

Study or Subgroup	Antimicrobial Events	Total	Control Events	Total	Weight	Risk Ratio M–H, Random, 95% CI
Craig et al⁵⁵ (2009)	0	27	1	23	6.3%	0.29 [0.01–6.69]
Garin et al⁵² (2006)	1	12	0	10	6.5%	2.54 [0.11–56.25]
Montini et al⁵³ (2008)	3	31	2	18	21.7%	0.87 [0.16–4.73]
Pennesi et al⁵¹ (2008)	1	11	0	10	6.5%	2.75 [0.12–60.70]
Roussey-Kesler et al⁵⁴ (2008)	6	52	7	63	59.0%	1.04 [0.37–2.90]
Total (95% CI)		**133**		**124**	**100.0%**	**1.04 [0.47–2.29]**
Total events	11		10			

Heterogeneity: τ² = 0.00; χ² = 1.38, df = 4 (P = .85); I² = 0%
Test for overall effect: z = 0.10 (P = .92)

Risk Ratio M–H, Random, 95% CI — 0.01 0.1 1 10 100 — Favors antimicrobial Favors control

D

Study or Subgroup	Antimicrobial Events	Total	Control Events	Total	Weight	Risk Ratio M–H, Random, 95% CI
Brandström et al⁵⁶ (2010)	5	41	14	43	20.9%	0.37 [0.15–0.95]
Craig et al⁵⁵ (2009)	1	24	4	29	7.1%	0.30 [0.04–2.53]
Garin et al⁵² (2006)	4	8	0	12	4.5%	13.00 [0.79–212.80]
Montini et al⁵³ (2008)	6	22	6	13	21.5%	0.59 [0.24–1.45]
Pennesi et al⁵¹ (2008)	9	22	7	24	23.6%	1.40 [0.63–3.12]
Roussey-Kesler et al⁵⁴ (2008)	6	23	9	24	22.3%	0.70 [0.29–1.64]
Total (95% CI)		**140**		**145**	**100.0%**	**0.75 [0.40–1.40]**
Total events	31		40			

Heterogeneity: τ² = 0.27; χ² = 9.54, df = 5 (P = .09); I² = 48%
Test for overall effect: z = 0.90 (P = .37)

Risk Ratio M–H, Random, 95% CI — 0.01 0.1 1 10 100 — Favors antimicrobial Favors control

E

Study or Subgroup	Antimicrobial Events	Total	Control Events	Total	Weight	Risk Ratio M–H, Random, 95% CI
Brandström et al⁵⁶ (2010)	5	28	11	25	35.0%	0.41 [0.16–1.01]
Craig et al⁵⁵ (2009)	3	10	2	8	14.8%	1.20 [0.26–5.53]
Pennesi et al⁵¹ (2008)	8	17	8	16	50.2%	0.94 [0.47–1.90]
Total (95% CI)		**55**		**49**	**100.0%**	**0.73 [0.39–1.35]**
Total events	16		21			

Heterogeneity: τ² = 0.07; χ² = 2.57, df = 2 (P = .28); I² = 22%
Test for overall effect: z = 1.01 (P = .31)

Risk Ratio M–H, Random, 95% CI — 0.01 0.1 1 10 100 — Favors antimicrobial Favors control

FIGURE 3

A, Recurrences of febrile UTI/pyelonephritis in 373 infants 2 to 24 months of age without VUR, with and without antimicrobial prophylaxis (based on 3 studies; data provided by Drs Craig, Garin, and Montini). B, Recurrences of febrile UTI/pyelonephritis in 72 infants 2 to 24 months of age with grade I VUR, with and without antimicrobial prophylaxis (based on 4 studies; data provided by Drs Craig, Garin, Montini, and Roussey-Kesler). C, Recurrences of febrile UTI/pyelonephritis in 257 infants 2 to 24 months of age with grade II VUR, with and without antimicrobial prophylaxis (based on 5 studies; data provided by Drs Craig, Garin, Montini, Pennesi, and Roussey-Kesler). D, Recurrences of febrile UTI/ pyelonephritis in 285 infants 2 to 24 months of age with grade III VUR, with and without antimicrobial prophylaxis (based on 6 studies; data provided by Drs Brandström, Craig, Garin, Montini, Pennesi, and Roussey-Kesler). E, Recurrences of febrile UTI/pyelonephritis in 104 infants 2 to 24 months of age with grade IV VUR, with and without antimicrobial prophylaxis (based on 3 studies; data provided by Drs Brandström, Craig, and Pennesi). M-H indicates Mantel-Haenszel; CI, confidence interval.

TABLE 5 Rates of VUR According to Grade in Hypothetical Cohort of Infants After First UTI and After Recurrence

	Rate, %	
	After First UTI (N = 100)	After Recurrence (N = 10)
No VUR	65	26
Grades I–III VUR	29	56
Grade IV VUR	5	12
Grade V VUR	1	6

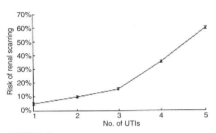

FIGURE 4

Relationship between renal scarring and number of bouts of pyelonephritis. Adapted from Jodal.⁵⁹

- Intentional vagueness: None.
- Policy level: Recommendation.

Action Statement 6b

- Aggregate quality of evidence: X (exceptional situation).
- Benefits: VCUG after a second UTI should identify infants with very high-grade reflux.
- Harms/risks/costs: VCUG is an uncomfortable, costly procedure that involves radiation, including to the ovaries of girls.
- Benefit-harms assessment: Preponderance of benefit over harm.
- Value judgments: The committee judged that patients with high-grade reflux and other abnormalities may benefit from interventions to prevent further scarring. Further studies of treatment for grade V VUR are not underway and are unlikely in the near future, because the condition is uncommon and randomization of treatment in this group generally has been considered unethical.

- Role of patient preferences: As mentioned previously, the judgment of parents may come into play, because VCUG is an uncomfortable procedure involving radiation exposure. In some cases, parents may prefer to subject their children to the procedure even when the chance of benefit is both small and uncertain. The benefits of treatment of VUR remain unproven, but the point estimates suggest a small potential benefit. Similarly, parents may want to avoid VCUG even after the second UTI. Because the benefit of identifying high-grade reflux is still in some doubt, these preferences should be considered. It is the judgment of the committee that VCUG is indicated after the second UTI.

- Exclusions: None.

- Intentional vagueness: Further evaluation will likely start with VCUG but may entail additional studies depending on the findings. The details of further evaluation are beyond the scope of this guideline.

- Policy level: Recommendation.

Action Statement 7

After confirmation of UTI, the clinician should instruct parents or guardians to seek prompt medical evaluation (ideally within 48 hours) for future febrile illnesses, to ensure that recurrent infections can be detected and treated promptly (evidence quality: C; recommendation).

Early treatment limits renal damage better than late treatment,[1,2] and the risk of renal scarring increases as the number of recurrences increase (Fig 4).[59] For these reasons, all infants who have sustained a febrile UTI should have a urine specimen obtained at the onset of subsequent febrile illnesses, so that a UTI can be diagnosed and treated promptly.

- Aggregate quality of evidence: C (observational studies).

- Benefits: Studies suggest that early treatment of UTI reduces the risk of renal scarring.

- Harms/risks/costs: There may be additional costs and inconvenience to parents with more-frequent visits to the clinician for evaluation of fever.

- Benefit-harms assessment: Preponderance of benefit over harm.

- Value judgments: None.

- Role of patient preferences: Parents will ultimately make the judgment to seek medical care.

- Exclusions: None.

- Intentional vagueness: None.

- Policy level: Recommendation.

CONCLUSIONS

The committee formulated 7 key action statements for the diagnosis and treatment of infants and young children 2 to 24 months of age with UTI and unexplained fever. Strategies for diagnosis and treatment depend on whether the clinician determines that antimicrobial therapy is warranted immediately or can be delayed safely until urine culture and urinalysis results are available. Diagnosis is based on the presence of pyuria and at least 50 000 CFUs per mL of a single uropathogen in an appropriately collected specimen of urine; urinalysis alone does not provide a definitive diagnosis. After 7 to 14 days of antimicrobial treatment, close clinical follow-up monitoring should be maintained, with evaluation of the urine during subsequent febrile episodes to permit prompt diagnosis and treatment of recurrent infections. Ultrasonography of the kidneys and bladder should be performed to detect anatomic abnormalities that require further evaluation (eg, additional imaging or urologic consultation). Routine VCUG after the

first UTI is not recommended; VCUG is indicated if RBUS reveals hydronephrosis, scarring, or other findings that would suggest either high-grade VUR or obstructive uropathy, as well as in other atypical or complex clinical circumstances. VCUG also should be performed if there is a recurrence of febrile UTI.

AREAS FOR RESEARCH

One of the major values of a comprehensive literature review is the identification of areas in which evidence is lacking. The following 8 areas are presented in an order that parallels the previous discussion.

1. The relationship between UTIs in infants and young children and reduced renal function in adults has been established but is not well characterized in quantitative terms. The ideal prospective cohort study from birth to 40 to 50 years of age has not been conducted and is unlikely to be conducted. Therefore, estimates of undesirable outcomes in adulthood, such as hypertension and end-stage renal disease, are based on the mathematical product of probabilities at several steps, each of which is subject to bias and error. Other attempts at decision analysis and thoughtful literature review have recognized the same limitations. Until recently, imaging tools available for assessment of the effects of UTIs have been insensitive. With the imaging techniques now available, it may be possible to identify the relationship of scarring to renal impairment and hypertension.

2. The development of techniques that would permit an alternative to invasive sampling and culture would be valuable for general use. Special attention should be given to infant girls and uncircumcised boys, because urethral catheterization may

be difficult and can produce contaminated specimens and SPA now is not commonly performed. Incubation time, which is inherent in the culture process, results in delayed treatment or presumptive treatment on the basis of tests that lack the desired sensitivity and specificity to replace culture.

3. The role of VUR (and therefore of VCUG) is incompletely understood. It is recognized that pyelonephritis (defined through cortical scintigraphy) can occur in the absence of VUR (defined through VCUG) and that progressive renal scarring (defined through cortical scintigraphy) can occur in the absence of demonstrated VUR.[52,53] The presumption that antimicrobial prophylaxis is of benefit for individuals with VUR to prevent recurrences of UTI or the development of renal scars is not supported by the aggregate of data from recent studies and currently is the subject of the Randomized Intervention for Children With Vesicoureteral Reflux study.[58]

4. Although the effectiveness of antimicrobial prophylaxis for the prevention of UTI has not been demonstrated, the concept has biological plausibility. Virtually all antimicrobial agents used to treat or to prevent infections of the urinary tract are excreted in the urine in high concentrations. Barriers to the effectiveness of antimicrobial prophylaxis are adherence to a daily regimen, adverse effects associated with the various agents, and the potential for emergence of anti-

microbial resistance. To overcome these issues, evidence of effectiveness with a well-tolerated, safe product would be required, and parents would need sufficient education to understand the value and importance of adherence. A urinary antiseptic, rather than an antimicrobial agent, would be particularly desirable, because it could be taken indefinitely without concern that bacteria would develop resistance. Another possible strategy might be the use of probiotics.

5. Better understanding of the genome (human and bacterial) may provide insight into risk factors (VUR and others) that lead to increased scarring. Blood specimens will be retained from children enrolled in the Randomized Intervention for Children With Vesicoureteral Reflux study, for future examination of genetic determinants of VUR, recurrent UTI, and renal scarring.[58] VUR is recognized to "run in families,"[60,61] and multiple investigators are currently engaged in research to identify a genetic basis for VUR. Studies may also be able to distinguish the contribution of congenital dysplasia from acquired scarring attributable to UTI.

6. One of the factors used to assess the likelihood of UTI in febrile infants is race. Data regarding rates among Hispanic individuals are limited and would be useful for prediction rules.

7. This guideline is limited to the initial management of the first UTI in febrile infants 2 to 24 months of age. Some of

the infants will have recurrent UTIs; some will be identified as having VUR or other abnormalities. Further research addressing the optimal course of management in specific situations would be valuable.

8. The optimal duration of antimicrobial treatment has not been determined. RCTs of head-to-head comparisons of various duration would be valuable, enabling clinicians to limit antimicrobial exposure to what is needed to eradicate the offending uropathogen.

LEAD AUTHOR

Kenneth B. Roberts, MD

SUBCOMMITTEE ON URINARY TRACT INFECTION, 2009–2011

Kenneth B. Roberts, MD, Chair
Stephen M. Downs, MD, MS
S. Maria E. Finnell, MD, MS
Stanley Hellerstein, MD
Linda D. Shortliffe, MD
Ellen R. Wald, MD
J. Michael Zerin, MD

OVERSIGHT BY THE STEERING COMMITTEE ON QUALITY IMPROVEMENT AND MANAGEMENT, 2009–2011

STAFF

Caryn Davidson, MA

ACKNOWLEDGMENTS

The committee gratefully acknowledges the generosity of the researchers who graciously shared their data to permit the data set with data for 1091 infants aged 2 to 24 months according to grade of VUR to be compiled, that is, Drs Per Brandström, Jonathan Craig, Eduardo Garin, Giovanni Montini, Marco Pennesi, and Gwenaelle Roussey-Kesler.

REFERENCES

1. Winter AL, Hardy BE, Alton DJ, Arbus GS, Churchill BM. Acquired renal scars in children. *J Urol.* 1983;129(6):1190–1194

2. Smellie JM, Poulton A, Prescod NP. Retrospective study of children with renal scarring associated with reflux and urinary infection. *BMJ.* 1994;308(6938):1193–1196

3. American Academy of Pediatrics, Committee on Quality Improvement, Subcommittee on Urinary Tract Infection. Practice parameter: the diagnosis, treatment, and evaluation of the initial urinary tract infection in febrile infants and young children. *Pediatrics.* 1999;103(4):843–852

4. Finnell SM, Carroll AE, Downs SM, et al. Technical report: diagnosis and management of an initial urinary tract infection in febrile infants and young children. *Pediatrics.* 2011;128(3):e749

5. American Academy of Pediatrics, Steering Committee on Quality Improvement and Management. Classifying recommenda-

tions for clinical practice guidelines. *Pediatrics*. 2004;114(3):874–877

6. Leong YY, Tan KW. Bladder aspiration for diagnosis of urinary tract infection in infants and young children. *J Singapore Paediatr Soc*. 1976;18(1):43–47

7. Pryles CV, Atkin MD, Morse TS, Welch KJ. Comparative bacteriologic study of urine obtained from children by percutaneous suprapubic aspiration of the bladder and by catheter. *Pediatrics*. 1959;24(6):983–991

8. Djojohadipringgo S, Abdul Hamid RH, Thahir S, Karim A, Darsono I. Bladder puncture in newborns: a bacteriological study. *Paediatr Indones*. 1976;16(11–12):527–534

9. Gochman RF, Karasic RB, Heller MB. Use of portable ultrasound to assist urine collection by suprapubic aspiration. *Ann Emerg Med*. 1991;20(6):631–635

10. Buys H, Pead L, Hallett R, Maskell R. Suprapubic aspiration under ultrasound guidance in children with fever of undiagnosed cause. *BMJ*. 1994;308(6930):690–692

11. Kramer MS, Tange SM, Drummond KN, Mills EL. Urine testing in young febrile children: a risk-benefit analysis. *J Pediatr*. 1994;125(1):6–13

12. Bonadio WA. Urine culturing technique in febrile infants. *Pediatr Emerg Care*. 1987;3(2):75–78

13. Lohr J. *Pediatric Outpatient Procedures*. Philadelphia, PA: Lippincott; 1991

14. Taylor CM, White RH. The feasibility of screening preschool children for urinary tract infection using dipslides. *Int J Pediatr Nephrol*. 1983;4(2):113–114

15. Sørensen K, Lose G, Nathan E. Urinary tract infections and diurnal incontinence in girls. *Eur J Pediatr*. 1988;148(2):146–147

16. Shannon F, Sepp E, Rose G. The diagnosis of bacteriuria by bladder puncture in infancy and childhood. *Aust Pediatr J*. 1969;5(2):97–100

17. Hoberman A, Chao HP, Keller DM, Hickey R, Davis HW, Ellis D. Prevalence of urinary tract infection in febrile infants. *J Pediatr*. 1993;123(1):17–23

18. Haddon RA, Barnett PL, Grimwood K, Hogg GG. Bacteraemia in febrile children presenting to a paediatric emergency department. *Med J Aust*. 1999;170(10):475–478

19. Wiswell TE, Roscelli JD. Corroborative evidence for the decreased incidence of urinary tract infections in circumcised male infants. *Pediatrics*. 1986;78(1):96–99

20. To T, Agha M, Dick PT, Feldman W. Cohort study on circumcision of newborn boys and subsequent risk of urinary-tract infection. *Lancet*. 1998;352(9143):1813–1816

21. Wiswell TE, Hachey WE. Urinary tract infections and the uncircumcised state: an update. *Clin Pediatr (Phila)*. 1993;32(3):130–134

22. Wiswell TE, Smith FR, Bass JW. Decreased incidence of urinary tract infections in circumcised male infants. *Pediatrics*. 1985;75(5):901–903

23. Ginsburg CM, McCracken GH Jr. Urinary tract infections in young infants. *Pediatrics*. 1982;69(4):409–412

24. Craig JC, Knight JF, Sureshkumar P, Mantz E, Roy LP. Effect of circumcision on incidence of urinary tract infection in preschool boys. *J Pediatr*. 1996;128(1):23–27

25. Levine DA, Platt SL, Dayan PS, et al. Risk of serious bacterial infection in young febrile infants with respiratory syncytial virus infections. *Pediatrics*. 2004;113(6):1728–1734

26. Roberts KB, Charney E, Sweren RJ, et al. Urinary tract infection in infants with unexplained fever: a collaborative study. *J Pediatr*. 1983;103(6):864–867

27. Gorelick MH, Hoberman A, Kearney D, Wald E, Shaw KN. Validation of a decision rule identifying febrile young girls at high risk for urinary tract infection. *Pediatr Emerg Care*. 2003;19(3):162–164

28. Gorelick MH, Shaw KN. Clinical decision rule to identify febrile young girls at risk for urinary tract infection. *Arch Pediatr Adolesc Med*. 2000;154(4):386–390

29. Shaw KN, Gorelick M, McGowan KL, Yakscoe NM, Schwartz JS. Prevalence of urinary tract infection in febrile young children in the emergency department. *Pediatrics*. 1998;102(2). Available at: www.pediatrics.org/cgi/content/full/102/2/e16

30. Shaikh N, Morone NE, Lopez J, et al. Does this child have a urinary tract infection? *JAMA*. 2007;298(24):2895–2904

31. Powell HR, McCredie DA, Ritchie MA. Urinary nitrite in symptomatic and asymptomatic urinary infection. *Arch Dis Child*. 1987;62(2):138–140

32. Kunin CM, DeGroot JE. Sensitivity of a nitrite indicator strip method in detecting bacteriuria in preschool girls. *Pediatrics*. 1977;60(2):244–245

33. Hoberman A, Wald ER, Reynolds EA, Penchansky L, Charron M. Is urine culture necessary to rule out urinary tract infection in young febrile children? *Pediatr Infect Dis J*. 1996;15(4):304–309

34. Herr SM, Wald ER, Pitetti RD, Choi SS. Enhanced urinalysis improves identification of febrile infants ages 60 days and younger at low risk for serious bacterial illness. *Pediatrics*. 2001;108(4):866–871

35. Kunin C. A ten-year study of bacteriuria in schoolgirls: final report of bacteriologic, urologic, and epidemiologic findings. *J Infect Dis*. 1970;122(5):382–393

36. Kemper K, Avner E. The case against screening urinalyses for asymptomatic bacteriuria in children. *Am J Dis Child*. 1992;146(3):343–346

37. Wald E. Genitourinary tract infections: cystitis and pyelonephritis. In: Feigin R, Cherry JD, Demmler GJ, Kaplan SL, eds. *Textbook of Pediatric Infectious Diseases*. 5th ed. Philadelphia, PA: Saunders; 2004:541–555

38. Mayo S, Acevedo D, Quiñones-Torrelo C, Canós I, Sancho M. Clinical laboratory automated urinalysis: comparison among automated microscopy, flow cytometry, two test strips analyzers, and manual microscopic examination of the urine sediments. *J Clin Lab Anal*. 2008;22(4):262–270

39. Kass E. Asymptomatic infections of the urinary tract. *Trans Assoc Am Phys*. 1956;69:56–64

40. Hoberman A, Wald ER, Reynolds EA, Penchansky L, Charron M. Pyuria and bacteriuria in urine specimens obtained by catheter from young children with fever. *J Pediatr*. 1994;124(4):513–519

41. Downs SM. Technical report: urinary tract infections in febrile infants and young children. *Pediatrics*. 1999;103(4). Available at: www.pediatrics.org/cgi/content/full/103/4/e54

42. Hoberman A, Wald ER, Hickey RW, et al. Oral versus initial intravenous therapy for urinary tract infections in young febrile children. *Pediatrics*. 1999;104(1):79–86

43. Hodson EM, Willis NS, Craig JC. Antibiotics for acute pyelonephritis in children. *Cochrane Database Syst Rev*. 2007;(4):CD003772

44. Bloomfield P, Hodson EM, Craig JC. Antibiotics for acute pyelonephritis in children. *Cochrane Database Syst Rev*. 2005;(1):CD003772

45. Hoberman A, Charron M, Hickey RW, Baskin M, Kearney DH, Wald ER. Imaging studies after a first febrile urinary tract infection in young children. *N Engl J Med*. 2003;348(3):195–202

46. Jahnukainen T, Honkinen O, Ruuskanen O, Mertsola J. Ultrasonography after the first febrile urinary tract infection in children. *Eur J Pediatr*. 2006;165(8):556–559

47. Economou G, Egginton J, Brookfield D. The importance of late pregnancy scans for renal tract abnormalities. *Prenat Diagn*. 1994;14(3):177–180

48. Roberts J. Experimental pyelonephritis in the monkey, part III: pathophysiology of ure-

teral malfunction induced by bacteria. *Invest Urol.* 1975;13(2):117–120

49. Smith T, Evans K, Lythgoe MF, Anderson PJ, Gordon I. Radiation dosimetry of technetium-99m-DMSA in children. *J Nucl Med.* 1996;37(8):1336–1342

50. Ward VL. Patient dose reduction during voiding cystourethrography. *Pediatr Radiol.* 2006;36(suppl 2):168–172

51. Pennesi M, Travan L, Peratoner L, et al. Is antibiotic prophylaxis in children with vesicoureteral reflux effective in preventing pyelonephritis and renal scars? A randomized, controlled trial. *Pediatrics.* 2008; 121(6). Available at: www.pediatrics.org/cgi/content/full/121/6/e1489

52. Garin EH, Olavarria F, Garcia Nieto V, Valenciano B, Campos A, Young L. Clinical significance of primary vesicoureteral reflux and urinary antibiotic prophylaxis after acute pyelonephritis: a multicenter, randomized, controlled study. *Pediatrics.* 2006;117(3): 626–632

53. Montini G, Rigon L, Zucchetta P, et al. Prophylaxis after first febrile urinary tract infection in children? A multicenter, randomized, controlled, noninferiority trial. *Pediatrics.* 2008;122(5):1064–1071

54. Roussey-Kesler G, Gadjos V, Idres N, et al. Antibiotic prophylaxis for the prevention of recurrent urinary tract infection in children with low grade vesicoureteral reflux: results from a prospective randomized study. *J Urol.* 2008;179(2):674–679

55. Craig J, Simpson J, Williams G. Antibiotic prophylaxis and recurrent urinary tract infection in children. *N Engl J Med.* 2009; 361(18):1748–1759

56. Brandström P, Esbjorner E, Herthelius M, Swerkersson S, Jodal U, Hansson S. The Swedish Reflux Trial in Children, part III: urinary tract infection pattern. *J Urol.* 2010; 184(1):286–291

57. National Institute for Health and Clinical Excellence. *Urinary Tract Infection in Children: Diagnosis, Treatment, and Long-term Management: NICE Clinical Guideline 54.* London, England: National Institute for Health and Clinical Excellence; 2007. Available at: www.nice.org.uk/nicemedia/live/11819/36032/36032.pdf. Accessed March 14, 2011

58. Keren R, Carpenter MA, Hoberman A, et al. Rationale and design issues of the Randomized Intervention for Children With Vesicoureteral Reflux (RIVUR) study. *Pediatrics.* 2008;122(suppl 5):S240–S250

59. Jodal U. The natural history of bacteriuria in childhood. *Infect Dis Clin North Am.* 1987; 1(4):713–729

60. Eccles MR, Bailey RR, Abbott GD, Sullivan MJ. Unravelling the genetics of vesicoureteric reflux: a common familial disorder. *Hum Mol Genet.* 1996;5(Spec No.):1425–1429

61. Scott JE, Swallow V, Coulthard MG, Lambert HJ, Lee RE. Screening of newborn babies for familial ureteric reflux. *Lancet.* 1997; 350(9075):396–400

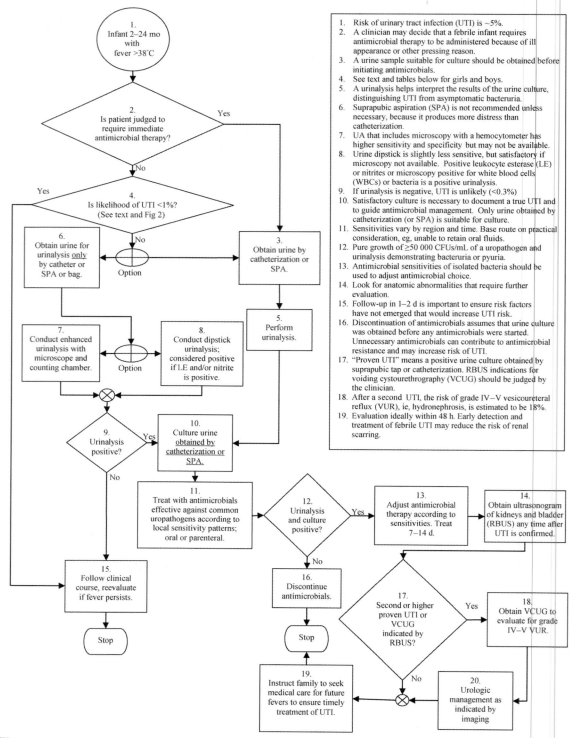

1. Risk of urinary tract infection (UTI) is ~5%.
2. A clinician may decide that a febrile infant requires antimicrobial therapy to be administered because of ill appearance or other pressing reason.
3. A urine sample suitable for culture should be obtained before initiating antimicrobials.
4. See text and tables below for girls and boys.
5. A urinalysis helps interpret the results of the urine culture, distinguishing UTI from asymptomatic bacteriuria.
6. Suprapubic aspiration (SPA) is not recommended unless necessary, because it produces more distress than catheterization.
7. UA that includes microscopy with a hemocytometer has higher sensitivity and specificity but may not be available.
8. Urine dipstick is slightly less sensitive, but satisfactory if microscopy not available. Positive leukocyte esterase (LE) or nitrites or microscopy positive for white blood cells (WBCs) or bacteria is a positive urinalysis.
9. If urinalysis is negative, UTI is unlikely (<0.3%)
10. Satisfactory culture is necessary to document a true UTI and to guide antimicrobial management. Only urine obtained by catheterization (or SPA) is suitable for culture.
11. Sensitivities vary by region and time. Base route on practical consideration, eg, unable to retain oral fluids.
12. Pure growth of ≥50 000 CFUs/mL of a uropathogen and urinalysis demonstrating bacteriuria or pyuria.
13. Antimicrobial sensitivities of isolated bacteria should be used to adjust antimicrobial choice.
14. Look for anatomic abnormalities that require further evaluation.
15. Follow-up in 1–2 d is important to ensure risk factors have not emerged that would increase UTI risk.
16. Discontinuation of antimicrobials assumes that urine culture was obtained before any antimicrobials were started. Unnecessary antimicrobials can contribute to antimicrobial resistance and may increase risk of UTI.
17. "Proven UTI" means a positive urine culture obtained by suprapubic tap or catheterization. RBUS indications for voiding cystourethrography (VCUG) should be judged by the clinician.
18. After a second UTI, the risk of grade IV–V vesicoureteral reflux (VUR), ie, hydronephrosis, is estimated to be 18%.
19. Evaluation ideally within 48 h. Early detection and treatment of febrile UTI may reduce the risk of renal scarring.

APPENDIX
Clinical practice guideline algorithm.

Urinary Tract Infection Clinical Practice Guideline Quick Reference Tools

• •

- Action Statement Summary
  — Urinary Tract Infection: Clinical Practice Guideline for the Diagnosis and Management of the Initial UTI in Febrile Infants and Children 2 to 24 Months
- *ICD-10-CM* Coding Quick Reference for Urinary Tract Infection
- AAP Patient Education Handout
  — *Urinary Tract Infections in Young Children*

Action Statement Summary

Urinary Tract Infection: Clinical Practice Guideline for the Diagnosis and Management of the Initial UTI in Febrile Infants and Children 2 to 24 Months

Action Statement 1

If a clinician decides that a febrile infant with no apparent source for the fever requires antimicrobial therapy to be administered because of ill appearance or another pressing reason, the clinician should ensure that a urine specimen is obtained for both culture and urinalysis before an antimicrobial agent is administered; the specimen needs to be obtained through catheterization or SPA, because the diagnosis of UTI cannot be established reliably through culture of urine collected in a bag (evidence quality: A; strong recommendation).

Action Statement 2

If a clinician assesses a febrile infant with no apparent source for the fever as not being so ill as to require immediate antimicrobial therapy, then the clinician should assess the likelihood of UTI (see below for how to assess likelihood).

Action Statement 2a

If the clinician determines the febrile infant to have a low likelihood of UTI (see text), then clinical follow-up monitoring without testing is sufficient (evidence quality: A; strong recommendation).

Action Statement 2b

If the clinician determines that the febrile infant is not in a low-risk group (see below), then there are 2 choices (evidence quality: A; strong recommendation). Option 1 is to obtain a urine specimen through catheterization or SPA for culture and urinalysis. Option 2 is to obtain a urine specimen through the most convenient means and to perform a urinalysis. If the urinalysis results suggest a UTI (positive leukocyte esterase test results or nitrite test or microscopic analysis results positive for leukocytes or bacteria), then a urine specimen should be obtained through catheterization or SPA and cultured; if urinalysis of fresh (<1 hour since void) urine yields negative leukocyte esterase and nitrite test results, then it is reasonable to monitor the clinical course without initiating antimicrobial therapy, recognizing that negative urinalysis results do not rule out a UTI with certainty.

Action Statement 3

To establish the diagnosis of UTI, clinicians should require *both* urinalysis results that suggest infection (pyuria and/or bacteriuria) *and* the presence of at least 50 000 colony-forming units (CFUs) per mL of a uropathogen cultured from a urine specimen obtained through catheterization or SPA (evidence quality: C; recommendation).

Action Statement 4a

When initiating treatment, the clinician should base the choice of route of administration on practical considerations. Initiating treatment orally or parenterally is equally efficacious. The clinician should base the choice of agent on local antimicrobial sensitivity patterns (if available) and should adjust the choice according to sensitivity testing of the isolated uropathogen (evidence quality: A; strong recommendation).

Action Statement 4b

The clinician should choose 7 to 14 days as the duration of antimicrobial therapy (evidence quality: B; recommendation).

Action Statement 5

Febrile infants with UTIs should undergo renal and bladder ultrasonography (RBUS) (evidence quality: C; recommendation).

Action Statement 6a

VCUG should not be performed routinely after the first febrile UTI; VCUG is indicated if RBUS reveals hydronephrosis, scarring, or other findings that would suggest either high-grade VUR or obstructive uropathy, as well as in other atypical or complex clinical circumstances (evidence quality B; recommendation).

Action Statement 6b

Further evaluation should be conducted if there is a recurrence of febrile UTI (evidence quality: X; recommendation).

Action Statement 7

After confirmation of UTI, the clinician should instruct parents or guardians to seek prompt medical evaluation (ideally within 48 hours) for future febrile illnesses, to ensure that recurrent infections can be detected and treated promptly (evidence quality: C; recommendation).

Coding Quick Reference for Urinary Tract Infection

ICD-10-CM

N39.0 Urinary tract infection, site not specified

P39.3 Neonatal urinary tract infection

Urinary Tract Infections in Young Children

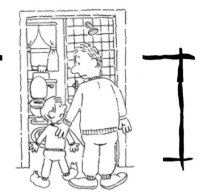

Urinary tract infections (UTIs) are common in young children. These infections can lead to serious health problems. UTIs may go untreated because the symptoms may not be obvious to the child or the parents. The following is information from the American Academy of Pediatrics about UTIs—what they are, how children get them, and how they are treated.

The urinary tract

The urinary tract makes and stores urine. It is made up of the kidneys, ureters, bladder, and urethra (see illustration on the next page). The kidneys produce urine. Urine travels from the kidneys down 2 narrow tubes called the ureters to the bladder. The bladder is a thin muscular bag that stores urine until it is time to empty urine out of the body. When it is time to empty the bladder, a muscle at the bottom of the bladder relaxes. Urine then flows out of the body through a tube called the urethra. The opening of the urethra is at the end of the penis in boys and above the vaginal opening in girls.

Urinary tract infections

Normal urine has no germs (bacteria). However, bacteria can get into the urinary tract from 2 sources: (1) the skin around the rectum and genitals and (2) the bloodstream from other parts of the body. Bacteria may cause infections in any or all parts of the urinary tract, including the following:

- Urethra (called urethritis)
- Bladder (called cystitis)
- Kidneys (called pyelonephritis)

UTIs are common in infants and young children. The frequency of UTIs in girls is much greater than in boys. About 3% of girls and 1% of boys will have a UTI by 11 years of age. A young child with a high fever and no other symptoms has a 1 in 20 chance of having a UTI. Uncircumcised boys have more UTIs than those who have been circumcised.

Symptoms

Symptoms of UTIs may include the following:

- Fever
- Pain or burning during urination
- Need to urinate more often, or difficulty getting urine out
- Urgent need to urinate, or wetting of underwear or bedding by a child who knows how to use the toilet
- Vomiting, refusal to eat
- Abdominal pain
- Side or back pain
- Foul-smelling urine
- Cloudy or bloody urine
- Unexplained and persistent irritability in an infant
- Poor growth in an infant

Diagnosis

If your child has symptoms of a UTI, your child's doctor will do the following:

- Ask about your child's symptoms.
- Ask about any family history of urinary tract problems.
- Ask about what your child has been eating and drinking.
- Examine your child.
- Get a urine sample from your child.

Your child's doctor will need to test your child's urine to see if there are bacteria or other abnormalities.

Ways urine is collected

Urine must be collected and analyzed to determine if there is a bacterial infection. Older children are asked to urinate into a container.

There are 3 ways to collect urine from a young child:

1. The preferred method is to place a small tube, called a catheter, through the urethra into the bladder. Urine flows through the tube into a special urine container.
2. Another method is to insert a needle through the skin of the lower abdomen to draw urine from the bladder. This is called needle aspiration.
3. If your child is very young or not yet toilet trained, the child's doctor may place a plastic bag over the genitals to collect the urine. Since bacteria on the skin can contaminate the urine and give a false test result, this method is used only to screen for infection. If an infection seems to be present, the doctor will need to collect urine through 1 of the first 2 methods in order to determine if bacteria are present.

Your child's doctor will discuss with you the best way to collect your child's urine.

Treatment

UTIs are treated with antibiotics. The way your child receives the antibiotic depends on the severity and type of infection. Antibiotics are usually given by mouth, as liquid or pills. If your child has a fever or is vomiting and is unable to keep fluids down, the antibiotics may be put directly into a vein or injected into a muscle.

UTIs need to be treated right away to

- Get rid of the infection.
- Prevent the spread of the infection outside of the urinary tract.
- Reduce the chances of kidney damage.

Infants and young children with UTIs usually need to take antibiotics for 7 to 14 days, sometimes longer. Make sure your child takes all the medicine your child's doctor prescribes. Do not stop giving your child the medicine until the child's doctor says the treatment is finished, even if your child feels better. UTIs can return if not fully treated.

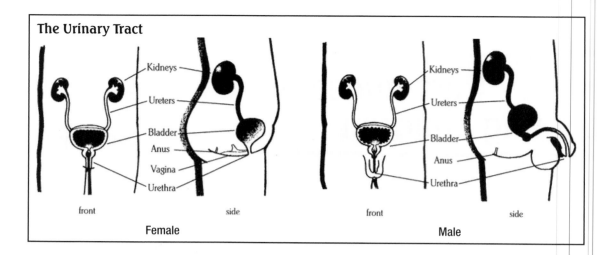

The Urinary Tract

Female

Male

Follow-up

If the UTI occurs early in life, your child's doctor will probably want to make sure the urinary tract is normal with a kidney and bladder ultrasound. This test uses sound waves to examine the bladder and kidneys.

In addition, your child's doctor may want to make sure that the urinary tract is functioning normally and is free of any damage. Several tests are available to do this, including the following:

Voiding cystourethrogram (VCUG). A catheter is placed into the urethra and the bladder is filled with a liquid that can be seen on x-rays. This test shows whether the urine is flowing back from the bladder toward the kidneys instead of all of it coming out through the urethra as it should.

Nuclear scans. Radioactive material is injected into a vein to see if the kidneys are normal. There are many kinds of nuclear scans, each giving different information about the kidneys and bladder. The radioactive material gives no more radiation than any other kind of x-ray.

Remember

UTIs are common and most are easy to treat. Early diagnosis and prompt treatment are important because untreated or repeated infections can cause long-term medical problems. Children who have had one UTI are more likely to have another. Be sure to see your child's doctor early if your child has had a UTI in the past and has fever. Talk with your child's doctor if you suspect that your child might have a UTI.

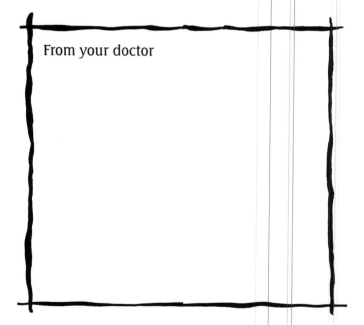

From your doctor

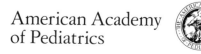

American Academy of Pediatrics

DEDICATED TO THE HEALTH OF ALL CHILDREN™

The American Academy of Pediatrics is an organization of 66,000 primary care pediatricians, pediatric medical subspecialists, and pediatric surgical specialists dedicated to the health, safety, and well-being of infants, children, adolescents, and young adults.

American Academy of Pediatrics
Web site — www.HealthyChildren.org

Section 2

Endorsed Clinical Practice Guidelines

The American Academy of Pediatrics endorses and accepts as its policy the following guidelines from other organizations.

AUTISM SPECTRUM DISORDER

Screening and Diagnosis of Autism
Quality Standards Subcommittee of the American Academy of Neurology and the Child Neurology Society

ABSTRACT. Autism is a common disorder of childhood, affecting 1 in 500 children. Yet, it often remains unrecognized and undiagnosed until or after late preschool age because appropriate tools for routine developmental screening and screening specifically for autism have not been available. Early identification of children with autism and intensive, early intervention during the toddler and preschool years improves outcome for most young children with autism. This practice parameter reviews the available empirical evidence and gives specific recommendations for the identification of children with autism. This approach requires a dual process: (1) routine developmental surveillance and screening specifically for autism to be performed on all children to first identify those at risk for any type of atypical development, and to identify those specifically at risk for autism; and (2) to diagnose and evaluate autism, to differentiate autism from other developmental disorders. (8/00)

CARDIOVASCULAR HEALTH

Expert Panel on Integrated Guidelines for Cardiovascular Health and Risk Reduction in Children and Adolescents: Summary Report
National Heart, Lung, and Blood Institute

INTRODUCTION (EXCERPT). Atherosclerotic cardiovascular disease (CVD) remains the leading cause of death in North Americans, but manifest disease in childhood and adolescence is rare. By contrast, risk factors and risk behaviors that accelerate the development of atherosclerosis begin in childhood, and there is increasing evidence that risk reduction delays progression toward clinical disease. In response, the former director of the National Heart, Lung, and Blood Institute (NHLBI), Dr Elizabeth Nabel, initiated development of cardiovascular health guidelines for pediatric care providers based on a formal evidence review of the science with an integrated format addressing all the major cardiovascular risk factors simultaneously. An expert panel was appointed to develop the guidelines in the fall of 2006. (10/12)

CEREBRAL PALSY

Diagnostic Assessment of the Child With Cerebral Palsy
Quality Standards Subcommittee of the American Academy of Neurology and the Practice Committee of the Child Neurology Society

ABSTRACT. *Objective.* The Quality Standards Subcommittee of the American Academy of Neurology and the Practice Committee of the Child Neurology Society develop practice parameters as strategies for patient management based on analysis of evidence. For this parameter the authors reviewed available evidence on the assessment of a child suspected of having cerebral palsy (CP), a nonprogressive disorder of posture or movement due to a lesion of the developing brain.

Methods. Relevant literature was reviewed, abstracted, and classified. Recommendations were based on a four-tiered scheme of evidence classification.

Results. CP is a common problem, occurring in about 2 to 2.5 per 1,000 live births. In order to establish that a brain abnormality exists in children with CP that may, in turn, suggest an etiology and prognosis, neuroimaging is recommended with MRI preferred to CT (Level A). Metabolic and genetic studies should not be routinely obtained in the evaluation of the child with CP (Level B). If the clinical history or findings on neuroimaging do not determine a specific structural abnormality or if there are additional and atypical features in the history or clinical examination, metabolic and genetic testing should be considered (Level C). Detection of a brain malformation in a child with CP warrants consideration of an underlying genetic or metabolic etiology. Because the incidence of cerebral infarction is high in children with hemiplegic CP, diagnostic testing for coagulation disorders should be considered (Level B). However, there is insufficient evidence at present to be precise as to what studies should be ordered. An EEG is not recommended unless there are features suggestive of epilepsy or a specific epileptic syndrome (Level A). Because children with CP may have associated deficits of mental retardation, ophthalmologic and hearing impairments, speech and language disorders, and oral-motor dysfunction, screening for these conditions should be part of the initial assessment (Level A).

Conclusions. Neuroimaging results in children with CP are commonly abnormal and may help determine the etiology. Screening for associated conditions is warranted as part of the initial evaluation. (3/04)

CERUMEN IMPACTION

Cerumen Impaction
American Academy of Otolaryngology—Head and Neck Surgery Foundation

ABSTRACT. This update of the 2008 American Academy of Otolaryngology—Head and Neck Surgery Foundation cerumen impaction clinical practice guideline provides evidence-based recommendations on managing cerumen impaction. Cerumen impaction is defined as an accumulation of cerumen that causes symptoms, prevents assessment of the ear, or both. Changes from the prior guideline include

- a consumer added to the development group;

- new evidence (3 guidelines, 5 systematic reviews, and 6 randomized controlled trials);

- enhanced information on patient education and counseling;

- a new algorithm to clarify action statement relationships;

- expanded action statement profiles to explicitly state quality improvement opportunities, confidence in the evidence, intentional vagueness, and differences of opinion;

- an enhanced external review process to include public comment and journal peer review; and

- new key action statements on managing cerumen impaction that focus on primary prevention, contraindicated intervention, and referral and coordination of care. (1/17)

CONGENITAL ADRENAL HYPERPLASIA

Congenital Adrenal Hyperplasia Due to Steroid 21-hydroxylase Deficiency: An Endocrine Society Clinical Practice Guideline
The Endocrine Society

CONCLUSIONS. We recommend universal newborn screening for severe steroid 21-hydroxylase deficiency followed by confirmatory tests. We recommend that prenatal treatment of CAH continue to be regarded as experimental. The diagnosis rests on clinical and hormonal data; genotyping is reserved for equivocal cases and genetic counseling. Glucocorticoid dosage should be minimized to avoid iatrogenic Cushing's syndrome. Mineralocorticoids and, in infants, supplemental sodium are recommended in classic CAH patients. We recommend against the routine use of experimental therapies to promote growth and delay puberty; we suggest patients avoid adrenalectomy. Surgical guidelines emphasize early single-stage genital repair for severely virilized girls, performed by experienced surgeons. Clinicians should consider patients' quality of life, consulting mental health professionals as appropriate. At the transition to adulthood, we recommend monitoring for potential complications of CAH. Finally, we recommend judicious use of medication during pregnancy and in symptomatic patients with nonclassic CAH. (9/10)

CONGENITAL MUSCULAR DYSTROPHY

Evidence-based Guideline Summary: Evaluation, Diagnosis, and Management of Congenital Muscular Dystrophy. Report of the Guideline Development Subcommittee of the American Academy of Neurology and the Practice Issues Review Panel of the American Association of Neuromuscular & Electrodiagnostic Medicine

American Academy of Neurology and American Association of Neuro-muscular & Electrodiagnostic Medicine

ABSTRACT. *Objective.* To delineate optimal diagnostic and therapeutic approaches to congenital muscular dystrophy (CMD) through a systematic review and analysis of the currently available literature.

Methods. Relevant, peer-reviewed research articles were identified using a literature search of the MEDLINE, EMBASE, and Scopus databases. Diagnostic and therapeutic data from these articles were extracted and analyzed in accordance with the American Academy of Neurology classification of evidence schemes for diagnostic, prognostic, and therapeutic studies. Recommendations were linked to the strength of the evidence, other related literature, and general principles of care.

Results. The geographic and ethnic backgrounds, clinical features, brain imaging studies, muscle imaging studies, and muscle biopsies of children with suspected CMD help predict subtype-specific diagnoses. Genetic testing can confirm some subtype-specific diagnoses, but not all causative genes for CMD have been described. Seizures and respiratory complications occur in specific subtypes. There is insufficient evidence to determine the efficacy of various treatment interventions to optimize respiratory, orthopedic, and nutritional outcomes, and more data are needed regarding complications.

Recommendations. Multidisciplinary care by experienced teams is important for diagnosing and promoting the health of children with CMD. Accurate assessment of clinical presentations and genetic data will help in identifying the correct subtype-specific diagnosis in many cases. Multiorgan system complications occur frequently; surveillance and prompt interventions are likely to be beneficial for affected children. More research is needed to fill gaps in knowledge regarding this category of muscular dystrophies. (3/15)

DEPRESSION

Guidelines for Adolescent Depression in Primary Care (GLAD-PC): Part I. Practice Preparation, Identification, Assessment, and Initial Management

Rachel A. Zuckerbrot, MD; Amy Cheung, MD; Peter S. Jensen, MD; Ruth E.K. Stein, MD; Danielle Laraque, MD; and GLAD-PC Steering Group

ABSTRACT. *Objectives.* To update clinical practice guidelines to assist primary care (PC) clinicians in the management of adolescent depression. This part of the updated guidelines is used to address practice preparation, identification, assessment, and initial management of adolescent depression in PC settings.

Methods. By using a combination of evidence- and consensus-based methodologies, guidelines were developed by an expert steering committee in 2 phases as informed by (1) current scientific evidence (published and unpublished) and (2) draft revision and iteration among the steering committee, which included experts, clinicians, and youth and families with lived experience.

Results. Guidelines were updated for youth aged 10 to 21 years and correspond to initial phases of adolescent depression management in PC, including the identification of at-risk youth, assessment and diagnosis, and initial management. The strength of each recommendation and its evidence base are summarized. The practice preparation, identification, assessment, and initial management section of the guidelines include recommendations for (1) the preparation of the PC practice for improved care of adolescents with depression; (2) annual universal screening of youth 12 and over at health maintenance visits; (3) the identification of depression in youth who are at high risk; (4) systematic assessment procedures by using reliable depression scales, patient and caregiver interviews, and *Diagnostic and Statistical Manual of Mental Disorders, Fifth Edition* criteria; (5) patient and family psychoeducation; (6) the establishment of relevant links in the community; and (7) the establishment of a safety plan.

Conclusions. This part of the guidelines is intended to assist PC clinicians in the identification and initial management of adolescents with depression in an era of great clinical need and shortage of mental health specialists, but they cannot replace clinical judgment; these guidelines are not meant to be the sole source of guidance for depression management in adolescents. Additional research that addresses the identification and initial management of youth with depression in PC is needed, including empirical testing of these guidelines. (2/18)

Guidelines for Adolescent Depression in Primary Care (GLAD-PC): Part II. Treatment and Ongoing Management

Amy H. Cheung, MD; Rachel A. Zuckerbrot, MD; Peter S. Jensen, MD; Danielle Laraque, MD; Ruth E.K. Stein, MD; and GLAD-PC Steering Group

ABSTRACT. *Objectives.* To update clinical practice guidelines to assist primary care (PC) in the screening and assessment of depression. In this second part of the updated guidelines, we address treatment and ongoing management of adolescent depression in the PC setting.

Methods. By using a combination of evidence- and consensus-based methodologies, the guidelines were updated in 2 phases as informed by (1) current scientific evidence (published and unpublished) and (2) revision and iteration among the steering committee, including youth and families with lived experience.

Results. These updated guidelines are targeted for youth aged 10 to 21 years and offer recommendations for the management of adolescent depression in PC, including (1) active monitoring of mildly depressed youth, (2) treatment with evidence-based medication and psychotherapeutic approaches in cases of moderate and/or severe depression, (3) close monitoring of side effects, (4) consultation and comanagement of care with mental health specialists, (5) ongoing tracking of outcomes, and (6) specific steps to be taken in instances of partial or no improvement after an initial treatment has begun. The strength of each recommendation and the grade of its evidence base are summarized.

Conclusions. The Guidelines for Adolescent Depression in Primary Care cannot replace clinical judgment, and they should not be the sole source of guidance for adolescent depression management. Nonetheless, the guidelines may assist PC clinicians in the management of depressed adolescents in an era of great clinical need and a shortage of mental health specialists. Additional research concerning the management of depressed youth in PC is needed, including the usability, feasibility, and sustainability of guidelines, and determination of the extent to which the guidelines actually improve outcomes of depressed youth. (2/18)

DUCHENNE MUSCULAR DYSTROPHY

Practice Guideline Update Summary: Corticosteroid Treatment of Duchenne Muscular Dystrophy

David Gloss, MD, MPH&TM; Richard T. Moxley III, MD; Stephen Ashwal, MD; and Maryam Oskoui, MD, for the American Academy of Neurology Guideline Development Subcommittee

ABSTRACT. **Objective.** To update the 2005 American Academy of Neurology (AAN) guideline on corticosteroid treatment of Duchenne muscular dystrophy (DMD).

Methods. We systematically reviewed the literature from January 2004 to July 2014 using the AAN classification scheme for therapeutic articles and predicated recommendations on the strength of the evidence.

Results. Thirty-four studies met inclusion criteria.

Recommendations. In children with DMD, prednisone should be offered for improving strength (Level B) and pulmonary function (Level B). Prednisone may be offered for improving timed motor function (Level C), reducing the need for scoliosis surgery (Level C), and delaying cardiomyopathy onset by 18 years of age (Level C). Deflazacort may be offered for improving strength and timed motor function and delaying age at loss of ambulation by 1.4–2.5 years (Level C). Deflazacort may be offered for improving pulmonary function, reducing the need for scoliosis surgery, delaying cardiomyopathy onset, and increasing survival at 5–15 years of follow-up (Level C for each). Deflazacort and prednisone may be equivalent in improving motor function (Level C). Prednisone may be associated with greater weight gain in the first years of treatment than deflazacort (Level C). Deflazacort may be associated with a greater risk of cataracts than prednisone (Level C). The preferred dosing regimen of prednisone is 0.75 mg/kg/d (Level B). Over 12 months, prednisone 10 mg/kg/weekend is equally effective (Level B), with no long-term data available. Prednisone 0.75 mg/kg/d is associated with significant risk of weight gain, hirsutism, and cushingoid appearance (Level B). *Neurology*® 2016;86:465–472 (2/16)

DYSPLASIA OF THE HIP

Guideline on Detection and Nonoperative Management of Pediatric Developmental Dysplasia of the Hip in Infants up to Six Months of Age: Evidence-based Clinical Practice Guideline
American Academy of Orthopaedic Surgeons

OVERVIEW. This clinical practice guideline is based upon a systematic review of published articles related to the detection and early management of hip instability and dysplasia in typically developing children less than 6 months of age. This guideline provides practice recommendations for the early screening and detection of hip instability and dysplasia and also highlights gaps in the published literature that should stimulate additional research. This guideline is intended towards appropriately trained practitioners involved in the early examination and assessment of typically developing children for hip instability and dysplasia. (9/14)

EMERGENCY MEDICAL SERVICES

National Model EMS Clinical Guidelines
National Association of State EMS Officials

ABSTRACT. These guidelines will be maintained by NASEMSO to facilitate the creation of state and local EMS system clinical guidelines, protocols or operating procedures. System medical directors and other leaders are invited to harvest content as will be useful. These guidelines are either evidence-based or consensus-based and have been formatted for use by field EMS professionals. (10/14)

ENDOCARDITIS

Prevention of Infective Endocarditis: Guidelines From the American Heart Association

Walter Wilson, MD, Chair; Kathryn A. Taubert, PhD, FAHA; Michael Gewitz, MD, FAHA; Peter B. Lockhart, DDS; Larry M. Baddour, MD; Matthew Levison, MD; Ann Bolger, MD, FAHA; Christopher H. Cabell, MD, MHS; Masato Takahashi, MD, FAHA; Robert S. Baltimore, MD; Jane W. Newburger, MD, MPH, FAHA; Brian L. Strom, MD; Lloyd Y. Tani, MD; Michael Gerber, MD; Robert O. Bonow, MD, FAHA; Thomas Pallasch, DDS, MS; Stanford T. Shulman, MD, FAHA; Anne H. Rowley, MD; Jane C. Burns, MD; Patricia Ferrieri, MD; Timothy Gardner, MD, FAHA; David Goff, MD, PhD, FAHA; and David T. Durack, MD, PhD

ABSTRACT. **Background.** The purpose of this statement is to update the recommendations by the American Heart Association (AHA) for the prevention of infective endocarditis that were last published in 1997.

Methods and Results. A writing group was appointed by the AHA for their expertise in prevention and treatment of infective endocarditis, with liaison members representing the American Dental Association, the Infectious Diseases Society of America, and the American Academy of Pediatrics. The writing group reviewed input from national and international experts on infective endocarditis. The recommendations in this document reflect analyses of relevant literature regarding procedure-related bacteremia and infective endocarditis, in vitro susceptibility data of the most common microorganisms that cause infective endocarditis, results of prophylactic studies in animal models of experimental endocarditis, and retrospective and prospective studies of prevention of infective endocarditis. MEDLINE database searches from 1950 to 2006 were done for English-language papers using the following search terms: endocarditis, infective endocarditis, prophylaxis, prevention, antibiotic, antimicrobial, pathogens, organisms, dental, gastrointestinal, genitourinary, streptococcus, enterococcus, staphylococcus, respiratory, dental surgery, pathogenesis, vaccine, immunization, and bacteremia. The reference lists of the identified papers were also searched. We also searched the AHA online library. The American College of Cardiology/AHA classification of recommendations and levels of evidence for practice guidelines were used. The paper was subsequently reviewed by outside experts not affiliated with the writing group and by the AHA Science Advisory and Coordinating Committee.

Conclusions. The major changes in the updated recommendations include the following: (1) The Committee concluded that only an extremely small number of cases of infective endocarditis might be prevented by antibiotic prophylaxis for dental procedures even if such prophylactic therapy were 100% effective. (2) Infective endocarditis prophylaxis for dental procedures should be recommended only for patients with underlying cardiac conditions associated with the highest risk of adverse outcome from infective endocarditis. (3) For patients with these underlying cardiac conditions, prophylaxis is recommended for all dental procedures that involve manipulation of gingival tissue or the periapical region of teeth or perforation of the oral mucosa. (4) Prophylaxis is not recommended based solely on an increased lifetime risk of acquisition of infective endocarditis. (5) Administration of antibiotics solely to prevent endocarditis is not recommended for patients who undergo a genitourinary or gastrointestinal tract procedure. These changes are intended to define more clearly when infective endocarditis prophylaxis is or is not recommended and to provide more uniform and consistent global recommendations. (*Circulation.* 2007;116: 1736–1754.) (5/07)

FLUORIDE

Recommendations for Using Fluoride to Prevent and Control Dental Caries in the United States
Centers for Disease Control and Prevention (8/01)

FOOD ALLERGY

Guidelines for the Diagnosis and Management of Food Allergy in the United States: Report of the NIAID-Sponsored Expert Panel
National Institute of Allergy and Infectious Diseases

ABSTRACT. Food allergy is an important public health problem that affects children and adults and may be increasing in prevalence. Despite the risk of severe allergic reactions and even death, there is no current treatment for food allergy: the disease can only be managed by allergen avoidance or treatment of symptoms. The diagnosis and management of food allergy also may vary from one clinical practice setting to another. Finally, because patients frequently confuse nonallergic food reactions, such as food intolerance, with food allergies, there is an unfounded belief among the public that food allergy prevalence is higher than it truly is. In response to these concerns, the National Institute of Allergy and Infectious Diseases, working with 34 professional organizations, federal agencies, and patient advocacy groups, led the development of clinical guidelines for the diagnosis and management of food allergy. These Guidelines are intended for use by a wide variety of health care professionals, including family practice physicians, clinical specialists, and nurse practitioners. The Guidelines include a consensus definition for food allergy, discuss comorbid conditions often associated with food allergy, and focus on both IgE-mediated and non-IgE-mediated reactions to food. Topics addressed include the epidemiology, natural history, diagnosis, and management of food allergy, as well as the management of severe symptoms and anaphylaxis. These Guidelines provide 43 concise clinical recommendations and additional guidance on points of current controversy in patient management. They also identify gaps in the current scientific knowledge to be addressed through future research. (12/10)

GASTROENTERITIS

Managing Acute Gastroenteritis Among Children: Oral Rehydration, Maintenance, and Nutritional Therapy
Centers for Disease Control and Prevention (11/03)

HEMORRHAGE

An Evidence-based Prehospital Guideline for External Hemorrhage Control
American College of Surgeons Committee on Trauma

ABSTRACT. This report describes the development of an evidence-based guideline for external hemorrhage control in the prehospital setting. This project included a systematic review of the literature regarding the use of tourniquets and hemostatic agents for management of life-threatening extremity and junctional hemorrhage. Using the GRADE methodology to define the key clinical questions, an expert panel then reviewed the results of the literature review, established the quality of the evidence and made recommendations for EMS care. A clinical care guideline is proposed for adoption by EMS systems. (3/14)

HIV

Guidelines for the Prevention and Treatment of Opportunistic Infections in HIV-Exposed and HIV-Infected Children
US Department of Health and Human Services

SUMMARY. This report updates the last version of the Guidelines for the Prevention and Treatment of Opportunistic Infections (OIs) in HIV-Exposed and HIV-Infected Children, published in 2009. These guidelines are intended for use by clinicians and other health-care workers providing medical care for HIV-exposed and HIV-infected children in the United States. The guidelines discuss opportunistic pathogens that occur in the United States and ones that might be acquired during international travel, such as malaria. Topic areas covered for each OI include a brief description of the epidemiology, clinical presentation, and diagnosis of the OI in children; prevention of exposure; prevention of first episode of disease; discontinuation of primary prophylaxis after immune reconstitution; treatment of disease; monitoring for adverse effects during treatment, including immune reconstitution inflammatory syndrome (IRIS); management of treatment failure; prevention of disease recurrence; and discontinuation of secondary prophylaxis after immune reconstitution. A separate document providing recommendations for prevention and treatment of OIs among HIV-infected adults and post-pubertal adolescents (*Guidelines for the Prevention and Treatment of Opportunistic Infections in HIV-Infected Adults and Adolescents*) was prepared by a panel of adult HIV and infectious disease specialists (see http://aidsinfo.nih.gov/guidelines).

These guidelines were developed by a panel of specialists in pediatric HIV infection and infectious diseases (the Panel on Opportunistic Infections in HIV-Exposed and HIV-Infected Children) from the U.S. government and academic institutions. For each OI, one or more pediatric specialists with subject-matter expertise reviewed the literature for new information since the last guidelines were published and then proposed revised recommendations for review by the full Panel. After these reviews and discussions, the guidelines underwent further revision, with review and approval by the Panel, and final endorsement by the National Institutes of Health (NIH), Centers for Disease Control and Prevention (CDC), the HIV Medicine Association (HIVMA) of the Infectious Diseases Society of America (IDSA), the Pediatric Infectious Disease Society (PIDS), and the American Academy of Pediatrics (AAP). So that readers can ascertain how best to apply the recommendations in their practice environments, the recommendations are rated by a letter that indicates the strength of the recommendation, a Roman numeral that indicates the quality of the evidence supporting the recommendation, and where applicable, a * notation that signifies a hybrid of higher-quality adult study evidence and consistent but lower-quality pediatric study evidence.

More detailed methodologic considerations are listed in Appendix 1 (Important Guidelines Considerations), including a description of the make-up and organizational structure of the Panel, definition of financial disclosure and management of conflict of interest, funding sources for the guidelines, methods of collecting and synthesizing evidence and formulating recommendations, public commentary, and plans for updating the guidelines. The names and financial disclosures for each of the Panel members are listed in Appendices 2 and 3, respectively.

An important mode of childhood acquisition of OIs and HIV infection is from infected mothers. HIV-infected women may be more likely to have coinfections with opportunistic pathogens (e.g., hepatitis C) and more likely than women who are not HIV-infected to transmit these infections to their infants. In addition, HIV-infected women or HIV-infected family members coinfected with certain opportunistic pathogens may be more likely to transmit these infections horizontally to their children, resulting in increased likelihood of primary acquisition of such infections in young children. Furthermore, transplacental transfer of antibodies that protect infants against serious infections may be lower in HIV-infected women than in women who are HIV-uninfected. Therefore, infections with opportunistic pathogens may affect not just HIV-infected infants but also HIV-exposed, uninfected infants. These guidelines for treating OIs in children, therefore, consider treatment of infections in all children—HIV-infected and HIV-uninfected—born to HIV-infected women.

In addition, HIV infection increasingly is seen in adolescents with perinatal infection who are now surviving into their teens and in youth with behaviorally acquired HIV infection. Guidelines for postpubertal adolescents can be found in the adult OI guidelines, but drug pharmacokinetics (PK) and response to treatment may differ in younger prepubertal or pubertal adolescents. Therefore, these guidelines also apply to treatment of HIV-infected youth who have not yet completed pubertal development.

Major changes in the guidelines from the previous version in 2009 include:

- Greater emphasis on the importance of antiretroviral therapy (ART) for prevention and treatment of OIs, especially those OIs for which no specific therapy exists;

- Increased information about diagnosis and management of IRIS;

- Information about managing ART in children with OIs, including potential drug-drug interactions;

- Updated immunization recommendations for HIV-exposed and HIV-infected children, including pneumococcal, human papillomavirus, meningococcal, and rotavirus vaccines;

- Addition of sections on influenza, giardiasis, and isosporiasis;

- Elimination of sections on aspergillosis, bartonellosis, and HHV-6 and HHV-7 infections; and

- Updated recommendations on discontinuation of OI prophylaxis after immune reconstitution in children.

The most important recommendations are highlighted in boxed major recommendations preceding each section, and a table of dosing recommendations appears at the end of each section. The guidelines conclude with summary tables that display dosing recommendations for all of the conditions, drug toxicities and drug interactions, and 2 figures describing immunization recommendations for children aged 0 to 6 years and 7 to 18 years.

The terminology for describing use of antiretroviral (ARV) drugs for treatment of HIV infection has been standardized to ensure consistency within the sections of these guidelines and with the *Guidelines for the Use of Antiretroviral Agents in Pediatric HIV Infection*. Combination antiretroviral therapy (cART) indicates use of multiple (generally 3 or more) ARV drugs as part of an HIV treatment regimen that is designed to achieve virologic suppression; highly active antiretroviral therapy (HAART), synonymous with cART, is no longer used and has been replaced by cART; the term ART has been used when referring to use of ARV drugs for HIV treatment more generally, including (mostly historical) use of one- or two-agent ARV regimens that do not meet criteria for cART.

Because treatment of OIs is an evolving science, and availability of new agents or clinical data on existing agents may change therapeutic options and preferences, these recommendations will be periodically updated and will be available at http://AIDSinfo.nih.gov. (11/13)

IMMUNOCOMPROMISED HOST

2013 Infectious Diseases Society of America Clinical Practice Guidelines for the Immunization of the Immunocompromised Host

Infectious Diseases Society of America

EXECUTIVE SUMMARY. These guidelines were created to provide primary care and specialty clinicians with evidence-based guidelines for active immunization of patients with altered immunocompetence and their household contacts in order to safely prevent vaccine-preventable infections. They do not represent the only approach to vaccination. Recommended immunization schedules for normal adults and children as well as certain adults and children at high risk for vaccine-preventable infections are updated and published annually by the Centers for Disease Control and Prevention (CDC) and partner organizations. Some recommendations have not been addressed by the Advisory Committee on Immunization Practices (ACIP) to the CDC or they deviate from recommendations. The goal of presenting these guidelines is to decrease morbidity and mortality from vaccine-preventable infections in immunocompromised patients. Summarized below are the recommendations made by the panel. Supporting tables that provide additional information are available in the electronic version. The panel followed a process used in the development of other Infectious Diseases Society of America guidelines, which included a systematic weighting of the quality of the evidence and the grade of the recommendation. The key clinical questions and recommendations are summarized in this executive summary. A detailed description of the methods, background, and evidence summaries that support each recommendation can be found in the full text of the guidelines. (1/14)

INFANTILE SPASMS

Evidence-based Guideline Update: Medical Treatment of Infantile Spasms

American Academy of Neurology and Child Neurology Society

ABSTRACT. *Objective.* To update the 2004 American Academy of Neurology/Child Neurology Society practice parameter on treatment of infantile spasms in children.

Methods. MEDLINE and EMBASE were searched from 2002 to 2011 and searches of reference lists of retrieved articles were performed. Sixty-eight articles were selected for detailed review; 26 were included in the analysis. Recommendations were based on a 4-tiered classification scheme combining pre-2002 evidence and more recent evidence.

Results. There is insufficient evidence to determine whether other forms of corticosteroids are as effective as adrenocorticotropic hormone (ACTH) for short-term treatment of infantile spasms. However, low-dose ACTH is probably as effective as high-dose ACTH. ACTH is more effective than vigabatrin (VGB) for short-term treatment of children with infantile spasms (excluding those with tuberous sclerosis complex). There is insufficient evidence to show that other agents and combination therapy are effective for short-term treatment of infantile spasms. Short lag time to treatment leads to better long-term developmental outcome. Successful short-term treatment of cryptogenic infantile spasms with ACTH or prednisolone leads to better long-term developmental outcome than treatment with VGB.

Recommendations. Low-dose ACTH should be considered for treatment of infantile spasms. ACTH or VGB may be useful for short-term treatment of infantile spasms, with ACTH considered preferentially over VGB. Hormonal therapy (ACTH or prednisolone) may be considered for use in preference to VGB in infants with cryptogenic infantile spasms, to possibly improve developmental outcome. A shorter lag time to treatment of infantile spasms with either hormonal therapy or VGB possibly improves long-term developmental outcomes. (6/12)

INTRAVASCULAR CATHETER-RELATED INFECTIONS

Guidelines for the Prevention of Intravascular Catheter-Related Infections

Society of Critical Care Medicine, Infectious Diseases Society of America, Society for Healthcare Epidemiology of America, Surgical Infection Society, American College of Chest Physicians, American Thoracic Society, American Society of Critical Care Anesthesiologists, Association for Professionals in Infection Control and Epidemiology, Infusion Nurses Society, Oncology Nursing Society, Society of Cardiovascular and Interventional Radiology, American Academy of Pediatrics, and the Healthcare Infection Control Practices Advisory Committee of the Centers for Disease Control and Prevention

ABSTRACT. These guidelines have been developed for practitioners who insert catheters and for persons responsible for surveillance and control of infections in hospital, outpatient, and home health-care settings. This report was prepared by a working group comprising members from professional organizations representing the disciplines of critical care medicine, infectious diseases, health-care infection control, surgery, anesthesiology, interventional radiology, pulmonary medicine, pediatric medicine, and nursing. The working group was led by the Society of Critical Care Medicine (SCCM), in collaboration with the Infectious Disease Society of America (IDSA), Society for Healthcare Epidemiology of America (SHEA), Surgical Infection Society (SIS), American College of Chest Physicians (ACCP), American Thoracic Society (ATS), American Society of Critical Care Anesthesiologists (ASCCA), Association for Professionals in Infection Control and Epidemiology (APIC), Infusion Nurses Society (INS), Oncology Nursing Society (ONS), Society of Cardiovascular and Interventional Radiology (SCVIR), American Academy of Pediatrics (AAP), and the Healthcare Infection Control Practices Advisory Committee (HICPAC) of the Centers for Disease Control and Prevention (CDC) and is intended to replace the *Guideline for Prevention of Intravascular Device-Related Infections* published in 1996. These guidelines are intended to provide evidence-based recommendations for preventing catheter-related infections. Major areas of emphasis include (1) educating and training health-care providers who insert and maintain catheters; (2) using maximal sterile barrier precautions during central venous catheter insertion; (3) using a 2% chlorhexidine preparation for skin antisepsis; (4) avoiding routine replacement of central venous catheters as a strategy to prevent infection; and (5) using antiseptic/antibiotic impregnated short-term central venous catheters if the rate of infection is high despite adherence to other strategies (ie, education and training, maximal sterile barrier precautions, and 2% chlorhexidine for skin antisepsis). These guidelines also identify performance indicators that can be used locally by health-care institutions or organizations to monitor their success in implementing these evidence-based recommendations. (11/02)

JAUNDICE

Guideline for the Evaluation of Cholestatic Jaundice in Infants

North American Society for Pediatric Gastroenterology, Hepatology, and Nutrition

ABSTRACT. For the primary care provider, cholestatic jaundice in infancy, defined as jaundice caused by an elevated conjugated bilirubin, is an uncommon but potentially serious problem that indicates hepatobiliary dysfunction. Early detection of cholestatic jaundice by the primary care physician and timely, accurate diagnosis by the pediatric gastroenterologist are important for successful treatment and a favorable prognosis. The Cholestasis Guideline Committee of the North American Society for Pediatric Gastroenterology, Hepatology and Nutrition has formulated a clinical practice guideline for the diagnostic evaluation of cholestatic jaundice in the infant. The Cholestasis Guideline Committee, consisting of a primary care pediatrician, a clinical epidemiologist (who also practices primary care pediatrics), and five pediatric gastroenterologists, based its recommendations on a comprehensive and systematic review of the medical literature integrated with expert opinion. Consensus was achieved through the Nominal Group Technique, a structured quantitative method.

The Committee examined the value of diagnostic tests commonly used for the evaluation of cholestatic jaundice and how those interventions can be applied to clinical situations in the infant. The guideline provides recommendations for management by the primary care provider, indications for consultation by a pediatric gastroenterologist, and recommendations for management by the pediatric gastroenterologist.

The Cholestasis Guideline Committee recommends that any infant noted to be jaundiced at 2 weeks of age be evaluated for cholestasis with measurement of total and direct serum bilirubin. However, breast-fed infants who can be reliably monitored and who have an otherwise normal history (no dark urine or light stools) and physical examination may be asked to return at 3 weeks of age and, if jaundice persists, have measurement of total and direct serum bilirubin at that time.

This document represents the official recommendations of the North American Society for Pediatric Gastroenterology, Hepatology and Nutrition on the evaluation of cholestatic jaundice in infants. The American Academy of Pediatrics has also endorsed these recommendations. These recommendations are a general guideline and are not intended as a substitute for clinical judgment or as a protocol for the care of all patients with this problem. (8/04)

MEDULLARY THYROID CARCINOMA

Revised American Thyroid Association Guidelines for the Management of Medullary Thyroid Carcinoma

American Thyroid Association Guidelines Task Force on Medullary Thyroid Carcinoma

ABSTRACT. ***Introduction.*** The American Thyroid Association appointed a Task Force of experts to revise the original Medullary Thyroid Carcinoma: Management Guidelines of the American Thyroid Association.

Methods. The Task Force identified relevant articles using a systematic PubMed search, supplemented with additional published materials, and then created evidence-based recommendations, which were set in categories using criteria adapted from the United States Preventive Services Task Force Agency for Healthcare Research and Quality. The original guidelines provided abundant source material and an excellent organizational structure that served as the basis for the current revised document.

Results. The revised guidelines are focused primarily on the diagnosis and treatment of patients with sporadic medullary thyroid carcinoma (MTC) and hereditary MTC.

Conclusions. The Task Force developed 67 evidence-based recommendations to assist clinicians in the care of patients with MTC. The Task Force considers the recommendations to represent current, rational, and optimal medical practice. (6/15)

MIGRAINE HEADACHE

Pharmacological Treatment of Migraine Headache in Children and Adolescents

Quality Standards Subcommittee of the American Academy of Neurology and the Practice Committee of the Child Neurology Society (12/04)

PALLIATIVE CARE
Clinical Practice Guidelines for Quality Palliative Care, Third Edition
National Consensus Project for Quality Palliative Care (2013)

RADIOLOGY
Neuroimaging of the Neonate
Quality Standards Subcommittee of the American Academy of Neurology and the Practice Committee of the Child Neurology Society

ABSTRACT. **Objective.** The authors reviewed available evidence on neonatal neuroimaging strategies for evaluating both very low birth weight preterm infants and encephalopathic term neonates.

Imaging for the Preterm Neonate. Routine screening cranial ultrasonography (US) should be performed on all infants of <30 weeks' gestation once between 7 and 14 days of age and should be optimally repeated between 36 and 40 weeks' post-menstrual age. This strategy detects lesions such as intraventricular hemorrhage, which influences clinical care, and those such as periventricular leukomalacia and low-pressure ventriculomegaly, which provide information about long-term neurodevelopmental outcome. There is insufficient evidence for routine MRI of all very low birth weight preterm infants with abnormal results of cranial US.

Imaging for the Term Infant. Noncontrast CT should be performed to detect hemorrhagic lesions in the encephalopathic term infant with a history of birth trauma, low hematocrit, or coagulopathy. If CT findings are inconclusive, MRI should be performed between days 2 and 8 to assess the location and extent of injury. The pattern of injury identified with conventional MRI may provide diagnostic and prognostic information for term infants with evidence of encephalopathy. In particular, basal ganglia and thalamic lesions detected by conventional MRI are associated with poor neurodevelopmental outcome. Diffusion-weighted imaging may allow earlier detection of these cerebral injuries.

Recommendations. US plays an established role in the management of preterm neonates of <30 weeks' gestation. US also provides valuable prognostic information when the infant reaches 40 weeks' postmenstrual age. For encephalopathic term infants, early CT should be used to exclude hemorrhage; MRI should be performed later in the first postnatal week to establish the pattern of injury and predict neurologic outcome. (6/02)

RHINOPLASTY
Improving Nasal Form and Function after Rhinoplasty
American Academy of Otolaryngology—Head and Neck Surgery Foundation

ABSTRACT. Rhinoplasty, a surgical procedure that alters the shape or appearance of the nose while preserving or enhancing the nasal airway, ranks among the most commonly performed cosmetic procedures in the United States, with >200,000 procedures reported in 2014. While it is difficult to calculate the exact economic burden incurred by rhinoplasty patients following surgery with or without complications, the average rhinoplasty procedure typically exceeds $4000. The costs incurred due to complications, infections, or revision surgery may include the cost of long-term antibiotics, hospitalization, or lost revenue from hours/days of missed work.

The resultant psychological impact of rhinoplasty can also be significant. Furthermore, the health care burden from psychological pressures of nasal deformities/aesthetic shortcomings, surgical infections, surgical pain, side effects from antibiotics, and nasal packing materials must also be considered for these patients. Prior to this guideline, limited literature existed on standard care considerations for pre- and postsurgical management and for standard surgical practice to ensure optimal outcomes for patients undergoing rhinoplasty. The impetus for this guideline is to utilize current evidence-based medicine practices and data to build unanimity regarding the peri- and postoperative strategies to maximize patient safety and to optimize surgical results for patients. (2/17)

SEDATION AND ANALGESIA
Clinical Policy: Evidence-based Approach to Pharmacologic Agents Used in Pediatric Sedation and Analgesia in the Emergency Department
American College of Emergency Physicians (10/04)

SEIZURE
Evaluating a First Nonfebrile Seizure in Children
Quality Standards Subcommittee of the American Academy of Neurology, the Child Neurology Society, and the American Epilepsy Society

ABSTRACT. **Objective.** The Quality Standards Subcommittee of the American Academy of Neurology develops practice parameters as strategies for patient management based on analysis of evidence. For this practice parameter, the authors reviewed available evidence on evaluation of the first nonfebrile seizure in children in order to make practice recommendations based on this available evidence.

Methods. Multiple searches revealed relevant literature and each article was reviewed, abstracted, and classified. Recommendations were based on a three-tiered scheme of classification of the evidence.

Results. Routine EEG as part of the diagnostic evaluation was recommended; other studies such as laboratory evaluations and neuroimaging studies were recommended as based on specific clinical circumstances.

Conclusions. Further studies are needed using large, well-characterized samples and standardized data collection instruments. Collection of data regarding appropriate timing of evaluations would be important. (8/00)

Treatment of the Child With a First Unprovoked Seizure
Quality Standards Subcommittee of the American Academy of Neurology and the Practice Committee of the Child Neurology Society

ABSTRACT. The Quality Standards Subcommittee of the American Academy of Neurology and the Practice Committee of the Child Neurology Society develop practice parameters as strategies for patient management based on analysis of evidence regarding risks and benefits. This parameter reviews published literature relevant to the decision to begin treatment after a child or adolescent experiences a first unprovoked seizure and presents evidence-based practice recommendations. Reasons why treatment may be considered are discussed. Evidence is reviewed concerning risk of recurrence as well as effect of treatment on prevention of recurrence and development of chronic epilepsy. Studies of side effects of anticonvulsants commonly used to treat seizures in children are also reviewed. Relevant articles are classified according to the Quality Standards Subcommittee classification scheme. Treatment after a first unprovoked seizure appears to decrease the risk of a second seizure, but there are few data from studies involving only children. There appears to be no benefit of treatment with regard to the prognosis for long-term seizure remission. Antiepileptic drugs (AED) carry risks of side effects that are particularly important in children. The decision as to whether or not to treat children and adolescents who have experienced a first unprovoked seizure must be based on a risk–benefit assessment that weighs the risk of having another seizure against the risk of chronic AED therapy. The decision should be individualized and take into account both medical issues and patient and family preference. (1/03)

STATUS EPILEPTICUS

Diagnostic Assessment of the Child With Status Epilepticus (An Evidence-based Review)

Quality Standards Subcommittee of the American Academy of Neurology and the Practice Committee of the Child Neurology Society

ABSTRACT. **Objective.** To review evidence on the assessment of the child with status epilepticus (SE).

Methods. Relevant literature were reviewed, abstracted, and classified. When data were missing, a minimum diagnostic yield was calculated. Recommendations were based on a four-tiered scheme of evidence classification.

Results. Laboratory studies (Na^{++} or other electrolytes, Ca^{++}, glucose) were abnormal in approximately 6% and are generally ordered as routine practice. When blood or spinal fluid cultures were done on these children, blood cultures were abnormal in at least 2.5% and a CNS infection was found in at least 12.8%. When antiepileptic drug (AED) levels were ordered in known epileptic children already taking AEDs, the levels were low in 32%. A total of 3.6% of children had evidence of ingestion. When studies for inborn errors of metabolism were done, an abnormality was found in 4.2%. Epileptiform abnormalities occurred in 43% of EEGs of children with SE and helped determine the nature and location of precipitating electroconvulsive events (8% generalized, 16% focal, and 19% both). Abnormalities on neuroimaging studies that may explain the etiology of SE were found in at least 8% of children.

Recommendations. Although common clinical practice is that blood cultures and lumbar puncture are obtained if there is a clinical suspicion of a systemic or CNS infection, there are insufficient data to support or refute recommendations as to whether blood cultures or lumbar puncture should be done on a routine basis in children in whom there is no clinical suspicion of a systemic or CNS infection (Level U). AED levels should be considered when a child with treated epilepsy develops SE (Level B). Toxicology studies and metabolic studies for inborn errors of metabolism may be considered in children with SE when there are clinical indicators for concern or when the initial evaluation reveals no etiology (Level C). An EEG may be considered in a child with SE as it may be helpful in determining whether there are focal or generalized epileptiform abnormalities that may guide further testing for the etiology of SE, when there is a suspicion of pseudostatus epilepticus (nonepileptic SE), or nonconvulsive SE, and may guide treatment (Level C). Neuroimaging may be considered after the child with SE has been stabilized if there are clinical indications or if the etiology is unknown (Level C). There is insufficient evidence to support or refute routine neuroimaging in a child presenting with SE (Level U). (11/06)

TELEHEALTH

Operating Procedures for Pediatric Telehealth

American Telemedicine Association

INTRODUCTION. Children represent one of our most vulnerable populations, and, as such, require special considerations when participating in telehealth encounters. Some services provided to adult patients by telehealth may not be easily adapted to or appropriate for pediatric patients due to physical factors (patient size), legal factors (consent, confidentiality), the ability to communicate and provide a history, developmental stage, unique pediatric conditions, and age-specific differences in both normal and disease states (AHRQ, n.d.; Alverson, 2008). These operating procedures for pediatric telehealth aim to improve the overall telehealth experience for pediatric patients, providers, and patient families. Telehealth holds particular promise in facilitating the management and coordination of care for medically complex children and those with chronic conditions, such as asthma, chronic lung disease, autism, diabetes, and behavioral health conditions.

Through the use of telehealth, providers can provide appointment flexibility, increase access, promote continuity of care, and improve quality, either as a part of or as a complement to care delivered through the patient-centered medical home (PCMH). Whether telehealth services are delivered through the PCMH or as a complement to it, telehealth providers **should** routinely communicate with a patient's primary care provider and any relevant specialists regarding a telehealth encounter. Telehealth providers **shall** have a standard mechanism in place to share secure documentation of the encounter with the PCMH (AAP, 2015) in a timely manner.

These operating procedures do reference general telehealth operating principles that apply beyond pediatrics and that warrant particular emphasis, but they are not meant to serve as a comprehensive stand-alone guide to the development and operation of a telemedicine service. ATA has developed and published core standards for telehealth operations that provide overarching guidance for clinical, technical and administrative standards (ATA, 2014a). The Pediatric Operating Procedures complement existing professional organization guidance from the American Academy of Pediatrics, the American Psychological Association, the American Association of Family Physicians and the Society of Adolescent Health and Medicine. (4/17)

THYROID NODULES AND DIFFERENTIATED THYROID CANCER

Management Guidelines for Children With Thyroid Nodules and Differentiated Thyroid Cancer

American Thyroid Association Guidelines Task Force on Pediatric Thyroid Cancer

ABSTRACT. **Background.** Previous guidelines for the management of thyroid nodules and cancers were geared toward adults. Compared with thyroid neoplasms in adults, however, those in the pediatric population exhibit differences in pathophysiology, clinical presentation, and long-term outcomes. Furthermore, therapy that may be recommended for an adult may not be appropriate for a child who is at low risk for death but at higher risk for long-term harm from overly aggressive treatment. For these reasons, unique guidelines for children and adolescents with thyroid tumors are needed.

Methods. A task force commissioned by the American Thyroid Association (ATA) developed a series of clinically relevant questions pertaining to the management of children with thyroid nodules and differentiated thyroid cancer (DTC). Using an extensive literature search, primarily focused on studies that included subjects ≤18 years of age, the task force identified and reviewed relevant articles through April 2014. Recommendations were made based upon scientific evidence and expert opinion and were graded using a modified schema from the United States Preventive Services Task Force.

Results. These inaugural guidelines provide recommendations for the evaluation and management of thyroid nodules in children and adolescents, including the role and interpretation of ultrasound, fine-needle aspiration cytology, and the management of benign nodules. Recommendations for the evaluation, treatment, and follow-up of children and adolescents with DTC are outlined and include preoperative staging, surgical management, postoperative staging, the role of radioactive iodine therapy, and goals for thyrotropin suppression. Management algorithms are proposed and separate recommendations for papillary and follicular thyroid cancers are provided.

Conclusions. In response to our charge as an independent task force appointed by the ATA, we developed recommendations based on scientific evidence and expert opinion for the management of thyroid nodules and DTC in children and adolescents. In our opinion, these represent the current optimal care for children and adolescents with these conditions. (7/15)

TOBACCO USE

Treating Tobacco Use and Dependence: 2008 Update
US Department of Health and Human Services

ABSTRACT. *Treating Tobacco Use and Dependence: 2008 Update,* a Public Health Service-sponsored Clinical Practice Guideline, is a product of the Tobacco Use and Dependence Guideline Panel ("the Panel"), consortium representatives, consultants, and staff. These 37 individuals were charged with the responsibility of identifying effective, experimentally validated tobacco dependence treatments and practices. The updated Guideline was sponsored by a consortium of eight Federal Government and nonprofit organizations: the Agency for Healthcare Research and Quality (AHRQ); Centers for Disease Control and Prevention (CDC); National Cancer Institute (NCI); National Heart, Lung, and Blood Institute (NHLBI); National Institute on Drug Abuse (NIDA); American Legacy Foundation; Robert Wood Johnson Foundation (RWJF); and University of Wisconsin School of Medicine and Public Health's Center for Tobacco Research and Intervention (UW-CTRI). This Guideline is an updated version of the 2000 *Treating Tobacco Use and Dependence: Clinical Practice Guideline* that was sponsored by the U.S. Public Health Service, U. S. Department of Health and Human Services.

An impetus for this Guideline update was the expanding literature on tobacco dependence and its treatment. The original 1996 Guideline was based on some 3,000 articles on tobacco treatment published between 1975 and 1994. The 2000 Guideline entailed the collection and screening of an additional 3,000 articles published between 1995 and 1999. The 2008 Guideline update screened an additional 2,700 articles; thus, the present Guideline update reflects the distillation of a literature base of more than 8,700 research articles. Of course, this body of research was further reviewed to identify a much smaller group of articles that served as the basis for focused Guideline data analyses and review.

This Guideline contains strategies and recommendations designed to assist clinicians; tobacco dependence treatment specialists; and health care administrators, insurers, and purchasers in delivering and supporting effective treatments for tobacco use and dependence. The recommendations were made as a result of a systematic review and meta-analysis of 11 specific topics identified by the Panel (proactive quitlines; combining counseling and medication relative to either counseling or medication alone; varenicline; various medication combinations; long-term medications; cessation interventions for individuals with low socioeconomic status/limited formal education; cessation interventions for adolescent smokers; cessation interventions for pregnant smokers; cessation interventions for individuals with psychiatric disorders, including substance use disorders; providing cessation interventions as a health benefit; and systems interventions, including provider training and the combination of training and systems interventions). The strength of evidence that served as the basis for each recommendation is indicated clearly in the Guideline update. A draft of the Guideline update was peer reviewed prior to publication, and the input of 81 external reviewers was considered by the Panel prior to preparing the final document. In addition, the public had an opportunity to comment through a *Federal Register* review process. The key recommendations of the updated Guideline, *Treating Tobacco Use and Dependence: 2008 Update,* based on the literature review and expert Panel opinion, are as follows:

Ten Key Guideline Recommendations

The overarching goal of these recommendations is that clinicians strongly recommend the use of effective tobacco dependence counseling and medication treatments to their patients who use tobacco, and that health systems, insurers, and purchasers assist clinicians in making such effective treatments available.

1. Tobacco dependence is a chronic disease that often requires repeated intervention and multiple attempts to quit. Effective treatments exist, however, that can significantly increase rates of long-term abstinence.

2. It is essential that clinicians and health care delivery systems consistently identify and document tobacco use status and treat every tobacco user seen in a health care setting.

3. Tobacco dependence treatments are effective across a broad range of populations. Clinicians should encourage every patient willing to make a quit attempt to use the counseling treatments and medications recommended in this Guideline.

4. Brief tobacco dependence treatment is effective. Clinicians should offer every patient who uses tobacco at least the brief treatments shown to be effective in this Guideline.

5. Individual, group, and telephone counseling are effective, and their effectiveness increases with treatment intensity. Two components of counseling are especially effective, and clinicians should use these when counseling patients making a quit attempt:
   - Practical counseling (problem solving/skills training)
   - Social support delivered as part of treatment

6. Numerous effective medications are available for tobacco dependence, and clinicians should encourage their use by all patients attempting to quit smoking—except when medically contraindicated or with specific populations for which there is insufficient evidence of effectiveness (i.e., pregnant women, smokeless tobacco users, light smokers, and adolescents).
   - Seven first-line medications (5 nicotine and 2 non-nicotine) reliably increase long-term smoking abstinence rates:
     – Bupropion SR
     – Nicotine gum
     – Nicotine inhaler
     – Nicotine lozenge
     – Nicotine nasal spray
     – Nicotine patch
     – Varenicline
     – Clinicians also should consider the use of certain combinations of medications identified as effective in this Guideline.

7. Counseling and medication are effective when used by themselves for treating tobacco dependence. The combination of counseling and medication, however, is more effective than either alone. Thus, clinicians should encourage all individuals making a quit attempt to use both counseling and medication.

8. Telephone quitline counseling is effective with diverse populations and has broad reach. Therefore, both clinicians and health care delivery systems should ensure patient access to quitlines and promote quitline use.

9. If a tobacco user currently is unwilling to make a quit attempt, clinicians should use the motivational treatments shown in this Guideline to be effective in increasing future quit attempts.

10. Tobacco dependence treatments are both clinically effective and highly cost-effective relative to interventions for other clinical disorders. Providing coverage for these treatments increases quit rates. Insurers and purchasers should ensure that all insurance plans include the counseling and medication identified as effective in this Guideline as covered benefits.

The updated Guideline is divided into seven chapters that provide an overview, including methods (Chapter 1); information on the assessment of tobacco use (Chapter 2); clinical interventions, both for patients willing and unwilling to make a quit attempt at this time (Chapter 3); intensive interventions (Chapter 4); systems interventions for health care administrators, insurers, and purchasers (Chapter 5); the scientific evidence supporting the Guideline recommendations (Chapter 6); and information relevant to specific populations and other topics (Chapter 7).

A comparison of the findings of the updated Guideline with the 2000 Guideline reveals the considerable progress made in tobacco research over the brief period separating these two publications. Tobacco dependence increasingly is recognized as a chronic disease, one that typically requires ongoing assessment and repeated intervention. In addition, the updated Guideline offers the clinician many more effective treatment strategies than were identified in the original Guideline. There now are seven different first-line effective agents in the smoking cessation pharmacopoeia, allowing the clinician and patient many different medication options. In addition, recent evidence provides even stronger support for counseling (both when used alone and with other treatments) as an effective tobacco cessation strategy; counseling adds to the effectiveness of tobacco cessation medications, quitline counseling is an effective intervention with a broad reach, and counseling increases tobacco cessation among adolescent smokers.

Finally, there is increasing evidence that the success of any tobacco dependence treatment strategy cannot be divorced from the health care system in which it is embedded. The updated Guideline contains new evidence that health care policies significantly affect the likelihood that smokers will receive effective tobacco dependence treatment and successfully stop tobacco use. For instance, making tobacco dependence treatment a covered benefit of insurance plans increases the likelihood that a tobacco user will receive treatment and quit successfully. Data strongly indicate that effective tobacco interventions require coordinated interventions. Just as the clinician must intervene with his or her patient, so must the health care administrator, insurer, and purchaser foster and support tobacco intervention as an integral element of health care delivery. Health care administrators and insurers should ensure that clinicians have the training and support to deliver consistent, effective intervention to tobacco users.

One important conclusion of this Guideline update is that the most effective way to move clinicians to intervene is to provide them with information regarding multiple effective treatment options and to ensure that they have ample institutional support to use these options. Joint actions by clinicians, administrators, insurers, and purchasers can encourage a culture of health care in which failure to intervene with a tobacco user is inconsistent with standards of care. (5/08)

TURNER SYNDROME

Clinical Practice Guidelines for the Care of Girls and Women With Turner Syndrome: Proceedings From the 2016 Cincinnati International Turner Syndrome Meeting

Claus H. Gravholt; Niels H. Andersen; Gerard S. Conway; Olaf M. Dekkers; Mitchell E. Geffner; Karen O. Klein; Angela E. Lin; Nelly Mauras; Charmian A. Quigley; Karen Rubin; David E. Sandberg; Theo C. J. Sas; Michael Silberbach; Viveca Söderström-Anttila; Kirstine Stochholm; Janielle A. van Alfen-van derVelden; Joachim Woelfle; and Philippe F. Backeljauw (on behalf of the International Turner Syndrome Consensus Group)

ABSTRACT. Turner syndrome affects 25–50 per 100,000 females and can involve multiple organs through all stages of life, necessitating multidisciplinary approach to care. Previous guidelines have highlighted this, but numerous important advances have been noted recently. These advances cover all specialty fields involved in the care of girls and women with TS. This paper is based on an international effort that started with exploratory meetings in 2014 in both Europe and the USA, and culminated with a Consensus Meeting held in Cincinnati, Ohio, USA in July 2016. Prior to this meeting, five groups each addressed important areas in TS care: 1) diagnostic and genetic issues, 2) growth and development during childhood and adolescence, 3) congenital and acquired cardiovascular disease, 4) transition and adult care, and 5) other comorbidities and neurocognitive issues. These groups produced proposals for the present guidelines. Additionally, four pertinent questions were submitted for formal GRADE (Grading of Recommendations, Assessment, Development and Evaluation) evaluation with a separate systematic review of the literature. These four questions related to the efficacy and most optimal treatment of short stature, infertility, hypertension, and hormonal replacement therapy. The guidelines project was initiated by the European Society of Endocrinology and the Pediatric Endocrine Society, in collaboration with the European Society for Paediatric Endocrinology, the Endocrine Society, the European Society of Human Reproduction and Embryology, the American Heart Association, the Society for Endocrinology, and the European Society of Cardiology. The guideline has been formally endorsed by the European Society of Endocrinology, the Pediatric Endocrine Society, the European Society for Paediatric Endocrinology, the European Society of Human Reproduction and Embryology and the Endocrine Society. Advocacy groups appointed representatives who participated in pre-meeting discussions and in the consensus meeting. (9/17)

VESICOURETERAL REFLUX

Report on the Management of Primary Vesicoureteral Reflux in Children

American Urological Association (5/97)

Section 3

Affirmation of Value
Clinical Practice Guidelines

*These guidelines are not endorsed as policy of the
American Academy of Pediatrics (AAP). Documents that lack
a clear description of the process for identifying, assessing,
and incorporating research evidence are not eligible for
AAP endorsement as practice guidelines. However, such
documents may be of educational value to members of the AAP.*

ASTHMA

Environmental Management of Pediatric Asthma: Guidelines for Health Care Providers
National Environmental Education Foundation

INTRODUCTION (EXCERPT). These guidelines are the product of a new Pediatric Asthma Initiative aimed at integrating environmental management of asthma into pediatric health care. This document outlines competencies in environmental health relevant to pediatric asthma that should be mastered by primary health care providers, and outlines the environmental interventions that should be communicated to patients.

These environmental management guidelines were developed for pediatricians, family physicians, internists, pediatric nurse practitioners, pediatric nurses, and physician assistants. In addition, these guidelines should be integrated into respiratory therapists' and licensed case/care (LICSW) management professionals' education and training.

The guidelines contain three components:

- Competencies: An outline of the knowledge and skills that health care providers and health professional students should master and demonstrate in order to incorporate management of environmental asthma triggers into pediatric practice.
- Environmental History Form: A quick, easy, user-friendly document that can be utilized as an intake tool by the health care provider to help determine pediatric patients' environmental asthma triggers.
- Environmental Intervention Guidelines: Follow-up questions and intervention solutions to environmental asthma triggers. (8/05)

PALLIATIVE CARE AND HOSPICE

Standards of Practice for Pediatric Palliative Care and Hospice
National Hospice and Palliative Care Organization (2/09)

SLEEP APNEA

Practice Guidelines for the Perioperative Management of Patients with Obstructive Sleep Apnea
American Society of Anesthesiologists (5/06)

TURNER SYNDROME

Care of Girls and Women With Turner Syndrome: A Guideline of the Turner Syndrome Study Group
Turner Syndrome Consensus Study Group

ABSTRACT. *Objectives.* The objective of this work is to provide updated guidelines for the evaluation and treatment of girls and women with Turner syndrome (TS).

Participants. The Turner Syndrome Consensus Study Group is a multidisciplinary panel of experts with relevant clinical and research experience with TS that met in Bethesda, Maryland, April 2006. The meeting was supported by the National Institute of Child Health and unrestricted educational grants from pharmaceutical companies.

Evidence. The study group used peer-reviewed published information to form its principal recommendations. Expert opinion was used where good evidence was lacking.

Consensus. The study group met for 3 d to discuss key issues. Breakout groups focused on genetic, cardiological, auxological, psychological, gynecological, and general medical concerns and drafted recommendations for presentation to the whole group. Draft reports were available for additional comment on the meeting web site. Synthesis of the section reports and final revisions were reviewed by e-mail and approved by whole-group consensus.

Conclusions. We suggest that parents receiving a prenatal diagnosis of TS be advised of the broad phenotypic spectrum and the good quality of life observed in TS in recent years. We recommend that magnetic resonance angiography be used in addition to echocardiography to evaluate the cardiovascular system and suggest that patients with defined cardiovascular defects be cautioned in regard to pregnancy and certain types of exercise. We recommend that puberty should not be delayed to promote statural growth. We suggest a comprehensive educational evaluation in early childhood to identify potential attention-deficit or nonverbal learning disorders. We suggest that caregivers address the prospect of premature ovarian failure in an open and sensitive manner and emphasize the critical importance of estrogen treatment for feminization and for bone health during the adult years. All individuals with TS require continued monitoring of hearing and thyroid function throughout the lifespan. We suggest that adults with TS be monitored for aortic enlargement, hypertension, diabetes, and dyslipidemia. (1/07)

SECTION 4

2018 Policies

From the American Academy of Pediatrics

• •

- *Policy Statements*
  ORGANIZATIONAL PRINCIPLES TO GUIDE AND DEFINE THE CHILD HEALTH CARE SYSTEM
  AND TO IMPROVE THE HEALTH OF ALL CHILDREN

- *Clinical Reports*
  GUIDANCE FOR THE CLINICIAN IN RENDERING PEDIATRIC CARE

- *Technical Reports*
  BACKGROUND INFORMATION TO SUPPORT AMERICAN ACADEMY OF PEDIATRICS POLICY

Includes policy statements, clinical reports, and technical reports published between January 1, 2018, and December 31, 2018

INTRODUCTION

This section of *Pediatric Clinical Practice Guidelines & Policies: A Compendium of Evidence-based Research for Pediatric Practice* is composed of policy statements, clinical reports, and technical reports issued by the American Academy of Pediatrics (AAP) and is designed as a quick reference tool for AAP members, AAP staff, and other interested parties. Section 4 includes the full text of all AAP policies published in 2018. Section 5 is a compilation of all active AAP policies (through December 31, 2018) arranged alphabetically, with abstracts where applicable. A subject index is also available. These materials should help answer questions that arise about the AAP position on child health care issues. **However, remember that AAP policy statements, clinical reports, and technical reports do not indicate an exclusive course of treatment or serve as a standard of medical care. Variations, taking into account individual circumstances, may be appropriate.**

Policy statements have been written by AAP committees, councils, task forces, or sections and approved by the AAP Board of Directors. Most of these statements have appeared previously in *Pediatrics, AAP News, or News & Comments* (the forerunner of *AAP News*).

This section does not contain all AAP policies. It does not include
- Press releases.
- Motions and resolutions that were approved by the Board of Directors. These can be found in the Board of Directors' minutes.
- Policies in manuals, pamphlets, booklets, or other AAP publications. These items can be ordered through the AAP. To order, visit http://shop.aap.org/books or call 866/843-2271.
- Testimony before Congress or government agencies.

All policy statements, clinical reports, and technical reports from the American Academy of Pediatrics automatically expire 5 years after publication unless reaffirmed, revised, or retired at or before that time. Please check the American Academy of Pediatrics website at www.aap.org for up-to-date reaffirmations, revisions, and retirements.

AAP Diversity and Inclusion Statement

- *Policy Statement*

POLICY STATEMENT Organizational Principles to Guide and Define the Child Health Care System and/or Improve the Health of all Children

American Academy
of Pediatrics

DEDICATED TO THE HEALTH OF ALL CHILDREN™

AAP Diversity and Inclusion Statement

The vision of the American Academy of Pediatrics (AAP) is that all children have optimal health and well-being and are valued by society and that AAP members practice the highest quality health care and experience professional satisfaction and personal well-being. From the founding of the AAP, pursuing this vision has included treasuring the uniqueness of each child and fostering a profession, health care system, and communities that celebrate all aspects of the diversity of each child and family.

The AAP appreciates that children are increasingly diverse, with differences that may include race, ethnicity, language spoken at home, religion, disability and special health care need, socioeconomic status, sexual orientation, gender identity, and other attributes.

The AAP, as an organization of pediatricians, pediatric medical subspecialists, and pediatric surgical specialists, recognizes that our membership is composed of a broad and diverse community. The AAP is strengthened by our diversity. The variety of skills, characteristics, and attributes offered by our members creates the vitality and success of the Academy and improves the care of all children and youth. Maximizing the diversity of our members and leaders allows the AAP to benefit from the rich talents and different perspectives of these individuals.

The AAP, as a national nonprofit organization, fervently respects, values, and promotes diversity and inclusiveness among all the individuals, groups, and vendors with whom we interact, collaborate, and partner.

The AAP is committed to being a learning organization that recruits, supports, and promotes talented, diverse individuals as employees and to fostering a work environment that embraces and celebrates diversity, promotes inclusiveness, and treats all employees with dignity and respect.

Celebrating the diversity of children and families and promoting nurturing, inclusive environments means actively opposing intolerance, bigotry, bias, and discrimination. The AAP is committed to using policy, advocacy, and education to encourage inclusivity and cultural effectiveness for all.

DOI: https://doi.org/10.1542/peds.2018-0193

PEDIATRICS (ISSN Numbers: Print, 0031-4005; Online, 1098-4275).

Copyright © 2018 by the American Academy of Pediatrics

COMPANION PAPER: A companion to this article can be found online at www.pediatrics.org/cgi/doi/10.1542/peds.2018-0177.

ABBREVIATION

AAP: American Academy of Pediatrics

To cite: AAP Diversity and Inclusion Statement. *Pediatrics.* 2018;141(4):e20180193

Advocacy for Improving Nutrition in the First 1000 Days to Support Childhood Development and Adult Health

• •

- *Policy Statement*

POLICY STATEMENT Organizational Principles to Guide and Define the Child Health Care System and/or Improve the Health of all Children

American Academy
of Pediatrics

DEDICATED TO THE HEALTH OF ALL CHILDREN™

Advocacy for Improving Nutrition in the First 1000 Days To Support Childhood Development and Adult Health

Sarah Jane Schwarzenberg, MD, FAAP, Michael K. Georgieff, MD, FAAP, COMMITTEE ON NUTRITION

abstract

Maternal prenatal nutrition and the child's nutrition in the first 2 years of life (1000 days) are crucial factors in a child's neurodevelopment and lifelong mental health. Child and adult health risks, including obesity, hypertension, and diabetes, may be programmed by nutritional status during this period. Calories are essential for growth of both fetus and child but are not sufficient for normal brain development. Although all nutrients are necessary for brain growth, key nutrients that support neurodevelopment include protein; zinc; iron; choline; folate; iodine; vitamins A, D, B_6, and B_{12}; and long-chain polyunsaturated fatty acids. Failure to provide key nutrients during this critical period of brain development may result in lifelong deficits in brain function despite subsequent nutrient repletion. Understanding the complex interplay of micro- and macronutrients and neurodevelopment is key to moving beyond simply recommending a "good diet" to optimizing nutrient delivery for the developing child. Leaders in pediatric health and policy makers must be aware of this research given its implications for public policy at the federal and state level. Pediatricians should refer to existing services for nutrition support for pregnant and breastfeeding women, infants, and toddlers. Finally, all providers caring for children can advocate for healthy diets for mothers, infants, and young children in the first 1000 days. Prioritizing public policies that ensure the provision of adequate nutrients and healthy eating during this crucial time would ensure that all children have an early foundation for optimal neurodevelopment, a key factor in long-term health.

University of Minnesota Masonic Children's Hospital, Minneapolis, Minnesota

Drs Schwarzenberg and Georgieff both contributed to the writing and editing of this policy statement and approved the final manuscript as submitted.

This document is copyrighted and is property of the American Academy of Pediatrics and its Board of Directors. All authors have filed conflict of interest statements with the American Academy of Pediatrics. Any conflicts have been resolved through a process approved by the Board of Directors. The American Academy of Pediatrics has neither solicited nor accepted any commercial involvement in the development of the content of this publication.

Policy statements from the American Academy of Pediatrics benefit from expertise and resources of liaisons and internal (AAP) and external reviewers. However, policy statements from the American Academy of Pediatrics may not reflect the views of the liaisons or the organizations or government agencies that they represent.

The guidance in this statement does not indicate an exclusive course of treatment or serve as a standard of medical care. Variations, taking into account individual circumstances, may be appropriate.

All policy statements from the American Academy of Pediatrics automatically expire 5 years after publication unless reaffirmed, revised, or retired at or before that time.

1,000 Days® is a trademark of 1,000 Days, a 501(c)(3) nonprofit organization. The 1,000 Days mark is used with permission from 1, 000 Days.

DOI: https://doi.org/10.1542/peds.2017-3716

To cite: Schwarzenberg SJ, Georgieff MK, AAP COMMITTEE ON NUTRITION. Advocacy for Improving Nutrition in the First 1000 Days To Support Childhood Development and Adult Health. *Pediatrics.* 2018;141(2):e20173716

INTRODUCTION

Healthy, normal neurodevelopment is a complex process involving cellular and structural changes in the brain that proceed in a specified sequence.[1,2] Changes that are too rapid or too slow in one part of the brain may result in the failure of crucial pathway connections to other parts of the brain. Timing is crucial; once a particular developmental sequence fails, it may not be possible to retrieve all the lost function. Moreover, neurodevelopment proceeds by a scaffolding process in which the development of increasingly complex neural circuits (and the behaviors they support) relies on successful completion of previous stages of development. Thus, optimal, healthy neurobehavioral development requires that all necessary factors be present at their biologically defined time points and that no inhibitory factors be present.

The most active period of neurologic development occurs in the first 1000 days of life, the period beginning at conception and ending at the start of the third postnatal year.[3] Rapid change occurs from the first development of a structure recognizable as the brain (postconception day 18) to age 2 years.[4] Important primary structures and processes that support fundamental behaviors and provide scaffolds for later-developing structures form during this time period. These structures and processes include the sensory systems (especially auditory and visual), the hippocampus (declarative learning and memory), myelination (speed of processing), and the monoamine neurotransmitter systems (affect, reward). Even the prefrontal cortex (planning, attention, inhibition, multitasking) and brain circuits involved in social development have the onset of rapid development in the first 1000 days. Although neurodevelopment continues throughout the life of a healthy person, by age 2 years the brain has undergone tremendous restructuring. Many of the developmental changes expected to occur during this period will not be able to occur in later life.

The period of fetal life and the first 2 years postpartum may be seen as a time of tremendous opportunity for neurodevelopment and a time of great vulnerability.[5] Healthy neurodevelopment is dependent on socioeconomic, interpersonal and/or family, and nutritional factors.[6] In the presence of a supportive environment, an attached primary caregiver, and a healthy diet, the brain typically thrives. In infants and children, toxic stress, emotional deprivation, and infection or inflammation have been shown to be associated with less optimal brain development, and a deficient diet for the child can worsen this. The effects of early adverse experiences may be a lifetime of medical and psychosocial problems, lost academic achievement and productivity, and possible effects on the next generation.[7–9] These long-term issues are the true cost to society, a cost that exceeds that of preventing them, and we again emphasize the importance of recognizing the developmental origins of adult health and disease.

For the purposes of this discussion, our focus is on the nutritional environment of the fetus, infant, and toddler. The nutritional environment has an effect on whether brain growth and differentiation proceed normally or abnormally. Both adequate overall nutrition (ie, absence of malnutrition) and provision of adequate amounts of key macro- and micronutrients at critical periods in development are necessary for normal brain development. Importantly, the definition of malnutrition includes both undernutrition (provision of inadequate amounts of macro- and/or micronutrients) and also obesity (provision of excessive calories, often at the expense of other crucial nutrients). It is important to recognize that many nutrients exhibit a U-shaped risk curve, whereby inadequate or excessive amounts both place the individual at risk. Each of these 2 forms of malnutrition affects neurodevelopment, and they may coexist in an individual.[10]

In this Policy Statement, we seek to inform pediatricians and other health care providers of the key role of nutrition in brain development in the first 1000 days of life (conception to 2 years of age). It is not meant as a comprehensive review of the data on brain-nutrient interaction (for this, see Rao and Georgieff[11]). With this policy statement, we intend to support pediatricians and other health care providers in promoting healthy nutrition and advocating for the expansion of programs that affect early life nutrition as a means of providing scaffolding for later nutritional programs and preventing early developmental loss. In this way, offered in this policy is an opportunity to improve each child's chance for the healthiest and most productive life possible.

Macronutrient (protein, fat, glucose) sufficiency is essential for normal brain development. Early macronutrient undernutrition is associated with lower IQ scores, reduced school success, and more behavioral dysregulation.[12] Intervention in early nutritional deficiency can be effective, and the full effects may be felt for many years.[13] In a study unlikely to be replicated, investigators in rural Guatemala between 1969 and 1989 provided protein-calorie supplementation of different degrees to different rural villages. Two villages received a high-calorie, high-protein supplement, and 2 villages received a low-calorie supplement without protein. Both supplements contained vitamins and minerals. The supplements were provided for pregnant and lactating women and children up to age 7 years. The investigators measured locally relevant outcomes over a period longer than 10 years, assessing children between 13 and 19 years of age. Children who had received high-calorie, high-protein supplementation before age 2 years scored higher on tests of knowledge, numeracy, reading, and vocabulary and had faster reaction times in information-processing tasks than age-matched children who received the low-calorie supplement. In villages receiving the high-calorie, high-protein supplement, there were no differences in test scores between children of high and low socioeconomic status, but in villages receiving the low-calorie supplements, children in the higher socioeconomic group had higher test scores. In summary, early supplementation of nutrients to children at risk for macronutrient deficiency improved neurodevelopmental outcomes over an extended period of life, beyond the period of supplementation.

There are populations in the United States that, similar to the villages in Guatemala, have inadequate access to macronutrients or only access to low-quality macronutrients. A food-insecure household, as defined by the US Department of Agriculture (USDA), is one in which "access to adequate food is limited by a lack of money and other resources."[14] In 2015, among US households with children, 16.6% (or 6.4 million households) were food insecure at some time during the year.[14] Of households with children with incomes below 185% of the poverty line, 36.8% were food insecure.[14] Impoverished households are at increased risk of food insecurity, but sudden social changes (for example, divorce, loss of job) can introduce food insecurity into households that are not impoverished. Although parents shield children from the worst effects of food insecurity, in approximately half of these food-insecure households, children were food insecure. In ~274 000 households in the United States in

2015, children were reported to be hungry, to have skipped a meal, or to have not eaten all day as a result of the severity of the food insecurity.[14] The researchers who conducted studies in Guatemala demonstrated the potential long-term efficacy (in terms of school performance) of targeting these households with low or very low food security for supplementation.

The failure to provide adequate macronutrients or key micronutrients at critical periods in brain development can have lifelong effects on a child. In addition to generalized macronutrient undernutrition, deficiencies of individual nutrients may have a substantial effect on neurodevelopment (Table 1). Prenatal and early infancy iron deficiency is associated with long-term neurobehavioral damage that may not be reversible, even with iron treatment.[15] Severe maternal iron deficiency, limited maternal-fetal iron transport (associated, for example, with cigarette smoking or maternal hypertension), or conditions that increase fetal iron demand (such as maternal diabetes) may lead to newborn iron deficiency and associated long-term cognitive deficits.[5] Adolescent iron deficiency is also associated with neurocognitive impairment but is reversible with iron treatment, suggesting differential effects of timing on brain function.[15] The earlier the timing of the deficiency, the more likely long-term effects will occur, probably because structure and regulation of genes involved in neural plasticity have been significantly altered.[5] Iodine is essential for synthesis of thyroid hormone, which is in turn crucial in neurodevelopment. Deficiency of iodine in pregnant women leads to cretinism in the child, with attendant severe, irreversible developmental delays. Mild to moderate postnatal chronic iodine deficiency is

TABLE 1 Nutrients That Particularly Affect Early Brain Development and Demonstrate a Critical or Sensitive Period

Macronutrients
Protein[a]
Specific fats (eg, LC-PUFAs)[a]
Glucose
Micronutrients
Zinc[a]
Copper[a]
Iodine[a]
Iron[a]
Selenium
Vitamins and cofactors
B vitamins (B$_6$, B$_{12}$)
Vitamin A
Vitamin K
Folate[a]
Choline[a]

LC-PUFA, long-chain polyunsaturated fatty acid. Reprinted with permission from Georgieff MK, Brunette KE, Tran PV. Early life nutrition and neural plasticity. *Dev Psychopathol*. 2015;27(2):415.

[a] Nutrients that meet the principles for demonstrating a critical or sensitive period during development.

associated with reduced performance on IQ tests.[1] Women living in iodine-deficient areas of the world require attention to supplementation during pregnancy.[16] Long-chain polyunsaturated fatty acids, which include docosahexaenoic acid and arachidonic acid, are important for normal development of vision and may also affect neurocognitive development.[17] Importantly in, some studies of supplementation of these fatty acids in early life, researchers did not demonstrate an effect on development until 6 years after supplementation. Traditions in complementary feeding or restricted diets because of poverty or neglect may reduce infant intake of many key factors in normal neurodevelopment, including zinc, protein, and iron.[18]

As the normative infant feeding, human milk and breastfeeding play a crucial role in neurodevelopment. Although randomized trials are not feasible, improved cognitive function in term and preterm infants who are fed human milk compared with those who are fed formula is supported by the weight of evidence on this topic.[19–21] Despite ongoing attempts to mimic human milk with infant formula, human milk may contain nutrients, growth factors, and cells important for brain development that formula lacks.[21] A role for the intestinal microbiome in brain development and behavior is supported by increasing evidence, and human milk and breastfeeding produce a microbiome with increased beneficial microbial communities.[22] Some micronutrient supplementation is needed in the breastfeeding infant (eg, zinc, iron, and vitamin D), and breastfeeding mothers need information about optimal nutrition.[23]

OBESITY

Although there is evidence that obesity in children and adolescents is associated with poorer educational success, studies are often complicated by small sample size, failure to control for confounding factors, and other aspects of study design.[24] In children born preterm with very low birth weights, body composition is correlated with neurodevelopment, and infants with greater fat-free mass (as opposed to fat mass) show improved neurodevelopment at 1 year of age. Weight gain alone, particularly when excessive weight is gained, may not achieve the desired goal of preserving brain development in the very low birth weight preterm infant.[25] Obesity of the expectant mother affects her offspring's health throughout the life span, including an increased risk for diabetes and obesity as well as an increased risk of adverse neurodevelopment.[26] Maternal obesity is also associated with decreased breastfeeding initiation rates, delayed onset of full milk production, and insufficient milk supply, resulting in a shortened duration of breastfeeding.[27–29] The introduction of complementary foods before 4 months of age may increase the risk of obesity in later

childhood.[30] In emerging but still limited evidence, it is suggested that childhood obesity may impact neurodevelopment.[10] If this is true, improving infant feeding patterns, including breastfeeding duration, age of complementary food introduction, and types of foods introduced, may protect neurodevelopment by reducing the risk of obesity in young children.[31–33] Although further studies will be important, obesity of mother or child appears to be a form of malnutrition affecting neurodevelopment in the first 1000 days.

In summary, nutrition is 1 of several factors affecting early neurodevelopment and is a factor that pediatricians and other health care providers have the capacity to improve by application of well-described, well-piloted, effective interventions.[5] Improved nutrition in the prenatal period, broad support for breastfeeding, and improved transitional and toddler nutrition all contribute to optimal neurocognitive development in the first 1000 days. Failure to provide adequate essential nutrients during the first 1000 days of life may result in increased expenditures later in the form of medical care, psychiatric and psychological care, remedial education, loss of wages, and management of behavior.[26,34] Conversely, the positive effects of improved early nutrition may not be apparent in short-term studies; indeed, because neurodevelopment is a biologic process across the life span in which changes are built on previous changes, the positive effects of an intervention may be seen after many years and may continue for many years. Thus, early nutritional intervention provides enormous potential advantages across the life span and, if nutritional needs are unmet in this period, developmental losses occur that are difficult to recover.

MEETING THE NUTRITIONAL NEEDS OF YOUNG CHILDREN FOR NEURODEVELOPMENT

Opportunities to improve early child nutrition, and thus neurodevelopment, are currently focused in 2 areas: first and foremost, programs directed at supporting breastfeeding and provision of nutritious food to young children; and second, guidelines that inform providers of the best practices in early childhood nutrition. It should be noted that programs that serve the nutritional needs of children after the first 1000 days form a crucial link from this early period to adulthood and are most effective when building on a scaffolding of optimal early nutrition.

Programs

Special Supplemental Nutrition Program for Women, Infants, and Children

The Special Supplemental Nutrition Program for Women, Infants, and Children (WIC) serves pregnant women, breastfeeding women (up to the child's first birthday), nonbreastfeeding postpartum women (up to 6 months postpartum), infants (up to their first birthday), and children up to their fifth birthday. As such, it is the most important program providing nutritional support in the first 1000 days. In the United States, 53% of all infants younger than 1 year are served by WIC. WIC supports breastfeeding prenatally through education and postpartum by helping mothers breastfeed, and they perform screening for anemia in women and children receiving services through the program.

Published evidence supports the impact of WIC on the health of children: prenatal WIC participation has been consistently associated with higher birth weight and longer gestation, particularly among mothers at highest risk,[35] and WIC participation has been linked to better infant health and less infant overweight and underweight.[36]

Despite the impact of WIC, children in many families who do not qualify under current guidelines would benefit from the nutrients and educational support of this program. Children whose families are on the margin of qualification for WIC may, for economic reasons, subsist on cheaper, less nutritionally replete diets. Many families fail to take advantage of the program after the first year of life, in part because of the challenge of access. Keeping families in the program longer (for example, through the elimination of the requirement to recertify eligibility at 1 year of age and extending eligibility for WIC through 6 years of age) will make supplemental food available to the growing toddler. WIC is a crucial program in providing food and education to support neurodevelopment.

Supplemental Nutrition Assistance Program

The Supplemental Nutrition Assistance Program (SNAP, formerly "Food Stamps") is a food and nutrition program of the USDA. It provides a modest benefit (just $1.35 on average per person per meal for households with children) to all who qualify. Seventy-two percent of households served are families with children. In addition to the antipoverty effects of the SNAP benefit (SNAP kept ~10.3 million people out of poverty in 2012, including nearly 4.9 million children), SNAP Nutrition Education, a partnership between the USDA and states, is intended to provide SNAP participants or eligible nonparticipants with the skills and knowledge to make healthy choices within a limited budget and choose active lifestyles consistent with federal dietary guidance. In fiscal year 2016, the USDA Food and Nutrition Service authorized $408 million to all 50 states, the District of Columbia, Guam, and the Virgin Islands to provide nutrition education and obesity prevention services using interventions that include direct education, social marketing, and policy, systems, and environmental changes.[37]

The USDA, in partnership with states, has supported the use of bonus incentives within SNAP, such as the use of "bonus dollars" in the form of tokens or paper coupons, for purchases made with SNAP benefits at farmer's markets.[38] Nutrition education or incentive programs that are specifically targeted to families with infants and young children would be valuable. In addition, many families receiving SNAP live in areas with limited grocery store options ("food deserts"), making it difficult to use their benefit optimally.

Child and Adult Care Food Program

The Child and Adult Care Food Program (CACFP) is administered by the USDA and, among other things, provides money to assist child care institutions and family or group day care homes in providing nutritious foods that contribute to the wellness, healthy growth, and development of children. In fiscal year 2013, CACFP served more than 3 million children. Completion of the revision of CACFP meal requirements to make them more consistent with the *Dietary Guidelines for Americans* (DGA)[39] should improve the nutritional quality of these meals for young children.

Food Pantries and Soup Kitchens

Food pantries and soup kitchens are generally community-supported programs that serve as a safety net for children and families struggling with inadequate food. However, many charitable food providers are not consistently able to provide healthful food in general, nutritional items appropriate for infants and toddlers, or amounts adequate to protect children from inadequate nutrition for more than a few days.

Maternal, Infant, and Early Childhood Home Visiting Program

Congress established the Maternal, Infant, and Early Childhood Home Visiting Program in 2010 to provide funds for states and tribes providing voluntary, evidence-based home visiting to at-risk families.[40] Although

not specifically aimed at nutrition, the services include education on parenting and health.

Baby-Friendly Hospital Initiative

The Baby-Friendly Hospital Initiative was developed by the United Nations Children's Fund and the World Health Organization in 1991 to increase hospital and/or birthing centers' attention to initiation of breastfeeding. Centers who qualify for this designation have implemented the "Ten Steps to Successful Breastfeeding" and adhere to the International Code of Marketing Breast-Milk Substitutes.[41] In a meta-analysis of programs created to improve many aspects of breastfeeding, Baby-Friendly Hospital support interventions had the greatest effect on promoting any breastfeeding.[42]

Guidelines

National Guidelines

The USDA and Department of Health and Human Services are responsible for developing and maintaining evidence-based guidelines for good nutrition, the DGA.[39] These guidelines focus on children 2 years and older. In 2014, the Birth to 24 Months project was started to develop guidelines for children in that age group.[43] This process is an evidence-based review of the existing literature on feeding children from birth to age 24 months. It begins with the formulation of questions, systematic reviews through the Nutrition Evidence Library at the USDA, and the grading of evidence on the basis of study quality, consistency of findings, number of studies and subjects, impact of outcome, and generalizability of findings.[44] Pediatricians with expertise in nutrition in these age groups are members of the committees currently doing this work. The final report and incorporation of these guidelines into the overall DGA is expected in 2020.

Because these guidelines are the reference point for state and federal policies and programs, pediatricians

TABLE 2 Resources To Help Pediatricians Optimize Nutrition in the First 1000 Days

Resource	Crucial Period	Major Points
The American College of Obstetrics and Gynecologists. Available at: http://www.acog.org	Prenatal, immediate postnatal	Breastfeeding toolkit, obesity toolkit
Guidelines for Perinatal Care. 8th ed. American Academy of Pediatrics and American College of Obstetrics and Gynecologists; 2017	Prenatal, immediate postnatal	Chapters on prenatal and postnatal care
Kleinman RE and Greer FR, eds. *Pediatric Nutrition*. 7th ed. American Academy of Pediatrics; 2014	From birth	Chapters that make recommendations on breastfeeding, complementary feeding, feeding the child, and macro- and micronutrients
Hagan JF, Shaw JS, Duncan PM, eds. *Bright Futures: Guidelines for Health Supervision of Infants, Children and Adolescents*. 4th ed. American Academy of Pediatrics; 2017	From birth	Chapters on healthy wt and healthy nutrition
Schanler RJ, Krebs NF, Mass SB, eds. *Breastfeeding Handbook for Physicians*. 2nd ed. American Academy of Pediatrics and The American College of Obstetrics and Gynecologists; 2013	From birth	Guide to rationale for breastfeeding, implementation, and maintenance
Policy statement: breastfeeding and the use of human milk. Section on breastfeeding. *Pediatrics*. 2012;129(3). Available at: www.pediatrics.org/cgi/content/full/129/3/e827	From birth	AAP policy on breastfeeding
Baker RD, Greer FR, and the Committee on Nutrition. Clinical report: diagnosis and prevention of iron deficiency and iron-deficiency anemia in infants and young children (0–3 y of age). *Pediatrics*. 2010;126(5):1–11	Birth to 3 y of age	AAP policy on iron supplementation

should be aware of the importance of these guidelines. The 2015 DGA saw an organized and concerted effort by special interest groups to subvert or dilute the results of the guideline process and the process itself. It is important that pediatricians, who are familiar with using evidence-based clinical guidelines, advocate for the scientific foundations of this process and support implementation of the guidelines.

American Academy of Pediatrics

The American Academy of Pediatrics (AAP) provides substantial information on the nutritional needs and support of children from birth to age 2 years, including information and guidance on breastfeeding[45] and on feeding infants and toddlers.[46] AAP policies on breastfeeding[21] and iron supplementation[47] directly address key issues in nutrition and cognition.

RECOMMENDATIONS

1. Pediatricians, family physicians, obstetricians, and other child health care providers need to be knowledgeable about breastfeeding to educate pregnant women about breastfeeding and be prepared to help breastfeeding mothers and their infants when problems occur. The AAP recommends exclusive breastfeeding for approximately the first 6 months of life and continuation after complementary foods have been introduced for at least the first year of life and beyond, as long as mutually desired by mother and child. Several organizations have reviewed interventions to support breastfeeding.[48,49] Despite the known advantages of human milk in early life, estimates are that 19% of children receive no human milk in infancy and only 22% breastfeed exclusively for the recommended 6 months;[50]

2. Pediatricians, family physicians, obstetricians, and other child health care providers can advocate at the local, state, and federal levels to preserve and strengthen nutrition programs with a focus on maternal, fetal, and neonatal nutrition. Interventions to ensure normal neurodevelopment include programs to minimize adverse environmental influences and programs to mitigate the effects of adverse environmental influences. These interventions begin with nutritional health for the pregnant woman, including adequate protein-energy intake, appropriate gestational weight gain, and iron sufficiency. To some degree, the placenta protects the fetus in terms of prioritization of nutrients from the mother. After birth, human milk provides optimal neurodevelopmental nutrition for at least the first 6 months.[21] After 6 months, pediatricians and other health care providers can support policies that advocate for optimal protein-calorie and micronutrient administration to infants and young children

TABLE 3 Organizations Focused on Hunger

Name	Web Site	Focus	Comments
Bread for the World	www.bread.org	Nonpartisan policy analysis and strategies to end hunger in the United States and the world. Provides education for opinion leaders, policy makers, and the public on hunger	Yearly report on key issues in hunger, often focused on the United States. Offers strategies for engaging churches and communities in advocacy. Faith-based, Christian organization
Feeding America	http://www.feedingamerica.org/	Nationwide network of food banks; develops and stocks food banks and other emergency food distribution systems	E-mail newsletter, annual report. Volunteer opportunities locally at many levels
Mazon	http://mazon.org	Policy change, strategy, and education to end hunger	Works to improve nutritious food choices in food banks, provides food for seniors, and impacts hunger in rural areas. Places a high priority on the support of child nutrition programs. Faith-based, Jewish organization
Community for Zero Hunger	http://www.zerohungercommunity.org	Supports UN Zero Hunger Challenge; focused on world hunger	High-level policy oriented
Share Our Strength	https://www.nokidhungry.org	Runs the No Kid Hungry Campaign; teaches cooking to low-income families, supports and teaches MyPlate	Guides volunteers to hunger-based opportunities in their communities
Food and Research Action Center	http://frac.org	National nonprofit organization that works on policy and research with hundreds of national, state, and local nonprofit organizations, public agencies, corporations, and labor organizations to address hunger, food insecurity, and their root cause: poverty	Maintains a list of state antihunger organizations, which can be found at: http://frac.org/about/1303-2
1,000 Days	www.thousanddays.org	Focuses on nutrition and all forms of malnutrition in the first 1000 d of life. Works in the United States and globally to promote action and investment in maternal, infant, and young child nutrition	1,000 Days is "high-level policy oriented" in both the global and domestic contexts, and the organization has a large grassroots constituency of advocates (primarily mothers) in the United States

UN, United Nations.

(eg, AAP iron policy[47]) as well as programs that provide high-quality nutrition to infants and young children (eg, WIC);

3. Pediatricians and other child health care providers can become conversant about food sources that supply the critical nutrients necessary for brain development during particularly important times. Although most pediatricians are aware that exclusive breastfeeding is the best source of nutrition for the first 6 months, dietary advice thereafter is less robust. Awareness of which foods are "healthy," not just as alternatives to unhealthy or junk food but as positive factors targeting optimal development, would allow pediatricians to make more appropriate dietary recommendations. As the infant's nutritional intake moves from the relative protection of breastfeeding to dependence on choices made by his or her parents, pediatrician guidance for informed food choices becomes increasingly important. Moreover, knowing which nutrients are at risk in the breastfed infant after 6 months (eg, zinc, iron, vitamin D) will guide dietary recommendations in the clinic or practice. Guidance for pediatricians is provided in existing documents (Tables 1 and 2) but over a spectrum of resources and chapters, and it is often without clear prescriptive recommendations;

4. Leaders in childhood nutrition can advocate for incorporating into existing nutritional advice an actionable guide to healthy eating as a positive choice rather than an avoidance of unhealthy foods. This would give pediatricians and families more prescriptive advice as to optimal dietary choices. Additionally, it is important that families understand that no 1 food is alone adequate to ensure optimal neurodevelopment and health (ie, a "superfood");

5. Pediatricians and other child health care providers can focus the attention of existing programs on improving micro- and macronutrient offerings for infants and young children. For example, providing information to existing food pantries and soup kitchens to create food packages and meals

that target the specific needs of pregnant women, breastfeeding women, and children in the first 2 years of life;

6. Pediatricians and other child health care providers can encourage families to take advantage of programs providing early childhood nutrition and advocate for eliminating barriers that families face to enrolling and remaining enrolled in such programs. Many families do not take advantage of WIC services after the first year of life. Encouraging the use of services and benefits for which the family is eligible and eliminating the requirement to recertify eligibility for young children at 1 year of age can improve early life nutrition for children;

7. Pediatricians and other child health care providers can oppose changes in eligibility or financing structures that would adversely affect key programs providing early childhood nutrition. Such changes include changing funding to block grants or delinking nutrition and health assistance programs, such as the adjunctive eligibility between WIC and Medicaid. Federal nutrition programs such as SNAP are successful because of eligibility rules and a funding structure that makes benefits available to children in almost all families with little income and few resources;

8. Pediatricians and other child health care providers can

anticipate neurodevelopmental concerns in children with early nutrient deficiency. Pediatricians can educate themselves as to which nutrients are at risk for deficiency and at what age as well as about appropriate screening for children at high risk. For example, the risk of iron deficiency is not equal throughout the pediatric life span. Pediatricians can be aware that the newborn, the toddler, and the adolescent are at highest risk and should be aware of factors that increase those risks;

9. Pediatricians and other child health care providers can partner with obstetricians and family physicians to encourage improvements in maternal diet and attention to clinical situations that may limit the fetus's access to crucial micronutrients; and

10. Pediatricians and other child health care providers can become advocates in the "Hunger Community." Many organizations work to reduce hunger at the local level, across the United States, and in the global community. As pediatricians consider their personal contribution to social action, involvement in 1 of these organizations is an excellent option (see Table 3).

LEAD AUTHORS

Sarah Jane Schwarzenberg, MD, FAAP
Michael K. Georgieff, MD, FAAP

COMMITTEE ON NUTRITION, 2016–2017

Stephen Daniels, MD, PhD, FAAP, Chairperson
Mark Corkins, MD, FAAP
Neville H. Golden, MD, FAAP
Jae H. Kim, MD, PhD, FAAP
C. Wesley Lindsey, MD, FAAP
Sheela N. Magge, MD, MSCE, FAAP
Sarah Jane Schwarzenberg, MD, FAAP

PAST COMMITTEE MEMBERS

Steven Abrams, MD, FAAP
Sarah de Ferranti, MD, FAAP

LIAISONS

Carrie L. Assar, PharmD, MS – *Food and Drug Administration*
Janet de Jesus, MS, RD – *National Institutes of Health*
Cria Perrine, PhD – *Centers for Disease Control and Prevention*
Valery Soto, MS, RD, LD – *USDA*

STAFF

Debra Burrowes, MHA
Madeline Curtis
Tamar Magarik Haro

ABBREVIATIONS	
AAP:	American Academy of Pediatrics
CACFP:	Child and Adult Care Food Program
DGA:	*Dietary Guidelines for Americans*
SNAP:	Supplemental Nutrition Assistance Program
USDA:	US Department of Agriculture
WIC:	Special Supplemental Nutrition Program for Women, Infants, and Children

Address correspondence to Sarah Jane Schwarzenberg, MD, FAAP. E-mail: schwa005@umn.edu

PEDIATRICS (ISSN Numbers: Print, 0031-4005; Online, 1098-4275).

FINANCIAL DISCLOSURE: The authors have indicated they have no financial relationships relevant to this article to disclose.

FUNDING: No external funding.

POTENTIAL CONFLICT OF INTEREST: The authors have indicated they have no potential conflicts of interest to disclose.

REFERENCES

1. Prado EL, Dewey KG. Nutrition and brain development in early life. *Nutr Rev.* 2014;72(4):267–284

2. Wachs TD, Georgieff M, Cusick S, McEwen BS. Issues in the timing of integrated early interventions: contributions from nutrition, neuroscience, and psychological research. *Ann N Y Acad Sci.* 2014;1308:89–106

3. Fox SE, Levitt P, Nelson CA III. How the timing and quality of early experiences influence the development of brain architecture. *Child Dev.* 2010;81(1):28–40

4. Thompson RA, Nelson CA. Developmental science and the media. Early brain development. *Am Psychol.* 2001;56(1):5–15

5. Georgieff MK, Brunette KE, Tran PV. Early life nutrition and neural plasticity. *Dev Psychopathol.* 2015;27(2):411–423

6. Bick J, Nelson CA. Early adverse experiences and the developing brain. *Neuropsychopharmacology.* 2016;41(1):177–196

7. Danese A, Pariante CM, Caspi A, Taylor A, Poulton R. Childhood maltreatment predicts adult inflammation in a life-course study. *Proc Natl Acad Sci USA.* 2007;104(4):1319–1324

8. Galobardes B, Lynch JW, Smith GD. Is the association between childhood socioeconomic circumstances and cause-specific mortality established? Update of a systematic review. *J Epidemiol Community Health.* 2008;62(5):387–390

9. Ngure FM, Reid BM, Humphrey JH, Mbuya MN, Pelto G, Stoltzfus RJ. Water, sanitation, and hygiene (WASH), environmental enteropathy, nutrition, and early child development: making the links. *Ann N Y Acad Sci.* 2014;1308:118–128

10. Martin A, Booth JN, Young D, et al. Associations between obesity and cognition in the pre-school years. *Obesity (Silver Spring).* 2016;24(1):207–214

11. Rao R, Georgieff MK. The nutritionally deprived fetus and newborn infant. In: Shevell M, Miller S, ed. *International Reviews of Child Neurology Series: Acquired Brain Injury in the Fetus & Newborn.* London, England: Mac Keith Press; 2012:277–287

12. Grantham-McGregor S. A review of studies of the effect of severe malnutrition on mental development. *J Nutr.* 1995;125(suppl 8):2233S–2238S

13. Pollitt E, Gorman KS, Engle PL, Rivera JA, Martorell R. Nutrition in early life and the fulfillment of intellectual potential. *J Nutr.* 1995;125(suppl 4):1111S–1118S

14. Coleman-Jensen A, Rabbitt MP, Gregory CA, Singh A. *Household Food Security in the United States in 2015, ERR-215.* Washington, DC: US Department of Agriculture, Economic Research Service; 2016

15. Georgieff MK. Long-term brain and behavioral consequences of early iron deficiency. *Nutr Rev.* 2011;69(suppl 1):S43–S48

16. Monk C, Georgieff MK, Osterholm EA. Research review: maternal prenatal distress and poor nutrition—mutually influencing risk factors affecting infant neurocognitive development. *J Child Psychol Psychiatry.* 2013;54(2):115–130

17. Colombo J, Carlson SE, Cheatham CL, et al. Long-term effects of LCPUFA supplementation on childhood cognitive outcomes. *Am J Clin Nutr.* 2013;98(2):403–412

18. Young BE, Krebs NF. Complementary feeding: critical considerations to optimize growth, nutrition, and feeding behavior. *Curr Pediatr Rep.* 2013;1(4):247–256

19. Bar S, Milanaik R, Adesman A. Long-term neurodevelopmental benefits of breastfeeding. *Curr Opin Pediatr.* 2016;28(4):559–566

20. Belfort MB, Anderson PJ, Nowak VA, et al. Breast milk feeding, brain development, and neurocognitive outcomes: a 7-year longitudinal study in infants born at less than 30 weeks' gestation. *J Pediatr.* 2016;177:133–139.e1

21. Section on Breastfeeding. Breastfeeding and the use of human milk. *Pediatrics.* 2012;129(3). Available at: www.pediatrics.org/cgi/content/full/129/3/e827

22. Diaz Heijtz R. Fetal, neonatal, and infant microbiome: perturbations and subsequent effects on brain development and behavior. *Semin Fetal Neonatal Med.* 2016;21(6):410–417

23. Cusick SE, Georgieff MK. The role of nutrition in brain development: the golden opportunity of the "first 1000 days". *J Pediatr.* 2016;175:16–21

24. Liang J, Matheson BE, Kaye WH, Boutelle KN. Neurocognitive correlates of obesity and obesity-related behaviors in children and adolescents. *Int J Obes (Lond).* 2014;38(4):494–506

25. Ramel SE, Gray HL, Christiansen E, Boys C, Georgieff MK, Demerath EW. Greater early gains in fat-free mass, but not fat mass, are associated with improved neurodevelopment at 1 year corrected age for prematurity in very low birth weight preterm infants. *J Pediatr.* 2016;173:108–115

26. Zambrano E, Ibáñez C, Martínez-Samayoa PM, Lomas-Soria C, Durand-Carbajal M, Rodríguez-González GL. Maternal obesity: lifelong metabolic outcomes for offspring from poor developmental trajectories during the perinatal period. *Arch Med Res.* 2016;47(1):1–12

27. O'Sullivan EJ, Perrine CG, Rasmussen KM. Early breastfeeding problems mediate the negative association between maternal obesity and exclusive breastfeeding at 1 and 2 months postpartum. *J Nutr.* 2015;145(10):2369–2378

28. Verret-Chalifour J, Giguère Y, Forest JC, Croteau J, Zhang P, Marc I. Breastfeeding initiation: impact of obesity in a large Canadian perinatal cohort study. *PLoS One.* 2015;10(2):e0117512

29. Winkvist A, Brantsæter AL, Brandhagen M, Haugen M, Meltzer HM, Lissner L. Maternal prepregnant body mass index and gestational weight gain are associated with initiation and duration of breastfeeding among Norwegian mothers. *J Nutr.* 2015;145(6):1263–1270

30. Daniels L, Mallan KM, Fildes A, Wilson J. The timing of solid introduction in an 'obesogenic' environment: a narrative review of the evidence and

methodological issues. *Aust N Z J Public Health.* 2015;39(4):366–373

31. Betoko A, Lioret S, Heude B, et al; EDEN Mother-Child Cohort Study Group. Influence of infant feeding patterns over the first year of life on growth from birth to 5 years. *Pediatr Obes.* 2017;12(suppl 1):94–101

32. Huh SY, Rifas-Shiman SL, Taveras EM, Oken E, Gillman MW. Timing of solid food introduction and risk of obesity in preschool-aged children. *Pediatrics.* 2011;127(3). Available at: www.pediatrics.org/cgi/content/full/127/3/e544

33. Victora CG, Bahl R, Barros AJ, et al; Lancet Breastfeeding Series Group. Breastfeeding in the 21st century: epidemiology, mechanisms, and lifelong effect. *Lancet.* 2016;387(10017):475–490

34. Walker SP, Wachs TD, Gardner JM, et al; International Child Development Steering Group. Child development: risk factors for adverse outcomes in developing countries. *Lancet.* 2007;369(9556):145–157

35. Colman S, Nichols-Barrer IP, Redline JE, Devaney BL, Ansell SV, Joyce T. *Effects of the Special Supplemental Nutrition Program for Women, Infants, and Children (WIC): A Review of Recent Research.* Washington, DC: US Department of Agriculture, Food, and Nutrition Service, Office of Research and Analysis; 2012

36. Black MM, Cutts DB, Frank DA, et al; Children's Sentinel Nutritional Assessment Program Study Group. Special supplemental nutrition program for women, infants, and children participation and infants' growth and health: a multisite surveillance study. *Pediatrics.* 2004;114(1):169–176

37. USDA. 2016. Available at: https://www.fns.usda.gov/snap/supplemental-nutrition-assistance-program-snap. Accessed December 26, 2017

38. USDA. 2016. Bonus incentives. Available at: https://www.fns.usda.gov/ebt/bonus-incentives. Accessed December 26, 2017

39. USDA. *2015–2020 Dietary Guidelines for Americans.* 8th ed. Washington, DC: US Department of Health and Human Services and US Department of Agriculture; 2015

40. Zero to Three. Maternal, infant, and early childhood visiting program. 2016. Available at: https://www.zerotothree.org/resources/1033-the-miechy-program. Accessed December 26, 2017

41. Baby-Friendly USA. Baby-friendly hospital initiative. 2017. Available at: https://www.babyfriendlyusa.org/about-us. Accessed February 11, 2017

42. Sinha B, Chowdhury R, Sankar MJ, et al. Interventions to improve breastfeeding outcomes: a systematic review and meta-analysis. *Acta Paediatr.* 2015;104(467):114–134

43. USDA. Pregnancy and birth to 24 months project. Available at: https://www.cnpp.usda.gov/birthto24months. Accessed December 26, 2017

44. Schneeman B. Science-based regulatory and policy considerations in nutrition. *Adv Nutr.* 2015;6(3):361S–367S

45. Schanler RJ, Krebs NF, Mass SB, eds. *Breastfeeding Handbook for Physicians.* 2nd ed. Elk Grove Village, IL: American Academy of Pediatrics; 2013

46. Kleinman RE, Greer FR, eds. *Pediatric Nutrition.* 7th ed. Elk Grove Village, IL: American Academy of Pediatrics; 2013

47. Baker RD, Greer FR; Committee on Nutrition American Academy of Pediatrics. Diagnosis and prevention of iron deficiency and iron-deficiency anemia in infants and young children (0-3 years of age). *Pediatrics.* 2010;126(5):1040–1050

48. US Preventive Services Task Force, Bibbins-Domingo K, Grossman DC, et al. Primary care interventions to support breastfeeding: US Preventive Services Task Force recommendation statement. *JAMA.* 2016;316(16):1688–1693

49. Rollins NC, Bhandari N, Hajeebhoy N, et al; Lancet Breastfeeding Series Group. Why invest, and what it will take to improve breastfeeding practices? *Lancet.* 2016;387(10017):491–504

50. Centers for Disease Control and Prevention. National immunization survey (NIS). 2016. Available at: https://www.cdc.gov/breastfeeding/data/NIS_data/. Accessed February 11, 2017

Advocating for Life Support Training of Children, Parents, Caregivers, School Personnel, and the Public

- *Policy Statement*

POLICY STATEMENT Organizational Principles to Guide and Define the Child Health Care System and/or Improve the Health of all Children

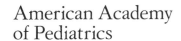

American Academy of Pediatrics
DEDICATED TO THE HEALTH OF ALL CHILDREN™

Advocating for Life Support Training of Children, Parents, Caregivers, School Personnel, and the Public

James M. Callahan, MD, FAAP,[a] Susan M. Fuchs, MD, FAAP,[b] COMMITTEE ON PEDIATRIC EMERGENCY MEDICINE

abstract

Out-of-hospital cardiac arrest occurs frequently among people of all ages, including more than 6000 children annually. Pediatric cardiac arrest in the out-of-hospital setting is a stressful event for family, friends, caregivers, classmates, school personnel, and witnesses. Immediate bystander cardiopulmonary resuscitation and the use of automated external defibrillators are associated with improved survival in adults. There is some evidence in which improved survival in children who receive immediate bystander cardiopulmonary resuscitation is shown. Pediatricians, in their role as advocates to improve the health of all children, are uniquely positioned to strongly encourage the training of children, parents, caregivers, school personnel, and the lay public in the provision of basic life support, including pediatric basic life support, as well as the appropriate use of automated external defibrillators.

[a]Division of Emergency Medicine, Department of Pediatrics, Children's Hospital of Philadelphia and Raymond and Ruth Perelman School of Medicine, University of Pennsylvania, Philadelphia, Pennsylvania; and [b]Department of Pediatrics, Feinberg School of Medicine, Northwestern University, Evanston, Illinois, and Division of Emergency Medicine, Ann & Robert H Lurie Children's Hospital of Chicago, Chicago, Illinois

Drs Callahan and Fuchs were responsible for all aspects of writing and editing this statement and reviewing and responding to questions and comments from reviewers and the Board of Directors.

DOI: https://doi.org/10.1542/peds.2018-0704

Address correspondence to James M. Callahan, MD, FAAP. E-mail: callahanj@email.chop.edu

To cite: Callahan JM, Fuchs SM, AAP COMMITTEE ON PEDIATRIC EMERGENCY MEDICINE. Advocating for Life Support Training of Children, Parents, Caregivers, School Personnel, and the Public. Pediatrics. 2018;141(6):e20180704

INTRODUCTION

Each year, more than 300 000 adults and 6000 children experience out-of-hospital cardiac arrest (OHCA).[1] Although survival rates in OHCA in both adults and children are low, the provision of bystander cardiopulmonary resuscitation (CPR) has been shown to increase the rate of survival, with favorable neurologic outcome in OHCA victims of all ages.[2] Schools are a potential setting for OHCA in children, adolescents, and adults. OHCA is frequently associated with an initial cardiac rhythm that is potentially treatable by using an automated external defibrillator (AED) in adults (ie, a "shockable rhythm"). Shockable rhythms, although less common in children, do occur with an increasing prevalence in older children and adolescents. The American Heart Association recommends the use of AEDs in children of all ages who have experienced OHCA until a manual defibrillator is available. Researchers have shown that the presence of AEDs in the community, training of lay people in their use, and their use during OHCA is associated with increased survival among adults with OHCA.[3–5] Training of the public is associated with increased rates of bystander CPR when OHCA occurs. Children can be taught from a young age how to seek assistance for victims of OHCA, and older children and adolescents can be taught CPR and how to use AEDs effectively.[6–8] More than 30 states currently require CPR training as a prerequisite for high school graduation. Although funding is a potential obstacle to more widespread implementation of CPR training in schools and AED installation, many innovative solutions to this have been used to overcome this barrier. Relatively small investments may yield significant improvement in survival after OHCA. Pediatricians are recognized as advocates for the health of all children and are in a unique position to advocate for increased life support training of children, parents, caregivers, school personnel, and the public, including the use of AEDs, and to be sources of such training and role models for its implementation.

RECOMMENDATIONS

1. Pediatricians should stay up-to-date on recommendations for CPR performance and pediatric basic and advanced life support, including recommendations for bystander CPR and AED use in out-of-hospital settings;

2. Pediatricians should support and advocate for:

   o Including age-appropriate life support training for children (eg, teaching young children how to seek assistance for victims of OHCA, teaching CPR to older children, and teaching CPR and AED use to adolescents) as part of the curriculum in schools beginning in the primary grades;

   o Providing life support training to all school personnel;

   o Programs that provide life support training for parents, caregivers, and the public that could be taught in schools, hospitals, and other health care organizations and by community groups;

   o Placement of an AED appropriate for the treatment of adults and children in every school in the community as well as training for proper AED use for school personnel and older children. AED should be placed in high schools first, and if funding is available, this could be expanded to other schools;

   o Placement of an AED appropriate for the treatment of adults and children near every school athletic facility and training for proper AED use for school personnel and older children; and

   o Funding to promote the above; and

3. Pediatricians should work with parents and legislators to mandate CPR training and AED placement in all public and private schools if those laws do not already exist in their state.

LEAD AUTHORS

James M. Callahan, MD, FAAP
Susan M. Fuchs, MD, FAAP

AMERICAN ACADEMY OF PEDIATRICS COMMITTEE ON PEDIATRIC EMERGENCY MEDICINE, 2017–2018

Joseph Wright, MD, MPH, FAAP, Chairperson
Terry Adirim, MD, MPH, FAAP
Michael S.D. Agus, MD, FAAP
James M. Callahan, MD, FAAP
Toni Gross, MD, MPH, FAAP
Natalie Lane, MD, FAAP
Lois Lee, MD, MPH, FAAP
Suzan Mazor, MD, FAAP
Prashant Mahajan, MD, MPH, MBA, FAAP
Nathan Timm, MD, FAAP

LIAISONS

Andrew Eisenberg, MD – *American Academy of Family Physicians*
Cynthia Wright Johnson, MSN, RN – *National Association of State EMS Officials*
Cynthiana Lightfoot, BFA, NRP – *American Academy of Pediatrics Family Partnerships Network*
Charles Macias, MD, MPH, FAAP – *National EMS for Children Innovation and Improvement Center*
Brian Moore, MD, MPH, FAAP – *National Association of Emergency Medical Services Physicians*
Diane Pilkey, RN, MPH – *Health Resources and Services Administration*
Katherine Remick, MD, FAAP – *National Association of Emergency Medical Technicians*
Mohsen Saidinejad, MD, MBA, FAAP, FACEP – *American College of Emergency Physicians*
Sally Snow, RN, BSN, CPEN, FAEN – *Emergency Nurses Association*
Mary Fallat, MD, FAAP – *American College of Surgeons*

OTHER FORMER COMMITTEE MEMBERS WITH INPUT DURING STATEMENT DEVELOPMENT

Joan E. Shook, MD, MBA, FAAP, Immediate Past Chairperson
Lee Benjamin, MD, FAAP, FACEP
Thomas H. Chun, MD, MPH, FAAP
Gregory P. Conners, MD, MPH, MBA, FAAP
Edward E. Conway Jr, MD, MS, FAAP
Nanette C. Dudley, MD, FAAP
Susan M. Fuchs, MD, FAAP
Brian R. Moore, MD, FAAP
Paul Sirbaugh, DO, MBA, FAAP

STAFF

Sue Tellez

ABBREVIATIONS

AED: automated external defibrillator
CPR: cardiopulmonary resuscitation
OHCA: out-of-hospital cardiac arrest

PEDIATRICS (ISSN Numbers: Print, 0031-4005; Online, 1098-4275).

FINANCIAL DISCLOSURE: The authors have indicated they have no financial relationships relevant to this article to disclose.

FUNDING: No external funding.

POTENTIAL CONFLICT OF INTEREST: The authors have indicated they have no potential conflicts of interest to disclose.

COMPANION PAPER: A companion to this article can be found online at www.pediatrics.org/cgi/doi/10.1542/peds.2018-0705.

REFERENCES

1. Mozaffarian D, Benjamin EJ, Go AS, et al; American Heart Association Statistics Committee and Stroke Statistics Subcommittee. Heart disease and stroke statistics—2015 update: a report from the American Heart Association. *Circulation.* 2015;131(4):e29–e322

2. Goto Y, Maeda T, Goto Y. Impact of dispatcher-assisted bystander cardiopulmonary resuscitation on neurological outcomes in children with out-of-hospital cardiac arrests: a prospective, nationwide, population-based cohort study. *J Am Heart Assoc.* 2014;3(3):e000499

3. Cave DM, Aufderheide TP, Beeson J, et al; American Heart Association Emergency Cardiovascular Care Committee; Council on Cardiopulmonary, Critical Care, Perioperative and Resuscitation; Council on Cardiovascular Diseases in the Young; Council on Cardiovascular Nursing; Council on Clinical Cardiology, and Advocacy Coordinating Committee. Importance and implementation of training in cardiopulmonary resuscitation and automated external defibrillation in schools: a science advisory from the American Heart Association. *Circulation.* 2011;123(6):691–706

4. Hallstrom AP, Ornato JP, Weisfeldt M, et al; Public Access Defibrillation Trial Investigators. Public-access defibrillation and survival after out-of-hospital cardiac arrest. *N Engl J Med.* 2004;351(7):637–646

5. Weisfeldt ML, Sitlani CM, Ornato JP, et al; ROC Investigators. Survival after application of automatic external defibrillators before arrival of the emergency medical system: evaluation in the resuscitation outcomes consortium population of 21 million. *J Am Coll Cardiol.* 2010;55(16): 1713–1720

6. Plant N, Taylor K. How best to teach CPR to schoolchildren: a systematic review. *Resuscitation.* 2013;84(4):415–421

7. Uray T, Lunzer A, Ochsenhofer A, et al. Feasibility of life-supporting first-aid (LSFA) training as a mandatory subject in primary schools. *Resuscitation.* 2003;59(2):211–220

8. Bollig G, Wahl HA, Svendsen MV. Primary school children are able to perform basic life-saving first aid measures. *Resuscitation.* 2009;80(6):689–692

Advocating for Life Support Training of Children, Parents, Caregivers, School Personnel, and the Public

- *Technical Report*

TECHNICAL REPORT

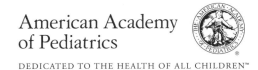

American Academy
of Pediatrics

DEDICATED TO THE HEALTH OF ALL CHILDREN™

Advocating for Life Support Training of Children, Parents, Caregivers, School Personnel, and the Public

Susan M. Fuchs, MD, FAAP, COMMITTEE ON PEDIATRIC EMERGENCY MEDICINE

abstract

Pediatric cardiac arrest in the out-of-hospital setting is a traumatic event for family, friends, caregivers, classmates, and school personnel. Immediate bystander cardiopulmonary resuscitation and the use of automatic external defibrillators have been shown to improve survival in adults. There is some evidence to show improved survival in children who receive immediate bystander cardiopulmonary resuscitation. Pediatricians, in their role as advocates to improve the health of all children, are uniquely positioned to strongly encourage the training of children, parents, caregivers, school personnel, and the lay public in the provision of basic life support, including pediatric basic life support, as well as the appropriate use of automated external defibrillators.

Pediatrics, Feinberg School of Medicine, Northwestern University, Evanston, Illinois; and Division of Emergency Medicine, Ann & Robert H Lurie Children's Hospital of Chicago, Chicago, Illinois

Dr Fuchs was responsible for all aspects of writing and editing this statement and reviewing and responding to questions and comments from reviewers and the Board of Directors.

Technical reports from the American Academy of Pediatrics benefit from expertise and resources of liaisons and internal (AAP) and external reviewers. However, technical reports from the American Academy of Pediatrics may not reflect the views of the liaisons or the organizations or government agencies that they represent.

The guidance in this report does not indicate an exclusive course of treatment or serve as a standard of medical care. Variations, taking into account individual circumstances, may be appropriate.

All technical reports from the American Academy of Pediatrics automatically expire 5 years after publication unless reaffirmed, revised, or retired at or before that time.

DOI: https://doi.org/10.1542/peds.2018-0705

Address correspondence to Susan M. Fuchs, MD, FAAP. E-mail: s-fuchs@northwestern.edu

PEDIATRICS (ISSN Numbers: Print, 0031-4005; Online, 1098-4275).

INTRODUCTION

Each year, 347 322 adults and 7037 children experience out-of-hospital cardiac arrest (OHCA).[1] Survival in children from nontraumatic OHCA remains dismal at 6.4%, and many survivors have poor neurologic outcomes.[2,3] Although the overall incidence of 8.04 per 100 000 person years of pediatric OHCA is less than that of adults, the incidence in infants younger than 1 year is actually higher (72 per 10 000 person years for infants vs 50–55 per 100 000 person years for adults). According to the Resuscitation Outcomes Consortium, the incidence for children 1 to 12 years of age is 3.73 per 10 000 person years and for adolescents (12–19 years) is 6.37 per 100 000 person years.[2,4] Infants also have the greatest mortality rate, with only 3.3% surviving to hospital discharge.[2] The survival rate of children and adolescents, however, surpasses that of adults (4.5%), with 9.1% of children and 8.9% of adolescents surviving to hospital discharge.[2,4] The most common cause of OHCA in infants includes sudden unexpected infant death (previously called sudden infant death syndrome) and congenital anomalies, whereas the most common cause of OHCA in children was drowning.[2,5] In adolescents, hanging and poisoning

To cite: Fuchs SM and AAP COMMITTEE ON PEDIATRIC EMERGENCY MEDICINE. Advocating for Life Support Training of Children, Parents, Caregivers, School Personnel, and the Public. *Pediatrics.* 2018;141(6):e20180705

were the most common causes of OHCA.[2] The authors of 1 study noted that survival was lower in Canadian children, with only 1.9% of survivors 1 to 19 years of age achieving hospital discharge, but included in this study were traumatic etiologies for OHCA, such as motor vehicle collisions, which had not been part of the data set in the studies referenced previously.[6]

In the Resuscitation Outcomes Consortium Epistry-Cardiac Arrest, emergency medical services (EMS) providers treated approximately 81% of pediatric patients suffering from OHCA; interventions included bag mask ventilation, advanced airway placement, vascular access, and drug therapy.[2] When available, the initial cardiac rhythm was documented as asystole or pulseless electrical activity in 82% of patients, and pulseless ventricular fibrillation or ventricular tachycardia (VF/VT) in 7%.[2,4] Adolescents were more likely than younger children or infants to have an initial VF/VT rhythm (15% vs 5% and 4%, respectively) but in percentages below the 23% of VF/VT seen in adults.[2,4] Predictors of a better outcome included witnessed arrest, bystander cardiopulmonary resuscitation (CPR), and initial rhythm of VF/VT.[2,4] These outcomes were further demonstrated in a literature review by Donoghue et al[3] in which witnessed arrest and submersion injury were also associated with increased survival in children younger than 18 years. A Japanese study of OHCA in children revealed that CPR instruction by dispatchers increased the CPR provision rate (adjusted odds ratio [OR] 7.51), and dispatcher-assisted bystander CPR was associated with improved neurologic outcomes at 1 month (adjusted OR 1.81) when compared with no bystander CPR.[7] The poorer outcomes associated with pediatric OHCA may be attributable to the fact that these events often occur in nonpublic locations, such as

a residence (88% of total), and are rarely witnessed (19%). In addition, bystander CPR occurs infrequently (35%), and automated external defibrillator (AED) use is rare.[2]

The American Heart Association (AHA) pediatric chain of survival includes the following links: (1) prevention of injury or arrest, (2) early and effective CPR, (3) prompt access to EMS, (4) rapid pediatric advanced life support, and (5) integrated postcardiac arrest care.[8] As stated previously, a key component of this chain is early and effective bystander CPR. The pediatric chain of survival varies slightly from the adult version, which includes (1) immediate recognition of cardiac arrest and activation of EMS, (2) early CPR with an emphasis on chest compressions, (3) rapid defibrillation, (4) effective advanced life support, and (5) integrated postcardiac arrest care.[9] The AHA considers victims in puberty and beyond to be adults for the purposes of CPR. Therefore, addressing the needs of adolescent victims would involve the adult algorithm instead of the pediatric approach. Step 3 in the adult algorithm, effective defibrillation, which includes the use of an AED, can be critical in adolescents because they have a higher rate of VF/VT arrests than infants and children.[2,4]

2010 AHA Guidelines

In 2010, the AHA released revised CPR recommendations, which changed the sequence to compressions, airway, breathing/ventilation. The revised recommendations called for 30 chest compressions followed by 2 breaths for adults with either 1 or 2 rescuers, a ratio of 30:2 for children with 1 rescuer, and a ratio of 15:2 for children with 2 rescuers.[9] These changes resulted from the discovery that high-quality chest compressions are needed to restore blood flow during cardiac arrest. The previous

sequence had delayed the initiation of crucial chest compressions. Additionally, some potential rescuers had difficulty completing the airway and breathing components, and others were reluctant to initiate CPR at all because of concern about giving mouth-to-mouth breaths.[8]

In infants and children, respiratory arrest is a frequent cause of cardiopulmonary arrest, so the airway and breathing/ventilation components remain important, but the new sequence only delays the first breath by 18 seconds.[10] The authors of a Japanese study demonstrated that traditional CPR (compressions followed by breathing) was associated with increased odds of a favorable neurologic outcome in children 1 month after an OHCA (adjusted OR, 2.30 vs 1.05) compared with chest compression–only CPR.[7] Therefore, although the AHA still recommends traditional CPR compared with chest compression–only CPR for children, if rescuers cannot provide rescue breaths, they should at least perform chest compressions.[10]

Importance of AED Training

The revised AHA guidelines also include a recommendation to extend the use of AEDs to children of any age experiencing an OHCA.[9] A manual defibrillator is preferred to treat infants and children with pulseless VF/VT, and an AED with a pediatric attenuator and pads is preferred for children younger than 8 years, but if neither are available, an AED without a dose attenuator can be used.[8,11] Extending AED training and use to the pediatric population provides a better opportunity to treat those infants and children with presenting heart rhythms that might respond to electrical therapy (eg, pulseless VF/VT). AEDs can also prompt rescuers to continue chest compressions in children with nonshockable rhythms, such as asystole and pulseless electrical activity.

The prevalence of readily available AEDs in public locations (eg, in airports, office buildings, malls, sports facilities, and schools) has been spurred by research literature demonstrating improved survival in adults treated with early defibrillation.[12] In the Public Access Defibrillation trial, survival rates for victims of OHCA doubled when AEDs were available and volunteers were trained in their use, and no inappropriate shocks were given.[12,13] An evaluation of OHCA in the Resuscitation Outcomes Consortium also found a near doubling of survival in those communities where an AED was used before the arrival of EMS.[14]

In 2000, the Cardiac Arrest Survival Act (Public Law 106-505) was signed into federal law. The intent was to reduce barriers to the placement and use of AEDs in public areas.[12] Since then, all 50 states have passed laws promoting lay rescuer programs and providing "Good Samaritan" protection for lay rescuers who use AEDs.[12] Although legal concerns are reduced by Good Samaritan laws, which are designed to encourage volunteers to provide emergency assistance to victims, the protections vary by state.[15] In 2003, the AHA International Liaison Committee on Resuscitation recommended that CPR training be incorporated into the school curriculum and encouraged inclusion of AED skills practice during CPR training.[16,17] The expectation was that over the long-term, training students in CPR would yield more potential responders in the population. Although the number of OHCAs witnessed by students in school is low, students may be able to assist OHCA victims in a nonschool location.

Basic Life Support Training for Parents, Caregivers, and the Public

Parents of high-risk infants often receive CPR training before their infant's discharge from the hospital. The methods used include one-on-one training, classroom training, and self-instruction. In a study in which the effectiveness of a self-instructional DVD to provide CPR training for parents of high-risk infants (eg, preterm infants or those with congenital heart disease) was evaluated, parents who watched the DVD not only were able to perform CPR but also shared the DVD with an additional 3 people in their environment. Parents were also able to review the DVD over the next 12 months; several parents in the study reported performing CPR on their own child in emergency situations, with 75% survival of those children.[18] A separate study in Denmark demonstrated that after laypeople were trained in basic life support and/or AED use, the rates of bystander CPR being performed increased from 22% to 74%.[19] Survival after OHCA in children with all presenting rhythms increased from 0% to 5.4%.[19] The authors of a study from Sweden demonstrated similar results; those who received bystander CPR had a 30-day survival of 10.5% versus only 4.0% when CPR was not performed.[20] Because research has shown improved outcomes with the performance of early bystander CPR, it is prudent for pediatricians to advocate for life support training for parents and caregivers. This training could occur in hospitals, physician offices, other health care facilities, schools, as well as be offered by professional and community groups.

Basic Life Support Training for School Personnel, Children, and Adolescents

In addition to students, who typically attend school 5 days a week, a substantial number of adults, such as teachers, parents, school personnel, and visitors, can be found on school grounds. In the United States, approximately 356 000 people experience OHCA each year; 1 out of every 250 to 600 occurs in a school.[1,21–23] The majority of these incidents occur in adults, often in an athletic setting. Training students and school personnel in CPR and having an accessible AED in higher-risk areas of the school, such as the gymnasium or athletic field, protects both students and adults. A study by Swor et al[23] using data from the Cardiac Arrest Registry to Enhance Survival revealed that of 30 603 cardiac arrests identified in communities studied, 47 (0.15%) occurred in K–12 schools, and 45.7% of those were in high schools. Of those 47 arrests, 66% occurred in adults and 34% occurred in children (younger than 19 years). Eighty-three percent were witnessed arrests. CPR was provided in 76% of cases, and 31.9% of victims survived to hospital discharge. An AED was applied in 58% of cases in which it was available, and victim survival increased to 36%.[23]

With the large numbers of children involved in school sports, having an AED on site can be life-saving. The estimated occurrence of sudden cardiac arrest in young athletes is 1:50 000 athletes[24] or approximately 1 in 70 high schools per year.[25] The Inter-Association Task Force of the National Athletic Trainers Association recommends the following preventive measures: effective communication, training of anticipated responders in performing CPR and using an AED, access to an AED, acquisition of necessary emergency equipment, and coordination and integration with EMS.[26] A study of the National Registry for AED Use in Sports involving 2149 high schools revealed that 87% of schools had AED programs. Over a 2-year period, researchers identified 59 cases of sudden cardiac arrest, of which 44% occurred among students and 66% occurred on an athletic field during training or a competition. Ninety-three percent of victims were given prompt CPR, and 85% had an AED applied. The overall survival to hospital discharge was

71%, including 85% of victims who were students.[25] This should prompt pediatricians to encourage the presence of an AED in high schools, especially at athletic events.

Can Children Be Taught CPR and AED Skills?

In their systematic review, Plant and Taylor[27] reviewed how to best teach CPR to schoolchildren. Children as young as 6 to 7 years can learn to call for an ambulance and how to use an AED.[28] They can also be taught to give basic first aid to an unconscious patient.[29] Older children (aged 11–15 years) performed better than younger children (aged 8–11 years) when assessed for their CPR knowledge and skills.[27,30] However, natural physical factors may have played a role in this variance; for example, a younger child may not have the size or strength to provide effective chest compressions. Children with a weight of >50 kg (approximately 13 years of age or older) and 9- to 18-year-old children and adolescents with a BMI >15 provided adequate compression depth more effectively than those who weighed less or had a lower BMI.[27,31,32] Because of the importance of delivering high-quality chest compressions, it might be reasonable to teach adult and pediatric CPR to those in middle school (13 years and older),[12] but age-appropriate messages (eg, how to recognize an unconsciousness victim and call for help) could be taught earlier.[27] The Basic Emergency Lifesaving Skills framework and curriculum developed by the Maternal and Child Health Bureau of the Health Resources and Services Administration implements this approach by teaching children on the basis of their attainment of developmental milestones.[33] Children in kindergarten (age 6 years) are taught how to recognize an emergency and get help, tell an adult or other responsible person, and stay safe. These skills

are reintroduced and reinforced in grades 1 through 12. In grade 3 (ages 9–10 years), skills of airway, breathing, and circulation, including CPR, were taught and acquired and then reinforced in subsequent grades 5 through 12 (ages 11–18 years).[34] The goals of these efforts are to encourage students trained in CPR to continue their refresher training and become adults skilled in CPR.

AED skills, on the other hand, do not require physical strength; research studies have revealed that children 6 to 7 years of age can effectively deliver simulated AED defibrillation.[27,28] Gundry et al[35] demonstrated that 11- to 12-year-old children could properly apply AED pads and use the AED within 90 seconds after receiving verbal instructions.

What Is the Best Way to Teach CPR and AED Training?

There are various ways in which to teach parents, caregivers, school personnel, the public, and students some or all of these skills. The AHA and American Red Cross provide instructional courses and materials. A local children's hospital may have CPR instructors on staff to help provide their personnel and parents CPR education. These courses may be open to local pediatricians and their staff. There are instructor-led courses as well as video and/or computer and self-instruction methods that interested learners can access. Although there are also online courses, the most important aspect of CPR is the practice of the skills of compressions and breathing, which are not part of these courses, unless coupled with an in-person practice session. The instructor-led courses vary in length from 1.25 to 4 hours, whereas self-directed programs range from 22 minutes to 2 hours.[12,36] High school students who received interactive computer-based training and practical training about CPR and AEDs demonstrated greater

knowledge and skills initially and at a 2 month follow-up than those who only had computer-based training.[27,37] However, children and adults who used self-instruction kits also showed improvement in performance after training.[38] Not only can a large number of children and adolescents learn CPR skills thorough these programs, but these programs can also facilitate the training of additional family members at home, which has been demonstrated in studies.[27,38,39] Short self-instruction programs in basic life support that include synchronous hands-on practice were demonstrated to be as effective as instructor-led courses.[36,40] Brief video and/or computer self-instruction training of laypeople in AED use that included synchronous hands-on AED practice was shown to be an effective alternative to instructor-led AED courses.[36,41,42]

What Are Barriers and Enablers to Life Support Training and Implementation?

Barriers to training in schools identified included time, funding, equipment, instructor training, and difficulty with class scheduling. Fortunately, researchers have demonstrated that classroom teachers can be as effective as health care instructors, and community volunteer trainers are also effective trainers.[27] Additionally, self-directed learning has been shown to be as successful as instructor-based learning; if instructor training can be reduced or eliminated, both staffing and funding concerns can be mitigated. Tight class time was the barrier cited most often in a study by Reder and Quan.[43] Self-directed video-based learning requiring less than 30 minutes to complete and that is focused on practical skills may reduce the need for extended classroom time commitment.

Costs of training vary depending on the method selected; unfortunately, funding for classes or self-directed videos remains a barrier for most schools. External sources of donations, such as local foundations, businesses, and civic organizations, may be able to contribute needed resources. Collaboration among schools, local fire departments, and EMS systems has also been productive in this regard.[12] Programs such as project Automated Defibrillators in Adam's Memory (launched in 1999 in Wisconsin) have provided educational programs for high school students and placed AEDs within high schools in the state.[44] This program has resulted in a total of 94 lives saved, of which 49% were children younger than 18 years.[45] In Canada, the Advanced Coronary Treatment (ACT) Foundation (a public-private partnership) helped to deliver training to more than 3.8 million students.[46] Thirty-seven states require CPR training for high school graduation. Unfortunately, only 2 states have passed legislation that addresses funding.[12,47,48] Recently, the Institute of Medicine (now the National Academy of Medicine) recommended CPR training as a requirement for graduation from middle school.[49] In addition, 21 states mandate the placement of AEDs in public schools, only 2 states (OR and NJ) mandate AEDs in all public and private schools, and only 4 states (OR, AL, RI, TX) have state funding.[48,50] Parents, teachers, coaches, and pediatricians can join together to advocate for funded mandates to save lives.

Another potential challenge is the retention of learned skills. Research has shown that CPR skills begin to deteriorate within 3 to 6 months, but AED skills are retained longer.[36,51] However, training children 10 to 13 years of age in CPR twice a year did not improve performance more than annual training.[52] Six-month CPR and AED skill retention in those taught via a self-directed video was slightly better than the retention associated with attendance at a 3- to 4-hour

training course.[41] Once trained, skills should be practiced annually.

Infection concerns, especially the provision of breaths, have also been a barrier for effective adult CPR. Although traditional CPR is still recommended in children, if a rescuer is unwilling or unable to provide ventilations, chest compression–only CPR is preferred over no CPR; chest compressions alone do improve outcomes over no CPR.[7,10]

Finally, legal concerns about malpractice or lawsuits should not be a barrier to performing CPR; Good Samaritan laws provide protection to laypeople who provide first aid to victims in the United States. Health care workers are also typically protected as well, except in the case of gross negligence.[15,53,54]

CONCLUSIONS

The overall rate of survival after pediatric OHCA is poor. Improved survival rates in adults attributable to the implementation of early bystander CPR and the use of AEDs have been documented in adults. There is some evidence showing improved survival in children who receive immediate bystander CPR. Early and effective CPR is essential for survival after pediatric OHCA. Additionally, although the majority of pediatric OHCAs are not the result of primary cardiac causes, as many as 15% of adolescents and 5% of children experiencing OHCA may present with an initial cardiac rhythm, as identified by an AED, that may be responsive to electrical treatment.[2,4]

Pediatricians should advocate for the institution of age-appropriate basic life support training in schools (eg, teaching young children how to seek help for victims of OHCA, teaching CPR to older children, and CPR and AED use to adolescents) and assist in the process by suggesting

avenues for funding of CPR training, by becoming certified AHA or American Red Cross instructors themselves to be able to teach target groups, and by minimizing barriers to learning and implementing CPR training. Pediatricians can encourage their staff to become providers or instructors, hold training classes in their office, provide literature to parents, play CPR videos in the waiting room, and have an AED in their office. Pediatricians should also advocate for the presence of AEDS in high schools, especially near gyms and athletic facilities and at athletic events. Many children can effectively learn how to perform CPR and use an AED and could subsequently provide care or assist in the care of a victim of OHCA, including teachers, coaches, parents, siblings, or classmates. Educating and certifying children in these skills and providing periodic refresher training will result in a more informed and effective population. Basic life support training, including the performance of CPR should be in the skills toolkit for children, with the additional skill of the use of an AED for adolescents, parents, caregivers, school personnel, and the general public.

LEAD AUTHOR

Susan M. Fuchs, MD, FAAP

AMERICAN ACADEMY OF PEDIATRICS COMMITTEE ON PEDIATRIC EMERGENCY MEDICINE, 2017–2018

Joseph Wright, MD, MPH, FAAP, Chairperson
Terry Adirim, MD, MPH, FAAP
Michael S.D. Agus, MD, FAAP
James M. Callahan, MD, FAAP
Toni Gross, MD, MPH, FAAP
Natalie Lane, MD, FAAP
Lois Lee, MD, MPH, FAAP
Suzan Mazor, MD, FAAP
Prashant Mahajan, MD, MPH, MBA, FAAP
Nathan Timm, MD, FAAP

LIAISONS

Andrew Eisenberg, MD – *American Academy of Family Physicians*
Cynthia Wright Johnson, MSN, RN – *National Association of State EMS Officials*

Cynthiana Lightfoot, BFA, NRP – *American Academy of Pediatrics Family Partnerships Network*
Charles Macias, MD, MPH, FAAP – *National EMS for Children Innovation and Improvement Center*
Brian Moore, MD, MPH, FAAP – *National Association of EMS Physicians*
Diane Pilkey, RN, MPH – *Health Resources and Services Administration*
Katherine Remick, MD, FAAP – *National Association of Emergency Medical Technicians*
Mohsen Saidinejad, MD, MBA, FAAP, FACEP – *American College of Emergency Physicians*
Sally Snow, RN, BSN, CPEN, FAEN – *Emergency Nurses Association*
Mary Fallat, MD, FAAP – *American College of Surgeons*

OTHER FORMER COMMITTEE MEMBERS WITH INPUT DURING STATEMENT DEVELOPMENT

Joan E. Shook, MD, MBA, FAAP, Immediate Past Chairperson
Lee Benjamin, MD, FAAP, FACEP
Thomas H. Chun, MD, MPH, FAAP
Gregory P. Conners, MD, MPH, MBA, FAAP
Edward E. Conway Jr, MD, MS, FAAP
Nanette C. Dudley, MD, FAAP
Susan M. Fuchs, MD, FAAP
Brian R. Moore, MD, FAAP
Paul Sirbaugh, DO, MBA, FAAP

STAFF

Sue Tellez

APPENDIX 1: AHA GUIDELINES

The AHA now encourages the compressions, airway, and breathing approach. Although pediatric cardiac arrests tend to be asphyxial in nature, the delay in providing breaths by starting with compressions should be only 18 seconds for a solo rescuer and less with 2 rescuers.[10] There are also key differences in the ratio of compressions to ventilations (breaths) in child victims based on their age and the number of rescuers.

In their CPR guidelines, the AHA defines a neonate as a new born (ie, an infant at the time of delivery, an infant as being a baby <1 year of age, and a child as being age 1 until puberty [breast development in girls, axillary hair in boys]). Victims beyond puberty (eg, adolescents) are considered adults.[8,55]

AHA basic life support guidelines for infants and children set the compression ratio 30 compressions to 2 breaths for a single rescuer, whereas the ratio becomes 15 compressions to 2 breaths if 2 rescuers are present. In the CPR sequence for lay providers, the AHA recommends a quick check for responsiveness and a check for breathing. If the victim is not responsive and not breathing or only gasping, chest compression should be initiated and no pulse check needed. (For health care providers, there is a 10-second pulse check before chest compressions are started.) Chest compressions should be performed at a rate of 100 to 120 compressions per minute.[10] Compression depth should be at least one-third of the anterior-posterior diameter of the chest or ~1.5 inches (4 cm) in infants and 2 inches (5 cm) in children. Once the child has reached puberty, the depth is at least 2 in (5 cm) but no more than 2.4 in (6 cm).[10] Complete chest recoil should occur after each compression (do not leave pressure on the chest). After 30 compressions, the single rescuer should open the airway and give 2 breaths, with each breath taking 1 second and making the chest rise. If the chest does not rise, the rescuer should reposition the head and try 2 breaths again, then resume chest compressions. This cycle of 30:2 should continue for 5 cycles or ~2 minutes before leaving the child to activate the emergency response system and obtain an AED if one is nearby. EMS is typically activated by calling 911. On returning with an AED, a single rescuer should use the AED (preferably with pediatric pads, if available) and follow its prompts (shock or resume CPR) until emergency responders arrive or the child begins breathing. If a rescuer is not trained in providing ventilations, or cannot perform them, the rescuer should continue with compression-only CPR until additional help arrives.[10]

If 2 rescuers are available, 1 rescuer should start chest compressions immediately while the other rescuer activates the emergency response system (call 911 or local EMS number) and gets an AED if one is available. Use the AED as soon as it is available and follow its prompts (shock or resume CPR).[10] When resuming CPR with 2 rescuers, the ratio should be 15 compressions to 2 breaths for 5 cycles (2 minutes). The chest compressor role should be rotated every 2 minutes to minimize rescuer fatigue.[8,10] CPR should be continued until the child begins to breathe or emergency responders arrive.

ABBREVIATIONS

AED: automated external defibrillator
AHA: American Heart Association
CPR: cardiopulmonary resuscitation
EMS: emergency medical services
OHCA: out-of-hospital cardiac arrest
OR: odds ratio
VF/VT: ventricular fibrillation or ventricular tachycardia

FINANCIAL DISCLOSURE: The authors have indicated they have no financial relationships relevant to this article to disclose.

FUNDING: No external funding.

POTENTIAL CONFLICT OF INTEREST: The authors have indicated they have no potential conflicts of interest to disclose.

COMPANION PAPER: A companion to this article can be found online at www.pediatrics.org/cgi/doi/10.1542/peds.2018-0704.

REFERENCES

1. Benjamin EJ, Blaha MJ, Chiuve SE, et al; American Heart Association Statistics Committee and Stroke Statistics Subcommittee. Heart disease and stroke statistics-2017 update: a report from the American Heart Association. *Circulation.* 2017;135(10):e146–e603

2. Atkins DL, Everson-Stewart S, Sears GK, et al; Resuscitation Outcomes Consortium Investigators. Epidemiology and outcomes from out-of-hospital cardiac arrest in children: the Resuscitation Outcomes Consortium Epistry-Cardiac Arrest. *Circulation.* 2009;119(11):1484–1491

3. Donoghue AJ, Nadkarni V, Berg RA, et al; CanAm Pediatric Cardiac Arrest Investigators. Out-of-hospital pediatric cardiac arrest: an epidemiologic review and assessment of current knowledge. *Ann Emerg Med.* 2005;46(6):512–522

4. Atkins DL, Berger S. Improving outcomes from out-of-hospital cardiac arrest in young children and adolescents. *Pediatr Cardiol.* 2012;33(3):474–483

5. Meyer L, Stubbs B, Fahrenbruch C, et al. Incidence, causes, and survival trends from cardiovascular-related sudden cardiac arrest in children and young adults 0 to 35 years of age: a 30-year review. *Circulation.* 2012;126(11):1363–1372

6. Ong MEH, Stiell I, Osmond MH, et al; OPALS Study Group. Etiology of pediatric out-of-hospital cardiac arrest by coroner's diagnosis. *Resuscitation.* 2006;68(3):335–342

7. Goto Y, Maeda T, Goto Y. Impact of dispatcher-assisted bystander cardiopulmonary resuscitation on neurological outcomes in children with out-of-hospital cardiac arrests: a prospective, nationwide, population-based cohort study. *J Am Heart Assoc.* 2014;3(3):e000499

8. Berg MD, Schexnayder SM, Chameides L, et al. Part 13: pediatric basic life support: 2010 American Heart Association guidelines for cardiopulmonary resuscitation and emergency cardiovascular care. *Circulation.* 2010;122(18, suppl 3):S862–S875

9. Travers AH, Rea TD, Bobrow BJ, et al. Part 4: CPR overview: 2010 American Heart Association guidelines for cardiopulmonary resuscitation and emergency cardiovascular care. *Circulation.* 2010;122(18 suppl 3):S676–S684

10. de Caen AR, Maconochie IK, Aickin R, et al; Pediatric Basic Life Support and Pediatric Advanced Life Support Chapter Collaborators. Part 6: pediatric basic life support and pediatric advanced life support: 2015 international consensus on cardiopulmonary resuscitation and emergency cardiovascular care science with treatment recommendations. *Circulation.* 2015;132(16 suppl 1):S177–S203

11. Link MS, Atkins DL, Passman RS, et al. Part 6: electrical therapies: automated external defibrillators, defibrillation, cardioversion, and pacing: 2010 American Heart Association guidelines for cardiopulmonary resuscitation and emergency cardiovascular care [published correction appears in *Circulation.* 2011;123(6):e235]. *Circulation.* 2010;122(18 suppl 3):S706–S719

12. Cave DM, Aufderheide TP, Beeson J, et al; American Heart Association Emergency Cardiovascular Care Committee; Council on Cardiopulmonary, Critical Care, Perioperative and Resuscitation; Council on Cardiovascular Diseases in the Young; Council on Cardiovascular Nursing; Council on Clinical Cardiology, and Advocacy Coordinating Committee. Importance and implementation of training in cardiopulmonary resuscitation and automated external defibrillation in schools: a science advisory from the American Heart Association. *Circulation.* 2011;123(6):691–706

13. Hallstrom AP, Ornato JP, Weisfeldt M, et al; Public Access Defibrillation Trial Investigators. Public-access defibrillation and survival after out-of-hospital cardiac arrest. *N Engl J Med.* 2004;351(7):637–646

14. Weisfeldt ML, Sitlani CM, Ornato JP, et al; ROC Investigators. Survival after application of automatic external defibrillators before arrival of the emergency medical system: evaluation in the resuscitation outcomes consortium population of 21 million. *J Am Coll Cardiol.* 2010;55(16):1713–1720

15. Stewart PH, Agin WS, Douglas SP. What does the law say to Good Samaritans?: a review of Good Samaritan statutes in 50 states and on US airlines. *Chest.* 2013;143(6):1774–1783

16. Hazinski MF, Markenson D, Neish S, et al; American Heart Association; American Academy of Pediatrics; American College of Emergency Physicians; American National Red Cross; National Association of School Nurses; National Association of State EMS Directors; National Association of EMS Physicians; National Association of Emergency Medical Technicians; Program for School Preparedness and Planning; National Center for Disaster Preparedness; Columbia University Mailman School of Public Health. Response to cardiac arrest and selected life-threatening medical emergencies: the medical emergency response plan for schools: a statement for healthcare providers, policymakers, school administrators, and community leaders. *Circulation.* 2004;109(2):278–291

17. Chamberlain DA, Hazinski MF; European Resuscitation Council; American Heart Association; Heart and Stroke Foundation of Canada; Resuscitation Council of Southern Africa; Australia and New Zealand Resuscitation Council; Consejo Latino-Americano de Resusucitación. Education in resuscitation: an ILCOR symposium: Utstein Abbey: Stavanger, Norway: June 22-24, 2001. *Circulation.* 2003;108(20):2575–2594

18. Pierick TA, Van Waning N, Patel SS, Atkins DL. Self-instructional CPR training for parents of high risk infants. *Resuscitation.* 2012;83(9):1140–1144

19. Møller Nielsen A, Lou Isbye D, Knudsen Lippert F, Rasmussen LS. Engaging a whole community in resuscitation. *Resuscitation.* 2012;83(9):1067–1071

20. Hasselqvist-Ax I, Riva G, Herlitz J, et al. Early cardiopulmonary resuscitation in

out-of-hospital cardiac arrest. *N Engl J Med.* 2015;372(24):2307–2315

21. Mosesso VN Jr. AEDs in schools: lessons learned and to be learned. *Resuscitation.* 2013;84(4):401–402

22. Lotfi K, White L, Rea T, et al. Cardiac arrest in schools. *Circulation.* 2007;116(12):1374–1379

23. Swor R, Grace H, McGovern H, Weiner M, Walton E. Cardiac arrests in schools: assessing use of automated external defibrillators (AED) on school campuses. *Resuscitation.* 2013;84(4):426–429

24. Drezner JA, Chun JSDY, Harmon KG, Derminer L. Survival trends in the United States following exercise-related sudden cardiac arrest in the youth: 2000-2006. *Heart Rhythm.* 2008;5(6):794–799

25. Drezner JA, Toresdahl BG, Rao AL, Huszti E, Harmon KG. Outcomes from sudden cardiac arrest in US high schools: a 2-year prospective study from the National Registry for AED Use in Sports. *Br J Sports Med.* 2013;47(18):1179–1183

26. Drezner JA, Courson RW, Roberts WO, Mosesso VN Jr, Link MS, Maron BJ. Inter-association task force recommendations on emergency preparedness and management of sudden cardiac arrest in high school and college athletic programs: a consensus statement. *Clin J Sport Med.* 2007;17(2):87–103

27. Plant N, Taylor K. How best to teach CPR to schoolchildren: a systematic review. *Resuscitation.* 2013;84(4):415–421

28. Uray T, Lunzer A, Ochsenhofer A, et al. Feasibility of life-supporting first-aid (LSFA) training as a mandatory subject in primary schools. *Resuscitation.* 2003;59(2):211–220

29. Bollig G, Wahl HA, Svendsen MV. Primary school children are able to perform basic life-saving first aid measures. *Resuscitation.* 2009;80(6):689–692

30. Lubrano R, Romero S, Scoppi P, et al. How to become an under 11 rescuer: a practical method to teach first aid to primary schoolchildren. *Resuscitation.* 2005;64(3):303–307

31. Jones I, Whitfield R, Colquhoun M, Chamberlain D, Vetter N, Newcombe R. At what age can schoolchildren provide effective chest compressions? An observational study from the Heartstart UK schools training programme. *BMJ.* 2007;334(7605):1201

32. Fleischhackl R, Nuernberger A, Sterz F, et al. School children sufficiently apply life supporting first aid: a prospective investigation. *Crit Care.* 2009;13(4):R127

33. Bernardo LM, Doyle C, Bryn S. Basic emergency lifesaving skills (BELS): a framework for teaching skills to children and adolescents. *Int J Trauma Nurs.* 2002;8(2):48–50

34. Maternal & Child Health Bureau. *Basic Emergency Lifesaving Skills (BELS): A Framework for Teaching Skills to Children and Adolescents.* Newton, MA: Children's Safety Network, Education Development Center, Inc; 1999. Available at: https://issuu.com/emscnrc/docs/bels. Accessed January 22, 2015

35. Gundry JW, Comess KA, DeRook FA, Jorgenson D, Bardy GH. Comparison of naive sixth-grade children with trained professionals in the use of an automated external defibrillator. *Circulation.* 1999;100(16):1703–1707

36. Mancini ME, Soar J, Bhanji F, et al; Education, Implementation, and Teams Chapter Collaborators. Part 12: education, implementation, and teams: 2010 international consensus on cardiopulmonary resuscitation and emergency cardiovascular care science with treatment recommendations. *Circulation.* 2010;122(16 suppl 2):S539–S581

37. Reder S, Cummings P, Quan L. Comparison of three instructional methods for teaching cardiopulmonary resuscitation and use of an automatic external defibrillator to high school students. *Resuscitation.* 2006;69(3):443–453

38. Lorem T, Palm A, Wik L. Impact of a self-instruction CPR kit on 7th graders' and adults' skills and CPR performance. *Resuscitation.* 2008;79(1):103–108

39. Isbye DL, Rasmussen LS, Ringsted C, Lippert FK. Disseminating cardiopulmonary resuscitation training by distributing 35,000

personal manikins among school children. *Circulation.* 2007;116(12):1380–1385

40. Cason CL, Kardong-Edgren S, Cazzell M, Behan D, Mancini ME. Innovations in basic life support education for healthcare providers: improving competence in cardiopulmonary resuscitation through self-directed learning. *J Nurses Staff Dev.* 2009;25(3):E1–E13

41. Roppolo LP, Pepe PE, Campbell L, et al. Prospective, randomized trial of the effectiveness and retention of 30-min layperson training for cardiopulmonary resuscitation and automated external defibrillators: the American Airlines study. *Resuscitation.* 2007;74(2):276–285

42. Bhanji F, Finn JC, Lockey A, et al; Education, Implementation, and Teams Chapter Collaborators. Part 8: education, implementation, and teams: 2015 international consensus on cardiopulmonary resuscitation and emergency cardiovascular care science with treatment recommendations. *Circulation.* 2015;132(16 suppl 1):S242–S268

43. Reder S, Quan L. Cardiopulmonary resuscitation training in Washington state public high schools. *Resuscitation.* 2003;56(3):283–288

44. Berger S, Whitstone BN, Frisbee SJ, et al. Cost-effectiveness of Project ADAM: a project to prevent sudden cardiac death in high school students. *Pediatr Cardiol.* 2004;25(6):660–667

45. Children's Hospital of Wisconsin. Project ADAM website. Available at: https://www.chw.org/childrens-and-the-community/resources-for-schools/cardiac-arrest-project-adam. Accessed November 27, 2017

46. Advance Coronary Treatment Foundation. ACT programs: high school CPR and defibrillator program. Available at: www.actfoundation.ca/act-programs. Accessed November 27, 2017

47. National Conference of State Legislatures. State laws of cardiac arrest and defibrillators. Available at: www.ncsl.org/research/health/laws-on-cardiac-arrest-and-defibrillators-aeds.aspx. Accessed November 22, 2017

48. Sudden Cardiac Arrest Foundation. AED laws. Available at: www.sca-aware.org/cpr-aed-laws. Accessed November 26, 2017

49. Institute of Medicine. In: Graham R, McCoy MA, Schultz AM, eds. *Strategies to Improve Cardiac Arrest Survival: A Time to Act*. Washington, DC: National Academies Press; 2015:374

50. Parent Heart Watch. AED legislation for schools. Available at: www.parentheartwatch.org/resources/legislation. Accessed November 27, 2017

51. Isbye DL, Meyhoff CS, Lippert FK, Rasmussen LS. Skill retention in adults and in children 3 months after basic life support training using a simple personal resuscitation manikin. *Resuscitation*. 2007;74(2):296–302

52. Bohn A, Van Aken HK, Möllhoff T, et al. Teaching resuscitation in schools: annual tuition by trained teachers is effective starting at age 10. A four-year prospective cohort study. *Resuscitation*. 2012;83(5):619–625

53. Daniels S. Good Samaritan acts. *Emerg Med Clin North Am*. 1999;17(2):491–504, xiii

54. Readiness Systems. Get to know the AED program rules. Available at: www.readisys.com/get-to-know-the-aed-program-rules/. Accessed November 27, 2017

55. Kattwinkel J, Perlman JM, Aziz K, et al. Part 15: neonatal resuscitation: 2010 American Heart Association guidelines for cardiopulmonary resuscitation and emergency cardiovascular care [published correction appears in *Circulation*. 2011;124(15):e406]. *Circulation*. 2010;122(18 suppl 3):S909–S919

Child Passenger Safety

- *Policy Statement*
  - *PPI: AAP Partnership for Policy Implementation*
    See Appendix 1 for more information.

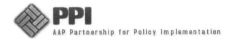

POLICY STATEMENT Organizational Principles to Guide and Define the Child Health Care System and/or Improve the Health of all Children

American Academy of Pediatrics

DEDICATED TO THE HEALTH OF ALL CHILDREN™

Child Passenger Safety

Dennis R. Durbin, MD, MSCE, FAAP,[a] Benjamin D. Hoffman, MD, FAAP,[b] COUNCIL ON INJURY, VIOLENCE, AND POISON PREVENTION

abstract

Child passenger safety has dramatically evolved over the past decade; however, motor vehicle crashes continue to be the leading cause of death for children 4 years and older. This policy statement provides 4 evidence-based recommendations for best practices in the choice of a child restraint system to optimize safety in passenger vehicles for children from birth through adolescence: (1) rear-facing car safety seats as long as possible; (2) forward-facing car safety seats from the time they outgrow rear-facing seats for most children through at least 4 years of age; (3) belt-positioning booster seats from the time they outgrow forward-facing seats for most children through at least 8 years of age; and (4) lap and shoulder seat belts for all who have outgrown booster seats. In addition, a fifth evidence-based recommendation is for all children younger than 13 years to ride in the rear seats of vehicles. It is important to note that every transition is associated with some decrease in protection; therefore, parents should be encouraged to delay these transitions for as long as possible. These recommendations are presented in the form of an algorithm that is intended to facilitate implementation of the recommendations by pediatricians to their patients and families and should cover most situations that pediatricians will encounter in practice. The American Academy of Pediatrics urges all pediatricians to know and promote these recommendations as part of child passenger safety anticipatory guidance at every health supervision visit.

[a]Department of Pediatrics, The Ohio State University College of Medicine and Nationwide Children's Hospital, Columbus, Ohio; and [b]Department of Pediatrics, Oregon Health and Science University, Portland, Oregon

Drs Durbin and Hoffman were equally responsible for conception and design of the revision, drafting, and editing of the manuscript.

This document is copyrighted and is property of the American Academy of Pediatrics and its Board of Directors. All authors have filed conflict of interest statements with the American Academy of Pediatrics. Any conflicts have been resolved through a process approved by the Board of Directors. The American Academy of Pediatrics has neither solicited nor accepted any commercial involvement in the development of the content of this publication.

Policy statements from the American Academy of Pediatrics benefit from expertise and resources of liaisons and internal (AAP) and external reviewers. However, policy statements from the American Academy of Pediatrics may not reflect the views of the liaisons or the organizations or government agencies that they represent.

The guidance in this statement does not indicate an exclusive course of treatment or serve as a standard of medical care. Variations, taking into account individual circumstances, may be appropriate.

All policy statements from the American Academy of Pediatrics automatically expire 5 years after publication unless reaffirmed, revised, or retired at or before that time.

DOI: https://doi.org/10.1542/peds.2018-2460

Address correspondence to Benjamin D. Hoffman, MD, FAAP. E-mail: hoffmanb@ohsu.edu

PEDIATRICS (ISSN Numbers: Print, 0031-4005; Online, 1098-4275).

Copyright © 2018 by the American Academy of Pediatrics

FINANCIAL DISCLOSURE: The authors have indicated they do not have a financial relationship relevant to this article to disclose.

FUNDING: No external funding.

POTENTIAL CONFLICT OF INTEREST: The authors have indicated they have no potential conflicts of interest to disclose.

To cite: Durbin DR, Hoffman BD, AAP COUNCIL ON INJURY, VIOLENCE, AND POISON PREVENTION. Child Passenger Safety. Pediatrics. 2018;142(5):e20182460

Improved vehicle crashworthiness and greater use of child restraint systems have significantly affected the safety of children in automobiles. Major shifts in child restraint use, particularly the use of booster seats among older children, have occurred in response to public education programs and enhancements to child restraint laws in nearly every state.[1–3] In addition, there has been a substantial increase in scientific evidence on which to base recommendations for best practices in child passenger safety. Current estimates of child restraint effectiveness indicate that child safety seats reduce the risk of injury by 71% to 82%[4,5] and reduce the risk of death by 28% when compared with children of similar ages in seat belts.[6] Booster seats reduce the risk of nonfatal injury among 4- to 8-year-olds by 45% compared with seat belts.[7] Despite this

TABLE 1 Summary of Best Practice Recommendations

Best Practice Recommendation	Complementary Information
1) Best practice recommendation: infant-only or convertible CSS used rear facing All infants and toddlers should ride in a rear-facing CSS as long as possible, until they reach the highest weight or height allowed by their CSS's manufacturer.	Rear-facing-only seats usually have a handle for carrying and can be snapped in and out of a base that is installed in the vehicle. They can only be used rear facing. Convertible CSSs can be used either forward or rear facing and typically have higher rear-facing weight and height limits than rear-facing-only seats. When children using rear-facing-only seats reach the highest weight for their seat, they should continue to ride rear-facing in a convertible seat for as long as possible. Most currently available convertible seats can be used rear facing to at least 40 lb.
2) Best practice recommendation: convertible or combination CSS used forward facing All children who have outgrown the rear-facing weight or height limit for their CSS should use a forward-facing CSS with a harness for as long as possible, up to the highest weight or height allowed by their CSS's manufacturer.	Combination CSSs are seats that can be used forward facing with a harness system and then, when the child exceeds the height or weight limit for the harness, as a booster seat with the harness removed. Most models of convertible and combination CSSs can accommodate children up to 65 lb and some up to 70–90 lb when used forward facing. The lowest maximum weight limit for currently available forward-facing car safety seats is 40 lb.
3) Best practice recommendation: belt-positioning booster seat All children whose weight or height is above the forward-facing limit for their CSS should use a belt-positioning booster seat until the vehicle lap and shoulder seat belt fits properly, typically when they have reached 4 ft 9 inches in height and are between 8 and 12 y of age.	A few vehicle models offer integrated forward-facing seats with a harness system. The vehicle owner's manual provides instructions for use of integrated seats when they are present. A crash-tested travel vest may be considered for children with special needs or in situations where a traditional CSS cannot be installed correctly. There is a safety advantage for young children to remain in car safety seats with a harness for as long as possible before transitioning to booster seats. Booster seats function by positioning the child so that both the lap and shoulder portions of the vehicle seat belt fit properly: the lap portion of the belt should fit low across the hips and pelvis, and the shoulder portion should fit across the middle of the shoulder and chest. They come in both high-back (a seat back that extends up beyond the child's head) and backless models. A few vehicle models offer integrated booster seats.
4) Best practice recommendation: Lap and shoulder vehicle seat belt When children are old enough and large enough to use the vehicle seat belt alone, they should always use lap and shoulder seat belts for optimal protection	The lap portion of the belt should fit low across the hips and pelvis, and the shoulder portion should fit across the middle of the shoulder and chest when the child sits with his back against the vehicle seat back. If they don't, the child is likely too small to use the vehicle seat belt alone and should continue to use a belt-positioning booster seat.
5) Best practice recommendation: all children <13 years of age should be restrained in the rear seats of vehicles for optimal protection All children <13 y should be restrained in the rear seats of vehicles for optimal protection	CSSs should be installed tightly either with the vehicle seat belt or with the LATCH system, if available. LATCH is a system of attaching a CSS to the vehicle that does not use the seat belt. It was designed to ease installation of the CSS. Whether parents use LATCH or the seat belt, they should always ensure a tight installation of the CSS into the vehicle.

LATCH, Lower Anchors and Tethers for Children.

progress, each year, nearly 1000 children younger than 16 years die in motor vehicle crashes in the United States.[8]

The American Academy of Pediatrics (AAP) strongly supports optimal safety for children and adolescents of all ages during all forms of travel. This policy statement provides 5 evidence-based recommendations for best practices to optimize safety in passenger vehicles for all children, from birth through adolescence (summary of recommendations in Table 1):

1. All infants and toddlers should ride in a rear-facing car safety seat (CSS) as long as possible, until they reach the highest weight or height allowed by their CSS's manufacturer. Most convertible seats have limits that will permit children to ride rear-facing for 2 years or more.

2. All children who have outgrown the rear-facing weight or height limit for their CSS should use a forward-facing CSS with a harness for as long as possible, up to the highest weight or height allowed by their CSS's manufacturer.

3. All children whose weight or height is above the forward-facing limit for their CSS should use a belt-positioning booster seat until the vehicle lap and shoulder seat belt fits properly, typically when they have reached 4 ft 9 inches in height and are between 8 and 12 years of age.

4. When children are old enough and large enough to use the vehicle seat belt alone, they should always use lap and shoulder seat belts for optimal protection.

5. All children younger than 13 years should be restrained in the rear seats of vehicles for optimal protection.

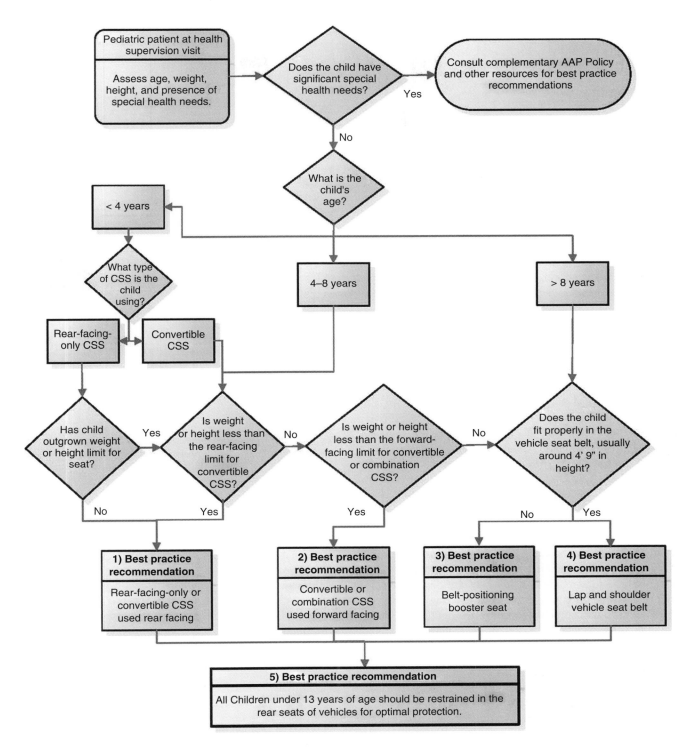

FIGURE 1

Algorithm to guide implementation of best practice recommendations for optimal child passenger safety. (See Table 1 for summary of recommendations and Table 2 for definitions and explanations.)

TABLE 2 Explanations of Decision Points and Additional Resources

Does the child have significant health needs?	Children with certain temporary or permanent physical and behavioral conditions such as altered muscle tone, decreased neurologic control, skeletal abnormalities, or airway compromise that may preclude the use of regular CSSs may require specialized restraint systems.
Consult complementary AAP Policy and other resources for best practice recommendations	The AAP has a Policy Statement providing specific guidance on best practice recommendations for children with special health care needs (http://aappolicy.aappublications.org/cgi/content/full/pediatrics%3B104/4/988). To locate a child passenger safety technician in your area with special training in special health needs, go to http://cert.safekids.org.
<4 y	Infants and toddlers have relatively large heads and several structural features of their neck and spine that place them at particularly high risk of head and spine injuries in motor vehicle crashes. Rear-facing CSSs provide optimal support to the head and spine in the event of a crash. Children who are small for their age may need to be evaluated like younger children. Consult a child passenger safety technician with enhanced training in special needs or other resources for assistance.
Has the child outgrown weight or height limit for seat? Is weight or height less than rear-facing limit for convertible CSS? Is weight or height less than forward-facing limit for convertible combination CSS?	The AAP annually updates information on child restraint systems currently available in the United States (www.healthychildren.org/carseatguide). The weight thresholds provided in the algorithm are considered minimum standards. More recent products have higher weight limits and should be used when possible. In general, children should remain in a child restraint system until they outgrow the weight or height limits for its intended use.
4–8 y	Most children 4–8 years of age are not large enough to fit properly in the vehicle seat belt and will require a CSS or booster seat for optimal restraint. A belt-positioning booster seat positions a child so that the lap and shoulder portions of the seat belt fit properly: the lap portion low across the hips and pelvis and the shoulder portion across the middle of the shoulder and chest.
8 y	Most children under 4 ft 9 inches in height will not fit properly in vehicle lap and shoulder seat belts.
Does child fit properly in the vehicle seat belt, usually around 4 ft 9 inches in height?	These 3 questions are an evaluation to determine whether a child is ready to be restrained by the vehicle seat belt without a booster seat. If the answer is "no" to any of these questions, the child should use a booster seat: 1. Is the child tall enough to sit against the vehicle seat back with her knees bent at the edge of the vehicle seat without slouching and stay in this position comfortably throughout the trip? 2. Does the shoulder belt lie across the middle of the chest and shoulder, not against the neck or face? 3. Is the lap belt low across the hips and pelvis?

Of note, the recommendation that all children be restrained in a rear-facing-only or convertible CSS used rear facing as long as possible represents a significant change from previous AAP policy and is based on data from the United States[9] as well as extensive experience in Sweden.[10,11] It is important to note that nearly all currently available CSSs have weight limits for rear-facing use that can accommodate children 35 to 40 lb.[12]

Certain considerations contained in this policy statement are relevant to commercial airline travel as well and are noted in the accompanying technical report. Additional AAP policy statements provide specific recommendations to optimize safety for preterm and low birth weight infants,[13] children in school buses,[14] and children using other forms of travel and recreational vehicles.[15–17] In addition, complementary AAP policy statements provide recommendations for teen drivers[18] and for the safe transport of newborn infants[19] and children with special health care needs.[20,21]

Pediatricians play a critical role in promoting child passenger safety. To facilitate their widespread implementation in practice, evidence-based recommendations for optimal protection of children of all ages in passenger vehicles are presented in the form of an algorithm (Fig 1) with an accompanying table of explanations and definitions (Table 2). A summary of the evidence in support of these recommendations is provided in the accompanying technical report.[22] Because pediatricians are a trusted source of information to parents, pediatricians need to maintain a basic level of knowledge of these best practice recommendations and promote and document them at every health supervision visit. Prevention of motor vehicle crash injury is unique in health supervision topics, as it is the only topic recommended at every health supervision visit by *Bright Futures*.[23] Pediatricians can also use this information to promote child passenger safety public education, legislation, and regulation at local, state, and national levels through a variety of advocacy activities, including aligning their state's child passenger safety law with the best practice recommendations promoted in this policy statement.

Pediatricians are urged to keep abreast of the evolving and multifaceted guidance and resources on motor vehicle safety for children. In particular, many communities have child passenger safety technicians who have completed a standardized National Highway Traffic Safety Administration course and who can provide hands-on advice and guidance to families. In most communities, child passenger safety technicians work at formal inspection stations; a list of these is available at https://www.nhtsa.gov/equipment/car-seats-and-booster-seats#install-inspection. If your community does not have an inspection station, you can find a child passenger safety technician in your area via the National Child Passenger Safety Certification Web site at http://cert.safekids.org or via the National Highway Traffic Safety Administration Child Safety Seat Inspection Station Locator at http://www.nhtsa.dot.gov/cps/cpsfitting/index.cfm. Car Seat Check Up Events are updated at https://www.safekids.org/events/field_type/check-event. In addition, additional resources for pediatricians and families can be found at www.aap.org or www.healthychildren.org.

LEAD AUTHORS

Dennis R. Durbin, MD, MSCE, FAAP

Benjamin D. Hoffman, MD, FAAP

COUNCIL ON INJURY, VIOLENCE AND POISON PREVENTION, 2018–2019

Benjamin D. Hoffman, MD, FAAP, Chairperson
Phyllis F. Agran, MD, MPH, FAAP
Sarah A. Denny, MD, FAAP
Michael Hirsh, MD, FAAP
Brian Johnston, MD, MPH, FAAP
Lois K. Lee, MD, MPH, FAAP
Kathy Monroe, MD, FAAP
Judy Schaechter, MD, MBA, FAAP
Milton Tenenbein, MD, FAAP
Mark R. Zonfrillo, MD, MSCE, FAAP
Kyran Quinlan, MD, MPH, FAAP, ex-officio

CONTRIBUTOR

Stuart Weinberg, MD, FAAP, Partnership for Policy Implementation

LIAISONS

Lynne Janecek Haverkos, MD, MPH, FAAP – *National Institute of Child Health and Human Development*
Jonathan D. Midgett, PhD – *Consumer Product Safety Commission*
Alexander W. (Sandy) Sinclair – *National Highway Traffic Safety Administration*
Richard Stanwick, MD, FAAP – *Canadian Paediatric Society*

STAFF

Bonnie Kozial

ABBREVIATIONS

AAP: American Academy of Pediatrics
CSS: car safety seat

REFERENCES

1. Durbin DR, Kallan MJ, Winston FK. Trends in booster seat use among young children in crashes. *Pediatrics*. 2001;108(6). Available at: www.pediatrics.org/cgi/content/full/108/6/e109

2. Winston FK, Chen IG, Elliott MR, Arbogast KB, Durbin DR. Recent trends in child restraint practices in the United States. *Pediatrics*. 2004;113(5). Available at: www.pediatrics.org/cgi/content/full/113/5/e458

3. Insurance Institute for Highway Safety. Child Restraint/Belt Use Laws. Arlington, VA: Insurance Institute for Highway Safety, Highway Loss Data Institute. Available at: http://www.iihs.org/iihs/topics/laws/safetybeltuse. Accessed August 17, 2010

4. Arbogast KB, Durbin DR, Cornejo RA, Kallan MJ, Winston FK. An evaluation of the effectiveness of forward facing child restraint systems. *Accid Anal Prev*. 2004;36(4):585–589

5. Zaloshnja E, Miller TR, Hendrie D. Effectiveness of child safety seats vs safety belts for children aged 2 to 3 years. *Arch Pediatr Adolesc Med*. 2007;161(1):65–68

6. Elliott MR, Kallan MJ, Durbin DR, Winston FK. Effectiveness of child safety seats vs seat belts in reducing risk for death in children in passenger vehicle crashes. *Arch Pediatr Adolesc Med*. 2006;160(6):617–621

7. Arbogast KB, Jermakian JS, Kallan MJ, Durbin DR. Effectiveness of belt positioning booster seats: an updated assessment. *Pediatrics*. 2009;124(5):1281–1286

8. National Highway Traffic Safety Administration. Fatality analysis reporting system (FARS) encyclopedia. Available at: http://www-fars.nhtsa.dot.gov/. Accessed August 21, 2018

9. McMurry TL, Arbogast KB, Sherwood CP, et al. Rear-facing versus forward-facing child restraints: an updated assessment. *Inj Prev*. 2018;24(1):55–59

10. Isaksson-Hellman I, Jakobsson L, Gustafsson C, Norin HA. Trends and effects of child restraint systems based on Volvo's Swedish accident database. In: *Proceedings of Child Occupant Protection 2nd Symposium*; November 12, 1997; Warrendale, PA

11. Jakobsson L, Isaksson-Hellman I, Lundell B. Safety for the growing child: experiences from Swedish accident data. In: *Proceedings from the 19th International Technical Conference on the Enhanced Safety of Vehicles*; June 6–9, 2005; Washington, DC. Abstr 05-0330

12. American Academy of Pediatrics. *Car Safety Seats: Product Listing for 2018*. Elk Grove Village, IL: Healthy Children, American Academy of Pediatrics; 2018. Available at: www.healthychildren.org/carseatlist. Accessed June 8, 2018

13. Bull MJ, Engle WA; Committee on Injury, Violence, and Poison Prevention and Committee on Fetus and Newborn; American Academy of Pediatrics. Safe transportation of preterm and low birth weight infants at hospital discharge. *Pediatrics*. 2009;123(5):1424–1429

14. Agran PF; American Academy of Pediatrics Committee on Injury, Violence, and Poison Prevention; American Academy of Pediatrics

Council on School Health. School transportation safety. *Pediatrics*. 2007;120(1):213–220

15. American Academy of Pediatrics, Committee on Injury and Poison. All-terrain vehicle injury prevention: two-, three-, and four-wheeled unlicensed motor vehicles. *Pediatrics*. 2000;105(6):1352–1354

16. American Academy of Pediatrics, Committee on Injury and Poison Prevention. Bicycle helmets. *Pediatrics*. 2001;108(4):1030–1032

17. American Academy of Pediatrics, Committee on Injury and Poison Prevention. Personal watercraft use by children and adolescents. *Pediatrics*. 2000;105(2):452–453

18. Weiss JC; Committee on Injury, Violence, and Poison Prevention, American Academy of Pediatrics; Committee on Adolescence, American Academy of Pediatrics. The teen driver. *Pediatrics*. 2006;118(6):2570–2581

19. Bull M, Agran P, Laraque D, et al; American Academy of Pediatrics, Committee on Injury and Poison Prevention. Safe transportation of newborns at hospital discharge. *Pediatrics*. 1999;104(4, pt 1):986–987

20. O'Neil J, Hoffman BD; Council on Injury, Violence, and Poison Prevention. School bus transportation of children with special health care needs [published correction appears in *Pediatrics*. 2018;142(1):e20181221]. *Pediatrics*. 2018;141(5):e20180513

21. Bull M, Agran P, Laraque D, et al; American Academy of Pediatrics, Committee on Injury and Poison Prevention. Transporting children with special health care needs. *Pediatrics*. 1999;104(4, pt 1):988–992

22. Durbin DR, Hoffman B; American Academy of Pediatrics, Committee on Injury, Violence, and Poison Prevention. Child passenger safety. *Pediatrics*. 2018;142(5):e20182461

23. American Academy of Pediatrics. Bright futures: health care professionals tools and resources web site. Available at: http://brightfutures. aap.org/materials-and-tools/ guidelines-and-pocket-guide/Pages/ default.aspx. Accessed August 17, 2010

Child Passenger Safety

- *Technical Report*

  - *PPI: AAP Partnership for Policy Implementation*
    See Appendix 1 for more information.

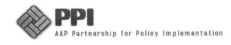

TECHNICAL REPORT

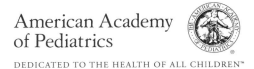

American Academy
of Pediatrics
DEDICATED TO THE HEALTH OF ALL CHILDREN™

Child Passenger Safety

Dennis R. Durbin, MD, MSCE, FAAP,[a] Benjamin D. Hoffman, MD, FAAP,[b] COUNCIL ON INJURY, VIOLENCE, AND POISON PREVENTION

abstract

Despite significant reductions in the number of children killed in motor vehicle crashes over the past decade, crashes continue to be the leading cause of death to children 4 years and older. Therefore, the American Academy of Pediatrics continues to recommend the inclusion of child passenger safety anticipatory guidance at every health supervision visit. This technical report provides a summary of the evidence in support of 5 recommendations for best practices to optimize safety in passenger vehicles for children from birth through adolescence that all pediatricians should know and promote in their routine practice. These recommendations are presented in the revised policy statement on child passenger safety in the form of an algorithm that is intended to facilitate their implementation by pediatricians with their patients and families. The algorithm is designed to cover the majority of situations that pediatricians will encounter in practice. In addition, a summary of evidence on a number of additional issues affecting the safety of children in motor vehicles, including the proper use and installation of child restraints, exposure to air bags, travel in pickup trucks, children left in or around vehicles, and the importance of restraint laws, is provided. Finally, this technical report provides pediatricians with a number of resources for additional information to use when providing anticipatory guidance to families.

[a]The Department of Pediatrics, The Ohio State University College of Medicine and Nationwide Children's Hospital in Columbus, Ohio; and [b]Department of Pediatrics, Oregon Health and Science University, Portland, Oregon

Drs Durbin and Hoffman were equally responsible for conception and design of the revision, drafting, and editing of the manuscript.

DOI: https://doi.org/10.1542/peds.2018-2461

Address correspondence to Benjamin D. Hoffman, MD. E-mail: hoffmanb@ohsu.edu

PEDIATRICS (ISSN Numbers: Print, 0031-4005; Online, 1098-4275).

FINANCIAL DISCLOSURE: The authors have indicated they do not have a financial relationship relevant to this article to disclose.

FUNDING: No external funding.

POTENTIAL CONFLICT OF INTEREST: The authors have indicated they have no potential conflicts of interest to disclose.

To cite: Durbin DR, Hoffman BD, AAP COUNCIL ON INJURY, VIOLENCE, AND POISON PREVENTION. Child Passenger Safety. *Pediatrics.* 2018;142(5):e20182461

I. INTRODUCTION

Magnitude of the Problem of Motor Vehicle Crashes

Motor vehicle crashes represent the leading cause of death for children and youth older than 4 years in the United States.[1] Each year, more than 5000 children and adolescents under the age of 21 years die in crashes, representing approximately 15% of people killed each year in crashes.[2] Fatalities represent only the tip of the motor vehicle crash problem for children and youth. For every fatality, approximately 18 children are hospitalized and more than 400 receive medical treatment of injuries sustained in a crash.[1] Current estimates of injuries and fatalities are updated annually and can be found on the Centers for Disease Control and Prevention's Web-based Injury Statistics Query and Reporting System at www.cdc.gov/injury/wisqars.

In the United States, motor vehicle traffic-related mortality rates are highest in African American, American Indian, and Alaskan native children, lowest among Asian American and Pacific Islander children, and intermediate for Hispanic and white children.[3] Examining trends over a 20-year period through 2003 reveals significantly declining rates for child occupant deaths among all race and ethnic groups examined. However, among infants (age 0–12 months), improvements in mortality rates among African American children have slowed more recently. Occupant mortality among children 1 to 4 years of age revealed a tendency toward increased mortality in African American, Hispanic, American Indian, and Alaskan native children. Although there were significant declines in total motor vehicle mortality across all racial groups, improvement in occupant injury was greater for white children, and disparities actually widened for both African American and American Indian and Alaskan native children, compared with white children.

The racial and ethnic disparities in motor vehicle occupant death rates are likely explained in large part by the lower use of restraints, including child restraint systems, by people of racial minorities. Seat belt and child restraint use among African American adults and children are lower than the national average.[4,5] Similarly, seat belt use among Hispanic (85%) and non-Hispanic African American (80%) adults traveling with children was lower than for white (96%) adults traveling with children.[6] The reasons for these disparities in restraint use are not completely known but may be related to a lack of knowledge as well as a lack of culturally appropriate messages from generalized public education intervention programs.[7] More culturally sensitive intervention programs designed to increase child restraint use among minority populations have shown significant increases in restraint use among target populations.[8]

Through the early 1990s, child occupant fatality rates remained relatively stagnant at approximately 3.5 deaths per 100 000 population.[9] Beginning in 1995, when children killed by deploying passenger air bags were first reported clinically, attention began to focus on the unique needs of children in automotive safety. Subsequently in the United States, the number of motor vehicle fatalities and serious injuries has been reduced through a combination of increased attention to age-appropriate restraint use and rear seating position[10–15] as well as enhanced child restraint laws and enforcement of these laws.[16,17] In the 10 years from 1999 to 2008, the number of children younger than 15 years who died in motor vehicle crashes in the United States declined by 45%.[2] Annual updates on the number of children killed in motor vehicle crashes can be obtained from the National Highway Traffic Safety Administration (NHTSA) at http://www-fars.nhtsa.dot.gov/Main/index.aspx.

Although significant progress has been made in reducing the number of children killed in crashes, the exposure of children to motor vehicle travel and, thus, to potential crashes is great. Children younger than 16 years travel nearly as much as adults, with an average of 3.4 trips per day and an average of 45 to 50 minutes per day spent in a vehicle, emphasizing the importance of age-appropriate restraint use on every trip.[18]

II. THE IMPORTANCE OF AGE-APPROPRIATE RESTRAINT USE

Mechanism of Action of Restraint Systems

Restraint systems are designed to reduce the risk of ejection during a crash, better distribute the energy load of the crash through structurally stronger bones rather than soft tissues, limit the crash forces experienced by the vehicle occupant by prolonging the time of deceleration, and limit the contact of the occupant with interior vehicle structures. Optimal performance of restraint systems depends on an adequate fit between the restraint system and the occupant at the time of the crash. Restraint systems can be generally categorized as vehicle restraints (air bags and seat belts) or add-on restraints specifically made for children (child restraint systems). Child restraint systems include rear-facing-only car safety seats (CSSs), convertible and combination CSSs, integrated seats, travel vests, and belt-positioning booster seats. A description of each type of restraint is provided below as well as in Table 1 of the accompanying policy statement.[19]

Age-Specific Prevalence of Restraint Use

In large part because of the increased attention paid to the needs of children in motor vehicle safety beginning in the mid-1990s, large increases in restraint use (including CSSs and booster seats) by children have been observed over the past decade. Data from the National Occupant Protection Use Survey and the National Survey of the Use of Booster Seats indicate that restraint use for children in the United States in 2008 stood at 99% among infants younger than 1 year, 92% among 1- to 3-year-olds, and 89% among 4- to 7-year-olds.[20] Restraint use for children driven by a belted driver was significantly higher (92%) than for those driven by an unbelted driver (54%). Importantly, although child restraint use is high among the youngest children, improper use of the restraint may limit the effectiveness of the system. Among children either younger than 1 year or weighing under 20 lb, a group that has traditionally been recommended to ride in a rear-facing CSS, 21% were not compliant with these recommendations.[21] Similarly, although overall restraint use among older children is relatively high, nearly half of children 12 years and younger who are under 54 inches in height are not using a CSS or booster seat, their recommended form of optimal restraint.[21] Although the prevalence of use by race and ethnicity varied somewhat among age groups, use rates tended to be higher among white and Asian American non-Hispanic children (at least 90% for all age groups) and lower among African American non-Hispanic children (ranging from 72% for 8- to 12-year-olds to 94% for infants <1 year of age).[22] Of note, child restraint use among African American children 4 to 7 years of age increased from 73% in 2007 to 84% in 2008.

Among children 8 years and younger in crashes, overall reported use of child restraint systems has increased nearly threefold since 1999 to 80% of children in a large sample of children in crashes by 2007.[23] The largest relative increase in child restraint use among children in crashes was among 6- to 8-year-olds, yet 57% of these children continued to be inappropriately restrained in 2007. Forward-facing car safety seats (FFCSSs) were primarily used by children 3 years and younger, whereas belt-positioning booster seats have become the most common restraints for 4- to 5-year-olds.[24]

Pediatric obesity has become a major public health concern in the United States, with the prevalence of being overweight among children tripling over the past 2 decades.[25] Currently, 34% of children are categorized as being "overweight" (BMI ≥95th percentile) or "at risk for overweight" (BMI ≥85th to <95th percentile).[26] Childhood obesity has significant implications for child passenger safety, because young children who are overweight may not

properly fit in CSSs or booster seats that would otherwise be appropriate for their age.[27] Fortunately, over the past several years, increasing numbers of CSSs and booster seats with higher weight and height limits have been introduced into the market in response to this challenge. Among currently available products listed in the American Academy of Pediatrics (AAP) pamphlet "2018 Car Safety Seats: A Guide for Families" (available at www.healthychildren. org/carseatlist), nearly all (53 of 58) of rear-facing-only seats can accommodate children to 30 lb or more, which represents at least the 75th percentile for girls and boys 24 months of age. Nearly all (85 of 87) currently available convertible and 3-in-1 CSSs can accommodate children to 35 lb or more (a weight that exceeds the 95th percentile for boys and girls 24 months of age) when used in a rear-facing manner. Similarly, for children 2 to 8 years of age, 105 of 117 currently available forward-facing seats used with a harness can accommodate children to at least 50 lb, which exceeds the 95th percentile for boys and girls younger than 5 years. Therefore, there are sufficient products available to consumers to accommodate larger children in the correct restraint. Limited data exist on the risk of injury to overweight children in motor vehicle crashes but suggest that overweight children may be at an increased risk of particular types of injuries, particularly lower-extremity fractures, as compared with children of normal weight.[28–30] Further research is needed to establish motor vehicle safety as yet another public health burden imposed by childhood obesity as well as to ensure that overweight children are properly protected in motor vehicles.

Seat belt use among all front-seat occupants (drivers and front passenger-seat occupants) in the United States has increased to 84%

in 2009.[31] Among older children, restraint use in any seating location in the vehicle in 2008 was 85% among 8- to 12-year-olds and 83% among 13- to 15-year-olds.[6,20] Seat belt use anywhere in the vehicle among 13- to 15-year-olds varied by race and ethnicity, with white adolescents having higher seat belt use rates (89%) than either Hispanic (82%) or African American non-Hispanic (46%) youth.

It is important to note that CSSs were designed as occupant safety devices in motor vehicles and not as general child seating devices. Authors of a recent study who used data from the National Electronic Injury Surveillance System operated by the US Consumer Product Safety Commission estimated that over 8000 infants under 1 year of age are evaluated in hospital emergency departments each year for car seat–related (non–motor vehicle crash) injuries suffered when the car seats were used improperly or for unintended purposes.[32] The majority (85%) of injuries were related to falls, either infants falling out of car seats or car seats falling from elevated surfaces such as countertops and tables. Nearly half of injuries occurred at home, and head and neck injuries accounted for 84% of the injuries to infants. Prolonged use of CSSs by young infants for positioning also contributes to the increased incidence of plagiocephaly, exacerbates gastroesophageal reflux, and increases risk of respiratory compromise.[33] Families should be encouraged to use CSSs only as occupant protection devices for travel as they were intended.

Installation of Child Restraint Systems

CSSs must be installed tightly to derive the optimum benefit of both the crashworthiness of the vehicle (eg, crumple zones that dissipate the energy of the crash and prolong the time of deceleration of the vehicle) as well as the design of the seat itself. As a general rule, if a CSS can be moved >1 in from side to side or front to back when grasped at the bottom of the seat near the belt or Lower Anchors and Tethers for Children (LATCH) attachment points, it is not installed tightly enough. Improper installation of a CSS may result in an increased likelihood of excessive movement of the child in the event of a crash, thus increasing the child's risk of injury.

The most recent estimates of CSS misuse are derived from an observational study of more than 5000 children, in which 72.6% of CSSs were observed to have some form of misuse.[34,35] The most common critical misuses were loose harness straps and a loose attachment of the CSS to the vehicle when using the seat belt. Authors of several studies have indicated that misused CSSs may increase a child's risk of serious injury in a crash.[13,14,36,37]

An issue specific to installing rear-facing CSSs relates to the recline angle of the seat. Proper installation results in a semireclined angle of approximately 45°, which enables the infant's head to lie against the back of the CSS, as opposed to potentially falling forward, compromising the infant's airway if the seat is angled too upright. Preterm infants are particularly vulnerable to an increased risk of oxygen desaturation, apnea, and/ or bradycardia, especially when placed in a semireclined position in CSSs.[38–41] Therefore, CSS monitoring in the infant's own CSS before discharge from the hospital should be considered for any infant less than 37 weeks' gestation at birth to determine whether the infant is physiologically mature and has stable cardiorespiratory function. More specific information on car seat testing of preterm newborn infants and recommendations based on

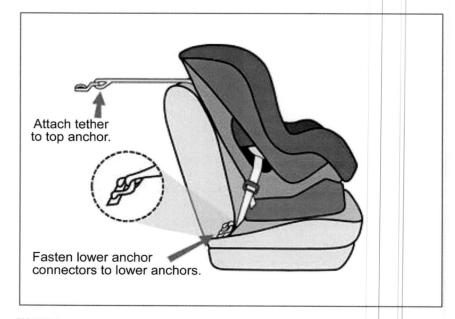

FIGURE 1
Schematic of the LATCH system.

results of testing are available in an AAP clinical report on the subject.[33]

A relatively new way by which CSSs can be installed in passenger vehicles, known as LATCH, was designed to reduce the difficulty associated with installing CSSs. This system uses dedicated attachment points in the vehicle, rather than using the vehicle seat belt, for CSS installation. All vehicles and child restraints manufactured and sold in the United States after September 2002 are required to have this anchoring system. For rear-facing CSSs, there are 2 points of attachment at the base of the CSS. For FFCSSs, a third dedicated attachment point near the top of the CSS is used for a top tether to attach to a separate anchor point in the vehicle (see Fig 1).

Researchers of previous work have evaluated the performance of LATCH (or its European counterpart ISOFIX) in laboratory sled-test environments[42–44] and demonstrated improved kinematics and reduced injury measures on crash test dummies, in particular with the use of the top tether, when compared with using a seat belt to attach the

CSS. To date, there are no real-world data being used to evaluate the performance of LATCH, although its theoretical advantages in ensuring proper installation suggest that families should use it when available.

Arbogast and Jermakian[45] have reviewed cases of CSSs attached using LATCH and illustrated examples of LATCH misuse. In 2005, a large-scale observation study in which authors examined LATCH use and misuse in the United States was conducted at 66 sites across 7 states.[46] The study indicated that many parents purchasing newer vehicles did not update their CSS to take advantage of the available LATCH attachment system. Approximately one-fifth of CSSs in vehicles equipped with LATCH did not have tether straps, and one-sixth did not have lower attachments. Even when their CSSs were LATCH equipped, approximately one-third of drivers with LATCH-equipped vehicles stated that they could not use LATCH because there were no anchors in their vehicles. Much of the nonuse of lower anchors in this study related to the fact that the vehicle safety belt was the only method available in the center rear-seating position for installing a CSS. The rear seats of most passenger vehicles typically are equipped with lower LATCH anchors only in the outboard seating positions. When parents had experience attaching CSSs using the safety belt and LATCH system, three-fourths reported a preference for LATCH, because they found it easier to use, obtained a tighter fit, and felt that the child was more secure.

EVIDENCE FOR BEST PRACTICE RECOMMENDATIONS

The following section of this technical report will provide a summary of the evidence in support of each of the best practice recommendations included in the accompanying policy statement.[19]

Children with certain physical and behavioral conditions may require specialized restraint systems and other considerations. Relevant conditions may include prematurity, cerebral palsy, the presence of a tracheostomy, muscle tone abnormalities, skeletal abnormalities, and certain behavioral or emotional conditions as well as temporary conditions, such as fractures requiring spica casts. Therefore, the AAP has developed a separate policy statement that reviews important considerations for transporting children with special health care needs and provides current guidelines for the protection of children with specific health care needs, including those transported in wheelchairs.[47]

Best Practice Recommendation

All infants and toddlers should ride in a rear-facing CSS as long as possible, until they reach the highest weight or height allowed by their CSS's manufacturer.

This best practice results from the need to support the young child's posterior torso, neck, head, and pelvis and to distribute crash forces over the entire body. Developmental considerations, including incomplete vertebral ossification, more horizontally oriented spinal facet joints, and excessive ligamentous laxity put young children at risk for head and spinal cord injury. Rear-facing CSSs address this risk by supporting the child's head, preventing the relatively large head from moving independently of the proportionately smaller neck.

In the United States, although the majority of children use rear-facing CSSs during the first year of life, 21% of infants either younger than 1 year or weighing less than 20 lb have been turned forward facing.[21] In Sweden, many children remain rear facing up to the age of 4 years and transition directly from the rear-facing CSS to a booster seat. Swedish researchers have reported that rear-facing CSSs reduce the risk of significant injuries (those with an Abbreviated Injury Scale score of 2 or greater) by 90%, relative to unrestrained children, reinforcing their policy of children remaining in a rear-facing CSS up to the age of 4 years.[48,49]

In 2007, Henary et al[50] reviewed US crash data to calculate the relative effectiveness of rear-facing CSSs compared with FFCSSs for children aged 0 to 23 months in crashes from 1988 to 2003. The authors reported that children in FFCSSs were significantly more likely to be seriously injured when compared with children in rear-facing CSSs in all crash types. That study, along with similar data from biomechanical studies and the Swedish experience,[48,49] provided the bases for the 2011 AAP policy recommendation that specifically called for children under age 2 years to remain in rear-facing CSSs. However, in 2016 the Henary et al[51] study was called into question, and after further analysis, the article

was retracted by the journal *Injury Prevention*, because the survey weights in the original analysis were thought to be improperly handled.

In 2017, a revised analysis of the 1988–2003 data, along with an extended analysis of the data through 2015, was published by a subset of the original authorship group. Their findings reveal that, although children 0 to 23 months still had lower rates of injury while rear facing compared with forward facing, the sample size was too small to achieve statistical significance.[52]

It should be noted that no analysis suggests any increased risk for infants in rear-facing CSSs compared with FFCSSs. Combined with biomechanical data and the Swedish experience, it remains evident that a recommendation that children remain rear facing as long as possible up to the manufacturer's limits for weight and length continues to be best practice and is consistent with NHTSA recommendations.[53]

Best Practice Recommendation

All children who have outgrown the rear-facing weight or height limit for their CSS should use a FFCSS with a harness for as long as possible, up to the highest weight or height allowed by their CSS's manufacturer.

The recommendation for FFCSSs has been based, in part, on an analysis by Kahane[54] of laboratory sled tests, observational studies, and police-reported crash data from the early 1980s that estimated that correctly used FFCSSs reduce the risk of death and injury by approximately 71%, compared with unrestrained children. The engineering tests documented the biomechanical benefits of the CSS in spreading the crash forces over the shoulders and hips and by controlling the excursion of the head during a crash. The study further estimated the effectiveness of a partially misused CSS as providing a 45% reduction in risk of fatality and serious injury. Using Fatality Analysis Reporting System (FARS) data from 1988 to 1994, NHTSA found that, among children between 1 and 4 years of age in passenger cars, those in FFCSSs had a 54% reduction in risk of death, compared with unrestrained children.[55] Given the currently high rates of restraint use among children in the United States, it is no longer meaningful to quote effectiveness estimates in comparison with unrestrained children.

Estimates of the effectiveness of FFCSSs in comparison with children using seat belts, on the basis of real-world crash data, vary depending on the source of data used, the time period studied, and the analytical approach taken. Estimating effectiveness of child restraint systems through analysis of crash databases is challenging because of the association between how passengers are restrained in a given crash and whether that crash will be in a specific database. For example, FARS, operated by NHTSA, is a census of vehicle crashes in the United States in which at least 1 person died. FARS has a sufficient number of outcomes of fatal child injuries for analyses but has a biased selection of crashes in that inclusion of crashes is associated with the outcome of interest, mortality. Several different analytic techniques, described hereafter, have been developed to minimize the effects of this bias.

Most studies to date indicate that FFCSSs are effective at preventing nonfatal injuries when compared with seat belts, with effectiveness estimates ranging from 71% to 82% reduction in serious injury risk.[13,56] Elliott and colleagues[14] compared the effectiveness of child restraints to seat belts in preventing fatal injuries for 2- to 6-year-old children in crashes by combining data from FARS with data from the National Automotive Sampling System–Crashworthiness Data System. The combined data set, in

theory, overcame several of the known limitations of using either data source alone. Compared with seat belts, child restraints, when not seriously misused (eg, unattached restraint, child restraint system harness not used) were associated with a 28% reduction in risk of death (relative risk [RR], 0.72; 95% confidence interval [CI], 0.54–0.97) after adjusting for seating position, vehicle type, model year, driver and passenger ages, and driver survival status. When including cases of serious misuse, the effectiveness estimate was slightly lower (21%) and not statistically significant (RR, 0.79; 95% CI, 0.59–1.05).[14]

In a controversial analysis, Levitt[57] used FARS data from 1975 to 2003 and, by various methods, directly compared the mortality rates for child restraints and for seat belts for children ages 2 to 6 and could not demonstrate a difference in effectiveness. Levitt[57] restricted the FARS data set to 2-vehicle crashes in which someone in the other vehicle (ie, the vehicle without the index child occupant) died, under the assumption that the distribution of restraint use among children in potentially fatal crashes is independent of whether someone in the other vehicle dies, after adjusting for various crash-related characteristics. In a subsequent study using a marginal structural model–type estimator in an attempt to explore the relationship between various biases inherent in data sources and the estimates of CSS restraint effectiveness, Elliott et al[58] suggest a 17% reduction in fatality risk for children 2 through 6 years of age in child restraint systems relative to seat belts. This reduction is estimated at 22% when severe misuse of the restraint is excluded.

Best Practice Recommendation

All children whose weight or height is above the forward-facing limit for their CSS should use a

belt-positioning booster seat until the vehicle lap and shoulder seat belt fits properly, typically when they have reached 4 ft 9 inches in height and are between 8 and 12 years of age.

Children who have outgrown a FFCSS (based on the height or weight limit of the seat) should be restrained in belt-positioning booster seats using the lap and shoulder belts in the back seat of a vehicle. Booster seats position the child so that the lap and shoulder belts fit properly. A correct fit of the belt is defined as the following:

- The shoulder belt lies across the middle of the chest and shoulder, not the neck or face.

- The lap belt is low across the hips and pelvis, not the abdomen.

- The child is tall enough to sit against the vehicle seat back with his or her knees bent without slouching and can stay in this position comfortably throughout the trip.

Although seat belt geometry varies from vehicle to vehicle depending on the depth of the seat bottom and placement of the upper and lower anchor points of the belt, most vehicle seat belts will not fit correctly until a child reaches about 4 ft 9 inches in height and is between 8 and 12 years of age. This height threshold was derived from a study of 155 children 6 to 12 years of age who were assessed for the fit of the vehicle seat belt in 3 different types of vehicles in 1993.[59] The minimum height of a child who could fit properly in the vehicle seat belts was 148 cm (58 in). It is important to note that this study is nearly 20 years old, and significant changes have been made to the vehicle fleet during this time.

Cases of serious cervical and lumbar spinal cord injury, as well as intraabdominal injuries, to children in motor vehicle crashes resulting from poorly fitting seat belts have been described for many years and are known as the "seat belt syndrome."[60] First described by Kulowski and Rost[61] in 1956, the term seat belt syndrome was coined by Garrett and Braunstein[62] in 1962 to describe a distinctive pattern of injuries associated with lap seat belts in serious crashes. Two predominant factors have been hypothesized to explain this constellation of injuries: the immaturity of the pediatric pelvis to properly anchor the lap portion of the belt and the tendency of children to scoot forward in the seat so their knees bend at the edge of the vehicle seat. From this position, in a rapid deceleration, the belt can directly compress abdominal organs against the spinal column, and the child's body may "jack-knife" around the belt, putting high tension forces on the lumbar spine, which may lead to distraction injuries of the posterior elements of the spine, such as Chance-type fractures.

Durbin et al[12] published the first real-world evaluation of the performance of booster seats as compared with seat belts for young children. These authors determined that the risk of injury after adjusting for child, crash, driver, and vehicle characteristics was 59% lower for 4- to 7-year-olds in belt-positioning booster seats than those using only seat belts. Applying these results to Wisconsin state data from 1998 to 2002, Corden[63] determined that there would be an approximate 57% reduction in deaths and hospitalizations if all 4- to 7-year-olds were in booster seats. A recent updated analysis of booster effectiveness in preventing nonfatal injuries was able to examine a greater percentage of older children using booster seats; 37% of the more recent study sample using booster seats were 6 to 8 years of age.[24] In this study, children 4 to 8 years of age using belt-positioning booster seats were 45% (95% CI, 4%–68%) less likely to sustain nonfatal injuries than children of similar ages using

the vehicle seat belt. Among children restrained in belt-positioning booster seats, there was no detectable difference in the risk of injury between the children in backless versus high-back boosters.

Rice et al[64] extended the data on booster seat performance by estimating the effectiveness of booster seats in reducing the risk of fatal injuries to children 4 to 8 years of age. Using a matched cohort analysis of data from FARS, Rice et al[64] determined that booster seats reduced the risk of fatal injuries by 67% for 4- to 5-year-olds and 55% for 6- to 8-year-olds, compared with unrestrained adults and children. They also determined that seat belts alone reduced the risk of fatal injury by approximately 62% for 4- to 8-year-olds, compared with unrestrained adults and children. They did not demonstrate a significant difference in fatality risk reduction for booster seats when compared with seat belts (RR, 0.92; 95% CI, 0.79–1.08). The authors postulated that although booster seats, which improve seat belt fit, may reduce the risk of nonfatal injuries (some of which may be attributable to improperly fitting seat belts), they may not improve the likelihood that children will survive a severe crash with major occupant compartment intrusion or during rollovers. It may be that properly fitting seat belts are no better than poorly fitting seat belts at preventing fatal injuries in these severe crashes.

Although most newer vehicles include lap and shoulder belts in all rear seating positions, many older vehicles still in use may have only lap belts available in some seating positions, typically in the center of the rear seat. Laboratory tests have been used to document increased head excursions when booster seats are used with lap belts, compared with when only lap belts are used.[65,66] Other research indicates that booster-aged children using only

lap belts are likely to strike their heads on vehicle seat backs or other interior components in front of them, even without booster seats.[67,68] A recent study using 2 real-world data sources suggested that children restrained in booster seats with lap belts had a lower injury risk when compared with children restrained in lap belts only, although the possibility of no difference could not be excluded.[69] For families faced with frequently transporting booster-aged children in lap belt–only seating positions, there are other restraint options (eg, FFCSSs with higher weight limits and safety vests) that, although typically more expensive than booster seats, are more likely to provide optimal protection if children ride regularly in these seating positions. Of note, the number of children in this scenario will decrease over time as vehicles equipped with lap belt–only restraints in rear seats are phased out of the US vehicle fleet.

Best Practice Recommendation

When children are old enough and large enough to use the vehicle seat belt alone, they should always use lap and shoulder seat belts for optimal protection.

Lap and shoulder belts have been required in rear outboard positions of vehicles since 1989. However, it was not until 2005 that lap and shoulder belts were required in the center rear seat position. Many manufacturers introduced center rear lap and shoulder belts in advance of this requirement, and by model year 2001, most vehicles provided them as standard equipment.[70] Arbogast et al[71] determined that the presence of a shoulder belt reduced the risk of injury by 81% for children seated in the center rear in seat belts, with the primary benefit seen in reductions in abdominal injuries. Parenteau et al[72] had previously documented a similar shift in the pattern of injury to children in lap-only belt restraints to lap and shoulder belts. Their study, however, looked at the rear seat as a whole and did not separate the rear seating positions.

Using data from FARS, NHTSA has evaluated the performance of lap and shoulder belts in the rear rows and found them to be effective (as compared with unrestrained occupants) in all crash directions for children and adult occupants 5 years and older. The estimated fatality reduction, as compared with unrestrained occupants, was 77% in rollover crashes, 42% in side impacts, 29% in frontal impacts, and 31% in rear impacts and other crashes.[73] Two studies have evaluated seat belt effectiveness specifically for children. Chipman,[74] using a database of fatal crashes in Ontario, estimated that seat belts reduced the risk of serious injury or death by 40% for children 4 to 14 years of age. Data from Wisconsin suggested that 100% seat belt use by children 8 to 15 years of age (as compared with the current 72% use) would result in reductions of 45% and 32% for deaths and hospitalizations, respectively.[63]

Best Practice Recommendation

All children younger than 13 years should be restrained in the rear seats of vehicles for optimal protection.

In large part because of the attention resulting from the tragedy of children killed by passenger air bags, significant declines in front seating of children in vehicles have occurred since the mid-1990s. By 2008, 95% of infants, 98% of children 1 to 3 years of age, and 88% of children 4 to 7 years of age rode in the rear seat.[20] This compares with rates of 85%, 90%, and 71%, respectively, in 2002, the first year that these data were available from direct observation studies.[75] Of note, rear seating does not appear to vary on the basis of whether there is a state law requiring children to ride in the rear. In 2008, 92% of children who live in states where such a law

exists were observed in the rear versus 93% of children from states where no such law exists.[20] Children using child restraint systems were more likely to sit in the rear ($\geq$93%) than were those in seat belts (89%) or riding unrestrained (84%). In a study of children involved in nonfatal crashes, children were more likely to be seated in the front if the vehicle was driven by a man or by someone other than the child's parent or if the vehicle was not equipped with a passenger air bag.[76] Among children younger than 4 years of age in CSSs who have been in crashes, there appears to be a preference for placing the CSS in the right outboard seating position in the rear row (41%), as compared with the center rear (31%) or left outboard (28%).[77] This likely has to do with the increased ability for the driver to directly observe the child more easily when in the right outboard rear seating position.

Several studies have documented the benefits of rear seating for children. Estimates of the elevated risk of injury for children in the front seat compared with children in the rear range from 40% to 70%, depending on the time period and characteristics of the group studied.[10,78,79] One of these studies specifically noted that the beneficial effects of the rear seat were no longer seen for children 13 years and older.[10] Thus, the AAP continues to recommend that all children younger than 13 years ride in the rear seat. Of interest, the benefits of rear seating for child occupants extend to side impacts as well, with children in the rear 62% less likely to sustain an injury.[80] Not only is the overall risk higher, but the severity of injury is also greater in the front seat. An analysis of crashes identified through the Crash Injury Research and Engineering Network revealed that front seat child occupants sustained more severe injuries than those seated in the rear rows as measured by an injury severity score >16.[81]

Two recent studies have specifically evaluated the potential incremental benefits of the center rear seating position as compared with the rear outboard positions. Lund[82] used data from the National Automotive Sampling System–General Estimates System from 1992 to 2000 to evaluate the effect of seating position on the risk of injury for children in child restraints. Lund[82] reported that children in the center rear seat had a similar risk of injury to children in the outboard rear seats. In contrast, Kallan et al[77] used data from the Partners for Child Passenger Safety project, a large, child-focused crash surveillance system, from 1998 to 2006 and found that children restrained in FFCSSs and seated in the center rear had an injury risk 43% lower than similarly restrained children in either of the rear outboard positions (adjusted odds ratio [OR], 0.57; 95% CI, 0.38–0.86). These contrasting findings are likely attributable to how injuries were defined in the 2 studies. Lund defined injury as any police-reported injury, which includes those of a relatively minor nature.[82] The threshold for injury was higher in Kallan's analysis, which included only injuries involving internal organs and fractures of the extremities.[77]

CHILDREN AND AIR BAGS

In November 1995, the *Morbidity and Mortality Weekly Report* of the Centers for Disease Control and Prevention described 8 deaths of child occupants involving air bag deployment that were of special concern, because they involved low-speed crashes in which the children otherwise should have survived.[83] As passenger air bags diffused into the market, numerous case reports began appearing in the medical literature in which authors described brain and skull injuries sustained by children in rear-facing CSSs and brain and cervical spine injuries sustained by older children who were often unrestrained or restrained in seat belts inappropriately for their age.[84–88]

Several researchers reviewed case series of children exposed to deploying passenger air bags to elucidate the mechanisms of injury.[89–93] For children killed in a rear-facing CSSs, the air bag typically deployed into the rear surface of the child restraint near the child's head, causing fatal skull and brain injuries. For older children who were either unrestrained or restrained in seat belts inappropriately for their age, braking before impact caused the child to pitch forward so that they were in the path of the air bag as it deployed. On deployment, the air bag caused a spectrum of injuries to the brain and cervical spine, including atlanto-occipital fractures, brain stem injuries, and diffuse axonal injury. Case series of other less serious injuries to child occupants associated with air bag deployment continue to appear in the literature, including injuries to the eye[94] and upper extremities[95] as well as respiratory and hearing problems related to the sound wave and cloud of fine particulate matter released during an air bag deployment.[96]

Several population-based estimates of the effects of air bags on young children in crashes have consistently indicated an increased risk of fatal and nonfatal injuries to both restrained and unrestrained child occupants.[11,12,97–101] Exposure to passenger air bags increased the risk of both minor injuries, including facial and chest abrasions, and moderate and more serious injuries, particularly head injuries and upper-extremity fractures.

On the basis of this evidence, NHTSA initiated a 2-pronged program of education and regulation in response to the initial reports of deaths and serious injuries to children from air bags. First, NHTSA, joined by many national organizations, including the AAP, recommended that all child passengers younger than 13 years sit in the rear seats of vehicles. Second, in 1997, NHTSA enacted a substantial regulatory change to Federal Motor Vehicle Safety Standard (FMVSS) 208, the safety standard used to govern the protection of motor vehicle occupants in frontal impact crashes. Because frontal air bags are designed to primarily protect occupants in frontal impact crashes, their performance is certified through FMVSS 208. The change provided automakers a choice in the type of test that could be used to certify frontal crash performance for unbelted adults.[102] This change in the standard resulted in the redesign of frontal air bags to reduce the force with which they deploy. These new air bags are often referred to as "second-generation air bags" and were generally present in all vehicles beginning with model year 1998.

Several studies have examined the effect of these design changes on child occupants in real-world crashes. Olson et al[103] found that second-generation air bags reduced the risk of death among right front-seated children 6 to 12 years of age by 29% compared with no air bag. For children younger than 6 years, both first- and second-generation air bags increased the risk of death compared with no air bag; however, the increased risk of death was less for second-generation air bags (10%) compared with first-generation air bags (66%). Arbogast et al[104] quantified the risk of serious nonfatal injuries in frontal crashes among belted children in the front seat of vehicles in which second-generation versus first-generation passenger air bags deployed. Serious injuries were reported in 14.9% in the first-generation group versus 9.9% in the second-generation group. In particular, children in the second-generation group sustained fewer head injuries, including concussions and other serious brain injuries, than in the first generation group.[104]

Braver et al[105] examined federal crash data to determine the effect of second- versus first-generation air bags on the risk of fatal injuries to children in the right front seat. Right-front passengers younger than 10 years in vehicles with second-generation air bags had statistically significant reductions in risk of dying in frontal collisions, as compared with children of similar ages in vehicles with first-generation air bags, including a 65% reduced risk among children 0 to 4 years of age (RR, 0.35; 95% CI, 0.21–0.60). Nonsignificant decreases in risk of death were observed among children 10 to 14 years of age.

Kuppa et al[106] evaluated the influence of the air bag on the effectiveness of rear seating using a double-pair comparison study of frontal impact crashes identified in FARS. Two pairs were analyzed: the first group consisted of fatal crashes in which a driver and front outboard seat passenger were present and at least 1 of them was killed; the second group consisted of fatal crashes in which a driver and a rear outboard seat passenger were present and at least 1 of them was killed. This analysis was used to examine vehicles with and without a passenger air bag separately. For restrained children 5 years or younger, the presence of a passenger air bag increased the benefit, in terms of reduced fatalities, associated with rear seating. For restrained child occupants older than 8 years, the rear seat was still associated with a lower risk of death than the front, but its benefit was less in vehicles with a passenger air bag than in vehicles without.

Air bags continue to undergo significant redesigns in an effort to optimize their effectiveness in serious crashes while minimizing their risk of adverse injuries in minor crashes. In 2001, additional revisions were made to FMVSS 208, which now requires the testing of air bag systems for all sizes of occupants, including children. At this time, no studies have evaluated the benefits of these designs, often termed "certified advanced compliant air bags," for child occupants.

There have been limited studies that have attempted to examine age-specific effects of air bags on risk of injury to children. Newgard and Lewis[100] used data from the National Automotive Sampling System–Crashworthiness Data System to evaluate specific cutoff points for age, height, and weight as effect modifiers of the association between the presence of a passenger air bag and serious injury among children involved in motor vehicle crashes. The time period studied, 1995–2002, preceded the time when second-generation air bags were generally available in the vehicle fleet. Newgard and Lewis[100] found that children 0 to 14 years of age involved in frontal collisions appeared to be at increased risk of serious injury from air bag presence (OR, 2.66; 95% CI, 0.23–30.9) and deployment (OR, 6.13; 95% CI, 0.30–126), although these values did not reach statistical significance. Among children 15 to 18 years of age involved in frontal collisions, there was a protective effect on injury from both air bag presence (OR, 0.19; 95% CI, 0.05–0.75) and deployment (OR, 0.31; 95% CI, 0.09–0.99). A similar analysis has not been replicated to determine whether different age cutoffs might be identified with children in vehicles equipped with second-generation air bags. Therefore, the AAP continues to strongly recommend that all children younger than 13 years sit in the rear seat. In vehicles with only a single row of seats, such as compact pickup trucks, the frontal air bag can be deactivated, or an on-off switch can be installed, to prevent its deployment in the event of a crash,

thus allowing either the installation of a CSS in the front seat or the ability of a child younger than 13 years to ride in the front if necessary.[107]

Side air bags were introduced in the mid-1990s as a safety strategy to reduce serious injuries and fatalities occurring in side-impact crashes. Initial crash tests involving vehicles equipped with so-called torso side air bags in the front seats revealed that the head was still at risk for serious injury in side-impact crashes.[108,109] To maximize the protection of the head for adult front and rear seat occupants of a variety of statures and seating postures, the roof-rail or head curtain air bag was developed and has become the preferred head protection system for side-impact crashes. These systems, frequently accompanied by a separate torso side air bag, provide more extensive coverage of the upper vehicle side interior, often extending the entire length of the vehicle, including the rear rows. Side air bags have become a common safety technology in the vehicle; 79% of model year 2006 vehicles have some type of side air bag either as standard or optional equipment.[110] NHTSA recently conducted an analysis of side-impact protection with a focus on side air bag technology.[111] They determined that side air bags resulted in a reduction in struck-side fatality risk of 18% in multivehicle crashes and substantial improvement in a thoracic injury metric, the Thoracic Trauma Index, in laboratory assessments. Benefits were greater for head side air bags than those with torso side air bags alone. However, these analyses were primarily focused on the protection of adult drivers and front-seat occupants. Arbogast and Kallan[112] used the Partners for Child Passenger Safety database to estimate the prevalence of side air bag exposure to children in crashes and to provide estimates of injury risk among those exposed. In the study sample, 2.7%

of children in crashes were exposed to a deployed side air bag. More than 75% of these children were seated in the rear seat, and 65% of those exposed were younger than 9 years. Of those exposed, 10.6% sustained an Abbreviated Injury Scale 2 injury to the head or upper extremity, a rate similar to that of children exposed to second-generation frontal air bags. These limited field data on the performance of side air bags with respect to child occupant protection suggest that, although a significant number of children are exposed to side air bag deployments, there is no evidence that these air bags pose a particular risk of serious or fatal injuries to children.

SPECIAL CONSIDERATIONS

The Safety of Children Left in or Around Vehicles

Children should never be left unattended in or around parked cars. Among the safety risks that have been described, being backed over when the vehicle is set in motion, hyperthermia, and strangulation from entrapment in power windows are among the most serious and preventable injuries. In 2008, Kids and Cars,[113] a safety advocacy group dedicated to the prevention of such injuries, amassed reports of a wide range of safety incidents involving nearly 1000 children and resulting in more than 200 deaths. In response to the Cameron Gulbransen Kids Transportation Safety Act of 2007 (public law number 110-189), the NHTSA created a virtual database called the Not in Traffic Surveillance system to ascertain population-based estimates of the prevalence of noncrash deaths and injuries. Not in Traffic Surveillance data indicate that approximately 35 to 40 occupants (primarily children) die of hyperthermia, and 5 die of power window strangulation each year, highlighting the importance of never leaving children unsupervised in or around cars.[114]

The Safety of Children in Pickup Trucks

Pickup trucks are popular vehicles in the United States, accounting for approximately 13% of new vehicle sales in 2008.[115] Although many have only a single row of seats, extended-cab models have a second row of seats and may be viewed as family vehicles by parents who want to follow safety recommendations that children be placed in the rear seat. Compact extended-cab pickup trucks, which typically have a smaller rear seat compartment, sometimes with side-facing, fold-down seats, present a particular safety hazard to children. Winston et al[116] found that children in the rear seat of compact extended-cab pickup trucks were more than 4 times as likely to be injured (adjusted OR, 4.69; 95% CI, 2.44–9.01) as were rear row–seated children in other vehicles. A substantial portion of the increased risk was mediated by contact with the vehicle interior during the crash, because the rear seat compartment in these trucks is typically not as well padded as in other vehicles. It is important to note that full-size extended-cab pickup trucks, which typically have a rear seat compartment similar in size and configuration to other vehicles, demonstrated injury risks similar to those of other passenger vehicles.

Of particular concern regarding the safety of pickup trucks for children is the use of the cargo area of pickup trucks for the transport of children and youth. Because the cargo area is not intended for passenger use, it is neither required nor designed to meet occupant safety standards applicable to passenger locations. The fatality risk to children in the cargo area of pickup trucks has been well described.[117,118] The most significant hazard of travel in the cargo area of a pickup truck is ejection of a passenger in a crash

or noncrash event (eg, sudden stop, turn, swerve, or loss of balance, as well as intentional or unintentional jumps and falls). Fortunately, the number of children and adolescents younger than 18 years killed as passengers in the cargo area of pickup trucks has declined by more than 50% over the past decade, from more than 40 per year to fewer than 20 per year more recently.[2] The most effective prevention strategies to reduce the number of deaths and injuries to children in pickup trucks are the prohibition of travel in the cargo area and age-appropriate restraint use in an appropriate rear-seat location in the cab.

The Safety of Children on Commercial Airlines

Currently, the Federal Aviation Administration (FAA) exempts children younger than 2 years from the requirement that all aircraft passengers occupy a seat with a separate safety belt.[119] The FAA and NHTSA agreed on a single government performance standard, FMVSS 213, that would satisfy both aviation and highway safety requirements for child restraint systems.[120] The FAA has also approved a harness-type restraint appropriate for children weighing between 22 and 44 lb. This type of device provides an alternative to using a hard-backed seat and is approved only for use on aircraft. It is not approved for use in motor vehicles.[121] Newman et al[122] examined the potential impact and costs of a requirement for the use of child restraint systems by young children on aircraft. The potential impact of such a regulation requires a number of assumptions, primarily regarding the effectiveness of child restraint systems in survivable aircraft crashes, and the proportion of families who would switch from air to ground travel if required to assume the added cost of an additional aircraft seat and the child restraint system for their children

younger than 2 years. Using available data on the risk of fatalities from air travel and the survivability of crashes and reasonable assumptions for RRs of death for restrained and unrestrained young children involved in crashes, Newman et al[122] found that the number of deaths that could be prevented in the United States with mandatory child restraint system use in commercial aircraft is small (less than 1 per year). The number of deaths that could be prevented by mandatory child restraint system use is limited because the number of deaths of unrestrained young children in survivable aircraft crashes is already low. Newman et al[122] suggested that a policy of requiring child restraint system use for airplane travel is likely to lead to a net increase in deaths caused by increased motor vehicle travel if the proportion of families switching to automobile travel exceeds about 5% to 10%. This threshold varied with the estimated number of lives saved by child restraint system use on airplanes, the average length of the added round trips by car, and the risk profile of the drivers but was unlikely to exceed 15%. The National Transportation Safety Board disputed the "diversion" claim made by Newman et al,[122] suggesting that available data did not indicate that diversion to road travel has previously occurred when circumstances made it likely (eg, immediately following the terrorist attacks in September 2001).[123]

An alternative approach supported by the FAA is to encourage families to inquire about the availability of open seats on less crowded flights so that parents could put their child in a child restraint system in a seat next to them without needing to buy a ticket and without revenue loss to the airline. This approach was also advocated by Bishai[124] in an editorial accompanying the Newman et al[122] study. If open seats are not available, families would be required to check the CSS as luggage. In 2008, the Department of Federal Affairs surveyed all major US airlines on their baggage policies and learned that with 1 exception, airlines have adopted policies that do not count CSSs toward checked baggage allowances.[125]

Data fundamental to creating an evidence-based policy, including information on the number of children under 2 years of age currently flying unrestrained, as well as data on the number of children sustaining injuries in turbulence are not available. Until data systems are created and used to provide evidence to inform the policy debate, and ticket pricing policies and security screening procedures are enhanced to make it easier for families to follow best practice recommendations for correct child restraint use during commercial airline travel and to have their own CSS or booster seat available to them following airline travel, the current situation of allowing young children to travel in a manner inconsistent with best practice recommendations is likely to continue.

CHILD RESTRAINT LAWS

The first state child occupant restraint law was passed in Tennessee in 1978, primarily attributable to the efforts of pediatrician Robert Sanders. By 1985, all 50 states and the District of Columbia had passed laws requiring child restraints for young children. However, these initial child passenger safety laws were generally inconsistent with best practice recommendations at the time, creating several gaps in coverage of children and resulting in poor compliance with the provisions of the laws.[126] Recognizing the importance of laws in both changing restraint behavior and educating the public about recommended restraint practices, most states

have recently enhanced their child occupant restraint laws through the enactment of booster seat use provisions for older children. Current information on all child restraint laws in the United States is updated by the Insurance Institute for Highway Safety and can be found at http://www.iihs.org/iihs/topics/laws/safetybeltuse?topicName=child-safety. Although the laws aim to ensure the appropriate use of all forms of child restraints (eg, CSSs and belt-positioning booster seats), the revised laws generally became known as "booster seat laws." Subsequent study of the association of a booster seat provision in a state child restraint law with changes in child restraint use in that state indicated that booster seat provisions covering children from 4 through 7 years of age increase the use of child restraints by 39% among children in this age range.[16] Children 4 to 5 years of age in states with booster seat laws were 23% more likely to be reported as appropriately restrained than were children in other states, and those 6 to 7 years of age were twice as likely to be reported as appropriately restrained. For 6- to 7-year-olds, the effect was much stronger when the law included children through 7 years of age than when it included only those 4 to 5 years of age.

A focus-group study of violators of California's child restraint law revealed that multiple complex factors influence consistent use of a CSS.[127] At the time of the study, the California law required children younger than 4 years and weighing less than 40 lb to be properly secured in a CSS meeting federal standards. Parents who violated the law described a number of factors, including unreliable access to a vehicle, the trip circumstances, parenting style, and child refusal that affected the use of a CSS at the time of parent citation. Among parents who had been ticketed for not restraining

their children, participation in a class in which child passenger safety information was provided revealed some benefit in their subsequent knowledge of child passenger safety issues, compared with a fine alone.

Seat belt laws have played a critical role in increasing seat belt use to 83% of front seat occupants by 2008.[128] However, seat belt use continues to be lower (at 80% in 2008) among drivers and front seat occupants 16 to 24 years of age. There are 2 different types of seat belt laws, based on the type of enforcement allowed by the law: primary and secondary enforcement. "Primary" enforcement laws allow a citation to be issued whenever a law enforcement officer observes an unbelted driver or passenger. "Secondary" enforcement seat belt laws require the officer to stop a violator for another traffic infraction before being able to issue a citation for not using a seat belt. Previous studies have revealed that, on average, the effects of primary laws are larger and more consistent than secondary laws in increasing seat belt use and decreasing injuries among adult drivers and passengers.[129–132]

Gaps between adult seat belt laws and child restraint laws result in a lack of coverage for many older children (5–15 years of age) in all seating positions. For example, in some states, a 15-year-old can ride legally in the back seat without a restraint because the laws in those states apply only to front seat occupants. To gain insight on the potential effect of primary enforcement safety belt laws on older child passengers, Durbin et al[133] compared reported use of seat belts among 13- to 15-year-old passengers in crashes in states with a primary enforcement seat belt law versus states with a secondary enforcement law. Restraint use was 7.2% (95% CI, 4.3%–10.1%) higher among 13- to 15-year-olds in primary enforcement states versus those in secondary enforcement states. Restraint use among 13- to 15-year-olds was significantly lower in secondary enforcement versus primary enforcement states, particularly when the driver was unrestrained. For 13- to 15-year-olds in a secondary state with an unrestrained driver, 65.8% were unrestrained, as compared with 22.8% in a primary enforcement state (adjusted RR, 3.0; 95% CI, 1.5–15.7). After adjusting for both driver age and restraint use, a 13- to 15-year-old was more than twice as likely to be unrestrained in a secondary enforcement state as compared with a primary enforcement state (RR, 2.2; 95% CI, 1.4–3.5). The authors concluded that primary enforcement laws were associated with higher rates of seat belt use compared with secondary enforcement laws among children 13 to 15 years of age, a group not generally covered by restraint laws.

RESOURCES FOR PEDIATRICIANS AND FAMILIES

NHTSA began a standardized child passenger safety training and certification program in 1998. Since then, tens of thousands of individuals have been certified as child passenger safety technicians.[134] These individuals participate in community-based child safety seat clinics and are a source of information to families on appropriate use and installation of all types of CSSs and booster seats. Although the algorithm to guide implementation of best practice recommendations by pediatricians provided in the policy statement is designed to cover the majority of situations that pediatricians will encounter in practice, pediatricians should consider child passenger safety technicians as sources of information when atypical circumstances may be encountered that are not adequately managed by the algorithm. In most communities, technicians work at formal inspection stations; a list of these is available at

https://www.nhtsa.gov/equipment/car-seats-and-booster-seats#install-inspection. If your community does not have an inspection station, you can find a technician in your area via the National Child Passenger Safety Certification Web site at http://cert.safekids.org or via the NHTSA Child Safety Seat Inspection Station Locator at http://www.nhtsa.dot.gov/cps/cpsfitting/index.cfm. Technicians with enhanced training in restraining children with special health needs, as well as those with Spanish language proficiency, can be identified at http://cert.safekids.org. In addition, additional resources for pediatricians and families can be found at www.aap.org and www.healthychildren.org/carseatguide.

LEAD AUTHORS

Dennis R. Durbin, MD, MSCE, FAAP
Benjamin Hoffman, MD, FAAP

COUNCIL ON INJURY, VIOLENCE, AND POISON PREVENTION, 2018–2019

Benjamin Hoffman, MD, FAAP, Chairperson
Phyllis F. Agran, MD, MPH, FAAP
Sarah A. Denny, MD, FAAP
Michael Hirsh, MD, FAAP
Brian Johnston, MD, MPH, FAAP
Lois K. Lee, MD, MPH, FAAP
Kathy Monroe, MD, FAAP
Judy Schaechter, MD, MBA, FAAP
Milton Tenenbein, MD, FAAP
Mark R. Zonfrillo, MD, MSCE, FAAP
Kyran Quinlan, MD, MPH, FAAP, ex-officio

CONTRIBUTOR

Stuart Weinberg, MD, FAAP, Partnership for Policy Implementation (PPI)

LIAISONS

Lynne Janecek Haverkos, MD, MPH, FAAP – *National Institute of Child Health and Human Development*
Jonathan D. Midgett, PhD – *Consumer Product Safety Commission*
Alexander W. (Sandy) Sinclair – *National Highway Traffic Safety Administration*
Richard Stanwick, MD, FAAP – *Canadian Paediatric Society*

STAFF

Bonnie Kozial

ABBREVIATIONS

AAP: American Academy of Pediatrics
CI: confidence interval
CSS: car safety seat
FAA: Federal Aviation Administration
FARS: Fatality Analysis Reporting System
FFCSS: forward-facing car safety seat
FMVSS: Federal Motor Vehicle Safety Standards
LATCH: Lower Anchors and Tethers for Children
NHTSA: National Highway Traffic Safety Administration
OR: odds ratio
RR: relative risk

REFERENCES

1. Center for Disease Control and Prevention. Injury prevention and control, web-based injury statistics query and reporting system (WISQARS). Available at: www.cdc.gov/injury/wisqars/index.html. Accessed August 17, 2010

2. National Highway Traffic Safety Administration. Fatality analysis reporting system (FARS) encyclopedia. Available at: http://www-fars.nhtsa.dot.gov/. Accessed August 17, 2010

3. Pressley JC, Barlow B, Kendig T, Paneth-Pollak R. Twenty-year trends in fatal injuries to very young children: the persistence of racial disparities. *Pediatrics.* 2007;119(4). Available at: www.pediatrics.org/cgi/content/full/119/4/e875

4. Garcia AN, Patel KV, Guralnik JM. Seat belt use among American Indians/Alaska Natives and non-Hispanic whites. *Am J Prev Med.* 2007;33(3):200–206

5. Daniels F, Moore W, Conti C, et al. The role of the African-American physician in reducing traffic-related injury and death among African Americans: consensus report of the National Medical Association. *J Natl Med Assoc.* 2002;94(2):108–118

6. National Highway Traffic Safety Administration, National Center for Statistics and Analysis. Seat belt use in 2008—race and ethnicity results among occupants traveling with children. DOT HS 811 107. Traffic safety facts, research note. 2009. Available at: http://www.nrd.nhtsa.dot.gov/Pubs/811107.PDF. Accessed August 17, 2010

7. Falcone RA Jr, Brentley AL, Ricketts CD, Allen SE, Garcia VF. Development, implementation and evaluation of a unique African-American faith-based approach to increase automobile restraint use. J Natl Med Assoc. 2006;98(8):1335–1341

8. Ebel BE, Koepsell TD, Bennett EE, Rivara FP. Use of child booster seats in motor vehicles following a community campaign: a controlled trial. JAMA. 2003;289(7):879–884

9. National Highway Traffic Safety Administration. Traffic Safety Facts 1999. A Compilation of Motor Vehicle Crash Data From the Fatality Analysis Reporting System and the General Estimates System. Washington, DC: National Highway Traffic Safety Administration. 2000. Available at: https://crashstats.nhtsa.dot.gov/Api/Public/ViewPublication/809100. Accessed August 17, 2010

10. Durbin DR, Chen I, Smith R, Elliott MR, Winston FK. Effects of seating position and appropriate restraint use on the risk of injury to children in motor vehicle crashes. Pediatrics. 2005;115(3). Available at: www.pediatrics.org/cgi/content/full/115/3/e305

11. Braver ER, Ferguson SA, Greene MA, Lund AK. Reductions in deaths in frontal crashes among right front passengers in vehicles equipped with passenger air bags. JAMA. 1997;278(17):1437–1439

12. Durbin DR, Elliott MR, Winston FK. Belt-positioning booster seats and reduction in risk of injury among children in vehicle crashes. JAMA. 2003;289(21):2835–2840

13. Arbogast KB, Durbin DR, Cornejo RA, Kallan MJ, Winston FK. An evaluation of the effectiveness of forward facing child restraint systems. Accid Anal Prev. 2004;36(4):585–589

14. Elliott MR, Kallan MJ, Durbin DR, Winston FK. Effectiveness of child safety seats vs seat belts in reducing risk for death in children in passenger vehicle crashes. Arch Pediatr Adolesc Med. 2006;160(6):617–621

15. Nichols JL, Glassbrenner D, Compton RP. The impact of a nationwide effort to reduce airbag-related deaths among children: an examination of fatality trends among younger and older age groups. J Safety Res. 2005;36(4):309–320

16. Winston FK, Kallan MJ, Elliott MR, Xie D, Durbin DR. Effect of booster seat laws on appropriate restraint use by children 4 to 7 years old involved in crashes. Arch Pediatr Adolesc Med. 2007;161(3):270–275

17. Segui-Gomez M, Wittenberg E, Glass R, Levenson S, Hingson R, Graham JD. Where children sit in cars: the impact of Rhode Island's new legislation. Am J Public Health. 2001;91(2):311–313

18. US Department of Transportation; Federal Highway Administration. National household travel survey. 2001. Available at: http://nhts.ornl.gov/. Accessed August 17, 2010

19. Durbin DR, Hoffman B; American Academy of Pediatrics, Council on Injury, Violence, and Poison Prevention. Child passenger safety. Pediatrics. 2018;142(5):e20182460

20. National Highway Traffic Safety Administration. Child Restraint Use in 2008—Overall Results. DOT HS 811 135. Traffic Safety Facts, Research Note. Washington, DC: National Highway Traffic Safety Administration, National Center for Statistics and Analysis; 2009. Available at: http://www-nrd.nhtsa.dot.gov/Pubs/811135.PDF. Accessed August 17, 2010

21. National Highway Traffic Safety Administration. Child Restraint Use in 2008—Use of Correct Restraint Types. DOT HS 811 132. Traffic Safety Facts, Research Note. Washington, DC: National Highway Traffic Safety Administration, National Center for Statistics and Analysis; 2009. Available at: http://www-nrd.nhtsa.dot.gov/Pubs/811132.PDF. Accessed August 17, 2010

22. National Highway Traffic Safety Administration. Child Restraint Use in 2008—Demographic Results. DOT HS 811 148. Traffic Safety Facts, Research Note. Washington, DC: National Highway Traffic Safety Administration, National Center for Statistics and Analysis; 2009. Available at: http://www-nrd.nhtsa.dot.gov/Pubs/811148.PDF. Accessed August 17, 2010

23. Partners for Child Passenger Safety. Fact and Trend Report. Philadelphia, PA: Children's Hospital of Philadelphia; 2008

24. Arbogast KB, Jermakian JS, Kallan MJ, Durbin DR. Effectiveness of belt positioning booster seats: an updated assessment. Pediatrics. 2009;124(5):1281–1286

25. Flegal KM. Epidemiologic aspects of overweight and obesity in the United States. Physiol Behav. 2005;86(5):599–602

26. Ogden CL, Carroll MD, Curtin LR, McDowell MA, Tabak CJ, Flegal KM. Prevalence of overweight and obesity in the United States, 1999-2004. JAMA. 2006;295(13):1549–1555

27. Trifiletti LB, Shields W, Bishai D, McDonald E, Reynaud F, Gielen A. Tipping the scales: obese children and child safety seats. Pediatrics. 2006;117(4):1197–1202

28. Pollack KM, Xie D, Arbogast KB, Durbin DR. Body mass index and injury risk among US children 9-15 years old in motor vehicle crashes. Inj Prev. 2008;14(6):366–371

29. Haricharan RN, Griffin RL, Barnhart DC, Harmon CM, McGwin G. Injury patterns among obese children involved in motor vehicle collisions. J Pediatr Surg. 2009;44(6):1218–1222; discussion 1222

30. Zonfrillo MR, Nelson KA, Durbin DR, Kallan MJ. The association of weight percentile and motor vehicle crash injury among 3 to 8 year old children. Ann Adv Automot Med. 2010;54:193–199

31. National Highway Traffic Safety Administration. Seat Belt Use in 2009 - Overall Results. DOT HS 811 100. Traffic Safety Facts, Research Note. Washington, DC: National Highway Traffic Safety Administration, National Center for Statistics and Analysis; 2009. Available at: https://crashstats.nhtsa.dot.gov/Api/Public/ViewPublication/811200. Accessed August 17, 2010

32. Parikh SN, Wilson L. Hazardous use of car seats outside the car in the United States, 2003-2007. *Pediatrics.* 2010;126(2):352–357

33. Bull MJ, Engle WA; Committee on Injury, Violence, and Poison Prevention and Committee on Fetus and Newborn; American Academy of Pediatrics. Safe transportation of preterm and low birth weight infants at hospital discharge. *Pediatrics.* 2009;123(5):1424–1429

34. Decina LE, Lococo KH. Child restraint system use and misuse in six states. *Accid Anal Prev.* 2005;37(3):583–590

35. Bulger EM, Kaufman R, Mock C. Childhood crash injury patterns associated with restraint misuse: implications for field triage. *Prehosp Disaster Med.* 2008;23(1):9–15

36. Sherwood CP, Ferguson SA, Crandall JR. Factors leading to crash fatalities to children in child restraints. *Annu Proc Assoc Adv Automot Med.* 2003;47:343–359

37. Czernakowski W, Müller M. Misuse mode and effects analysis—an approach to predict and quantify misuse of child restraint systems. *Accid Anal Prev.* 1993;25(3):323–333

38. Willett LD, Leuschen MP, Nelson LS, Nelson RM Jr. Risk of hypoventilation in premature infants in car seats. *J Pediatr.* 1986;109(2):245–248

39. Willett LD, Leuschen MP, Nelson LS, Nelson RM Jr. Ventilatory changes in convalescent infants positioned in car seats. *J Pediatr.* 1989;115(3):451–455

40. Merchant JR, Worwa C, Porter S, Coleman JM, deRegnier RA. Respiratory instability of term and near-term healthy newborn infants in car safety seats. *Pediatrics.* 2001;108(3):647–652

41. Bass JL, Mehta KA, Camara J. Monitoring premature infants in car seats: implementing the American Academy of Pediatrics policy in a community hospital. *Pediatrics.* 1993;91(6):1137–1141

42. Charlton JL, Fildes B, Laemmle R, Smith S, Douglas F. A preliminary evaluation of child restraints and anchorage systems for an Australian car. *Annu Proc Assoc Adv Automot Med.* 2004;48:73–86

43. Sherwood CP, Abdelilah Y, Crandall JR, Stevens SL, Saggese JM, Eichelberger MR. The performance of various rear facing child restraint systems in a frontal crash. *Annu Proc Assoc Adv Automot Med.* 2004;48:303–321

44. Bilston LE, Brown J, Kelly P. Improved protection for children in forward-facing restraints during side impacts. *Traffic Inj Prev.* 2005;6(2):135–146

45. Arbogast KB, Jermakian JS. Field use patterns and performance of child restraints secured by lower anchors and tethers for children (LATCH). *Accid Anal Prev.* 2007;39(3):530–535

46. Decina LE, Lococo KH. Observed LATCH use and misuse characteristics of child restraint systems in seven states. *J Safety Res.* 2007;38(3):273–281

47. Bull M, Agran P, Laraque D, et al. American Academy of Pediatrics. Committee on Injury and Poison Prevention. Transporting children with special health care needs. *Pediatrics.* 1999;104(4, pt 1):988–992

48. Isaksson-Hellman I, Jakobsson L, Gustafsson C, Norin HA. Trends and effects of child restraint systems based on Volvo's Swedish accident database. In: Proceedings of Child Occupant Protection 2nd Symposium; November 12, 1997; Warrendale, PA.

49. Jakobsson L, Isaksson-Hellman I, Lundell B. Safety for the growing child: experiences from Swedish accident data. In: *Proceedings of the 19th International Technical Conference on the Enhanced Safety of Vehicles*; June 6–9, 2005; Washington, DC. [abstract 05-0330]

50. Henary B, Sherwood CP, Crandall JR, et al. Car safety seats for children: rear facing for best protection [retraction appears in *Inj Prev.* 2018;24(1):e2]. *Inj Prev.* 2007;13(6):398–402

51. Henary B, Sherwood CP, Crandall JR, et al. Retraction: car safety seats for children: rear facing for best protection. *Inj Prev.* 2018;24(1):e2

52. McMurry TL, Arbogast KB, Sherwood CP, et al. Rear-facing versus forward-facing child restraints: an updated assessment. *Inj Prev.* 2018;24(1):55–59

53. National Highway Traffic Safety Administration. Car seat recommendations for children. Available at: https://www.nhtsa.gov/sites/nhtsa.dot.gov/files/documents/carseatrecommendationsforchildren.pdf. Accessed June 8, 2018

54. Kahane CJ. *An Evaluation of Child Passenger Safety: The Effectiveness and Benefits of Safety Seats. DOT HS 806 890.* Washington, DC: National Highway Traffic Safety Administration; 1986

55. National Highway Traffic Safety Administration. Revised Estimates of Child Restraint Effectiveness. Washington, DC: National Highway Traffic Safety Administration.1996. Available at: https://crashstats.nhtsa.dot.gov/Api/Public/ViewPublication/96855. Accessed August 17, 2010

56. Zaloshnja E, Miller TR, Hendrie D. Effectiveness of child safety seats vs safety belts for children aged 2 to 3 years. *Arch Pediatr Adolesc Med.* 2007;161(1):65–68

57. Levitt SD. Evidence that seat belts are as effective as child safety seats in preventing death for children aged two and up. *Rev Econ Stat.* 2008;90(1):158–163

58. Elliott MR, Durbin DR, Winston FK. A propensity score approach to estimating child restraint effectiveness in preventing mortality. *Stat Interface.* 2009;2(4):437–447

59. Klinich KD, Pritz HB, Beebe MS, Welty K, Burton RW. *Study of Older Child Restraint/Booster Seat Fit and NASS Injury Analysis. DOT HS 808 248.* Washington, DC: National Highway Traffic Safety Administration; 1994

60. Durbin DR, Arbogast KB, Moll EK. Seat belt syndrome in children: a case report and review of the literature. *Pediatr Emerg Care.* 2001;17(6):474–477

61. Kulowski J, Rost WB. Intra-abdominal injury from safety belt in auto accident; report of a case. *AMA Arch Surg.* 1956;73(6):970–971

62. Garrett JW, Braunstein PW. The seat belt syndrome. *J Trauma.* 1962;2:220–238

63. Corden TE. Analysis of booster seat and seat belt use: how many Wisconsin childhood deaths and hospitalizations could have been prevented in 1998–2002? *WMJ.* 2005;104(1):42–45

64. Rice TM, Anderson CL, Lee AS. The association between booster seat use and risk of death among motor vehicle occupants aged 4-8: a matched cohort study. *Inj Prev.* 2009;15(6):379–383

65. Weber K, Melvin JW. Injury potential with misused child restraining systems. In: Proceedings of the 27th Stapp Car Crash Conference; October 17–19, 1983; Warrendale, PA

66. Henderson M, Brown J, Paine M. Injuries to restrained children. In: *38th Annual Proceedings, Association for the Advancement of Automotive Medicine*; September 21-23, 1994; Lyon, France

67. Sherwood CP, Abdelilah Y, Crandall JR. Quantifying the relationship between vehicle interior geometry and child restraint systems. *Annu Proc Assoc Adv Automot Med.* 2006;50:381–396

68. Sherwood CP, Crandall JR, Stevens SL, Saggese JM, Eichelberger MR. Sled tests and CIREN data illustrating the benefits of booster seats. *Int J Crashworthiness.* 2005;10(4):351–358

69. Kirley BB, Teoh ER, Lund AK, Arbogast KB, Kallan MJ, Durbin DR. Making the most of the worst-case scenario: should belt-positioning booster seats be used in lap-belt-only seating positions? *Traffic Inj Prev.* 2009;10(6):580–583

70. Kahane CJ. *Lives Saved by the Federal Motor Vehicle Safety Standards and Other Vehicle Safety Technologies, 1960-2002. DOT HS 809 833.* Washington, DC: National Highway Traffic Safety Administration, National Center for Statistics and Analysis, Evaluation Division; 2004. Available at: http://www-nrd.nhtsa.dot.gov/Pubs/809833.PDF. Accessed August 17, 2010

71. Arbogast KB, Durbin DR, Kallan MJ, Winston FK. Evaluation of pediatric use patterns and performance of lap shoulder belt systems in the center rear. *Annu Proc Assoc Adv Automot Med.* 2004;48:57–72

72. Parenteau CS, Viano DC, Shah M, et al. Field relevance of a suite of rollover tests to real-world crashes and injuries. *Accid Anal Prev.* 2003;35(1):103–110

73. Morgan C. *Effectiveness of Lap/Shoulder Belts in the Back Outboard Seating Positions. DOT HS 808 945.* Washington, DC: National Highway Traffic Safety Administration, Evaluation Division, Plans and Policy; 1999. Available at: http://www-nrd.nhtsa.dot.gov/Pubs/808945.PDF. Accessed August 17, 2010

74. Chipman ML. Risk factors for injury: similarities and differences for traffic crashes and other causes. *Accid Anal Prev.* 1995;27(5):699–706

75. Kindelberger J, Starnes M. *Moving Children From the Front Seat to the Back Seat: The Influence of Child Safety Campaigns. DOT HS 809 698. Traffic Safety Facts, Research Note.* Washington, DC: National Highway Traffic Safety Administration, National Center for Statistics and Analysis; 2003. Available at: https://crashstats.nhtsa.dot.gov/Api/Public/ViewPublication/809698. Accessed August 17, 2010

76. Durbin DR, Chen I, Elliott M, Winston FK. Factors associated with front row seating of children in motor vehicle crashes. *Epidemiology.* 2004;15(3):345–349

77. Kallan MJ, Durbin DR, Arbogast KB. Seating patterns and corresponding risk of injury among 0- to 3-year-old children in child safety seats. *Pediatrics.* 2008;121(5). Available at: www.pediatrics.org/cgi/content/full/121/5/e1342

78. Berg MD, Cook L, Corneli HM, Vernon DD, Dean JM. Effect of seating position and restraint use on injuries to children in motor vehicle crashes. *Pediatrics.* 2000;105(4 pt 1):831–835

79. Lennon A, Siskind V, Haworth N. Rear seat safer: seating position, restraint use and injuries in children in traffic crashes in Victoria, Australia. *Accid Anal Prev.* 2008;40(2):829–834

80. Durbin DR, Elliott M, Arbogast KB, Anderko RL, Winston FK. The effect of seating position on risk of injury for children in side impact collisions. *Annu Proc Assoc Adv Automot Med.* 2001;45:61–72

81. Ehrlich PF, Brown JK, Sochor MR, Wang SC, Eichelberger ME. Factors influencing pediatric injury severity score and Glasgow Coma Scale in pediatric automobile crashes: results from the Crash Injury Research Engineering Network. *J Pediatr Surg.* 2006;41(11):1854–1858

82. Lund UJ. The effect of seating location on the injury of properly restrained children in child safety seats. *Accid Anal Prev.* 2005;37(3):435–439

83. Centers for Disease Control and Prevention (CDC). Air-bag-associated fatal injuries to infants and children riding in front passenger seats—United States. *MMWR Morb Mortal Wkly Rep.* 1995;44(45):845–847

84. Huff GF, Bagwell SP, Bachman D. Airbag injuries in infants and children: a case report and review of the literature. *Pediatrics.* 1998;102(1). Available at: www.pediatrics.org/cgi/content/full/102/1/e2

85. Willis BK, Smith JL, Falkner LD, Vernon DD, Walker ML. Fatal air bag mediated craniocervical trauma in a child. *Pediatr Neurosurg.* 1996;24(6):323–327

86. Hollands CM, Winston FK, Stafford PW, Shochat SJ. Severe head injury caused by airbag deployment. *J Trauma.* 1996;41(5):920–922

87. Centers for Disease Control and Prevention (CDC). Update: fatal air bag-related injuries to children—United States, 1993-1996. *MMWR Morb Mortal Wkly Rep.* 1996;45(49):1073–1076

88. Marshall KW, Koch BL, Egelhoff JC. Air bag-related deaths and serious injuries in children: injury patterns and imaging findings. *AJNR Am J Neuroradiol.* 1998;19(9):1599–1607

89. Winston FK, Reed R. Airbags and children: results of a National Highway Traffic Administration special investigation into actual crashes. In: Proceedings of the 40th Stapp Car Crash Conference; November 4–6, 1996; Albuquerque, NM

90. Mikhail JN, Huelke DF. Air bags: an update. *J Emerg Nurs.* 1997;23(5):439–445

91. Augenstein JS, Digges KH, Lombardo LV, et al. Occult abdominal injuries to airbag-protected crash victims: a challenge to trauma systems. *J Trauma*. 1995;38(4):502–508

92. McKay MP, Jolly BT. A retrospective review of air bag deaths. *Acad Emerg Med*. 1999;6(7):708–714

93. Shkrum MJ, McClafferty KJ, Nowak ES, German A. Driver and front seat passenger fatalities associated with air bag deployment. Part 2: a review of injury patterns and investigative issues. *J Forensic Sci*. 2002;47(5):1035–1040

94. Ball DC, Bouchard CS. Ocular morbidity associated with airbag deployment: a report of seven cases and a review of the literature. *Cornea*. 2001;20(2):159–163

95. Arbogast KB, DeNardo MB, Xavier AM, Kallan MJ, Durbin DR, Winston FK. Upper extremity fractures in restrained children exposed to passenger airbags. In: SAE World Congress and Exhibition; March 3-6, 2003; Detroit, MI

96. Mittal MK, Kallan MJ, Durbin DR. Breathing difficulty and tinnitus among children exposed to airbag deployment. *Accid Anal Prev*. 2007;39(3):624–628

97. Kahane CJ. *Fatality Reduction by Air Bags: Analysis of Accident Data Through Early 1996*. Washington, DC: National Highway Traffic Safety Administration, Evaluation Division, Plans and Policy; 1996

98. Braver ER, Whitfield R, Ferguson SA. Seating positions and children's risk of dying in motor vehicle crashes. *Inj Prev*. 1998;4(3):181–187

99. Cummings P, Koepsell TD, Rivara FP, McKnight B, Mack C. Air bags and passenger fatality according to passenger age and restraint use. *Epidemiology*. 2002;13(5):525–532

100. Newgard CD, Lewis RJ. Effects of child age and body size on serious injury from passenger air-bag presence in motor vehicle crashes. *Pediatrics*. 2005;115(6):1579–1585

101. Smith KM, Cummings P. Passenger seating position and the risk of passenger death in traffic crashes: a matched cohort study. *Inj Prev*. 2006;12(2):83–86

102. Federal Motor Vehicle Safety Standard and Regulation. *Part 571, Federal Motor Vehicle Safety Standards: Crashworthiness, No. 208*. Washington, DC: Department of Transportation; 1998

103. Olson CM, Cummings P, Rivara FP. Association of first- and second-generation air bags with front occupant death in car crashes: a matched cohort study. *Am J Epidemiol*. 2006;164(2):161–169

104. Arbogast KB, Durbin DR, Kallan MJ, Winston FK. Effect of vehicle type on the performance of second generation air bags for child occupants. *Annu Proc Assoc Adv Automot Med*. 2003;47:85–99

105. Braver ER, Scerbo M, Kufera JA, Alexander MT, Volpini K, Lloyd JP. Deaths among drivers and right-front passengers in frontal collisions: redesigned air bags relative to first-generation air bags. *Traffic Inj Prev*. 2008;9(1):48–58

106. Kuppa S, Saunders J, Fessahaie O. *Rear Seat Occupant Protection in Frontal Crashes*. Washington, DC: National Highway Traffic Safety Administration. Available at: https://pdfs.semanticscholar.org/174d/a2fef0352495de5a155bb9f1105c1f67d8aa.pdf. Accessed August 17, 2010

107. Department of Transportation; National Highway Traffic Safety Administration. Air bag deactivation. 1997. Available at: www.nhtsa.gov/cars/rules/rulings/deactnpr.n21.html. Accessed August 17, 2010

108. Dalmotas D, German A, Tylko S. The crash and field performance of side-mounted airbag systems. In: *17th Enhanced Safety of Vehicles Conference*; June 4–7, 2001; Amsterdam, Netherlands

109. Prasad A, Samaha R, Louden A. Evaluation of injury risk from side impact air bags. In: *17th Enhanced Safety of Vehicles Conference*; June 4–7, 2001; Amsterdam, Netherlands

110. McCartt AT, Kyrychenko SY. Efficacy of side air bags in reducing driver deaths in driver-side car and SUV collisions. *Traffic Inj Prev*. 2007;8(2):162–170

111. Kahane CJ. *An Evaluation of Side Impact Protection*. Washington, DC: National Highway Traffic Safety Administration, Evaluation Division; 2007. Available at: http://www-nrd.nhtsa.dot.gov/Pubs/810748.PDF. Accessed August 17, 2010

112. Arbogast KB, Kallan MJ. The exposure of children to deploying side air bags: an initial field assessment. *Annu Proc Assoc Adv Automot Med*. 2007;51:245–259

113. Kids and Cars Statistics. Available at: https://www.kidsandcars.org/media/statistics/. Accessed August 21, 2018

114. National Highway Traffic Safety Administration. *Not-in-Traffic Surveillance 2007 – Highlights. Traffic Safety Facts, Crash Stats. DOT HS 811 085*. Washington, DC: National Highway Traffic Safety Administration, National Center for Statistics and Analysis; 2009. Available at: http://www-nrd.nhtsa.dot.gov/Pubs/811085.PDF. Accessed August 17, 2010

115. US Environmental Protection Agency. Light-Duty Automotive Technology and Fuel Economy Trends: 1975 Through 2008. Appendix D: Data Stratified by Vehicle Type. Washington, DC: US Environmental Protection Agency; 2008. Available at: https://nepis.epa.gov/Exe/ZyPDF.cgi/P1004N5Y.PDF?Dockey=P1004N5Y.PDF. Accessed August 17, 2010

116. Winston FK, Durbin DR, Kallan MJ, Elliott MR. Rear seating and risk of injury to child occupants by vehicle type. *Annu Proc Assoc Adv Automot Med*. 2001;45:51–60

117. Agran PF, Winn DG, Castillo DN. Pediatric injuries in the back of pickup trucks. *JAMA*. 1990;264(6):712–716

118. Anderson CL, Agran PF, Winn DG, Greenland S. Fatalities to occupants of cargo areas of pickup trucks. *Accid Anal Prev*. 2000;32(4):533–540

119. Federal Aviation Administration. 14 CFR 135.128. Available at: https://www.law.cornell.edu/cfr/text/14/135.128. Accessed August 17, 2010

120. Federal Motor Vehicle Safety. Standard No. 213. 49 CFR 571.213. Available at: http://edocket.access.gpo.gov/cfr_2004/octqtr/49cfr571.213.htm. Accessed August 17, 2010

121. Federal Aviation Authority. Flying with Children: About Child Restraint Systems. Available at: https://www.faa.gov/travelers/fly_children/#aboutCRS. Accessed August 17, 2010

122. Newman TB, Johnston BD, Grossman DC. Effects and costs of requiring child-restraint systems for young children traveling on commercial airplanes. *Arch Pediatr Adolesc Med.* 2003;157(10):969–974

123. National Transportation Safety Board, Office of Research and Engineering, Safety Studies and Statistical Analysis Division. Analysis of diversion to automobile in regard to the disposition of Safety Recommendation A-95-51. August 3, 2004. Available at: https://www.ntsb.gov/safety/safety-recs/RecLetters/sr_a-95-51_diversion_analysis.pdf. Accessed August 22, 2018

124. Bishai D. Hearts and minds and child restraints in airplanes. *Arch Pediatr Adolesc Med.* 2003;157(10):953–954

125. Expedia. Airline fee chart. Available at: https://www.expedia.com/p/info-other/airline-fees.htm. Accessed August 17, 2010

126. Staunton C, Davidson S, Kegler S, Dawson L, Powell K, Dellinger A. Critical gaps in child passenger safety practices, surveillance, and legislation: Georgia, 2001. *Pediatrics.* 2005;115(2):372–379

127. Agran PF, Anderson CL, Winn DG. Violators of a child passenger safety law. *Pediatrics.* 2004;114(1):109–115

128. National Highway Traffic Safety Administration. *Seat Belt Use in 2008—Demographic Results. DOT HS 811 183. Traffic Safety Facts, Research Note.* National Highway Traffic Safety Administration, National Center for Statistics and Analysis; 2009. Available at: http://www-nrd.nhtsa.dot.gov/Pubs/811183.PDF. Accessed August 17, 2010

129. Rivara FP, Thompson DC, Cummings P. Effectiveness of primary and secondary enforced seat belt laws. *Am J Prev Med.* 1999;16(suppl 1):30–39

130. Eby DW, Fordyce TA, Vivoda JM. A comparison of safety belt use between commercial and noncommercial light-vehicle occupants. *Accid Anal Prev.* 2002;34(3):285–291

131. Houston DJ, Richardson LE Jr. Traffic safety and the switch to a primary seat belt law: the California experience. *Accid Anal Prev.* 2002;34(6):743–751

132. Centers for Disease Control and Prevention (CDC). Impact of primary laws on adult use of safety belts—United States, 2002. *MMWR Morb Mortal Wkly Rep.* 2004;53(12):257–260

133. Durbin DR, Smith R, Kallan MJ, Elliott MR, Winston FK. Seat belt use among 13-15 year olds in primary and secondary enforcement law states. *Accid Anal Prev.* 2007;39(3):524–529

134. National Child Passenger Safety. About CPS certification. Available at: www.safekids.org/certification/. Accessed August 17, 2010

Counseling in Pediatric Populations at Risk for Infertility and/or Sexual Function Concerns

- *Clinical Report*

CLINICAL REPORT Guidance for the Clinician in Rendering Pediatric Care

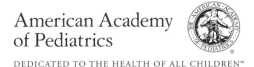

American Academy
of Pediatrics
DEDICATED TO THE HEALTH OF ALL CHILDREN™

Counseling in Pediatric Populations at Risk for Infertility and/or Sexual Function Concerns

Leena Nahata, MD, FAAP,[a] Gwendolyn P. Quinn, PhD,[b] Amy C. Tishelman, PhD,[c] SECTION ON ENDOCRINOLOGY

abstract

Reproductive health is an important yet often overlooked topic in pediatric health care; when addressed, the focus is generally on prevention of sexually transmitted infections and unwanted pregnancy. Two aspects of reproductive health counseling that have received minimal attention in pediatrics are fertility and sexual function for at-risk pediatric populations, and youth across many disciplines are affected. Although professional organizations, such as the American Academy of Pediatrics and the American Society of Clinical Oncology, have published recommendations about fertility preservation discussions, none of these guidelines address how to have ongoing conversations with at-risk youth and their families about the potential for future infertility and sexual dysfunction in developmentally appropriate ways. Researchers suggest many pediatric patients at risk for reproductive problems remain uncertain and confused about their fertility or sexual function status well into young adulthood. Potential infertility may cause distress and anxiety, has been shown to affect formation of romantic relationships, and may lead to unplanned pregnancy in those who incorrectly assumed they were infertile. Sexual dysfunction is also common and may lead to problems with intimacy and self-esteem; survivors of pediatric conditions consistently report inadequate guidance from clinicians in this area. Health care providers and parents report challenges in knowing how and when to discuss these issues. In this context, the goal of this clinical report is to review evidence and considerations for providers related to information sharing about impaired fertility and sexual function in pediatric patients attributable to congenital and acquired conditions or treatments.

[a]Division of Endocrinology and Center for Biobehavioral Health, The Ohio State University and Nationwide Children's Hospital, Columbus, Ohio; [b]Department of Obstetrics and Gynecology, New York University Langone Medical Center, New York University New York, New York; and Departments of [c]Endocrinology and Psychiatry, Boston Children's Hospital and Harvard Medical School, Harvard University, Boston, Massachusetts

Drs Nahata, Quinn, and Tishelman conceptualized this article, drafted the initial manuscript, edited and revised the manuscript, approved the final manuscript as submitted, and agree to be accountable for all aspects of the work.

Clinical reports from the American Academy of Pediatrics benefit from expertise and resources of liaisons and internal (AAP) and external reviewers. However, clinical reports from the American Academy of Pediatrics may not reflect the views of the liaisons or the organizations or government agencies that they represent.

The guidance in this report does not indicate an exclusive course of treatment or serve as a standard of medical care. Variations, taking into account individual circumstances, may be appropriate.

All clinical reports from the American Academy of Pediatrics automatically expire 5 years after publication unless reaffirmed, revised, or retired at or before that time.

DOI: https://doi.org/10.1542/peds.2018-1435

Address correspondence to Leena Nahata, MD, FAAP. E-mail: leena.nahata@nationwidechildrens.org

To cite: Nahata L, Quinn GP, Tishelman AC; AAP SECTION ON ENDOCRINOLOGY. Counseling in Pediatric Populations at Risk for Infertility and/or Sexual Function Concerns. *Pediatrics.* 2018;142(2):e20181435

INTRODUCTION

Reproductive and sexual health are important yet often overlooked topics in pediatric health care; when addressed, the focus is generally on prevention of sexually transmitted infections (STIs) and unwanted

TABLE 1 Examples of Pediatric Populations at Risk for Infertility and/or Sexual Dysfunction (1 or Both May be Affected)

Discipline[a]	Condition or Treatment
Hematology, oncology, and/or immunology	Gonadotoxic chemotherapy
	Gonadotoxic radiation
	Genitourinary surgery
	Genitourinary cancer
	Sickle cell disease
	Hemochromatosis
	Any condition treated with chronic transfusions
	Any condition treated with stem cell transplantation
Genetics	Galactosemia
	Turner syndrome
	Klinefelter syndrome
	Down syndrome
	Fragile X
	Cystic fibrosis
Rheumatology and/or nephrology	Lupus and/or mixed connective tissue disease
	Vasculitis
	Steroid-dependent nephrotic syndrome
	Rheumatoid arthritis
	End-stage renal disease
Gastroenterology, cardiology, and/or pulmonary	Inflammatory bowel disease
	End-stage liver disease
	End-stage cardiac disease
	End-stage lung disease
Urology, gynecology, and/or anatomic	Spina bifida
	Cerebral palsy
	Disorders of sex development
	Bilateral cryptorchidism
	Anorchia and/or testicular regression
	Prune Belly syndrome
	Hypospadias
	Mayer-Rokitansky-Küster-Hauser
	Bladder exstrophy-epispadias complex
	Spinal cord injuries
	Anorectal malformations
	Endometriosis
	Fibroids
Endocrinology	Hyperprolactinemia
	Thyroid dysfunction
	Diabetes mellitus
	Hypogonadotropic hypogonadism
	Polycystic ovarian syndrome
	Autoimmune ovarian insufficiency
	Transgender
Infectious diseases	Mumps
	HIV/AIDS
	STIs

[a] Some conditions may be associated with >1 category.

pregnancy.[1,2] An expanding body of literature has highlighted other important aspects, such as puberty, sexuality, and healthy relationships, in addition to emphasizing specific populations for whom extra guidance may be needed, such as lesbian, gay, bisexual, transgender, and questioning youth.[3,4] However, two aspects of reproductive health counseling that have received minimal attention in pediatrics are fertility and sexual function for at-risk populations, and pediatric patients across many disciplines are affected (Table 1).

Fertility is the ability to produce offspring from one's genetic material. Sexual function refers to the physical and emotional ability to experience sexual pleasure and satisfaction when desired.[5] Multiple medical conditions (eg, disorders of sex development) and treatments (eg, chemotherapy and radiation, hormonal treatments for transgender youth) occurring in childhood and/or adolescence may impair future fertility and sexual function (Table 1). Some patient populations may benefit from technologies developed to preserve gametes for future use, known as fertility preservation. (The American Academy of Pediatrics [AAP] has a technical report forthcoming on fertility preservation for pediatric and adolescent patients with cancer.) Briefly, established forms of fertility preservation include sperm cryopreservation for pubertal boys and oocyte cryopreservation for postmenarchal girls; experimental options, such as testicular and ovarian tissue preservation, may be considered for prepubertal boys and premenarchal girls, respectively. Although professional organizations such as the AAP and the American Society of Clinical Oncology have published recommendations about fertility preservation discussions for at-risk children and adolescents,[6–8] none of these publications address how to have ongoing conversations with children and adolescents and their families about the potential for future infertility and sexual dysfunction in developmentally appropriate ways.

Researchers suggest many pediatric patients at risk for reproductive problems remain uncertain and confused about their fertility or sexual function status well into young adulthood. Potential infertility may cause distress and anxiety, has been shown to affect formation of romantic relationships, and may lead to unplanned pregnancy in those who incorrectly assumed they were infertile.[9,10] Sexual dysfunction is also common in otherwise healthy and at-risk adolescents, leading to problems with intimacy and self-esteem[11,12]; young adult cancer survivors consistently report inadequate guidance from health care providers in this area.[11] Health care providers and parents of childhood cancer survivors, as well as other populations facing intellectual or physical disabilities affecting reproductive health, report challenges in knowing how and when to discuss these issues.[9,13,14]

In youth with conditions such as congenital adrenal hyperplasia and androgen insensitivity syndrome, critical decisions affecting fertility and sexual function were historically made in infancy, with adolescents and young adults later relying on their families and health care providers for ongoing counseling.[15] Individuals with these conditions report distress when information about their potential infertility or sexual dysfunction is kept from them and frequently ask their health care providers for guidance in how to share information about these sensitive topics with intimate partners.[16] Whenever relevant, families should be counseled about risks and controversies surrounding medically unnecessary surgeries without patient involvement in decision-making and be informed about fertility and sexual function implications on an ongoing basis.[15]

Some health care providers managing conditions that affect fertility and sexual function, such as pediatric rheumatologists, nephrologists, and oncologists, may lack knowledge and inconsistently provide counseling or referrals to reproductive health specialists.[17–20] A recent national survey revealed the majority of pediatric endocrinologists, urologists, and gynecologists felt inadequately trained in fertility and sexual function and desired additional guidance in these areas; many providers were unsure whose responsibility it was to provide such counsel to patients and families.[20] As a result, although at-risk patients may be seeing many different care providers, they may

not be counseled about fertility or sexual function in any of these encounters.[11,21] In this context, our goal with this clinical report is to review evidence and considerations for providers related to information sharing about impaired fertility and sexual function in pediatric patients resulting from congenital or acquired conditions or medical treatments.

ASSESSING RISK

In preparation for the clinical encounter, the first step is to become educated about fertility and sexual function concerns on the basis of a given patient's condition and/or treatment history. Initial questions to consider may include the following: (1) Is there a medical or surgical intervention taking place that may affect the patient's future fertility and/or sexual function? (2) Is there an opportunity now to protect or preserve fertility and/or sexual function? (3) What type of information can be shared about future fertility and/or sexual function implications?

Obtaining information about these topics may be challenging at times because there is little empirical evidence on reproductive and sexual health outcomes in many conditions, and there may not be an easily accessible source. Some medical conditions or groups of conditions have disease-specific guidelines and literature in which infertility risk, sexual function concerns, and interventions (see Resources) are discussed, but in other cases, one would need to research the specific condition or treatment agent itself. Ultimately, providers may need to work with parents to determine optimal approaches to care and communication, even in the absence of known information. Beyond fertility and sexual function, there may be concerns about pregnancy because of implications for the mother or teratogenicity of certain

medications. In such cases, involving a maternal-fetal medicine specialist may be of benefit.

INTERDISCIPLINARY APPROACH TO CARE

When possible, an interdisciplinary approach to care is helpful to incorporate expertise regarding (1) the primary medical conditions and treatment plan (oncologist, rheumatologist, geneticist, or other treating provider) and (2) optimal approaches for assessing gonadal function in male and female patients of different ages and pubertal stages (such as general and/or reproductive endocrinologist, gynecologist, or urologist). In addition, although team physicians may understand the relevant medical issues for a child or adolescent, a behavioral health professional will be best equipped to appreciate issues accounting for culture, child development and/or developmental limitations, family psychosocial issues, and the best way to engage a child in decision-making. The interdisciplinary team (including the primary care provider) should communicate before the patient encounter to share information and designate which members of the team are best suited to counsel the child and family about various aspects of fertility and sexual function. It is important to document the discussion and send it to all members of the health care team as a shared guide for future reproductive health planning.

Although a team approach is optimal, challenges occurring within interdisciplinary frameworks can impede care and ultimately result in suboptimal practices. Difficulties sometimes occur when encounters are rushed, precluding optimal communication between team members, and/or if consensus cannot be reached because of fundamentally different beliefs and approaches. Other challenges include inadvertent transmission of conflicting information by different team members, models in which some members may not be equally comfortable disagreeing with team leaders or across disciplines, and lack of clarity regarding parameters and/or responsibilities across members. Finally, poor access to pediatric specialists who are trained and comfortable counseling about fertility and sexual function or lack of insurance coverage for certain subspecialists, such as mental and/ or behavioral health professionals, may pose barriers to establishing optimal interdisciplinary care. Communication about these sensitive issues should be well documented so that all current and future providers (eg, in the transition to adult care) are informed about what has been discussed. Finally, when a comprehensive team cannot be established, a variety of disciplines could take the lead in providing counseling about fertility and sexual function.

ASSESS WHAT THE CHILD AND PARENTS KNOW AND INTERVENTIONS THAT MAY HAVE BEEN PERFORMED

Studies reveal families may not be aware of potential threats to fertility and/or sexual function or may not feel comfortable broaching the topic and thus rely on health care providers to initiate these conversations.[8,15] It is important to assess what parents and patients understand about previous medical or surgical interventions (eg, exposure to gonadotoxic therapies, fertility preservation attempts, and/or surgery involving the genitalia or gonads) and their fertility and/or sexual function implications. In many cases, information about fertility and sexual function may have initially been shared in the context of a new medical diagnosis that is life altering or life-threatening or when there is a pressing urgency to initiate treatment, which can affect retention

of information. Additionally, years may have passed, the child may have been too young to participate in the initial discussions or decisions, and there may be new information that has emerged since initial counseling occurred.

In some cases, parents may express a desire to withhold information about their child's condition and/or infertility risk. Families should be counseled that although nondisclosure was previously common in pediatric care, the literature on a vast array of subjects, from HIV[22] to adoption or informing offspring of their conception by gamete or embryo donation,[23] reveals the importance of developmentally appropriate disclosure at the earliest possible age. Studies in women with Turner syndrome reveal that an absence of communication about the condition can create tremendous distress later in life when infertility is discovered.[24] Researchers suggest many families desire the health care provider's input and support in decision-making about disclosure.[25] The health care provider may find it helpful to start the conversation about disclosure with families by addressing common misconceptions. For instance, a parent may believe the child is too young for such discussions. However, literature reveals that parental lack of disclosure does not mean the child is unaware, and the child may have unexpressed anxiety. Another common misconception is that if the child is not asking questions, he or she is not interested or concerned. However, the child may simply be following the emotional tone that has been established in the home when talking about the condition and its effects; if the child notices parental discomfort or anger when the condition is discussed, he or she may not feel safe to ask questions. A lack of information or living in uncertainty may also lead to inaccurate beliefs (eg, "I must not

have a problem because no one is talking to me about it"), or looking to suboptimal sources for information, such as the Internet.

COUNSELING CONSIDERATIONS

Time

Discussions about the decision-making process affecting fertility and sexual function most optimally occur when sufficient time is allotted. Often, these topics are discussed along with other complex health-related information, making them difficult to comprehend and digest. When possible, it is important to plan for ongoing counseling with families as they absorb information and continue to formulate questions and generate concerns. Patients old enough to be involved in the decision-making process (described in the next section) should have time to consider options, with ongoing discussions as the patient-provider relationship is solidified. Compensation for time spent on counseling should be provided by insurers as an integral component of managing the underlying condition.

Normalize the Stress of Ambiguity

Many families find it difficult to manage stress and decision-making when medical issues are unknown and unpredictable, as is frequently the case with fertility and sexual function concerns. It is important to acknowledge the stress and help the family and youth plan to manage it and build positive coping skills while giving guidance in avoiding catastrophizing.

Recognize and Acknowledge Stressors and Strengths

Family stressors, such as a patient's or parents' psychosocial issues or financial constraints, can affect a family's ability to make decisions or engage in discussions about fertility and sexual function. Parents and children with cognitive limitations or acute mental health issues may lack the ability to comprehend fertility and sexual function. Parents of children with limited survival may also experience difficulty considering future fertility or sexual function. Health care providers can help families navigate these issues, identify their strengths, and facilitate general means of coping.

Address Cultural, Linguistic, and Health Literacy Factors

Cultural factors, including religious beliefs, may affect a patient and caregiver's comfort in discussing or considering interventions related to fertility and/or sexual function, but these should not be barriers to sharing relevant information. It is also important to secure interpreter services when language proficiency may hinder communication, and the interpreter needs to be comfortable speaking directly about issues of a sensitive nature. In addition, health literacy may be low, and both parents and their children may need concise and simple explanations of risks and options.

Facilitate Connections With Others for Support

Youth may benefit from connecting with older adolescents and adults with similar conditions for support and guidance regarding fertility and sexual function. Parents may also benefit from peer advice about how to support their children and initiate age-appropriate discussions.

Talking Points Based on Age or Developmental Stage

Children, even at a young age, may begin to envision future parenthood. Even parents of infants may envision them as future parents and hope to be grandparents. However, pediatric patients may struggle to think about future fertility when facing life-threatening illnesses, such as cancer, or when uncomfortable in their own bodies, such as those with gender dysphoria. The health care

TABLE 2 Overview for the Clinician

Before encounter
Assess the patient's fertility and sexual function risk and/or implications
Develop a framework for counseling by using an interdisciplinary approach when possible
During the initial encounter
Assess what the parents and child have been told and what interventions (if any) have been offered
Consider cultural factors, ethical issues, and other special circumstances that may impact communication
Plan initial talking points for both the parents and patient on the basis of age or developmental stage
Ongoing care
Plan future talking points for both the parents and patient on the basis of age or developmental stage

provider can offer guidance about developmentally appropriate levels of information with more detail as the child matures.

Although health care provider–initiated discussions about fertility with both children and parents are appropriate starting at a young age, sexual function counseling generally takes place with adolescents and young adults without parents present. However, some youth may develop concerns at a younger age regarding body image and future romantic relationships, and parents may share these concerns as well, necessitating these discussions with families early in a child's life. It is important to emphasize to parents that the youth's fertility and sexual function are only 2 aspects of their child, and that families should foster positive development and relationships at every developmental stage. Suggestions for specific talking points by age or developmental stage are as follows (summary provided in Table 2):

Parents of Infants or Young Children

Inform parents about known and unknown fertility or sexual function outcomes relevant to the particular condition or treatment and when decisions about medical or surgical interventions are being made. Assess family supports and, when possible, connect families with others who have had similar experiences. Inform families about current fertility preservation (explain that

options for prepubertal children are experimental) and treatment strategies and that new fertility-related technologies may emerge. Inform families that medical and surgical approaches may evolve to preserve and/or improve sexual function. Even young children may show interest and curiosity about their bodies, and the topic of future parenthood can and should be discussed in an age-appropriate manner.

School-Aged Children

Developmentally, children's levels of cognitive maturity and self-awareness increase as they age; however, there is some variability from child to child, making it difficult to define an exact age at which different information should be shared with a child. In clinical research, assent is typically required at 7 years of age on the basis of assumptions of decision-making capacity in typically developing youth,[26] but younger children should be involved and provided with information. It is important to be sensitive to the changing perspectives of school-aged children, modify discussions accordingly to provide information geared toward a child's cognitive and emotional readiness, and set the stage for open communication. It can be helpful to give children permission to ask any questions of interest and let them know they have a right to all information they want to know about their bodies and medical conditions.

Talk with the parents to see whether they would prefer to start these discussions at home and provide guidance accordingly for these discussions. Children may be told "there are many different ways to become a parent and have a family." Check in periodically with children to assess their understanding and encourage continued conversation both with parents and providers. Although detailed discussions about sex may not be appropriate at this age, children should feel comfortable asking about their bodies regarding appearance and function at home and at doctors' visits; open-ended prompts, such as "How are you feeling about your body?" may be helpful. As children approach adolescence, they will have an increasing awareness of their sexuality, and counseling should be tailored accordingly.

Adolescents and Young Adults

Starting around 14 to 16 years of age in typically developing youth, pediatric patients should begin to take more responsibility for their own reproductive and sexual health in preparation for future transition to adult care.[27] Adolescents may feel more comfortable engaging in conversations with their health care providers than with their parents, and establishing patient-provider relationships at this stage provides an opportunity for recurring conversations over time. Optimally, counseling should take place with parents present and also with the youth alone. Asking open-ended questions is helpful, although being specific with regard to fertility, family building, and sexual function and health is important. Relevant topics may include anatomy, masturbation, erections, nocturnal emissions, sexual fantasies, sexual orientation, orgasms, sensation, and performance.[1] Adolescents and young adults may struggle with future thinking and long-term decision-making yet wonder and

worry about the impact of fertility and sexual impairment on dating and the formation of romantic relationships. Female adolescents may wonder whether carrying a pregnancy is an option regardless of ability to have a biological child. It is also critical to emphasize that even if an individual is likely to be infertile, barrier methods need to be used with every sexual encounter to prevent STIs, including human papillomavirus infection, and contraception should be used to prevent an unwanted pregnancy. These can be awkward conversations, and efforts should be made to create a safe and comfortable environment to facilitate discussions. It is also important to inquire where patients are getting their information (ie, friends, media) to better understand their level of knowledge and potential misconceptions.

SUMMARY AND RECOMMENDATIONS

Infertility and sexual dysfunction have a significant effect on quality of life. Given that numerous pediatric conditions and treatments impair reproductive capacity and sexual function, general pediatricians and pediatric medical subspecialists should provide ongoing counseling about these risks and potential management options as well as psychosocial support. Considering the sensitive nature of these topics, clear communication between health care providers and inclusion of youth in discussions and decisions are paramount. In summary, the AAP recommends the following:

- Counseling about fertility and sexual function for at-risk pediatric populations is essential and should begin with parents in infancy or at the earliest time point a patient may be affected.

- All children should have access to full information about their conditions using developmentally sensitive approaches as they

mature, understanding that perspectives, comprehension, and patient concerns are not static and can change with maturity.

- Treatment-specific fertility and sexual function risks and potential interventions and recommendations should be evidence-based; when evidence is unavailable, this information needs to be transmitted to families in the context of information sharing and decision-making.

- Interdisciplinary teams must develop a strategy to address issues of fertility and sexual function in a direct but sensitive manner, allotting enough time for questions and considerations and ensuring that a consistent message is relayed. Teams should also identify which provider will discuss each aspect of the risk and potential intervention and at what time point.

- Clear documentation about the content and outcomes of discussions is imperative to optimize communication among health care providers and also facilitate a smooth transition to adult care.

RESOURCES

The Children's Oncology Group. Long-term follow-up guidelines for survivors of childhood, adolescent, and young adult cancers. Available at: http://www.survivorshipguidelines.org/

American Society for Reproductive Medicine, Ethics Committee. Fertility preservation and reproduction in patients facing gonadotoxic therapies: a committee opinion. *Fertil Steril.* 2013;100(5):1224–1231. Available at: http://www.fertstert.org/article/S0015-0282(13)03007-0/fulltext

Oktay K, Harvey BE, Partridge AH, et al. Fertility preservation in patients with cancer: ASCO clinical practice guideline update. *J Clin Oncol*. 2018. Available at: http://ascopubs.org/doi/abs/10.1200/JCO.2018.78.1914

International Society for Sexual Medicine. Sexual function in childhood cancer survivors: a report from project REACH. Available at: http://www.issm.info/news/research-highlights/research-summaries/sexual-function-in-childhood-cancer-survivors-a-report-from-project-reach/

Hembree WC, Cohen-Kettenis PT, Gooren L, et al. Endocrine treatment of gender-dysphoric/gender-incongruent persons: an Endocrine Society Clinical Practice Guideline. *J Clin Endocrinol Metab*. 2017;102(11):3869–3903

Lee PA, Nordenström A, Houk CP, et al. Global disorders of sex development update since 2006: perceptions, approach and care. *Horm Res Paediatr*. 2016;85(3):158–180. Available at: https://www.karger.com/Article/FullText/442975

The Oncofertility Consortium (overview of fertility preservation,

includes information on some nonmalignant conditions as well). Available at: http://oncofertility.northwestern.edu/

Johnson EK, Finlayson C, Rowell EE, et al. Fertility preservation for pediatric patients: current state and future possibilities. *J Urol*. 2017;198(1):186–194. Available at: http://www.sciencedirect.com/science/article/pii/S0022534717302239

Alberta (Canada) Health Sciences. Sexuality and disability. Available at: https://teachingsexualhealth.ca/wp-content/uploads/sites/4/Sexual-and-Development-Disablity-Guide-2016.pdf

Advocates for Youth. Sexual health education for young people with disabilities: research and resources for parents/guardians. Available at: http://www.advocatesforyouth.org/publications/publications-a-z/2560

Wilson GN, Cooley WC. *Preventive Health Care for Children With Genetic Conditions*. 2nd ed. Cambridge, United

Kingdom: Cambridge University Press; 2006

Cassidy SB, Allanson JE. *Management of Genetic Syndromes*. Hoboken, NJ: John Wiley & Sons; 2010

LEAD AUTHORS

Leena Nahata, MD, FAAP
Gwendolyn P. Quinn, PhD
Amy C. Tishelman, PhD

SECTION ON ENDOCRINOLOGY EXECUTIVE COMMITTEE, 2017–2018

Jane L. Lynch, MD, FAAP, Chairperson
Jill L. Brodsky, MD, FAAP
Samuel J. Casella, MD, MSc, FAAP
Linda A. DiMeglio, MD, MPH, FAAP
Ximena Lopez, MD, FAAP
Kupper A. Wintergerst, MD, FAAP
Irene Sills, MD, FAAP, Immediate Past Chairperson

STAFF

Laura Laskosz, MPH

ABBREVIATIONS

AAP: American Academy of Pediatrics
STI: sexually transmitted infection

PEDIATRICS (ISSN Numbers: Print, 0031-4005; Online, 1098-4275).

FINANCIAL DISCLOSURE: The authors have indicated they have no financial relationships relevant to this article to disclose.

FUNDING: No external funding.

POTENTIAL CONFLICT OF INTEREST: The authors have indicated they have no potential conflicts of interest to disclose.

REFERENCES

1. Breuner CC, Mattson G; Committee on Adolescence; Committee on Psychosocial Aspects of Child and Family Health. Sexuality education for children and adolescents. *Pediatrics*. 2016;138(2):e20161348

2. Hagan JF, Shaw JS, Duncan PM. *Bright Futures for PDA: Guidelines for Health Supervision of Infants, Children, and Adolescents*. 3rd ed. Elk Grove Village, IL: American Academy of Pediatrics; 2008

3. Ott MA, Sucato GS; Committee on Adolescence. Contraception for adolescents. *Pediatrics*. 2014;134(4). Available at: www.pediatrics.org/cgi/content/full/134/4/e1257

4. Burke PJ, Coles MS, Di Meglio G, et al; Society for Adolescent Health and Medicine. Sexual and reproductive health care: a position paper of the Society for Adolescent Health and Medicine. *J Adolesc Health*. 2014;54(4):491–496

5. American Sexual Health Association. Sexual functioning. 2017. Available at: www.ashasexualhealth.org/sexual-health/sexual-functioning/. Accessed January 10, 2017

6. Ethics Committee of American Society for Reproductive Medicine. Fertility preservation and reproduction in patients facing gonadotoxic therapies:

a committee opinion. *Fertil Steril*. 2013;100(5):1224–1231

7. Fallat ME, Hutter J; American Academy of Pediatrics Committee on Bioethics; American Academy of Pediatrics Section on Hematology/Oncology; American Academy of Pediatrics Section on Surgery. Preservation of fertility in pediatric and adolescent patients with cancer. *Pediatrics*. 2008;121(5). Available at: www.pediatrics.org/cgi/content/full/121/5/e1461

8. Oktay K, Harvey BE, Partridge AH, et al. Fertility preservation in patients with cancer: ASCO clinical practice

guideline update [published online ahead of print April 5, 2018]. *J Clin Oncol.* doi:10.1200/JCO.2018.78.1914

9. Ellis SJ, Wakefield CE, McLoone JK, Robertson EG, Cohn RJ. Fertility concerns among child and adolescent cancer survivors and their parents: a qualitative analysis. *J Psychosoc Oncol.* 2016;34(5):347–362

10. Nilsson J, Jervaeus A, Lampic C, et al. 'Will I be able to have a baby?' Results from online focus group discussions with childhood cancer survivors in Sweden. *Hum Reprod.* 2014;29(12):2704–2711

11. Frederick NN, Recklitis CJ, Blackmon JE, Bober S. Sexual dysfunction in young adult survivors of childhood cancer. *Pediatr Blood Cancer.* 2016;63(9):1622–1628

12. Zebrack BJ, Foley S, Wittmann D, Leonard M. Sexual functioning in young adult survivors of childhood cancer. *Psychooncology.* 2010;19(8):814–822

13. East LJ, Orchard TR. Somebody else's job: experiences of sex education among health professionals, parents and adolescents with physical disabilities in Southwestern Ontario. *Sex Disabil.* 2014;32(3):335–350

14. Murphy C, Lincoln S, Meredith S, Cross EM, Rintell D. Sex education and intellectual disability: practices and insight from pediatric genetic counselors. *J Genet Couns.* 2016;25(3):552–560

15. Lee PA, Nordenström A, Houk CP, et al; Global DSD Update Consortium. Global disorders of sex development update since 2006: perceptions, approach and care [published correction appears in *Horm Res Paediatr.* 2016;85(3):180]. *Horm Res Paediatr.* 2016;85(3):158–180

16. Sutton EJ, Young J, McInerney-Leo A, Bondy CA, Gollust SE, Biesecker BB. Truth-telling and Turner syndrome: the importance of diagnostic disclosure. *J Pediatr.* 2006;148(1):102–107

17. Goodwin T, Elizabeth Oosterhuis B, Kiernan M, Hudson MM, Dahl GV. Attitudes and practices of pediatric oncology providers regarding fertility issues. *Pediatr Blood Cancer.* 2007;48(1):80–85

18. Miller SD, Li Y, Meyers KE, Caplan A, Miller VA, Ginsberg JP. Fertility preservation in paediatric nephrology: results of a physician survey. *J Ren Care.* 2014;40(4):257–262

19. Nahata L, Sivaraman V, Quinn GP. Fertility counseling and preservation practices in youth with lupus and vasculitis undergoing gonadotoxic therapy. *Fertil Steril.* 2016;106(6):1470–1474

20. Nahata L, Ziniel SI, Garvey KC, Yu RN, Cohen LE. Fertility and sexual function: a gap in training in pediatric endocrinology. *J Pediatr Endocrinol Metab.* 2016;30(1):3–10

21. Nahata L, Quinn GP, Tishelman A. A call for fertility and sexual function counseling in pediatrics. *Pediatrics.* 2016;137(6):e20160180

22. Delaney RO, Serovich JM, Lim JY. Reasons for and against maternal HIV disclosure to children and perceived child reaction. *AIDS Care.* 2008;20(7):876–880

23. Ethics Committee of American Society for Reproductive Medicine. Informing offspring of their conception by gamete or embryo donation: a committee opinion. *Fertil Steril.* 2013;100(1):45–49

24. King JE, Plamondon J, Counts D, Laney D, Dixon SD. Barriers in communication and available resources to facilitate conversation about infertility with girls diagnosed with Turner syndrome. *J Pediatr Endocrinol Metab.* 2016;29(2):185–191

25. Gallo AM, Angst DB, Knafl KA, Twomey JG, Hadley E. Health care professionals' views of sharing information with families who have a child with a genetic condition. *J Genet Couns.* 2010;19(3):296–304

26. Hein IM, De Vries MC, Troost PW, Meynen G, Van Goudoever JB, Lindauer RJL. Informed consent instead of assent is appropriate in children from the age of twelve: policy implications of new findings on children's competence to consent to clinical research. *BMC Med Ethics.* 2015;16(1):76

27. Cooley WC, Sagerman PJ; American Academy of Pediatrics; American Academy of Family Physicians; American College of Physicians; Transitions Clinical Report Authoring Group. Supporting the health care transition from adolescence to adulthood in the medical home. *Pediatrics.* 2011;128(1):182–200

Diagnosis, Evaluation, and Management of High Blood Pressure in Children and Adolescents

• •

- *Technical Report*

  - *PPI: AAP Partnership for Policy Implementation*
    See Appendix 1 for more information.

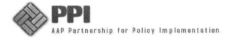

TECHNICAL REPORT

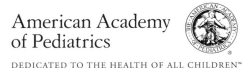

Diagnosis, Evaluation, and Management of High Blood Pressure in Children and Adolescents

Carissa M. Baker-Smith, MD, MS, MPH, FAAP, FAHA,[a] Susan K. Flinn, MA,[b] Joseph T. Flynn, MD, MS, FAAP,[c] David C. Kaelber, MD, PhD, MPH, FAAP, FACP, FACMI,[d] Douglas Blowey, MD,[e] Aaron E. Carroll, MD, MS, FAAP,[f] Stephen R. Daniels, MD, PhD, FAAP,[g] Sarah D. de Ferranti, MD, MPH, FAAP,[h] Janis M. Dionne, MD, FRCPC,[i] Bonita Falkner, MD,[j] Samuel S. Gidding, MD,[k] Celeste Goodwin,[l] Michael G. Leu, MD, MS, MHS, FAAP,[m] Makia E. Powers, MD, MPH, FAAP,[n] Corinna Rea, MD, MPH, FAAP,[o] Joshua Samuels, MD, MPH, FAAP,[p] Madeline Simasek, MD, MSCP, FAAP,[q] Vidhu V. Thaker, MD, FAAP,[r,s,t] Elaine M. Urbina, MD, MS, FAAP,[u] SUBCOMMITTEE ON SCREENING AND MANAGEMENT OF HIGH BP IN CHILDREN

abstract

Systemic hypertension is a major cause of morbidity and mortality in adulthood. High blood pressure (HBP) and repeated measures of HBP, hypertension (HTN), begin in youth. Knowledge of how best to diagnose, manage, and treat systemic HTN in children and adolescents is important for primary and subspecialty care providers.

OBJECTIVES: To provide a technical summary of the methodology used to generate the 2017 "Clinical Practice Guideline for Screening and Management of High Blood Pressure in Children and Adolescents," an update to the 2004 "Fourth Report on the Diagnosis, Evaluation, and Treatment of High Blood Pressure in Children and Adolescents."

DATA SOURCES: Medline, Cochrane Central Register of Controlled Trials, and Excerpta Medica Database references published between January 2003 and July 2015 followed by an additional search between August 2015 and July 2016.

STUDY SELECTION: English-language observational studies and randomized trials.

METHODS: Key action statements (KASs) and additional recommendations regarding the diagnosis, management, and treatment of HBP in youth were the product of a detailed systematic review of the literature. A content outline establishing the breadth and depth was followed by the generation of 4 patient, intervention, comparison, outcome, time questions. Key questions addressed: (1) diagnosis of systemic HTN, (2) recommended work-up of systemic HTN, (3) optimal blood pressure (BP) goals, and (4) impact of high BP on indirect markers of cardiovascular disease in youth. Once selected, references were subjected to a 2-person review of the abstract and title followed by a separate 2-person full-text review. Full citation information,

[a]Division of Cardiology, Department of Pediatrics, School of Medicine, University of Maryland, Baltimore, Maryland; [b]Consultant, Washington, District of Columbia; [c]Division of Nephrology, Department of Pediatrics, University of Washington and Seattle Children's Hospital, Seattle, Washington; Departments of [d]Division of General Internal Medicine, Pediatrics and Population and Quantitative Health Sciences, Case Western Reserve University and Center for Clinical Informatics Research and Education, The MetroHealth System, Cleveland, Ohio; [e]University of Missouri-Kansas City, Children's Mercy Kansas City, Children's Mercy Integrated Care Solutions, Kansas City, Missouri; [f]Department of Pediatrics, School of Medicine, Indiana University, Indianapolis, Indiana; [g]Department of Pediatrics, School of Medicine, University of Colorado, Children's Hospital Colorado, Aurora, Colorado; [h]Preventive Cardiology Clinic, [o]Primary Care at Longwood, and [r]Department of Medicine, Boston Children's Hospital, Harvard Medical School, Harvard University, Boston, Massachusetts; [i]Division of Nephrology, Department of Pediatrics, University of British Columbia and BC Children's Hospital, Vancouver, British Columbia, Canada; Departments of [j]Medicine and Pediatrics, Thomas Jefferson University, Philadelphia, Pennsylvania; [k]Cardiology Division, Nemours Cardiac Center, A. I. duPont Hospital for Children and Department of Pediatrics, Sidney Kimmel Medical College, Thomas Jefferson University, Philadelphia, Pennsylvania; [l]National Pediatric Blood Pressure Awareness Foundation, Prairieville, Louisiana; Departments of [m]Pediatrics and Biomedical Informatics and Medical Education, University of Washington, University of Washington Medicine Information Technology Services, and Seattle Children's Hospital, Seattle, Washington; [n]Department of Pediatrics, Morehouse School of Medicine, Atlanta, Georgia; Departments of [p]Pediatrics and Internal Medicine, McGovern School of Medicine, University of Texas, Houston, Texas; [q]Department of Pediatrics, UPMC Shadyside Family Medicine

To cite: Baker-Smith CM, Flinn SK, Flynn JT, et al. Diagnosis, Evaluation, and Management of High Blood Pressure in Children and Adolescents. *Pediatrics.* 2018;142(3):e20182096

population data, findings, benefits and harms of the findings, as well as other key reference information were archived. Selected primary references were then used for KAS generation. Level of evidence (LOE) scoring was assigned for each reference and then in aggregate. Appropriate language was used to generate each KAS based on the LOE and the balance of benefit versus harm of the findings. Topics that could not be researched via the stated approach were (1) definition of HTN in youth, and (2) definition of left ventricular hypertrophy. KASs related to these stated topics were generated via expert opinion.

RESULTS: Nearly 15 000 references were identified during an initial literature search. After a deduplication process, 14 382 references were available for title and abstract review, and 1379 underwent full text review. One hundred twenty-four experimental and observational studies published between 2003 and 2016 were selected as primary references for KAS generation, followed by an additional 269 primary references selected between August 2015 and July 2016. The LOE for the majority of references was C. In total, 30 KASs and 27 additional recommendations were generated; 12 were related to the diagnosis of HTN, 13 were related to management and additional diagnostic testing, 3 to treatment goals, and 2 to treatment options. Finally, special additions to the clinical practice guideline included creation of new BP tables based on BP values obtained solely from children with normal weight, creation of a simplified table to enhance screening and recognition of abnormal BP, and a revision of the criteria for diagnosing left ventricular hypertrophy.

CONCLUSIONS: An extensive and detailed systematic approach was used to generate evidence-based guidelines for the diagnosis, management, and treatment of youth with systemic HTN.

INTRODUCTION

The 2017 "Clinical Practice Guideline for Screening and Management of High Blood Pressure in Children and Adolescents" serves as an update to the 2004 "Fourth Report on the Diagnosis, Evaluation, and Treatment of High Blood Pressure in Children and Adolescents" (Fourth Report).[1] The Fourth Report was sponsored by the National Heart, Lung, and Blood Institute (NHLBI), whereas the 2017 Clinical Practice Guideline (CPG) is sponsored by the American Academy of Pediatrics (AAP) and has been endorsed by the American College of Cardiology and by the American Heart Association. The authors of the Fourth Report relied primarily on summary statements created by a panel of expert clinicians who carefully evaluated the existing published literature. However, since the publication of the Fourth Report, there has been a notable increase in the number of peer-reviewed primary references, review articles, and systematic reviews (SRs) related to high blood pressure (HBP) and systemic hypertension (HTN) in youth. Hence, the CPG was developed not only by including experts but also by using a reproducible, systematic search and reference archival process, detailed study design evaluation, and evidence strength determination. In developing the 30 key action statements (KASs) of the 2017 CPG, the subcommittee members assessed the individual and aggregate evidence quality and incorporated the balance of benefits and harms of the findings before assigning a recommendation strength.[2]

Systemic HTN is 1 of 7 markers of poor cardiovascular health, according to the American Heart Association.[3] The presence of systemic HTN in childhood and adolescence is 1 of the key risk factors predictive of HTN and cardiovascular disease (CVD) in adults.[4–6] Systemic hypertension in youth has been associated with increased left ventricular mass (LVM), greater carotid intima-media thickness (cIMT),[5] stiffer arteries,[7] reduced endothelial function,[8] and renal[9] as well as neurocognitive impairments.[10] HBP in children has been shown to track into adulthood,[11,12] and HTN in adulthood is a leading cause of morbidity and mortality.[13–15] For these reasons, appropriate diagnostic, management, and treatment strategies should be used in children. However, the diagnosis of HTN can be challenging and is often missed.[16,17]

Estimates of the prevalence of elevated blood pressure (BP) and HTN in children are largely based on analyses of weighted samples from the NHANES.[18] Analyses of more recent NHANES (1999–2012) data, as well as other cross-sectional and prospective study data, suggest a strong association between obesity and HBP in youth,[19,20] such that the prevalence of childhood HTN is higher among children with overweight and obese status.[21] Children and adolescents with specific chronic diseases, such as chronic kidney disease (CKD), also have an increased prevalence of elevated BP and HTN. According to the Chronic Kidney Disease (CKD) in Children study, 37% of youth with CKD had elevated systolic blood pressure (SBP) or diastolic blood pressure (DBP) (>90th percentile), and 14% are hypertensive (based on repeated BP assessment), with either a SBP and/or DBP greater than or equal to the 95th percentile.[22–24]

Stated Objective of the AAP Regarding the Preparation of Updated "Clinical Practice Guideline for Screening and Management of High Blood Pressure in Children and Adolescents"

On February 6, 2014, members of the AAP Sections on Nephrology, Nutrition, and Cardiology and Cardiac Surgery made a formal request to the Executive Committee of the AAP to sponsor a new pediatric HTN CPG focused on the evaluation and management of HBP in children and adolescents. Arguments made to support the generation of an updated guideline included the following:

1. recognition of the need for an update to the Fourth Report to reflect the breadth of new evidence related to HBP in children and adolescents; and

2. greater clarity for primary care providers regarding the utility of BP assessment and management of HTN in the pediatric population.

The request proposed a modification to the screening process and safeguards against both under- and overdiagnosis of HTN. New normative BP tables based on BP values obtained in children with normal BMI were proposed.[25] Furthermore, given increasing evidence to support the use of ambulatory blood pressure monitoring (ABPM) for more accurately assessing BP, it was proposed that the revision expand on the indications for ABPM.[26] The new CPG was intended to specifically incorporate methods for screening and diagnosing target organ damage (TOD), to include data from the pediatric antihypertensive clinical trials published since 2004, and to provide additional information regarding screening for secondary causes of HTN.

In spring 2014, the AAP Executive Committee authorized the formation of the Screening and Management of High Blood Pressure in Children Clinical Practice Guideline Subcommittee of the Council on Quality Improvement and Patient Safety (henceforth, "the subcommittee").

Composition of the Subcommittee Members and Meetings

The subcommittee comprised individuals with expertise in the field of systemic HTN in youth, including representatives from a variety of relevant AAP committees. The subcommittee was cochaired by a pediatric nephrologist, Joseph Flynn, MD, MS, FAAP, and a general pediatrician, David Kaelber, MD, PhD, MPH, FAAP. Carissa Baker-Smith, MD, MPH, MS, FAAP, FAHA, a pediatric cardiologist, served as epidemiologist and methodologist for the CPG. She created the original content outline, drafted the patient, intervention, comparison, outcome,

and treatment/time (PICOT) questions, organized the literature search, structured the article review and selection process, assisted with archiving all selected references, drafted the evidence table (ET) and the technical report (TR). Kymika Okechukwu, MPA, was the AAP staff representative for the project. Susan K. Flinn, MA, was the professional medical editor, who drafted and edited the text of the CPG and assisted with editing the TR. Two librarians, knowledgeable in the process of SR, Kimberly Yang and Emilie Ludeman, assisted the epidemiologist in identifying search terms and conducting the literature search for reference selection in Medline, Cochrane Central Register of Controlled Trials (CENTRAL), and Excerpta Medica dataBASE (Embase).

All subcommittee members played an active role in the process of title and abstract review, article retrieval and storage in Mendeley,[27] reference review, KAS generation, ET generation, and editing of the CPG document sections. All conflicts of interests were disclosed at the beginning of the process and updated throughout the process. Reported conflicts of interest can be found at the end of this TR.

The subcommittee met face-to-face in June 2015 and March 2016. Conference calls occurred every 2 to 4 weeks, along with frequent and regular e-mail correspondence. These meetings, calls, and e-mails were used to assess the evidence and to draft the CPG content. Given the broad range of representation and expertise, potential biases were managed through group discussion and review of the data throughout the process.

Definitions

- Children and adolescents: youth 1 to <18 years of age
- Infants: youth 1 to 12 months of age
- Neonates: youth 0 to 1 month of age

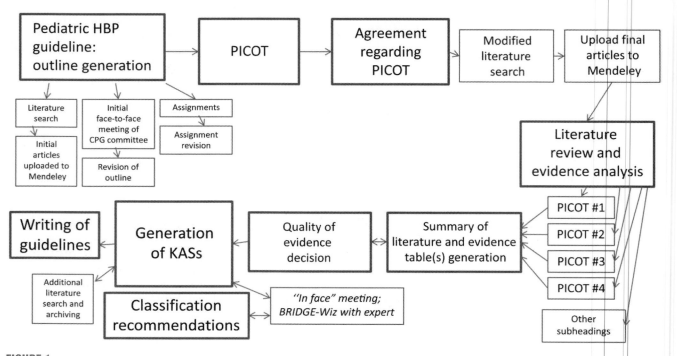

FIGURE 1

Process flow map used for creation of the 2017 "Clinical Practice Guideline for Screening and Management of High Blood Pressure in Children and Adolescents."

CHANGES IN THE DEFINITION OF HYPERTENSION IN YOUTH

According to the Fourth Report and its predecessors, the diagnosis of HTN in youth is purely a statistical determination based on the distribution of BP values obtained in youth. Unfortunately, BPs used for developing BP percentiles in the Fourth Report were obtained from children with both normal and unhealthy weight, skewing the mean. In addition, it was also appreciated that at approximately 13 years of age, the 90th percentile for BP is ~120/80 mm Hg. Previously, it was possible for youth, entering adult care at 18 years of age, to have a "normal" pediatric BP, but, unchanged, an "abnormal" adult BP categorization. As a result, the definition of HTN was revised in the 2017 CPG to reflect statistical definitions for HTN in children younger than 13 years and to use adult cutoff values for youth 13 years of age and older.

FORMULATION AND ARTICULATION OF THE QUESTIONS ADDRESSED BY THE CPG SUBCOMMITTEE

The process of creating the CPG involved ensuring that key topics related to HTN in youth were addressed, ensuring that the literature search was complete and unbiased in identifying the most relevant references, ensuring that data were extracted and analyzed correctly, and that the selected references were summarized fully and accurately. The subcommittee also sought to ensure that the process of KAS generation was transparent and based on the available evidence and that the language used to describe a particular KAS corresponded to the recommendation strength, level of evidence (LOE), and benefits versus harms of the published findings.[28] A process flow map of the steps taken to generate the CPG can be found in Fig 1.

Content Outline

The epidemiologist created a general topic outline. The original content outline included 16 main topics and a total of 100 subtopics that determined the breadth of topics to be addressed in the updated CPG. Agreement regarding outline content was obtained from all subcommittee members. Some of the originally selected topics were ultimately excluded because of lack of sufficient evidence, and other topics were combined to generate a more concise CPG.

SR Process

The SR was conducted in accordance with the Preferred Reporting Items for Systemic Reviews and Meta-Analysis guidelines.[29] The epidemiologist carefully drafted 4 PICOT questions to guide the literature search. These questions addressed how the diagnosis of systemic HTN should be made in infants, children, and adolescents; the recommended clinical and laboratory-based approach for identification of potential causes of systemic HTN (eg, evaluation for secondary causes); the target BP to be achieved with treatment; and the impact of BP severity on indirect markers of CVD in youth. Outcome measures, inclusion and exclusion criteria, and comparison groups were predetermined before the initiation of the literature search. The primary literature search was conducted by Emilie Ludeman and Kimberly Yang.

A line-by-line description of the search strategy is presented in Supplemental Appendix A, including the dates of the primary search for each PICOT. At the time of KAS generation, between August 2015 and July 2016, subcommittee members conducted additional searches. The epidemiologist was not directly involved in these additional literature searches but requested that search criteria, date, and time of each search be stored. All selected citations, including those identified during the initial and subsequent searches, were entered into 4 separate spreadsheets by PICOT (eg, PICOT 1, PICOT 2, PICOT 3, PICOT 4). Originally identified references, selected on the basis of the SR, were numbered. Added references, selected between August 2015 and July 2016, were labeled not with a number but as "added." All selected references, either chosen on the basis of title and abstract review or later chosen on the basis of separate searches conducted by subcommittee members during the KAS generation phase, were downloaded as a PDF from the Internet and then uploaded into Mendeley, a commercially available reference management software, used for reference storage and deduplication. Mendeley served as the subcommittee's central reference repository for easy access to selected articles during the article review and appraisal process.[27]

An ET was created for storage of data from references selected for inclusion in the CPG. The following information was entered for each reference in the ET: PICOT number, citation number in the CPG, original search reference number (identification number within the PICOT 1–4 spreadsheet), author(s), relevant KAS number, relevant CPG section number, year of publication, journal of publication, full citation, LOE assignment for the individual reference, type of study (eg, observational, randomized controlled trial [RCT], etc), primary population, reported sample size, subpopulations of interest, method of BP assessment (eg, manual, oscillometric, ABPM), intervention (if applicable), quality of BP measurements (at least 3 measurements made during a single visit), study findings, identified benefits of the study findings, potential harms related to the study findings, benefit versus harm analysis, and potential limitations of the study.

PICOT Questions Generation

Once the CPG subcommittee members agreed on the topics to be covered, 4 PICOT questions were created (see below). Nearly 80% of the topics included in the outline were amenable to a PICOT search strategy and included in the PICOT formatted search (see Supplemental Tables 1 through 4 for outline topics addressed by the 4 PICOT questions); 20% were not. Topics that were not amenable to the PICOT search format included the following: strategies for prevention, challenges in the implementation of pediatric hypertension guidelines, economic impact of BP management, patient perspective, parental perspective, evidence gaps, and proposed future directions. Definition of HTN in neonates (0–1 month), infants (1–12 months of age), children (1–13 years of age), adolescents (13–18 years of age), and the definition of left ventricular

hypertrophy (LVH) were also not searched via a PICOT format (see Supplemental Table 5). These topics were individually researched, and expert opinion was used to create statements relevant to these topics.

PICOT 1

How should systemic HTN (primary HTN, renovascular HTN) be diagnosed in neonates, infants, and children (0–18 years of age)? How should white coat hypertension (WCH) and masked hypertension (MH) be diagnosed in children and adolescents? What is the optimal approach to diagnosing HTN in children and adolescents?

PICOT 2

What is the recommended workup for evaluating children and adolescents with suspected or confirmed systemic HTN? How do we best identify the underlying etiologies of secondary HTN in children and adolescents, including renal-, endocrine-, environment-, medication-, and obesity-related causes? When should providers suspect a monogenic form of systemic HTN among children and adolescents?

PICOT 3

What is the optimal goal SBP and/ or DBP for children and adolescents? What nonpharmacologic and pharmacologic therapies are available for the treatment of HTN in children and adolescents?

PICOT 4

In children and adolescents 1 to 18 years of age, how does the presence and the severity of systemic HTN influence indirect markers of CVD and vascular dysfunction (eg, flow-mediated dilation [FMD], cIMT), and how does HTN in children impact long-term risk of HTN into adulthood? Among children and adolescents with systemic HTN, how does the presence and the

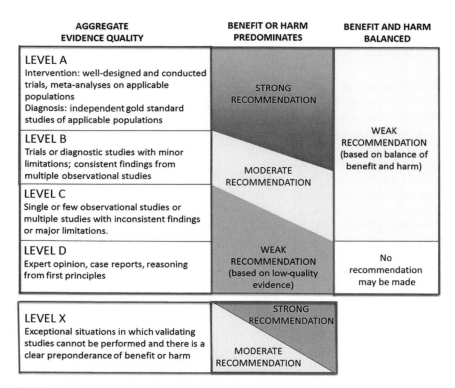

AGGREGATE EVIDENCE QUALITY	BENEFIT OR HARM PREDOMINATES	BENEFIT AND HARM BALANCED
LEVEL A Intervention: well-designed and conducted trials, meta-analyses on applicable populations Diagnosis: independent gold standard studies of applicable populations	STRONG RECOMMENDATION	WEAK RECOMMENDATION (based on balance of benefit and harm)
LEVEL B Trials or diagnostic studies with minor limitations; consistent findings from multiple observational studies	MODERATE RECOMMENDATION	
LEVEL C Single or few observational studies or multiple studies with inconsistent findings or major limitations.		
LEVEL D Expert opinion, case reports, reasoning from first principles	WEAK RECOMMENDATION (based on low-quality evidence)	No recommendation may be made
LEVEL X Exceptional situations in which validating studies cannot be performed and there is a clear preponderance of benefit or harm	STRONG RECOMMENDATION / MODERATE RECOMMENDATION	

FIGURE 2

Integrating evidence quality appraisal with anticipated benefits versus harms[27]: individual references were graded, benefits versus harms of the findings were assessed, and the aggregate evidence quality was used to generate a strong, moderate, or weak recommendation.

severity of systemic HTN influence comorbidities such as dyslipidemia, obstructive sleep apnea syndrome (OSAS), and cognition?

Search Strategy

The epidemiologist and 2 librarians created a list of appropriate search terms and strategies (see Appendix A). Search terms included keywords and database-specific terminology (eg, medical subject headings terms, Emtree). The primary literature review for all PICOT questions was limited to studies published between 2003 and 2015. PubMed, CENTRAL, and Embase database searches were conducted on September 1, 2015, for PICOT 1; September 2, 2015, for PICOT 2; September 15–16, 2015, for PICOT 3; and September 17, 2015 for PICOT 4.

Inclusion criteria (see Supplemental Table 6) included the following:

- neonates, infants, children, and adolescents;

- male and female sex;

- all races and/or ethnicities;

- RCTs and observational studies (eg, cross-sectional, retrospective cohort, and prospective cohort); and

- case series for rare conditions for which large population studies were unavailable.

Exclusion criteria included the following:

- abstract only;

- adult-only population (especially when relevant pediatric studies were available);

- duplicate studies (in some cases, the same data were presented in another reference, and submitted to a different journal);

- primary population was non-United States (unless there were an insufficient number of US studies to address the key question);

- non–English language studies;

- letters;

- commentaries; and

- references related to topics that were not included in the CPG.

The citation information and any reasons for study exclusion were recorded by the methodologist. Review articles, meta-analyses, and most SRs were included for background. Adult studies were excluded from KAS generation but may have been included for background or table content. Studies that took place outside of the United States were included only when US data regarding the topics were not available or were limited.

Evidence Review and Selection

Analysis of Available Evidence, Assignment of LOE, Assignment of Grade Strength

AAP policy stipulates that the evidence in support of each KAS be prospectively identified, appraised, and summarized and that an explicit link between the LOE and grade of recommendation be defined. A summary of the available grades is described in Fig 2.[28]

Strong Recommendation

A strong recommendation is the highest level of recommendation, reserved for recommendations supported by evidence with grade A or B that demonstrates a preponderance of benefit over harm. Interventions based on level X evidence might also be categorized as "strong" on the basis of their risk-benefit profile. A strong recommendation in favor of a particular action is made when the anticipated benefits of the recommended intervention clearly exceed the harms (as a strong recommendation against an action is made when the anticipated harms clearly exceed the benefits) and the quality of the supporting evidence is excellent. In some clearly identified circumstances, strong recommendations are made when high-quality evidence is impossible to obtain and the anticipated benefits strongly outweigh the harms. The implication for clinicians is that they should follow a strong recommendation unless a clear and compelling rationale for an alternative approach is present.

Moderate Recommendation

A moderate recommendation is made when the anticipated benefit exceeds the harms but the methodology used to generate the evidence is not sound. Moderately recommended KASs are to be supported by grade B or grade C evidence. Level X evidence may also be used to support a moderate recommendation depending on risk-benefit considerations. A recommendation in favor of a particular action is made when the anticipated benefit exceeds the harm but the quality of evidence is not as strong. In some clearly identified circumstances, moderate recommendations are made when high-quality evidence is impossible to obtain but the anticipated benefits outweigh the harms. The implication for clinicians is that they should be prudent when following a moderate recommendation but should remain alert to new information and sensitive to patient preferences.

Weak Recommendation and No Recommendation

When published evidence is lacking, and/or when the limited evidence available demonstrates an equivocal risk-benefit profile, no recommended key action is offered. No recommendation indicates that there is a lack of pertinent published evidence and that the anticipated balance of benefits and harms is presently unclear. The implication for clinicians is that they should be alert to new published evidence that clarify the balance of benefit versus harm. The classification of

recommendations for the 2017 CPG is depicted in Fig 2.

Evidence Selection Process

A 3-step process was used to select references for review. The first step included the selection of references from 3 databases (eg, Medline, CENTRAL, Embase). References were deduplicated. Next, by using preestablished written criteria for article selection for each PICOT, references were selected on the basis of title and abstract review. When the 2 reviewers disagreed, the epidemiologist provided the deciding vote on whether to include a particular reference. A third and final step involved full reference review.

A final search of articles published between August 2015 and July 2016 was completed at the time of KAS generation to identify any additional relevant references. Subcommittee teams also had the option of incorporating additional background references into the text preceding each KAS. Additional references were selected on the basis of expert opinion and familiarity with the literature. Background references selected for inclusion in the final document were also achieved in the ET.

Generation of KASs

KASs were actionable statements, drafted on the basis of the assembled evidence, intended to guide clinical practice. Writing teams consisting of 2 or more subcommittee members were established to generate KASs for each selected topic. The clinical expertise of subcommittee members was used during the KAS generation phase. Subcommittee members with expertise in the topic were selected to either review the references relevant to a particular topic or serve as primary author(s) of the KAS relevant to their clinical expertise. In other cases, authors for the KAS were selected on the basis of previous involvement in article selection for

the particular topic. In addition to the creation of KAS writing teams, expert work groups were established to address (1) the revision of the HTN definition (members were Flynn, Kaelber, Giddings, Falkner, and Urbina) and (2) defining LVH (members were Giddings, Urbina, De Ferranti, and Baker-Smith).[30]

Building Recommendations in a Developer's Guideline Editor

The language used for each KAS was specifically chosen to reflect the strength of recommendation by using Building Recommendations in a Developer's Guideline Editor (BRIDGE-Wiz),[31] an interactive clinical software application that has been adopted by the AAP to aid CPG authors. This application leads guideline writing teams through a series of questions intended to create clear, transparent, and actionable KASs. BRIDGE-Wiz incorporates LOE and benefit-harm assessment into a final determination of each recommendation strength. BRIDGE-Wiz provides safeguard against creating vague and/or underspecified recommendations. This software was used to generate KASs during an in-person meeting held at the AAP headquarters on March 21, 2016. BRIDGE-Wiz was also used to help generate the text for KASs generated after the March 21, 2016, meeting.

Generation of Recommended KAS

After considering the available LOE and recommendation grades, the subcommittee formulated 30 KASs.[32] Each KAS included the following:

- an aggregate evidence quality score;
- a list of the potential benefit(s) of the proposed KAS;
- a description of the risks, harms, and costs of the proposed KAS;
- a benefit-harm assessment;
- a description of any intentional vagueness;

- a description of the role of patient preference;
- any exclusions;
- an assessment of the strength of the recommendation; and
- key references used to generate the specific KAS.

RESULTS

Summary of Findings by PICOT

PICOT 1

How should systemic HTN (primary HTN, renovascular HTN) be diagnosed in neonates, infants, and children (0–18 years of age)? How should WCH and MH be diagnosed in children and adolescents? What is the optimal approach to diagnosing HTN in children and adolescents?

A comparison between central aortic or brachial artery BP and cuff BP was beyond the scope of this CPG but has been described in a recent SR.[33] Criteria for the diagnosis of systemic HTN in neonates and infants has not been prospectively studied, at least since 2003. Only review articles were identified to suggest appropriate BP cutoffs for neonates born at 26 to 44 weeks' gestation.[34,35] The gold standard method for BP assessment in the neonate is intra-arterial analysis; the estimated prevalence of HTN in the neonate is approximately 0.2% to 3% but is higher in those with bronchopulmonary dysplasia, persistent ductus arteriosus, intraventricular hemorrhage, or an indwelling umbilical artery catheter (eg, up to 9% develop HTN). BP patterns may vary depending on developmental stage and gestational age at birth. According to the available literature, it may be best to use gestational age at birth and days of life when determining appropriateness of BP.[35]

At the present time, specific BP levels in youth have not yet been linked to cardiovascular outcomes in adulthood. Current normative values for BP are based on auscultatory BP measurements for normal-weight children. Unchanged from the Fourth Report, defining abnormal BP in youth 1 to <13 years of age continues to rely on a statistical definition.[25,36] The methods involved in determining statistical BP cutoff values have been peer reviewed and published.[25] For youth 13 years of age and above, adult BP cutoff values were adopted.[36]

Regarding the methods used for diagnosis of systemic HTN in children 3 to <18 years of age, initial BPs in children may be assessed via use of an approved oscillometric device, an aneroid sphygmomanometer or mercury sphygmomanometer (HgS).[36,37] Proper technique is essential for proper BP assessment.[38,39] When possible, manual BP assessments are preferred over oscillometric assessments, given data suggesting that oscillometric BP assessments routinely overestimate BP.[40]

Repeated measurement of BP remains an important step in determining whether a child truly has HBP.[41–43] Existing evidence would suggest that not all providers, practices, and/or patients adhere to recommendations for follow-up BP assessment within the recommended time frame.[41] The BPs obtained when vital signs are initially assessed do not necessarily reflect the true BP.[38] By more recent estimates, 90.0% (*n* = 1569) of children undergoing repeated measure of BP within a single visit did not experience a change in BP. However, 6.2% (*n* = 107) experienced a decrease in BP category and 2.9% (*n* = 49) experienced an increase in BP category.[42] A single BP measurement may lead to a misclassification of BP category and inappropriate action. Repeated BP measurement remains a requirement for diagnosing HTN.

The electronic health record (EHR) may also be helpful in diagnosing HTN among youth. Challenges associated with use of a complex table may lead to lack of recognition.[44] However, the EHR may be a useful tool for improved recognition of abnormal BP.[45,46] Finally, ABPM is a reliable, although less accessible, method for distinguishing WCH and MH from systemic hypertension.[47] Limitations of ABPM include a lack of reference data for children <120 cm in height and BP cutoff values that differ from those used to define abnormal in-office BP. Use of ABPM is currently recommended for confirmation of diagnosis and measurements obtained via ABPM may be more reproducible than those obtained via office or home BP.[36,48]

PICOT 2

What is the recommended workup for evaluating children and adolescents with suspected or confirmed systemic HTN? How do we best identify the underlying etiologies of secondary HTN in children and adolescents, including renal-, endocrine-, environment-, medication-, and obesity-related causes? When should providers suspect a monogenic form of systemic HTN among children and adolescents?

The evaluation of children and adolescents with suspected HTN consists of confirmation of the diagnosis. Potential secondary causes of systemic HTN can be found in Table 14 of the CPG.[36] Additional diagnostic studies may be required.[36] It has been suggested that primary HTN accounts for most cases of HTN among children older than 6 years and among 90% of children older than 15 years.[49–51] Patients with secondary HTN tend to be younger and are more likely to have abnormal serum creatinine, renal ultrasonography, and echocardiography findings.[50] Youth with secondary causes of HTN may be at greater risk for hypertensive emergency and require more immediate management and intervention.[52]

PICOT 3

What is the optimal goal SBP and/or DBP for children and adolescents? What nonpharmacologic and pharmacologic therapies are available for the treatment of HBP in children and adolescents?

The optimal goal SBP and DBP for children and adolescents remain unknown. However, data from a recent survey study indicate that compared with normotension, elevated BP can be associated with the development of TOD in adults.[53] Additionally, more recent cross-sectional data demonstrate an association between elevated BP (>90th percentile) and TOD in youth.[7] Thus, the CPG recommends a target BP of <90th percentile, even for children and adolescents with primary HTN.

Nonpharmacologic treatment options include diets low in sodium (eg, Dietary Approaches to Stop Hypertension [DASH] diet) and fat and diets rich in low-fat dairy,[54] fresh fruits, vegetables, and legumes.[55] Pharmacologic treatment options include angiotensin-converting enzyme inhibitors (ACEi), long-acting calcium channel blockers (CCB), angiotensin receptor blockers (ARB), and thiazide diuretics. A detailed SR in which the roughly 21 antihypertensive trials conducted in 3454 hypertensive children with follow-up between 3 and 24 weeks are summarized has been published and has been referenced in the CPG.[56] α agonists and β-blockers are not routinely recommended for the initial treatment of hypertension in youth.

The PICOT 3 search was focused on identifying references that addressed the question of BP management, both nonpharmacologic and pharmacologic, in children and adolescents. It is well known that lifestyle modifications can have a significant and positive impact on BP management.[57] Furthermore, since the enactment of the 1997 Food and Drug Administration Modernization Act and passage of the Best Drugs for Children Act,[58] the path for assessing the pharmacokinetics, dose-effect, and safety of antihypertensive therapy in children has been cleared. The goals of PICOT 3 and its associated KASs were to both identify effective therapies (eg, lifestyle, noninvasive therapies, and antihypertensive therapies) and to evaluate response to therapy.

PICOT 4

In children and adolescents 1 to <18 years of age, how does the presence and the severity of systemic HTN influence indirect markers of CVD and vascular dysfunction (eg, FMD, cIMT), and how does HTN in children impact long-term risk of HTN into adulthood? Among children and adolescents with systemic HTN, what is the relationship between severity of systemic HTN comorbid conditions such as dyslipidemia, OSAS, and impaired cognition?

The question of hypertension's impact on long-term cardiovascular health in children has been debated. Indirect measures of CVD risk include cIMT, FMD, and LVH. PICOT 4 sought to address the question of hypertension's impact on these and other indirect markers of CVD risk. In particular, the subcommittee evaluated whether a change in BP was associated with a change in FMD, cIMT, and/or LVH. This PICOT also addressed other potential comorbidities associated with HTN, including obesity, diabetes mellitus, dyslipidemia, OSAS, metabolic syndrome, cognitive impairment, and proteinuria.

On the basis of cumulative data from 4 large prospective cohort studies, the Cardiovascular Risk in Young Finns Study, Childhood Determinants of Adult Health Study, the Bogalusa Heart Study, and the Muscatine Study, the strength of association between the presence of childhood risk factors for premature CVD and the presence of cIMT is dependent on age of onset of elevation in SBP in 6- to 18-year-olds, whereas elevations in DBP were not associated with abnormal cIMT.[5]

General Results From Full Search

A total of 14 763 references were selected after the initial PICOT search. After deduplication, 14 382 references were available for title and abstract review. The 2-person abstract and title review resulted in a total of 1379 references for full text review. A total of 124 references were selected for KAS generation (see Supplemental Table 7). An additional 269 primary references were selected for inclusion during the expanded search.

Primary Literature Search, PICOT 1

The primary questions used to conduct the literature search for PICOT 1 were as follows: How should HTN in children and adolescents be diagnosed and what is the optimal approach to diagnosing HTN in children and adolescents?

Of the 304 selected references, 266 were excluded (see Supplemental Table 8). An additional 58 references were selected during KAS generation (see Supplemental Table 9). Of the total 48 primary references used for KAS generation, there were 2 LOE A references, 19 LOE B references, 16 LOE C references, and 4 were SRs, and 7 were background references. Ten KASs were generated related to PICOT 1.

Primary Literature Search, PICOT 2

The primary questions used to conduct the literature search for PICOT 2 were as follows: What is the recommended workup for hypertension in neonates, infants, children, and adolescents? How do we best identify the underlying etiologies of secondary hypertension in the pediatric population?

The literature search for PICOT 2 was focused on the diagnostic approach for identifying renal, renovascular, cardiac, endocrine (including pheochromocytoma), medication-related, and genetic causes of HTN. A total of 1567 references were selected on the basis of initial search terms (see Supplemental Table 7). After the deduplication process, a total of 1565 references were selected. Abstract and title review led to the exclusion of 196 references after full reference review. See Supplemental Table 10 for the excluded PICOT 2 references.

Of a total of 225 references selected, 86 references (see Supplemental Table 11), 9 were selected for KAS generation. Seventy-two additional references that were added during the search conducted between August 2015 and July 2016 were also used to generate KASs related to PICOT 2.

Of the selected references used to generate PICOT 2–related KASs, 4 were LOE B and 24 were LOE C. Eight background references were selected at the discretion of the KAS authors.

Primary Literature Search, PICOT 3

The primary questions used to conduct the literature search for PICOT 3 were as follows: What is the optimal goal SBP and/or DBP for children and adolescents? What nonpharmacologic and pharmacologic therapies are available for the treatment of HBP in children?

A total of 6958 references were selected on the basis of initial search terms (see Supplemental Table 7). A minimum therapeutic follow-up period of 3 months was required for inclusion of a study. After a deduplication process conducted in Mendeley, a total of 6710 references were selected. Abstract and title

review led to the selection of 631 references for full reference review and data extraction. A total of 59 references were initially selected for inclusion in KAS generation. Some of the references were excluded because the topics covered were beyond the scope of the CPG (eg, RCTs of the use of dark chocolate, cocoa, beetroot juice, dietary fiber, dietary protein, diet rich in fish, or garlic to treat hypertension in children),[59–66] (see Supplemental Table 12 for the excluded PICOT 3 references), and other references were excluded because they pertained to a particular subset of children with hypertension (eg, pharmacologic management of hypertension in children with CKD).[67,68] There were many trials in which combination therapy in the adult population was addressed. Such topics were not explored in the CPG,[69–74] and such references were ultimately excluded. Some references considered to be duplicates (eg, reports of the pediatric candesartan trial) were excluded.[75,76] In total, 587 references were excluded (see Supplemental Table 12).

After the updated search and KAS generation, 45 additional references were selected for inclusion for a total of 60 references (see Supplemental Table 13). The majority of selected references were cross-sectional studies. A total of 60 primary references were used to generate KASs for PICOT 3: 10 were LOE A, 11 were LOE B, 31 were LOE C, and none were LOE D/EO. In addition, 5 background references and 3 SRs were selected for inclusion and KAS generation.

Primary Literature Search, PICOT 4

The primary question used to conduct the literature search for PICOT 4 was as follows: In children and adolescents 0 to 18 years of age, how does the presence and the severity of systemic hypertension influence indirect markers of CVD

and vascular dysfunction (eg, FMD, cIMT), and how does hypertension in children impact long-term risk of hypertension into adulthood?

A total of 3857 references were selected after a deduplication process was conducted in Mendeley. Abstract and title review led to the selection of 3744 references for full review and data extraction. In total, 219 references were selected for full review (see Supplemental Table 7), and 196 were excluded for the following reasons: 1 abstract only, 10 non-English language and/ or non-US population, 110 adult-only population, and 98 for other reasons (eg, review article, duplicate reference, etc; see Supplemental Table 14).

After the updated search, a total of 23 references were selected for inclusion in PICOT 4. The majority of selected references were cross-sectional studies or retrospective cohort studies.

SPECIAL ADDITIONS TO THE CPG

Creation of New BP Tables

The subcommittee engaged Bernard Rosner, PhD, the statistician previously consulted by the NHLBI on past pediatric BP guidelines, to generate new normative BP tables on the basis of values obtained only in children with normal BMI. The goal was to eliminate the effects of obesity on the normative values, which was a criticism of the normative BP tables published in the Fourth Report. Methods used to generate these tables have previously been published.[25]

Data included in this updated analysis were already presented in the National High Blood Pressure Education Program NHLBI database and consisted of 11 pediatric BP studies conducted between 1976 and 2000.[77–86] For the new normative BP table, only subjects with BMI <85th percentile based on Centers for

Disease Control and Prevention age- and sex-specific BMI growth charts were used. Separate sex-specific analyses were performed for SBP and DBP. Of note, the heights used in the new tables are those for children of x years, 6 months, and therefore may differ from height values found in standard growth charts.

To remove study effects, a restricted cubic spline linear regression model was run of BP on study age, height z score, and weight z score, represented as 10 dummy variables. Height and height z scores corresponding to height at age x years+ 6 months and not the CDC height percentiles, were used. The study effects from the regression model were used to compute "adjusted BP" (eg, BP_adj), which was the BP that would be obtained if a subject came from an average study. A second restricted cubic spline regression was then run of the adjusted BP on age, height, and age × height, with knots at the fifth, 27.5th, 50th, 75th, and 95th percentiles and residuals that were assumed to be normally distributed.

A cubic spline was used because it is considered to be more flexible than a single ordinary polynomial regression over the entire age and/ or height z score. The cubic spline is a concatenation of separate cubic polynomials with smooth intersections at the knots. The restricted cubic spline model assumes normal residuals, which implies that the effects of age and height are the same for all quantiles of BP. To relax this assumption, quantile regression methods were used. With quantile regression, mean BP was modeled by using restricted cubic spline. However, a separate set of regression coefficients was obtained for each quantile (s = 0.01, 0.05, 0.10, 0.25, 0.50, 0.75, 0.90, 0.95, and 0.99). The quantile regression approach, using separate restricted cubic splines for each quantile, offers the most flexibility in terms of

both specification of the regression function for a specific quantile and allowance for separate regression equations for different quantiles.

Complete tables for the 90th percentile are available in Table 4 of Rosner et al,[87] along with the regression equations used to generate each of the quantiles(s) in the restricted cubic spline in addition to a macro that ran 99 quantile regressions for s = 0.01, 0.99 (0.01) and estimated the closest quantile that agrees with a child's given BP, age, sex, and height. These percentiles, both in tabular form for assessment of BP of individual children and in a SAS macro for assessment of BP percentiles in batch mode for larger numbers of children, are available online.[88]

Information regarding how to incorporate 2017 CPG BP definitions into the EHR can be found in Supplemental Appendix B.[87]

Simplified BP Table

The CPG also includes a new, simplified table for initial BP screening based on the 90th percentile BP for age and sex for children at the fifth percentile for height. This gives the BP values in the simplified table a negative predictive value of more than 99%.[89] The simplified table was designed for use only as a screening tool to identify children and adolescents who need further BP evaluation.

It is not intended that one will use the simplified table to diagnose elevated BP or hypertension but rather to determine when a BP measurement should be repeated. To diagnose elevated BP or hypertension, it is important to use the actual BP values in the complete BP tables because these may be as much as 9 mm Hg higher than those in the simplified table, depending on the child's age and length or height. A typical use case for this simplified table is for nursing staff to quickly identify BP

that may need further evaluation either by the nurse himself or herself or by the clinician. For adolescents ≥13 years of age, a threshold of 120/80 mm Hg was used in the simplified table regardless of sex to align with adult guidelines for detection of elevated BP.[90]

New Definition of LVH

Echocardiography is used to assess the presence of left ventricular target organ injury related to hypertension in children.[1] The basis for this assessment is (1) the relationship of LVM to BP,[91] (2) the independent and strong relationship of LVH to adverse CVD outcomes in adults,[92–94] and (3) the fact that a significant percentage of children and adolescents with hypertension demonstrate a degree of LVH associated with adverse outcomes in adults.[95–97]

The left ventricle (LV) structure in the CPG is stratified into 4 groups on the basis of LVM (normal or hypertrophied) and relative LV wall thickness (normal or increased). The 4 stratified groups proposed for LVM include (1) normal geometry with normal LVM and normal relative wall thickness (RWT), (2) concentric geometry with normal LVM and increased RWT, (3) eccentric LVH with increased LVM and normal RWT, and (4) concentric LVH with both increased LVM and increased RWT[98,99] (see Supplemental Table 15).

Because the heart increases in size in relation to body size, indexing LVM is required.[100]

For the 2017 CPG, the following definitions for LV target organ injury were chosen regarding hypertrophy, RWT, and ejection fraction (EF). These definitions are based on published guidelines from the American Society of Echocardiography and associations of thresholds for indexed LVM with adverse outcomes in adults[92,93,98,100]:

- LVH is defined as left ventricular mass, indexed >51 g/m$^{2.7}$ or LVM >115 g/body surface area (BSA) for boys and LVM >95 g/BSA for girls. (Note that the values for LVH are well above the 95th percentile for distributions of LVM in children and adolescents.[98] The clinical significance of values between the 95th percentile of a population-based distribution and these thresholds is uncertain.[101])

- An LV RWT >0.42 indicates concentric geometry. LV wall thickness >1.4 cm is abnormal.[102]

- Decreased LV EF is a value <53%.

CONCLUSIONS

The 2017 "Clinical Practice Guideline for Screening and Management of High Blood Pressure in Children in Adolescents" is a comprehensive, evidence-based guideline intended for use by primary and subspecialty care providers. In this TR, we review the methodology used to generate the guideline. A systematic approach was used to generate evidence-based guidelines for the diagnosis, management, and treatment of youth with HBP.

ACKNOWLEDGMENTS

We thank Kimberly Yang, Emilie Ludeman, and Bernard Rosner, PhD.

LEAD AUTHORS

Carissa M. Baker-Smith, MD, MS, MPH, FAAP, FAHA
Susan K. Flinn, MA
Joseph T. Flynn, MD, MS, FAAP
David C. Kaelber, MD, PhD, MPH, FAAP, FACP, FACMI
Douglas Blowey, MD
Aaron E. Carroll, MD, MS, FAAP
Stephen R. Daniels, MD, PhD, FAAP
Sarah D. de Ferranti, MD, MPH, FAAP
Janis M. Dionne, MD, FRCPC
Bonita Falkner, MD
Samuel S. Gidding, MD
Celeste Goodwin
Michael G. Leu, MD, MS, MHS, FAAP
Makia E. Powers, MD, MPH, FAAP
Corinna Rea, MD, MPH, FAAP
Joshua Samuels, MD, MPH, FAAP
Madeline Simasek, MD, MSCP, FAAP
Vidhu V. Thaker, MD, FAAP
Elaine M. Urbina, MD, MS, FAAP

SUBCOMMITTEE ON SCREENING AND MANAGEMENT OF HIGH BLOOD PRESSURE IN CHILDREN (OVERSIGHT BY THE COUNCIL ON QUALITY IMPROVEMENT AND PATIENT SAFETY)

Joseph T. Flynn, MD, MS, FAAP, Co-chair, *Section on Nephrology*
David Kaelber, MD, PhD, FAAP, Co-chair, *Council on Clinical Information Technology and Section on Medicine-Pediatrics*
Carissa M. Baker-Smith, MD, MS, MPH, FAAP, *Fellow of the American Heart Association Epidemiologist*

Aaron Carroll, MD, MS, FAAP, *Partnership for Policy Implementation*
Stephen R. Daniels, MD, PhD, FAAP, *Committee on Nutrition*
Sarah D. de Ferranti, MD, MPH, FAAP, *Committee on Cardiology & Cardiac Surgery*
Michael G. Leu, MD, MS, MHS, FAAP, *Council on Quality Improvement and Patient Safety*
Makia Powers, MD, MPH, FAAP, *Committee on Adolescence*
Corinna Rea, MD, MPH, FAAP, *Section on Early Career Physicians*
Joshua Samuels, MD, MPH, FAAP, *Section on Nephrology*
Madeline Simasek, MD, FAAP, *Quality Improvement Innovation Networks*
Vidhu Thaker, MD, FAAP, *Section on Obesity*
Elaine Urbina, MD, FAAP, *American Heart Association, Atherosclerosis, Hypertension, & Obesity in the Young Committee*

LIAISONS

Douglas Blowey, MD — *American Society of Pediatric Nephrology*
Janis Dionne, MD, FRCPC — *Canadian Association of Paediatric Nephrologists*
Bonita Falkner, MD — *International Pediatric Hypertension Association*
Samuel Gidding, MD — *American College of Cardiology/American Heart Association*
Celeste Goodwin — *National Pediatric Blood Pressure Awareness Foundation*

MEDICAL WRITER

Susan K. Flinn, MA

STAFF

Kymika Okechukwu, MPA, Senior Manager, Evidence-Based Practice Initiatives

ABBREVIATIONS

AAP: American Academy of Pediatrics
ABPM: ambulatory blood pressure monitoring
ACEi: angiotensin-converting enzyme inhibitor
BP: blood pressure
BRIDGE-Wiz: Building Recommendations in a Developer's Guideline Editor
BSA: body surface area
CENTRAL: Cochrane Central Register of Controlled Trials
cIMT: carotid intima-media thickness

CKD: chronic kidney disease
CPG: Clinical Practice Guideline
CVD: cardiovascular disease
DASH: Dietary Approaches to Stop Hypertension
DBP: diastolic blood pressure
EF: ejection fraction
EHR: electronic health record
Embase: Excerpta Medica dataBASE
ET: evidence table
FMD: flow-mediated dilation
HBP: high blood pressure
HgS: mercury sphygmomanometer
KAS: key action statement
LOE: level of evidence
LV: left ventricle

LVH: left ventricular hypertrophy
LVM: left ventricular mass
MH: masked hypertension
NHLBI: National Heart, Lung, and Blood Institute
OSAS: obstructive sleep apnea syndrome
PICOT: patient, intervention, comparison, outcome, and treatment/time
RCT: randomized controlled trial
RWT: relative wall thickness
SBP: systolic blood pressure
SR: systematic review
TOD: target organ damage
TR: technical report
WCH: white coat hypertension

Residency, University of Pittsburgh Medical Center, Children's Hospital of Pittsburgh and School of Medicine, University of Pittsburgh, Pittsburgh, Pennsylvania; ^sDivision of Molecular Genetics, Department of Pediatrics, Columbia University Irving Medical Center, Columbia University, New York, New York; ^tBroad Institute, Cambridge, Massachusetts; and ^uPreventive Cardiology, Cincinnati Children's Hospital Medical Center, Cincinnati, Ohio

DOI: https://doi.org/10.1542/peds.2018-2096

Address correspondence to Carissa M. Baker-Smith. Email: cbaker-smith@som.umaryland.edu

PEDIATRICS (ISSN Numbers: Print, 0031-4005; Online, 1098-4275).

Copyright © 2018 by the American Academy of Pediatrics

FINANCIAL DISCLOSURE: The authors have indicated they have no financial relationships relevant to this article to disclose.

FUNDING: No external funding.

POTENTIAL CONFLICT OF INTEREST: The authors have indicated they have no potential conflicts of interest to disclose.

REFERENCES

1. National High Blood Pressure Education Program Working Group on High Blood Pressure in Children and Adolescents. The fourth report on the diagnosis, evaluation, and treatment of high blood pressure in children and adolescents. *Pediatrics.* 2004;114(2 suppl 4th report):555–576

2. American Academy of Pediatrics Steering Committee on Quality Improvement and Management. Classifying recommendations for clinical practice guidelines. *Pediatrics.* 2004;114(3):874–877

3. Benjamin EJ, Blaha MJ, Chiuve SE, et al; American Heart Association Statistics Committee and Stroke Statistics Subcommittee. Heart disease and stroke statistics-2017 update: a report from the American Heart Association [published correction appears in *Circulation.* 2017;135(10):e646; *Circulation.* 2017;136(10):e196]. *Circulation.* 2017;135(10):e146–e603

4. Sun SS, Grave GD, Siervogel RM, Pickoff AA, Arslanian SS, Daniels SR. Systolic blood pressure in childhood predicts hypertension and metabolic syndrome later in life. *Pediatrics.* 2007;119(2):237–246

5. Juonala M, Magnussen CG, Venn A, et al. Influence of age on associations between childhood risk factors and carotid intima-media thickness in adulthood: the Cardiovascular Risk in Young Finns Study, the Childhood Determinants of Adult Health Study, the Bogalusa Heart Study, and the Muscatine Study for the International Childhood Cardiovascular Cohort (i3C) Consortium. *Circulation.* 2010;122(24):2514–2520

6. Shen W, Zhang T, Li S, et al. Race and sex differences of long-term blood pressure profiles from childhood and adult hypertension: the Bogalusa Heart Study. *Hypertension.* 2017;70(1):66–74

7. Urbina EM, Khoury PR, McCoy C, Daniels SR, Kimball TR, Dolan LM. Cardiac and vascular consequences of pre-hypertension in youth. *J Clin Hypertens (Greenwich).* 2011;13(5):332–342

8. Garanty-Bogacka B, Syrenicz M, Syrenicz A, Gebala A, Lulka D, Walczak M. Serum markers of inflammation and endothelial activation in children with obesity-related hypertension. *Neuroendocrinol Lett.* 2005;26(3):242–246

9. Lubrano R, Travasso E, Raggi C, Guido G, Masciangelo R, Elli M. Blood pressure load, proteinuria and renal function in pre-hypertensive children. *Pediatr Nephrol.* 2009;24(4):823–831

10. Adams HR, Szilagyi PG, Gebhardt L, Lande MB. Learning and attention problems among children with pediatric primary hypertension. *Pediatrics.* 2010;126(6). Available at: www.pediatrics.org/cgi/content/full/126/6/e1425

11. Bao W, Threefoot SA, Srinivasan SR, Berenson GS. Essential hypertension predicted by tracking of elevated blood pressure from childhood to adulthood: the Bogalusa Heart Study. *Am J Hypertens.* 1995;8(7):657–665

12. Theodore RF, Broadbent J, Nagin D, et al. Childhood to Early-Midlife Systolic Blood Pressure Trajectories: Early-Life Predictors, Effect Modifiers, and Adult Cardiovascular Outcomes. *Hypertension.* 2015;66(6):1108–1115

13. Chen X, Wang Y. Tracking of blood pressure from childhood to adulthood: a systematic review and meta-regression analysis. *Circulation.* 2008;117(25):3171–3180

14. Theodore RF, Broadbent J, Nagin D, et al. Childhood to early-midlife systolic blood pressure trajectories: early-life predictors, effect modifiers, and adult cardiovascular outcomes. *Hypertension.* 2015;66(6):1108–1115

15. Chobanian AV, Bakris GL, Black HR, et al; Joint National Committee on Prevention, Detection, Evaluation, and Treatment of High Blood Pressure; National Heart, Lung, and Blood Institute; National High Blood Pressure Education Program Coordinating Committee. Seventh report of the Joint National Committee on Prevention, Detection, Evaluation, and Treatment of High Blood Pressure. *Hypertension.* 2003;42(6):1206–1252

16. Hansen ML, Gunn PW, Kaelber DC. Underdiagnosis of hypertension in children and adolescents. *JAMA.* 2007;298(8):874–879

17. Kaelber DC, Liu W, Ross M, et al; Comparative Effectiveness Research Through Collaborative Electronic Reporting (CER2) Consortium. Diagnosis and medication treatment of pediatric hypertension: a retrospective cohort study. *Pediatrics.* 2016;138(6):e20162195

18. Din-Dzietham R, Liu Y, Bielo MV, Shamsa F. High blood pressure trends in children and adolescents in national surveys, 1963 to 2002. *Circulation.* 2007;116(13):1488–1496

19. Skinner AC, Perrin EM, Moss LA, Skelton JA. Cardiometabolic risks and severity of obesity in children and young adults. *N Engl J Med.* 2015;373(14):1307–1317

20. Graf C, Rost SV, Koch B, et al. Data from the StEP TWO programme showing the effect on blood pressure and different parameters for obesity in overweight and obese primary school children. *Cardiol Young.* 2005;15(3):291–298

21. Falkner B. Recent clinical and translational advances in pediatric hypertension. *Hypertension.* 2015;65(5):926–931

22. Flynn JT, Mitsnefes M, Pierce C, et al; Chronic Kidney Disease in Children Study Group. Blood pressure in children with chronic kidney disease: a report from the Chronic Kidney Disease in Children study. *Hypertension.* 2008;52(4):631–637

23. Samuels J, Ng D, Flynn JT, et al; Chronic Kidney Disease in Children Study Group. Ambulatory blood pressure patterns in children with chronic kidney disease. *Hypertension.* 2012;60(1):43–50

24. Shatat IF, Flynn JT. Hypertension in children with chronic kidney disease. *Adv Chronic Kidney Dis.* 2005;12(4):378–384

25. Rosner B, Cook N, Portman R, Daniels S, Falkner B. Determination of blood pressure percentiles in normal-weight children: some methodological issues. *Am J Epidemiol.* 2008;167(6):653–666

26. Flynn JT, Urbina EM. Pediatric ambulatory blood pressure monitoring: indications and interpretations. *J Clin Hypertens (Greenwich).* 2012;14(6):372–382

27. Mendeley [computer program]. New York, NY: Elsevier; 2008

28. American Academy of Pediatrics Steering Committee on Quality Improvement and Management. Classifying recommendations for clinical practice guidelines. *Pediatrics.* 2004;114(3):874–877

29. Preferred reporting items for systematic reviews and meta-analyses (PRISMA) web site. Available at: www.prisma-statement.org/. Accessed April 24, 2018

30. Flynn JT, Kaelber DC, Baker-Smith CM; Subcommittee on Screening and Management of High Blood Pressure in Children, et al. Clinical practice guideline for screening and management of high blood pressure in children and adolescents [published correction appears in Pediatrics. 2017;140(6):e20173035]. *Pediatrics.* 2017;140(3):e20171904

31. BRIDGE-Wiz. Available versions of BridgeWiz. Available at: http://gem.med.yale.edu/BRIDGE-Wiz/ . Accessed April 24, 2018

32. BRIDGE-Wiz. Available versions of BridgeWiz. Available at: http://gem.med.yale.edu/BRIDGE-Wiz/. Accessed April 24, 2018

33. Picone DS, Schultz MG, Otahal P, et al. Accuracy of cuff-measured blood pressure: systematic reviews and meta-analyses. *J Am Coll Cardiol.* 2017;70(5):572–586

34. Kent AL, Chaudhari T. Determinants of neonatal blood pressure. *Curr Hypertens Rep.* 2013;15(5):426–432

35. Dionne JM, Abitbol CL, Flynn JT. Hypertension in infancy: diagnosis, management and outcome [published correction appears in *Pediatr Nephrol.* 2012;27(1):159–160]. *Pediatr Nephrol.* 2012;27(1):17–32

36. Flynn JT, Kaelber DC, Baker-Smith CM, et al; Subcommittee on Screening and Management of High Blood Pressure in Children. Clinical practice guideline for screening and management of high blood pressure in children and adolescents [published correction appears in *Pediatrics.* 2017;140(6):e20173035]. *Pediatrics.* 2017;140(3):e20171904

37. Ostchega Y, Prineas RJ, Nwankwo T, Zipf G. Assessing blood pressure accuracy of an aneroid sphygmomanometer in a national survey environment. *Am J Hypertens.* 2011;24(3):322–327

38. Podoll A, Grenier M, Croix B, Feig DI. Inaccuracy in pediatric outpatient blood pressure measurement. *Pediatrics.* 2007;119(3). Available at: www.pediatrics.org/cgi/content/full/119/3/e538

39. Mourad A, Carney S. Arm position and blood pressure: an audit. *Intern Med J.* 2004;34(5):290–291

40. Flynn JT, Pierce CB, Miller ER III, et al; Chronic Kidney Disease in Children Study Group. Reliability of resting blood pressure measurement and classification using an oscillometric device in children with chronic kidney disease. *J Pediatr.* 2012;160(3):434–440.e1

41. Daley MF, Sinaiko AR, Reifler LM, et al. Patterns of care and persistence after incident elevated blood pressure. *Pediatrics.* 2013;132(2). Available at: www.pediatrics.org/cgi/content/full/132/2/e349

42. Becton LJ, Egan BM, Hailpern SM, Shatat IF. Blood pressure reclassification in adolescents based on repeat clinic blood pressure measurements. *J Clin Hypertens (Greenwich).* 2013;15(10):717–722

43. Chiolero A, Cachat F, Burnier M, Paccaud F, Bovet P. Prevalence of hypertension in schoolchildren based on repeated measurements and association with overweight. *J Hypertens.* 2007;25(11):2209–2217

44. Bijlsma MW, Blufpand HN, Kaspers GJ, Bökenkamp A. Why pediatricians fail to diagnose hypertension: a multicenter survey. *J Pediatr.* 2014;164(1):173–177.e7

45. Chaudhry B, Wang J, Wu S, et al. Systematic review: impact of health information technology on quality, efficiency, and costs of medical care. *Ann Intern Med.* 2006;144(10):742–752

46. Shojania KG, Jennings A, Mayhew A, Ramsay CR, Eccles MP, Grimshaw J. The effects of on-screen, point of care

computer reminders on processes and outcomes of care. *Cochrane Database Syst Rev.* 2009;(3):CD001096

47. Furusawa ÉA, Filho UD, Junior DM, Koch VH. Home and ambulatory blood pressure to identify white coat and masked hypertension in the pediatric patient. *Am J Hypertens.* 2011;24(8):893–897

48. Stergiou GS, Alamara CV, Salgami EV, Vaindirlis IN, Dacou-Voutetakis C, Mountokalakis TD. Reproducibility of home and ambulatory blood pressure in children and adolescents. *Blood Press Monit.* 2005;10(3):143–147

49. Patel HP, Mitsnefes M. Advances in the pathogenesis and management of hypertensive crisis. *Curr Opin Pediatr.* 2005;17(2):210–214

50. Flynn JT. Evaluation and management of hypertension in childhood. *Prog Pediatr Cardiol.* 2001;12(2):177–188

51. Seeman T, Dusek J, Vondrichová H, et al. Ambulatory blood pressure correlates with renal volume and number of renal cysts in children with autosomal dominant polycystic kidney disease. *Blood Press Monit.* 2003;8(3):107–110

52. Baracco R, Mattoo TK. Pediatric hypertensive emergencies. *Curr Hypertens Rep.* 2014;16(8):456

53. Markus MR, Stritzke J, Lieb W, et al. Implications of persistent prehypertension for ageing-related changes in left ventricular geometry and function: the MONICA/KORA Augsburg study. *J Hypertens.* 2008;26(10):2040–2049

54. Yuan WL, Kakinami L, Gray-Donald K, Czernichow S, Lambert M, Paradis G. Influence of dairy product consumption on children's blood pressure: results from the QUALITY cohort. *J Acad Nutr Diet.* 2013;113(7):936–941

55. Damasceno MM, de Araújo MF, de Freitas RW, de Almeida PC, Zanetti ML. The association between blood pressure in adolescents and the consumption of fruits, vegetables and fruit juice—an exploratory study. *J Clin Nurs.* 2011;20(11–12):1553–1560

56. Chaturvedi S, Lipszyc DH, Licht C, Craig JC, Parekh R. Pharmacological interventions for hypertension in children. *Evid Based Child Health.* 2014;9(3):498–580

57. Kim N, Seo DC, King MH, Lederer AM, Sovinski D. Long-term predictors of blood pressure among adolescents during an 18-month school-based obesity prevention intervention. *J Adolesc Health.* 2014;55(4):521–527

58. Eunice Kennedy Shriver National Institutes of Child Health and Human Development. Best Pharmaceuticals for Children Act (BPCA). Available at: https://bpca.nichd.nih.gov/about/Pages/default.aspx. Accessed April 24, 2018

59. Chan EK, Quach J, Mensah FK, Sung V, Cheung M, Wake M. Dark chocolate for children's blood pressure: randomised trial. *Arch Dis Child.* 2012;97(7):637–640

60. Ried K, Frank OR, Stocks NP. Aged garlic extract lowers blood pressure in patients with treated but uncontrolled hypertension: a randomised controlled trial. *Maturitas.* 2010;67(2):144–150

61. Davison K, Berry NM, Misan G, Coates AM, Buckley JD, Howe PR. Dose-related effects of flavanol-rich cocoa on blood pressure. *J Hum Hypertens.* 2010;24(9):568–576

62. Coles LT, Clifton PM. Effect of beetroot juice on lowering blood pressure in free-living, disease-free adults: a randomized, placebo-controlled trial. *Nutr J.* 2012;11:106

63. He J, Streiffer RH, Muntner P, Krousel-Wood MA, Whelton PK. Effect of dietary fiber intake on blood pressure: a randomized, double-blind, placebo-controlled trial. *J Hypertens.* 2004;22(1):73–80

64. He J, Wofford MR, Reynolds K, et al. Effect of dietary protein supplementation on blood pressure: a randomized, controlled trial. *Circulation.* 2011;124(5):589–595

65. Ashraf R, Khan RA, Ashraf I, Qureshi AA. Effects of Allium sativum (garlic) on systolic and diastolic blood pressure in patients with essential hypertension. *Pak J Pharm Sci.* 2013;26(5):859–863

66. Ramel A, Martinez JA, Kiely M, Bandarra NM, Thorsdottir I. Moderate consumption of fatty fish reduces diastolic blood pressure in overweight and obese European young adults during energy restriction. *Nutrition.* 2010;26(2):168–174

67. Litwin M, Grenda R, Sladowska J, Antoniewicz J. Add-on therapy with angiotensin II receptor 1 blocker in children with chronic kidney disease already treated with angiotensin-converting enzyme inhibitors. *Pediatr Nephrol.* 2006;21(11):1716–1722

68. Ellis D, Moritz ML, Vats A, Janosky JE. Antihypertensive and renoprotective efficacy and safety of losartan. A long-term study in children with renal disorders. *Am J Hypertens.* 2004;17(10):928–935

69. Neutel JM, Rotenberg K. Comparison of a chronotherapeutically administered beta blocker vs. a traditionally administered beta blocker in patients with hypertension. *J Clin Hypertens (Greenwich).* 2005;7(7):395–400; quiz 401–402

70. Izzo JL Jr, Purkayastha D, Hall D, Hilkert RJ. Comparative efficacy and safety of amlodipine/benazepril combination therapy and amlodipine monotherapy in severe hypertension. *J Hum Hypertens.* 2010;24(6):403–409

71. Beitelshees AL, Gong Y, Bailey KR, et al. Comparison of office, ambulatory, and home blood pressure antihypertensive response to atenolol and hydrochlorthiazide. *J Clin Hypertens (Greenwich).* 2010;12(1):14–21

72. Asmar R, Oparil S. Comparison of the antihypertensive efficacy of irbesartan/HCTZ and valsartan/HCTZ combination therapy: impact of age and gender. *Clin Exp Hypertens.* 2010;32(8):499–503

73. Matsui Y, Eguchi K, O'Rourke MF, et al. Differential effects between a calcium channel blocker and a diuretic when used in combination with angiotensin II receptor blocker on central aortic pressure in hypertensive patients. *Hypertension.* 2009;54(4):716–723

74. Bakris GL, Iyengar M, Lukas MA, Ordronneau P, Weber MA. Effect of combining extended-release carvedilol and lisinopril in hypertension: results of the COSMOS study. *J Clin Hypertens (Greenwich).* 2010;12(9):678–686

75. Franks AM, O'Brien CE, Stowe CD, Wells TG, Gardner SF. Candesartan cilexetil effectively reduces blood

pressure in hypertensive children. *Ann Pharmacother*. 2008;42(10):1388–1395

76. Hoy SM, Keating GM. Candesartan cilexetil: in children and adolescents aged 1 to <17 years with hypertension. *Am J Cardiovasc Drugs*. 2010;10(5):335–342

77. Schachter J, Kuller LH, Perfetti C. Blood pressure during the first five years of life: relation to ethnic group (black or white) and to parental hypertension. *Am J Epidemiol*. 1984;119(4):541–553

78. Barón AE, Freyer B, Fixler DE. Longitudinal blood pressures in blacks, whites, and Mexican Americans during adolescence and early adulthood. *Am J Epidemiol*. 1986;123(5):809–817

79. Voors AW, Foster TA, Frerichs RR, Webber LS, Berenson GS. Studies of blood pressures in children, ages 5-14 years, in a total biracial community: the Bogalusa Heart Study. *Circulation*. 1976;54(2):319–327

80. Gutgesell M, Terrell G, Labarthe D. Pediatric blood pressure: ethnic comparisons in a primary care center. *Hypertension*. 1981;3(1):39–47

81. Fixler DE, Laird WP. Validity of mass blood pressure screening in children. *Pediatrics*. 1983;72(4):459–463

82. Clarke WR, Schrott HG, Leaverton PE, Connor WE, Lauer RM. Tracking of blood lipids and blood pressures in school age children: the Muscatine study. *Circulation*. 1978;58(4):626–634

83. Lauer RM, Clarke WR, Beaglehole R. Level, trend, and variability of blood pressure during childhood: the Muscatine study. *Circulation*. 1984;69(2):242–249

84. McGarvey ST, Zinner SH, Willett WC, Rosner B. Maternal prenatal dietary potassium, calcium, magnesium, and infant blood pressure. *Hypertension*. 1991;17(2):218–224

85. Gómez-Marín O, Prineas RJ, Sinaiko AR. The sodium-potassium blood pressure trial in children. Design, recruitment, and randomization: the children and adolescent blood pressure program. *Control Clin Trials*. 1991;12(3):408–423

86. Lackland DT, Riopel DA, Shepard DM, et al. *Blood Pressure and Anthropometric Measurement Results of the South Carolina Dental Health and Pediatric Blood Pressure Study*. Columbia, SC: South Carolina Department of Health and Environmental Control; 1985

87. Rosner B, Cook N, Portman R, Daniels S, Falkner B. Determination of blood pressure percentiles in normal-weight children: some methodological issues. *Am J Epidemiol*. 2008;167(6):653–666

88. Rosner B. Pediatric blood pressure. Available at: http://sites.google.com/a/channing.harvard.edu/bernardrosner/pediatric-blood-press. Accessed March 1, 2018

89. Kaelber DC, Pickett F. Simple table to identify children and adolescents needing further evaluation of blood pressure. *Pediatrics*. 2009;123(6). Available at: www.pediatrics.org/cgi/content/full/123/6/e972

90. Whelton PK, Carey RM, Aranow WS, et al. 2017 ACC/AHA/AAPA/ABC/ACPM/AGS/APhA/ASH/ASPC/NMA/PCNA guideline for the prevention, detection, evaluation, and management of high blood pressure in adults: executive summary: a report of the American College of Cardiology/American Heart Association Task Force on Clinical Practice Guidelines. *Hypertension*. 2018;71(6):1269–1324

91. Urbina EM, Gidding SS, Bao W, Pickoff AS, Berdusis K, Berenson GS. Effect of body size, ponderosity, and blood pressure on left ventricular growth in children and young adults in the Bogalusa Heart Study. *Circulation*. 1995;91(9):2400–2406

92. Kuznetsova T, Haddad F, Tikhonoff V, et al; European Project on Genes in Hypertension (EPOGH) Investigators. Impact and pitfalls of scaling of left ventricular and atrial structure in population-based studies. *J Hypertens*. 2016;34(6):1186–1194

93. Armstrong AC, Gidding S, Gjesdal O, Wu C, Bluemke DA, Lima JA. LV mass assessed by echocardiography and CMR, cardiovascular outcomes, and medical practice. *JACC Cardiovasc Imaging*. 2012;5(8):837–848

94. Armstrong AC, Jacobs DR Jr, Gidding SS, et al. Framingham score and LV mass predict events in young adults: CARDIA study. *Int J Cardiol*. 2014;172(2):350–355

95. Gidding SS, Palermo RA, DeLoach SS, Keith SW, Falkner B. Associations of cardiac structure with obesity, blood pressure, inflammation, and insulin resistance in African-American adolescents. *Pediatr Cardiol*. 2014;35(2):307–314

96. Hanevold C, Waller J, Daniels S, Portman R, Sorof J; International Pediatric Hypertension Association. The effects of obesity, gender, and ethnic group on left ventricular hypertrophy and geometry in hypertensive children: a collaborative study of the International Pediatric Hypertension Association [published correction appears in *Pediatrics*. 2005;115(4):1118]. *Pediatrics*. 2004;113(2):328–333

97. Daniels SR, Loggie JM, Khoury P, Kimball TR. Left ventricular geometry and severe left ventricular hypertrophy in children and adolescents with essential hypertension. *Circulation*. 1998;97(19):1907–1911

98. Lang RM, Badano LP, Mor-Avi V, et al. Recommendations for cardiac chamber quantification by echocardiography in adults: an update from the American Society of Echocardiography and the European Association of Cardiovascular Imaging. *J Am Soc Echocardiogr*. 2015;28(1):1–39.e14

99. Daniels SR, Kimball TR, Morrison JA, Khoury P, Witt S, Meyer RA. Effect of lean body mass, fat mass, blood pressure, and sexual maturation on left ventricular mass in children and adolescents. Statistical, biological, and clinical significance. *Circulation*. 1995;92(11):3249–3254

100. de Simone G, Devereux RB, Daniels SR, Koren MJ, Meyer RA, Laragh JH. Effect of growth on variability of left ventricular mass: assessment of allometric signals in adults and children and their capacity to predict cardiovascular risk. *J Am Coll Cardiol*. 1995;25(5):1056–1062

101. Foster BJ, Khoury PR, Kimball TR, Mackie AS, Mitsnefes M. New reference centiles for left ventricular mass relative to lean body mass in children. *J Am Soc Echocardiogr*. 2016;29(5):441–447.e2

102. Khoury PR, Mitsnefes M, Daniels SR, Kimball TR. Age-specific reference intervals for indexed left ventricular mass in children. *J Am Soc Echocardiogr*. 2009;22(6):709–714

Diagnosis and Management of Gastroesophageal Reflux in Preterm Infants

- *Clinical Report*

CLINICAL REPORT   Guidance for the Clinician in Rendering Pediatric Care

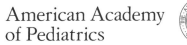

American Academy
of Pediatrics

DEDICATED TO THE HEALTH OF ALL CHILDREN™

Diagnosis and Management of Gastroesophageal Reflux in Preterm Infants

Eric C. Eichenwald, MD, FAAP, COMMITTEE ON FETUS AND NEWBORN

abstract

Gastroesophageal reflux (GER), generally defined as the passage of gastric contents into the esophagus, is an almost universal phenomenon in preterm infants. It is a common diagnosis in the NICU; however, there is large variation in its treatment across NICU sites. In this clinical report, the physiology, diagnosis, and symptomatology in preterm infants as well as currently used treatment strategies in the NICU are examined. Conservative measures to control reflux, such as left lateral body position, head elevation, and feeding regimen manipulation, have not been shown to reduce clinically assessed signs of GER in the preterm infant. In addition, preterm infants with clinically diagnosed GER are often treated with pharmacologic agents; however, a lack of evidence of efficacy together with emerging evidence of significant harm (particularly with gastric acid blockade) strongly suggest that these agents should be used sparingly, if at all, in preterm infants.

Department of Pediatrics, Children's Hospital of Philadelphia, Philadelphia, Pennsylvania

Dr Eichenwald is the primary author of the policy and approved the final manuscript as submitted.

This document is copyrighted and is property of the American Academy of Pediatrics and its Board of Directors. All authors have filed conflict of interest statements with the American Academy of Pediatrics. Any conflicts have been resolved through a process approved by the Board of Directors. The American Academy of Pediatrics has neither solicited nor accepted any commercial involvement in the development of the content of this publication.

Clinical reports from the American Academy of Pediatrics benefit from expertise and resources of liaisons and internal (AAP) and external reviewers. However, clinical reports from the American Academy of Pediatrics may not reflect the views of the liaisons or the organizations or government agencies that they represent.

The guidance in this report does not indicate an exclusive course of treatment or serve as a standard of medical care. Variations, taking into account individual circumstances, may be appropriate.

All clinical reports from the American Academy of Pediatrics automatically expire 5 years after publication unless reaffirmed, revised, or retired at or before that time.

DOI: https://doi.org/10.1542/peds.2018-1061

Address correspondence to Eric C. Eichenwald, MD, FAAP. E-mail: eichenwald@email.chop.edu

PEDIATRICS (ISSN Numbers: Print, 0031-4005; Online, 1098-4275).

Copyright © 2018 by the American Academy of Pediatrics

FINANCIAL DISCLOSURE: The author has indicated he has no financial relationships relevant to this article to disclose.

To cite: Eichenwald EC and AAP COMMITTEE ON FETUS AND NEWBORN. Diagnosis and Management of Gastroesophageal Reflux in Preterm Infants. *Pediatrics.* 2018;142(1):e20181061

INTRODUCTION

Gastroesophageal reflux (GER), generally defined as the passage of gastric contents into the esophagus,[1] is an almost universal phenomenon in preterm infants. The normal physiologic occurrence of GER in infants can be distinguished from pathologic GER disease, which includes troublesome symptoms or complications associated with GER.[2] GER occurs commonly in infants, in part because of relatively large volumes ingested during feeding and supine positioning, which frequently place the gastroesophageal junction in a liquid environment. Whether GER becomes clinically significant depends on both the quality (eg, degree of acidity) and quantity of reflux[3,4] as well as potential injury to the esophageal mucosa. GER is a common diagnosis in the NICU; however, there is as much as a 13-fold variation in its diagnosis and treatment across sites.[5,6] Preterm infants who are diagnosed with GER have longer hospital stays and higher hospital costs than infants without GER,[5,7,8] making it an important clinical phenomenon in the NICU.

GER in preterm infants is most often diagnosed and treated on the basis of clinical and behavioral signs rather than on specific testing to prove or disprove pathology,[6] and many infants continue to be treated after they are discharged from the hospital.[9] However, evidence that GER causes harm in preterm infants is scant.[10,11] Indeed, routine use of antireflux medications for the treatment of symptomatic GER in preterm infants was 1 of the therapies singled out as being of questionable value in the recent American Academy of Pediatrics (AAP) Choosing Wisely campaign.[12]

In this clinical report, the following will be reviewed: (1) the physiology of GER in preterm infants, (2) methods for its diagnosis, (3) evidence that it is associated with the signs frequently attributed to GER, and (4) the safety and efficacy of nonpharmacologic and pharmacologic therapy.

PHYSIOLOGY

The primary mechanism of GER in preterm infants is transient lower esophageal sphincter relaxation (TLESR). TLESR is an abrupt reflex decrease in lower esophageal sphincter (LES) pressure to levels at or below intragastric pressure, unrelated to swallowing. Preterm infants have dozens of episodes of TLESR each day,[13] many of which are associated with some degree of GER. As such, GER is a normal phenomenon in preterm infants, which is exacerbated by a pure liquid diet and age-specific body position.[3] In addition, the presence of an indwelling gastric tube through the esophageal sphincter increases the frequency of GER, presumably secondary to impaired closure of the LES.[14] Delayed gastric emptying does not appear to play a contributory role in GER in preterm infants, in that infants with symptomatic GER do not have delayed gastric emptying

compared with other infants.[15,16] However, GER is more common immediately after a feeding, likely because of gastric distension.[15] Body position also influences TLESR and GER in preterm infants. Infants placed in the right-side-down lateral position after a feeding have more TLESR episodes and liquid reflux compared with the left-side-down lateral position, despite gastric emptying being enhanced in the right lateral position.[17,18] Prone position also decreases episodes of GER versus supine position, likely because of more optimal positioning of the LES relative to the distended stomach.[17]

Mechanisms to protect the esophagus and airway from GER appear to be intact in the preterm infant. These include reflex forward peristalsis of the esophagus in response to distention from refluxate in the lower esophagus with closure of the upper esophageal sphincter to prevent refluxate reaching the pharynx. Despite these mechanisms, if refluxed material does reach the upper esophagus, the upper esophageal sphincter will reflexively open to allow the material into the pharynx, which results in the frequent episodes of "spitting" or emesis observed in infants.

DIAGNOSIS

Several methods have been used to diagnose GER in the preterm population, including contrast fluoroscopy, pH monitoring, and multichannel intraesophageal impedance (MII) monitoring. Although contrast fluoroscopy can be used to show episodes of reflux, it cannot be used to differentiate clinically significant GER from insignificant GER. Monitoring of pH in the lower esophagus has classically been used to diagnose GER in older children and adults. Reflux of acidic gastric contents results in transient periods of acidity in the

lower esophagus. Common measures obtained from pH probe monitoring include the total number of reflux episodes, the duration of the longest reflux episode, and the "reflux index" (RI), which is the percentage of the total recording time with an esophageal pH <4. In pH studies, an RI >7% is considered abnormal, an RI <3% considered normal, and RIs between 3% and 7% are considered indeterminate.[2] However, labeling a study "abnormal" does not prove that it is causing the symptoms in question.

Measurement of esophageal pH is not a reliable method to diagnose GER in preterm infants[19] because their stomach pH is rarely <4 owing to frequent milk feedings and a higher baseline pH. In addition, abnormal esophageal pH does not correlate well with symptom severity.[20] Other measures that have been investigated include the presence of pepsin in saliva[21] and the pH of oropharyngeal secretions.[22] Although these measures may correlate with acidic reflux, it is unknown whether they correlate with symptom severity.

Currently, the most accurate method for detecting GER is MII monitoring, which is frequently combined with simultaneous measurement of pH.[2] MII can be used to track the movement of fluids, solids, and air in the esophagus by measuring changes in electrical impedance between multiple electrodes along an esophageal catheter. MII can be used to discern whether a fluid bolus is traveling antegrade (swallow) or retrograde (reflux) in the esophagus and can be used to determine the height of the retrograde bolus. It is a reliable and reproducible technique for diagnosing GER in preterm infants[14] and can be combined with a pH sensor to determine if GER is acidic, mildly acidic, or alkaline. López-Alonso et al[23] measured 24-hour MII and pH in 26 healthy preterm infants with a median postmenstrual age of 32 weeks.

The median number of reflux episodes recorded in 24 hours was 71; 25.4% were acidic, 72.9% were weakly acidic, and 2.7% were alkaline. Of note, the gastric pH was higher than 4 for almost 70% of the recording time. Not surprisingly, periods of feeding were associated with a higher number of total reflux events per hour.

In practice, GER is diagnosed most often in infants on the basis of clinical and behavioral signs and/or response to a trial of pharmacologic or nonpharmacologic interventions.[6] Signs attributed to GER include feeding intolerance, poor growth, apnea, desaturation and bradycardia, and worsening pulmonary disease as well as nonspecific behavioral signs including arching, irritability, and apparent discomfort associated with feedings. There is no evidence, however, that these signs are temporally associated with measured GER episodes.[20,24,25] In 1 study of 40 preterm and 18 term infants evaluated with combined MII/pH testing for a clinical suspicion of GER, signs (including irritability, bradycardia and desaturations, or feeding intolerance) were rarely associated with documented reflux events.[20] In another study of 14 healthy preterm infants, Snel et al[24] recorded both esophageal pH and infant behaviors. General behavior scores did not change during esophageal acidification episodes. In addition, infants frequently demonstrated behaviors ascribed to GER (apparent discomfort, head retraction, and "mouthing") unrelated to pH-documented GER episodes. In these results, it is suggested that preterm infant behaviors commonly ascribed to reflux are, in reality, not associated with GER and that treatment should not be based solely on clinical signs.

GER IN THE PRETERM INFANT

Several clinical conditions are thought to be associated with GER in the preterm infant, although analyses are hampered because most cases of GER are diagnosed clinically.

Apnea, Desaturation, and Bradycardia

Preterm infants have a hyperreactive laryngeal response to chemoreceptor stimulation that precipitates apnea or bradycardia. In addition, as previously noted, almost all preterm infants have some GER. These 2 observations have led to speculation that GER can precipitate apnea, oxygen desaturation, and bradycardia episodes in preterm infants and that pharmacologic treatment of GER might decrease the incidence or severity of these events.[26] However, researchers examining the timing of reflux episodes in relation to apneic events have found that they are rarely temporally related[14,27] and that GER does not prolong or worsen apnea.[28] In 1 study, small amounts of normal saline were infused into the pharynx of sleeping preterm infants at term-equivalent age. The investigators found that swallow frequency increased, but apnea did not occur,[29] and they suggested that apnea is provoked when the larynx, not the pharynx, is stimulated. The larynx is not usually stimulated by reflux of small amounts of liquid. Finally, there is no evidence that pharmacologic treatment of GER with agents that decrease gastric acidity or promote gastrointestinal motility decrease the risk of recurrent apnea or bradycardia in preterm infants.[30,31]

Respiratory Disease and Bronchopulmonary Dysplasia

Proving a causal relationship between GER and respiratory symptoms in children has been difficult. Suggested methods of diagnostics, such as GER scintigraphy and the presence of lipid-laden macrophages in bronchoalveolar lavage, lack specificity[32] or correlate poorly with esophageal impedance and fail to differentiate reflux-related

aspiration from primary aspiration from above.[33] In 1 study, children with a heterogeneous array of chronic lung problems who had documented GER had higher concentrations of pepsin and inflammatory interleukins in their bronchoalveolar lavage fluid than those without GER, suggesting microaspiration may contribute to their lung disease.[34]

It is not clear whether GER causes "silent" microaspiration in mechanically ventilated preterm infants that worsens lung disease, particularly in infants with developing or established bronchopulmonary dysplasia (BPD). In 1 study, it was reported that pepsin was detected in 93% of tracheal aspirates obtained from intubated preterm infants during the first postnatal month,[35] and in addition, that ventilated preterm infants who developed BPD had higher levels of tracheal aspirate pepsin than those who did not. In addition, these investigators reported that increased concentrations of pepsin were associated with increased severity of BPD[36] and speculated that chronic aspiration of gastric contents may contribute to the development of BPD. However, these results should be interpreted with caution because of emerging data on the low sensitivity and specificity of pepsin in bronchoalveolar lavage assays for the detection of GER-related aspiration.[37]

In contrast, Akinola et al[38] reported no relationship between the diagnosis of BPD and the clinical diagnosis of GER confirmed by esophageal pH monitoring.[38] In a small study comparing combined MII and pH monitoring in 12 infants with BPD and 34 without who were evaluated for clinical signs believed to be attributable to GER, infants with BPD had a similar number of documented reflux events as infants without BPD.[25] In both groups, fewer than 10% of the documented reflux events were temporally associated with reflux symptoms as assessed by nursing observation. However, infants with BPD were more likely to have "pH only events" (acidic pH in the lower esophagus without an associated MII determined reflux event), which were more often associated with symptoms, but at a low frequency (9% vs 4.9% in infants without BPD). Although infants with evolving BPD are more likely to have a diagnosis of and receive therapy for GER,[39] with these results, it is suggested that these infants do not have an increased incidence of symptomatic GER.

Feeding Problems

Some infants and children with GER may exhibit feeding problems, including feeding resistance, failure to thrive, or food aversion.[40,41] Although preterm infants may have frequent regurgitation, there is no evidence that this leads to poor growth or other nutritional difficulties.[7,42] Although preterm infants with a diagnosis of GER are sometimes treated with prokinetic agents to enhance gastric emptying,[6] there are no data to suggest that delayed gastric emptying is a physiologic mechanism for GER in this population.[15] As noted previously, other feeding-related behaviors in preterm infants often attributed to GER, including feeding-associated arching or irritability and oral feeding aversion, are not temporally associated with MII or lower pH documented reflux events and, thus, are not reliable markers of clinically significant reflux.[20,24]

TREATMENT

Although preterm infants frequently receive nonpharmacologic and pharmacologic therapy for GER, there is a paucity of data about the effect of treatment on symptoms or short- and long-term outcomes. Furthermore, the lack of randomized

placebo-controlled trials of GER therapies in preterm infants makes it difficult to assess the efficacy of long-term therapy versus the expected natural history of GER. Despite the lack of data, in recent years, the use of antireflux medications both in the NICU and after discharge has substantially increased.[9,43]

Nonpharmacologic Management

Body Positioning

Body positioning is widely used as a conservative management approach to infants believed to have GER. Placing infants on a head-up angle is a common initial approach to management; however, head elevation is ineffective in reducing acid reflux in older infants. In addition, car seat placement was found to elicit worse acid GER in term infants.[44–46] This position has not been studied in preterm infants to prevent symptomatic GER, but there is no reason to expect the physiologic result would be different from term infants. Placing preterm infants in the left lateral versus right lateral position after feeding and in prone versus supine position may reduce TLESRs and reflux episodes.[15,17,18] However, although placement in the right lateral position may increase reflux episodes after feeding, van Wijk et al[18] showed that this position also enhanced gastric emptying. These authors suggested placing infants in the right lateral position immediately after feeding, followed in 1 hour by placing them in the left lateral position to decrease acid reflux. However, 1 small MII and pH study of term infants at a mean postnatal age of 13 weeks revealed that, despite a reduction in reflux episodes in the left lateral position, behavioral manifestations of reflux (crying and/or irritability) did not improve.[47] Thus, whether positioning techniques can reduce signs of GER in infants with reflux remains uncertain. Given that lateral and prone positioning also

increase the risk of sudden infant death syndrome (SIDS),[48] the AAP and the North American Society for Pediatric Gastroenterology and Nutrition have concurred that infants with GER should be placed for sleep in the supine position, with the exception of the rare infants for whom the risk of death from GER is greater than the risk of SIDS.[2] The AAP Task Force on SIDS, after conferring with the authors of the North American Society for Pediatric Gastroenterology and Nutrition statement, provided additional guidance: "Examples of such upper airway disorders are those in which airway-protective mechanisms are impaired, including infants with anatomic abnormalities, such as type 3 or 4 laryngeal clefts, who have not undergone antireflux surgery."[48] Safe sleep approaches, including supine positioning on a flat and firm surface and avoidance of commercial devices designed to maintain head elevation in the crib, should be paramount as a model for parents of infants approaching discharge (ie, infants greater than 32 weeks' postmenstrual age) from the hospital.[49]

Feeding Strategies

If GER results from increased intragastric pressure, smaller-volume feedings given more frequently might result in fewer GER episodes. Omari et al[15] reported that feeding hourly, compared with feeding every 2 or 3 hours, resulted in fewer total GER episodes but more frequent acidic reflux episodes. Jadcherla et al[50] reported that longer feeding duration and slower milk flow rates were associated with fewer GER events, diagnosed by MII and pH study, although nutrient composition of expressed human milk may be compromised with this approach. No randomized trials have been used to compare the effects of continuous intragastric or transpyloric versus bolus intragastric tube feedings on GER symptom severity.[51]

Another feeding strategy has been to thicken feedings with agents including xanthan gum, starch, or rice cereal.[52] Unfortunately, in recent data, researchers have linked thickening with a xanthan gum product to late-onset necrotizing enterocolitis[53]; as such, it is recommended that xanthan gum or similar thickeners not be used in preterm or former preterm infants in the first year of life. Commercially available formula products that thicken on acidification in the stomach are not nutritionally appropriate for preterm infants. A systematic review of randomized controlled trials of thickened formulas in term infants with GER revealed that although these agents reduced episodes of regurgitation, they were ineffective in reducing acidic GER.[54] Only small trials of thickeners have been performed in the preterm population. In 1 trial of a starch-thickened preterm formula, the total number of GER episodes was unchanged compared with a standard formula feeding; however, total lower esophageal acid exposure was less with the thickened formula feeding. No assessment was made about whether the reduction in acid exposure had an effect on associated symptoms.[55]

In the data, it is suggested that elemental or extensively hydrolyzed protein formulas reduce gastrointestinal transit time and reduce symptoms in term infants with symptomatic GER.[56] These observations in term infants may be an overlap of signs of cow milk protein allergy and those attributed to GER, including vomiting, failure to thrive, and irritability.[57] In contrast, in small studies of preterm infants, although feeding with extensively hydrolyzed protein formula compared with standard formula or human milk resulted in fewer reflux episodes as measured by MII and pH study,[58,59] it did not reduce behavioral signs of GER.[59]

It is unclear what role cow milk protein allergy may play in preterm infants with signs of GER; a trial of extensively hydrolyzed protein-based formula may be reasonable in age-appropriate preterm infants with signs of severe reflux.

Pharmacologic Management

Prokinetic Agents

Prokinetic (promotility) agents include metoclopramide, domperidone, and erythromycin. Prokinetic agents have been widely used in older infants to reduce the symptoms of GER. These drugs appear to improve gastric emptying, reduce regurgitation, and enhance LES tone. None of these drugs has been shown to reduce GER symptoms in preterm infants,[60,61] and all have the potential for significant adverse effects, including a higher risk of infantile pyloric stenosis (erythromycin), cardiac arrhythmia (erythromycin), and neurologic side effects (domperidone and metoclopramide). Because of a lack of data about efficacy and a concerning safety profile, these drugs should not be used in preterm infants if the only indication is the treatment of GER.

Sodium Alginate

In older infants and children, researchers in several studies have revealed that alginate-containing formulations, which are frequently combined with sodium bicarbonate, may reduce the symptoms of GER.[61] In the presence of gastric acid, alginate formulations precipitate into a low-density viscous gel that acts as a physical barrier to the gastric mucosa; when combined with sodium bicarbonate (Gaviscon), a carbon dioxide foam forms, which preferentially is refluxed into the esophagus during GER events, protecting the lower esophagus from acidification. In preterm infants in small studies, sodium alginate preparations decreased the number of acidic GER episodes and

total esophageal acid exposure[62] and decreased the frequency of regurgitation.[63] However, the long-term safety of these preparations in preterm infants has not been evaluated.

Histamine-2 Receptor Blockers

Histamine-2 (H_2) receptor blockers (eg, ranitidine, famotidine) compete with histamine for the H_2 receptor in the parietal cells in the stomach, decreasing hydrochloric acid secretion and increasing intragastric pH. H_2 receptor blockers are frequently prescribed for infants in whom GER is clinically diagnosed[6,9] on the theory that these symptoms are secondary to acidic reflux into the lower esophagus. However, no researchers have assessed the efficacy of H_2 blockers on the symptom profile of preterm infants with presumed reflux. In addition, use of these drugs in preterm infants has been linked to an increased incidence of necrotizing enterocolitis in several studies[64] and a higher incidence of late-onset infections and death,[65] possibly resulting from alteration of the intestinal microbiome.[66]

Proton Pump Inhibitors

Proton pump inhibitors (PPIs) block the gastric proton pump, decreasing both basal and stimulated parietal cell acid secretion. PPIs in older children have been associated with a higher risk of gastric bacterial overgrowth, gastroenteritis, and community-acquired pneumonia.[67–69] PPIs are used less often than H_2 blockers in preterm infants but are used for similar indications.[9] Given their effect on gastric acid secretion, it is likely that PPIs would have similar potential adverse effects as H_2 blockers, although this has not been investigated. Although there is evidence that administration of PPIs will consistently maintain the stomach pH >4 in preterm infants, they are largely ineffective in relieving clinical signs of GER. In randomized double-blind placebo-controlled trials, both omeprazole and lansoprazole were ineffective in reducing GER signs in infants. In addition, lansoprazole was associated with a higher rate of adverse events.[70]

SUMMARY AND RECOMMENDATIONS

1. GER is almost universal in preterm infants. It is a physiologic process secondary to frequent TLESR, relatively large-volume liquid diet, and age-specific body positioning. As such, it is a normal developmental phenomenon that will resolve with maturation.

2. Pathologic GER occurs when reflux of acidic gastric contents causes injury to the lower esophageal mucosa. Although preterm infants do have some acidic GER episodes, most GER episodes in this population are only weakly acidic because of their lower gastric acidity and frequent milk feedings, making such esophageal injury unlikely to occur.

3. Signs commonly ascribed to GER in preterm infants include feeding intolerance or aversion, poor weight gain, frequent regurgitation, apnea, and desaturation and bradycardia and behavioral signs, including irritability and perceived postprandial discomfort. In the data, the temporal association of these perceived signs of GER with either acidic or nonacidic reflux episodes as measured by MII and pH is not supported, and the signs will usually improve with time without treatment.

4. Data regarding the possible association between worsening lung disease attributable to GER and microaspiration in mechanically ventilated preterm infants are sparse. Further studies to elucidate such an association and to assess the effect of GER treatment on the severity of lung disease are needed.

5. There is marked variability in the diagnosis and treatment of GER in preterm infants among NICUs, perhaps because the diagnosis is usually made by clinical assessment of signs and symptoms and/or a trial of nonpharmacologic or pharmacologic treatment rather than definitive tests.

6. Conservative measures to control reflux, such as left lateral body position, head elevation, and feeding regimen manipulation, have not been shown to reduce clinically assessed signs of GER in the preterm infant; for infants greater than 32 weeks' postmenstrual age, safe sleep approaches, including supine positioning on a flat and firm surface and avoidance of commercial devices designed to maintain head elevation in the crib, should be paramount as a model for parents of infants approaching discharge from the hospital.

7. Preterm infants with clinically diagnosed GER are often treated with pharmacologic agents; however, a lack of evidence of efficacy together with emerging evidence of significant harm (particularly with gastric acid blockade) strongly suggest that these agents should be used sparingly, if at all, in preterm infants.

LEAD AUTHOR

Eric C. Eichenwald, MD, FAAP

COMMITTEE ON FETUS AND NEWBORN, 2017–2018

James J. Cummings, MD, FAAP, Chairperson
Susan Wright Aucott, MD, FAAP
Eric C. Eichenwald, MD, FAAP
Jay P. Goldsmith, MD, FAAP
Ivan L. Hand, MD, FAAP
Sandra E. Juul, MD, PhD, FAAP
Brenda Bradley Poindexter, MD, MS, FAAP
Karen M. Puopolo, MD, PhD, FAAP
Dan L. Stewart, MD, FAAP

LIAISONS

RADM Wanda D. Barfield, MD, MPH, FAAP – *Centers for Disease Control and Prevention*
Thierry Lacaze, MD – *Canadian Paediatric Society*
Maria A. Mascola, MD – *American College of Obstetricians and Gynecologists*
Meredith Mowitz, MD, MS, FAAP – *Section on Neonatal-Perinatal Medicine*
Tonse N. K. Raju, MD, DCH, FAAP – *National Institutes of Health*

STAFF

Jim Couto, MA

ABBREVIATIONS

AAP: American Academy of Pediatrics
BPD: bronchopulmonary dysplasia
GER: gastroesophageal reflux
H_2: histamine-2
LES: lower esophageal sphincter
MII: multichannel intraesophageal impedance
PPI: proton pump inhibitor
RI: reflux index
SIDS: sudden infant death syndrome
TLESR: transient lower esophageal sphincter relaxation

FUNDING: No external funding.

POTENTIAL CONFLICT OF INTEREST: The author has indicated he has no potential conflicts of interest to disclose.

REFERENCES

1. Lightdale JR, Gremse DA; Section on Gastroenterology, Hepatology, and Nutrition. Gastroesophageal reflux: management guidance for the pediatrician. *Pediatrics*. 2013;131(5). Available at: www.pediatrics.org/cgi/content/full/131/5/e1684

2. Vandenplas Y, Rudolph CD, Di Lorenzo C, et al; North American Society for Pediatric Gastroenterology Hepatology and Nutrition; European Society for Pediatric Gastroenterology Hepatology and Nutrition. Pediatric gastroesophageal reflux clinical practice guidelines: joint recommendations of the North American Society for Pediatric Gastroenterology, Hepatology, and Nutrition (NASPGHAN) and the European Society for Pediatric Gastroenterology, Hepatology, and Nutrition (ESPGHAN). *J Pediatr Gastroenterol Nutr*. 2009;49(4):498–547

3. Poets CF. Gastroesophageal reflux: a critical review of its role in preterm infants. *Pediatrics*. 2004;113(2). Available at: www.pediatrics.org/cgi/content/full/113/2/e128

4. Poets CF, Brockmann PE. Myth: gastroesophageal reflux is a pathological entity in the preterm infant. *Semin Fetal Neonatal Med*. 2011;16(5):259–263

5. Jadcherla SR, Slaughter JL, Stenger MR, Klebanoff M, Kelleher K, Gardner W. Practice variance, prevalence, and economic burden of premature infants diagnosed with GERD. *Hosp Pediatr*. 2013;3(4):335–341

6. Dhillon AS, Ewer AK. Diagnosis and management of gastro-oesophageal reflux in preterm infants in neonatal intensive care units. *Acta Paediatr*. 2004;93(1):88–93

7. Khalaf MN, Porat R, Brodsky NL, Bhandari V. Clinical correlations in infants in the neonatal intensive care unit with varying severity of gastroesophageal reflux. *J Pediatr Gastroenterol Nutr*. 2001;32(1):45–49

8. Ferlauto JJ, Walker MW, Martin MS. Clinically significant gastroesophageal reflux in the at-risk premature neonate: relation to cognitive scores, days in the NICU, and total hospital charges. *J Perinatol*. 1998;18(6, pt 1):455–459

9. Slaughter JL, Stenger MR, Reagan PB, Jadcherla SR. Neonatal histamine-2 receptor antagonist and proton pump inhibitor treatment at United States children's hospitals. *J Pediatr*. 2016;174:63–70.e3

10. Golski CA, Rome ES, Martin RJ, et al. Pediatric specialists' beliefs about gastroesophageal reflux disease in premature infants. *Pediatrics*. 2010;125(1):96–104

11. Tighe M, Afzal NA, Bevan A, Hayen A, Munro A, Beattie RM. Pharmacological treatment of children with gastro-oesophageal reflux. *Cochrane Database Syst Rev*. 2014;(11):CD008550

12. Ho T, Dukhovny D, Zupancic JA, Goldmann DA, Horbar JD, Pursley DM. Choosing wisely in newborn medicine: five opportunities to increase value. *Pediatrics*. 2015;136(2). Available at: www.pediatrics.org/cgi/content/full/136/2/e482

13. Omari TI, Barnett C, Snel A, et al. Mechanisms of gastroesophageal reflux in healthy premature infants. *J Pediatr*. 1998;133(5):650–654

14. Peter CS, Sprodowski N, Bohnhorst B, Silny J, Poets CF. Gastroesophageal reflux and apnea of prematurity: no temporal relationship. *Pediatrics*. 2002;109(1):8–11

15. Omari TI, Barnett CP, Benninga MA, et al. Mechanisms of gastro-oesophageal reflux in preterm and term infants with reflux disease. *Gut*. 2002;51(4):475–479

16. Ewer AK, Durbin GM, Morgan ME, Booth IW. Gastric emptying and gastro-oesophageal reflux in preterm infants. *Arch Dis Child Fetal Neonatal Ed*. 1996;75(2):F117–F121

17. Corvaglia L, Rotatori R, Ferlini M, Aceti A, Ancora G, Faldella G. The effect of body positioning on gastroesophageal reflux in premature infants: evaluation by combined impedance and pH monitoring. *J Pediatr*. 2007;151(6):591–596, 596.e1

18. van Wijk MP, Benninga MA, Dent J, et al. Effect of body position changes on postprandial gastroesophageal reflux and gastric emptying in the healthy premature neonate. *J Pediatr*. 2007;151(6):585–590, 590.e1–e2

19. Mitchell DJ, McClure BG, Tubman TR. Simultaneous monitoring of gastric and oesophageal pH reveals limitations of conventional oesophageal pH monitoring in milk fed infants. *Arch Dis Child*. 2001;84(3):273–276

20. Funderburk A, Nawab U, Abraham S, et al. Temporal association between reflux-like behaviors and gastroesophageal reflux in preterm and term infants. *J Pediatr Gastroenterol Nutr*. 2016;62(4):556–561

21. Farhath S, He Z, Saslow J, et al. Detection of pepsin in mouth swab: correlation with clinical gastroesophageal reflux in preterm infants. *J Matern Fetal Neonatal Med*. 2013;26(8):819–824

22. James ME, Ewer AK. Acid oropharyngeal secretions can predict gastro-oesophageal reflux in preterm infants. *Eur J Pediatr*. 1999;158(5):371–374

23. López-Alonso M, Moya MJ, Cabo JA, et al. Twenty-four-hour esophageal impedance-pH monitoring in healthy preterm neonates: rate and characteristics of acid, weakly acidic, and weakly alkaline gastroesophageal reflux. *Pediatrics*. 2006;118(2). Available at: www.pediatrics.org/cgi/content/full/118/2/e299

24. Snel A, Barnett CP, Cresp TL, et al. Behavior and gastroesophageal reflux in the premature neonate. *J Pediatr Gastroenterol Nutr*. 2000;30(1):18–21

25. Nobile S, Noviello C, Cobellis G, Carnielli VP. Are infants with bronchopulmonary dysplasia prone to gastroesophageal reflux? A prospective observational study with esophageal pH-impedance monitoring. *J Pediatr*. 2015;167(2):279–285.e1

26. Eichenwald EC; Committee on Fetus and Newborn, American Academy of Pediatrics. Apnea of Prematurity. *Pediatrics*. 2016;137(1):e20153757

27. Poets CF. Gastroesophageal reflux and apnea of prematurity—coincidence, not causation. Commentary on L. Corvaglia et Al.: a thickened formula does not reduce apneas related to

gastroesophageal reflux in preterm infants (Neonatology 2013;103;98-102). *Neonatology.* 2013;103(2):103–104

28. Di Fiore JM, Arko M, Whitehouse M, Kimball A, Martin RJ. Apnea is not prolonged by acid gastroesophageal reflux in preterm infants. *Pediatrics.* 2005;116(5):1059–1063

29. Page M, Jeffery HE. Airway protection in sleeping infants in response to pharyngeal fluid stimulation in the supine position. *Pediatr Res.* 1998;44(5):691–698

30. Wheatley E, Kennedy KA. Cross-over trial of treatment for bradycardia attributed to gastroesophageal reflux in preterm infants. *J Pediatr.* 2009;155(4):516–521

31. Kimball AL, Carlton DP. Gastroesophageal reflux medications in the treatment of apnea in premature infants. *J Pediatr.* 2001;138(3):355–360

32. Kazachkov MY, Muhlebach MS, Livasy CA, Noah TL. Lipid-laden macrophage index and inflammation in bronchoalveolar lavage fluids in children. *Eur Respir J.* 2001;18(5):790–795

33. Bar-Sever Z. Scintigraphic evaluation of gastroesophageal reflux and pulmonary aspiration in children. *Semin Nucl Med.* 2017;47(3):275–285

34. Starosta V, Kitz R, Hartl D, Marcos V, Reinhardt D, Griese M. Bronchoalveolar pepsin, bile acids, oxidation, and inflammation in children with gastroesophageal reflux disease. *Chest.* 2007;132(5):1557–1564

35. Farhath S, Aghai ZH, Nakhla T, et al. Pepsin, a reliable marker of gastric aspiration, is frequently detected in tracheal aspirates from premature ventilated neonates: relationship with feeding and methylxanthine therapy. *J Pediatr Gastroenterol Nutr.* 2006;43(3):336–341

36. Farhath S, He Z, Nakhla T, et al. Pepsin, a marker of gastric contents, is increased in tracheal aspirates from preterm infants who develop bronchopulmonary dysplasia. *Pediatrics.* 2008;121(2). Available at: www.pediatrics.org/cgi/content/full/121/2/e253

37. Abdallah AF, El-Desoky T, Fathi K, Elkashef WF, Zaki A. Clinical utility of bronchoalveolar lavage pepsin in diagnosis of gastroesophageal reflux among wheezy infants. *Can Respir J.* 2016;2016:9480843

38. Akinola E, Rosenkrantz TS, Pappagallo M, McKay K, Hussain N. Gastroesophageal reflux in infants < 32 weeks gestational age at birth: lack of relationship to chronic lung disease. *Am J Perinatol.* 2004;21(2):57–62

39. Fuloria M, Hiatt D, Dillard RG, O'Shea TM. Gastroesophageal reflux in very low birth weight infants: association with chronic lung disease and outcomes through 1 year of age. *J Perinatol.* 2000;20(4):235–239

40. Dellert SF, Hyams JS, Treem WR, Geertsma MA. Feeding resistance and gastroesophageal reflux in infancy. *J Pediatr Gastroenterol Nutr.* 1993;17(1):66–71

41. Mathisen B, Worrall L, Masel J, Wall C, Shepherd RW. Feeding problems in infants with gastro-oesophageal reflux disease: a controlled study. *J Paediatr Child Health.* 1999;35(2):163–169

42. Frakaloss G, Burke G, Sanders MR. Impact of gastroesophageal reflux on growth and hospital stay in premature infants. *J Pediatr Gastroenterol Nutr.* 1998;26(2):146–150

43. Malcolm WF, Gantz M, Martin RJ, Goldstein RF, Goldberg RN, Cotten CM; National Institute of Child Health and Human Development Neonatal Research Network. Use of medications for gastroesophageal reflux at discharge among extremely low birth weight infants. *Pediatrics.* 2008;121(1):22–27

44. Orenstein SR, Whitington PF, Orenstein DM. The infant seat as treatment for gastroesophageal reflux. *N Engl J Med.* 1983;309(13):760–763

45. Orenstein SR. Effects on behavior state of prone versus seated positioning for infants with gastroesophageal reflux. *Pediatrics.* 1990;85(5):765–767

46. Bagucka B, De Schepper J, Peelman M, Van de Maele K, Vandenplas Y. Acid gastro-esophageal reflux in the 10 degrees-reversed-Trendelenburg-position in supine sleeping infants. *Acta Paediatr Taiwan.* 1999;40(5):298–301

47. Loots C, Kritas S, van Wijk M, et al. Body positioning and medical therapy for infantile gastroesophageal reflux symptoms. *J Pediatr Gastroenterol Nutr.* 2014;59(2):237–243

48. Moon RY; Task Force on Sudden Infant Death Syndrome. SIDS and other sleep-related infant deaths: evidence base for 2016 updated recommendations for a safe infant sleeping environment. *Pediatrics.* 2016;138(5):e20162940

49. American Academy of Pediatrics Committee on Fetus and Newborn. Hospital discharge of the high-risk neonate. *Pediatrics.* 2008;122(5):1119–1126

50. Jadcherla SR, Chan CY, Moore R, Malkar M, Timan CJ, Valentine CJ. Impact of feeding strategies on the frequency and clearance of acid and nonacid gastroesophageal reflux events in dysphagic neonates. *JPEN J Parenter Enteral Nutr.* 2012;36(4):449–455

51. Richards R, Foster JP, Psaila K. Continuous versus bolus intragastric tube feeding for preterm and low birth weight infants with gastro-oesophageal reflux disease. *Cochrane Database Syst Rev.* 2014;(7):CD009719

52. Madhoun LL, Siler-Wurst KK, Sitaram S, Jadcherla SR. Feed-thickening practices in NICUs in the current era: variability in prescription and implementation patterns. *J Neonatal Nurs.* 2015;21(6):255–262

53. Beal J, Silverman B, Bellant J, Young TE, Klontz K. Late onset necrotizing enterocolitis in infants following use of a xanthan gum-containing thickening agent. *J Pediatr.* 2012;161(2):354–356

54. Horvath A, Dziechciarz P, Szajewska H. The effect of thickened-feed interventions on gastroesophageal reflux in infants: systematic review and meta-analysis of randomized, controlled trials. *Pediatrics.* 2008;122(6). Available at: www.pediatrics.org/cgi/content/full/122/6/e1268

55. Corvaglia L, Aceti A, Mariani E, et al. Lack of efficacy of a starch-thickened preterm formula on gastro-oesophageal reflux in preterm infants: a pilot study. *J Matern Fetal Neonatal Med.* 2012;25(12):2735–2738

56. Garzi A, Messina M, Frati F, et al. An extensively hydrolysed cow's milk formula improves clinical symptoms of gastroesophageal reflux and reduces the gastric emptying time in infants. *Allergol Immunopathol (Madr)*. 2002;30(1):36–41

57. Salvatore S, Vandenplas Y. Gastroesophageal reflux and cow milk allergy: is there a link? *Pediatrics*. 2002;110(5):972–984

58. Corvaglia L, Mariani E, Aceti A, Galletti S, Faldella G. Extensively hydrolyzed protein formula reduces acid gastro-esophageal reflux in symptomatic preterm infants. *Early Hum Dev*. 2013;89(7):453–455

59. Logarajaha V, Onga C, Jayagobib PA, et al. PP-15 the effect of extensively hydrolyzed protein formula in preterm infants with symptomatic gastro-oesophageal reflux. *J Pediatr Gastroenterol Nutr*. 2015;61(4):526

60. Hibbs AM, Lorch SA. Metoclopramide for the treatment of gastroesophageal reflux disease in infants: a systematic review. *Pediatrics*. 2006;118(2):746–752

61. Corvaglia L, Monari C, Martini S, Aceti A, Faldella G. Pharmacological therapy of gastroesophageal reflux in preterm infants. *Gastroenterol Res Pract*. 2013;2013:714564

62. Corvaglia L, Aceti A, Mariani E, De Giorgi M, Capretti MG, Faldella G. The efficacy of sodium alginate (Gaviscon) for the treatment of gastro-oesophageal reflux in preterm infants. *Aliment Pharmacol Ther*. 2011;33(4):466–470

63. Atasay B, Erdeve O, Arsan S, Türmen T. Effect of sodium alginate on acid gastroesophageal reflux disease in preterm infants: a pilot study. *J Clin Pharmacol*. 2010;50(11):1267–1272

64. Guillet R, Stoll BJ, Cotten CM, et al; National Institute of Child Health and Human Development Neonatal Research Network. Association of H2-blocker therapy and higher incidence of necrotizing enterocolitis in very low birth weight infants. *Pediatrics*. 2006;117(2). Available at: www.pediatrics.org/cgi/content/full/117/2/e137

65. Terrin G, Passariello A, De Curtis M, et al. Ranitidine is associated with infections, necrotizing enterocolitis, and fatal outcome in newborns. *Pediatrics*. 2012;129(1). Available at: www.pediatrics.org/cgi/content/full/129/1/e40

66. Gupta RW, Tran L, Norori J, et al. Histamine-2 receptor blockers alter the fecal microbiota in premature infants. *J Pediatr Gastroenterol Nutr*. 2013;56(4):397–400

67. Wang K, Lin HJ, Perng CL, et al. The effect of H2-receptor antagonist and proton pump inhibitor on microbial proliferation in the stomach. *Hepatogastroenterology*. 2004;51(59):1540–1543

68. Laheij RJ, Sturkenboom MC, Hassing RJ, Dieleman J, Stricker BH, Jansen JB. Risk of community-acquired pneumonia and use of gastric acid-suppressive drugs. *JAMA*. 2004;292(16):1955–1960

69. Canani RB, Cirillo P, Roggero P, et al; Working Group on Intestinal Infections of the Italian Society of Pediatric Gastroenterology, Hepatology and Nutrition (SIGENP). Therapy with gastric acidity inhibitors increases the risk of acute gastroenteritis and community-acquired pneumonia in children. *Pediatrics*. 2006; 117(5). Available at: www.pediatrics.org/cgi/content/full/117/5/e817

70. Orenstein SR, Hassall E, Furmaga-Jablonska W, Atkinson S, Raanan M. Multicenter, double-blind, randomized, placebo-controlled trial assessing the efficacy and safety of proton pump inhibitor lansoprazole in infants with symptoms of gastroesophageal reflux disease. *J Pediatr*. 2009; 154(4):514–520.e4

Effective Discipline to Raise Healthy Children

- *Policy Statement*

POLICY STATEMENT Organizational Principles to Guide and Define the Child Health Care System
and/or Improve the Health of all Children

American Academy
of Pediatrics

DEDICATED TO THE HEALTH OF ALL CHILDREN™

Effective Discipline to Raise Healthy Children

Robert D. Sege, MD, PhD, FAAP,[a] Benjamin S. Siegel, MD, FAAP,[b,c] COUNCIL ON CHILD ABUSE AND NEGLECT, COMMITTEE ON PSYCHOSOCIAL ASPECTS OF CHILD AND FAMILY HEALTH

abstract

Pediatricians are a source of advice for parents and guardians concerning the management of child behavior, including discipline strategies that are used to teach appropriate behavior and protect their children and others from the adverse effects of challenging behavior. Aversive disciplinary strategies, including all forms of corporal punishment and yelling at or shaming children, are minimally effective in the short-term and not effective in the long-term. With new evidence, researchers link corporal punishment to an increased risk of negative behavioral, cognitive, psychosocial, and emotional outcomes for children. In this Policy Statement, the American Academy of Pediatrics provides guidance for pediatricians and other child health care providers on educating parents about positive and effective parenting strategies of discipline for children at each stage of development as well as references to educational materials. This statement supports the need for adults to avoid physical punishment and verbal abuse of children.

[a]Center for Community Engaged Medicine, Institute for Clinical Research and Health Policy Studies, Tufts Medical Center, Boston, Massachusetts; and Departments of [b]Pediatrics and [c]Psychiatry, Boston Medical Center and School of Medicine, Boston University, Boston, Massachusetts

Drs Sege and Siegel created the first draft of this statement, responded to committee and Board comments, and edited the Policy Statement; and all authors approved the final manuscript as submitted.

This document is copyrighted and is property of the American Academy of Pediatrics and its Board of Directors. All authors have filed conflict of interest statements with the American Academy of Pediatrics. Any conflicts have been resolved through a process approved by the Board of Directors. The American Academy of Pediatrics has neither solicited nor accepted any commercial involvement in the development of the content of this publication.

Policy statements from the American Academy of Pediatrics benefit from expertise and resources of liaisons and internal (AAP) and external reviewers. However, policy statements from the American Academy of Pediatrics may not reflect the views of the liaisons or the organizations or government agencies that they represent.

The guidance in this statement does not indicate an exclusive course of treatment or serve as a standard of medical care. Variations, taking into account individual circumstances, may be appropriate.

All policy statements from the American Academy of Pediatrics automatically expire 5 years after publication unless reaffirmed, revised, or retired at or before that time.

DOI: https://doi.org/10.1542/peds.2018-3112

Address correspondence to Robert D. Sege, MD, PhD, FAAP. E-mail: rsege@tuftsmedicalcenter.org

PEDIATRICS (ISSN Numbers: Print, 0031-4005; Online, 1098-4275).

To cite: Sege RD, Siegel BS, AAP COUNCIL ON CHILD ABUSE AND NEGLECT, AAP COMMITTEE ON PSYCHOSOCIAL ASPECTS OF CHILD AND FAMILY HEALTH. Effective Discipline to Raise Healthy Children. Pediatrics. 2018;142(6):e20183112

INTRODUCTION

Pediatricians are an important source of information for parents.[1] They are often asked by parents and guardians about nutrition, development, safety, and overall health maintenance. Pediatricians form a relationship with parents, within which they partner with parents to achieve optimal health, growth, and development in their children, including childhood behavior management. Duncan et al[2] reviewed periodic surveys of members of the American Academy of Pediatrics (AAP) and noted that between 2003 and 2012, pediatricians had increased their discussions of discipline with parents. By 2012, more than half (51%) of the pediatricians surveyed responded that they discussed discipline in 75% to 100% of health supervision visits with parents of children ages 0 through 10 years.

A recent survey (2016) indicated that US pediatricians do not endorse corporal punishment. Only 6% of 787 US pediatricians (92% in primary care) who responded to this survey held positive attitudes toward spanking, and only 2.5% expected positive outcomes from spanking. Respondents did not believe that spanking was the "only way to get the child to behave" (78% disagreed) or that "spanking is a normal part of parenting" (75% disagreed).[3]

This policy statement incorporates new research and updates the 1998 AAP clinical report titled "Guidance for Effective Discipline,"[4] which suggested, "Parents should be encouraged and assisted in developing methods other than spanking in response to undesired behaviors."

BACKGROUND

In 1989, the United Nations (UN) Convention on the Rights of the Child, through its Committee on the Rights of the Child, called on all member states to ban corporal punishment of children and institute educational programs on positive discipline.[5] In the UN report, article 19 reads, "Parties shall take all appropriate legislative, administrative, social, and educational measures to protect the child from all forms of physical or mental violence, injury or abuse, neglect or negligent treatment, maltreatment or exploitation, including sexual abuse, while in the care of [the] parent(s) [or] legal guardian(s) or any other person who has the care of the child."

The Global Initiative to End all Corporal Punishment of Children provided a comprehensive definition of spanking and corporal punishment: "The definition of corporal or physical punishment adopted by the Committee on the Rights of the Child in its *General Comment No. 8* (2006) has the key reference point, 'any punishment in which physical force issued and intended to cause some degree of pain or discomfort, however light.' According to the committee, this mostly involves hitting ("smacking," "slapping," or "spanking") children

with the hand or with an implement (a whip, stick, belt, shoe, wooden spoon, or similar), but it can also involve, for example, kicking, shaking, or throwing children; scratching, pinching, biting, pulling hair, or boxing ears; forcing children to stay in uncomfortable positions; burning, scalding, or forced ingestion (for example, washing a child's mouth out with soap or forcing them to swallow hot spices). Nonphysical forms of punishment that are cruel and degrading and thus incompatible with the convention include, for example, punishment which belittles, humiliates, denigrates, scapegoats, threatens, scares, or ridicules the child. In the view of the committee, corporal punishment is invariably degrading."[6]

For the purpose of this policy statement, corporal punishment is the "noninjurious, open-handed hitting with the intention of modifying child behavior."[7] Spanking can be considered a form of physical punishment. As Gershoff and Grogan-Kaylor[7] noted, most people understand "corporal punishment, physical punishment, and spanking as synonymous." The term "verbal abuse" is used to mean nonphysical forms of punishment as defined above.

This policy statement incorporates results accrued from research and new knowledge of brain development and recommend that pediatricians advise parents against the use of any form of corporal punishment. Verbal abuse (for a definition, see above: the Global Initiative to End All Corporal Punishment of Children) by parents intended to cause shame and humiliation of the child also has deleterious effects on children's self-esteem. This policy statement complements a previous AAP policy statement that recommended the abolishment of corporal punishment in schools.[8]

EFFECTIVE DISCIPLINE SUPPORTS NORMAL CHILD DEVELOPMENT

Optimal child development requires the active engagement of adults who, among other functions, teach children about acceptable behavior. The word "discipline" is derived from the Latin word "disciplinare," meaning to teach or train, as in disciple (a follower or student of a teacher, leader, or philosopher). Effective disciplinary strategies, appropriate to a child's age and development, teach the child to regulate his or her own behavior; keep him or her from harm; enhance his or her cognitive, socioemotional, and executive functioning skills; and reinforce the behavioral patterns taught by the child's parents and caregivers.

There are a number of approaches to discipline that pediatricians may discuss with parents during well-child visits and those visits that are designed to address discipline issues. These approaches are reviewed in *Bright Futures Guidelines for Health Supervision of Infants, Children, and Adolescents*,[9] on the AAP Web site HealthyChildren.org,[10] and in the AAP program Connected Kids: Safe, Strong, Secure.[11] *Bright Futures* includes sections on discipline for each age group. Each of these recommended approaches to discipline is based on the broad concepts of child development and related common behavioral concerns.

CORPORAL PUNISHMENT

Use of Corporal Punishment

There is evidence that support for corporal punishment among parents is declining in the United States. According to a 2004 survey,[12] approximately two-thirds of parents of young children reported using some sort of physical punishment. These parents reported that by fifth grade, 80% of children had been physically punished, and 85% of teenagers reported exposure to physical punishment, with 51% having been hit with a belt or similar object.[12–15] These findings suggest that, in 2004, many parents considered spanking to be a socially acceptable form of discipline. In contrast, a more recent national survey of adults shows declining support for spanking (or hitting), particularly among young parents. A 2013 poll[16] conducted by Harris Interactive found that support for the statement "good, hard spanking is sometimes necessary to discipline a child" had dropped from 84% in 1986 to 70% in 2012. Parents younger than 36 years more often believed that spanking was never appropriate, and only half reported ever spanking their own children. An analysis of a 2016 national survey conducted by yougov.com revealed that respondents with young children in the home, regardless of race and ethnicity, did not support corporal punishment, "suggesting the possibility that a generational shift in social norms [about corporal punishment] may be taking place."[17]

Direct Observations of Corporal Punishment

Although some studies of discipline practices used observations during home visits,[1] a small study published in 2014[18] used voice recordings to explore parent-child interactions during daily activities. The recordings of 15 of the 33 families in the study (45%) included the use of corporal punishment. Most parents used a verbal disciplinary strategy before corporal punishment. Corporal punishment then occurred at a mean of 30 seconds later, suggesting that parents may have been "responding either impulsively or emotionally rather than instrumentally and intentionally." The effects of corporal punishment were transient: within 10 minutes, most children (73%) had resumed the same behavior for which they had been punished.

Ineffectiveness of Corporal Punishment

A 2016 meta-analysis showed that current literature does not support the finding of benefit from physical punishment in the long-term.[7] Several small, older studies (including meta-analyses),[19–22] largely of parents who were referred for help with child behavior problems, demonstrated apparent short-term effectiveness of spanking. Only a single 1981 study of 24 children showed statistically significant short-term improvement in compliance compared with alternative strategies (time-out and a control group).[23]

Cycle of Corporal Punishment and Aggressive Child Behavior

Evidence obtained from a longitudinal cohort study suggested that corporal punishment of toddlers was associated with subsequent aggressive behavior. The Fragile Families and Child Wellbeing Study was based on a population-based birth cohort of approximately 5000 children from 20 large US cities between 1998 and 2000[24]; data were collected at birth and 1, 3, 5, and 9 years of age. Young children who were spanked more than twice per month at age 3 years were more aggressive at age 5 even when the researchers controlled for the child's aggressive behavior at age 3, maternal parenting and risk factors, and demographic factors.[25] A follow-up study[26] assessed these children at 9 years of age and noted correlations between spanking at age 5 years and higher levels of externalizing behavior and lower receptive vocabulary scores at age 9. A subsequent study analyzed data from all 4 waves and concluded that an increased frequency of spanking was associated with a subsequent increased frequency of externalizing behaviors, which were then associated with more spanking in response.[27] This interaction between spanking and misbehavior occurs

over time; each negative interaction reinforces previous negative interactions as a complex negative spiral.

In a study that explored parental discipline approaches,[28] researchers noted that both European American and African American parents used an escalation strategy in disciplining their 6- to 8-year-old children. Both groups of parents used reasoning more frequently than yelling. The next most frequent strategy was denying privileges, and spanking was the least frequent method reported by all parents. Similarly, in focus groups conducted around the country in 2002 during the development of the AAP Connected Kids materials, participating parents reported the use of corporal punishment as a last resort.[11,29]

Special Populations

Children in foster care who have experienced abuse or neglect may exhibit challenging behaviors. Programs exist that assist foster parents in addressing discipline. A recent AAP clinical report describes the behavioral effects of maltreatment and offers suggestions for helping these children heal.[30] Pediatricians may advise foster parents to consider the behavioral consequences of past abuse in understanding how these children may respond differently to their foster parents' attempts to correct their behavior.[31]

Parents of children with special health care needs may need additional assistance regarding discipline strategies. These strategies begin with an understanding of a child's physical, emotional, and cognitive capacities. In some cases, consultation with a developmental-behavioral pediatrician may be helpful.[32]

Parental Factors Associated With Reliance on Corporal Punishment

Parental Depression

A longitudinal study examined the interactions between parental corporal punishment, parental depression, negative perceptions of a child's behavior, and the child's externalizing behavior.[33] The sample included 245 children and parents in stable relationships from mostly middle-class, married, European American parents. Depressive symptoms for both mothers and fathers were related to more negative appraisals of the child's behavior and more frequent corporal punishment and predicted higher levels of child externalizing problems at 5.5 years of age.

Influence of Past Parental Trauma

A recent article, Kistin et al[34] reported interviews with 30 low-income mothers and provided an important perspective on the complexity of disciplinary strategies used by mothers who had themselves experienced trauma. They reported that mothers related their children's negative behaviors to their own past experiences; harsh discipline was used in an attempt to prevent future behavioral problems.

Corporal Punishment As a Risk Factor for Nonoptimal Child Development

There appears to be a strong association between spanking children and subsequent adverse outcomes.[35–53] Reports published since the previous 1998 AAP report have provided further evidence that has deepened the understanding of the effects of corporal punishment. The consequences associated with parental corporal punishment are summarized as follows[7,19,21,27,35,54–62]:

- corporal punishment of children younger than 18 months of age increases the likelihood of physical injury;

- repeated use of corporal punishment may lead to aggressive behavior and altercations between the parent and child and may negatively affect the parent-child relationship;

- corporal punishment is associated with increased aggression in preschool and school-aged children;

- experiencing corporal punishment makes it more, not less, likely that children will be defiant and aggressive in the future;

- corporal punishment is associated with an increased risk of mental health disorders and cognition problems;

- the risk of harsh punishment is increased when the family is experiencing stressors, such as family economic challenges, mental health problems, intimate partner violence, or substance abuse; and

- spanking alone is associated with adverse outcomes, and these outcomes are similar to those in children who experience physical abuse.

The association between corporal punishment and adverse adult health outcomes was examined in a 2017 report that analyzed original data from the 1998 Adverse Childhood Experiences Study, which recommended that spanking be considered as an additional independent risk factor, similar in nature and effect to other adverse childhood experiences.[63] In their analysis of the original 1998 Adverse Childhood Experiences study data, the investigators found that spanking was associated with increased odds of suicide attempts, moderate-to-heavy drinking, and substance use disorder in adulthood independent of the risks associated with having experienced physical and emotional abuse.

Physiologic Changes Associated With Corporal Punishment and Verbal Abuse

A history of parental corporal punishment and parental verbal abuse has been associated with changes in brain anatomy that can be visualized by using MRI. Researchers studied a group of young adults (N = 23; ages 18–25) who had prolonged and repeated exposure to harsh corporal punishment and compared the results of brain MRIs to those from a matched control group (N = 22). They reported reduced prefrontal cortical gray matter volume and performance IQ.[64] A similar study from this group noted MRI results that revealed differences in white matter tracts in young adults (N = 16) who were exposed to parental verbal abuse and had no history of trauma.[65] A more recent review noted relationships between physical punishment and cortisol levels.[66] Elevated cortisol levels reflect stress and have been associated with toxic stress and subsequent changes in brain architecture.

Harsh Verbal Abuse Associated With Child and Adolescent Mental Health Problems

In 2009, the UN Children's Fund defined "yelling and other harsh verbal discipline as psychologically aggressive towards children."[28] In a longitudinal study investigating the relationship between harsh verbal abuse by parents and child outcomes, researchers noted that harsh verbal abuse before age 13 years was associated with an increase in adolescent conduct problems and depressive symptoms between ages 13 and 14. Adolescent behavior affected parental behavior as well; misconduct predicted increases in parents' use of harsh discipline between ages 13 and 14 years. Furthermore, parental warmth did not moderate the longitudinal associations between harsh discipline by parents and adolescent conduct and depressive symptoms.[67]

STRATEGIES FOR PROMOTING EFFECTIVE DISCIPLINE

Effective disciplinary techniques grow from an understanding of normal child development. Parents value advice from their pediatricians, as illustrated by a 2012 study[1] involving 500 parents in New Orleans, Louisiana. The investigators found that parents were more likely to follow the advice of pediatricians compared with other professionals, and nearly half (48%) indicated that they were most likely to consult their pediatricians for advice on corporal punishment. In a second article,[68] these investigators further noted that perceived social norms were the strongest predictor of having a positive attitude toward corporal punishment, with the second-strongest predictor being perceived approval of corporal punishment by professionals.

Clinical Setting

Pediatricians may assist parents by providing information about child development and effective parenting strategies. Although parents often seek information and hold their pediatricians in a position of trust, discussions of discipline may prove challenging. This section presents approaches to counseling.

Anticipatory Guidance

A direct discussion advising against any form of corporal punishment may be useful. When appropriate, the pediatrician may counsel family members that spanking is not an appropriate or effective disciplinary strategy. Parents may be counseled that although spanking seems to interrupt a child's misbehavior, it is ineffective in the longer-term. For many children, spanking increases aggression and anger instead of teaching responsibility

and self-control. This advice will be most helpful if it is combined with teaching parents new strategies to replace their previous use of corporal punishment. Appropriate methods for addressing children's behavior will change as the children grow and develop increased cognitive and executive function abilities.[9]

Teaching parents effective strategies may allow them to avoid escalating to the point of using corporal punishment. In a randomized trial, Barkin et al[69] demonstrated that it was possible to teach parents to use time-outs within the constraints of an office visit. Clinicians used motivational interviewing techniques to help parents learn to discipline using other techniques.

When discussing corporal punishment, pediatricians may explore and acknowledge parents' current experiences, past social-emotional development, attitudes, and beliefs. Because parents may use spanking as a last resort, they may spank less (or not at all) if they have learned effective discipline techniques.[11] Specific discussions of behavior problems and behavior management strategies allow pediatricians to provide useful advice that is based on an understanding of child behavior.

Educational Resources

Pediatric providers may reinforce behavioral counseling through recommending or distributing parent education materials. For example, studies have shown that in-office videos may be able to deliver messages to multicultural parents.[70,71] Having parents read brief research summaries of problems associated with corporal punishment decreased positive attitudes about it.[72] Each of these approaches reinforced verbal advice with other means of supporting caregivers in learning new parenting techniques.

The Centers for Disease Control and Prevention has posted positive parenting tips on its Web site.[73] The AAP provides content for parents through its HealthyChildren.org Web site and its Connected Kids: Safe, Strong, Secure[11] and Bright Futures[9] programs. Each of these resources encourages parents to use positive reinforcement as a primary means of teaching acceptable behavior. For example, parents can learn that young children crave attention, and telling a child, "I love it when you . . ." is an easy means of reinforcing desired behavior.

Community Resources

Although pediatricians offer anticipatory guidance, many parents will want or need more assistance in developing strong parenting skills. The medical home can link parents to community resources. Health care sites may implement the Safe Environment for Every Kid[74,75] program. The program includes a brief questionnaire that examines family risk factors. Parents who identify needs, including parenting challenges, meet with a colocated social worker who can link them to parent supports in the community. This program also has online educational modules.[76,77]

A variety of national and community-based organizations offer parents support through Triple P,[78] which is one example of an evidence-based parent education program. In another program, HealthySteps,[79] a developmental specialist is placed in the office setting to help support families of children ages 0 to 3 years. In most states, Children's Trust Funds and child welfare agencies sponsor parent resource centers. Help Me Grow,[80] a state-based information and referral network, has been implemented in the majority of the United States. The Center for the Improvement of Child Caring offers resources specifically tailored to African American families.[81–83]

Many clinic- and community-based programs are specifically oriented toward helping parents effectively address their children's behavior.[84] Examples include *The Incredible Years*,[85] a brief office-based video intervention in the office that is used to discuss discipline issues[86]; Safety Check, which is used to teach time-outs[69]; the Family Nurturing Program, which is used to improve parenting attitudes and knowledge[87]; and the Chicago Parent Program, a comprehensive 12-week parenting skills training program.[88] The Video Intervention Project is an evidence-based parenting program that involves feedback on parent-child interactions by trained child development staff in a primary care office setting.[89]

The 2012 AAP clinical report was focused on the psychological maltreatment of children and adolescents and contained a comprehensive review of preventive measures that provide alternatives to the use of corporal punishment.[90] The literature describe other resources and programs, such as Internet-based training and group-based parent training programs.[91–93] This list of resources is not intended to be comprehensive; many national organizations and local communities also offer effective parenting resources.

CONCLUSIONS

Parents look to pediatric providers for guidance concerning a variety of parenting issues, including discipline. Keeping in mind that the evidence that corporal punishment is both ineffective in the long-term and associated with cognitive and mental health problems can guide these discussions. When parents want guidance about the use of spanking, pediatricians can explore parental feelings, help them better define the goals of discipline, and offer specific behavior management strategies. In addition to providing appropriate education to families, providers can refer them to community resources, including parenting groups, classes, and mental health services.[94]

The AAP recommends that adults caring for children use healthy forms of discipline, such as positive reinforcement of appropriate behaviors, setting limits, redirecting, and setting future expectations. The AAP recommends that parents do not use spanking, hitting, slapping, threatening, insulting, humiliating, or shaming.

POLICY RECOMMENDATIONS

Parents value pediatricians' discussion of and guidance about child behavior and parenting practices.

1. Parents, other caregivers, and adults interacting with children and adolescents should not use corporal punishment (including hitting and spanking), either in anger or as a punishment for or consequence of misbehavior, nor should they use any disciplinary strategy, including verbal abuse, that causes shame or humiliation.

2. When pediatricians offer guidance about child behavior and parenting practices, they may choose to offer the following:

   a. guidance on effective discipline strategies to help parents teach their children acceptable behaviors and protect them from harm;

   b. information concerning the risks of harmful effects and the ineffectiveness of using corporal punishment; and

   c. the insight that although many children who were spanked become happy, healthy adults, current evidence suggests that spanking is not necessary and may result in long-term harm.

3. Agencies that offer family support, such as state- or community-supported family resource centers, schools, or other public health agencies, are strongly encouraged to provide information about effective alternatives to corporal punishment to parents and families, including links to materials offered by the AAP.

4. In their roles as child advocates, pediatricians are encouraged to assume roles at local and state levels to advance this policy as being in the best interest of children.

LEAD AUTHORS

Robert D. Sege, MD, PhD, FAAP
Benjamin S. Siegel, MD, FAAP

COUNCIL ON CHILD ABUSE AND NEGLECT EXECUTIVE COMMITTEE, 2015–2017

Emalee G. Flaherty, MD, FAAP
CAPT Amy R. Gavril, MD, FAAP
Sheila M. Idzerda, MD, FAAP
Antoinette Laskey, MD, MPH, MBA, FAAP
Lori Anne Legano, MD, FAAP
John M. Leventhal, MD, FAAP
James Louis Lukefahr, MD, FAAP
Robert D. Sege, MD, PhD, FAAP

LIAISONS

Beverly Fortson, PhD – *Centers for Disease Control and Prevention*
Harriet MacMillan, MD, FRCPC – *American Academy of Child and Adolescent Psychiatry*
Elaine Stedt, MSW – *Office on Child Abuse and Neglect, Administration for Children, Youth and Families*

STAFF

Tammy Piazza Hurley

COMMITTEE ON PSYCHOSOCIAL ASPECTS OF CHILD AND FAMILY HEALTH, 2016–2017

Michael W. Yogman, MD, FAAP, Chairperson
Rebecca Baum, MD, FAAP
Thresia B. Gambon, MD, FAAP
Arthur Lavin, MD, FAAP
Gerri Mattson, MD, FAAP
Raul Montiel-Esparza, MD
Lawrence Sagin Wissow, MD, MPH, FAAP

LIAISONS

Terry Carmichael, MSW — *National Association of Social Workers*

Edward Christophersen, PhD, FAAP (hon) — *Society of Pediatric Psychology*

Norah Johnson, PhD, RN, NP-BC — *National Association of Pediatric Nurse Practitioners*

Leonard Read Sulik, MD — *American Academy of Child and Adolescent Psychiatry*

STAFF

Stephanie Domain, MS

ABBREVIATIONS

AAP: American Academy of Pediatrics

UN: United Nations

Copyright © 2018 by the American Academy of Pediatrics

FINANCIAL DISCLOSURE: The authors have indicated they have no financial relationships relevant to this article to disclose.

FUNDING: No external funding.

POTENTIAL CONFLICT OF INTEREST: The authors have indicated they have no potential conflicts of interest to disclose.

REFERENCES

1. Taylor CA, Moeller W, Hamvas L, Rice JC. Parents' professional sources of advice regarding child discipline and their use of corporal punishment. *Clin Pediatr (Phila)*. 2013;52(2):147–155

2. Duncan PM, Kemper AR, Shaw JS, et al. What do pediatricians discuss during health supervision visits? National surveys comparing 2003 to 2012. In: *Pediatric Academic Societies Annual Meeting*; May 4–7, 2013; Washington, DC

3. Taylor CA, Fleckman JM, Scholer SJ, Branco N. US pediatricians' attitudes, beliefs, and perceived injunctive norms about spanking. *J Dev Behav Pediatr*. 2018;39(7):564–572

4. American Academy of Pediatrics, Committee on Psychosocial Aspects of Child and Family Health. Guidance for effective discipline. American Academy of Pediatrics. Committee on Psychosocial Aspects of Child and Family Health [published correction appears in *Pediatrics*. 1998;102(2, pt 1):433]. *Pediatrics*. 1998;101(4, pt 1):723–728. Reaffirmed April 2014

5. United Nations Committee on the Rights of the Child. *General Comment No. 8: The Right of the Child to Protection From Corporal Punishment and Other Cruel or Degrading Forms of Punishment (Arts. 19; 28, Para. 2; and 37, Inter Alia)*. Geneva, Switzerland: UN Committee on the Rights of the Child; 2007. Available at: www.refworld.org/docid/460bc7772.html. Accessed July 19, 2018

6. Global Initiative to End All Corporal Punishment of Children. *Prohibiting and Eliminating Corporal Punishment: A Key Health Issue in Addressing Violence Against Children*. Geneva, Switzerland: World Health Organization; 2015. Available at: www.who.int/topics/violence/Global-Initiative-End-All-Corporal-Punishment-children.pdf. Accessed July 19, 2018

7. Gershoff ET, Grogan-Kaylor A. Spanking and child outcomes: old controversies and new meta-analyses. *J Fam Psychol*. 2016;30(4):453–469

8. American Academy of Pediatrics, Committee on School Health. American Academy of Pediatrics. Committee on School Health. Corporal punishment in schools. *Pediatrics*. 2000;106(2, pt 1):343

9. Hagan JF, Shaw JS, Duncan PM, eds. *Bright Futures: Guidelines for Health Supervision of Infants, Children, and Adolescents*. 4th ed. Elk Grove Village, IL: American Academy of Pediatrics; 2017

10. American Academy of Pediatrics. HealthyChildren.org. Available at: www.healthychildren.org/English/Pages/default.aspx. Accessed July 19, 2018

11. American Academy of Pediatrics. Connected Kids: Safe, Strong, Secure. Available at: https://www.aap.org/en-us/advocacy-and-policy/aap-health-initiatives/Pages/Connected-Kids.aspx. Accessed July 19, 2018

12. Regalado M, Sareen H, Inkelas M, Wissow LS, Halfon N. Parents' discipline of young children: results from the National Survey of Early Childhood Health. *Pediatrics*. 2004;113(suppl 6):1952–1958

13. Socolar RR, Savage E, Evans H. A longitudinal study of parental discipline of young children. *South Med J*. 2007;100(5):472–477

14. Gershoff ET, Bitensky SH. The case against corporal punishment of children: converging evidence from social science research and international human rights law and implications for U.S. public policy. *Psychol Public Policy Law*. 2007;13(4):231–272

15. Bender HL, Allen JP, McElhaney KB, et al. Use of harsh physical discipline and developmental outcomes in adolescence. *Dev Psychopathol*. 2007;19(1):227–242

16. The Harris Poll. *Four in Five Americans Believe Parents Spanking Their Children is Sometimes Appropriate*. New York, NY: Harris Insights and Analytics; 2013. Available at: https://theharrispoll.com/new-york-n-y-september-26-2013-to-spank-or-not-to-spank-its-an-age-old-question-that-every-parent-must-face-some-parents-may-start-off-with-the-notion-that-i-will-never-spank-my-child-bu/. Accessed July 19, 2018

17. Sege R, Bethell C, Linkenbach J, Jones J, Klika B, Pecora PJ. *Balancing Adverse Childhood Experiences With HOPE: New Insights Into the Role of Positive Experience on Child and Family Development*. Boston, MA: The Medical Foundation; 2017. Available at: www.cssp.org/publications/documents/Balancing-ACEs-with-HOPE-FINAL.pdf. Accessed July 19, 2018

18. Holden GW, Williamson PA, Holland GW. Eavesdropping on the family: a pilot

investigation of corporal punishment in the home. *J Fam Psychol.* 2014;28(3):401–406

19. Larzelere RE. A review of the outcomes of parental use of nonabusive or customary physical punishment. *Pediatrics.* 1996;98(4, pt 2):824–828

20. Baumrind D. A blanket injunction against disciplinary use of spanking is not warranted by the data. *Pediatrics.* 1996;98(4, pt 2):828–831

21. Paolucci EO, Violato C. A meta-analysis of the published research on the affective, cognitive, and behavioral effects of corporal punishment. *J Psychol.* 2004;138(3):197–221

22. Baumrind D, Larzelere RE, Cowan PA. Ordinary physical punishment: is it harmful? Comment on Gershoff (2002). *Psychol Bull.* 2002;128(4):580–589; discussion 602–611

23. Bean AW, Roberts MW. The effect of time-out release contingencies on changes in child noncompliance. *J Abnorm Child Psychol.* 1981;9(1):95–105

24. Reichman NE, Teitler JO, Garfinkel I, McLanahan SS. Fragile families: sample and design. *Child Youth Serv Rev.* 2001;23(4–5):303–326

25. Taylor CA, Manganello JA, Lee SJ, Rice JC. Mothers' spanking of 3-year-old children and subsequent risk of children's aggressive behavior. *Pediatrics.* 2010;125(5). Available at: www.pediatrics.org/cgi/content/full/125/5/e1057

26. MacKenzie MJ, Nicklas E, Waldfogel J, Brooks-Gunn J. Spanking and child development across the first decade of life. *Pediatrics.* 2013;132(5). Available at: www.pediatrics.org/cgi/content/full/132/5/e1118

27. MacKenzie MJ, Nicklas E, Brooks-Gunn J, Waldfogel J. Spanking and children's externalizing behavior across the first decade of life: evidence for transactional processes. *J Youth Adolesc.* 2015;44(3):658–669

28. Lansford JE, Wager LB, Bates JE, Dodge KA, Pettit GS. Parental reasoning, denying privileges, yelling, and spanking: ethnic differences and associations with child externalizing behavior. *Parent Sci Pract.* 2012;12(1):42–56

29. Sege RD, Hatmaker-Flanigan E, De Vos E, Levin-Goodman R, Spivak H. Anticipatory guidance and violence prevention: results from family and pediatrician focus groups. *Pediatrics.* 2006;117(2):455–463

30. Sege RD, Amaya-Jackson L; American Academy of Pediatrics Committee on Child Abuse and Neglect, Council on Foster Care, Adoption, and Kinship Care; American Academy of Child and Adolescent Psychiatry Committee on Child Maltreatment and Violence; National Center for Child Traumatic Stress. Clinical considerations related to the behavioral manifestations of child maltreatment. *Pediatrics.* 2017;139(4):e20170100

31. Council on Foster Care; Adoption, and Kinship Care; Committee on Adolescence, and Council on Early Childhood. Health care issues for children and adolescents in foster care and kinship care. *Pediatrics.* 2015;136(4). Available at: www.pediatrics.org/cgi/content/full/136/4/e1131

32. Kistin CJ, Tompson MC, Cabral HJ, Sege RD, Winter MR, Silverstein M. Subsequent maltreatment in children with disabilities after an unsubstantiated report for neglect. *JAMA.* 2016;315(1):85–87

33. Callender KA, Olson SL, Choe DE, Sameroff AJ. The effects of parental depressive symptoms, appraisals, and physical punishment on later child externalizing behavior. *J Abnorm Child Psychol.* 2012;40(3):471–483

34. Kistin CJ, Radesky J, Diaz-Linhart Y, Tompson MC, O'Connor E, Silverstein M. A qualitative study of parenting stress, coping, and discipline approaches among low-income traumatized mothers. *J Dev Behav Pediatr.* 2014;35(3):189–196

35. Durrant JE. Physical punishment, culture, and rights: current issues for professionals. *J Dev Behav Pediatr.* 2008;29(1):55–66

36. Mackenzie MJ, Nicklas E, Brooks-Gunn J, Waldfogel J. Who spanks infants and toddlers? Evidence from the fragile families and child well-being study. *Child Youth Serv Rev.* 2011;33(8):1364–1373

37. Evans SZ, Simons LG, Simons RL. The effect of corporal punishment and verbal abuse on delinquency: mediating mechanisms. *J Youth Adolesc.* 2012;41(8):1095–1110

38. Donovan KL, Brassard MR. Trajectories of maternal verbal aggression across the middle school years: associations with negative view of self and social problems. *Child Abuse Negl.* 2011;35(10):814–830

39. Surjadi FF, Lorenz FO, Conger RD, Wickrama KA. Harsh, inconsistent parental discipline and romantic relationships: mediating processes of behavioral problems and ambivalence. *J Fam Psychol.* 2013;27(5):762–772

40. Maguire-Jack K, Gromoske AN, Berger LM. Spanking and child development during the first 5 years of life. *Child Dev.* 2012;83(6):1960–1977

41. Lansford JE, Criss MM, Laird RD, et al. Reciprocal relations between parents' physical discipline and children's externalizing behavior during middle childhood and adolescence. *Dev Psychopathol.* 2011;23(1):225–238

42. Olson SL, Lopez-Duran N, Lunkenheimer ES, Chang H, Sameroff AJ. Individual differences in the development of early peer aggression: integrating contributions of self-regulation, theory of mind, and parenting. *Dev Psychopathol.* 2011;23(1):253–266

43. Lee SJ, Altschul I, Gershoff ET. Does warmth moderate longitudinal associations between maternal spanking and child aggression in early childhood? *Dev Psychol.* 2013;49(11):2017–2028

44. McCoy KP, George MR, Cummings EM, Davies PT. Constructive and destructive marital conflict, parenting, and children's school and social adjustment. *Soc Dev.* 2013;22(4):641–662

45. Gunnoe ML. Associations between parenting style, physical discipline, and adjustment in adolescents' reports. *Psychol Rep.* 2013;112(3):933–975

46. Lee SJ, Grogan-Kaylor A, Berger LM. Parental spanking of 1-year-old children and subsequent child protective services involvement. *Child Abuse Negl.* 2014;38(5):875–883

47. McCurdy K. The influence of support and stress on maternal attitudes. *Child Abuse Negl.* 2005;29(3):251–268

48. MacKenzie MJ, Nicklas E, Brooks-Gunn J, Waldfogel J. Repeated exposure to high-frequency spanking and child externalizing behavior across the first decade: a moderating role for cumulative risk. *Child Abuse Negl.* 2014;38(12):1895–1901

49. Lee SJ, Perron BE, Taylor CA, Guterman NB. Paternal psychosocial characteristics and corporal punishment of their 3-year-old children. *J Interpers Violence.* 2011;26(1):71–87

50. Turner HA, Muller PA. Long-term effects of child corporal punishment on depressive symptoms in young adults: potential moderators and mediators. *J Fam Issues.* 2004;25(6):761–782

51. Berzenski SR, Yates TM. Preschoolers' emotion knowledge and the differential effects of harsh punishment. *J Fam Psychol.* 2013;27(3):463–472

52. Owen DJ, Slep AM, Heyman RE. The effect of praise, positive nonverbal response, reprimand, and negative nonverbal response on child compliance: a systematic review. *Clin Child Fam Psychol Rev.* 2012;15(4):364–385

53. Kochanska G, Kim S. Toward a new understanding of legacy of early attachments for future antisocial trajectories: evidence from two longitudinal studies. *Dev Psychopathol.* 2012;24(3):783–806

54. Gershoff ET. *Report on Physical Punishment in the United States: What Research Tells Us About Its Effects on Children.* Columbus, OH: Center for Effective Discipline; 2008

55. Gershoff ET. Spanking and child development: we know enough now to stop hitting our children. *Child Dev Perspect.* 2013;7(3):133–137

56. Zolotor AJ. Corporal punishment. *Pediatr Clin North Am.* 2014;61(5):971–978

57. Durrant J, Ensom R. Physical punishment of children: lessons from 20 years of research. *CMAJ.* 2012;184(12):1373–1377

58. Ferguson CJ. Spanking, corporal punishment and negative long-term outcomes: a meta-analytic review of longitudinal studies. *Clin Psychol Rev.* 2013;33(1):196–208

59. Straus MA, Paschall MJ. Corporal punishment by mothers and development of children's cognitive ability: a longitudinal study of two nationally representative age cohorts. *J Aggress Maltreat Trauma.* 2009;18(5):459–483

60. Flaherty EG, Stirling J Jr; American Academy of Pediatrics; Committee on Child Abuse and Neglect. Clinical report—the pediatrician's role in child maltreatment prevention. *Pediatrics.* 2010;126(4):833–841

61. Taylor CA, Lee SJ, Guterman NB, Rice JC. Use of spanking for 3-year-old children and associated intimate partner aggression or violence. *Pediatrics.* 2010;126(3):415–424

62. Brooks-Gunn J, Schneider W, Waldfogel J. The Great Recession and the risk for child maltreatment. *Child Abuse Negl.* 2013;37(10):721–729

63. Afifi TO, Ford D, Gershoff ET, et al. Spanking and adult mental health impairment: the case for the designation of spanking as an adverse childhood experience. *Child Abuse Negl.* 2017;71:24–31

64. Tomoda A, Suzuki H, Rabi K, Sheu YS, Polcari A, Teicher MH. Reduced prefrontal cortical gray matter volume in young adults exposed to harsh corporal punishment. *Neuroimage.* 2009;47(suppl 2):T66–T71

65. Choi J, Jeong B, Rohan ML, Polcari AM, Teicher MH. Preliminary evidence for white matter tract abnormalities in young adults exposed to parental verbal abuse. *Biol Psychiatry.* 2009;65(3):227–234

66. Gershoff ET. Should parents' physical punishment of children be considered a source of toxic stress that affects brain development? *Fam Relat.* 2016;65(1):151–162

67. Wang MT, Kenny S. Longitudinal links between fathers' and mothers' harsh verbal discipline and adolescents' conduct problems and depressive symptoms. *Child Dev.* 2014;85(3):908–923

68. Taylor CA, Hamvas L, Rice J, Newman DL, DeJong W. Perceived social norms, expectations, and attitudes toward corporal punishment among an urban community sample of parents. *J Urban Health.* 2011;88(2):254–269

69. Barkin SL, Finch SA, Ip EH, et al. Is office-based counseling about media use, timeouts, and firearm storage effective? Results from a cluster-randomized, controlled trial. *Pediatrics.* 2008;122(1). Available at: www.pediatrics.org/cgi/content/full/122/1/e15

70. Scholer SJ, Hudnut-Beumler J, Dietrich MS. A brief primary care intervention helps parents develop plans to discipline. *Pediatrics.* 2010;125(2). Available at: www.pediatrics.org/cgi/content/full/125/2/e242

71. Smith AE, Hudnut-Beumler J, Scholer SJ. Can discipline education be culturally sensitive? *Matern Child Health J.* 2017;21(1):177–186

72. Holden GW, Brown AS, Baldwin AS, Croft Caderao K. Research findings can change attitudes about corporal punishment. *Child Abuse Negl.* 2014;38(5):902–908

73. Centers for Disease Control and Prevention. Positive parenting tips. Available at: www.cdc.gov/ncbddd/childdevelopment/positiveparenting/index.html. Accessed July 19, 2018

74. Dubowitz H, Lane WG, Semiatin JN, Magder LS, Venepally M, Jans M. The safe environment for every kid model: impact on pediatric primary care professionals. *Pediatrics.* 2011;127(4). Available at: www.pediatrics.org/cgi/content/full/127/4/e962

75. Dubowitz H, Lane WG, Semiatin JN, Magder LS. The SEEK model of pediatric primary care: can child maltreatment be prevented in a low-risk population? *Acad Pediatr.* 2012;12(4):259–268

76. Safe Environment for Every Kid. SEEK online training activity description. Available at: https://www.seekwellbeing.org/the-seek-online-training-description. Accessed July 19, 2018

77. Maryland Department of Health. Clinical innovations. Title: SEEK (Safe Environment for Every Kid) Program. Available at: https://health.maryland.gov/innovations/Pages/seekprogram.aspx. Accessed July 19, 2018

78. Sanders MR, Kirby JN, Tellegen CL, Day JJ. The Triple P-Positive Parenting Program: a systematic review and meta-analysis of a multi-level system

of parenting support. *Clin Psychol Rev.* 2014;34(4):337–357

79. HealthySteps. HealthySteps for young children. Available at: http://healthysteps.org/. Accessed July 19, 2018

80. Help Me Grow National Center. Help Me Grow. Available at: www.helpmegrownational.org/index.php. Accessed July 19, 2018

81. Center for the Improvement of Child Caring. CICC's Confident Parenting Program. Available at: www.ciccparenting.org/ConfidentParentingDesc.aspx. Accessed July 19, 2018

82. Center for the Improvement of Child Caring. CICC's Effective Black Parenting Program. Available at: www.ciccparenting.org/EffBlackParentingDesc.aspx. Accessed July 19, 2018

83. New York Charter Parent Action Network. Resources for parents raising a black male child. Available at: http://nycpan.org/sites/default/files/resources/resources_for_raising_a_black_male_child.pdf. Accessed July 19, 2018

84. Oberklaid F, Baird G, Blair M, Melhuish E, Hall D. Children's health and development: approaches to early identification and intervention. *Arch Dis Child.* 2013;98(12):1008–1011

85. Perrin EC, Sheldrick RC, McMenamy JM, Henson BS, Carter AS. Improving parenting skills for families of young children in pediatric settings: a randomized clinical trial. *JAMA Pediatr.* 2014;168(1):16–24

86. Scholer SJ, Hudnut-Beumler J, Mukherjee A, Dietrich MS. A brief intervention facilitates discussions about discipline in pediatric primary care. *Clin Pediatr (Phila).* 2015;54(8):732–737

87. Palusci VJ, Crum P, Bliss R, Bavolek SJ. Changes in parenting attitudes and knowledge among inmates and other at-risk populations after a family nurturing program. *Child Youth Serv Rev.* 2008;30(1):79–89

88. Breitenstein SM, Gross D, Fogg L, et al. The Chicago Parent Program: comparing 1-year outcomes for African American and Latino parents of young children. *Res Nurs Health.* 2012;35(5):475–489

89. Video Interaction Project. Available at: www.videointeractionproject.org/. Accessed July 19, 2018

90. Hibbard R, Barlow J, Macmillan H; Child Abuse and Neglect; American Academy of Child and Adolescent Psychiatry; Child Maltreatment and Violence. Psychological maltreatment. *Pediatrics.* 2012;130(2):372–378

91. Enebrink P, Högström J, Forster M, Ghaderi A. Internet-based parent management training: a randomized controlled study. *Behav Res Ther.* 2012;50(4):240–249

92. Reed A, Snyder J, Staats S, et al. Duration and mutual entrainment of changes in parenting practices engendered by behavioral parent training targeting recently separated mothers. *J Fam Psychol.* 2013;27(3):343–354

93. Barlow J, Smailagic N, Ferriter M, Bennett C, Jones H. Group-based parent-training programmes for improving emotional and behavioural adjustment in children from birth to three years old. *Cochrane Database Syst Rev.* 2010;(3):CD003680

94. American Academy of Pediatrics. *Strategies for System Change in Children's Mental Health: A Chapter Action Kit.* Elk Grove Village, IL: American Academy of Pediatrics; 2007. Available at: https://www.aap.org/en-us/advocacy-and-policy/aap-health-initiatives/healthy-foster-care-america/Documents/mh2ch.pdf#search=Mental%20Health%20task%20force. Accessed July 19, 2018

The Effects of Armed Conflict on Children

- *Policy Statement*

POLICY STATEMENT Organizational Principles to Guide and Define the Child Health Care System and/or Improve the Health of all Children

American Academy
of Pediatrics

DEDICATED TO THE HEALTH OF ALL CHILDREN™

The Effects of Armed Conflict on Children

Sherry Shenoda, MD, FAAP,[a] Ayesha Kadir, MD, MSc, FAAP,[b] Shelly Pitterman, PhD,[c]
Jeffrey Goldhagen, MD, MPH, FAAP,[a] SECTION ON INTERNATIONAL CHILD HEALTH

abstract

Children are increasingly exposed to armed conflict and targeted by governmental and nongovernmental combatants. Armed conflict directly and indirectly affects children's physical, mental, and behavioral health. It can affect every organ system, and its impact can persist throughout the life course. In addition, children are disproportionately impacted by morbidity and mortality associated with armed conflict. A children's rights–based approach provides a framework for collaboration by the American Academy of Pediatrics, child health professionals, and national and international partners to respond in the domains of clinical care, systems development, and policy formulation. The American Academy of Pediatrics and child health professionals have critical and synergistic roles to play in the global response to the impact of armed conflict on children.

[a]Division of Community and Societal Pediatrics, University of Florida College of Medicine–Jacksonville, Jacksonville, Florida; [b]Centre for Social Paediatrics, Herlev Hospital, Herlev, Denmark; and [c]United Nations High Commissioner for Refugees, Washington, District of Columbia

Dr Shenoda identified the need to write this policy statement, conducted the supporting literature review, and wrote the first draft of the manuscript; Dr Goldhagen identified the need to write this policy statement and wrote the first draft of the manuscript; Dr Kadir and Mr Pitterman contributed to revisions; and all authors approved the final manuscript as submitted.

DOI: https://doi.org/10.1542/peds.2018-2585

Address correspondence to Sherry Shenoda, MD, FAAP. E-mail: sshenoda@thechildrensclinic.org.

If we are to reach real peace in this world, and if we are to carry on a real war against war, we shall have to begin with the children.

Mahatma Gandhi

To cite: Shenoda S, Kadir A, Pitterman S, et al. The Effects of Armed Conflict on Children. *Pediatrics.* 2018;142(6): e20182585

BACKGROUND

The acute and chronic effects of armed conflict on child health and well-being are among the greatest children's rights violations of the 21st century. For the purpose of this policy statement and the associated technical report,[1] armed conflict is defined as any organized dispute that involves the use of weapons, violence, or force, whether within national borders or beyond and whether involving state actors or nongovernmental entities (Table 1). Examples include international wars, civil wars, and conflicts between other kinds of groups, such as ethnic conflicts and violence associated with narcotics trafficking and gang violence involving narcotics. Civilian casualties have increased such that 90% of deaths from armed conflicts in the first decade of the 21st century were civilians,[2] a significant number of whom were children.[3–5] Children

TABLE 1 Selected Definitions

	Definition
Armed conflict	Any organized dispute that involves the use of weapons, violence, or force, whether within national borders or beyond and whether involving state actors or nongovernmental entities.
Asylum seeker	A person who seeks safety from persecution or serious harm in a country other than his or her own and awaits a decision on the application for refugee status under relevant international and national instruments. In case of a negative decision, the person must leave the country and may be expelled, as may any nonnational in an irregular or unlawful situation, unless permission to stay is provided on humanitarian or other related grounds.[7]
Internally displaced people	People or groups of people who have been forced or obliged to flee or to leave their homes or places of habitual residence, in particular as a result of or to avoid the effects of armed conflict, situations of generalized violence, violations of human rights, or natural or human-made disasters, and who have not crossed an internationally recognized state border[7]
Refugee	A person, who "owing to well-founded fear of persecution for reasons of race, religion, nationality, membership of a particular social group or political opinions, is outside the country of his nationality and is unable or, owing to such fear, is unwilling to avail himself of the protection of that country."[7]
Social determinants of health	The circumstances in which people are born, grow up, live, work, and age and the systems put in place to deal with illness. These circumstances are in turn shaped by a wider set of forces: economics, social policies, and politics.[8]
Stateless person	A person who is not considered as a national by any state under the operation of its law. As such, a stateless person lacks those rights attributable to nationality: the diplomatic protection of a state, the inherent right of sojourn in the state of residence, and the right of return in case he or she travels.[7]

are no longer considered as simply collateral damage in many armed conflicts. Instead, they are targeted by combatants.[6]

As a result, children bear a significant burden of conflict-associated morbidity and mortality.[3–5] The effects on the physical, mental, developmental, and behavioral health of children are profound, with all organ systems in the developing child affected as a result of direct injury. Children are also affected indirectly through deprivation and toxic stress, which can have a lasting effect on health across the life course. For example, children affected by armed conflict have an increased prevalence of posttraumatic stress disorder, depression, anxiety, and behavioral and psychosomatic complaints, which persist long after cessation of hostilities.[9–11]

Given the global prevalence of armed conflict and its pervasive effects on children, it is critically important that child health professionals understand these effects and respond both domestically and globally.

EFFECTS OF ARMED CONFLICT ON CHILDREN

The effects of armed conflict on children are both direct and indirect.[1] Direct effects take the form of

physical injury, developmental delay, disability, mental and behavioral health sequelae, and death. Military actions, violence associated with drug trafficking, indiscriminate airstrikes, and other forms of armed conflict have the intended and unintended consequence of killing and maiming children.[12] Indirect effects relate to the destruction of infrastructure required by children for their optimal survival and development, environmental exposures, and other downstream effects on social determinants of health, such as worsened living conditions and ill health of caregivers.[6,13–17] For example, the destruction of health infrastructure and the disruption of health systems result in breakdowns in vaccination programs, disease surveillance, and access to health and dental care.[14,18] Traditionally safe spaces for children (eg, schools, hospitals, and play areas) are increasingly affected by armed groups as a result of indiscriminate crossfire, looting, or direct targeting. The results are disruptions in schooling and impaired economic growth and development.[6,12,16,19] Besieged populations or those whose farms and fields have been destroyed are vulnerable to acute and chronic malnutrition, with subsequent effects on growth, immune and metabolic

systems functioning, and cognitive development.[20]

Many children affected by armed conflict are forcibly displaced from their homes.[21] Of the 68.5 million people forcibly displaced worldwide in 2017, more than 25 million were refugees living outside of their countries of origin; over half of these refugees were children, many of whom had spent their entire childhoods as people displaced.[21] The number of unaccompanied immigrant children has also reached record numbers, and this group is at a high risk for exploitation, trafficking, and psychological problems.[21–25]

Hundreds of thousands of children worldwide are also thought to be involved in armed conflict as combatants.[26,27] Children associated with armed groups (child soldiers) are victims of severe human rights violations. They may be threatened with death, deprived of food, given drugs, or forced to take part in armed combat in other ways.[26,27] They are at risk for physical and mental injury, death, sexual exploitation, rape, and sexually transmitted infections. After escaping, these children are also at risk for prolonged detention, during which they are treated as perpetrators rather than victims.[12]

RECOMMENDATIONS FOR MITIGATING THE EFFECTS OF ARMED CONFLICT ON CHILDREN

The American Academy of Pediatrics (AAP) and pediatric health professionals play critical and synergistic roles in responding to the impact of armed conflict on children. A children's rights–based approach provides a framework for addressing the breadth of these effects. Armed conflicts violate multiple children's rights, as enumerated in the United Nations Convention on the Rights of the Child (UNCRC).[17] Among these violations, the United Nations has identified 6 constituting grave human rights violations that constitute a breach of international humanitarian law: (1) recruitment and use of children, (2) killing or maiming of children,[28] (3) sexual violence against children, (4) attacks against schools or hospitals, (5) abduction of children, and (6) denial of humanitarian access.[28]

Informed by the articles of the UNCRC and by the human rights principle of indivisibility and interdependence, it is important for child health professionals to address all rights relevant to children affected by armed conflict if optimal health and development are to be realized. Toward this end, the AAP offers the below recommendations.

Opportunities for Clinical Practice

Clinicians caring for immigrant children in the United States should be prepared to address the physical, mental, and behavioral health effects of armed conflict. Child health professionals working in many settings outside the United States will also need to be prepared to respond to the direct and indirect effects of armed conflict.[29,30]

1. Child health professionals and staff who care for children affected by armed conflict should have access to training in trauma-informed care and to the development of trauma-informed practices.[31] In trauma-informed care, child health professionals recognize the realities of children's traumatic life experiences and respond to the effects of this trauma on children's health, development, and well-being.[32] They seek to mitigate the harmful effects of these experiences by providing multidisciplinary and age-appropriate services that reflect children's need for physical, mental, emotional, and sexual and reproductive health care as well as providing social work and legal services. Child health professionals with a trauma-informed practice are knowledgeable regarding the effects of trauma, sensitive in their response to trauma, and function to help mitigate the effects of trauma.

2. Child health professionals should be prepared to diagnose and provide initial management for prevalent mental health conditions among children exposed to armed conflict, such as depression, anxiety, and behavioral and psychosomatic complaints.[9,10] When possible, management strategies may include partnership with mental and behavioral health providers in the community to promote collaborative networks to care for these children as well as partnerships with organizations promoting resilience and social integration.[33–36] Referring parents or caregivers who are affected for care can also mitigate the effect of parental stress on child health.

3. Child health professionals should be trained to provide culturally effective care.[37] As affirmed in previous policy statements, the AAP defines culturally effective pediatric care as "the delivery of care within the context of appropriate physician knowledge, understanding, and appreciation of all cultural distinctions, leading to optimal health outcomes."[38] This includes working effectively with language services and with families with limited literacy.[1]

4. Child health professionals in the United States and abroad are encouraged to collaborate with local refugee resettlement organizations and other public and private sector organizations, such as schools, health systems, and social services, to facilitate the integration of children and families into their communities and to help families meet unmet needs.[25,39] Multisector collaboration plays a critical role in supporting (a) children in maintaining a sense of their identity and the ability to associate with peers; (b) the integrity of families and swift family reunification; (c) protection from abuse and neglect; (d) special care and education for children with disabilities; (e) the highest standard of medical care; (f) enrollment in eligible social programs and services; (g) an adequate standard of living; (h) access to educational opportunities that meet the special needs of the child; (i) access to play and cultural activities; (j) protection from child labor, drug abuse, sexual exploitation, trafficking, and other forms of exploitation; and (k) access to rehabilitative care.

5. Child health professionals working with refugees in camps or in conflict settings should have access to special preparation to do so. In addition to general preparation for international work[40] (such as credentialing, establishing clear roles and responsibilities, and understanding conditions that are locally prevalent), clinicians working in camps or conflict settings will be more effective if they are familiar

with internationally recognized standards for child protection and the care of children in humanitarian emergencies in addition to having preparation to manage physical injuries caused by armed conflict, sequelae of sexual violence, psychological trauma, and malnutrition, as appropriate within their scope of practice.[41–44]

Opportunities for Systems Strengthening

Optimal health and development for children exposed to armed conflict require community, health, and social systems equipped to fulfill the protection, promotion, and participation rights of these children (Tables 2 and 3). The structure and scope of systems will vary depending on the place in which they are being implemented and the vulnerabilities of the children being served.

1. Systems serving children exposed to armed conflict should provide access to physical, mental, behavioral, developmental, oral, and rehabilitation health services.[17] In secure environments, such as countries where children have received asylum, pediatricians may contribute to the development of policies, protocols, and resources to implement systems of care in which the holistic needs of each child are addressed. As affirmed in previous AAP policy statements, this includes advocating for insurance coverage and mental health parity as well as close collaboration with government agencies and community organizations to ensure that newly arrived child refugees or those seeking asylum are referred to medical, behavioral, and dental health homes and receive legal representation when needed.[25,39,46,49]

2. Systems should protect children from abuse and exploitation. As

TABLE 2 Summary of Key Articles of the UNCRC in the Areas of Protection, Promotion, and Participation

Articles	Rights
Rights of Protection: Keeping Safe From Harm	
6	Right to life
9	Right not to be separated from parents
19	Right to be protected from all forms of abuse
20	Right to special attention (eg, adoption and fostering if deprived of family)
32	Right to be protected from economic exploitation
33	Right to be protected from illicit drugs
34	Right to be protected from all forms of sexual exploitation
Rights of Promotion: Life, Survival, and Development to Full Potential	
24	Right to the highest standard of health care
27	Right to a standard of living adequate for the child's physical, mental, spiritual, moral, and social development
Rights of Participation: Having an Active Voice	
7, 8	Right to an identity (name, family, and nationality)
12,13	Right to express views freely and to be listened to
17	Right to access to information
23	Right for children with disabilities to enjoy life and participate actively in society

articulated in the UNCRC, children have special and extensive rights of protection from all forms of abuse and exploitation. As such, domestic and global systems, such as government border agencies and state departments, must protect children (displaced and nondisplaced) affected by armed violence from (a) kidnapping in secure and nonsecure zones, (b) all forms of violence (including sexual violence and child marriage), (c) inappropriate placement and adoption practices, (d) child labor, (e) drug abuse, (f) trafficking and other forms of exploitation, and (g) unjust detention or punishment.[17]

3. Systems should enhance environments capable of promoting optimal health and well-being. Governments should develop systems so that all children are registered at birth, no children are stateless, and children separated from their parents or caregivers by national borders have opportunities for reunification. Governments should also prohibit separation of children from their families (except in limited circumstances, such as abuse and neglect cases), regularly review care plans for children in state custody so that

these plans remain in the best interest of the child, provide special care for children with disabilities so they may lead full and independent lives, protect children from sexual violence and exploitation, provide all children with an adequate standard of living that meets their needs (particularly with regard to food, clothing, and housing), and ensure that all children may attend school.[17]

4. Child health professionals should work individually and within systems to enhance the participation of children and youth in their communities. Children and youth have the right to (a) respect for their views; (b) freedom of expression of thought, conscience, and religion; (c) freedom of association; (d) respect for privacy; and (e) access to information.[17] It is important to refrain from viewing children affected by armed conflict as helpless victims. Not only do they have the capacity for resilience in the face of seemingly debilitating circumstances but they are also agents for peace in their own right.[17] The active participation of children should be encouraged in their care, in their communities, and in the development of

TABLE 3 Resources (Online)

	Resource
Resources for clinicians	AAP Immigrant Child Health Toolkit
	AAP Trauma Toolbox for Primary Care
	AAP Enhancing Cultural Competence in Pediatric Medical Homes
	AAP clinical report: Health and Mental Health Needs of Children in US Military Families
	Canadian Pediatric Society: Caring for Kids New to Canada
	CDC Refugee Health Guidelines
	EthnoMed
	National Child Traumatic Stress Network: Refugee Trauma
	National Immigration Law Center
	Department of Health and Human Services, Office of Refugee Resettlement
	The Sphere Project
AAP policy statements	Early Childhood Adversity, Toxic Stress, and the Role of the Pediatrician: Translating Developmental Science into Lifelong Health (2012)
	Ensuring Culturally Effective Pediatric Care: Implications for Education and Health Policy (2004)[37]
	Health Equity and Children's Rights (2010)[45]
	The Pediatrician's Role in Community Pediatrics (2005)
	Providing Care for Immigrant, Migrant, and Border Children (2013)[25]
	Detention of Immigrant Children (2017)[46]
Legal context	Geneva Convention (1949)
	UNCRC (1989)[33] and accompanying Optional Protocol on the Involvement of Children in Armed Conflict (2000)[47]
	United Nations Refugee Convention (1951) and Protocol Relating to the Status of Refugees (1967)
Nongovernmental organizations	World Health Organization
	International Organization for Migrations
	Physicians for Human Rights
	International Physicians for the Prevention of Nuclear War
	Physicians for Social Responsibility
	Save the Children
	War Child
	Child Rights Information Network
	Human Rights Watch
Selected other resources	American Psychological Association: *Resilience of Refugee Children After War* (2011)
	Education Cannot Wait[48]
	Physicians for Human Rights: *Introduction to Medical Neutrality*
	Save the Children: *Stolen Futures: The Reintegration of Children Affected by Armed Conflict* (2007)
	UNHCR: *Global Report* (annual)
	UNICEF: *Uprooted: The Growing Crisis for Refugee and Migrant Children* (2016)
	Uppsala Conflict Data Program: Department of Peace and Conflict Research

CDC, Centers for Disease Control and Prevention; UNICEF, United Nations Children's Fund.

programs and policies directed toward them.

5. More research is needed to advance our understanding of the health and developmental sequelae of armed conflict as well as of the mitigating factors and evidence-based interventions to promote health and well-being. Domains for additional research include the physical, developmental, and psychosocial health effects of exposure to armed conflict on children; the contributions of social determinants to these effects; the burden of pediatric morbidity and mortality attributable to armed conflict; intervention strategies;

and optimal child health metrics for humanitarian response. Pediatricians may collaborate with academic institutions, pediatric societies, governments, and international nongovernmental organizations to support this research.

Opportunities for Public Policy Advocacy

A precedent exists for the involvement of physicians and health organizations in the prevention of and response to armed conflict and war.[50–52] The AAP supports the generation and implementation of policies that advance the health, development, well-being, and rights

of children affected by armed conflict and displacement.[45]

1. Core human rights principles should be integrated into US policy. In addition, the AAP reaffirms its commitment to advocate for policies that conform to the principles of the UNCRC and supports US ratification.

2. The participation of children younger than 18 years of age in armed conflict should be ended. This recommendation is consistent with both the recommendation of the 26th International Conference of the Red Cross and Red

Crescent and the Optional Protocol to the UNCRC on the Involvement of Children in Armed Conflict.[47,53] The United States, as a signatory of the Optional Protocol, should continue to work with international partners to eliminate the participation of children in direct hostilities.[47,54]

3. All children affected by armed conflict, including children associated with armed groups and children displaced, should be protected from all forms of torture and deprivation of liberty, including extended or arbitrary detention. Former child combatants, including children conscripted as gang members, are among the victims of armed conflict and should be treated as such. It is imperative to recognize the physical, mental, and behavioral health effects of their experiences and to prevent their further traumatization in detention centers and extrajudicial proceedings.[55,56]

4. Governments and nongovernmental entities have an obligation to uphold the Geneva Conventions with respect to maintaining the sanctity of safe places for children and ensuring medical and educational neutrality. Civilian homes, schools, playgrounds, and health facilities must be safe places for children to live, learn, and receive medical care. Child health professionals are also charged to uphold human rights norms, such as nondiscrimination, in these safe places.[54]

5. Special protection and humanitarian assistance should be afforded to child refugees and children displaced. Children fleeing armed conflict should be allowed to petition for asylum and should be screened for evidence of human trafficking.[46,57] Governments should prevent statelessness and family separation by ensuring rights to a name, nationality, and identity by registering all children. Doing so overcomes the barriers to accessing education, health care, and employment, which result from statelessness.[58]

6. Children should not be separated from their families during displacement and resettlement. An intact family is the optimal environment for children's health and well-being. In the event of separation, family reunification should be prioritized.

7. Children should be protected from landmines, unexploded ordnances, small arms, and light weapons through clearing efforts and strict control on their sale, ownership, and safe storage. Environmental hazards, such as unexploded ordnances and landmines, injure and kill children long after conflicts have ended.[59,60] The availability and durability of small arms facilitates the use of children by armed groups, heightens levels of violence, and results in greater levels of violence postconflict.[61]

8. Children should be afforded a voice in creating policy and programs that prevent and mitigate harmful effects of armed conflict. Children affected by armed conflict are often from minority groups whose history, language, or culture has been suppressed. They have a right to be heard, to have their opinions considered in decisions affecting them, to access nonbiased information, to associate with peers, and to have freedom of expression, association, and culture. These rights should be implicitly and explicitly integrated into the principles and into the implementation and evaluation strategies of all policies.

9. Children affected by armed conflict should have access to educational opportunities as part of an environment conducive to their reintegration into society. There is strong evidence to suggest that education for boys and girls at all levels reduces most forms of political violence.[62] However, education currently receives less than 2% of all humanitarian funding, and girls are more likely than boys to be excluded from education.[48] Because education is a priority for many children[63] and essential for their well-being, child health providers may advocate for their educational rights and access, especially during humanitarian emergencies.

LEAD AUTHORS

Sherry Shenoda, MD, FAAP
Ayesha Kadir, MD, MSc, FAAP
Shelly Pitterman, PhD
Jeffrey Goldhagen, MD, MPH, FAAP

SECTION ON INTERNATIONAL CHILD HEALTH EXECUTIVE COMMITTEE, 2017–2018

Parminder S. Suchdev, MD, MPH, FAAP, Chairperson
Kevin J. Chan, MD, MPH, FAAP
Cynthia R. Howard, MD, MPH, FAAP
Patrick McGann, MD, FAAP
Nicole E. St Clair, MD, FAAP
Katherine Yun, MD, MHS, FAAP
Linda D. Arnold, MD, FAAP, Immediate Past Chairperson

STAFF

Vayram Nyadroh

ABBREVIATIONS

AAP: American Academy of
          Pediatrics
UNCRC: United Nations
              Convention on the
              Rights of the Child

PEDIATRICS (ISSN Numbers: Print, 0031-4005; Online, 1098-4275).

Copyright © 2018 by the American Academy of Pediatrics

FINANCIAL DISCLOSURE: The authors have indicated they have no financial relationships relevant to this article to disclose.

FUNDING: No external funding.

POTENTIAL CONFLICT OF INTEREST: The authors have indicated they have no potential conflicts of interest to disclose.

COMPANION PAPER: A companion to this article can be found online at www.pediatrics.org/cgi/doi/10.1542/peds.2018-2586.

REFERENCES

1. Kadir A, Shenoda S, Goldhagen J, Pitterman S; Section on International Child Health. The effects of armed conflict on children. *Pediatrics.* 2018;142(6):e20182586

2. Garfield R. The epidemiology of war. In: Levy BS, Sidel VW, eds. *War and Public Health.* 2nd ed. New York, NY: Oxford University Press; 2008:23–36

3. Toole MJ, Waldman RJ. The public health aspects of complex emergencies and refugee situations. *Annu Rev Public Health.* 1997;18:283–312

4. Zwi AB, Grove NJ, Kelly P, Gayer M, Ramos-Jimenez P, Sommerfeld J. Child health in armed conflict: time to rethink. *Lancet.* 2006;367(9526):1886–1888

5. Kruk ME, Freedman LP, Anglin GA, Waldman RJ. Rebuilding health systems to improve health and promote statebuilding in post-conflict countries: a theoretical framework and research agenda. *Soc Sci Med.* 2010;70(1):89–97

6. Global Coalition to Protect Education From Attack. Lessons in war 2015: military use of schools and universities during armed conflict. 2015. Available at: https://www.scholarsatrisk.org/wp-content/uploads/2016/05/Lessons_in_War_2015.pdf. Accessed May 14, 2018

7. Institute of Medicine. Key migration terms. 2004. Available at:https://www.iom.int/key-migration-terms. Accessed May 14, 2018

8. World Health Organization. Social determinants of health: key concepts. 2017. Available at: www.who.int/social_determinants/thecommission/finalreport/key_concepts/en/. Accessed May 14, 2018

9. World Health Organization. Collective violence. In: Krug EG, Dahlberg LL, Mercy JA, Zwi AB, Lozano R, eds. *World Report on Violence and Health.* Geneva, Switzerland: World Health Organization; 2002:213–239. Available at: www.who.int/violence_injury_prevention/violence/global_campaign/en/chap8.pdf. Accessed May 14, 2018

10. Attanayake V, McKay R, Joffres M, Singh S, Burkle F Jr, Mills E. Prevalence of mental disorders among children exposed to war: a systematic review of 7,920 children. *Med Confl Surviv.* 2009;25(1):4–19

11. Betancourt TS, Meyers-Ohki SE, Charrow AP, Tol WA. Interventions for children affected by war: an ecological perspective on psychosocial support and mental health care. *Harv Rev Psychiatry.* 2013;21(2):70–91

12. Zerrougui L. *Annual Report of the Special Representative of the Secretary-General for Children and Armed Conflict.* New York, NY: United Nations; 2015

13. Left J, Moestue H. Large and small: impacts of armed violence on children and youth. In: McDonald G, LeBrun E, eds. *Small Arms Survey 2009: Shadows of War.* Cambridge, UK: Cambridge University Press; 2009:193–217. Available at: www.smallarmssurvey.org/fileadmin/docs/A-Yearbook/2009/en/Small-Arms-Survey-2009-Chapter-06-EN.pdf. Accessed May 14, 2018

14. Guha-Sapir D, D'Aoust O. *Demographic and Health Consequences of Civil Conflict.* Washington, DC: World Bank; 2011. Available at: http://hdl.handle.net/10986/9083. Accessed May 14, 2018

15. Levy BS, Sidel VW. War and public health: an overview. In: Levy BS, Sidel VW, eds. *War and Public Health.* 2nd ed. New York, NY: Oxford University Press; 2008:3–20

16. Safeguarding Health in Conflict Coalition. No protection, no respect: health workers and health facilities under attack. Available at: https://www.safeguardinghealth.org/sites/shcc/files/SHCC2016final.pdf. Accessed May 14, 2018

17. Hodgkin R, Newell P. *Implementation Handbook for the Convention on the Rights of the Child.* 3rd ed. New York, NY: United Nations Children's Fund; 2007

18. Requejo JH, Bryce J, Barros AJ, et al. Countdown to 2015 and beyond: fulfilling the health agenda for women and children. *Lancet.* 2015;385(9966):466–476

19. Office of the Special Representative of the Secretary-General for Children and Armed Conflict. *Protect Schools + Hospitals: Guidance Note on Security Council Resolution 1998.* New York, NY: United Nations; 2014

20. Das JK, Salam RA, Imdad A, Bhutta ZA. Infant and young child growth. In: Black RE, Laxminarayan R, Temmerman M, Walker N, eds. *Disease Control Priorities: Reproductive, Maternal, Newborn, and Child Health.* Vol 2. 3rd ed. Washington, DC: International Bank for Reconstruction and Development / The World Bank; 2016:225–239

21. United Nations High Commissioner for Refugees. Global trends: forced displacement in 2017. Available at: http://www.unhcr.org/5b27be547.pdf. Accessed June 19, 2018

22. Bhabha J. Seeking asylum alone: treatment of separated and trafficked children in need of refugee protection. *Int Migr.* 2004;42(1):141–148

23. Danish Red Cross. Unaccompanied minor asylum seekers with street behaviour. Seven presentations from the Danish Red Cross Conference. 2014. Available at: https://www.rodekors.dk/media/869917/Unaccompanied-minor-asylum-seekers-w-street-behaviour.pdf. Accessed May 14, 2018

24. International Organization for Migration. Unaccompanied children on the move. 2011. Available at: https://publications.iom.int/system/files/pdf/uam_report_11812.pdf. Accessed May 14, 2018

25. Council on Community Pediatrics. Providing care for immigrant, migrant, and border children. *Pediatrics*. 2013;131(6). Available at: www.pediatrics.org/cgi/content/full/131/6/e2028

26. Betancourt TS, Borisova II, de la Soudière M, Williamson J. Sierra Leone's child soldiers: war exposures and mental health problems by gender. *J Adolesc Health*. 2011;49(1):21–28

27. United Nations Children's Fund. The Paris principles: principles and guidelines on children associated with armed forces or armed groups. 2007. Available at: https://www.unicef.org/emerg/files/ParisPrinciples31 0107English.pdf. Accessed May 14, 2018

28. United Nations; Office of the Special Representative of the Secretary-General for Children and Armed Conflict. Working Paper No 1: the six grave violations against children during armed conflict: the legal foundation. 2013. Available at: https://childrenandarmedconflict.un.org/publications/WorkingPaper-1_SixGraveViolationsLegalFoundation.pdf. Accessed May 14, 2018

29. Palfrey JS, Sofis LA, Davidson EJ, Liu J, Freeman L, Ganz ML; Pediatric Alliance for Coordinated Care. The Pediatric Alliance for Coordinated Care: evaluation of a medical home model. *Pediatrics*. 2004;113(suppl 5):1507–1516

30. Medical Home Initiatives for Children With Special Needs Project Advisory Committee. The medical home. *Pediatrics*. 2002;110(1, pt 1):184–186

31. American Academy of Pediatrics. The resilience project: we can stop toxic stress. Training toolkit. 2017. Available at: https://www.aap.org/en-us/advocacy-and-policy/aap-health-initiatives/resilience/Pages/Training-Toolkit.aspx. Accessed May 14, 2018

32. Marsac ML, Kassam-Adams N, Hildenbrand AK, et al. Implementing a trauma-informed approach in pediatric health care networks. *JAMA Pediatr*. 2016;170(1):70–77

33. United Nations Human Rights Office of the High Commissioner. Convention on the rights of the child. 1989. Available at: www.ohchr.org/en/professionalinterest/pages/crc.aspx. Accessed May 14, 2018

34. Fazel M, Reed RV, Panter-Brick C, Stein A. Mental health of displaced and refugee children resettled in high-income countries: risk and protective factors. *Lancet*. 2012;379(9812):266–282

35. Luthar SS, Cicchetti D, Becker B. The construct of resilience: a critical evaluation and guidelines for future work. *Child Dev*. 2000;71(3):543–562

36. Betancourt TS, Khan KT. The mental health of children affected by armed conflict: protective processes and pathways to resilience. *Int Rev Psychiatry*. 2008;20(3):317–328

37. Britton CV; American Academy of Pediatrics Committee on Pediatric Workforce. Ensuring culturally effective pediatric care: implications for education and health policy. *Pediatrics*. 2004;114(6):1677–1685

38. Committee on Pediatric Workforce. Enhancing pediatric workforce diversity and providing culturally effective pediatric care: implications for practice, education, and policy making. *Pediatrics*. 2013;132(4). Available at: www.pediatrics.org/cgi/content/full/132/4/e1105

39. Council on Community Pediatrics. Poverty and child health in the United States. *Pediatrics*. 2016;137(4):e20160339

40. St Clair NE, Pitt MB, Bakeera-Kitaka S, et al; Global Health Task Force of the American Board of Pediatrics. Global health: preparation for working in resource-limited settings. *Pediatrics*. 2017;140(5):e20163783

41. Disaster Preparedness Advisory Council; Committee on Pediatric Emergency Medicine. Ensuring the health of children in disasters. *Pediatrics*. 2015;136(5). Available at: www.pediatrics.org/cgi/content/full/136/5/e1407

42. Save the Children International. Child protection. Available at: https://www.savethechildren.net/what-we-do/child-protection. Accessed May 14, 2018

43. United Nations Children's Fund. Child protection from violence, exploitation and abuse: armed violence reduction. Available at: www.unicef.org/protection/57929_58011.html. Accessed May 14, 2018

44. War Child. No child in war. Available at: www.warchild.org.uk. Accessed May 14, 2018

45. Council on Community Pediatrics; Committee on Native American Child Health. Health equity and children's rights. *Pediatrics*. 2010;125(4):838–849

46. Linton JM, Griffin M, Shapiro AJ; Council on Community Pediatrics. Detention of immigrant children. *Pediatrics*. 2017;139(5):e20170483

47. United Nations Human Rights Office of the High Commissioner. Optional protocol to the convention on the rights of the child on the involvement of children in armed conflict. 2000. Available at: www.ohchr.org/EN/ProfessionalInterest/Pages/OPACCRC.aspx. Accessed May 14, 2018

48. United Nations Children's Fund. Education cannot wait: a fund for education in emergencies. Available at: www.educationcannotwait.org/. Accessed May 14, 2018

49. American Academy of Pediatrics. Blueprint for children: how the next president can build a foundation for a healthy future. 2016. Available at: https://www.aap.org/en-us/Documents/BluePrintForChildren.pdf. Accessed May 14, 2018

50. International Physicians for the Prevention of Nuclear War. Available at: www.ippnw.org. Accessed May 14, 2018

51. Physicians for Social Responsibility. Available at: www.psr.org. Accessed May 14, 2018

52. Physicians for Human Rights. Available at: http://physiciansforhumanrights.org. Accessed May 14, 2018

53. Office of the Special Representative of the Secretary-General for Children and Armed Conflict. Ratification status of the optional protocol. Available at: https://treaties.un.org/pages/

viewdetails.aspx?src=ind&mtdsg_no=
iv-11-b&chapter=4&lang=en. Accessed
May 14, 2018

54. International Committee of the Red
    Cross. *Respecting and Protecting
    Health Care in Armed Conflicts and in
    Situations Not Covered by International
    Humanitarian Law*. Geneva,
    Switzerland: International Committee
    of the Red Cross; 2012

55. United Nations Office of the Special
    Representative of the Secretary-
    General for Children Affected by
    Armed Conflict. Working paper no.
    3, children and justice during and in
    the aftermath of armed conflict. 2011.
    Available at: www.refworld.org/docid/
    4e6f2f132.html. Accessed May 14, 2018

56. Hamilton C, Anderson K, Barnes R,
    Dorling K. *Administrative Detention
    of Children: A Global Report*. New

York, NY: United Nations Children's
Fund; 2011. Available at: https://www.
unicef.org/protection/Administrative_
detention_discussion_paper_
April2011.pdf. Accessed May 14, 2018

57. Greenbaum J, Bodrick N; Committee
    on Child Abuse and Neglect;
    Section on International Child
    Health. Global human trafficking
    and child victimization. *Pediatrics*.
    2017;140(6):e20173138

58. United Nations High Commissioner for
    Refugees. *I Am Here, I Belong: The Urgent
    Need to End Childhood Statelessness*.
    Geneva, Switzerland: United Nations High
    Commissioner for Refugees Division of
    International Protection; 2015

59. Bilukha OO, Brennan M, Anderson M.
    The lasting legacy of war: epidemiology
    of injuries from landmines and
    unexploded ordnance in Afghanistan,

2002-2006. *Prehosp Disaster Med*.
2008;23(6):493–499

60. Walsh NE, Walsh WS. Rehabilitation
    of landmine victims—the ultimate
    challenge. *Bull World Health Organ*.
    2003;81(9):665–670

61. United Nations Children's Fund. No
    guns, please: we are children! 2001.
    Available at: https://www.unicef.org/
    publications/files/No_Guns_Please_-_
    We_Are_Children(1).pdf. Accessed May
    14, 2018

62. Østby G, Urdal H. *Education and Civil
    Conflict: A Review of the Quantitative,
    Empirical Literature*. Paris, France:
    United Nations Educational, Scientific
    and Cultural Organization; 2010

63. Save the Children. *What Do Children
    Want in Times of Emergency and
    Crisis? They Want an Education*.
    London, UK: Save the Children; 2015

The Effects of Armed Conflict on Children

• •

• *Technical Report*

TECHNICAL REPORT

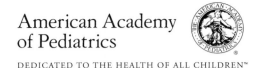

American Academy
of Pediatrics

DEDICATED TO THE HEALTH OF ALL CHILDREN™

The Effects of Armed Conflict on Children

Ayesha Kadir, MD, MSc, FAAP,[a] Sherry Shenoda, MD, FAAP,[b] Jeffrey Goldhagen, MD, MPH, FAAP,[b] Shelly Pitterman, PhD,[c] SECTION ON INTERNATIONAL CHILD HEALTH

abstract

More than 1 in 10 children worldwide are affected by armed conflict. The effects are both direct and indirect and are associated with immediate and long-term harm. The direct effects of conflict include death, physical and psychological trauma, and displacement. Indirect effects are related to a large number of factors, including inadequate and unsafe living conditions, environmental hazards, caregiver mental health, separation from family, displacement-related health risks, and the destruction of health, public health, education, and economic infrastructure. Children and health workers are targeted by combatants during attacks, and children are recruited or forced to take part in combat in a variety of ways. Armed conflict is both a toxic stress and a significant social determinant of child health. In this Technical Report, we review the available knowledge on the effects of armed conflict on children and support the recommendations in the accompanying Policy Statement on children and armed conflict.

[a]Centre for Social Paediatrics, Herlev Hospital, Herlev, Denmark; [b]Division of Community and Societal Pediatrics, University of Florida College of Medicine–Jacksonville, Jacksonville, Florida; and [c]United Nations High Commissioner for Refugees Regional Representative for the United States and the Caribbean, Washington, District of Columbia

Dr Kadir identified the need to write this Technical Report, conducted the literature review to support it, and wrote the first draft; Dr Shenoda identified the need to write this Technical Report, conducted the literature review to support it, and contributed to revisions; Dr Goldhagen contributed to revisions; Mr Pitterman contributed to revisions and the figure; and all authors approved the final manuscript as submitted.

The guidance in this report does not indicate an exclusive course of treatment or serve as a standard of medical care. Variations, taking into account individual circumstances, may be appropriate.

All Technical Reports from the American Academy of Pediatrics automatically expire 5 years after publication unless reaffirmed, revised, or retired at or before that time.

Technical Reports from the American Academy of Pediatrics benefit from expertise and resources of liaisons and internal (AAP) and external reviewers. However, Technical Reports from the American Academy of Pediatrics may not reflect the views of the liaisons or the organizations or government agencies that they represent.

This Technical Report does not reflect the views of United Nations High Commissioner for Refugees.

DOI: https://doi.org/10.1542/peds.2018-2586

To cite: Kadir A, Shenoda S, Goldhagen J, et al. The Effects of Armed Conflict on Children. *Pediatrics.* 2018;142(6): e20182586

INTRODUCTION

More than 1 in 10 children worldwide are affected by armed conflict.[1] Combat activities and population displacement caused by conflict have direct effects on child mortality and morbidity. In addition, there are long-lasting indirect effects that are mediated by complex political, social, economic, and environmental changes. In 2015, there were 223 violent conflicts, of which 43 were limited- or full-scale wars.[2]

The nature of war has changed. Combat zones are increasingly widespread, weapons cause destruction on a larger scale,[3,4] conflicts are more protracted (waxing and waning over lengthier periods of time),[5] and the availability and use of small arms facilitates the use of children as combatants.[6] These changes have led to geographically widespread, complex, and nuanced effects on children's physical, developmental, and mental health and wellbeing. Furthermore, the effects of armed conflict continue long after hostilities have ceased. Unexploded ordnances, such as landmines and cluster bombs, result in injuries and death for decades after combat has ended.[7] Similarly, the adverse effects of population displacement, the destruction of health systems and social infrastructure, environmental damage, and economic sanctions may compromise children's access to basic necessities, such as food, health care, and education, for decades. As a result, even short-lived armed conflicts affect child health and wellbeing across the life course and through adulthood.

The rules of war have also changed. Schools, which have been traditionally safe places, are targeted, and children are often attacked while on their way to or from school.[8,9] In many armed conflicts, schools and educational facilities are used by combatant forces, including government forces, as bases for combat and to recruit children.[8,9] The result is reduced school enrollment, high dropout rates, lower educational attainment, poor schooling conditions, and the exploitation of children.[9,10] Similarly, attacks on both government and nongovernmental health facilities and mobile clinics are increasingly prevalent.[11] These attacks violate the Geneva Conventions[12] and result in the death of patients and health workers, the destruction of health infrastructure,[11] and increasing barriers to care because of people's fear of being injured or killed while seeking treatment.[11]

DEFINITION OF ARMED CONFLICT

For the purpose of this Technical Report and the associated Policy Statement,[13] armed conflict is defined as any organized dispute that involves the use of weapons, violence, or force, whether within national borders or beyond them, and whether involving state actors or nongovernment entities. Examples include international wars, civil wars, and conflicts between other kinds of groups, such as ethnic conflicts and

TABLE 1 Timeline of International Agreements and Treaties Protecting Children and Medical Personnel From Armed Conflict

Year	Agreements and Treaties
1948	Universal Declaration of Human Rights
1949	The Geneva Conventions I–IV: The Geneva Conventions comprise 4 treaties and 3 protocols that regulate the conduct of armed conflict. Together, they form the basis of international humanitarian law. Aspects of the conventions of particular relevance to child health include the protection of the wounded and the sick, health and public health personnel, and humanitarian aid; the protected status of health facilities; the free passage of essential food, clothing, and medical supplies to the civilian population; and the protection of children who are orphaned or separated.[12]
1951	The UN Convention Relating to the Status of Refugees: The UN Convention Relating to the Status of Refugees (1951) and the Protocol Relating to the Status of Refugees (1967), known collectively as the Refugee Convention, are the foundation for the protection of refugees in international law. The convention defines the term refugee and establishes specific rights of refugees and the obligations of states for the provision and protection of these rights. Because people who are internally displaced have not crossed an international border, they do not fall under the protection of the Refugee Convention. However, people who are internally displaced retain all their rights and protection afforded under human rights and international humanitarian law.[16,17]
1959	UN Declaration of the Rights of the Child
1967	UN Protocol Relating to the Status of Refugees
1977	Protocols I and II of the Geneva Conventions
1989	UNCRC: After the adoption of the Universal Declaration of Human Rights in 1948 and in recognition of the special need for protection of children, the UN adopted the Declaration of the Rights of the Child (1959). The declaration forms the basis for the UNCRC (1989), which is a legally binding treaty in which 40 substantive rights of children are established. Particular attention is given to children who are affected by armed conflict, setting out a basic minimum standard for their care and the promotion of their health and wellbeing. This includes the right to protection from violence and sexual exploitation; the right to freedom of thought and education, health services, and welfare services; and specific rights of children who are refugees, separated, and unaccompanied.[14,15] In 2000, the Optional Protocol on the Involvement of Children in Armed Conflict was adopted and aimed at preventing children <18 years old from being recruited for or taking part in hostilities.[18,19] The United States ratified the optional protocol in 2002 but remains the only country that has not ratified the UNCRC.
2000	Optional Protocol to the UNCRC on the Involvement of Children in Armed Conflict

violence associated with narcotics trafficking and narco-gang violence.

HISTORICAL AND LEGAL CONTEXT

Several legal declarations and treaties protect the health of children and health workers and preserve access to health care during armed conflict. The most important of these include the Geneva Conventions (1949), the United Nations (UN) Refugee Convention (1951) and 1967 Protocol, and the United Nations Convention on the Rights of the Child (UNCRC) (1989) with its accompanying Optional Protocol on the Involvement of Children in Armed Conflict (2000; Table 1). According to international law, the involvement of children in armed

conflict and the targeting of health workers and facilities by combatants are human rights violations. Of particular relevance is the UNCRC, a legally binding treaty in which 40 substantive rights for children are outlined and grouped into 3 categories: protection, promotion, and participation (Table 2). Specific child rights include protection from violence and sexual exploitation, freedom of thought, education, health services, welfare services, and specific rights of children who are refugees, separated, and unaccompanied.[14,15] The United States remains the only country that has not ratified the UNCRC.

To strengthen the legal protection of children during armed conflict, the Optional Protocol to the UNCRC

TABLE 2 Summary of Key Articles of the UNCRC in the Areas of Protection, Promotion, and Participation

Articles	Rights
Rights of Protection: Keeping Safe From Harm	
6	Right to life
9	Right not to be separated from parents
19	Right to be protected from all forms of abuse
20	Right to special attention (eg, adoption and fostering if deprived of family)
32	Right to be protected from economic exploitation
33	Right to be protected from illicit drugs
34	Right to be protected from all forms of sexual exploitation
Rights of Promotion: Life, Survival, and Development to Full Potential	
24	Right to the highest standard of health care
27	Right to a standard of living adequate for a child's physical, mental, spiritual, moral, and social development
Rights of Participation: Having an Active Voice	
7, 8	Right to an identity (name, family, and nationality)
12, 13	Right to express views freely and be listened to
17	Right to have access to information
23	Right for children who are disabled to enjoy life and participate actively in society

was adopted by the UN to prevent children younger than 18 years old from being recruited into or participating as combatants in hostilities.[18] In the optional protocol, 16 years old is established as the absolute minimum age for voluntary recruitment, and signatories are required to take all feasible measures to ensure that 16- and 17-year-old members of the armed forces do not take part in hostilities. The optional protocol was ratified by the US Senate in 2002.[20] The United States has also passed a law stipulating that 16-year-old children may not enlist and specifying that the voluntary enlistment of 17-year-old children requires the consent of a parent or guardian.[21] Furthermore, as of 2007, US policy has been that 17-year-olds may not be deployed to combat zones.

The UN has identified 6 categories of human rights violations against children, known as the 6 grave violations. These violations include the killing and maiming of children, the abduction of children, the recruitment or use of children as soldiers, sexual violence against children, attacks against schools or hospitals, and the denial of humanitarian access.[22] The first 4 are direct acts of violence against children, and the last 2 are indirect actions that cause harm to children and directly relate to health care and health workers. The commission of any of these violations constitutes a breach of international humanitarian law.[22]

GLOBAL BURDEN OF ARMED CONFLICT ON CHILD HEALTH

Armed conflict is a public health issue.[23] An estimated 246 million children live in areas affected by conflict (Fig 1).[1,24–26] Forced displacement is at a record high: more than 68.5 million people, including 28 million children, are currently living as refugees, asylum seekers, stateless people, or internally displaced people (see Table 3 for definitions).[27–31] Of the world's 25 million refugees, half are children: nearly 1 in 200 children across the globe.[27,30] The authors of the 2005 State of the World's Children report, "Childhood Under Threat," suggested that 90% of conflict-related deaths from 1990 to 2005 were civilians, many of whom were children.[32]

However, the precise effect of any given armed conflict on child health is difficult to determine.[34–36] Conflicts disrupt the health information systems that report morbidity and mortality under typical circumstances.[23] As a result, most published estimates of the population health effects of armed conflict are based on media reports and official pronouncements from governments and combating parties, which may politicize or intentionally misrepresent information.[23,37] Deaths are also difficult to verify, and this may lead to underestimation. For example, in a report by the UN special rapporteur on children and armed conflict, it was estimated that thousands of children had died in the Syrian conflict in 2015.[38] However, only 591 child deaths were verified by the UN, which accounts for barely 0.01% of the 50 000 deaths that other analysts had estimated to have occurred during that year.[2,34] Other problems in estimating the child health impact of armed conflict include the near absence of population-level data on morbidity and the tendency to aggregate child and adult data. As a result, there are no pooled estimates for the total number of children killed, injured, orphaned, handicapped, and/or psychologically traumatized by exposure to armed conflicts.

Given the challenges described, it is not surprising that there are few prevalence studies on the indirect causes of mortality or morbidity among children affected by armed conflict. Most of the literature is in the form of case reports in which researchers describe the type and distribution of injuries treated or smaller studies on communicable disease transmission, perinatal health, nutrition, or environmental contamination. Nonetheless, it is clear that the conditions created by armed conflict (social determinants of health, such as population displacement, the destruction of infrastructure, and the deterioration of heath and public health systems) significantly increase childhood mortality and morbidity. Although

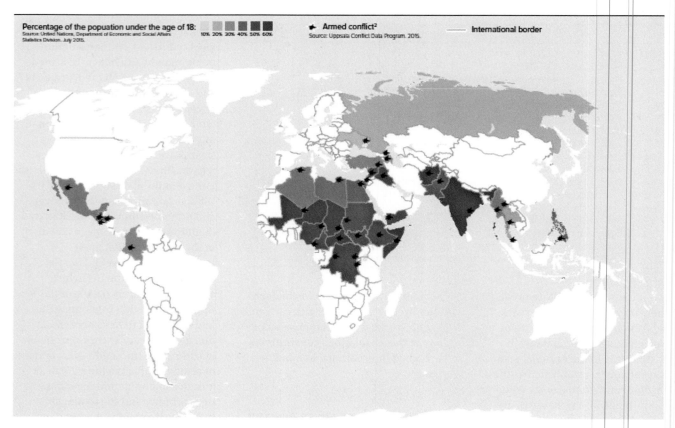

Percentage of the popuation under the age of 18: 10% 20% 30% 40% 50% 60%   ✦ Armed conflict²   —— International border
Source: United Nations, Department of Economic and Social Affairs Statistics Division. July 2015.   Source: Uppsala Conflict Data Program. 2015.

FIGURE 1

Children living in countries affected by armed conflict. Percentage of the overall population <18 years of age in countries affected by armed conflict, which is defined as any organized dispute that involves the use of weapons, violence, or force, whether within national borders or beyond them, and whether involving state actors or nongovernment entities.The boundaries and names shown and the designations used on this map do not imply official endorsement or acceptance by the United Nations. Source: United Nations, Department of Economic and Social Affairs, Population Division (2015). World Population Prospects: The 2015 Revision. Source: Melander, Erik, Therése Pettersson, and Lotta Themnér (2016) Organized violence, 1989–2015. *Journal of Peace Research* 53(5):727–742.

there are no studies in which researchers examine changes in the hypothalamic-pituitary-adrenal axis after exposure to armed conflict, it can be argued that the severity and chronicity of the stresses that children endure rise to the level of toxic stress[39] with its well-documented impact on physical and mental health across the life course.

Data on neonatal and infant health can provide insight into how the conditions created by armed conflict indirectly affect children's health. In conflict zones, there are higher rates of stillbirth, low birth weight, preterm birth, and perinatal mortality than during peacetime or in peaceful areas of the same country.[40–42] Mortality

rates in infants and children younger than 5 years old are also higher in areas affected by conflict when compared with prewar data or data from peaceful areas of the same country.[43–45]

Health facilities and health workers are increasingly becoming casualties of armed conflict, including targeted attacks. Reports from Syria, Yemen, Afghanistan, Nigeria, and Pakistan offer just a few examples.[46–48] In 2014, 603 health workers were killed and an additional 958 were injured in attacks in 32 countries.[49] The trend has become so common that the World Health Organization has developed a monitoring system to track these attacks and their effects.[49]

EFFECT OF ARMED CONFLICT ON CHILDREN'S PHYSICAL HEALTH

Direct Effects of Combat on Child Health

The kinds of injuries children sustain from armed conflict vary depending on the nature of combat, with all age groups being affected. In Iraq and Afghanistan, the most common forms of war trauma in children are blast and bullet injuries.[50] Blast injuries are caused by explosions and result in shockwave and shearing injuries, penetrating trauma, burns, crush injuries, and contamination injuries from the explosive device or environment.[51] Children suffering from blast injuries usually present with multiple injury sites and types. Burns and severe head and neck

TABLE 3 Selected Definitions

	Definition
Armed conflict	Any organized dispute that involves the use of weapons, violence, or force, whether within national borders or beyond them, and whether involving state actors or nongovernment entities
Asylum seeker	A person who seeks safety from persecution or serious harm in a country other than his or her own and awaits a decision on the application for refugee status under relevant international and national instruments; in case of a negative decision, the person must leave the country and may be expelled, as may any nonnational in an irregular or unlawful situation, unless permission to stay is provided on humanitarian or other related grounds[31]
Internally displaced people	People or groups of people who have been forced or obliged to flee or to leave their homes or places of habitual residence, in particular as a result of or to avoid the effects of armed conflict, situations of generalized violence, violations of human rights, or natural or human-made disasters and who have not crossed an internationally recognized state border[31]
Refugee	A person who "owing to well-founded fear of persecution for reasons of race, religion, nationality, membership of a particular social group, or political opinions is outside the country of his [or her] nationality and is unable or, owing to such fear, is unwilling to avail himself [or herself] of the protection of that country"[31]
Social determinants of health	The circumstances in which people are born, grow up, live, work, and age and the systems put in place to deal with illness. These circumstances are in turn shaped by a wider set of forces: economics, social policies, and politics.[33]
Stateless person	A person who is not considered as a national by any state under the operation of its law. As such, a stateless person lacks those rights attributable to nationality: the diplomatic protection of a state, no inherent right of sojourn in the state of residence, and no right of return in case he or she travels.[31]

injuries, and particularly penetrating head trauma,[52] are the most common and the most lethal.[53] This pattern differs from blast injury in adults, who more often suffer injuries to the extremities.[53] The high prevalence of penetrating trauma sustained by children in combat zones also differs markedly from pediatric trauma in the United States, where blunt trauma is more common and mortality is significantly lower.[54] Pediatric trauma patients in combat zones have high mortality rates, which are likely attributable to both the severity of the injuries sustained as well as barriers in accessing adequate and timely care.[54]

Chemical warfare has been documented in numerous conflicts dating back to Word War I.[55–58] Despite international law banning the development, stockpiling, and use of chemical weapons,[59] reports of the continued use of these weapons

against civilian populations have been issued as recently as May 2018.[60] Children are thought to be at higher risk of toxicity from chemical weapons because of their smaller mass, higher respiratory rate and minute volume, smaller airway diameter, lower fluid reserve, lower seizure threshold, and more limited cardiovascular stress response when compared with adults.[61]

Estimates suggest that the prevalence of rape and sexual exploitation of children in armed conflict is increasing.[62] In addition to the psychological trauma of sexual violence during armed conflict, girls who suffer rape are less likely than adults to seek medical attention and are at increased risk for sexually transmitted infections (STIs), pregnancy, obstetric or gynecologic complications (eg, vesicovaginal fistulas), and subsequent infertility.[63,64] Boys also experience rape and

STIs, although they are less likely than girls to report these violations because of stigma.[64] Those who survive their experiences suffer from psychological trauma and often face stigma and exclusion when they return to their communities.[65] Children born of rape during armed conflicts are a population that requires special attention. Girls who become pregnant as a result of rape may have ambivalent feelings toward their children, and the children may not be accepted into their communities.[63]

Environmental Hazards

Armed conflict creates environmental hazards that continue to affect children long after hostilities have ended. Landmines and unexploded ordnances pose a major risk for death and disability for decades.[7] Studies from Afghanistan, Eritrea, Laos, and Nepal revealed that children accounted for approximately half of all injuries caused by explosive remnants of war.[66–70] Children are most likely to sustain injuries to the upper extremities, face, and torso.[67,71,72] These injury patterns are seen because children are most often injured while playing, tampering with an explosive device, or performing economic activities, such as herding livestock.[66–68,73,74] Chemical weapons and other chemical contaminants can also have long-term effects. A recent systematic review and meta-analysis of the association between Agent Orange and birth defects in Vietnam revealed that children born to individuals who had been exposed to Agent Orange were nearly twice as likely to have birth defects than children of individuals who were unexposed.[75] The destruction of buildings, water supplies, wastewater systems, factories, fuel stations, and farms has been shown to limit access to potable water and sanitation and release infectious and chemical contaminants into the air, water, and soil.[76] The long-term effects of these hazards on child health have not been well studied.

Damage to Health and Public Health Infrastructure and the Targeting of Health Facilities

The destruction of health care and public health systems is a major cause of morbidity and mortality in children affected by armed conflict. Children, especially those younger than 5 years old, bear the highest burden of indirect conflict-related death.[77–79] Lower respiratory tract infections, diarrhea, measles, malaria, and malnutrition are among the leading causes of mortality in children in conflict-affected areas.[9,80]

The deterioration of health systems during armed conflict is characterized by the destruction of physical infrastructure, disruptions in supply chains, and the diversion of state funds from health to the military.[9,81–84] Health workers and health care facilities are increasingly targeted by combatants, resulting in the killing and flight of the health workforce.[85] In some recent instances, military operations have been conducted under the guise of public health services, thus undermining local trust in health workers and placing health teams at risk for attack.[86] Families may be increasingly reluctant to seek medical care at both formal and informal health facilities,[87] fearing that children in the facilities will be targeted by attacks.[81,83] Sieges, snipers, and active fighting may also prevent families from traveling to health facilities.

The conditions created by armed conflict compromise key public health functions, including vaccine delivery, health surveillance, and disease outbreak investigation,[82,88] resulting in increased rates of infectious disease transmission.[89] Previously eradicated, vaccine-preventable diseases may reemerge in conflict-affected areas, as evidenced by an outbreak of polio

in the Syrian Arab Republic in 2013.[89,90] Similarly, there is a clear relationship between violent conflict and the incidence of HIV and/or AIDS, tuberculosis, and malaria.[89] Countries experiencing high levels of armed conflict or political terror are also vulnerable to other diseases associated with crowding, population displacement, and lack of access to health care, such as the neglected tropical disease leishmaniasis.[82] Indeed, there is a direct dose-response relationship between the intensity of violent conflict and the incidence of cutaneous and visceral leishmaniasis.[82]

Food may be used as a weapon of war, and the effect of food insecurity on child health is exacerbated by the destruction of health and public health programs used to target malnutrition. Attacks on crops and livestock, food stores and shops, and transport links compromise the food supply during periods of conflict, and infrastructure and agriculture may require years to recover after the cessation of hostilities.[9,77,91] Children in conflict and humanitarian settings have high levels of moderate and severe acute malnutrition, anemia, and other nutritional deficiencies.[77,92–94] For example, a report on South Sudanese refugee children living in camps in Ethiopia described global acute malnutrition rates of 25% to 30% in children 6 months to 5 years of age with a severe acute malnutrition prevalence of 5.7% to 10%.[93]

Forced Displacement

Displacement, whether within the borders of the country or across international boundaries, carries with it specific health risks and needs that are influenced by conditions before the journey, during travel, and in the place of arrival.[95–97] Low-income regions host 85% of refugees worldwide.[27] Children who are forcibly displaced have more limited access to health care and basic

services when compared with local populations even in countries with longstanding refugee resettlement programs.[98–100] In addition, children who are forcibly displaced often lack access to other basic needs, such as food, potable water, adequate sanitation, and education.[9] Crowding of people who are displaced in camps and urban areas has been associated with outbreaks of cholera and other communicable diseases.[84,101] Disruptions in immunization programs and a simultaneous worsening of sanitary and living conditions are associated with outbreaks of vaccine-preventable diseases, such as measles, meningitis, and pertussis.[84] Children who are displaced are at high risk for trafficking, violence, and exploitation, including sexual violence, labor, detention by government authorities, xenophobic attacks from the general public, bullying in schools, and domestic violence.[30] Half of primary school–aged children who are refugees and 75% of adolescent refugees are out of school.[102]

EFFECT OF ARMED CONFLICT ON CHILDREN'S MENTAL AND PSYCHOSOCIAL HEALTH

Exposure to armed conflict has social and psychological repercussions that endure long after the termination of hostilities.[103] As with physical health, postconflict mental health is dependent on multiple factors, including mental health status before the conflict, the nature of the conflict, exposure to stressors, and the cultural and community context.[104]

Children who are affected by war have an increased prevalence of posttraumatic stress disorder (PTSD), depression, anxiety, and behavioral and psychosomatic complaints.[104] Pooled estimates from a systematic review of nearly 8000 children who were exposed to war revealed that the prevalence of PTSD is 47%, that of depression is 43%, and that of anxiety is 27%, although rates are lower among children with more remote exposures.[105] Young children ages 0 to 6 years exhibit increased anxiety, fear, startling, attention seeking, temper tantrums, sadness, and crying as well as difficulty sleeping alone and frequent awakenings.[106] They are more likely to suffer psychosomatic symptoms, such as stomach aches and irregular bowel movements, and they demonstrate alterations in their play, which can become either more aggressive or more withdrawn.[106] Parental mental health has an important influence on the mental health of children affected by conflict, particularly in young children.[106] Adolescents with cumulative exposure to war events and those with PTSD resulting from war events have also been found have significantly higher rates of substance abuse.[107]

The mental health impact of displacement appears to vary depending on where children are resettled. Factors that negatively affect mental health and social wellbeing among children who are displaced in low- and middle-income countries (LMICs) include exposure to mass trauma and family violence,[108] displacement,[109] social isolation, loss of social status, and perceived discrimination.[104,109] Among children who are resettled in high-income countries, risk factors for negative mental health outcomes include exposure to postmigration violence, multiple changes of residence in host countries, parental exposure to violence, poor financial support, having a single parent, and having a parent with a psychiatric disorder.[110] Learning problems in these children have been associated with traumatic experiences, detention, barriers in communication, low expectations from teachers, bullying, and discrimination.[111]

Protective influences on the mental health and social wellbeing of children who are refugees in high-income countries include parental support and family cohesion, self-reported support from friends, self-reported positive school experience, and same–ethnic origin foster care.[110] In LMICs, children who are displaced benefit from repatriation to their countries of origin once it is safe to do so.[109]

SPECIAL GROUPS

Children Associated With Armed Groups

Children are recruited or forced to participate in armed conflict in many different ways, including as soldiers, cooks, domestic workers, porters, human shields, mine sweepers, gang members, and sex slaves.[19,32,62,112,113] The number of children associated with armed forces and armed groups worldwide is unknown but is thought to run into the hundreds of thousands,[113] suggesting a pervasive violation of the UNCRC optional protocol on the involvement of children in armed conflict.[18] Children are recruited into armed conflict because they are easier to condition and control in part because their cognitive and social development is not yet complete.[32] The description given by children released from the Lord's Resistance Army in Uganda and the Democratic Republic of the Congo provides insight into the harrowing process of turning a child into a soldier: newly abducted children are placed in strictly controlled environments, socially isolated, forced to deidentify with their families and communities, and made to develop new identities.[114] To force the acquisition of these new identities, children may be required to kill members of their own families.[19,32] A more recent phenomenon is the use of children as young as 8 years old to conduct suicide bombings.[115] This phenomenon has a disproportionate impact on girls, who constitute up to 40% of children associated with armed groups[116] but three-quarters of child suicide bombers.[115]

Children who were associated with armed groups experience particular physical, developmental, and mental health risks; barriers in access to health services; and significant obstacles to social reintegration. In addition to physical injury and death, they are at high risk for HIV and other STIs, obstetric complications, and substance abuse.[64] Social isolation, loss of identity, and being forced to act in strictly defined gendered roles negatively affect mental health and can result in a disconnect between these children and their families and communities on return to civilian life.[114] Abduction, younger age of conscription, exposure to violence, female sex, and community stigma are associated with PTSD, depression, anxiety, and hostility.[113] Those who have lost parents and/or were involved in raping, injuring, or killing have worse mental health outcomes than those who have not.[62] Children associated with armed groups display gendered differences in mental health outcomes, with girls being more likely to have anxiety, depression, and feelings of hostility than boys.[112] Protective factors for psychosocial adjustment include perceptions of respect, understanding, and acceptance from family members; social support; and educational and economic opportunities.[113,117] Despite growing knowledge about their health risks and needs, children who were associated with armed groups continue to face social stigma and have limited access to treatment and rehabilitative care.[32,64,113] Furthermore, states are increasingly arresting and detaining children who are perceived to be associated or potentially associated with armed groups,[118] and these children are often held in conditions that violate their rights as articulated in the UNCRC and do not meet international standards for juvenile justice.[118]

Children Who Are Unaccompanied and Separated

Armed conflict separates children from their families, as evidenced by the increasing numbers of children fleeing conflict between both state and nonstate actors without parents or guardians. The number of children who are unaccompanied and separated who applied for asylum worldwide nearly tripled in 2015 to a staggering 98 400 children.[27] These children often do not possess official documents, making it challenging for authorities to identify their age, risks, needs, and rights to protection.[119] Health workers may be asked to assess their age, but a lack of reliable methods and the use of arbitrary practices place these children at risk for inappropriate treatment by authorities.[120] When they are identified by authorities and brought into state care, children who are unaccompanied and separated may face migration detention, discriminatory treatment, long delays in family reunification (if reunification is possible), and limited access to health care, social services, and education.[30,121] Health issues of particular concern include infections, nutritional deficiencies, and mental health problems relating to their traumatic experiences, particularly anxiety, depression, and PTSD.[122–125] Their young age, lack of documentation, and subsequent barriers in access to care and protection place children who are unaccompanied and separated at a high risk for trafficking and exploitation even after they are in the care of responsible authorities in the destination country.[126] Of the nearly 90 000 unaccompanied minors who applied for asylum in Europe in 2015,[127] at least 10 000 have gone missing.[128]

Children With Remote Exposure to Armed Conflict

Children who are not in close proximity to or are displaced by armed conflict may also face health and social risks related to the conflict. News and media coverage of war and extreme violence events have been shown to increase PTSD symptoms among US school children.[129] Children of deployed US military personnel have higher rates of emotional and behavioral problems and substance abuse[130,131] and are at a higher risk for physical abuse and neglect both during and after parental return from deployment.[131–133]

INTERVENTIONS TO PREVENT AND MITIGATE THE EFFECTS OF ARMED CONFLICT ON CHILDREN

Many interventions have been undertaken by individuals, groups, and societies to protect children and treat those who have been affected by armed conflict. Despite a wealth of experience, few studies have been conducted, and the evidence base for interventions used to prevent and mitigate the effects of conflict on children remains limited.

Interventions to Protect and Promote Physical Health

Children who are affected by armed conflict require care from clinicians who are familiar with their health risks and needs and who are skilled in providing care to children from different cultural and language backgrounds. There is some evidence for a positive effect of cultural competence training on patient outcomes.[134] Conversely, studies on migrant health have revealed that providers' lack of familiarity with migrant health conditions and health determinants can negatively affect the effectiveness of care.[135,136] In some settings, medical interpreters serve in a dual role of language mediators and cultural mediators; they translate between languages and also identify and explain health concepts and cultural needs that are relevant to the encounter and the care of the patient. The use of professional interpreters improves the quality of translations,[137] reduces unnecessary diagnostic investigations and treatments,[138] reduces the cost of care, and increases patient satisfaction.[139,140] The use of informal or untrained interpreters has been found to be detrimental to care.[139]

Disaster training courses are available for clinicians in the United States. These courses can be useful for providers who work in conflict settings as well as for general pediatricians who are involved in the care of children who are refugees and children who are remote from armed conflict.[141,142] Such courses can assist providers in understanding the context-specific health needs of children, the management of chronic conditions, and the care of children with special health care needs in conflict and postconflict settings.

Child-focused nongovernmental organizations, multilateral international organizations, and the US military have a wealth of experience in trauma-informed care.[131,143–146] Providing trauma-informed care involves making specific alterations in the care setting and the delivery of care that take into account the traumatic experiences of patients and caregivers and the way trauma has affected them.[147] Promoting the participation of children and their caregivers in their health care provides them with a sense of control over their situations, which is critical to promote healing and avoid exacerbating or causing further trauma.[148] Measures such as the creation of child-friendly spaces, communicating with the help of trained cultural mediators, the use of play in care provision, and informing children and their caregivers of what will take place during health care visits can alleviate fear, promote mutual trust, and ultimately improve care, follow-up, and adherence to therapy.[139,148,149] Simple measures such as asking the patients what would make them most comfortable during consultations, leaving the door slightly ajar when feasible, or allowing the patients to sit closer to the door may alleviate feelings of powerlessness or imprisonment.[148]

The use of child-friendly spaces can be adapted to the medical home model for the provision of trauma-informed care in the United States. Child-friendly spaces are defined by the UN Children's Fund as spaces that "support the resilience and wellbeing of children and young people through community-organized, structured activities conducted in a safe, child-friendly, and stimulating environment."[150] Such spaces, whether they are in schools, community settings, or health facilities, are specifically adapted to meet the needs of children. They may include colorful decorations directed toward a child audience, toys and child-sized furniture, and relevant equipment that is designed for use by children. The use of child-friendly spaces is one approach to mitigate traumatic stressors while addressing the physical, psychological, and behavioral health needs of these children.

In addition, pediatricians caring for children who are affected by conflict often find that it is important to recognize the health needs of caregivers and families, facilitate access to care when necessary, and ensure that children and their families have access to relevant social and legal assistance. This is consistent with guidance from the American Academy of Pediatrics, which states that children should have access to care in a medical home that is "continuous, comprehensive, family centered, coordinated, compassionate, and culturally effective."[151] In a study of the feasibility of using a medical home model in children with special health care needs (60% of whom had ≥5 medical problems and >40% of whom were dependent

on technology), researchers found that the medical home model was feasible with dedicated primary care leadership, adequate financial resources, cultural and language expertise, and family buy-in.[152] As a population with special health and social care needs, children who are affected by armed conflict and their families stand to benefit from the trauma-informed services of a pediatrician housed in a compassionate medical home.

Interventions to Protect and Promote Mental Health

Psychosocial interventions are used during complex humanitarian emergencies to restore stability in the lives of children who are affected by armed conflict.[153] This is achieved by establishing routines and engaging young people and their caregivers in activities to support the wellbeing of the community. In postconflict environments, this may be accomplished by rebuilding homes, schools, and health care centers.[153] In settings that are remote from conflict, such as asylum centers, this is accomplished by reuniting families, providing them with their own shelters, and enrolling children in school.[154] The use of child-friendly spaces for psychosocial and educational interventions has been successful in promoting child mental health both during and after conflict.[149]

Psychosocial interventions have been used successfully to complement psychiatric interventions in children with diagnosed mental illnesses.[103] Coordinated psychosocial and mental health interventions in schools have been found to be beneficial, especially in LMICs.[103,155–157] School-based programs help children overcome difficulties that are associated with forced migration and positively affect self-esteem, motivation, and self-efficacy.[155,156] Studies conducted with children who have experienced armed conflict universally reveal that

these children look toward education to improve their lives and futures.[158] In light of this and in consideration of the cultural stigma associated with mental illness,[159] providing mental health services in a school setting may be more socially and culturally acceptable.[160]

In addition to addressing psychological trauma and promoting mental health in children who are affected by armed conflict, psychosocial and mental health programs are a means to promote resilience in children.[161] Resilience is a positive adaptive process in the face of exposure to negative events or threats.[162] Children who are affected by war often exhibit immense adaptability, which can be cultivated to mitigate the toxic stress effects of armed conflict. Intelligence, emotional regulation, and coping contribute to resilience and should be viewed as dynamic processes rather than as personal traits.[163] Factors that enhance resilience may include social support, caregiver mental health, membership in a religious community, cultural values, and access to child care and schools in war-affected regions.[163]

Studies of resilience among children who are affected by war reveal the importance of context in the kinds of factors that are protective and how these factors influence resilience outcomes. Community acceptance has a protective effect on adaptive behaviors and mental health outcomes in children who have been associated with armed groups[112]; however, this effect has not been generally observed in other children who are affected by conflict.[164] Parental support has been associated with better school performance,[165] life satisfaction, and positive perceptions of health in 2 large cross-sectional studies of adolescents in the occupied Palestinian territories.[166] Among unaccompanied minors, well-supported living arrangements,[125] religious faith,[167] strong social support systems, and healthy interpersonal relationships[168] have protective effects on mental health and adaptation to new environments. Researchers in studies of resilience provide insight into promising ways to protect and promote the wellbeing of children who are affected by armed conflict. However, interventions used to promote resilience should not be considered as a replacement for mental health interventions in children who are traumatized.[163]

Public Health and Health System Interventions

In conflict zones and refugee settings, public health work is typically focused on rapid epidemiologic assessment, the development of early warning systems for infectious disease surveillance, and response to potential and actual outbreaks of infectious diseases.[77] In addition, in public health responses, disease prevention, including vaccination campaigns, the establishment of sanitation systems and potable water supplies, and mass food distribution, is prioritized.[77,169] In cases of protracted displacement, the administration of routine vaccinations may also be implemented.[170]

Other prevention measures include the establishment of surveillance systems to detect conflict- and displacement-related morbidity and the development of interventions to mitigate their effects on population health.[77] Supplementary feeding programs and targeted food distribution may be established in areas where there is a demonstrated burden of micronutrient deficiency or acute malnutrition.[169] Contingency planning and the training of frontline staff can be used to facilitate the early detection of disease and the implementation of needed interventions.[77] Finally, support may be provided to repair or improve the capacity of existing medical facilities or establish new facilities.[4,169]

Experience has shown that strong collaboration between the health sector and other sectors, including immigration, civil protection authorities, education, and nongovernmental organizations, results in a more effective management of complex emergencies and better health outcomes for people who are displaced and for receiving populations.[171] On the basis of experience in work in Europe with the ongoing migration crisis and the US Centers for Disease Control and Prevention's Refugee Health Program, adequate preparedness also requires good health surveillance in sending, transit, and receiving countries and effective communication of this information to health care providers.[171,172]

To inform clinical and public health preparedness and interventions, data on short- and long-term pediatric morbidity and mortality attributable to armed conflict are critical. Although several databases are used to track mortality directly from armed conflict, these do not include disaggregated data on children. There are numerous case reports and descriptive studies of child health outcomes in conflict settings that are used to help characterize specific groups, but these do not provide a broad or nuanced understanding of the effects of a given conflict on children. There is an urgent need to establish methods of data collection that can be used during armed conflict to monitor short- and long-term morbidity, mortality, and the effects of interventions.

CONCLUSIONS

Armed conflict is a neglected social determinant of child health, and the acute and chronic effects of armed conflict on child health and wellbeing are among the greatest child rights violations of the 21st century. The destructive effects of conflict include all 6 grave child rights violations as well as a broad range of both direct and indirect effects that follow children through the life course and into adulthood. Despite the extraordinary number of children living in areas affected by conflict, our understanding of the scale of conflict's effects on children, the nuances of these effects, and ways to mitigate and treat them remain limited. It is incumbent on pediatricians, allied child health care providers, public health professionals, researchers, and policy makers to address the impact of armed conflict on children as a critical and priority issue. Children must be counted.

LEAD AUTHORS

Ayesha Kadir, MD, MSc, FAAP
Sherry Shenoda, MD, FAAP
Jeffrey Goldhagen, MD, MPH, FAAP
Shelly Pitterman, PhD

SECTION ON INTERNATIONAL CHILD HEALTH EXECUTIVE COMMITTEE, 2017–2018

Parminder S. Suchdev, MD, MPH, FAAP, Chairperson
Kevin J. Chan, MD, MPH, FAAP
Cynthia R. Howard, MD, MPH, FAAP
Patrick McGann, MD, FAAP
Nicole E. St Clair, MD, FAAP
Katherine Yun, MD, MHS, FAAP
Linda D. Arnold, MD, FAAP, Immediate-Past Chairperson

STAFF

Vayram Nyadroh

ABBREVIATIONS

LMIC: low- and middle-income country
PTSD: posttraumatic stress disorder
STI: sexually transmitted infection
UN: United Nations
UNCRC: United Nations Convention on the Rights of the Child

Address correspondence to Ayesha Kadir, MD, MSc, FAAP. E-mail: kadira@gmail.com

PEDIATRICS (ISSN Numbers: Print, 0031-4005; Online, 1098-4275).

Copyright © 2018 by the American Academy of Pediatrics

FINANCIAL DISCLOSURE: The authors have indicated they have no financial relationships relevant to this article to disclose.

FUNDING: No external funding.

POTENTIAL CONFLICT OF INTEREST: The authors have indicated they have no potential conflicts of interest to disclose.

COMPANION PAPER: A companion to this article can be found online at www.pediatrics.org/cgi/doi/10.1542/peds.2018-2585.

REFERENCES

1. UNICEF. *More Than 1 in 10 Children Living in Countries and Areas Affected by Armed Conflict.* New York, NY: UNICEF; 2015

2. Heidelberg Institute for International Conflict Research. *Conflict Barometer 2015.* Heidelberg, Germany: Department of Political Science, University of Heidelberg; 2016

3. Garfield R. The epidemiology of war. In: Levy BS, Sidel VW, eds. *War and Public Health.* 2nd ed. Oxford, United Kingdom: Oxford University Press; 2008:23

4. Levy BS, Sidel VW, Levy B, Sidel V, eds. *War and Public Health: An Overview.* 2nd ed. Oxford, United Kingdom: Oxford University Press; 2008

5. Smith D. Trends and causes of armed conflict. In: Austin A, Fischer M, Ropers N, eds. *Transforming Ethnopolitical Conflict: The Berghof Handbook.* New York, NY: Springer; 2004:111–127

6. UNICEF. No guns, please. We are children! 2001. Available at: https://www.unicef.org/publications/files/No_Guns_Please_-_We_Are_Children(1).pdf. Accessed May 14, 2018

7. World Health Organization. *Guidance for Surveillance of Injuries Due to Landmines and Unexploded Ordnance.* Geneva, Switzerland: World Health Organization; 2000

8. Global Coalition to Protect Education From Attack. Education under attack 2014. 2014. Available at: www.protectingeducation.org/education-under-attack-2014. Accessed May 14, 2018

9. Guha-Sapir D, D'Aoust O. *Demographic and Health Consequences of Civil Conflict. World Development Report.* Washington, DC: World Bank; 2011. Available at: http://hdl.handle.net/10986/9083. Accessed May 14, 2018

10. Poirier T. The effects of armed conflict on schooling in Sub-Saharan Africa. *Int J Educ Dev.* 2012;32(2):341–351

11. Safeguarding Health in Conflict Coalition. No protection, no respect: health workers and health facilities under attack. Available at: https://www.safeguardinghealth.org/sites/shcc/files/SHCC2016final.pdf. Accessed May 14, 2018

12. International Committee of the Red Cross. The Geneva Conventions and commentaries. Available at: https://www.icrc.org/en/war-and-law/treaties-customary-law/geneva-conventions. Accessed October 1, 2018

13. Shenoda S, Kadir A, Pitterman S, Goldhagen J; American Academy of Pediatrics, Section on International Child Health. The effects of armed conflict on children. *Pediatrics.* 2018;142(6):e20182585

14. United Nations Human Rights Office of the High Commissioner. Convention on the Rights of the Child. 1989. Available at: www.ohchr.org/en/professionalinterest/pages/crc.aspx. Accessed May 14, 2018

15. Shenoda S, Kadir A, Goldhagen J. Children and armed conflict. *Pediatrics.* 2015;136(2). Available at: www.pediatrics.org/cgi/content/full/136/2/e309

16. United Nations High Commissioner for Refugees. Convention and protocol relating to the status of refugees. Available at: www.unhcr.org/3b66c2aa10.html. Accessed May 14, 2018

17. Levy BS, Sidel VW. Protecting non-combatant civilians during war. *Med Confl Surviv.* 2015;31(2):1–4

18. United Nations Human Rights Office of the High Commissioner. Optional Protocol to the Convention on the Rights of the Child on the Involvement of Children in Armed Conflict. 2000. Available at: www.ohchr.org/EN/ProfessionalInterest/Pages/OPACCRC.aspx. Accessed May 14, 2018

19. UN Office of the Special Representative of the Secretary-General for Children Affected by Armed Conflict. Working paper no. 3, children and justice during and in the aftermath of armed conflict. 2011. Available at: www.refworld.org/docid/4e6f2f132.html. Accessed May 14, 2018

20. United States Senate Committee on Foreign Relations. Executive report 107-4. The Optional Protocol to the Convention on the Rights of the Child on the Sale of Children, Child Prostitution, and Child Pornography and the Optional Protocol to the Convention on the Rights of the Child on the Involvement of Children in armed Conflict. 2002. Available at: https://www.congress.gov/congressional-report/107th-congress/executive-report/4. Accessed May 14, 2018

21. Cornell Law School Legal Information Institute. U.S. code, title 10, subtitle A, part II, chapter 31, 10 USC § 505(a). Regular components: qualifications, term, grade. Available at: https://www.law.cornell.edu/uscode/text/10/505. Accessed May 14, 2018

22. United Nations; Office of the Special Representatives of the Secretary General for Children and Armed Conflict. Working paper no 1: the six grave violations against children during armed conflict. 2013. Available at: https://childrenandarmedconflict.un.org/publications/WorkingPaper-1_SixGraveViolationsLegalFoundation.pdf. Accessed May 14, 2018

23. Murray CJ, King G, Lopez AD, Tomijima N, Krug EG. Armed conflict as a public health problem. *BMJ.* 2002;324(7333):346–349

24. UNICEF. Children and emergencies in 2014: facts and figures. 2015. Available at: www.unicef.org/media/files/UNICEF_Children_and_Emergencies_2014_fact_sheet.pdf. Accessed May 14, 2018

25. UNICEF, United Nations Office of the Special Representative of the Secretary-General for Children and Armed Conflict. Machel study 10-year strategic review: children and conflict in a changing world. 2009. Available at: https://www.unicef.org/publications/index_49985.html. Accessed May 14, 2018

26. Lake A. Development must target the millions of children affected by humanitarian crises. *The Guardian.* September 11, 2015. Available at: https://www.theguardian.com/global-development/2015/sep/11/sustainable-development-goals-target-millions-children-humanitarian-crises. Accessed October 1, 2018

27. United Nations High Commissioner for Refugees. Global trends: forced displacement in 2017. Available at: http://www.unhcr.org/globaltrends2017/. Accessed June 19, 2018

28. United Nations. *The Millennium Development Goals Report 2015.* New York, NY: United Nations; 2015

29. United Nations High Commissioner for Refugees. Figures at a glance. Available at: www.unhcr.org/figures-at-a-glance.html. Accessed May 14, 2018

30. UNICEF. Uprooted: the growing crisis for refugee and migrant children. 2016. Available at: https://www.unicef.org/publications/files/Uprooted_growing_crisis_for_refugee_and_migrant_children.pdf. Accessed May 14, 2018

31. Institute of Medicine. Key migration terms. 2004. Available at: https://www.iom.int/key-migration-terms. Accessed May 14, 2018

32. UNICEF. *State of the World's Children: Childhood Under Threat.* New York, NY: UNICEF; 2005

33. World Health Organization. *Social Determinants of Health: Key Concepts.* Geneva, Switzerland: World Health Organization; 2017. Available at: www.who.int/social_determinants/thecommission/finalreport/key_concepts/en/. Accessed May 14, 2018

34. Uppsala Conflict Data Program. Number of conflicts: 1975–2017. Available at: http://ucdp.uu.se/. Accessed May 14, 2018

35. International Institute for Strategic Studies. The armed conflict database. Available at: https://www.iiss.org/en/Publications/ACD. Accessed May 14, 2018

36. Armed Conflict Event Location and Event Data Project. Available at: https://www.acleddata.com/. Accessed May 14, 2018

37. Uppsala Conflict Data Program. How are UCDP data collected? 2016. Available at: www.pcr.uu.se/research/ucdp/faq/#How_are_UCDP_data_collected_. Accessed May 14, 2018

38. Children and Armed Conflict. *Report of the UN Secretary General.* General Assembly Seventieth Session. Agenda Item 68. New York, NY: United Nations; 2016

39. Shonkoff JP, Garner AS; Committee on Psychosocial Aspects of Child and Family Health; Committee on Early Childhood, Adoption, and Dependent Care; Section on Developmental and Behavioral Pediatrics. The lifelong effects of early childhood adversity and toxic stress. *Pediatrics.* 2012;129(1). Available at: www.pediatrics.org/cgi/content/full/129/1/e232

40. Radoncić F, Hudić I, Balić A, Fatusić Z. Perinatal outcomes during 1986-2005 in Tuzla Canton, Bosnia and Herzegovina. *J Matern Fetal Neonatal Med.* 2008;21(8):567–572

41. Bodalal Z, Agnaeber K, Nagelkerke N, Stirling B, Temmerman M, Degomme O. Pregnancy outcomes in Benghazi, Libya, before and during the armed conflict in 2011. *East Mediterr Health J.* 2014;20(3):175–180

42. Simetka O, Reilley B, Joseph M, Collie M, Leidinger J. Obstetrics during Civil War: six months on a maternity ward in Mallavi, northern Sri Lanka. *Med Confl Surviv.* 2002;18(3):258–270

43. Lee TJ, Mullany LC, Richards AK, Kuiper HK, Maung C, Beyrer C. Mortality rates in conflict zones in Karen, Karenni, and Mon states in eastern Burma. *Trop Med Int Health.* 2006;11(7):1119–1127

44. Garfield R, Leu CS. A multivariate method for estimating mortality rates among children under 5 years from health and social indicators in Iraq. *Int J Epidemiol.* 2000;29(3):510–515

45. Guha-Sapir D, van Panhuis WG. The importance of conflict-related mortality in civilian populations. *Lancet.* 2003;361(9375):2126–2128

46. McNeil DG Jr. Gunmen kill Nigerian polio vaccine workers in echo of Pakistan attacks. *New York Times.* February 8, 2013. Available at: https://www.nytimes.com/2013/02/09/world/africa/in-nigeria-polio-vaccine-workers-are-killed-by-gunmen.html?mtrref=www.google.com&gwh=5003C2BCD0EDDED0AECBBEBA4FC3FD03&gwt=pay. Accessed October 1, 2018

47. Médecins Sans Frontières. Kunduz hospital airstrike. Available at: www.msf.org/en/topics/kunduz-hospital-airstrike. Accessed May 14, 2018

48. Trelles M, Stewart BT, Kushner AL. Attacks on civilians and hospitals must stop. *Lancet Glob Health.* 2016;4(5):e298–e299

49. World Health Organization. Tracking attacks on health workers – don't let them go unnoticed. 2015. Available at: www.who.int/features/2015/healthworkers-in-emergencies/en/. Accessed May 14, 2018

50. Creamer KM, Edwards MJ, Shields CH, Thompson MW, Yu CE, Adelman W. Pediatric wartime admissions to US military combat support hospitals in Afghanistan and Iraq: learning from the first 2,000 admissions. *J Trauma.* 2009;67(4):762–768

51. Champion HR, Holcomb JB, Young LA. Injuries from explosions: physics, biophysics, pathology, and required research focus. *J Trauma.* 2009;66(5):1468–1477; discussion 1477

52. Klimo P Jr, Ragel BT, Jones GM, McCafferty R. Severe pediatric head injury during the Iraq and Afghanistan conflicts. *Neurosurgery.* 2015;77(1):1–7; discussion 7

53. Edwards MJ, Lustik M, Eichelberger MR, Elster E, Azarow K, Coppola C. Blast injury in children: an analysis from Afghanistan and Iraq, 2002-2010. *J Trauma Acute Care Surg.* 2012;73(5):1278–1283

54. Borgman M, Matos RI, Blackbourne LH, Spinella PC. Ten years of military pediatric care in Afghanistan and Iraq. *J Trauma Acute Care Surg.* 2012;73(6, suppl 5):S509–S513

55. Fitzgerald GJ. Chemical warfare and medical response during World War I. *Am J Public Health.* 2008;98(4):611–625

56. Cook-Deegan R, Hu H, Shukri A. *Winds of Death: Iraq's Use of Poison Gas Against its Kurdish Population.* Boston, MA: Physicians for Human Rights; 1989

57. Leaning J, Barron RA, Rumack BH. *Bloody Sunday: Trauma in Tbilisi.* Boston, MA: Physicians for Human Rights; 1990

58. Middle East Watch; Physicians for Human Rights. *Unquiet Graves: The Search for the Disappeared in Iraqi Kurdistan.* New York, NY: Human Rights Watch; 1992

59. Organization for the Prohibition of Chemical Weapons. Chemical weapons convention. Available at: https://www.opcw.org/chemical-weapons-convention/. Accessed May 14, 2018

60. Organization for the Prohibition of Chemical Weapons. Report of the OPCW fact-finding mission in Syria regarding an alleged incident in Saraqib, Syrian Arab Republic on February 4, 2018. 2018. Available at: https://www.opcw.org/fileadmin/OPCW/S_series/2018/en/s-1626-2018_e_.pdf. Accessed May 22, 2018

61. Rotenberg JS, Newmark J. Nerve agent attacks on children: diagnosis and management. *Pediatrics.* 2003;112(3, pt 1):648–658

62. Betancourt TS, Borisova II, de la Soudière M, Williamson J. Sierra Leone's child soldiers: war exposures and mental health problems by gender. *J Adolesc Health.* 2011;49(1):21–28

63. Malemo Kalisya L, Lussy Justin P, Kimona C, et al. Sexual violence toward children and youth in war-torn eastern Democratic Republic of Congo. *PLoS One.* 2011;6(1):e15911

64. Humphreys G. Healing child soldiers. *Bull World Health Organ.* 2009;87(5):330–331

65. Betancourt TS, Agnew-Blais J, Gilman SE, Williams DR, Ellis BH. Past horrors, present struggles: the role of stigma in the association between war experiences and psychosocial adjustment among former child soldiers in Sierra Leone. *Soc Sci Med.* 2010;70(1):17–26

66. Bilukha OO, Brennan M. Injuries and deaths caused by unexploded ordnance in Afghanistan: review of surveillance data, 1997-2002. *BMJ.* 2005;330(7483):127–128

67. Bilukha OO, Brennan M, Anderson M. The lasting legacy of war: epidemiology of injuries from landmines and unexploded ordnance in Afghanistan, 2002-2006. *Prehosp Disaster Med.* 2008;23(6):493–499

68. Bilukha OO, Laurenge H, Danee L, Subedi KP, Becknell K. Injuries and deaths due to victim-activated improvised explosive devices, landmines and other explosive remnants of war in Nepal. *Inj Prev.* 2011;17(5):326–331

69. Morikawa M, Taylor S, Persons M. Deaths and injuries due to unexploded ordnance (UXO) in northern Lao PDR (Laos). *Injury.* 1998;29(4):301–304

70. Hanevik K, Kvåle G. Landmine injuries in Eritrea. *BMJ.* 2000;321(7270):1189

71. Mousavi B, Soroush MR, Masoumi M, et al. Epidemiological study of child casualties of landmines and unexploded ordnances: a national study from Iran. *Prehosp Disaster Med.* 2015;30(5):472–477

72. Bendinelli C. Effects of land mines and unexploded ordnance on the pediatric population and comparison with adults in rural Cambodia. *World J Surg.* 2009;33(5):1070–1074

73. Bilukha OO, Brennan M, Anderson M, Tsitsaev Z, Murtazaeva E, Ibragimov R. Seen but not heard: injuries and deaths from landmines and unexploded ordnance in Chechnya, 1994-2005. *Prehosp Disaster Med.* 2007;22(6):507–512

74. Save the Children; UNICEF. *Small Hands Heavy Burden: How the Syria Conflict Is Driving More Children Into the Workforce.* Amman, Jordan: Save the Children; 2015

75. Ngo AD, Taylor R, Roberts CL, Nguyen TV. Association between Agent Orange and birth defects: systematic review and meta-analysis. *Int J Epidemiol.* 2006;35(5):1220–1230

76. United Nations Environment Programme. *Environmental Assessment of the Gaza Strip Following the Escalation of Hostilities in December 2008 – January 2009.* Nairobi, Kenya: United Nations Environment Programme; 2009

77. Toole MJ, Waldman RJ. The public health aspects of complex emergencies and refugee situations. *Annu Rev Public Health.* 1997;18:283–312

78. Zwi AB, Grove NJ, Kelly P, Gayer M, Ramos-Jimenez P, Sommerfeld J. Child health in armed conflict: time to rethink. *Lancet.* 2006;367(9526):1886–1888

79. Kruk ME, Freedman LP, Anglin GA, Waldman RJ. Rebuilding health systems to improve health and promote statebuilding in post-conflict countries: a theoretical framework and research agenda. *Soc Sci Med.* 2010;70(1):89–97

80. Requejo JH, Bryce J, Barros AJ, et al. Countdown to 2015 and beyond: fulfilling the health agenda for women and children. *Lancet.* 2015;385(9966):466–476

81. Human Rights Watch; Safeguarding Health in Conflict Coalition. *Attacks on Health: Global Report.* New York, NY: Human Rights Watch; 2015

82. Berry I, Berrang-Ford L. Leishmaniasis, conflict, and political terror: a spatio-temporal analysis. *Soc Sci Med.* 2016;167:140–149

83. Physicians for Human Rights. A map of attacks on health care in Syria. Available at: http://physiciansforhumanrights.org/library/multimedia/a-map-of-attacks-on-health-care-in-syria.html. Accessed May 14, 2018

84. Connolly MA, Gayer M, Ryan MJ, Salama P, Spiegel P, Heymann DL. Communicable diseases in complex emergencies: impact and challenges. *Lancet.* 2004;364(9449):1974–1983

85. Chan M, Lake A. *Statement on Attacks on Medical Facilities and Personnel in the Syrian Arab Republic*. Geneva, Switzerland: World Health Organization; 2016

86. Riaz H, Rehman A. Polio vaccination workers gunned down in Pakistan. *Lancet Infect Dis*. 2013;13(2):120

87. World Health Organization. *Donor Update 2016*. Damascus, Syria: World Health Organization; 2016

88. Beyrer C, Villar JC, Suwanvanichkij V, Singh S, Baral SD, Mills EJ. Neglected diseases, civil conflicts, and the right to health. *Lancet*. 2007;370(9587):619–627

89. Ghobarah HA, Huth P, Russett B. The post-war public health effects of civil conflict. *Soc Sci Med*. 2004;59(4):869–884

90. Akil L, Ahmad HA. The recent outbreaks and reemergence of poliovirus in war and conflict-affected areas. *Int J Infect Dis*. 2016;49:40–46

91. Medecins Sans Frontieres. Syria: starvation continues in Madaya - MSF denounces continued blockage of essential aid and medical evacuations. 2016. Available at: www.msf.org/en/article/syria-starvation-continues-madaya-msf-denounces-continued-blockage-essential-aid-and-medical. Accessed May 14, 2018

92. Bilukha OO, Jayasekaran D, Burton A, et al; Division of Global Health Protection, Center for Global Health; Centers for Disease Control and Prevention (CDC). Nutritional status of women and child refugees from Syria-Jordan, April-May 2014. *MMWR Morb Mortal Wkly Rep*. 2014;63(29):638–639

93. Andresen E, Bilukha OO, Menkir Z, et al; Centers for Disease Control and Prevention. Notes from the field: malnutrition and elevated mortality among refugees from South Sudan - Ethiopia, June-July 2014. *MMWR Morb Mortal Wkly Rep*. 2014;63(32):700–701

94. Centers for Disease Control (CDC). Nutritional status of Somali refugees—eastern Ethiopia, September 1988-May 1989. *MMWR Morb Mortal Wkly Rep*. 1989;38(26):455–456, 461–463

95. Gushulak BD, MacPherson DW. Health aspects of the pre-departure phase of migration. *PLoS Med*. 2011;8(5):e1001035

96. Lynch C, Roper C. The transit phase of migration: circulation of malaria and its multidrug-resistant forms in Africa. *PLoS Med*. 2011;8(5):e1001040

97. Zimmerman C, Kiss L, Hossain M. Migration and health: a framework for 21st century policy-making. *PLoS Med*. 2011;8(5):e1001034

98. Habib RR, Hojeij S, Elzein K, Chaaban J, Seyfert K. Associations between life conditions and multi-morbidity in marginalized populations: the case of Palestinian refugees. *Eur J Public Health*. 2014;24(5):727–733

99. Davidson N, Skull S, Burgner D, et al. An issue of access: delivering equitable health care for newly arrived refugee children in Australia. *J Paediatr Child Health*. 2004;40(9–10):569–575

100. Cáceres DC, Izquierdo VF, Mantilla L, Jara J, Velandia M. Epidemiologic profile of the population displaced by the internal armed conflict of the country in a neighborhood of Cartagena, Colombia, 2000 [in Spanish]. *Biomedica*. 2002;22(suppl 2):425–444

101. Goma Epidemiology Group. Public health impact of Rwandan refugee crisis: what happened in Goma, Zaire, in July, 1994? Goma Epidemiology Group. *Lancet*. 1995;345(8946):339–344

102. United Nations High Commissioner for Refugees, Global Education Monitoring Report. *No More Excuses: Provide Education to All Forcibly Displaced People*. Paris, France: United Nations Educational, Scientific and Cultural Organization; 2016

103. Betancourt TS, Meyers-Ohki SE, Charrow AP, Tol WA. Interventions for children affected by war: an ecological perspective on psychosocial support and mental health care. *Harv Rev Psychiatry*. 2013;21(2):70–91

104. Krug E, Dahlberg L, Mercy J, Zwi A, Lozano R, eds. Collective violence. In: *World Report on Violence and Health*. Geneva, Switzerland: World Health Organization; 2002

105. Attanayake V, McKay R, Joffres M, Singh S, Burkle F Jr, Mills E. Prevalence of mental disorders among children exposed to war: a systematic review of 7,920 children. *Med Confl Surviv*. 2009;25(1):4–19

106. Slone M, Mann S. Effects of war, terrorism and armed conflict on young children: a systematic review. *Child Psychiatry Hum Dev*. 2016;47(6):950–965

107. Schiff M, Pat-Horenczyk R, Benbenishty R, Brom D, Baum N, Astor RA. High school students' posttraumatic symptoms, substance abuse and involvement in violence in the aftermath of war. *Soc Sci Med*. 2012;75(7):1321–1328

108. Sriskandarajah V, Neuner F, Catani C. Parental care protects traumatized Sri Lankan children from internalizing behavior problems. *BMC Psychiatry*. 2015;15:203

109. Reed RV, Fazel M, Jones L, Panter-Brick C, Stein A. Mental health of displaced and refugee children resettled in low-income and middle-income countries: risk and protective factors. *Lancet*. 2012;379(9812):250–265

110. Fazel M, Reed RV, Panter-Brick C, Stein A. Mental health of displaced and refugee children resettled in high-income countries: risk and protective factors. *Lancet*. 2012;379(9812):266–282

111. Graham HR, Minhas RS, Paxton G. Learning problems in children of refugee background: a systematic review. *Pediatrics*. 2016;137(6):e20153994

112. Betancourt TS, Borisova I, Williams TP, et al. Psychosocial adjustment and mental health in former child soldiers—systematic review of the literature and recommendations for future research. *J Child Psychol Psychiatry*. 2013;54(1):17–36

113. UNICEF. *The Paris Principles: Principles and Guidelines on Children Associated With Armed Forces or Armed Groups*. New York, NY: UNICEF; 2007

114. Kelly JT, Branham L, Decker MR. Abducted children and youth in Lord's Resistance Army in Northeastern Democratic Republic of the Congo (DRC): mechanisms of indoctrination and control. *Confl Health*. 2016;10(1):11

115. UNICEF Regional Office for West and Central Africa. Beyond Chibok. 2016. Available at: https://www.unicef.org/

infobycountry/files/Beyond_Chibok.pdf. Accessed May 14, 2018

116. War Child. Key facts and statistics about child soldiers. Available at: https://www.warchild.org.uk/issues/child-soldiers. Accessed May 14, 2018

117. Betancourt TS, Borisova II, Williams TP, et al. Sierra Leone's former child soldiers: a follow-up study of psychosocial adjustment and community reintegration. *Child Dev*. 2010;81(4):1077–1095

118. Hamilton C, Anderson K, Barnes R, Dorling K. *Administrative Detention of Children: A Global Report*. New York, NY: UNICEF; 2011

119. Aynsley-Green A, Cole TJ, Crawley H, Lessof N, Boag LR, Wallace RM. Medical, statistical, ethical and human rights considerations in the assessment of age in children and young people subject to immigration control. *Br Med Bull*. 2012;102:17–42

120. Hjern A, Brendler-Lindqvist M, Norredam M. Age assessment of young asylum seekers. *Acta Paediatr*. 2012;101(1):4–7

121. Linton JM, Griffin M, Shapiro AJ; Council on Community Pediatrics. Detention of immigrant children. *Pediatrics*. 2017;139(5):e20170483

122. Marquardt L, Krämer A, Fischer F, Prüfer-Krämer L. Health status and disease burden of unaccompanied asylum-seeking adolescents in Bielefeld, Germany: cross-sectional pilot study. *Trop Med Int Health*. 2016;21(2):210–218

123. Jensen TK, Skårdalsmo EM, Fjermestad KW. Development of mental health problems - a follow-up study of unaccompanied refugee minors. *Child Adolesc Psychiatry Ment Health*. 2014;8:29

124. Bean T, Derluyn I, Eurelings-Bontekoe E, Broekaert E, Spinhoven P. Comparing psychological distress, traumatic stress reactions, and experiences of unaccompanied refugee minors with experiences of adolescents accompanied by parents. *J Nerv Ment Dis*. 2007;195(4):288–297

125. Hodes M, Jagdev D, Chandra N, Cunniff A. Risk and resilience for psychological distress amongst unaccompanied asylum seeking adolescents. *J Child Psychol Psychiatry*. 2008;49(7):723–732

126. Bhabha J. Seeking asylum alone: treatment of separated and trafficked children in need of refugee protection. *Int Migr*. 2004;42(1):141–148

127. Eurostat. *Almost 90 000 Unaccompanied Minors Among Asylum Seekers Registered in the EU in 2015*. Auchan, Luxembourg: Eurostat Press Office; 2016

128. European Parliament Press Release. Fate of 10,000 missing refugee children debated in Civil Liberties Committee. 2016. Available at: www.europarl.europa.eu/pdfs/news/expert/infopress/20160419IPR23951/20160419IPR23951_en.pdf. Accessed May 14, 2018

129. Pfefferbaum B, Seale TW, Brandt EN Jr, Pfefferbaum RL, Doughty DE, Rainwater SM. Media exposure in children one hundred miles from a terrorist bombing. *Ann Clin Psychiatry*. 2003;15(1):1–8

130. White CJ, de Burgh HT, Fear NT, Iversen AC. The impact of deployment to Iraq or Afghanistan on military children: a review of the literature. *Int Rev Psychiatry*. 2011;23(2):210–217

131. Siegel BS, Davis BE; Committee on Psychosocial Aspects of Child and Family Health and Section on Uniformed Services. Health and mental health needs of children in US military families. *Pediatrics*. 2013;131(6). Available at: www.pediatrics.org/cgi/content/full/131/6/e2002

132. Taylor CM, Ross ME, Wood JN, et al. Differential child maltreatment risk across deployment periods of US Army soldiers. *Am J Public Health*. 2016;106(1):153–158

133. Rabenhorst MM, McCarthy RJ, Thomsen CJ, Milner JS, Travis WJ, Colasanti MP. Child maltreatment among U.S. Air Force parents deployed in support of Operation Iraqi Freedom/Operation Enduring Freedom. *Child Maltreat*. 2015;20(1):61–71

134. Lie DA, Lee-Rey E, Gomez A, Bereknyei S, Braddock CH III. Does cultural competency training of health professionals improve patient outcomes? A systematic review and proposed algorithm for future research. *J Gen Intern Med*. 2011;26(3):317–325

135. Gushulak B, Weekers J, Macpherson D. Migrants and emerging public health issues in a globalized world: threats, risks and challenges, an evidence-based framework. *Emerg Health Threats J*. 2009;2:e10

136. Bradby H, Humphris R, Newall D, Phillimore J. *Public Health Aspects of Migrant Health: A Review of the Evidence on Health Status for Refugees and Asylum Seekers in the European Region*. Geneva, Switzerland: World Health Organization Regional Office for Europe; 2015

137. Flores G, Laws MB, Mayo SJ, et al. Errors in medical interpretation and their potential clinical consequences in pediatric encounters. *Pediatrics*. 2003;111(1):6–14

138. Hampers LC, McNulty JE. Professional interpreters and bilingual physicians in a pediatric emergency department: effect on resource utilization. *Arch Pediatr Adolesc Med*. 2002;156(11):1108–1113

139. Bischoff A. *Caring for Migrant and Minority Patients in European Hospitals: A Review of Effective Interventions*. Neuchâtel, Switzerland: Swiss Forum for Migration and Population Studies; 2006

140. Garcia EA, Roy LC, Okada PJ, Perkins SD, Wiebe RA. A comparison of the influence of hospital-trained, ad hoc, and telephone interpreters on perceived satisfaction of limited English-proficient parents presenting to a pediatric emergency department. *Pediatr Emerg Care*. 2004;20(6):373–378

141. Olness K, Sinha M, Herran M, Cheren M, Pairojkul S. Training of health care professionals on the special needs of children in the management of disasters: experience in Asia, Africa, and Latin America. *Ambul Pediatr*. 2005;5(4):244–248

142. Disaster Preparedness Advisory Council; Committee on Pediatric Emergency Medicine. Ensuring the health of children in disasters. *Pediatrics*. 2015;136(5). Available at: www.pediatrics.org/cgi/content/full/136/5/e1407

143. War Child. Available at: www.warchild. org. Accessed May 14, 2018

144. UNICEF. Children, not soldiers. 2014. Available at: https:// childrenandarmedconflict.un.org/ children-not-soldiers. Accessed May 14, 2018

145. Save the Children. Child protection. Available at: https://www. savethechildren.net/what-we-do/child-protection. Accessed May 14, 2018

146. Save the Children. *Child Friendly Spaces in Emergencies: A Handbook for Save the Children Staff*. London, UK: Save the Children; 2013

147. Marsac ML, Kassam-Adams N, Hildenbrand AK, et al. Implementing a trauma-informed approach in pediatric health care networks. *JAMA Pediatr*. 2016;170(1):70–77

148. Raja S, Hasnain M, Hoersch M, Gove-Yin S, Rajagopalan C. Trauma informed care in medicine: current knowledge and future research directions. *Fam Community Health*. 2015;38(3):216–226

149. Browne E. *Child Friendly Spaces for Adolescent Girls in Emergency Settings*. Birmingham, United Kingdom: GSDRC; 2013. Available at: www.gsdrc. org/docs/open/hdq932.pdf. Accessed May 14, 2018

150. UNICEF. *Guidelines for Child Friendly Spaces in Emergencies*. New York, NY: UNICEF; 2011

151. Medical Home Initiatives for Children With Special Needs Project Advisory Committee; American Academy of Pediatrics. The medical home. *Pediatrics*. 2002;110(1, pt 1):184–186

152. Palfrey JS, Sofis LA, Davidson EJ, Liu J, Freeman L, Ganz ML; Pediatric Alliance for Coordinated Care. The pediatric alliance for coordinated care: evaluation of a medical home model. *Pediatrics*. 2004;113(suppl 5): 1507–1516

153. Betancourt TS, Williams T. Building an evidence base on mental health interventions for children affected by armed conflict. *Intervention (Amstelveen)*. 2008;6(1):39–56

154. United Nations High Commissioner for Refugees. Discussion paper on recommended reception standards for asylum-seekers in the context of the harmonisation of refugee and asylum policies of the European Union. 2000. Available at: www.refworld.org/docid/ 3ae6b3378.html. Accessed May 14, 2018

155. Barry MM, Clarke AM, Jenkins R, Patel V. A systematic review of the effectiveness of mental health promotion interventions for young people in low and middle income countries. *BMC Public Health*. 2013;13:835

156. Tyrer RA, Fazel M. School and community-based interventions for refugee and asylum seeking children: a systematic review. *PLoS One*. 2014;9(2):e89359

157. American Psychological Association. *Resilience and Recovery After War: Refugee Children and Families in the US*. Washington, DC: American Psychological Association; 2010

158. Save the Children UK. *What Do Children Want in Times of Emergency and Crisis? They Want an Education*. London, UK: Save the Children; 2015

159. Seeman N, Tang S, Brown AD, Ing A. World survey of mental illness stigma. *J Affect Disord*. 2016;190:115–121

160. Fazel M, Garcia J, Stein A. The right location? Experiences of refugee adolescents seen by school-based mental health services. *Clin Child Psychol Psychiatry*. 2016;21(3):368–380

161. Masten AS. Global perspectives on resilience in children and youth. *Child Dev*. 2014;85(1):6–20

162. Luthar SS, Cicchetti D, Becker B. The construct of resilience: a critical evaluation and guidelines for future work. *Child Dev*. 2000;71(3):543–562

163. Betancourt TS, Khan KT. The mental health of children affected by armed conflict: protective processes and pathways to resilience. *Int Rev Psychiatry*. 2008;20(3):317–328

164. Tol WA, Song S, Jordans MJ. Annual research review: resilience and mental health in children and adolescents living in areas of armed conflict—a systematic review of findings in low- and middle-income countries. *J Child Psychol Psychiatry*. 2013;54(4):445–460

165. Barber BK. Political violence, family relations, and Palestinian youth functioning. *J Adolesc Res*. 1999;14(2):206–230

166. Harel-Fisch Y, Radwan Q, Walsh SD, et al. Psychosocial outcomes related to subjective threat from armed conflict events (STACE): findings from the Israeli-Palestinian cross-cultural HBSC study. *Child Abuse Negl*. 2010;34(9):623–638

167. Ní Raghallaigh M, Gilligan R. Active survival in the lives of unaccompanied minors: coping strategies, resilience, and the relevance of religion. *Child Fam Soc Work*. 2010;15(2):226–237

168. Oppedal B, Idsoe T. The role of social support in the acculturation and mental health of unaccompanied minor asylum seekers. *Scand J Psychol*. 2015;56(2):203–211

169. Young H, Borrel A, Holland D, Salama P. Public nutrition in complex emergencies. *Lancet*. 2004;364(9448):1899–1909

170. Lam E, McCarthy A, Brennan M. Vaccine-preventable diseases in humanitarian emergencies among refugee and internally-displaced populations. *Hum Vaccin Immunother*. 2015;11(11):2627–2636

171. Oberoi P, Sotomayor J, Pace P, Rijks B, Weekers J, Walilegne YT. *International Migration, Health and Human Rights*. Geneva, Switzerland: Institute of Medicine, World Health Organization, United Nations High Commissioner for Refugees; 2013

172. World Health Organization. *Stepping Up Action on Refugee and Migrant Health: Towards a WHO European Framework for Collaborative Action*. Outcome document of the High-level Meeting on Refugee and Migrant Health 23-24 November, 2015. Geneva, Switzerland: World Health Organization Regional Office for Europe; 2015

Ensuring Comprehensive Care and Support for Transgender and Gender-Diverse Children and Adolescents

• •

- *Policy Statement*

POLICY STATEMENT Organizational Principles to Guide and Define the Child Health Care System and/or Improve the Health of all Children

American Academy
of Pediatrics

DEDICATED TO THE HEALTH OF ALL CHILDREN™

Ensuring Comprehensive Care and Support for Transgender and Gender-Diverse Children and Adolescents

Jason Rafferty, MD, MPH, EdM, FAAP, COMMITTEE ON PSYCHOSOCIAL ASPECTS OF CHILD AND FAMILY HEALTH, COMMITTEE ON ADOLESCENCE, SECTION ON LESBIAN, GAY, BISEXUAL, AND TRANSGENDER HEALTH AND WELLNESS

As a traditionally underserved population that faces numerous health disparities, youth who identify as transgender and gender diverse (TGD) and their families are increasingly presenting to pediatric providers for education, care, and referrals. The need for more formal training, standardized treatment, and research on safety and medical outcomes often leaves providers feeling ill equipped to support and care for patients that identify as TGD and families. In this policy statement, we review relevant concepts and challenges and provide suggestions for pediatric providers that are focused on promoting the health and positive development of youth that identify as TGD while eliminating discrimination and stigma.

abstract

Department of Pediatrics, Hasbro Children's Hospital, Providence, Rhode Island; Thundermist Health Centers, Providence, Rhode Island; and Department of Child Psychiatry, Emma Pendleton Bradley Hospital, East Providence, Rhode Island

Dr Rafferty conceptualized the statement, drafted the initial manuscript, reviewed and revised the manuscript, approved the final manuscript as submitted, and agrees to be accountable for all aspects of the work.

Policy statements from the American Academy of Pediatrics benefit from expertise and resources of liaisons and internal (AAP) and external reviewers. However, policy statements from the American Academy of Pediatrics may not reflect the views of the liaisons or the organizations or government agencies that they represent.

The guidance in this statement does not indicate an exclusive course of treatment or serve as a standard of medical care. Variations, taking into account individual circumstances, may be appropriate.

All policy statements from the American Academy of Pediatrics automatically expire 5 years after publication unless reaffirmed, revised, or retired at or before that time.

INTRODUCTION

In its dedication to the health of all children, the American Academy of Pediatrics (AAP) strives to improve health care access and eliminate disparities for children and teenagers who identify as lesbian, gay, bisexual, transgender, or questioning (LGBTQ) of their sexual or gender identity.[1,2] Despite some advances in public awareness and legal protections, youth who identify as LGBTQ continue to face disparities that stem from multiple sources, including inequitable laws and policies, societal discrimination, and a lack of access to quality health care, including mental health care. Such challenges are often more intense for youth who do not conform to social expectations and norms regarding gender. Pediatric providers are increasingly encountering such youth and their families, who seek medical advice and interventions, yet they may lack the formal training to care for youth that identify as transgender and gender diverse (TGD) and their families.[3]

This policy statement is focused specifically on children and youth that identify as TGD rather than the larger LGBTQ population, providing brief, relevant background on the basis of current available research

To cite: Rafferty J, AAP COMMITTEE ON PSYCHOSOCIAL ASPECTS OF CHILD AND FAMILY HEALTH, AAP COMMITTEE ON ADOLESCENCE, AAP SECTION ON LESBIAN, GAY, BISEXUAL, AND TRANSGENDER HEALTH AND WELLNESS. Ensuring Comprehensive Care and Support for Transgender and Gender-Diverse Children and Adolescents. *Pediatrics.* 2018;142(4): e20182162

TABLE 1 Relevant Terms and Definitions Related to Gender Care

Term	Definition
Sex	An assignment that is made at birth, usually male or female, typically on the basis of external genital anatomy but sometimes on the basis of internal gonads, chromosomes, or hormone levels
Gender identity	A person's deep internal sense of being female, male, a combination of both, somewhere in between, or neither, resulting from a multifaceted interaction of biological traits, environmental factors, self-understanding, and cultural expectations
Gender expression	The external way a person expresses their gender, such as with clothing, hair, mannerisms, activities, or social roles
Gender perception	The way others interpret a person's gender expression
Gender diverse	A term that is used to describe people with gender behaviors, appearances, or identities that are incongruent with those culturally assigned to their birth sex; gender-diverse individuals may refer to themselves with many different terms, such as transgender, nonbinary, genderqueer,[7] gender fluid, gender creative, gender independent, or noncisgender. "Gender diverse" is used to acknowledge and include the vast diversity of gender identities that exists. It replaces the former term, "gender nonconforming," which has a negative and exclusionary connotation.
Transgender	A subset of gender-diverse youth whose gender identity does not match their assigned sex and generally remains persistent, consistent, and insistent over time; the term "transgender" also encompasses many other labels individuals may use to refer to themselves.
Cisgender	A term that is used to describe a person who identifies and expresses a gender that is consistent with the culturally defined norms of the sex they were assigned at birth
Agender	A term that is used to describe a person who does not identify as having a particular gender
Affirmed gender	When a person's true gender identity, or concern about their gender identity, is communicated to and validated from others as authentic
MTF; affirmed female; trans female	Terms that are used to describe individuals who were assigned male sex at birth but who have a gender identity and/or expression that is asserted to be more feminine
FTM; affirmed male; trans male	Terms that are used to describe individuals who were assigned female sex at birth but who have a gender identity and/or expression that is asserted to be more masculine
Gender dysphoria	A clinical symptom that is characterized by a sense of alienation to some or all of the physical characteristics or social roles of one's assigned gender; also, gender dysphoria is the psychiatric diagnosis in the *DSM-5*, which has focus on the distress that stems from the incongruence between one's expressed or experienced (affirmed) gender and the gender assigned at birth.
Gender identity disorder	A psychiatric diagnosis defined previously in the *DSM-IV* (changed to "gender dysphoria" in the *DSM-5*); the primary criteria include a strong, persistent cross-sex identification and significant distress and social impairment. This diagnosis is no longer appropriate for use and may lead to stigma, but the term may be found in older research.
Sexual orientation	A person's sexual identity in relation to the gender(s) to which they are attracted; sexual orientation and gender identity develop separately.

This list is not intended to be all inclusive. The pronouns "they" and "their" are used intentionally to be inclusive rather than the binary pronouns "he" and "she" and "his" and "her." Adapted from Bonifacio HJ, Rosenthal SM. Gender variance and dysphoria in children and adolescents. *Pediatr Clin North Am*. 2015;62(4):1001–1016. Adapted from Vance SR Jr, Ehrensaft D, Rosenthal SM. Psychological and medical care of gender nonconforming youth. *Pediatrics*. 2014;134(6):1184–1192. DSM-5, *Diagnostic and Statistical Manual of Mental Disorders, Fifth Edition*; DSM-IV, *Diagnostic and Statistical Manual of Mental Disorders, Fourth Edition*; FTM, female to male; MTF, male to female.

and expert opinion from clinical and research leaders, which will serve as the basis for recommendations. It is not a comprehensive review of clinical approaches and nuances to pediatric care for children and youth that identify as TGD. Professional understanding of youth that identify as TGD is a rapidly evolving clinical field in which research on appropriate clinical management is limited by insufficient funding.[3,4]

DEFINITIONS

To clarify recommendations and discussions in this policy statement, some definitions are provided. However, brief descriptions of human behavior or identities may not capture nuance in this evolving field.

"Sex," or "natal gender," is a label, generally "male" or "female," that is typically assigned at birth on the basis of genetic and anatomic characteristics, such as genital anatomy, chromosomes, and sex hormone levels. Meanwhile, "gender identity" is one's internal sense of who one is, which results from a multifaceted interaction of biological traits, developmental influences, and environmental conditions. It may be male, female, somewhere in between, a combination of both, or neither (ie, not conforming to a binary conceptualization of gender). Self-recognition of gender identity develops over time, much the same way as a child's physical body does. For some people, gender identity can be fluid, shifting in different contexts. "Gender expression"

refers to the wide array of ways people display their gender through clothing, hair styles, mannerisms, or social roles. Exploring different ways of expressing gender is common for children and may challenge social expectations. The way others interpret this expression is referred to as "gender perception" (Table 1).[5,6]

These labels may or may not be congruent. The term "cisgender" is used if someone identifies and expresses a gender that is consistent with the culturally defined norms of the sex that was assigned at birth. "Gender diverse" is an umbrella term to describe an ever-evolving array of labels that people may apply when their gender identity, expression, or even perception does not conform to the norms and stereotypes others expect of their assigned sex. "Transgender" is usually reserved for a subset of such youth whose gender identity does not match their assigned sex and generally remains persistent, consistent, and insistent over time. These terms are not diagnoses; rather, they are personal and often dynamic ways of describing one's own gender experience.

Gender identity is not synonymous with "sexual orientation," which refers to a person's identity in relation to the gender(s) to which they are sexually and romantically attracted. Gender identity and sexual orientation are distinct but interrelated constructs.[8] Therefore, being transgender does not imply a sexual orientation, and people who identify as transgender still identify as straight, gay, bisexual, etc, on the basis of their attractions. (For more information, *The Gender Book*, found at www.thegenderbook.com, is a resource with illustrations that are used to highlight these core terms and concepts.)

EPIDEMIOLOGY

In population-based surveys, questions related to gender identity are rarely asked, which makes it difficult to assess the size and characteristics of the population that is TGD. In the 2014 Behavioral Risk Factor Surveillance System of the Centers for Disease Control and Prevention, only 19 states elected to include optional questions on gender identity. Extrapolation from these data suggests that the US prevalence of adults who identify as transgender or "gender nonconforming" is 0.6% (1.4 million), ranging from 0.3% in North Dakota to 0.8% in Hawaii.[9] On the basis of these data, it has been estimated that 0.7% of youth ages 13 to 17 years (~150 000) identify as transgender.[10] This number is much higher than previous estimates, which were

extrapolated from individual states or specialty clinics, and is likely an underestimate given the stigma regarding those who openly identify as transgender and the difficulty in defining "transgender" in a way that is inclusive of all gender-diverse identities.[11]

There have been no large-scale prevalence studies among children and adolescents, and there is no evidence that adult statistics reflect young children or adolescents. In the 2014 Behavioral Risk Factor Surveillance System, those 18 to 24 years of age were more likely than older age groups to identify as transgender (0.7%).[9] Children report being aware of gender incongruence at young ages. Children who later identify as TGD report first having recognized their gender as "different" at an average age of 8.5 years; however, they did not disclose such feelings until an average of 10 years later.[12]

MENTAL HEALTH IMPLICATIONS

Adolescents and adults who identify as transgender have high rates of depression, anxiety, eating disorders, self-harm, and suicide.[13–20] Evidence suggests that an identity of TGD has an increased prevalence among individuals with autism spectrum disorder, but this association is not yet well understood.[21,22] In 1 retrospective cohort study, 56% of youth who identified as transgender reported previous suicidal ideation, and 31% reported a previous suicide attempt, compared with 20% and 11% among matched youth who identified as cisgender, respectively.[13] Some youth who identify as TGD also experience gender dysphoria, which is a specific diagnosis given to those who experience impairment in peer and/or family relationships, school performance, or other aspects of their life as a consequence of the

incongruence between their assigned sex and their gender identity.[23]

There is no evidence that risk for mental illness is inherently attributable to one's identity of TGD. Rather, it is believed to be multifactorial, stemming from an internal conflict between one's appearance and identity, limited availability of mental health services, low access to health care providers with expertise in caring for youth who identify as TGD, discrimination, stigma, and social rejection.[24] This was affirmed by the American Psychological Association in 2008[25] (with practice guidelines released in 2015[8]) and the American Psychiatric Association, which made the following statement in 2012:

Being transgender or gender variant implies no impairment in judgment, stability, reliability, or general social or vocational capabilities; however, these individuals often experience discrimination due to a lack of civil rights protections for their gender identity or expression…. [Such] discrimination and lack of equal civil rights is damaging to the mental health of transgender and gender variant individuals.[26]

Youth who identify as TGD often confront stigma and discrimination, which contribute to feelings of rejection and isolation that can adversely affect physical and emotional well-being. For example, many youth believe that they must hide their gender identity and expression to avoid bullying, harassment, or victimization. Youth who identify as TGD experience disproportionately high rates of homelessness, physical violence (at home and in the community), substance abuse, and high-risk sexual behaviors.[5,6,12,27–31] Among the 3 million HIV testing events that were reported in 2015, the highest percentages of new infections were among women who identified as transgender[32] and were also at particular risk for not knowing their HIV status.[30]

GENDER-AFFIRMATIVE CARE

In a gender-affirmative care model (GACM), pediatric providers offer developmentally appropriate care that is oriented toward understanding and appreciating the youth's gender experience. A strong, nonjudgmental partnership with youth and their families can facilitate exploration of complicated emotions and gender-diverse expressions while allowing questions and concerns to be raised in a supportive environment.[5] In a GACM, the following messages are conveyed:

- transgender identities and diverse gender expressions do not constitute a mental disorder;

- variations in gender identity and expression are normal aspects of human diversity, and binary definitions of gender do not always reflect emerging gender identities;

- gender identity evolves as an interplay of biology, development, socialization, and culture; and

- if a mental health issue exists, it most often stems from stigma and negative experiences rather than being intrinsic to the child.[27,33]

The GACM is best facilitated through the integration of medical, mental health, and social services, including specific resources and supports for parents and families.[24] Providers work together to destigmatize gender variance, promote the child's self-worth, facilitate access to care, educate families, and advocate for safer community spaces where children are free to develop and explore their gender.[5] A specialized gender-affirmative therapist, when available, may be an asset in helping children and their families build skills for dealing with gender-based stigma, address symptoms of anxiety or depression, and reinforce the child's overall resiliency.[34,35] There is a limited but growing body

of evidence that suggests that using an integrated affirmative model results in young people having fewer mental health concerns whether they ultimately identify as transgender.[24,36,37]

In contrast, "conversion" or "reparative" treatment models are used to prevent children and adolescents from identifying as transgender or to dissuade them from exhibiting gender-diverse expressions. The Substance Abuse and Mental Health Services Administration has concluded that any therapeutic intervention with the goal of changing a youth's gender expression or identity is inappropriate.[33] Reparative approaches have been proven to be not only unsuccessful[38] but also deleterious and are considered outside the mainstream of traditional medical practice.[29,39–42] The AAP described reparative approaches as "unfair and deceptive."[43] At the time of this writing,* conversion therapy was banned by executive regulation in New York and by legislative statutes in 9 other states as well as the District of Columbia.[44]

Pediatric providers have an essential role in assessing gender concerns and providing evidence-based information to assist youth and families in medical decision-making. Not doing so can prolong or exacerbate gender dysphoria and contribute to abuse and stigmatization.[35] If a pediatric provider does not feel prepared to address gender concerns when they occur, then referral to a pediatric or mental health provider with more expertise is appropriate. There is little research on communication and efficacy with transfers in care for youth who identify as TGD,

---

* For more information regarding state-specific laws, please contact the AAP Division of State Government Affairs at stgov@ aap.org.

particularly from pediatric to adult providers.

DEVELOPMENTAL CONSIDERATIONS

Acknowledging that the capacity for emerging abstract thinking in childhood is important to conceptualize and reflect on identity, gender-affirmation guidelines are being focused on individually tailored interventions on the basis of the physical and cognitive development of youth who identify as TGD.[45] Accordingly, research substantiates that children who are prepubertal and assert an identity of TGD know their gender as clearly and as consistently as their developmentally equivalent peers who identify as cisgender and benefit from the same level of social acceptance.[46] This developmental approach to gender affirmation is in contrast to the outdated approach in which a child's gender-diverse assertions are held as "possibly true" until an arbitrary age (often after pubertal onset) when they can be considered valid, an approach that authors of the literature have termed "watchful waiting." This outdated approach does not serve the child because critical support is withheld. Watchful waiting is based on binary notions of gender in which gender diversity and fluidity is pathologized; in watchful waiting, it is also assumed that notions of gender identity become fixed at a certain age. The approach is also influenced by a group of early studies with validity concerns, methodologic flaws, and limited follow-up on children who identified as TGD and, by adolescence, did not seek further treatment ("desisters").[45,47] More robust and current research suggests that, rather than focusing on who a child will become, valuing them for who they are, even at a young age, fosters secure attachment and resilience, not only for the child but also for the whole family.[5,45,48,49]

MEDICAL MANAGEMENT

Pediatric primary care providers are in a unique position to routinely inquire about gender development in children and adolescents as part of recommended well-child visits[50] and to be a reliable source of validation, support, and reassurance. They are often the first provider to be aware that a child may not identify as cisgender or that there may be distress related to a gender-diverse identity. The best way to approach gender with patients is to inquire directly and nonjudgmentally about their experience and feelings before applying any labels.[27,51]

Many medical interventions can be offered to youth who identify as TGD and their families. The decision of whether and when to initiate gender-affirmative treatment is personal and involves careful consideration of risks, benefits, and other factors unique to each patient and family. Many protocols suggest that clinical assessment of youth who identify as TGD is ideally conducted on an ongoing basis in the setting of a collaborative, multidisciplinary approach, which, in addition to the patient and family, may include the pediatric provider, a mental health provider (preferably with expertise in caring for youth who identify as TGD), social and legal supports, and a pediatric endocrinologist or adolescent-medicine gender specialist, if available.[6,28] There is no prescribed path, sequence, or end point. Providers can make every effort to be aware of the influence of their own biases. The medical options also vary depending on pubertal and developmental progression.

Clinical Setting

In the past year, 1 in 4 adults who identified as transgender avoided a necessary doctor's visit because of fear of being mistreated.[31] All clinical office staff have a role in affirming a patient's gender identity. Making flyers available or displaying posters related to LGBTQ health issues, including information for children who identify as TGD and families, reveals inclusivity and awareness. Generally, patients who identify as TGD feel most comfortable when they have access to a gender-neutral restroom. Diversity training that encompasses sensitivity when caring for youth who identify as TGD and their families can be helpful in educating clinical and administrative staff. A patient-asserted name and pronouns are used by staff and are ideally reflected in the electronic medical record without creating duplicate charts.[52,53] The US Centers for Medicare and Medicaid Services and the National Coordinator for Health Information Technology require all electronic health record systems certified under the Meaningful Use incentive program to have the capacity to confidentially collect information on gender identity.[54,55] Explaining and maintaining confidentiality procedures promotes openness and trust, particularly with youth who identify as LGBTQ.[1] Maintaining a safe clinical space can provide at least 1 consistent, protective refuge for patients and families, allowing authentic gender expression and exploration that builds resiliency.

Pubertal Suppression

Gonadotrophin-releasing hormones have been used to delay puberty since the 1980s for central precocious puberty.[56] These reversible treatments can also be used in adolescents who experience gender dysphoria to prevent development of secondary sex characteristics and provide time up until 16 years of age for the individual and the family to explore gender identity, access psychosocial supports, develop coping skills, and further define appropriate treatment goals. If pubertal suppression treatment is suspended, then endogenous puberty will resume.[20,57,58]

Often, pubertal suppression creates an opportunity to reduce distress that may occur with the development of secondary sexual characteristics and allow for gender-affirming care, including mental health support for the adolescent and the family. It reduces the need for later surgery because physical changes that are otherwise irreversible (protrusion of the Adam's apple, male pattern baldness, voice change, breast growth, etc) are prevented. The available data reveal that pubertal suppression in children who identify as TGD generally leads to improved psychological functioning in adolescence and young adulthood.[20,57–59]

Pubertal suppression is not without risks. Delaying puberty beyond one's peers can also be stressful and can lead to lower self-esteem and increased risk taking.[60] Some experts believe that genital underdevelopment may limit some potential reconstructive options.[61] Research on long-term risks, particularly in terms of bone metabolism[62] and fertility,[63] is currently limited and provides varied results.[57,64,65] Families often look to pediatric providers for help in considering whether pubertal suppression is indicated in the context of their child's overall well-being as gender diverse.

Gender Affirmation

As youth who identify as TGD reflect on and evaluate their gender identity, various interventions may be considered to better align their gender expression with their underlying identity. This process of reflection, acceptance, and, for some, intervention is known as "gender affirmation." It was formerly referred to as "transitioning," but many view the process as an affirmation and acceptance of who they have always been rather than a transition

TABLE 2 The Process of Gender Affirmation May Include ≥1 of the Following Components

Component	Definition	General Age Range[a]	Reversibility[a]
Social affirmation	Adopting gender-affirming hairstyles, clothing, name, gender pronouns, and restrooms and other facilities	Any	Reversible
Puberty blockers	Gonadotropin-releasing hormone analogues, such as leuprolide and histrelin	During puberty (Tanner stage 2–5)[b]	Reversible[c]
Cross-sex hormone therapy	Testosterone (for those who were assigned female at birth and are masculinizing); estrogen plus androgen inhibitor (for those who were assigned male at birth and are feminizing)	Early adolescence onward	Partially reversible (skin texture, muscle mass, and fat deposition); irreversible once developed (testosterone: Adam's apple protrusion, voice changes, and male pattern baldness; estrogen: breast development); unknown reversibility (effect on fertility)
Gender-affirming surgeries	"Top" surgery (to create a male-typical chest shape or enhance breasts); "bottom" surgery (surgery on genitals or reproductive organs); facial feminization and other procedures	Typically adults (adolescents on case-by-case basis[d])	Not reversible
Legal affirmation	Changing gender and name recorded on birth certificate, school records, and other documents	Any	Reversible

[a] Note that the provided age range and reversibility is based on the little data that are currently available.

[b] There is limited benefit to starting gonadotropin-releasing hormone after Tanner stage 5 for pubertal suppression. However, when cross-sex hormones are initiated with a gradually increasing schedule, the initial levels are often not high enough to suppress endogenous sex hormone secretion. Therefore, gonadotropin-releasing hormone may be continued in accordance with the Endocrine Society Guidelines.[68]

[c] The effect of sustained puberty suppression on fertility is unknown. Pubertal suppression can be, and often is indicated to be, followed by cross-sex hormone treatment. However, when cross-sex hormones are initiated without endogenous hormones, then fertility may be decreased.[68]

[d] Eligibility criteria for gender-affirmative surgical interventions among adolescents are not clearly defined between established protocols and practice. When applicable, eligibility is usually determined on a case-by-case basis with the adolescent and the family along with input from medical, mental health, and surgical providers.[68–71]

from 1 gender identity to another. Accordingly, some people who have gone through the process prefer to call themselves "affirmed females, males, etc" (or just "females, males, etc"), rather than using the prefix "trans-." Gender affirmation is also used to acknowledge that some individuals who identify as TGD may feel affirmed in their gender without pursuing medical or surgical interventions.[7,66]

Supportive involvement of parents and family is associated with better mental and physical health outcomes.[67] Gender affirmation among adolescents with gender dysphoria often reduces the emphasis on gender in their lives, allowing them to attend to other developmental tasks, such as academic success, relationship building, and future-oriented planning.[64] Most protocols for gender-affirming interventions incorporate World Professional Association of Transgender

Health[35] and Endocrine Society[68] recommendations and include ≥1 of the following elements (Table 2):

1. Social Affirmation: This is a reversible intervention in which children and adolescents express partially or completely in their asserted gender identity by adapting hairstyle, clothing, pronouns, name, etc. Children who identify as transgender and socially affirm and are supported in their asserted gender show no increase in depression and only minimal (clinically insignificant) increases in anxiety compared with age-matched averages.[48] Social affirmation can be complicated given the wide range of social interactions children have (eg, extended families, peers, school, community, etc). There is little guidance on the best approach (eg, all at once, gradual, creating new social networks, or affirming within existing networks, etc). Pediatric providers

can best support families by anticipating and discussing such complexity proactively, either in their own practice or through enlisting a qualified mental health provider.

2. Legal Affirmation: Elements of a social affirmation, such as a name and gender marker, become official on legal documents, such as birth certificates, passports, identification cards, school documents, etc. The processes for making these changes depend on state laws and may require specific documentation from pediatric providers.

3. Medical Affirmation: This is the process of using cross-sex hormones to allow adolescents who have initiated puberty to develop secondary sex characteristics of the opposite biological sex. Some changes are partially reversible if hormones are stopped, but others become

irreversible once they are fully developed (Table 2).

4. Surgical Affirmation: Surgical approaches may be used to feminize or masculinize features, such as hair distribution, chest, or genitalia, and may include removal of internal organs, such as ovaries or the uterus (affecting fertility). These changes are irreversible. Although current protocols typically reserve surgical interventions for adults,[35,68] they are occasionally pursued during adolescence on a case-by-case basis, considering the necessity and benefit to the adolescent's overall health and often including multidisciplinary input from medical, mental health, and surgical providers as well as from the adolescent and family.[69–71]

For some youth who identify as TGD whose natal gender is female, menstruation, breakthrough bleeding, and dysmenorrhea can lead to significant distress before or during gender affirmation. The American College of Obstetrics and Gynecology suggests that, although limited data are available to outline management, menstruation can be managed without exogenous estrogens by using a progesterone-only pill, a medroxyprogesterone acetate shot, or a progesterone-containing intrauterine or implantable device.[72] If estrogen can be tolerated, oral contraceptives that contain both progesterone and estrogen are more effective at suppressing menses.[73] The Endocrine Society guidelines also suggest that gonadotrophin-releasing hormones can be used for menstrual suppression before the anticipated initiation of testosterone or in combination with testosterone for breakthrough bleeding (enables phenotypic masculinization at a lower dose than if testosterone is used alone).[68] Masculinizing hormones in natal female patients may lead to a cessation of menses,

but unplanned pregnancies have been reported, which emphasizes the need for ongoing contraceptive counseling with youth who identify as TGD.[72]

HEALTH DISPARITIES

In addition to societal challenges, youth who identify as TGD face several barriers within the health care system, especially regarding access to care. In 2015, a focus group of youth who identified as transgender in Seattle, Washington, revealed 4 problematic areas related to health care:

1. safety issues, including the lack of safe clinical environments and fear of discrimination by providers;

2. poor access to physical health services, including testing for sexually transmitted infections;

3. inadequate resources to address mental health concerns; and

4. lack of continuity with providers.[74]

This study reveals the obstacles many youth who identify as TGD face in accessing essential services, including the limited supply of appropriately trained medical and psychological providers, fertility options, and insurance coverage denials for gender-related treatments.[74]

Insurance denials for services related to the care of patients who identify as TGD are a significant barrier. Although the Office for Civil Rights of the US Department of Health and Human Services explicitly stated in 2012 that the nondiscrimination provision in the Patient Protection and Affordable Care Act includes people who identify as gender diverse,[75,76] insurance claims for gender affirmation, particularly among youth who identify as TGD, are frequently denied.[54,77] In 1 study, it was found that approximately 25% of individuals

who identified as transgender were denied insurance coverage because of being transgender.[31] The burden of covering medical expenses that are not covered by insurance can be financially devastating, and even when expenses are covered, families describe high levels of stress in navigating and submitting claims appropriately.[78] In 2012, a large gender center in Boston, Massachusetts, reported that most young patients who identified as transgender and were deemed appropriate candidates for recommended gender care were unable to obtain it because of such denials, which were based on the premise that gender dysphoria was a mental disorder, not a physical one, and that treatment was not medically or surgically necessary.[24] This practice not only contributes to stigma, prolonged gender dysphoria, and poor mental health outcomes,[77] but it may also lead patients to seek nonmedically supervised treatments that are potentially dangerous.[24] Furthermore, insurance denials can reinforce a socioeconomic divide between those who can finance the high costs of uncovered care and those who cannot.[24,77]

The transgender youth group in Seattle likely reflected the larger TGD population when they described how obstacles adversely affect self-esteem and contribute to the perception that they are undervalued by society and the health care system.[74,77] Professional medical associations, including the AAP, are increasingly calling for equity in health care provisions regardless of gender identity or expression.[1,8,23,72] There is a critical need for investments in research on the prevalence, disparities, biological underpinnings, and standards of care relating to gender-diverse populations. Pediatric providers who work with state government and insurance officials can play an essential role in advocating for stronger nondiscrimination policies and improved coverage.

There is a lack of quality research on the experience of youth of color who identify as transgender. One theory suggests that the intersection of racism, transphobia, and sexism may result in the extreme marginalization that is experienced among many women of color who identify as transgender,[79] including rejection from their family and dropping out of school at younger ages (often in the setting of rigid religious beliefs regarding gender),[80] increased levels of violence and body objectification,[81] 3 times the risk of poverty compared with the general population,[31] and the highest prevalence of HIV compared with other risk groups (estimated as high as 56.3% in 1 meta-analysis).[30] One model suggests that pervasive stigma and oppression can be associated with psychological distress (anxiety, depression, and suicide) and adoption of risk behaviors by such youth to obtain a sense of validation toward their complex identities.[79]

FAMILY ACCEPTANCE

Research increasingly suggests that familial acceptance or rejection ultimately has little influence on the gender identity of youth; however, it may profoundly affect young people's ability to openly discuss or disclose concerns about their identity. Suppressing such concerns can affect mental health.[82] Families often find it hard to understand and accept their child's gender-diverse traits because of personal beliefs, social pressure, and stigma.[49,83] Legitimate fears may exist for their child's welfare, safety, and acceptance that pediatric providers need to appreciate and address. Families can be encouraged to communicate their concerns and questions. Unacknowledged concerns can contribute to shame and hesitation in regard to offering support and understanding,[84]

which is essential for the child's self-esteem, social involvement, and overall health as TGD.[48,85–87] Some caution has been expressed that unquestioning acceptance per se may not best serve questioning youth or their families. Instead, psychological evidence suggests that the most benefit comes when family members and youth are supported and encouraged to engage in reflective perspective taking and validate their own and the other's thoughts and feelings despite divergent views.[49,82]

In this regard, suicide attempt rates among 433 adolescents in Ontario who identified as "trans" were 4% among those with strongly supportive parents and as high as 60% among those whose parents were not supportive.[85] Adolescents who identify as transgender and endorse at least 1 supportive person in their life report significantly less distress than those who only experience rejection. In communities with high levels of support, it was found that nonsupportive families tended to increase their support over time, leading to dramatic improvement in mental health outcomes among their children who identified as transgender.[88]

Pediatric providers can create a safe environment for parents and families to better understand and listen to the needs of their children while receiving reassurance and education.[83] It is often appropriate to assist the child in understanding the parents' concerns as well. Despite expectations by some youth with transgender identity for immediate acceptance after "coming out," family members often proceed through a process of becoming more comfortable and understanding of the youth's gender identity, thoughts, and feelings. One model suggests that the process resembles grieving, wherein the family separates from their expectations for their child to embrace a new reality. This process may proceed through stages of shock,

denial, anger, feelings of betrayal, fear, self-discovery, and pride.[89] The amount of time spent in any of these stages and the overall pace varies widely. Many family members also struggle as they are pushed to reflect on their own gender experience and assumptions throughout this process. In some situations, youth who identify as TGD may be at risk for internalizing the difficult emotions that family members may be experiencing. In these cases, individual and group therapy for the family members may be helpful.[49,78]

Family dynamics can be complex, involving disagreement among legal guardians or between guardians and their children, which may affect the ability to obtain consent for any medical management or interventions. Even in states where minors may access care without parental consent for mental health services, contraception, and sexually transmitted infections, parental or guardian consent is required for hormonal and surgical care of patients who identify as TGD.[72,90] Some families may take issue with providers who address gender concerns or offer gender-affirming care. In rare cases, a family may deny access to care that raises concerns about the youth's welfare and safety; in those cases, additional legal or ethical support may be useful to consider. In such rare situations, pediatric providers may want to familiarize themselves with relevant local consent laws and maintain their primary responsibility for the welfare of the child.

SAFE SCHOOLS AND COMMUNITIES

Youth who identify as TGD are becoming more visible because gender-diverse expression is increasingly admissible in the media, on social media, and in schools and communities. Regardless of whether a youth with a gender-diverse identity ultimately identifies as transgender, challenges exist in nearly every social context, from lack of understanding to outright rejection, isolation, discrimination, and victimization. In the US Transgender Survey of nearly 28 000 respondents, it was found that among those who were out as or perceived to be TGD between kindergarten and eighth grade, 54% were verbally harassed, 24% were physically assaulted, and 13% were sexually assaulted; 17% left school because of maltreatment.[31] Education and advocacy from the medical community on the importance of safe schools for youth who identify as TGD can have a significant effect.

At the time of this writing,* only 18 states and the District of Columbia had laws that prohibited discrimination based on gender expression when it comes to employment, housing, public accommodations, and insurance benefits. Over 200 US cities have such legislation. In addition to basic protections, many youth who identify as TGD also have to navigate legal obstacles when it comes to legally changing their name and/or gender marker.[54] In addition to advocating and working with policy makers to promote equal protections for youth who identify as TGD, pediatric providers can play an important role by developing a familiarity with local laws and organizations that provide social work and legal assistance to youth who identify as TGD and their families.

School environments play a significant role in the social and emotional development of children. Every child has a right to feel safe

* For more information regarding state-specific laws, please contact the AAP Division of State Government Affairs at stgov@ aap.org.

and respected at school, but for youth who identify as TGD, this can be challenging. Nearly every aspect of school life may present safety concerns and require negotiations regarding their gender expression, including name/pronoun use, use of bathrooms and locker rooms, sports teams, dances and activities, overnight activities, and even peer groups. Conflicts in any of these areas can quickly escalate beyond the school's control to larger debates among the community and even on a national stage.

The formerly known Gay, Lesbian, and Straight Education Network (GLSEN), an advocacy organization for youth who identify as LGBTQ, conducts an annual national survey to measure LGBTQ well-being in US schools. In 2015, students who identified as LGBTQ reported high rates of being discouraged from participation in extracurricular activities. One in 5 students who identified as LGBTQ reported being hindered from forming or participating in a club to support lesbian, gay, bisexual, or transgender students (eg, a gay straight alliance, now often referred to as a genders and sexualities alliance) despite such clubs at schools being associated with decreased reports of negative remarks about sexual orientation or gender expression, increased feelings of safety and connectedness at school, and lower levels of victimization. In addition, >20% of students who identified as LGBTQ reported being blocked from writing about LGBTQ issues in school yearbooks or school newspapers or being prevented or discouraged by coaches and school staff from participating in sports because of their sexual orientation or gender expression.[91]

One strategy to prevent conflict is to proactively support policies and protections that promote inclusion and safety of all students. However, such policies are far from

consistent across districts. In 2015, GLSEN found that 43% of children who identified as LGBTQ reported feeling unsafe at school because of their gender expression, but only 6% reported that their school had official policies to support youth who identified as TGD, and only 11% reported that their school's antibullying policies had specific protections for gender expression.[91] Consequently, more than half of the students who identified as transgender in the study were prevented from using the bathroom, names, or pronouns that aligned with their asserted gender at school. A lack of explicit policies that protected youth who identified as TGD was associated with increased reported victimization, with more than half of students who identified as LGBTQ reporting verbal harassment because of their gender expression. Educators and school administrators play an essential role in advocating for and enforcing such policies. GLSEN found that when students recognized actions to reduce gender-based harassment, both students who identified as transgender and cisgender reported a greater connection to staff and feelings of safety.[91] In another study, schools were open to education regarding gender diversity and were willing to implement policies when they were supported by external agencies, such as medical professionals.[92]

Academic content plays an important role in building a safe school environment as well. The 2015 GLSEN survey revealed that when positive representations of people who identified as LGBTQ were included in the curriculum, students who identified as LGBTQ reported less hostile school environments, less victimization and greater feelings of safety, fewer school absences because of feeling unsafe, greater feelings of connectedness to their school community, and an increased interest in high school graduation and postsecondary education.[91] At the time of this writing,* 8 states had laws that explicitly forbade teachers from even discussing LGBTQ issues.[54]

MEDICAL EDUCATION

One of the most important ways to promote high-quality health care for youth who identify as TGD and their families is increasing the knowledge base and clinical experience of pediatric providers in providing culturally competent care to such populations, as recommended by the recently released guidelines by the Association of American Medical Colleges.[93] This begins with the medical school curriculum in areas such as human development, sexual health, endocrinology, pediatrics, and psychiatry. In a 2009–2010 survey of US medical schools, it was found that the median number of hours dedicated to LGBTQ health was 5, with one-third of US medical schools reporting no LGBTQ curriculum during the clinical years.[94]

During residency training, there is potential for gender diversity to be emphasized in core rotations, especially in pediatrics, psychiatry, family medicine, and obstetrics and gynecology. Awareness could be promoted through the inclusion of topics relevant to caring for children who identify as TGD in the list of core competencies published by the American Board of Pediatrics, certifying examinations, and relevant study materials. Continuing education and maintenance of certification activities can include topics relevant to TGD populations as well.

---

* For more information regarding state-specific laws, please contact the AAP Division of State Government Affairs at stgov@ aap.org.

RECOMMENDATIONS

The AAP works toward all children and adolescents, regardless of gender identity or expression, receiving care to promote optimal physical, mental, and social well-being. Any discrimination based on gender identity or expression, real or perceived, is damaging to the socioemotional health of children, families, and society. In particular, the AAP recommends the following:

1. that youth who identify as TGD have access to comprehensive, gender-affirming, and developmentally appropriate health care that is provided in a safe and inclusive clinical space;

2. that family-based therapy and support be available to recognize and respond to the emotional and mental health needs of parents, caregivers, and siblings of youth who identify as TGD;

3. that electronic health records, billing systems, patient-centered notification systems, and clinical research be designed to respect the asserted gender identity of each patient while maintaining confidentiality and avoiding duplicate charts;

4. that insurance plans offer coverage for health care that is specific to the needs of youth who identify as TGD, including coverage for medical, psychological, and, when indicated, surgical gender-affirming interventions;

5. that provider education, including medical school, residency, and continuing education, integrate core competencies on the emotional and physical health needs and best practices for the care of youth who identify as TGD and their families;

6. that pediatricians have a role in advocating for, educating, and developing liaison relationships with school districts and other community organizations to promote acceptance and inclusion of all children without fear of harassment, exclusion, or bullying because of gender expression;

7. that pediatricians have a role in advocating for policies and laws that protect youth who identify as TGD from discrimination and violence;

8. that the health care workforce protects diversity by offering equal employment opportunities and workplace protections, regardless of gender identity or expression; and

9. that the medical field and federal government prioritize research that is dedicated to improving the quality of evidence-based care for youth who identify as TGD.

LEAD AUTHOR

Jason Richard Rafferty, MD, MPH, EdM, FAAP

CONTRIBUTOR

Robert Garofalo, MD, FAAP

COMMITTEE ON PSYCHOSOCIAL ASPECTS OF CHILD AND FAMILY HEALTH, 2017–2018

Michael Yogman, MD, FAAP, Chairperson
Rebecca Baum, MD, FAAP
Thresia B. Gambon, MD, FAAP
Arthur Lavin, MD, FAAP
Gerri Mattson, MD, FAAP
Lawrence Sagin Wissow, MD, MPH, FAAP

LIAISONS

Sharon Berry, PhD, LP – *Society of Pediatric Psychology*
Ed Christophersen, PhD, FAAP – *Society of Pediatric Psychology*
Norah Johnson, PhD, RN, CPNP-BC – *National Association of Pediatric Nurse Practitioners*
Amy Starin, PhD, LCSW – *National Association of Social Workers*
Abigail Schlesinger, MD – *American Academy of Child and Adolescent Psychiatry*

STAFF

Karen S. Smith
James Baumberger

COMMITTEE ON ADOLESCENCE, 2017–2018

Cora Breuner, MD, MPH, FAAP, Chairperson
Elizabeth M. Alderman, MD, FSAHM, FAAP
Laura K. Grubb, MD, MPH, FAAP
Makia E. Powers, MD, MPH, FAAP
Krishna Upadhya, MD, FAAP
Stephenie B. Wallace, MD, FAAP

LIAISONS

Laurie Hornberger, MD, MPH, FAAP – *Section on Adolescent Health*
Liwei L. Hua, MD, PhD – *American Academy of Child and Adolescent Psychiatry*
Margo A. Lane, MD, FRCPC, FAAP – *Canadian Paediatric Society*
Meredith Loveless, MD, FACOG – *American College of Obstetricians and Gynecologists*
Seema Menon, MD – *North American Society of Pediatric and Adolescent Gynecology*
CDR Lauren B. Zapata, PhD, MSPH – *Centers for Disease Control and Prevention*

STAFF

Karen Smith

SECTION ON LESBIAN, GAY, BISEXUAL, AND TRANSGENDER HEALTH AND WELLNESS EXECUTIVE COMMITTEE, 2016–2017

Lynn Hunt, MD, FAAP, Chairperson
Anne Teresa Gearhart, MD, FAAP
Christopher Harris, MD, FAAP
Kathryn Melland Lowe, MD, FAAP
Chadwick Taylor Rodgers, MD, FAAP
Ilana Michelle Sherer, MD, FAAP

FORMER EXECUTIVE COMMITTEE MEMBERS

Ellen Perrin, MD, MA, FAAP

LIAISON

Joseph H. Waters, MD – *AAP Section on Pediatric Trainees*

STAFF

Renee Jarrett, MPH

ACKNOWLEDGMENTS

We thank Isaac Albanese, MPA, and Jayeson Watts, LICSW, for their thoughtful reviews and contributions.

ABBREVIATIONS

AAP: American Academy of Pediatrics
GACM: gender-affirmative care model
GLSEN: Gay, Lesbian, and Straight Education Network
LGBTQ: lesbian, gay, bisexual, transgender, or questioning
TGD: transgender and gender diverse

DOI: https://doi.org/10.1542/peds.2018-2162

Address correspondence to Jason Rafferty, MD, MPH, EdM, FAAP. E-mail: Jason_Rafferty@mail.harvard.edu

PEDIATRICS (ISSN Numbers: Print, 0031-4005; Online, 1098-4275).

Copyright © 2018 by the American Academy of Pediatrics

FINANCIAL DISCLOSURE: The author has indicated he has no financial relationships relevant to this article to disclose.

FUNDING: No external funding.

POTENTIAL CONFLICT OF INTEREST: The author has indicated he has no potential conflicts of interest to disclose.

REFERENCES

1. Levine DA; Committee on Adolescence. Office-based care for lesbian, gay, bisexual, transgender, and questioning youth. *Pediatrics*. 2013;132(1). Available at: www.pediatrics.org/cgi/content/full/132/1/e297

2. American Academy of Pediatrics Committee on Adolescence. Homosexuality and adolescence. *Pediatrics*. 1983;72(2):249–250

3. Institute of Medicine; Committee on Lesbian Gay Bisexual, and Transgender Health Issues and Research Gaps and Opportunities. *The Health of Lesbian, Gay, Bisexual, and Transgender People: Building a Foundation for Better Understanding*. Washington, DC: National Academies Press; 2011. Available at: https://www.ncbi.nlm.nih.gov/books/NBK64806. Accessed May 19, 2017

4. Deutsch MB, Radix A, Reisner S. What's in a guideline? Developing collaborative and sound research designs that substantiate best practice recommendations for transgender health care. *AMA J Ethics*. 2016;18(11):1098–1106

5. Bonifacio HJ, Rosenthal SM. Gender variance and dysphoria in children and adolescents. *Pediatr Clin North Am*. 2015;62(4):1001–1016

6. Vance SR Jr, Ehrensaft D, Rosenthal SM. Psychological and medical care of gender nonconforming youth. *Pediatrics*. 2014;134(6):1184–1192

7. Richards C, Bouman WP, Seal L, Barker MJ, Nieder TO, T'Sjoen G. Non-binary or genderqueer genders. *Int Rev Psychiatry*. 2016;28(1):95–102

8. American Psychological Association. Guidelines for psychological practice with transgender and gender nonconforming people. *Am Psychol*. 2015;70(9):832–864

9. Flores AR, Herman JL, Gates GJ, Brown TNT. *How Many Adults Identify as Transgender in the United States*. Los Angeles, CA: The Williams Institute; 2016

10. Herman JL, Flores AR, Brown TNT, Wilson BDM, Conron KJ. *Age of Individuals Who Identify as Transgender in the United States*. Los Angeles, CA: The Williams Institute; 2017

11. Gates GJ. *How Many People are Lesbian, Gay, Bisexual, and Transgender?* Los Angeles, CA: The Williams Institute; 2011

12. Olson J, Schrager SM, Belzer M, Simons LK, Clark LF. Baseline physiologic and psychosocial characteristics of transgender youth seeking care for gender dysphoria. *J Adolesc Health*. 2015;57(4):374–380

13. Almeida J, Johnson RM, Corliss HL, Molnar BE, Azrael D. Emotional distress

among LGBT youth: the influence of perceived discrimination based on sexual orientation. *J Youth Adolesc.* 2009;38(7):1001–1014

14. Clements-Nolle K, Marx R, Katz M. Attempted suicide among transgender persons: the influence of gender-based discrimination and victimization. *J Homosex.* 2006;51(3):53–69

15. Colizzi M, Costa R, Todarello O. Transsexual patients' psychiatric comorbidity and positive effect of cross-sex hormonal treatment on mental health: results from a longitudinal study. *Psychoneuroendocrinology.* 2014;39:65–73

16. Haas AP, Eliason M, Mays VM, et al. Suicide and suicide risk in lesbian, gay, bisexual, and transgender populations: review and recommendations. *J Homosex.* 2011;58(1):10–51

17. Maguen S, Shipherd JC. Suicide risk among transgender individuals. *Psychol Sex.* 2010;1(1):34–43

18. Connolly MD, Zervos MJ, Barone CJ II, Johnson CC, Joseph CL. The mental health of transgender youth: advances in understanding. *J Adolesc Health.* 2016;59(5):489–495

19. Grossman AH, D'Augelli AR. Transgender youth and life-threatening behaviors. *Suicide Life Threat Behav.* 2007;37(5):527–537

20. Spack NP, Edwards-Leeper L, Feldman HA, et al. Children and adolescents with gender identity disorder referred to a pediatric medical center. *Pediatrics.* 2012;129(3):418–425

21. van Schalkwyk GI, Klingensmith K, Volkmar FR. Gender identity and autism spectrum disorders. *Yale J Biol Med.* 2015;88(1):81–83

22. Jacobs LA, Rachlin K, Erickson-Schroth L, Janssen A. Gender dysphoria and co-occurring autism spectrum disorders: review, case examples, and treatment considerations. *LGBT Health.* 2014;1(4):277–282

23. American Psychiatric Association. *Diagnostic and Statistical Manual of Mental Disorders.* 5th ed. Arlington, VA: American Psychiatric Association; 2013

24. Edwards-Leeper L, Spack NP. Psychological evaluation and medical treatment of transgender youth in an interdisciplinary "Gender Management Service" (GeMS) in a major pediatric center. *J Homosex.* 2012;59(3):321–336

25. Anton BS. Proceedings of the American Psychological Association for the legislative year 2008: minutes of the annual meeting of the Council of Representatives, February 22–24, 2008, Washington, DC, and August 13 and 17, 2008, Boston, MA, and minutes of the February, June, August, and December 2008 meetings of the Board of Directors. *Am Psychol.* 2009;64(5):372–453

26. Drescher J, Haller E; American Psychiatric Association Caucus of Lesbian, Gay and Bisexual Psychiatrists. *Position Statement on Discrimination Against Transgender and Gender Variant Individuals.* Washington, DC: American Psychiatric Association; 2012

27. Hidalgo MA, Ehrensaft D, Tishelman AC, et al. The gender affirmative model: what we know and what we aim to learn. *Hum Dev.* 2013;56(5):285–290

28. Tishelman AC, Kaufman R, Edwards-Leeper L, Mandel FH, Shumer DE, Spack NP. Serving transgender youth: challenges, dilemmas and clinical examples. *Prof Psychol Res Pr.* 2015;46(1):37–45

29. Adelson SL; American Academy of Child and Adolescent Psychiatry (AACAP) Committee on Quality Issues (CQI). Practice parameter on gay, lesbian, or bisexual sexual orientation, gender nonconformity, and gender discordance in children and adolescents. *J Am Acad Child Adolesc Psychiatry.* 2012;51(9):957–974

30. Herbst JH, Jacobs ED, Finlayson TJ, McKleroy VS, Neumann MS, Crepaz N; HIV/AIDS Prevention Research Synthesis Team. Estimating HIV prevalence and risk behaviors of transgender persons in the United States: a systematic review. *AIDS Behav.* 2008;12(1):1–17

31. James SE, Herman JL, Rankin S, Keisling M, Mottet L, Anafi M. *The Report of the 2015 U.S. Transgender Survey.* Washington, DC: National Center for Transgender Equality; 2016

32. Centers for Disease Control and Prevention. *CDC-Funded HIV Testing:* *United States, Puerto Rico, and the U.S. Virgin Islands.* Atlanta, GA: Centers for Disease Control and Prevention; 2015. Available at: https://www.cdc.gov/hiv/pdf/library/reports/cdc-hiv-funded-testing-us-puerto-rico-2015.pdf. Accessed August 2, 2018

33. Substance Abuse and Mental Health Services Administration. *Ending Conversion Therapy: Supporting and Affirming LGBTQ Youth.* Rockville, MD: Substance Abuse and Mental Health Services Administration; 2015

34. Korell SC, Lorah P. An overview of affirmative psychotherapy and counseling with transgender clients. In: Bieschke KJ, Perez RM, DeBord KA, eds. *Handbook of Counseling and Psychotherapy With Lesbian, Gay, Bisexual, and Transgender Clients.* 2nd ed. Washington, DC: American Psychological Association; 2007:271–288

35. World Professional Association for Transgender Health. *Standards of Care for the Health of Transsexual, Transgender, and Gender Nonconforming People.* 7th ed. Minneapolis, MN: World Professional Association for Transgender Health; 2011. Available at: https://www.wpath.org/publications/soc. Accessed April 15, 2018

36. Menvielle E. A comprehensive program for children with gender variant behaviors and gender identity disorders. *J Homosex.* 2012;59(3):357–368

37. Hill DB, Menvielle E, Sica KM, Johnson A. An affirmative intervention for families with gender variant children: parental ratings of child mental health and gender. *J Sex Marital Ther.* 2010;36(1):6–23

38. Haldeman DC. The practice and ethics of sexual orientation conversion therapy. *J Consult Clin Psychol.* 1994;62(2):221–227

39. Byne W. Regulations restrict practice of conversion therapy. *LGBT Health.* 2016;3(2):97–99

40. Cohen-Kettenis PT, Delemarre-van de Waal HA, Gooren LJ. The treatment of adolescent transsexuals: changing insights. *J Sex Med.* 2008;5(8):1892–1897

41. Bryant K. Making gender identity disorder of childhood: historical lessons for contemporary debates. *Sex Res Soc Policy.* 2006;3(3):23–39

42. World Professional Association for Transgender Health. *WPATH De-Psychopathologisation Statement.* Minneapolis, MN: World Professional Association for Transgender Health; 2010. Available at: https://www.wpath.org/policies. Accessed April 16, 2017

43. American Academy of Pediatrics. AAP support letter conversion therapy ban [letter]. 2015. Available at: https://www.aap.org/en-us/advocacy-and-policy/federal-advocacy/Documents/AAPsupportletterconversiontherapyban.pdf. Accessed August 1, 2018

44. Movement Advancement Project. *LGBT Policy Spotlight: Conversion Therapy Bans.* Boulder, CO: Movement Advancement Project; 2017. Available at: http://www.lgbtmap.org/policy-and-issue-analysis/policy-spotlight-conversion-therapy-bans. Accessed August 6, 2017

45. Ehrensaft D, Giammattei SV, Storck K, Tishelman AC, Keo-Meier C. Prepubertal social gender transitions: what we know; what we can learn—a view from a gender affirmative lens. *Int J Transgend.* 2018;19(2):251–268

46. Olson KR, Key AC, Eaton NR. Gender cognition in transgender children. *Psychol Sci.* 2015;26(4):467–474

47. Olson KR. Prepubescent transgender children: what we do and do not know. *J Am Acad Child Adolesc Psychiatry.* 2016;55(3):155–156.e3

48. Olson KR, Durwood L, DeMeules M, McLaughlin KA. Mental health of transgender children who are supported in their identities. *Pediatrics.* 2016;137(3):e20153223

49. Malpas J. Between pink and blue: a multi-dimensional family approach to gender nonconforming children and their families. *Fam Process.* 2011;50(4):453–470

50. Hagan JF Jr, Shaw JS, Duncan PM, eds. *Bright Futures: Guidelines for Health Supervision of Infants, Children, and Adolescents.* 4th ed. Elk Grove, IL: American Academy of Pediatrics; 2016

51. Minter SP. Supporting transgender children: new legal, social, and medical approaches. *J Homosex.* 2012;59(3):422–433

52. AHIMA Work Group. Improved patient engagement for LGBT populations: addressing factors related to sexual orientation/gender identity for effective health information management. *J AHIMA.* 2017;88(3):34–39

53. Deutsch MB, Green J, Keatley J, Mayer G, Hastings J, Hall AM; World Professional Association for Transgender Health EMR Working Group. Electronic medical records and the transgender patient: recommendations from the World Professional Association for Transgender Health EMR Working Group. *J Am Med Inform Assoc.* 2013;20(4):700–703

54. Dowshen N, Meadows R, Byrnes M, Hawkins L, Eder J, Noonan K. Policy perspective: ensuring comprehensive care and support for gender nonconforming children and adolescents. *Transgend Health.* 2016;1(1):75–85

55. Cahill SR, Baker K, Deutsch MB, Keatley J, Makadon HJ. Inclusion of sexual orientation and gender identity in stage 3 meaningful use guidelines: a huge step forward for LGBT health. *LGBT Health.* 2016;3(2):100–102

56. Mansfield MJ, Beardsworth DE, Loughlin JS, et al. Long-term treatment of central precocious puberty with a long-acting analogue of luteinizing hormone-releasing hormone. Effects on somatic growth and skeletal maturation. *N Engl J Med.* 1983;309(21):1286–1290

57. Olson J, Garofalo R. The peripubertal gender-dysphoric child: puberty suppression and treatment paradigms. *Pediatr Ann.* 2014;43(6):e132–e137

58. de Vries AL, Steensma TD, Doreleijers TA, Cohen-Kettenis PT. Puberty suppression in adolescents with gender identity disorder: a prospective follow-up study. *J Sex Med.* 2011;8(8):2276–2283

59. Wallien MS, Cohen-Kettenis PT. Psychosexual outcome of gender-dysphoric children. *J Am Acad Child Adolesc Psychiatry.* 2008;47(12):1413–1423

60. Waylen A, Wolke D. Sex 'n' drugs 'n' rock 'n' roll: the meaning and social consequences of pubertal timing. *Eur J Endocrinol.* 2004;151(suppl 3):U151–U159

61. de Vries AL, Klink D, Cohen-Kettenis PT. What the primary care pediatrician needs to know about gender incongruence and gender dysphoria in children and adolescents. *Pediatr Clin North Am.* 2016;63(6):1121–1135

62. Vlot MC, Klink DT, den Heijer M, Blankenstein MA, Rotteveel J, Heijboer AC. Effect of pubertal suppression and cross-sex hormone therapy on bone turnover markers and bone mineral apparent density (BMAD) in transgender adolescents. *Bone.* 2017;95:11–19

63. Finlayson C, Johnson EK, Chen D, et al. Proceedings of the working group session on fertility preservation for individuals with gender and sex diversity. *Transgend Health.* 2016;1(1):99–107

64. Kreukels BP, Cohen-Kettenis PT. Puberty suppression in gender identity disorder: the Amsterdam experience. *Nat Rev Endocrinol.* 2011;7(8):466–472

65. Rosenthal SM. Approach to the patient: transgender youth: endocrine considerations. *J Clin Endocrinol Metab.* 2014;99(12):4379–4389

66. Fenway Health. *Glossary of Gender and Transgender Terms.* Boston, MA: Fenway Health; 2010. Available at: http://fenwayhealth.org/documents/the-fenway-institute/handouts/Handout_7-C_Glossary_of_Gender_and_Transgender_Terms__fi.pdf. Accessed August 16, 2017

67. de Vries AL, McGuire JK, Steensma TD, Wagenaar EC, Doreleijers TA, Cohen-Kettenis PT. Young adult psychological outcome after puberty suppression and gender reassignment. *Pediatrics.* 2014;134(4):696–704

68. Hembree WC, Cohen-Kettenis PT, Gooren L, et al. Endocrine treatment of gender-dysphoric/gender-incongruent persons: an endocrine society clinical practice guideline. *J Clin Endocrinol Metab.* 2017;102(11):3869–3903

69. Milrod C, Karasic DH. Age is just a number: WPATH-affiliated surgeons' experiences and attitudes toward

vaginoplasty in transgender females under 18 years of age in the United States. *J Sex Med.* 2017;14(4):624–634

70. Milrod C. How young is too young: ethical concerns in genital surgery of the transgender MTF adolescent. *J Sex Med.* 2014;11(2):338–346

71. Olson-Kennedy J, Warus J, Okonta V, Belzer M, Clark LF. Chest reconstruction and chest dysphoria in transmasculine minors and young adults: comparisons of nonsurgical and postsurgical cohorts. *JAMA Pediatr.* 2018;172(5):431–436

72. Committee on Adolescent Health Care. Committee opinion no. 685: care for transgender adolescents. *Obstet Gynecol.* 2017;129(1):e11–e16

73. Greydanus DE, Patel DR, Rimsza ME. Contraception in the adolescent: an update. *Pediatrics.* 2001;107(3):562–573

74. Gridley SJ, Crouch JM, Evans Y, et al. Youth and caregiver perspectives on barriers to gender-affirming health care for transgender youth. *J Adolesc Health.* 2016;59(3):254–261

75. Sanchez NF, Sanchez JP, Danoff A. Health care utilization, barriers to care, and hormone usage among male-to-female transgender persons in New York City. *Am J Public Health.* 2009;99(4):713–719

76. Transgender Law Center. *Affordable Care Act Fact Sheet.* Oakland, CA: Transgender Law Center; 2016. Available at: https://transgenderlawcenter.org/resources/health/aca-fact-sheet. Accessed August 8, 2016

77. Nahata L, Quinn GP, Caltabellotta NM, Tishelman AC. Mental health concerns and insurance denials among transgender adolescents. *LGBT Health.* 2017;4(3):188–193

78. Grant JM, Mottet LA, Tanis J, Harrison J, Herman JL, Keisling M. *Injustice at Every Turn: A Report of the National Transgender Discrimination Survey.* Washington, DC: National Center for Transgender Equality and National Gay and Lesbian Task Force; 2011 Available at: http://www.thetaskforce.org/static_

html/downloads/reports/reports/ntds_full.pdf. Accessed August 6, 2018

79. Sevelius JM. Gender affirmation: a framework for conceptualizing risk behavior among transgender women of color. *Sex Roles.* 2013;68(11–12):675–689

80. Koken JA, Bimbi DS, Parsons JT. Experiences of familial acceptance-rejection among transwomen of color. *J Fam Psychol.* 2009;23(6):853–860

81. Lombardi EL, Wilchins RA, Priesing D, Malouf D. Gender violence: transgender experiences with violence and discrimination. *J Homosex.* 2001;42(1):89–101

82. Wren B. 'I can accept my child is transsexual but if I ever see him in a dress I'll hit him': dilemmas in parenting a transgendered adolescent. *Clin Child Psychol Psychiatry.* 2002;7(3):377–397

83. Riley EA, Sitharthan G, Clemson L, Diamond M. The needs of gender-variant children and their parents: a parent survey. *Int J Sex Health.* 2011;23(3):181–195

84. Whitley CT. Trans-kin undoing and redoing gender: negotiating relational identity among friends and family of transgender persons. *Sociol Perspect.* 2013;56(4):597–621

85. Travers R, Bauer G, Pyne J, Bradley K, Gale L, Papadimitriou M; Trans PULSE; Children's Aid Society of Toronto; Delisle Youth Services. *Impacts of Strong Parental Support for Trans Youth: A Report Prepared for Children's Aid Society of Toronto and Delisle Youth Services.* Toronto, ON: Trans PULSE; 2012. Available at: http://transpulseproject.ca/wp-content/uploads/2012/10/Impacts-of-Strong-Parental-Support-for-Trans-Youth-vFINAL.pdf

86. Ryan C, Russell ST, Huebner D, Diaz R, Sanchez J. Family acceptance in adolescence and the health of LGBT young adults. *J Child Adolesc Psychiatr Nurs.* 2010;23(4):205–213

87. Grossman AH, D'augelli AR, Frank JA. Aspects of psychological resilience among transgender youth. *J LGBT Youth.* 2011;8(2):103–115

88. McConnell EA, Birkett M, Mustanski B. Families matter: social support and mental health trajectories among lesbian, gay, bisexual, and transgender youth. *J Adolesc Health.* 2016;59(6):674–680

89. Ellis KM, Eriksen K. Transsexual and transgenderist experiences and treatment options. *Fam J Alex Va.* 2002;10(3):289–299

90. Lamda Legal. *Transgender Rights Toolkit: A Legal Guide for Trans People and Their Advocates.* New York, NY: Lambda Legal; 2016 Available at: https://www.lambdalegal.org/publications/trans-toolkit. Accessed August 6, 2018

91. Kosciw JG, Greytak EA, Giga NM, Villenas C, Danischewski DJ. *The 2015 National School Climate Survey: The Experiences of Lesbian, Gay, Bisexual, Transgender, and Queer Youth in Our Nation's Schools.* New York, NY: GLSEN; 2016. Available at: https://www.glsen.org/article/2015-national-school-climate-survey. Accessed August 8, 2018

92. McGuire JK, Anderson CR, Toomey RB, Russell ST. School climate for transgender youth: a mixed method investigation of student experiences and school responses. *J Youth Adolesc.* 2010;39(10):1175–1188

93. Association of American Medical Colleges Advisory Committee on Sexual Orientation, Gender Identity, and Sex Development. In: Hollenback AD, Eckstrand KL, Dreger A, eds. *Implementing Curricular and Institutional Climate Changes to Improve Health Care for Individuals Who Are LGBT, Gender Nonconforming, or Born With DSD: A Resource for Medical Educators.* Washington, DC: Association of American Medical Colleges; 2014. Available at: https://members.aamc.org/eweb/upload/Executive LGBT FINAL.pdf. Accessed August 8, 2018

94. Obedin-Maliver J, Goldsmith ES, Stewart L, et al. Lesbian, gay, bisexual, and transgender-related content in undergraduate medical education. *JAMA.* 2011;306(9):971–977

The Eye Examination in the Evaluation of Child Abuse

• *Clinical Report*

CLINICAL REPORT Guidance for the Clinician in Rendering Pediatric Care

American Academy
of Pediatrics

DEDICATED TO THE HEALTH OF ALL CHILDREN™

The Eye Examination in the Evaluation of Child Abuse

Cindy W. Christian, MD, FAAP,[a] Alex V. Levin, MD, MHSc, FAAO, FRCSC, FAAP,[b] COUNCIL ON CHILD ABUSE AND NEGLECT, SECTION ON OPHTHALMOLOGY, AMERICAN ASSOCIATION OF CERTIFIED ORTHOPTISTS, AMERICAN ASSOCIATION FOR PEDIATRIC OPHTHALMOLOGY AND STRABISMUS, AMERICAN ACADEMY OF OPHTHALMOLOGY

abstract

Child abuse can cause injury to any part of the eye. The most common manifestations are retinal hemorrhages (RHs) in infants and young children with abusive head trauma (AHT). Although RHs are an important indicator of possible AHT, they are also found in other conditions. Distinguishing the number, type, location, and pattern of RHs is important in evaluating a differential diagnosis. Eye trauma can be seen in cases of physical abuse or AHT and may prompt referral for ophthalmologic assessment. Physicians have a responsibility to consider abuse in the differential diagnosis of pediatric eye trauma. Identification and documentation of inflicted ocular trauma requires a thorough examination by an ophthalmologist, including indirect ophthalmoscopy, most optimally through a dilated pupil, especially for the evaluation of possible RHs. An eye examination is helpful in detecting abnormalities that can help identify a medical or traumatic etiology for previously well young children who experience unexpected and unexplained mental status changes with no obvious cause, children with head trauma that results in significant intracranial hemorrhage and brain injury, and children with unexplained death.

[a]Department of Pediatrics, Perelman School of Medicine, University of Pennsylvania and Children's Hospital of Philadelphia, Philadelphia, Pennsylvania; and [b]Departments of Pediatric Ophthalmology and Ocular Genetics, Wills Eye Hospital and Ophthalmology and Pediatrics, Sidney Kimmel Medical College, Thomas Jefferson University, Philadelphia, Pennsylvania

Drs Christian and Levin were involved in all aspects of the drafting, editing, and finalizing of this manuscript and approved the final manuscript as submitted.

DOI: https://doi.org/10.1542/peds.2018-1411

To cite: Christian CW, Levin AV, AAP COUNCIL ON CHILD ABUSE AND NEGLECT, AAP SECTION ON OPHTHALMOLOGY, AMERICAN ASSOCIATION OF CERTIFIED ORTHOPTISTS, AMERICAN ASSOCIATION FOR PEDIATRIC OPHTHALMOLOGY AND STRABISMUS, AMERICAN ACADEMY OF OPHTHALMOLOGY. The Eye Examination in the Evaluation of Child Abuse. *Pediatrics.* 2018; 142(2):e20181411

INTRODUCTION

Direct or indirect trauma to the eye may be caused by child physical abuse. The most common manifestations are retinal hemorrhages (RHs), seen in approximately 75% of children who are victims of abusive head trauma (AHT), and are thought by many authors to be associated with the child experiencing repeated acceleration or deceleration forces with or without blunt force head impact.[1] Ophthalmologists are often asked to examine children when there is a concern of AHT. Such concern arises when there are signs of head and body injury, such as intracranial hemorrhage, but ocular injury is also a consideration when children present with unexplained alterations of consciousness or unexplained seizures. Ophthalmologists also have an independent duty to conduct a full eye examination when they have a concern about possible abuse as a cause of ocular injury. Ophthalmologists have an obligation to report their suspicions to the appropriate child protective service agency and, when available, consult with child abuse pediatricians or other professionals in the field of child abuse for guidance and additional assistance.

INDICATIONS FOR OPHTHALMOLOGY CONSULTATION

Eye abnormalities can be caused by direct blunt trauma or can be associated with more global brain injury. Children with inflicted injury to the eye come to the attention of the ophthalmologist in a number of ways. Most often, an ophthalmologist is consulted by colleagues because of a concern of AHT in a child with neurologic or other concerning injury. On occasion, an infant or child may present directly to an ophthalmologist with symptoms of neurologic or eye pathology that has resulted from an undisclosed inflicted injury. Examples include infants or children with an acquired strabismus from elevated intracranial pressure resulting from trauma or a child with a hyphema from an inflicted eye injury. Uncommonly, RHs may be discovered unexpectedly during a routine ophthalmologic examination. In children with AHT, the absence of visual compromise or the lack of external indicators of eye injury does not rule out the possibility of significant RHs. Therefore, one cannot rely on ocular signs or symptoms to determine which children might benefit from ophthalmologic consultation. Rather, ophthalmologic consultation is based on objective indicators of possible eye pathology, including findings that raise concern of possible AHT (eg, increased intracranial pressure, intracranial hemorrhage, or unexplained coma). An ophthalmologic examination is

not an appropriate screening test for AHT in neurologically well-appearing infants who have an extracranial injury suggestive of abuse because RHs are uncommonly identified in this setting.[2]

The ophthalmologist is in a unique position to give a detailed clinical description of the patient's hemorrhagic retinopathy. The indirect ophthalmoscope provides a wide and stereoscopic field of view and enables the ophthalmologist to examine the anterior retinal edges (ora serrata), which is not possible using the direct ophthalmoscope even if the pupils are dilated. Eye examination for this purpose is best performed by an ophthalmologist. When indicated, a slit lamp inspection of the anterior segment to identify signs of trauma (eg, hyphema) can be helpful. Examination for an afferent pupillary defect (Marcus Gunn pupil) before pharmacologic pupillary dilation can be performed to identify optic nerve injury. Ophthalmologic consultation in the setting of suspected abuse is recommended for any child with visible injury to the eye, unexplained alterations of consciousness, intracranial hemorrhage, coagulopathy, or possible medical disease that might mimic abuse.

THE EYE EXAMINATION

Although health care professionals other than ophthalmologists may be skilled at detecting the absence or presence of RHs,[3] a full view of the retina and characterization of the number, type, location, and pattern of the hemorrhages require consultation by an ophthalmologist by using indirect ophthalmoscopy, preferably with a dilated pupil. When there is a concern about transiently stopping pupillary reactivity, which affects the ability to monitor neurologic status, techniques such as dilation of 1 eye at a time, use of short-acting

mydriatics, and use of a lens that affords some view through an undilated pupil can be used to allow indirect ophthalmoscopy, preferably within the first 24 hours and ideally within 72 hours after the child's acute presentation because some RHs resolve quickly. Even if the need for an eye examination is realized after 72 hours, ophthalmologic consultation may still be useful to identify persistent abnormalities, such as hemorrhages, retinoschisis, chorioretinal scars, and papilledema. Ophthalmologists can recognize characteristic findings of diseases of the eye and retina that are in the differential diagnosis of RHs, such as patterns suggestive of vasculitis, the peripapillary hemorrhages of papilledema, retinal infection, or leukemic infiltrates. Although not required, photodocumentation may enhance but not replace detailed written descriptions and drawings of eye findings when available. Regardless, a detailed documentation of the eye examination is essential.[4] Although several documentation and grading tools have been suggested, there is not yet a standard accepted tool.[5] Diagnostic impressions should objectively address the level of concern for abuse, relevant differential diagnosis, additional recommendations, and suggestions for further medical or ophthalmologic evaluation and possible reporting. As appropriate, acceptable terminology to describe the hemorrhages might include "nonspecific" (with differential diagnosis), "suggestive," or "highly suggestive" of AHT. It may even be appropriate in some situations to indicate that there is no other reported cause of the retinal picture in the specific circumstance of historical and medical findings.

In recent years, researchers using techniques such as optical coherence tomography have documented the vitreoretinal interface and schisis cavities in victims with AHT.[6] Intravenous fluorescein angiography may detect characteristic areas of peripheral retinal nonperfusion, especially in the months after the incident.[7,8] These ancillary tests also have the potential to improve the understanding of pathophysiologic mechanisms of RHs and enable the ophthalmologist to identify retinal details not previously documented by clinical examination.

ORBITAL AND OCULAR INJURIES RESULTING FROM ABUSE

Injuries to the globe and surrounding structures are well described in child abuse and usually result from blunt trauma. Periorbital ecchymosis may result from abusive or accidental trauma to the forehead or periorbital tissues. Bilateral periorbital ecchymosis may be secondary to forehead trauma, basilar skull fractures, or subgaleal hematoma and can be seen in neuroblastoma and leukemia.[9] Frontal bone and orbital roof fractures are uncommon injuries in infants and young children and are even less common in those abused.[10,11] In children, these fractures are the result of significant blunt force injury and are best identified with computed tomography (CT), including a three-dimensional CT.[12]

Subconjunctival hemorrhages are well described in infants who are abused, who often but may not always have additional manifestations of abuse at the time of diagnosis.[13] Causes of subconjunctival hemorrhage in young children include direct eye trauma, indirect forces to the vessels from sudden increases in intrathoracic pressure, birth, or medical disease, including hemorrhagic conjunctivitis, pertussis, or hematologic disorders (thrombocytopenia in particular).

Traumatic hyphema can result from either blunt or penetrating trauma to the eye. In an older child, hyphema is commonly the result of an accidental high-energy blow to the globe rather than abuse.[14] Traumatic cataract

may present in association with a hyphema at the time of injury or even weeks or months thereafter. Direct injury to the eye can also cause corneal abrasions or lacerations, globe rupture, or damage to the iris. Globe rupture may occur from blunt impact or contact with a sharp object. Any significant injury to the eye or orbit is best referred to an ophthalmologist for complete eye examination and management.

RHs AND AHT

RHs have been recognized as a key indicator of abusive head injury for more than 30 years.[15] Although mild and moderate RHs can be seen in a number of medical and traumatic conditions in children,[16] prospective and retrospective clinical studies have revealed that severe RH is strongly associated with AHT.[17,18] Approximately 25% of victims of AHT have no RH, and one-third of all cases have mild to moderate RH.[18] In 2 recent systematic reviews comprising over 30 clinical studies and thousands of children, the strong association of severe RH with AHT was confirmed.[1,19] In general, the number and severity of RHs correlate with the severity of neurologic injury.[20,21] For example, RHs are found infrequently in neurologically normal patients and are most frequently identified at autopsy in cases of fatal AHT. RHs in AHT can vary in number, size, and location within the retina. They can be bilateral or unilateral, confined to the peripapillary area or posterior pole, or can extend to the ora serrata. RHs can be subretinal, intraretinal, or preretinal and may extend into the vitreous.[1] Retinal folds, retinoschisis (splitting of the retinal layers), and retinal detachment (less common) are caused by trauma, although rare exceptions are reported.[22] RHs that are too numerous to count, are multilayered, bilateral, and extend to the ora serrata are highly specific

for AHT.[1,23] Traumatic macular retinoschisis and folds are usually specific for AHT, although they have been reported after fatal accidental trauma, including head crush injuries, motor vehicle accidents, and falls.[1,24–27] Lesions similar to retinal folds and retinoschisis have been seen in leukemia, sickle cell anemia, and infantile aneurysm. In such cases, there may be isolated elevation of the internal limiting membrane of the retina with sub–internal limiting membrane blood, usually without surrounding retinal folds. These entities are readily excluded from the differential diagnosis by history, epidemiologic factors, or diagnostic testing. There are many causes of retinal detachment, which is uncommon in AHT; history and examination along with diagnostic testing assist in the differential diagnosis. On occasion, traumatic RH can occur in the absence of intracranial injury identified by imaging.[28,29]

Postnatal traumatic RHs cannot be accurately dated. One recent study reveals that intra-RHs resolve more quickly than pre-RHs, and hemorrhages that are too numerous to count only last for a few days after injury.[30] For example, these data reveal that the presence of pre-RHs without intra-RHs indicates an injury of at least a few days to 1 week in age. Although 1 article revealed that RH may worsen after admission,[31] this was not observed in another study.[32] The degree of RH worsening after admission would not turn a mild retinopathy into severe RH, retinoschisis, or retinal folds.

RHs IN OTHER DISEASES

Although extensive, multilayered RHs that extend to the ora serrata, macular retinoschisis, and retinal folds are each highly suggestive of AHT, the diagnosis of AHT is not made on the basis of eye examination alone. History, physical examination, and diagnostic testing are always critical in establishing and working through a reasonable differential diagnosis. RHs have other etiologies, especially in critically ill children, including meningitis, leukemia, coagulopathy, and retinal disorders, all of which are identified by history, general and ocular examination, and appropriate medical evaluation. RHs in these diagnoses are almost always few in number and are confined to the posterior retina, although exceptions exist.[16,33] Hyperacute elevations of intracranial pressure, as seen in crush injuries or ruptured aneurysms, can also occasionally result in severe RHs.[34] Occipital impact or epidural hemorrhage may lead to RH and is usually intraretinal and confined to the posterior pole.[35,36]

The birth process often results in RHs, in part influenced by the delivery method. RHs that result from birth are most common after vacuum-assisted vaginal delivery (>70%) and are least common after routine cesarean delivery (<20%).[37,38] Severe RHs, macular retinoschisis, and retinal folds have not been reported in association with birth. Timing of birth RHs to resolution is well established, with flame hemorrhages resolving by 2 weeks (usually by 72 hours) and dot or blot hemorrhages by 6 weeks (but usually by 2 weeks).[39–41] Pre-RHs, foveal RHs, and the rarely present sub-RHs that result from birth may take many weeks or several months to resorb.[37]

Findings of systemic illness can be identified in an ocular fundus examination and may shed light on the etiology of a child's symptoms, such as necrotic retinitis from infection, retinal vascular abnormalities in Menkes disease, papilledema, or retinal manifestations of leukemia or bacterial endocarditis. There are no retinal ocular findings in sudden infant death syndrome, although routine ocular examination has

not been common practice in these cases.[4,42] Perhaps such eye examinations would be useful, but further study is needed. Studies have revealed that seizures, cough, apnea, and childhood vaccinations do not cause RH.[43–45] Elevated intracranial pressure, except when hyperacute (eg, ruptured aneurysm, severe sudden head injury), does not result in extensive RH beyond the peripapillary area nor macular retinoschisis or folds.[34,46]

Excluding RHs that are associated with birth, AHT is the leading cause of RHs in infants. Victims of AHT present to medical care with a wide range of symptoms, from mild irritability and vomiting to unexplained coma or seizures. Some present with a false history of trauma (most often a short fall), and others present with only the symptoms that resulted from their abuse. Unsuspecting physicians misdiagnose up to one-third of victims with AHT presenting symptoms depending on the child's age, severity of symptoms, and family composition.[47] A retinal examination is not a substitute for brain imaging when assessing infants who have been physically abused who have no neurologic symptoms of AHT.[2]

MECHANISMS AND PATHOPHYSIOLOGY OF RHs

The pathogenesis of RHs is multifactorial. In recent years, important trends have emerged in the understanding of RHs attributable to AHT in young children. Evidence has continued to increase in support of the diagnostic specificity of severe RH as an indicator of AHT in children with and without evidence of blunt impact injury to the head.[1,17,48] Extensive literature, including clinical studies and computer modeling, support this observation.[49] This research, along with clinical experience, support the role of vitreoretinal traction

sustained during the repetitive acceleration or deceleration mechanism that characterizes shaking as an important contributory factor in causing RH and macular retinoschisis.[4,6,49,50] Although the abusive traumatic event is the primary etiology of the RH, factors such as hypoxia, anemia, reperfusion, autonomic vascular dysregulation, significant shifts in sodium balance, coagulopathy, and intracranial pressure elevation may modulate the appearance of RHs.[51] Further research is needed to better define the role of these and other factors as the understanding of the pathophysiology and diagnostic specificity of RH continues to evolve.

OUTCOMES

Visual morbidity from physical child abuse is significant, affecting more than 40% of children with severe AHT.[52] In AHT, visual outcome is not usually related to direct ocular trauma but is instead related to occipital cortical damage and/or optic nerve injury.[53] RHs generally resolve without sequelae and, depending on the type of hemorrhage, can resolve quickly.[30] Retinal causes of visual loss from AHT include retinal detachment, macular scarring or fibrosis, and vitreous hemorrhage, which can lead to amblyopia if the hemorrhage does not resorb without surgery. Infants and children with ocular injury from any cause require careful ophthalmologic follow-up to maximize their visual outcome.

THE POSTMORTEM EYE EXAMINATION

An autopsy is a unique opportunity for examination not only of the eye and its contents but also of the orbital tissues, which may yield findings helpful in determining the cause of the child's death. Although ophthalmology consultation can be obtained after death and before an autopsy and the use of monocular indirect ophthalmoscopy has been reported by nonophthalmologists,[54] proper autopsy techniques provide a more accurate assessment of ocular and retinal findings. Even when premortem ophthalmoscopy is performed, postmortem examination is necessary to view the orbital tissues. When possible, an examination by a trained ocular pathologist is ideal. Postmortem eye and orbital tissue examination is another means of documenting RH and retinoschisis but may also reveal hemosiderin deposition from previous events, such as hemorrhages into fat, muscles, or cranial nerve sheaths as well as intradural optic nerve sheath hemorrhages, all of which have diagnostic significance in identifying abused children.[55]

One obstacle to postmortem examination of the eyes and orbits has been a societal distaste or resistance, which in some cases has led to fear among pathologists of legal repercussion.[56] This may reflect a cultural or emotional objection specifically to eye removal. There might be a misconception that eye or orbital removal will alter the appearance of the body postmortem at a funeral viewing when in fact this is not the case. Techniques are now detailed to allow for proper removal of the eye and orbits without disfigurement. En bloc removal of the globe with all orbital tissues is recommended.[56] Although consent is not routinely obtained for coroner cases or forensic autopsies, there may be situations or jurisdictions in which specific consent for eye and orbital tissue removal is required. If a parent or guardian refuses this procedure, it may be necessary to seek legal intervention, such as a court order or intervention by child protective services, to allow the procedure to be performed.

CHALLENGES AND FUTURE DIRECTIONS

Although a retinal examination may assist in identifying the cause of unexplained mental status changes, seizures, intracranial hemorrhage, or unexplained early childhood deaths, premortem clinical ophthalmologic consultation and postmortem removal of the eyes and orbital tissues are not routine practices in some centers. Failure to conduct these procedures, particularly when there is no other explanation for a life-threatening event or death, risks losing an important opportunity to gain valuable information. Information gained in such an evaluation might lead to identifying an etiology and in the case of a surviving child, prevent death by identifying potential risks of abuse or recognizing other diseases.

There continue to be reports of novel, unsubstantiated causes of RH and other ocular findings in young children, such as vitamin D deficiency or vaccination.[57] Although there is no credible evidence that vitamin D deficiency or routine childhood vaccinations cause RH,[44] practitioners should be open to reports that broaden and at the same time narrow the RH differential diagnosis. For example, mild posterior pole RHs now have been described in osteogenesis imperfecta.[58] Cardiopulmonary resuscitation is not a cause of widespread RH.[59,60] Only with more widespread use of ophthalmologic consultation and postmortem ocular and orbital examination can such possibilities be discovered or refuted and then appropriately fit into the differential diagnostic process.

Photodocumentation and other emerging technologies, when available, have also proven to be potentially important ophthalmic procedures in documenting retinal abnormalities for both clinical and educational purposes.[61] Further research regarding these new technologies will lead to advances in the understanding of RHs and improve clinical evaluation.

GUIDANCE FOR PHYSICIANS

Ophthalmologic consultation is an important part of the diagnostic evaluation of all previously well children younger than 5 years old who experience unexplained coma, seizures, intracranial hemorrhage or injury, or have a systemic disorder known to have ocular manifestations. A complete eye examination is also important in the evaluation of unexplained death in infants and children. As mandated reporters, all physicians have a legal and ethical duty to report suspected abuse to local or state child protective service agencies. Reports can be made by calling their state's toll-free child abuse reporting hotline. Whenever possible, the accompanying parent(s) or guardian(s) should be notified about the concern and the need to report. It can be helpful to raise concern about the finding and, while not apportioning blame, inform the family that because of the nature and circumstance of the examination findings, a report for further investigation is mandated by law and serves to prevent the child from being injured again should that prove to be the cause of the observed findings. Additional guidance about reporting is available from the American Academy of Pediatrics.[62]

Specific guidance for the eye examination in the evaluation of child abuse is as follows:

- Retinal examination by an ophthalmologist is particularly important when there is a suspicion of AHT, although RHs may occasionally be found in infants and children with other causes of intracranial hemorrhage. Multiple (too numerous to count), bilateral, and multilayered hemorrhages that extend to the periphery of the retina are highly specific for AHT, and when identified, a complete evaluation for additional injuries is warranted.

- Full indirect ophthalmoscopic examination through a dilated pupil is the optimal method of examining the retina in these circumstances. Examiners should include a detailed description of findings, such as the number, type, location, and pattern of RHs when present. Retinal abnormalities may be photographed after the clinical examination when a camera is available. When indicated, a slit lamp inspection of the anterior segment to identify signs of trauma (eg, hyphema) can be helpful. Examinations for an afferent pupillary defect (Marcus Gunn pupil) before pharmacologic pupillary dilation should be performed to identify possible optic nerve injury.

- Because findings such as RH may be transient, it is desirable that the ophthalmologic consultation take place within 24 hours of the patient's presentation for medical care but certainly within 72 hours.

- In potential victims of abuse who are neurologically asymptomatic, a retinal examination is not an appropriate screening test for brain injury; rather, such children should undergo brain imaging (such as an MRI or CT) as the appropriate screen if indicated. If the neuroimaging result is normal, yet concern still exists about possible AHT, then eye examination may still be considered.

- Pediatricians who suspect a diagnosis of AHT should make a prompt referral to an ophthalmologist, who should be available for prompt evaluation of the patient because important safety and medical issues are dependent on determining an appropriate diagnosis.

- When pharmacologic pupillary dilation is believed to be undesirable, as in children with severe central nervous system injury, timely ophthalmologic consultation is still helpful. An attempt to view the retina and optic nerve through the use of direct ophthalmoscopy, small pupil indirect ophthalmoscopic techniques, sequential pharmacologic dilation, and/ or fast-acting mydriatics (eg, phenylephrine 2.5%) can still yield important information.

- When a previously well child younger than 5 years old dies without explanation, regardless of whether a premortem retinal examination was conducted, examination of the eyes and orbital tissues as part of the autopsy may shed light on the cause of death. When possible, an ocular pathologist should perform the examination.

- Postmortem eye removal is not necessary in children who have clearly died of witnessed severe accidental head trauma or otherwise readily diagnosed systemic medical conditions.

LEAD AUTHORS

Cindy W. Christian, MD, FAAP
Alex V. Levin, MD, MHSc, FAAO, FRCSC, FAAP

COUNCIL ON CHILD ABUSE AND NEGLECT, 2017–2018

Emalee G. Flaherty, MD, FAAP, Co-Chairperson
Andrew P. Sirotnak, MD, FAAP, Co-Chairperson
Ann E. Budzak, MD, FAAP
CAPT Amy R. Gavril, MD, MSCI, FAAP
Suzanne Breen Haney, MD, FAAP
Sheila M. Idzerda, MD, FAAP
Antoinette Laskey, MD, MPH, MBA, FAAP
Lori A. Legano, MD, FAAP
Stephen A. Messner, MD, FAAP
Rebecca L. Moles, MD, FAAP
Vincent J. Palusci, MD, MS, FAAP

LIAISONS

Beverly Fortson, PhD – *Centers for Disease Control and Prevention*
Sara Lark Harmon, MD – *Section on Pediatric Trainees*
Harriet MacMillan, MD – *American Academy of Child and Adolescent Psychiatry*
Elaine Stedt, MSW – *Administration for Children, Youth, and Families*

STAFF

Tammy Piazza Hurley

SECTION ON OPHTHALMOLOGY, 2017–2018

Daniel J. Karr, MD, FAAP, Chairperson
Geoffrey E. Bradford, MD, MS, FAAP, Chairperson-Elect
Sharon Lehman, MD, FAAP, Immediate Past Chairperson
Kanwal Nischal, MD, FAAP
John Denis Roarty, MD, FAAP
Steven E. Rubin, MD, FAAP
Donny Won Suh, MD, FAAP

LIAISONS

Gregg T. Lueder, MD, FAAP – *American Academy of Ophthalmology Council*
Sarah MacKinnon, MSc, OC(C), COMT – *American Association of Certified Orthoptists*
Christie L. Morse, MD, FAAP – *American Association for Pediatric Ophthalmology and Strabismus*
Pamela Erskine Williams, MD, FAAP – *American Academy of Ophthalmology*

STAFF

Jennifer Riefe

> **ABBREVIATIONS**
>
> AHT: abusive head trauma
> CT: computed tomography
> RH: retinal hemorrhage

Address correspondence to Cindy W. Christian, MD, FAAP. E-mail: christian@email.chop.edu

PEDIATRICS (ISSN Numbers: Print, 0031-4005; Online, 1098-4275).

Copyright © 2018 by the American Academy of Pediatrics

FINANCIAL DISCLOSURE: The authors have indicated they have no financial relationships relevant to this article to disclose.

FUNDING: No external funding.

POTENTIAL CONFLICT OF INTEREST: Drs Christian and Levin have provided medicolegal expert work for both the defense and the prosecution or plaintiff for both criminal and civil matters involving child abuse.

REFERENCES

1. Bhardwaj G, Chowdhury V, Jacobs MB, Moran KT, Martin FJ, Coroneo MT. A systematic review of the diagnostic accuracy of ocular signs in pediatric abusive head trauma. *Ophthalmology.* 2010;117(5):983–992.e17

2. Rubin DM, Christian CW, Bilaniuk LT, Zazyczny KA, Durbin DR. Occult head injury in high-risk abused children. *Pediatrics.* 2003;111(6, pt 1):1382–1386

3. Morad Y, Kim YM, Mian M, Huyer D, Capra L, Levin AV. Nonophthalmologist accuracy in diagnosing retinal hemorrhages in the shaken baby syndrome. *J Pediatr.* 2003;142(4):431–434

4. Levin AV. Retinal hemorrhages: advances in understanding. *Pediatr Clin North Am.* 2009;56(2):333–344

5. Levin AV, Cordovez JA, Leiby BE, Pequignot E, Tandon A. Retinal hemorrhage in abusive head trauma: finding a common language. *Trans Am Ophthalmol Soc.* 2014;112:1–10

6. Sturm V, Landau K, Menke MN. Optical coherence tomography findings in shaken baby syndrome. *Am J Ophthalmol.* 2008;146(3):363–368

7. Bielory BP, Dubovy SR, Olmos LC, Hess DJ, Berrocal AM. Fluorescein angiographic and histopathologic findings of bilateral peripheral retinal nonperfusion in nonaccidental injury: a case series. *Arch Ophthalmol.* 2012;130(3):383–387

8. Goldenberg DT, Wu D, Capone A Jr, Drenser KA, Trese MT. Nonaccidental trauma and peripheral retinal nonperfusion. *Ophthalmology.* 2010;117(3):561–566

9. Gumus K. A child with raccoon eyes masquerading as trauma. *Int Ophthalmol.* 2007;27(6):379–381

10. Oppenheimer AJ, Monson LA, Buchman SR. Pediatric orbital fractures. *Craniomaxillofac Trauma Reconstr.* 2013;6(1):9–20

11. Losee JE, Afifi A, Jiang S, et al. Pediatric orbital fractures: classification, management, and early follow-up. *Plast Reconstr Surg.* 2008;122(3):886–897

12. Parisi MT, Wiester RT, Done SL, Sugar NF, Feldman KW. Three-dimensional computed tomography skull reconstructions as an aid to child abuse evaluations. *Pediatr Emerg Care.* 2015;31(11):779–786

13. DeRidder CA, Berkowitz CD, Hicks RA, Laskey AL. Subconjunctival hemorrhages in infants and children: a sign of nonaccidental trauma. *Pediatr Emerg Care.* 2013;29(2):222–226

14. SooHoo JR, Davies BW, Braverman RS, Enzenauer RW, McCourt EA. Pediatric traumatic hyphema: a review of 138 consecutive cases. *J AAPOS.* 2013;17(6):565–567

15. Al-Holou WN, O'Hara EA, Cohen-Gadol AA, Maher CO. Nonaccidental head injury in children. Historical vignette. *J Neurosurg Pediatr.* 2009;3(6):474–483

16. Agrawal S, Peters MJ, Adams GG, Pierce CM. Prevalence of retinal hemorrhages in critically ill children. *Pediatrics.* 2012;129(6). Available at: www.pediatrics.org/cgi/content/full/129/6/e1388

17. Binenbaum G, Mirza-George N, Christian CW, Forbes BJ. Odds of abuse associated with retinal hemorrhages in children suspected of child abuse. *J AAPOS.* 2009;13(3):268–272

18. Vinchon M, de Foort-Dhellemmes S, Desurmont M, Delestret I. Confessed abuse versus witnessed accidents in infants: comparison of clinical, radiological, and ophthalmological data in corroborated cases. *Childs Nerv Syst.* 2010;26(5):637–645

19. Maguire S, Pickerd N, Farewell D, Mann M, Tempest V, Kemp AM. Which clinical features distinguish inflicted from non-inflicted brain injury? A systematic review. *Arch Dis Child.* 2009;94(11):860–867

20. Morad Y, Kim YM, Armstrong DC, Huyer D, Mian M, Levin AV. Correlation between retinal abnormalities and intracranial abnormalities in the shaken baby syndrome. *Am J Ophthalmol.* 2002;134(3):354–359

21. Binenbaum G, Christian CW, Ichord RN, et al. Retinal hemorrhage and brain injury patterns on diffusion-weighted magnetic resonance imaging in children with head trauma. *J AAPOS.* 2013;17(6):603–608

22. George ND, Yates JR, Bradshaw K, Moore AT. Infantile presentation of X linked retinoschisis. *Br J Ophthalmol.* 1995;79(7):653–657

23. Forbes BJ, Rubin SE, Margolin E, Levin AV. Evaluation and management of retinal hemorrhages in infants with and without abusive head trauma. *J AAPOS.* 2010;14(3):267–273

24. Lueder GT, Turner JW, Paschall R. Perimacular retinal folds simulating nonaccidental injury in an infant. *Arch Ophthalmol.* 2006;124(12):1782–1783

25. Lantz PE, Sinal SH, Stanton CA, Weaver RG Jr. Perimacular retinal folds from childhood head trauma. *BMJ.* 2004;328(7442):754–756

26. Kivlin JD, Currie ML, Greenbaum VJ, Simons KB, Jentzen J. Retinal hemorrhages in children following fatal motor vehicle crashes: a case series. *Arch Ophthalmol.* 2008;126(6):800–804

27. Reddie IC, Bhardwaj G, Dauber SL, Jacobs MB, Moran KT. Bilateral retinoschisis in a 2-year-old following a three-storey fall. *Eye (Lond).* 2010;24(8):1426–1427

28. Morad Y, Avni I, Capra L, et al. Shaken baby syndrome without intracranial hemorrhage on initial computed tomography. *J AAPOS.* 2004;8(6):521–527

29. Morad Y, Avni I, Benton SA, et al. Normal computerized tomography of brain in children with shaken baby syndrome. *J AAPOS.* 2004;8(5):445–450

30. Binenbaum G, Chen W, Huang J, Ying GS, Forbes BJ. The natural history of retinal hemorrhage in pediatric head trauma. *J AAPOS.* 2016;20(2):131–135

31. Gilles EE, McGregor ML, Levy-Clarke G. Retinal hemorrhage asymmetry in inflicted head injury: a clue to pathogenesis? *J Pediatr.* 2003;143(4):494–499

32. Gnanaraj L, Gilliland MG, Yahya RR, et al. Ocular manifestations of crush head injury in children. *Eye (Lond).* 2007;21(1):5–10

33. Levinson JD, Pasquale MA, Lambert SR. Diffuse bilateral retinal hemorrhages in an infant with a coagulopathy and prolonged cardiopulmonary resuscitation. *J AAPOS.* 2016;20(2):166–168

34. Shiau T, Levin AV. Retinal hemorrhages in children: the role of intracranial pressure. *Arch Pediatr Adolesc Med.* 2012;166(7):623–628

35. Forbes BJ, Cox M, Christian CW. Retinal hemorrhages in patients with epidural hematomas. *J AAPOS.* 2008;12(2):177–180

36. Duhaime AC, Christian C, Armonda R, Hunter J, Hertle R. Disappearing subdural hematomas in children. *Pediatr Neurosurg.* 1996;25(3):116–122

37. Hughes LA, May K, Talbot JF, Parsons MA. Incidence, distribution, and duration of birth-related retinal hemorrhages: a prospective study. *J AAPOS.* 2006;10(2):102–106

38. Laghmari M, Skiker H, Handor H, et al. Birth-related retinal hemorrhages in the newborn: incidence and relationship with maternal, obstetric and neonatal factors. Prospective study of 2,031 cases [in French]. *J Fr Ophtalmol.* 2014;37(4):313–319

39. Callaway NF, Ludwig CA, Blumenkranz MS, Jones JM, Fredrick DR, Moshfeghi DM. Retinal and optic nerve hemorrhages in the newborn infant: one-year results of the Newborn Eye Screen Test Study. *Ophthalmology.* 2016;123(5):1043–1052

40. Watts P, Maguire S, Kwok T, et al. Newborn retinal hemorrhages: a systematic review. *J AAPOS.* 2013;17(1):70–78

41. Emerson MV, Pieramici DJ, Stoessel KM, Berreen JP, Gariano RF. Incidence and rate of disappearance of retinal hemorrhage in newborns. *Ophthalmology.* 2001;108(1):36–39

42. Altman RL, Brand DA, Forman S, et al. Abusive head injury as a cause of apparent life-threatening events in infancy. *Arch Pediatr Adolesc Med.* 2003;157(10):1011–1015

43. Curcoy AI, Trenchs V, Morales M, Serra A, Pineda M, Pou J. Do retinal haemorrhages occur in infants with convulsions? *Arch Dis Child.* 2009;94(11):873–875

44. Binenbaum G, Christian CW, Guttmann K, Huang J, Ying GS, Forbes BJ. Evaluation of temporal association between vaccinations and retinal hemorrhage in children. *JAMA Ophthalmol.* 2015;133(11):1261–1265

45. Goldman M, Dagan Z, Yair M, Elbaz U, Lahat E, Yair M. Severe cough and retinal hemorrhage in infants and young children. *J Pediatr.* 2006;148(6):835–836

46. Binenbaum G, Rogers DL, Forbes BJ, et al. Patterns of retinal hemorrhage associated with increased intracranial pressure in children. *Pediatrics.* 2013;132(2). Available at: www.pediatrics.org/cgi/content/full/132/2/e430

47. Jenny C, Hymel KP, Ritzen A, Reinert SE, Hay TC. Analysis of missed cases of abusive head trauma. *JAMA.* 1999;281(7):621–626

48. Maguire SA, Watts PO, Shaw AD, et al. Retinal haemorrhages and related findings in abusive and non-abusive head trauma: a systematic review. *Eye (Lond).* 2013;27(1):28–36

49. Levin AV. Retinal hemorrhage in abusive head trauma. *Pediatrics.* 2010;126(5):961–970

50. Muni RH, Kohly RP, Sohn EH, Lee TC. Hand-held spectral domain optical coherence tomography finding in shaken-baby syndrome. *Retina.* 2010;30(suppl 4):S45–S50

51. Levin A. In: David TJ, ed. *Recent Advances in Paediatrics*, vol. 18. London, England: Churchill Livingstone; 2000:151–219

52. Lind K, Toure H, Brugel D, Meyer P, Laurent-Vannier A, Chevignard M. Extended follow-up of neurological, cognitive, behavioral and academic outcomes after severe abusive head trauma. *Child Abuse Negl.* 2016;51:358–367

53. Barlow KM, Thomson E, Johnson D, Minns RA. Late neurologic and cognitive sequelae of inflicted traumatic brain injury in infancy. *Pediatrics.* 2005;116(2). Available at: www.pediatrics.org/cgi/content/full/116/2/e174

54. Lantz PE, Adams GG. Postmortem monocular indirect ophthalmoscopy. *J Forensic Sci.* 2005;50(6):1450–1452

55. Wygnanski-Jaffe T, Levin AV, Shafiq A, et al. Postmortem orbital findings in shaken baby syndrome. *Am J Ophthalmol.* 2006;142(2):233–240

56. Gilliland MG, Levin AV, Enzenauer RW, et al. Guidelines for postmortem protocol for ocular investigation of sudden unexplained infant death and suspected physical child abuse. *Am J Forensic Med Pathol.* 2007;28(4):323–329

57. Squier W. The "Shaken Baby" syndrome: pathology and mechanisms. *Acta Neuropathol.* 2011;122(5):519–542

58. Ganesh A, Jenny C, Geyer J, Shouldice M, Levin AV. Retinal hemorrhages in type I osteogenesis imperfecta after minor trauma. *Ophthalmology.* 2004;111(7):1428–1431

59. Odom A, Christ E, Kerr N, et al. Prevalence of retinal hemorrhages in pediatric patients after in-hospital cardiopulmonary resuscitation: a prospective study. *Pediatrics.* 1997;99(6). Available at: www.pediatrics.org/cgi/content/full/99/6/e3

60. Pham H, Enzenauer RW, Elder JE, Levin AV. Retinal hemorrhage after cardiopulmonary resuscitation with chest compressions. *Am J Forensic Med Pathol.* 2013;34(2):122–124

61. Riggs BJ, Trimboli-Heidler C, Spaeder MC, Miller MM, Dean NP, Cohen JS. The use of ophthalmic ultrasonography to identify retinal injuries associated with abusive head trauma. *Ann Emerg Med.* 2016;67(5):620–624

62. Christian CW; Committee on Child Abuse and Neglect, American Academy of Pediatrics. The evaluation of suspected child physical abuse. *Pediatrics.* 2015;135(5). Available at: www.pediatrics.org/cgi/content/full/135/5/e1337

Food Additives and Child Health

● ●

- *Policy Statement*

POLICY STATEMENT Organizational Principles to Guide and Define the Child Health Care System and/or Improve the Health of all Children

American Academy
of Pediatrics

DEDICATED TO THE HEALTH OF ALL CHILDREN™

Food Additives and Child Health

Leonardo Trasande, MD, MPP, FAAP,[a] Rachel M. Shaffer, MPH,[b] Sheela Sathyanarayana, MD, MPH,[b,c]
COUNCIL ON ENVIRONMENTAL HEALTH

abstract

Our purposes with this policy statement and its accompanying technical report are to review and highlight emerging child health concerns related to the use of colorings, flavorings, and chemicals deliberately added to food during processing (direct food additives) as well as substances in food contact materials, including adhesives, dyes, coatings, paper, paperboard, plastic, and other polymers, which may contaminate food as part of packaging or manufacturing equipment (indirect food additives); to make reasonable recommendations that the pediatrician might be able to adopt into the guidance provided during pediatric visits; and to propose urgently needed reforms to the current regulatory process at the US Food and Drug Administration (FDA) for food additives. Concern regarding food additives has increased in the past 2 decades, in part because of studies in which authors document endocrine disruption and other adverse health effects. In some cases, exposure to these chemicals is disproportionate among minority and low-income populations. Regulation and oversight of many food additives is inadequate because of several key problems in the Federal Food, Drug, and Cosmetic Act. Current requirements for a "generally recognized as safe" (GRAS) designation are insufficient to ensure the safety of food additives and do not contain sufficient protections against conflict of interest. Additionally, the FDA does not have adequate authority to acquire data on chemicals on the market or reassess their safety for human health. These are critical weaknesses in the current regulatory system for food additives. Data about health effects of food additives on infants and children are limited or missing; however, in general, infants and children are more vulnerable to chemical exposures. Substantial improvements to the food additives regulatory system are urgently needed, including greatly strengthening or replacing the "generally recognized as safe" (GRAS) determination process, updating the scientific foundation of the FDA's safety assessment program, retesting all previously approved chemicals, and labeling direct additives with limited or no toxicity data.

[a]Pediatrics, Environmental Medicine, and Health Policy, School of Medicine, New York University, New York, New York; and [b]Department of Environmental and Occupational Health Sciences, School of Public Health, and [c]Pediatrics, University of Washington, Seattle, Washington

Dr Trasande developed the initial idea for the document. Ms. Shaffer and Dr. Trasande researched, wrote, and revised the statement. Dr. Sathyanarayana critically reviewed the document; and all authors approved the final manuscript as submitted.

DOI: https://doi.org/10.1542/peds.2018-1408

Address correspondence to Leonardo Trasande, MD, MPP, FAAP. E-mail: Leonardo.Trasande@nyumc.org

PEDIATRICS (ISSN Numbers: Print, 0031-4005; Online, 1098-4275).

FINANCIAL DISCLOSURE: The authors have indicated they have no financial relationships relevant to this article to disclose.

FUNDING: Dr Trasande is supported by R01ES022972, R56ES027256, UG30D023305, R01DK100307, and U01OH011299. Ms Shaffer is

To cite: Trasande L, Shaffer RM, Sathyanarayana S; AAP COUNCIL ON ENVIRONMENTAL HEALTH. Food Additives and Child Health. *Pediatrics.* 2018;142(2):e20181408

TABLE 1 Summary of Food-Related Uses and Health Concerns for the Compounds Discussed in This Statement

Category	Chemical	Food-Related Use	Selected Health Concerns
Indirect food additives	Bisphenols	Polycarbonate plastic containers	Endocrine disruption[3–8]
		Polymeric, epoxy resins in food and beverage cans	Obesogenic activity,[9–12] neurodevelopmental disruption[13–16]
	Phthalates	Clear plastic food wrap	Endocrine disruption[17–20]
		Plastic tubing, storage containers used in industrial food production	Obesogenic activity[21,22]
		Multiple uses in food manufacturing equipment	Oxidative stress,[23,24] cardiotoxicity[25,26]
	Perfluoroalkyl chemicals (PFCs)	Grease-proof paper and paperboard	Immunosupression,[27,28] endocrine disruption,[29–31] obesogenic activity,[32] decreased birth wt[33]
	Perchlorate	Food packaging	Thyroid hormone disruption[34–36]
Direct food additives	Nitrates and nitrites	Direct additive as preservative and color enhancer, especially to meats	Carcinogenicity,[37–39] thyroid hormone disruption[40,41]

INTRODUCTION

Today, more than 10 000 chemicals are allowed to be added to food and food contact materials in the United States, either directly or indirectly, under the 1958 Food Additives Amendment to the 1938 Federal Food, Drug, and Cosmetic Act (FFDCA) (public law number 85-929). Many of these were grandfathered in for use by the federal government before the 1958 amendment, and an estimated 1000 chemicals are used under a "generally recognized as safe" (GRAS) designation process without US Food and Drug Administration (FDA) approval.[1] Yet, suggested in accumulating evidence from nonhuman laboratory and human epidemiological studies is that chemicals used in food and food contact materials may contribute to disease and disability, as described in the accompanying technical report and summarized in Table 1. Children may be particularly susceptible to the effects of these compounds, given that they have higher relative exposures compared with adults (because of greater dietary intake per pound), their metabolic (ie, detoxification) systems are still developing, and key organ systems are undergoing substantial changes and maturation that are vulnerable to disruptions.[2] In this policy statement and accompanying technical report, we will not address other contaminants that

inadvertently enter the food and water supply, such as aflatoxins, polychlorinated biphenyls, dioxins, metals including mercury, pesticide residues such as DDT, and vomitoxin. In this statement, we will not focus on genetically modified foods, because they involve a separate set of regulatory and biomedical issues. Caffeine or other stimulants intentionally added to food products will not be covered.

The potential for endocrine system disruption is of great concern, especially in early life, when developmental programming of organ systems is susceptible to permanent and lifelong disruption. The international medical and scientific communities have called attention to these issues in several recent landmark reports, including a scientific statement from the Endocrine Society in 2009,[42] which was updated in 2015 to reflect rapidly accumulating knowledge[3]; a joint report from the World Health Organization and United Nations Environment Program in 2013[43]; and a statement from the International Federation of Gynecology and Obstetrics in 2015.[44] Chemicals of increasing concern include the following:

- bisphenols, which are used in the lining of metal cans to prevent corrosion[45];

- phthalates, which are esters of diphthalic acid that are often

used in adhesives, lubricants, and plasticizers during the manufacturing process[17];

- nonpersistent pesticides, which have been addressed in a previous policy statement from the American Academy of Pediatrics and, thus, will not be discussed in this statement[46];

- perfluoroalkyl chemicals (PFCs), which are used in grease-proof paper and packaging[47]; and

- perchlorate, an antistatic agent used for plastic packaging in contact with dry foods with surfaces that do not contain free fat or oil and also present as a degradation product of bleach used to clean food manufacturing equipment.[48]

Additional compounds of concern discussed in the accompanying technical report include artificial food colors, nitrates, and nitrites.

Environmentally relevant doses (ie, low nanomolar concentrations that people are likely to encounter in daily life) of bisphenol A (BPA)[4] trigger the conversion of cells to adipocytes,[9] disrupt pancreatic β-cell function in vivo,[49] and affect glucose transport in adipocytes.[9–11] Phthalates are metabolized to chemicals that influence the expression of master regulators of lipid and carbohydrate metabolism, the peroxisome proliferator-activated receptors,[21] with specific effects that produce insulin resistance in nonhuman laboratory studies. Some studies have documented similar metabolic effects in human populations.[22] Some phthalates are well known to be antiandrogenic and can affect fetal reproductive development.[18,19,50] Authors of recent studies have linked perfluoroalkyl chemicals with reduced immune response to vaccine[27,28] and thyroid hormone alterations,[29,51,52] among other adverse health end points. Perchlorate is known to disrupt thyroid hormone[34] and, along with exposures to other food contaminants, such as polybrominated diphenyl ethers,[53–55] may be contributing to the increase in neonatal hypothyroidism that has been documented in the United States.[56] Artificial food colors may be associated with exacerbation of attention-deficit/hyperactivity disorder symptoms.[57] Nitrates and nitrites can interfere with thyroid hormone production[40] and, under specific endogenous conditions, may result in the increased production of carcinogenic N-nitroso compounds.[37,38]

Racial and ethnic differences in food additive exposures are well documented.[58,59] Higher urinary concentrations of BPA have been documented in African American individuals,[60] and BPA concentrations have been inversely associated with family income.[61] Given that obesity is well recognized to be more prevalent among low-income and minority children in the United States,[62] disproportionate exposures to obesogenic chemicals such as BPA partially explain sociodemographic disparities in health.

REGULATORY FRAMEWORK FOR DIRECT AND INDIRECT FOOD ADDITIVES

The Food Additives Amendment of 1958 was passed as an amendment to the FFDCA and was used to provide specific guidance for food additives. The legislation required a formal agency review, public comment, and open rulemaking process for new chemical additives. It also contained an exemption for common food additives, such as oil or vinegar, when used in ways that were GRAS.[63] Under these specific scenarios, a formal rulemaking process was not required.

Despite this framework, there remain substantial gaps in data about potential health effects of food additives. A recent evaluation of 3941 direct food additives revealed that 63.9% of these had no feeding data whatsoever (either a study of the lethal dose in 50% of animals or an oral toxicology study). Only 263 (6.7%) had reproductive toxicology data, and 2 had developmental toxicology data.[64]

This lack of data on food additives stems from 2 critical problems within the food regulatory system. First, the GRAS process, although intended to be used in limited situations, has become the process by which virtually all new food additives enter the market. Consequently, neither the FDA nor the public have adequate notice or review. The Government Accountability Office conducted an extensive review of the FDA GRAS program in 2010 and determined that the FDA is not able to ensure the safety of existing or new additives through this approval mechanism.[65] Concerns also have been raised about conflicts of interest in the scientific review of food additives leading to GRAS designation. A recent evaluation of 451 GRAS evaluations voluntarily submitted to the FDA revealed that 22.4% of evaluations were made by an employee of the manufacturer, 13.3% were made by an employee of a consulting firm selected by the manufacturer, and 64.3% were made by an expert panel selected by the consulting firm or manufacturer. None were made by a third party.[66]

Second, the FDA does not have authority to obtain data on or reassess the safety of chemicals already on the market.[1] This issue is of great importance and concern for chemicals approved decades ago on the basis of limited and sometimes antiquated testing methods. For instance, some compounds, such as styrene and eugenol methyl ether, remain approved for use as flavoring agents, although they have been subsequently classified as reasonably anticipated to be human carcinogens by the US National Toxicology Program.[67]

Further compounding the problems noted above are other shortcomings within agency procedures. For example, the FDA does not regularly consider cumulative effects of food additives in the context of other chemical exposures that may affect the same biological receptor or mechanism, despite their legal requirement to do so.[68–70] Synergistic effects of chemicals found in foods are also not considered. Synergistic and cumulative effects are especially important, given that multiple food contaminants, such as polybrominated diphenyl ethers, perchlorate, and organophosphate pesticides, can disrupt various aspects of the thyroid hormone system.[71] Dietary interactions may also be important, given that iodine sufficiency is essential for thyroid function.[72]

In addition, the FDA's toxicological testing recommendations have not been updated on the basis of new scientific information. Testing guidelines for food contact materials are based on estimated dietary exposure, and only genotoxicity tests are recommended for exposures estimated to be less than 150 µg per person per day, regardless of body weight.[73] Thus, toxicological testing may not account for behavioral or other end points that may be more likely to be impaired by early life exposures, especially to additives that act at low doses to disrupt endocrine pathways. Furthermore, these guidelines may not be adequately protective for children, given that they may receive higher relative doses than adults because of their lower body weights.

RECOMMENDATIONS FOR PEDIATRICIANS AND THE HEALTH SECTOR

It is difficult to know how to reduce exposures to many of these chemicals, but some recommendations are cited here.[74–76] Insofar as these modifications can pose additional costs, barriers may exist for low-income families to reduce their exposure to food additives of concern. Pediatricians may wish to tailor guidance in the context of practicality, especially because food insecurity remains a substantial child health concern. Pediatricians also can advocate for modernization of the FFDCA, as described in the subsequent section, which is of unique importance for low-income populations who may not be as readily able to reduce exposure to food additives.

- Prioritize consumption of fresh or frozen fruits and vegetables when possible, and support that effort by developing a list of low-cost sources for fresh fruits and vegetables.

- Avoid processed meats, especially maternal consumption during pregnancy.

- Avoid microwaving food or beverages (including infant formula and pumped human milk) in plastic, if possible.

- Avoid placing plastics in the dishwasher.

- Use alternatives to plastic, such as glass or stainless steel, when possible.

- Look at the recycling code on the bottom of products to find the plastic type, and avoid plastics with recycling codes 3 (phthalates), 6 (styrene), and 7 (bisphenols) unless plastics are labeled as "biobased" or "greenware,"

indicating that they are made from corn and do not contain bisphenols.

- Encourage hand-washing before handling foods and/or drinks, and wash all fruits and vegetables that cannot be peeled.

RECOMMENDATIONS FOR POLICY MAKERS

Just as the American Academy of Pediatrics had recommended principles for the modernization of the Toxic Substances Control Act (TSCA) to strengthen regulation of chemicals in nonfood products to protect children's health,[77] the Academy endorses previously described priority areas for improvements to the food additive regulatory program[78] and provides additional recommendations below, some of which could be accomplished by the FDA, whereas others may require congressional action to change the current law.

RECOMMENDATIONS FOR GOVERNMENT

1. The GRAS process is in need of substantial revision. A more robust and transparent process of evaluation is needed, including additional requirements for toxicity testing before approval of chemicals for the marketplace. The GRAS system should be revised as soon as possible and should fully document and disclose conflicts of interest in the evaluation process.

2. The FDA should leverage expertise and technical evaluations from other agencies to gather missing data and identify knowledge gaps, while the current GRAS process remains in place.

3. The FDA should establish requirements for prioritization and retesting of previously approved chemicals.

4. Congress should provide the FDA authority to collect information

about the use of food additives and to require additional data from the industry when gaps in knowledge and potential safety concerns are raised.

5. There should be dedicated resources for research and testing that will allow for a more effective evidence-based database to support a revised FDA safety review process.

6. The FDA should update the scientific foundation for the FDA safety assessment process, including but not limited to the following: expand the scope of recommended testing battery to cover endocrine-related and neurobehavioral effects, ensure adequate safety factors for pregnant and breastfeeding women and additional vulnerable populations, and develop strategies to integrate emerging testing techniques.

7. The FDA should consider cumulative and mixture effects from dietary sources, including other additives and contaminants that interact with relevant biological pathways.

8. The FDA should establish requirements for labeling of additives with limited or no toxicity data and those not reviewed for safety by the FDA.

9. The federal government should encourage provisions that ensure transparency and public access to information, including potential conflicts of interest.

The changes described above can be used to help restore public confidence in the safety of food additives. The FDA can and should make improvements within the scope of current agency authority. Ultimately, congressional action may be required to reform the food additives regulatory process. To aid in this process, the pediatrician community should come together on these issues to advocate for the protection of children's health.

LEAD AUTHORS

Leonardo Trasande, MD, MPP, FAAP
Rachel M. Shaffer, MPH
Sheela Sathyanarayana, MD, MPH

COUNCIL ON ENVIRONMENTAL HEALTH EXECUTIVE COMMITTEE, 2016–2017

Jennifer A. Lowry, MD, FAAP, Chairperson
Samantha Ahdoot, MD, FAAP
Carl R. Baum, MD, FACMT, FAAP
Aaron S. Bernstein, MD, MPH, FAAP
Aparna Bole, MD, FAAP
Carla C. Campbell, MD, MS, FAAP
Philip J. Landrigan, MD, FAAP
Susan E. Pacheco, MD, FAAP

Adam J. Spanier, MD, PhD, MPH, FAAP
Leonardo Trasande, MD, MPP, FAAP
Alan D. Woolf, MD, MPH, FAAP

FORMER EXECUTIVE COMMITTEE MEMBERS

Heather Lynn Brumberg, MD, MPH, FAAP
Bruce P. Lanphear, MD, MPH, FAAP
Jerome A. Paulson, MD, FAAP

LIAISONS

John M. Balbus, MD, MPH – *National Institute of Environmental Health Sciences*
Diane E. Hindman, MD, FAAP – *Section on Pediatric Trainees*
Nathaniel G. DeNicola, MD, MSc – *American College of Obstetricians and Gynecologists*
Ruth Ann Etzel, MD, PhD, FAAP – *US Environmental Protection Agency*

Mary Ellen Mortensen, MD, MS – *Centers for Disease Control and Prevention/National Center for Environmental Health*
Mary H. Ward, PhD – *National Cancer Institute*

STAFF

Paul Spire

ABBREVIATIONS

BPA: bisphenol A
FDA: US Food and Drug Administration
FFDCA: Federal Food, Drug, and Cosmetic Act
GRAS: generally recognized as safe

---

supported by T32ES015459. The content is solely the responsibility of the authors and does not necessarily represent the official views of the National Institutes of Health or the Centers of Disease Control and Prevention.

POTENTIAL CONFLICT OF INTEREST: The authors have indicated they have no potential conflicts of interest to disclose.

REFERENCES

1. Neltner TG, Kulkarni NR, Alger HM, et al. Navigating the U.S. Food Additive Regulatory Program. *Compr Rev Food Sci Food Saf.* 2011;10(6):342–368

2. Landrigan PJ, Goldman LR. Children's vulnerability to toxic chemicals: a challenge and opportunity to strengthen health and environmental policy. *Health Aff (Millwood).* 2011;30(5):842–850

3. Gore AC, Chappell VA, Fenton SE, et al. Executive summary to EDC-2: the Endocrine Society's second scientific statement on endocrine-disrupting chemicals. *Endocr Rev.* 2015;36(6):593–602

4. Howdeshell KL, Hotchkiss AK, Thayer KA, Vandenbergh JG, vom Saal FS. Exposure to bisphenol A advances puberty. *Nature.* 1999;401(6755):763–764

5. Rubin BS. Bisphenol A: an endocrine disruptor with widespread exposure and multiple effects. *J Steroid Biochem Mol Biol.* 2011;127(1–2):27–34

6. Welshons WV, Nagel SC, vom Saal FS. Large effects from small exposures. III. Endocrine mechanisms mediating effects of bisphenol A at levels of human exposure. *Endocrinology.* 2006;147(suppl 6):S56–S69

7. Jukic AM, Calafat AM, McConnaughey DR, et al. Urinary concentrations of phthalate metabolites and bisphenol a and associations with follicular-phase length, luteal-phase length, fecundability, and early pregnancy loss. *Environ Health Perspect.* 2016;124(3):321–328

8. Ehrlich S, Williams PL, Missmer SA, et al. Urinary bisphenol A concentrations and early reproductive health outcomes among women undergoing IVF. *Hum Reprod.* 2012;27(12):3583–3592

9. Masuno H, Kidani T, Sekiya K, et al. Bisphenol A in combination with insulin can accelerate the conversion of 3T3-L1 fibroblasts to adipocytes. *J Lipid Res.* 2002;43(5):676–684

10. Sakurai K, Kawazuma M, Adachi T, et al. Bisphenol A affects glucose transport in mouse 3T3-F442A adipocytes. *Br J Pharmacol.* 2004;141(2):209–214

11. Hugo ER, Brandebourg TD, Woo JG, Loftus J, Alexander JW, Ben-Jonathan N. Bisphenol A at environmentally relevant doses inhibits adiponectin release from human adipose tissue explants and adipocytes. *Environ Health Perspect.* 2008;116(12):1642–1647

12. Vom Saal FS, Nagel SC, Coe BL, Angle BM, Taylor JA. The estrogenic endocrine disrupting chemical bisphenol A (BPA) and obesity. *Mol Cell Endocrinol.* 2012;354(1–2):74–84

13. Braun JM, Kalkbrenner AE, Calafat AM, et al. Impact of early-life bisphenol A exposure on behavior and executive function in children. *Pediatrics.* 2011;128(5):873–882

14. Sathyanarayana S, Braun JM, Yolton K, Liddy S, Lanphear BP. Case report: high prenatal bisphenol a exposure and infant neonatal neurobehavior. *Environ Health Perspect.* 2011;119(8):1170–1175

15. Ejaredar M, Lee Y, Roberts DJ, Sauve R, Dewey D. Bisphenol A exposure and children's behavior: a systematic review. *J Expo Sci Environ Epidemiol.* 2017;27(2):175–183

16. Mustieles V, Pérez-Lobato R, Olea N, Fernández MF. Bisphenol A: human exposure and neurobehavior. *Neurotoxicology.* 2015;49:174–184

17. Sathyanarayana S. Phthalates and children's health. *Curr Probl Pediatr Adolesc Health Care.* 2008;38(2):34–49

18. Swan SH, Sathyanarayana S, Barrett ES, et al; TIDES Study Team. First trimester phthalate exposure and

anogenital distance in newborns. *Hum Reprod.* 2015;30(4):963–972

19. Gray LE Jr, Ostby J, Furr J, Price M, Veeramachaneni DN, Parks L. Perinatal exposure to the phthalates DEHP, BBP, and DINP, but not DEP, DMP, or DOTP, alters sexual differentiation of the male rat. *Toxicol Sci.* 2000;58(2):350–365

20. Meeker JD, Ferguson KK. Urinary phthalate metabolites are associated with decreased serum testosterone in men, women, and children from NHANES 2011-2012. *J Clin Endocrinol Metab.* 2014;99(11):4346–4352

21. Desvergne B, Feige JN, Casals-Casas C. PPAR-mediated activity of phthalates: a link to the obesity epidemic? *Mol Cell Endocrinol.* 2009;304(1–2):43–48

22. Attina TM, Trasande L. Association of exposure to di-2-ethylhexylphthalate replacements with increased insulin resistance in adolescents from NHANES 2009-2012. *J Clin Endocrinol Metab.* 2015;100(7):2640–2650

23. Ferguson KK, McElrath TF, Chen YH, Mukherjee B, Meeker JD. Urinary phthalate metabolites and biomarkers of oxidative stress in pregnant women: a repeated measures analysis. *Environ Health Perspect.* 2015;123(3):210–216

24. Ferguson KK, Loch-Caruso R, Meeker JD. Urinary phthalate metabolites in relation to biomarkers of inflammation and oxidative stress: NHANES 1999-2006. *Environ Res.* 2011;111(5):718–726

25. Posnack NG, Lee NH, Brown R, Sarvazyan N. Gene expression profiling of DEHP-treated cardiomyocytes reveals potential causes of phthalate arrhythmogenicity. *Toxicology.* 2011;279(1–3):54–64

26. Posnack NG, Swift LM, Kay MW, Lee NH, Sarvazyan N. Phthalate exposure changes the metabolic profile of cardiac muscle cells. *Environ Health Perspect.* 2012;120(9):1243–1251

27. Grandjean P, Andersen EW, Budtz-Jørgensen E, et al. Serum vaccine antibody concentrations in children exposed to perfluorinated compounds. *JAMA.* 2012;307(4):391–397

28. Granum B, Haug LS, Namork E, et al. Pre-natal exposure to perfluoroalkyl substances may be associated with altered vaccine antibody levels and immune-related health outcomes in early childhood. *J Immunotoxicol.* 2013;10(4):373–379

29. Wang Y, Rogan WJ, Chen PC, et al. Association between maternal serum perfluoroalkyl substances during pregnancy and maternal and cord thyroid hormones: Taiwan maternal and infant cohort study. *Environ Health Perspect.* 2014;122(5):529–534

30. Vélez MP, Arbuckle TE, Fraser WD. Maternal exposure to perfluorinated chemicals and reduced fecundity: the MIREC study. *Hum Reprod.* 2015;30(3):701–709

31. Fei C, McLaughlin JK, Lipworth L, Olsen J. Maternal levels of perfluorinated chemicals and subfecundity. *Hum Reprod.* 2009;24(5):1200–1205

32. Halldorsson TI, Rytter D, Haug LS, et al. Prenatal exposure to perfluorooctanoate and risk of overweight at 20 years of age: a prospective cohort study. *Environ Health Perspect.* 2012;120(5):668–673

33. Lam J, Koustas E, Sutton P, et al. The Navigation Guide - evidence-based medicine meets environmental health: integration of animal and human evidence for PFOA effects on fetal growth. *Environ Health Perspect.* 2014;122(10):1040–1051

34. Centers for Disease Control and Prevention; Agency for Toxic Substances and Disease Registry. Public health statement for perchlorates. 2008. Available at: www. atsdr.cdc.gov/phs/phs.asp?id=892& tid=181. Accessed May 18, 2017

35. Steinmaus CM. Perchlorate in water supplies: sources, exposures, and health effects. *Curr Environ Health Rep.* 2016;3(2):136–143

36. Ghassabian A, Trasande L. Disruption in thyroid signaling pathway: a mechanism for the effect of endocrine-disrupting chemicals on child neurodevelopment. *Front Endocrinol (Lausanne).* 2018;9:204

37. IARC Working Group on the Evaluation of Carcinogenic Risks to Humans. IARC monographs on the evaluation of carcinogenic risks to humans. Ingested nitrate and nitrite, and cyanobacterial peptide toxins. *IARC Monogr Eval Carcinog Risks Hum.* 2010;94:v–vii, 1–412

38. Bouvard V, Loomis D, Guyton KZ, et al; International Agency for Research on Cancer Monograph Working Group. Carcinogenicity of consumption of red and processed meat. *Lancet Oncol.* 2015;16(16):1599–1600

39. Pogoda JM, Preston-Martin S, Howe G, et al. An international case-control study of maternal diet during pregnancy and childhood brain tumor risk: a histology-specific analysis by food group. *Ann Epidemiol.* 2009;19(3):148–160

40. De Groef B, Decallonne BR, Van der Geyten S, Darras VM, Bouillon R. Perchlorate versus other environmental sodium/iodide symporter inhibitors: potential thyroid-related health effects. *Eur J Endocrinol.* 2006;155(1):17–25

41. Tonacchera M, Pinchera A, Dimida A, et al. Relative potencies and additivity of perchlorate, thiocyanate, nitrate, and iodide on the inhibition of radioactive iodide uptake by the human sodium iodide symporter. *Thyroid.* 2004;14(12):1012–1019

42. Diamanti-Kandarakis E, Bourguignon JP, Giudice LC, et al. Endocrine-disrupting chemicals: an Endocrine Society scientific statement. *Endocr Rev.* 2009;30(4):293–342

43. Bergman Å, Heindel JJ, Jobling S, Kidd KA, Zoeller RT, eds; United Nations Environment Programme; World Health Organization. *State of the Science of Endocrine Disrupting Chemicals – 2012.* Geneva, Switzerland: WHO and UNEP; 2013. Available at: www.who.int/ ceh/publications/endocrine/. Accessed May 18, 2017

44. Di Renzo GC, Conry JA, Blake J, et al. International Federation of Gynecology and Obstetrics opinion on reproductive health impacts of exposure to toxic environmental chemicals. *Int J Gynaecol Obstet.* 2015;131(3):219–225

45. US Food and Drug Administration. Update on bisphenol A for use in food contact applications: January 2010. Available at: https://www. fda.gov/downloads/NewsEvents/ PublicHealthFocus/UCM197778.pdf. Accessed May 18, 2017

46. Forman J, Silverstein J; Committee on Nutrition; Council on Environmental Health; American Academy of Pediatrics. Organic foods: health and environmental advantages and disadvantages. *Pediatrics*. 2012;130(5). Available at: www.pediatrics.org/cgi/content/full/130/5/e1406

47. Buck RC, Franklin J, Berger U, et al. Perfluoroalkyl and polyfluoroalkyl substances in the environment: terminology, classification, and origins. *Integr Environ Assess Manag*. 2011;7(4):513–541

48. US Food and Drug Administration. Filing of food additive petition. Available at: www.gpo.gov/fdsys/pkg/FR-2015-03-16/html/2015-05937.htm. Accessed May 18, 2017

49. Alonso-Magdalena P, Laribi O, Ropero AB, et al. Low doses of bisphenol A and diethylstilbestrol impair Ca2+ signals in pancreatic alpha-cells through a nonclassical membrane estrogen receptor within intact islets of Langerhans. *Environ Health Perspect*. 2005;113(8):969–977

50. Hauser R, Skakkebaek NE, Hass U, et al. Male reproductive disorders, diseases, and costs of exposure to endocrine-disrupting chemicals in the European Union. *J Clin Endocrinol Metab*. 2015;100(4):1267–1277

51. C8 Science Panel. Probable link evaluation of thyroid disease. *C8 Probable Link Reports*. 2012. Available at: www.c8sciencepanel.org/pdfs/Probable_Link_C8_Thyroid_30Jul2012.pdf. Accessed May 18, 2017

52. Melzer D, Rice N, Depledge MH, Henley WE, Galloway TS. Association between serum perfluorooctanoic acid (PFOA) and thyroid disease in the U.S. National Health and Nutrition Examination Survey. *Environ Health Perspect*. 2010;118(5):686–692

53. Jacobson MH, Barr DB, Marcus M, et al. Serum polybrominated diphenyl ether concentrations and thyroid function in young children. *Environ Res*. 2016;149:222–230

54. Schecter A, Päpke O, Harris TR, et al. Polybrominated diphenyl ether (PBDE) levels in an expanded market basket survey of U.S. food and estimated PBDE dietary intake by age and

sex. *Environ Health Perspect*. 2006;114(10):1515–1520

55. Wu N, Herrmann T, Paepke O, et al. Human exposure to PBDEs: associations of PBDE body burdens with food consumption and house dust concentrations. *Environ Sci Technol*. 2007;41(5):1584–1589

56. Hinton CF, Harris KB, Borgfeld L, et al. Trends in incidence rates of congenital hypothyroidism related to select demographic factors: data from the United States, California, Massachusetts, New York, and Texas. *Pediatrics*. 2010;125(suppl 2):S37–S47

57. Nigg JT, Lewis K, Edinger T, Falk M. Meta-analysis of attention-deficit/hyperactivity disorder or attention-deficit/hyperactivity disorder symptoms, restriction diet, and synthetic food color additives. *J Am Acad Child Adolesc Psychiatry*. 2012;51(1):86–97.e8

58. Wolff MS, Teitelbaum SL, Windham G, et al. Pilot study of urinary biomarkers of phytoestrogens, phthalates, and phenols in girls. *Environ Health Perspect*. 2007;115(1):116–121

59. Silva MJ, Barr DB, Reidy JA, et al. Urinary levels of seven phthalate metabolites in the U.S. population from the National Health and Nutrition Examination Survey (NHANES) 1999-2000. *Environ Health Perspect*. 2004;112(3):331–338

60. Trasande L, Attina TM, Blustein J. Association between urinary bisphenol A concentration and obesity prevalence in children and adolescents. *JAMA*. 2012;308(11):1113–1121

61. Nelson JW, Scammell MK, Hatch EE, Webster TF. Social disparities in exposures to bisphenol A and polyfluoroalkyl chemicals: a cross-sectional study within NHANES 2003-2006. *Environ Health*. 2012;11:10

62. Flegal KM, Carroll MD, Kit BK, Ogden CL. Prevalence of obesity and trends in the distribution of body mass index among US adults, 1999-2010. *JAMA*. 2012;307(5):491–497

63. Maffini MV, Alger HM, Olson ED, Neltner TG. Looking back to look forward: a review of FDA's food additives safety assessment and recommendations for

modernizing its program. *Compr Rev Food Sci Food Saf*. 2013;12(4):439–453

64. Neltner TG, Alger HM, Leonard JE, Maffini MV. Data gaps in toxicity testing of chemicals allowed in food in the United States. *Reprod Toxicol*. 2013;42:85–94

65. Government Accountability Office. Food safety: FDA should strengthen its oversight of food ingredients determined to be generally recognized as safe (GRAS). 2010. Available at: www.gao.gov/products/GAO-10-246. Accessed May 18, 2017

66. Neltner TG, Alger HM, O'Reilly JT, Krimsky S, Bero LA, Maffini MV. Conflicts of interest in approvals of additives to food determined to be generally recognized as safe: out of balance. *JAMA Intern Med*. 2013;173(22):2032–2036

67. Huff J, Center for Science in the Public Interest; Natural Resources Defense Council; Center for Food Safety; Consumers Union; Improving Kids' Environment; Center for Environmental Health; Environmental Working Group. Food additive petition pursuant to 21 USC § 348 seeking amended food additive regulation to: 1) remove FDA's approval at 21 CFR § 172.515 of seven synthetic flavors; and 2) add to that section a prohibition on use of these seven flavors and one additional flavor approved as GRAS by the flavor industry because all eight have been found by the National Toxicology Program to induce cancer in man or animal. 2015. Available at: https://www.nrdc.org/sites/default/files/hea_15060901a.pdf. Accessed May 18, 2017

68. Maffini MV, Trasande L, Neltner TG. Perchlorate and diet: human exposures, risks, and mitigation strategies. *Curr Environ Health Rep*. 2016;3(2):107–117

69. Maffini MV, Neltner TG. Brain drain: the cost of neglected responsibilities in evaluating cumulative effects of environmental chemicals. *J Epidemiol Community Health*. 2015;69(5):496–499

70. Food additives, 21 USC 348(c)(5) (1997)

71. Shimizu R, Yamaguchi M, Uramaru N, et al. Structure-activity relationships of 44 halogenated compounds for iodotyrosine deiodinase-inhibitory activity. *Toxicology*. 2013;314(1):22–29

72. Rogan WJ, Paulson JA, Baum C, et al; Council on Environmental Health. Iodine deficiency, pollutant chemicals, and the thyroid: new information on an old problem. *Pediatrics*. 2014;133(6):1163–1166

73. Sotomayor RE, Arvidson KB, Mayer JN, McDougal AJ, Sheu C. Regulatory report: assessing the safety of food contact substances. 2007. Available at: http://wayback.archive-it.org/7993/20171114191242/https://www.fda.gov/Food/IngredientsPackagingLabeling/PackagingFCS/ucm064166.htm. Accessed May 18, 2017

74. Otter D, Sathyanarayana S, Galvez M, Sheffield PE; National Pediatric Environmental Health Specialty Unit Education Committee. Consumer guide: phthalates and bisphenol A. 2014. Available at: www.pehsu.net/_Phthalates_and_Bisphenol_A_Advisory.html. Accessed May 18, 2017

75. Rudel RA, Gray JM, Engel CL, et al. Food packaging and bisphenol A and bis(2-ethyhexyl) phthalate exposure: findings from a dietary intervention. *Environ Health Perspect*. 2011;119(7):914–920

76. Zota AR, Phillips CA, Mitro SD. Recent fast food consumption and bisphenol A and phthalates exposures among the U.S. population in NHANES, 2003-2010. *Environ Health Perspect*. 2016;124(10):1521–1528

77. Council on Environmental Health. Chemical-management policy: prioritizing children's health. *Pediatrics*. 2011;127(5):983–990

78. The Pew Charitable Trusts. *Fixing the Oversight of Chemicals Added to Our Food. Findings and Recommendations of Pew's Assessment of the US Food Additives Program*. Philadelphia, PA: The Pew Charitable Trusts; 2013. Available at: www.pewtrusts.org/en/research-and-analysis/reports/2013/11/07/fixing-the-oversight-of-chemicals-added-to-our-food. Accessed May 18, 2017

Food Additives and Child Health

• •

- *Technical Report*

TECHNICAL REPORT

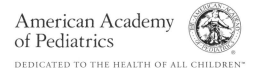

DEDICATED TO THE HEALTH OF ALL CHILDREN™

Food Additives and Child Health

Leonardo Trasande, MD, MPP, FAAP,[a] Rachel M. Shaffer, MPH,[b] Sheela Sathyanarayana, MD, MPH,[b,c]
COUNCIL ON ENVIRONMENTAL HEALTH

abstract

Increasing scientific evidence suggests potential adverse effects on children's health from synthetic chemicals used as food additives, both those deliberately added to food during processing (direct) and those used in materials that may contaminate food as part of packaging or manufacturing (indirect). Concern regarding food additives has increased in the past 2 decades in part because of studies that increasingly document endocrine disruption and other adverse health effects. In some cases, exposure to these chemicals is disproportionate among minority and low-income populations. This report focuses on those food additives with the strongest scientific evidence for concern. Further research is needed to study effects of exposure over various points in the life course, and toxicity testing must be advanced to be able to better identify health concerns prior to widespread population exposure. The accompanying policy statement describes approaches policy makers and pediatricians can take to prevent the disease and disability that are increasingly being identified in relation to chemicals used as food additives, among other uses.

[a]Departments of Pediatrics, Environmental Medicine, and Health Policy, School of Medicine, New York University, New York, New York; [b]Department of Environmental and Occupational Health Sciences, School of Public Health, and [c]Department of Pediatrics, University of Washington, Seattle, Washington

Dr Trasande developed the initial idea for the document. Ms Shaffer and Dr Trasande researched, wrote, and revised the statement. Dr Sathyanarayana critically reviewed the document; all authors approved the final manuscript as submitted.

The authors are grateful to Dr. Mary Ward for her insights and comments regarding the literature on nitrates, which enhanced that section of the technical report.

DOI: https://doi.org/10.1542/peds.2018-1410

Address correspondence to Leonardo Trasande, MD, MPP, FAAP. E-mail: Leonardo.Trasande@nyumc.org

PEDIATRICS (ISSN Numbers: Print, 0031-4005; Online, 1098-4275).

FINANCIAL DISCLOSURE: The authors have indicated they have no financial relationships relevant to this article to disclose.

To cite: Trasande L, Shaffer RM, Sathyanarayana S, AAP COUNCIL ON ENVIRONMENTAL HEALTH. Food Additives and Child Health. *Pediatrics.* 2018;142(2):e20181410

More than 10 000 chemicals are allowed to be added to food in the United States, either directly or indirectly, under the 1958 Food Additives Amendment to the 1938 Federal Food Drug and Cosmetic Act (Public Law 85-929). An estimated 1000 chemicals are used under a "Generally Recognized as Safe" (GRAS) designation without US Food and Drug Administration (FDA) approval or notification.[1] Many chemical uses have been designated as GRAS by company employees or hired consultants.[2] Because of the overuse of the GRAS process and other key failings within the food safety system, there are substantial gaps in data about potential health effects of food additives. Of the 3941 food additives listed on the "Everything Added to Food in the United States" Web site, reproductive toxicology data were available for only 263 (6.7%), and developmental toxicology data were available for only 2.[3]

Accumulating evidence from nonhuman laboratory and human epidemiologic studies suggests that colorings, flavorings, chemicals deliberately added to food during processing (direct food additives), and substances in food contact materials (including adhesives, dyes,

TABLE 1 Summary of Food-Related Uses and Health Concerns for the Compounds Discussed in This Report

Category	Chemical	Food-Related Use	Selected Health Concerns
Indirect food additives	Bisphenols	Polycarbonate plastic containers	Endocrine disruption[11–18]
		Polymeric, epoxy resins in food and beverage cans	Obesogenic activity,[19–22] neurodevelopmental disruption[23–26]
	Phthalates	Clear plastic food wrap	Endocrine disruption[6,27–29]
		Plastic tubing, storage containers used in industrial food production	Obesogenic activity[30–32]
		Multiple uses in food manufacturing equipment	Oxidative stress,[33,34] cardiotoxicity[35,36]
	Perfluoroalkyl chemicals (PFCs)	Grease-proof paper and paperboard	Immunosupression,[37,38] endocrine disruption,[39–41] obesogenic activity,[42] decreased birth wt[43]
	Perchlorate	Food packaging	Thyroid hormone disruption[44–46]
Direct food additives	Nitrates and nitrites	Direct additive as preservative and color enhancer, especially to meats	Carcinogenicity,[10,47,48] thyroid hormone disruption[49,50]

coatings, paper, paperboard, plastic, and other polymers) that may come into contact with food as part of packaging or processing equipment but are not intended to be added directly to food (indirect food additives) may contribute to disease and disability in the population (Table 1). Children may be particularly susceptible to the effects of these compounds because they have higher relative exposures compared with adults (because of greater dietary intake per pound), their metabolic (ie, detoxification) systems are still developing, and key organ systems are undergoing substantial changes and maturations that are vulnerable to disruptions.[4] Chemicals of increasing concern include bisphenols, which are used in the lining of metal cans to prevent corrosion[5]; phthalates, which are esters of diphthalic acid that are used in adhesives and plasticizers during the manufacturing process[6]; nonpersistent pesticides, which have been addressed in a previous American Academy of Pediatrics (AAP) policy statement and thus are not discussed in this report[7]; perfluoroalkyl chemicals (PFCs), which are used in grease-proof paper and paperboard food packaging[8]; and perchlorate, an antistatic agent used for packaging in contact with dry foods with surfaces that do not contain free fat or oil.[9] Nitrates and nitrites, which have been the subject of previous international reviews,[10] and artificial food coloring also are addressed in this report.

This technical report will not address other contaminants that inadvertently enter the food and water supply (such as aflatoxins), polychlorinated biphenyls, dioxins, metals (including mercury), persistent pesticide residues (such as DDT), and vomitoxin. This report will not focus on genetically modified foods because they involve a separate set of regulatory and biomedical issues. Caffeine or other stimulants intentionally added to food products will not be covered.

The AAP is particularly concerned about food contact substances associated with the disruption of the endocrine system in early life, when the developmental programming of organ systems is susceptible to permanent and lifelong disruption. The international medical and scientific communities have called attention to these issues in several recent landmark reports, including a scientific statement from the Endocrine Society in 2009,[51] which was updated in 2015 to account for rapidly accumulating evidence[11]; a joint report from the World Health Organization and United Nations Environment Programme in 2013[52]; and a statement from the International Federation of Gynaecology and Obstetrics in 2015.[53] Subsequent sections of this technical report focus on individual categories of chemicals and provide evidence on potential effects on children's health to support the accompanying AAP policy statement.[54]

INDIRECT FOOD ADDITIVES

Bisphenols

The use of bisphenols as food additives accelerated in the 1960s, when bisphenol A (BPA) was identified as a useful ingredient in the manufacture of polycarbonate plastics and polymeric metal can coatings.[55] BPA has recently been banned from infant bottles,[56] and plastic beverage containers are increasingly designated as BPA free. However, BPA and related compounds are still used in polymeric resin coatings to prevent metal corrosion in food and beverage containers.[57]

BPA has been the focus of significant research and attention. It can bind to the estrogen receptor and cause tissues to respond as if estradiol is present; thus, it is classified as an "endocrine disruptor."[12] Nonhuman laboratory studies and human epidemiologic studies suggest links between BPA exposure and numerous endocrine-related end points, including reduced fertility,[13,14] altered timing of puberty,[15] changes in mammary gland development,[16,58] and development of neoplasias.[59] Environmentally relevant doses of BPA trigger the conversion of cells to adipocytes,[19,60] disrupt pancreatic β-cell function in vivo,[61] and affect glucose transportation in adipocytes.[19–21] BPA exposure in utero has been associated with adverse neurodevelopmental outcomes,[23–25] and cross-sectional studies have associated BPA with decrements in fetal growth,[62] childhood obesity,[63,64] and low-grade albuminuria,[65] although longitudinal studies of prenatal exposure have yielded less consistent relationships with postnatal body mass.[66–69]

A comprehensive, cross-sectional study of dust, indoor and outdoor air, and solid and liquid food in preschool-aged children suggested that dietary sources constitute 99% of BPA exposure.[70] Dental sealants and thermal copy paper are also sources.[71,72] Higher urinary concentrations of BPA have been documented in African American individuals,[63] and BPA concentrations have been inversely associated with family income.[73] Given that obesity is well documented to be more prevalent among low-income and minority children,[74] disproportionate exposure to endocrine-disrupting chemicals, such as BPA, may partially explain sociodemographic disparities in health.[75]

The FDA recently banned the use of BPA in infant bottles and sippy cups,[5] and numerous companies are voluntarily removing BPA from their products because of consumer pressure. Yet, in many cases, it has been replaced with closely related alternatives, such as bisphenol S. These emerging alternatives have been identified in paper products and human urine.[76,77] The few studies focused on evaluating bisphenol S have identified similar genotoxicity and estrogenicity to BPA[78–82] and greater resistance to environmental degradation than BPA.[83,84] Efforts to remove BPA from plastics and metal cans will only provide health and economic benefits if it is replaced with a safe alternative.[55]

Phthalates

Phthalate esters have a diverse array of uses in consumer products, and they can be classified into 2 categories: low–molecular weight phthalates are frequently added to shampoos, cosmetics, lotions, and other personal care products to preserve scent,[6]

whereas high–molecular weight phthalates are used to produce vinyl plastics for diverse settings ranging from flooring, clear food wrap, and flexible plastic tubing commonly used in food manufaturing.[85] Within the high–molecular weight category, di-2-ethylhexylphthalate (DEHP) is of particular interest because industrial processes to produce food frequently use plastic products containing DEHP.[86] Racial and/or ethnic differences in phthalate exposures are well documented.[87,88]

A robust literature, including numerous animal and human studies, shows that DEHP, benzyl butyl phthalate, and dibutyl phthalate are antiandrogenic and adversely affect male fetal genital development. These chemicals exert direct testicular toxicity, thereby reducing circulating testosterone concentrations within the body and increasing the risk of hypospadias and cryptorchidism at birth. These phthalates are also associated with changes in men's hormone concentrations and changes in sperm motility and quantity.[6,27–29,89–91] Mono-(2-ethylhexyl)phthalate, a DEHP metabolite, also interacts with 3 peroxisome proliferator–activated receptors,[30] which play key roles in lipid and carbohydrate metabolism, providing biological plausibility for DEHP metabolites in contributing to childhood obesity and insulin resistance.[92] Epidemiologic studies have also demonstrated an association between urinary phthalate metabolites and markers of oxidative stress.[33,34] Laboratory studies have found that metabolites of phthalates are linked to oxidative stress.[93,94] Oxidative stress appears to diminish the insulin-dependent stimulation of insulin-signaling elements and glucose transport activity[95] and modify the endothelial relaxant nitric oxide, promoting vasoconstriction, platelet adhesion, and the release of proinflammatory cytokines, such as interleukin-1.[96,97] Therefore, if phthalates are proinflammatory and increase oxidative stress, these effects

could lead to changes to metabolic health outcomes. Emerging animal evidence also suggests that DEHP may produce arrhythmia,[35] change metabolic profiles, and produce dysfunction in cardiac myocytes.[36]

Data from the National Health and Nutrition Examination Survey (NHANES) indicate that DEHP metabolites decreased by approximately 37% between 2001 and 2010.[98] These decreases are attributable to the replacement of DEHP with diisodecyl (DIDP) and diisononylphthalate (DINP), phthalates that have not been banned or restricted by regulatory agencies and are increasingly detected within the population. Urinary metabolites of DIDP and DINP were detected in 94% and 98% of the population, respectively, in the 2009–2010 NHANES.[98] DIDP and DINP have been widely identified as food contaminants,[99] and cross-sectional data from NHANES from 2009 to 2012 show positive associations of DIDP and DINP metabolite concentrations with insulin resistance and systolic blood pressure z scores in children and adolescents.[31,32]

PFCs

PFCs are synthetic organic fluorinated compounds whose carbon–fluorine bonds impart high stability and thermal resistance. PFCs have wide utility in stain-resistant sprays for carpets and upholstery, fire-retarding foams, nonstick cooking surfaces, and grease-proofing of paper and paperboard used in food packaging.[100,101] The 2003–2004 NHANES revealed that >98% of the US population has detectable concentrations of PFCs in their blood, including perfluorooctane sulfonic acid (PFOS), perfluorooctanoic acid (PFOA), perfluorohexane sulfonic acid (PFHxS), and perfluorononanoic acid (PFNA).[102] Although exposure can occur through dermal contact and inhalation, consumption of contaminated food is a major route of exposure to PFOS and PFOA for most people.[100] Studies have associated PFOA and PFOS exposure with adverse health outcomes, such as reduced immune response to vaccines,[37,38] metabolic changes,[42] and decreased birth weight.[43] There is also growing concern regarding the endocrine-disrupting potential of PFCs; studies have linked PFOA and PFOS to reduced fertility[39,40] and thyroid alterations[41,103–105] among other effects. These compounds are also extremely persistent and bioaccumulative, with half-lives between 2 and 9 years in the human body.[106]

Because of health and environmental concerns, US production of PFOS was phased out in 2002, and PFOA was phased out in 2015.[107] However, these particular compounds are only 2 of more than a dozen members of the parent family. For example, closely related PFNA chiefly replaced PFOA; increasing PFNA concentrations were detected in the 2003–2004 NHANES and have remained stable thereafter.[102]

In January 2016, the FDA banned the use of 3 classes of long-chain PFCs as indirect food additives.[108] Yet, structurally similar short-chain PFCs, such as PFHxS, may continue to be used. Median levels of PFHxS have been measured since NHANES 2003–2004 and have remained stable through NHANES 2009–2010.[109] A Swedish study of perfluoroalkyl acid trends between 1996 and 2010 confirmed increases in PFHxS concentrations (8.3% per year) but also noted increases of 11% per year in another short-chain PFC substitute for PFOS, perfluoroalkylbutane sulfonate (PFBS), which is increasingly found in food.[110] Modest, infrequently (2%) detectable concentrations of PFBS were identified among the US population in NHANES 2011–2012. Although studies have not sufficiently evaluated the human health consequences of exposure to short-chain PFCs, the structural similarity to banned compounds suggests that they may also pose human health risks.[111,112]

Perchlorate

Perchlorate most commonly enters the food supply through its presence as a contaminant in water or as a component of nitrate fertilizers.[44,45,113] Exposed crops may retain elevated levels of the compound, as described in exploratory studies conducted by the FDA.[114] In addition, perchlorate is an indirect food additive. Contamination in food occurs through its use as an antistatic agent for plastic packaging in contact with dry foods with surfaces that do not contain free fat or oil (such as sugar, flour, and starches) or through degradation from hypochlorite bleach, which is used as a cleaning solution in food manufacturing.[115]

Perchlorate is known to disrupt thyroid hormone production through interference with the sodium iodide symporter (NIS), which allows essential iodide uptake in the thyroid gland.[44,116] The thyroid hormone is critical for early life brain development, among other processes, and alterations to normal hormone concentrations can have lifelong cognitive consequences.[117–121] Exposure to perchlorate among pregnant women, especially those who are iodine deficient, raises particular concern given that the developing fetus is entirely reliant on the maternal thyroid hormone during the first trimester of pregnancy.[117,122,123] Maternal hypothyroidism during pregnancy has been associated with cognitive deficits in children.[120,121] Infants represent another important susceptible population, and the intake of powdered formula may result in high perchlorate exposure from associated packaging materials. Perchlorate and other food contaminants that alter thyroid hormone homeostasis, such as polybrominated diphenyl ethers,[124–126] may be contributing to the increase in neonatal hypothyroidism and other thyroid system perturbations that have been documented in the United States.[127,128] In addition, the thyroid hormone is critical for normal growth processes, and recent evidence suggests that high exposure to multiple compounds that interfere with iodide uptake is associated with poor growth outcomes.[49]

DIRECT FOOD ADDITIVES

Artificial Food Colors

Synthetic artificial food colors (AFCs) are added to foods and beverages for aesthetic reasons, and the resulting brightly colored products are appealing to young children in particular. In some cases, AFCs serve as substitutes for nutritious ingredients, such as in fruit juice drinks that contain little or no actual fruit. Nine AFCs currently are approved for use in the United States: Blue 1, Blue 2, Green 3, Yellow 5, Yellow 6, Red 3, Red 40, Citrus Red 2, and Orange B.[129] FDA data indicate that the use of AFCs increased more than fivefold between 1950 and 2012, from 12 to 68 mg per capita per day.[130]

Over the last several decades, studies have raised concerns regarding the effect of AFCs on child behavior and their role in exacerbating attention-deficit/hyperactivity disorder symptoms.[131–136] Elimination of AFCs from the diet may provide benefits to children with attention-deficit/hyperactivity disorder.[131,137–139] Although the mechanisms of action have not yet been fully elucidated, at least one AFC, Blue 1, may cross the blood-brain barrier.[135,140] Overall, however, further work is needed to better understand the implications of AFC exposure and resolve the uncertainties across the scientific evidence. The available literature should be interpreted with caution because of the absence of information about the ingredients for a number of reasons, including patent protection.

The FDA has set acceptable daily intakes for each of the AFCs.[141] However, these standards, as well as original safety approval for the color additives, are based on animal studies that do not include neurologic or neurobehavioral end points.[140,142]

Given that such effects have been observed in children, a thorough reassessment of AFCs is warranted to determine whether they meet the agency's benchmark of safety: "convincing evidence that establishes with reasonable certainty that no harm will result from the intended use of the color additive."[142]

Nitrates and Nitrites

There has been longstanding concern regarding the use of nitrates and nitrites as preservatives in cured and processed meats, fish, and cheese.[143] In a 2004 statement, the American Medical Association emphasized that infants are particularly vulnerable to methemoglobinemia from nitrates and nitrites because of the chemical composition of their gastric tracts.[144] The American Medical Association statement also highlighted the risk of gastrointestinal or neural cancer from the ingestion of nitrates and nitrites, which (although not carcinogenic themselves) may react with secondary amines or amides to form carcinogenic N-nitroso compounds (NOCs) in the body. In 2006, the International Agency for Research on Cancer classified ingested nitrates and nitrites, in situations that would lead to endogenous nitrosation (production of NOCs), as "probable human carcinogens" (Group 2A).[10,145] In 2015, the International Agency for Research on Cancer specifically classified processed meat (which includes meat that has been salted, cured, or otherwise altered to improve flavor and preservation) as "carcinogenic to humans" (Group 1).[47] Such processing can result in the increased formation of NOCs, and there is convincing evidence linking consumption of processed meats with colorectal cancer.[47] High maternal intake of nitrite-cured meats has also been linked to an increased risk of childhood brain tumors in the offspring, especially tumors of the astroglia.[48,145] Current FDA regulations currently allow up to 500 ppm of sodium nitrate and 200 ppm of sodium nitrite in final meat products. However, no nitrates or nitrites can be used in food produced specifically for infants or young children.[146] Nitrates, like perchlorate, can also disrupt thyroid function by blocking the NIS and thereby interfering with essential iodide uptake. Although its relative potency is much lower than that of other common NIS inhibitors, nitrate is still a significant concern, given that (1) combined exposures from food and water may account for a larger proportion of NIS inhibition than from perchlorate exposure and (2) NIS inhibitors may act together additively.[50,147] Thyroid hormones are essential for many physiologic processes in the body, including normal growth, and recent evidence suggests that high exposure to NIS inhibitors, including nitrate, is associated with reductions in growth measures.[49] In addition, as noted above with regard to perchlorate, maternal thyroid disruption during pregnancy is of particular concern because the fetus is entirely reliant on the maternal thyroid hormone during the first trimester. Thyroid hormone is critical for neurologic developmental processes, and early life deficiencies can result in lifelong adverse effects on cognitive health.[117–121]

In recent years, there has been increasing use of alternative sources of nitrate and nitrite preservatives, such as celery powder, in products labeled as "natural" and "organic."[148,149] These products may contain nitrates and nitrites in concentrations that can be equivalent to or higher than those found in traditional products using sodium-based sources.[149,150] Thus, consumers should be aware that with respect to nitrates and nitrites alone, natural and organic products may not provide advantages over conventional products.

LEAD AUTHORS

Leonardo Trasande, MD, MPP, FAAP
Rachel M. Shaffer, MPH
Sheela Sathyanarayana, MD, MPH

COUNCIL ON ENVIRONMENTAL HEALTH EXECUTIVE COMMITTEE, 2016–2017

Jennifer A. Lowry, MD, FAAP, Chairperson
Samantha Ahdoot, MD, FAAP
Carl R. Baum, MD, FACMT, FAAP
Aaron S. Bernstein, MD, MPH, FAAP
Aparna Bole, MD, FAAP
Carla C. Campbell, MD, MS, FAAP
Philip J. Landrigan, MD, FAAP
Susan E. Pacheco, MD, FAAP
Adam J. Spanier, MD, PhD, MPH, FAAP
Leonardo Trasande, MD, MPP, FAAP
Alan D. Woolf, MD, MPH, FAAP

FORMER EXECUTIVE COMMITTEE MEMBERS

Heather Lynn Brumberg, MD, MPH, FAAP
Bruce P. Lanphear, MD, MPH, FAAP
Jerome A. Paulson, MD, FAAP

LIAISONS

John M. Balbus, MD, MPH – *National Institute of Environmental Health Sciences*
Diane E. Hindman, MD, FAAP – *American Academy of Pediatrics Section on Pediatric Trainees*
Nathaniel G. DeNicola, MD, MSc – *American College of Obstetricians and Gynecologists*
Ruth Ann Etzel, MD, PhD, FAAP – *US Environmental Protection Agency*
Mary Ellen Mortensen, MD, MS – *Centers for Disease Control and Prevention and National Center for Environmental Health*
Mary H. Ward, PhD – *National Cancer Institute*

STAFF

Paul Spire

ABBREVIATIONS

AAP: American Academy of Pediatrics
AFC: artificial food color
BPA: bisphenol A
DEHP: di-2-ethylhexylphthalate
DIDP: diisodecyl
DINP: diisononylphthalate
FDA: Food and Drug Administration
GRAS: generally recognized as safe
NHANES: National Health and Nutrition Examination Survey
NIS: sodium iodide symporter
NOC: N-nitroso compound
PFC: perfluoroalkyl chemical
PFHxS: perfluorohexane sulfonic acid
PFNA: perfluorononanoic acid
PFOA: perfluorooctanoic acid
PFOS: perfluorooctane sulfonic acid

FUNDING: Dr Trasande is supported by R01ES022972, R56ES027256, UG30D023305, R01DK100307, and U01OH011299. Ms Shaffer is supported by T32ES015459. The content is solely the responsibility of the authors and does not necessarily represent the official views of the National Institutes of Health or the Centers of Disease Control and Prevention.

POTENTIAL CONFLICT OF INTEREST: The authors have indicated they have no potential conflicts of interest to disclose.

REFERENCES

1. Neltner TG, Kulkarni NR, Alger HM, et al. Navigating the U.S. Food Additive Regulatory Program. *Compr Rev Food Sci Food Saf.* 2011;10(6):342–368

2. Neltner TG, Alger HM, O'Reilly JT, Krimsky S, Bero LA, Maffini MV. Conflicts of interest in approvals of additives to food determined to be generally recognized as safe: out of balance. *JAMA Intern Med.* 2013;173(22):2032–2036

3. Neltner TG, Alger HM, Leonard JE, Maffini MV. Data gaps in toxicity testing of chemicals allowed in food in the United States. *Reprod Toxicol.* 2013;42:85–94

4. Landrigan PJ, Goldman LR. Children's vulnerability to toxic chemicals: a challenge and opportunity to strengthen health and environmental policy. *Health Aff (Millwood).* 2011;30(5):842–850

5. US Food and Drug Administration. Update on bisphenol A for use in food contact applications: January 2010. Available at: https://www.fda.gov/downloads/NewsEvents/PublicHealthFocus/UCM197778.pdf. Accessed May 18, 2017

6. Sathyanarayana S. Phthalates and children's health. *Curr Probl Pediatr Adolesc Health Care.* 2008;38(2):34–49

7. Forman J, Silverstein J; Committee on Nutrition; Council on Environmental Health; American Academy of Pediatrics. Organic foods: health and environmental advantages and disadvantages. *Pediatrics.* 2012;130(5): Available at: www.pediatrics.org/cgi/content/full/130/5/e1406

8. Buck RC, Franklin J, Berger U, et al. Perfluoroalkyl and polyfluoroalkyl substances in the environment: terminology, classification, and origins. *Integr Environ Assess Manag.* 2011;7(4):513–541

9. US Food and Drug Administration. Filing of food additive petition. *Fed Regist.* 2015;80(50):13508–13510

10. IARC Working Group on the Evaluation of Carcinogenic Risks to Humans. IARC monographs on the evaluation of carcinogenic risks to humans. Ingested nitrate and nitrite, and cyanobacterial peptide toxins. *IARC Monogr Eval Carcinog Risks Hum.* 2010;94:v–vii, 1–412

11. Gore AC, Chappell VA, Fenton SE, et al. Executive summary to EDC-2: the Endocrine Society's second scientific statement on endocrine-disrupting chemicals. *Endocr Rev.* 2015;36(6):593–602

12. Rubin BS. Bisphenol A: an endocrine disruptor with widespread exposure and multiple effects. *J Steroid Biochem Mol Biol.* 2011;127(1–2):27–34

13. Ehrlich S, Williams PL, Missmer SA, et al. Urinary bisphenol A concentrations and early reproductive health outcomes among women undergoing IVF. *Hum Reprod.* 2012;27(12):3583–3592

14. Cantonwine DE, Hauser R, Meeker JD. Bisphenol A and human reproductive health. *Expert Rev Obstet Gynecol.* 2013;8(4)

15. Howdeshell KL, Hotchkiss AK, Thayer KA, Vandenbergh JG, vom Saal FS. Exposure to bisphenol A advances puberty. *Nature.* 1999;401(6755):763–764

16. Vandenberg LN, Maffini MV, Wadia PR, Sonnenschein C, Rubin BS, Soto AM. Exposure to environmentally relevant doses of the xenoestrogen bisphenol-A alters development of the fetal mouse mammary gland. *Endocrinology.* 2007;148(1):116–127

17. Welshons WV, Nagel SC, vom Saal FS. Large effects from small exposures. III. Endocrine mechanisms mediating effects of bisphenol A at levels of human exposure. *Endocrinology.* 2006;147(6 Suppl):S56–S69

18. Jukic AM, Calafat AM, McConnaughey DR, et al. Urinary concentrations of phthalate metabolites and bisphenol A and associations with follicular-phase length, luteal-phase length, fecundability, and early pregnancy loss. *Environ Health Perspect.* 2016;124(3):321–328

19. Masuno H, Kidani T, Sekiya K, et al. Bisphenol A in combination with insulin can accelerate the conversion of 3T3-L1 fibroblasts to adipocytes. *J Lipid Res.* 2002;43(5):676–684

20. Hugo ER, Brandebourg TD, Woo JG, Loftus J, Alexander JW, Ben-Jonathan N. Bisphenol A at environmentally relevant doses inhibits adiponectin release from human adipose tissue explants and adipocytes. *Environ Health Perspect.* 2008;116(12):1642–1647

21. Sakurai K, Kawazuma M, Adachi T, et al. Bisphenol A affects glucose transport in mouse 3T3-F442A adipocytes. *Br J Pharmacol.* 2004;141(2):209–214

22. Vom Saal FS, Nagel SC, Coe BL, Angle BM, Taylor JA. The estrogenic endocrine disrupting chemical bisphenol A (BPA) and obesity. *Mol Cell Endocrinol.* 2012;354(1–2):74–84

23. Braun JM, Kalkbrenner AE, Calafat AM, et al. Impact of early-life bisphenol A exposure on behavior and executive function in children. *Pediatrics.* 2011;128(5):873–882

24. Sathyanarayana S, Braun JM, Yolton K, Liddy S, Lanphear BP. Case report: high prenatal bisphenol A exposure and infant neonatal neurobehavior. *Environ Health Perspect.* 2011;119(8):1170–1175

25. Ejaredar M, Lee Y, Roberts DJ, Sauve R, Dewey D. Bisphenol A exposure and children's behavior: A systematic review. *J Expo Sci Environ Epidemiol.* 2017;27(2):175–183

26. Mustieles V, Pérez-Lobato R, Olea N, Fernández MF. Bisphenol A: Human exposure and neurobehavior. *Neurotoxicology.* 2015;49:174–184

27. Gray LE Jr, Ostby J, Furr J, Price M, Veeramachaneni DN, Parks L. Perinatal

exposure to the phthalates DEHP, BBP, and DINP, but not DEP, DMP, or DOTP, alters sexual differentiation of the male rat. *Toxicol Sci.* 2000;58(2):350–365

28. Meeker JD, Ferguson KK. Urinary phthalate metabolites are associated with decreased serum testosterone in men, women, and children from NHANES 2011-2012. *J Clin Endocrinol Metab.* 2014;99(11):4346–4352

29. Swan SH, Main KM, Liu F, et al; Study for Future Families Research Team. Decrease in anogenital distance among male infants with prenatal phthalate exposure. *Environ Health Perspect.* 2005;113(8):1056–1061

30. Desvergne B, Feige JN, Casals-Casas C. PPAR-mediated activity of phthalates: a link to the obesity epidemic? *Mol Cell Endocrinol.* 2009;304(1–2):43–48

31. Trasande L, Attina TM. Association of exposure to di-2-ethylhexylphthalate replacements with increased blood pressure in children and adolescents. *Hypertension.* 2015;66(2):301–308

32. Attina TM, Trasande L. Association of exposure to di-2-ethylhexylphthalate replacements with increased insulin resistance in adolescents from NHANES 2009-2012. *J Clin Endocrinol Metab.* 2015;100(7):2640–2650

33. Ferguson KK, Loch-Caruso R, Meeker JD. Urinary phthalate metabolites in relation to biomarkers of inflammation and oxidative stress: NHANES 1999-2006. *Environ Res.* 2011;111(5):718–726

34. Ferguson KK, McElrath TF, Chen YH, Mukherjee B, Meeker JD. Urinary phthalate metabolites and biomarkers of oxidative stress in pregnant women: a repeated measures analysis. *Environ Health Perspect.* 2015;123(3):210–216

35. Posnack NG, Lee NH, Brown R, Sarvazyan N. Gene expression profiling of DEHP-treated cardiomyocytes reveals potential causes of phthalate arrhythmogenicity. *Toxicology.* 2011;279(1–3):54–64

36. Posnack NG, Swift LM, Kay MW, Lee NH, Sarvazyan N. Phthalate exposure changes the metabolic profile of cardiac muscle cells. *Environ Health Perspect.* 2012;120(9):1243–1251

37. Grandjean P, Andersen EW, Budtz-Jørgensen E, et al. Serum vaccine antibody concentrations in children exposed to perfluorinated compounds. *JAMA.* 2012;307(4):391–397

38. Granum B, Haug LS, Namork E, et al. Pre-natal exposure to perfluoroalkyl substances may be associated with altered vaccine antibody levels and immune-related health outcomes in early childhood. *J Immunotoxicol.* 2013;10(4):373–379

39. Vélez MP, Arbuckle TE, Fraser WD. Maternal exposure to perfluorinated chemicals and reduced fecundity: the MIREC study. *Hum Reprod.* 2015;30(3):701–709

40. Fei C, McLaughlin JK, Lipworth L, Olsen J. Maternal levels of perfluorinated chemicals and subfecundity. *Hum Reprod.* 2009;24(5):1200–1205

41. Wang Y, Rogan WJ, Chen PC, et al. Association between maternal serum perfluoroalkyl substances during pregnancy and maternal and cord thyroid hormones: Taiwan maternal and infant cohort study. *Environ Health Perspect.* 2014;122(5):529–534

42. Halldorsson TI, Rytter D, Haug LS, et al. Prenatal exposure to perfluorooctanoate and risk of overweight at 20 years of age: a prospective cohort study. *Environ Health Perspect.* 2012;120(5):668–673

43. Lam J, Koustas E, Sutton P, et al. The navigation guide - evidence-based medicine meets environmental health: integration of animal and human evidence for PFOA effects on fetal growth. *Environ Health Perspect.* 2014;122(10):1040–1051

44. Centers for Disease Control and Prevention; Agency for Toxic Substances and Disease Registry. Public health statement for perchlorates. 2008. Available at: www.atsdr.cdc.gov/phs/phs.asp?id=892&tid=181. Accessed May 18, 2017

45. Steinmaus CM. Perchlorate in water supplies: sources, exposures, and health effects. *Curr Environ Health Rep.* 2016;3(2):136–143

46. Ghassabian A, Trasande L. Disruption in thyroid signaling pathway: a mechanism for the effect of endocrine-disrupting chemicals on child

neurodevelopment. *Front Endocrinol (Lausanne).* 2018;9:204

47. Bouvard V, Loomis D, Guyton KZ, et al; International Agency for Research on Cancer Monograph Working Group. Carcinogenicity of consumption of red and processed meat. *Lancet Oncol.* 2015;16(16):1599–1600

48. Pogoda JM, Preston-Martin S, Howe G, et al. An international case-control study of maternal diet during pregnancy and childhood brain tumor risk: a histology-specific analysis by food group. *Ann Epidemiol.* 2009;19(3):148–160

49. Mervish NA, Pajak A, Teitelbaum SL, et al; Breast Cancer and Environment Research Project (BCERP). Thyroid antagonists (perchlorate, thiocyanate, and nitrate) and childhood growth in a longitudinal study of U.S. girls. *Environ Health Perspect.* 2016;124(4):542–549

50. Tonacchera M, Pinchera A, Dimida A, et al. Relative potencies and additivity of perchlorate, thiocyanate, nitrate, and iodide on the inhibition of radioactive iodide uptake by the human sodium iodide symporter. *Thyroid.* 2004;14(12):1012–1019

51. Diamanti-Kandarakis E, Bourguignon J-P, Giudice LC, et al. Endocrine-disrupting chemicals: an Endocrine Society scientific statement. *Endocr Rev.* 2009;30(4):293–342

52. Bergman Å, Heindel JJ, Jobling S, Kidd KA, Zoeller RT, eds. United Nations Environment Programme, World Health Organization. *State of the Science of Endocrine Disrupting Chemicals – 2012.* Geneva, Switzerland: WHO and UNEP; 2013, Available at www.who.int/ceh/publications/endocrine/. Accessed May 18, 2017

53. Di Renzo GC, Conry JA, Blake J, et al. International Federation of Gynecology and Obstetrics opinion on reproductive health impacts of exposure to toxic environmental chemicals. *Int J Gynaecol Obstet.* 2015;131(3):219–225

54. Trasande L, Shaffer RM, Sathyanarayana S; American Academy of Pediatrics Council on Environmental Health. Technical report: Food additives and child health. *Pediatrics.* 2018;142(2):e20181408

55. Trasande L. Further limiting bisphenol A in food uses could provide health

and economic benefits. *Health Aff (Millwood)*. 2014;33(2):316–323

56. Tavernise S. F.D.A. makes it official: BPA can't be used in baby bottles and cups. *New York Times*. July 17, 2012. Available at: www.nytimes.com/2012/07/18/science/fda-bans-bpa-from-baby-bottles-and-sippy-cups.html. Accessed July 18, 2012

57. Schecter A, Malik N, Haffner D, et al. Bisphenol A (BPA) in U.S. food. *Environ Sci Technol*. 2010;44(24):9425–9430

58. Muñoz-de-Toro M, Markey CM, Wadia PR, et al. Perinatal exposure to bisphenol-A alters peripubertal mammary gland development in mice. *Endocrinology*. 2005;146(9):4138–4147

59. Seachrist DD, Bonk KW, Ho SM, Prins GS, Soto AM, Keri RA. A review of the carcinogenic potential of bisphenol A. *Reprod Toxicol*. 2016;59:167–182

60. Masuno H, Iwanami J, Kidani T, Sakayama K, Honda K. Bisphenol a accelerates terminal differentiation of 3T3-L1 cells into adipocytes through the phosphatidylinositol 3-kinase pathway. *Toxicol Sci*. 2005;84(2):319–327

61. Alonso-Magdalena P, Laribi O, Ropero AB, et al. Low doses of bisphenol A and diethylstilbestrol impair Ca2+ signals in pancreatic alpha-cells through a nonclassical membrane estrogen receptor within intact islets of Langerhans. *Environ Health Perspect*. 2005;113(8):969–977

62. Snijder CA, Heederik D, Pierik FH, et al. Fetal growth and prenatal exposure to bisphenol A: the generation R study. *Environ Health Perspect*. 2013;121(3):393–398

63. Trasande L, Attina TM, Blustein J. Association between urinary bisphenol A concentration and obesity prevalence in children and adolescents. *JAMA*. 2012;308(11):1113–1121

64. Wang T, Li M, Chen B, et al. Urinary bisphenol A (BPA) concentration associates with obesity and insulin resistance. *J Clin Endocrinol Metab*. 2012;97(2):E223–E227

65. Trasande L, Attina TM, Trachtman H. Bisphenol A exposure is associated with low-grade urinary albumin excretion in children of the United States. *Kidney Int*. 2013;83(4):741–748

66. Braun JM, Lanphear BP, Calafat AM, et al. Early-life bisphenol A exposure and child body mass index: a prospective cohort study. *Environ Health Perspect*. 2014;122(11):1239–1245

67. Valvi D, Casas M, Mendez MA, et al. Prenatal bisphenol A urine concentrations and early rapid growth and overweight risk in the offspring. *Epidemiology*. 2013;24(6):791–799

68. Harley KG, Aguilar Schall R, Chevrier J, et al. Prenatal and postnatal bisphenol A exposure and body mass index in childhood in the CHAMACOS cohort. *Environ Health Perspect*. 2013;121(4):514–520

69. Legler J, Fletcher T, Govarts E, et al. Obesity, diabetes, and associated costs of exposure to endocrine-disrupting chemicals in the European Union. *J Clin Endocrinol Metab*. 2015;100(4):1278–1288

70. Wilson NK, Chuang JC, Morgan MK, Lordo RA, Sheldon LS. An observational study of the potential exposures of preschool children to pentachlorophenol, bisphenol-A, and nonylphenol at home and daycare. *Environ Res*. 2007;103(1):9–20

71. Fleisch AF, Sheffield PE, Chinn C, Edelstein BL, Landrigan PJ. Bisphenol A and related compounds in dental materials. *Pediatrics*. 2010;126(4):760–768

72. Schwartz AW, Landrigan PJ. Bisphenol A in thermal paper receipts: an opportunity for evidence-based prevention. *Environ Health Perspect*. 2012;120(1):A14–A15, author reply A15

73. Nelson JW, Scammell MK, Hatch EE, Webster TF. Social disparities in exposures to bisphenol A and polyfluoroalkyl chemicals: a cross-sectional study within NHANES 2003-2006. *Environ Health*. 2012;11:10

74. Flegal KM, Carroll MD, Kit BK, Ogden CL. Prevalence of obesity and trends in the distribution of body mass index among US adults, 1999-2010. *JAMA*. 2012;307(5):491–497

75. Patel CJ, Ioannidis JP, Cullen MR, Rehkopf DH. Systematic assessment of the correlations of household income with infectious, biochemical, physiological, and environmental factors in the United States, 1999-2006. *Am J Epidemiol*. 2015;181(3):171–179

76. Liao C, Liu F, Alomirah H, et al. Bisphenol S in urine from the United States and seven Asian countries: occurrence and human exposures. *Environ Sci Technol*. 2012;46(12):6860–6866

77. Liao C, Liu F, Kannan K. Bisphenol s, a new bisphenol analogue, in paper products and currency bills and its association with bisphenol A residues. *Environ Sci Technol*. 2012;46(12):6515–6522

78. Kuruto-Niwa R, Nozawa R, Miyakoshi T, Shiozawa T, Terao Y. Estrogenic activity of alkylphenols, bisphenol S, and their chlorinated derivatives using a GFP expression system. *Environ Toxicol Pharmacol*. 2005;19(1):121–130

79. Chen MY, Ike M, Fujita M. Acute toxicity, mutagenicity, and estrogenicity of bisphenol-A and other bisphenols. *Environ Toxicol*. 2002;17(1):80–86

80. Yoshihara S, Mizutare T, Makishima M, et al. Potent estrogenic metabolites of bisphenol A and bisphenol B formed by rat liver S9 fraction: their structures and estrogenic potency. *Toxicol Sci*. 2004;78(1):50–59

81. Okuda K, Fukuuchi T, Takiguchi M, Yoshihara S. Novel pathway of metabolic activation of bisphenol A-related compounds for estrogenic activity. *Drug Metab Dispos*. 2011;39(9):1696–1703

82. Audebert M, Dolo L, Perdu E, Cravedi JP, Zalko D. Use of the γH2AX assay for assessing the genotoxicity of bisphenol A and bisphenol F in human cell lines. *Arch Toxicol*. 2011;85(11):1463–1473

83. Danzl E, Sei K, Soda S, Ike M, Fujita M. Biodegradation of bisphenol A, bisphenol F and bisphenol S in seawater. *Int J Environ Res Public Health*. 2009;6(4):1472–1484

84. Ike M, Chen MY, Danzl E, Sei K, Fujita M. Biodegradation of a variety of bisphenols under aerobic and anaerobic conditions. *Water Sci Technol*. 2006;53(6):153–159

85. Schettler T. Human exposure to phthalates via consumer products. *Int J Androl*. 2006;29(1):134–139, discussion 181–185

86. Fromme H, Gruber L, Schlummer M, et al. Intake of phthalates and di(2-ethylhexyl)adipate: results of the Integrated Exposure Assessment Survey based on duplicate diet samples and biomonitoring data. *Environ Int.* 2007;33(8):1012–1020

87. Wolff MS, Teitelbaum SL, Windham G, et al. Pilot study of urinary biomarkers of phytoestrogens, phthalates, and phenols in girls. *Environ Health Perspect.* 2007;115(1):116–121

88. Silva MJ, Barr DB, Reidy JA, et al. Urinary levels of seven phthalate metabolites in the U.S. population from the National Health and Nutrition Examination Survey (NHANES) 1999-2000. *Environ Health Perspect.* 2004;112(3):331–338

89. Gray LE Jr, Wilson VS, Stoker T, et al. Adverse effects of environmental antiandrogens and androgens on reproductive development in mammals. *Int J Androl.* 2006;29(1):96–104, discussion 105–108

90. Hauser R, Meeker JD, Singh NP, et al. DNA damage in human sperm is related to urinary levels of phthalate monoester and oxidative metabolites. *Hum Reprod.* 2007;22(3):688–695

91. Hauser R, Skakkebaek NE, Hass U, et al. Male reproductive disorders, diseases, and costs of exposure to endocrine-disrupting chemicals in the European Union. *J Clin Endocrinol Metab.* 2015;100(4):1267–1277

92. Trasande L, Attina TM, Sathyanarayana S, Spanier AJ, Blustein J. Race/ethnicity-specific associations of urinary phthalates with childhood body mass in a nationally representative sample. *Environ Health Perspect.* 2018;121(4):501

93. Jepsen KF, Abildtrup A, Larsen ST. Monophthalates promote IL-6 and IL-8 production in the human epithelial cell line A549. *Toxicol In Vitro.* 2004;18(3):265–269

94. Seo KW, Kim KB, Kim YJ, Choi JY, Lee KT, Choi KS. Comparison of oxidative stress and changes of xenobiotic metabolizing enzymes induced by phthalates in rats. *Food Chem Toxicol.* 2004;42(1):107–114

95. Henriksen EJ, Diamond-Stanic MK, Marchionne EM. Oxidative stress and the etiology of insulin resistance and type 2 diabetes. *Free Radic Biol Med.* 2011;51(5):993–999

96. Singh U, Jialal I. Oxidative stress and atherosclerosis. *Pathophysiology.* 2006;13(3):129–142

97. Harrison D, Griendling KK, Landmesser U, Hornig B, Drexler H. Role of oxidative stress in atherosclerosis. *Am J Cardiol.* 2003;91(3A):7A–11A

98. Zota AR, Calafat AM, Woodruff TJ. Temporal trends in phthalate exposures: findings from the National Health and Nutrition Examination Survey, 2001-2010. *Environ Health Perspect.* 2014;122(3):235–241

99. Serrano SE, Braun J, Trasande L, Dills R, Sathyanarayana S. Phthalates and diet: a review of the food monitoring and epidemiology data. *Environ Health.* 2014;13(1):43

100. Trudel D, Horowitz L, Wormuth M, Scheringer M, Cousins IT, Hungerbühler K. Estimating consumer exposure to PFOS and PFOA. *Risk Anal.* 2008;28(2):251–269

101. Centers for Disease Control and Prevention; Agency for Toxic Substances and Disease Registry. Public health statement: perfluoroalkyls. 2009. Available at: www.atsdr.cdc.gov/toxprofiles/tp200-c1-b.pdf. Accessed May 18, 2017

102. Calafat AM, Wong LY, Kuklenyik Z, Reidy JA, Needham LL. Polyfluoroalkyl chemicals in the U.S. population: data from the National Health and Nutrition Examination Survey (NHANES) 2003-2004 and comparisons with NHANES 1999-2000. *Environ Health Perspect.* 2007;115(11):1596–1602

103. Wen L-L, Lin L-Y, Su T-C, Chen P-C, Lin C-Y. Association between serum perfluorinated chemicals and thyroid function in U.S. adults: the National Health and Nutrition Examination Survey 2007-2010. *J Clin Endocrinol Metab.* 2013;98(9):E1456–E1464

104. C8 Science Panel. Probable link evaluation of thyroid disease. July 20, 2012. Available at: www.c8sciencepanel.org/pdfs/Probable_Link_C8_Thyroid_30Jul2012.pdf. Accessed May 18, 2017

105. Melzer D, Rice N, Depledge MH, Henley WE, Galloway TS. Association between serum perfluorooctanoic acid (PFOA) and thyroid disease in the U.S. National Health and Nutrition Examination Survey. *Environ Health Perspect.* 2010;118(5):686–692

106. US Environmental Protection Agency. Emerging contaminants - perfluorooctane sulfonate (PFOS) and perfluorooctanoic acid (PFOA). 2014

107. US Environmental Protection Agency. Long-chain perfluorinated chemicals (PFCs) action plan. 2009. Available at: https://www.epa.gov/sites/production/files/2016-01/documents/pfcs_action_plan1230_09.pdf. Accessed May 18, 2017

108. US Food and Drug Administration. Indirect food additives: paper and paperboard components. 2016. Available at: https://www.federalregister.gov/documents/2016/01/04/2015-33026/indirect-food-additives-paper-and-paperboard-components. Accessed May 18, 2017

109. Calafat AM, Wong LY, Kuklenyik Z, Reidy JA, Needham LL. Polyfluoroalkyl chemicals in the U.S. population: data from the National Health and Nutrition Examination Survey (NHANES) 2003-2004 and comparisons with NHANES 1999-2000. *Environ Health Perspect.* 2007;115(11):1596–1602

110. Glynn A, Berger U, Bignert A, et al. Perfluorinated alkyl acids in blood serum from primiparous women in Sweden: serial sampling during pregnancy and nursing, and temporal trends 1996-2010. *Environ Sci Technol.* 2012;46(16):9071–9079

111. Scheringer M, Trier X, Cousins IT, et al. Helsingør statement on poly- and perfluorinated alkyl substances (PFASs). *Chemosphere.* 2014;114:337–339

112. Blum A, Balan SA, Scheringer M, et al. The Madrid statement on poly- and perfluoroalkyl substances (PFASs). *Environ Health Perspect.* 2015;123(5):A107–A111

113. European Commission. Food contaminants. 2015. Available at: http://ec.europa.eu/food/food/chemicalsafety/contaminants/index_en.htm. Accessed May 18, 2017

114. US Food and Drug Administration. Preliminary estimation of perchlorate

dietary exposure based on FDA 2004/2005 exploratory data. Available at: www.fda.gov/Food/ FoodborneIllnessContaminants/ ChemicalContaminants/ucm077653. htm. Accessed May 18, 2017

115. Maffini MV, Trasande L, Neltner TG. Perchlorate and diet: human exposures, risks, and mitigation strategies. *Curr Environ Health Rep.* 2016;3(2):107–117

116. Rogan WJ, Paulson JA, Baum C, et al; Council on Environmental Health. Iodine deficiency, pollutant chemicals, and the thyroid: new information on an old problem. *Pediatrics.* 2014;133(6):1163–1166

117. Zoeller RT, Rovet J. Timing of thyroid hormone action in the developing brain: clinical observations and experimental findings. *J Neuroendocrinol.* 2004;16(10):809–818

118. Miller MD, Crofton KM, Rice DC, Zoeller RT. Thyroid-disrupting chemicals: interpreting upstream biomarkers of adverse outcomes. *Environ Health Perspect.* 2009;117(7):1033–1041

119. Moog NK, Entringer S, Heim C, Wadhwa PD, Kathmann N, Buss C. Influence of maternal thyroid hormones during gestation on fetal brain development. *Neuroscience.* 2017;342:68–100

120. Päkkilä F, Männistö T, Hartikainen AL, et al. Maternal and child's thyroid function and child's intellect and scholastic performance. *Thyroid.* 2015;25(12):1363–1374

121. Haddow JE, Palomaki GE, Allan WC, et al. Maternal thyroid deficiency during pregnancy and subsequent neuropsychological development of the child. *N Engl J Med.* 1999;341(8):549–555

122. US Environmental Protection Agency; Science Advisory Board. Perchlorate - Approaches for Deriving Maximum Contaminant Level Goals for Drinking Water. 2013. Available at: https://yosemite.epa.gov/sab/ sabproduct.nsf/02ad90b136fc21ef8 5256eba00436459/d3bb75d4297ca4698 525794300522ace!OpenDocument& TableRow=2.2. Accessed May 18, 2017

123. Steinmaus C, Pearl M, Kharrazi M, et al. Thyroid hormones and moderate exposure to perchlorate during pregnancy in women in southern California. *Environ Health Perspect.* 2016;124(6):861–867

124. Abdelouahab N, Langlois MF, Lavoie L, Corbin F, Pasquier JC, Takser L. Maternal and cord-blood thyroid hormone levels and exposure to polybrominated diphenyl ethers and polychlorinated biphenyls during early pregnancy. *Am J Epidemiol.* 2013;178(5):701–713

125. Schecter A, Päpke O, Harris TR, et al. Polybrominated diphenyl ether (PBDE) levels in an expanded market basket survey of U.S. food and estimated PBDE dietary intake by age and sex. *Environ Health Perspect.* 2006;114(10):1515–1520

126. Wu N, Herrmann T, Paepke O, et al. Human exposure to PBDEs: associations of PBDE body burdens with food consumption and house dust concentrations. *Environ Sci Technol.* 2007;41(5):1584–1589

127. Hinton CF, Harris KB, Borgfeld L, et al. Trends in incidence rates of congenital hypothyroidism related to select demographic factors: data from the United States, California, Massachusetts, New York, and Texas. *Pediatrics.* 2010;125(suppl 2):S37–S47

128. Cao Y, Blount BC, Valentin-Blasini L, Bernbaum JC, Phillips TM, Rogan WJ. Goitrogenic anions, thyroid-stimulating hormone, and thyroid hormone in infants. *Environ Health Perspect.* 2010;118(9):1332–1337

129. US Food and Drug Administration. Summary of color additives for use in the United States in foods, drugs, cosmetics, and medical devices. Available at: www.fda.gov/ForIndustry/ ColorAdditives/ColorAdditiveInve ntories/ucm115641.htm. Accessed May 18, 2017

130. Stevens LJ, Burgess JR, Stochelski MA, Kuczek T. Amounts of artificial food colors in commonly consumed beverages and potential behavioral implications for consumption in children. *Clin Pediatr (Phila).* 2014;53(2):133–140

131. Nigg JT, Lewis K, Edinger T, Falk M. Meta-analysis of attention-deficit/ hyperactivity disorder or attention-deficit/hyperactivity disorder symptoms, restriction diet, and synthetic food color additives. *J Am Acad Child Adolesc Psychiatry.* 2012;51(1):86–97.e8

132. Stevens LJ, Kuczek T, Burgess JR, Stochelski MA, Arnold LE, Galland L. Mechanisms of behavioral, atopic, and other reactions to artificial food colors in children. *Nutr Rev.* 2013;71(5):268–281

133. Millichap JG, Yee MM. The diet factor in attention-deficit/hyperactivity disorder. *Pediatrics.* 2012;129(2):330–337

134. Weiss B. Synthetic food colors and neurobehavioral hazards: the view from environmental health research. *Environ Health Perspect.* 2012;120(1):1–5

135. Arnold LE, Lofthouse N, Hurt E. Artificial food colors and attention-deficit/ hyperactivity symptoms: conclusions to dye for. *Neurotherapeutics.* 2012;9(3):599–609

136. Kleinman RE, Brown RT, Cutter GR, Dupaul GJ, Clydesdale FM. A research model for investigating the effects of artificial food colorings on children with ADHD. *Pediatrics.* 2011;127(6):e1575–e1584

137. Nigg JT, Holton K. Restriction and elimination diets in ADHD treatment. *Child Adolesc Psychiatr Clin N Am.* 2014;23(4):937–953

138. Arnold LE, Hurt E, Lofthouse N. Attention-deficit/hyperactivity disorder: dietary and nutritional treatments. *Child Adolesc Psychiatr Clin N Am.* 2013;22(3):381–402, v

139. Stevenson J, Buitelaar J, Cortese S, et al. Research review: the role of diet in the treatment of attention-deficit/hyperactivity disorder—an appraisal of the evidence on efficacy and recommendations on the design of future studies. *J Child Psychol Psychiatry.* 2014;55(5):416–427

140. US Food and Drug Administration. Food advisory committee meeting. March 30-31, 2011. Available at: https:// wayback.archive-it.org/org-1137/ 20170406211705/https://www.fda. gov/downloads/AdvisoryCommittee s/CommitteesMeetingMaterials/ FoodAdvisoryCommittee/UCM255119. pdf. Accessed May 18, 2017

141. US Food and Drug Administration; Background Document for the

Food Advisory Committee. Certified color additives in food and possible association with attention deficit hyperactivity disorder in children. March 30–31, 2011. Available at: https://wayback.archive-it.org/org-1137/20170406211659/https://www.fda.gov/downloads/AdvisoryCommittees/CommitteesMeetingMaterials/FoodAdvisoryCommittee/UCM248549.pdf. Accessed May 18, 2017

142. Food and drugs color additives. *Fed Regist.* 1977; Codified as 21 CFR 70

143. Tricker AR, Preussmann R. Carcinogenic N-nitrosamines in the diet: occurrence, formation, mechanisms and carcinogenic potential. *Mutat Res.* 1991;259(3–4):277–289

144. American Medical Association; Council on Scientific Affairs. *Labeling of Nitrite Content of Processed Foods.* Chicago, IL: American Medical Association; 2004

145. Grosse Y, Baan R, Straif K, Secretan B, El Ghissassi F, Cogliano V; WHO International Agency for Research on Cancer Monograph Working Group. Carcinogenicity of nitrate, nitrite, and cyanobacterial peptide toxins. *Lancet Oncol.* 2006;7(8):628–629

146. Food additives permitted for direct addition to food for human consumption - food preservatives - sodium nitrite. *Fed Regist.* 2005; Codified as 21 CFR 1721.175

147. De Groef B, Decallonne BR, Van der Geyten S, Darras VM, Bouillon R. Perchlorate versus other environmental sodium/iodide symporter inhibitors: potential thyroid-related health effects. *Eur J Endocrinol.* 2006;155(1):17–25

148. Sebranek JG, Jackson-Davis AL, Myers KL, Lavieri NA. Beyond celery and starter culture: advances in natural/organic curing processes in the United States. *Meat Sci.* 2012;92(3):267–273

149. Neuman W. What's inside the bun? *New York Times.* July 1, 2011. Available at www.nytimes.com/2011/07/02/business/02hotdog.html. Accessed May 18, 2017

150. Nuñez De González MT, Osburn WN, Hardin MD, et al. Survey of residual nitrite and nitrate in conventional and organic/natural/uncured/indirectly cured meats available at retail in the United States. *J Agric Food Chem.* 2012;60(15):3981–3990

Interpretation of Do Not Attempt Resuscitation Orders for Children Requiring Anesthesia and Surgery

• *Clinical Report*

CLINICAL REPORT   Guidance for the Clinician in Rendering Pediatric Care

American Academy
of Pediatrics

DEDICATED TO THE HEALTH OF ALL CHILDREN™

Interpretation of Do Not Attempt Resuscitation Orders for Children Requiring Anesthesia and Surgery

Mary E. Fallat, MD, FAAP,[a] Courtney Hardy, MD, MBA, FAAP,[b] SECTION ON SURGERY, SECTION ON ANESTHESIOLOGY AND PAIN MEDICINE, COMMITTEE ON BIOETHICS

abstract

This clinical report addresses the topic of pre-existing do not attempt resuscitation or limited resuscitation orders for children and adolescents undergoing anesthesia and surgery. Pertinent considerations for the clinician include the rights of children, decision-making by parents or legally approved representatives, the process of informed consent, and the roles of surgeon and anesthesiologist. A process of re-evaluation of the do not attempt resuscitation orders, called "required reconsideration," should be incorporated into the process of informed consent for surgery and anesthesia, distinguishing between goal-directed and procedure-directed approaches. The child's individual needs are best served by allowing the parent or legally approved representative and involved clinicians to consider whether full resuscitation, limitations based on procedures, or limitations based on goals is most appropriate.

[a]Department of Surgery, University of Louisville, Louisville, Kentucky; and [b]Division of Pediatric Anesthesiology, Washington University in St Louis, St Louis, Missouri

Dr Fallat developed the outline, revised the original publication as a draft, responded to all queries and comments generated by reviewing sections and committees, developed the next draft, twice vetted the paper with the Committee on Bioethics and attended a conference call with the committee members to interpret and add their edits, developed the final draft, and responded to the board member's comments. Dr Hardy's contributions included writing and reviewing, and he approves the final manuscript.

This document is copyrighted and is property of the American Academy of Pediatrics and its Board of Directors. All authors have filed conflict of interest statements with the American Academy of Pediatrics. Any conflicts have been resolved through a process approved by the Board of Directors. The American Academy of Pediatrics has neither solicited nor accepted any commercial involvement in the development of the content of this publication.

Clinical reports from the American Academy of Pediatrics benefit from expertise and resources of liaisons and internal (AAP) and external reviewers. However, clinical reports from the American Academy of Pediatrics may not reflect the views of the liaisons or the organizations or government agencies that they represent.

The guidance in this report does not indicate an exclusive course of treatment or serve as a standard of medical care. Variations, taking into account individual circumstances, may be appropriate.

All clinical reports from the American Academy of Pediatrics automatically expire 5 years after publication unless reaffirmed, revised, or retired at or before that time.

To cite: Fallat ME, Hardy C, , AAP SECTION ON SURGERY, AAP SECTION ON ANESTHESIOLOGY AND PAIN MEDICINE, AAP COMMITTEE ON BIOETHICS. Interpretation of Do Not Attempt Resuscitation Orders for Children Requiring Anesthesia and Surgery. Pediatrics. 2018;141(5):e20180598

CONSIDERATIONS FOR CHILDREN WITH DO NOT RESUSCITATE OR LIMITED RESUSCITATION ORDERS WHO REQUIRE ANESTHESIA AND SURGERY

Origin of Do Not Resuscitate Orders

In the 1970s, the Critical Care Committee at Massachusetts General Hospital developed the original do not resuscitate (DNR) guidelines in response to nursing requests for clarification of what should be done when cardiopulmonary resuscitation (CPR) was unwanted or believed to be unwarranted by a patient, parent, or legally approved representative (hereafter referred to as representative).[1] Alternative names or abbreviations for a DNR policy vary geographically, with some including the letter "A," as in "do not attempt resuscitation" or "DNAR."[2,3] For purposes of this document, the term DNAR will be used, recognizing that neither of these terms carries a universal meaning. Both DNR and DNAR terms imply the omission of action, historically synonymous and sometimes misperceived as "giving up," and some have advocated for the term "allow natural death," to emphasize that the order is to allow the natural consequences of a disease or injury and to emphasize ongoing end-of-life care.[2] Partial DNR or limited resuscitation orders are also described.[4–6] DNAR orders may be clinically and ethically appropriate when the burdens of resuscitation exceed the expected benefit. A common misunderstanding that patients and families have is that CPR (calling a code) will keep patients alive and living exactly as they were before the code, not recognizing that the need for CPR can result in ischemia to the brain and resultant long-term disability.

Currently, all hospitals seeking accreditation from The Joint Commission are required to have a DNAR or resuscitation limits policy in place.[7] The policy should define a DNAR order and describe the guidelines for its inclusion in a patient's medical record. A DNAR order implies a documented discussion with the patient, family, or representative, addressing the patient's wishes about resuscitation interventions. DNAR orders specify what interventions are permitted and what interventions are not permitted. The orders need to be documented in the medical record in a standardized fashion such that they are clearly identified and are uniformly accessible by all medical care providers. In some institutions, they will be featured in some way, such as color-coding. Hard copies may be printed if the patient is traveling to another location in the hospital. Some jurisdictions may require confirmation by a witness or a second treating physician. DNAR orders should not have implications regarding the use of other therapeutic interventions that may be appropriate for the patient, including surgery and anesthesia.[8–10]

Origin of DNAR Orders for Patients Undergoing Surgery and Anesthesia

The controversial topic of DNAR orders for patients undergoing surgery and anesthesia has received growing attention in the medical literature since the early 1990s. Authors began to more specifically address the pediatric age group, beginning with the publication of the predecessor of this clinical report in 2004, "Do-Not-Resuscitate Orders for Pediatric Patients Who Require Anesthesia and Surgery."[11] For children, contemporary DNAR orders are generally written when (1) in the judgment of the treating physician, an attempt to resuscitate the child will not benefit the child (this may be with or without parent or representative concurrence; for example, if the child has satisfied state criteria for brain death); or (2) the parent or representative (with the assent of a developmentally appropriate child) expresses his or her preference that CPR be withheld in the event the child suffers a cardiopulmonary arrest, and the physician concurs.[8,12,13] DNAR orders usually are written with the assumption that cardiopulmonary arrest will be a spontaneous event that is the culmination of the dying process of a child who has a terminal or life-limiting illness with an expected decline in bodily function over time. The dilemma with which surgeons and anesthesiologists are confronted regarding children with DNAR orders undergoing an operative procedure is twofold: (1) anesthesia promotes some degree of hemodynamic abnormality that may result in cardiopulmonary arrest, and (2) many routine anesthetic manipulations can be classified as resuscitative measures.

A number of hospitals across the nation still do not have a policy that specifically addresses the extent to which DNAR orders apply in the operating room. Hospital and anesthesia staff continue to

advocate suspension of the DNAR in the operating room.[14–16] There is persistent reticence by some specialty surgeons to routinely discuss advance directives preoperatively or to perform surgery on adult patients whose directives limit postoperative care.[17] The American Academy of Pediatrics and the American Society of Anesthesiologists (ASA) have issued guidelines on forgoing life-sustaining medical treatment, issues of informed consent,[18,19] and evaluation and preparation of pediatric patients undergoing anesthesia.[20] None of these policies offers a detailed approach for operative procedures considered for children with an existing DNAR order. In the current statement, we address the dilemmas of who should assume responsibility (ie, the primary care physician, the surgeon, or the anesthesiologist) for discussing with the parent or representative the potential risks of cardiopulmonary arrest during surgery and anesthesia, whether the DNAR order should be temporarily suspended during the procedure, and how long a temporary suspension should last if this option is chosen. Early involvement of palliative care may help families and the medical team better gauge the need for operative procedures, their goals, and what to do if there is an intraoperative change in status.[21]

DISCUSSION

Physicians caring for children have a duty to respect the wishes of the child and family, to do good (beneficence), and to avoid harm (nonmaleficence). This may lead to conflicting considerations for a child with a DNAR order. Some physicians believe that honoring a DNAR request harms a child by allowing a potentially preventable death to occur. Others believe that the child's welfare is best served by not having a sustained and poor health-related quality of life and not having to endure nonbeneficial therapy, which may be painful or unpleasant.[14,15,21] Older children and adolescents should be included in the decision-making process (patient assent) when their neurologic status, development, and level of maturity allow. However, state laws usually require that a parent or legal representative make these decisions on the child's behalf[18] because this individual generally will be the person presumed to be the most appropriate and capable to determine what actions would be in the best interest of the child. Conflicts arise when the parent or representative and/or child and the physician fail to agree on what would be optimal care under a given set of circumstances.

Resuscitative interventions outside of the operating room setting are those used to prevent or reverse cardiopulmonary arrest.[22] The operative setting complicates a discussion of resuscitative interventions because anesthetic agents routinely promote cardiovascular instability.[11,12,14,22] During the perioperative period, resuscitative measures only refer to the measures undertaken to restore spontaneous respiration and circulation once a cardiopulmonary arrest has occurred.[9,23] Surveys of physicians and patients with DNAR orders confirm that clarification is needed on the interpretation of a DNAR order, especially its applicability in the operating room.[24,25]

Informed Permission

Physicians generally must obtain informed permission from a parent or representative before a child can undergo any medical intervention, including surgery.[19] For resuscitation efforts, consent may often be inferred from emergency circumstances, unless the patient's representative is available to provide or refuse consent or unless there is evidence that consent would be refused if sought.

However, the parents of terminally ill children or children with life-limiting severe disabilities may have already been asked to address whether resuscitation should be attempted in the event the child's underlying disease results in cardiopulmonary arrest.

Customarily, physicians will approach the parent or representative about instituting a DNAR or the limits of resuscitation order when it is believed that resuscitation of the child would not be beneficial and would only prolong the dying process.[25] When a parent or representative agrees to a DNAR order, it is generally a decision guided by information a physician or medical team has provided, anticipating that cardiopulmonary arrest will be a direct consequence of the child's underlying disease. Surgery and anesthesia each introduce additional risks to the patient and may lead to different probabilities of a successful outcome, depending on the strategy. For example, local or regional anesthesia might be a good strategy for some procedures, but only in a cooperative patient. Because surgeons and anesthesiologists are rarely involved in the original DNAR decision, they cannot be certain that the implications of the DNAR status in the perioperative setting were discussed with the patient's parent or representative.[15] Therefore, it is appropriate for the parent or representative, the surgeon, and the anesthesiologist to re-evaluate the DNAR order for a child who requires an operative procedure. This re-evaluation process is called "required reconsideration"[15] and may be incorporated into the process of informed consent for surgery and anesthesia. Discussions with families and patients regarding consent under these circumstances may be initiated by attending staff, particularly in hospitals with residency teaching programs, where residents may be routinely involved in the consent process.

There is often no previous relationship established between the patient, parents, and surgical team, with the exception of a brief preoperative assessment. Active listening and compassionate understanding are essential and are a critical part of patient- and family-centered care.[26] Using an integrated approach by including the hospitalist, intensive care, or palliative care team in the discussion is appropriate and may be more comfortable for the family. Including the primary care physician is also an option if he or she is available and willing to be part of the discussion. The parent or representative is asked about specific interventions and his or her understanding of the relative merits of each of these interventions during anesthesia and surgery (Table 1).[20] Airway management is determined by what is mandated by the child's condition and the surgical procedure. Specific prohibition of tracheal intubation is problematic, and beliefs and concerns of the patient and family are carefully elicited and discussed. Exceptions to the injunctions against intervention are specifically noted in the patient's medical record. The parent or representative may agree to a temporary suspension of the DNAR order during the perioperative period. If so, the temporal end point to the DNAR suspension needs to be recorded. If an agreement cannot be obtained after thorough discussion, the wishes of the informed parent or representative will prevail. In some cases, the parents may believe that the burden of a therapy is not worth the potential benefits and decline the procedure. When an individual physician believes that the parent's wishes are inconsistent with his or her medical, ethical, or moral views, the physician's professional refusal of participation in care may be appropriate, with withdrawal from the case after ensuring continuity of care.[11,18] Consultation with the institutional ethics committee may be beneficial.[27]

TABLE 1 Perioperative Interventions

Airway management
    Bag and mask ventilation
    Intubation
Needle thoracentesis
Chest tube insertion
Blood product transfusion
Invasive monitoring (eg, central venous,
    arterial)
Chest compressions
Defibrillation
Cardiac pacing
Point-of-care arrest medications (epinephrine,
    atropine, sodium bicarbonate, calcium,
    other vasoactive drugs)
Postoperative ventilation support

Optimum care for hopelessly ill patients. A report of the Clinical Care Committee of the Massachusetts General Hospital. *N Engl J Med.* 1976;295(7):362–364.

Role of the Surgeon or Proceduralist

The following are representative operative interventions that might be considered for a pediatric patient with a DNAR order. Some of these are procedures that might be performed in interventional radiology by a radiologist, in the endoscopy suite by a gastroenterologist or pulmonologist, or at the bedside:

1. Provision of a support device that will enable the child to be discharged from the hospital (eg, gastrostomy tube or tracheostomy);

2. Urgent surgery for a condition unrelated to the underlying chronic problem (eg, acute appendicitis in a patient with terminal cancer);

3. Urgent surgery for a condition related to the underlying chronic problem but not believed to be a terminal event (eg, a pathologic fracture or bowel obstruction);

4. A procedure to decrease pain;

5. A procedure to provide vascular access; and

6. An endoscopic procedure to investigate gastrointestinal tract bleeding.

As part of the expected professional role, the operating surgeon is required to discuss the risks of a procedure with the parent or representative of any pediatric patient, including how the patient's condition might influence the risk of anesthesia. The American College of Surgeons issued a statement to guide surgeons in operating on patients with an active DNAR order.[28] The Association of periOperative Registered Nurses also has a similar statement to guide the essential members of the perioperative team.[29] It is expected that the surgeon will advise the parent or representative and the child (if developmentally appropriate) regarding the operative risks and benefits and recommend a policy of required reconsideration of previous DNAR orders. The results of all discussions are documented in the patient's medical record. The surgeon will ultimately convey the patient's and/or representative's wishes to the members of the entire surgical team, help team members understand the wishes of the patient, parent, or representative, and replace individuals who find that the family's wishes conflict with their personal values. The difficulty arises when there is no one who is willing to honor a family's wish to continue the DNAR status during anesthesia and surgery. Stalemates such as this may be referred to the ethics committee of the institution.

Role of the Anesthesiologist

As early as 1994, the ASA released recommendations on caring for surgical patients with active DNAR orders, explicitly rejecting the practice of automatically rescinding the DNAR order before procedures involving the use of anesthesia because this practice "may not sufficiently address a patient's rights to self-determination in a responsible and ethical manner."[20] The purpose of required reconsideration of DNAR orders is to determine what is best for the patient under the circumstances, not to convince the patient and family to have the DNAR order suspended. The guidelines proposed by the ASA clearly recommend that all physicians involved in the case (primary physician, surgeon, and anesthesiologist) discuss together with the patient (and parent or representative) the appropriateness of maintaining the DNAR order during the operation, distinguishing between goal-directed and procedure-directed DNAR orders. This integrated approach is a hallmark of patient- and family-centered care.[26] Model procedure-specific DNAR documentation forms are published and may be modified for individual hospital use.[12]

A common concern of families is that the preoperative anesthesiologist is often not the one who will perform the procedure, making specific communication with the anesthesiologist of record optimal, if at all possible. A number of procedures are also now performed by using "sedation" and may be performed outside of the operating room environment. For purposes of this statement, the considerations regarding pre-existing DNAR orders are the same.

Goal-Directed Approach

A goal-directed approach is used to focus on the patient's goals, values, and preferences rather than on individual procedures that may be used in resuscitation. The primary goal is to do everything to prevent the need for resuscitation, but if it is indicated, this approach is used to recognize that patients are often less concerned with technical details of the resuscitation than with more subjective and personal issues regarding quality of life before and after resuscitation. An approach that honors the family's treatment goals while reflecting the reality and unique aspects of the perioperative environment is promulgated with this model. However, some anesthesiologists are uncomfortable with the indeterminate nature of a goal-directed DNAR order and have ethical or legal concerns about having such crucial decisions rest solely on their best judgment at the time of an arrest. In addition, goal-directed DNAR orders may be less feasible if the anesthesiologist and surgeon caring for the child have not established a relationship with the family before surgery.

Procedure-Directed Approach

A procedure-directed approach may be more appropriate in these circumstances, which involves careful consideration of a series of specific interventions that are more likely to be used (Table 1). This checklist is not unlike what might be used if a child has resuscitation limits. Each procedure must be placed in the context of the child's usual quality of life and likelihood of the ability of the procedure to produce the desired effect, given his or her unique physiology. This approach has limited flexibility when an unexpected situation occurs.[12] In addition, many of the procedures listed are not resuscitative by nature, but circumstance and the ability of the medical team to convey this effectively and without misunderstanding may be difficult. Critics of this approach believe that parents or caregivers often lack the capacity to truly understand the plan being developed, whereas proponents believe that at least some parents can make thoughtful decisions about specific interventions, and their wishes should be respected.[4–6,10] Although the goal-directed approach can conceivably be integrated with a procedure-directed approach (ie, formulating a procedure-directed plan based on the parent and patient goals), this often requires the luxury of time and is not always feasible. However, many of the procedures that might be considered in this group of children also are not emergencies, and there is time for thoughtful discussion and decision.

Perioperative suspension of the DNAR order is considered by some anesthesiologists to be the ideal compromise because it enables the physician to act without restraint while providing the patient with a realistic chance of achieving the operative goals.[30,31] Anesthetic agents and techniques may promote some degree of hemodynamic and respiratory instability, especially in patients with a deteriorated health condition.[16,32] The deliberate depression of vital functions by the anesthetic may require resuscitative measures to stabilize the patient.[33] Consequently, controversy about the use of these interventions arises when the patient has a written DNAR order. Many of the routine anesthetic interventions performed as part of operative support are considered resuscitative measures under different circumstances. These include the use of paralytic agents, vasoactive drugs, blood products, and positive-pressure ventilation. This overlap in terminology promotes confusion and inconsistencies among physicians in the interpretation of a patient's DNAR order and what it implies in an operative setting. Keffer and Keffer[23] have proposed that resuscitation in the operating room be defined as "those measures undertaken to re-establish cardiac rhythm once a cardiac arrest has occurred." This definition establishes a simple end point beyond which a patient's desire to not be resuscitated would come into play.

For a fragile patient, providing anesthesia can be a fine balance between controlling pain and supporting hemodynamic stability, for example, in a preterm newborn infant or a septic patient. The anesthesiologist's concern for patient comfort during the procedure may support perioperative suspension of DNAR orders. An active DNAR order restricts the physicians' ability to treat any complications of their own procedure during anesthesia. Faced with this dilemma, anesthesiologists

are forced to decrease the risk of cardiopulmonary arrest by increasing hemodynamic stability through the use of less anesthetic.[33,34] For the patient, this may potentially result in more discomfort and suffering.

One reason to distinguish DNAR in the operating room from DNAR in other settings is the difference in the success rate of CPR administered for a spontaneous cardiopulmonary arrest versus one that results from anesthesia. Anesthetic-related arrests are believed to be more easily reversible because of the immediate ability to respond and the controlled nature of the event.[35–37] When a cardiac arrest is ascribed to anesthesia, there is a better chance of successful resuscitation.[38] This increased chance of recovery is likely based on the fact that the arrest is not attributable to the underlying disease and does not necessarily presage death. A relevant survey was conducted on 4301 seriously ill adult patients, of which 745 underwent an operative procedure and 57 had previously written DNAR orders in their medical records. Only 3 of the 57 patients with preoperative DNAR orders (5%) experienced an intraoperative cardiopulmonary arrest, 2 of whom had the DNAR order reversed before surgery and 1 who did not and died in the operating room without an attempt at resuscitation. All 3 patients died within 5 days of operation.[38] Overall, 31 (54%) of the patients with DNAR orders who underwent surgery survived to leave the hospital, and 30% survived at least 4 months.

A more recent review of 4128 adult patients with a DNAR order and 4128 age-matched and procedure-matched patients without a DNAR order in 120 hospitals participating in the American College of Surgeons National Surgical Quality Improvement Program from 2005 to 2008 reported that surgical patients with DNAR orders have significant comorbidities; many patients sustain postoperative complications, and nearly 1 in 4 die within 30 days of surgery. DNR status was an independent risk factor for poor surgical outcome.[16,32] The multivariate logistic regression model was adjusted for more than 30 risk factors, including ASA class 3 to 5, ascites, albumin level <3.5 g/dL, impaired sensorium, preoperative sepsis, disseminated cancer, and dialysis dependence.

The possibility of legal action or investigation exists when withholding or withdrawing care at the end of a patient's life. Standard and accepted practices of communication, collaboration, and a well-documented DNAR order, with documentation of the conversation and decision from the patient and family, will be legally protective.[39]

Traditionally, CPR has been considered a success if the patient survives the initial resuscitation effort. For patients with pre-existing DNAR orders who consider rescinding this status perioperatively, the utility of CPR may be better gauged on the length of patient survival and health care–related quality of life after resuscitation. By using this definition, CPR may be inappropriate from the parent or representative viewpoint if resuscitation has the overwhelming probability of resulting in patient suffering and only prolonging the time to death.[8] The anesthesiologist will need to inform the parent or representative of the risks and potential benefits of intraoperative resuscitation. Required reconsideration as part of the process of informed consent for anesthesia may reduce ambiguities and misunderstandings associated with patients who have DNAR orders. It will provide anesthesiologists with the opportunity to educate the parent or representative and become familiar with their values and perceptions of the child's quality of life and together clarify how the child's DNAR order should be interpreted perioperatively. By giving parents or representatives and clinicians the option of choosing from among full resuscitation, limitations based on procedures, or limitations based on goals, the child's needs are individualized and better served. Regardless of the decision made by the parent or representative, the individual acting on behalf of the child must be readily available for consultation during the procedure. The ASA, like the American College of Surgeons, advocates that physicians withdraw from a case if they are unwilling or unable to respect and implement the decision of the patient (or parent or representative) to limit the use of resuscitation.[20,28]

If DNAR Orders Are Suspended

If the decision is made to suspend DNAR orders during anesthesia and surgery, it is necessary to define the duration of suspension.[20,40] The physiologic effects of anesthesia and surgery rarely terminate at the end of the procedure, but the duration thereafter depends on the anesthetic technique used and the type of surgical procedure performed. The acute effects of most anesthetic medications generally resolve within several hours or a day after surgery. It is a requirement of the Centers for Medicaid & Medicare Services that an inpatient have a postoperative visit within 48 hours of a procedure involving anesthesia and that there be documentation in the medical record.[41] Recovery of respiratory function after surgery is dependent on preoperative pulmonary function, chronicity of illness, and length of the procedure. Some patients will experience cardiopulmonary arrest during or immediately after surgery resulting from an acute and reversible complication. It may be appropriate to use mechanical ventilation after surgery as long as the patient continues to show significant and sustained improvement in pulmonary function. Once the patient ceases to recover or deteriorates, withdrawal of ventilatory support may be considered. This might include compassionate extubation for end-of-life comfort care with family present. Generally speaking, the suspension of DNAR orders continue until the postanesthetic visit, until the patient has been weaned from mechanical ventilation, or until the primary physician involved in the patient's care and the family agree to reinstate the DNAR order.

The surgeon and anesthesiologist may, in consultation with the family, reinstate a DNAR order intraoperatively. For example, if cardiac arrest occurs during surgery, and it is apparent that the arrest is the result of an irreversible underlying disease or complication and that CPR would only allow continued deterioration, the DNAR order may be reinstated.

If resuscitation measures are withheld and intraoperative arrest occurs, such a death may be classified as "expected" for quality assurance purposes, rather than "unexpected." Expected deaths do not require root cause analysis or the in-depth quality assurance review of the individual providers or program required when the death is unexpected, but expected deaths will still require notification of the medical examiner and organ procurement organization.[14,22,41,42] Discussion of the death for educational purposes is valuable and allows staff debriefing of the event to prevent secondary psychological trauma and to examine the appropriateness of the patient's refusal of aggressive treatment, whether documentation was adequate, and whether care was consistent with the patient's wishes.[14,22,41]

IMPLEMENTING REQUIRED RECONSIDERATION

Hospitals are encouraged to develop and maintain written

policies permitting the forgoing of life-sustaining treatment of patients, including the child or adolescent patient, in appropriate circumstances.[18,19] Once a DNAR order is in place according to accepted standards, it is important that it be reviewed before surgery to determine applicability in the operating room and the postoperative recovery period. Table 2 lists the ideal elements of a required reconsideration policy for children with a DNAR or limited resuscitation orders, and the following represents a summary of the essential elements of discussion and documentation:

- A preoperative discussion with the child's parent or representative and the developmentally appropriate child or adolescent, including information about the likelihood of requiring resuscitation, the potential causes of an arrest and their reversibility, the chance of success, and possible outcomes with and without resuscitation;

- An agreement about what, if any, resuscitative measures will be instituted during the procedure;

- A decision to uphold or suspend a DNAR order on the basis of the planned procedure, the anticipated benefit for the child, and the likelihood of patient compromise as a result of the procedure;

- Documentation of the salient features of the physician-family discussion in the medical record;

- Communication by the surgeon of plans to honor an intraoperative DNAR order to relevant staff;

- Allowing a physician or other health care professional who is unwilling to honor a family's refusal of resuscitation to withdraw from the case and allow others to assume care. Ideally, the withdrawing

TABLE 2 Required Reconsideration Options for Pediatric Patients With DNAR Orders Who Require Anesthesia and Surgery

Full resuscitation
　Perioperative suspension of DNAR orders with qualification of perioperative interval
Goal-directed approach
　Focuses on patient goals, values, and preferences
　Implies personal relationship between physician and patient and family with understanding of quality-of-life concerns
　Most subjective approach
Procedure-directed approach
　Specific interventions (see Table 1) placed in context of child's quality of life are each reviewed before procedure

physician or health care professional will make a conscientious effort to identify another health care professional to replace him or her with someone who is willing to honor the DNAR request[11,14];

- Recognition that the decision of a patient, parent, or representative to refuse intraoperative resuscitation can be compatible with the provision of therapeutic measures (including those listed in Table 1, with the exception of chest compressions and defibrillation) to treat conditions other than arrest. This decision does not necessarily imply limits on other forms of care, such as intensive care; and

- If the family chooses to rescind the DNAR order in the operating room and arrest culminates in successful resuscitation, but the patient's process of dying has only been prolonged, make a provision to discuss withdrawal of life support after a determined amount of time.[20,40]

LEAD AUTHORS

Mary E. Fallat, MD, FAAP
Courtney Hardy, MD, MBA, FAAP

SECTION ON SURGERY, 2017–2018

Rebecka L. Meyers, MD, FAAP, Chairperson
Gail Ellen Besner, MD, FAAP
Andrew Davidoff, MD, FACS, FAAP

Mary E. Fallat, MD, FAAP
Kurt F. Heiss, MD, FAAP

STAFF

Vivian Baldassari Thorne

SECTION ON ANESTHESIOLOGY AND PAIN MEDICINE, 2017–2018

Rita Agarwal, MD, FAAP, Chairperson
Joseph Tobias, MD, FAAP, Immediate Past Chairperson
Raeford Eugene Brown Jr, MD, FAAP
Nina A. Guzzetta, MD, FAAP
Courtney Hardy, MD, FAAP
Anita Honkanen, MD, FAAP
Mary Landrigan-Ossar, MD, PhD, FAAP

LIAISONS

Randall P. Flick, MD, MPH, FAAP – *American Society of Anesthesiologists*
Constance Susan Houck, MD, FAAP – *American Academy of Pediatrics Committee on Drugs*

STAFF

Jennifer Riefe

COMMITTEE ON BIOETHICS, 2017–2018

Aviva L. Katz, MD, MA, FAAP, Chairperson
Naomi Tricot Laventhal, MD, FAAP
Robert C. Macauley, MD, MDiv, FAAP
Margaret Rusha Moon, MD, FAAP
Alexander L. Okun, MD, FAAP
Douglas J. Opel, MD, MPH, FAAP
Mindy B. Statter, MD, FAAP

LIAISONS

Dawn Davies, MD, FRCPC, MA – *Canadian Paediatric Society*
Mary Lynn Dell, MD, DMin – *American Academy of Child and Adolescent Psychiatry*
Douglas S. Diekema, MD, MPH, FAAP – *American Board of Pediatrics*
Sigal Klipstein, MD – *American College of Obstetricians and Gynecologists*

CONSULTANT

Nanette Elster, JD, MPH – *Legal Consultant*

STAFF

Florence Rivera

ABBREVIATIONS

ASA: American Society of Anesthesiologists
CPR: cardiopulmonary resuscitation
DNAR: do not attempt resuscitation
DNR: do not resuscitate

DOI: https://doi.org/10.1542/peds.2018-0598

Address correspondence to Mary E. Fallat. E-mail: mefall01@louisville.edu

PEDIATRICS (ISSN Numbers: Print, 0031-4005; Online, 1098-4275).

FINANCIAL DISCLOSURE: The authors have indicated they have no financial relationships relevant to this article to disclose.

FUNDING: No external funding.

POTENTIAL CONFLICT OF INTEREST: The authors have indicated they have no potential conflicts of interest to disclose.

REFERENCES

1. Optimum care for hopelessly ill patients. A report of the Clinical Care Committee of the Massachusetts General Hospital. *N Engl J Med*. 1976;295(7):362–364

2. Breault JL. DNR, DNAR, or AND? Is language important? *Ochsner J*. 2011;11(4):302–306

3. Morrison W, Berkowitz I. Do not attempt resuscitation orders in pediatrics. *Pediatr Clin North Am*. 2007;54(5):757–771, xi–xii

4. Sanders A, Schepp M, Baird M. Partial do-not-resuscitate orders: a hazard to patient safety and clinical outcomes? *Crit Care Med*. 2011;39(1):14–18

5. Berger JT. Ethical challenges of partial do-not-resuscitate (DNR) orders: placing DNR orders in the context of a life-threatening conditions care plan. *Arch Intern Med*. 2003;163(19):2270–2275

6. Dumot JA, Burval DJ, Sprung J, et al. Outcome of adult cardiopulmonary resuscitations at a tertiary referral center including results of "limited" resuscitations. *Arch Intern Med*. 2001;161(14):1751–1758

7. The Joint Commission. Patient rights. In: *Manual of the Joint Commission on Accreditation of Health Care Organizations*. Chicago, IL: The Joint Commission; 1994

8. American Medical Association. *Code of Medical Ethics*. Chicago, IL: American Medical Association; 2016

9. Keffer MJ, Keffer HL. The do-not-resuscitate order. Moral responsibilities of the perioperative nurse. *AORN J*. 1994;59(3):641–645, 648–650

10. Gelbman BD, Gelbman JM. Deconstructing DNR. *J Med Ethics*. 2008;34(9):640–641

11. Fallat ME, Deshpande JK; American Academy of Pediatrics; Section on Surgery; Section on Anesthesia and Pain Medicine; Committee on Bioethics. Do-not-resuscitate orders for pediatric patients who require anesthesia and surgery. *Pediatrics*. 2004;114(6):1686–1692

12. Truog RD, Waisel DB, Burns JP. DNR in the OR: a goal-directed approach. *Anesthesiology*. 1999;90(1):289–295

13. Jackson S. Perioperative do-not-resuscitate orders. *AMA J Ethics*. 2015;17(3):229–235

14. Ewanchuk M, Brindley PG. Perioperative do-not-resuscitate orders—doing 'nothing' when 'something' can be done. *Crit Care*. 2006;10(4):219

15. Truog RD, Waisel DB, Burns JP. Do-not-resuscitate orders in the surgical setting. *Lancet*. 2005;365(9461):733–735

16. McCoy KL, Carty SE. Surgery and do-not-resuscitate orders: the real risks defined. Comment on "high mortality in surgical patients with do-not-resuscitate orders". *Arch Surg*. 2011;146(8):928–929

17. Redmann AJ, Brasel KJ, Alexander CG, Schwarze ML. Use of advance directives for high-risk operations: a national survey of surgeons. *Ann Surg*. 2012;255(3):418–423

18. Weise KL, Okun AL, Carter BS, Christian CW; Committee on Bioethics; Section on Hospice and Palliative Medicine; Committee on Child Abuse and Neglect. Guidance on forgoing life-sustaining medical treatment. *Pediatrics*. 2017;140(3):e20171905

19. Committee on Bioethics. Informed consent in decision-making in pediatric practice. *Pediatrics*. 2016;138(2):e20161484

20. American Society of Anesthesiologists; Committee on Ethics. *Ethical Guidelines for the Anesthesia Care of Patients With Do-Not-Resuscitate Orders or Other Directives That Limit Treatment*. Park Ridge, IL: American Society of Anesthesiologists. Available at: https://www.asahq.org/~/media/sites/asahq/files/public/resources/standards-guidelines/ethical-guidelines-for-the-anesthesia-care-of-patients.pdf. Accessed June 12, 2017

21. American Academy of Pediatrics; Committee on Bioethics and Committee on Hospital Care. Palliative care for children. *Pediatrics*. 2000;106(2, pt 1):351–357

22. Walker RM. DNR in the OR. Resuscitation as an operative risk. *JAMA*. 1991;266(17):2407–2412

23. Keffer MJ, Keffer HL. Do-not-resuscitate in the operating room: moral obligations of anesthesiologists. *Anesth Analg*. 1992;74(6):901–905

24. La Puma J, Silverstein MD, Stocking CB, Roland D, Siegler M. Life-sustaining treatment. A prospective study of patients with DNR orders in a teaching hospital. *Arch Intern Med*. 1988;148(10):2193–2198

25. Sanderson A, Zurakowski D, Wolfe J. Clinician perspectives regarding the do-not-resuscitate order. *JAMA Pediatr*. 2013;167(10):954–958

26. Committee on Hospital Care and Institute for Patient- and Family-Centered Care. Patient- and

family-centered care and the pediatrician's role. *Pediatrics.* 2012;129(2):394–404

27. American Academy of Pediatrics; Committee on Bioethics. Institutional ethics committees. Committee on Bioethics. *Pediatrics.* 2001;107(1):205–209

28. American College of Surgeons. Statement on advance directives by patients: "do not resuscitate" in the operating room. *Bull Am Coll Surg.* 2014;99(1):42–43

29. Association of periOperative Registered Nurses. *Position Statement on Perioperative Care of Patients With Do-Not-Resuscitate or Allow-Natural-Death Orders.* Denver, CO: Association of periOperative Registered Nurses; 2014

30. Cohen NH. Do not resuscitate orders in the operating room: the birth of a policy. *Camb Q Healthc Ethics.* 1995;4(1):103–110

31. Fine PG, Jackson SH. Do not resuscitate in the operating room: more than rights and wrongs. *Am J Anesthesiol.* 1995;22(1):46–51

32. Kazaure H, Roman S, Sosa JA. High mortality in surgical patients with do-not-resuscitate orders: analysis of 8256 patients. *Arch Surg.* 2011;146(8):922–928

33. Truog RD. "Do-not-resuscitate" orders during anesthesia and surgery. *Anesthesiology.* 1991;74(3):606–608

34. Bernat JL, Grabowski EW. Suspending do-not-resuscitate orders during anesthesia and surgery. *Surg Neurol.* 1993;40(1):7–9

35. Cohen CB, Cohen PJ. Do-not-resuscitate orders in the operating room. *N Engl J Med.* 1991;325(26):1879–1882

36. Martin RL, Soifer BE, Stevens WC. Ethical issues in anesthesia: management of the do-not-resuscitate patient. *Anesth Analg.* 1991;73(2):221–225

37. Olsson GL, Hallén B. Cardiac arrest during anaesthesia. A computer-aided study in 250,543 anaesthetics. *Acta Anaesthesiol Scand.* 1988;32(8):653–664

38. Wenger NS, Greengold NL, Oye RK, et al. Patients with DNR orders in the operating room: surgery, resuscitation, and outcomes. SUPPORT investigators. Study to understand prognoses and preferences for outcomes and risks of treatments. *J Clin Ethics.* 1997;8(3):250–257

39. Waisel D, Jackson S, Fine P. Should do-not-resuscitate orders be suspended for surgical cases? *Curr Opin Anaesthesiol.* 2003;16(2):209–213

40. Bernat JL. Ethical issues in the perioperative management of neurologic patients. *Neurol Clin.* 2004;22(2):viii–ix, 457–471

41. CMS Manual System. Department of Health & Human Services (DHHS) Centers for Medicare & Medicaid Services (CMS). Transmittal 74. Effective/Implementation Date: 12/2/2011. Interpretive Guidelines §482.52(b)(3)

42. Youngner SJ, Cascorbi HF, Shuck JM. DNR in the operating room. Not really a paradox. *JAMA.* 1991;266(17):2433–2434

Management of Neonates Born at ≥35 0/7 Weeks' Gestation With Suspected or Proven Early-Onset Bacterial Sepsis

• *Clinical Report*

CLINICAL REPORT   Guidance for the Clinician in Rendering Pediatric Care

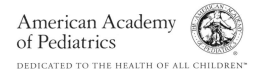

American Academy
of Pediatrics

DEDICATED TO THE HEALTH OF ALL CHILDREN™

Management of Neonates Born at ≥35 0/7 Weeks' Gestation With Suspected or Proven Early-Onset Bacterial Sepsis

Karen M. Puopolo, MD, PhD, FAAP,[a,b] William E. Benitz, MD, FAAP,[c] Theoklis E. Zaoutis, MD, MSCE, FAAP,[a,d]
COMMITTEE ON FETUS AND NEWBORN, COMMITTEE ON INFECTIOUS DISEASES

abstract

The incidence of neonatal early-onset sepsis (EOS) has declined substantially over the last 2 decades, primarily because of the implementation of evidence-based intrapartum antimicrobial therapy. However, EOS remains a serious and potentially fatal illness. Laboratory tests alone are neither sensitive nor specific enough to guide EOS management decisions. Maternal and infant clinical characteristics can help identify newborn infants who are at risk and guide the administration of empirical antibiotic therapy. The incidence of EOS, the prevalence and implications of established risk factors, the predictive value of commonly used laboratory tests, and the uncertainties in the risk/benefit balance of antibiotic exposures all vary significantly with gestational age at birth. Our purpose in this clinical report is to provide a summary of the current epidemiology of neonatal sepsis among infants born at ≥35 0/7 weeks' gestation and a framework for the development of evidence-based approaches to sepsis risk assessment among these infants.

[a]Department of Pediatrics, Perelman School of Medicine, University of Pennsylvania, Philadelphia, Pennsylvania; [b]Children's Hospital of Philadelphia, and [d]Roberts Center for Pediatric Research, Philadelphia, Pennsylvania; and [c]Division of Neonatal and Developmental Medicine, Department of Pediatrics, School of Medicine, Stanford University, Palo Alto, California

This document is copyrighted and is property of the American Academy of Pediatrics and its Board of Directors. All authors have filed conflict of interest statements with the American Academy of Pediatrics. Any conflicts have been resolved through a process approved by the Board of Directors. The American Academy of Pediatrics has neither solicited nor accepted any commercial involvement in the development of the content of this publication.

Clinical reports from the American Academy of Pediatrics benefit from expertise and resources of liaisons and internal (AAP) and external reviewers. However, clinical reports from the American Academy of Pediatrics may not reflect the views of the liaisons or the organizations or government agencies that they represent.

The guidance in this report does not indicate an exclusive course of treatment or serve as a standard of medical care. Variations, taking into account individual circumstances, may be appropriate.

All clinical reports from the American Academy of Pediatrics automatically expire 5 years after publication unless reaffirmed, revised, or retired at or before that time.

DOI: https://doi.org/10.1542/peds.2018-2894

Address correspondence to Karen M. Puopolo, MD, PhD, FAAP. E-mail: puopolok@email.chop.edu

PEDIATRICS (ISSN Numbers: Print, 0031-4005; Online, 1098-4275).

To cite: Puopolo KM, Benitz WE, Zaoutis TE, AAP COMMITTEE ON FETUS AND NEWBORN, AAP COMMITTEE ON INFECTIOUS DISEASES. Management of Neonates Born at ≥35 0/7 Weeks' Gestation With Suspected or Proven Early-Onset Bacterial Sepsis. Pediatrics. 2018;142(6):e20182894

Early-onset sepsis (EOS) is a serious and potentially fatal complication of birth. Assessing term and late-preterm newborn infants for risk of EOS is one of the most common clinical tasks conducted by pediatric providers.[1] As the use of preventive intrapartum antibiotic therapies has increased and the incidence of EOS has decreased, physicians are challenged to identify those newborn infants who are at the highest risk of infection. Pediatric providers are particularly concerned about initially well-appearing infants with identified risk factors for EOS for fear of missing the opportunity to intervene before infants become critically ill. The need to (1) assess a newborn infant's risk of EOS, (2) determine which steps should be taken at particular levels of risk (including the administration of empirical, broad-spectrum antibiotic therapies), and (3) decide when to discontinue empirical antibiotic therapies are critically important decisions that are made daily by physicians caring for neonates.

Depending on the local structure of pediatric care, these decisions are made by community pediatricians, family physicians, emergency department physicians, newborn hospitalists, and/or neonatal intensive care specialists.

PATHOGENESIS AND CURRENT EPIDEMIOLOGY OF NEONATAL EOS

EOS is defined as a blood or cerebrospinal fluid (CSF) culture obtained within 72 hours after birth growing a pathogenic bacterial species. This microbiologic definition stands in contrast to the functional definitions of sepsis that are used in pediatric and adult patients, for whom the definition is used to specify a series of time-sensitive interventions. Before the first national guidelines were published in which researchers recommended intrapartum antibiotic prophylaxis (IAP) to prevent perinatal group B *Streptococcus* (GBS) disease,[2] the overall incidence of EOS in the United States was 3 to 4 cases per 1000 live births.[3] Currently, the incidence of EOS among infants who are born at term has declined to approximately 0.5 in 1000 live births.[4,5] The EOS incidence is higher (approximately 1 in 1000 live births) among late-preterm infants but still an order of magnitude lower than the incidence among preterm, very low birth weight infants.[4–7] Culture-confirmed meningitis among term infants is even more rare, with an incidence of 0.01 to 0.02 cases per 1000 live births.[4,8] Morbidity and mortality from EOS remain substantial; approximately 60% of term infants with EOS require neonatal intensive care for respiratory distress and/or blood pressure support.[8] Mortality is approximately 2% to 3% among infants with EOS born at ≥35 weeks' gestation.[4,5,8]

EOS primarily begins in utero and was originally described as amniotic infection syndrome.[9,10] Among term infants, the pathogenesis of EOS is most commonly that of ascending colonization and infection of the uterine compartment with maternal gastrointestinal and genitourinary flora during labor with subsequent colonization and invasive infection of the fetus and/or fetal aspiration of infected amniotic fluid. Rarely, EOS may develop at or near term before the onset of labor. Whether acquired hematogenously across the placenta or via an ascending route, bacterial infection can be a cause of stillbirth in the third trimester.[11,12] *Listeria monocytogenes*, which is usually transmitted from the mother to the fetus by the transplacental hematogenous spread of infection before the onset of labor, is an infrequent but notable cause of EOS.[13]

RISK FACTORS FOR EOS

The occurrence, severity, and duration of specific clinical risk factors can be used to assess the risk of EOS among term and late-preterm infants. Evidence has supported the predictive value of gestational age, maternal intraamniotic infection (represented either by intrapartum fever or the obstetric clinical diagnosis of chorioamnionitis), the duration of rupture of membranes (ROM), maternal GBS colonization, the administration of appropriate intrapartum antibiotic therapy, and the newborn clinical condition.[2,14–16] Surveillance studies in the United States reveal higher rates of EOS among infants who are born to mothers of African American race compared with those who are not of African American race, but race is not an independent predictor in multivariable analyses.[4,5,7] Multiple other factors associated with an increased risk of EOS (eg, twin gestation, fetal tachycardia, meconium-stained amniotic fluid) also are not independent predictors of infection.

The clinical diagnosis of chorioamnionitis has been used as a primary risk factor for identifying infants who are at risk for EOS, presenting multiple difficulties for obstetric and neonatal providers. Although most infants with EOS are born to women with this clinical diagnosis, specificity is poor; only a small proportion of infants who are born in the setting of chorioamnionitis develop EOS.[16–19] In a review of nearly 400 000 newborn infants, researchers confirmed the high rate of chorioamnionitis diagnosis among the mothers of infants with EOS but estimated that approximately 450 term infants who were exposed to chorioamnionitis would have to be treated per case of confirmed EOS.[20] These data are used to provide a strong argument against using the clinical diagnosis of chorioamnionitis as a sole indicator of risk for EOS in term infants. The identification of chorioamnionitis itself is challenging, particularly among women who are laboring at or near term. The American College of Obstetricians and Gynecologists (ACOG) has recently opted to transition away from the use of the term chorioamnionitis to the use of intraamniotic infection and has published guidance for its diagnosis and management.[21] The ACOG aligned with the recommendations of a multispecialty workshop sponsored by the *Eunice Kennedy Shriver* National Institute of Child Health and Human Development in defining a confirmed diagnosis of intraamniotic infection as 1 made by using positive amniotic fluid Gram-stain and/or culture results or by using placental histopathology.[21,22] Suspected intraamniotic infection is defined as maternal intrapartum fever (either a single maternal intrapartum temperature ≥39.0°C or a temperature of 38.0°C–38.9°C that persists for >30 minutes) and 1 or more of the following: maternal leukocytosis, purulent cervical drainage, and fetal tachycardia. The

ACOG recommends that intrapartum antibiotic therapy be administered whenever intraamniotic infection is diagnosed or suspected and when otherwise unexplained maternal fever occurs in isolation. These recommendations are based on data revealing the protective effect of intrapartum antibiotic therapy for both the mother and fetus when infection is present while acknowledging frequent uncertainty about the presence of intraamniotic infection.

ANTIBIOTIC STEWARDSHIP IN EOS MANAGEMENT

Newborn infants may be exposed to antibiotic drugs before birth in the form of GBS IAP, maternal surgical prophylaxis in cesarean deliveries, or intrapartum antibiotic therapy administered because of suspected or confirmed intraamniotic infection or other maternal infections. Combined, these indications result in an antibiotic exposure of 32% to 45% of all newborn infants.[23–25] Administered to protect mothers and newborn infants, such early antibiotic exposures may also have negative consequences for term and late-preterm infants. Researchers in retrospective studies conducted primarily among term infants have associated antibiotic administration in infancy with increased risks of later childhood health problems, such as wheezing, asthma, food allergy, inflammatory bowel disease, and childhood obesity.[26–32] Although the biologic basis of such associations is not firmly established, researchers suggest that neonatal antibiotic administration alters the developing gut microbiome.[33–35] Intrapartum antibiotic administration has been associated with changes in stool bacterial composition at 1 week, 3 months, and 12 months of age.[34,35] The impact of breastfeeding on gut dysbiosis may be important given that mother-infant separation for EOS evaluation can delay the initiation of

breastfeeding and increase formula supplementation.[36] Although the relationship between early neonatal antibiotic exposure and subsequent childhood health remains to be defined, current evidence reveals that such exposures do affect newborn infants in the short-term; therefore, physicians should consider the risk/benefit balance of initiating antibiotic therapy for the risk of EOS as well as for continuing empirical antibiotic therapy in the absence of a culture-confirmed infection.

RISK STRATIFICATION FOR TERM AND LATE-PRETERM INFANTS

Three approaches currently exist for the use of risk factors to identify infants who are at increased risk of EOS, as detailed in the following sections. Each approach has merits and limitations, and each is a reasonable approach to risk assessment among infants who are born at ≥35 weeks' gestation. No strategy can be used to immediately identify all infants who will develop EOS or avoid the treatment of a substantial number of infants who are uninfected. Therefore, each strategy must include measures to monitor infants who are not initially identified and to minimize the duration of antibiotic administration to infants who are uninfected. Those at birth centers should develop institutional approaches that are best suited to their local resources and structures. Optimally, the effect of the chosen approach should be measured to identify low-frequency adverse events and to affirm efficacy.

Categorical Risk Factor Assessment

A categorical risk factor assessment includes risk factor threshold values to identify infants who are at increased risk for EOS. Algorithms for the management of GBS-specific EOS have been used as a general framework for the prevention of all EOS.[3,37,38] Risk factors used in such algorithms included (1) any

newborn infant who is ill appearing; (2) a mother with a clinical diagnosis of chorioamnionitis; (3) a mother who is colonized with GBS and who received inadequate IAP, with a duration of ROM being >18 hours or birth before 37 weeks' gestation; or (4) a mother who is colonized with GBS who received inadequate IAP but with no additional risk factors. Recommendations in these algorithms include the following: laboratory testing and empirical antibiotic therapy for infants in categories 1 and 2, laboratory testing for category 3, and observation in the hospital for ≥48 hours for category 4.

Different versions of this approach have been published since 1996 and have been incorporated by physicians into local algorithms. An advantage of using categorical risk factors is that substantial data have been reported that are used to address the effects on GBS-specific disease and on the frequency of neonatal EOS evaluation.[3,39–45] Limitations of this approach include a lack of clear definitions for newborn clinical illness, difficulties in establishing the clinical diagnosis of maternal chorioamnionitis, an inconsistent consideration of intrapartum antibiotics, and the absence of guidance on what is used to define abnormal laboratory test results in the newborn infant.

Multivariate Risk Assessment

A multivariate risk assessment includes an individualized synthesis of established risk factors and the newborn clinical condition to estimate each infant's risk of EOS. A cohort of 608 000 newborn infants was used to develop predictive models for culture-confirmed EOS based on objective data that are known at the moment of birth[7] and the evolving newborn condition during the first 6 to 12 hours after birth.[46] The objective data include gestational age, the highest maternal intrapartum temperature, the maternal GBS colonization status, the duration of ROM, and the type and duration of intrapartum antibiotic therapies. The predictive models were used to develop a Web-based Neonatal Early-Onset Sepsis Risk Calculator with recommended clinical algorithms that are based on the final risk estimate.[47] Blood culture and enhanced clinical observation are recommended for infants with an EOS risk estimated at ≥1 per 1000 live births, and blood culture and empirical antibiotic therapy are recommended for infants with an EOS risk estimated at ≥3 per 1000 live births. A prospective validation in 204 685 infants revealed that blood culture testing declined by 66%, and empirical antibiotic administration declined by 48% with this approach compared with the previous use of a categorical risk algorithm based on recommendations by the Centers for Disease Control and Prevention (CDC).[44] No adverse effects of the multivariate risk approach were noted during birth hospitalization. Readmissions for culture-confirmed infection during the week after discharge from the birth hospital were rare (approximately 5 in 100 000 births) and did not differ by the approach (sepsis risk calculator versus CDC risk algorithm) used at birth.

The advantages of the multivariate approach are that it (1) is used to provide differential information on an individual infant's risk rather than place infants in categories with a wide range of risk, (2) includes only objective data and not a clinical diagnosis of maternal chorioamnionitis, and (3) results in relatively few well-appearing newborn infants being treated empirically with antibiotic agents. Potential concerns are derived from the anticipated effect on birth hospitals because this multivariate approach necessitates increased clinical surveillance for some

infants in the well nursery and/or postpartum care unit. The classification of infants as clinically ill, equivocal, or well appearing requires ongoing clinical assessment over the first 12 hours after birth.[44,46,48] Workflow changes could be needed to accommodate changes in the frequency of vital signs and other clinical assessments for infants who are identified as being at moderate risk of EOS. Those at institutions opting for this approach may set different risk thresholds for specific actions other than those that are validated[44,48] but should also consider quantifying the effect of the chosen risk thresholds to affirm safety and efficacy.

Risk Assessment Primarily Based on Newborn Clinical Condition

A third strategy consists of the reliance on clinical signs of illness to identify infants with EOS. Under this approach, regardless of any estimation of neonatal or maternal risk factors for EOS, infants who appear ill at birth and those who develop signs of illness over the first 48 hours after birth are either treated empirically with antibiotic agents or further evaluated by laboratory screening. Among term and late-preterm infants, good clinical condition at birth is associated with a reduction in risk for EOS of approximately 60% to 70%.[44,46] A multidisciplinary panel sponsored by the *Eunice Kennedy Shriver* National Institute of Child Health and Human Development advocated that infants be flagged for risk of EOS on the basis of the obstetric diagnosis of suspected intraamniotic infection but that those conducting newborn evaluation primarily rely on clinical observation alone for well-appearing term and late-preterm infants.[22] Those at several centers have reported experience with strategies based on the identification of at-risk newborn infants using categorical or multivariate approaches to risk accompanied by laboratory tests

and serial examinations of at-risk newborn infants.[42,49–53] Researchers at 1 center in Italy reported a cohort of 7628 term infants who were managed with a categorical approach to risk identification and compared the outcomes with a cohort of 7611 infants who were managed with serial physical examinations every 4 to 6 hours through 48 hours of age. Significant decreases in the use of laboratory tests, blood cultures, and empirical antibiotic agents were observed in the second cohort. Two infants who developed EOS in the second cohort were identified as they developed signs of illness.[42]

The primary advantage of this approach is a significant reduction in the rate of antibiotic use. Those at institutions adopting such an approach will need to decide whether to adopt a categorical or multivariate approach for the identification of infants who are at risk. Alternatively, providers can decide to conduct serial clinical evaluations on all newborn infants without regard to risk of EOS. The latter approach would provide a means of identifying infants who develop EOS despite a low estimate of risk and initially reassuring clinical condition. Such cases occur at rate of approximately 1 in 10 000 live births among term and late-preterm infants.[46] Potential disadvantages of this approach are that it can require significant changes to newborn care at birth hospitals, including the establishment of processes to ensure universal serial, structured, documented examinations and the development of clear criteria for additional evaluation and empirical antibiotic administration. Frequent medical examinations of all newborn infants may be variably acceptable to families and may add significantly to the cost of well nursery care. Importantly, physicians and families must understand that the identification of initially well-appearing infants who develop clinical illness is not a failure of care but rather an anticipated outcome of this approach to EOS risk management.

LABORATORY TESTING

Blood Culture

In the absence of validated, clinically available molecular diagnostics, blood culture remains the diagnostic standard for EOS. Newborn surface cultures and gastric aspirate analysis cannot be used to diagnose EOS, and urine culture is not indicated in sepsis evaluations performed at <72 hours of age. In modern blood culture systems, optimized enriched culture media with antimicrobial neutralization properties, continuous-read detection systems, and specialized pediatric culture bottles are used. Concerns have been raised about the incomplete detection of low-level bacteremia and the effect of intrapartum antibiotic administration.[22,54] However, these systems are used to reliably detect bacteremia at a level of 1 to 10 colony-forming units per mL if a minimum blood volume of 1 mL is inoculated. Furthermore, researchers in several studies have reported no effect of intrapartum antibiotic therapy on time to positivity.[55–59] Culture media containing antimicrobial neutralization elements efficiently neutralize β-lactam antibiotic agents and gentamicin.[55] A median blood culture time to positivity of <24 hours is reported among term infants when using contemporary blood culture techniques.[60–63] Despite the performance characteristics of modern blood cultures, a prolonged empirical antibiotic treatment of term newborn infants who are critically ill may occasionally be appropriate despite negative culture results.

Pediatric blood culture bottles generally require a minimum inoculum of 1 mL of blood for optimal recovery of organisms.[64,65] The use of 2 separate culture bottles may provide the opportunity to determine if commensal species are true infections by comparing growth in the 2 cultures.[66,67] The use of 1 aerobic and 1 anaerobic culture bottle may be done to optimize the organism recovery of rare strict anaerobic species,[68] and most neonatal pathogens, including GBS, *Escherichia coli*, and *Staphylococcus aureus*, will grow under anaerobic conditions. Anaerobic blood culture is routinely performed as part of sepsis evaluation among obstetric and other adult patients. Those at individual centers may benefit from collaborative discussion with those at the laboratory where cultures are processed to optimize local processes.

CSF Culture

CSF culture should ideally be performed along with blood culture and before the initiation of empirical antibiotic therapy for infants who are at the highest risk of EOS. Among infants born at ≥35 weeks' gestation, those at the highest risk include those with critical illness. CSF cell counts obtained after the initiation of empirical antibiotic therapy may be difficult to interpret.[69,70] However, physicians must balance the challenges of CSF interpretation with the realities of care: lumbar puncture should not be performed if the newborn infant's clinical condition would be compromised or antibiotic initiation would be delayed by the procedure. Meningitis was diagnosed clinically in 4% of EOS cases in CDC surveillance, but only half of the diagnoses were made by using CSF culture, reflecting the practical difficulties in performing lumbar puncture.[4] CSF culture and analysis should be performed if blood cultures grow a pathogen to optimize the type and duration of antibiotic therapy. CSF culture and analysis do not need to be performed in the vast majority of term infants for whom blood cultures are sterile. The incidence of culture-confirmed meningitis in the absence of culture-confirmed bacteremia is approximately 1 to 2 cases per 100 000 live births.[4,8] Physicians may, therefore, use their best judgment to determine when CSF analysis should be performed in the absence of documented bacteremia.

White Blood Cell Count

The white blood cell (WBC) count, immature/total neutrophil ratio (I/T), and absolute neutrophil count (ANC) are commonly used to assess the risk of EOS. Multiple clinical factors can affect the WBC count and differential, including gestational age at birth, sex, and mode of delivery.[71–74] Fetal bone marrow depression attributable to maternal preeclampsia or placental insufficiency and prolonged exposure to inflammatory signals, such as those associated with the premature ROM, frequently result in abnormal values in the absence of infection. As the incidence of EOS declines, the clinical utility of the WBC count also declines. Researchers in 2 large, multicenter studies applied the likelihood ratio, a test characteristic that is independent of disease incidence, to assess the relationship between WBC count and culture-confirmed EOS among term and late-preterm infants and found that none of the components (WBC count, I/T, nor ANC) performed well. Extreme values (total WBC count <5000/μL [I/T >0.3; ANC <2000/μL] in one study[73] and WBC count <1000/μL [ANC <100/μL; and I/T >0.5] in the other[75]) were associated with the highest likelihood ratios but very low sensitivities. WBC count >20 000/μL and platelet counts were not associated with EOS in either study. The I/T squared (I/T divided by the ANC) performed better than any of the more traditional tests and was independent of age in hours but also had modest sensitivity and specificity.[76]

Other Inflammatory Markers

Researchers in multiple studies address other markers of inflammation, including C-reactive protein (CRP), procalcitonin, interleukins (ILs) (soluble IL-2 receptor, IL-6, and IL-8), tumor necrosis factor α, and CD64.[77–80] Both CRP and procalcitonin concentrations increase in newborn infants in response to a variety of inflammatory stimuli, including infection, asphyxia, and pneumothorax. Procalcitonin concentrations also increase naturally over the first 24 to 36 hours after birth.[79] Single values of CRP or procalcitonin obtained after birth to assess the risk of EOS are neither sensitive nor specific to guide EOS care decisions. Consistently normal values of CRP and procalcitonin over the first 48 hours of age are associated with the absence of EOS, but serial abnormal values alone should not be used to decide whether to administer antibiotics in the absence of culture-confirmed infection. Additionally, at this time, a serial evaluation of inflammatory markers should not be used to assess well-appearing term newborn infants for risk of EOS.

TREATMENT OF EOS

The microbial causes of EOS in the United States have been unchanged over the past 10 years. Researchers in national surveillance studies continue to identify GBS as the most common bacteria isolated in EOS cases among term and late-preterm infants, accounting for approximately 40% to 45% of all cases,[4,5] followed by E coli in approximately 10% to 15% of cases. The remaining cases are caused primarily by other Gram-positive organisms (predominantly viridans group streptococci and enterococci), and approximately 5% are caused by other Gram-negative

organisms. S aureus (approximately 3%–4%) and L monocytogenes (approximately 1%–2%) are less common causes of EOS among term infants.[4,5]

Ampicillin and gentamicin, in combination, is the first choice for empirical therapy for EOS. This combination will be effective against GBS, most other streptococcal and enterococcal species, and L monocytogenes. Although two-thirds of E coli EOS isolates and most other Gram-negative EOS isolates are resistant to ampicillin, the majority remain sensitive to gentamicin.[4] Extended-spectrum β-lactamase–producing organisms are rarely reported among EOS cases in the United States. Therefore, the routine empirical use of broader-spectrum antibiotic agents is typically not justified and may be harmful.[81] Nonetheless, approximately 7% of E coli cases (1.7% of all EOS cases) were resistant to both ampicillin and gentamicin in recent CDC surveillance studies.[4] Among term newborn infants who are critically ill, the empirical addition of broader-spectrum therapy should be considered until culture results are available.

When EOS is confirmed by using blood culture, lumbar puncture should be performed if not previously done. Serial daily blood cultures should be performed until microbiological sterility is documented. In definitive antibiotic therapy, providers should use the narrowest spectrum of appropriate antibiotics. The duration of therapy should be guided by expert references (eg, the American Academy of Pediatrics *Red Book: Report of the Committee on Infectious Diseases*) and informed by using CSF analysis results and the achievement of sterile cultures. Consultation with infectious disease specialists can be considered for cases that are complicated by meningitis or other site-specific infections and for

cases that are caused by resistant or atypical organisms. Among term infants with unexplained critical cardiorespiratory illness, an empirical course of antibiotic therapy may be justified even in the absence of culture-confirmed infection. Most often, however, antibiotic therapy should be discontinued when blood cultures are sterile at 36 to 48 hours of incubation unless there is evidence of site-specific infection. Continuing empirical antibiotic therapy in response to laboratory test abnormalities alone is rarely justified, particularly among well-appearing term infants.

PREVENTION STRATEGIES

The only proven preventive strategy for EOS is the appropriate administration of maternal IAP. Recommendations from national professional organizations should be followed for the administration of GBS intrapartum prophylaxis as well as for the administration of intrapartum antibiotic therapy when there is suspected or confirmed intraamniotic infection. Neonatal practices are focused on the identification and empirical antibiotic treatment of newborn infants who are at risk for EOS; these practices cannot prevent EOS. The empirical administration of intramuscular penicillin to all newborn infants to prevent neonatal GBS-specific EOS is not justified and is not endorsed by the American Academy of Pediatrics. Neither GBS IAP nor any neonatal EOS practice will prevent late-onset GBS infection[3,82,83] or any other form of late-onset bacterial infection.

SUMMARY POINTS

We include the following summary points:

1. The epidemiology of EOS differs substantially between term and/ or late-preterm infants and very preterm infants.

2. Infants born at ≥35 0/7 weeks' gestation can be stratified by the level of risk for EOS. Acceptable approaches to risk stratification include the following:

   o categorical algorithms in which threshold values for intrapartum risk factors are used;

   o multivariate risk assessment based on both intrapartum risk factors and infant examinations. The Neonatal Early-Onset Sepsis Risk Calculator[47] is an example of this approach; and

   o serial physical examination to detect the presence of clinical signs of illness after birth. This approach may begin with a categorical or multivariate assessment to identify newborn infants who are at risk and will be subjected to serial monitoring, or this may be applied to all newborn infants.

3. Birth centers should consider the development of locally tailored, documented guidelines for EOS risk assessment and clinical management. Ongoing surveillance once guidelines are implemented is recommended.

4. The diagnosis of EOS is made by using blood or CSF cultures. EOS cannot be diagnosed by using laboratory tests, such as a complete blood cell count or CRP or by using surface cultures, gastric aspirate analysis, or urine culture.

5. The combination of ampicillin and gentamicin is the appropriate empirical antibiotic regimen for most infants who are at risk for EOS. The empirical administration of additional broad-spectrum agents may be indicated in term infants who are critically ill until appropriate culture results are known.

6. When blood cultures are sterile, antibiotic therapy should be discontinued by 36 to 48 hours of incubation unless there is clear evidence of site-specific infection.

LEAD AUTHORS

Karen M. Puopolo, MD, PhD, FAAP
William E. Benitz, MD, FAAP
Theoklis E. Zaoutis, MD, MSCE, FAAP

COMMITTEE ON FETUS AND NEWBORN, 2017–2018

James Cummings, MD, Chairperson
Sandra Juul, MD
Ivan Hand, MD
Eric Eichenwald, MD
Brenda Poindexter, MD
Dan L. Stewart, MD
Susan W. Aucott, MD
Karen M. Puopolo, MD
Jay P. Goldsmith, MD
Kristi Watterberg, MD, Immediate Past Chairperson

LIAISONS

Kasper S. Wang, MD – *American Academy of Pediatrics Section on Surgery*
Thierry Lacaze, MD – *Canadian Paediatric Society*
Joseph Wax, MD – *American College of Obstetricians and Gynecologists*
Tonse N.K. Raju, MD, DCH – *National Institutes of Health*
Wanda Barfield, MD, MPH, CAPT USPHS – *Centers for Disease Control and Prevention*
Erin Keels, MS, APRN, NNP-BC – *National Association of Neonatal Nurses*

STAFF

Jim Couto, MA

COMMITTEE ON INFECTIOUS DISEASES, 2017–2018

Carrie L. Byington, MD, FAAP, Chairperson
Yvonne A. Maldonado, MD, FAAP, Vice Chairperson
Ritu Banerjee, MD, PhD, FAAP
Elizabeth D. Barnett, MD, FAAP
James D. Campbell, MD, MS, FAAP
Jeffrey S. Gerber, MD, PhD, FAAP
Ruth Lynfield, MD, FAAP
Flor M. Munoz, MD, MSc, FAAP
Dawn Nolt, MD, MPH, FAAP
Ann-Christine Nyquist, MD, MSPH, FAAP
Sean T. O'Leary, MD, MPH, FAAP
Mobeen H. Rathore, MD, FAAP
Mark H. Sawyer, MD, FAAP
William J. Steinbach, MD, FAAP
Tina Q. Tan, MD, FAAP
Theoklis E. Zaoutis, MD, MSCE, FAAP

EX OFFICIO

David W. Kimberlin, MD, FAAP – *Red Book* Editor
Michael T. Brady, MD, FAAP – *Red Book* Associate Editor
Mary Anne Jackson, MD, FAAP – *Red Book* Associate Editor
Sarah S. Long, MD, FAAP – *Red Book* Associate Editor
Henry H. Bernstein, DO, MHCM, FAAP – *Red Book* Online Associate Editor
H. Cody Meissner, MD, FAAP – Visual *Red Book* Associate Editor

LIAISONS

Amanda C. Cohn, MD, FAAP – *Centers for Disease Control and Prevention*
Jamie Deseda-Tous, MD – *Sociedad Latinoamericana de Infectologia Pediatrica*
Karen M. Farizo, MD – *United States Food and Drug Administration*
Marc Fischer, MD, FAAP – *Centers for Disease Control and Prevention*
Natasha Halasa, MD, MPH, FAAP – *Pediatric Infectious Diseases Society*
Nicole Le Saux, MD – *Canadian Paediatric Society*
Scot Moore, MD, FAAP – *Committee on Practice Ambulatory Medicine*
Angela K. Shen, ScD, MPH – *National Vaccine Program Office*
Neil S. Silverman, MD – *American College of Obstetricians and Gynecologists*
James J. Stevermer, MD, MSPH, FAAFP – *American Academy of Family Physicians*
Jeffrey R. Starke, MD, FAAP – *American Thoracic Society*
Kay M. Tomashek, MD, MPH, DTM – *National Institutes of Health*

STAFF

Jennifer M. Frantz, MPH

ABBREVIATIONS

ACOG: American College of Obstetricians and Gynecologists
ANC: absolute neutrophil count
CDC: Centers for Disease Control and Prevention
CRP: C-reactive protein
CSF: cerebrospinal fluid
EOS: early-onset sepsis
GBS: group B *Streptococcus*
IAP: intrapartum antibiotic prophylaxis
IL: interleukin
I/T: immature/total neutrophil ratio
ROM: rupture of membranes
WBC: white blood cell

FINANCIAL DISCLOSURE: The authors have indicated they have no financial relationships relevant to this article to disclose.

FUNDING: No external funding.

POTENTIAL CONFLICT OF INTEREST: The authors have indicated they have no potential conflicts of interest to disclose.

COMPANION PAPER: A companion to this article can be found online at www.pediatrics.org/cgi/doi/10.1542/peds.2018-2896.

REFERENCES

1. Mukhopadhyay S, Taylor JA, Von Kohorn I, et al. Variation in sepsis evaluation across a national network of nurseries. *Pediatrics*. 2017;139(3):e20162845

2. Verani JR, McGee L, Schrag SJ; Division of Bacterial Diseases, National Center for Immunization and Respiratory Diseases, Centers for Disease Control and Prevention (CDC). Prevention of perinatal group B streptococcal disease–revised guidelines from CDC, 2010. *MMWR Recomm Rep*. 2010;59(RR-10):1–36

3. Schuchat A, Zywicki SS, Dinsmoor MJ, et al. Risk factors and opportunities for prevention of early-onset neonatal sepsis: a multicenter case-control study. *Pediatrics*. 2000;105(1, pt 1):21–26

4. Schrag SJ, Farley MM, Petit S, et al. Epidemiology of invasive early-onset neonatal sepsis, 2005 to 2014. *Pediatrics*. 2016;138(6):e20162013

5. Weston EJ, Pondo T, Lewis MM, et al. The burden of invasive early-onset neonatal sepsis in the United States, 2005-2008. *Pediatr Infect Dis J*. 2011;30(11):937–941

6. Stoll BJ, Hansen NI, Bell EF, et al; Eunice Kennedy Shriver National Institute of Child Health and Human Development Neonatal Research Network. Trends in care practices, morbidity, and mortality of extremely preterm neonates, 1993-2012. *JAMA*. 2015;314(10):1039–1051

7. Puopolo KM, Draper D, Wi S, et al. Estimating the probability of neonatal early-onset infection on the basis of maternal risk factors. *Pediatrics*. 2011;128(5). Available at: www.pediatrics.org/cgi/content/full/128/5/e1155

8. Stoll BJ, Hansen NI, Sánchez PJ, et al; Eunice Kennedy Shriver National Institute of Child Health and Human Development Neonatal Research Network. Early onset neonatal sepsis: the burden of group B Streptococcal and *E. coli* disease continues. *Pediatrics*. 2011;127(5):817–826

9. Benirschke K. Routes and types of infection in the fetus and the newborn. *AMA J Dis Child*. 1960;99(6):714–721

10. Blanc WA. Pathways of fetal and early neonatal infection. Viral placentitis, bacterial and fungal chorioamnionitis. *J Pediatr*. 1961;59(4):473–496

11. Goldenberg RL, McClure EM, Saleem S, Reddy UM. Infection-related stillbirths. *Lancet*. 2010;375(9724):1482–1490

12. Gibbs RS, Roberts DJ. Case records of the Massachusetts General Hospital. Case 27-2007. A 30-year-old pregnant woman with intrauterine fetal death. *N Engl J Med*. 2007;357(9):918–925

13. Lamont RF, Sobel J, Mazaki-Tovi S, et al. Listeriosis in human pregnancy: a systematic review. *J Perinat Med*. 2011;39(3):227–236

14. Escobar GJ, Li DK, Armstrong MA, et al. Neonatal sepsis workups in infants >/=2000 grams at birth: a population-based study. *Pediatrics*. 2000;106(2, pt 1):256–263

15. Benitz WE, Gould JB, Druzin ML. Risk factors for early-onset group B streptococcal sepsis: estimation of odds ratios by critical literature review. *Pediatrics*. 1999;103(6). Available at: www.pediatrics.org/cgi/content/full/103/6/e77

16. Mukhopadhyay S, Puopolo KM. Risk assessment in neonatal early onset sepsis. *Semin Perinatol*. 2012;36(6):408–415

17. Jackson GL, Engle WD, Sendelbach DM, et al. Are complete blood cell counts useful in the evaluation of asymptomatic neonates exposed to suspected chorioamnionitis? *Pediatrics*. 2004;113(5):1173–1180

18. Jackson GL, Rawiki P, Sendelbach D, Manning MD, Engle WD. Hospital course and short-term outcomes of term and late preterm neonates following exposure to prolonged rupture of membranes and/or chorioamnionitis. *Pediatr Infect Dis J*. 2012;31(1):89–90

19. Kiser C, Nawab U, McKenna K, Aghai ZH. Role of guidelines on length of therapy in chorioamnionitis and neonatal sepsis. *Pediatrics*. 2014;133(6):992–998

20. Wortham JM, Hansen NI, Schrag SJ, et al; Eunice Kennedy Shriver NICHD Neonatal Research Network. Chorioamnionitis and culture-confirmed, early-onset neonatal infections. *Pediatrics*. 2016;137(1):e20152316

21. Heine RP, Puopolo KM, Beigi R, Silverman NS, El-Sayed YY; Committee on Obstetric Practice. Committee opinion no. 712: intrapartum management of intraamniotic infection. *Obstet Gynecol*. 2017;130(2):e95–e101

22. Higgins RD, Saade G, Polin RA, et al; Chorioamnionitis Workshop Participants. Evaluation and management of women and newborns with a maternal diagnosis of chorioamnionitis: summary of a workshop. *Obstet Gynecol*. 2016;127(3):426–436

23. Van Dyke MK, Phares CR, Lynfield R, et al. Evaluation of universal antenatal screening for group B streptococcus. *N Engl J Med*. 2009;360(25):2626–2636

24. Persaud RR, Azad MB, Chari RS, Sears MR, Becker AB, Kozyrskyj AL; CHILD Study Investigators. Perinatal antibiotic exposure of neonates in Canada and associated risk factors: a population-based study. *J Matern Fetal Neonatal Med*. 2015;28(10):1190–1195

25. Stokholm J, Schjørring S, Pedersen L, et al. Prevalence and predictors of antibiotic administration during

pregnancy and birth. *PLoS One.* 2013;8(12):e82932

26. Ajslev TA, Andersen CS, Gamborg M, Sørensen TI, Jess T. Childhood overweight after establishment of the gut microbiota: the role of delivery mode, pre-pregnancy weight and early administration of antibiotics. *Int J Obes.* 2011;35(4):522–529

27. Alm B, Erdes L, Möllborg P, et al. Neonatal antibiotic treatment is a risk factor for early wheezing. *Pediatrics.* 2008;121(4):697–702

28. Alm B, Goksör E, Pettersson R, et al. Antibiotics in the first week of life is a risk factor for allergic rhinitis at school age. *Pediatr Allergy Immunol.* 2014;25(5):468–472

29. Risnes KR, Belanger K, Murk W, Bracken MB. Antibiotic exposure by 6 months and asthma and allergy at 6 years: findings in a cohort of 1, 401 US children. *Am J Epidemiol.* 2011;173(3):310–318

30. Russell SL, Gold MJ, Hartmann M, et al. Early life antibiotic-driven changes in microbiota enhance susceptibility to allergic asthma. *EMBO Rep.* 2012;13(5):440–447

31. Saari A, Virta LJ, Sankilampi U, Dunkel L, Saxen H. Antibiotic exposure in infancy and risk of being overweight in the first 24 months of life. *Pediatrics.* 2015;135(4):617–626

32. Trasande L, Blustein J, Liu M, Corwin E, Cox LM, Blaser MJ. Infant antibiotic exposures and early-life body mass. *Int J Obes.* 2013;37(1):16–23

33. Greenwood C, Morrow AL, Lagomarcino AJ, et al. Early empiric antibiotic use in preterm infants is associated with lower bacterial diversity and higher relative abundance of *Enterobacter. J Pediatr.* 2014;165(1):23–29

34. Corvaglia L, Tonti G, Martini S, et al. Influence of intrapartum antibiotic prophylaxis for group B *Streptococcus* on gut microbiota in the first month of life. *J Pediatr Gastroenterol Nutr.* 2016;62(2):304–308

35. Azad MB, Konya T, Persaud RR, et al; CHILD Study Investigators. Impact of maternal intrapartum antibiotics, method of birth and breastfeeding on gut microbiota during the first year of

life: a prospective cohort study. *BJOG.* 2016;123(6):983–993

36. Mukhopadhyay S, Lieberman ES, Puopolo KM, Riley LE, Johnson LC. Effect of early-onset sepsis evaluations on in-hospital breastfeeding practices among asymptomatic term neonates. *Hosp Pediatr.* 2015;5(4):203–210

37. Centers for Disease Control and Prevention. Prevention of perinatal group B streptococcal disease: a public health perspective. Centers for Disease Control and Prevention [published correction appears in *MMWR Morb Mortal Wkly Rep.* 1996;45(31):679]. *MMWR Recomm Rep.* 1996;45(RR-7):1–24

38. Schrag S, Gorwitz R, Fultz-Butts K, Schuchat A. Prevention of perinatal group B streptococcal disease. Revised guidelines from CDC. *MMWR Recomm Rep.* 2002;51(RR-11):1–22

39. Schrag SJ, Zywicki S, Farley MM, et al. Group B streptococcal disease in the era of intrapartum antibiotic prophylaxis. *N Engl J Med.* 2000;342(1):15–20

40. Schrag SJ, Zell ER, Lynfield R, et al; Active Bacterial Core Surveillance Team. A population-based comparison of strategies to prevent early-onset group B streptococcal disease in neonates. *N Engl J Med.* 2002;347(4):233–239

41. Puopolo KM, Escobar GJ. Early-onset sepsis: a predictive model based on maternal risk factors. *Curr Opin Pediatr.* 2013;25(2):161–166

42. Cantoni L, Ronfani L, Da Riol R, Demarini S; Perinatal Study Group of the Region Friuli-Venezia Giulia. Physical examination instead of laboratory tests for most infants born to mothers colonized with group B *Streptococcus*: support for the Centers for Disease Control and Prevention's 2010 recommendations. *J Pediatr.* 2013;163(2):568–573

43. Mukhopadhyay S, Dukhovny D, Mao W, Eichenwald EC, Puopolo KM. 2010 perinatal GBS prevention guideline and resource utilization. *Pediatrics.* 2014;133(2):196–203

44. Kuzniewicz MW, Puopolo KM, Fischer A, et al. A quantitative, risk-based approach to the management of

neonatal early-onset sepsis. *JAMA Pediatr.* 2017;171(4):365–371

45. Mukhopadhyay S, Eichenwald EC, Puopolo KM. Neonatal early-onset sepsis evaluations among well-appearing infants: projected impact of changes in CDC GBS guidelines. *J Perinatol.* 2013;33(3):198–205

46. Escobar GJ, Puopolo KM, Wi S, et al. Stratification of risk of early-onset sepsis in newborns ≥ 34 weeks' gestation. *Pediatrics.* 2014;133(1):30–36

47. Northern California Kaiser-Permanente. Neonatal Early-Onset Sepsis Calculator. Available at: https://neonatalsepsiscalculator.kaiserpermanente.org. Accessed April 5, 2018

48. Dhudasia MB, Mukhopadhyay S, Puopolo KM. Implementation of the sepsis risk calculator at an academic birth hospital. *Hosp Pediatr.* 2018;8(5):243–250

49. Ottolini MC, Lundgren K, Mirkinson LJ, Cason S, Ottolini MG. Utility of complete blood count and blood culture screening to diagnose neonatal sepsis in the asymptomatic at risk newborn. *Pediatr Infect Dis J.* 2003;22(5):430–434

50. Flidel-Rimon O, Galstyan S, Juster-Reicher A, Rozin I, Shinwell ES. Limitations of the risk factor based approach in early neonatal sepsis evaluations. *Acta Paediatr.* 2012;101(12):e540–e544

51. Hashavya S, Benenson S, Ergaz-Shaltiel Z, Bar-Oz B, Averbuch D, Eventov-Friedman S. The use of blood counts and blood cultures to screen neonates born to partially treated group B *Streptococcus*-carrier mothers for early-onset sepsis: is it justified? *Pediatr Infect Dis J.* 2011;30(10):840–843

52. Berardi A, Fornaciari S, Rossi C, et al. Safety of physical examination alone for managing well-appearing neonates ≥ 35 weeks' gestation at risk for early-onset sepsis. *J Matern Fetal Neonatal Med.* 2015;28(10):1123–1127

53. Joshi NS, Gupta A, Allan JM, et al. Clinical monitoring of well-appearing infants born to mothers with chorioamnionitis. *Pediatrics.* 2018;141(4):e20172056

54. Wynn JL, Wong HR, Shanley TP, Bizzarro MJ, Saiman L, Polin RA. Time for a neonatal-specific consensus definition

for sepsis. *Pediatr Crit Care Med.* 2014;15(6):523–528

55. Dunne WM Jr, Case LK, Isgriggs L, Lublin DM. In-house validation of the BACTEC 9240 blood culture system for detection of bacterial contamination in platelet concentrates. *Transfusion.* 2005;45(7):1138–1142

56. Flayhart D, Borek AP, Wakefield T, Dick J, Carroll KC. Comparison of BACTEC PLUS blood culture media to BacT/Alert FA blood culture media for detection of bacterial pathogens in samples containing therapeutic levels of antibiotics. *J Clin Microbiol.* 2007;45(3):816–821

57. Jorgensen JH, Mirrett S, McDonald LC, et al. Controlled clinical laboratory comparison of BACTEC plus aerobic/F resin medium with BacT/Alert aerobic FAN medium for detection of bacteremia and fungemia. *J Clin Microbiol.* 1997;35(1):53–58

58. Krisher KK, Gibb P, Corbett S, Church D. Comparison of the BacT/Alert PF pediatric FAN blood culture bottle with the standard pediatric blood culture bottle, the Pedi-BacT. *J Clin Microbiol.* 2001;39(8):2880–2883

59. Nanua S, Weber C, Isgriggs L, Dunne WM Jr. Performance evaluation of the VersaTREK blood culture system for quality control testing of platelet units. *J Clin Microbiol.* 2009;47(3):817–818

60. Garcia-Prats JA, Cooper TR, Schneider VF, Stager CE, Hansen TN. Rapid detection of microorganisms in blood cultures of newborn infants utilizing an automated blood culture system. *Pediatrics.* 2000;105(3, pt 1):523–527

61. Sarkar SS, Bhagat I, Bhatt-Mehta V, Sarkar S. Does maternal intrapartum antibiotic treatment prolong the incubation time required for blood cultures to become positive for infants with early-onset sepsis? *Am J Perinatol.* 2015;32(4):357–362

62. Guerti K, Devos H, Ieven MM, Mahieu LM. Time to positivity of neonatal blood cultures: fast and furious? *J Med Microbiol.* 2011;60(pt 4):446–453

63. Jardine L, Davies MW, Faoagali J. Incubation time required for neonatal blood cultures to become positive. *J Paediatr Child Health.* 2006;42(12):797–802

64. Schelonka RL, Chai MK, Yoder BA, Hensley D, Brockett RM, Ascher DP. Volume of blood required to detect common neonatal pathogens. *J Pediatr.* 1996;129(2):275–278

65. Yaacobi N, Bar-Meir M, Shchors I, Bromiker R. A prospective controlled trial of the optimal volume for neonatal blood cultures. *Pediatr Infect Dis J.* 2015;34(4):351–354

66. Sarkar S, Bhagat I, DeCristofaro JD, Wiswell TE, Spitzer AR. A study of the role of multiple site blood cultures in the evaluation of neonatal sepsis. *J Perinatol.* 2006;26(1):18–22

67. Struthers S, Underhill H, Albersheim S, Greenberg D, Dobson S. A comparison of two versus one blood culture in the diagnosis and treatment of coagulase-negative *staphylococcus* in the neonatal intensive care unit. *J Perinatol.* 2002;22(7):547–549

68. Mukhopadhyay S, Puopolo KM. Clinical and microbiologic characteristics of early-onset sepsis among very low birth weight infants: opportunities for antibiotic stewardship. *Pediatr Infect Dis J.* 2017;36(5):477–481

69. Garges HP, Moody MA, Cotten CM, et al. Neonatal meningitis: what is the correlation among cerebrospinal fluid cultures, blood cultures, and cerebrospinal fluid parameters? *Pediatrics.* 2006;117(4):1094–1100

70. Greenberg RG, Smith PB, Cotten CM, Moody MA, Clark RH, Benjamin DK Jr. Traumatic lumbar punctures in neonates: test performance of the cerebrospinal fluid white blood cell count. *Pediatr Infect Dis J.* 2008;27(12):1047–1051

71. Christensen RD, Henry E, Jopling J, Wiedmeier SE. The CBC: reference ranges for neonates. *Semin Perinatol.* 2009;33(1):3–11

72. Manroe BL, Weinberg AG, Rosenfeld CR, Browne R. The neonatal blood count in health and disease. I. Reference values for neutrophilic cells. *J Pediatr.* 1979;95(1):89–98

73. Newman TB, Puopolo KM, Wi S, Draper D, Escobar GJ. Interpreting complete blood counts soon after birth in newborns at risk for sepsis. *Pediatrics.* 2010;126(5):903–909

74. Schmutz N, Henry E, Jopling J, Christensen RD. Expected ranges for blood neutrophil concentrations of neonates: the Manroe and Mouzinho charts revisited. *J Perinatol.* 2008;28(4):275–281

75. Hornik CP, Benjamin DK, Becker KC, et al. Use of the complete blood cell count in early-onset neonatal sepsis. *Pediatr Infect Dis J.* 2012;31(8):799–802

76. Newman TB, Draper D, Puopolo KM, Wi S, Escobar GJ. Combining immature and total neutrophil counts to predict early onset sepsis in term and late preterm newborns: use of the I/T^2. *Pediatr Infect Dis J.* 2014;33(8):798–802

77. Benitz WE. Adjunct laboratory tests in the diagnosis of early-onset neonatal sepsis. *Clin Perinatol.* 2010;37(2):421–438

78. Lynema S, Marmer D, Hall ES, Meinzen-Derr J, Kingma PS. Neutrophil CD64 as a diagnostic marker of sepsis: impact on neonatal care. *Am J Perinatol.* 2015;32(4):331–336

79. Su H, Chang SS, Han CM, et al. Inflammatory markers in cord blood or maternal serum for early detection of neonatal sepsis-a systemic review and meta-analysis. *J Perinatol.* 2014;34(4):268–274

80. Chiesa C, Panero A, Rossi N, et al. Reliability of procalcitonin concentrations for the diagnosis of sepsis in critically ill neonates. *Clin Infect Dis.* 1998;26(3):664–672

81. Clark RH, Bloom BT, Spitzer AR, Gerstmann DR. Empiric use of ampicillin and cefotaxime, compared with ampicillin and gentamicin, for neonates at risk for sepsis is associated with an increased risk of neonatal death. *Pediatrics.* 2006;117(1):67–74

82. Jordan HT, Farley MM, Craig A, et al; Active Bacterial Core Surveillance (ABCs), Emerging Infections Program Network, CDC. Revisiting the need for vaccine prevention of late-onset neonatal group B streptococcal disease: a multistate, population-based analysis. *Pediatr Infect Dis J.* 2008;27(12):1057–1064

83. Phares CR, Lynfield R, Farley MM, et al; Active Bacterial Core Surveillance/ Emerging Infections Program Network. Epidemiology of invasive group B streptococcal disease in the United States, 1999-2005. *JAMA.* 2008;299(17):2056–2065

Management of Neonates Born at ≤34 6/7 Weeks' Gestation With Suspected or Proven Early-Onset Bacterial Sepsis

• *Clinical Report*

CLINICAL REPORT Guidance for the Clinician in Rendering Pediatric Care

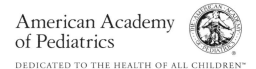

American Academy
of Pediatrics

DEDICATED TO THE HEALTH OF ALL CHILDREN™

Management of Neonates Born at ≤34 6/7 Weeks' Gestation With Suspected or Proven Early-Onset Bacterial Sepsis

Karen M. Puopolo, MD, PhD, FAAP,[a,b] William E. Benitz, MD, FAAP,[c] Theoklis E. Zaoutis, MD, MSCE, FAAP,[a,d]
COMMITTEE ON FETUS AND NEWBORN, COMMITTEE ON INFECTIOUS DISEASES

abstract

Early-onset sepsis (EOS) remains a serious and often fatal illness among infants born preterm, particularly among newborn infants of the lowest gestational age. Currently, most preterm infants with very low birth weight are treated empirically with antibiotics for risk of EOS, often for prolonged periods, in the absence of a culture-confirmed infection. Retrospective studies have revealed that antibiotic exposures after birth are associated with multiple subsequent poor outcomes among preterm infants, making the risk/benefit balance of these antibiotic treatments uncertain. Gestational age is the strongest single predictor of EOS, and the majority of preterm births occur in the setting of other factors associated with risk of EOS, making it difficult to apply risk stratification strategies to preterm infants. Laboratory tests alone have a poor predictive value in preterm EOS. Delivery characteristics of extremely preterm infants present an opportunity to identify those with a lower risk of EOS and may inform decisions to initiate or extend antibiotic therapies. Our purpose for this clinical report is to provide a summary of the current epidemiology of preterm neonatal sepsis and provide guidance for the development of evidence-based approaches to sepsis risk assessment among preterm newborn infants.

[a]Department of Pediatrics, Perelman School of Medicine, University of Pennsylvania, Philadelphia, Pennsylvania; [b]Children's Hospital of Philadelphia, and [d]Roberts Center for Pediatric Research, Philadelphia, Pennsylvania; and [c]Division of Neonatal and Developmental Medicine, Department of Pediatrics, School of Medicine, Stanford University, Palo Alto, California

DOI: https://doi.org/10.1542/peds.2018-2896

Address correspondence to Karen M. Puopolo, MD, PhD, FAAP. E-mail: puopolok@email.chop.edu

PEDIATRICS (ISSN Numbers: Print, 0031-4005; Online, 1098-4275).

To cite: Puopolo KM, Benitz WE, Zaoutis TE, AAP COMMITTEE ON FETUS AND NEWBORN, AAP COMMITTEE ON INFECTIOUS DISEASES. Management of Neonates Born at ≤34 6/7 Weeks' Gestation With Suspected or Proven Early-Onset Bacterial Sepsis. *Pediatrics.* 2018;142(6):e20182896

Antibiotics are administered shortly after birth to nearly all preterm infants with very low birth weight (VLBW) (birth weight <1500 g) because of the risk of early-onset sepsis (EOS).[1–4] Physicians are often reluctant to discontinue antibiotics once initiated for many reasons, including the relatively high risk of EOS among preterm infants and the relatively high rate of mortality attributable to infection. Particularly among infants with VLBW, neonatal clinicians must determine which infants are most likely to have EOS when nearly all have some degree of respiratory or systemic instability. Poor predictive performance of common laboratory tests and concerns regarding the unreliability of blood cultures add to the difficulty in discriminating at-risk infants. Because gestational age is the strongest predictor of EOS and approximately two-thirds of preterm births are associated with preterm labor, premature rupture of membranes (PROM), or clinical chorioamnionitis,[5] risk stratification strategies cannot be applied to preterm newborn infants in the same manner as for term neonates.

PATHOGENESIS AND CURRENT EPIDEMIOLOGY OF PRETERM NEONATAL EOS

Preterm EOS is defined as a blood or cerebrospinal fluid (CSF) culture obtained within 72 hours after birth that is growing a pathogenic bacterial species. This microbiological definition stands in contrast to the functional definitions of sepsis used in pediatric and adult patients, for whom the definition is used to specify a series of time-sensitive interventions. The current overall incidence of EOS in the United States is approximately 0.8 cases per 1000 live births.[6] A disproportionate number of cases occur among infants born preterm in a manner that is inversely proportional to gestational age at birth. The incidence of EOS is approximately 0.5 cases per 1000 infants born at ≥37 weeks' gestation, compared with approximately 1 case per 1000 infants born at 34 to 36 weeks' gestation, 6 cases per 1000 infants born at <34 weeks' gestation, 20 cases per 1000 infants born at <29 weeks' gestation, and 32 cases per 1000 infants born at 22 to 24 weeks' gestation.[6–10] The incidence of EOS has declined among term infants over the past 25 years, a change attributed to the implementation of evidence-based intrapartum antimicrobial therapy. The impact of such therapies on preterm infants is less clear. Authors of the most recent studies report an EOS incidence among infants with VLBW ranging from 9 to 11 cases per 1000 infants with VLBW,

whereas studies from the early 1990s revealed rates of 19 to 32 per 1000 infants.[10,11] Improvements among VLBW incidence may be limited to those born at older gestational ages. No significant change over time was observed in a study of 34 636 infants born from 1993 to 2012 at 22 to 28 weeks' gestation, with the reported incidence ranging from 20.5 to 24.4 per 1000 infants.[8] Morbidity and mortality from EOS remain substantial: 95% of preterm infants with EOS require neonatal intensive care for respiratory distress and/or blood pressure support, and 75% of deaths from EOS occur among infants with VLBW.[6,10] The mortality rate among those with EOS is an order of magnitude higher among preterm compared with term infants, whether measured by gestational age (1.6% at ≥37 weeks, 30% at 25–28 weeks, and approximately 50% at 22–24 weeks)[7,8,10] or birth weight (3.5% among those born at ≥1500 g vs 35% for those born at <1500 g).[6]

The pathogenesis of preterm EOS is complex. EOS primarily begins in utero and was originally described as the "amniotic infection syndrome."[12,13] Among term infants, EOS pathogenesis most commonly develops during labor and involves ascending colonization and infection of the uterine compartment with maternal gastrointestinal and genitourinary flora, with subsequent colonization and invasive infection of the fetus and/or fetal aspiration of infected amniotic fluid. This intrapartum sequence may be responsible for EOS that develops after PROM or during preterm labor that is induced for maternal indications. However, the pathogenesis of preterm EOS likely begins before the onset of labor in many cases of preterm labor and/or PROM. Intraamniotic infection (IAI) may cause stillbirth in the second and third trimesters.[14] In approximately 25% of cases, IAI is the cause of preterm labor and PROM, particularly

when these occur at the lowest gestational ages; evidence suggests that microbial-induced maternal inflammation can initiate parturition and elicit fetal inflammatory responses.[5,15–18] Organisms isolated from the intrauterine compartment of women with preterm labor, PROM, or both are primarily vaginal in origin and include low-virulence species, such as *Ureaplasma*, as well as anaerobic species and well-recognized neonatal pathogens, such as *Escherichia coli* and group B *Streptococcus* (GBS).[16–18] The isolation of maternal oral flora and, more rarely, *Listeria monocytogenes*, suggests a transplacental pathway for some IAIs.[16,18–20] Inflammation inciting parturition may not, however, always be attributable to IAI. Inflammation resulting from immune-mediated rejection of the fetal or placental compartment (from maternal extrauterine infection), as well as that incited by reproductive or nonreproductive microbiota, may all contribute to the pathogenesis of preterm labor and PROM, complicating the interpretation of placental pathology.[15,20]

RISK FACTORS FOR PRETERM EOS

Multiple clinical risk factors have been used to assess the risk of EOS among infants born at ≤34 6/7 weeks' gestation. Univariate analyses of risk factors for EOS among preterm infants have been used to identify gestational age, birth weight, PROM and prolonged rupture of membranes (ROM), preterm onset of labor, maternal age and race, maternal intrapartum fever, mode of delivery, and administration of intrapartum antibiotics to be associated with risk of EOS; however, the independent contribution of any specific factor other than gestational age has been difficult to quantify. For example, among term infants, there is a linear relationship between the duration of ROM and the risk of EOS.[9]

In contrast, the relationship between PROM and the risk of EOS is not simply described by its occurrence or duration but modified by gestational age as well as by the additional presence of clinical chorioamnionitis and the administration of latency and intrapartum antibiotics.[17,21-24] These observations are likely related to uncertainty regarding the role of intrauterine infection and cervical structural defects in the pathogenesis of spontaneous PROM.[24,25]

The clinical diagnosis of chorioamnionitis has been used as a primary risk factor for identifying infants at risk for EOS. Most preterm infants with EOS are born to women with this clinical diagnosis.[4,26-29] The American College of Obstetricians and Gynecologists (ACOG) recently advocated for using the term "intraamniotic infection" rather than chorioamnionitis (which is primarily a histologic diagnosis) and published guidance for its diagnosis and management.[30] A confirmed diagnosis of IAI is made by a positive result on an amniotic fluid Gram-stain, culture, or placental histopathology. Suspected IAI is diagnosed by maternal intrapartum fever (either a single documented maternal intrapartum temperature of ≥39.0°C or a temperature of 38.0–38.9°C that persists for >30 minutes) and 1 or more of the following: (1) maternal leukocytosis, (2) purulent cervical drainage, and (3) fetal tachycardia. The ACOG recommends that intrapartum antibiotics be administered whenever IAI is diagnosed or suspected and when otherwise unexplained maternal fever occurs during labor. Chorioamnionitis or IAI is strongly associated with EOS in preterm infants, with a number needed to treat of only 6 to 40 infants per case of confirmed EOS.[4,26-29] Conversely, the absence of clinical and histologic chorioamnionitis may be used to identify a group of preterm infants who are at a lower

risk for EOS. In a study of 15 318 infants born at 22 to 28 weeks' gestation, those born by cesarean delivery with membrane rupture at delivery and without clinical chorioamnionitis were significantly less likely to have EOS or die before 12 hours of age.[4] The number needed to treat for infants born in these circumstances was approximately 200; with the additional absence of histologic chorioamnionitis, the number needed to treat is approximately 380.[4] Another study of 109 cases of EOS occurring among 5313 infants with VLBW over a 25-year period revealed that 97% of cases occurred in infants born with some combination of PROM, preterm labor, or concern for IAI.[29] In that report, 2 cases of listeriosis occurred in the context of unexplained fetal distress in otherwise uncomplicated pregnancies.

ANTIBIOTIC STEWARDSHIP IN PRETERM EOS MANAGEMENT

Currently, most premature infants with VLBW are treated empirically with antibiotics for risk of EOS, often for prolonged periods, even in the absence of a culture-confirmed infection. Prolonged empirical antibiotics are administered to approximately 35% to 50% of infants with a low gestational age, with significant center-specific variation.[1-4] Antibiotic drugs are administered for many reasons, including the relatively high incidence of EOS among preterm infants, the relatively high rate of mortality attributable to infection, and the frequency of clinical instability after birth. Empirical antibiotics administered to very preterm infants in the first days after birth have been associated with an increased risk of subsequent poor outcomes.[1,4,31-33] One multicenter study of 4039 infants born from 1998 to 2001 with a birth weight of <1000 g revealed that those infants who died or had a diagnosis of necrotizing

enterocolitis (NEC) before hospital discharge were significantly more likely to have received prolonged empirical antibiotic therapy in the first week after birth.[1] The authors of the study estimated that the risk of NEC increased by 7% for each additional day of antibiotics administered in the absence of culture-confirmed EOS. Authors of a single-center study of infants with VLBW estimated that the risk of NEC increased by 20% for each additional day of antibiotics administered in the absence of a culture-confirmed infection.[31] Authors of another study of 11 669 infants with VLBW assessed the overall rate of antibiotic use and found that higher rates during the first week after birth or during the entire hospitalization were both associated with increased mortality, even when adjusted for multiple predictors of neonatal morbidity and mortality.[33] One concern in each of these studies is that some infants categorized as uninfected may in fact have suffered from EOS. Yet, even among 5640 infants born at 22 to 28 weeks' gestation at a lower risk for EOS, those who received prolonged empirical antibiotic therapy during the first week after birth had higher rates of death and bronchopulmonary dysplasia.[4] Several explanations are possible for all of these findings, including simply that physicians administer the most antibiotics to the sickest infants. Other potential mechanisms include the role of antibiotics in promoting dysbiosis of the gut, skin, and respiratory tract, affecting the interactions between colonizing flora in maintaining health and promoting immunity; it is also possible that antibiotics and dysbiosis function as modulators of vascular development.[34,35] Although the full relationship between early neonatal antibiotic exposures and subsequent childhood health remains to be defined, current evidence suggests that such exposures do affect preterm infants. Physicians should consider the risk/benefit balance of initiating antibiotic therapy for risk of EOS as well as for continuing empirical antibiotic therapy in the absence of a culture-confirmed infection.

RISK CATEGORIZATION FOR PRETERM INFANTS

Perhaps the greatest contributor to the nearly universal practice of empirical antibiotic administration to preterm infants is the uncertainty in EOS risk assessment. Because gestational age is the strongest predictor of EOS, and two-thirds of preterm births are associated with preterm labor, PROM, or clinical concern for intrauterine infection,[5] risk stratification strategies cannot be applied to preterm infants in the same manner as for term neonates. In particular, the Neonatal Early-Onset Sepsis Risk Calculator does not apply to infants born before 34 0/7 weeks' gestation.[36] The objective of EOS risk assessment among preterm infants is, therefore, to determine which infants are at the lowest risk for infection and who, despite clinical instability, may be spared administration of empirical antibiotics. The circumstances of preterm birth may provide the best current approach to EOS management for preterm infants.

Preterm Infants at Lower Risk for EOS

Criteria for preterm infants to be considered at a lower risk for EOS include the following: (1) obstetric indications for preterm birth (such as maternal preeclampsia or other noninfectious medical illness or placental insufficiency), (2) birth by cesarean delivery, and (3) absence of labor, attempts to induce labor, or any ROM before delivery. Acceptable initial approaches to these infants might include (1) no laboratory evaluation and no empirical antibiotic therapy, or (2) a blood culture and clinical monitoring. For infants who do not improve after initial stabilization and/or those

who have severe systemic instability, the administration of empirical antibiotics may be reasonable but is not mandatory.

Infants in this category who are born by vaginal or cesarean delivery after efforts to induce labor and/or ROM before delivery are subject to factors associated with the pathogenesis of EOS during delivery. If any concern for infection arises during the process of delivery, the infant should be managed as recommended below for preterm infants at a higher risk for EOS. Otherwise, an acceptable approach to these infants is to obtain a blood culture and to initiate antibiotic therapy for infants with respiratory and/or cardiovascular instability after birth.

Preterm Infants at Higher Risk for EOS

Infants born preterm because of cervical incompetence, preterm labor, PROM, chorioamnionitis or IAI, and/or acute and otherwise unexplained onset of nonreassuring fetal status are at the highest risk for EOS. In these cases, IAI may be the cause of preterm birth or a secondary complication of PROM and cervical dilatation. IAI may also be the cause of unexplained fetal distress. The most reasonable approach to these infants is to perform a blood culture and start empirical antibiotic treatment. Obtaining CSF for culture before the administration of antibiotics should be considered if the infant will tolerate the procedure and if it will not delay the initiation of antibiotic therapy.

LABORATORY TESTING

Blood Culture

In the absence of validated, clinically available molecular diagnostic tests, a blood culture remains the diagnostic standard for EOS. Newborn surface cultures and gastric aspirate analysis cannot be used to diagnose EOS, and a urine culture is not indicated in

sepsis evaluations performed at <72 hours of age. Modern blood culture systems use optimized enriched culture media with antimicrobial neutralization properties, continuous-read detection systems, and specialized pediatric culture bottles. Although concerns have been raised regarding incomplete detection of low-level bacteremia and the effects of intrapartum antibiotic administration,[27,37] these systems reliably detect bacteremia at a level of 1 to 10 colony-forming units if a minimum of 1 mL of blood is inoculated; authors of several studies report no effect of intrapartum antibiotics on time to positivity.[38–42] Culture media containing antimicrobial neutralization elements efficiently neutralize β-lactam antibiotics and gentamicin.[39] A median blood culture time to positivity <24 hours is reported among VLBW infants when using contemporary blood culture techniques.[29,43–46] Pediatric blood culture bottles generally require a minimum of 1 mL of blood for optimal recovery of organisms.[47,48] The use of 2 separate bottles may provide the opportunity to determine if commensal species are true infections by comparing growth in the two.[49,50] Use of 1 aerobic and 1 anaerobic culture bottle may optimize organism recovery. Most neonatal pathogens, including GBS, *E coli*, coagulase-negative *Staphylococcus*, and *Staphylococcus aureus*, will grow in anaerobic conditions. One study revealed that with routine use of both pediatric aerobic and adult anaerobic blood cultures, strict anaerobic species (primarily *Bacteroides fragilis*) were isolated in 16% of EOS cases in preterm infants with VLBW.[29] An anaerobic blood culture is routinely performed among adult patients at risk for infection and can be used for neonatal blood cultures. Individual centers may benefit from collaborative discussion with the laboratory where cultures are processed to optimize local processes.

CSF Culture

The incidence of meningitis is higher among preterm infants (approximately 0.7 cases per 1000 live births at 22–28 weeks' gestation)[4] compared with the incidence in the overall birth population (approximately 0.02–0.04 cases per 1000 live births).[6,10] In the study of differential EOS risk among very preterm infants, meningitis did not occur at all among lower-risk preterm infants.[4] The true incidence of meningitis among preterm infants may be underestimated because of the common practice of performing a lumbar puncture after the initiation of empirical antibiotic therapy. Although most preterm infants with culture-confirmed early-onset meningitis grow the same organism from blood cultures, the concordance is not 100%, and CSF cell count parameters may not always identify meningitis.[51] If a CSF culture has not been obtained before the initiation of empirical antibiotics, physicians should balance the physiologic stability of the infant, the risk of EOS, and the potential harms associated with prolonged antibiotic therapy when making the decision to perform a lumbar puncture in preterm infants who are critically ill.

White Blood Cell Count

The white blood cell (WBC) count, differential (immature-to-total neutrophil ratio), and absolute neutrophil count are commonly used to assess risk of EOS. Multiple clinical factors can affect the WBC count and differential, including gestational age at birth, sex, and mode of delivery.[52–55] Fetal bone marrow depression attributable to maternal preeclampsia or placental insufficiency, as well as prolonged exposure to inflammatory signals (such as PROM), frequently result in abnormal values in the absence

of infection. Most studies in which the performance characteristics of the complete blood cell (CBC) count in predicting infection is addressed have been focused on term infants. In 1 large multicenter study, the authors assessed the relationship between the WBC count and culture-confirmed EOS and analyzed data separately for infants born at <34 weeks' gestation.[56] They found that all components of the CBC count lacked sensitivity for predicting EOS. The highest likelihood ratios (LRs) for EOS were associated with extreme values. A positive LR of >3 (ie, a likelihood of infection at least 3 times higher than the entire group of infants born at <34 weeks' gestation) was associated with a WBC count of <1000 cells per μL, an absolute neutrophil count of <1000, and an immature-to-total neutrophil ratio of >0.25. A total WBC count of >50 000 cells per μL (LR, 2.3) and a platelet count of <50 000 (LR, 2.2) had a modest relationship to EOS.

Other Inflammatory Markers

Other markers of inflammation, including C-reactive protein (CRP), procalcitonin, interleukins (soluble interleukin 2 receptor, interleukin 6, and interleukin 8), tumor necrosis factor α, and CD64 are addressed in multiple studies.[57–60] Both CRP and procalcitonin concentrations increase in newborn infants in response to a variety of inflammatory stimuli, including infection, asphyxia, and pneumothorax. Procalcitonin concentrations also increase naturally over the first 24 to 36 hours after birth.[60] Single values of CRP or procalcitonin obtained after birth to assess the risk of EOS are neither sufficiently sensitive nor specific to guide EOS care decisions. Consistently normal values of CRP and procalcitonin over the first 48 hours of age are associated with the absence of EOS, but serial abnormal values alone should not be used to extend antibiotic therapy in the

absence of a culture-confirmed infection.

TREATMENT OF PRETERM EOS

The microbiology of EOS in the United States is largely unchanged over the past 10 years. Authors of national surveillance studies continue to identify *E coli* as the most common bacteria isolated in EOS cases that occur among preterm infants, whether defined by a gestational age of <34 weeks or by a birth weight of <1500 g. Overall, *E coli* is isolated in approximately 50%, and GBS is isolated in approximately 20% of all EOS cases occurring among infants born at <34 weeks' gestation.[6] Fungal organisms are isolated in <1% of cases. Approximately 10% of cases are caused by other Gram-positive organisms (predominantly viridans group streptococci and enterococci), and approximately 20% of cases are caused by other Gram-negative organisms. *S aureus* (approximately 1%–2%) and *L monocytogenes* (approximately 1%) are uncommon causes of preterm EOS.[4,6,11] If an anaerobic culture is routinely performed, strict anaerobic bacteria are isolated in up to 15% of EOS cases among preterm infants with VLBW, with *B fragilis* being the predominant anaerobic species isolated.[29]

Ampicillin and gentamicin are the first choice for empirical therapy for EOS. This combination will be effective against GBS, most other streptococcal and enterococcal species, and *L monocytogenes*. Although two-thirds of *E coli* EOS isolates and most other Gram-negative EOS isolates are resistant to ampicillin, the majority remain sensitive to gentamicin.[6] Extended-spectrum, β-lactamase-producing organisms are only rarely reported among EOS cases in the United States. Therefore, the routine empirical use of broader-spectrum antibiotics is not warranted and may be harmful.[61]

Nonetheless, 1% to 2% of *E coli* cases were resistant to both ampicillin and gentamicin in recent surveillance studies by the Centers for Disease Control and Prevention, and *B fragilis* is not uniformly sensitive to these medications.[6,62] Therefore, among preterm infants who are severely ill and at the highest risk for Gram-negative EOS (such as infants with VLBW born after prolonged PROM and infants exposed to prolonged courses of antepartum antibiotic therapy[63–65]), the empirical addition of broader-spectrum antibiotic therapy may be considered until culture results are available. The choice of additional therapy should be guided by local antibiotic resistance data.

When EOS is confirmed by a blood culture, a lumbar puncture should be performed if not previously done. Antibiotic therapy should use the narrowest spectrum of appropriate agents once antimicrobial sensitivities are known. The duration of therapy should be guided by expert references (eg, the American Academy of Pediatrics [AAP] *Red Book: Report of the Committee on Infectious Diseases*) and informed by the results of a CSF analysis and the achievement of sterile blood and CSF cultures. Consultation with infectious disease specialists should be considered for cases complicated by meningitis or other site-specific infections and for cases with complex antibiotic resistance patterns.

When initial blood culture results are negative, antibiotic therapy should be discontinued by 36 to 48 hours of incubation, unless there is evidence of site-specific infection. Persistent cardiorespiratory instability is common among infants with VLBW and is not alone an indication for prolonged empirical antibiotic administration. Continuing empirical antibiotic administration in response to laboratory test abnormalities alone is rarely justified, particularly among preterm infants born in the setting of maternal obstetric conditions known to affect fetal hematopoiesis.

PREVENTION STRATEGIES

The only proven preventive strategy for EOS is the appropriate administration of maternal intrapartum antibiotic prophylaxis. The most current recommendations from national organizations, such as the AAP, ACOG, and Centers for Disease Control and Prevention, should be followed for the administration of GBS intrapartum prophylaxis as well as for the administration of intrapartum antibiotic therapy when there is suspected or confirmed IAI. Neonatal practices are focused on the identification and empirical antibiotic treatment of preterm neonates at risk for EOS; these practices cannot prevent EOS. The empirical administration of intramuscular penicillin to all newborn infants to prevent neonatal, GBS-specific EOS is not justified and is not endorsed by the AAP. Neither GBS intrapartum antibiotic prophylaxis nor any neonatal EOS practice will prevent late-onset GBS infection or any other form of late-onset bacterial infection. Preterm infants are particularly susceptible to late-onset GBS infection, with approximately 40% of late-onset GBS cases occurring among infants born at ≤34 6/7 weeks' gestation.[66,67]

SUMMARY POINTS

1. The epidemiology, microbiology, and pathogenesis of EOS differ substantially between term infants and preterm infants with VLBW.

2. Infants born at ≤34 6/7 weeks' gestation can be categorized by level of risk for EOS by the circumstances of their preterm birth.

   o Infants born preterm by cesarean delivery because of maternal noninfectious illness or placental insufficiency in the absence of labor, attempts to induce labor, or ROM before delivery are at a relatively low risk for EOS. Depending on the clinical condition of the neonate, physicians should consider the risk/benefit balance of an EOS evaluation and empirical antibiotic therapy.

   o Infants born preterm because of maternal cervical incompetence, preterm labor, PROM, clinical concern for IAI, or acute onset of unexplained nonreassuring fetal status are at the highest risk for EOS. Such neonates should undergo EOS evaluation with a blood culture and empirical antibiotic treatment.

   o Obstetric and neonatal care providers should communicate and document the circumstances of preterm birth to facilitate EOS risk assessment among preterm infants.

3. Clinical centers should consider the development of locally appropriate written guidelines for preterm EOS risk assessment and clinical management. After guidelines are implemented, ongoing surveillance, designed to identify low-frequency adverse events and affirm efficacy, is recommended.

4. The diagnosis of EOS is made by a blood or CSF culture. EOS cannot be diagnosed by laboratory tests alone, such as CBC count or CRP levels.

5. The combination of ampicillin and gentamicin is the most appropriate empirical antibiotic regimen for infants at risk for EOS. Empirical administration of additional broad-spectrum antibiotics may be indicated in preterm infants who are severely ill and at a high risk for EOS, particularly after prolonged antepartum maternal antibiotic treatment.

6. When blood cultures are sterile, antibiotic therapy should be discontinued by 36 to 48 hours of incubation, unless there is clear evidence of site-specific infection. Persistent cardiorespiratory instability is common among preterm infants with VLBW and is not alone an indication for prolonged empirical antibiotic administration. Laboratory test abnormalities alone rarely justify prolonged empirical antibiotic administration, particularly among preterm infants at a lower risk for EOS.

LEAD AUTHORS

Karen M. Puopolo, MD, PhD, FAAP
William E. Benitz, MD, FAAP
Theoklis E. Zaoutis, MD, MSCE, FAAP

COMMITTEE ON FETUS AND NEWBORN, 2017–2018

James Cummings, MD, Chairperson
Sandra Juul, MD
Ivan Hand, MD
Eric Eichenwald, MD
Brenda Poindexter, MD
Dan L. Stewart, MD
Susan W. Aucott, MD
Karen M. Puopolo, MD, PhD, FAAP
Jay P. Goldsmith, MD
Kristi Watterberg, MD, Immediate Past Chairperson

LIAISONS

Kasper S. Wang, MD – *American Academy of Pediatrics Section on Surgery*
Thierry Lacaze, MD – *Canadian Paediatric Society*
Joseph Wax, MD – *American College of Obstetricians and Gynecologists*
Tonse N.K. Raju, MD, DCH – *National Institutes of Health*

Wanda Barfield, MD, MPH, CAPT USPHS – *Centers for Disease Control and Prevention*
Erin Keels, MS, APRN, NNP-BC – *National Association of Neonatal Nurses*

STAFF

Jim Couto, MA

COMMITTEE ON INFECTIOUS DISEASES, 2017–2018

Carrie L. Byington, MD, FAAP, Chairperson
Yvonne A. Maldonado, MD, FAAP, Vice Chairperson
Ritu Banerjee, MD, PhD, FAAP
Elizabeth D. Barnett, MD, FAAP
James D. Campbell, MD, MS, FAAP
Jeffrey S. Gerber, MD, PhD, FAAP
Ruth Lynfield, MD, FAAP
Flor M. Munoz, MD, MSc, FAAP
Dawn Nolt, MD, MPH, FAAP
Ann-Christine Nyquist, MD, MSPH, FAAP
Sean T. O'Leary, MD, MPH, FAAP
Mobeen H. Rathore, MD, FAAP
Mark H. Sawyer, MD, FAAP
William J. Steinbach, MD, FAAP
Tina Q. Tan, MD, FAAP
Theoklis E. Zaoutis, MD, MSCE, FAAP

EX OFFICIO

David W. Kimberlin, MD, FAAP – *Red Book* Editor
Michael T. Brady, MD, FAAP – *Red Book* Associate Editor
Mary Anne Jackson, MD, FAAP – *Red Book* Associate Editor
Sarah S. Long, MD, FAAP – *Red Book* Associate Editor
Henry H. Bernstein, DO, MHCM, FAAP – *Red Book* Online Associate Editor
H. Cody Meissner, MD, FAAP – Visual *Red Book* Associate Editor

LIAISONS

Amanda C. Cohn, MD, FAAP – *Centers for Disease Control and Prevention*
Jamie Deseda-Tous, MD – *Sociedad Latinoamericana de Infectología Pediátrica*

Karen M. Farizo, MD – *US Food and Drug Administration*
Marc Fischer, MD, FAAP – *Centers for Disease Control and Prevention*
Natasha Halasa, MD, MPH, FAAP – *Pediatric Infectious Diseases Society*
Nicole Le Saux, MD – *Canadian Pediatric Society*
Scot Moore, MD, FAAP – *Committee on Practice Ambulatory Medicine*
Angela K. Shen, ScD, MPH – *National Vaccine Program Office*
Neil S. Silverman, MD – *American College of Obstetricians and Gynecologists*
James J. Stevermer, MD, MSPH, FAAFP – *American Academy of Family Physicians*
Jeffrey R. Starke, MD, FAAP – *American Thoracic Society*
Kay M. Tomashek, MD, MPH, DTM – *National Institutes of Health*

STAFF

Jennifer M. Frantz, MPH

ABBREVIATIONS

AAP: American Academy of Pediatrics
ACOG: American College of Obstetricians and Gynecologists
CBC: complete blood cell
CRP: C-reactive protein
CSF: cerebrospinal fluid
EOS: early-onset sepsis
GBS: group B *Streptococcus*
IAI: intraamniotic infection
LR: likelihood ratio
NEC: necrotizing enterocolitis
PROM: premature rupture of membranes
ROM: rupture of membranes
VLBW: very low birth weight
WBC: white blood cell

FINANCIAL DISCLOSURE: The authors have indicated they have no financial relationships relevant to this article to disclose.

FUNDING: No external funding.

POTENTIAL CONFLICT OF INTEREST: The authors have indicated they have no potential conflicts of interest to disclose.

COMPANION PAPER: A companion to this article can be found online at www.pediatrics.org/cgi/doi/10.1542/peds.2018-2894.

REFERENCES

1. Cotten CM, Taylor S, Stoll B, et al; NICHD Neonatal Research Network. Prolonged duration of initial empirical antibiotic treatment is associated with increased rates of necrotizing enterocolitis and death for extremely low birth weight infants. *Pediatrics.* 2009;123(1):58–66

2. Cordero L, Ayers LW. Duration of empiric antibiotics for suspected early-onset sepsis in extremely low birth weight infants. *Infect Control Hosp Epidemiol.* 2003;24(9):662–666

3. Oliver EA, Reagan PB, Slaughter JL, Buhimschi CS, Buhimschi IA. Patterns of empiric antibiotic administration

for presumed early-onset neonatal sepsis in neonatal intensive care units in the United States. *Am J Perinatol.* 2017;34(7):640–647

4. Puopolo KM, Mukhopadhyay S, Hansen NI, et al; NICHD Neonatal Research Network. Identification of extremely premature infants at low risk for early-onset sepsis. *Pediatrics.* 2017;140(5):e20170925

5. Goldenberg RL, Culhane JF, Iams JD, Romero R. Epidemiology and causes of preterm birth. *Lancet.* 2008;371(9606):75–84

6. Schrag SJ, Farley MM, Petit S, et al. Epidemiology of invasive early-onset neonatal sepsis, 2005 to 2014. *Pediatrics.* 2016;138(6):e20162013

7. Weston EJ, Pondo T, Lewis MM, et al. The burden of invasive early-onset neonatal sepsis in the United States, 2005-2008. *Pediatr Infect Dis J.* 2011;30(11):937–941

8. Stoll BJ, Hansen NI, Bell EF, et al; Eunice Kennedy Shriver National Institute of Child Health and Human Development Neonatal Research Network. Trends in care practices, morbidity, and mortality of extremely preterm neonates, 1993-2012. *JAMA.* 2015;314(10):1039–1051

9. Puopolo KM, Draper D, Wi S, et al. Estimating the probability of neonatal early-onset infection on the basis of maternal risk factors. *Pediatrics.* 2011;128(5). Available at: www.pediatrics. org/cgi/content/full/128/5/e1155

10. Stoll BJ, Hansen NI, Sánchez PJ, et al; Eunice Kennedy Shriver National Institute of Child Health and Human Development Neonatal Research Network. Early onset neonatal sepsis: the burden of group B streptococcal and *E. coli* disease continues. *Pediatrics.* 2011;127(5):817–826

11. Stoll BJ, Hansen NI, Higgins RD, et al; National Institute of Child Health and Human Development. Very low birth weight preterm infants with early onset neonatal sepsis: the predominance of gram-negative infections continues in the National Institute of Child Health and Human Development Neonatal Research Network, 2002-2003. *Pediatr Infect Dis J.* 2005;24(7):635–639

12. Benirschke K. Routes and types of infection in the fetus and the newborn. *AMA J Dis Child.* 1960;99(6):714–721

13. Blanc WA. Pathways of fetal and early neonatal infection. Viral placentitis, bacterial and fungal chorioamnionitis. *J Pediatr.* 1961;59:473–496

14. Goldenberg RL, McClure EM, Saleem S, Reddy UM. Infection-related stillbirths. *Lancet.* 2010;375(9724):1482–1490

15. Romero R, Dey SK, Fisher SJ. Preterm labor: one syndrome, many causes. *Science.* 2014;345(6198):760–765

16. Goldenberg RL, Hauth JC, Andrews WW. Intrauterine infection and preterm delivery. *N Engl J Med.* 2000;342(20):1500–1507

17. Carroll SG, Ville Y, Greenough A, et al. Preterm prelabour amniorrhexis: intrauterine infection and interval between membrane rupture and delivery. *Arch Dis Child Fetal Neonatal Ed.* 1995;72(1):F43–F46

18. Muglia LJ, Katz M. The enigma of spontaneous preterm birth. *N Engl J Med.* 2010;362(6):529–535

19. Lamont RF, Sobel J, Mazaki-Tovi S, et al. Listeriosis in human pregnancy: a systematic review. *J Perinat Med.* 2011;39(3):227–236

20. Vinturache AE, Gyamfi-Bannerman C, Hwang J, Mysorekar IU, Jacobsson B; Preterm Birth International Collaborative (PREBIC). Maternal microbiome - a pathway to preterm birth. *Semin Fetal Neonatal Med.* 2016;21(2):94–99

21. Hanke K, Hartz A, Manz M, et al; German Neonatal Network (GNN). Preterm prelabor rupture of membranes and outcome of very-low-birth-weight infants in the German Neonatal Network. *PLoS One.* 2015;10(4):e0122564

22. Ofman G, Vasco N, Cantey JB. Risk of early-onset sepsis following preterm, prolonged rupture of membranes with or without chorioamnionitis. *Am J Perinatol.* 2016;33(4):339–342

23. Dutta S, Reddy R, Sheikh S, Kalra J, Ray P, Narang A. Intrapartum antibiotics and risk factors for early onset sepsis. *Arch Dis Child Fetal Neonatal Ed.* 2010;95(2):F99–F103

24. Parry S, Strauss JF III. Premature rupture of the fetal membranes. *N Engl J Med.* 1998;338(10):663–670

25. American College of Obstetricians and Gynecologists' Committee on Practice Bulletins—Obstetrics. Practice bulletin no. 172: premature rupture of membranes. *Obstet Gynecol.* 2016;128(4):e165–e177

26. Benitz WE, Gould JB, Druzin ML. Risk factors for early-onset group B streptococcal sepsis: estimation of odds ratios by critical literature review. *Pediatrics.* 1999;103(6). Available at: www.pediatrics.org/cgi/content/full/103/6/e77

27. Higgins RD, Saade G, Polin RA, et al; Chorioamnionitis Workshop Participants. Evaluation and management of women and newborns with a maternal diagnosis of chorioamnionitis: summary of a workshop. *Obstet Gynecol.* 2016;127(3):426–436

28. Wortham JM, Hansen NI, Schrag SJ, et al; Eunice Kennedy Shriver NICHD Neonatal Research Network. Chorioamnionitis and culture-confirmed, early-onset neonatal infections. *Pediatrics.* 2016;137(1):e20152323

29. Mukhopadhyay S, Puopolo KM. Clinical and microbiologic characteristics of early-onset sepsis among very low birth weight infants: opportunities for antibiotic stewardship. *Pediatr Infect Dis J.* 2017;36(5):477–481

30. Committee on Obstetric Practice. Committee opinion no. 712: intrapartum management of intraamniotic infection. *Obstet Gynecol.* 2017;130(2):e95–e101

31. Alexander VN, Northrup V, Bizzarro MJ. Antibiotic exposure in the newborn intensive care unit and the risk of necrotizing enterocolitis. *J Pediatr.* 2011;159(3):392–397

32. Kuppala VS, Meinzen-Derr J, Morrow AL, Schibler KR. Prolonged initial empirical antibiotic treatment is associated with adverse outcomes in premature infants. *J Pediatr.* 2011;159(5):720–725

33. Ting JY, Synnes A, Roberts A, et al; Canadian Neonatal Network Investigators. Association between

antibiotic use and neonatal mortality and morbidities in very low-birth-weight infants without culture-proven sepsis or necrotizing enterocolitis. *JAMA Pediatr.* 2016;170(12):1181–1187

34. Vangay P, Ward T, Gerber JS, Knights D. Antibiotics, pediatric dysbiosis, and disease. *Cell Host Microbe.* 2015;17(5):553–564

35. Kinlay S, Michel T, Leopold JA. The future of vascular biology and medicine. *Circulation.* 2016;133(25):2603–2609

36. Kaiser Permanente Division of Research. Neonatal early-onset sepsis calculator. Available at: https://neonatalsepsiscalculator. kaiserpermanente.org. Accessed April 5, 2018

37. Wynn JL, Wong HR, Shanley TP, Bizzarro MJ, Saiman L, Polin RA. Time for a neonatal-specific consensus definition for sepsis. *Pediatr Crit Care Med.* 2014;15(6):523–528

38. Dunne WM Jr, Case LK, Isgriggs L, Lublin DM. In-house validation of the BACTEC 9240 blood culture system for detection of bacterial contamination in platelet concentrates. *Transfusion.* 2005;45(7):1138–1142

39. Flayhart D, Borek AP, Wakefield T, Dick J, Carroll KC. Comparison of BACTEC PLUS blood culture media to BacT/Alert FA blood culture media for detection of bacterial pathogens in samples containing therapeutic levels of antibiotics. *J Clin Microbiol.* 2007;45(3):816–821

40. Jorgensen JH, Mirrett S, McDonald LC, et al. Controlled clinical laboratory comparison of BACTEC plus aerobic/F resin medium with BacT/Alert aerobic FAN medium for detection of bacteremia and fungemia. *J Clin Microbiol.* 1997;35(1):53–58

41. Krisher KK, Gibb P, Corbett S, Church D. Comparison of the BacT/Alert PF pediatric FAN blood culture bottle with the standard pediatric blood culture bottle, the Pedi-BacT. *J Clin Microbiol.* 2001;39(8):2880–2883

42. Nanua S, Weber C, Isgriggs L, Dunne WM Jr. Performance evaluation of the VersaTREK blood culture system for

quality control testing of platelet units. *J Clin Microbiol.* 2009;47(3):817–818

43. Garcia-Prats JA, Cooper TR, Schneider VF, Stager CE, Hansen TN. Rapid detection of microorganisms in blood cultures of newborn infants utilizing an automated blood culture system. *Pediatrics.* 2000;105(3 pt 1):523–527

44. Sarkar SS, Bhagat I, Bhatt-Mehta V, Sarkar S. Does maternal intrapartum antibiotic treatment prolong the incubation time required for blood cultures to become positive for infants with early-onset sepsis? *Am J Perinatol.* 2015;32(4):357–362

45. Guerti K, Devos H, Ieven MM, Mahieu LM. Time to positivity of neonatal blood cultures: fast and furious? *J Med Microbiol.* 2011;60(pt 4):446–453

46. Jardine L, Davies MW, Faoagali J. Incubation time required for neonatal blood cultures to become positive. *J Paediatr Child Health.* 2006;42(12):797–802

47. Schelonka RL, Chai MK, Yoder BA, Hensley D, Brockett RM, Ascher DP. Volume of blood required to detect common neonatal pathogens. *J Pediatr.* 1996;129(2):275–278

48. Yaacobi N, Bar-Meir M, Shchors I, Bromiker R. A prospective controlled trial of the optimal volume for neonatal blood cultures. *Pediatr Infect Dis J.* 2015;34(4):351–354

49. Sarkar S, Bhagat I, DeCristofaro JD, Wiswell TE, Spitzer AR. A study of the role of multiple site blood cultures in the evaluation of neonatal sepsis. *J Perinatol.* 2006;26(1):18–22

50. Struthers S, Underhill H, Albersheim S, Greenberg D, Dobson S. A comparison of two versus one blood culture in the diagnosis and treatment of coagulase-negative *staphylococcus* in the neonatal intensive care unit. *J Perinatol.* 2002;22(7):547–549

51. Garges HP, Moody MA, Cotten CM, et al. Neonatal meningitis: what is the correlation among cerebrospinal fluid cultures, blood cultures, and cerebrospinal fluid parameters? *Pediatrics.* 2006;117(4):1094–1100

52. Manroe BL, Weinberg AG, Rosenfeld CR, Browne R. The neonatal blood count in health and disease. I. Reference

values for neutrophilic cells. *J Pediatr.* 1979;95(1):89–98

53. Schmutz N, Henry E, Jopling J, Christensen RD. Expected ranges for blood neutrophil concentrations of neonates: the Manroe and Mouzinho charts revisited. *J Perinatol.* 2008;28(4):275–281

54. Christensen RD, Henry E, Jopling J, Wiedmeier SE. The CBC: reference ranges for neonates. *Semin Perinatol.* 2009;33(1):3–11

55. Newman TB, Puopolo KM, Wi S, Draper D, Escobar GJ. Interpreting complete blood counts soon after birth in newborns at risk for sepsis. *Pediatrics.* 2010;126(5):903–909

56. Hornik CP, Benjamin DK, Becker KC, et al. Use of the complete blood cell count in early-onset neonatal sepsis. *Pediatr Infect Dis J.* 2012;31(8): 799–802

57. Benitz WE. Adjunct laboratory tests in the diagnosis of early-onset neonatal sepsis. *Clin Perinatol.* 2010;37(2):421–438

58. Lynema S, Marmer D, Hall ES, Meinzen-Derr J, Kingma PS. Neutrophil CD64 as a diagnostic marker of sepsis: impact on neonatal care. *Am J Perinatol.* 2015;32(4):331–336

59. Su H, Chang SS, Han CM, et al. Inflammatory markers in cord blood or maternal serum for early detection of neonatal sepsis-a systemic review and meta-analysis. *J Perinatol.* 2014;34(4):268–274

60. Chiesa C, Panero A, Rossi N, et al. Reliability of procalcitonin concentrations for the diagnosis of sepsis in critically ill neonates. *Clin Infect Dis.* 1998;26(3):664–672

61. Clark RH, Bloom BT, Spitzer AR, Gerstmann DR. Empiric use of ampicillin and cefotaxime, compared with ampicillin and gentamicin, for neonates at risk for sepsis is associated with an increased risk of neonatal death. *Pediatrics.* 2006;117(1):67–74

62. Snydman DR, Jacobus NV, McDermott LA, et al. Lessons learned from the anaerobe survey: historical perspective and review of the most recent data (2005-2007). *Clin Infect Dis.* 2010;50(suppl 1):S26–S33

63. Stoll BJ, Hansen N, Fanaroff AA, et al. Changes in pathogens causing early-onset sepsis in very-low-birth-weight infants. *N Engl J Med.* 2002;347(4):240–247

64. Schrag SJ, Hadler JL, Arnold KE, Martell-Cleary P, Reingold A, Schuchat A. Risk factors for invasive, early-onset *Escherichia coli* infections in the era of widespread intrapartum antibiotic use. *Pediatrics.* 2006;118(2):570–576

65. Puopolo KM, Eichenwald EC. No change in the incidence of ampicillin-resistant, neonatal, early-onset sepsis over 18 years. *Pediatrics.* 2010;125(5). Available at: www.pediatrics.org/cgi/content/full/125/5/e1031

66. Jordan HT, Farley MM, Craig A, et al; Active Bacterial Core Surveillance (ABCs)/Emerging Infections Program Network, CDC. Revisiting the need for vaccine prevention of late-onset neonatal group B streptococcal disease: a multistate, population-based analysis. *Pediatr Infect Dis J.* 2008;27(12):1057–1064

67. Phares CR, Lynfield R, Farley MM, et al; Active Bacterial Core Surveillance/Emerging Infections Program Network. Epidemiology of invasive group B streptococcal disease in the United States, 1999-2005. *JAMA.* 2008;299(17):2056–2065

Marijuana Use During Pregnancy and Breastfeeding: Implications for Neonatal and Childhood Outcomes

- *Clinical Report*

CLINICAL REPORT Guidance for the Clinician in Rendering Pediatric Care

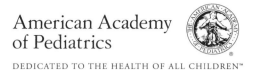

DEDICATED TO THE HEALTH OF ALL CHILDREN™

Marijuana Use During Pregnancy and Breastfeeding: Implications for Neonatal and Childhood Outcomes

Sheryl A. Ryan, MD, FAAP,[a] Seth D. Ammerman, MD, FAAP, FSAHM, DABAM,[b] Mary E. O'Connor, MD, MPH, FAAP,[c,d]
COMMITTEE ON SUBSTANCE USE AND PREVENTION, SECTION ON BREASTFEEDING

abstract

Marijuana is one of the most widely used substances during pregnancy in the United States. Emerging data on the ability of cannabinoids to cross the placenta and affect the development of the fetus raise concerns about both pregnancy outcomes and long-term consequences for the infant or child. Social media is used to tout the use of marijuana for severe nausea associated with pregnancy. Concerns have also been raised about marijuana use by breastfeeding mothers. With this clinical report, we provide data on the current rates of marijuana use among pregnant and lactating women, discuss what is known about the effects of marijuana on fetal development and later neurodevelopmental and behavioral outcomes, and address implications for education and policy.

[a]Department of Pediatrics, Penn State Health Milton S. Hershey Medical Center, Hershey, Pennsylvania; [b]Division of Adolescent Medicine, Department of Pediatrics, Stanford University and Teen Health Van, Stanford Children's Health, Palo Alto, California; [c]Department of Pediatrics, School of Medicine, University of Colorado, Aurora, Colorado; and [d]Dartmouth-Hitchcock Medical Center, Lebanon, New Hampshire

Dr Ammerman helped draft and revise the manuscript and critically reviewed the manuscript; Dr Ryan took the lead on drafting the manuscript and helped revise and critically reviewed the manuscript; Dr O'Connor helped draft and revise the manuscript and critically reviewed the manuscript with a focus on the breastfeeding portion; and all authors approved the final manuscript as submitted.

PREGNANCY AND MARIJUANA USE

Epidemiology

Data from 2016 reported in the National Survey on Drug Use and Health (NSDUH) revealed that 4.9% of pregnant women 15 through 44 years of age reported use of marijuana* in the past month, compared with 11% of nonpregnant women in the same age group.[1] This was an increase from the prior year, 3.4% and 10.3%, respectively. Among 18- through 25-year-old pregnant women, 8.5% reported past month marijuana use in 2016, compared with 3.3% of pregnant 26- through 44-year-old women.

---

* For the purposes of this report, the word "marijuana" is used intentionally to denote all substances derived from the cannabis plant, in lieu of the word cannabis, even when specifically designated as such by cited research to avoid confusion; the exception is when the term cannabis is part of a quotation. "Cannabis" is less typically used in most clinical settings and currently refers more to commercial products. Using the term marijuana also is consistent with many previous publications on this topic.

To cite: Ryan SA, Ammerman SD, O'Connor ME, AAP COMMITTEE ON SUBSTANCE USE AND PREVENTION, AAP SECTION ON BREASTFEEDING. Marijuana Use During Pregnancy and Breastfeeding: Implications for Neonatal and Childhood Outcomes. *Pediatrics.* 2018;142(3):e20181889

Although 2016 data are not available for pregnant 15- through 17-year-old women, 2012–2013 data revealed 14.6% reporting use of illicit† drugs in the past month. Among these illicit substances, marijuana is the substance most commonly used by pregnant women. Widely variable rates are reported among published studies in both the United States and the United Kingdom. Authors of a US multicenter lifestyle study in 2001 reported a prevalence of δ-9-tetrahydrocannabinol (THC), the psychoactive substance in marijuana, in infant meconium samples to be 7.2%.[2] Authors of a 2006 United Kingdom–based pilot study found that 13.25% of a cohort of Scottish newborn infants had meconium samples that had positive results for tetrahydrocannabinol and/or tetrahydrocannabinol-9-carboxylic acid.[3] In studies of urban, young, and socioeconomically disadvantaged pregnant women, reported rates of marijuana use ranged between 15% and 28%.[4–6] Using NSDUH data from 2002 to 2014, Brown et al[7] reported that the prevalence of "past month" marijuana use among pregnant women 18 through 44 years of age increased from 2.37% to 3.84%, with the highest use rates reported in 18- through 25-year-old women (7.47% in 2014). Several state-specific surveys have also been used to document increasing rates of marijuana use among pregnant women. The Pregnancy Risk Assessment Monitoring System (PRAMS), a surveillance project of the Centers for Disease Control and Prevention and state health departments, collects state-specific, population-based data on maternal attitudes and experiences before, during, and after pregnancy

(available at cdc.gov/prams). PRAMS has conducted surveys on a sample of women in Vermont with live births since 2001 and has included questions about marijuana use during pregnancy since 2009.[8] In 2013, 9.4% of women in Vermont reported marijuana use during their pregnancy, with no significant change in rates since 2009. PRAMS data from Hawaii revealed that women who reported experiencing significant nausea during their pregnancy reported higher rates of marijuana use (3.7%) compared with pregnant women without nausea (2.3%).[9] The 2012 NSDUH found that pregnant women reported a decrease in their marijuana use from 9.0% to 4.8% in the first and second trimesters, respectively, to 2.4% by the third trimester. Reported rates of tobacco use during pregnancy decreased from 19.9% to 13.4% and to 12.8% in the first, second, and third trimesters, respectively. Authors of other studies have found that 48% to 60% of marijuana users report continuing use during their entire pregnancy, believing it to be safer than tobacco.[4,10,11] In the Longitudinal Development and Infancy Study from the United Kingdom, Moore et al[11] found that most pregnant women who used cocaine, ecstasy, methylenedioxymethamphetamine, and other stimulants stopped using these substances by the second trimester, but 48% of previous marijuana users continued to use marijuana as well as alcohol (64%) and tobacco (46%) throughout their entire pregnancy. In addition, the Longitudinal Development and Infancy Study revealed that the frequency and amounts of both marijuana and tobacco use were sustained throughout the entire pregnancy, similar to prepregnancy levels, whereas the extent of reported alcohol use was reduced. PRAMS data from Vermont also revealed that for 2013 births, 44.6% of women who reported being marijuana smokers before pregnancy continued to use

marijuana during their pregnancy.[8] In contrast to these studies, Forray et al[12] found that, of 101 women who reported using marijuana at the beginning of pregnancy and who received substance abuse counseling, 78% were abstinent at a mean of 151 days later and remained abstinent until delivery.

Mark et al[13] demonstrated in a retrospective cohort study of urban, predominantly African American women that, of patients receiving prenatal care and delivering at their institution, 21.8% initially had positive screen results for marijuana use (by either self-report or urine toxicology), but only 1.9% had positive urine screen results for marijuana at the time of delivery. They attributed their high rate of cessation of marijuana use during pregnancy to be related to opportunities for education about adverse effects of drug use, including tobacco and marijuana, during prenatal visits.[13]

Marijuana use during pregnancy has been found to be associated with higher rates of licit and illicit substance use and certain socioeconomic and demographic characteristics. For example, in the Vermont PRAMS study, researchers found that pregnant women who reported marijuana use were more likely to be younger (<25 years of age), to be from households with lower income, to smoke cigarettes, and to report having experienced a significant emotional stressor (traumatic, financial, or partner related) before or during the pregnancy.[8] Mark et al[13] found that use of marijuana was more common in women who reported being unemployed, without a high school diploma, users of either alcohol or cigarettes, depressed, or a victim of abuse. In the Generation R study in the Netherlands, El Marroun et al[14] found in a sample of more than 7000 pregnant women that 85% of marijuana smokers were also

---

† The NSDUH defined illicit drug use to include marijuana/hashish, cocaine (including crack), heroin, hallucinogens, inhalants, or prescription-type psychotherapeutics used nonmedically.

cigarette smokers. Schempf and Strobino[6] found that marijuana use was not independently related to prenatal care. In their population of poor, urban women, lack of adequate prenatal care, defined as 1 or no prenatal visits, was significantly more likely among cocaine and opiate users but not marijuana users.[6] Reasons reported for this correlation with cocaine and opiate use included fear of being reported to police or child protective services and lower perceived benefit of prenatal care. Emphasized in these studies is the importance of considering the potential confounding of additional demographic and behavioral variables when evaluating the independent role of marijuana on pregnancy and fetal and infant outcomes.[15,16]

It is important to note that reported marijuana use rates can vary depending on the method of screening used. Current guidance recommends routine screening of all pregnant women for substance use by way of validated questionnaires or conversations with patients.[5,17] Authors of most studies to date have relied predominantly on self-report, which may have resulted in significant underestimation compared with questionnaires or objective measures using urine screening or meconium samples. However, even these objective measures will provide variable results, depending on the chronicity and intensity of use and the recency of use related to the time that a urine sample is obtained. With the increasing number of states legalizing marijuana use and with marijuana being touted on the Internet as a safe treatment of nausea during pregnancy, current rates of use of marijuana during pregnancy are a concern. Health care providers may see increases in the number of pregnant women using marijuana during at least a portion of their pregnancy.[18]

It is unclear why pregnant women are choosing to use marijuana during their pregnancy, because there are few data available on the benefits of marijuana use during pregnancy. Roberson et al[9] found that women reporting marijuana use during pregnancy were more likely to report experiencing severe nausea and vomiting (3.7%) compared with those not experiencing these severe symptoms (2.7%). In a second study of women using marijuana during their pregnancy, 51% reported using it for relief of nausea and vomiting, and 92% of those women reported its effectiveness; no controls were included in this study.[19] Although the use of marijuana is being touted on social media as an effective and safe treatment of nausea and vomiting of pregnancy, there are currently no indications for its use during pregnancy; the American College of Obstetricians and Gynecologists (ACOG) clearly stated this in its Committee Opinion in 2015.[5] Of note, none of the states with legal medicinal marijuana laws list pregnancy as a contraindication for recommending or dispensing medicinal marijuana.[18]

Pharmacokinetics of Cannabinoids During Pregnancy

Marijuana can affect the normal transport functions and physiologic status of the placenta throughout pregnancy.[20] One study has revealed that short-term exposure to cannabidiol, a nonpsychoactive substance found in marijuana, can enhance the placental barrier permeability to pharmacologic agents and recreational substances, potentially placing the fetus at risk from these agents or drugs.[21] El Marroun et al[22] found that marijuana use during pregnancy, as compared with either no marijuana use or tobacco use, results in increased resistance index and pulsatility index of the uterine artery, with resulting potential effects on uterine blood flow, such as increased placental resistance and reduced placental circulation.

Studies that have been used to assess the ability of metabolites of drugs of abuse, including marijuana, to cross the placenta are not recent and have revealed that recreational and licit substances directly cross the placenta, either through passive diffusion or, less commonly, through active transport or pinocytosis.[23] Among the numerous cannabinoids present in marijuana, the substance most responsible for the psychoactive effects, THC, has been shown to readily cross the placenta.[24] The THC molecule is highly lipophilic and is distributed rapidly to the brain and fat of the fetus after ingestion or inhalation by the pregnant woman. After maternal ingestion, concentrations of THC in fetal blood are approximately one-third to one-tenth of maternal concentrations.[24,25] These concentrations can vary depending on the permeability and biological capacity of the placenta.[26] In addition, when marijuana is smoked, serum carbon monoxide concentrations in the pregnant woman are 5 times higher than those when tobacco is smoked, resulting potentially in impaired maternal respiratory gas exchange and subsequent adverse effect on the fetus.[27] Given these known effects of marijuana on the placenta and placental transport, it is biologically plausible that marijuana use during pregnancy could affect both maternal and fetal outcomes.

Adverse Effects of Marijuana on Pregnancy and on the Neonate, Infant, Child, and Adolescent

Outcomes During the Neonatal Period

Two recent systematic reviews and meta-analyses have been published to determine the independent effect of marijuana use during pregnancy on both maternal and early neonatal outcomes. The first study by Gunn et al[28] was used to review 24 studies to determine the effect of marijuana use on maternal anemia; neonatal growth parameters, such as birth weight, head circumference, and length; admission to the NICU;

gestational age; and preterm birth. They found that women who used any marijuana during pregnancy had a higher likelihood of developing anemia, and infants exposed prenatally to marijuana had a decrease in birth weight (mean difference in weight of 110 g for exposed versus unexposed neonates) and a higher likelihood of needing admission to an NICU. They found no relationship between marijuana use and any of their other selected outcomes. The authors pointed out, however, that a major limitation of their study was their inability to determine the independent effect of marijuana, given that most of the studies assessed did not exclude individuals with polysubstance use, including tobacco or alcohol, or measure use of those substances. The authors also cited additional limitations, such as how the use of marijuana was identified mainly by self-report, and few of the outcomes assessed were standardized across studies.

Conner et al[29] has attempted to address the limitations cited in the review by Gunn et al[28] by adjusting the effects of marijuana exposure during pregnancy for tobacco use and other confounders, such as other drug use, wherever possible, in a second meta-analysis. Their study included the systematic review of 31 studies (from 1982 to 2015) in which they specifically evaluated the effect of maternal marijuana use on neonatal outcomes that included low birth weight (<2500 g), preterm delivery (<37 weeks' gestation), birth weight, gestational age at delivery, admission to the NICU, small-for-gestational-age status, stillbirth, spontaneous abortion, low Apgar scores, placental abruption, and perinatal death.[29] A major strength of this review was the inclusion of cohort studies used to measure use of other substances, such as tobacco and other recreational drugs, and socioeconomic and demographic factors to control for these confounders and determine the independent role of marijuana use. Exposure to marijuana was defined as any amount, frequency, or duration during the pregnancy, assessed through self-report or objective means when available; comparison groups were women who did not use any marijuana during their pregnancy. When analyses controlled for concomitant tobacco use, women who smoked marijuana only were not at risk for preterm delivery, but those who smoked both tobacco and marijuana did experience higher rates of preterm delivery compared with those not using either marijuana or tobacco. They also found no independent relationship between marijuana use and small-for-gestational-age status, placental abruption, need for NICU admission, or spontaneous abortion. They did find that women using marijuana during pregnancy were more likely to deliver an infant with lower mean birth weight or lower Apgar scores and to experience stillbirth, but these results were unadjusted, because the authors were limited in their analytic ability to provide adjusted relative risk rates for these outcomes. They concluded that maternal marijuana use during pregnancy was not an independent risk factor for several outcomes, given the confounding effect with factors such as tobacco use. They stated that the "increasing frequency of marijuana use during pregnancy may play a role in risk for adverse neonatal outcomes" but cautioned that "women who use marijuana more frequently are also more likely to use higher amounts of tobacco and other drugs," which could not be accounted for completely in their review.

Both systematic reviews included longitudinal cohort studies used to provide data that are mixed in terms of adverse outcomes in infants exposed to prenatal marijuana during pregnancy. These include the Ottawa Prenatal Prospective Study (OPPS), a longitudinal cohort study of low-risk, white, predominantly middle-class families[30,31]; the Maternal Health Practices and Child Development Study (MHPCD), a cohort study of high-risk, low socioeconomic–status women, representing both white and African American women[32]; the Generation R study, a population-based study from the Netherlands[14]; and the United Kingdom–based Avon Longitudinal Study of Pregnancy and Childhood.[33] Researchers of the OPPS and the MHPCD found no independent relationship between prenatal marijuana use and preterm births, miscarriages, pregnancy complications, or Apgar scores or physical anomalies in the neonates, but researchers of the OPPS did find a decrease in the length of gestation by 0.8 weeks associated with heavy marijuana use.[34,35] Researchers of the MPHCD study found that weight at birth was increased for neonates prenatally exposed to marijuana in the third trimester of pregnancy.[35] In the Generation R study, fetal growth was measured by using ultrasonography, and the researchers found an independent effect of marijuana use, over and above the effect observed with concomitant tobacco use, on decreased fetal growth that was observed beginning in the second trimester and resulted in lower birth weight, specifically when marijuana use was begun early in pregnancy and continued throughout the entire pregnancy.[14] The Generation R study was also used to assess the role of paternal marijuana use, and no independent association with fetal growth was found. In the Avon Longitudinal Study, Fergusson et al[33] found an association between prenatal marijuana use and smaller birth lengths, smaller head circumferences, and lower birth weights among those reporting marijuana use in pregnancy, compared with women in the control group who did not report use.

Authors of another recent large, population-based cohort study found that self-reported marijuana use, without concomitant use of nicotine and/or tobacco, was not associated with pregnancy complications, preterm birth, or changes in neonatal outcomes such as Apgar scores and growth parameters.[36] However, concomitant use of both marijuana and tobacco, compared with tobacco use alone, resulted in an increased risk of multiple adverse perinatal outcomes, higher rates of maternal asthma and preeclampsia, preterm births, and infants with decreased (<25th percentile) head circumferences and decreased (<25th percentile) birth weights. Less than 1% of the total sample of 12 069 women reported use of marijuana, which raises concerns about the representativeness of the sample or validity of self-reported use of substances.

A small number of studies have been used to assess the role of marijuana in outcomes not addressed in the 2 systematic reviews above, such as outcomes in preterm infants, neonatal behavioral outcomes, and fetal anomalies. Dotters-Katz et al[37] published a secondary data analysis on a group of preterm infants born before 35 weeks' gestation comparing the neonatal outcomes of those with prenatal marijuana exposure by maternal report or drug screening ($n = 138$) versus infants with no marijuana exposure ($n = 1732$). They found that prenatal marijuana exposure had no detrimental effect on death before hospital discharge, grade 3 or 4 intraventricular hemorrhage, periventricular leukomalacia, necrotizing enterocolitis, bronchopulmonary dysplasia, cerebral palsy, and/or a Bayley Scales of Infant Development–II <70 at 2 years of age.[37] van Gelder et al[38] found a higher rate of anencephaly in fetuses of women who smoked marijuana immediately before and during the first trimester of pregnancy, although the authors did not control for whether these women took supplemental folic acid during early pregnancy. Immediate newborn behaviors that have been observed in those infants who were exposed to marijuana in utero include altered arousal patterns, regulation, and excitability, as measured by the NICU Network Neurobehavioral Scale.[39] Increased tremors and prolonged and exaggerated startle reflexes, as measured by the Neonatal Behavioral Assessment Scale, were observed in the first week and persisted at 9 and 30 days of life.[40] Poor habituation and responses to visual but not auditory stimuli,[41] abnormal high-pitched cries,[42] and abnormal sleep patterns with decreased quiet sleep and increased sleep motility[43] have also been noted in the first week of life. A study by Dreher et al[44] of Jamaican infants exposed to marijuana prenatally did not reveal any abnormalities. Although researchers have suggested that these behaviors share some similarities with symptoms observed in the neonatal abstinence syndrome as well as with opioid withdrawal, there are no data being used now to support a clinical withdrawal syndrome with marijuana exposure.

In summary, the evidence for independent, adverse effects of marijuana on human neonatal outcomes and prenatal development is limited, and inconsistency in findings may be the result of the potential confounding caused by the high correlation between marijuana use and use of other substances such as cigarettes and alcohol, as well as sociodemographic risk factors. However, the evidence from the available research studies indicate reason for concern, particularly in fetal growth and early neonatal behaviors.

Later Effects During Childhood, Adolescence, and Early Adulthood

Two longitudinal studies (the OPPS and the MHPCD, which have been described in the previous section) have been used to observe cohorts of prenatally exposed individuals from infancy through adolescence and early adulthood, and these provide most of the limited available evidence on the long-term adverse neurodevelopmental effects resulting from prenatal exposure to marijuana.[30,32] Authors of both studies have assessed long-term outcomes in the areas of executive function, cognition, academic achievement, and behavior.

Researchers of OPPS have observed its cohort since 1978 (original total of 84 pregnant women who use marijuana) and have demonstrated that, independent of tobacco and other drugs, marijuana exposure has significant and pervasive effects that are noticeable in children beginning at 4 years of age and continuing into young adulthood. Initial observable effects at 4 years of age included lower scores in verbal reasoning and memory tasks.[45] At 6 years of age, children exposed to marijuana, compared with nonexposed children in the control group, showed deficits in global measures of language comprehension, memory, visual and/or perceptual function, and reading tasks that require sustained attention, with a dose response observed, in that those exposed to higher amounts of marijuana prenatally demonstrated higher dysfunction on impulsive and hyperactive scales.[46–48] At 9 through 12 years of age, marijuana exposure was not independently associated with global intelligence or verbal subscales on intelligence testing but was associated with deficits in executive function tasks, such as impulse control and visual problem-solving.[49–52] At 13 through 16 years of age, problems were seen in attention, problem-solving, visual integration, and analytic skills requiring sustained attention.[51,53–55] A functional MRI study of this cohort at ages 18 through 22 years revealed changes in neural activity with working memory tasks that were not observed in unexposed matched children in the control group.[56] Fried et al have postulated that the behavioral problems and decreased performance on global measures observed throughout childhood and into early adulthood reflect deficits in executive functioning, not overall intelligence.[31,54,57,58]

Researchers of the MHPCD have observed a cohort of exposed infants since 1982 to determine the independent effects of marijuana on cognition, behavior, temperament, mental health disorders, and substance use from infancy through adolescence and early adulthood. At 9 months of age, impaired mental development was seen.[59] At 3, 4, and 6 years of age, deficits in executive function tasks similar to those observed in the OPPS, with poorer memory and verbal measures were found[60,61]; at 6 years of age, impaired sustained attention on vigilance tasks and verbal reasoning and increased impulsivity and hyperactivity was observed with those exposed during the first trimester whose mothers smoked at least 1 joint per day.[61] Adverse consequences in later childhood included impaired executive functioning and visual problem-solving at 9 through 12 years of age and increased hyperactivity, impulsivity, and inattention at 10 years of age for those whose mothers had smoked marijuana during both the first and third trimesters.[62] Unlike the OPPS, whose authors did not find deficits in intellectual abilities and on measurements of standardized academic tests at ages 6 through 9 or 13 through 16 years, authors of the MHPCD did find lower reading and spelling scores in 10-year-old children whose mothers reported smoking at least 1 joint per day during the first trimester of pregnancy and deficits in reading comprehension and underachievement, as measured by the Wide Range Achievement

Test–Revised, with mothers who reported smoking marijuana during the second trimester.[62] Lower global achievement, reading, spelling, and math scores were also seen at 14 years of age.[63] Measures of problem behaviors and mental health symptoms were also reported in both cohort studies. The authors of the OPPS found higher rates of reported problem behaviors at 6 through 9 years of age[64] and higher rates of depressive symptoms at 16 through 21 years of age.[65] Authors of the MHPCD also found higher rates of depressive symptoms and externalizing behaviors via parent and teacher report in the exposed cohort at 10 years of age and an increased risk of psychosis in young adults.[66,67] Higher rates of substance use were also reported by these 2 cohort studies. Authors of the OPPS found earlier onset and greater use of both marijuana and tobacco in the exposed cohorts, observed at ages 16 through 21 years,[65] and authors of the MHPCD found higher rates of marijuana and tobacco use across the ages of 14 through 21 years, even after controlling for home environment and parental substance use.[66,68] Sonon et al[69] have also demonstrated higher rates of marijuana use in young adulthood after prenatal exposure to marijuana.

In summary, it is essential to note that the studies discussed above have limitations that may threaten the validity of the findings. For example, the studies in which authors look at proximal results, such as fetal or early neonatal outcomes, rely in most part on self-report of marijuana use, and there is little standardization across studies in the amount of marijuana used and frequency of use. Many of these studies included pregnant women who used other substances in addition to marijuana, such as tobacco, alcohol, or other drugs, and analytic methods were used to control for the confounding effects of these other substances.

For more distal outcomes, such as later childhood and adolescent cognition and behavior, studies were limited in the environmental and sociodemographic variables that the authors could control, which could be expected to influence development across childhood and adolescence.[70,71] Despite these limitations and the relative paucity of research in this area, the findings regarding growth variables[72] and neurodevelopmental and behavioral outcomes can be used to suggest that marijuana use during pregnancy may not be harmless. In addition, the existing cohort studies were conducted when the available marijuana had a much lower potency than what is available today, which raises concern that the adverse consequences of prenatal exposure in currently pregnant women may be much greater than what has been reported to date.[18] (See the "Other Considerations" section for discussion on potency.) Rigorous research is needed to determine the independent effects of marijuana, as well as tobacco and other drugs, on neonatal and later childhood and adult outcomes.

Mechanisms Used to Explain Underlying Effects on the Developing Fetus

Cannabinoids mediate their effects through the cannabinoid receptors, type 1 and 2. The endocannabinoid system (ECS) comprises these receptors, along with the neurochemical cannabinoids anandamide and 2-arachidonoylglycerol. This has been studied in both animal as well as human models, specifically for its effect on the immune system and the central nervous system.[23] Although the consequences of prenatal marijuana exposure in pregnant women, both behavioral and developmental, have been documented in epidemiological studies, the molecular mechanisms that are postulated to be associated with these effects of prenatal drug exposure are only now being elucidated. The ECS is detectable from the early stages of embryonic development (as early as 5 weeks' gestation) and has been found to play an essential role in the early stages of neuronal development and cell survival.[73] Researchers of new data elucidate how this system is involved in the control of neuronal developmental processes such as cell proliferation, migration, and differentiation; thus, it is not surprising that cannabinoid exposure during early developmental stages can result in the long-term neurobehavioral consequences described previously.

Although authors of early studies relied on animal models, authors of recent studies conducted on electively aborted fetuses have provided specific human data, which have been used to support findings observed with animal models. Tortoriello et al[20] have used sophisticated quantitative and qualitative molecular analyses and pharmacologic methods to study human fetuses electively aborted during the second trimester, in both pregnant women who smoked marijuana and pregnant women in a control group who did not use marijuana.[19] They found that in fetuses exposed prenatally to marijuana, levels of molecular substances essential for neuronal cell axonal elongation (SCG10) are significantly reduced, which affects the disassembly of microtubules essential for axonal elongation and the "pathfinding" essential for the development of normal neuronal circuitry during early brain development. THC acts as a partial agonist and binds to the cannabinoid receptors (CB1) during fetal development by reducing endogenous endocannabinoid synthesis (especially 2-arachidonoylglycerol) and subsequent CB1 expression. This results in a functional "hijacking" or supraphysiological modulation of the normal ECS during early

fetal brain development. The result is a disruption of the precisely orchestrated signaling and sequencing functions of the ECS, affected by the CB1 receptors, and mediated through the excessive degradation of the intracellular substances such as SCG10 and JNK1.[74] Researchers have also found that unlike the adult brain, in which CB1 receptors are widely distributed throughout most areas of the brain, in the fetus, CB1 receptors are found primarily in the mesocorticolimbic structures such as the amygdaloid complex, the hippocampus, and the ventral striatum, all areas that are important for emotional regulation, cognition, and memory.[75] Researchers have also found that male fetuses may have a greater vulnerability to early developmental effects of prenatal marijuana exposure.[65,76] It is still unclear to what extent this disruption or alteration of developmental synaptic organization is responsible for early neonatal birth effects, longer-term neurodevelopmental effects, or increased vulnerability of later teenagers and adults for addiction or psychiatric illness. With the limited data, it is suggested that the neuronal systems involved in early development need to be studied further for us to understand more fully the molecular mechanism underlying the effects of maternal marijuana on the human fetal brain and specifically for those systems involved in neurocognition, impulsivity, and addiction vulnerability.[76]

Epigenetic mechanisms are also being proposed as one of the explanations for the consequences of prenatal marijuana exposure on fetal neurodevelopment and to explain why adolescents and adults who have been exposed to marijuana prenatally demonstrate an increased vulnerability to later addiction and psychiatric disorders.[77] Epigenetics refers to the mechanism by which gene expression is altered without

changes to the genetic code that occur after the genetic makeup of the individual is determined, either prenatally or postnatally. These genetic alterations include microRNAs, DNA methylation, and posttranslational modifications of nucleosomal histones.[77] They are stable alterations that occur during critical developmental periods and result in enduring phenotypical abnormalities.[77] For example, researchers have found that marijuana exposure in early fetal life decreases the expression of genes (through histone lysine methylation) for dopamine receptors (DRD2) in those areas of the brain important for reward recognition (ventral striatum, nucleus accumbens), which may explain higher rates of drug addiction in adults exposed prenatally to marijuana.[78] THC also causes substantial changes in gene expression levels of several other significant systems in the brain that are linked to the ECS, such as the opioid, glutamate, and γ-aminobutyric acid systems, which may persist well into adulthood.[79]

Linkages of the ECS to Other Neurotransmitter Systems

The ECS has been found to have a strong interaction with the opioid systems, through the μ, δ, and κ opioid receptors,[80] Jutras-Aswad et al[79] have found that early marijuana exposure influenced the expression and activity of opioid receptors that have been found to be important in reward and subsequent addictive behaviors. The ECS has also been found to be associated with the serotonergic, adrenergic, glutamate, and γ-aminobutyric acid systems.[78]

Issues for the Clinician

The American Academy of Pediatrics (AAP), the ACOG, and the American Society of Addiction Medicine recommend that all women considering pregnancy, pregnant women throughout their pregnancy, and those attending predelivery pediatric visits be screened routinely for alcohol and other drug use, including marijuana, by using a validated screening questionnaire.[17,81] Screening and brief intervention techniques are recommended to counsel abstinence for individuals using substances and to refer for treatment those individuals meeting criteria for any substance use disorder.[81] Despite these recommendations, in 1 study, Holland et al[82] found that of the 19% of women reporting current marijuana use (53%) or past marijuana use at their initial prenatal visit, only 52% received any kind of counseling. In addition, the counseling that was provided was focused mainly on legal and child protective consequences of detection at delivery, rather than specific medical or health effects of marijuana use. In July 2015, the ACOG published a position statement that was specifically used to advise against the "prescribing or suggesting the use of marijuana for medicinal purposes during preconception, pregnancy and lactation."[5] Most states that have legalized medicinal marijuana have not specifically limited its dispensing to pregnant women. Oregon is the only state that has legislated specific point-of-sale warnings to dispensaries for women who are pregnant or breastfeeding.[83] It is beyond the scope of this report to discuss specific validated questionnaires that are available or various means for objective screening.

Health care providers are mandated to report to child protective services any cases of suspected child abuse or neglect. The 2010 Child Abuse and Prevention and Treatment Act requires all states to have policies and procedures for reporting newborns and other children who are exposed to illicit substances under the definition of child abuse and/or neglect. Because marijuana is

still an illicit substance under federal law, this law applies to marijuana exposure in all states regardless of the legal status of marijuana use by adults in each state. Individual states may have other requirements for the reporting of newborn infants exposed to drugs and other exposures to children.[84]

Given these legal requirements, it is advisable for all health care providers who see pregnant women to be aware of the specific reporting requirements of their state and the potential adverse legal and social consequences of identifying substance use in their patients. When a legal or medical obligation exists for a health care provider to test a patient, he or she should counsel patients about these potential consequences before ordering drug tests and make a reasonable effort to obtain informed consent.[5] Of note, in states with requirements for the reporting of newborn infants exposed to drugs, these supersede federal law on confidential protection of patient records when receiving addiction treatment (42 Code of Federal Regulations Part 2).[81]

BREASTFEEDING AND MARIJUANA USE

Breastfeeding is recognized as the ideal feeding method for infants because of the numerous short-term and long-term benefits of breastfeeding for the mother and the infant. These benefits include but are not limited to decreased infections, such as gastroenteritis, ear infections, and severe respiratory diseases; decreased obesity and diabetes mellitus; decreased rate of sudden infant death syndrome; improved intellectual development; decreased postpartum blood loss; increased child spacing; and decreased risk of type 2 diabetes mellitus for the mother.[85]

When pregnant mothers take medications prescribed or

recreationally, the benefits of breastfeeding must be weighed against the effects of the drug on the infant to make a decision that is in the infant's and mother's best interests. Many medications that mothers use while breastfeeding are also taken during pregnancy. It can be difficult to determine whether effects of the drug on the infant are attributable to exposure during pregnancy or from breastfeeding. Additionally, a mother's ability to care for her infant may be impaired because of her use of marijuana. Infants can also be exposed to marijuana through inhalation of marijuana smoked in the presence of the infant.[86,87]

Epidemiology

There are few data about the frequency of use of marijuana by women while breastfeeding. A report from Colorado, where marijuana is legal for some, surveyed women attending the Special Supplemental Nutrition Program for Women, Infants, and Children program in the state's largest local health department. It revealed that 7.4% of mothers younger than 30 years of age and 4% of mothers older than 30 years of age were current marijuana users. Of all marijuana users (past, ever, current), 35.8% said that they had used at some point during pregnancy, 41% had used since the infant was born, and 18% had used while breastfeeding.[88]

Pharmacokinetics of Marijuana in Human Milk

The excretion of medications into human milk depends on chemical factors about the drug, including ionization, the molecular weight, the solubility in lipids and water, and the pH of the drug. The major psychoactive cannabinoid of marijuana, THC, is 99% protein bound, is lipid soluble, and has a molecular weight of 314.[89] The low molecular weight and high lipid solubility combine to cause marijuana transfer into human milk. It also causes storage of THC in lipid-filled tissues such as the brain. Little is known about the other cannabinoids in marijuana and their transfer into human milk. There are few data about the transfer of THC into human milk. With Table 1, we list the results from the only 2 primary references about concentrations of THC in human milk. These limited data by Perez-Reyes and Wall[90] and Marchei et al[91] reveal that THC transfers into human milk. There is no information about how the amount transferred is related to the concentration of THC in the marijuana, the frequency of use, or the concentration in maternal plasma.

The Effect of Marijuana on Breastfed Infants

There are 2 small studies by Tennes et al[92] and Astley and Little[93] from the 1980s in which the authors attempt to evaluate the effect of maternal marijuana use while breastfeeding on the infant. Both studies included mothers who also used alcohol, other drugs, and tobacco. Tennes et al[92] studied 258 mothers using marijuana and compared them to mothers who did not use marijuana. They examined the infants at 24 to 72 hours of age and a subgroup at 1 year of age. They found the following results: (1) marijuana users were more likely to use illicit drugs and alcohol with a significant linear dose-response relationship between the use of marijuana and alcohol ($R = 0.45$; $P < .01$); (2) infants exposed to marijuana were slightly shorter; (3) most mothers decreased use of marijuana during pregnancy; and (4) no differences were noted in the 1-year growth and scores on the Bayley Scales of Infant Development; however, only 27 of the infants tested at 1 year were exposed to marijuana while being breastfed. These results are limited by the small number

TABLE 1 Primary Sources for the Concentrations of THC Transmission Into Human Milk

Mother	Maternal Marijuana Dose	Amount of THC in Maternal Plasma	Amount of THC in Human Milk
A[91]	Smoked in pipe 1 time per day	—	105 ng/mL
B[91]	Smoked in pipe 7 times per day	7.2 ng/mL	60.3 ng/mL
C[90]	No information	—	86 ng/mL

—, not applicable.

of infants exposed to marijuana through breastfeeding, self-selection of mothers who participated in the 1-year follow-up, and lack of control for use of other substances, particularly alcohol.[92]

Astley and Little[93] studied diet, alcohol, and tobacco use during lactation in a group of middle-class mothers. Developmental evaluation at 1 year was completed on 68 infants whose mothers used marijuana while breastfeeding who were matched with mothers with similar alcohol and tobacco use who did not use marijuana while breastfeeding. Of the breastfeeding mothers, 79% reported marijuana use while pregnant, compared with 15% of mothers of infants who were fed formula. In multivariate regression analysis, the infant's exposure to marijuana during breastfeeding in the first month was associated with 14 ± 5 points decrease in motor scores after controlling for tobacco, alcohol, and cocaine use during pregnancy and lactation. There was no effect of marijuana use in the third month of life while breastfeeding. Marijuana use in the first trimester of pregnancy confounded these results, and it was not clear whether exposure prenatally or during breastfeeding had more association. The studies by Tennes et al[92] and Astley and Little[93] had small sample sizes, were completed more than 30 years ago, were associated with use of marijuana during the mother's pregnancy, and had no long-term follow-up. These limitations make it difficult to separate independent effects of marijuana use during

breastfeeding from prenatal exposure.

Another area of concern is the use of expressed maternal milk for feeding preterm infants when the mother has reported marijuana use or receives positive test results for marijuana. Expressed maternal milk has been shown to significantly improve outcomes in preterm infants by decreasing the rate of necrotizing enterocolitis (both surgical and nonsurgical), contributing to earlier attainment of full enteral feeds, decreasing the rate of sepsis, and improving neurodevelopmental outcomes, especially for the preterm infants with a birth weight of less than 1500 g.[85]

Published Recommendations From Other Organizations

The 2012 AAP policy statement, "Breastfeeding and the Use of Human Milk," included the following guidance: "maternal substance abuse is not a categorical contraindication to breastfeeding." "Street drugs such as PCP (phencyclidine), cocaine, and cannabis can be detected in human milk, and their use by breastfeeding mothers is of concern, particularly regarding the infant's long-term neurobehavioral development and thus are contraindicated."[85] Although this has been interpreted by some professional organizations to indicate that in the parent using marijuana, the choice to breastfeed is "contraindicated," this was not the intent of that statement. It is suggested instead that the mother be encouraged to breastfeed while, at the same time, it is strongly encouraged that she abstain completely from using marijuana as well as other drugs, alcohol, and tobacco. This position has been supported by several other professional organizations and resources. For example, LactMed (a free searchable database from the National Library of Medicine) recommends that mothers be encouraged to abstain from or reduce their marijuana use while breastfeeding and to minimize infant exposure to marijuana smoke. The LactMed peer review panel, which reviews published data to ensure scientific validity and currency, recommends continuing breastfeeding.[86] This is similar to the recommendations of the ACOG, which state, "There are insufficient data to evaluate the effects of marijuana use on infants during lactation and breastfeeding, and in the absence of such data, marijuana use is discouraged."[5] The Academy of Breastfeeding Medicine states "A recommendation of abstaining from any marijuana use is warranted. At this time, although the data are not strong enough to recommend not breastfeeding with any marijuana use, we urge caution."[94] After Colorado legalized the use of marijuana by adults ≥21 years old, the Colorado Department of Public Health and Environment developed educational material about marijuana use during pregnancy and while breastfeeding. These materials include patient education handouts that may be helpful to pediatricians and families and are available at the following link: www.colorado.gov/ pacific/sites/default/files/MJ_RMEP_ Pregnancy-Breastfeeding-Clinical-Guidelines.pdf. Other states that have legalized marijuana may have similar educational information for health care providers and families.

OTHER CONSIDERATIONS

The potency of marijuana now routinely available is much higher than what was available a decade ago. The potency of THC in samples studied in 1983 averaged 3.2%, and the average in 2008 was 13.2%; the authors of that same study identified isolated samples with THC contents as high as 27.3% and 37.2%.[95] These higher potencies as well as new practices of marijuana use, such as dabbing or vaping, can significantly increase the concentration of THC being consumed. Studies have revealed that the development of marijuana strains with higher THC concentrations has reduced the concentration of cannabidiol, possibly decreasing the medicinal benefits for a select number of conditions. There are many other substances contained in the marijuana plant in addition to THC and cannabidiol about which little is known. Additionally, marijuana is often grown with the use of pesticides, herbicides, rodenticides, and fertilizers, many of which are toxic.[96,97] Exposure to marijuana may also expose the fetus and infant to these toxins.

CONCLUSIONS AND RECOMMENDATIONS

Pediatricians are in a unique position to counsel women of childbearing age about the potential negative consequences of marijuana use during pregnancy and breastfeeding. Discussing what is known about adverse consequences of marijuana use during pregnancy and breastfeeding at prenatal visits with either the pediatrician or the obstetric provider is an important component of promoting the best health outcomes for both the pregnant woman and the infant. Legalization of marijuana may give the false impression that marijuana is safe. Given ethical concerns, there are no randomized controlled trials on the effect of marijuana use by pregnant and lactating women, and the available longitudinal studies must be viewed with caution

given the potential confounding of the effect of marijuana during pregnancy by other licit and illicit substances and sociodemographic and environmental risks factors. However, highlighted in the available epidemiological and animal data are concerns regarding both short-term growth and long-term neurodevelopmental and behavioral consequences of prenatal exposure to marijuana. Our current understanding of the ECS and its role in the development of neural circuitry early in fetal life also provides "theoretical justification" for the potential of marijuana substances, particularly THC, to affect neurodevelopment.[18]

Breastfeeding has numerous valuable health benefits for the mother and the infant, particularly the preterm infant. Limited data reveal that THC does transfer into human milk, and there is no evidence for the safety or harm of marijuana use during lactation. Therefore, women also need to be counseled about what is known about the adverse effects of THC on brain development during early infancy, when brain growth and development are rapid.

The importance of the published findings and the emerging research regarding the potential negative effects of marijuana on brain development are a cause for concern despite the limited research and are the basis for the following recommendations:

1. Women who are considering becoming pregnant or who are of reproductive age need to be informed about the lack of definitive research and counseled about the current concerns regarding potential adverse effects of THC use on the woman and on fetal, infant, and child development. Marijuana can be included as part of a discussion about the use of tobacco, alcohol, and other

drugs and medications during pregnancy.

2. As part of routine anticipatory guidance and in addition to contraception counseling, it is important to advise all adolescents and young women that if they become pregnant, marijuana should not be used during pregnancy.

3. Pregnant women who are using marijuana or other cannabinoid-containing products to treat a medical condition or to treat nausea and vomiting during pregnancy should be counseled about the lack of safety data and the possible adverse effects of THC in these products on the developing fetus and referred to their health care provider for alternative treatments that have better pregnancy-specific safety data.

4. Women of reproductive age who are pregnant or planning to become pregnant and are identified through universal screening as using marijuana should be counseled and, as clinically indicated, receive brief intervention and be referred to treatment.

5. Although marijuana is legal in some states, pregnant women who use marijuana can be subject to child welfare investigations if they have a positive marijuana screen result. Health care providers should emphasize that the purpose of screening is to allow treatment of the woman's substance use, not to punish or prosecute her.

6. Present data are insufficient to assess the effects of exposure of infants to maternal marijuana use during breastfeeding. As a result, maternal marijuana use while breastfeeding is discouraged. Because the potential risks of infant exposure to marijuana metabolites are

unknown, women should be informed of the potential risk of exposure during lactation and encouraged to abstain from using any marijuana products while breastfeeding.

7. Pregnant or breastfeeding women should be cautioned about infant exposure to smoke from marijuana in the environment, given emerging data on the effects of passive marijuana smoke.

8. Women who have become abstinent from previous marijuana use should be encouraged to remain abstinent while pregnant and breastfeeding.

9. Further research regarding the use of and effects of marijuana during pregnancy and breastfeeding is needed.

10. Pediatricians are urged to work with their state and/or local health departments if legalization of marijuana is being considered or has occurred in their state to help with constructive, nonpunitive policy and education for families.

RESOURCES

Additional resources include the AAP Resources on Marijuana (www.aap/marijuana), the AAP Section on Breastfeeding (www.aap.org/breastfeeding), the Academy of Breastfeeding Medicine (www.bfmed.org), the ACOG (www.acog.org/About-ACOG/ACOG-Departments/Breastfeeding), and LactMed (toxnet.nlm.nih.gov/newtoxnet/lactmed.htm).

LEAD AUTHORS

Sheryl A. Ryan, MD, FAAP
Seth D. Ammerman, MD, FAAP, FSAHM, DABAM
Mary E. O'Connor, MD, MPH, FAAP

COMMITTEE ON SUBSTANCE USE AND PREVENTION, 2017–2018

Sheryl A. Ryan, MD, FAAP, Chairperson

Stephen W. Patrick, MD, MPH, MS, FAAP
Jennifer Plumb, MD, MPH, FAAP
Joanna Quigley, MD, FAAP
Leslie R. Walker-Harding, MD, FAAP

FORMER COMMITTEE MEMBERS

Seth D. Ammerman, MD, FAAP, FSAHM, DABAM
Lucien Gonzalez, MD, MS, FAAP

LIAISON

Gregory Tau, MD, PhD – *American Academy of Child and Adolescent Psychiatry*

STAFF

Renee Jarrett, MPH

SECTION ON BREASTFEEDING EXECUTIVE COMMITTEE, 2017–2018

Joan Younger Meek, MD, MS, RD, FAAP, IBCLC, Chairperson
Maya Bunik, MD, MSPH, FAAP
Mary E. O'Connor, MD, MPH, FAAP
Lisa Stellwagen, MD, FAAP
Jennifer Thomas, MD, MPH, FAAP
Julie Ware, MD, FAAP

SUBCOMMITTEE CHAIRPERSONS

Lawrence Noble, MD, FAAP – *Policy Chairperson*
Krystal Revai, MD, MPH, FAAP – *Chief Chapter Breastfeeding Coordinator*
Margaret Parker, MD, MPH, FAAP – *Education Program Chairperson*

FORMER EXECUTIVE COMMITTEE MEMBER

Margreete Johnston, MD, MPH, FAAP

STAFF

Ngozi Onyema-Melton, MPH, CHES

ABBREVIATIONS

AAP: American Academy of Pediatrics
ACOG: American College of Obstetricians and Gynecologists
ECS: endocannabinoid system
MHPCD: Maternal Health Practices and Child Development Study
NSDUH: National Survey on Drug Use and Health
OPPS: Ottawa Prenatal Prospective Study
PRAMS: Pregnancy Risk Assessment Monitoring System
THC: δ-9-tetrahydrocannabinol

All clinical reports from the American Academy of Pediatrics automatically expire 5 years after publication unless reaffirmed, revised, or retired at or before that time.

DOI: https://doi.org/10.1542/peds.2018-1889

Address correspondence to Seth D. Ammerman, MD, FAAP, FSAHM, DABAM. E-mail: seth.ammerman@stanford.edu

PEDIATRICS (ISSN Numbers: Print, 0031-4005; Online, 1098-4275).

Copyright © 2018 by the American Academy of Pediatrics

FINANCIAL DISCLOSURE: The authors have indicated they have no financial relationships relevant to this article to disclose.

FUNDING: No external funding.

POTENTIAL CONFLICT OF INTEREST: The authors have indicated they have no potential conflicts of interest to disclose.

REFERENCES

1. National Survey on Drug Use and Health. Available at: https://www.samhsa.gov/data/data-we-collect/nsduh-national-survey-drug-use-and-health. Accessed September 7, 2017

2. Lester BM, ElSohly M, Wright LL, et al. The Maternal Lifestyle Study: drug use by meconium toxicology and maternal self-report. *Pediatrics.* 2001;107(2):309–317

3. Williamson S, Jackson L, Skeoch C, Azzim G, Anderson R. Determination of the prevalence of drug misuse by meconium analysis. *Arch Dis Child Fetal Neonatal Ed.* 2006;91(4):F291–F292

4. Passey ME, Sanson-Fisher RW, D'Este CA, Stirling JM. Tobacco, alcohol and cannabis use during pregnancy: clustering of risks. *Drug Alcohol Depend.* 2014;134:44–50

5. Committee on Obstetric Practice. Committee opinion no. 722: marijuana use during pregnancy and lactation. *Obstet Gynecol.* 2017;130(4):e205–e209

6. Schempf AH, Strobino DM. Drug use and limited prenatal care: an examination of responsible barriers. *Am J Obstet Gynecol.* 2009;200(4):412.e1–412.e10

7. Brown QL, Sarvet AL, Shmulewitz D, Martins SS, Wall MM, Hasin DS. Trends in marijuana use among pregnant and nonpregnant reproductive-aged women, 2002-2014. *JAMA.* 2017;317(2):207–209

8. Vermont Department of Health. Marijuana use before, during, and after pregnancy. Available at: http://www.healthvermont.gov/sites/default/files/documents/2017/02/PRAMS_Marijuana_2009_2013_corrected.pdf. Accessed October 19, 2017

9. Roberson EK, Patrick WK, Hurwitz EL. Marijuana use and maternal experiences of severe nausea during pregnancy in Hawai'i. *Hawaii J Med Public Health.* 2014;73(9):283–287

10. Beatty JR, Svikis DS, Ondersma SJ. Prevalence and perceived financial costs of marijuana versus tobacco use among urban low-income pregnant women. *J Addict Res Ther.* 2012;3(4):100–135

11. Moore DG, Turner JD, Parrott AC, et al. During pregnancy, recreational drug-using women stop taking ecstasy (3,4-methylenedioxy-N-methylamphetamine) and reduce alcohol consumption, but continue to smoke tobacco and cannabis: initial findings from the Development and Infancy Study. *J Psychopharmacol.* 2010;24(9):1403–1410

12. Forray A, Merry B, Lin H, Ruger JP, Yonkers KA. Perinatal substance use: a prospective evaluation of abstinence and relapse. *Drug Alcohol Depend.* 2015;150:147–155

13. Mark K, Desai A, Terplan M. Marijuana use and pregnancy: prevalence, associated characteristics, and birth outcomes. *Arch Women Ment Health.* 2016;19(1):105–111

14. El Marroun H, Tiemeier H, Steegers EA, et al. Intrauterine cannabis exposure affects fetal growth trajectories: the Generation R Study. *J Am Acad Child Adolesc Psychiatry.* 2009;48(12):1173–1181

15. van Gelder MM, Reefhuis J, Caton AR, Werler MM, Druschel CM, Roeleveld N; National Birth Defects Prevention Study. Characteristics of pregnant illicit drug users and associations between cannabis use and perinatal outcome in a population-based study. *Drug Alcohol Depend.* 2010;109(1–3):243–247

16. Alhusen JL, Lucea MB, Bullock L, Sharps P. Intimate partner violence, substance use, and adverse neonatal outcomes among urban women. *J Pediatr.* 2013;163(2):471–476

17. American Academy of Pediatrics; American College of Obstetricians and Gynecologists. *Guidelines for Perinatal Care.* 8th ed. Elk Grove Village, IL: American Academy of Pediatrics; and Washington, DC: American College of Obstetricians and Gynecologists; 2017

18. Volkow ND, Compton WM, Wargo EM. The risks of marijuana use during pregnancy. *JAMA.* 2017;317(2):129–130

19. Westfall RE, Janssen PA, Lucas P, Capler R. Survey of medicinal cannabis use among childbearing women: patterns of its use in pregnancy and retroactive self-assessment of its efficacy against 'morning sickness'. *Complement Ther Clin Pract.* 2006;12(1):27–33

20. Tortoriello G, Morris CV, Alpar A, et al. Miswiring the brain: Δ9-tetrahydrocannabinol disrupts cortical development by inducing an SCG10/stathmin-2 degradation pathway. *EMBO J.* 2014;33(7):668–685

21. Feinshtein V, Erez O, Ben-Zvi Z, et al. Cannabidiol enhances xenobiotic permeability through the human placental barrier by direct inhibition of breast cancer resistance protein: an ex vivo study. *Am J Obstet Gynecol.* 2013;209(6):573.e1–573.e15

22. El Marroun H, Tiemeier H, Steegers EA, et al. A prospective study on intrauterine cannabis exposure and fetal blood flow. *Early Hum Dev.* 2010;86(4):231–236

23. Loebstein R, Lalkin A, Koren G. Pharmacokinetic changes during pregnancy and their clinical relevance. *Clin Pharmacokinet.* 1997;33(5):328–343

24. Grotenhermen F. Pharmacokinetics and pharmacodynamics of cannabinoids. *Clin Pharmacokinet.* 2003;42(4):327–360

25. Hutchings DE, Martin BR, Gamagaris Z, Miller N, Fico T. Plasma concentrations of delta-9-tetrahydrocannabinol in dams and fetuses following acute or multiple prenatal dosing in rats. *Life Sci.* 1989;44(11):697–701

26. Boskovic R, Klein J, Woodland C, Karaskov T, Koren G. The role of the placenta in variability of fetal exposure to cocaine and cannabinoids: a twin study. *Can J Physiol Pharmacol.* 2001;79(11):942–945

27. Wu TC, Tashkin DP, Djahed B, Rose JE. Pulmonary hazards of smoking marijuana as compared with tobacco. *N Engl J Med.* 1988;318(6):347–351

28. Gunn JK, Rosales CB, Center KE, et al. Prenatal exposure to cannabis and maternal and child health outcomes: a systematic review and meta-analysis. *BMJ Open.* 2016;6(4):e009986

29. Conner SN, Bedell V, Lipsey K, Macones GA, Cahill AG, Tuuli MG. Maternal marijuana use and adverse neonatal outcomes: a systematic review and meta-analysis. *Obstet Gynecol.* 2016;128(4):713–723

30. Fried PA. Marihuana use by pregnant women and effects on offspring: an update. *Neurobehav Toxicol Teratol.* 1982;4(4):451–454

31. Fried PA. The Ottawa Prenatal Prospective Study (OPPS): methodological issues and findings—it's easy to throw the baby out with the bath water. *Life Sci.* 1995;56(23–24):2159–2168

32. Richardson GA, Day NL, Taylor PM. The effect of prenatal alcohol, marijuana and tobacco exposure on neonatal behavior. *Infant Behav Dev.* 1989;12(2):199–209

33. Fergusson DM, Horwood LJ, Northstone K; Avon Longitudinal Study of Pregnancy and Childhood (ALSPAC) Study Team. Maternal use of cannabis and pregnancy outcome. *BJOG.* 2002;109(1):21–27

34. Fried PA, Watkinson B, Willan A. Marijuana use during pregnancy and decreased length of gestation. *Am J Obstet Gynecol.* 1984;150(1):23–27

35. Day N, Sambamoorthi U, Taylor P, et al. Prenatal marijuana use and neonatal outcome. *Neurotoxicol Teratol.* 1991;13(3):329–334

36. Chabarria KC, Racusin DA, Antony KM, et al. Marijuana use and its effects in pregnancy. *Am J Obstet Gynecol.* 2016;215(4):506.e1–506.e7

37. Dotters-Katz SK, Smid MC, Manuck TA, Metz TD. Risk of neonatal and childhood morbidity among preterm infants exposed to marijuana. *J Matern Fetal Neonatal Med.* 2017;30(24):2933–2939

38. van Gelder MM, Reefhuis J, Caton AR, Werler MM, Druschel CM, Roeleveld N; National Birth Defects Prevention Study. Maternal periconceptional illicit drug use and the risk of congenital malformations. *Epidemiology.* 2009;20(1):60–66

39. de Moraes Barros MC, Guinsburg R, de Araújo Peres C, Mitsuhiro S, Chalem E, Laranjeira RR. Exposure to marijuana during pregnancy alters neurobehavior in the early neonatal period. *J Pediatr.* 2006;149(6):781–787

40. Fried PA, Watkinson B, Dillon RF, Dulberg CS. Neonatal neurological status in a low-risk population after prenatal exposure to cigarettes, marijuana, and alcohol. *J Dev Behav Pediatr.* 1987;8(6):318–326

41. Fried PA, Makin JE. Neonatal behavioural correlates of prenatal exposure to marihuana, cigarettes and alcohol in a low risk population. *Neurotoxicol Teratol.* 1987;9(1):1–7

42. Lester BM, Dreher M. Effects of marijuana use during pregnancy on newborn cry. *Child Dev.* 1989;60(4):765–771

43. Scher MS, Richardson GA, Coble PA, Day NL, Stoffer DS. The effects of prenatal alcohol and marijuana exposure: disturbances in neonatal sleep cycling and arousal. *Pediatr Res.* 1988;24(1):101–105

44. Dreher MC, Nugent K, Hudgins R. Prenatal marijuana exposure and neonatal outcomes in Jamaica: an ethnographic study. *Pediatrics.* 1994;93(2):254–260

45. Fried PA, Watkinson B. 36- and 48-month neurobehavioral follow-up of children prenatally exposed to marijuana, cigarettes, and alcohol. *J Dev Behav Pediatr.* 1990;11(2):49–58

46. Fried PA, O'Connell CM, Watkinson B. 60- and 72-month follow-up of children prenatally exposed to marijuana, cigarettes, and alcohol: cognitive and language assessment. *J Dev Behav Pediatr.* 1992;13(6):383–391

47. Fried PA, Watkinson B, Gray R. A follow-up study of attentional behavior in 6-year-old children exposed prenatally to marihuana, cigarettes, and alcohol. *Neurotoxicol Teratol.* 1992;14(5):299–311

48. Fried PA. Behavioral outcomes in preschool and school-age children exposed prenatally to marijuana: a review and speculative interpretation. *NIDA Res Monogr.* 1996;164:242–260

49. Fried PA, Watkinson B, Siegel LS. Reading and language in 9- to 12-year olds prenatally exposed to cigarettes and marijuana. *Neurotoxicol Teratol.* 1997;19(3):171–183

50. Fried PA, Watkinson B, Gray R. Differential effects on cognitive functioning in 9- to 12-year olds prenatally exposed to cigarettes and marihuana. *Neurotoxicol Teratol.* 1998;20(3):293–306

51. Fried PA, Watkinson B. Visuoperceptual functioning differs in 9- to 12-year olds prenatally exposed to cigarettes and marihuana. *Neurotoxicol Teratol.* 2000;22(1):11–20

52. Fried PA. Conceptual issues in behavioral teratology and their application in determining long-term sequelae of prenatal marihuana exposure. *J Child Psychol Psychiatry.* 2002;43(1):81–102

53. Fried PA, Watkinson B. Differential effects on facets of attention in adolescents prenatally exposed to cigarettes and

marihuana. *Neurotoxicol Teratol.* 2001;23(5):421–430

54. Fried PA. Adolescents prenatally exposed to marijuana: examination of facets of complex behaviors and comparisons with the influence of in utero cigarettes. *J Clin Pharmacol.* 2002;42(S1):97S–102S

55. Fried PA, Watkinson B, Gray R. Differential effects on cognitive functioning in 13- to 16-year-olds prenatally exposed to cigarettes and marihuana. *Neurotoxicol Teratol.* 2003;25(4):427–436

56. Smith AM, Fried PA, Hogan MJ, Cameron I. Effects of prenatal marijuana on visuospatial working memory: an fMRI study in young adults. *Neurotoxicol Teratol.* 2006;28(2):286–295

57. Fried PA, Smith AM. A literature review of the consequences of prenatal marihuana exposure. An emerging theme of a deficiency in aspects of executive function. *Neurotoxicol Teratol.* 2001;23(1):1–11

58. Fried P, Watkinson B, James D, Gray R. Current and former marijuana use: preliminary findings of a longitudinal study of effects on IQ in young adults. *CMAJ.* 2002;166(7):887–891

59. Richardson GA, Day NL, Goldschmidt L. Prenatal alcohol, marijuana, and tobacco use: infant mental and motor development. *Neurotoxicol Teratol.* 1995;17(4):479–487

60. Day NL, Richardson GA, Goldschmidt L, et al. Effect of prenatal marijuana exposure on the cognitive development of offspring at age three. *Neurotoxicol Teratol.* 1994;16(2):169–175

61. Goldschmidt L, Richardson GA, Willford J, Day NL. Prenatal marijuana exposure and intelligence test performance at age 6. *J Am Acad Child Adolesc Psychiatry.* 2008;47(3):254–263

62. Goldschmidt L, Richardson GA, Cornelius MD, Day NL. Prenatal marijuana and alcohol exposure and academic achievement at age 10. *Neurotoxicol Teratol.* 2004;26(4):521–532

63. Goldschmidt L, Richardson GA, Willford JA, Severtson SG, Day NL. School achievement in 14-year-old

youths prenatally exposed to marijuana. *Neurotoxicol Teratol.* 2012;34(1):161–167

64. O'Connell CM, Fried PA. Prenatal exposure to cannabis: a preliminary report of postnatal consequences in school-age children. *Neurotoxicol Teratol.* 1991;13(6):631–639

65. Porath AJ, Fried PA. Effects of prenatal cigarette and marijuana exposure on drug use among offspring. *Neurotoxicol Teratol.* 2005;27(2):267–277

66. Day NL, Leech SL, Goldschmidt L. The effects of prenatal marijuana exposure on delinquent behaviors are mediated by measures of neurocognitive functioning. *Neurotoxicol Teratol.* 2011;33(1):129–136

67. Day NL, Goldschmidt L, Day R, Larkby C, Richardson GA. Prenatal marijuana exposure, age of marijuana initiation, and the development of psychotic symptoms in young adults. *Psychol Med.* 2015;45(8):1779–1787

68. Day NL, Goldschmidt L, Thomas CA. Prenatal marijuana exposure contributes to the prediction of marijuana use at age 14. *Addiction.* 2006;101(9):1313–1322

69. Sonon KE, Richardson GA, Cornelius JR, Kim KH, Day NL. Prenatal marijuana exposure predicts marijuana use in young adulthood. *Neurotoxicol Teratol.* 2015;47:10–15

70. Metz TD, Stickrath EH. Marijuana use in pregnancy and lactation: a review of the evidence. *Am J Obstet Gynecol.* 2015;213(6):761–778

71. Warner TD, Roussos-Ross D, Behnke M. It's not your mother's marijuana: effects on maternal-fetal health and the developing child. *Clin Perinatol.* 2014;41(4):877–894

72. National Academies of Sciences, Engineering, and Medicine. *The Health Effects of Cannabis and Cannabinoids: The Current State of Evidence and Recommendations for Research.* Washington, DC: National Academies Press; 2017. Available at: https://www.nap.edu/catalog/24625/the-health-effects-of-cannabis-and-cannabinoids-the-current-state. Accessed August 10, 2017

73. Schneider M. Cannabis use in pregnancy and early life and its consequences: animal models. *Eur Arch Psychiatry Clin Neurosci.* 2009;259(7):383–393

74. Keimpema E, Mackie K, Harkany T. Molecular model of cannabis sensitivity in developing neuronal circuits. *Trends Pharmacol Sci.* 2011;32(9):551–561

75. Wang X, Dow-Edwards D, Anderson V, Minkoff H, Hurd YL. In utero marijuana exposure associated with abnormal amygdala dopamine D2 gene expression in the human fetus. *Biol Psychiatry.* 2004;56(12):909–915

76. Sundram S. Cannabis and neurodevelopment: implications for psychiatric disorders. *Hum Psychopharmacol.* 2006;21(4):245–254

77. Morris CV, DiNieri JA, Szutorisz H, Hurd YL. Molecular mechanisms of maternal cannabis and cigarette use on human neurodevelopment. *Eur J Neurosci.* 2011;34(10):1574–1583

78. DiNieri JA, Wang X, Szutorisz H, et al. Maternal cannabis use alters ventral striatal dopamine D2 gene regulation in the offspring. *Biol Psychiatry.* 2011;70(8):763–769

79. Jutras-Aswad D, DiNieri JA, Harkany T, Hurd YL. Neurobiological consequences of maternal cannabis on human fetal development and its neuropsychiatric outcome. *Eur Arch Psychiatry Clin Neurosci.* 2009;259(7):395–412

80. Wang X, Dow-Edwards D, Anderson V, Minkoff H, Hurd YL. Discrete opioid gene expression impairment in the human fetal brain associated with maternal marijuana use. *Pharmacogenomics J.* 2006;6(4):255–264

81. American Society of Addiction Medicine. *Public Policy Statement on Substance Use, Misuse, and Use Disorders During and Following Pregnancy, With an Emphasis on Opioids.* Rockville, MD: American Society of Addiction Medicine; 2017. Available at: www.asam.org/advocacy/find-a-policy-statement/view-policy-statement/public-policy-statements/2017/01/19/substance-use-misuse-and-use-disorders-during-and-following-pregnancy-with-an-emphasis-on-opioids. Accessed August 10, 2017

82. Holland CL, Rubio D, Rodriguez KL, et al. Obstetric health care providers' counseling responses to pregnant patient disclosures of marijuana use. *Obstet Gynecol.* 2016;127(4):681–687

83. Oregon Health Authority Public Health Division. Medical marijuana dispensary program. Information bulletin 2015-04. 2015. Available at: www.oregon. gov/oha/PH/DISEASESCONDITIONS/ CHRONICDISEASE/MEDICALMARIJUANAP ROGRAM/documents/bulletins/ Informational%20Bulletin%202015-04%20Early%20Retail%20Sales.pdf. Accessed August 10, 2017

84. Child Welfare Information Gateway. *Parental Drug Use as Child Abuse.* Washington, DC: US Department of Health and Human Services, Children's Bureau; 2016. Available at: https://www. childwelfare.gov/topics/systemwide/ laws-policies/statutes/drugexposed/. Accessed August 10, 2017

85. Section on Breastfeeding. Breastfeeding and the use of human milk. *Pediatrics.* 2012;129(3). Available at: www.pediatrics.org/cgi/content/ full/129/3/e827

86. US National Library of Medicine. LactMed. Available at: https://toxnet. nlm.nih.gov. Accessed August 10, 2017

87. Sachs HC; Committee on Drugs. The transfer of drugs and therapeutics into human breast milk: an update on selected topics. *Pediatrics.* 2013;132(3). Available at: www. pediatrics.org/cgi/content/full/132/3/ e796

88. Wang GS. Pediatric concerns due to expanded cannabis use: unintended consequences of legalization. *J Med Toxicol.* 2017;13(1):99–105

89. Hale TW, Rowe HE. Cannabis. In: Hale TW, Rowe HE, eds. *Medications and Mother's Milk.* 17th ed. New York, NY: Springer Publishing Co; 2017:146–148

90. Perez-Reyes M, Wall ME. Presence of delta9-tetrahydrocannabinol in human milk. *N Engl J Med.* 1982;307(13):819–820

91. Marchei E, Escuder D, Pallas CR, et al. Simultaneous analysis of frequently used licit and illicit psychoactive drugs in breast milk by liquid chromatography tandem mass spectrometry. *J Pharm Biomed Anal.* 2011;55(2):309–316

92. Tennes K, Avitable N, Blackard C, et al. Marijuana: prenatal and postnatal exposure in the human. *NIDA Res Monogr.* 1985;59:48–60

93. Astley SJ, Little RE. Maternal marijuana use during lactation and infant development at one year. *Neurotoxicol Teratol.* 1990;12(2):161–168

94. Reece-Stremtan S, Marinelli KA. ABM clinical protocol #21: guidelines for breastfeeding and substance use or substance use disorder, revised 2015. *Breastfeed Med.* 2015;10(3):135–141

95. National Criminal Justice Reference Service. *Quarterly Report: Potency Monitoring Project.* Report 104. Washington, DC: National Center for Natural Products Research; 2009. Available at: www.ncjrs.gov. Accessed March 22, 2017

96. Migoya D, Baca R. Colorado yields to marijuana industry pressure on pesticides. *Denver Post.* 2015. Available at: https://www.denverpost.com/2015/ 10/03/colorado-yields-to-marijuana-industry-pressure-on-pesticides/. Accessed August 10, 2017

97. Slater D. The legal marijuana industry needs to be regulated. *Sierra Magazine.* 2017:–. Available at: https:// www.sierraclub.org/sierra/2017-2-march-april/grapple/legal-marijuana-industry-needs-be-regulated. Accessed August 19, 2017

Pediatric Considerations Before, During, and After Radiological or Nuclear Emergencies

- *Policy Statement*

POLICY STATEMENT Organizational Principles to Guide and Define the Child Health Care System and/or Improve the Health of all Children

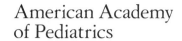

DEDICATED TO THE HEALTH OF ALL CHILDREN™

Pediatric Considerations Before, During, and After Radiological or Nuclear Emergencies

Jerome A. Paulson, MD, FAAP, COUNCIL ON ENVIRONMENTAL HEALTH

abstract

Infants, children, and adolescents can be exposed unexpectedly to ionizing radiation from nuclear power plant events, improvised nuclear or radiologic dispersal device explosions, or inappropriate disposal of radiotherapy equipment. Children are likely to experience higher external and internal radiation exposure levels than adults because of their smaller body and organ size and other physiologic characteristics, by picking up contaminated items, and through consumption of contaminated milk or foodstuffs. This policy statement and accompanying technical report update the 2003 American Academy of Pediatrics policy statement on pediatric radiation emergencies by summarizing newer scientific knowledge from studies of the Chernobyl and Fukushima Daiichi nuclear power plant events, use of improvised radiologic dispersal devices, exposures from inappropriate disposal of radiotherapy equipment, and potential health effects from residential proximity to nuclear plants. Policy recommendations are made for providers and governments to improve future responses to these types of events.

Department of Pediatrics, School of Medicine and Health Sciences and Department of Environmental and Occupational Health, Milken Institute School of Public Health, George Washington University, Washington, DC

Dr Paulson was responsible for all aspects of writing and revising this statement and has approved the final manuscript as submitted.

This document is copyrighted and is property of the American Academy of Pediatrics and its Board of Directors. All authors have filed conflict of interest statements with the American Academy of Pediatrics. Any conflicts have been resolved through a process approved by the Board of Directors. The American Academy of Pediatrics has neither solicited nor accepted any commercial involvement in the development of the content of this publication.

Policy statements from the American Academy of Pediatrics benefit from expertise and resources of liaisons and internal (AAP) and external reviewers. However, policy statements from the American Academy of Pediatrics may not reflect the views of the liaisons or the organizations or government agencies that they represent.

The guidance in this statement does not indicate an exclusive course of treatment or serve as a standard of medical care. Variations, taking into account individual circumstances, may be appropriate.

All policy statements from the American Academy of Pediatrics automatically expire 5 years after publication unless reaffirmed, revised, or retired at or before that time.

DOI: https://doi.org/10.1542/peds.2018-3000

Address correspondence to Jerome A. Paulson, MD, FAAP. E-mail: jerry@envirohealthdoctor.com.

PEDIATRICS (ISSN Numbers: Print, 0031-4005; Online, 1098-4275).

To cite: Paulson JA and AAP COUNCIL ON ENVIRONMENTAL HEALTH. Pediatric Considerations Before, During, and After Radiological or Nuclear Emergencies. *Pediatrics.* 2018;142(6): e20183000

BACKGROUND

Children can be exposed to environmental radiation as a result of nuclear power, fuels reprocessing, and weapons production plant (hereafter designated "nuclear plant") events; from an improvised nuclear device or radiologic dispersal device; or from abandoned medical radiation equipment that could potentially result in substantial levels of radiation exposure and associated health effects. Because the radiation levels from these sources could lead to a radiation emergency, this term is used to refer to these types of exposures hereafter in this report. Children and their families are likely to be extremely anxious about such events and may turn to their medical professional for advice. Parents may also ask providers about concerns related to residential and school proximity to nuclear power plants. Health professionals are concerned about these exposures because, in general, children are more sensitive to radiation and are more likely to develop the short-term and some of the long-term effects of radiation exposure. Children are likely to experience higher external and internal radiation exposure levels than adults because children are shorter and have smaller body diameters and organ sizes.[1] Children have a longer time to live, and, thus, more time in which to develop adverse outcomes. In addition, children may ingest radioactive material from picking up contaminated items and putting hands in their mouths when crawling,[2] ingesting soil,[3] or consuming milk from cows feeding on contaminated pastures or feed.[4]

An updated policy statement and a technical report[5] are needed that incorporate (1) new scientific knowledge from late effects studies of the Chernobyl accident, (2) lessons from the 2011 Fukushima Daiichi Japanese nuclear power plant accident, (3) information pertinent to the use of improvised radiologic dispersal devices and the specter of nuclear detonation in heavily populated regions, (4) radiation exposures from lack of appropriate disposal of older radiation therapy equipment, and (5) recommendations based on new knowledge from epidemiologic studies and from biokinetic models to address mitigation efforts. Although concerns have been raised about potential health effects associated with radiation exposures of children living or going to schools in proximity to nuclear power plants, the data related to these exposures and the outcome of leukemia are inconclusive and tend toward no association.[6]

Four major nuclear plant accidents have occurred: Windscale in Seascale, Cumbria, in the United Kingdom (1957); Three Mile Island in Pennsylvania (1979); Chernobyl in Ukraine (1986); and Fukushima

Daiichi nuclear power plant in Fukushima Prefecture, Japan (2011). There were 504 open-air nuclear weapons tests in 13 sites around the globe between the years of 1945 and 1980. Events involving abandoned medical radiation equipment have resulted in acute radiation sickness and deaths as well as contamination of thousands of people and homes.[7]

It is important to recognize that some mental health effects of a radiation event may begin as soon as the public becomes aware of the event, but other mental health effects may be delayed. Physical health effects after radiation exposure include short-term effects that appear within days to months after radiation exposure and long-term effects that generally appear 18 months to many years later.[8] The types and severity of short-term effects are related in part to the level of exposure and the tissues exposed. In general, children are more sensitive to radiation and are more likely to develop the short-term and some of the long-term effects of radiation exposure.

TYPES OF RADIATION EMERGENCIES AND RELATED EXPOSURES

Detailed information about types of radiation emergencies and other types of exposures to radiologic materials can be found in the technical report.[5]

RECOMMENDATIONS TO PEDIATRICIANS AND THE HEALTH SECTOR

1. Much of the preparedness planning for radiologic or nuclear events is the same as the preparedness for all emergency events. Pediatricians and other providers should refer to information on the National Pediatric Readiness Project Web site (https://emscimprovement.center/

projects/pediatricreadiness/) and on many American Academy of Pediatrics Web pages (https://www.aap.org/en-us/advocacy-and-policy/aap-health-initiatives/Children-and-Disasters/Pages/default.aspx);

2. Because mental health effects have been demonstrated to be among the most clinically important adverse outcomes subsequent to radiation and other disasters in subsets of the general population, but data are limited on short- and long-term health effects in exposed children, pediatricians should provide ongoing assessment, treatment, and specialist referrals for the mental health, behavioral, and developmental needs of patients and their parents or caregivers exposed to radiation emergencies and disasters;

3. Because the management of exposed children can potentially require monitoring for contamination, decontamination, and determination of the extent of contamination or exposure, this will need to be performed at a center equipped to perform these functions for a large number of victims. Pediatric providers should inquire from their local and state health departments about the location of community reception centers that may be designated, depending on the type of emergency, in real time. More information about population monitoring and community reception centers can be found at http://emergency.cdc.gov/radiation/pdf/population-monitoring-guide.pdf;

4. Information about when and how to use potassium iodide (KI) should be downloaded and kept in a place that will be accessible during an emergency. KI, like all medications, has risks as well

as benefits and should be given when there are, and according to, instructions from public health agencies. Information is available in Table 3 of the accompanying technical report.[5] Information about crushing and mixing KI tablets can be found on the US Food and Drug Administration Web site (https://www.fda.gov/Drugs/EmergencyPreparedness/BioterrorismandDrugPreparedness/ucm063814.htm);

5. When the risk of exposure to radioactive iodine is temporary, mothers can continue to breastfeed if appropriate doses of KI are given to her and the infant within 4 hours of the contamination; if not, mother and infant should then be prioritized to receive other protective measures like evacuation. Mothers who are breastfeeding should consider temporarily stopping breastfeeding and switching to either expressed milk (that was pumped and stored before the exposure) or ready-to-feed infant formula until the mother can be seen by a doctor for appropriate treatment with KI.[9,10] If no other source of food is available for the infant, the mother should continue to breastfeed after washing the nipple and breast thoroughly with soap and warm water and gently wiping around and away from the infant's mouth;

6. Pediatric medical centers should ensure that their facilities are properly equipped to receive and manage contaminated children. Planning also needs to consider adults who will accompany children and may be likewise contaminated;

7. Providers in the emergency department, the ICU, and other inpatient settings should have access to an application developed by the Centers for Disease Control and Prevention, the Internal Contamination Clinical Reference Application, which can be downloaded to a mobile device free of charge at http://emergency.cdc.gov/radiation/iccr.asp.[11] It would be prudent to download this information in hard copy and arrange to keep the material easily available before a radiologic emergency, when communication problems may make it difficult to do so;

8. Providers should refer to additional information on Radiation Emergency Medical Management at http://www.remm.nlm.gov/[12];

9. Accrediting agencies such as the Accreditation Association for Ambulatory Health Care and The Joint Commission should include a requirement for office training and preparedness for radiation emergencies, including KI administration to exposed children, in their accrediting standards; and

10. Training of all health professionals in the management of mental health issues associated with all emergency events should be expanded because demand will outstrip supply of mental health professionals.

RECOMMENDATIONS TO GOVERNMENT

1. Primary care providers are the medical home for children and families; therefore, these providers must be included in all aspects of preparedness training undertaken or funded by government entities;

2. Likewise, training in triage, acute management, and more importantly, long-term management of exposed children must be provided to primary care providers who create medical homes for children and families;

3. Because treatment with KI should be commenced immediately before or during the passage of a radioactive cloud in an event in which radioiodines are released, KI supplies need to be stored where readily available to the public. Storage in the National Strategic Stockpile will not allow for timely distribution of materials; KI should be stored in hospitals, public health departments, and other local sites;

4. Storage of KI should be standardized among the states to avoid confusion and miscommunication among people living near state borders who may receive information through the media from multiple state health departments;

5. Funding should be expanded for mental health services to meet the need for all types of disasters, including radiologic or nuclear emergencies; and

6. A list of child-appropriate decontamination procedures and service providers should be developed and disseminated to primary care providers, first responders, and emergency departments.

RECOMMENDATIONS FOR FAMILIES

1. Families should review the recommendations for preparation and behavior during major emergency events. The American Academy of Pediatrics and government agencies have prepared comprehensive information for families (https://www.healthychildren.org/English/safety-prevention/at-home/Pages/Family-Disaster-Supplies-List.aspx and https://www.ready.gov/nuclear-blast);

2. Preparations before a nuclear event are consistent with preparations for all types of major emergencies:

   ○ Build an emergency supply kit (nonperishable foods, water, flashlight, medical supplies), collect copies of prescriptions, and collect copies of important documents (driver's license, social security numbers, proof of residence, insurance policies, immunization records, etc);

   ○ Make a family emergency plan of a place to shelter; make plans for an out-of-town contact if not possible to connect by phone in a location; learn emergency plans for workplace, school, and child care; notify caregivers of plans; and make plans for pets; and

   ○ Obtain information from utility companies about emergency contact information if a power outage occurs;

3. Activities during a nuclear event are advised as follows:

   ○ Minimize exposure by increasing the distance between people and the source of radiation; this may involve remaining indoors or evacuating. Follow the recommendations of local public health authorities;

   ○ If told to evacuate, keep car windows and vents closed and use recirculation;

   ○ If advised to remain indoors, turn off air conditioners, ventilation fans, furnaces, and other air intakes;

   ○ Shield people by placing heavy, dense material between people and the radiation source; go to a basement or other underground area, if possible. Select an

appropriate shelter location (http://emergency.cdc.gov/radiation/pdf/infographic_where_to_go.pdf)[13];

   ○ Do not use phones unless absolutely necessary so network congestion is decreased;

   ○ Stay out of the incident zone;

   ○ Take KI on the basis of advice from regional and local government sources;

   ○ Do not take KI unless advised to because of the potential for serious adverse effects;

   ○ If shelter is not possible in the family residence because of destruction or the family is far away from a residence, go to the designated public shelter (text SHELTER and zip code to 43312 (4FEMA) to find the nearest shelter;

   ○ Follow decontamination instructions from local authorities;

   ○ Change clothes and shoes and place contaminated clothes in plastic bags, which should be sealed and placed out of the way; and

   ○ Take a thorough shower, washing body and hair;

4. Activities after a nuclear or radiologic event are advised as follows:

   ○ Seek medical treatment of unusual symptoms (eg, nausea, vomiting, bleeding, etc);

   ○ Help neighbors, infants, children, the elderly, those with disabilities, and those with access problems;

   ○ Return home only when authorities say it is safe to do so; and

   ○ Keep food in covered containers or in the refrigerator, wash the outside of containers before use, only eat food in covered

containers, and seek advice from local authorities on the consumption of uncovered foodstuffs.

ACKNOWLEDGMENTS

Dr Paulson thanks Martha S. Linet, MD, MPH, and Ziad Kazzi, MD, for their help in providing the technical information in the accompanying technical report, which informed the recommendations in this policy statement, and for their thoughtful input and reviews.

LEAD AUTHOR

Jerome A. Paulson, MD, FAAP

COUNCIL ON ENVIRONMENTAL HEALTH EXECUTIVE COMMITTEE, 2017–2018

Jennifer Ann Lowry, MD, FAAP, Chairperson
Samantha Ahdoot, MD, FAAP
Carl R. Baum, MD, FACMT, FAAP
Aaron S. Bernstein, MD, FAAP
Aparna Bole, MD, FAAP
Lori G. Byron, MD, FAAP
Philip J. Landrigan, MD, MSc, FAAP
Steven M. Marcus, MD, FAAP
Susan E. Pacheco, MD, FAAP
Adam J. Spanier, MD, PhD, MPH, FAAP
Alan D. Woolf, MD, MPH, FAAP

FORMER EXECUTIVE COMMITTEE MEMBERS

Heather Lynn Brumberg, MD, MPH, FAAP
Leonardo Trasande, MD, MPP, FAAP

LIAISONS

John M. Balbus, MD, MPH – *National Institute of Environmental Health Sciences*
Nathaniel G. DeNicola, MD, MSc – *American Congress of Obstetricians and Gynecologists*
Ruth A. Etzel, MD, PhD, FAAP – *US Environmental Protection Agency*
Diane E. Hindman, MD, FAAP – *Section on Pediatric Trainees*
Mary Ellen Mortensen, MD, MS – *Centers for Disease Control and Prevention and National Center for Environmental Health*
Mary H. Ward, PhD – *National Cancer Institute*

STAFF

Paul Spire

ABBREVIATION
KI: potassium iodide

FINANCIAL DISCLOSURE: The author has indicated he has no financial relationships relevant to this article to disclose.

FUNDING: No external funding.

POTENTIAL CONFLICT OF INTEREST: The author has indicated he has no potential conflicts of interest to disclose.

COMPANION PAPER: A companion to this article can be found online at www.pediatrics.org/cgi/doi/10.1542/peds.2018-3001.

REFERENCES

1. Tracy BL. Would children be adequately protected by existing intervention levels during a radionuclear emergency? *Radiat Prot Dosimetry.* 2010;142(1):40–45

2. Binder S, Sokal D, Maughan D. Estimating soil ingestion: the use of tracer elements in estimating the amount of soil ingested by young children. *Arch Environ Health.* 1986;41(6):341–345

3. Simon SL. Soil ingestion by humans: a review of history, data, and etiology with application to risk assessment of radioactively contaminated soil. *Health Phys.* 1998;74(6):647–672

4. Simon SL, Bouville A, Land CE. Fallout from nuclear weapons tests and cancer risks: exposures 50 years ago still have health implications today that will continue into the future. *Am Sci.* 2006;94(1):48–57

5. Linet MA, Kazzi Z, Paulson JA; American Academy of Pediatrics, Council on Environmental Health. Pediatric considerations before, during, and after radiological/ nuclear emergencies. *Pediatrics.* 2018;142(6):e20183001

6. Stather JW. Childhood leukaemia near nuclear sites: fourteenth report of the Committee on Medical Aspects of Radiation in the Environment (COMARE). *Radiat Prot Dosimetry.* 2011;147(3):351–354

7. Biddle W. *A Field Guide to Radiation.* New York, NY: Penguin Books; 2012

8. Mabuchi K, Fujiwara S, Preston DL, et al. Long-term health effects of radiation. In: Shrieve DC, Loeffler JS, eds. *Radiation Injury.* Philadelphia, PA: Lippincott, Williams and Wilkins; 2011:89–113

9. Centers for Disease Control and Prevention. Radiation emergencies: breastfeeding. Available at: http://emergency.cdc.gov/radiation/breastfeeding.asp. Accessed August 22, 2017

10. American Academy of Pediatrics. Infant feeding in disasters and emergencies. 2015. Available at: https://www.aap.org/en-us/advocacy-and-policy/aap-health-initiatives/Breastfeeding/Documents/InfantNutritionDisaster.pdf. Accessed May 10, 2017

11. Centers for Disease Control and Prevention. Internal contamination clinical reference application. Available at: http://emergency.cdc.gov/radiation/iccr.asp. Accessed August 22, 2017

12. US Department of Health and Human Services; Radiation Emergency Medical Management. Guidance on diagnosis and treatment for healthcare providers. Available at: www.remm.nlm.gov/. Accessed August 22, 2017

13. Centers for Disease Control and Prevention. Where to go in a radiation emergency. Available at: http://emergency.cdc.gov/radiation/pdf/infographic_where_to_go.pdf. Accessed August 22, 2017

Pediatric Considerations Before, During, and After Radiological or Nuclear Emergencies

• *Technical Report*

TECHNICAL REPORT

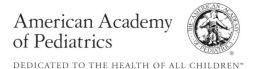

American Academy of Pediatrics

DEDICATED TO THE HEALTH OF ALL CHILDREN™

Pediatric Considerations Before, During, and After Radiological or Nuclear Emergencies

Martha S. Linet, MD, MPH,[a,b] Ziad Kazzi, MD,[c,d] Jerome A. Paulson, MD, FAAP,[e] COUNCIL ON ENVIRONMENTAL HEALTH

Infants, children, and adolescents can be exposed unexpectedly to ionizing radiation from nuclear power plant events, improvised nuclear or radiologic dispersal device explosions, or inappropriate disposal of radiotherapy equipment. Children are likely to experience higher external and internal radiation exposure levels than adults because of their smaller body and organ size and other physiologic characteristics as well as their tendency to pick up contaminated items and consume contaminated milk or foodstuffs. This technical report accompanies the revision of the 2003 American Academy of Pediatrics policy statement on pediatric radiation emergencies by summarizing newer scientific data from studies of the Chernobyl and the Fukushima Daiichi nuclear power plant events, use of improvised radiologic dispersal devices, exposures from inappropriate disposal of radiotherapy equipment, and potential health effects from residential proximity to nuclear plants. Also included are recommendations from epidemiological studies and biokinetic models to address mitigation efforts. The report includes major emphases on acute radiation syndrome, acute and long-term psychological effects, cancer risks, and other late tissue reactions after low-to-high levels of radiation exposure. Results, along with public health and clinical implications, are described from studies of the Japanese atomic bomb survivors, nuclear plant accidents (eg, Three Mile Island, Chernobyl, and Fukushima), improper disposal of radiotherapy equipment in Goiania, Brazil, and residence in proximity to nuclear plants. Measures to reduce radiation exposure in the immediate aftermath of a radiologic or nuclear disaster are described, including the diagnosis and management of external and internal contamination, use of potassium iodide, and actions in relation to breastfeeding.

abstract

[a]Radiation Epidemiology Branch, Division of Cancer Epidemiology and Genetics, National Cancer Institute, Bethesda, Maryland; [b]Agency for Toxic Substances and Disease Registry, Centers for Disease Control and Prevention, Atlanta, Georgia; [c]National Center for Environmental Health, Centers for Disease Control and Prevention, Atlanta, Georgia; [d]Department of Emergency Medicine, Emory University, Atlanta, Georgia; and [e]Department of Pediatrics, School of Medicine and Health Sciences, and Department of Environmental and Occupational Health, Milken Institute School of Public Health, George Washington University, Washington, District of Columbia

Drs Linet and Kazzi contributed much of the technical information in this report, and Dr Paulson was responsible for drafting the document; and all authors approved the final manuscript as submitted.

DOI: https://doi.org/10.1542/peds.2018-3001

To cite: Linet MS, Kazzi Z, Paulson JA. Pediatric Considerations Before, During, and After Radiological or Nuclear Emergencies. Pediatrics. 2018;142(6):e20183001

BACKGROUND AND RATIONALE FOR UPDATE

Children can be exposed to environmental radiation as a result of nuclear power, fuels reprocessing, and weapons production plant (hereafter designated "nuclear plant") events; from an improvised nuclear device or radiologic dispersal device; or from abandoned medical radiation equipment that could potentially result in substantial levels of radiation exposure and associated health effects. Because the radiation levels from these sources could lead to a radiation emergency, this term is used to refer to these types of exposures hereafter in this report. Children and their families are likely to be extremely anxious about such events and about residential proximity to nuclear plants (the latter being associated with very low or no radiation exposure) and may turn to their medical professional for advice. Health care professionals are concerned about these exposures because, in general, children are more sensitive to radiation and are more likely to develop the short-term and some of the long-term effects of radiation exposure. Children are likely to experience higher external and internal radiation exposure levels than adults because children are shorter and have smaller body diameters and organ sizes.[1] Children have a longer time to live and, thus, more time in which to develop adverse outcomes. In addition, children may ingest radioactive material from picking up contaminated items and putting hands in their mouths when crawling,[2] ingesting soil,[3] or consuming milk from cows feeding on contaminated pastures or feed.[4]

In a policy statement published in 2003,[5] the American Academy of Pediatrics (AAP) Council on Environmental Health summarized the history, features, and health effects associated with radiation emergencies in children and provided recommendations for treating, mitigating, and preventing serious health effects in children. An update to the policy statement is needed that incorporates (1) new scientific knowledge from late-effects studies of the Chernobyl event, (2) lessons from the 2011 Fukushima Daiichi Japanese nuclear power plant event, (3) information pertinent to the use of improvised radiologic dispersal devices and the specter of nuclear detonation in heavily populated regions, (4) radiation exposures from the inappropriate disposal of radiotherapy equipment, (5) reports of potential health effects associated with radiation exposures of children living in proximity to nuclear plants, and (6) recommendations based on new knowledge from epidemiological studies and from biokinetic models to address mitigation efforts.

A number of AAP publications are related to the material in this technical report, including (1) "Medical Countermeasures for Children in Public Health Emergencies, Disasters, or Terrorism"[6]; (2) "Ensuring the Health of Children in Disasters"[7]; and (3) "Providing Psychosocial Support to Children and Families in the Aftermath of Disasters and Crises."[8] This technical report presents detailed information that supports the recommendations of the accompanying policy statement.[9]

TYPES OF RADIATION EMERGENCIES AND RELATED EXPOSURES

The description and findings from epidemiological studies of the most important types of radiation emergencies and related exposures are summarized in Table 1. Concern about health effects associated with radiation emergencies began with the atomic bombings in Hiroshima and Nagasaki in 1945 that killed more than 100 000 people and injured nearly as many. Concern about adverse health and genetic effects led to long-term follow-up studies of mortality (established in 1950) and cancer incidence (begun in 1958) that continue to the present day and have yielded critically important data.[10]

Four major nuclear plant accidents have occurred: Windscale in Seascale, Cumbria, in the United Kingdom (1957); Three Mile Island in Pennsylvania (1979); Chernobyl in Ukraine (1986); and Fukushima Daiichi nuclear power plant in Fukushima Prefecture, Japan (2011).

Beginning in 1945, atmospheric nuclear testing was undertaken by the United States (New Mexico, Nevada, and the Marshall Islands), the Soviet Union (Kazakhstan), the United Kingdom (Australian territories and some Pacific Islands), France (French Polynesia), and China (Gobi Desert in Xinjiang Province) and resulted in 504 devices exploding at 13 sites. A 1963 treaty led to a limited test ban by the Soviet Union, the United States, and the United Kingdom, but atmospheric testing continued until 1974 by France and until 1980 by China.[4] Health studies have been focused on cancer risks in military participants and/ or observers and on thyroid cancer and leukemia occurring among the general population living in proximity to the testing sites.[19,24]

Events involving abandoned medical radiation equipment have resulted in acute radiation sickness and deaths as well as contamination of thousands of people and homes.[22]

Since 1983, concerns about excess leukemia among children living in proximity to nuclear power, fuels reprocessing, and weapons-production facilities have led to epidemiological studies of more than 200 nuclear facilities in 10 countries.[23] Most of the studies reveal no association. Confounding cannot be ruled out in the few studies that have revealed an association, particularly because small

TABLE 1 Characteristics of Physical Health Outcomes From Radiation Disasters and Related Events

Disaster or Event Category; Publication	Exposed Populations	Radiation Released	Population Studied	Radiation Levels	Health Outcomes
Atomic bombings, Hiroshima and Nagasaki, 1945					
Preston et al[11]	Hiroshima, Nagasaki	Detonation at high altitudes produced minimal fallout; direct radiation was important only within 3 km	2452 in utero	0.005–3 Sv	Significant excess of all solid cancers was first observed after 5 decades of follow-up.
Preston et al[11]	Hiroshima, Nagasaki	Detonation at high altitudes produced minimal fallout; direct radiation was important only within 3 km	15 388 <6 y	0.005–3 Sv	Significant excess of all solid cancers after 5 decades of follow-up; risks were higher than those in utero at the time of the bombings.
Preston et al[12]	Hiroshima, Nagasaki	Detonation at high altitudes produced minimal fallout; direct radiation was important only within 3 km	30 000 children	0.005–3 Sv	Significant excess risks for cancers of most anatomic sites; risks were highest for those exposed at youngest ages; risks declined 17% per decade of age at exposure; excess cancer risks persist throughout life.
Nuclear plant accidents, 1957–2013					
Cooper et al[13]	Windscale, 1957	750 TBq of radioactive materials were released, including 22 TBq of ^{137}Cs and 740 TBq of ^{131}I	No epidemiological study of children residing in proximity	NA	Risk projection assessment only, without validation; accident may have resulted in 240 excess cases of thyroid cancer.
Report of the President's Commission on the Three Mile Island accident[14]	Three Mile Island, 1979	The highest radiation doses were from krypton and xenon; iodine was released in barely measurable quantities	Dose data were not available separately for those exposed as children.	Doses were estimated to be about the same as natural background radiation exposure	No measurable differences between 3582 exposed (within 10 miles of Three Mile Island) versus 4000 unexposed pregnant women for prematurity, congenital abnormalities, hypothyroidism, neonatal deaths, or other factors. No excess leukemia or cancer was noted in entire exposed population or offspring.
Brenner et al[15]	Chernobyl, 1986	1760 PBq radioiodines, 85 PBq ^{137}Cs, 1150 PBq tellurium-132, 5200 PBq ^{133}Xe, and particulate radionuclides	12 514 people <18 y residentially proximate in Ukraine at exposure; 65 incident thyroid cancers	<0.05–≥3 Gy	Incidence of thyroid cancer significantly increased twofold at 15–22 y; no downturn.
Harada et al[16]	Fukushima Daiichi nuclear accident, 2011	340–800 PBq released into the atmosphere as of 2014, with 80% falling into the Pacific Ocean	Epidemiological study under development	Measurements in 3 nearby locations ranged from 1.03 to 1.66 mSv/y from external radiation and 0.0058–0.019 mSv/y from internal radiation.	Risk projection suggests that lifetime increases in risk from solid cancer, leukemia, and breast cancer will be increased by 1.06%, 0.03%, and 0.28%, respectively.

TABLE 1 Continued

Disaster or Event Category; Publication	Exposed Populations	Radiation Released	Population Studied	Radiation Levels	Health Outcomes
Aboveground nuclear tests, 1949–1980					
Lyon et al[17]	Nevada test site	86 atmospheric tests during 1951–1962	2497 children ages 12–18 y	0–400+ mGy; mean = 120 mGy	Incidence of thyroiditis 20 y after baseline assessment was fivefold increased; too few thyroid cancers were present to estimate risks.
Simon et al[18]	Marshall Islands	66 atmospheric tests during 1946–1958	No epidemiological study, risk projection	Whole-body doses ranged from 5 to 2000 mGy; thyroid doses ranged from 12 to 7600 mGy.	Estimated that 1.6% of all cancers among Marshall Islands residents alive between 1948 and 1970 were attributable to the radiation from the testing
de Vathaire et al[19]	French Polynesia	41 atmospheric tests during 1966–1974	Case-control study: 229 thyroid cancer cases versus 373 controls	Thyroid doses ranged from 0 to 39 mGy for cases and 0–36 mGy for controls. Average dose to cases for those <15 y of age was 1.8 mGy.	Significant dose-response relationship observed; high excess risk of thyroid cancer with wide confidence intervals
Land et al[20,21]	Semipalatinsk	456 atmospheric tests during 1949–1989	Prevalence of ultrasound-detected thyroid nodules in 2376 people <21 y from nuclear tests, 1949–1962	Estimated doses, Gy External: range = 0–0.55, and mean = 0.056; internal: range = 0–3.1, and mean = 0.20	Significant dose response for thyroid nodules; risk was fivefold increase in male individuals, but only 27% (and nonsignificantly) higher in female individuals.
Inappropriately discarded radiation medical equipment					
International Atomic Energy Agency[22]	Goiania, Brazil	Old radiotherapy source was stolen, dismantled, and handled by many people; contained ^{137}Cs	No systematic epidemiological study	Most had estimated doses of <0.5 Gy, but several had substantially higher doses up to 6 Gy.	4 people died, 112 000 people were screened, 249 had significant radiation levels; 42 homes were decontaminated or destroyed.
Residence in proximity to nuclear plant, 1983–present					
Laurier et al[23]	Populations in proximity in United Kingdom, United States, France, Germany, and other countries	Studies of close to 200 geographic sites in proximity to nuclear plants in 10 countries; 25 multisite studies	Some variation, but generally leukemia in people <25 y (most studied younger ages)	Measured radiation levels were lower than levels from natural background radioactivity.	Some clusters were observed including in proximity to Sellafield and Dounreay nuclear reprocessing plants in the United Kingdom and in Elbmarsch near Krümmel plant in Germany and perhaps Aldermaston and Burghfield (United Kingdom) and La Hague (France), but multisite studies reveal no increase in risk.

^{133}Xe, xenon-133; NA, not applicable; PB, petabecquerel; TB, terabecquerel.

increases in risk were observed with distance from sites for proposed nuclear power stations that were never built.[25]

CHARACTERISTICS, UNITS, SOURCES, AND BIOLOGICAL EFFECTS OF RADIATION EXPOSURE

Terminology

Ionizing radiation, a type of high-frequency energy that can produce adverse effects through damage to DNA and cells, includes electromagnetic (eg, radiographs and γ-rays, involving streams of photons or "packets" of energy) and particulate forms (eg, electrons, protons, α-particles, neutrons, muons, and heavy-charged ions). Radionuclides (often referred to as radioactive isotopes) are atoms with unstable nuclei that release excess energy by the emission of γ-rays or α- or β-particles when they undergo radioactive decay.[26]

Units

Energy from radiation is measured in several types of units. The international system (Systéme International d'Unités [SI]) unit Gy (1 Gy = 100 rad) is the radiation absorbed dose. The SI unit Sv (1 Sv = 100 rem) takes into account a weighting or quality factor that is based on the relative biological effectiveness of doses from particulate radiation (eg, Sv = Gy × relative biological effectiveness). The SI unit of activity for radiation emission of a radionuclide is Bq, which is defined as 1 atomic disintegration per second (for conversion, 1 Bq = $1/3.7 \times 10^{10}$ Ci). The most important radionuclides and radioactive emissions associated with radiation emergencies are shown in Table 2.

Characteristics and Sources

Children can be exposed to radiation emitted from sources that are external or internal to the body.

Exposure may occur to the whole body (eg, external radiation from natural background exposures or radiation emergencies) or may involve partial body exposure (eg, radiographs from medical radiography and most forms of radiotherapy). Sources of exposure may include natural background exposure (eg, radon, natural background γ-rays, cosmic rays) or manmade exposures (eg, radiographs from medical radiography, radionuclides administered in nuclear medicine procedures, and the radioactive materials used in nuclear power or weapons plants). Several key forms of ionizing radiation are encountered in radiation-related emergencies. β-particles are emitted from radionuclides that are created as by-products of nuclear reactors (such as radioactive iodines) or may be released from radionuclides used in medicine (such as xenon). γ-Rays are emitted from various radionuclides like isotopes of cesium and cobalt and after a nuclear detonation. Neutrons are mostly emitted after a nuclear detonation and are more effective at producing tissue damage than γ-rays. Other forms of radiation, such as α-particles, which are emitted from radon or from polonium-210, have a shorter range.[4]

Children can become internally contaminated with radioactive material in a number of scenarios, such as the detonation of an improvised nuclear device (a device that incorporates radioactive materials designed to result in dispersal of radioactive material). Other examples include the release of radioactive material in the environment from a radiologic dispersal device (a bomb made from radioactive material combined with conventional explosives that is capable of spreading radioactive material over a wide area) or from a nuclear plant accident. The radioactive material may enter the body through

inhalation, by ingestion, or by blast injection into a wound. Dermal absorption is usually limited, except in cases of skin contamination with tritium. The clinical consequences of internal contamination depend on the type and amount of radioactive material that is taken up by the body and its chemical and physical (radioactive) properties.

Biological Effects

Ionizing radiation may interact directly with target tissues or indirectly through the production of free radicals from its interaction with water molecules. Effects of radiation on cells differ depending on the cell's rate of division and with the level of cell differentiation. Tissue sensitivity to radiation varies from highest to lowest as follows: lymphocytes, erythroblasts, spermatogonia, epidermal stem cells, and gastrointestinal stem cells. Other types of cells (muscle, bone, and nerve cells) are less sensitive to the effects of radiation. DNA appears to be the principal target for biological effects of radiation, including cell death, mutation, and carcinogenesis. If cells are irradiated with ionizing radiation, single-strand or double-strand DNA breaks or other DNA changes may occur. This can be followed by error-free DNA repair, but if the repair is incorrect, it can result in cell death, chromosomal instability, mutation, and/or carcinogenesis.[26] Indirect effects may occur through the production of free radicals in living tissue and nontargeted effects, such as release of cytokines and other products of inflammation.

EXAMPLES OF MEASURES TO REDUCE RADIATION EXPOSURES DURING AN EMERGENCY

Below are examples of strategies to reduce exposure to radiation and associated health risks.

TABLE 2 Radionuclides Potentially Released From a Radiation Disaster, Routes of Absorption and Treatments

Element, Symbol, Source	Type of Radiation; Half-life	Respiratory Absorption	Gastrointestinal Absorption	Primary Toxicity	Treatment
Americium [241]Am	α; 432 y	75%	Minimal	—	Calcium or zinc DTPA[a]
Californium [252]Cf	α, strong neutron emitter; 2.4 y	—	25% absorbed in liver	65% absorbed in bone; half deposited in skeleton and liver are gone in 50 and 20 y, respectively	Calcium or zinc DTPA
Carbon [14]C	Weak β emitter; 5730 y	Yes	Yes	Can cross placenta, becomes organically bound to developing cells and hence endangers fetuses	No treatment available
Cesium [137]Cs	β, γ; 30 y	Complete	Complete	—	Prussian blue[a]
Cobalt [60]Co	β, γ; 5.3 y	High	<5%	—	—
Iodine ^{131}I, [125]I	β, γ; 8 d, 60 d, respectively	High	High	—	KI[a] immediately before or within 4 h of exposure
Plutonium [238][239]Pu	α, radiographs; 24 400 y	High	Minimal	—	Calcium or zinc DTPA[a]
Strontium [90]Sr	β, γ; 28 y	Limited	Moderate	—	Aluminum hydroxide; calcium chloride suspension; calcium gluconate
Thallium [201]Tl	Potassium analog, when injected emits 80 keV radiographs; 73 h	—	—	—	Prussian blue
Tritium [3]H	Hydrogen isotope, decays with emission of low-energy electron; 10 d	—	—	Tritiated water is taken easily into the body by inhalation, ingestion, or transdermal absorption; instantaneously absorbed and mixes with body water	Force fluids; water diuresis
Uranium [235]U and radon daughters	α; 4.47 billion y	Inhalation can cause lung cancer	Ingestion can cause bone and liver cancer	—	Bicarbonate to alkalinize the urine

Other important radionuclides in radioactive fallout that may contribute to internal dose and are not included in the table are as follows: iron-55 ([55]Fe), ruthenium-106 ([106]Ru), antimony-125 ([125]Sb), cerium-144 ([144]Ce), neptunium-239 ([239]Np), technetium-132 ([132]Te), barium-140 ([140]Ba), molybdenum-99 ([99]Mo), lanthanum-140 ([140]La), rhodium-105 ([105]Rh), promethium-149 ([149]Pm), praseodymium-143 ([143]Pr). Adapted from American Academy of Pediatrics Committee on Environmental Health. Radiation disasters and children. *Pediatrics*. 2003;111(6 pt 1):1455–1466. Adapted from Goans RE. *Medical Management of Radiological Casualties*. 4th ed. Bethesda, MD: Armed Forces Radiobiology Research Institute, Uniformed Services University of the Health Science; 2013.[27] [3]H, tritium-3; ^{14}C, carbon-14; ^{60}Co, cobalt-60; ^{90}Sr, strontium-90; ^{125}I, iodine-125; ^{201}Tl, thallium-201; [235]U, uranium-235; [238]PU, plutonium-238; [239]Pu, plutonium-239; [241]Am, americium-241; [252]Cf, californium-252; DFOA, deferoxamine; DMSA, dimercaptosuccinic acid; DTPA, diethylenetriaminepentacetic acid; EDTA, edetic acid (ethylene-dinitrillo tetraacetic acid); NAC, N-acetyl cysteine. —, not applicable.
[a] Approved by the FDA for this indication.

Measures to Reduce Contamination Immediately After an Incident

Guidance to individuals and professionals on measures to reduce contamination in the immediate aftermath of a radiologic or nuclear disaster is provided by the US Department of Health and Human Services[28,29] and the National Council on Radiation Protection and Measurements.[30] The immediate measures, summarized in Table 3, include specific actions to be undertaken by children and parents to reduce external and internal contamination according to the person's location at the time of the emergency. More detailed information on many different aspects of responding to a nuclear event was published in 2010 by a federal interagency expert committee led by the Executive Office of the President.[31] Information in the document produced by the Federal Interagency Committee addresses such topics as identifying an expanded zone for management of activities, selecting appropriate radiation detection devices, decontaminating critical infrastructure, conducting waste management, and many other key elements.

Potassium Iodide

In the event that radioactive iodine is released into the environment, potassium iodide (KI) is a supplementary or secondary protective measure. The primary protection is sheltering in place or evacuation (as instructed by local public health officials) to prevent

TABLE 3 Guidance to Parents on Individual Measures Immediately After a Radiation Emergency

Location or Topic	Actions to Be Taken
If outside or close to the location of the incident	Cover nose and mouth to reduce particulate exposures
	Do not touch objects thrown off by incident or dust
	Quickly go to nearest intact building with thick walls
	Once inside, take off outer clothes, place in a sealed bag, and place bag where others will not touch
	Shower and wash body and hair with soap and water
	Turn on radio and/or television for further instructions
If inside building	If building is not intact (ie, there are broken windows or walls), go to the nearest intact building
	Shut all windows, doors, and fireplace dampers
	Turn off all fans and heating and air conditioning units
	Turn on radio and/or television for further instructions
If in car	Close windows and vents and turn off heat and air conditioner
	Cover nose and mouth with a cloth
	If you cannot get to home or another intact building safely, stay in car and park in a safe place
	Turn off engine
	Turn on radio and listen for instructions
	Stay in car until told it is safe to get back on the road
Children and family	If with children and family, stay together
	If children are in another building or school, children should stay there, and parents should not travel to children until told it is safe to travel
	Children should stay in emergency shelter at school
Pets	Bring pets inside an intact building
	Wash pets with soap and water
Food and water	Do not consume any food or water out in the open air
	Food inside cans and sealed containers is safe, but food outside of cans and/or containers should be washed to remove dust
	Obtain guidance from authorities about other food and/or water

exposure in the first place. Guidance to federal agencies and state and local governments on safe and effective use of KI is provided by the US Food and Drug Administration (FDA).[32] The adoption and implementation of the recommendations are at the discretion of the state and local governments responsible for developing regional emergency response plans related to radiation emergencies. KI has been well established to block thyroid radioiodine uptake and is effective in reducing the risk of development of thyroid cancer in individuals and populations at risk after inhalation or ingestion of radioiodines.[32,33] The mechanism of action involves KI saturating the thyroid gland with nonradioactive iodine, thereby preventing uptake of the radioiodines, which are then excreted in urine. KI only prevents the uptake of radioiodines not the uptake of other radionuclides and is, therefore, not a general radioprotective agent. The FDA prioritizes treatment with KI on the basis of age, focusing on

infants, children, and pregnant and breastfeeding women, because they are at the highest risk of developing thyroid cancer. Treatment should be commenced immediately before or during the passage of a radioactive cloud in an event in which radioiodines are released, although treatment may still have a substantial protective effect even if 3 or 4 hours have passed. If the release of radioiodines and secondary exposure is protracted, then even delayed administration may result in benefits.

Shown in Table 4 are the threshold thyroid radioactive exposures and recommended doses of KI for different risk groups. At the time of the preparation of this document, there are 5 FDA-approved over-the-counter KI products:

- iOSAT tablets (65 and 130 mg; Anbex, Inc, Williamsburg, VA; www.anbex.com)[34];

- Thyrosafe tablets (65 mg; Recipharm, Jordbro, Sweden; www.thyrosafe.com)[35];

- Thyroshield solution (65 mg/mL; Arco Pharmaceuticals, LLC, St Louis, MO; www.thyroshield.com)[36]; and

- KI oral solution (65 mg/mL; Mission Pharmacal, San Antonio, TX).

KI provides protection for approximately 24 hours and should be given daily until the risk of exposure no longer exists. Pregnant women and neonates should not receive repeated doses of KI, because it has the potential to suppress thyroid function in the fetus and neonate (they must be prioritized for other protective measures, such as evacuation). The benefits of KI treatment to reduce the risk of thyroid cancer outweigh risks of transient hypothyroidism. However, given the potential sequelae of transient hypothyroidism for intellectual development, the FDA recommends that neonates treated with 1 dose or more of KI be monitored for this effect by measurement of thyroid-stimulating

TABLE 4 Guidance on Use of KI

Age Group	Predicted Thyroid Gland Exposure, mGy	KI Dose, mg	No. or Fraction of 130-mg Tablets	No. or Fraction of 65-mg Tablets	Milliliters of Oral Solution, 65 mg/mL
>40 y	≥5000	130	1	2	2
18–40 y	≥100	130	1	2	2
Pregnant or lactating women	≥50	130	1	2	2
12–18 y[a]	≥50	65	0.5	1	1
3–12 y	≥50	65	0.5	1	1
1 mo–3 y	≥50	32	Use KI oral solution[b]	0.5	0.5
0–1 mo	≥50	16	Use KI oral solution[b]	Use KI oral solution[b]	0.25

[a] Adolescents approaching adult size (≥150 lb) should receive the full adult dose (130 mg).
[b] KI oral solution is supplied in 1-oz (30-mL) bottles with a dropper marked for 1-, 0.5-, and 0.25-mL dosing. Each milliliter contains 65 mg of KI iodide.

hormone and be treated with thyroid hormone therapy if hypothyroidism occurs.[37–39] Allergy to seafood, radiocontrast media, and povidone-iodine preparations should not be considered iodine allergy and are not a contraindication to the administration of KI. People with true iodine sensitivity should avoid KI, as should individuals with dermatitis herpetiformis and hypocomplementemic vasculitis, both rare conditions associated with increased risk of iodine hypersensitivity. People with Graves' disease and autoimmune thyroiditis should be treated with caution, especially if treatment extends beyond a few days. Adverse effects of KI may include skin rashes that can be severe (iododerma), swelling of salivary glands, and iodism (metallic taste, burning mouth and throat, sore teeth and gums, upper respiratory congestion, and occasionally gastrointestinal symptoms and diarrhea). Although KI is available over the counter, people should check with their doctors if there are any health concerns.[32]

Measures Related to Breastfeeding

Data are limited on quantitative estimates of human milk activity from iodine-131 (^{131}I) administered for nuclear medicine diagnostic or therapeutic procedures and from radionuclides resulting from radiation emergencies. Estimates based on biokinetic and other modeling data suggest that internal contamination from such sources could reach substantial concentrations in human milk and result in significant radiation exposures to nursing children.[40–43] Higher levels of ^{131}I may be transferred to infants from breastfeeding than to the fetus from intake of the pregnant mother.[44,45] When the risk of exposure to radioactive iodine is temporary, mothers who are at risk for becoming internally contaminated can continue to breastfeed on the first day of exposure if appropriate doses of KI are administered to her and to the infant within 4 hours of the contamination. If not, the mother and infant should then be prioritized to receive other protective measures like evacuation.

According to the Centers for Disease Control and Prevention, women who are breastfeeding should take only 1 dose of KI if they have been internally contaminated with (or are likely to be internally contaminated with) radioactive iodine.[46] They should be prioritized to receive other protective action measures (https://emergency.cdc.gov/radiation/ki.asp). If the situation is such that the exposure to radioactive iodine is prolonged and more than 1 dose of KI is indicated for the mother and the infant, then breastfeeding must be temporarily suspended because of the risks associated with KI therapy in infants and neonates.[47] Mothers must be supported to express their milk to maintain their milk supply until the infant can resume breastfeeding. Safe human milk (that was pumped and stored before the exposure) or ready-to-feed infant formula, to avoid potentially contaminated tap water, should be provided as a temporary solution. Breastfeeding can resume once public health officials indicate that it is safe.

If the mother's internal contamination with radioactive iodine is high or if repeat doses of KI to the infant are necessary (because of lack of availability of noncontaminated food sources), the infant should be evaluated for secondary hypothyroidism that could have resulted from the repeat dosing of KI.[48]

As a general measure, the mother should wash the nipple and breast thoroughly with soap and warm water and gently wipe around and away from the infant's mouth before breastfeeding.

Again, as noted above, it is important to reiterate that KI will not be protective if the exposure has been to radionuclides other than the radioiodines. Many radiation events will be a mix of radionuclides and/or not contain radioactive iodine. Public health officials will provide breastfeeding guidance after considering the risks and benefits that are particular to the specific event and radionuclides.

DIAGNOSIS AND MANAGEMENT OF CONTAMINATION

The Radiation Emergency Medical Management Web site

(https://www.remm.nlm.gov/) provides a wealth of information on management of radiologic emergency incidents for both clinicians and managers. The Radiation Injury Treatment Network is another important resource (https://ritn.net/default.aspx). Pediatric patients and their accompanying family members who may have been contaminated from fallout and related radionuclides from radiation emergency events should be referred (or redirected if they appear at a pediatric practice) to hospital emergency departments with staff trained in decontamination, evaluation, and treatment measures for acute radiation syndrome (ARS), associated injuries, and related problems in patients, as well as protective measures for staff.

External Contamination

Initial efforts to manage external contamination of parents and children at the community level are described in previous sections of this report and in Table 3. If parents and children have not removed and bagged clothing in sealed plastic bags and showered with soap and water before arriving at a central location or medical facility, they should do so.

Internal Contamination

The diagnosis of internal contamination can be made by direct measurement of radiation emissions by using an external detector for radionuclides that decay by emitting γ-rays, such as ^{131}I and cesium-137 (^{137}Cs). Alternatively, analysis of urine or feces can be used to detect the radionuclides inside the body for radionuclides that do not emit γ-rays, such as polonium-210 and strontium-90. Performing these measurements in children will be more challenging than adults because of different body sizes that affect the radiation detector instrument calibration and because of greater difficulty in obtaining urine or fecal samples.

TABLE 5 Guidance to Professionals on Drugs Available for the Treatment of Internal Contamination

Medical Countermeasure	Indication	Comment
Prussian blue	Enhances the fecal elimination of radioactive cesium or thallium by interrupting their enterohepatic circulation	Considered safe in children because it is not absorbed into the body. Not approved for ages <2 y. Use preemergency use authorization for ages 6 mo–2 y. Causes constipation and blue feces.
Pentetate calcium trisodium	Enhances the renal elimination of plutonium, americium, and curium	Approved in children. If >1 dose is needed, the zinc form is preferred.
Pentetate zinc trisodium	Enhances the renal elimination of plutonium, americium, and curium	Approved in children.
KI	Saturates the thyroid with stable iodine, which prevents the uptake of radioiodine.	See Table 3 and text.

Once the amount of radioactive material inside the body is estimated, it is compared with the corresponding radionuclide-specific Clinical Decision Guide.[30] The Clinical Decision Guide is meant to assist clinicians in determining whether the level of internal radionuclides is clinically significant. If the amount of radionuclide measured inside the body is greater than or equal to the corresponding Clinical Decision Guide, further medical management is warranted.[49] For radionuclides other than the isotopes of iodine, the Clinical Decision Guide values for children are 20% of those for adults because of their increased radiosensitivity.[50]

The medical management of patients with internal contamination consists primarily of supportive care and long-term monitoring for cancer and other health outcomes. Additional management strategies attempt to decrease the radiation dose received over the lifetime of the patient by enhancing the elimination of the radionuclide through diuresis or chelation therapy or by preventing uptake into the target organ. Specific drug therapies are available for a limited number of radionuclides and are listed in Table 5. The Centers for Disease Control and Prevention has developed an application to assist clinicians in assessing and managing internal contamination. This tool, the Internal Contamination Clinical Reference application, can be downloaded to a mobile device free of charge at http://emergency.cdc.gov/radiation/iccr.asp.[51] It would be prudent to download and print this information in hard copy and arrange to keep the material easily available before a radiologic emergency, when communication problems may make it difficult to do so.

Many of the drugs and equipment specifically for use in disasters of all types, including nuclear and radiation disasters, are not used for other purposes and are therefore not routinely stocked in hospitals, pharmacies, or physician offices. The US government has created the Strategic National Stockpile, a national repository of antibiotics, vaccines, chemical antidotes, antitoxins, and other critical medical equipment and supplies. Material can be shipped to locations of need on short notice. Some individual states, particularly those with nuclear reactors, may have their own stocks of KI.

HEALTH OUTCOMES

Some mental health effects of a radiation event may begin as soon as the public becomes aware of the event; other mental health effects will be delayed. Physical health effects after radiation exposure include short-term effects that appear within days to months after radiation exposure and long-term effects that generally appear 18 months to many years later. The intervals between first exposure and long-term effects may be decades in length.[10] The types and severity of short-term effects are related in part to the level of exposure and the tissues exposed. In general, children are more sensitive to radiation and are more likely to develop both the short-term and some of the long-term effects of radiation exposure.

Mental health effects have long been known to be a major clinical problem associated with most types of radiation and other types of disasters.[8,52] Psychological effects potentially include anxiety; depression; fear; somatic complaints; and social, thought, and behavioral problems and other elements of posttraumatic stress disorder. Overall, the excess adverse psychological effects attributable to natural and manmade disasters is approximately 20% after the first 12 months.[53] Radiation-related disasters are of particular concern because of the intangible nature of radiation exposure, lack of information about the actual level of radiation exposure to individuals in the exposed population, conflicting reports about the details of the event by authorities and the media, widespread rumors about adverse effects on humans and animals, a tendency to attribute all subsequent short- and long-term health problems to radiation exposure, fears about health effects in future generations, nonsystematic health monitoring after the event, and social and economic disruptions.[52] Risk factors for adults that are associated with mental health consequences include the severity of the disaster;

postdisaster circumstances, such as adequacy of emotional support and access to professional interventions; and personal characteristics that increase susceptibility, including being female, having young children, and having previous psychiatric problems.[53] Long-standing research on the psychological effects of radiation disasters has been focused primarily on adults and has revealed acute as well as long-term anxiety, depressive symptoms, and somatic symptoms, particularly in mothers of young children.[54] Although short- and long-term effects on psychological functioning, emotional adjustment, and developmental trajectory of children subsequent to nonradiation disasters have been studied extensively,[8,55] mental health effects in children exposed to radiation disasters were not evaluated in methodologically rigorous longitudinal epidemiological studies until after the Three Mile Island[54] and Chernobyl accidents,[53] as described in more detail later in this report.

Short-term Outcomes

ARS

ARS is an acute illness caused by irradiation of the whole or a large part of the body by a high dose of penetrating radiation over a short period of time (usually a few minutes). The time course of ARS can be divided into 4 nondiscrete phases: prodrome (occurring within minutes to hours of the radiation exposure and characterized by nausea, vomiting, fever, diarrhea, and fatigue); a latent phase (beginning a few hours after the exposure and lasting up to 2–5 weeks, during which patients may feel well but adverse effects occur at the tissue level); a manifest illness stage (potentially beginning as soon as a few hours after the exposure and lasting up to a few months); and recovery (beginning a few weeks after the event and lasting up to

2 years) or death.[56] ARS may also be conceptualized as a clinical continuum of manifestations that encompass multiple organs or systems and feature an important role for inflammation. This clinical continuum encompasses multiorgan injury, multiorgan dysfunction syndrome, and multiorgan failure, the latter being irreversible.[57] Treatments for emesis include ondansetron (approved for children of all ages) or granisetron (approved for children 2 years and older); bone marrow depression is treated with colony-stimulating factors like filgrastim, sargramostim, and pegfilgrastim.[58] These drugs are available, in some cases in limited quantities, in the Strategic National Stockpile.

Symptoms, Outcomes, and Exposure Level

The type, severity, and rate of appearance of clinical symptoms depend on the radiation dose received and the part of the body exposed. The larger the radiation dose absorbed by the body above the levels at which clinical symptoms are manifest, the more compressed the timeline of these phases and the more severe the clinical manifestation. The threshold whole-body dose for developing clinically apparent ARS is 1 Gy, although children may have a lower threshold than adults (Table 6). At whole-body doses of approximately 4.5 Gy, approximately 50% to 60% of exposed untreated patients will die. At doses of 8 Gy or more, virtually no patients will survive.

A patient's survival will depend on the dose of radiation received, the presence of other injuries (eg, trauma and burns), and comorbid medical conditions. During a mass-casualty incident, limited treatment resources will be allocated to patients who have survivable injuries, whereas others will be triaged for palliative care, highlighting the importance of determining the radiation dose received by a patient. This dose can be estimated by using time to emesis and absolute lymphocyte counts based on data in adults. The Radiation Emergency Medical Management Web site provides tools to estimate radiation dose[64] Using the history and physical examination in addition to these estimation tools, health care providers can identify patients who are likely to develop the potentially survivable form of the ARS and therefore benefit from available medical countermeasures (Table 7).

Short- and Long-term Effects: Mental Health Conditions

As noted previously, a major clinical problem associated with most types of radiation disasters is occurrence of mental health effects, including depression, anxiety, posttraumatic stress disorder, and medically unexplained somatic symptoms.[67] These problems may affect populations for many years after the event. As 1 example, long-term psychological effects have been documented among atomic bomb survivors.[68–70] Another example is the twofold increased lifetime depression rates among women living in proximity to Chernobyl

TABLE 6 Clinical Effects in Relation to Whole-body Radiation Dose

Clinical Effect	Whole-body Dose, Gy
Threshold for developing clinically apparent ARS	1 (children may have a lower threshold than adults)
$LD_{50/60}$ without significant medical therapy[59–63] (http://www.remm.nlm.gov/LD50-60.htm)	~4.5
LD_{100}	8
Hematopoietic syndrome	2–6
Gastrointestinal syndrome	6–10
Cerebrovascular syndrome	>20
Cutaneous syndrome	>2 (to the skin)

$LD_{50/60}$, lethal dose that will kill 50% of the exposed population within 60 days; LD_{100}, lethal dose, 100%.

compared with the general population of women in Ukraine.[71] In both the Three Mile Island and Chernobyl (Ukraine) accidents, mothers of young children were 3 times as likely as women without young children to describe their health as "fair" or "poor," which the investigators observed to be notable, given the differences in the levels of radiation exposure, evacuation, culture, and postdisaster sociopolitical environment.[67] The President's Commission review of the health outcomes associated with the Three Mile Island accident concluded that the greatest public health problem was mental health,[14] similar to the conclusion of the Chernobyl Forum 20 years after the Chernobyl accident.[72] Psychosocial issues are addressed in much more

detail in a separate AAP clinical report titled "Providing Psychosocial Support to Children and Families in the Aftermath of Disasters and Crises."[8]

Long-term Effects: Cancer and Related Conditions

Several tissues (eg, thyroid, bone marrow, breast, and brain) are more sensitive to radiation in children than in adults, and children are at higher risk of radiation-related cancers of these tissues.[73] Other tissues do not appear to be more sensitive in children than in adults (eg, lung and bladder). Table 1 lists the key types of radiation emergencies considered, the affected populations, exposure information, whether a risk projection or epidemiological study was conducted, and key physical health outcomes.

TABLE 7 Medical Countermeasures for Treating the Hematopoietic Subsyndrome of ARS

Medical Countermeasure	Indication	Comment
Granulocyte colony-stimulating factor (filgrastim and pegfilgrastim)	Neutropenia	Approved for use in adults and children.
Granulocyte-macrophage colony-stimulating factor (sargramostim)	Neutropenia	The liquid formulations containing benzyl alcohol or lyophilized formulations reconstituted with bacteriostatic water for injection, USP (0.9% benzyl alcohol), should not be administered to neonates and young infants.
Antibacterials	Neutropenia	Follow guidelines provided by professional societies (eg, Infectious Diseases Society of America and the American Society of Clinical Oncology[65,66]).
Antivirals	Neutropenia	Follow guidelines provided by professional societies (eg, Infectious Diseases Society of America and the American Society of Clinical Oncology[65,66]).
Antifungals	Neutropenia	Follow guidelines provided by professional societies (eg, Infectious Diseases Society of America and the American Society of Clinical Oncology[65,66]).
Platelets	Thrombocytopenia	Irradiated and leukocyte reduced.
Packed red blood cells	Anemia	Irradiated and leukocyte reduced.
Stem cell transplant	Failure to respond to other therapies	Contact the Radiation Injury Treatment Network (https://ritn.net/default.aspx)
	Absence of significant combined injuries or comorbid conditions	

USP, US Pharmacopeia.

Japanese Atomic Bomb Survivors: Life Span Study

Much of our understanding of health effects from radiation disasters and emergencies is based on results of long-term follow-up of the survivors of the bombings in 1945 of Hiroshima and Nagasaki. The populations in these 2 cities each experienced a single high–dose-rate external radiation exposure.[10] The Life Span Study includes mortality follow-up since 1950 and cancer incidence follow-up since 1958 of 120 000 survivors, including approximately 30 000 children. The wide dose range (<0.005 Gy to 2–4 Gy; mean dose = 0.2 Gy), broad variation in age at exposure, and long-term follow-up has led to several key results (see Table 1). First, the radiation-related risks of solid cancers, and to a lesser extent the leukemias, except for acute myeloid leukemia, has persisted for more than 5 decades after exposure and may persist during the entire lifetime. Second, there is evidence of a linear dose response for all solid tumors combined, including a statistically significant dose response for survivors with cumulative estimated doses under 0.15 Gy. Significant radiation-associated excess risks were observed for most, but not all, specific types of solid cancers and for all types of leukemia except chronic lymphocytic leukemia, although the level of the excess relative risks per Gy and the excess absolute rates varied according to organ or tissue and by age at exposure. Third, the relative and absolute patterns of occurrence of solid tumors have been shown to be strongly modified by age at exposure, with children and adolescents demonstrating the highest risks.[10]

Japanese Atomic Bomb Survivors: In Utero Study

The solid cancer incidence among atomic bomb survivors who were in utero at the time of the bombings (based on 94 incident cancers) was compared with risks among survivors exposed postnatally at younger than 6 years (based on 649 incident cancers) and followed-up during 1958–1999. The excess relative risks at 50 years of age for a given dose was substantially higher for those exposed postnatally than for those exposed in utero. Excess absolute rates were markedly higher for a given attained age among those exposed in early childhood compared with a substantially lower increase for a given attained age among those exposed in utero (see Table 1).[11] Researchers of this study could not, however, provide cancer incidence risk estimates during childhood in the absence of complete cancer incidence data during 1945–1957 (the period after bombings but before the establishment of population-based cancer registries in Hiroshima and Nagasaki).

Nuclear Plant Accidents: Windscale, Three Mile Island, Chernobyl, Fukushima

No epidemiological studies were conducted in the population residentially proximate to the Windscale nuclear plant after the accident. An investigation of cancer incidence in the population living in proximity to the Three Mile Island facility revealed no association for childhood cancers overall; an increased risk for childhood leukemia was based on only 4 cases, but incidence rates were low compared with regional and national rates.[74]

After the release of radioactivity from the Fukushima Daiichi nuclear power plant in March 2011 resulting from the Great East Japan Earthquake and tsunami, an effort was undertaken to estimate internal radiation levels, but information is limited because of initial organizational difficulties, high natural background radiation, and contamination of radiation measuring devices.[75] Direct measurements in a small number of early responders and evacuees who stayed in Fukushima for several days after the accident revealed low maximum effective doses and thyroid equivalent doses. A large thyroid disease clinical ultrasonographic screening of approximately 300 000 residents 18 years or younger residing in the Fukushima Prefecture was conducted during 2011–2014.[76] The investigators reported a 50-fold excess incidence rate ratio when compared with the Japanese national thyroid cancer incidence for people of the same age. Despite the absence of individual organ radiation doses, the investigators indicated that the findings suggested a notable increase in thyroid cancer incidence attributable to the accident. However, many other radiation experts have concluded that this screening program identified the thyroid cancer incidence rates expected after screening. Other criticisms of the conclusions included the use of an inappropriate external comparison of a screened population with national rates not based on screening; absence of a statistical difference of the internal comparisons among the low, intermediate, and highly contaminated areas within the Fukushima Prefecture; low measured thyroid radiation levels that are inconsistent with the high risk estimates reported; lack of broad-based individual thyroid organ measurements; and the ecologic nature of the screening study (eg, no individual thyroid radiation doses were reported, so it is unclear whether thyroid cancer cases had higher radiation exposures than noncases).[77–79]

Approximately 5% to 7% of children from the Fukushima Prefecture who participated in the mental health surveys (participation rates ranging from 55% to 66%) required immediate support and counseling.[80]

Compared with other nuclear plant accidents, the dose estimation effort and assessment of long-term health risks conducted after the Chernobyl accident have been much more comprehensive. From follow-up studies of children and adolescents exposed to radioiodines in the fallout from Chernobyl, studies have consistently revealed sizeable dose-related increases in thyroid cancer, with risks greatest in those youngest at exposure and potentially among those with a deficiency of stable iodine levels.[81] Studies of pediatric leukemia in Ukraine, Belarus, and Russia after the Chernobyl accident have shown inconsistent results, but there was no evidence of excess leukemia in European countries after the accident.[82]

Aboveground Nuclear Testing

Thyroid cancer and other thyroid diseases have been evaluated in children and adolescents exposed to the fallout from aboveground testing in Nevada, the Marshall Islands, French Polynesia, and Kazakhstan. Most of these studies have revealed dose-response increases in the risk of these outcomes (Table 1).[17–20]

Inappropriately Discarded Medical Radiation Equipment

For the most part, there has been little systematic study and no long-term follow-up of populations exposed to radiation from events involving abandoned medical radiation equipment. The incident in Goiania, Brazil, has been described in detail (see Table 1). An old ^{137}Cs teletherapy source stolen from an abandoned hospital in 1987 in Goiania, Brazil, was dismantled, and many people handled the pieces. As a result of this event, among the 112 000 people that were monitored, 4 people died, 1 person had an arm amputated, 249 people were contaminated with ^{137}Cs, and 42 homes had to be decontaminated or destroyed.[22]

Residential Proximity to Nuclear Plants

Extensive investigations quantifying risks of childhood leukemia in proximity to approximately 200 nuclear power plants and weapons facilities in 10 countries have mostly shown no increase in risk, with a small number of exceptions.[23,25] Pediatric leukemia clusters have been identified in proximity to Sellafield and Dounreay nuclear fuels reprocessing plants in the United Kingdom, in Elbmarsch near the Krümmel plant in Germany, and perhaps in proximity to the Aldermaston and Burghfield weapons production plants in the United Kingdom and the La Hague nuclear power plant in France.[23] There is no clear evidence of increased risk based on multisite studies.[23] Alternate hypotheses used to explain these childhood leukemia clusters have been proposed, but to date there is no confirmatory evidence that can be used to support these hypotheses. The limitations of many of the studies conducted to date include inadequate study designs, residence information restricted to the location at the diagnosis of childhood leukemia and absence of complete address histories, low statistical power because of the low levels of radiation exposure and small numbers of childhood leukemia outcomes, limited understanding of the etiology of childhood leukemia (including relevant time windows of exposure and latency), and inability to adjust for potential confounders.[83]

Long-term Effects: Tissue Reactions and Conditions Other Than Cancer

Tissue Effects After High-Dose Radiotherapy

Compared with adults, children undergoing radiotherapy appear to experience higher risks of the harmful tissue reactions, other than cancer, that occur at relatively high radiation exposure levels. Valuable sources of data about adverse effects other than cancer associated with high-dose radiation exposures include follow-up studies of childhood cancer survivors.[84–94] These studies have identified impairment of growth and maturation, neurologic effects (attributable to loss of brain volume or interference with myelinization of nerve axons or development of synapses), cardiovascular system abnormalities, decreased pulmonary function, thyroid and other neuroendocrine effects (attributable to hypothyroidism, reduction in growth hormone secretion, other hormonal deficiencies, and primary gonadal failure in male individuals), reproductive effects, cataracts and cortical opacities, hearing and vestibular abnormalities, and a range of effects on teeth (the latter particularly notable among children younger than 5 years at exposure). Many of these studies lack detailed information on estimated organ doses.

Tissue Effects After Low-to-Moderate Doses of Radiation Exposure

Data are more limited on late effects, other than cancer, in relation to low-to-moderate doses of radiation exposure. Adverse effects on mental and cognitive function have been observed among children and adolescents undergoing scalp irradiation for tinea capitis[95] and among infants treated with radiation for hemangiomas on the face, head, or other sites.[96] Increased risks of lens opacities (eg, cortical and posterior subscapular opacities) have been associated with low-to-moderate doses of radiation among infants irradiated for hemangiomas[97] and atomic bomb survivors exposed at young ages.[98–101] Internal exposure of children and adolescents to radioiodines from the Chernobyl nuclear accident has been associated with subsequent increased risks of nonmalignant thyroid nodules.[102] Similar increased risks of nonmalignant thyroid nodules have been observed among those exposed as children or adolescents to radioiodines from the fallout from the Semipalatinsk Test Site in Kazakhstan at the time of the aboveground testing[20] as well as in those exposed at ages younger than 20 years to the atomic bombings in Hiroshima and Nagasaki.[103] Findings were inconsistent for radiation exposure and risk of hypothyroidism, hyperthyroidism, and measures of thyroid autoimmune disease from studies of Chernobyl residents exposed in childhood or adolescence.[104–108] High doses of ionizing radiation have long been associated with circulatory disease, but evidence for an association at lower exposure is more controversial. Authors of a meta-analysis of populations exposed in adulthood support a relationship between circulatory disease mortality and low and moderate doses of ionizing radiation.[109] Growing evidence has been used to link radiation exposure from the atomic bombings during childhood with subsequent risk of hypertension, stroke, and heart disease.[110–112] A few studies have evaluated health effects among those exposed in utero to radioiodines.[113,114]

CONCLUSIONS

This technical report summarizes clinically relevant information about the characteristics, sources, and biological effects of radiation exposure to clarify the rationale for the specific measures to reduce radiation exposures and adverse health effects from a radiation emergency. Clinical and related features of radiation-related health outcomes are described for short-term (eg, ARS), short- and long-term (eg, mental health conditions), and long-term (eg, cancer and tissue reactions and conditions other than cancer) effects. This report summarizes newer scientific data on cancer and other serious health effects from long-term follow-up of the Japanese atomic bomb survivors and the Chernobyl nuclear accident and populations exposed to aboveground nuclear testing. The health outcomes reported since the 2011 Fukushima Daiichi nuclear plant event are critically evaluated. Also described are short-term health effects from inappropriately discarded medical radiation equipment, of which there have been no long-term studies. In addition, results are scrutinized for the large number of studies of health effects among populations living in proximity to nuclear plants. Recommendations for pediatricians and the health care sector, government, and families can be found in the accompanying policy statement.[9]

ACKNOWLEDGMENTS

We thank Dr Steve Simon for scientific review and Ms Ka Lai Lou for technical assistance with the article preparation.

LEAD AUTHORS

Martha S. Linet, MD, MPH
Ziad Kazzi, MD, FACMT, FAACT, FAAEM, FACEP
Jerome A. Paulson, MD, FAAP

ABBREVIATIONS

^{131}I: iodine-131
^{137}Cs: cesium-137
AAP: American Academy of Pediatrics
ARS: acute radiation syndrome
FDA: US Food and Drug Administration
KI: potassium iodide
SI: Systéme International d'Unités

Address correspondence to Jerome A. Paulson, MD, FAAP. E-mail: jerry@envirohealthdoctor.com

PEDIATRICS (ISSN Numbers: Print, 0031-4005; Online, 1098-4275).

FINANCIAL DISCLOSURE: The authors have indicated they have no financial relationships relevant to this article to disclose.

FUNDING: Supported by the intra-agency agreement between the National Institute of Allergy and Infectious Diseases and the National Cancer Institute, National Institute of Allergy and Infectious Diseases agreement Y2-A1-5077 and National Cancer Institute agreement Y3-CO-5117.

POTENTIAL CONFLICT OF INTEREST: The authors have indicated they have no potential conflicts of interest to disclose.

COMPANION PAPER: A companion to this article can be found online at www.pediatrics.org/cgi/doi/10.1542/peds.2018-3000.

REFERENCES

1. Tracy BL. Would children be adequately protected by existing intervention levels during a radionuclear emergency? *Radiat Prot Dosimetry.* 2010;142(1):40–45

2. Binder S, Sokal D, Maughan D. Estimating soil ingestion: the use of tracer elements in estimating the amount of soil ingested by young children. *Arch Environ Health.* 1986;41(6):341–345

3. Simon SL. Soil ingestion by humans: a review of history, data, and etiology with application to risk assessment of radioactively contaminated soil. *Health Phys.* 1998;74(6):647–672

4. Simon SL, Bouville A, Land CE. Fallout from nuclear weapons tests and cancer risks: exposures 50 years ago still have health implications today that will continue into the future. *Am Sci.* 2006;94(1):48–57

5. American Academy of Pediatrics Committee on Environmental Health. Radiation disasters and children. *Pediatrics.* 2003;111(6 pt 1):1455–1466

6. Disaster Preparedness Advisory Council. Medical countermeasures for children in public health emergencies, disasters, or terrorism. *Pediatrics.* 2016;137(2):e20154273

7. Disaster Preparedness Advisory Council; Committee on Pediatric Emergency Medicine. Ensuring the health of children in disasters. *Pediatrics.* 2015;136(5). Available at: www.pediatrics.org/cgi/content/full/136/5/e1407

8. Schonfeld DJ, Demaria T; Disaster Preparedness Advisory Council and Committee on Psychosocial Aspects of Child and Family Health. Providing psychosocial support to children and families in the aftermath of disasters and crises. *Pediatrics.* 2015;136(4). Available at: www.pediatrics.org/cgi/content/full/136/4/e1120

9. Paulson JA, Council on Environmental Health. Pediatric considerations before, during, and after radiological or nuclear emergencies. *Pediatrics.* 2018;142(6):e20183000

10. Mabuchi K, Fujiwara S, Preston DL, Shimizu Y, Nakamura N, Shore RE. Atomic bomb survivors: long-term health effects of radiation. In: Shrieve DC, Loeffler JS, eds. *Human Radiation Injury.* Philadelphia, PA: Wolter Kluwer/Lippincott Williams and Wilkins; 2011:89–113

11. Preston DL, Cullings H, Suyama A, et al. Solid cancer incidence in atomic bomb survivors exposed in utero or as young children. *J Natl Cancer Inst.* 2008;100(6):428–436

12. Preston DL, Ron E, Tokuoka S, et al. Solid cancer incidence in atomic bomb survivors: 1958-1998. *Radiat Res.* 2007;168(1):1–64

13. Cooper RJ, Randle K, Sokhi RS. *Radioactive Releases in the Environment: Impact and Assessment.* New York, NY: Wiley; 2003

14. Kemeny J. *Report of the President's Commission on the Accident at Three Mile Island: The Need for Change in the Legacy of TMI.* Washington, DC: The President's Committee on the Accident at Three Mile Island; 1979

15. Brenner AV, Tronko MD, Hatch M, et al. I-131 dose response for incident thyroid cancers in Ukraine related to the Chornobyl accident. *Environ Health Perspect.* 2011;119(7):933–939

16. Harada KH, Niisoe T, Imanaka M, et al. Radiation dose rates now and in the future for residents neighboring restricted areas of the Fukushima Daiichi Nuclear Power Plant. *Proc Natl Acad Sci USA.* 2014;111(10):E914–E923

17. Lyon JL, Alder SC, Stone MB, et al. Thyroid disease associated with exposure to the Nevada nuclear weapons test site radiation: a reevaluation based on corrected dosimetry and examination data. *Epidemiology.* 2006;17(6):604–614

18. Simon SL, Bouville A, Land CE, Beck HL. Radiation doses and cancer risks in the Marshall Islands associated with exposure to radioactive fallout from Bikini and Enewetak nuclear weapons tests: summary. *Health Phys.* 2010;99(2):105–123

19. de Vathaire F, Drozdovitch V, Brindel P, et al. Thyroid cancer following nuclear tests in French Polynesia. *Br J Cancer.* 2010;103(7):1115–1121

20. Land CE, Zhumadilov Z, Gusev BI, et al. Ultrasound-detected thyroid nodule prevalence and radiation dose from fallout. *Radiat Res.* 2008;169(4):373–383

21. Land CE, Kwon D, Hoffman FO, et al. Accounting for shared and unshared dosimetric uncertainties in the dose response for ultrasound-detected thyroid nodules after exposure to radioactive fallout. *Radiat Res.* 2015;183(2):159–173

22. International Atomic Energy Agency. The radiological accident in Goiania. 1988. Available at: http://www-pub.iaea.org/mtcd/publications/pdf/pub815_web.pdf. Accessed May 5, 2014

23. Laurier D, Jacob S, Bernier MO, et al. Epidemiological studies of leukaemia in children and young adults around nuclear facilities: a critical review. *Radiat Prot Dosimetry.* 2008;132(2):182–190

24. Gilbert ES, Land CE, Simon SL. Health effects from fallout. *Health Phys.* 2002;82(5):726–735

25. Stather JW. Childhood leukaemia near nuclear sites: fourteenth report of the Committee on Medical Aspects of Radiation in the Environment (COMARE). *Radiat Prot Dosimetry.* 2011;147(3):351–354

26. Hall EJ, Gaccia AJ. *Radiobiology for the Radiologist.* 7th ed. Philadelphia, PA: Lippincott Williams and Wilkins; 2011

27. Goans RE. *Medical Management of Radiological Casualties.* 4th ed. Bethesda, MD: Armed Forces Radiobiology Research Institute, Uniformed Services University of the Health Science; 2013

28. Centers for Disease Control and Prevention. Frequently asked questions (FAQ) about radiation emergencies. 2015. Available at: http://emergency.cdc.gov/radiation/emergencyfaq.asp. Accessed February 15, 2015

29. US Department of Health and Human Services. Decontamination procedures. 2015. Available at: www.remm.nlm.gov/ext_contamination.htm. Accessed February 15, 2015

30. National Council on Radiation Protection and Measurements.

Management of Persons Contaminated With Radionuclides: Handbook. NCRP Report No. 161. Vol 1. Bethesda, MD: National Council on Radiation Protection and Measurements; 2008

31. National Security Staff Interagency Policy Coordination Subcommittee for Preparedness and Response to Radiological and Nuclear Threats. Planning guidance for response to a nuclear detonation: second edition. 2010. Available at: https://asprtracie.hhs.gov/technical-resources/resource/1432/planning-guidance-for-response-to-a-nuclear-detonation-second-edition. Accessed February 15, 2015

32. US Department of Health and Human Services; US Food and Drug Administration. Guidance potassium iodide as a thyroid blocking agent in radiation emergencies. Available at: https://www.fda.gov/downloads/Drugs/.../Guidances/ucm080542.pdf. Accessed October 16, 2018

33. Spallek L, Krille L, Reiners C, Schneider R, Yamashita S, Zeeb H. Adverse effects of iodine thyroid blocking: a systematic review. *Radiat Prot Dosimetry.* 2012;150(3):267–277

34. ANBEX. iOSAT: potassium iodide for thyroid blocking in a radiation emergency. Available at: www.anbex.com. Accessed September 23, 2014

35. Thyrosafe. Thyrosafe. Available at: www.thyrosafe.com/. Accessed September 23, 2014

36. Thyroshield. Thyroshield. Available at: www.thyroshield.com/. Accessed September 23, 2014

37. Bongers-Schokking JJ, Koot HM, Wiersma D, Verkerk PH, de Muinck Keizer-Schrama SM. Influence of timing and dose of thyroid hormone replacement on development in infants with congenital hypothyroidism. *J Pediatr.* 2000;136(3):292–297

38. Calaciura F, Mendorla G, Distefano M, et al. Childhood IQ measurements in infants with transient congenital hypothyroidism. *Clin Endocrinol (Oxf).* 1995;43(4):473–477

39. Fisher DA. The importance of early management in optimizing IQ in infants with congenital hypothyroidism. *J Pediatr.* 2000;136(3):273–274

40. Ahlgren L, Ivarsson S, Johansson L, Mattsson S, Nosslin B. Excretion of radionuclides in human breast milk after the administration of radiopharmaceuticals. *J Nucl Med.* 1985;26(9):1085–1090

41. Romney BM, Nickoloff EL, Esser PD, Alderson PO. Radionuclide administration to nursing mothers: mathematically derived guidelines. *Radiology.* 1986;160(2):549–554

42. Mountford PJ, Coakley AJ. A review of the secretion of radioactivity in human breast milk: data, quantitative analysis and recommendations. *Nucl Med Commun.* 1989;10(1):15–27

43. Rubow S, Klopper J, Wasserman H, Baard B, van Niekerk M. The excretion of radiopharmaceuticals in human breast milk: additional data and dosimetry. *Eur J Nucl Med.* 1994;21(2):144–153

44. International Commission on Radiation Protection. Doses to infants from ingestion of radionuclides in mothers' milk. ICRP publication 95. [published correction appears in *Ann ICRP.* 2006;36(1–2):329–336]. *Ann ICRP.* 2004;34(3–4):iii, 15–267, 269–280

45. Simon SL, Luckyanov N, Bouville A, VanMiddlesworth L, Weinstock RM. Transfer of 131I into human breast milk and transfer coefficients for radiological dose assessments. *Health Phys.* 2002;82(6):796–806

46. Centers for Disease Control and Prevention. Potassium iodide (KI). Available at: https://emergency.cdc.gov/radiation/ki.asp. Accessed October 16, 2018

47. American Academy of Pediatrics. Infant feeding in disasters and emergencies. 2015. Available at: https://www.aap.org/en-us/advocacy-and-policy/aap-health-initiatives/Breastfeeding/Documents/InfantNutritionDisaster.pdf. Accessed May 10, 2017

48. National Council on Radiation Protection and Measurements. *Preconception and Prenatal Radiation Exposure: Health Effects and Protective Guide.* NCRP Report 174. Bethesda, MD: National Council on Radiation Protection Measurements; 2013

49. Kazzi Z, Buzzell J, Bertelli L, Christensen D. Emergency department

management of patients internally contaminated with radioactive material. *Emerg Med Clin North Am.* 2015;33(1):179–196

50. National Council on Radiation Protection and Measurements. *Management of Persons Contaminated With Radionuclides.* NCRP Report 161. Vol 2. Bethesda, MD: National Council on Radiation Protection and Measurements; 2008

51. Centers for Disease Control and Prevention. Internal Contamination Clinical Reference (ICCR) application. Available at: http://emergency.cdc.gov/radiation/iccr.asp. Accessed February 15, 2015

52. Neria Y, Nandi A, Galea S. Post-traumatic stress disorder following disasters: a systematic review. *Psychol Med.* 2008;38(4):467–480

53. Bromet EJ, Havenaar JM, Guey LTA. A 25 year retrospective review of the psychological consequences of the Chernobyl accident. *Clin Oncol (R Coll Radiol).* 2011;23(4):297–305

54. Bromet EJ, Goldgaber D, Carlson G, et al. Children's well-being 11 years after the Chornobyl catastrophe. *Arch Gen Psychiatry.* 2000;57(6):563–571

55. Butler AS, Panzer AM, Goldfrank LR, Institute of Medicine; Board on Neuroscience and Behavioral Health; Committee on Responding to the Psychological Consequences of Terrorism. *Preparing for the Psychological Consequences of Terrorism: A Public Health Strategy.* Washington, DC: The National Academies Press; 2003

56. Radiation Emergency Medical Management. Time phases of acute radiation syndrome - dose >8 Gy. Available at: www.remm.nlm.gov/ars_timephases5.htm. Accessed February 15, 2015

57. Radiation Emergency Medical Management. Multi-organ injury, multi-organ dysfunction syndrome, multi-organ failure: a new hypothesis of whole body radiation effects. Available at: www.remm.nlm.gov/multiorganinjury.htm. Accessed February 15, 2015

58. Singh VK, Romaine PL, Newman VL, Seed TM. Medical countermeasures

for unwanted CBRN exposures: part II radiological and nuclear threats with review of recent countermeasure patents. *Expert Opin Ther Pat.* 2016;26(12):1399–1408

59. Burchfield LA. *Radiation Safety: Protection and Management for Homeland Security and Emergency Response.* Hoboken, NJ: Wiley; 2009

60. Centers for Disease Control and Prevention. Acute radiation syndrome: fact sheet for clinicians. Available at: https://emergency.cdc.gov/radiation/arsphysicianfactsheet.asp. Accessed October 18, 2018

61. Christodouleas JP, Forrest RD, Ainsley CG, Tochner Z, Hahn SM, Glatstein E. Short-term and long-term health risks of nuclear-power-plant accidents. *N Engl J Med.* 2011;364(24):2334–2341

62. Melnick AL. *Biological, Chemical, and Radiological Terrorism: Emergency Preparedness and Response for the Primary Care Physician.* 1st ed. New York, NY: Springer Sciences and Business Media; 2008

63. Yamamoto LG. Risks and management of radiation exposure. *Pediatr Emerg Care.* 2013;29(9):1016–1026; quiz 1027–1029

64. Radiation Emergency Medical Management. Dose estimator for exposure: 3 biodosimetry tools. Available at: www.remm.nlm.gov/ars_wbd.htm. Accessed February 15, 2015

65. Flowers CR, Seidenfeld J, Bow EJ, et al. Antimicrobial prophylaxis and outpatient management of fever and neutropenia in adults treated for malignancy: American Society of Clinical Oncology clinical practice guideline. *J Clin Oncol.* 2013;31(6):794–810

66. Freifeld AG, Bow EJ, Sepkowitz KA, et al; Infectious Diseases Society of America. Clinical practice guideline for the use of antimicrobial agents in neutropenic patients with cancer: 2010 update by the Infectious Diseases Society of America. *Clin Infect Dis.* 2011;52(4):e56–e93

67. Bromet EJ. Emotional consequences of nuclear power plant disasters. *Health Phys.* 2014;106(2):206–210

68. Honda S, Shibata Y, Mine M, et al. Mental health conditions

among atomic bomb survivors in Nagasaki. *Psychiatry Clin Neurosci.* 2002;56(5):575–583

69. Lifton RJ. *Death in Life: Survivors of Hiroshima.* 1st ed. New York, NY: Random House; 1967

70. Kim Y, Tsutsumi A, Izutsu T, Kawamura N, Miyazaki T, Kikkawa T. Persistent distress after psychological exposure to the Nagasaki atomic bomb explosion. *Br J Psychiatry.* 2011;199(5):411–416

71. Bromet EJ, Gluzman SF, Paniotto VI, et al. Epidemiology of psychiatric and alcohol disorders in Ukraine: findings from the Ukraine World Mental Health survey. *Soc Psychiatry Psychiatr Epidemiol.* 2005;40(9):681–690

72. United Nations. *The Chernobyl Forum: 2003-2005.* 2nd edition.Vienna, Austria: International Atomic Energy Agency; 2006

73. United Nations Scientific Committee on the Effects of Atomic Radiation. *Scientific Annex B: Effects of Radiation Exposure of Children.* Vol 2. New York, NY: United Nations Scientific Committee on the Effects of Atomic Radiation; 2013

74. Hatch MC, Beyea J, Nieves JW, Susser M. Cancer near the Three Mile Island nuclear plant: radiation emissions. *Am J Epidemiol.* 1990;132(3):397–412; discussion 413–417

75. Matsuda N, Kumagai A, Ohtsuru A, et al. Assessment of internal exposure doses in Fukushima by a whole body counter within one month after the nuclear power plant accident. *Radiat Res.* 2013;179(6):663–668

76. Tsuda T, Tokinobu A, Yamamoto E, Suzuki E. Thyroid cancer detection by ultrasound among residents ages 18 years and younger in Fukushima, Japan: 2011 to 2014. *Epidemiology.* 2016;27(3):316–322

77. Wakeford R, Auvinen A, Gent RN, et al. Re: thyroid cancer among young people in Fukushima. *Epidemiology.* 2016;27(3):e20–e21

78. Nagataki S, Takamura N, Kamiya K, Akashi M. Measurements of individual radiation doses in residents living around the Fukushima Nuclear Power Plant. *Radiat Res.* 2013;180(5):439–447

79. Jorgensen TJ. Re: thyroid cancer among young people in Fukushima. *Epidemiology.* 2016;27(3):e17

80. Yasumura S, Hosoya M, Yamashita S, et al; Fukushima Health Management Survey Group. Study protocol for the Fukushima Health Management Survey. *J Epidemiol.* 2012;22(5):375–383

81. Cardis E, Hatch M. The Chernobyl accident—an epidemiological perspective. *Clin Oncol (R Coll Radiol).* 2011;23(4):251–260

82. Parkin DM, Clayton D, Black RJ, et al. Childhood leukaemia in Europe after Chernobyl: 5 year follow-up. *Br J Cancer.* 1996;73(8):1006–1012

83. Kuehni C, Spycher BD. Nuclear power plants and childhood leukaemia: lessons from the past and future directions. *Swiss Med Wkly.* 2014;144:w13912

84. Armstrong GT, Liu Q, Yasui Y, et al. Long-term outcomes among adult survivors of childhood central nervous system malignancies in the Childhood Cancer Survivor Study. *J Natl Cancer Inst.* 2009;101(13):946–958

85. Brouwer CA, Postma A, Hooimeijer HL, et al. Endothelial damage in long-term survivors of childhood cancer. *J Clin Oncol.* 2013;31(31):3906–3913

86. de Fine Licht S, Winther JF, Gudmundsdottir T, et al. Hospital contacts for endocrine disorders in Adult Life after Childhood Cancer in Scandinavia (ALiCCS): a population-based cohort study. *Lancet.* 2014;383(9933):1981–1989

87. Gawade PL, Hudson MM, Kaste SC, et al. A systematic review of dental late effects in survivors of childhood cancer. *Pediatr Blood Cancer.* 2014;61(3):407–416

88. Mertens AC, Yasui Y, Liu Y, et al; Childhood Cancer Survivor Study. Pulmonary complications in survivors of childhood and adolescent cancer. A report from the Childhood Cancer Survivor Study. *Cancer.* 2002;95(11):2431–2441

89. Oeffinger KC, Mertens AC, Sklar CA, et al; Childhood Cancer Survivor Study. Chronic health conditions in adult survivors of childhood cancer. *N Engl J Med.* 2006;355(15):1572–1582

90. Paulino AC, Constine LS, Rubin P, Williams JP. Normal tissue development, homeostasis, senescence, and the sensitivity to radiation injury across the age spectrum. *Semin Radiat Oncol.* 2010;20(1):12–20

91. Signorello LB, Mulvihill JJ, Green DM, et al. Congenital anomalies in the children of cancer survivors: a report from the childhood cancer survivor study. *J Clin Oncol.* 2012;30(3):239–245

92. Stewart FA, Seemann I, Hoving S, Russell NS. Understanding radiation-induced cardiovascular damage and strategies for intervention. *Clin Oncol (R Coll Radiol).* 2013;25(10):617–624

93. Whelan K, Stratton K, Kawashima T, et al. Auditory complications in childhood cancer survivors: a report from the childhood cancer survivor study. *Pediatr Blood Cancer.* 2011;57(1):126–134

94. Whelan KF, Stratton K, Kawashima T, et al. Ocular late effects in childhood and adolescent cancer survivors: a report from the childhood cancer survivor study. *Pediatr Blood Cancer.* 2010;54(1):103–109

95. Ron E, Modan B, Floro S, Harkedar I, Gurewitz R. Mental function following scalp irradiation during childhood. *Am J Epidemiol.* 1982;116(1):149–160

96. Hall P, Adami HO, Trichopoulos D, et al. Effect of low doses of ionising radiation in infancy on cognitive function in adulthood: Swedish population based cohort study. *BMJ.* 2004;328(7430):19

97. Hall P, Granath F, Lundell M, Olsson K, Holm LE. Lenticular opacities in individuals exposed to ionizing radiation in infancy. *Radiat Res.* 1999;152(2):190–195

98. Minamoto A, Taniguchi H, Yoshitani N, et al. Cataract in atomic bomb survivors. *Int J Radiat Biol.* 2004;80(5):339–345

99. Nakashima E, Neriishi K, Minamoto A. A reanalysis of atomic-bomb cataract data, 2000-2002: a threshold analysis. *Health Phys.* 2006;90(2):154–160

100. Neriishi K, Nakashima E, Akahoshi M, et al. Radiation dose and cataract surgery incidence in atomic bomb survivors, 1986-2005. *Radiology.* 2012;265(1):167–174

101. Shore RE, Neriishi K, Nakashima E. Epidemiological studies of cataract risk at low to moderate radiation doses: (not) seeing is believing. *Radiat Res.* 2010;174(6):889–894

102. Zablotska LB, Bogdanova TI, Ron E, et al. A cohort study of thyroid cancer and other thyroid diseases after the Chornobyl accident: dose-response analysis of thyroid follicular adenomas detected during first screening in Ukraine (1998-2000). *Am J Epidemiol.* 2008;167(3):305–312

103. Imaizumi M, Usa T, Tominaga T, et al. Radiation dose-response relationships for thyroid nodules and autoimmune thyroid diseases in Hiroshima and Nagasaki atomic bomb survivors 55-58 years after radiation exposure. *JAMA.* 2006;295(9):1011–1022

104. Cahoon EK, Rozhko A, Hatch M, et al. Factors associated with serum thyroglobulin levels in a population living in Belarus. *Clin Endocrinol (Oxf).* 2013;79(1):120–127

105. Hatch M, Furukawa K, Brenner A, et al. Prevalence of hyperthyroidism after exposure during childhood or adolescence to radioiodines from the chornobyl nuclear accident: dose-response results from the Ukrainian-American Cohort Study. *Radiat Res.* 2010;174(6):763–772

106. McConnell RJ, Brenner AV, Oliynyk VA, et al. Factors associated with elevated serum concentrations of anti-TPO antibodies in subjects with and without diffuse goitre. Results from the Ukrainian-American Cohort Study of thyroid cancer and other thyroid diseases following the Chornobyl accident. *Clin Endocrinol (Oxf).* 2007;67(6):879–890

107. Ostroumova E, Brenner A, Oliynyk V, et al. Subclinical hypothyroidism after radioiodine exposure: Ukrainian-American cohort study of thyroid cancer and other thyroid diseases after the Chornobyl accident (1998-2000). *Environ Health Perspect.* 2009;117(5):745–750

108. Ostroumova E, Rozhko A, Hatch M, et al. Measures of thyroid function among Belarusian children and adolescents exposed to iodine-131 from the accident at the Chernobyl nuclear plant. *Environ Health Perspect.* 2013;121(7):865–871

109. Little MP, Azizova TV, Bazyka D, et al. Systematic review and meta-analysis of circulatory disease from exposure to low-level ionizing radiation and estimates of potential population mortality risks. *Environ Health Perspect.* 2012;120(11):1503–1511

110. Sasaki H, Wong FL, Yamada M, Kodama K. The effects of aging and radiation exposure on blood pressure levels of atomic bomb survivors. *J Clin Epidemiol.* 2002;55(10):974–981

111. Tatsukawa Y, Nakashima E, Yamada M, et al. Cardiovascular disease risk among atomic bomb survivors exposed in utero, 1978-2003. *Radiat Res.* 2008;170(3):269–274

112. Yamada M, Wong FL, Fujiwara S, Akahoshi M, Suzuki G. Noncancer disease incidence in atomic bomb survivors, 1958-1998. *Radiat Res.* 2004;161(6):622–632

113. Hatch M, Brenner A, Bogdanova T, et al. A screening study of thyroid cancer and other thyroid diseases among individuals exposed in utero to iodine-131 from Chernobyl fallout. *J Clin Endocrinol Metab.* 2009;94(3):899–906

114. Neta G, Hatch M, Kitahara CM, et al. In utero exposure to iodine-131 from Chernobyl fallout and anthropometric characteristics in adolescence. *Radiat Res.* 2014;181(3):293–301

Pediatric Medication Safety in the Emergency Department

· ·

- *Policy Statement*

POLICY STATEMENT Organizational Principles to Guide and Define the Child Health Care System and/or Improve the Health of all Children

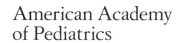

American Academy
of Pediatrics

DEDICATED TO THE HEALTH OF ALL CHILDREN™

Pediatric Medication Safety in the Emergency Department

Lee Benjamin, MD, FAAP, FACEP,[a] Karen Frush, MD, FAAP,[b] Kathy Shaw, MD, MSCE, FAAP,[c] Joan E. Shook, MD, MBA, FAAP,[d] Sally K. Snow, BSN, RN, CPEN, FAEN,[e] AMERICAN ACADEMY OF PEDIATRICS Committee on Pediatric Emergency Medicine, AMERICAN COLLEGE OF EMERGENCY PHYSICIANS Pediatric Emergency Medicine Committee, EMERGENCY NURSES ASSOCIATION Pediatric Emergency Medicine Committee

abstract

Pediatric patients cared for in emergency departments (EDs) are at high risk of medication errors for a variety of reasons. A multidisciplinary panel was convened by the Emergency Medical Services for Children program and the American Academy of Pediatrics Committee on Pediatric Emergency Medicine to initiate a discussion on medication safety in the ED. Top opportunities identified to improve medication safety include using kilogram-only weight-based dosing, optimizing computerized physician order entry by using clinical decision support, developing a standard formulary for pediatric patients while limiting variability of medication concentrations, using pharmacist support within EDs, enhancing training of medical professionals, systematizing the dispensing and administration of medications within the ED, and addressing challenges for home medication administration before discharge.

[a]Department of Emergency Medicine, St Joseph Mercy Ann Arbor, Ypsilanti, Michigan; [b]Department of Pediatrics, School of Medicine, Duke University, Durham, North Carolina; [c]Department of Pediatrics, Children's Hospital of Philadelphia, Philadelphia, Pennsylvania; [d]Section of Emergency Medicine, Department of Pediatrics, Baylor College of Medicine, Houston, Texas; and [e]Retired; Former Trauma Program Director, Cook Children's Medical Center, Fort Worth, Texas

All authors contributed to the writing and organization of the policy statement and reviewed and support the final submission.

Jointly published in the Annals of Emergency Medicine.

BACKGROUND

Despite a national focus on patient safety since the publication of the Institute of Medicine (now the National Academy of Medicine) report "To Err is Human" in 1999, medical errors remain a leading cause of morbidity and mortality across the United States.[1] Medication errors are by far the most common type of medical error occurring in hospitalized patients,[2] and the medication error rate in pediatric patients has been found to be as much as 3 times the rate in adult patients.[3,4] Because many medication errors and adverse drug events (ADEs) are preventable,[1] strategies to improve medication safety are an essential component of an overall approach to providing quality care to children.

The pediatric emergency care setting is recognized as a high-risk environment for medication errors because of a number of factors, including medically complex patients with multiple medications who are unknown to emergency department (ED) staff, a lack of standard pediatric drug dosing and formulations,[5] weight-based dosing,[6,7] verbal

To cite: Benjamin L, Frush K, Shaw K, et al. AMERICAN ACADEMY OF PEDIATRICS Committee on Pediatric Emergency Medicine, AMERICAN COLLEGE OF EMERGENCY PHYSICIANS Pediatric Emergency Medicine Committee, EMERGENCY NURSES ASSOCIATION Pediatric Emergency Medicine Committee. Pediatric Medication Safety in the Emergency Department. Pediatrics. 2018;141(3):e20174066

orders, a hectic environment with frequent interruptions,[8] a lack of clinical pharmacists on the ED care team,[9,10] inpatient boarding status,[11] the use of information technology systems that lack pediatric safety features,[12] and numerous transitions in care. In addition, the vast majority of pediatric patients seeking care in EDs are not seen in pediatric hospitals but rather in community hospitals, which may treat a low number of pediatric patients.[13] Studies also outline the problem of medication errors in children in the prehospital setting. A study of 8 Michigan emergency medical services agencies revealed errors for commonly used medications, with up to one-third of medications being dosed incorrectly.[14] Medication error rates reported from single institutions with dedicated pediatric EDs range from 10% to 31%,[15,16] and in a study from a pediatric tertiary care center network, Shaw et al[6] showed that medication errors accounted for almost 20% of all incident reports, with 13% of the medication errors causing patient harm. The authors of another study examined medication errors in children at 4 rural EDs in northern California and found an error rate of 39%, with 16% of these errors having the potential to cause harm.[17] The following discussion adds to the broad topic of medication safety by introducing specific opportunities unique to pediatric patients within EDs to facilitate local intervention on the basis of institutional experience and resources.

STRATEGIES FOR IMPROVEMENT

A multidisciplinary expert panel was convened by the Emergency Medical Services for Children program and the American Academy of Pediatrics (AAP), through its Committee on Pediatric Emergency Medicine, to discuss challenges related to pediatric medication safety in

the emergency setting. The panel included emergency care providers, nurses, pharmacists, electronic health record industry representatives, patient safety organization leaders, hospital accreditation organizations, and parents of children who suffered ADEs. The panel outlined numerous opportunities for improvement, including raising awareness of risks for emergency care providers, trainees, children, and their families; developing policies and processes that support improved pediatric medication safety; and implementing best practices to reduce pediatric ADEs. Specific strategies discussed by the panel, as well as recent advances in improving pediatric medication safety, are described.

Decreasing Pediatric Medication Prescribing Errors in the ED

Computerized Physician Order Entry

Historically, the majority of pediatric medication errors were associated with the ordering phase of the medication process. Specific risks related to pediatric weight-based dosing include not using the appropriate weight,[6] performing medication calculations based on pounds instead of the recognized standard of kilograms,[6] and making inappropriate calculations, including tenfold dosing errors.[18–20] Childhood obesity introduces further opportunity for dosing error. In addition to the lack of science to guide medication dosing in patients with obesity,[21] frequent underdosing[22] is reported, and currently available resuscitation tools are commonly imprecise.[23] Furthermore, there are limited opportunities for prescription monitoring or double-checking in the ED setting, and many times calculations are performed in the clinical area without input from a pharmacist.[9] The implementation of computerized physician order entry (CPOE) and clinical decision support (CDS) with electronic prescribing

have reduced many of these errors, because most CPOE systems obviate the need for simple dose calculation. However, CPOE systems have not fully eliminated medication errors. Commercial or independently developed CPOE systems may fail to address critical unique pediatric dosing requirements.[12,24] Kilogram-only scales are recommended for obtaining weights, yet conversion to pounds either by the operator or electronic health record may introduce opportunity for error into the system. In addition, providers may override CDS, despite its proven success in reducing errors.[16,25] Prescribers frequently choose to ignore or override CDS prescribing alerts, with reported override rates as high as 96%.[26] Allowing for free text justification to override alerts for nonformulary drugs may introduce errors. The development of an override algorithm can help reduce user variability.[27] As the use of CPOE increases, one can expect that millions of medication errors will be prevented.[28] For EDs that do not use CPOE, preprinted medication order forms have been shown to significantly reduce medication errors in a variety of settings and serve as a low-cost substitute for CPOE.[29–32]

Standardized Formulary

The Institute of Medicine (now the National Academy of Medicine) recommends development of medication dosage guidelines, formulations, labeling, and administration techniques for the pediatric emergency care setting.[5] Unfortunately, there are currently no universally accepted, pediatric-specific standards with regard to dose suggestion and limits, and dosing guidelines and alerts found in CPOE are commonly provided by third-party vendors that supply platforms to both children's and general hospitals. The development of a standard pediatric formulary, independent of an adult-focused system, can reduce opportunities for error by specifying limited concentrations and standard dosage of high-risk and frequently used medications, such as resuscitation medications, vasoactive infusions, narcotics, and antibiotics, as well as look-alike and sound-alike medications.[33] A standard formulary will allow for consistent education during initial training and continuing medical education for emergency care providers, creating a consistent measure of provider competency. At least 1 large hospital organization has successfully implemented this type of change.[34] In addition, the American Society of Health-System Pharmacists is working with the Food and Drug Administration to develop and implement national standardized concentrations for both intravenous and oral liquid medications.[35]

ED Pharmacists

Currently, many medications are prepared and dispensed in the ED without pharmacist verification or preparation because many EDs lack consistent on-site pharmacist coverage.[9,36] In a survey of pharmacists, 68% reported at least 8 hours of ED coverage on weekdays, but fewer than half of EDs see this support on weekends, with a drastic reduction in coverage during overnight and morning hours.[37] The American College of Emergency Physicians (ACEP) supports the integration of pharmacists within the ED team, specifically recognizing the pediatric population as a high-risk group that may benefit from pharmacist presence.[38] The Emergency Nurses Association (ENA) supports the role of the emergency nurse as well as pharmacy staff to efficiently complete the best possible medication history and reduce medication discrepencies.[39,40] The American Society of Health-System Pharmacists suggests that ED pharmacists may help verify and prepare high-risk medications, be available to

prepare and double-check dosing of medications during resuscitation, and provide valuable input in medication reconciliation, especially of medically complex children whose medications and dosing may be unknown to ED staff and who present without a medication list or portable emergency information form.[41] Medically complex patients typify the difficulty with medication reconciliation, with an error rate of 21% in a tertiary care facility.[42] In this study, no 1 source from the parent, pharmacy, and primary provider group was both available and appropriately sensitive or specific in completing medication reconciliation. Pharmacist-managed reconciliation has had a positive impact for admitted pediatric patients and may translate to the emergency setting.[43,44] ED pharmacists can also help monitor for ADEs, provide drug information, and provide information regarding medication ingestions to both providers and patients and/or families.[45]

Dedicated pharmacists can be integrated through various methods, such as hiring dedicated pharmacy staff for the ED,[7] having these staff immediately available when consulted, or having remote telepharmacy review of medication orders by a central pharmacist.[46,47] Although further research is needed on the potential outcomes on medication safety and return on investment when a pharmacist is placed in the ED, current experience reveals improvements in medication safety when a pharmacist is present.[48] Studies from general EDs reveal significant cost savings as well,[49] with the authors of 1 study in a single urban adult ED identifying more than $1 million dollars of cost avoidance in only 4 months.[50]

Training in Pediatric Medication Safety

Dedicated training in pediatric medication safety is highly variable in

the curricula of professional training programs in medical, nursing, and pharmacy schools.[51] Although national guidelines support the training of prehospital personnel with specific pediatric content and safety and error-reduction training,[52] a nearly 35% prehospital medication error rate for critical medications for pediatric patients remains.[14] At the graduate medical education level, the curricula of pediatric and emergency medicine residency programs and pediatric emergency medicine fellowship programs do not define specific requirements for pediatric medication safety training.[53–55] The same is true for pharmacy programs.[56] Although schools of pharmacy include pediatric topics in their core curricula, pediatric safety advocates believe there is an opportunity for enhanced and improved training.[57]

Experts in pediatric emergency care from the multidisciplinary panel recommend development of a curriculum on pediatric medication safety that could be offered to all caregivers of children in emergency settings. A standard curriculum may include content such as common medication errors in children, systems-improvement tools to avoid or abate errors, and the effects of developmental differences in pediatric patients. Demonstrating competency on the basis of this curriculum is 1 means by which institutions may reduce risks of medication errors.

Decreasing Pediatric Medication Administration Errors in the ED

The dispensing and administration phases serve as final opportunities to optimize medication safety. Strategies to reduce errors include standardizing the concentrations available for a given drug, having readily available and up-to-date medication reference materials, using premixed intravenous preparations when possible, having automated dispensing cabinets with appropriate pediatric dosage formulations, using barcoded medication administration,[58] having pharmacists and ED care providers work effectively as a team, and having policies to guide medication use.[59,60] Although yet to be studied in the ED environment, smart infusion pumps have shown promise in other arenas in reducing administration errors for infusions.[61]

Nurses are held accountable by each state's nurse practice act for the appropriateness of all medications given. Nursing schools teach the 5 rights of medication administration: the right patient, the right medication, the right dose, the right time, and the right route.[62] Elliott and Liu[63] expand the 5 rights to include right documentation, right action, right form, and right response to further improve medication safety. Simulated medication administration addresses opportunities beyond those captured within these rights and may have implications within the ED.[64] Additionally, given the association of medication preparation interruptions and administration errors,[65] the use of a distraction-free medication safety zone has been shown to enhance medication safety.[66,67] Implementation of an independent 2-provider check process for high-alert medications, as suggested by The Joint Commission, also reduces administration errors.[68] Both the Institute for Safe Medication Practices and The Joint Commission provide excellent guidance on these topics.[69]

Decreasing Pediatric Medication Errors in the Home

Recognizing and addressing language barriers and health literacy variability in the ED can affect medication safety in the home. Nonstandardized delivery devices continue to be used in the home, and dosing error rates of greater than 40% are reported.[70] Advanced counseling and instrument provision

in the ED are proven to decrease dosing errors at home.[71] Pictograms provided to aide in medication measurement have also been shown to decrease errors and may be considered as part of discharge instructions.[72] The AAP supports policy on the use of milliliter-only dosing for liquid medications used in the home and suggests that standardized delivery devices be distributed from the ED for use with these medications.[73] As the body of literature regarding health literacy evolves, further addressing these issues in real time may influence out-of-hospital care.

SUMMARY

Pediatric medication safety requires a multidisciplinary approach across the continuum of emergency care, starting in the prehospital setting, during emergency care, and beyond. Key areas for medication safety specific to pediatric care in the ED include the creation of standardized medication dosing guidelines, better integration and use of information technology to support patient safety, and increased education standards across health care disciplines. The following is a list of specific recommendations that can lead to improved pediatric medication safety in the emergency care setting.

RECOMMENDATIONS

1. Create a standard formulary for pediatric high-risk and commonly used medications;

2. standardize concentrations of high-risk medications;

3. reduce the number of available concentrations to the smallest possible number;

4. provide recommended precalculated doses;

5. measure and record weight in kilograms only;

6. use length-based dosing tools when a scale is unavailable or use is not feasible;

7. implement and support the availability of pharmacists in the ED;

8. use standardized order sets with embedded best practice prescribing and dosing range maximums;

9. promote the development of distraction-free medication safety zones for medication preparation;

10. implement process screening, such as a 2-provider independent check for high-alert medications;

11. implement and use CPOE and CDS with pediatric-specific kilogram-only dosing rules, including upper dosing limits within ED information systems;

12. encourage community providers of children with medical complexity to maintain a current medication list and an emergency information form to be available for emergency care;

13. create and integrate a dedicated pediatric medication safety curriculum into training programs for nurses, physicians, respiratory therapists, nurse practitioners, physician assistants, prehospital providers, and pharmacists;

14. develop tools for competency assessment;

15. dispense standardized delivery devices for home administration of liquid medications;

16. dispense milliliter-only dosing for liquid medications used in the home;

17. employ advanced counseling such as teach-back when sharing medication instructions for home use; and

18. use pictogram-based dosing instruction sheets for use of home medications.

LEAD AUTHORS

Lee Benjamin, MD, FAAP, FACEP
Karen Frush, MD, FAAP
Kathy Shaw, MD, MSCE, FAAP
Joan E. Shook, MD, MBA, FAAP
Sally K. Snow, BSN, RN, CPEN, FAEN

AAP COMMITTEE ON PEDIATRIC EMERGENCY MEDICINE, 2017–2018

Joseph Wright, MD, MPH, FAAP, Chairperson
Terry Adirim, MD, MPH, FAAP
Michael S.D. Agus, MD, FAAP
James Callahan, MD, FAAP
Toni Gross, MD, MPH, FAAP
Natalie Lane, MD, FAAP
Lois Lee, MD, MPH, FAAP
Suzan Mazor, MD, FAAP
Prashant Mahajan, MD, MPH, MBA, FAAP
Nathan Timm, MD

LIAISONS

Andrew Eisenberg, MD — *American Academy of Family Physicians*
Cynthia Wright Johnson, MSN, RN — *National Association of State Emergency Medical Service Officials*
Cynthiana Lightfoot, BFA, NRP — *AAP Family Partnerships Network*
Charles Macias, MD, MPH, FAAP — *Emergency Medical Service for Children Innovation and Improvement Center*
Brian Moore, MD, MPH, FAAP — *National Association of Emergency Medical Service Physicians*
Diane Pilkey, RN, MPH — *Maternal and Child Health Bureau*
Katherine Remick, MD, FAAP — *National Association of Emergency Medical Technicians*
Mohsen Saidinejad, MD, MBA, FAAP, FACEP — *ACEP*
Sally Snow, RN, BSN, CPEN, FAEN — *ENA*
David Tuggle, MD, FAAP — *American College of Surgeons*

FORMER AAP COMMITTEE ON PEDIATRIC EMERGENCY MEDICINE MEMBERS, 2012–2016

Alice Ackerman, MD, MBA
Thomas Chun, MD, MPH, FAAP
Gregory Conners, MD, MPH, MBA, FAAP
Edward Conway, Jr, MD, MS, FAAP
Nanette Dudley, MD, FAAP
Joel Fein, MD
Susan Fuchs, MD, FAAP
Marc Gorelick, MD, MSCE
Natalie Lane, MD, FAAP
Charles Macias, MD, MPH, FAAP
Brian Moore, MD, FAAP

Steven Selbst, MD
Kathy Shaw, MD, MSCE, Chair (2008–2012)
Joan Shook, MD, MBA, FAAP, Chair (2012–2016)
Joseph Wright, MD, MPH, FAAP

STAFF

Sue Tellez
Tamar Margarik Haro

ACEP PEDIATRIC EMERGENCY MEDICINE COMMITTEE, 2016–2017

Madeline Joseph, MD, FACEP, Chair
Kiyetta Alade, MD
Christopher Amato, MD, FACEP
Jahn T. Avarello, MD, FACEP
Steven Baldwin, MD
Isabel A. Barata, MD, FACEP, FAAP
Lee S. Benjamin, MD, FACEP
Kathleen Berg, MD
Kathleen Brown, MD, FACEP
Jeffrey Bullard-Berent, MD, FACEP
Ann Marie Dietrich, MD, FACEP
Phillip Friesen, DO
Michael Gerardi, MD, FACEP, FAAP
Alan Heins, MD, FACEP
Doug K. Holtzman, MD, FACEP
Jeffrey Homme, MD, FACEP
Timothy Horeczko, MD, MSCR
Paul Ishimine, MD, FACEP
Samuel Lam, MD, RDMS
Katharine Long
Kurtis Mayz, JD, MD, MBA
Sanjay Mehta, MD, Med, FACEP
Larry Mellick, MD
Aderonke Ojo, MD, MBBS
Audrey Z. Paul, MD, PhD
Denis R. Pauze, MD, FACEP
Nadia M. Pearson, DO
Debra Perina, MD, FACEP
Emory Petrack, MD
David Rayburn, MD, MPH
Emily Rose, MD
W. Scott Russell, MD, FACEP
Timothy Ruttan, MD, FACEP
Mohsen Saidinejad, MD, MBA, FACEP
Brian Sanders, MD
Joelle Simpson, MD, MPH
Patrick Solari, MD
Michael Stoner, MD
Jonathan H. Valente, MD, FACEP
Jessica Wall, MD
Dina Wallin, MD
Muhammad Waseem, MD, MS, FACEP
Paula J. Whiteman, MD, FACEP
Dale Woolridge, MD, PhD, FACEP

FORMER ACEP PEDIATRIC EMERGENCY MEDICINE COMMITTEE MEMBERS, 2012–2016

Joseph Arms, MD
Richard M. Cantor, MD, FACEP
Ariel Cohen, MD

Carrie DeMoor, MD
James M. Dy, MD
Paul J. Eakin, MD
Sean Fox, MD
Marianne Gausche-Hill, MD, FACEP, FAAP
Timothy Givens, MD
Charles J. Graham, MD, FACEP
Robert J. Hoffman, MD, FACEP
Mark Hostetler, MD, FACEP
Hasmig Jinivizian, MD
David Markenson, MD, MBA, FACEP
Joshua Rocker, MD, FACEP
Brett Rosen, MD
Gerald R. Schwartz, MD, FACEP
Harold A. Sloas, DO
Annalise Sorrentino, MD, FACEP
Orel Swenson, MD
Michael Witt, MD, MPH, FACEP

STAFF

Loren Rives, MNA
Dan Sullivan
Stephanie Wauson

ENA PEDIATRIC COMMITTEE, 2016–2017

Tiffany Young, BSN, RN, CPNP, 2016 Chair
Joyce Foresman-Capuzzi, MSN, RN, CNS, 2017 Chair
Rose Johnson, RN
Heather Martin, DNP, MS RN, PNP-BC
Justin Milici, MSN, RN
Cam Brandt, MS, RN
Nicholas Nelson, MS RN, EMT-P

BOARD LIAISONS

Maureen Curtis-Cooper, BSN, RN, 2016 Board Liaison
Kathleen Carlson, MSN, RN, 2017 Board Liaison

STAFF

Marlene Bokholdt, MSN, RN

ABBREVIATIONS

AAP: American Academy of Pediatrics
ACEP: American College of Emergency Physicians
ADE: adverse drug event
CDS: clinical decision support
CPOE: computerized physician order entry
ED: emergency department
ENA: Emergency Nurses Association

All policy statements from the American Academy of Pediatrics automatically expire 5 years after publication unless reaffirmed, revised, or retired at or before that time.

DOI: https://doi.org/10.1542/peds.2017-4066

Address correspondence to Lee Benjamin, MD, FAAP, FACEP. E-mail: lbenjamin@epmg.com

PEDIATRICS (ISSN Numbers: Print, 0031-4005; Online, 1098-4275).

FINANCIAL DISCLOSURE: The authors have indicated they have no financial relationships relevant to this article to disclose.

FUNDING: No external funding.

POTENTIAL CONFLICT OF INTEREST: The authors have indicated they have no potential conflicts of interest to disclose.

REFERENCES

1. Institute of Medicine, Committee on Quality of Health Care in America. In: Kohn LT, Corrigan JM, Donaldson MS, eds. *To Err is Human: Building a Safer Health System.* Washington, DC: National Academies Press; 1999

2. Leape LL, Brennan TA, Laird N, et al. The nature of adverse events in hospitalized patients. Results of the Harvard Medical Practice Study II. *N Engl J Med.* 1991;324(6):377–384

3. Kaushal R, Bates DW, Landrigan C, et al. Medication errors and adverse drug events in pediatric inpatients. *JAMA.* 2001;285(16):2114–2120

4. Woo Y, Kim HE, Chung S, Park BJ. Pediatric medication error reports in Korea adverse event reporting system database, 1989-2012: comparing with adult reports. *J Korean Med Sci.* 2015;30(4):371–377

5. Institute of Medicine, Committee of the Future of Emergency Care in the US Health System. *Emergency Care for Children: Growing Pains.* Washington, DC: National Academies Press; 2006

6. Shaw KN, Lillis KA, Ruddy RM, et al; Pediatric Emergency Care Applied Research Network. Reported medication events in a paediatric emergency research network: sharing to improve patient safety. *Emerg Med J.* 2013;30(10):815–819

7. Rinke ML, Moon M, Clark JS, Mudd S, Miller MR. Prescribing errors in a pediatric emergency department. *Pediatr Emerg Care.* 2008;24(1):1–8

8. Berg LM, Källberg AS, Göransson KE, Östergren J, Florin J, Ehrenberg A. Interruptions in emergency department work: an observational and interview study. *BMJ Qual Saf.* 2013;22(8):656–663

9. Thomasset KB, Faris R. Survey of pharmacy services provision in the emergency department. *Am J Health Syst Pharm.* 2003;60(15):1561–1564

10. Cesarz JL, Steffenhagen AL, Svenson J, Hamedani AG. Emergency department discharge prescription interventions by emergency medicine pharmacists. *Ann Emerg Med.* 2013;61(2):209–14.e1

11. Patanwala AE, Warholak TL, Sanders AB, Erstad BL. A prospective observational study of medication errors in a tertiary care emergency department. *Ann Emerg Med.* 2010;55(6):522–526

12. American Academy of Pediatrics: Task Force on Medical Informatics. Special requirements for electronic medical record systems in pediatrics. *Pediatrics.* 2001;108(2):513–515

13. Gausche-Hill M, Schmitz C, Lewis RJ. Pediatric preparedness of US emergency departments: a 2003 survey. *Pediatrics.* 2007;120(6):1229–1237

14. Hoyle JD, Davis AT, Putman KK, Trytko JA, Fales WD. Medication dosing errors in pediatric patients treated by emergency medical services. *Prehosp Emerg Care.* 2012;16(1):59–66

15. Kozer E, Scolnik D, Macpherson A, et al. Variables associated with medication errors in pediatric emergency medicine. *Pediatrics.* 2002;110(4):737–742

16. Sard BE, Walsh KE, Doros G, Hannon M, Moschetti W, Bauchner H. Retrospective evaluation of a computerized physician order entry adaptation to prevent prescribing errors in a pediatric emergency department. *Pediatrics.* 2008;122(4):782–787

17. Marcin JP, Dharmar M, Cho M, et al. Medication errors among acutely ill and injured children treated in rural emergency departments. *Ann Emerg Med.* 2007;50(4):361–367, 367.e1–367.e2

18. Glover ML, Sussmane JB. Assessing pediatrics residents' mathematical skills for prescribing medication: a need for improved training. *Acad Med.* 2002;77(10):1007–1010

19. Lesar TS. Tenfold medication dose prescribing errors. *Ann Pharmacother.* 2002;36(12):1833–1839

20. Doherty C, Mc Donnell C. Tenfold medication errors: 5 years' experience at a university-affiliated pediatric hospital. *Pediatrics.* 2012;129(5):916–924

21. Harskamp-van Ginkel MW, Hill KD, Becker KC, et al; Best Pharmaceuticals for Children Act–Pediatric Trials Network Administrative Core Committee. Drug dosing and pharmacokinetics in children with obesity: a systematic review [published correction appears in *JAMA Pediatr.* 2015;169(12):1179]. *JAMA Pediatr.* 2015;169(7):678–685

22. Miller JL, Johnson PN, Harrison DL, Hagemann TM. Evaluation of inpatient admissions and potential antimicrobial and analgesic dosing errors in overweight children. *Ann Pharmacother.* 2010;44(1):35–42

23. Young KD, Korotzer NC. Weight estimation methods in children: a systematic review. *Ann Emerg Med.* 2016;68(4):441–451.e10

24. Zorc JJ, Hoffman JM, Harper MB. IT in the ED: a new section of Pediatric Emergency Care. *Pediatr Emerg Care.* 2012;28(12):1399–1401

25. Kirk RC, Li-Meng Goh D, Packia J, Min Kam H, Ong BK. Computer calculated dose in paediatric prescribing. *Drug Saf.* 2005;28(9):817–824

26. van der Sijs H, Aarts J, Vulto A, Berg M. Overriding of drug safety alerts in computerized physician order entry. *J Am Med Inform Assoc.* 2006;13(2):138–147

27. Her QL, Seger DL, Amato MG, et al. Development of an algorithm to assess appropriateness of overriding alerts for nonformulary medications in a computerized prescriber-order-entry system. *Am J Health Syst Pharm.* 2016;73(1):e34–e45

28. Radley DC, Wasserman MR, Olsho LE, Shoemaker SJ, Spranca MD, Bradshaw B. Reduction in medication errors in hospitals due to adoption of computerized provider order entry systems. *J Am Med Inform Assoc.* 2013;20(3):470–476

29. Kozer E, Scolnik D, MacPherson A, Rauchwerger D, Koren G. Using a preprinted order sheet to reduce prescription errors in a pediatric emergency department: a randomized, controlled trial. *Pediatrics.* 2005;116(6):1299–1302

30. Larose G, Bailey B, Lebel D. Quality of orders for medication in the resuscitation room of a pediatric emergency department. *Pediatr Emerg Care.* 2008;24(9):609–614

31. Broussard M, Bass PF III, Arnold CL, McLarty JW, Bocchini JA Jr. Preprinted order sets as a safety intervention in pediatric sedation. *J Pediatr.* 2009;154(6):865–868

32. Burmester MK, Dionne R, Thiagarajan RR, Laussen PC. Interventions to reduce medication prescribing errors in a paediatric cardiac intensive care unit. *Intensive Care Med.* 2008;34(6):1083–1090

33. Institute for Safe Medication Practices. ISMP medication safety alert. Progress with preventing name confusion errors. 2007. Available at: https://www.ismp.org/newsletters/acutecare/articles/20070809.asp. Accessed November 16, 2016

34. Murray KL, Wright D, Laxton B, Miller KM, Meyers J, Englebright J. Implementation of standardized pediatric i.v. medication concentrations. *Am J Health Syst Pharm.* 2014;71(17):1500–1508

35. American Society of Health-System Pharmacists. ASHP awarded FDA contract to improve safety of intravenous and oral liquid medications: standardization contract is part of FDA's Safe Use Initiative [press release]. Available at: https://www.ashp.org/news/2017/02/09/16/44/standardize-4-safety-initiative-releases-final-iv-recommendations-for-medication-safety. Accessed November 16, 2016

36. Shaw KN, Ruddy RM, Olsen CS, et al; Pediatric Emergency Care Applied Research Network. Pediatric patient safety in emergency departments: unit characteristics and staff perceptions. *Pediatrics.* 2009;124(2):485–493

37. Thomas MC, Acquisto NM, Shirk MB, Patanwala AE. A national survey of emergency pharmacy practice in the United States. *Am J Health Syst Pharm.* 2016;73(6):386–394

38. American College of Emergency Physicians. Clinical pharmacist services in the emergency department. 2015. Available at: https://www.acep.org/clinical---practice-management/clinical-pharmacist-services-in-the-emergency-department/. Accessed November 16, 2016

39. Johnston R, Saulnier L, Gould O. Best possible medication history in the emergency department: comparing pharmacy technicians and pharmacists. *Can J Hosp Pharm.* 2010;63(5):359–365

40. Emergency Nurses Association. Position statement: role of the emergency nurse in medication reconciliation. Des Plaines, IL: Emergency Nurses Association; 2015. Available at: https://www.ena.org/docs/default-source/resource-library/practice-resources/position-statements/roleofednurseinmedicationreconcilation.pdf?sfvrsn=8c413f53_8. Accessed November 29, 2016

41. American Academy of Pediatrics; Committee on Pediatric Emergency Medicine and Council on Clinical Information Technology; American College of Emergency Physicians; Pediatric Emergency Medicine Committee. Policy statement—emergency information forms and emergency preparedness for children with special health care needs. *Pediatrics.* 2010;125(4):829–837

42. Stone BL, Boehme S, Mundorff MB, Maloney CG, Srivastava R. Hospital admission medication reconciliation in medically complex children: an observational study. *Arch Dis Child.* 2010;95(4):250–255

43. Provine AD, Simmons EM, Bhagat PH. Establishment and evaluation of pharmacist-managed admission medication history and reconciliation process for pediatric patients. *J Pediatr Pharmacol Ther.* 2014;19(2):98–102

44. Gardner B, Graner K. Pharmacists' medication reconciliation-related clinical interventions in a children's hospital. *Jt Comm J Qual Patient Saf.* 2009;35(5):278–282

45. American Society of Health-System Pharmacists. ASHP guidelines on emergency medicine pharmacist services. Available at: https://www.ashp.org/-/media/assets/policy-guidelines/docs/guidelines/emergency-medicine-pharmacist-services.ashx?la=en&hash=6503B2C3B0F5382A00FD3FCC9190E803D6C4BA2F. Accessed November 16, 2016

46. Scott DM, Friesner DL, Rathke AM, Doherty-Johnsen S. Medication error reporting in rural critical access hospitals in the North Dakota Telepharmacy Project. *Am J Health Syst Pharm.* 2014;71(1):58–67

47. Cole SL, Grubbs JH, Din C, Nesbitt TS. Rural inpatient telepharmacy consultation demonstration for after-hours medication review. *Telemed J E Health.* 2012;18(7):530–537

48. Patanwala AE, Sanders AB, Thomas MC, et al. A prospective, multicenter study of pharmacist activities resulting in medication error interception in the emergency department. *Ann Emerg Med.* 2012;59(5):369–373

49. Aldridge VE, Park HK, Bounthavong M, Morreale AP. Implementing a comprehensive, 24-hour emergency department pharmacy program. *Am J Health Syst Pharm.* 2009;66(21):1943–1947

50. Lada P, Delgado G Jr. Documentation of pharmacists' interventions in an emergency department and associated cost avoidance. *Am J Health Syst Pharm*. 2007;64(1):63–68

51. Warholak TL, Queiruga C, Roush R, Phan H. Medication error identification rates by pharmacy, medical, and nursing students. *Am J Pharm Educ*. 2011;75(2):24

52. US Department of Transportation, National Highway Traffic Safety Administration. National emergency medical services education standards. DOT HS 811 077A. Available at: www.ems.gov/pdf/811077a.pdf. Accessed November 16, 2016

53. Accreditation Council for Graduate Medical Education. ACGME program requirements for graduate medical education in pediatrics. Available at: https://www.acgme.org/Portals/0/PFAssets/ProgramRequirements/320_pediatrics_2017-07-01.pdf. Accessed January 10, 2018

54. Accreditation Council for Graduate Medical Education. ACGME program requirements for graduate medical education in emergency medicine. Available at: ttps://www.acgme.org/Portals/0/PFAssets/ProgramRequirements/110_emergency_medicine_2017-07-01.pdf. Accessed January 10, 2018

55. Accreditation Council for Graduate Medical Education. ACGME program requirements for graduate medical education in pediatric emergency medicine. Available at: https://www.acgme.org/Portals/0/PFAssets/ProgramRequirements/114_emergency_med_peds_2017-07-01.pdf?ver=2017-05-18-091501-330. Accessed January 10, 2018

56. Accreditation Council for Pharmacy Education. ACPE accreditation standards and guidelines for the professional program in pharmacy leading to the doctor of pharmacy degree. Available at: https://acpe-accredit.org/pdf/FinalS2007Guidelines2.0.pdf. Accessed November 16, 2016

57. Emergency Medical Services for Children/National Resource Center. Pediatric patient safety toolbox. Available at: https://emscimprovement.center/resources/toolboxes/pediatric-patient-safety-toolbox/. Accessed November 16, 2016

58. Poon EG, Cina JL, Churchill W, et al. Medication dispensing errors and potential adverse drug events before and after implementing bar code technology in the pharmacy. *Ann Intern Med*. 2006;145(6):426–434

59. Rinke ML, Bundy DG, Velasquez CA, et al. Interventions to reduce pediatric medication errors: a systematic review. *Pediatrics*. 2014;134(2):338–360

60. ED-based pharmacists make a big dent in medication errors. *ED Manag*. 2014;26(8):91–94

61. Manrique-Rodríguez S, Sánchez-Galindo AC, López-Herce J, et al. Impact of implementing smart infusion pumps in a pediatric intensive care unit. *Am J Health Syst Pharm*. 2013;70(21):1897–1906

62. Nugent P, Vitale BA. In: Nugent PM, Vitale BA, eds. *Fundamentals of Nursing: Content Review Plus Practice Questions*. Philadelphia, PA: F.A. Davis Company; 2013:361–362

63. Elliott M, Liu Y. The nine rights of medication administration: an overview. *Br J Nurs*. 2010;19(5):300–305

64. Pauly-O'Neill S. Beyond the five rights: improving patient safety in pediatric medication administration through simulation. *Clin Simul Nurs*. 2009;5(5):e181–e186

65. Westbrook JI, Woods A, Rob MI, Dunsmuir WT, Day RO. Association of interruptions with an increased risk and severity of medication administration errors. *Arch Intern Med*. 2010;170(8):683–690

66. Anthony K, Wiencek C, Bauer C, Daly B, Anthony MK. No interruptions please: impact of a No Interruption Zone on medication safety in intensive care units. *Crit Care Nurse*. 2010;30(3):21–29

67. United States Pharmacopeial Convention. Physical environments that promote safe medication use. Revision bulletin. 2010. Available at: http://www.uspnf.com/sites/default/files/usp_pdf/EN/USPNF/c1066.pdf. Accessed November 16, 2016

68. The Joint Commission. Preventing pediatric medication errors. *Sentinel Event Alert*. 2008;(39):1–4

69. American Hospital Association, Health Research and Educational Trust, Institute for Safe Medication Practices. Pathways for medication safety: looking collectively at risk. Available at: www.ismp.org/tools/pathwaysection2.pdf. Accessed November 16, 2016

70. Yin HS, Dreyer BP, Ugboaja DC, et al. Unit of measurement used and parent medication dosing errors. *Pediatrics*. 2014;134(2). Available at: www.pediatrics.org/cgi/content/full/134/2/e354

71. Yin HS, Dreyer BP, Moreira HA, et al. Liquid medication dosing errors in children: role of provider counseling strategies. *Acad Pediatr*. 2014;14(3):262–270

72. Chan HK, Hassali MA, Lim CJ, Saleem F, Tan WL. Using pictograms to assist caregivers in liquid medication administration: a systematic review. *J Clin Pharm Ther*. 2015;40(3):266–272

73. American Academy of Pediatrics, Committee on Drugs. Metric units and the preferred dosing of orally administered liquid medications. *Pediatrics*. 2015;135(4):784–787

Pediatric Readiness in the Emergency Department

- *Policy Statement*

POLICY STATEMENT

Organizational Principles to Guide and Define the Child Health Care System and/or Improve the Health of all Children

American Academy
of Pediatrics

DEDICATED TO THE HEALTH OF ALL CHILDREN™

Pediatric Readiness in the Emergency Department

Katherine Remick, MD, FAAP, FACEP, FAEMS,[a,b,c] Marianne Gausche-Hill, MD, FAAP, FACEP, FAEMS,[d,e,f] Madeline M. Joseph, MD, FAAP, FACEP,[g,h] Kathleen Brown, MD, FAAP, FACEP,[i] Sally K. Snow, BSN, RN, CPEN,[j] Joseph L. Wright, MD, MPH, FAAP,[k,l] AMERICAN ACADEMY OF PEDIATRICS Committee on Pediatric Emergency Medicine and Section on Surgery, AMERICAN COLLEGE OF EMERGENCY PHYSICIANS Pediatric Emergency Medicine Committee, EMERGENCY NURSES ASSOCIATION Pediatric Committee

abstract

This is a revision of the previous joint Policy Statement titled "Guidelines for Care of Children in the Emergency Department." Children have unique physical and psychosocial needs that are heightened in the setting of serious or life-threatening emergencies. The majority of children who are ill and injured are brought to community hospital emergency departments (EDs) by virtue of proximity. It is therefore imperative that all EDs have the appropriate resources (medications, equipment, policies, and education) and capable staff to provide effective emergency care for children. In this Policy Statement, we outline the resources necessary for EDs to stand ready to care for children of all ages. These recommendations are consistent with the recommendations of the Institute of Medicine (now called the National Academy of Medicine) in its report "The Future of Emergency Care in the US Health System." Although resources within emergency and trauma care systems vary locally, regionally, and nationally, it is essential that ED staff, administrators, and medical directors seek to meet or exceed these recommendations to ensure that high-quality emergency care is available for all children. These updated recommendations are intended to serve as a resource for clinical and administrative leadership in EDs as they strive to improve their readiness for children of all ages.

[a]National Emergency Medical Services for Children Innovation and Improvement Center, Baylor College of Medicine, Houston, Texas; [b]Department of Pediatrics, Dell Medical School, The University of Texas at Austin, Austin, Texas; [c]Dell Children's Medical Center, Austin, Texas; [d]Los Angeles County Emergency Medical Services Agency, Santa Fe Springs, California; [e]Department of Emergency Medicine and Pediatrics, David Geffen School of Medicine and Harbor–University of California, Los Angeles Medical Center, University of California, Los Angeles, Los Angeles, California; [f]Department of Emergency Medicine, Los Angeles Biomedical Research Institute, Los Angeles, California; [g]Division of Pediatric Emergency Medicine, Department of Emergency Medicine and Pediatrics, University of Florida College of Medicine–Jacksonville, Jacksonville, Florida; [h]University of Florida Health Sciences Center–Jacksonville, Jacksonville, Florida; Departments of [i]Pediatrics and Emergency Medicine, School of Medicine and Health Sciences, George Washington University and Children's National Medical Center, Washington, District of Columbia; [j]Emergency Nurses Association, Des Plaines, Illinois; [k]University of Maryland Capital Region Health, University of Maryland Medical System, Cheverly, Maryland; and [l]Department of Family Science, University of Maryland School of Public Health, College Park, Maryland

Drs Gausche-Hill, Remick, Joseph, Brown, and Wright and Ms Snow were each responsible for all aspects of writing and editing the document and reviewing and responding to questions and comments from reviewers and the Board of Directors; and all authors approved the final manuscript as submitted.

Published simultaneously on November 1, 2018, by the Annals of Emergency Medicine and Journal of Emergency Nursing.

To cite: Remick K, Gausche-Hill M, Joseph MM, et al; AMERICAN ACADEMY OF PEDIATRICS Committee on Pediatric Emergency Medicine and Section on Surgery, AMERICAN COLLEGE OF EMERGENCY PHYSICIANS Pediatric Emergency Medicine Committee, EMERGENCY NURSES ASSOCIATION Pediatric Committee. Pediatric Readiness in the Emergency Department. Pediatrics. 2018;142(5):e20182459

INTRODUCTION

In this Policy Statement, we delineate the recommended resources necessary to prepare emergency departments (EDs) to care for pediatric patients. Adoption of the recommendations in this Policy Statement will facilitate the delivery of emergency care for children of all ages and, when appropriate, timely transfer to a facility with specialized pediatric services. This joint Policy Statement is an update of previously published guidelines.[1–4]

These recommendations are intended to apply to all EDs that provide care for children. In the United States, most children who seek emergency care (83%) present to general EDs versus specialized pediatric EDs.[5] Intended users of these recommendations include all EDs that are open 24 hours per day, 7 days per week, including freestanding EDs and critical access hospital EDs. This Policy Statement is not intended to address urgent care centers because other recommendations are available to address those settings.[6]

BACKGROUND

In the National Hospital Ambulatory Medical Care Survey, it was reported that in 2014, there were approximately 5000 EDs in the United States. Of the more than 141 million ED visits in the United States in 2014, approximately 20% were for children younger than 15 years old.[7] Children have unique anatomic, physiologic, developmental, and medical needs that differ from those of adults. These differences must be considered when developing emergency services, training ED staff, and stocking equipment, medication, and supplies.

Improving Pediatric Readiness in US EDs

In 2006 in the "Future of Emergency Care" series, the Institute of Medicine (IOM) (now the National Academy of Medicine) noted ongoing deficiencies in both the prehospital and ED settings, including the availability of pediatric equipment, access to supplies and medications, training for staff, and policies in which the unique needs of children are incorporated.[8] Although there have been marked improvements in many areas of everyday pediatric readiness, persistent variability and a need for improvement remain across the continuum of care.[5,9-12]

One of the specific recommendations from the 2006 IOM report was that hospitals appoint coordinators for pediatric emergency care. At that time, only 18% of EDs in the United States reported having a physician coordinator, and only 12% had a nursing coordinator for pediatric emergency care. A national assessment performed in 2003[13] revealed that EDs that have staff in these positions tend to be more prepared, as measured by using compliance with the "Guidelines for the Care of Children in the ED" published by the American College of Emergency Physicians (ACEP) and American Academy of Pediatrics (AAP) in 2001.[1] In 2009, the AAP, ACEP, and Emergency Nurses Association (ENA), with the support of the Emergency Medical Services for Children (EMSC) program, undertook a major revision of these guidelines.[3,4] The 2009 joint Policy Statement is the subject for this policy revision.

The National Pediatric Readiness Project, launched in 2013, is an ongoing quality improvement (QI) initiative among the federal EMSC program, AAP, ACEP, and ENA to ensure pediatric readiness of EDs.[9] In phase 1 of the project, hospital ED leaders in all US states and territories were asked to complete a comprehensive Web-based assessment of their readiness to care for children. The assessment was based on the 2009 joint Policy Statement.[3,4] The response rate was 83%, representing more than 4000 EDs.[5] The data from this project reveal a snapshot of the nation's readiness to provide care to children in the ED. They also provide information on gaps in readiness at the state and national levels, confidential site-specific needs, and recommendations to improve readiness. Key findings include the following:

1. The majority of children who seek emergency care (69.4%) are cared for in EDs that see fewer than 15 pediatric patients per day, highlighting the need to provide additional pediatric emergency resources to smaller and often rural EDs.

2. The overall median score for the nation was 70 (of 100 possible points). This represents an improvement when compared with a similar survey completed in 2003 (median score of 55 points).[5,13]

3. The median score for EDs with a high volume of pediatric patients (>27 pediatric visits per day) was greater than that of EDs with medium, medium-high (5–27 pediatric visits per day), or low pediatric volume (<5 pediatric visits per day).

4. Approximately half of EDs lacked a physician (52.5%) or nurse (40.7%) pediatric emergency care coordinator (PECC). The presence of a PECC is strongly correlated with improved pediatric readiness, independent of other factors.[5] Another analysis of hospital-based EDs in the state of California also revealed that the presence of a PECC was associated with improved overall pediatric readiness scores.[14]

5. Fifty-five percent of EDs reported the absence of a QI plan in which they address pediatric care, and of those that had a QI plan, 41.7% lacked specific quality indicators for children. The presence of a QI plan that included pediatric-specific indicators was independently associated with improved overall readiness scores in California.[14]

6. In the absence of participation in a pediatric verification program, trauma center status was not predictive of higher pediatric readiness scores.[14]

7. Approximately half of hospitals reported lacking disaster plans

(53.2%) that include specific care needs for children.[5]

8. A process to ensure that weights are measured and recorded in kilograms only, which is a pediatric safety concern, was also lacking in 32.3% of EDs completing the assessment.[5]

Pediatric Readiness and Pediatric Facility Recognition

The EMSC program has long promoted improved preparedness and recognition of prepared EDs. Current EMSC program performance measures address pediatric readiness for children with both traumatic and medical emergencies.[10] Performance Measure 04 reads as follows: "the percent[age] of hospitals recognized through a statewide, territorial, or regional[ly] standardized system that are able to stabilize and/or manage pediatric medical emergencies." At this time, 11 states have developed such a system (recognizing 8% of all US hospital-based EDs),[15] and all have used the 2009 joint Policy Statement as the basis of their recognition criteria. Some states have published descriptions of the process they used to establish and maintain a pediatric recognition system.[14,16]

Recognition and verification have been associated with improved readiness scores. Remick et al[14] described an association between higher hospital readiness scores and an on-site verification program in California. National data reveal that states that have a recognition and/or verification system and have achieved EMSC program Performance Measure 04 have readiness scores that are an average of 10 points higher than those that do not have such a system.[15] In addition, hospitals that have been recognized scored, on average, 22 points higher on the assessment than those that had not been recognized as pediatric ready by their states (National EMSC Data Analysis and Resource Center, unpublished observations, 2014).

Pediatric Readiness: Improving the Safety and Quality of Pediatric Emergency Care

Over the past 15 years, patient safety has become a key priority for health systems.[17] In 2014, the AAP released the revised Policy Statement "Patient Safety in the Pediatric Emergency Care Setting."[18] This statement and other recent work have revealed the value of specific structural and process measures on improved patient safety and quality of care. For example, a weight-based, color-coded medication safety system can be used to decrease dosing errors and improve the timeliness of dosing,[19,20] and order sets, reminders, and clinical practice recommendations embedded within information systems can be used to increase adherence to best practices.[21,22]

Although previous guidelines[1,2] were consensus based, several recent studies have revealed the effects of pediatric readiness on outcomes for children treated in EDs. Some investigators have examined the effect of improved pediatric readiness and/or facility recognition on the quality of pediatric emergency care. Ball et al[23] compared outcomes in children with extremity immobilization and a pain score of 5 or greater in a state with a medical facility recognition program to similar facilities in a state without a facility recognition program. The children in the state with the recognition system had improved timeliness of the management of pain for fractures and decreased exposure to radiation use.[23] Kessler et al[24] demonstrated that teams of health care providers who practiced in EDs with higher pediatric readiness scores performed better in a standardized simulation of the care of children with sepsis. A statewide program in Arizona to improve the pediatric readiness of EDs has been associated with a decreased pediatric mortality rate after participation in a verification

process based on compliance with published guidelines.[25] Shared resources and coordination of care in emergency care systems is a strategy that may be used to improve pediatric readiness locally, regionally, and nationally. Further research should be supported to evaluate the effects of each of the recommended components of the guidelines on the quality of pediatric emergency care.

The information from the pediatric readiness assessment, research described earlier in this Policy Statement, and expert opinion from the coauthoring organizations were used to inform this revised Policy Statement. These recommendations include current information on equipment, medications, supplies, and personnel that are considered critical for managing pediatric emergencies in EDs. In this Policy Statement, we also offer recommendations for the administration and coordination of pediatric care in the ED; pediatric emergency care QI, performance improvement (PI), and patient safety activities; policies, procedures, and protocols for pediatric care; and key ED support services. It is believed that all EDs in the United States can meet or exceed these recommendations and that some hospitals, such as those with pediatric critical care capabilities or children's hospitals with greater resources, will develop and implement even more comprehensive recommendations and share their expertise with their local and regional communities. These updated recommendations are intended to serve as a resource for clinical and administrative leadership of EDs as they strive to improve their readiness for children of all ages.

ADMINISTRATION AND COORDINATION FOR THE CARE OF CHILDREN IN THE ED

A pediatric emergency care coordinator (PECC) is a physician coordinator identified by the ED medical director or a registered nurse coordinator identified by the ED nurse director. Identification of a physician and nurse PECC is central to the readiness of any ED that cares for children. Recommendations include the following:

1. The physician and nurse PECCs may be concurrently assigned other roles in the ED (eg, frontline staff designated by leadership) or may oversee more than 1 program in the ED (ie, medical or nursing director or as coordinator for trauma, stroke, or cardiac [STEMI]). PECC roles may be shared through formal agreements with administrative entities, such as within hospital systems, when there is another ED capable of providing definitive pediatric care.

2. Facilitate the following qualifications for physician and nurse PECCs:

   a. the physician PECC is qualified by the facility to provide emergency care. Optimally, the physician PECC is a board-certified and/or eligible specialist in emergency medicine or pediatric emergency medicine. Otherwise, the physician PECC must meet the qualifications for credentialing of the hospital as an emergency clinician specialist with special training and experience in the evaluation and management of the child who is critically ill. The physician PECC is credentialed by the facility and has verified competency in the care of children, including resuscitation, per the hospital policy. For EDs with limited resources, this administrative role may be shared with a clinical nurse specialist, nurse practitioner, or physician assistant (ie, advanced practice provider) who is credentialed

   to care for patients in the ED; and

   b. the nurse PECC is a registered nurse who possesses special interest, knowledge, and skill in the emergency nursing care of children through clinical experience and has demonstrated competence in critical thinking and clinical skills. When available, a certified emergency nurse or, preferably, a certified pediatric emergency nurse is desirable. Otherwise, the nurse coordinator has verified competency per hospital policy and may have other credentials, such as certified pediatric nurse or certified critical care registered nurse.

3. The physician and nurse PECCs work collaboratively and are responsible for the following:

   a. promoting adequate skill and knowledge of ED staff physicians, nurses, and other health care providers and staff (ie, physician assistants, advanced practice nurses, paramedics, and technicians) in the emergency care and resuscitation of infants and children. PECCs should have significant input into the methods of demonstrating competency in pediatric emergency care for their respective disciplines;

   b. participating in the development of the pediatric components of the QI plan and facilitating QI activities related to pediatric emergency care;

   c. assisting with the development and periodic review of ED policies and procedures and standards for medications, equipment, and supplies to ensure adequate resources for children of all ages;

   d. serving as liaisons and/or coordinators in collaboration with appropriate in-hospital and

   out-of-hospital pediatric care committees in the community and/or region and emergency medical services (EMS), trauma, and emergency preparedness coordinators (if they exist);

   e. serving as liaisons to definitive-care hospitals, such as regional pediatric referral hospitals and trauma centers, EMS agencies, primary care providers, health insurers, and any other care resources needed to integrate services along the pediatric care continuum, such as pediatric injury prevention, chronic disease management, and community education programs;

   f. facilitating pediatric emergency medical and nursing education for ED health care providers and staff, including but not limited to the identification of continuing pediatric emergency education resources;

   g. facilitating the inclusion of pediatric-specific elements in physician and nursing orientation in the ED;

   h. in coordination with the local credentialing processes, facilitating competency evaluations for staff that are pertinent to children of all ages. When available, simulation (ie, pediatric scenario–based mock codes) has been revealed to improve pediatric care in resuscitation and team settings[26–28];

   i. facilitating the integration of pediatric needs in hospital disaster and/or emergency preparedness plans and promoting the inclusion of pediatric patients in disaster drills[29];

   j. collaborating with ED leadership to enable adequate staffing, medications, equipment, supplies, and other resources for children in the ED; and

k. communicating with ED and hospital leadership on efforts to facilitate pediatric emergency care.

COMPETENCIES FOR PHYSICIANS, ADVANCED PRACTICE PROVIDERS, NURSES, AND OTHER ED HEALTH CARE PROVIDERS

Recommendations include the following:

A. Physicians, advanced practice providers, nurses, and other ED health care providers, on the basis of their level of training and scope of practice, should have the necessary skill, knowledge, and training in the emergency evaluation and treatment of children of all ages consistent with the services provided by the hospital.

B. Baseline and periodic competency evaluations completed for all ED clinical staff, including physicians, advanced practice providers, nurses, and other health care providers are age specific and include neonates, infants, children, adolescents, and children with special health care needs. Competencies are determined by each institution's hospital policy and medical staff privileges as a part of the local credentialing process for all licensed ED staff.

C. The demonstration and maintenance of pediatric clinical competencies may be achieved through continuing education, including participation in local educational programs, professional organization conferences, or national pediatric emergency care courses, or scheduled mock codes or patient simulation, team training exercises, or experiences in other clinical settings, such as the operating room (ie, airway management). The evaluation of such competencies may be achieved through direct observation, chart reviews,

written knowledge tests, and/ or the maintenance of physician or advanced practice provider board certification or nurse certification when pediatric emergency medicine is a significant component of annual continuing education requirements.

D. Potential areas for pediatric competency and professional performance evaluations may include but are not limited to the following:

1. assessment and treatment, including the following: (a) triage, (b) illness and injury assessment and management, and (c) pain assessment and treatment, including nonpharmacologic pain management (eg, distraction techniques and comfort holds);

2. medication administration and delivery;

3. device and/or equipment safety (eg, low-volume infusion pumps);

4. procedures, including the following: (a) airway management, (b) vascular access, and (c) sedation and analgesia;

5. resuscitation, including the following: (a) critical care monitoring, (b) neonatal resuscitation, and (c) pediatric resuscitation;

6. trauma resuscitation and stabilization,[30] including the following: (a) burn management, (b) traumatic brain injury, (c) fracture management, (d) hemorrhage control, and (e) recognition and reporting of nonaccidental trauma;

7. disaster drills that include a triage of pediatric victims, the tracking and identification of unaccompanied children, family reunification, and the

determination of pediatric surge capacity[29];

8. patient- and family-centered care, including cultural competency; and

9. team training and effective communication, including the following: (a) transitions of care and/or handoffs[31] and (b) closed-loop communication.

QI AND/OR PI IN THE ED

Quality is best ensured by evaluating each of the 6 domains addressed by the IOM[31,32]: safe, equitable, patient centered, timely, efficient, and effective. PI processes are essential to evaluating the quality of care, and measurement is integral to PI activities. Pediatric-specific metrics should be carefully identified to assess the quality of care throughout each phase of health care delivery across the emergency care continuum. A pediatric patient care review process is integrated into the QI and/or PI plan of the ED according to the following recommendations:

A. The potential framework for QI efforts may be focused on the effectiveness of structural elements, processes, and clinical outcomes relative to pediatric emergency care. Minimum components of the QI and/or PI process should include collecting and analyzing data to discover variances, defining a plan for improvement, and evaluating the success of the QI and/or PI plan with measures that are outcome based. High-level QI efforts are used to facilitate education and training, the implementation of targeted system change, and the measurement of system performance over time until steady, high-level performance is achieved.

B. The QI and/or PI plan of the ED shall include pediatric-specific indicators. Pediatric emergency

TABLE 1 Sample Performance Measures for Pediatric Emergency Care

Measures	Description
System based	
Patient triage	Measurement of wt in kilograms for pediatric patients; method to identify age-based abnormal pediatric vital signs
Infrastructure and personnel	Presence of all recommended pediatric equipment in the ED; presence of physician and nurse coordinators for pediatric emergency care
Patient-centered care	Patient and/or caregiver understanding of discharge instructions
ED flow	Door-to-provider time; total length of stay
Pain management	Pain assessment and reassessment for children with acute fractures
Quality and safety	Number of return visits within 48 h resulting in hospitalization; medication error rates
Disease specific	
Trauma	Use of head computed tomography in children with minor head trauma; protocol for suspected child maltreatment
Respiratory diseases	Administration of systemic steroids for pediatric asthma exacerbations; use of an evidence-based guideline to manage bronchiolitis
Infectious diseases	Use of antibiotics in children with suspected viral illness

Based on the work of Alessandrini E, Varadarajan K, Alpern ER, et al. Emergency department quality: an analysis of existing pediatric measures. *Acad Emerg Med.* 2011;18(5):519–526.

care metrics have been identified (Table 1) and should be strongly considered for inclusion in the overall QI plan. In addition, performance bundles may be used to assess the quality of care provided for specific clinical conditions (eg, pediatric septic shock, pediatric asthma, and pediatric closed head injury).

C. Components of the process are used to integrate out-of-hospital, ED, trauma, inpatient pediatrics, pediatric critical care, and hospital-wide QI or PI activities and may be interfaced with regional, state, or national QI collaboratives, including injury prevention efforts.[33–36]

D. Mechanisms are in place to monitor professional performance, credentialing, continuing education, and clinical competencies, including the integration of findings from QI audits and case reviews for pediatric emergency care.

Numerous resources are available to assist ED staff with implementing QI and/or PI activities (Table 2).

POLICIES, PROCEDURES, AND PROTOCOLS FOR THE ED

Recommendations include the following:

A. Policies, procedures, and protocols for the emergency care of children are age specific and include neonates, infants, children, adolescents, and children with special health care needs. Staff are educated accordingly and monitored for compliance and periodically updated. These include, but are not limited to, the following:

1. illness and injury triage;

2. pediatric patient assessment and reassessment;

3. documentation of a full set of pediatric vital signs, including core temperature, respiratory rate, pulse oximetry, heart rate, blood pressure (including manual confirmation), pain, and mental status when indicated;

4. identification and notification of the responsible provider of abnormal vital signs (age or weight based);

5. immunization assessment and management (eg, tetanus and

TABLE 2 Examples of Pediatric Emergency Care PI Activities and Resources

Clinical ED Registry (https://www.acep.org/cedr/)

Committee on Quality Transformation, Section on Emergency Medicine (https://www.aap.org/en-us/about-the-aap/Committees-Councils-Sections/Section-on-Emergency-Medicine/Pages/About-Us.aspx)

EMSC Innovation and Improvement Center (https://emscimprovement.center)

ENA (https://www.ena.org/#practice-resources)

Education in QI for Pediatric Practice (https://eqipp.aap.org/)

The National Pediatric Readiness Assessment (https://www.pedsready.org)

PediaLink: The AAP Online Learning Center (https://pedialink.aap.org/visitor)

Pediatric Readiness Toolkit (www.pediatricreadiness.org)

Pediatric Trauma Society (http://pediatrictraumasociety.org/)

Interfacility Tool Kit for the Pediatric Patient (http://www.traumanurses.org/inter-facility-tool-kit-for-the-pediatric-patient)

Pediatric TQIP (https://www.facs.org/quality-programs/trauma/tqip/pediatric-tqip)

PECARN guidelines (http://www.pecarn.org)

PECARN, Pediatric Emergency Care Applied Research Network; TQIP, Trauma Quality Improvement Program.

rabies) of the patient who is underimmunized[37];

6. sedation and analgesia (including nonpharmacologic interventions for comfort) for procedures, including medical imaging[38,39];

7. consent (including situations in which a parent or legal guardian is not immediately available)[40];

8. social and behavioral health issues, including parents and patients who are belligerent, impaired, or violent[41–43];

9. physical or chemical restraint of patients;

10. child maltreatment mandated reporting and assessment (physical and sexual abuse, sexual assault, human trafficking, and neglect)[44];

11. death of a child in the ED[45,46];

12. do-not-resuscitate orders;

13. lack of a medical home;

14. children with special health care needs, including developmental disabilities (eg, autism spectrum disorders and ventilator dependence);

15. family-centered care,[47–52] including the following:

a. involving families and guardians in patient care decision-making and medication safety processes;

b. family and guardian presence during all aspects of emergency care, including resuscitation;

c. education of the patient, family, and caregivers and guardians;

d. discharge planning and education; and

e. bereavement counseling;

16. communication with a patient's medical home or primary health care provider at the time of the ED visit (this can help ensure that a judicious and appropriate approach to examination, testing, imaging, and treatment is coordinated and follow-up is arranged in the most cost-effective and up-to-date manner)[53];

17. telehealth and telecommunications[54]; and

18. an all-hazard disaster preparedness plan in which the following pediatric issues are addressed[55]:

a. availability of medications, vaccines (eg, tetanus and rabies), equipment, supplies, and appropriately trained providers for children in disasters;

b. pediatric surge capacity for both children who are injured and noninjured;

c. decontamination, isolation, and quarantine of families and children of all ages;

d. minimization of parent-child separation and improved methods for reuniting separated children with their families;

e. access to specific medical and behavioral health therapies, as well as social services, for children in the event of a disaster;

f. disaster drills that include a pediatric mass casualty incident at least once every 2 years; all drills include pediatric patients; and

g. the care of children with special health care needs, including children with developmental disabilities.

B. Evidence-based clinical pathways, order sets, or decision support should be available to providers in real time. These may be systematically derived, consensus driven, or locally developed on the basis of available evidence. Many children's hospitals and/or academic centers have developed such clinical pathways. Collaboration with regional pediatric centers and trauma centers may facilitate the use of standard, evidence-based guidelines. An updated and complete list is available on the National Pediatric Readiness Project Web site.[56–60]

C. Hospitals should have written pediatric interfacility transfer procedures and/or agreements that include the following pediatric components[61–63]:

1. defined processes for the initiation of transfer, including the roles and responsibilities of the referring facility and referral center (including responsibilities for requesting transfer, method of transport, and communication);

2. a transport plan to deliver children safely (including the use of child passenger–restraint devices) and in a timely manner to the appropriate facility that is capable of providing definitive care;

3. processes for selecting the appropriate care facility for pediatric specialty services that are not available at the hospital; these specialty services may include the following: (a) medical and surgical specialty care, (b) critical care, (c) reimplantation (replacement of severed digits or limbs), (d) trauma and burn care, (e) psychiatric emergencies, (f) obstetric and perinatal emergencies, (g) child maltreatment (physical and sexual abuse and assault), (h) rehabilitation for recovery from critical medical or traumatic conditions, (i) orthopedic emergencies, and (j) neurosurgical emergencies;

4. processes for selecting the appropriately staffed transport service to match a patient's acuity level (ie, level of care required and equipment needed for transport) and that are appropriate for children with special health care needs;

5. processes for patient transfer (including obtaining informed consent)[64];

6. a plan for the transfer of critical patient information (ie, medical record, imaging, and copy of signed transport consent) as well as personal belongings and the provision of directions and referral institution information to the family;

7. processes for the return transfer of the pediatric patient to the referring facility as appropriate; and

8. integration with telehealth and/or telecommunications processes and mobile-integrated health and/or community paramedicine as appropriate.[54]

PEDIATRIC PATIENT AND MEDICATION SAFETY IN THE ED

The delivery of pediatric care should reflect an awareness of unique pediatric patient safety concerns and should include the following policies or practices[65,66]:

A. Children should be weighed in kilograms, with the exception of children who require emergency stabilization, and the weight should be recorded in a prominent place on the medical record, preferably with the vital signs.

   1. For children who require resuscitation or emergency stabilization, a standard method for estimating weight in kilograms should be used.

B. A full set of vital signs should be recorded and reassessed per hospital policy for all children.

C. The following processes for safe medication (including blood products) prescribing, delivery, and disposal should be established[67,68]:

   1. use precalculated dosing guidelines for children of all ages;

   2. consider adding a pharmacist with pediatric competency to the ED team, especially in large EDs, during times of higher volume;

   3. identify the administration phase as a high-risk practice (eg, the simple misplacement of a decimal point can result in a 10-fold medication error);

   4. promote distraction-free zones for medication preparation[69,70];

5. implement and use computerized physician order entry and clinical decision support with pediatric-specific, kilogram-only dosing rules, including upper dosing limits, within ED information systems;

6. implement and use computerized physician order entry to create allergy alerts for all prescribed medications;

7. practice vigilance for all administered or prescribed medications and consider developing standardized order sets, particularly for high-risk medications, such as opioids and antibiotics;

8. implement an independent 2-provider cross-check process for high-alert medications;

9. create a standard formulary for pediatric high-risk and commonly used medications;

10. standardize concentrations of high-risk medications;

11. reduce the number of available concentrations to the smallest possible number;

12. implement systems in which weight-based calculations are bypassed during pediatric resuscitations and treatment to reduce potentially harmful mistakes;

13. establish a culture of safety surrounding pediatric medication administration that encourages the reporting of near-miss or adverse medication events that can then be analyzed as feedback into the system in a continuous QI model;

14. ensure that caregivers are well instructed on medication administration, particularly for pain and antipyretic medications, before being discharged from the ED; and

15. promote the integration of health literacy concepts and skills, including the use of plain language, the teach-back method, pictograms, and lower-literacy instructions.[71–75]

D. Pediatric emergency services should be culturally and linguistically appropriate,[76] and the ED should provide an environment that is safe for children and supports patient- and family-centered care.[48,49,77]

   1. Enhance family-centered care by actively engaging patients and families in safety at all points of care, and address issues of ethnic culture, language, and literacy.

   2. Direct families to appropriate resources, and review patients' rights and responsibilities from the perspective of safety.

   3. Include shared decision-making.

   4. Use trained language interpreter services rather than bilingual relatives.

E. Patient-identification policies, consistent with The Joint Commission's National Patient Safety Goals, should be implemented and monitored.[78]

F. Policies for the timely tracking, reporting, and evaluation of patient safety events and for the disclosure of medical errors or unanticipated outcomes should be implemented and monitored, and education and training in disclosure should be available to care providers who are assigned this responsibility.[65,66]

SUPPORT SERVICES FOR THE ED

Recommendations include the following:

A. The radiology department should have the skills and capability to provide imaging studies of children, the equipment necessary to do so, and guidelines to reduce radiation exposure that are age and size specific.[79–81]

1. The radiology capability of hospitals may vary from 1 institution to another; however, every ED should promote on-site radiology capabilities to meet the needs of children in the community.

2. Medical imaging protocols that are used to address age- or weight-appropriate dose reductions for children receiving studies in which ionizing radiation is imparted, consistent with "as low as reasonably achievable" principles, are necessary.[82]

3. A process should be established for the referral of children to appropriate facilities for radiologic procedures that exceed the capability of the hospital.

4. A process should be in place for timely review and interpretation reporting by a qualified radiologist for medical imaging studies in children.

5. When a patient is transferred from 1 facility to another, to avoid unnecessary radiation exposure, all efforts should be made to transfer completed images. New technology (eg, Cloud file sharing or Health Insurance Portability and Accountability Act protection) may facilitate image sharing between facilities.[83]

B. The laboratory should have the skills and capability to perform laboratory tests for children of all ages, including obtaining samples, and have available microtechnology for small or limited sample sizes.

1. The clinical laboratory capability must meet the needs of the children in the community it serves.

2. There should be a clear understanding of what the laboratory capability is for any given community, and definitive plans for referring children to the appropriate facility for laboratory studies should be in place.

3. Protocols should be developed for the screening and administration of blood and blood products for children who are ill or injured.

EQUIPMENT, SUPPLIES, AND MEDICATIONS

Pediatric equipment, supplies, and medications shall be easily accessible, labeled, and logically organized (eg, kilogram weight, weight-based color coding, etc).

A. Medication chart, color-based coding, medical software, or other systems shall be readily available to ED staff to ensure proper sizing of resuscitation equipment and proper dosing of medications based on patient weight in kilograms.

B. Resuscitation equipment and supplies shall be located in the ED; trays and other items may be housed in other departments (such as the newborn nursery or central supply) with a process to ensure immediate accessibility to ED staff. A mobile or portable appropriately stocked pediatric crash cart should be available in the ED at all times.

C. ED staff shall be appropriately educated as to the location of all items (Supplemental Figs 1 and 2).

D. Each ED shall have a daily method to verify the proper location and function of equipment and expiration of medications and supplies.

E. Tables 3 and 4 and Supplemental Figs 1 and 2 outline medications, equipment, and supplies necessary for the care of children in the ED by qualified health care providers.[84]

TABLE 3 Resuscitation Medications for Use in Pediatric Patients in EDs

Adenosine
Amiodarone
Atropine
Calcium chloride and/or calcium gluconate
Epinephrine (1 mg/mL [IM] and 0.1 mg/mL [IV] solutions)[a]
Lidocaine
Procainamide
Sodium bicarbonate (4.2%)[b]
Vasopressor agents (eg, dopamine, epinephrine, and norepinephrine)

For a more complete list of medications used in a pediatric ED, see Winkelman et al.[75] IM, intramuscular; IV, intravenous.

[a] The formerly epinephrine 1:1000 solution is now 1 mg/mL for IM use or inhalation; the 1:10 000 solution is now 0.1 mg/mL for IV use.

[b] If only sodium bicarbonate 8.4% is available, may dilute 1:1 with normal saline before administration in children <2 y of age.

CONCLUSIONS

In the 2006 report, "Emergency Care for Children: Growing Pains," the IOM uses the word "uneven" to describe the current status of pediatric emergency care in the United States.[8] Although much progress has been made to improve pediatric readiness across communities,[5] there remains a significant opportunity for further progress nationwide. An important first step in ensuring readiness is the identification of a physician and nurse coordinator for pediatric emergency care.

All EDs must be continually prepared to receive; accurately assess; and, at a minimum, stabilize and safely transfer children who are acutely ill or injured. This is necessary even for hospitals located in communities with readily accessible pediatric tertiary-care centers and regionalized systems for pediatric trauma and critical care. The vast majority of children requiring emergency services in the United States receive this care in a non–children's hospital ED, with 69% of EDs providing care for fewer than 15 children per day.[5] This relatively infrequent exposure of hospital-based emergency care professionals to children who are seriously ill or injured represents

TABLE 4 Medications to Be Used in the ED for the Care of Children

Analgesics (oral, intranasal, and parenteral)
Anesthetics (eg, eutectic mixture of local anesthetics; lidocaine 2.5% and prilocaine 2.5%; lidocaine, epinephrine, and tetracaine; and LMX 4 [4% lidocaine])
Anticonvulsants (eg, levetiracetam, valproate, carbamazepine, fosphenytoin, and phenobarbital)
Antidotes (common antidotes should be accessible to the ED)[a]
Antiemetics (eg, ondansetron and prochlorperazine)
Antihypertensives (eg, labetalol, nicardipine, and sodium nitroprusside)
Antimicrobials (parenteral and oral)
Antipsychotics (eg, olanzapine and haloperidol)
Antipyretics (eg, acetaminophen and ibuprofen)
Benzodiazepines (eg, midazolam and lorazepam)
Bronchodilators
Corticosteroids (eg, dexamethasone, methylprednisolone, and hydrocortisone)
Dextrose ($D_{10}W$)
Diphenhydramine
Furosemide
Glucagon
Insulin
Lidocaine
Magnesium sulfate
Mannitol
Naloxone hydrochloride
Neuromuscular blockers (eg, rocuronium and succinylcholine)
Oral glucose
Sucrose solutions for pain control in infants
Sedation medications (eg, etomidate and ketamine)
Vaccines
3% hypertonic saline

$D_{10}W$, dextrose 10% in water.
[a] For less frequently used antidotes, a procedure for obtaining them should be in place.

a substantial barrier to the maintenance of essential skills and clinical competency. Recognition of the unique needs of children who are ill and/or injured and served by an emergency care facility, including children with special health care needs; the commitment to better meet those needs through the adoption of these recommendations; and an ongoing commitment to evaluate care quality and safety and maintain pediatric competencies should provide a strong foundation for pediatric emergency care.

Resources that can be used to assist with the implementation of all aspects of this document can be found at www.pediatricreadiness.org.

LEAD AUTHORS

Katherine Remick, MD, FAAP, FACEP, FAEMS
Marianne Gausche-Hill, MD, FAAP, FACEP
Madeline M. Joseph, MD, FAAP, FACEP
Kathleen Brown, MD, FAAP, FACEP
Sally K. Snow, BSN, RN, CPEN
Joseph L. Wright, MD, MPH, FAAP

AAP COMMITTEE ON PEDIATRIC EMERGENCY MEDICINE, 2017–2018

Joseph Wright, MD, MPH, FAAP, Chairperson
Terry Adirim, MD, MPH, FAAP
Michael S.D. Agus, MD, FAAP
James Callahan, MD, FAAP
Toni Gross, MD, MPH, FAAP
Natalie Lane, MD, FAAP
Lois Lee, MD, MPH, FAAP
Suzan Mazor, MD, FAAP
Prashant Mahajan, MD, MPH, MBA, FAAP
Nathan Timm, MD, FAAP

LIAISONS

Andrew Eisenberg, MD, MHA – *American Academy of Family Physicians*
Cynthia Wright Johnson, MSN, RN – *National Association of State EMS Officials*
Cynthiana Lightfoot, BFA, NRP – *American Academy of Pediatrics Family Partnerships Network*
Charles Macias, MD, MPH, FAAP – *Emergency Medical Services for Children Innovation and Improvement Center*
Brian Moore, MD, MPH, FAAP – *National Association of EMS Physicians*
Diane Pilkey, RN, MPH – *Health Resources and Services Administration*
Katherine Remick, MD, FAAP – *National Association of Emergency Medical Technicians*
Mohsen Saidinejad, MD, MBA, FAAP, FACEP – *American College of Emergency Physicians*
Sally Snow, RN, BSN, CPEN, FAEN – *Emergency Nurses Association*
Mary Fallat, MD, FAAP – *American College of Surgeons*

FORMER AAP COMMITTEE ON PEDIATRIC EMERGENCY MEDICINE MEMBERS, 2012–2016

Alice Ackerman, MD, MBA, FAAP
Thomas Chun, MD, MPH, FAAP
Gregory Conners, MD, MPH, MBA, FAAP
Edward Conway Jr, MD, MS, FAAP
Nanette Dudley, MD, FAAP
Joel Fein, MD, FAAP
Susan Fuchs, MD, FAAP
Marc Gorelick, MD, MSCE, FAAP
Natalie Lane, MD, FAAP

Steven Selbst, MD, FAAP
Kathy Shaw, MD, MSCE, FAAP, Chairperson (2008–2012)
Joan Shook, MD, MBA, FAAP, Chairperson (2012–2016)

STAFF

Sue Tellez

AAP SECTION ON SURGERY EXECUTIVE COMMITTEE, 2016–2017

Kurt F. Heiss, MD, Chairperson
Elizabeth Beierle, MD
Gail Ellen Besner, MD
Cynthia D. Downard, MD
Mary Elizabeth Fallat, MD
Kenneth William Gow, MD

STAFF

Vivian Baldassari Thorne

ACEP PEDIATRIC EMERGENCY MEDICINE COMMITTEE, 2016–2017

Madeline Joseph, MD, FACEP, Chairperson
Kiyetta Alade, MD
Christopher Amato, MD, FACEP
Jahn T. Avarello, MD, FACEP
Steven Baldwin, MD
Isabel A. Barata, MD, FACEP, FAAP
Lee S. Benjamin, MD, FACEP
Kathleen Berg, MD
Kathleen Brown, MD, FACEP
Jeffrey Bullard-Berent, MD, FACEP
Ann Marie Dietrich, MD, FACEP
Phillip Friesen, DO
Michael Gerardi, MD, FACEP, FAAP
Alan Heins, MD, FACEP
Doug K. Holtzman, MD, FACEP
Jeffrey Homme, MD, FACEP
Timothy Horeczko, MD, MSCR
Paul Ishimine, MD, FACEP
Samuel Lam, MD, RDMS
Katharine Long
Kurtis Mayz, JD, MD, MBA
Sanjay Mehta, MD, Med, FACEP
Larry Mellick, MD
Aderonke Ojo, MD, MBBS
Audrey Z. Paul, MD, PhD
Denis R. Pauze, MD, FACEP
Nadia M. Pearson, DO
Debra Perina, MD, FACEP
Emory Petrack, MD
David Rayburn, MD, MPH
Emily Rose, MD
W. Scott Russell, MD, FACEP
Timothy Ruttan, MD, FACEP
Mohsen Saidinejad, MD, MBA, FACEP
Brian Sanders, MD
Joelle Simpson, MD, MPH
Patrick Solari, MD
Michael Stoner, MD
Jonathan H. Valente, MD, FACEP
Jessica Wall, MD
Dina Wallin, MD

Muhammad Waseem, MD, MS, FACEP
Paula J. Whiteman, MD, FACEP
Dale Woolridge, MD, PhD, FACEP

**FORMER ACEP PEDIATRIC EMERGENCY
MEDICINE COMMITTEE MEMBERS,
2012–2016**

Joseph Arms, MD
Richard M. Cantor, MD, FACEP
Ariel Cohen, MD
Carrie DeMoor, MD
James M. Dy, MD
Paul J. Eakin, MD
Sean Fox, MD
Marianne Gausche-Hill, MD, FACEP, FAAP
Timothy Givens, MD
Charles J. Graham, MD, FACEP
Robert J. Hoffman, MD, FACEP
Mark Hostetler, MD, FACEP
Hasmig Jinivizian, MD
David Markenson, MD, MBA, FACEP
Joshua Rocker, MD, FACEP
Brett Rosen, MD
Gerald R. Schwartz, MD, FACEP

Harold A. Sloas, DO
Annalise Sorrentino, MD, FACEP
Orel Swenson, MD
Michael Witt, MD, MPH, FACEP

STAFF

Loren Rives, MNA
Dan Sullivan
Stephanie Wauson

ENA PEDIATRIC COMMITTEE, 2016–2017

Tiffany Young, BSN, RN, CPNP, 2016 Chairperson
Joyce Foresman-Capuzzi, MSN, RN, CNS, 2017
Chairperson
Rose Johnson, RN
Heather Martin, DNP, MS, RN, PNP-BC
Justin Milici, MSN, RN
Cam Brandt, MS, RN
Nicholas Nelson, MS, RN, EMT-P

BOARD LIAISONS

Maureen Curtis-Cooper, BSN, RN, 2016 Board
Liaison
Kathleen Carlson, MSN, RN, 2017 Board Liaison

STAFF

Marlene Bokholdt, MSN, RN

ABBREVIATIONS

AAP: American Academy of
      Pediatrics
ACEP: American College of
       Emergency Physicians
ED: emergency department
EMS: emergency medical
      services
EMSC: Emergency Medical
       Services for Children
ENA: Emergency Nurses
      Association
IOM: Institute of Medicine
PECC: pediatric emergency care
       coordinator
PI: performance improvement
QI: quality improvement

the Emergency Nurses Association and its Board of Directors. All authors have filed conflict of interest statements with the American Academy of Pediatrics. Any conflicts have been resolved through a process approved by the Board of Directors. The American Academy of Pediatrics has neither solicited nor accepted any commercial involvement in the development of the content of this publication.

Policy statements from the American Academy of Pediatrics benefit from expertise and resources of liaisons and internal (AAP) and external reviewers. However, policy statements from the American Academy of Pediatrics may not reflect the views of the liaisons or the organizations or government agencies that they represent.

The guidance in this statement does not indicate an exclusive course of treatment or serve as a standard of medical care. Variations, taking into account individual circumstances, may be appropriate.

All policy statements from the American Academy of Pediatrics automatically expire 5 years after publication unless reaffirmed, revised, or retired at or before that time.

DOI: https://doi.org/10.1542/peds.2018-2459

Address correspondence to Katherine Remick, MD. E-mail: kate.remick@gmail.com

PEDIATRICS (ISSN Numbers: Print, 0031-4005; Online, 1098-4275).

FINANCIAL DISCLOSURE: The authors have indicated they have no financial relationships relevant to this article to disclose.

FUNDING: No external funding.

POTENTIAL CONFLICT OF INTEREST: The authors have indicated they have no potential conflicts of interest to disclose.

REFERENCES

1. American Academy of Pediatrics, Committee on Pediatric Emergency Medicine ; American College of Emergency Physicians, Pediatric Committee. Care of children in the emergency department: guidelines for preparedness. *Pediatrics.* 2001;107(4):777–781

2. Gausche-Hill M, Wiebe RA. Guidelines for preparedness of emergency departments that care for children: a call to action. *Ann Emerg Med.* 2001;37(4):389–391

3. American Academy of Pediatrics, Committee on Pediatric Emergency Medicine; American College of Emergency Physicians, Pediatric Committee; Emergency Nurses Association, Pediatric Committee. Joint policy statement—guidelines for care of children in the emergency department. *Pediatrics.* 2009;124(4):1233–1243

4. American Academy of Pediatrics Committee on Pediatric Emergency Medicine; American College of Emergency Physicians, Pediatric Committee; Emergency Nurses Association, Pediatric Committee. Joint policy statement—guidelines for care of children in the emergency department. *Ann Emerg Med.* 2009;54(4):543–552

5. Gausche-Hill M, Ely M, Schmuhl P, et al. A national assessment of pediatric readiness of emergency departments. *JAMA Pediatr.* 2015;169(6):527–534

6. Committee on Pediatric Emergency Medicine. Pediatric care recommendations for freestanding

urgent care facilities. *Pediatrics.* 2014;133(5):950–953

7. US Department of Health and Human Services; Centers for Disease Control and Prevention; National Center for Health Statistics. National Hospital Ambulatory Medical Care Survey: 2014 emergency department summary tables. Available at: https://www.cdc.gov/nchs/data/nhamcs/web_tables/2014_ed_web_tables.pdf. Accessed December 6, 2017

8. Institute of Medicine, Committee of the Future of Emergency Care in the US Health System. *Emergency Care for Children: Growing Pains.* Washington, DC: National Academies Press; 2006

9. National Pediatric Readiness Project. National pediatric readiness project. 2014. Available at: www.pediatricreadiness.org/State_Results/National_Results.aspx. Accessed April 10, 2014

10. US Department of Health and Human Services, Health Resources and Services Administration. Performance measures. Available at: https://emscimprovement.center/emsc/performance-measures/. Accessed August 31, 2017

11. Alessandrini EA, Wright JL. The continuing evolution of pediatric emergency care. *JAMA Pediatr.* 2015;169(6):523–524

12. Sacchetti A. Is it still an emergency department if it can't treat children? *Ann Emerg Med.* 2016;67(3): 329–331

13. Gausche-Hill M, Schmitz C, Lewis RJ. Pediatric preparedness of US emergency departments: a 2003 survey. *Pediatrics.* 2007;120(6):1229–1237

14. Remick K, Kaji AH, Olson L, et al. Pediatric readiness and facility verification. *Ann Emerg Med.* 2016;67(3):320–328.e1

15. Emergency Medical Services for Children. Pediatric medical recognition systems fact sheet. 2016. Available at: www.nedarc.org/documents/medicalRecognition_030416.pdf. Accessed June 7, 2018

16. Hohenhaus SM, Lyons E, Phillippi RG. Emergency departments and pediatric categorization, approval, and recognition: a review of two states. *J Emerg Nurs.* 2008;34(3):236–237

17. Institute of Medicine. *To Err Is Human: Building a Safer Health System.* Washington, DC: National Academies Press; 2000

18. Krug SE, Frush K; Committee on Pediatric Emergency Medicine, American Academy of Pediatrics. Patient safety in the pediatric emergency care setting. *Pediatrics.* 2007;120(6):1367–1375. Reaffirmed June 2011 and July 2014

19. Stevens AD, Hernandez C, Jones S, et al. Color-coded prefilled medication syringes decrease time to delivery and dosing errors in simulated prehospital pediatric resuscitations: a randomized crossover trial. *Resuscitation.* 2015;96:85–91

20. Feleke R, Kalynych CJ, Lundblom B, Wears R, Luten R, Kling D. Color coded medication safety system reduces community pediatric emergency nursing medication errors. *J Patient Saf.* 2009;5(2):79–85

21. Cabana MD, Rand CS, Powe NR, et al. Why don't physicians follow clinical practice guidelines? A framework for improvement. *JAMA.* 1999;282(15):1458–1465

22. Gandhi TK, Sequist TD, Poon EG, et al. Primary care clinician attitudes towards electronic clinical reminders and clinical practice guidelines. *AMIA Annu Symp Proc.* 2003:848

23. Ball JW, Sanddal ND, Mann NC, et al. Emergency department recognition program for pediatric services: does it make a difference? *Pediatr Emerg Care.* 2014;30(9):608–612

24. Kessler DO, Walsh B, Whitfill T, et al; INSPIRE ImPACTS Investigators. Disparities in adherence to pediatric sepsis guidelines across a spectrum of emergency departments: a multicenter, cross-sectional observational in situ simulation study. *J Emerg Med.* 2016;50(3):403–415.e1–e3

25. Rice A, Dudek J, Gross T, St Mars T, Woolridge D. The impact of a pediatric emergency department facility verification system on pediatric mortality rates in Arizona. *J Emerg Med.* 2017;52(6):894–901

26. Weinberg ER, Auerbach MA, Shah NB. The use of simulation for pediatric training and assessment. *Curr Opin Pediatr.* 2009;21(3):282–287

27. Lasater K. High-fidelity simulation and the development of clinical judgment: students' experiences. *J Nurs Educ.* 2007;46(6):269–276

28. Decker S, Sportsman S, Puetz L, Billings L. The evolution of simulation and its contribution to competency. *J Contin Educ Nurs.* 2008;39(2):74–80

29. Gardner AH, Fitzgerald MR, Schwartz HP, Timm NL. Evaluation of regional hospitals' use of children in disaster drills. *Am J Disaster Med.* 2013;8(2):137–143

30. Bulger EM, Snyder D, Schoelles K, et al; American College of Surgeons, Committee on Trauma. An evidence-based prehospital guideline for external hemorrhage control: American College of Surgeons Committee on Trauma. *Prehosp Emerg Care.* 2014;18(2):163–173

31. American Academy of Pediatrics, Committee on Pediatric Emergency Medicine; American College of Emergency Physicians, Pediatric Emergency Medicine Committee; Emergency Nurses Association, Pediatric Committee. Handoffs: transitions of care for children in the emergency department. *Pediatrics.* 2016;138(5):e20162680

32. Institute of Medicine. *Crossing the Quality Chasm: A New Health System for the 21st Century.* Washington, DC: National Academies Press; 2001

33. Children's Hospital Association. Sepsis collaborative. Available at: https://www.childrenshospitals.org/sepsiscollaborative. Accessed May 8, 2017

34. American Academy of Pediatrics. Collaborative initiatives. Available at: https://www.aap.org/en-us/advocacy-and-policy/aap-health-initiatives/Children-and-Disasters/Pages/Collaborative-Initiatives.aspx. Accessed May 8, 2017

35. EMS for Children Innovation and Improvement Center. Collaboratives. Available at: https://emscimprovement.center/collaboratives/. Accessed May 8, 2017

36. EMS for Children Innovation and Improvement Center. Pediatric readiness quality collaborative (PRQC). Available at: https://emscimprovement. center/collaboratives/PRQuality-collaborative/. Accessed June 13, 2018

37. American College of Emergency Physicians. Immunization of adults and children in the emergency department. *Ann Emerg Med.* 2008;51(5):695

38. Fein JA, Zempsky WT, Cravero JP; American Academy of Pediatrics, Committee on Pediatric Emergency Medicine, Section on Anesthesiology and Pain Medicine. Relief of pain and anxiety in pediatric patients in emergency medical systems. *Pediatrics.* 2012;130(5). Available at: www.pediatrics.org/cgi/content/full/130/5/e1391

39. Mace SE, Brown LA, Francis L, et al; EMSC Panel (Writing Committee) on Critical Issues in the Sedation of Pediatric Patients in the Emergency. Clinical policy: critical issues in the sedation of pediatric patients in the emergency department. *Ann Emerg Med.* 2008;51(4):378–399, 399.e1–e57

40. Committee on Pediatric Emergency Medicine; Committee on Bioethics. Consent for emergency medical services for children and adolescents. *Pediatrics.* 2011;128(2):427–433

41. Dolan MA, Fein JA; Committee on Pediatric Emergency Medicine. Pediatric and adolescent mental health emergencies in the emergency medical services system. *Pediatrics.* 2011;127(5). Available at: www.pediatrics.org/cgi/content/full/127/5/e1356

42. US Department of Labor, Occupation Safety and Health Administration. Guidelines for preventing workplace violence for healthcare and social service workers. 2016. Available at: https://www.osha.gov/Publications/osha3148.pdf. Accessed December 6, 2017

43. US Department of Labor, Occupation Safety and Health Administration. Preventing workplace violence: a roadmap for healthcare facilities. 2015. Available at: https://www.osha.gov/Publications/OSHA3827.pdf. Accessed December 6, 2017

44. Greenbaum J, Bodrick N; Committee on Child Abuse and Neglect; Section on International Child Health. Global human trafficking and child victimization. *Pediatrics.* 2017;140(6):e20173138

45. American Academy of Pediatrics, Committee on Pediatric Emergency Medicine; American College of Emergency Physicians, Pediatric Emergency Medicine Committee; Emergency Nurses Association, Pediatric Committee. Death of a child in the emergency department. *Pediatrics.* 2014;134(1):198–201

46. O'Malley P, Barata I, Snow S; American Academy of Pediatrics, Committee on Pediatric Emergency Medicine; American College of Emergency Physicians, Pediatric Emergency Medicine Committee; Emergency Nurses Association, Pediatric Committee. Death of a child in the emergency department. *Pediatrics.* 2014;134(1). Available at: www.pediatrics.org/cgi/content/full/134/1/e313

47. Committee on Hospital Care; American Academy of Pediatrics. Family-centered care and the pediatrician's role. *Pediatrics.* 2003;112(3, pt 1):691–697

48. O'Malley P, Mace SE, Brown K; American Academy of Pediatrics; American College of Emergency Physicians. Patient- and family-centered care and the role of the emergency physician providing care to a child in the emergency department. *Ann Emerg Med.* 2006;48(5):643–645

49. O'Malley P, Brown K, Mace SE; American Academy of Pediatrics, Committee on Pediatric Emergency Medicine; American College of Emergency Physicians, Pediatric Emergency Medicine Committee. Patient- and family-centered care and the role of the emergency physician providing care to a child in the emergency department. *Pediatrics.* 2006;118(5):2242–2244

50. Emergency Nurses Association. *ENA Position Statement: Care of the Pediatric Patient in the Emergency Care Setting.* Des Plaines, IL: Emergency Nurses Association; 2007

51. Guzzetta CE, Clark AP, Wright JL. Family presence in emergency medical

services for children. *Clin Pediatr Emerg Med.* 2006;7(1):15–24

52. Emergency Nurses Association. *ENA Position Statement: Family Presence at the Bedside During Invasive Procedures and Cardiopulmonary Resuscitation.* Des Plaines, IL: Emergency Nurses Association; 2005

53. Medical Home Initiatives for Children With Special Needs Project Advisory Committee; American Academy of Pediatrics. The medical home. *Pediatrics.* 2002;110(1, pt 1): 184–186

54. Marcin JP, Rimsza ME, Moskowitz WB; Committee on Pediatric Workforce. The use of telemedicine to address access and physician workforce shortages. *Pediatrics.* 2015;136(1):202–209

55. Disaster Preparedness Advisory Council; Committee on Pediatric Emergency Medicine. Ensuring the health of children in disasters. *Pediatrics.* 2015;136(5). Available at: www.pediatrics.org/cgi/content/full/136/5/e1407

56. Kuppermann N, Holmes JF, Dayan PS, et al; Pediatric Emergency Care Applied Research Network (PECARN). Identification of children at very low risk of clinically-important brain injuries after head trauma: a prospective cohort study. *Lancet.* 2009;374(9696):1160–1170

57. Gray MP, Keeney GE, Grahl MJ, Gorelick MH, Spahr CD. Improving guideline-based care of acute asthma in a pediatric emergency department. *Pediatrics.* 2016;138(5):e20153339

58. American Academy of Pediatrics, Section on Emergency Medicine; Children's Hospital Association of Texas. Pediatric Septic Shock Collaborative septic shock identification tool. Available at: http://chatexas.com/wp-content/uploads/2016/12/Septic-Shock-Identification-Tool-1.pdf. Accessed May 8, 2017

59. Tieder JS, Bonkowsky JL, Etzel RA, et al; Subcommittee on Apparent Life Threatening Events. Brief resolved unexplained events (formerly apparent life-threatening events) and evaluation of lower-risk infants: executive summary. *Pediatrics.* 2016;137(5):e20160591

60. Harrison D, Beggs S, Stevens B. Sucrose for procedural pain management in infants. *Pediatrics.* 2012;130(5):918–925

61. Emergency Medical Services for Children. Interfacility transfer tool kit for the pediatric patient. Available at: https://emscimprovement.center/resources/publications/interfacility-transfer-tool-kit/. Accessed June 13, 2018

62. Emergency Nurses Association, Position Statement Committee. Interfacility transfer of emergency care patients. 2015. Available at: https://www.ena.org/docs/default-source/resource-library/practice-resources/position-statements/facilitatingtheinterfacilitytransfer.pdf?sfvrsn=d3d9c8f4_14. Accessed June 13, 2018

63. American College of Surgeons, Committee on Trauma. Resources for optimal care of the injured patient. 2014. Available at: https://www.facs.org/~/media/files/quality%20programs/trauma/vrc%20resources/resources%20for%20optimal%20care.ashx. Accessed May 8, 2017

64. Benjamin L, Ishimine P, Joseph M, Mehta S. Evaluation and treatment of minors. *Ann Emerg Med.* 2018;71(2):225–232

65. Lannon CM, Coven BJ, Lane France F, et al; National Initiative for Children's Health Care Quality Project Advisory Committee. Principles of patient safety in pediatrics. *Pediatrics.* 2001;107(6):1473–1475

66. Krug SE, Frush K; American Academy of Pediatrics, Committee on Pediatric Emergency Medicine. Patient safety in the pediatric emergency care setting. *Pediatrics.* 2007;120(6):1367–1375

67. Stucky ER; American Academy of Pediatrics, Committee on Drugs; American Academy of Pediatrics, Committee on Hospital Care. Prevention of medication errors in the pediatric inpatient setting. *Pediatrics.* 2003;112(2):431–436

68. Lesar TS, Mitchell A, Sommo P. Medication safety in critically ill children. *Clin Pediatr Emerg Med.* 2006;7(4):215–225

69. Westbrook JI, Woods A, Rob MI, Dunsmuir WT, Day RO. Association of interruptions with an increased risk and severity of medication administration errors. *Arch Intern Med.* 2010;170(8):683–690

70. The Joint Commission. Preventing pediatric medication errors. *Sentinel Event Alert.* 2008;39(39):1–4

71. American Academy of Pediatrics. Abrams MA, Dreyer BP, eds. *Plain Language Pediatrics: Health Literacy Strategies and Communication Resources for Common Pediatric Topics.* Elk Grove Village, IL: American Academy of Pediatrics; 2008

72. Institute of Medicine. *Toward Health Equity and Patient-Centeredness: Integrating Health Literacy, Disparities Reduction, and Quality Improvement: Workshop Summary.* Washington, DC: National Academies Press; 2009

73. Cheng TL, Dreyer BP, Jenkins RR. Introduction: child health disparities and health literacy. *Pediatrics.* 2009;124(suppl 3):S161–S162

74. DeWalt DA, Hink A. Health literacy and child health outcomes: a systematic review of the literature. *Pediatrics.* 2009;124(suppl 3):S265–S274

75. Winkelman TNA, Caldwell MT, Bertram B, Davis MM. Promoting health literacy for children and adolescents. *Pediatrics.* 2016;138(6):e20161937

76. Taveras EM, Flores G. Why culture and language matter: the clinical consequences of providing culturally and linguistically appropriate services to children in the emergency department. *Clin Pediatr Emerg Med.* 2004;5(2):76–84

77. Sadler BL, Joseph A. *Evidence for Innovation: Transforming Children's Health Through the Physical Environment.* Alexandria, VA: National Association of Children's Hospitals and Related Institutions; 2008

78. The Joint Commission. National patient safety goals effective January 2017: hospital accreditation program. 2017. Available at: https://www.jointcommission.org/assets/1/6/NPSG_Chapter_HAP_Jan2017.pdf. Accessed May 8, 2017

79. Brody AS, Frush DP, Huda W, Brent RL; American Academy of Pediatrics, Section on Radiology. Radiation risk to children from computed tomography. *Pediatrics.* 2007;120(3):677–682

80. Goske MJ, Applegate KE, Boylan J, et al. The 'Image Gently' campaign: increasing CT radiation dose awareness through a national education and awareness program. *Pediatr Radiol.* 2008;38(3):265–269

81. Strauss KJ, Goske MJ. Estimated pediatric radiation dose during CT. *Pediatr Radiol.* 2011;41(suppl 2):472–482

82. Furlow B. Radiation protection in pediatric imaging. *Radiol Technol.* 2011;82(5):421–439

83. Vest JR, Jung H, Ostrovsky A, Tanmoy Das L, McGinty GB. Image sharing technologies and reduction of imaging utilization: A systematic review and meta-analysis. *J Am Coll Radiol.* 2015;12(12):1371–1379.e3

84. Hegenbarth MA; American Academy of Pediatrics, Committee on Drugs. Preparing for pediatric emergencies: drugs to consider. *Pediatrics.* 2008;121(2):433–443

Pediatricians and Public Health: Optimizing the Health and Well-Being of the Nation's Children

- *Policy Statement*

POLICY STATEMENT Organizational Principles to Guide and Define the Child Health Care System and/or Improve the Health of all Children

American Academy of Pediatrics

DEDICATED TO THE HEALTH OF ALL CHILDREN™

Pediatricians and Public Health: Optimizing the Health and Well-Being of the Nation's Children

Alice A. Kuo, MD, PhD, FAAP,[a] Pauline A. Thomas, MD, FAAP,[b,c] Lance A. Chilton, MD, FAAP,[d] Laurene Mascola, MD, MPH,[e] COUNCIL ON COMMUNITY PEDIATRICS, SECTION ON EPIDEMIOLOGY, PUBLIC HEALTH, AND EVIDENCE

abstract

Ensuring optimal health for children requires a population-based approach and collaboration between pediatrics and public health. The prevention of major threats to children's health (such as behavioral health issues) and the control and management of chronic diseases, obesity, injury, communicable diseases, and other problems cannot be managed solely in the pediatric office. The integration of clinical practice with public health actions is necessary for multiple levels of disease prevention that involve the child, family, and community. Although pediatricians and public health professionals interact frequently to the benefit of children and their families, increased integration of the 2 disciplines is critical to improving child health at the individual and population levels. Effective collaboration is necessary to ensure that population health activities include children and that the child health priorities of the American Academy of Pediatrics (AAP), such as poverty and child health, early brain and child development, obesity, and mental health, can engage federal, state, and local public health initiatives. In this policy statement, we build on the 2013 AAP Policy Statement on community pediatrics by identifying specific opportunities for collaboration between pediatricians and public health professionals that are likely to improve the health of children in communities. In the statement, we provide recommendations for pediatricians, public health professionals, and the AAP and its chapters.

[a]David Geffen School of Medicine, University of California, Los Angeles, Los Angeles, California; [b]Department of Medicine, New Jersey Medical School, Rutgers University, Newark, New Jersey; [c]Summit Medical Group, New Brunswick, New Jersey; [d]School of Medicine, University of New Mexico, Albuquerque, New Mexico; and [e]Los Angeles County Department of Public Health, Los Angeles, California

Drs Kuo, Chilton, Thomas and Mascola conceptually outlined this statement, each wrote sections of the draft, and all authors reviewed and revised subsequent drafts (in conjunction with American Academy of Pediatrics staff) and approved the final manuscript as submitted.

DOI: https://doi.org/10.1542/peds.2017-3848

To cite: Kuo AA, Thomas PA, Chilton LA, et alAAP COUNCIL ON COMMUNITY PEDIATRICS, AAP SECTION ON EPIDEMIOLOGY, PUBLIC HEALTH, AND EVIDENCE. Pediatricians and Public Health: Optimizing the Health and Well-Being of the Nation's Children. Pediatrics. 2018;141(2):e20173848

THE HEALTH OF A NATION CAN BE JUDGED BY THE HEALTH OF ITS YOUNGEST MEMBERS

Many children and youth in the United States are not thriving. For example, in 2015, 19.7% of US children lived in families with incomes below the federal poverty level.[1] Of children and teenagers in the United States from 2011 to 2014, ~1 in 3 was overweight or obese; 17% were obese.[2,3] Of children 9 to 17 years old, ~1 in 5 may have a diagnosable mental or addictive disorder that could cause at least minimal impairment.[4] As of early 2017, ~4.8% of US children remained uninsured.[5] In 2014, 4042 children and youth aged 0 to 21 years were killed by firearms in the United States.[6]

Although children's health outcomes are influenced by access to quality health care in a medical home, social, economic, and environmental factors are critical determinants of child health.[7] Pediatricians and public health professionals are particularly well suited to address these multifaceted issues in the community setting. Grounded in a shared commitment to prevention and population health, the 2 groups must leverage each profession's strengths and expertise to promote prevention, improve the delivery of health services, and advance health at the community level. In the 2013 American Academy of Pediatrics (AAP) Policy Statement "Community Pediatrics: Navigating the Intersection of Medicine, Public Health, and Social Determinants of Children's Health," researchers briefly described partnership with public health as a key component of practicing community pediatrics. However, it is critical for all pediatricians to recognize the importance and value of collaboration with public health colleagues to improve children's health. In recent years, there has been a growing movement to increase collaboration between the fields of clinical medicine and public health.[8,9] Recent child health emergencies (such as the 2015 measles outbreak that was associated with exposures in Disneyland; the water crisis in Flint, Michigan; and the emergence of Zika virus) further reinforce the need for medical and public health expertise to approach an urgent child health issue. The enhancement of this relationship is also critical because of the health care system's increased focus on reducing

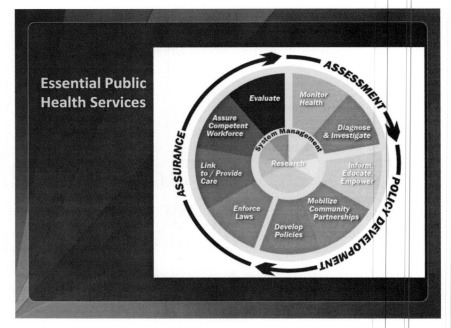

FIGURE 1

Ten essential public health services include the following: (1) monitor health status to identify and solve community health problems; (2) diagnose and investigate health problems and health hazards in the community; (3) inform, educate, and empower people about health issues; (4) mobilize community partnerships and action to identify and solve health problems; (5) develop policies and plans that support individual and community health efforts; (6) enforce laws and regulations that protect health and ensure safety; (7) link people to needed personal health services and ensure the provision of health care when otherwise unavailable; (8) ensure the presence of a competent public and personal health care workforce; (9) evaluate the effectiveness, accessibility, and quality of personal and population-based health services; and (10) research for new insights and innovative solutions to health problems. (Reprinted with permission from the Centers for Disease Control and Prevention. The public health system and the 10 essential public health services. Available at: https://www.cdc.gov/nphpsp/essentialservices.html. Accessed March 21, 2017.)

health care costs by improving population health outcomes.

A DEFINITION OF PUBLIC HEALTH FOR PEDIATRICIANS

In the National Academy of Medicine (formerly the Institute of Medicine) report "The Future of Public Health," researchers describe public health as "fulfilling society's interest in assuring conditions in which people can be healthy." They further identify 3 core functions for public health: assessment, assurance, and policy development.[10] In 1994, a consensus list of essential public health services was developed by federal health agencies in partnership with major national public health organizations and adopted by the Public Health Functions Steering Committee.

These services, mapped to the 3 core functions, are illustrated in Fig 1.[11]

Many public health activities are conducted by local, state, and federal government agencies.[12–14] The primary roles of these agencies are to monitor health and disease, provide strategies for disease prevention, and promote healthy practices. Public health practitioners contribute to these functions by informing, educating, and mobilizing members of the public about current and emerging health issues; advocating for and enforcing laws and regulations that protect health and ensure safety; and addressing a number of specific conditions (Table 1).

However, many other entities (public and private, local and national)

TABLE 1 Examples of Threats to Children's Health Requiring Pediatrics and Public Health Collaboration to Prevent or Alleviate

Environmental health concerns, including climate disruption, air quality, water safety, environmental toxins, and natural disasters
Food safety
Vaccine refusal
Communicable diseases
Obesity epidemic
Adverse childhood experiences resulting in toxic stress, including poverty, social isolation, and violence
Health care access, especially for underserved groups (eg, children of undocumented immigrants)
Injury prevention (including gun violence), education, regulation, and anticipatory guidance
Substance abuse (including smoking, alcohol, and illicit drugs)

participate in maintaining and supporting public health.

PEDIATRICIANS' UNDERSTANDING OF THE WORK OF MAJOR ENTITIES PROVIDING RECOMMENDATIONS IN PUBLIC HEALTH

Public health entities such as the Advisory Committee on Immunization Practices of the Centers for Disease Control and Prevention (CDC),[15] the CDC Community Preventive Services Task Force,[16] the Maternal and Child Health Bureau, and the US Preventive Services Task Force[17] provide a portion of the evidence base for the content of well-child care. These public health entities synthesize, review, and provide information and recommendations about preventive care and policies. They often provide easily accessed, up-to-date information for children and families and can provide information to pediatricians about the monitoring of diseases and disease-prevention activities in communities. The efforts of these groups inform and assist AAP efforts to improve child health. The AAP informs pediatricians about the information and recommendations that many of these entities produce. Although individual pediatricians in primary-care practice and medical and surgical subspecialties need not maintain expertise in the work of these public health entities, they should be aware of the public health data and resources that they

provide to support population health improvement.

PEDIATRICIANS' ROLE IN PUBLIC HEALTH

Pediatricians function as an arm of public health by preventing diseases in their patients (eg, by promoting immunizations), treating diseases, and promoting healthy lifestyles (eg, by striving toward tobacco and substance abuse prevention and promoting healthy nutrition and physical activity). Pediatricians are often the first to know about a public health issue and must report it to the local or state department of health (eg, a child with meningitis, a family testing positive for tuberculosis, or a child in day care with lead poisoning). Starting with individual patient occurrences, these may be considered sentinel events, signaling problems that may require action by a public health agency. Additionally, pediatricians typically participate in ≥1 of the 3 core public health practice functions by assessing an individual's health status and health needs, ensuring that necessary services are provided, or developing policy.[10]

However, the pediatrician can only partially address population health issues within the examination room.[18] Pediatricians can also participate in a variety of population-based efforts that promote child health. The Title V Maternal and Child Health Block Grant Program

needs assessment process is a key opportunity.[19] This process is used to foster collaboration between the federal Maternal and Child Health Bureau, each state's Department of Health, families, practitioners, and community organizations to work toward improving community-wide child and maternal health outcomes.

Pediatricians can also serve on the advisory boards of public health programs, school boards, and school-based clinics and partner with health-promotion projects in communities. Individual prevention approaches that are based in the pediatric examination room and population-based activities are complementary strategies that help advance the health and well-being of all children.

PEDIATRIC AND PUBLIC HEALTH COLLABORATIONS

Public health and pediatrics are professions with a shared commitment to disease and injury prevention, anticipatory guidance, and early recognition and response to threats to lifelong health. Historically, the fields of pediatrics and public health have successfully collaborated on a variety of children's health issues (Table 2). Collaborations can include a range of activities, including sharing information and data, developing joint health-promotion and planning initiatives, coordinating health care services, and implementing education and/or training activities.[20]

Case Examples

The following cases are recent child health scenarios that required collaboration between pediatrics and public health.

Disneyland Measles Outbreak (December 2014 to February 2015)

During the 2014–2015 measles outbreak that was linked to exposures at Disneyland theme parks in Southern California, 125

TABLE 2 Examples of Activities in Which Pediatrics and Public Health Practitioners Currently Collaborate

Epidemic response and emergency preparedness
Immunization endeavors, including education, administration, and tracking through registries
Lead poisoning prevention
Newborn screening
Perinatal hepatitis B prevention
Promotion of healthy lifestyles
Protecting the health of travelers
Recognition and reporting of new illness and outbreaks by pediatricians
Substance use prevention and reduction, including tobacco, alcohol, and illicit drugs

confirmed cases were identified by the California Department of Public Health, 110 of which were in California residents. State Senator Richard Pan, MD, FAAP (Democrat-Sacramento) and State Senator Ben Allen (Democrat-Santa Monica) coauthored a bill (SB 277) that was introduced in the California State Legislature in early February 2015 (with support from AAP, California) that mandated that all children be vaccinated on school entry. This bill in effect only allowed for medical exemptions and did not allow parents to exempt their children from vaccinations on the basis of religious or personal beliefs. Hundreds of pediatricians across the state were joined by thousands of nonpediatrician physicians, all of whom educated legislators about the importance of this bill. California's governor signed the bill into law in June 2015, and the law went into effect on January 1, 2016.[21]

Flint Water Contamination Crisis (April 2014 to Present)

Contamination of the drinking water in the city of Flint, Michigan, occurred after city officials changed the water supply to a local river without applying corrosion inhibitors. Pediatrician Mona Hana-Attisha, MD, MPH, FAAP, noticed that the number of children <5 years old with blood lead concentrations of >5 µg/dL[22] increased after the change in water supply. By using hospital records, she was able to determine the percentage of Flint children with blood lead concentrations of >5 µg/dL (which is the concentration, based

on the US population, of children ages 1–5 years who are in the top 2.5% of children when tested for lead in their blood). The percentage increased from 2.4% to 4.9%, and in areas with higher water-lead content, it increased from 4% to 10.6%.[23] Because of her data and efforts by environmental advocates, in January 2016, both the state and federal governments declared the Flint water crisis a state of emergency and authorized aid toward resolving the crisis and ameliorating the effects on child development. At the time of this publication, efforts are ongoing.

Emergence of the Zika Virus (September 2015 to Present)

After a Zika virus outbreak was identified in January 2015 in northeast Brazil, 35 newborn infants with microcephaly were identified who were born between September and November 2015 to mothers from that area; by summer 2016, >1700 infants with microcephaly had been born in northeast Brazil since the beginning of the outbreak. The link between microcephaly in infants and Zika virus infection has been established with certainty.[24] Zika is a *Flavivirus* that is transmitted by *Aedes* mosquitoes, the same kind of mosquito that transmits yellow fever, dengue, and chikungunya virus infections. The CDC issued a report[25] in January 2016 cautioning pregnant women who travel to areas with endemic Zika virus infection and recommending protection against mosquito bites, such as the use of mosquito nets while sleeping and the use of Environmental Protection

Agency–approved insect repellents. The CDC has issued several updated guidance documents[26] about the epidemic, which has reached many countries in the Caribbean and Central America as well as Puerto Rico and the Southern United States. In a summary of knowledge about Zika virus published in August 2016, Tom Frieden, MD, MPH, who was the director of the CDC at the time, and his colleagues[24] cited work with the AAP on developing guidance for pediatricians on dealing with infants who are born to mothers who were exposed to the virus. Efforts to develop a Zika vaccine were showing early signs of success as of the summer of 2016.

Keys to Successful Collaborations

Many factors can influence the strength and effectiveness of primary care and public health collaborations. The 2012 report "Primary Care and Public Health: Exploring Integration to Improve Population Health"[20] includes a series of principles for the successful integration of primary care and public health, including the following:

- A shared goal of population health improvement;

- Community engagement in defining and addressing population health needs;

- Aligned leadership;

- Sustainability; and

- Sharing and collaborating in the use of data and analysis.

Pediatricians and public health professionals can draw on these principles for collaborative activities and use resources such as *The Practical Playbook: Public Health and Primary Care Together* (practicalplaybook.org) to help refine their collaboration strategies. This resource provides step-by-step guidance to assist public health and primary-care professionals in working together to improve population health.

PEDIATRIC ADVOCACY FOR CHILD PUBLIC HEALTH ISSUES

Pediatricians' voices are important for effective advocacy on issues that affect children's health. As described in the AAP Policy Statement "Community Pediatrics: Navigating the Intersection of Medicine, Public Health, and Social Determinants of Children's Health,"[27] pediatricians are well positioned to advocate for access to health care in a medical home as well as for the social, economic, educational, and environmental resources that are essential for every child's healthy development. This advocacy is needed at local, state, and federal levels. Pediatricians can also serve as critical allies and advocates to support the public health infrastructure as part of the overall child health care system in the United States. Public health funding at the federal level has remained flat for the last several years, whereas most local and state public health department budgets have declined.[28] A lack of investment in public health systems, services, and programs can hinder important activities for child health, including disease surveillance and reporting, health promotion, and emergency preparedness. Pediatricians can provide important insights about the need for public health investments to optimize child health at the individual and population levels.

TRAINING PEDIATRICIANS IN PUBLIC HEALTH PRINCIPLES

Many medical school and residency training programs have recently incorporated teaching into their curricula on the functions and activities of public health entities, such as epidemiologic investigation, public health surveillance, and assurance of safety. Targeted educational instruction in public health is important for pediatricians to address issues from the wider society and environment that affect the health of their individual patients. Pediatricians need training to understand the importance of the identification of sentinel public health events, understanding that such events may signal public health problems that require intervention. Pediatric residents should also know whom to notify of potential sentinel events and how to get support for their elucidation. To understand and help address community health issues, pediatricians should also have access to training on how to use community health data.

The Residency Review Committee of the Accreditation Council for Graduate Medical Education continues to strengthen pediatric training program requirements for education in community health and child advocacy.[29,30] The Academic Pediatric Association,[31] the AAP Community Pediatrics Training Initiative,[32] the Council on Community Pediatrics, and others have developed educational goals and objectives, curricula, and other resources to support this training. After the publication of the 2012 National Academy of Medicine (formerly Institute of Medicine) recommendations in "Primary Care and Public Health: Exploring Integration to Improve Population Health,"[20] the CDC launched a Primary Care and Public Health Initiative[33] to foster relationships between physicians and local and state public health professionals through collaborations with residency program educators.

COLLABORATION TO IMPROVE POPULATION HEALTH AND REDUCE HEALTH CARE COSTS

The Patient Protection and Affordable Care Act (ACA) (Public Law Number 111-148 [2010]) includes a number of insurance reforms and provisions that promote population health. The ACA also provides potential opportunities for pediatricians and public health professionals to collaborate more closely through provisions that focus on health promotion and the prevention of diseases in all individuals, including children. Although not an exhaustive list, some related ACA provisions include the following:

- Requiring nonprofit, tax-exempt hospitals to conduct community health needs assessments every 3 years and involve those with expertise in public health;[34]

- Funding the Maternal, Infant, and Early Childhood Home Visiting Program, which can provide support and education to individuals to promote positive parenting and early child development. Each state must complete a needs assessment to identify at-risk communities to receive any Title V Maternal and Child Health Block Grant funds;

- Requiring private insurance plans to cover preventive services, prohibiting copayments and deductibles for preventive services, and allowing families the opportunity to access age-appropriate benefits for children, including coverage for all Bright Futures–recommended services with no cost sharing; and

- Creating the National Prevention Council to coordinate and promote health and disease-prevention efforts among federal-level agencies and departments and develop a National Prevention Strategy.[35]

Children benefit from these provisions, and the continued implementation of these efforts will be improved by the involvement and collaboration of pediatricians and public health professionals. Any changes made to the ACA should maintain these important reforms.

An additional and critical opportunity for collaboration lies in the US health care system's increased focus on improving the health of populations while reducing health care costs. As the system evolves to address this challenge through new models of payment, systems integrations, and the broader use of population health data, pediatricians and public health professionals must collaborate and participate in these efforts. Together, they can promote investments in prevention and attention to the social determinants of child health as strategies for developing a strong foundation for lifelong health. A strong foundation established in childhood can potentially reduce chronic disease, improve health outcomes, and ultimately, decrease health care costs across the life course.

A definition change in the provision of preventive services in Medicaid serves as an example of how new models of payment can strengthen the ties between clinical medicine and public health toward the improvement of population health. As of January 2014, the Preventive Services Rule Change issued by the Centers for Medicare and Medicaid Services provides an opportunity for nonphysicians, such as community health workers, to become eligible for Medicaid payment as long as the services provided are recommended by a physician or other licensed practitioner within their states' scope of practice.[36] A state must proactively allow this change by submitting a state Medicaid plan amendment to the Centers for Medicare and Medicaid Services. For example, if the state permits it, this rule would allow asthma educators who are not licensed practitioners but provide services in a home or community setting to be eligible to be paid for their services by Medicaid if those services are recommended by a physician or other state-licensed

practitioner as an extension of the medical home. Asthma educators have been shown to provide cost-effective asthma education and management services, working with children and families in their social and environmental contexts.[37] This is an example of how an evolving model of payment may support a population health approach and collaborations between pediatricians and public health professionals.

RECOMMENDATIONS

The following recommendations are aimed at helping pediatricians and public health professionals work together optimally to improve child health at the individual and population levels.

Recommendations for Individual Pediatricians

- Pediatricians should remain aware of reporting requirements for individual diseases, outbreaks, and vaccine adverse events that require reporting to public health agencies. They should also be aware of local and state health department resources (newsletters, Web sites, social media, etc) for information on diseases and outbreaks;

- Pediatricians should make use of the resources and recommendations that are provided by public health agencies and organizations, including local and state health departments, the CDC and its Advisory Committee on Immunization Practices, the US Preventive Services Task Force, the Maternal and Child Health Bureau, and the National Academy of Medicine;

- Pediatricians should be aware of how to access local and state public health data to identify population health needs and trends;

- Pediatricians can identify opportunities to collaborate with public health entities on community disease prevention and

health promotion programs for children and adolescents;

- Pediatricians can serve as advisors to public health entities, such as the Maternal and Child Health Bureau Title V Block Grant Program;

- Pediatricians should consider advocating for population-based approaches to health within their own health care institutions and systems; and

- Pediatricians who are training pediatric residents should include public health and population health curricula and incorporate public health practitioners into the training.

Recommendations for Collaboration Between Pediatricians and Public Health Professionals

- Pediatricians and public health professionals can work together on sharing data and information about children's health issues, including access to quality health care and health disparities. In partnership with public health and health care systems, they can also work together on mapping and analyzing community health data to identify geographic hot spots of health problems that are in need of targeted interventions;

- Pediatricians and public health professionals should partner on prevention and health-promotion projects to address chronic disease and disability through complementary clinical and community-based approaches;

- Pediatricians and public health professionals should collaborate with families to advocate for healthy environments in which children learn, live, and play;

- Pediatricians and public health entities should work together to ensure that children and adolescents are specifically considered in disaster planning, including the development of strategic plans for communication, and in the management of the children, particularly children with special health care needs;

- Pediatricians and public health professionals can partner to advocate for investments in public health systems and infrastructure at the local, state, and federal levels. Advocacy should emphasize the importance of public health investments for improving both individual and population health;

- Pediatricians and public health professionals can partner to promote public and private efforts at the local, state, and federal levels that promote healthy community development; and

- Public health professionals and pediatricians should work together to disseminate important public health information, such as immunization messages, to parents and families.

Recommendations for the AAP and AAP Chapters

The following recommendations address opportunities for the AAP and its chapters to promote pediatric and public health collaborations for child health and well-being:

- The AAP and its chapters should include pediatrician members who serve in public health departments, National Health Service Corps facilities, Indian Health Service facilities, and federally qualified health care centers in AAP and chapter-level communications and activities;

- AAP chapters should develop working relationships with state and local health departments so that important matters of joint interest (eg, outbreaks of infectious disease, disaster planning,

newborn screening changes, needs assessments, and planning for anticipated health effects of climate change) are effectively communicated and, when a crisis occurs, they can work together effectively; and

- The AAP should consider making continuing medical education opportunities in public health practice and priorities available to all of its members.

CONCLUSIONS

In the seminal report "Primary Care and Public Health: Exploring Integration to Improve Population Health,"[20] researchers noted that "actors in both primary care and public health contribute to the promotion of health and well-being; the assurance of conditions in which people can be healthy; and the provision of timely, effective, and coordinated health care." This is particularly relevant and important regarding issues of child health. Pediatricians and their public health colleagues are important actors in addressing the social determinants of health that have major consequences on childhood health and well-being. Greater communication, collaboration, and partnership between pediatricians and the public health sector have the potential to improve individual- and population-level child health outcomes.

AUTHORS

Alice A. Kuo, MD, PhD, FAAP
Pauline A. Thomas, MD, FAAP
Lance A. Chilton, MD, FAAP
Laurene Mascola, MD, MPH

COUNCIL ON COMMUNITY PEDIATRICS EXECUTIVE COMMITTEE, 2016–2017

Lance A. Chilton, MD, FAAP, Chairperson

Patricia J. Flanagan, MD, FAAP, Vice Chairperson
Kimberley J. Dilley, MD, MPH, FAAP
James H. Duffee, MD, MPH, FAAP
Andrea E. Green, MD, FAAP
J. Raul Gutierrez, MD, MPH, FAAP
Virginia A. Keane, MD, FAAP
Scott D. Krugman, MD, MS, FAAP
Julie M. Linton, MD, FAAP
Carla D. McKelvey, MD, MPH, FAAP
Jacqueline L. Nelson, MD, FAAP

LIAISONS

Jacqueline R. Dougé, MD, MPH, FAAP, Chairperson, *Public Health Special Interest Group*
Kathleen Rooney-Otero, MD, MPH, *Section on Pediatric Trainees*

STAFF

Camille Watson, MS

SECTION ON EPIDEMIOLOGY EXECUTIVE COMMITTEE, 2016–2017

Charles R. Woods Jr, MD, MS, FAAP, Chairperson
Ameth A. Aguirre, MD, MPH, FAAP
Mona A. Eissa, MD, FAAP
Lillianne M. Lewis, MD, MPH, FAAP
Christina A. Nelson, MD, MPH, FAAP
Sheila L. Palevsky, MD, MPH, FAAP
Michael J. Smith, MD, FAAP

LIAISONS

Michael Leu, MD, MS, MHS, FAAP, *Council on Quality Improvement and Patient Safety*
Wade Harrison, MD, MPH, *Section on Pediatric Trainees*
Patty A. Vitale, MD, MPH, FAAP, *US Preventive Services Task Force*
Alex R. Kemper, MD, MPH, MS, FAAP, *Pediatric Research in Office Settings*

STAFF

Kymika Okechukwu, MPA

ABBREVIATIONS

AAP: American Academy of Pediatrics
ACA: Patient Protection and Affordable Care Act
CDC: Centers for Disease Control and Prevention

Address correspondence to Alice A. Kuo, MD, PhD, FAAP. E-mail: akuo@mednet.ucla.edu

PEDIATRICS (ISSN Numbers: Print, 0031-4005; Online, 1098-4275).

FINANCIAL DISCLOSURE: Dr Chilton has indicated he has an advisory board relationship with Sanofi Pasteur. The other authors have indicated they have no financial relationships relevant to this article to disclose.

FUNDING: No external funding.

POTENTIAL CONFLICT OF INTEREST: The authors have indicated they have no potential conflicts of interest to disclose.

REFERENCES

1. Barnett JC, Vornovitsky M. *Income and Poverty in the United States: 2015. Report No. P60-256*. Washington, DC: US Census Bureau; 2016:60–256. Available at: https://www.census.gov/library/publications/2016/demo/p60-256.html. Accessed March 21, 2017

2. Ogden CL, Carroll MD, Fryar CD, Flegal KM. Prevalence of obesity among adults and youth: United States, 2011–2014. *NCHS Data Brief*. 2015;(219):1–8

3. Ogden CL, Carroll MD, Curtin LR, Lamb MM, Flegal KM. Prevalence of high body mass index in US children and adolescents, 2007-2008. *JAMA*. 2010;303(3):242–249

4. National Advisory Mental Health Council; Workgroup on Child and Adolescent Mental Health Intervention Development and Deployment. *Blueprint for Change: Research on Child and Adolescent Mental Health*. Washington, DC: National Institute of Mental Health; 2001. Available at: www.nimh.nih.gov/about/advisory-boards-and-groups/namhc/reports/blueprint-for-change-research-on-child-and-adolescent-mental-health.shtml. Accessed March 21, 2017

5. Proctor BD, Semega JL, Kollar MA. *Poverty in the United States: 2015. Report No. P60-257*. Washington, DC: US Census Bureau; 2016:60–257. Available at: https://www.census.gov/content/dam/Census/library/publications/2016/demo/p60-257.pdf. Accessed March 21, 2017

6. Centers for Disease Control and Prevention. WISQARS. Fatal injury reports, national, regional and state (RESTRICTED), 1999-2015. Available at: http://webappa.cdc.gov/sasweb/ncipc/dataRestriction_inj.html. Accessed March 21, 2017

7. Braveman PA, Egerter SA, Mockenhaupt RE. Broadening the focus: the need to address the social determinants of health. *Am J Prev Med*. 2011;40(1, suppl 1):S4–S18

8. American Academy of Family Physicians. *Integration of Primary Care and Public Health (Position Paper)*. Leawood, KS: American Academy of Family Physicians; 2015. Available at: www.aafp.org/about/policies/all/integprimarycareandpublichealth.html. Accessed August 2, 2017

9. National Academy of Medicine. *Collaboration Between Health Care and Public Health: Workshop Summary*. Washington, DC: National Academies Press; 2015. Available at: http://nationalacademies.org/hmd/Reports/2015/Collaboration-between-Health-Care-and-Public-Health.aspx. Accessed August 2, 2017

10. National Academy of Medicine; Committee for the Study of the Future of Public Health; Division of Health Care Services. *The Future of Public Health*. Washington, DC: National Academy Press; 1988

11. Centers for Disease Control and Prevention. The public health system and the 10 essential public health services. Available at: https://www.cdc.gov/stlpublichealth/publichealthservices/essentialhealthservices.html. Accessed March 21, 2017

12. National Association of County and City Health Officials. Directory of local health departments. Available at: http://www.naccho.org/resources/lhd-directory. Accessed March 21, 2017

13. Centers for Disease Control and Prevention. Public health resources: state health departments. Available at: www.cdc.gov/mmwr/international/relres.html. Accessed March 21, 2017

14. American Public Health Association. State and regional public health organizations. Available at: www.apha.org/apha-communities/affiliates/state-and-regional-public-health-associations. Accessed March 21, 2017

15. Advisory Committee on Immunization Practices. Vaccines. Available at: www.cdc.gov/vaccines/acip/index.html. Accessed March 21, 2017

16. Community Preventive Services Task Force. The community guide. Available at: www.thecommunityguide.org/index.html. Accessed March 21, 2017

17. US Preventive Services Task Force Web site. Available at: https://www.uspreventiveservicestaskforce.org/Page/Name/about-the-uspstf. Accessed March 21, 2017

18. McGinnis JM, Foege WH. Actual causes of death in the United States. *JAMA*. 1993;270(18):2207–2212

19. US Department of Health and Human Services; Health Resources and Services Administration. *Title V Maternal and Child Health Services Block Grant to States Program. Guidance and Forms for the Title V Application/Annual Report*. Rockville, MD: Health Resources and Services Administration; 2017. Available at: http://mchb.hrsa.gov/sites/default/files/mchb/MaternalChildHealthInitiatives/TitleV/blockgrantguidanceappendix.pdf. Accessed March 21, 2017

20. National Academy of Medicine. *Primary Care and Public Health: Exploring Integration to Improve Population Health*. Washington, DC: The National Academies Press; 2012. Available at: https://www.nap.edu/catalog/13381/primary-care-and-public-health-exploring-integration-to-improve-population. Accessed August 2, 2017

21. California State Legislature. Senate Bill 277. Public health: vaccinations. 2015 Available at: https://leginfo.legislature.ca.gov/faces/billNavClient.xhtml?bill_id=201520160SB277. Accessed March 21, 2017

22. Centers for Disease Control and Prevention. What do parents need to know to protect their children? Blood lead levels in children. Available at: www.cdc.gov/nceh/lead/ACCLPP/

blood_lead_levels.htm. Accessed March 21, 2017

23. Hanna-Attisha M, LaChance J, Sadler RC, Champney Schnepp A. Elevated blood lead levels in children associated with the flint drinking water crisis: a spatial analysis of risk and public health response. *Am J Public Health*. 2016;106(2):283–290

24. Frieden TR, Schuchat A, Petersen LR. Zika virus 6 months later. *JAMA*. 2016;316(14):1443–1444

25. Petersen EE, Staples JE, Meaney-Delman D, et al. Interim guidelines for pregnant women during a Zika virus outbreak—United States, 2016. *MMWR Morb Mortal Wkly Rep*. 2016;65(2):30–33

26. Oduyebo T, Igbinosa I, Petersen EE, et al. Update: interim guidance for health care providers caring for pregnant women with possible Zika virus exposure—United States, July 2016. *MMWR Morb Mortal Wkly Rep*. 2016;65(29):739–744

27. American Academy of Pediatrics; Council on Community Pediatrics. Community pediatrics: navigating the intersection of medicine, public health, and social determinants of children's health. *Pediatrics*. 2013;131(3):623–628

28. Trust for America's Health. *Investing in America's Health: a State-by-State Look at Public Health Funding and Key Health Facts. Issue Report*. Washington, DC: Trust for America's Health; 2013. Available at: http://healthyamericans. org/assets/files/TFAH2013InvstgAmr csHlth05%20FINAL.pdf. Accessed March 21, 2017

29. Nader PR, Broyles SL, Brennan J, Taras H. Two national surveys on pediatric training and activities in school health: 1991 and 2001. *Pediatrics*. 2003;111(4, pt 1):730–734

30. Accreditation Council for Graduate Medical Education. *Program Requirements for Graduate Medical Education in Pediatrics*. Chicago, IL: Accreditation Council for Graduate Medical Education; 2011

31. Academic Pediatric Association. Educational guidelines for pediatric residency. Available at: http://www. academicpeds.org/egwebnew/index. cfm. Accessed March 21, 2017

32. Rezet B, Hoffman BD, Kaczorowski J. Pediatrics in the community: integrating community pediatrics into residency training. *Pediatr Rev*. 2010;31(4):159–160

33. Centers for Disease Control and Prevention. Primary care and public health initiative. Available at: www.cdc. gov/ostlts/medicineandpublichealth/ index.html. Accessed March 21, 2017

34. Somerville MH, Mueller CH, Boddie-Willis CL, Folkemer DC, Grossman ER. *Hospital Community Benefits After the ACA: Partnerships for Community Health Improvement. Hilltop Institute Issue Brief*. Baltimore, MD: The Hilltop Institute; 2012. Available at: www.rwjf.org/content/ dam/farm/reports/issue_briefs/ 2012/rwjf72344. Accessed March 21, 2017

35. US Department of Health and Human Services; Office of the Surgeon General; National Prevention Council. *National Prevention Strategy*. Washington, DC: US Department of Health and Human Services, Office of the Surgeon General; 2011. Available at: www. surgeongeneral.gov/priorities/ prevention/strategy/. Accessed March 21, 2017

36. Medicaid Preventive Services. Regulatory change. Available at: https://www.medicaid.gov/medicaid/ benefits/downloads/preventive-webinar-presentation-4-9-14.pdf. Accessed March 21, 2017

37. Markus AR, Andres E, West K, Gerstein MT, Lyons VS. Medicaid payment innovations to financially sustain comprehensive childhood asthma management programs at federally qualified health centers. *J Asthma Allergy Educ*. 2013;4(3):112–122

Physician's Role in Coordinating Care of Hospitalized Children

• *Clinical Report*

CLINICAL REPORT   Guidance for the Clinician in Rendering Pediatric Care

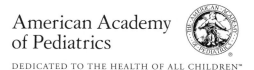

American Academy
of Pediatrics

DEDICATED TO THE HEALTH OF ALL CHILDREN™

Physician's Role in Coordinating Care of Hospitalized Children

Daniel A. Rauch, MD, FAAP, COMMITTEE ON HOSPITAL CARE, SECTION ON HOSPITAL MEDICINE

abstract

The hospitalization of a child is a stressful event for the child and family. The physician responsible for the admission has an important role in directing the care of the child, communicating with the child's providers (medical and primary caregivers), and advocating for the safety of the child during the hospitalization and transition out of the hospital. These challenges remain constant across the varied facilities in which children are hospitalized. The purpose of this revised clinical report is to update pediatricians about principles to improve the coordination of care and review expectations and practice.

Department of Pediatrics, Tufts University School of Medicine, The Floating Hospital for Children at Tufts Medical Center, Boston, Massachusetts

Dr Rauch was responsible for all aspects of revising, writing, and editing the document, reviewing and responding to questions and comments from reviewers and the Board of Directors, and approved the final manuscript as submitted.

Clinical reports from the American Academy of Pediatrics benefit from expertise and resources of liaisons and internal (AAP) and external reviewers. However, clinical reports from the American Academy of Pediatrics may not reflect the views of the liaisons or the organizations or government agencies that they represent.

The guidance in this report does not indicate an exclusive course of treatment or serve as a standard of medical care. Variations, taking into account individual circumstances, may be appropriate.

All clinical reports from the American Academy of Pediatrics automatically expire 5 years after publication unless reaffirmed, revised, or retired at or before that time.

DOI: https://doi.org/10.1542/peds.2018-1503

Address correspondence to Daniel Rauch, MD, FAAP. E-mail: darauch@aap.net

PEDIATRICS (ISSN Numbers: Print, 0031-4005; Online, 1098-4275).

Although infrequent, the hospitalization of a child is a stressful experience for the child and his or her family. Most children are hospitalized for an acute illness or injury.[1] Children can be cared for in freestanding children's hospitals, children's hospitals within general hospitals, or in nonchildren's hospital facilities.[2] The processes of care are different in each environment. In some facilities, children are cared for by a team of pediatricians and pediatric medical subspecialists, surgeons, or other providers, and in others, care is performed by the primary care physician. Some care models can result in fragmentation of care, with the potential loss of information that is vital to the care of the child. Children and youth with special health care needs are particularly vulnerable to these risks because of the complexity of their care, the multiple consultants involved, and a sometimes poor connection to a medical home.[3] Furthermore, overall satisfaction with the hospital experience from the patient and family perspective is an important element of quality of care and a metric that is being used to determine payment rates, so good coordination affects both patient outcomes and net earnings.

Physicians caring for hospitalized children need to direct systems that coordinate care of the hospitalized child at admission, throughout the stay, and on discharge through direct communication with the child's primary care physician. In addition, the hospitalization should be used as an opportunity to review the child's health history to identify unmet needs that may or may not contribute to the hospitalization, such

To cite: Rauch DA, AAP COMMITTEE ON HOSPITAL CARE, AAP SECTION ON HOSPITAL MEDICINE. Physician's Role in Coordinating Care of Hospitalized Children. *Pediatrics.* 2018; 142(2):e20181503

as the coordination of multiple subspecialty-care issues for the child or youth with special health care needs, incomplete immunizations, or dental needs. Admission also provides an opportunity to identify social determinants of health that may require nonmedical intervention, such as social work or even legal referrals. During the hospitalization, multiple sign-outs among care teams, residents in teaching venues, and hospitalists in other venues create additional opportunities for incomplete information transfer. A good quality sign-out system has been the focus of many recent investigations, such as the I-PASS study, which standardized the method and content of sign-outs.[4,5]

This clinical report is an update of the previous version published by the American Academy of Pediatrics Committee on Hospital Care in 2010.[6] The purpose of this revision is to update pediatricians about principles to improve coordination of care.

PHYSICIAN'S ROLE IN COORDINATING CARE OF HOSPITALIZED CHILDREN

Children are hospitalized in a wide variety of environments, from community hospitals to large quaternary-care children's hospitals. For a growing subset of children, especially children and youth with special health care needs, hospitalization is an expected part of their ongoing illness.[7] The physician of record can vary from the child's primary care physician to a hospitalist to a pediatric medical subspecialist to a surgeon, depending on both the reason for admission and the facility. Despite this variation in circumstances, there are similarities in the needs of every hospitalized child that must be addressed by the physician in charge of the child's care.

Care coordination, as an integral part of the medical home, is vitally important to ongoing care of the child and family. Care delivery is an important component of patient and/ or family satisfaction that can affect medical, social, and psychological outcomes. Attention to the processes of hospitalization, from admission to patient handoffs to discharge, is crucial because of the potential opportunities for miscommunication to adversely affect care.

Admission to the hospital may be planned or unplanned. For the scheduled admission, the goal of the hospitalization usually is clearly stated, and there has been previous communication between the referring physician and the hospital as well as approval by the child's insurance carrier. Unfortunately, scheduled admissions may not include real-time physician interaction. It is useful for hospitals to have a mechanism for the receiving physician to contact the referring physician. Health information technology can play a pivotal role in care coordination. Electronic health records (EHRs) and other communication tools can facilitate information sharing among patients and/or families and their health care teams. Unfortunately, many EHR systems do not interact, limiting the ability of some health information technology–facilitated communication. Scheduled admissions usually occur in the context of an ongoing treatment plan for the child, which implies that the child is engaged in ongoing medical care through which the child's health care maintenance is being addressed. However, in the case of children and youth with special health care needs or other children with medical complexity, there may be multiple outpatient providers focused on specific disease processes and less attention paid to general health care needs.

Many pediatric hospital admissions are unscheduled,[8] which presents several challenges to hospital providers. The child and family experience stress during such a medical emergency. Because the inciting incident was unplanned, the family may not have all the necessary information about the child's health at hand, such as immunization records. Shared EHRs, patient portal access, and patient databases (such as immunization registries) can be used to alleviate some of the challenges of unplanned admissions. The acute timing may have precluded a visit or even communication with the primary care physician, who may be unaware of the necessity for hospitalization. The history and physical examination performed by the inpatient physician are an important aspect of assessing the child's general health. Acute problems will be dealt with during the hospitalization, and other health care gaps may be directly addressed or referred back to the primary care physician. A mechanism should in place for the inpatient physician to contact the primary care physician as soon as possible after admission to give notice and share information. This initial contact establishes the foundation for communication that will continue throughout the hospitalization and the discharge process. Because most unscheduled admissions initiate in the emergency department, communication and coordination with the emergency physician are necessary to learn about all evaluations that have already been performed and any pending tests and to understand the need for hospitalization.

Every admission includes an initial assessment, which may begin before the child's arrival or during the discussion between the referring provider and the accepting service at the hospital. At this point, the receiving facility needs to confirm that it can manage the anticipated problem; otherwise, a higher level of care should be recommended. If the child is accepted for admission, then safe transport must be arranged. Once the child has arrived, a timely initial evaluation must be performed, which includes a history of the presenting illness, past medical history, allergies, medications, a review of systems, immunization history, growth and developmental history, family and social history (including an assessment of safety and HEADSS[9] assessment for teenagers), and a thorough physical examination that includes a pain assessment. Depending on the acuity and severity of the presenting illness as well as the time of admission, parts of the history may be deferred to the following day or a time when the child can be interviewed privately. When necessary, medical interpretation services (not a sibling or other patient)[10] should be used, and attention should be given to cultural issues. Attempts to secure a copy of any recent notes, testing, or treatments associated with the current problem should be made. Facilities should be equipped to send and receive necessary medical records in a reliable, timely, and confidential manner. However, direct communication with the referring physician and primary care physician should not be overlooked because this will help provide a context of the child's illness within the family, confirm current medication, and prevent unnecessary duplication of previous tests. Continuing this conversation during the hospitalization (particularly when the family is faced with difficult decisions) may help the family gain trust in a new, hospital-based provider.

Admission to the hospital also provides an opportunity to review the general health care of the child. Although most children in the United States have access to primary care, not all do. A hospital admission may come from a breakdown in outpatient care resulting from a lack of access. Additionally, a thorough history and physical examination may reveal issues that do not relate to the reason for admission but are significant. These issues may be addressed during the hospitalization, or the patient can be referred for outpatient management afterward.

Lastly but also importantly, discharge planning begins on admission. Every admission to the hospital should have a defined treatment end point or at least a critical fork in the decision tree (ie, for abdominal pain, go to the operating room or a trial of oral intake). Defining the discharge parameters at the time of admission helps focus the family on clinical parameters rather than the clock or calendar. Anticipating discharge needs at the time of admission helps involve services that can provide services during the hospitalization or arrange for appropriate outpatient follow-up, such as social work, occupational therapy, and physical therapy.

All pediatric patients admitted to the hospital are cared for by a team of providers on the inpatient service. It is likely that care will be handed off as shifts change or the physician leaves the inpatient area. It is the responsibility of the admitting physician service to provide for accurate and appropriate handoffs to other physician team members. There has been much recent literature about different handoff processes.[5,11,12] The key is that there is no single mnemonic or practice that ensures quality handoffs but a bundle of tactics and a commitment to a consistent standardized process. This coordination of care becomes more important as the care extends beyond the admitting provider to consulting services, and it then becomes the responsibility of the physician of record to acknowledge every consultant's recommendation and ensure that a care plan is achieved and that the care plan is communicated to the family and primary care physician. When necessary, the attending physician must consider the options when there is disagreement among consultants and call for care meetings to establish a clear care plan. These meetings may include the family when discussing treatment options or may be for providers only when the issue is communication between providers to attain an agreed-on plan. When comanagement is in effect, physicians need to respect protocols regarding the scope of their involvement and communicate regularly with the comanagers.[13,14] These protocols are institution specific and may even vary between services, but define the expected role of each service in patient care. When necessary, this communication should be verbal and not solely through the chart. Ultimately, there needs to be a single physician who has the final decision-making ability, and this should be decided at admission. Circumstances may arise during the hospitalization in which the physician of record changes so that there may be more than one over the hospital course, but there should be only one at any point in time. Patients boarded in the emergency department or being treated under observation status require the same amount of attention of the responsible attending physician as all other admitted patients. When the physician of record does not routinely care for pediatric patients or has a narrow clinical focus, consultation with a generalist (such as a hospitalist or general pediatrician) can provide a more holistic approach to the child and family as well as specific attention to pediatric issues, such as weight-dependent medication dosing and developmentally appropriate care. This is recommended for any child or youth with special health care needs or with behavioral issues.[15] Some hospitals have set age (<14 years), weight (<40 kg), or length of stay (>24 hours) criteria for mandatory consultation.[16]

Discharge should represent the achievement of the goal of admission agreed on by the family and medical team. Communication with the primary care physician during the course of the hospitalization prepares the patient for the transition back to the outpatient environment. To reduce potential errors, thorough medication reconciliation should be provided to the family in verbal and written form and be available in the discharge summary to providers who continue to care for the child (Table 1). Referrals should be provided at the time of discharge, including primary care if the child does not have a medical home. Robust education and ongoing family support via telephone or home-based visits have been shown to prevent subsequent acute-care utilization. Communication with the primary care physician does not end at discharge but continues until all pending test results are obtained, and this has been recognized by transitional care management *Current Procedural Terminology* codes published by the Centers for Medicare and Medicaid Services in 2015. Even in a shared EHR environment, tests originating during hospitalization are the joint responsibility of the inpatient physician of record[17] and medical home physician.

The ability to serve as an inpatient physician is determined by the hospital as part of the credentialing process.[18] This physician increasingly is not the primary care physician, thus the emphasis is on communication between the primary care physician and hospital staff and interoperability of EHRs. In many hospitals, the inpatient physician is a hospitalist. In teaching hospitals, residents, fellows, and students are part of the care team. In tertiary-care centers, subspecialists and surgeons may serve as the physician of record. There is always an attending-level physician responsible for the child.

TABLE 1 Key Elements of a Discharge Summary

- dates of admission and discharge
- discharge diagnoses
- brief hospital course, including procedures and test results
- discharge medications
- immunizations given during hospitalization
- pending laboratory or test results
- follow-up appointments

Coughlin DT, Leyenaar JK, Shen M, et al. Pediatric discharge content: a multisite assessment of physician preferences and experiences. *Hosp Pediatr.* 2014;4(1):9–15.

Resident work hour restrictions have created more handoffs of care and a team approach to care. This requires more attention to high-quality handoffs. The expectations enumerated in this report for communication and coordination ultimately fall on the attending physician. The expectations are no less for subspecialists or surgeons.

Coordinating care involves more than ensuring proper medical care. The treating physician is responsible for the patient's safety during the hospitalization. Although a safe hospital environment requires a commitment to safety from the hospital culture and often depends on systems of care, individual physicians should be aware of the safety initiatives at the hospital and be active participants. Safety initiatives include proven efforts, such as medication reconciliation and hand-washing. Performing handoffs properly and effectively[19] minimizes potential information loss. Other safety initiatives include attention to overuse of tests, pediatric dosing of medication and radiation, and adherence to practice pathways that reduce variation in care. It is important for physicians caring for hospitalized children to be strong advocates for children in the hospital environment, especially in nonchildren's hospital environments, where children are the minority of patients and systems for adult patients may be the default setup even if they are inappropriate for pediatric patients.

The American Academy of Pediatrics recommends patient- and family-centered rounds,[20] which require a multidisciplined commitment to participation in rounds, engagement of the family (with interpretation services as needed), and a physician leader who is skilled in patient- and family-centered care. There may be circumstances in which patient- and family-centered rounds are not performed either because of logistics (such as no available guardian) or family preference, but these should be exceptions to the standard of care.

CONCLUSIONS

The hospitalization of a child is a dramatic event for the child and the child's family. The physician's role in coordinating the hospitalization is to minimize the drama and trauma while maximizing the benefits to be gained from the hospitalization. Coordination of care should include careful attention to specific needs of the child and family and communication with all care providers to ensure safe transit from the outpatient arena, through the hospital, and back to the medical home.

LEAD AUTHOR

Daniel A. Rauch, MD, FAAP

COMMITTEE ON HOSPITAL CARE, 2017–2018

Jennifer Ann Jewell, MD, FAAP, Chairperson
Kimberly Dawn Ernst, MD, MSMI, FAAP
Vanessa Lynn Hill, MD, FAAP
Benson Shih-Han Hsu, MD, MBA, FAAP
Vinh Thuy Lam, MD, FAAP
Daniel A. Rauch, MD, FAAP
Charles David Vinocur, MD, FAAP

FORMER COMMITTEE MEMBER

Claudia K. Preuschoff, MD, FAAP

LIAISONS

Karen Castleberry – *Family Liaison*
Barbara Romito, MA, CCLS – *Association of Child Life Professionals*
Michael S. Leonard, MD, FAAP – *The Joint Commission Professional and Technical Advisory Council*

ABBREVIATION

EHR: electronic health record

FINANCIAL DISCLOSURE: Dr Rauch has indicated he serves as Chair of the American Board of Pediatrics Hospital Medicine Sub-board and receives $4800 annually as part of that position.

FUNDING: No external funding.

POTENTIAL CONFLICT OF INTEREST: The author has indicated he has no potential conflicts of interest to disclose.

REFERENCES

1. Berdahl TA, Friedman BS, McCormick MC, Simpson L. Annual report on health care for children and youth in the United States: trends in racial/ethnic, income, and insurance disparities over time, 2002-2009. *Acad Pediatr.* 2013;13(3):191–203

2. Friedman B, Berdahl T, Simpson LA, et al. Annual report on health care for children and youth in the United States: focus on trends in hospital use and quality. *Acad Pediatr.* 2011;11(4):263–279

3. Boudreau AA, Perrin JM, Goodman E, Kurowski D, Cooley WC, Kuhlthau K. Care coordination and unmet specialty care among children with special health care needs. *Pediatrics.* 2014;133(6):1046–1053

4. Starmer AJ, Sectish TC, Simon DW, et al. Rates of medical errors and preventable adverse events among hospitalized children following implementation of a resident handoff bundle. *JAMA.* 2013;310(21):2262–2270

5. Haig KM, Sutton S, Whittington J. SBAR: a shared mental model for improving communication between clinicians. *Jt Comm J Qual Patient Saf.* 2006;32(3):167–175

6. Lye PS; American Academy of Pediatrics; Committee on Hospital Care and Section on Hospital Medicine. Clinical report—physicians' roles in coordinating care of hospitalized children. *Pediatrics.* 2010;126(4):829–832

7. Elias ER, Murphy NA; Council on Children With Disabilities. Home care of children and youth with complex health care needs and technology dependencies. *Pediatrics.* 2012;129(5):996–1005

8. Merrill CT, Owens PL. *HCUP Statistical Brief No. 33: Reasons for Being Admitted to the Hospital Through the Emergency Department for Children and Adolescents, 2004.* Rockville, MD: Agency for Healthcare Research and Quality; 2007. Available at: www.hcup-us.ahrq.gov/reports/statbriefs/sb33.pdf. Accessed December 10, 2015

9. Goldenring J, Rosen D. Getting into adolescent heads: an essential update. *Contemp Pediatr.* 2004;21(1):64–90

10. Lindholm M, Hargraves JL, Ferguson WJ, Reed G. Professional language interpretation and inpatient length of stay and readmission rates. *J Gen Intern Med.* 2012;27(10):1294–1299

11. Horwitz LI, Moin T, Green ML. Development and implementation of an oral sign-out skills curriculum. *J Gen Intern Med.* 2007;22(10):1470–1474

12. Starmer AJ, Spector ND, Srivastava R, Allen AD, Landrigan CP, Sectish TC; I-PASS Study Group. I-pass, a mnemonic to standardize verbal handoffs. *Pediatrics.* 2012;129(2):201–204

13. Schaffzin JK, Simon TD. Pediatric hospital medicine role in the comanagement of the hospitalized surgical patient. *Pediatr Clin North Am.* 2014;61(4):653–661

14. Rappaport DI, Rosenberg RE, Shaughnessy EE, et al. Pediatric hospitalist comanagement of surgical patients: structural, quality, and financial considerations. *J Hosp Med.* 2014;9(11):737–742

15. Simon TD, Mahant S, Cohen E. Pediatric hospital medicine and children with medical complexity: past, present, and future. *Curr Probl Pediatr Adolesc Health Care.* 2012;42(5):113–119

16. California Department of Health Care Services; California Children's Services. Standards for hospitals. In: *California Children's Services Manual of Procedures.* Sacramento, CA: California Department of Health Care Services; 1999. Available at: www.dhcs.ca.gov/services/ccs/Documents/PedCommunity.pdf. Accessed December 10, 2015

17. Wachter RM, Auerbach AD. Filling the black hole of hospital discharge (editorial in response to article by Walz et al., *J Gen Intern Med* 2011). *J Gen Intern Med.* 2011;26(4):354–355

18. Rauch DA; Committee on Hospital Care; Section on Hospital Medicine. Medical staff appointment and delineation of pediatric privileges in hospitals. *Pediatrics*. 2012;129(4):784–787

19. American Academy of Pediatrics Committee on Hospital Care. Clinical report: standardization of inpatient handoff communication. *Pediatrics*.2016;138(5):e20162681

20. Committee on Hospital Care and Institute for Patient- and Family-Centered Care. Patient- and family-centered care and the pediatrician's role. *Pediatrics*. 2012;129(2):394–404

The Power of Play: A Pediatric Role in Enhancing Development in Young Children

- *Clinical Report*

CLINICAL REPORT   Guidance for the Clinician in Rendering Pediatric Care

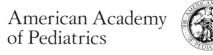

American Academy
of Pediatrics

DEDICATED TO THE HEALTH OF ALL CHILDREN™

The Power of Play: A Pediatric Role in Enhancing Development in Young Children

Michael Yogman, MD, FAAP,[a] Andrew Garner, MD, PhD, FAAP,[b] Jeffrey Hutchinson, MD, FAAP,[c] Kathy Hirsh-Pasek, PhD,[d] Roberta Michnick Golinkoff, PhD,[e] COMMITTEE ON PSYCHOSOCIAL ASPECTS OF CHILD AND FAMILY HEALTH, COUNCIL ON COMMUNICATIONS AND MEDIA

abstract

Children need to develop a variety of skill sets to optimize their development and manage toxic stress. Research demonstrates that developmentally appropriate play with parents and peers is a singular opportunity to promote the social-emotional, cognitive, language, and self-regulation skills that build executive function and a prosocial brain. Furthermore, play supports the formation of the safe, stable, and nurturing relationships with all caregivers that children need to thrive.

Play is not frivolous: it enhances brain structure and function and promotes executive function (ie, the process of learning, rather than the content), which allow us to pursue goals and ignore distractions.

When play and safe, stable, nurturing relationships are missing in a child's life, toxic stress can disrupt the development of executive function and the learning of prosocial behavior; in the presence of childhood adversity, play becomes even more important. The mutual joy and shared communication and attunement (harmonious serve and return interactions) that parents and children can experience during play regulate the body's stress response. This clinical report provides pediatric providers with the information they need to promote the benefits of play and and to write a prescription for play at well visits to complement reach out and read. At a time when early childhood programs are pressured to add more didactic components and less playful learning, pediatricians can play an important role in emphasizing the role of a balanced curriculum that includes the importance of playful learning for the promotion of healthy child development.

[a]Department of Pediatrics, Harvard Medical School, Harvard University and Mount Auburn Hospital, Cambridge, Massachusetts; [b]Department of Pediatrics, School of Medicine, Case Western Reserve University and University Hospitals Medical Practices, Cleveland, Ohio; [c]Department of Pediatrics, F. Edward Hebert School of Medicine, Uniformed Services University, Bethesda, Maryland; [d]Department of Psychology, Brookings Institution and Temple University, Philadelphia, Pennsylvania; and [e]School of Education, University of Delaware, Newark, Delaware

Dr Yogman prepared the first draft of this report and took the lead in reconciling the numerous edits, contributions, and suggestions from the other authors; Drs Garner, Hutchinson, Hirsh-Pasek, and Golinkoff made significant contributions to the manuscript by revising multiple drafts and responding to all reviewer concerns; and all authors approved the final manuscript as submitted.

To cite: Yogman M, Garner A, Hutchinson J, et al; AAP COMMITTEE ON PSYCHOSOCIAL ASPECTS OF CHILD AND FAMILY HEALTH, AAP COUNCIL ON COMMUNICATIONS AND MEDIA. The Power of Play: A Pediatric Role in Enhancing Development in Young Children. *Pediatrics.* 2018;142(3):e20182058

INTRODUCTION

Since the publication of the American Academy of Pediatrics (AAP) Clinical Reports on the importance of play in 2007,[1,2] newer research has provided additional evidence of the critical importance of play in facilitating parent engagement; promoting safe, stable, and nurturing relationships; encouraging the development of numerous competencies, including executive functioning skills; and improving life course trajectories.[3–5] An increasing societal focus on academic readiness (promulgated by the No Child Left Behind Act of 2001) has led to a focus on structured activities that are designed to promote academic results as early as preschool, with a corresponding decrease in playful learning. Social skills, which are part of playful learning, enable children to listen to directions, pay attention, solve disputes with words, and focus on tasks without constant supervision.[6] By contrast, a recent trial of an early mathematics intervention in preschool showed almost no gains in math achievement in later elementary school.[7] Despite criticism from early childhood experts, the 2003 Head Start Act reauthorization ended the program evaluation of social emotional skills and was focused almost exclusively on preliteracy and premath skills.[8] The AAP report on school readiness includes an emphasis on the importance of whole child readiness (including social–emotional, attentional, and cognitive skills).[9] Without that emphasis, children's ability to pay attention and behave appropriately in the classroom is disadvantaged.

The definition of play is elusive. However, there is a growing consensus that it is an activity that is intrinsically motivated, entails active engagement, and results in joyful discovery. Play is voluntary and often has no extrinsic goals; it is fun and often spontaneous. Children are often seen actively engaged in and passionately engrossed in play; this builds executive functioning skills and contributes to school readiness (bored children will not learn well).[10] Play often creates an imaginative private reality, contains elements of make believe, and is nonliteral.

Depending on the culture of the adults in their world, children learn different skills through play. Sociodramatic play is when children act out the roles of adulthood from having observed the activities of their elders. Extensive studies of animal play suggest that the function of play is to build a prosocial brain that can interact effectively with others.[11]

Play is fundamentally important for learning 21st century skills, such as problem solving, collaboration, and creativity, which require the executive functioning skills that are critical for adult success. The United Nations Convention on the Rights of the Child has enshrined the right to engage in play that is appropriate to the age of the child in Article 21.[12] In its 2012 exhibit "The Century of the Child: 1900–2000," the Museum of Modern Art noted, "Play is to the 21st century what work was to industrialization. It demonstrates a way of knowing, doing, and creating value."[13] Resnick[14] has described 4 guiding principles to support creative learning in children: projects, passion, peers, and play. Play is not just about having fun but about taking risks, experimenting, and testing boundaries. Pediatricians can be influential advocates by encouraging parents and child care providers to play with children and to allow children to have unstructured time to play as well as by encouraging educators to recognize playful learning as an important complement to didactic learning. Some studies[15–18] note that the new information economy, as opposed to the older industrial 1, demands more innovation and less imitation, more creativity and less conformity. Research on children's learning indicates that learning thrives when children are given some agency (control of their own actions) to play a role in their own learning.[19] The demands of today's world require that the teaching methods of the past 2 centuries, such as memorization, be replaced by innovation, application, and transfer.[18]

NATURE OF LEARNING AND PLAY

Bruner et al[20] stressed the fact that play is typically buffered from real-life consequences. Play is part of our evolutionary heritage, occurs in a wide spectrum of species, is fundamental to health, and gives us opportunities to practice and hone the skills needed to live in a complex world.[21] Although play is present in a large swath of species within the animal kingdom, from invertebrates (such as the octopus, lizard, turtle, and honey bee) to mammals (such as rats, monkeys, and humans),[22] social play is more prominent in animals with a large neocortex.[23] Studies of animal behavior suggests that play provides animals and humans with skills that will help them with survival and reproduction.[24] Locomotor skills learned through rough-and-tumble play enables escape from predators. However, animals play even when it puts them at risk of predation.[25] It is also suggested that play teaches young animals what they can and cannot do at times when they are relatively free from the survival pressures of adult life.[26] Play and learning are inextricably linked.[27] A Russian psychologist recognized that learning occurs when children actively engage in practical activities within a supportive social context. The accumulation of new knowledge is built on previous learning, but the acquisition of new skills is facilitated by social and often playful interactions. He was interested in what he called the "zone of proximal development," which consists of mastering skills that a child could not do alone but could be developed with minimal assistance.[28] Within the zone of proximal development, the "how" of learning occurs through a reiterative process called scaffolding, in which new skills are built on previous skills and are facilitated by a supportive social environment. The construct of scaffolding has been extrapolated to younger children. Consider how a social smile at 6 to 8 weeks of age invites cooing conversations, which leads to the reciprocal dance of social communication even before language emerges, followed by social referencing (the reading of a parent's face for nonverbal emotional content). The balance between facilitating unstructured playtime for children and encouraging adult scaffolding of play will vary depending on the competing needs in individual families, but the "serve-and-return" aspect of play requires caregiver engagement.[29]

Early learning and play are fundamentally social activities[30] and fuel the development of language and thought. Early learning also combines playful discovery with the development of social–emotional skills. It has been demonstrated that children playing with toys act like scientists and learn by looking and listening to those around them.[15–17] However, explicit instructions limit a child's creativity; it is argued that we should let children learn through observation and active engagement rather than passive memorization or direct instruction. Preschool children do benefit from learning content, but programs have many more didactic components than they did 20 years ago.[31] Successful programs are those that encourage playful learning in which children are actively engaged in meaningful discovery.[32] To encourage learning, we need to talk to children, let them play, and let them watch what we do as we go about our everyday lives. These opportunities foster the development of executive functioning skills that are critically important for the development of 21st century skills, such as collaboration, problem

solving, and creativity, according to the 2010 IBM's Global CEO Study.[33]

CATEGORIES OF PLAY

Play has been categorized in a variety of ways, each with its own developmental sequence.[32,34]

Object Play

This type of play occurs when an infant or child explores an object and learns about its properties. Object play progresses from early sensorimotor explorations, including the use of the mouth, to the use of symbolic objects (eg, when a child uses a banana as a telephone) for communication, language, and abstract thought.

Physical, Locomotor, or Rough-and-Tumble Play

This type of play progresses from pat-a-cake games in infants to the acquisition of foundational motor skills in toddlers[35] and the free play seen at school recess. The development of foundational motor skills in childhood is essential to promoting an active lifestyle and the prevention of obesity.[36–39] Learning to cooperate and negotiate promotes critical social skills. Extrapolation from animal data suggests that guided competition in the guise of rough-and-tumble play allows all participants to occasionally win and learn how to lose graciously.[40] Rough-and-tumble play, which is akin to the play seen in animals, enables children to take risks in a relatively safe environment, which fosters the acquisition of skills needed for communication, negotiation, and emotional balance and encourages the development of emotional intelligence. It enables risk taking and encourages the development of empathy because children are guided not to inflict harm on others.[25,30,40] The United Kingdom has modified its guidelines on play, arguing that the culture has gone too far by leaching

healthy risks out of childhood: new guidelines on play by the national commission state, "The goal is not to eliminate risk."[41]

Outdoor Play

Outdoor play provides the opportunity to improve sensory integration skills.[36,37,39] These activities involve the child as an active participant and address motor, cognitive, social, and linguistic domains. Viewed in this light, school recess becomes an essential part of a child's day.[42] It is not surprising that countries that offer more recess to young children see greater academic success among the children as they mature.[42,43] Supporting and implementing recess not only sends a message that exercise is fundamentally important for physical health but likely brings together children from diverse backgrounds to develop friendships as they learn and grow.[42]

Social or Pretend Play Alone or With Others

This type of play occurs when children experiment with different social roles in a nonliteral fashion. Play with other children enables them to negotiate "the rules" and learn to cooperate. Play with adults often involves scaffolding, as when an adult rotates a puzzle to help the child place a piece. Smiling and vocal attunement, in which infants learn turn taking, is the earliest example of social play. Older children can develop games and activities through which they negotiate relationships and guidelines with other players. Dress up, make believe, and imaginary play encourage the use of more sophisticated language to communicate with playmates and develop common rule-bound scenarios (eg, "You be the teacher, and I will be the student").

Play has also been grouped as self-directed versus adult guided. Self-directed play, or free play, is crucial to children's exploration of the world and understanding of their preferences and interests.[19,32,44] Guided play retains the child agency, such that the child initiates the play, but it occurs either in a setting that an adult carefully constructs with a learning goal in mind (eg, a children's museum exhibit or a Montessori task) or in an environment where adults supplement the child-led exploration with questions or comments that subtly guide the child toward a goal. Board games that have well-defined goals also fit into this category.[45] For example, if teachers want children to improve executive functioning skills (see the "Tools of the Mind" curriculum),[46] they could create drum-circle games, in which children coregulate their behavior. Familiar games such as "Simon Says" or "Head, Shoulders, Knees, and Toes" ask children to control their individual actions or impulses and have been shown to improve executive functioning skills.[47] Guided play has been defined as a child-led, joyful activity in which adults craft the environment to optimize learning.[4,48] This approach harkens back to Vygotsky[28] and the zone of proximal development, which represents the skills that children are unable to master on their own but are able to master in the context of a safe, stable, and nurturing relationship with an adult. The guidance and dialogue provided by the adult allow the child to master skills that would take longer to master alone and help children focus on the elements of the activity to guide learning. One way to think about guided play is as "constrained tinkering."[14,48] This logic also characterizes Italy's Emilio Reggio approach, which emphasizes the importance of teaching children to listen and look.

According to Vygotsky,[28] the most efficient learning occurs in a social context, where learning is scaffolded by the teacher into meaningful contexts that resonate with children's active engagement and previous experiences. Scaffolding is a part of guided play; caregivers are needed to provide the appropriate amount of input and guidance for children to develop optimal skills.

DEVELOPMENT OF PLAY

How does play develop? Play progresses from social smiling to reciprocal serve-and-return interactions; the development of babbling; games, such as "peek-a-boo"; hopping, jumping, skipping, and running; and fantasy or rough-and-tumble play. The human infant is born immature compared with infants of other species, with substantial brain development occurring after birth. Infants are entirely dependent on parents to regulate sleep–wake rhythms, feeding cycles, and many social interactions. Play facilitates the progression from dependence to independence and from parental regulation to self-regulation. It promotes a sense of agency in the child. This evolution begins in the first 3 months of life, when parents (both mothers and fathers) interact reciprocally with their infants by reading their nonverbal cues in a responsive, contingent manner.[49] Caregiver–infant interaction is the earliest form of play, known as attunement,[50] but it is quickly followed by other activities that also involve the taking of turns. These serve-and-return behaviors promote self-regulation and impulse control in children and form a strong foundation for understanding their interaction with adults. The back-and-forth episodes also feed into the development of language.

Reciprocal games occur with both mothers and fathers[51] and often begin in earnest with the emergence of social smiles at 6 weeks of age. Parents mimic their infant's "ooh" and "ah" in back-and-forth verbal games, which progress into conversations in which the parents utter pleasantries ("Oh, you had a good lunch!"), and the child responds by vocalizing back. Uncontrollable crying as a response to stress in a 1-year-old is replaced as the child reaches 2 to 3 years of age with the use of words to self-soothe, building on caregivers scaffolding their emotional responses. Already by 6 months of age, the introduction of solid foods requires the giving and receiving of reciprocal signals and communicative cues. During these activities, analyses of physiologic heart rate rhythms of infants with both their mothers and fathers have shown synchrony.[49,52]

By 9 months of age, mutual regulation is manifested in the way infants use their parents for social referencing.[53,54] In the classic visual cliff experiment, it was demonstrated that an infant will crawl across a Plexiglas dropoff to explore if the mother encourages the infant but not if she frowns. Nonverbal communication slowly leads to formal verbal language skills through which emotions such as happiness, sadness, and anger are identified for the child via words. Uncontrollable crying in the 1-year-old then becomes whining in the 2-year-old and verbal requests for assistance in the 3-year-old as parents scaffold the child's emotional responses and help him or her develop alternative, more adaptive behaviors. Repetitive games, such as peek-a-boo and "this little piggy," offer children the joy of being able to predict what is about to happen, and these games also enhance the infants' ability to solicit social stimulation.

By 12 months of age, a child's experiences are helping to lay the foundation for the ongoing development of social skills. The expression of true joy and mastery on children's faces when they take their first step is truly a magical moment that all parents remember. Infant memory, in Piagetian terms, develops as infants develop object permanence through visible and invisible displacements, such as repetitive games like peek-a-boo. With the advent of locomotor skills, rough-and-tumble play becomes increasingly available. During the second year, toddlers learn to explore their world, develop the beginnings of self-awareness, and use their parents as a home base (secure attachment), frequently checking to be sure that the world they are exploring is safe.[55] As children become independent, their ability to socially self-regulate becomes apparent: they can focus their attention and solve problems efficiently, they are less impulsive, and they can better manage the stress of strong emotions.[56] With increased executive functioning skills, they can begin to reflect on how they should respond to a situation rather than reacting impulsively. With the development of language and symbolic functioning, pretend play now becomes more prominent.[57] Fantasy play, dress up, and fort building now join the emotional and social repertoire of older children just as playground activities, tag, and hide and seek develop motor skills. In play, children are also solving problems and learning to focus attention, all of which promote the growth of executive functioning skills.

EFFECTS ON BRAIN STRUCTURE AND FUNCTIONING

Play is not frivolous; it is brain building. Play has been shown to have both direct and indirect effects on brain structure and functioning. Play leads to changes at the molecular (epigenetic), cellular (neuronal connectivity), and behavioral levels (socioemotional and executive functioning skills) that promote learning and adaptive and/or prosocial behavior. Most of this research on brain structure and functioning has been done with rats

and cannot be directly extrapolated to humans.

Jaak Panksepp,[11] a neuroscientist and psychologist who has extensively studied the neurologic basis of emotion in animals, suggests that play is 1 of 7 innate emotional systems in the midbrain.[58] Rats love rough-and-tumble play and produce a distinctive sound that Panksepp labeled "rat laughter."[42,59–64] When rats are young, play appears to initiate lasting changes in areas of the brain that are used for thinking and processing social interaction.

The dendritic length, complexity, and spine density of the medial prefrontal cortex (PFC) are refined by play.[64–67] The brain-derived neurotrophic factor (BDNF) is a member of the neurotrophin family of growth factors that acts to support the survival of existing neurons and encourage the growth and differentiation of new neurons and synapses. It is known to be important for long-term memory and social learning. Play stimulates the production of BDNF in RNA in the amygdala, dorsolateral frontal cortex, hippocampus, and pons.[65,68–70] Gene expression analyses indicate that the activities of approximately one-third of the 1200 genes in the frontal and posterior cortical regions were significantly modified by play within an hour after a 30-minute play session.[69,70] The gene that showed the largest effect was BDNF. Conversely, rat pup adversity, depression, and stress appear to result in the methylation and downregulation of the BDNF gene in the PFC.[71]

Two hours per day of play with objects predicted changes in brain weight and efficiency in experimental animals.[11,66] Rats that were deprived of play as pups (kept in sparse cages devoid of toys) not only were less competent at problem solving later on (negotiating mazes) but the medial PFC of the play-deprived rats was significantly more immature,

suggesting that play deprivation interfered with the process of synaptogenesis and pruning.[72] Rat pups that were isolated during peak play periods after birth (weeks 4 and 5) are much less socially active when they encounter other rats later in life.[73,74]

Play-deprived rats also showed impaired problem-solving skills, suggesting that through play, animals learn to try new things and develop behavioral flexibility.[73] Socially reared rats with damage to their PFC mimic the social deficiencies of rats with intact brains but who were deprived of play as juveniles.[66] The absence of the play experience leads to anatomically measurable changes in the neurons of the PFC. By refining the functional organization of the PFC, play enhances the executive functioning skills derived from this part of the brain.[66] Whether these effects are specific to play deprivation or merely reflect the generic effect of a lack of stimulation requires further study. Rats that were raised in experimental toy-filled cages had bigger brains and thicker cerebral cortices and completed mazes more quickly.[67,75]

Brain neurotransmitters, such as dopamine made by cells in the substantia nigra and ventral tegmentum, are also related to the reward quality of play: drugs that activate dopamine receptors increase play behavior in rats.[76]

Play and stress are closely linked. High amounts of play are associated with low levels of cortisol, suggesting either that play reduces stress or that unstressed animals play more.[23] Play also activates norepinephrine, which facilitates learning at synapses and improves brain plasticity. Play, especially when accompanied by nurturing caregiving, may indirectly affect brain functioning by modulating or buffering adversity and by reducing toxic stress to levels that are more compatible with coping and resilience.[77,78]

In human children, play usually enhances curiosity, which facilitates memory and learning. During states of high curiosity, functional MRI results showed enhanced activity in healthy humans in their early 20s in the midbrain and nucleus accumbens and functional connectivity to the hippocampus, which solidifies connections between intrinsic motivation and hippocampus-dependent learning.[79] Play helps children deal with stress, such as life transitions. When 3- to 4-year-old children who were anxious about entering preschool were randomly assigned to play with toys or peers for 15 minutes compared with listening to a teacher reading a story, the play group showed a twofold decrease in anxiety after the intervention.[24,80] In another study, preschool children with disruptive behavior who engaged with teachers in a yearlong 1-to-1 play session designed to foster warm, caring relationships (allowing children to lead, narrating the children's behavior out loud, and discussing the children's emotions as they played) showed reduced salivary cortisol stress levels during the day and improved behavior compared with children in the control group.[81] The notable exception is with increased stress experienced by children with autism spectrum disorders in new or social circumstances.[82] Animal studies suggest the role of play as a social buffer. Rats that were previously induced to be anxious became relaxed and calm after rough-and-tumble play with a nonanxious playful rat.[83] Extrapolating from these animal studies, one can suggest that play may serve as an effective buffer for toxic stress.

BENEFITS OF PLAY

The benefits of play are extensive and well documented and include improvements in executive functioning, language, early math skills (numerosity and spatial concepts), social development, peer relations, physical development and health, and enhanced sense of agency.[13,32,56,57,84–88] The opposite is also likely true; Panksepp[89] suggested that play deprivation is associated with the increasing prevalence of attention-deficit/hyperactivity disorder.[90]

Executive functioning, which is described as the process of how we learn over the content of what we learn, is a core benefit of play and can be characterized by 3 dimensions: cognitive flexibility, inhibitory control, and working memory. Collectively, these dimensions allow for sustained attention, the filtering of distracting details, improved self-regulation and self-control, better problem solving, and mental flexibility. Executive functioning helps children switch gears and transition from drawing with crayons to getting dressed for school. The development of the PFC and executive functioning balances and moderates the impulsiveness, emotionality, and aggression of the amygdala. In the presence of childhood adversity, the role of play becomes even more important in that the mutual joy and shared attunement that parents and children can experience during play downregulates the body's stress response.[91–94] Hence, play may be an effective antidote to the changes in amygdala size, impulsivity, aggression, and uncontrolled emotion that result from significant childhood adversity and toxic stress. Future research is needed to clarify this association.

Opportunities for peer engagement through play cultivate the ability to negotiate. Peer play usually involves problem solving about the rules of the game, which requires negotiation and cooperation. Through these encounters, children learn to use more sophisticated language when playing with peers.[95,96]

Play in a variety of forms (active physical play, pretend play, and play with traditional toys and shape sorters [rather than digital toys]) improves children's skills. When children were given blocks to play with at home with minimal adult direction, preschool children showed improvements in language acquisition at a 6-month follow-up, particularly low-income children. The authors suggest that the benefits of Reach Out and Play may promote development just as Reach Out and Read does.[97] When playing with objects under minimal adult direction, preschool children named an average of 3 times as many nonstandard uses for an object compared with children who were given specific instructions.[98] In Jamaica, toddlers with growth retardation who were given weekly play sessions to improve mother–child interactions for 2 years were followed to adulthood and showed better educational attainment, less depression, and less violent behavior.[3]

Children who were in active play for 1 hour per day were better able to think creatively and multitask.[22] Randomized trials of physical play in 7- to 9-year-olds revealed enhanced attentional inhibition, cognitive flexibility, and brain functioning that were indicative of enhanced executive control.[99] Play with traditional toys was associated with an increased quality and quantity of language compared with play with electronic toys,[100] particularly if the video toys did not encourage interaction.[101] Indeed, it has been shown that play with digital shape sorters rather than traditional shape sorters stunted the parent's use of spatial language.[102] Pretend play encourages self-regulation because children must collaborate on the imaginary environment and agree about pretending and conforming to roles, which improves their ability to reason about hypothetical events.[56,57,103–105] Social–emotional skills are increasingly viewed as related to academic and economic success.[106] Third-grade prosocial behavior correlated with eighth-grade reading and math better than with third-grade reading and math.[17,107]

The health benefits of play involving physical activity are many. Exercise not only promotes healthy weight and cardiovascular fitness but also can enhance the efficacy of the immune, endocrine, and cardiovascular systems.[37] Outdoor playtime for children in Head Start programs has been associated with decreased BMI.[39] Physical activity is associated with decreases in concurrent depressive symptoms.[108] Play decreases stress, fatigue, injury, and depression and increases range of motion, agility, coordination, balance, and flexibility.[109] Children pay more attention to class lessons after free play at recess than they do after physical education programs, which are more structured.[43] Perhaps they are more active during free play.

Play also reflects and transmits cultural values. In fact, recess began in the United States as a way to socially integrate immigrant children. Parents in the United States encourage children to play with toys and/or objects alone, which is typical of communities that emphasize the development of independence. Conversely, in Japan, peer social play with dolls is encouraged, which is typical of cultures that emphasize interdependence.[110]

BENEFITS TO ADULTS OF PLAYING WITH CHILDREN

Playing with children adds value not only for children but also for adult caregivers, who can reexperience or reawaken the joy of their own childhood and rejuvenate themselves. Through play and rereading their favorite childhood books, parents learn to see the world from their child's perspective and are likely to communicate more effectively with their child, even appreciating and sharing their child's sense of humor and individuality. Play enables children and adults to be passionately and totally immersed in an activity of their choice and to experience intense joy, much as athletes do when they are engaging in their optimal performance. Discovering their true passions is another critical strategy for helping both children and adults cope with adversity. One study documented that positive parenting activities, such as playing and shared reading, result in decreases in parental experiences of stress and enhancement in the parent–child relationship, and these effects mediate relations between the activities and social–emotional development.[111–113]

Most importantly, play is an opportunity for parents to engage with their children by observing and understanding nonverbal behavior in young infants, participating in serve-andreturn exchanges, or sharing the joy and witnessing the blossoming of the passions in each of their children.

Play not only provides opportunities for fostering children's curiosity,[14] self-regulation skills,[46] language development, and imagination but also promotes the dyadic reciprocal interactions between children and parents, which is a crucial element of healthy relationships.[114] Through the buffering capacity of caregivers, play can serve as an antidote to toxic stress, allowing the physiologic stress response to return to baseline.[77] Adult success in later life can be related to the experience of childhood play that cultivated creativity, problem solving, teamwork, flexibility, and innovations.[18,52,115]

Successful scaffolding (new skills built on previous skills facilitated by a supportive social environment) can be contrasted with interactions in which adults direct children's play. It has been shown that if a caregiver instructs a child in how a toy works, the child is less likely to discover other attributes of the toy in contrast to a child being left to explore the toy without direct input.[38,116–118] Adults who facilitate a child's play without being intrusive can encourage the child's independent exploration and learning.

IMPLICATIONS FOR PRESCHOOL EDUCATION

Scaffolding play activities facilitated by adults enable children to work in groups: to share, negotiate, develop decision-making and problem-solving skills, and discover their own interests. Children learn to resolve conflicts and develop self-advocacy skills and their own sense of agency. The false dichotomy between play versus formal learning is now being challenged by educational reformers who acknowledge the value of playful learning or guided play, which captures the strengths of both approaches and may be essential to improving executive functioning.[18,19,34,119] Hirsh-Pasek et al[34] report a similar finding: children have been shown to discover causal mechanisms more quickly when they drive their learning as opposed to when adults display solutions for them.

Executive functioning skills are foundational for school readiness and academic success, mandating a frame shift with regard to early education. The goal today is to support interventions that cultivate a range of skills, such as executive functioning, in all children so that the children enter preschool and kindergarten curious and knowing how to learn. Kindergarten should provide children with an opportunity for playful collaboration and tinkering,[14] a different approach from the model that promotes more exclusive didactic learning at the expense of playful learning. The emerging alternative model is to prevent toxic stress and build resilience by developing executive functioning skills. Ideally, we want to protect the brain to enable it to learn new skills, and we want to focus on learning those skills that will be used to buffer the brain from any future adversity.[18] The Center on the Developing Child at Harvard University offers an online resource on play and executive functioning with specific activities suggested for parents and children (http://developingchild.harvard.edu/wp-content/uploads/2015/05/Enhancing-and-Practicing-Executive-Function-Skills-with-Children-from-Infancy-to-Adolescence-1.pdf).[120]

Specific curricula have now been developed and tested in preschools to help children develop executive functioning skills. Many innovative programs are using either the Reggio Emilia philosophy or curricula such as Tools of the Mind (developed in California)[121] or Promoting Alternative Thinking Strategies–Preschool and/or Kindergarten.[122] Caregivers need to provide the appropriate amount of input and guidance for children to develop optimal problem-solving skills through guided play and scaffolding. Optimal learning can be depicted by a bell-shaped curve, which illustrates the optimal zone of arousal and stress for complex learning.[123]

Scaffolding is extensively used to support skills such as buddy reading, in which children take turns being lips and ears and learn to read and listen to each other as an example of guided play. A growing body of research shows that this curriculum not only improves executive functioning skills but also shows improvement in brain functioning on functional MRI.[6,124–126]

Focusing on cultivating executive functioning and other skills through playful learning in these early years

is an alternative and innovative way of thinking about early childhood education. Instead of focusing solely on academic skills, such as reciting the alphabet, early literacy, using flash cards, engaging with computer toys, and teaching to tests (which has been overemphasized to promote improved test results), cultivating the joy of learning through play is likely to better encourage long-term academic success. Collaboration, negotiation, conflict resolution, self-advocacy, decision-making, a sense of agency, creativity, leadership, and increased physical activity are just some of the skills and benefits children gain through play.

MODERN CHALLENGES

For many families, there are risks in the current focus only on achievement, after-school enrichment programs, increased homework, concerns about test performance, and college acceptance. The stressful effects of this approach often result in the later development of anxiety and depression and a lack of creativity. Parental guilt has led to competition over who can schedule more "enrichment opportunities" for their children. As a result, there is little time left in the day for children's free play, for parental reading to children, or for family meal times. Many schools have cut recess, physical education, art, and music to focus on preparing children for tests. Unsafe local neighborhoods and playgrounds have led to nature deficit disorder for many children.[127] A national survey of 8950 preschool children and parents found that only 51% of children went outside to walk or play once per day with either parent.[128] In part, this may reflect the local environment: 94% of parents have expressed safety concerns about outdoor play, and access may be limited. Only 20%

of homes are located within a half-mile of a park.[129,130] Cultural changes have also jeopardized the opportunities children have to play. From 1981 to 1997, children's playtime decreased by 25%. Children 3 to 11 years of age have lost 12 hours per week of free time. Because of increased academic pressure, 30% of US kindergarten children no longer have recess.[42,129] An innovative program begun in Philadelphia is using cities (on everyday walks and in everyday neighborhoods) as opportunities for creating learning landscapes that provide opportunities for parents and children to spark conversation and playful learning.[131,132] For example, Ridge et al[132] have placed conversational prompts throughout supermarkets and laundromats to promote language and lights at bus stops to project designs on the ground, enabling children to play a game of hopscotch that is specifically designed to foster impulse control. By promoting the learning of social and emotional skills, the development of emotional intelligence, and the enjoyment of active learning, protected time for free play and guided play can be used to help children improve their social skills, literacy, and school readiness. Children can then enter school with a stronger foundation for attentional disposition based on the skills and attitudes that are critical for academic success and the long-term enjoyment of learning and love of school.

ROLE OF MEDIA IN CHILDREN'S PLAY

Media (eg, television, video games, and smartphone and tablet applications) use often encourages passivity and the consumption of others' creativity rather than active learning and socially interactive play. Most importantly, immersion in electronic media takes away time from real play, either outdoors or indoors. Real learning happens better in person-to-person exchanges rather than machine-to-person interactions. Most parents are eager to do the right thing for their children. However, advertisers and the media can mislead parents about how to best support and encourage their children's growth and development as well as creativity. Parent surveys have revealed that many parents see media and technology as the best way to help their children learn.[133] However, researchers contradict this. Researchers have compared preschoolers playing with blocks independently with preschoolers watching Baby Einstein tapes and have shown that the children playing with blocks independently developed better language and cognitive skills than their peers watching videos.[34,134] Although active engagement with age-appropriate media, especially if supported by cowatching or coplay with peers or parents, may have some benefits,[135] real-time social interactions remain superior to digital media for home learning.[136]

It is important for parents to understand that media use often does not support their goals of encouraging curiosity and learning for their children.[137–141] Despite research that reveals an association between television watching and a sedentary lifestyle and greater risks of obesity, the typical preschooler watches 4.5 hours of television per day, which displaces conversation with parents and the practice of joint attention (focus by the parent and child on a common object) as well as physical activity. For economically challenged families, competing pressures make it harder for parents to find the time to play with children. Encouraging outdoor exercise may be more difficult for such families given unsafe playgrounds. Easy access to electronic media can be difficult for parents to compete with.

In the 2015 symposium,[137] the AAP clarified recommendations acknowledging the ubiquity and transformation of media from primarily television to other modalities, including video chatting. In 2016, the AAP published 2 new policies on digital media affecting young children, school-aged children, and adolescents. These policies included recommendations for parents, pediatricians, and researchers to promote healthy media use.[139,140] The AAP has also launched a Family Media Use Plan to help parents and families create healthy guidelines for their children's media use so as to avoid displacing activities such as active play, and guidelines can also be found on the HealthyChildren.org and Common Sense Media (commonsensemedia. org) Web sites.

BARRIERS TO PLAY

There are barriers to encouraging play. Our culture is preoccupied with marketing products to young children.[142] Parents of young children who cannot afford expensive toys may feel left out.[143] Parents who can afford expensive toys and electronic devices may think that allowing their children unfettered access to these objects is healthy and promotes learning. The reality is that children's creativity and play is enhanced by many inexpensive toys (eg, wooden spoons, blocks, balls, puzzles, crayons, boxes, and simple available household objects) and by parents who engage with their children by reading, watching, playing alongside their children, and talking with and listening to their children. It is parents' and caregivers' presence and attention that enrich children, not elaborate electronic gadgets. One-on-one play is a time-tested way of being fully present. Low-income families may have less time to play with their children while working long hours to

provide for their families, but a warm caregiver or extended family as well as a dynamic community program can help support parents' efforts.[144] The importance of playtime with children cannot be overemphasized to parents as well as schools and community organizations. Many children do not have safe places to play.[145] Neighborhood threats, such as violence, guns, drugs, and traffic, pose safety concerns in many neighborhoods, particularly low-income areas. Children in low-income, urban neighborhoods also may have less access to quality public spaces and recreational facilities in their communities.[145] Parents who feel that their neighborhoods are unsafe may also not permit their children to play outdoors or independently.

Public health professionals are increasingly partnering with other sectors, such as parks and recreation, public safety, and community development, to advocate for safe play environments in all communities. This includes efforts to reduce community violence, improve physical neighborhood infrastructure, and support planning and design decisions that foster safe, clean, and accessible public spaces.

ROLE OF PEDIATRICIANS

Pediatricians can advocate for the importance of all forms of play as well as for the role of play in the development of executive functioning, emotional intelligence, and social skills (Table 1). Pediatricians have a critical role to play in protecting the integrity of childhood by advocating for all children to have the opportunity to express their innate curiosity in the world and their great capacity for imagination. For children with special needs, it is especially important to create safe opportunities for play. A children's museum may offer

TABLE 1 Recommendations From Pediatricians to Parents

Use play to help meet milestones. From birth, infants use play to explore the world around them as
   well as to learn and develop important life skills.

0–6 mo
   Show your infant interesting objects, such as a brightly colored mobile or toy.
   Talk to your infant often to familiarize him or her with your voice, and respond when he or she coos
      and babbles.
   Place your infant in different positions so he or she can see the world from different angles.
   Let your infant bring safe objects to his or her mouth to explore and experience new textures.
   Vary facial expressions and gestures so that your infant can imitate them. Imitate your infant's
      sounds and engage in a back-and-forth conversation using your infant's sounds as a prompt.

7–12 mo
   Use a mirror to show faces to your infant.
   Provide your infant with a safe environment to crawl and explore.
   Place your infant in a variety of positions, such as on his or her tummy, side, etc.
   Give your infant opportunities to learn that his or her actions have effects (for example, when he or
      she drops a toy and it falls to the ground). Put a few toys within the reach of your infant so he or
      she can take toys out and play with them.
   Play peek-a-boo.

1–3 y
   Allow your child to spend time with objects and toys that he or she enjoys.
   Give your child pens, markers, or crayons and paper to practice scribbling.
   Encourage your child to interact with peers.
   Help your child explore his or her body through different movements (for example, walking,
      jumping, and standing on 1 leg).
   Provide opportunities to create make-believe situations with objects (for example, pretending to
      drink out of an empty cup or offering toys that enable pretend play).
   Respond when your child speaks, answer questions, and provide verbal encouragement.
   Provide blocks, plastic containers, wooden spoons, and puzzles.
   Read regularly to and with your child. Encourage pretend play based on these stories.
   Sing songs and play rhythms so that your child can learn and join in the fun.

4–6 y
   Provide opportunities for your child to sing and dance.
   Tell stories to your child and ask questions about what he or she remembers.
   Give your child time and space to act out imaginary scenes, roles, and activities.
   Allow your child to move between make-believe games and reality (for example, playing house and
      helping you with chores).
   Schedule time for your child to interact with friends to practice socializing and building friendships.
   Encourage your child to try a variety of movements in a safe environment (for example, hopping,
      swinging, climbing, and doing somersaults).

Adapted from www.pathway.org.

special mornings when it is open only to children with special needs. Extra staffing enables these children and their siblings to play in a safe environment because they may not be able to participate during crowded routine hours.

The AAP recommends that pediatricians:

1. Encourage parents to observe and respond to the nonverbal behavior of infants during their first few months of life (eg, responding to their children's emerging social smile) to help them better understand this unique form of communication.

For example, encouraging parents to recognize their children's emerging social smile and to respond with a smile of their own is a form of play that also teaches the infants a critical social–emotional skill: "You can get my attention and a smile from me anytime you want just by smiling yourself." By encouraging parents to observe the behavior of their children, pediatricians create opportunities to engage parents in discussions that are nonjudgmental and free from criticism (because they are grounded in the parents' own observations and interpretations

of how to promote early learning);

2. Advocate for the protection of children's unstructured playtime because of its numerous benefits, including the development of foundational motor skills that may have lifelong benefits for the prevention of obesity, hypertension, and type 2 diabetes;

3. Advocate with preschool educators to do the following: focus on playful rather than didactic learning by letting children take the lead and follow their own curiosity; put a premium on building social–emotional and executive functioning skills throughout the school year; and protect time for recess and physical activity;

4. Emphasize the importance of playful learning in preschool curricula for fostering stronger caregiver–infant relationships and promoting executive functioning skills. Communicating this message to policy makers, legislators, and educational administrators as well as the broader public is equally important; and

5. Just as pediatricians support Reach Out and Read, encourage playful learning for parents and infants by writing a "prescription for play" at every well-child visit in the first 2 years of life.

A recent randomized controlled trial of the Video Interaction Project (an enhancement of Reach Out and Read) has demonstrated that the promotion of reading and play during pediatric visits leads to enhancements in social–emotional development.[112] In today's world, many parents do not appreciate the importance of free play or guided play with their children and have come to think of worksheets and other highly structured activities as play.[146] Although many parents feel that they do not have time to play with their children, pediatricians can help parents understand that playful learning moments are everywhere, and even daily chores alongside parents can be turned into playful opportunities, especially if the children are actively interacting with parents and imitating chores. Young children typically seek more attention from parents.[46] Active play stimulates children's curiosity and helps them develop the physical and social skills needed for school and later life.[32]

CONCLUSIONS

- Cultural shifts, including less parent engagement because of parents working full-time, fewer safe places to play, and more digital distractions, have limited the opportunities for children to play. These factors may negatively affect school readiness, children's healthy adjustment, and the development of important executive functioning skills;

- Play is intrinsically motivated and leads to active engagement and joyful discovery. Although free play and recess need to remain integral aspects of a child's day, the essential components of play can also be learned and adopted by parents, teachers, and other caregivers to promote healthy child development and enhance learning;

- The optimal educational model for learning is for the teacher to engage the student in activities that promote skills within that child's zone of proximal development, which is best accomplished through dialogue and guidance, not via drills and passive rote learning. There is a current debate, particularly about preschool curricula, between an emphasis on content and attempts to build skills by introducing seat work earlier

versus seeking to encourage active engagement in learning through play. With our understanding of early brain development, we suggest that learning is better fueled by facilitating the child's intrinsic motivation through play rather than extrinsic motivations, such as test scores;

- An alternative model for learning is for teachers to develop a safe, stable, and nurturing relationship with the child to decrease stress, increase motivation, and ensure receptivity to activities that promote skills within each child's zone of proximal development. The emphasis in this preventive and developmental model is to promote resilience in the presence of adversity by enhancing executive functioning skills with free play and guided play;

- Play provides ample opportunities for adults to scaffold the foundational motor, social–emotional, language, executive functioning, math, and self-regulation skills needed to be successful in an increasingly complex and collaborative world. Play helps to build the skills required for our changing world; and

- Play provides a singular opportunity to build the executive functioning that underlies adaptive behaviors at home; improve language and math skills in school; build the safe, stable, and nurturing relationships that buffer against toxic stress; and build social–emotional resilience.

For more information, see Kearney et al's *Using Joyful Activity To Build Resiliency in Children in Response to Toxic Stress.*[147]

LEAD AUTHORS

Michael Yogman, MD, FAAP
Andrew Garner, MD, PhD, FAAP
Jeffrey Hutchinson, MD, FAAP
Kathy Hirsh-Pasek, PhD
Roberta Golinkoff, PhD

CONTRIBUTOR

Virginia Keane, MD, FAAP

COMMITTEE ON PSYCHOSOCIAL ASPECTS OF CHILD AND FAMILY HEALTH, 2017–2018

Michael Yogman, MD, FAAP, Chairperson
Rebecca Baum, MD, FAAP
Thresia Gambon, MD, FAAP
Arthur Lavin, MD, FAAP
Gerri Mattson, MD, FAAP
Lawrence Wissow, MD, MPH, FAAP

LIAISONS

Sharon Berry, PhD, LP – *Society of Pediatric Psychology*
Amy Starin, PhD, LCSW – *National Association of Social Workers*
Edward Christophersen, PhD, FAAP – *Society of Pediatric Psychology*
Norah Johnson, PhD, RN, CPNP-BC – *National Association of Pediatric Nurse Practitioners*
Abigail Schlesinger, MD – *American Academy of Child and Adolescent Psychiatry*

STAFF

Karen S. Smith

COUNCIL ON COMMUNICATIONS AND MEDIA, 2017–2018

David L Hill, MD, FAAP, Chairperson
Nusheen Ameenuddin, MD, MPH, FAAP
Yolanda (Linda) Reid Chassiakos, MD, FAAP
Corinn Cross, MD, FAAP
Rhea Boyd, MD, FAAP
Robert Mendelson, MD, FAAP
Megan A Moreno, MD, MSEd, MPH, FAAP
Jenny Radesky, MD, FAAP
Wendy Sue Swanson, MD, MBE, FAAP
Jeffrey Hutchinson, MD, FAAP
Justin Smith, MD, FAAP

LIAISONS

Kristopher Kaliebe, MD – *American Academy of Child and Adolescent Psychiatry*
Jennifer Pomeranz, JD, MPH – *American Public Health Association Health Law Special Interest Group*
Brian Wilcox, PhD – *American Psychological Association*

STAFF

Thomas McPheron

ABBREVIATIONS

AAP: American Academy of Pediatrics
BDNF: brain-derived neurotrophic factor
PFC: prefrontal cortex

All clinical reports from the American Academy of Pediatrics automatically expire 5 years after publication unless reaffirmed, revised, or retired at or before that time.

DOI: https://doi.org/10.1542/peds.2018-2058

Address correspondence to Michael Yogman, MD, FAAP. E-mail: myogman@massmed.org

PEDIATRICS (ISSN Numbers: Print, 0031-4005; Online, 1098-4275).

FINANCIAL DISCLOSURE: The authors have indicated they have no financial relationships relevant to this article to disclose.

FUNDING: No external funding.

POTENTIAL CONFLICT OF INTEREST: The authors have indicated they have no potential conflicts of interest to disclose.

REFERENCES

1. Ginsburg KR; American Academy of Pediatrics Committee on Communications; American Academy of Pediatrics Committee on Psychosocial Aspects of Child and Family Health. The importance of play in promoting healthy child development and maintaining strong parent-child bonds. *Pediatrics.* 2007;119(1):182–191

2. Milteer RM, Ginsburg KR; Council on Communications and Media; Committee on Psychosocial Aspects of Child and Family Health. The importance of play in promoting healthy child development and maintaining strong parent-child bond: focus on children in poverty. *Pediatrics.* 2012;129(1). Available at: www.pediatrics.org/cgi/content/full/129/1/e204

3. Walker SP, Chang SM, Vera-Hernández M, Grantham-McGregor S. Early childhood stimulation benefits adult competence and reduces violent behavior. *Pediatrics.* 2011;127(5):849–857

4. Weisberg DS, Hirsh-Pasek K, Golinkoff RM, Kittredge AK, Klahr D. Guided play: principles and practices. *Curr Dir Psychol Sci.* 2016;25(3):177–182

5. Zelazo PD, Blair CB, Willoughby MT. *Executive Function: Implications for Education (NCER 2017-2000).* Washington, DC: National Center for Education Research, Institute of Education Sciences; 2017. Available at: https://ies.ed.gov/ncer/pubs/20172000/pdf/20172000.pdf. Accessed October 24, 2017

6. Diamond A, Barnett WS, Thomas J, Munro S. Preschool program improves cognitive control. *Science.* 2007;318(5855):1387–1388

7. Watts TW, Duncan GJ, Clements DH, Sarama J. What is the long-run impact of learning mathematics during preschool? *Child Dev.* 2018;89(2):539–555

8. Meisels SJ, Atkins-Burnett S. The Head start national reporting system: a critique. *Young Child.* 2004;59:64–66

9. High PC; American Academy of Pediatrics, Committee on Early Childhood, Adoption, and Dependent Care and Council on School Health. School readiness. *Pediatrics.* 2008;121(4). Available at: www.pediatrics.org/cgi/content/full/121/4/e1008. Reaffirmed September 2013

10. Henderson TZ, Atencio DJ. Integration of play, learning, and experience: what museums afford young visitors. *Early Child Educ J.* 2007;35(3):245–251

11. Panksepp J. *Affective Neuroscience: The Foundations of Human and Animal Emotions.* 1st ed. New York, NY: Oxford University Press; 1998

12. United Nations Human Rights Office of the Commissioner. Convention on the Rights of the Child. 1989. Available at: www.ohchr.org/EN/ProfessionalInterest/Pages/CRC.aspx. Accessed October 24, 2017

13. Kinchin J, O'Connor A. *Century of the Child: Growing by Design 1900-2000.* New York, NY: Museum of Modern Art; 2012. Available at: https://www.moma.org/interactives/exhibitions/2012/centuryofthechild/. Accessed October 24, 2017

14. Resnick M. *Lifelong Kindergarten: Cultivate Creativity Through Projects, Passion, Peers, and Play.* Cambridge, MA: MIT Press; 2017

15. Gopnik A. What babies know. *New York Times.* 2016;(July 31):4

16. Gopnik A. *The Garden and the Carpenter.* New York, NY: Farrar Straus and Giroux; 2016

17. Gopnik A, Meltzoff AN, Kuhl PK. *The Scientist in the Crib.* 1st ed. New York, NY: William Morrow and Co; 1999

18. Golinkoff R, Hirsh-Pasek K. *Becoming Brilliant: What Science Tells us About Raising Successful Children.* Washington, DC: APA Press; 2016

19. Hirsh-Pasek K, Zosh JM, Golinkoff RM, Gray JH, Robb MB, Kaufman J. Putting education in "educational" apps: lessons from the science of learning. *Psychol Sci Public Interest.* 2015;16(1):3–34

20. Bruner JS, Jolly A, Sylva K, eds. *Play: Its Role in Development and Evolution.* 1st ed. New York, NY: Basic Books; 1976

21. Toub TS, Rajan V, Golinkoff R, Hirsh-Pasek K. Playful learning: a solution to the play versus learning dichotomy. In: Berch D, Geary D, eds. *Evolutionary Perspectives on Education and Child Development.* New York, NY: Springer; 2016:117–145

22. Mather JA, Anderson RC. Exploration, play and habituation in octopuses (*Octopus dofleini*). *J Comp Psychol.* 1999;113(3):333–338

23. Wang S, Aamodt S. *Welcome to Your Child's Brain: How the Mind Grows From Conception to College.* New York, NY: Bloomsbury USA; 2011

24. Wenner M. The serious need for play. *Sci Am Mind.* 2009;20(1):22–29

25. Burghardt GM. *The Genesis of Animal Play: Testing the Limits.* 1st ed. Cambridge, MA: MIT Press; 2005

26. Goodall J. *In the Shadow of Man.* Boston, MA: Houghton Mifflin; 2010

27. Dewar G. The cognitive benefits of play: effects on the learning brain. Available at: www.parentingscience.com/benefits-of-play.html. Accessed October 24, 2017

28. Vygotsky LS. Play and its role in the mental development of the child. In: Bruner J, Jolly A, Sylva K, eds. *Play.* New York, NY: Basic Books; 1976:609–618

29. Berk L, Meyers AB. *Infants and Children: Prenatal Through Middle Childhood.* 8th ed. New York, NY: Plenum; 2015

30. Pellis SM, Pellis VC, Bell HC. The function of play in the development of the social brain. *Am J Play.* 2010;2:278–296

31. Moore JL, Waltman K. Pressure to increase test scores in reaction to NCLB: an investigation of related factors. In: *Meeting of the American Educational Research and Evaluation Association;* September 2007; Chicago, IL

32. Hirsh-Pasek K, Golinkoff RM, Berk L, Singer DG. *A Mandate for Playful Learning in Preschool.* New York, NY: Oxford University Press; 2009

33. Tomasco S. IBM 2010 Global CEO Study: creativity selected as most crucial factor for future success. Available at: https://www.o3.ibm.com/press/us/en/pressrelease/31670.wss. Accessed April 27, 2018

34. Hirsh-Pasek K, Golinkoff RM, Eyer D. *Einstein Never Used Flashcards: How Our Children Really Learn—and Why They Need to Play More and Memorize Less.* Pleasant Valley, NY: Rosedale; 2003

35. Logan SW, Robinson LE, Wilson AE, Lucas WA. Getting the fundamentals of movement: a meta-analysis of the effectiveness of motor skill interventions in children. *Child Care Health Dev.* 2012;38(3):305–315

36. Pellegrini AD, Smith PK. Physical activity play: the nature and function of a neglected aspect of playing. *Child Dev.* 1998;69(3):577–598

37. Lubans DR, Morgan PJ, Cliff DP, Barnett LM, Okely AD. Fundamental movement skills in children and adolescents: review of associated health benefits. *Sports Med.* 2010;40(12):1019–1035

38. Gopnik A. How babies think. *Sci Am.* 2010;303(1):76–81

39. Ansari A, Pettit K, Gershoff E. Combating obesity in head start: outdoor play and change in children's body mass index. *J Dev Behav Pediatr.* 2015;36(8):605–612

40. Pellis SM, Pellis VC. Play fighting of rats in comparative perspective: a schema for neurobehavioral analyses. *Neurosci Biobehav Rev.* 1998;23(1):87–101

41. Barry E. In British playgrounds, bringing in risk to build resilience. *New York Times.* March 10, 2018. Available at: https://www.nytimes.com/2018/03/10/world/europe/britain-playgrounds-risk.html. Accessed April 27, 2018

42. Murray R, Ramstetter C; Council on School Health; American Academy of Pediatrics. The crucial role of recess in school. *Pediatrics.* 2013;131(1):183–188

43. Pelligrini AD, Holmes RM. The role of recess in primary school. In: Singer D, Golinkoff R, Hirsh-Pasek K, eds. *Play = Learning: How Play Motivates and Enhances Children's Cognitive and Socio-Emotional Growth.* New York, NY: Oxford University Press; 2006

44. Fisher KR, Hirsh-Pasek K, Golinkoff RM, Gryfe SG. Conceptual split? Parents and experts perceptions of play in the 21st century. *J Appl Dev Psychol.* 2008;29:305–316

45. Hassinger-Das B, Toub TS, Zosh JM, Michnick J, Golinkoff R, Hirsh-Pasek K. More than just fun: a place for games in joyful learning. *J Study Educ Dev.* 2017;40(2):191–218

46. Galinsky E. *Mind in the Making.* 1st ed. New York, NY: Harper Collins; 2010

47. McClelland MM, Tominey SL. *Stop, Act, Think: Integrating Self-Regulation in the Early Childhood Classroom.* London, United Kingdom: Taylor & Francis; 2016

48. Weisberg DS, Hirsh-Pasek K, Golinkoff RM. Guided play: where curricular goals meet a playful pedagogy. *Mind Brain Educ.* 2013;7(2):104–112

49. Yogman MW, Lester BM, Hoffman J. Behavioral and cardiac rhythmicity during mother-father-stranger infant social interaction. *Pediatr Res.* 1983;17(11):872–876

50. Stern D. *The Interpersonal World of the Infant: A View From Psychoanalysis and Developmental Psychology.* New York, NY: Basic Books; 1980

51. Yogman MW. Games fathers and mothers play with their infants. *Infant Ment Health J.* 1981;2(4):241–248

52. Feldman R, Magori-Cohen R, Galili G, Singer M, Louzoun Y. Mother and infant coordinate heart rhythms through episodes of interaction synchrony. *Infant Behav Dev.* 2011;34(4):569–577

53. Campos JJ, Klinnert MD, Sorce JF, Emde RN, Svejda M. Emotions as behavior regulators: social referencing in infancy. In: Plutchik R, Kellerman H, eds. *Emotion: Theory, Research, and Experience.* Vol 2. New York, NY: Academic Press; 1983:57–86

54. Sorce JF, Emde RN, Campos JJ, Klinnert MD. Maternal emotional signaling: its effect on the visual cliff behavior of 1-year-olds. *Dev Psychol.* 1985;21(1):195–200

55. Mahler M, Pine F, Bergman A. *The Psychological Birth of the Human Infant.* 1st ed. New York, NY: Basic Books; 1998

56. Bodrova E, Germeroth C, Leong DJ. Play and self-regulation: lessons from Vygotsky. *Am J Play.* 2013;6(1):111–123

57. Walker CM, Gopnik A. Pretense and possibility—a theoretical proposal about the effects of pretend play on development: comment on Lillard et al. (2013). *Psychol Bull.* 2013;139(1):40–44

58. Burgdorf J, Panksepp J. The neurobiology of positive emotions. *Neurosci Biobehav Rev.* 2006;30(2):173–187

59. Burgdorf J, Panksepp J, Moskal JR. Frequency-modulated 50 kHz ultrasonic vocalizations: a tool for uncovering the molecular substrates of positive affect. *Neurosci Biobehav Rev.* 2011;35(9):1831–1836

60. Panksepp J. Neuroevolutionary sources of laughter and social joy: modeling primal human laughter in laboratory rats. *Behav Brain Res.* 2007;182(2):231–244

61. Ishiyama S, Brecht M. Neural correlates of ticklishness in the rat somatosensory cortex. *Science.* 2016;354(6313):757–760

62. Panksepp J, Burgdorf J. "Laughing" rats and the evolutionary antecedents of human joy? *Physiol Behav.* 2003;79(3):533–547

63. Burgdorf J, Wood PL, Kroes RA, Moskal JR, Panksepp J. Neurobiology of 50-kHz ultrasonic vocalizations in rats: electrode mapping, lesion, and pharmacology studies. *Behav Brain Res.* 2007;182(2):274–283

64. Six S, Panksepp J. ADHD and play. *Scholarpedia.* 2012;7(10):30371

65. Gordon NS, Burke S, Akil H, Watson SJ, Panksepp J. Socially-induced brain 'fertilization': play promotes brain derived neurotrophic factor transcription in the amygdala and dorsolateral frontal cortex in juvenile rats. *Neurosci Lett.* 2003;341(1):17–20

66. Bell HC, Pellis SM, Kolb B. Juvenile peer play experience and the development of the orbitofrontal and medial prefrontal cortices. *Behav Brain Res.* 2010;207(1):7–13

67. Diamond MC, Krech D, Rosenzweig MR. The effects of an enriched environment on the histology of the rat cerebral cortex. *J Comp Neurol.* 1964;123:111–120

68. Huber R, Tononi G, Cirelli C. Exploratory behavior, cortical BDNF expression, and sleep homeostasis. *Sleep.* 2007;30(2):129–139

69. Burgdorf J, Kroes RA, Beinfeld MC, Panksepp J, Moskal JR. Uncovering the molecular basis of positive affect using rough-and-tumble play in rats: a role for insulin-like growth factor I. *Neuroscience.* 2010;168(3):769–777

70. Gordon NS, Kollack-Walker S, Akil H, Panksepp J. Expression of c-fos gene activation during rough and tumble play in juvenile rats. *Brain Res Bull.* 2002;57(5):651–659

71. Roth TL, Lubin FD, Funk AJ, Sweatt JD. Lasting epigenetic influence of early-life adversity on the BDNF gene. *Biol Psychiatry.* 2009;65(9):760–769

72. Pellis SM, Pellis VC, Himmler BT. How play makes for a more adaptable brain: a comparative and neural perspective. *Am J Play.* 2014;7(1):73–98

73. Einon DF, Morgan MJ, Kibbler CC. Brief periods of socialization and later behavior in the rat. *Dev Psychobiol.* 1978;11(3):213–225

74. Hol T, Van den Berg CL, Van Ree JM, Spruijt BM. Isolation during the play period in infancy decreases adult social interactions in rats. *Behav Brain Res.* 1999;100(1–2):91–97

75. Greenough WT, Black JE. Induction of brain structure by experience: substrates for cognitive development. In: Gunnar MR, Nelson CA, eds. *Developmental Behavioral Neuroscience: The Minnesota Symposia on Child Psychology.* Vol 24. Hillsdale, NJ: L Erlbaum; 1992:155–200

76. Vanderschuren LJ, Niesink RJ, Van Ree JM. The neurobiology of social play behavior in rats. *Neurosci Biobehav Rev.* 1997;21(3):309–326

77. Siviy SM. Effects of pre-pubertal social experiences on the responsiveness of juvenile rats to predator odors. *Neurosci Biobehav Rev.* 2008;32(7):1249–1258

78. Garner AS, Shonkoff JP, Siegel BS, et al; Committee on Psychosocial Aspects of Child and Family Health; Committee on Early Childhood, Adoption, and Dependent Care; Section on Developmental and Behavioral Pediatrics. Early childhood adversity, toxic stress, and the role of the pediatrician: translating developmental science into lifelong health. *Pediatrics.* 2012;129(1). Available at: www.pediatrics.org/cgi/content/full/129/1/e224

79. Gruber MJ, Gelman BD, Ranganath C. States of curiosity modulate hippocampus-dependent learning via the dopaminergic circuit. *Neuron.* 2014;84(2):486–496

80. Barnett LA. Research note: young children's resolution of distress through play. *J Child Psychol Psychiatry.* 1984;25(3):477–483

81. Hatfield BE, Williford AP. Cortisol patterns for young children displaying disruptive behavior: links to a teacher-child, relationship-focused intervention. *Prev Sci.* 2017;18(1):40–49

82. Corbett BA, Schupp CW, Simon D, Ryan N, Mendoza S. Elevated cortisol during play is associated with age and social engagement in children with autism. *Mol Autism.* 2010;1(1):13

83. Siviy SM. Play and adversity: how the playful mammalian brain withstands threats and anxieties. *Am J Play.* 2010;2(3):297–314

84. Pellis SM, Pellis VC. *The Playful Brain: Venturing to the Limits of Neuroscience.* Oxford, United Kingdom: Oneworld Publications; 2009

85. Wolfgang CH, Stannard LL, Jones I. Block play performance among preschoolers as a predictor of later school achievement in mathematics. *J Res Child Educ.* 2001;15(2):173–180

86. Lewis V, Boucher J, Lupton L, Watson S. Relationships between symbolic play, functional play, verbal and non-verbal ability in young children. *Int J Lang Commun Disord.* 2000;35(1):117–127

87. Fisher KR, Hirsh-Pasek K, Newcombe N, Golinkoff RM. Taking shape: supporting preschoolers' acquisition of geometric knowledge through guided play. *Child Dev.* 2013;84(6):1872–1878

88. Cheng YL, Mix KS. Spatial training improves children's mathematics ability. *J Cogn Dev.* 2012;15(1):2–11

89. Panksepp J. Can PLAY diminish ADHD and facilitate the construction of the social brain? *J Can Acad Child Adolesc Psychiatry.* 2007;16(2):57–66

90. Christakis DA. Rethinking attention-deficit/hyperactivity disorder. *JAMA Pediatr.* 2016;170(2):109–110

91. Atkinson L, Jamieson B, Khoury J, Ludmer J, Gonzalez A. Stress physiology in infancy and early childhood: cortisol flexibility, attunement and coordination. *J Neuroendocrinol.* 2016;28(8)

92. Blair C, Granger D, Willoughby M, Kivlighan K. Maternal sensitivity is related to hypothalamic-pituitary-adrenal axis stress reactivity and regulation in response to emotion challenge in 6-month-old infants. *Ann N Y Acad Sci.* 2006;1094:263–267

93. Laurent HK, Harold GT, Leve L, Shelton KH, Van Goozen SH. Understanding the unfolding of stress regulation in infants. *Dev Psychopathol.* 2016;28(4, pt 2):1431–1440

94. Hibel LC, Granger DA, Blair C, Finegood ED; Family Life Project Key Investigators. Maternal-child adrenocortical attunement in early childhood: continuity and change. *Dev Psychobiol.* 2015;57(1):83–95

95. Sutherland SL, Friedman O. Just pretending can be really learning: children use pretend play as a source for acquiring generic knowledge. *Dev Psychol.* 2013;49(9):1660–1668

96. Dickinson DK, Tabors PO, eds. *Beginning Literacy With Language: Young Children Learning at Home and School.* Baltimore, MD: Paul Brookes Publishing; 2001

97. Christakis DA, Zimmerman FJ, Garrison MM. Effect of block play on language acquisition and attention in toddlers: a pilot randomized controlled trial. *Arch Pediatr Adolesc Med.* 2007;161(10):967–971

98. Dansky JL, Silverman I. Effects of play on associative fluency in preschool-aged children. *Dev Psychol.* 1973;9(1):38–43

99. Hillman CH, Pontifex MB, Castelli DM, et al. Effects of the FITkids randomized controlled trial on executive control and brain function. *Pediatrics.* 2014;134(4). Available at: www.pediatrics.org/cgi/content/full/134/4/e1063

100. Przybylski AK. Electronic gaming and psychosocial adjustment. *Pediatrics.* 2014;134(3). Available at: www.pediatrics.org/cgi/content/full/134/3/e716

101. Sosa AV. Association of the type of toy used during play with the quantity and quality of parent-infant communication. *JAMA Pediatr.* 2016;170(2):132–137

102. Zosh J, Verdine B, Filipowicz A, Golinkoff R, Hirsh-Pasek K, Newcombe N. Talking shape: parental language with electronic versus traditional shape sorters. *Int Mind Brain Educ Soc.* 2015;9(3):136–144

103. Buchsbaum D, Bridgers S, Skolnick Weisberg D, Gopnik A. The power of possibility: causal learning, counterfactual reasoning, and pretend play. *Philos Trans R Soc Long B Biol Sci.* 2012;367(1599):2202–2212

104. Carlson SM, White RE, Davis-Unger AC. Evidence for a relation between executive function and pretense representation in preschool children. *Cogn Dev.* 2014;29:1–16

105. Lillard AS, Lerner MD, Hopkins EJ, Dore RA, Smith ED, Palmquist CM. The impact of pretend play on children's development: a review of the evidence. *Psychol Bull.* 2013;139(1):1–34

106. Heckman J. Keynote address. In: Winthrop R, ed. *Soft Skills for Workforce Success: From Research to Action.* Washington, DC: Brookings Institution; 2015. Available at: www.brookings.edu/~/media/events/2015/06/17-soft-skills-workforce-success/0617_transcript_softskills.pdf. Accessed October 24, 2017

107. Pellis SM, Iwaniuk AN. Evolving a playful brain: a levels of control approach. *Int J Comp Psychol.* 2004;17:90–116

108. Korczak DJ, Madigan S, Colasanto M. Children's physical activity and depression: a meta-analysis. *Pediatrics.* 2017;139(4):e20162266

109. Goldstein J. Play in children's development, health and well-being: technology and play. In: Pellegrini DA, ed. *Oxford Handbook of the Development of Play.* New York, NY: Oxford University Press; 2011

110. Rothbaum F, Pott M, Azuma H, Miyake K, Weisz J. The development of close relationships in Japan and the United States: paths of symbiotic harmony and generative tension. *Child Dev.* 2000;71(5):1121–1142

111. Berkule SB, Cates CB, Dreyer BP, et al. Reducing maternal depressive symptoms through promotion of parenting in pediatric primary care. *Clin Pediatr (Phila).* 2014;53(5):460–469

112. Weisleder A, Cates CB, Dreyer BP, et al. Reading is not just for language: promoting cognitive stimulation also enhances socioemotional development. In: *Pediatric Academic Societies Annual Conference*; April 30–May 4, 2016; Baltimore, MD

113. Cates CB, Weisleder A, Dreyer BP, et al. Leveraging healthcare to promote responsive parenting: impacts of the Video Interaction Project on parenting stress. *J Child Fam Stud.* 2016;25(3):827–835

114. Brazelton TB, Yogman M, Als H, Tronick E. The infant as a focus for family reciprocity. In: Lewis M, Rosenblum L, eds. *The Child and Its Family.* New York, NY: Plenum; 1980

115. Lieber R. Why planning for play deserves serious thought. *New York Times.* 2016;(January 2):B1

116. Bonawitz EB, Ferranti D, Saxe R, et al. Just do it? Investigating the gap between prediction and action in toddlers' causal inferences. *Cognition.* 2010;115(1):104–117

117. Bonawitz E, Shafto P, Gweon H, Goodman ND, Spelke E, Schulz L. The double-edged sword of pedagogy: instruction limits spontaneous exploration and discovery. *Cognition.* 2011;120(3):322–330

118. Schulz LE, Bonawitz EB. Serious fun: preschoolers engage in more exploratory play when evidence is confounded. *Dev Psychol.* 2007;43(4):1045–1050

119. Sobel DM, Sommerville JA. The importance of discovery in children's causal learning from interventions. *Front Psychol.* 2010;1:176

120. Center on the Developing Child. Enhancing and practicing executive function skills with children from infancy to adolescence. Available at: http://developingchild.harvard.edu/wp-content/uploads/2015/05/Enhancing-and-Practicing-Executive-Function-Skills-with-Children-from-Infancy-to-Adolescence-1.pdf

121. Bodrova E, Leong DJ. *Tools of the Mind: The Vygotskian Approach to Early Childhood Education.* 2nd ed. New York, NY: Merrill/Prentice Hall; 2007

122. Domitrovich CE, Cortes RC, Greenberg MT. Improving young children's social and emotional competence: a randomized trial of the preschool "PATHS" curriculum. *J Prim Prev.* 2007;28(2):67–91

123. Yerkes RM, Dodson JD. The relation of strength of stimulus to rapidity of habit-formation. *J Comp Neurol Psychol.* 1908;18(5):459–482

124. Blair C, Raver CC. Closing the achievement gap through modification of neurocognitive and neuroendocrine function: results from a cluster randomized controlled trial of an innovative approach to the education of children in kindergarten. *PLoS One.* 2014;9(11):e112393

125. Diamond A, Lee K. Interventions shown to aid executive function development

in children 4 to 12 years old. *Science.* 2011;333(6045):959–964

126. Blair C, Granger DA, Willoughby M, et al; FLP Investigators. Salivary cortisol mediates effects of poverty and parenting on executive functions in early childhood. *Child Dev.* 2011;82(6):1970–1984

127. Louv R. *Last Child in the Woods: Saving Our Children From Nature-Deficit Disorder.* Chapel Hill, NC: Algonquin Books; 2008

128. Tandon PS, Zhou C, Christakis DA. Frequency of parent-supervised outdoor play of US preschool-aged children. *Arch Pediatr Adolesc Med.* 2012;166(8):707–712

129. Hofferth SL, Sandberg JF. Changes in American children's time, 1981-1997. *Adv Life Course Res.* 2011;6:193–229

130. Bishop R. Go out and play, but mean it: using frame analysis to explore recent news media coverage of the rediscovery of unstructured play. *Soc Sci J.* 2013;50(4):510–520

131. Hirsh-Pasek K, Golinkoff RM. Transforming cities into learning landscapes. Available at: https://ssir.org/articles/entry/transforming_cities_into_learning_landscapes. Accessed October 24, 2017

132. Ridge KE, Skolnick Weisber D, Ilgaz H, Hirsh-Pasek KA, Golnikoff RM. Supermarket speak: increasing talk among low socio-economic status families. *Mind Brain Educ.* 2015;9(3):127–135

133. Radesky JS, Eisenberg S, Kistin CJ, et al. Overstimulated consumers or next-generation learners? Parent tensions about child mobile technology use. *Ann Fam Med.* 2016;14(6):503–508

134. Anderson DR, Pempek TA. Television and very young children. *Am Behav Sci.* 2005;48(5):505–522

135. Adachi PJ, Willoughby T. The link between playing video games and positive youth outcomes. *Child Dev Perspect.* 2017;11(3):202–206

136. Radesky JS, Zuckerman B. Learning from apps in the home: parents and play. In: Kucirkova N, Falloon G, eds. *Apps, Technology, and Younger Learners: International Evidence for Teaching.* Oxford, United Kingdom: Routledge; 2017

137. American Academy of Pediatrics. Growing up digital. In: *Media Research Symposium;* October 1, 2015; Berlin, Germany

138. Lillard AS, Peterson J. The immediate impact of different types of television on young children's executive function. *Pediatrics.* 2011;128(4):644–649

139. American Academy of Pediatrics Council on Communications and Media. Policy statement: children, adolescents, and the media. *Pediatrics.* 2016;132(5):958–961

140. American Academy of Pediatrics Council on Communications and Media. Policy statement: media and young minds. *Pediatrics.* 2016;138(5):89–92

141. Rich M. Health importance of media on children. In: *American Academy of Pediatrics National Conference and Exhibition;* October 2016; San Francisco, CA

142. Hirsh-Pasek K, Golinkoff RM. The great balancing act: optimizing core curricula through playful learning. In: Zigler E, Gilliam W, Barnett S, eds. *The Preschool Education Debates.* Baltimore, MD: Brookes Publishing Co; 2011:110–116

143. Christakis E. *The Importance of Being Little.* New York, NY: Viking Press; 2016

144. Bodrova E, Leong D. *Tools of the Mind: The Vygotskian Approach to Early Childhood Education,* 2nd ed. New York, NY: Pearson; 2006

145. Child Trends. Neighborhood safety. Available at: https://www.childtrends.org/indicators/neighborhood-safety/. Accessed October 24, 2017

146. Fisher EP. The impact of play on development: a meta-analysis. *Play Cult.* 1992;5(2):159–181

147. Kearney B, Ritzenthaler H, Gray G, Yoder W. *Using Joyful Activity To Build Resiliency in Children in Response to Toxic Stress.* Brook Park, OH: Ohio Guidestone; 2017

The Prenatal Visit

• •

- *Clinical Report*

CLINICAL REPORT Guidance for the Clinician in Rendering Pediatric Care

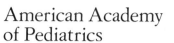

American Academy
of Pediatrics

DEDICATED TO THE HEALTH OF ALL CHILDREN™

The Prenatal Visit

Michael Yogman, MD, FAAP,[a] Arthur Lavin, MD, FAAP,[b] George Cohen, MD, FAAP,
COMMITTEE ON PSYCHOSOCIAL ASPECTS OF CHILD AND FAMILY HEALTH

abstract

A pediatric prenatal visit during the third trimester is recommended for all expectant families as an important first step in establishing a child's medical home, as recommended by *Bright Futures: Guidelines for Health Supervision of Infants, Children, and Adolescents, Fourth Edition*. As advocates for children and their families, pediatricians can support and guide expectant parents in the prenatal period. Prenatal visits allow general pediatricians to establish a supportive and trusting relationship with both parents, gather basic information from expectant parents, offer information and advice regarding the infant, and may identify psychosocial risks early and high-risk conditions that may require special care. There are several possible formats for this first visit. The one used depends on the experience and preference of the parents, the style of the pediatrician's practice, and pragmatic issues of payment.

^aHarvard Medical School and Mount Auburn Hospital, Boston, Massachusetts; and ^bAdvanced Pediatrics, Beachwood, Ohio

This document is copyrighted and is property of the American Academy of Pediatrics and its Board of Directors. All authors have filed conflict of interest statements with the American Academy of Pediatrics. Any conflicts have been resolved through a process approved by the Board of Directors. The American Academy of Pediatrics has neither solicited nor accepted any commercial involvement in the development of the content of this publication.

Clinical reports from the American Academy of Pediatrics benefit from expertise and resources of liaisons and internal (AAP) and external reviewers. However, clinical reports from the American Academy of Pediatrics may not reflect the views of the liaisons or the organizations or government agencies that they represent.

The guidance in this report does not indicate an exclusive course of treatment or serve as a standard of medical care. Variations, taking into account individual circumstances, may be appropriate.

All clinical reports from the American Academy of Pediatrics automatically expire 5 years after publication unless reaffirmed, revised, or retired at or before that time.

DOI: https://doi.org/10.1542/peds.2018-1218

Address correspondence to Michael Yogman, MD, FAAP. E-mail: myogman@massmed.org

PEDIATRICS (ISSN Numbers: Print, 0031-4005; Online, 1098-4275).

Copyright © 2018 by the American Academy of Pediatrics

FINANCIAL DISCLOSURE: The authors have indicated they have no financial relationships relevant to this article to disclose.

FUNDING: No external funding.

POTENTIAL CONFLICT OF INTEREST: The authors have indicated they have no potential conflicts of interest to disclose.

To cite: Yogman M, Lavin A, Cohen G. The Prenatal Visit. *Pediatrics.* 2018;142(1):e20181218

As the medical specialty that is entirely focused on the health and well-being of the child, embedded in the family, pediatric care ideally begins before pregnancy, with reproductive life planning of adolescents and young adults, and continues during the pregnancy, with an expectant mother and father of any age. This clinical report is an updated revision of the original clinical report from the American Academy of Pediatrics (AAP) on the prenatal visit.[1] Although survey results show that 78% of pediatricians offer a prenatal visit, only 5% to 39% of first-time parents actually attend a visit.[2] The prenatal visit offers the opportunity to create a lasting personal relationship between parents and the pediatrician, one of the most important values in all ongoing pediatric care. The AAP has put forward the rationale and standards for the prenatal visit for pediatricians in *Bright Futures: Guidelines for Health Supervision of Infants, Children, and Adolescents, Fourth Edition* (Bright Futures),[3] as well as for parents and families (www.healthychildren.org).[4] This clinical report augments these approaches to making the prenatal visit an important part of the practice of pediatrics.

Less than 5% of urban poor pregnant women see a pediatrician during the prenatal period although they are at higher risk of adverse pregnancy outcomes; pregnant women in rural areas may have even more difficulty accessing a prenatal visit.[5,6] To attempt to reduce disparities in pregnancy outcomes, encouraging nonresident prospective fathers to attend the prenatal visit along with expectant mothers is particularly important, albeit challenging.[7]

Prenatal contact with a pediatrician may begin with a contact from a prospective parent to the pediatrician's office to ask whether the practice is accepting new patients and to inquire about hours, fees, hospital affiliation, health insurance accepted, and emergency coverage. These questions may be answered by a member of the office staff or the pediatrician, and this exchange establishes an initial relationship between the office and the parent. During this conversation, the expectant parent can be encouraged to schedule a prenatal visit with the pediatric health care provider, and both parents can be encouraged to attend. The prenatal visit can be enhanced if the parents come prepared with questions. Optimally, this visit should occur at the beginning of the third trimester of pregnancy.

A prenatal visit with the pediatrician is especially important for first-time parents or families who are new to the practice; single parents; women with a high-risk pregnancy or who are experiencing pregnancy complications or multiple gestations; and parents whose previous pregnancies had a complication such as preterm delivery, an infant with a congenital anomaly, a prolonged course in the NICU, or a perinatal death. Same-sex couples and parents expecting via surrogacy may have questions unique to their circumstance. This visit also can be particularly valuable to parents who are planning to adopt a child, because they may have had previous experience with pregnancy complications and/or be sensitized to special vulnerabilities in their infant (see the AAP clinical report The Pediatrician's Role in Supporting Adoptive Families at http://pediatrics.aappublications.org/content/130/4/e1040). If adoption occurs or is to occur across states or internationally, review of records, need for waiting periods, scheduling of initial visits, concerns about potential fetal exposure (eg, maternal substance use or fetal alcohol spectrum disorders), and additional recommended screenings and/or tests can be discussed.[8,9] If needed, pediatricians can consult experts in international adoption or the AAP Council on Foster Care, Adoption, and Kinship Care.[10]

The most comprehensive prenatal visit is a full office visit, during which a trusting relationship can be established and expectant parents can have time to express their needs, interests, and concerns and receive initial anticipatory guidance. Most pediatricians believe that the prenatal visit is helpful in establishing a relationship with families that is essential for the medical home. Because they may not be able to initiate these visits, pediatricians can discuss the concept with referring obstetricians, family physicians, and internists, who can, in turn, encourage their patients to contact pediatricians for a prenatal visit. Office Web sites and social media can also be used to advertise this service to expectant parents.

The following objectives for a prenatal visit are suggested as important topics to be addressed.[2] The actual range of topics covered can be determined by the preference of the provider, the interest of the expectant parent(s), or the presence of an existing complication with the pregnancy or the fetus. Topics not covered prenatally can be presented to parents during the newborn or first postnatal visit.

OBJECTIVES

1. To provide a foundation on which to build a positive family-pediatric professional partnership, a crucial part of the patient-centered medical home.

2. To access pertinent aspects of the past obstetric and present prenatal history; to review family history of genetic or chromosomal disorders and to review fetal exposure to substances that may affect the infant.

3. To introduce anticipatory guidance about early infant care and infant safety practices.

4. To identify psychosocial factors (eg, perinatal depression) that may affect family function and family adjustment to the newborn (eg, social determinants of health, adverse child experiences, and promoting healthy social-emotional development and resiliency).

Establishing a Positive Pediatrician-Family Relationship, a Crucial Part of the Patient-Centered Medical Home

The prenatal period is an ideal time to start building the health care alliance that may last for many years, commonly until the patient reaches adulthood.[11] The prenatal visit often is an opportunity for the family to determine whether their relationship and their mutual philosophies will form the basis of a positive relationship.

The prenatal visit is also an opportunity for parents to invite other supportive adults, including grandparents,[12,13] to establish a relationship with the pediatrician and to encourage them to come to future visits and support the new parent(s). A prenatal visit can be used to introduce parents to the concept of a medical home for the child's health and development needs. Parental familiarity with the pediatric health care provider prenatally may be helpful if a referral or transfer of care occurs because of perinatal complications or the newborn infant's medical condition.[14] Adolescent parents[15] and older first-time parents may benefit from the opportunity to share their specific concerns with a knowledgeable professional.

Information From the Prenatal and Family History

Gathering information about pregnancy complications, parental depression, and family medical and social history (especially social determinants of health) is helpful as a background to the context of the pregnancy. This inquiry also conveys to parents an interest in the broader psychosocial environment of the infant, including areas in which support would be most useful, especially if there is any risk of domestic violence.[16–18] Answering parents' questions about the approach to pediatric care also is helpful. This is a good opportunity to review how the practice uses the tools of social media and e-mail to communicate with families.

Additional topics that may be addressed include:

- developmental dysplasia of the hip, early urinary tract infections, asthma, lipid disorders, cardiac disease, sickle cell disease, substance abuse, psychiatric illness, domestic violence, chronic medical conditions, and ongoing medications;

- plans for feeding, circumcision, child care, work schedules, and support systems;

- parents' plans regarding child care and expectations about work-life balance;

- cultural beliefs, values, and practices related to pregnancy and parenting;

- concerns regarding tobacco, alcohol, and other drug use[19,20] and exposure to environmental hazards; and

- parents' attitudes about and use of complementary and alternative medications and health care.

If there are other children in the family, pediatricians can provide helpful advice about managing the older sibling's adjustment. Managing parental expectations about their child is important in laying the foundation for positive attachment. Questions useful to consider as the pediatrician approaches the prenatal visit are listed in the chapter on the prenatal visit in *Bright Futures: Guidelines for Health Supervision of Infants, Children, and Adolescents, Fourth Edition.*[3]

Anticipatory Guidance and Enhanced Parenting Skills; Social Determinants of Health

The prenatal visit offers an opportunity to discuss a range of concerns that may be of great interest to the expectant parents and pediatric provider. The following areas for discussion are meant to be a helpful reference. The conversation, the specific concerns of the parents, and time allowed will define which of these issues are discussed at the prenatal visit. The prenatal visit also offers an opportunity for assessment of family risk factors and connections to key evidence-based and other early learning, health, and development programs in the community.

Positive Parenting

One of the pediatrician's tasks is to provide guidance to mothers, fathers, and other supportive adults to become more competent caregivers. This can begin with discussion of the parents' concerns, planned strategies, and cultural and family beliefs and values. Advice can be offered about shared roles in parenting, such as diapering, bathing, nighttime care, and helping with feeding. Pregnancy and delivery make the central importance of the mother in the newborn infant's

life clear, but it is important to talk about the special role fathers and same-sex partners play in good outcomes for children as well.[21] A key goal of positive parenting is the reliable provision of the infants' basic needs—food, shelter, love, and care—and in doing so, fostering the development of trust.[22,23] The adverse effects of poverty on child health have been well documented.[22,24] Optimal use of supports and resources (eg, the Special Supplemental Nutrition Program for Women, Infants, and Children [WIC]) can be discussed and information about access can be provided. Positive parenting also includes providing a steady emotional climate in which reasonable expectations are sustained consistently.[25] Avoiding and/or buffering adverse childhood experiences, such as parental postpartum depression, increasingly is seen as an evidence-based part of pediatric care, and this can begin by identifying prenatal risk factors.[26] It is important to share evidence-informed online information sources and other local resources about parenting and child development for families. Many excellent resources are available, such as the Building "Piece" of Mind program from the Ohio chapter of the AAP (http://ohioaap.org/tag/parenting/), the Zero to Three program (http://www.zerotothree.org/child-development/), the Triple P Positive Parenting Program (http://www.triplep-parenting.net/glo-en/home), and the Talk, Read, Sing tool kit available from the Clinton Foundation (Too Small to Fail [www.toosmall.org]).

The pediatrician can share with parents the knowledge that children, at an early age, can learn through playful serve-and-return interactions with adults and that playing with and daily reading, singing, and talking to children from birth onward are recommended, as is providing a language-rich environment and minimizing media exposure.

Connections to Community Resources

Office materials and Web sites can demonstrate provider awareness of key early childhood resources in the community, from home visiting, Early Head Start, child care resource and referral agencies, quality child care settings, local libraries, and parent support groups, as well as cardiopulmonary resuscitation courses. A discussion of the types of child care typically available (family care, in-home baby-sitting, family day care, child care centers) is helpful.

Delivery and Nursery Routines

A discussion of the hospital routines around delivery and nursery care may include: who will be in the delivery room and how new infants behave in the first hours and days; qualifying who will provide newborn care in the hospital and what will happen if there is (1) an unanticipated urgent delivery away from the expected hospital, (2) a home birth, or (3) an admission to a special care nursery is also helpful. This discussion might include the newborn infant's ability to seek and attach to the mother's breast right after delivery, the related concept of skin-to-skin care, and the 12-hour postdelivery sleep phase after the adrenaline rush of labor. Mothers often choose to have the infant with them continuously during the entire hospital stay, which aids successful lactation.

Thoughts on Feeding the Newborn Infant

This is an appropriate teaching moment for describing to both parents the many advantages of exclusive breastfeeding and how it improves outcomes for both the mother and infant.[27,28] Special breastfeeding training of expectant fathers or partners has been shown to increase their support of breastfeeding mothers as well as the duration of breastfeeding.[29] For parents living with food insecurity, breastfeeding offers economic advantages as well. Rooming in and avoiding unnecessary supplementation can be mentioned as ways to support nursing.

The benefits of breastfeeding can be reviewed if there are no contraindications, and lactation support services can be discussed.[30–33] However, ultimately, decisions about feeding the infant are made by the parents. If formula feeding is the parents' choice, they can be supported in their decision and given advice on formula type and preparation and proper bottle use. Ultimately, the goal is a growing, healthy infant and parents who enjoy feeding so that they can be supported in whatever decision they make. The Special Supplemental Nutrition Program for Women, Infants, and Children (WIC) also is available to help with nutrition discussion and support prenatally, and mothers can be referred to determine whether they are eligible for a nutrition package during pregnancy, if not already participating in the program.

Parental expectations can be shaped so that parents do not become overly concerned if infants take a few days to learn to latch to the breast and lose some weight before the mother's milk comes in. Infants commonly lose weight for a few days before the mother's milk comes in but typically regain birth weight at or before 2 weeks of age. If mothers who plan to breastfeed are taking any medication, a helpful reference for the pediatrician to evaluate safety is the LactMed Drugs and Lactation Database (http://toxnet.nlm.nih.gov/newtoxnet/lactmed.htm).[34]

Screening

Screening for various infections and conditions that can affect the fetus is an important part of pregnancy, delivery, and birth. The prenatal visit is an excellent time to discuss the benefit of screening and the specific screening tests prospective mothers will experience. For example, the mother is regularly screened by her obstetrician to assess fetal growth and development and may have fetal testing for genetic diseases and chromosomal abnormalities. In addition, the mother may be screened for conditions that may affect the fetus, such as gestational diabetes, pregnancy-induced hypertension, and the presence of infectious agents, such as hepatitis B, cytomegalovirus, group B streptococci, and HIV.

For the infant, the main universal screening programs are used to detect metabolic diseases, sickle cell disease, cystic fibrosis, newborn jaundice, critical congenital cardiac disease, and hearing impairments. Parents may seek more information about risk factors for the management of newborn jaundice. Some discussion of these conditions can be helpful to many families so they understand what is being looked for, how the tests are performed, and what the response to test results will be. Family history may have led to detailed genetic testing and counseling and may warrant special discussion.[35–38] Routine postpartum care can be discussed. The rationale for routine recommendations for vitamin K to prevent gastrointestinal or cerebral hemorrhage, eye ointment to prevent eye infection leading to blindness, and the birth hepatitis B vaccine can be explained.

Circumcision

Discussion of circumcision, including benefits, risks, the surgical process, and analgesia, can be presented at this visit, with particular attention to the family's religious, personal, and cultural views.[39]

Infant Visit Routines and Care Offered at the Office

Most parents are interested in understanding what to expect for a routine pediatric visit as well as information about office and telephone hours, the appointment scheduling process, and coverage for night, weekend, and emergency care. The prenatal visit also is a good time to establish the pediatrician's expectations of the family and explain the use of electronic communications during and after routine office hours, including billing for this service. The routine periodic schedule of well-child care visits from *Bright Futures: Guidelines for Health Supervision of Infants, Children, and Adolescents, Fourth Edition*[3] can be shared with the parents (http://brightfutures. aap.org/clinical_practice.html), along with information from *Bright Futures* about behavior, development, and the importance of social determinants of health.

The prenatal visit also is a good time to ask parents about their preferred approach to communication with the office, clarifying office policies on the availability of telephone and electronic communications. Preferred Web sites (HealthyChildren.org) for sharing information and other helpful resources and books can be recommended.

Safety

Safety is an important topic to discuss with the parents, particularly advice on "safe sleep"[40] and the importance of proper bedding,[40,41] proper holding of the infant, water temperature during bathing, the proper use of a pacifier, and hand washing. Encouraging a good family diet, regular checkups with the family physician or obstetrician[42] and dentist,[43,44] and appropriate rest and exercise also is important. Guidelines from the American College of Obstetricians and Gynecologists (ACOG) increasingly emphasize attention to oral health and smoking cessation during pregnancy, and pediatricians can reinforce these recommendations during the prenatal visit.[45,46] Specific safety issues to discuss include the use of car seats, gun safety in the home, smoke detectors and carbon monoxide monitors, and reducing exposures to toxins such as mold and lead.

Emotions in the Newborn Infant

For many families, including those with other children, the unique emotional life of a newborn infant is unfamiliar and can be challenging. It is key to manage expectations and raise parental awareness about the range of temperaments infants can have as well as the strengths and challenges of them. There can be some discussion on how crying can be a normal mode of communication, explaining that a common peak typically occurs during the evening hours at 6 weeks of age and giving advice on how best to respond to it. Parents can be given techniques for soothing fussy infants, such as holding, including cuddling and skin-to-skin contact[47]; rocking; singing; talking quietly; and dimming lights and playing soft music.

The prenatal visit provides an opportunity to discuss how to recognize when crying is an indicator of actual pain or illness. It is important to establish strategies for parental coping with the stress of an infant crying and the demands of infancy, including setting clear plans for strategies to deal with stress.

Emotions in the Parents

The experience of enhanced, powerful emotions of a wide variety is likely universal to most parents during and after delivery. Even if no serious difficulties with emotions emerge, it is helpful for expectant parents to be aware of the special power of both positive and negative emotions that surround a new person being born and entering their life.

It is also important for all expectant parents to be aware that it is common for many mothers, as many as 10% to 20%,[48] and some fathers to experience depression before, during, and/or after delivery. Postpartum depression is largely unappreciated, because stigma prevents a majority of parents from being identified and accessing services.[48] Several states have recommended universal postpartum depression screening by pediatricians, and insurers are increasingly paying for these screens. The prenatal visit offers mothers a valuable opportunity to become aware of the facts about depression so they know to call for help from their primary care physician or their obstetrician if they experience significant persistent sadness, which can be compounded by fatigue from lack of sleep.[49–51]

The pediatrician can instruct parents that infants usually awaken to feed every 3 hours during the night until approximately 3 months of age, when brain maturation enables one longer sleep stretch in every 24-hour cycle. To shape this longer stretch to the dark hours, parents can wake infants every 3 hours to feed during the day, keep the lights dim after dark to entrain circadian rhythms, and schedule a bedtime feeding at 11:00 PM right from birth so that the longer sleep stretch after 3 months of age begins then.

At the prenatal visit, pediatricians can listen for and make note of fathers' or partners' feelings about lack of parenting skills and decreased marital intimacy. This is an opportunity to lay the groundwork for pediatric providers to be available to fathers as well as mothers after the birth of the infant.

Decreasing the Risk of Serious Illness and Effective Response to Medical Problems Should They Occur

The prenatal visit is a good time to review family history of any illnesses or congenital diseases or any concerns the parents have had during the pregnancy. Adolescent parents often benefit from more guidance than more experienced parents, and older-than-usual parents also feel stressed and insecure. Single parents may not have family or other support systems and may benefit from postpartum referral to social service agencies, evidence-based home visiting programs, or parenting programs (Incredible Years, Triple P) in local communities, if available, for help. The absence of the father, parental conflict, a chronic parental physical condition or concern about mental health, and preterm birth or a birth defect in the infant may require additional medical visits and involvement of specialists[52–55] and can present physical, emotional, and financial burdens for the parents. Many expectant parents wish to discuss the value of cord blood banking and the relative merits of private– versus public–cord blood donation.[56]

During the pregnancy, maternal obesity and maternal drug use[8,9] are risk factors for labor complications, birth defects, and/or developmental impairment.[57–59] Maternal diet is important, and ACOG recommendations about the weight gain during pregnancy can be emphasized.

New data are increasingly available about the adverse health effects of environmental toxins during pregnancy (eg, mercury and fish), and pediatricians can work with obstetricians and the ACOG to knowledgably respond to parents' questions on this topic.[60–63] Pediatric providers may want to request direct contact with obstetric providers and request obstetric records to clarify prenatal complications, particularly regarding abnormalities detected on prenatal ultrasonography that may require postnatal follow-up. New understanding of the relationship between environmental toxins and epigenetic modifications have provided a stronger evidence-based recommendation highlighting the fetal programming of adult diseases.[64]

The prenatal visit also is a good time to give parents guidelines about the timing of taking their newborn infant out in crowded public places or inviting visitors/relatives to their home. With regard to preventing infections, this is a good moment to discuss and encourage parents and family members to be immunized against pertussis and, if during the right season, influenza. Tetanus-diphtheria-acellular pertussis (Tdap) immunization is recommended for every pregnant woman after 20 weeks' gestation, for every pregnancy, and for fathers as well.[65] Underimmunized siblings at home also present a risk to a newborn infant, and expectant parents can be encouraged to ensure siblings are fully immunized before the delivery.

Many parents have questions about the recommended schedule of immunizations. The prenatal visit is a valuable opportunity to discuss the value of immunizations and the reason for the recommended schedule. It is an opportunity to listen to any parental concerns well before the infant is born, and the decision is on the family. It is also important for the pediatric provider to outline office immunization policy with regard to parents who wish to alter the standard immunization schedule.

Information Sharing With the Family

Although the volume of information and advice may seem overwhelming to expectant parents, they can be given appropriate handouts to supplement and reinforce information provided at the prenatal visit. A follow-up visit or telephone call can be offered if they still have questions. A Web page can be a good source of information and can include parent questionnaires for subsequent visits.

TYPES OF PRENATAL VISITS

The Full Prenatal Visit

The most comprehensive form of prenatal visit is a scheduled office visit with both expectant parents.

Nurse practitioners can have a significant role in conducting prenatal visits. The objectives listed previously are accomplished through an in-person discussion with the provider. Discussion can include office and telephone hours; fees; office staff; hospital affiliations; coverage for night, weekend, and emergency care; arrangements for newborn care after delivery both at the hospital the pediatricians visit and at a hospital where the pediatrician is not on the staff; and the pediatrician's expectations of the family. A handout containing this information can be helpful for the family, including information on how and when to schedule the first visit after newborn discharge and how to retrieve the discharge summary if care was provided by a hospitalist. This type of visit is most important for first-time parents, for adolescent and other young parents, when pregnancy complications or newborn problems are anticipated, or when parents are unusually anxious for any reason. The establishment of a mutual commitment to a sound and rewarding family-physician relationship usually results from the visit.

If women with high-risk pregnancies require bed rest, there may be a need for a prenatal visit with only 1 parent and/or telephone calls. These contacts can include the same content as the full prenatal visit. The outcome should be the same mutual commitment as from the full prenatal visit in the office. If an infant is born prematurely, before a prenatal visit could occur, it is often helpful to meet with the parents in a modified prenatal visit before the infant is discharged from the NICU. In the tragic circumstance of a pregnancy loss after a prenatal visit, a follow-up expression of sympathy by the pediatric provider can feel supportive.

The Brief Visit To Get Acquainted

Some pediatricians may offer a less formal prenatal visit than a full consultation, and some parents also may prefer this option. A meet-and-greet session, individually or in a group, can include meeting key staff members such as the practice manager, taking a short tour of the office, and receiving other administrative information and handouts. This type of visit may be appropriate for parents before deciding on scheduling a full prenatal visit. Other models include group visits at the maternity hospital as part of a prenatal class or at community events for expectant parents.

The Basic Contact or Telephone Call

The initial prenatal contact often is an expectant parent's call to the pediatrician's office. The staff member can offer a brief description of the practice, basic information including a source of referral, expected delivery date, and type of insurance and can be invited to make an appointment for a full prenatal visit. An office information handout may be sent to the expectant parents, if requested.

No Prenatal Contact

If no prenatal contact has been made, the objectives and discussion of the prenatal visit can be presented to the parents in the newborn visit or first postnatal visit. Because of other priorities, the parents may not absorb some of this discussion; therefore, a handout containing pertinent information may be used at this type of visit. At the infant's first office visit, parents should be encouraged to have an additional family member accompany them to care for the infant while the parents and pediatrician confer.

Payment

Pediatricians or office staff can discuss with parents whether the visit will be covered by the expectant parent's insurance and whether a referral will be required. A discussion of insurance plans that the practice accepts may be included. Payment for a prenatal visit often requires advocacy with third-party payers, both individually and through pediatric councils. Both the recommendations of *Bright Futures: Guidelines for Health Supervision of Infants, Children, and Adolescents, Fourth Edition*[3] and this clinical report can provide further support for advocacy. Pediatric providers may seek advice from AAP coding resources and may review acceptable codes with their health plans.

RECOMMENDATIONS

1. A prenatal visit is an important first step to help expectant families (especially first-time parents) establish their child's medical home. The visit is a unique opportunity to address the relationship between the family and practice and for the bidirectional sharing of information between the parents and pediatric provider.

2. Pediatric practices can effectively incorporate prenatal visits into their routine. Services can be flexible and designed to meet the needs of expectant parents. A full prenatal visit is preferred, if feasible.

3. Payment for full prenatal visits is supported by the evidence in *Bright Futures* and this report. State chapters of the AAP (as through pediatric councils) and pediatric practices can advocate to payers the short-term and long-term benefits of prenatal visits on the health outcomes of infants and their parents.

4. Pediatricians can share their established practices on prenatal visits with local obstetricians, internists, and family physicians, and with expectant parents.

5. Pediatric residents can effectively be taught during residency about the content and importance of the prenatal visit.

6. Increased partnerships with colleagues in obstetrics and gynecology, who are now routinely screening mothers for perinatal depression, are encouraged. Whenever risk factors are identified, obstetric and gynecologic colleagues can be encouraged to refer expectant parents for prenatal pediatric visits so that postpartum family care is optimized.

7. A comprehensive review of this topic with suggested questions and specific suggestions for expectant parents can be found in the *Bright Futures: Guidelines for Health Supervision of Infants, Children, and Adolescents, Fourth Edition*.[3]

8. Parents can find resources of value during the prenatal period at www.healthychildren.org.[4]

EXAMPLES OF QUESTIONS TO USE IN THE PRENATAL VISIT[66]

1. What kinds of previous experience with infants have you had?

2. Are you working? Are you planning to return to work after delivery?

3. How are the siblings adjusting to the pregnancy?

4. Have you attended prenatal classes, and have they been helpful?

5. What kind of relationship did you have with your parents when you were growing up?

6. Are you planning to rear your infant in a manner similar to or different from the way your parents reared you?

7. What expectations do you have about this infant?

8. What worries and concerns do you have?

9. What are your plans about feeding the infant (offer support, whether for breast or formula feeding)?

10. To specifically engage the father/partner, when appropriate, address at least one question to just the father/partner, for example, if the infant is a boy, do you plan to have him circumcised?

11. Was this a convenient time for you to be pregnant?

12. How do you cope when you are stressed?

LEAD AUTHORS

Michael Yogman, MD, FAAP
Arthur Lavin, MD, FAAP
George Cohen, MD, FAAP

COMMITTEE ON PSYCHOSOCIAL ASPECTS OF CHILD AND FAMILY HEALTH, 2015–2016

Michael Yogman, MD, FAAP, Chairperson
Arthur Lavin, MD, FAAP
Keith M. Lemmon, MD, FAAP
Gerri Mattson, MD, FAAP
Jason Richard Rafferty, MD
Lawrence Sagin Wissow, MD, MPH, FAAP

CONSULTANT

George J. Cohen, MD, FAAP

LIAISONS

Sharon Berry, PhD — *Society of Pediatric Psychology*
Terry Carmichael, MSW — *National Association of Social Workers*
Edward R. Christophersen, PhD, FAAP (hon) — *Society of Pediatric Psychology*
Norah Johnson, PhD, RN, CPNP — *National Association of Pediatric Nurse Practitioners*
L. Read Sulik, MD — *American Academy of Child and Adolescent Psychiatry*

STAFF

Stephanie Domain, MS

ABBREVIATIONS

AAP: American Academy of Pediatrics
ACOG: American College of Obstetricians and Gynecologists

REFERENCES

1. Cohen GJ; Committee on Psychosocial Aspects of Child and Family Health. The prenatal visit. *Pediatrics.* 2009;124(4):1227–1232

2. Campbell DE. Prenatal visit. In: McInerny TK, Adam HM, Campbell DE, DeWitt TG, Foy JM, Kamat DM, eds. *Textbook of Pediatric Care.* 1st ed. Elk Grove Village, IL: American Academy of Pediatrics; 2009:797–800

3. Hagan JF, Shaw JS, Duncan P, eds. *Bright Futures: Guidelines for Health Supervision of Infants, Children and Adolescents.* 4th ed. Elk Grove Village, IL: American Academy of Pediatrics; 2017

4. American Academy of Pediatrics. HealthyChildren.org. Available at: https://www.healthychildren.org/English/Pages/default.aspx. Accessed March 7, 2018

5. Bryant AS, Worjoloh A, Caughey AB, Washington AE. Racial/ethnic disparities in obstetric outcomes and care: prevalence and determinants. *Am J Obstet Gynecol.* 2010;202(4):335–343

6. Tessema J, Jefferds ME, Cogswell M, Carlton E. Motivators and barriers to prenatal supplement use among minority women in the United States. *J Am Diet Assoc.* 2009;109(1):102–108

7. Alio AP, Mbah AK, Grunsten RA, Salihu HM. Teenage pregnancy and the influence of paternal involvement on fetal outcomes. *J Pediatr Adolesc Gynecol.* 2011;24(6):404–409

8. Williams JF, Smith VC; Committee on Substance Abuse. Fetal alcohol spectrum disorders. *Pediatrics.* 2015;136(5). Available at: www.pediatrics.org/cgi/content/full/136/5/e1395

9. Behnke M, Smith VC; Committee on Substance Abuse; Committee on Fetus and Newborn. Prenatal substance abuse: short- and long-term effects on the exposed fetus. *Pediatrics.* 2013;131(3). Available at: www.pediatrics.org/cgi/content/full/131/3/e1009

10. Jones VF; Committee on Early Childhood, Adoption, and Dependent Care. Comprehensive health evaluation of the newly adopted child. *Pediatrics.* 2012;129(1). Available at: www.pediatrics.org/cgi/content/full/129/1/e214

11. Regalado M, Halfon N. Primary care services promoting optimal child development from birth to age 3 years: review of the literature. *Arch Pediatr Adolesc Med.* 2001;155(12):1311–1322

12. Reitzes DC, Mutran EJ. Grandparenthood: factors influencing frequency of grandparent-grandchildren contact and grandparent role satisfaction. *J Gerontol B Psychol Sci Soc Sci.* 2004;59(1):S9–S16

13. McCallion P, Janicki MP, Kolomer SR. Controlled evaluation of support groups for grandparent caregivers of children with developmental disabilities and delays. *Am J Ment Retard.* 2004;109(5):352–361

14. American Academy of Pediatrics Committee on Fetus and Newborn. Hospital discharge of the high-risk neonate. *Pediatrics.* 2008;122(5):1119–1126

15. Dallas C. Family matters: how mothers of adolescent parents experience adolescent pregnancy and parenting. *Public Health Nurs.* 2004;21(4):347–353

16. Fonagy P, Steele H, Steele M. Maternal representations of attachment during pregnancy predict the organization of infant-mother attachment at one year of age. *Child Dev.* 1991;62(5):891–905

17. Luoma I, Kaukonen P, Mäntymaa M, Puura K, Tamminen T, Salmelin R. A longitudinal study of maternal depressive symptoms, negative expectations and perceptions of child problems. *Child Psychiatry Hum Dev.* 2004;35(1):37–53

18. McHale JP, Kazali C, Rotman T, Talbot J, Carleton M, Lieberson R. The transition to coparenthood: parents' pre-birth expectations and early coparental adjustment at 3 months postpartum. *Dev Psychopathol.* 2004;16(3):711–733

19. Kolobe TH. Childrearing practices and developmental expectations for Mexican-American mothers and the developmental status of their infants. *Phys Ther.* 2004;84(5):439–453

20. Mason R. Family support for first-time mothers in the Aleutians.

Int J Circumpolar Health. 2004; (suppl 1):39–42

21. Yogman MW, Garfield C; Committee on Psychosocial Aspects of Child and Family Health. Fathers' roles in the care and development of their children: the role of pediatricians. *Pediatrics.* 2016;138(1):e20161128

22. Council on Community Pediatrics. Poverty and child health in the United States. *Pediatrics.* 2016;137(4):e20160339

23. Council on Community Pediatrics; Committee on Nutrition. Promoting food security for all children. *Pediatrics.* 2015;136(5). Available at: www.pediatrics.org/cgi/content/full/136/5/e1431

24. Pascoe JM, Wood DL, Duffee JH, Kuo A; Committee on Psychosocial Aspects of Child and Family Health; Council on Community Pediatrics. Mediators and adverse effects of child poverty in the United States. *Pediatrics.* 2016;137(4):e20160340

25. Duong J, Bradshaw CP. Links between contexts and middle to late childhood social-emotional development. *Am J Community Psychol.* 2017;60(3–4):538–554

26. Garner AS, Shonkoff JP; Committee on Psychosocial Aspects of Child and Family Health; Committee on Early Childhood, Adoption, and Dependent Care; Section on Developmental and Behavioral Pediatrics. Early childhood adversity, toxic stress, and the role of the pediatrician: translating developmental science into lifelong health. *Pediatrics.* 2012;129(1). Available at: www.pediatrics.org/cgi/content/full/129/1/e224

27. Bachrach VR, Schwarz E, Bachrach LR. Breastfeeding and the risk of hospitalization for respiratory disease in infancy: a meta-analysis. *Arch Pediatr Adolesc Med.* 2003;157(3):237–243

28. Cloherty M, Alexander J, Holloway I. Supplementing breast-fed babies in the UK to protect their mothers from tiredness or distress. *Midwifery.* 2004;20(2):194–204

29. Pisacane A, Continisio GI, Aldinucci M, D'Amora S, Continisio P. A controlled trial of the father's role in breastfeeding promotion. *Pediatrics.* 2005;116(4). Available at: www.pediatrics.org/cgi/content/full/116/4/e494

30. Ishii KD, Heinig MJ. What grandparents can do to help a breastfeeding mother. *J Hum Lact.* 2005;21(1):67–68

31. Shakespeare J, Blake F, Garcia J. Breast-feeding difficulties experienced by women taking part in a qualitative interview study of postnatal depression. *Midwifery.* 2004;20(3):251–260

32. Guise JM, Palda V, Westhoff C, Chan BK, Helfand M, Lieu TA; U.S. Preventive Services Task Force. The effectiveness of primary care-based interventions to promote breastfeeding: systematic evidence review and meta-analysis for the US Preventive Services Task Force. *Ann Fam Med.* 2003;1(2):70–78

33. Section on Breastfeeding. Breastfeeding and the use of human milk. *Pediatrics.* 2012;129(3). Available at: www.pediatrics.org/cgi/content/full/129/3/e827

34. National Institutes of Health, US National Library of Medicine. LactMed: a new NLM database on drugs and lactation. Available at: https://www.nlm.nih.gov/news/lactmed_announce_06.html. Accessed April 7, 2016

35. Rappaport VJ. Prenatal diagnosis and genetic screening—integration into prenatal care. *Obstet Gynecol Clin North Am.* 2008;35(3):435–458, ix

36. Dolan SM, Moore C. Linking family history in obstetric and pediatric care: assessing risk for genetic disease and birth defects. *Pediatrics.* 2007;120(suppl 2):S66–S70

37. Kuppermann M, Pena S, Bishop JT, et al. Effect of enhanced information, values clarification, and removal of financial barriers on use of prenatal genetic testing: a randomized clinical trial. *JAMA.* 2014;312(12):1210–1217

38. Dolan SM. Personalized genomic medicine and prenatal genetic testing. *JAMA.* 2014;312(12):1203–1205

39. American Academy of Pediatrics Task Force on Circumcision. Circumcision policy statement. *Pediatrics.* 2012;130(3):585–586

40. Moon RY; Task Force on Sudden Infant Death Syndrome. SIDS and other sleep-related infant deaths: expansion of recommendations for a safe infant sleeping environment. *Pediatrics.* 2011;128(5). Available at: www.pediatrics.org/cgi/content/full/128/5/e1341

41. Jenni OG, Fuhrer HZ, Iglowstein I, Molinari L, Largo RH. A longitudinal study of bed sharing and sleep problems among Swiss children in the first 10 years of life. *Pediatrics.* 2005;115(suppl 1):233–240

42. Kirkham C, Harris S, Grzybowski S. Evidence-based prenatal care: part I. General prenatal care and counseling issues. *Am Fam Physician.* 2005;71(7):1307–1316

43. Bright Futures at Georgetown University. Pregnancy and postpartum. In: Casamassimo P, Holt K, eds. *Bright Futures in Practice: Oral Health-Pocket Guide.* Washington, DC: Georgetown University, National Maternal and Child Health Resource Center; 2004:18–23

44. Hujoel PP, Bollen AM, Noonan CJ, del Aguila MA. Antepartum dental radiography and infant low birth weight. *JAMA.* 2004;291(16):1987–1993

45. American College of Obstetricians and Gynecologists Women's Health Care Physicians; Committee on Health Care for Underserved Women. Committee opinion no. 569: oral health care during pregnancy and through the lifespan. *Obstet Gynecol.* 2013; 122(2 pt 1):417–422

46. Committee opinion no. 471: smoking cessation during pregnancy. *Obstet Gynecol.* 2010;116(5):1241–1244

47. Johnston CC, Stevens B, Pinelli J, et al. Kangaroo care is effective in diminishing pain response in preterm neonates. *Arch Pediatr Adolesc Med.* 2003;157(11):1084–1088

48. Earls MF; Committee on Psychosocial Aspects of Child and Family Health American Academy of Pediatrics. Incorporating recognition and management of perinatal and postpartum depression into pediatric practice. *Pediatrics.* 2010;126(5):1032–1039

49. Liberto TL. Screening for depression and help-seeking in postpartum women during well-baby pediatric visits: an integrated review. *J Pediatr Health Care.* 2012;26(2):109–117

50. Goodman P, Mackey MC, Tavakoli AS. Factors related to childbirth satisfaction. *J Adv Nurs.* 2004;46(2):212–219

51. George L. Lack of preparedness: experiences of first-time mothers. *MCN Am J Matern Child Nurs.* 2005;30(4):251–255

52. Rahman A, Iqbal Z, Bunn J, Lovel H, Harrington R. Impact of maternal depression on infant nutritional status and illness: a cohort study. *Arch Gen Psychiatry.* 2004;61(9):946–952

53. Sisson MC, Witcher PM, Stubsten C. The role of the maternal-fetal medicine specialist in high-risk obstetric care. *Crit Care Nurs Clin North Am.* 2004;16(2):187–191

54. Scher MS, Kidder BM, Shah D, Bangert BA, Judge NE. Pediatric neurology participation in a fetal diagnostic service. *Pediatr Neurol.* 2004;30(5):338–344

55. Hack M, Taylor HG, Drotar D, et al. Chronic conditions, functional limitations, and special health care needs of school-aged children born with extremely low-birth-weight in the 1990s. *JAMA.* 2005;294(3):318–325

56. Shearer WT, Lubin BH, Cairo MS, Notarangelo LD; Section on Hematology/Oncology; Section on Allergy and Immunology. Cord blood banking for potential future transplantation. *Pediatrics.* 2017;140(5):e20172695

57. Watkins ML, Rasmussen SA, Honein MA, Botto LD, Moore CA. Maternal obesity and risk for birth defects. *Pediatrics.* 2003; 111(5 pt 2):1152–1158

58. Schuler ME, Nair P, Kettinger L. Drug-exposed infants and developmental outcome: effects of a home intervention and ongoing maternal drug use. *Arch Pediatr Adolesc Med.* 2003;157(2):133–138

59. Narkowicz S, Płotka J, Polkowska Ż, Biziuk M, Namieśnik J. Prenatal exposure to substance of abuse: a worldwide problem. *Environ Int.* 2013;54:141–163

60. ACOG Committee Opinion No. 575. Exposure to toxic environmental agents. *Obstet Gynecol.* 2013;122(4):931–935

61. Abelsohn A, Gibson BL, Sanborn MD, Weir E. Identifying and managing adverse environmental health effects: 5. Persistent organic pollutants. *CMAJ.* 2002;166(12):1549–1554

62. Sathyanarayana S, Focareta J, Dailey T, Buchanan S. Environmental exposures: how to counsel preconception and prenatal patients in the clinical setting. *Am J Obstet Gynecol.* 2012;207(6):463–470

63. Mother to baby: medications and more during pregnancy and breastfeeding. Fact sheets. Available at: http://mothertobaby.org/fact-sheets-parent/. Accessed June 8, 2016

64. Lau C, Rogers JM, Desai M, Ross MG. Fetal programming of adult disease: implications for prenatal care. *Obstet Gynecol.* 2011;117(4):978–985

65. Návar AM, Halsey NA, Carter TC, Montgomery MP, Salmon DA. Prenatal immunization education the pediatric prenatal visit and routine obstetric care. *Am J Prev Med.* 2007;33(3):211–213

66. Yogman MW. Pediatric prenatal visit. In: Green M, Haggerty R, eds. *Ambulatory Pediatrics.* Philadelphia, PA: Saunders; 1990:92–94

Recommendations for Prevention and Control of Influenza in Children, 2018–2019

- *Policy Statement*

    - *PPI: AAP Partnership for Policy Implementation*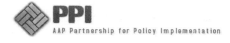
      See Appendix 1 for more information.

POLICY STATEMENT Organizational Principles to Guide and Define the Child Health Care System and/or Improve the Health of all Children

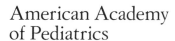

American Academy
of Pediatrics

DEDICATED TO THE HEALTH OF ALL CHILDREN™

Recommendations for Prevention and Control of Influenza in Children, 2018–2019

COMMITTEE ON INFECTIOUS DISEASES

The authors of this statement update the recommendations of the American Academy of Pediatrics for the routine use of influenza vaccine and antiviral medications in the prevention and treatment of influenza in children. Highlights for the upcoming 2018–2019 season include the following:

1. Annual influenza immunization is recommended for everyone 6 months and older, including children and adolescents.

2. The American Academy of Pediatrics recommends an inactivated influenza vaccine (IIV), trivalent or quadrivalent, as the primary choice for influenza vaccination in children because the effectiveness of a live attenuated influenza vaccine against influenza A(H1N1) was inferior during past influenza seasons and is unknown for this upcoming season.

3. A live attenuated influenza vaccine may be used for children who would not otherwise receive an influenza vaccine (eg, refusal of an IIV) and for whom it is appropriate because of age (2 years of age and older) and health status (ie, healthy and without any underlying chronic medical condition).

4. All 2018–2019 seasonal influenza vaccines contain an influenza A(H1N1) vaccine strain similar to that included in the 2017–2018 seasonal vaccines. In contrast, the influenza A(H3N2) and influenza B (Victoria lineage) vaccine strains included in the 2018–2019 trivalent and quadrivalent vaccines differ from those in the 2017–2018 seasonal vaccines.

 a. Trivalent vaccines contain an influenza A(Michigan/45/2015[H1N1]) pdm09–like virus, an influenza A(Singapore/INFIMH-16-0019/2016[H3N2])–like virus (updated), and an influenza B (Colorado/60/2017)–like virus (B/Victoria lineage; updated).

 b. Quadrivalent vaccines contain an additional B virus (Phuket/3073/2013–like virus; B/Yamagata lineage).

5. All children with egg allergy of any severity can receive an influenza vaccine without any additional precautions beyond those recommended for all vaccines.

DOI: https://doi.org/10.1542/peds.2018-2367

PEDIATRICS (ISSN Numbers: Print, 0031-4005; Online, 1098-4275).

Copyright © 2018 by the American Academy of Pediatrics

FINANCIAL DISCLOSURE: The authors have indicated they have no financial relationships relevant to this article to disclose.

FUNDING: No external funding.

POTENTIAL CONFLICT OF INTEREST: The authors have indicated they have no potential conflicts of interest to disclose.

To cite: AAP COMMITTEE ON INFECTIOUS DISEASES. Recommendations for Prevention and Control of Influenza in Children, 2018–2019. *Pediatrics.* 2018;142(4):e20182367

6. Pregnant women may receive an influenza vaccine (IIV only) at any time during pregnancy to protect themselves as well as their infants, who benefit from the transplacental transfer of antibodies. Postpartum women who did not receive vaccination during pregnancy should be encouraged to receive an influenza vaccine before discharge from the hospital. Influenza vaccination during breastfeeding is safe for mothers and their infants.

7. The vaccination of health care workers is a crucial step in preventing influenza and reducing health care-associated influenza infections because health care personnel often care for individuals at high risk for influenza-related complications.

8. Pediatricians should attempt to promptly identify their patients who are suspected of having an influenza infection for timely initiation of antiviral treatment when indicated and on the basis of shared decision-making between each pediatrician and child caregiver to reduce morbidity and mortality. Although best results are seen when a child is treated within 48 hours of symptom onset, antiviral therapy should still be considered beyond 48 hours of symptom onset in children with severe disease or those at high risk of complications (see Table 2 in the full policy statement).

KEY POINTS RELEVANT TO THE 2018–2019 INFLUENZA SEASON

1. The American Academy of Pediatrics (AAP) recommends annual influenza vaccination for everyone 6 months and older, including children and adolescents, during the 2018–2019 influenza season. Special effort should be made to vaccinate individuals in the following groups:

- all children, including infants born preterm, 6 months and older (based on chronologic age) with chronic medical conditions that increase the risk of complications from influenza, such as pulmonary diseases (eg, asthma), metabolic diseases (eg, diabetes mellitus), hemoglobinopathies (eg, sickle cell disease), hemodynamically significant cardiac disease, immunosuppression, renal and hepatic disorders, or neurologic and neurodevelopmental disorders;

- all household contacts and out-of-home care providers of children with high-risk conditions or younger than 5 years, especially infants younger than 6 months;

- children and adolescents (6 months–18 years of age) receiving an aspirin- or salicylate-containing medication, which places them at risk for Reye syndrome after influenza virus infection;

- children who are American Indians and/or Alaskan natives;

- all health care personnel (HCP);

- all child care providers and staff; and

- all women who are pregnant, are considering pregnancy, are in the postpartum period, or are breastfeeding during the influenza season.

Children often have the highest attack rates of influenza in the community during seasonal influenza epidemics, play a pivotal role in the transmission of influenza infection to household and other close contacts, and experience relatively elevated morbidity, including severe or fatal complications from influenza infection.[1] In the United States, almost two-thirds of children younger than 6 years and nearly all children 6 years and older spend significant time in child care or school settings outside the home. Exposure to groups of children increases the risk of contracting infectious diseases.[2] Children younger than 2 years are at increased risk of hospitalization and complications attributable to influenza.[1] School-aged children bear a large influenza disease burden and have a significantly higher chance of seeking influenza-related medical care compared with healthy adults.[1] Reducing influenza virus transmission (eg, by using appropriate hand hygiene and respiratory hygiene and/or cough etiquette) among children who attend out-of-home child care or school has been shown to decrease the burden of childhood influenza and transmission of influenza virus to household contacts and community members of all ages.[2]

2. The 2017–2018 influenza season was a high-severity season, with high levels of outpatient clinic and emergency department

Highlights for the 2018–2019 Influenza Season

- Vaccination remains the best available preventive measure to prevent influenza illness.

- Annual influenza vaccine is recommended for everyone 6 months and older.

- ACIP reintroduced LAIV4 as an option for the 2018–2019 influenza season.

- The AAP recommends an IIV (IIV3 or IIV4) as the primary choice for all children because the effectiveness of LAIV4 was inferior against influenza A (/H1N1) during past seasons and is unknown against influenza A (/H1N1) for this upcoming season.

- LAIV4 may be used for children who would not otherwise receive an influenza vaccine (eg, refusal of an IIV) and for whom it is appropriate according to age (ie, 2 years of age and older) and health status (ie, healthy and without any underlying chronic medical condition).

- As always, families should receive counseling on these revised recommendations for the 2018–2019 season.

- Children should receive the influenza vaccine as soon as possible after it is available in their community, preferably by the end of October.

- The No. recommended doses of an influenza vaccine depends on a child's age at the time of the first administered dose and vaccine history.

- All children with egg allergy of any severity can receive either an IIV or LAIV without any additional precautions beyond those recommended for any vaccine.

- Pregnant women may receive an IIV at any time during pregnancy. Postpartum women who did not receive vaccination during pregnancy should be encouraged to receive the vaccine before discharge from the hospital. Vaccination is safe during breastfeeding for mothers and their infants.

- All HCP should receive an annual influenza vaccine, which is a crucial step in preventing influenza and reducing health care–associated influenza infections.

- Antiviral medications are important in the control of influenza but are not a substitute for influenza vaccination.

visits for influenza-like illness (ILI), high influenza-related hospitalization rates, high numbers of pediatric deaths, and elevated and geographically widespread influenza activity across the country for an extended period.[3, 4] Influenza A(H3N2) viruses predominated overall for the season through February 2018; influenza B viruses predominated from March 2018 onward. The 2017–2018 season ranks as the third most severe since the 2003–2004 season and was the first to be classified as high severity for all age groups.[3] The peak percentage of outpatient visits for ILI was the third highest recorded since the 1997–1998 season. Although the hospitalization rates for children this season did not exceed the rates reported during the 2009 pandemic, hospitalization surpassed rates reported in previous high-severity influenza A(H3N2)–predominant seasons. Excluding the 2009 pandemic, the 179 pediatric deaths reported through August 18, 2018, during the 2017–2018 season (approximately half of which occurred in otherwise healthy children) are the highest reported since influenza-associated pediatric mortality became a nationally notifiable condition in 2004. Analyses of the influenza A(H1N1)pdm09, influenza A(H3N2), and influenza B (Yamagata lineage) viruses showed that circulating viruses were antigenically and genetically similar to the cell-grown reference viruses representing the 2017–2018 Northern Hemisphere influenza vaccine viruses. Although the overall number of circulating influenza B (Victoria lineage) viruses was low, a substantial amount of antigenic drift from the vaccine reference virus influenza B(Brisbane/60/2008) was observed.[3]

Pediatric hospitalizations and deaths caused by influenza vary by the predominant circulating strain and from one season to the next (Table 1). Historically, 80% to 85% of pediatric deaths have occurred in unvaccinated children 6 months and older. Among pediatric deaths of children 6 months and older who were eligible for influenza vaccination and for whom vaccination status was known, only 22% had received at least 1 dose of an influenza vaccine during the 2017–2018 season.[3] Influenza vaccination is associated with reduced risk of laboratory-confirmed influenza-related pediatric death.[5] In one case cohort analysis in which researchers compared vaccination uptake among laboratory-confirmed influenza-associated pediatric deaths with estimated vaccination coverage among pediatric cohorts in the United States from 2010 to 2014, Flannery et al[5] found that only 26% of case patients received a vaccine before illness onset compared with average vaccination coverage of 48%. The overall vaccine

TABLE 1 Pediatric Deaths and Hospitalizations by Season and Predominant Strain

Influenza Season	Predominant Strain	Pediatric Deaths	Hospitalizations (0–4 y Old) per 100 000	Hospitalizations (5–17 y Old) per 100 000
2017–2018 (preliminary data)	H3N2	179	71.4	19.7
2016–2017	H3N2	101	43.7	16.7
2015–2016	pH1N1	92	42.4	9.7
2014–2015[a]	H3N2	148	57.2	16.6
2013–2014	pH1N1	111	47.2	9.4
2012–2013	H3N2	171	67	14.6
2011–2012[a]	H3N2	37	16	4
2010–2011	H3N2	124	49.4	9.1
2009–2010	pH1N1	288	77.4	27.2
2008–2009	H1N1	137	28	5
2007–2008	H3N2	88	40.3	5.5

Adapted from Centers for Disease Control and Prevention. FluView 2017–2018 data as of August 18, 2018. Available at: www.cdc.gov/flu/weekly/fluviewinteractive.htm.
[a] Vaccine strains did not change from previous influenza season.

effectiveness against influenza-associated death in children was 65% (95% confidence interval [CI] 54% to 74%). More than one-half of pediatric deaths in this study had ≥1 underlying medical condition with increased risk of severe influenza-related complications; notably, only 1 in 3 of these at-risk children had been vaccinated, yet vaccine effectiveness against death in children with underlying conditions was 51% (95% CI 31% to 67%). Similarly, influenza vaccination reduces by three-fourths the risk of severe, life-threatening laboratory-confirmed influenza in children requiring admission to the ICU.[6] During the past 11 seasons, the rates of influenza-associated hospitalization for children younger than 5 years have always exceeded the rates for children 5 through 17 years of age.

As of August 18, 2018, the following data were reported by the Centers for Disease Control and Prevention (CDC) during the 2017–2018 influenza season:

179 laboratory-confirmed influenza-associated pediatric deaths occurred;

106 were associated with influenza A viruses, 68 were associated with influenza B viruses;

3 were associated with an undetermined type of influenza virus; and

2 were associated with both influenza A and influenza B viruses.

Among the 154 children with known medical history, 51% of the deaths occurred in children with at least one underlying medical condition that is recognized by the Advisory Committee on Immunization Practices (ACIP) to increase the risk of influenza-attributable disease severity. Among children hospitalized with influenza and for whom medical record data were available, approximately 43% had no recorded underlying condition, whereas 26.2% had asthma or a reactive airway disease, 16.8% had a neurologic disorder, and 10.5% had obesity (Fig 1).[3] In a recent study of hospitalizations for influenza A versus influenza B, the odds of mortality were significantly greater with influenza B than with influenza A and were not entirely explained by underlying health conditions.[7]

3. Vaccination remains the best available preventive measure against influenza illness. The universal administration of a seasonal vaccine to everyone 6 months and older is the best strategy available for preventing illness from influenza. Any licensed and age-appropriate inactivated influenza vaccine (IIV) available should be used to vaccinate children. There is notable room for improvement in

influenza vaccination because overall influenza vaccination rates have been suboptimal during past seasons in both children and adults. Children's likelihood of being immunized according to recommendations appears to be associated with the immunization practices of their parents. One study revealed that children were 2.77 times (95% CI 2.74 to 2.79) more likely to also be immunized for seasonal influenza if their parents were immunized.[8] When parents who were previously not immunized had received immunization for seasonal influenza, their children were 5.44 times (95% CI 5.35 to 5.53) more likely to receive an influenza vaccine.

4. The AAP recommends a trivalent inactivated influenza vaccine (IIV3) or quadrivalent inactivated influenza vaccine (IIV4) as the primary choice for influenza vaccination in children because the effectiveness of quadrivalent live attenuated influenza vaccine (LAIV4) against influenza A(H1N1) was inferior during past influenza seasons, and effectiveness is unknown for this upcoming season. Both the AAP Committee on Infectious Diseases and the ACIP of the CDC have reviewed and carefully considered all influenza vaccine efficacy data available to date as well as new information regarding the

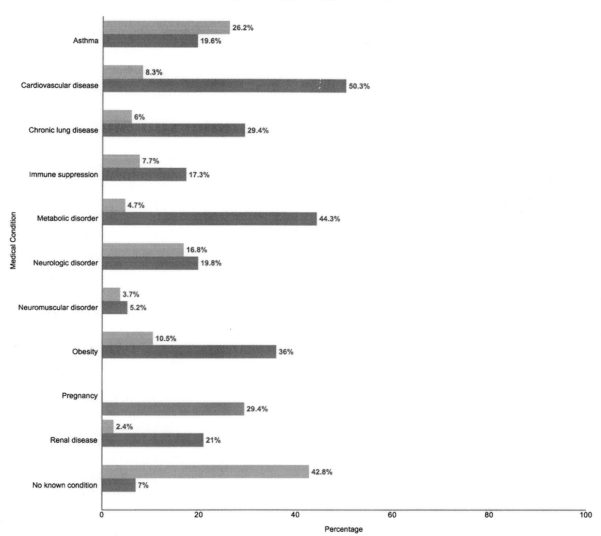

FIGURE 1

Selected underlying medical conditions in patients hospitalized with laboratory-confirmed influenza (Influenza Hospitalization Surveillance Network 2017–2018). Asthma includes a medical diagnosis of asthma or a reactive airway disease. Cardiovascular diseases include conditions such as coronary heart disease, cardiac valve disorders, congestive heart failure, pulmonary hypertension, and aortic stenosis; hypertension disease alone is not included. Chronic lung diseases include conditions such as chronic obstructive pulmonary disease, bronchiolitis obliterans, chronic aspiration pneumonia, and interstitial lung disease. Immune suppression includes conditions such as immunoglobulin deficiency, leukemia, lymphoma, HIV and/or AIDS, and individuals taking immunosuppressive medications. Metabolic disorders include conditions such as diabetes mellitus, thyroid dysfunction, adrenal insufficiency, and liver disease. Neurologic disorders include conditions such as seizure disorders, cerebral palsy, and cognitive dysfunction. Neuromuscular disorders include conditions such as multiple sclerosis and muscular dystrophy. Obesity was assigned if indicated in a patient's medical chart of if BMI was >30. Pregnancy percentage was calculated by using the number of female case patients between 15 and 44 years of age as the denominator. Renal diseases include conditions such as acute or chronic renal failure, nephrotic syndrome, glomerulonephritis, and impaired creatinine clearance. No known condition indicates that the case patient did not have any known underlying medical condition indicated in the medical chart at the time of hospitalization. (Reprinted from Centers for Disease Control and Prevention. FluView 2017–2018 preliminary data as of August 18, 2018. Available at: gis.cdc.gov/grasp/fluview/FluHospChars.html.)

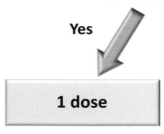

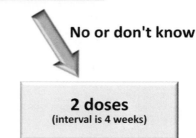

FIGURE 2

The number of 2018–2019 seasonal influenza vaccine doses for children 6 months through 8 years of age. ª The 2 doses need not have been received during the same season or consecutive seasons. ᵇ Receipt of LAIV4 in the past is still expected to have primed a child's immune system despite recent evidence for poor effectiveness. There currently are no data that suggest otherwise.

updated LAIV4 formulation available for the 2018–2019 season to provide their latest recommendations. Although the AAP and CDC each support the use of LAIV4 for the 2018–2019 influenza season with the aim of achieving adequate vaccination coverage and optimal protection in children of all ages, the AAP recommends vaccination with IIV3 or IIV4 for all children and LAIV4 for children who would not otherwise receive an influenza vaccine (eg, refusal of an IIV) and for whom it is appropriate according to age (ie, 2 years of age and older) and health status (ie, healthy and without any underlying chronic medical condition).

5. Both trivalent and quadrivalent influenza vaccines are available in the United States for the 2018–2019 season. To vaccinate as many people as possible for this influenza season, neither vaccine formulation is preferred over the other. Although manufacturers anticipate an adequate supply of the quadrivalent vaccine, pediatricians should administer whichever formulation is available in their communities. The trivalent vaccine contains an influenza

A(Michigan/45/2015[H1N1]) pdm09–like virus, an influenza A(Singapore/INFIMH-16-0019/2016[H3N2])–like virus, and an influenza B(Colorado/60/2017)–like virus (B/Victoria lineage). The influenza A(H3N2) virus component is updated because the egg-propagated influenza A (Singapore) vaccine virus is antigenically more similar to circulating viruses. The influenza B component is updated because of the increasing global circulation of an antigenically drifted influenza B (Victoria lineage) virus. The quadrivalent vaccine contains an additional influenza B(Phuket/3073/2013)–like virus (B/Yamagata lineage), which is the same as last season.

6. The number of seasonal influenza vaccine doses to be administered in the 2018–2019 influenza season remains the same and depends on a child's age at the time of the first administered dose and vaccine history (Fig 2):

- Influenza vaccines are not licensed for administration to infants younger than 6 months.

- Children 9 years and older need only 1 dose.

- Children 6 months through 8 years of age need the following:
  o 2 doses if they have received fewer than 2 doses of any trivalent or quadrivalent influenza vaccine (IIV or live attenuated influenza vaccine [LAIV]) before July 1, 2018. The interval between the 2 doses should be at least 4 weeks; or
  o Only 1 dose if they have previously received 2 or more total doses of any trivalent or quadrivalent influenza vaccine (IIV or LAIV) before July 1, 2018. The 2 previous doses do not need to have been received during the same influenza season or consecutive influenza seasons.

Vaccination should not be delayed to obtain a specific product for either dose. Any available age-appropriate trivalent or quadrivalent vaccine can be used. A child who receives only 1 of the 2 doses as a quadrivalent formulation is likely to be less primed against the additional influenza B virus.

7. Pediatric offices may choose to serve as a venue for providing influenza vaccination for parents and other care providers of children if the practice is acceptable to both pediatricians and the adults who are to be vaccinated.[1] Medical liability issues and medical record documentation requirements need to be considered before a pediatrician begins immunizing adults.[9] (see risk management guidance associated with adult immunizations at http://pediatrics.aappublications.org/content/129/1/e247). Pediatricians are reminded to document the recommendation for adult vaccination in the child's medical record. In addition, adults should still be encouraged to have a medical home and communicate their vaccination status to their primary care providers. Offering adult vaccinations in the pediatric

TABLE 2 People at High Risk of Influenza Complications and Thus Recommended for Antiviral Treatment of Suspected or Confirmed Influenza

Children <5 years and especially <2 years

Adults ≥50 years

People with chronic pulmonary (including asthma), cardiovascular (except hypertension alone), renal, hepatic, hematologic (including sickle cell disease), or metabolic disorders (including diabetes mellitus) or neurologic and neurodevelopment conditions (including disorders of the brain, spinal cord, peripheral nerve, and muscle such as cerebral palsy, epilepsy [seizure disorders], stroke, intellectual disability, moderate to severe developmental delay, muscular dystrophy, or spinal cord injury)

People with immunosuppression, including that caused by medications or by HIV infection

All women who are pregnant, are considering pregnancy, or are in the postpartum period during the influenza season

People <19 years old who are receiving long-term aspirin therapy

American Indian and/or Alaskan native people

People with extreme obesity (ie, BMI ≥40)

Residents of nursing homes and other chronic care facilities

Hospitalized patients at high risk of influenza complications

Adapted from Grohskopf LA, Sokolow LZ, Broder KR, et al. Prevention and control of seasonal influenza with vaccines: recommendations of the Advisory Committee on Immunization Practices—United States, 2018–19 influenza season. *MMWR Recomm Rep.* 2018;67(3):1–20.

practice setting would not be intended to undermine the adult medical home model but could serve as an additional venue for parents and other care providers of children to receive influenza vaccines. Vaccination of close contacts of children at high risk of influenza-related complications (Table 2) is intended to reduce children's risk of exposure to influenza (ie, "cocooning"). The practice of cocooning also may help protect infants younger than 6 months who are too young to be immunized with the influenza vaccine.

8. Pregnant women who are immunized against influenza at any time during their pregnancy can provide protection for infants during their first 6 months of life, when they are too young to receive the influenza vaccine themselves, through transplacental passage of antibodies. Postpartum women who did not receive an influenza vaccination during pregnancy should be encouraged to discuss with their obstetricians receipt of the vaccine before discharge from the hospital. Vaccination during breastfeeding is safe for mothers and their infants. Pregnant women are a population of special concern because they are at increased risk for complications from influenza. Influenza vaccination is recommended by the ACIP and the American College of Obstetricians

and Gynecologists for all women at any trimester of gestation for the protection of mothers against influenza and its complications.[1, 10] Substantial evidence has been accumulated regarding the efficacy of maternal influenza immunization in preventing laboratory-confirmed influenza disease and its complications in both mothers and their infants in the first 2 to 6 months of life.[11–17] Infants born to women who receive an influenza vaccination during pregnancy can have a risk reduction of 72% (95% CI 39% to 87%) for laboratory-confirmed influenza hospitalization in the first few months of life.[18]

Any licensed, recommended, and age-appropriate trivalent or quadrivalent inactivated vaccine may be used to vaccinate pregnant women, including quadrivalent recombinant inactivated vaccine (RIV4).[1] However, experience with the use of RIVs in pregnant women 18 years and older is limited because RIVs have been available only since the 2013–2014 influenza season. Substantial data indicate that an IIV does not cause fetal harm when administered to a pregnant woman, although data on the safety of influenza vaccination in the early first trimester are limited.[19] A cohort study from the Vaccines and Medications in Pregnancy Surveillance System of vaccine exposure during the 2010–2011 through 2013–2014 seasons

revealed no significant association of spontaneous abortion with influenza vaccine exposure in the first trimester or within the first 20 weeks of gestation.[20] Although researchers in previous studies have not noted any association between influenza vaccination and adverse pregnancy outcomes, one recent observational Vaccine Safety Datalink (VSD) study conducted during the 2010–2011 and 2011–2012 influenza seasons noted an association between the receipt of an IIV containing H1N1pdm09 and early spontaneous abortion when an H1N1pdm-09–containing vaccine had also been received the previous season.[21] A follow-up study is in progress. The ACIP influenza vaccine recommendations for pregnant women have not been changed for this coming season.

9. As soon as a seasonal influenza vaccine becomes available locally, pediatricians or vaccine administrators should encourage immunization of HCP, notify parents and caregivers of vaccine availability and the importance of annual vaccination, and immunize children 6 months and older per recommendations, especially those at high risk of complications from influenza. This strategy is particularly important for children who need 2 doses of the influenza vaccine to achieve optimal protection before the circulation of influenza viruses in the community. Children should receive the first dose as soon as possible after a vaccine becomes available to allow sufficient time for receipt of the second dose ≥4 weeks later, preferably by the end of October. The onset and duration of influenza circulation is unpredictable. To effectively protect children, prompt initiation of influenza vaccination and continuing to vaccinate throughout the influenza season, regardless of whether influenza is circulating (or has circulated) in the community, are important components of an effective vaccination strategy. Protective immune responses generally persist in children throughout the influenza season. Although there is limited evidence that waning immunity from early administration of the vaccine increases the risk of infection in children, authors of recent reports raise the possibility that early vaccination of adults, particularly the elderly, might contribute to reduced protection later in the influenza season. Older adults are recognized as having a less robust immune response to influenza vaccines. A multiseason analysis from the US Influenza Vaccine Effectiveness Network revealed that vaccine effectiveness declined by approximately 7% per month for H3N2 and influenza B and by 6% to 11% per month for H1N1pdm09 in individuals 9 years and older.[22] Vaccine effectiveness remained greater than zero for at least 5 to 6 months after vaccination. Further evaluation is needed before any policy change in timing is made. An early onset of the influenza season is another concern about delayed vaccination. Until there are definitive data that can be used to determine whether waning immunity influences vaccine effectiveness in children, the administration of the influenza vaccine should not be delayed to a later date because this increases the likelihood of missing influenza vaccination altogether.

10. To effectively protect children, providers may continue to offer the vaccine until June 30 of each year, when the seasonal influenza vaccine expires, because the duration of influenza circulation is unpredictable. Although peak influenza activity in the United States tends to occur from January through March, influenza activity can occur in early fall (October) or late spring (end of May) and may have more than one disease peak. Similarly, although influenza activity in the United States is typically low during the summer, influenza cases and outbreaks also can occur. Furthermore, this approach also allows for optimal ability to immunize travelers, particularly international travelers, who may be exposed to influenza yearround depending on their destinations.

11. HCP, influenza campaign organizers, and public health agencies are encouraged to collaborate to develop improved strategies for the planning, distribution, communication, and administration of vaccines. These include the following:

- Plan to make influenza vaccination easily accessible for all children. Examples include sending alerts to families that a vaccine is available (eg, e-mails, texts, letters, and patient portals); creating walk-in influenza vaccination clinics; extending hours beyond routine times during peak vaccination periods; administering an influenza vaccine during both well-child examinations and sick visits as well as to patients who are hospitalized, especially those at high risk of influenza complications, before discharge from the hospital (unless medically contraindicated); implementing standing orders for influenza vaccination; considering how to immunize parents, adult caregivers, and siblings (see risk management guidance associated with adult immunizations at

http://pediatrics.aappublications.org/content/129/1/e247)[9] at the same time in the same office setting as children; and working with other institutions (eg, schools, child care programs, local public health departments, and religious organizations) or alternative care sites, such as emergency departments, to expand venues for administering the vaccine. If a child receives the influenza vaccine outside of his or her medical home, such as at a pharmacy, retail-based clinic, or another practice setting, appropriate documentation of vaccination should be provided to the patient to be shared with his or her medical home and entered into the state or regional immunization information system (ie, registry).

- Concerted efforts among the aforementioned groups, plus vaccine manufacturers, distributors, and payers, are necessary to appropriately prioritize distribution to the primary care office setting and patient-centered medical homes before other venues, especially when vaccine supplies are delayed or limited. Similar efforts should be made to assuage the vaccine supply discrepancy between privately insured patients and those eligible for vaccination through the Vaccines for Children Program.

- Public health will benefit from pediatricians' discussions about vaccine safety, effectiveness, and indications. Pediatricians can influence vaccine acceptance by explaining the importance of annual influenza vaccination for children, emphasizing when a second dose of the vaccine is indicated, and explaining why the intranasal formulation is not recommended for routine use in all children. The AAP and CDC have created communication resources to convey these important messages and help the public understand influenza recommendations. Resources will be available in the *Red Book Online* (https://redbook. solutions.aap.org/selfserve/ ssPage.aspx?SelfServeContentId= influenza-resources).[23]

- The AAP supports mandatory influenza vaccination programs for all HCP in all settings, including outpatient settings. HCP should act as role models for both their patients and colleagues by receiving influenza vaccination annually and letting others know that they have received the vaccine, highlighting the safety and effectiveness of annual influenza vaccination. Influenza vaccination programs for HCP benefit the health of employees, their patients, and members of the community. Mandatory influenza immunization for all HCP is considered to be ethical, just, and necessary to improve patient safety. Employees of health care institutions are asked to act in the best interests of the health of their patients and to honor the requirement of causing no harm.

12. Antiviral medications are important in the control of influenza but are not a substitute for influenza vaccination. The neuraminidase inhibitors (NAIs) oral oseltamivir (Tamiflu) and inhaled zanamivir (Relenza) are the best-studied antiviral medications recommended for chemoprophylaxis or the treatment of influenza in children during the 2018–2019 season.[24] Intravenous peramivir (Rapivab), a third NAI, was approved in September 2017 as a treatment of acute uncomplicated influenza in children 2 years and older who are not hospitalized and have been symptomatic for no more than 2 days. Intravenous zanamivir is not approved in the United States and is not available for compassionate use.[25] Intravenous formulations are especially important as the only treatment option for serious

influenza infection in those children who cannot absorb orally or enterally administered oseltamivir or tolerate inhaled zanamivir.

Recent viral surveillance and resistance data from the CDC and the World Health Organization reveal that the majority of currently circulating influenza viruses likely to cause influenza in North America during the 2018–2019 season continue to be susceptible to oseltamivir, zanamivir, and peramivir.[1] If a newly emergent oseltamivir- or peramivir-resistant virus is a concern, recommendations for alternative system treatment, such as the use of intravenous zanamivir,[25,26] will be available from the CDC and AAP. Resistance characteristics can also change for an individual child over the duration of a treatment course, especially in those who are severely immunocompromised and may receive extended courses of antiviral medications because of prolonged viral shedding. Up-to-date information on current recommendations and therapeutic options can be found on the AAP Web site (www.aap.org) or in the *Red Book Online*, through state-specific AAP chapter Web sites, or on the CDC Web site.[27]

SEASONAL INFLUENZA VACCINES

Before the 2013–2014 influenza season, only trivalent influenza vaccines that included a single influenza B strain were available. Since the 1980s, 2 antigenically distinct lineages (ie, Victoria or Yamagata) of influenza B viruses have circulated globally. Vaccination against 1 influenza B viral lineage generally confers little cross-protection against the other influenza B viral lineage. Thus, trivalent vaccines offer limited immunity against circulating influenza B strains of the lineage not present in the vaccine. Furthermore, in recent

years, it has proven difficult to predict consistently which influenza B lineage will predominate during a given influenza season. Therefore, a quadrivalent vaccine with influenza B strains of both lineages would be predicted to offer additional protection, but there is no evidence at this time that a quadrivalent vaccine is more effective. Table 3 includes a summary of information on the types of influenza vaccines licensed for children and adults during the 2018–2019 season. More than 1 product may be appropriate for a given patient. Vaccination should not be delayed to obtain a specific product.

IIVs

For the 2018–2019 season, an IIV will be available for intramuscular injection in both IIV3 and IIV4 formulations. IIVs do not contain a live virus. The available IIV formulations and age groups for which use is approved are presented in Table 4. IIV formulations can be used in healthy children as well as those with underlying chronic medical conditions. The most common adverse events after IIV3 administration are local injection site pain and tenderness. Fever occurs within 24 hours after immunization in approximately 10% to 35% of children younger than 2 years but rarely in older children and adults. Mild systemic symptoms, such as nausea, lethargy, headache, muscle aches, and chills, may occur after the administration of IIV3. Several formulations of IIV4 are now available with specific age indications, including brands licensed for use in children as young as 6 months. In children, the most common injection site adverse reactions after the administration of IIV4 are pain, redness, and swelling. The most common systemic adverse events are drowsiness, irritability, loss of appetite, fatigue, muscle aches, headache, arthralgia, and gastrointestinal tract symptoms.

TABLE 3 Recommended Seasonal Influenza Vaccines for Different Age Groups: United States, 2018–2019 Influenza Season

Vaccine	Trade Name	Manufacturer	Presentation	Thimerosal Mercury Content (μm of Hg per 0.5 mL Dose)	Age Group	CPT Code
Inactivated						
IIV3	Fluzone high-dose	Sanofi Pasteur	0.5 mL prefilled syringe	0	≥65 y	90662
IIV3	Afluria	Seqirus	0.5 mL prefilled syringe	0	≥5 y	90656
			5.0 mL multidose vial	24.5	≥5 y	90658
aIIV3	Fluad	Seqirus	0.5 mL prefilled syringe	0	≥65 y	90653
ccIIV4	Flucelvax quadrivalent	Seqirus	0.5 mL prefilled syringe	0	≥4 y	90674
			5.0 mL multidose vial	25	≥4 y	90756
IIV4	Fluzone quadrivalent	Sanofi Pasteur	0.25 mL prefilled syringe	0	6–35 mo	90685
			0.5-mL prefilled syringe	0	≥36 mo	90686
			5.0 mL multidose vial	25	≥6 mo	90687, 90688
IIV4	Fluarix quadrivalent	GlaxoSmithKline	0.5 mL prefilled syringe	0	≥6 mo	90686
IIV4	FluLaval quadrivalent	ID Biomedical Corporation of Quebec	0.5 mL prefilled syringe	0	≥6 mo	90686
		Distributed by GlaxoSmithKline	5.0 mL multidose vial	<25	≥6 mo	90688
IIV4	Afluria quadrivalent	Seqirus	0.5 mL prefilled syringe	0	≥5 y	90686
			5.0 mL multidose vial	24.5	≥5 y	90688
Recombinant						
RIV4	Flublok quadrivalent	Protein Sciences Corporation (distributed by Sanofi Pasteur)	0.5 mL prefilled syringe	0	≥18 y	90682
Live attenuated						
LAIV4	FluMist quadrivalent	MedImmune	0.2 mL prefilled intranasal sprayer	0	2–49 y	90672

aIIV3, adjuvanted inactivated influenza vaccine trivalent; ccIIV4, quadrivalent cell culture–based inactivated influenza vaccine; CPT, *Current Procedural Terminology*. Implementation guidance on supply, pricing, payment, CPT coding, and liability issues can be found in the *Red Book Online*.[28] Adapted from American Academy of Pediatrics, Committee on Infectious Diseases. Recommendations for prevention and control of influenza in children, 2017–2018. *Pediatrics*. 2017;140(4):e20172550; and Grohskopf LA, Sokolow LZ, Broder KR, et al. Prevention and control of seasonal in uenza with vaccines: recommendations of the Advisory Committee on Immunization Practices—United States, 2018–19 influenza season. MMWR Recomm Rep. 2018;67(3):1–20.

These events are reported with comparable frequency with IIV3s. Therefore, an IIV4 is available for people ≥6 months old when otherwise appropriate and may offer broader protection against circulating influenza B strains than an IIV3.

This is the first influenza season during which several vaccine products are licensed for children 6 through 35 months of age, as listed in Table 3. All of these vaccines are quadrivalent, but the dose volumes and antigen amounts vary among different IIV products. In addition to the 0.25 mL (7.5 μg of hemagglutinin per vaccine virus) Fluzone vaccine, 2 other IIV4 vaccines containing 15 μg of hemagglutinin per vaccine virus per 0.5 mL dose (Fluarix and FluLaval) are now available for children 6 through 35 months of age.

TABLE 4 Summary of Antiviral Treatment of Clinical Influenza During the 2018–2019 Season

Offer Treatment ASAP to Children	Consider Treatment ASAP for
Hospitalized with suspected influenza	Any healthy child with suspected influenza
Hospitalized for severe, complicated, or progressive illness attributable to influenza regardless of duration of symptoms	Healthy children with suspected influenza who live at home with a sibling or household contact who is <6 months old or has a medical condition that predisposes to complications
With suspected influenza (of any severity) and at high risk of complications	

ASAP, as soon as possible.

Before November 2016, the only IIV formulations licensed for children 6 through 35 months of age were the 0.25 mL (containing 7.5 μg of hemagglutinin per vaccine virus) dose formulations of Fluzone and Fluzone Quadrivalent. The recommendation for the use of a reduced dose and volume for children in this age group (half of that recommended for people ≥3 years of age) was based on the increased reactogenicity noted among children (particularly younger children)

after older influenza vaccines, primarily whole-virus inactivated vaccines. Currently available split-virus inactivated products have demonstrated less reactogenicity.[1]

Given that the formulations of IIV4 vaccines for children 6 through 35 months of age are different, care should be taken to administer the appropriate, recommended volume and dose for each product. In each instance, the recommended volume may be administered from an appropriate prefilled syringe, a single-dose vial, or a multidose vial (a maximum of 10 doses can be withdrawn from a multidose vial) as supplied by the manufacturer. Note that for Fluzone, if a 0.5 mL single-use vial of Fluzone Quadrivalent is used for a child between 6 and 35 months of age, only half the volume (0.25 mL) should be administered to provide the currently approved dose for this product, and the other half should be discarded. A 0.5 mL unit dose of any IIV should not be split into 2 separate 0.25 mL doses because of safety concerns for lack of sterility, variance with the package insert, and potential compliance difficulties with vaccine excise taxes.

Children 36 months of age and older can receive any licensed IIV. All IIVs licensed for children of this age in the United States are split-product, egg-based, inactivated vaccines administered in a 0.5 mL dose and containing 15 µg of hemagglutinin from each strain in the vaccine.

Two quadrivalent influenza vaccines manufactured by using newer technologies will be available during the 2018–2019 season, 1 of which can be used in children. A recombinant baculovirus-expressed hemagglutinin influenza vaccine (RIV4) for people 18 years and older is produced in cell culture, and a quadrivalent cell culture–based IIV is available for individuals 4 years and older. Both of these vaccines are also administered intramuscularly. No preference is expressed for RIV4 versus IIVs within specified indications.

The US Food and Drug Administration (FDA) licensed a trivalent MF59 adjuvanted IIV for people 65 years and older in November 2015; it was the first adjuvanted influenza vaccine marketed in the United States. Adjuvants may be included in a vaccine to elicit a more robust immune response, which could lead to a reduction in the number of doses required for children. In 1 recent study of children, the relative vaccine efficacy of an MF-59 adjuvanted influenza vaccine was significantly greater than a nonadjuvanted vaccine in the 6- through 23-month age group.[29] However, adjuvanted seasonal influenza vaccines are not licensed for children at this time.

During the 2 influenza seasons spanning 2010 through 2012, there were increased reports of febrile seizures in the United States in young children who received an IIV3 and the 13-valent pneumococcal conjugate vaccine (PCV13) concomitantly. Subsequent retrospective analyses of past seasons revealed a slight increase in the risk of febrile seizures in children 6 through 23 months of age when PCV13 vaccines are administered concomitantly with an IIV.[30] The concomitant administration of an IIV3, PCV13, and the diphtheria-tetanus-acellular pertussis vaccine was associated with the greatest relative risk estimate, corresponding to a maximum additional 30 febrile seizure cases per 100 000 children vaccinated compared with the administration of the vaccines on separate days. In contrast, data from the Post-Licensure Rapid Immunization Safety Monitoring (PRISM) program of the FDA, the largest vaccine safety surveillance program in the United States, revealed that there was no significant increase in febrile seizures associated with the concomitant administration of these 3 vaccines in children 6 to 59 months of age during the 2010–2011 season.[31] In a subsequent sentinel Center for Biologics Evaluation and Research–Post-Licensure Rapid Immunization Safety Monitoring surveillance report looking at influenza vaccines and febrile seizures in the 2013–2014 and 2014–2015 influenza seasons, there was no evidence of an elevated risk of febrile seizures in children 6 to 23 months of age after IIV vaccination during the 2013–2014 and 2014–2015 seasons. It was concluded that the risk of seizures after PCV13 or concomitant PCV13 and IIV administration is low compared with a child's lifetime risk of febrile seizures due to other causes.[32] Although the possibility of increased risk for febrile seizures cannot be ruled out, the simultaneous administration of an IIV with PCV13 and/or other vaccines for the 2018–2019 influenza season continues to be recommended when these vaccines are indicated. Overall, the benefits of timely vaccination with same-day administration of an IIV and PCV13 or the diphtheria-tetanus-acellular pertussis vaccine outweigh the risk of febrile seizures, which rarely have any long-term sequelae.

A large body of scientific evidence reveals that thimerosal-containing vaccines are not associated with increased risk of autism spectrum disorders in children.[1] Thimerosal from vaccines has not been linked to any medical condition. As such, the AAP extends its strongest support to the current World Health Organization recommendations to retain the use of thimerosal as a preservative in multiuse vials in the global vaccine supply. Some people may still raise concerns about the trace amount of thimerosal in some IIV vaccine formulations (Table 3), and in some states, including California, Delaware, Illinois, Missouri, New York, and Washington, there is a legislated restriction on the use of thimerosal-containing vaccines. The benefits of protecting children against the known risks of influenza are clear. Therefore, to the extent authorized by state law, children should receive any available formulation of an IIV rather than delay vaccination while waiting for reduced thimerosal content or thimerosal-free vaccines. Although some IIV formulations contain a trace amount of thimerosal, thimerosal-free IIV products can be obtained (Table 3). To respond to consumer requests, vaccine manufacturers are delivering increasing amounts of thimerosal-free influenza vaccines each year.

Live Attenuated (Intranasal) Influenza Vaccine

For the 2018–2019 influenza season, the AAP recommends LAIV4 to be used for children who would not otherwise receive an influenza vaccine (eg, refusal of an IIV) and for whom it is appropriate according to age (ie, 2 years of age and older) and health status (ie, healthy and without any underlying chronic medical condition). This recommendation represents a change from the 2016–2017 and 2017–2018 influenza seasons, when intranasal LAIV4 was not recommended in any setting in light of the evidence of its poor effectiveness in previous seasons against influenza A(H1N1)pdm09 viruses. After reviewing studies on the effectiveness of LAIV4 during past seasons, the ACIP of the CDC recommended that LAIV4 be an option for influenza vaccination in people for whom it is appropriate for the 2018–2019 season.[1] Although the AAP and the CDC each support the use of LAIV4 for the 2018–2019 season with the aim of achieving adequate vaccination coverage and optimal protection in children of all ages and both acknowledge that efficacy data are not available for the current LAIV4 formulation, the AAP recommends IIV3 or IIV4 as the primary choice of influenza vaccine for all children.

LAIV was initially licensed in the United States in 2003 as a trivalent formulation. LAIV4 has been licensed in the United States since 2012 and was first available during the 2013–2014 influenza season, replacing trivalent live attenuated influenza vaccine (LAIV3). Recommended for people 2 through 49 years of age, LAIV4 is administered intranasally. The most commonly reported reactions in children were runny nose or nasal congestion, headache, decreased activity or lethargy, and sore throat. LAIV4 should not be administered to people with notable nasal congestion because that can impede vaccine delivery. The safety of LAIV in people with a history of asthma, diabetes mellitus, or other high-risk medical conditions associated with an elevated risk of complications from influenza (see the section on contraindications and precautions) has not been firmly established. In postlicensure surveillance of LAIV over 7 seasons, the Vaccine Adverse Event Reporting System, jointly sponsored by the FDA and CDC, did not identify any new or unexpected safety concerns, although there were reports of the use of LAIV in people with a contraindication or precaution. Although the use of LAIV in young children with chronic medical conditions, including asthma, has been implemented outside of the United States, data are considered insufficient to support an expanded recommendation in the United States.

The CDC conducted a systematic review of all published studies evaluating the effectiveness of LAIV3 and LAIV4 in children from the 2010–2011 to the 2016–2017 seasons, including data from United States and European studies.[1,33] The data revealed that the effectiveness of LAIV3 or LAIV4 for influenza strain A (H1N1) was lower than that of an IIV in children 2 to 17 years of age. A LAIV was more effective against influenza B strains and similarly effective against influenza A(H3N2) in some age groups compared with an IIV.

For the 2017–2018 season, a new influenza A(/H1N1) pdm09–like virus, influenza A/Slovenia/2903/2015, was included in LAIV4, replacing influenza A/Bolivia/559/2013. In a study conducted by the LAIV4 manufacturer, researchers evaluated viral shedding and immunogenicity associated with the LAIV4 formulation containing the new influenza A(/H1N1)pdm09–like virus among US children 24 months through 3 years of age. Shedding and immunogenicity data provided by the manufacturer reveal that the new influenza A(H1N1)pdm09–like virus included in its latest formulation has improved replicative fitness over previous LAIV4 influenza A(H1N1) pdm09–like vaccine strains, resulting in an improved immune response comparable to that of the LAIV3 available before the 2009 pandemic. Shedding and replicative fitness are not known to be correlated with efficacy, and no published effectiveness estimates for this formulation of the vaccine against influenza A(H1N1)pdm09 viruses are available because influenza A(H3N2) and influenza B viruses predominated during the 2017–2018 Northern Hemisphere season.

The effectiveness of influenza vaccines varies and is affected by many factors, including age and health status of the recipient, influenza type and subtype, previous vaccinations, and degree of antigenic match between the vaccine and circulating viruses. It is possible that vaccine effectiveness also differs among different individual vaccine products (for example, different IIVs); however, product-specific comparative effectiveness data are lacking for most vaccines. Although national influenza vaccination coverage among children did not decline during the past 2 seasons, when LAIV was not recommended in the United States, overall vaccination coverage remains suboptimal. Additional options for the vaccination of children may provide a means to improve coverage, particularly in school-based settings.

Particular focus should be placed on the administration of an IIV in all children and adolescents with underlying medical conditions associated with an elevated risk of complications from influenza. Achieving high coverage rates of influenza vaccine in infants and children is a priority to protect them against influenza disease and its complications. Additional experience over multiple influenza seasons will help to determine optimal use of the available vaccine formulations in children.

INFLUENZA VACCINES AND EGG ALLERGY

It is not necessary to inquire about egg allergy before the administration of any influenza vaccine, including on screening forms. There is strong evidence that individuals with egg allergy can safely receive an influenza vaccine without any additional precautions beyond those recommended for any vaccine.[1,34,] [35] The presence of egg allergy in an individual is not a contraindication to receive an IIV or LAIV. Influenza vaccine recipients with egg allergy are at no greater risk for a systemic allergic reaction than those without egg allergy. Precautions, such as choice of a particular vaccine, special observation periods, or restriction of administration to particular medical settings, are not warranted and constitute an unnecessary barrier to immunization. Standard vaccination practice for all vaccines in children should include the ability to respond to rare acute hypersensitivity reactions. Patients who refuse to receive an egg-based vaccine may be vaccinated with an age-appropriate recombinant or cell-cultured product. Children who have had a previous allergic reaction to any component of the influenza vaccine, for any reason, should be evaluated by an allergist to determine whether future receipt of the vaccine is appropriate.

VACCINE STORAGE AND ADMINISTRATION

The AAP Storage and Handling Tip Sheet provides resources for practices to develop comprehensive vaccine management protocols to keep the temperature for vaccine storage constant during a power failure or other disaster (https://www.aap.org/en-us/Documents/immunization_disasterplanning.pdf).[36] The AAP recommends the development of a written disaster plan for all practice settings. Additional information is available on the AAP Web site.[37]

Any of the influenza vaccines can be administered at the same visit with all other recommended routine vaccines.

Intramuscular Vaccine

IIVs for intramuscular injection are shipped and stored at 2°C to 8°C (36°F–46°F); frozen vaccines should not be used. These vaccines are administered intramuscularly into the anterolateral thigh of infants and young children and into the deltoid muscle of older children and adults. Most vaccines have variable immune responses in young children. This is the first influenza season for which 3 vaccine products are available for children 6 through 35 months of age, as listed in Table 3. The dose volume of the available vaccines, 2 of which contain twice the amount of antigen in this young age group, varies for these different brands, so care should be taken by clinicians to administer the correct dose. Clinical data reveal comparable immunogenicity and reactogenicity for these vaccines with the one used in this age group in recent seasons and administered as 0.25 mL per dose (Table 3). Although the amount of antigen differs, the number of doses required with either vaccine for this age group is the same. A 0.5 mL unit dose of any IIV should not be split into 2 separate 0.25 mL doses because of safety concerns for lack of sterility, variance

with the package insert, and potential compliance difficulties with vaccine excise taxes.

LAIV4

The cold-adapted, temperature-sensitive LAIV4 formulation currently licensed in the United States is shipped and stored at 2°C to 8°C (35°F–46°F) and administered intranasally in a prefilled, single-use sprayer containing 0.2 mL of the vaccine. A removable dose-divider clip is attached to the sprayer to facilitate the administration of 0.1 mL separately into each nostril. After the administration of any live virus vaccine, at least 4 weeks should pass before another live-virus vaccine is administered.

CURRENT AAP RECOMMENDATIONS

Seasonal influenza vaccination is recommended for all children 6 months and older. The AAP recommends an IIV (IIV3 or IIV4) as the primary influenza vaccine choice for all children because the effectiveness of LAIV4 was inferior against influenza A(H1N1) during past seasons, and effectiveness is unknown against influenza A(H1N1) for this upcoming season. LAIV4 may be used for children who would not otherwise receive an influenza vaccine (eg, refusal of an IIV) and for whom it is appropriate according to age (ie, 2 years of age and older) and health status (ie, healthy and without any underlying chronic medical condition). Additional details on the contraindications and precautions for the use of all influenza vaccines are listed below.

Children and adolescents with certain underlying medical conditions have an elevated risk of complications from influenza, including the following:

• asthma or other chronic pulmonary diseases, including cystic fibrosis;

- hemodynamically significant cardiac disease;
- immunosuppressive disorders or therapy;
- HIV infection;
- sickle cell anemia and other hemoglobinopathies;
- diseases that necessitate long-term aspirin therapy or salicylate-containing medication, including juvenile idiopathic arthritis or Kawasaki disease, that may place a child at increased risk of Reye syndrome if infected with influenza;
- chronic renal dysfunction;
- chronic metabolic disease, including diabetes mellitus;
- any condition that can compromise respiratory function or handling of secretions or increase the risk of aspiration, such as neurodevelopmental disorders, spinal cord injuries, seizure disorders, or neuromuscular abnormalities; and
- pregnancy.

Particular efforts should be made to ensure vaccination in the following groups to prevent the transmission of influenza to those at risk, unless contraindicated:

- household contacts and out-of-home care providers of children younger than 5 years and at-risk children of all ages;
- close contacts of people with immunosuppression;
- any woman who is pregnant or considering pregnancy, is in the postpartum period, or is breastfeeding during the influenza season. It is safe to administer an IIV to pregnant women during any trimester of gestation and postpartum. Any licensed, recommended, and age-appropriate trivalent or quadrivalent IIV or RIV4 may be used, although experience with the use of RIV4 in pregnant women is

limited. LAIV is contraindicated during pregnancy. Studies have shown that infants born to women who are immunized have better influenza-related health outcomes compared with infants of women who are unimmunized. However, according to Internet-based panel surveys conducted by the CDC, only approximately 47% of pregnant women during the 2016–2017 influenza season and 35.6% of pregnant women during the 2017–2018 season (according to preliminary data) reported receiving an influenza vaccine, although both pregnant women and their newborn infants are at a higher risk of complications. More data on the safety of influenza vaccination in the early first trimester are becoming available. In a 5-year retrospective cohort study from 2003 to 2008 of more than 10 000 women, influenza vaccination in the first trimester was not associated with an increase in the rates of major congenital malformations.[18] Similarly, a systematic review and meta-analysis of studies of congenital anomalies after vaccination during pregnancy including data from 15 studies (14 cohort studies and 1 case control study) did not reveal any association between congenital defects and influenza vaccination in any trimester, including the first trimester of gestation.[38] Assessments of any association with influenza vaccination and preterm birth and small-for-gestational-age infants have yielded inconsistent results, with most studies reporting a protective effect or no association with these outcomes. A cohort study from the Vaccines and Medications in Pregnancy Surveillance System of vaccine exposure during the 2010–2011 through 2013–2014 seasons revealed no significant association of spontaneous abortion with influenza vaccine

exposure in the first trimester or within the first 20 weeks of gestation.[20] Although researchers in most studies have not noted an association between influenza vaccination and adverse pregnancy outcomes, 1 recent observational Vaccine Safety Datalink study conducted during the 2010–2011 and 2011–2012 seasons revealed an association between receipt of an IIV containing H1N1pdm09 and risk of spontaneous abortion when an H1N1pdm-09–containing vaccine had also been received the previous season.[21] A follow-up study is in progress, and ACIP influenza vaccine recommendations for pregnant women have not been changed for this coming season;

- breastfeeding mothers. Breastfeeding is strongly recommended to protect against influenza viruses because it activates innate antiviral mechanisms, specifically type 1 interferons. Human milk from mothers vaccinated during the third trimester also contains higher levels of influenza-specific immunoglobulin A.[39] Greater exclusivity of breastfeeding in the first 6 months of life decreases the episodes of respiratory illness with fever in infants of mothers who are vaccinated mothers. For infants born to mothers with confirmed influenza illness at delivery, breastfeeding is encouraged, and guidance on breastfeeding practices can be found at https://www.cdc.gov/breastfeeding/breastfeeding-special-circumstances/maternal-or-infant-illnesses/influenza.html and https://www.cdc.gov/flu/professionals/infectioncontrol/peri-post-settings.htm.[40,][41] Breastfeeding should be encouraged even if the mother or infant has influenza. The mother should pump and feed expressed breast milk if she or her infant

TABLE 5 Recommended Dosage and Schedule of Influenza Antiviral Medications for Treatment and Chemoprophylaxis in Children for the 2018–2019 Influenza Season: United States

Medication	Treatment (5 d)	Chemoprophylaxis (10 d)
Oseltamivir[a]		
Adults	75 mg twice daily	75 mg once daily
Children ≥12 mo		
Body wt		
≤15 kg (≤33 lb)	30 mg twice daily	30 mg once daily
>15–23 kg (33–51 lb)	45 mg twice daily	45 mg once daily
>23–40 kg (>51–88 lb)	60 mg twice daily	60 mg once daily
>40 kg (>88 lb)	75 mg twice daily	75 mg once daily
Infants ages 9–11 mo[b]	3.5 mg/kg per dose twice daily	3.5 mg/kg per dose once daily
Term infants ages 0–8 mo[b]	3 mg/kg per dose twice daily	3 mg/kg per dose once daily for infants 3–8 mo old; not recommended for infants <3 mo old unless situation judged critical because of limited safety and efficacy data in this age group
Preterm infants	See details in footnote[c]	—
Zanamivir[d]		
Adults	10 mg (two 5 mg inhalations) twice daily	10 mg (two 5 mg inhalations) once daily
Children (≥7 y old for treatment; ≥5 y old for chemoprophylaxis)	10 mg (two 5 mg inhalations) twice daily	10 mg (two 5 mg inhalations) once daily
Peramivir		
Adults	600 mg intravenous infusion once given over 15–30 min	—
Children (2–12 y old)	One 12 mg/kg dose, up to 600 mg maximum, via intravenous infusion for 15–30 min	—
Children (13–17 y old)	One 600 mg dose via intravenous infusion for 15–30 min	—

Adapted from Centers for Disease Control and Prevention. Antiviral agents for the treatment and chemoprophylaxis of influenza: recommendations of the Advisory Committee on Immunization Practices (ACIP). *MMWR Recomm Rep.* 2011;60(RR–1):1–24; and Kimberlin DW, Acosta EP, Prichard MN, et al; National Institute of Allergy and Infectious Diseases Collaborative Antiviral Study Group. Oseltamivir pharmacokinetics, dosing, and resistance among children aged <2 y with influenza. *J Infect Dis.* 2013;207(5):709–720. — indicates not applicable.

[a] Oseltamivir is administered orally without regard to meals, although administration with meals may improve gastrointestinal tolerability. Oseltamivir is available as Tamiflu in 30 mg, 45 mg, and 75 mg capsules and as a powder for oral suspension that is reconstituted to provide a final concentration of 6 mg/mL. For the 6 mg/mL suspension, a 30 mg dose is given with 5 mL of oral suspension, a 45 mg dose is given with 7.5 mL oral suspension, a 60 mg dose is given with 10 mL oral suspension, and a 75 mg dose is given with 12.5 mL oral suspension. If the commercially manufactured oral suspension is not available, a suspension can be compounded by retail pharmacies (final concentration also 6 mg/mL) on the basis of instructions contained in the package label. In patients with renal insufficiency, the dose should be adjusted on the basis of creatinine clearance. For the treatment of patients with creatinine clearance 10 to 30 mL per min: 75 mg once daily for 5 days. For the chemoprophylaxis of patients with creatinine clearance 10 to 30 mL per min: 30 mg once daily for 10 days after exposure or 75 mg once every other day for 10 days after exposure (5 doses).

[b] Approved by the FDA for children as young as 2 wk of age. Given preliminary pharmacokinetic data and limited safety data, oseltamivir can be used to treat influenza in both term and preterm infants from birth because benefits of therapy are likely to outweigh possible risks of treatment.

[c] Oseltamivir dosing for preterm infants. The wt-based dosing recommendation for preterm infants is lower than for term infants. Preterm infants may have lower clearance of oseltamivir because of immature renal function, and doses recommended for term infants may lead to high drug concentrations in this age group. Limited data from the National Institute of Allergy and Infectious Diseases Collaborative Antiviral Study Group provide the basis for dosing preterm infants by using their postmenstrual age (gestational age plus chronological age): 1.0 mg/kg per dose orally twice daily for those <38 wk postmenstrual age; 1.5 mg/kg per dose orally twice daily for those 38 through 40 wk postmenstrual age; and 3.0 mg/kg per dose orally twice daily for those >40 wk postmenstrual age. For extremely preterm infants (<28 wk), please consult a pediatric infectious diseases physician.

[d] Zanamivir is administered by inhalation by using a proprietary Diskhaler device distributed together with the medication. Zanamivir is a dry powder, not an aerosol, and should not be administered by using nebulizers, ventilators, or other devices typically used for administering medications in aerosolized solutions. Zanamivir is not recommended for people with chronic respiratory diseases, such as asthma or chronic obstructive pulmonary disease, which increase the risk of bronchospasm.

are too sick to breastfeed. If the breastfeeding mother requires antiviral agents, treatment with oral oseltamivir is preferred. However, none of the antiviral agents are reasons to discontinue breastfeeding;

- American Indian and/or Alaskan native children and adolescents;

- HCP or health care volunteers. Despite the AAP recommendation for mandatory influenza immunization for all HCP, many HCP remain unvaccinated. With an increasing number of organizations mandating influenza vaccination, coverage among HCP was 78.6% for the 2016–2017 season, which is similar to the 79.0% in the 2015–2016 season. Early season 2017–2018 vaccine coverage among HCP was 67.6%, which is similar to the early season coverage during the 2016–2017 season. Optimal prevention of influenza in the health care setting depends on the vaccination of at least 90% of HCP, which is consistent with the national Healthy People 2020 target for annual influenza vaccination among HCP. However, overall vaccination rates for this group remain consistently below this goal. The AAP recently reaffirmed its support for a mandatory influenza vaccination policy for all HCP nationwide, including those in outpatient settings. Mandating influenza vaccination for all HCP is ethical, just, and necessary to

TABLE 6 Comparison of Types of Influenza Diagnostic Tests

Testing Category	Method	Influenza Viruses Detected	Distinguished Influenza A Virus Subtypes	Time to Results	Performance
Rapid molecular assay	Nucleic acid amplification	Influenza A or B viral RNA	No	15–30 min	High sensitivity; high specificity
Rapid influenza diagnostic test	Antigen detection	Influenza A or B virus antigens	No	10–15 min	Low-to-moderate sensitivity (higher with analyzer devise); high specificity
Direct and indirect immunofluorescence assays	Antigen detection	Influenza A or B virus antigens	No	1–4 h	Moderate sensitivity; high specificity
Molecular assays (including RT PCR)	Nucleic acid amplification	Influenza A or B viral RNA	Yes, if subtype primers are used	1–8 h	High sensitivity; high specificity
Multiplex molecular assays	Nucleic acid amplification	Influenza A or B viral RNA; other viral or bacterial targets (RNA or DNA)	Yes, if subtype primers are used	1–2 h	High sensitivity; high specificity
Rapid cell culture (shell vial and cell mixtures)	Virus isolation	Influenza A or B virus	Yes	1–3 d	High sensitivity; high specificity
Viral culture (tissue cell culture)	Virus isolation	Influenza A or B virus	Yes	3–10 d	High sensitivity; high specificity

Negative results may not be used to rule out influenza. Respiratory tract specimens should be collected as close to illness onset as possible for testing. Clinicians should consult the manufacturer's package insert for the specific test for the approved respiratory specimen(s). Specificities are generally high (>95%) for all tests compared with RT PCR. FDA-cleared rapid influenza diagnostic tests are Clinical Laboratory Improvement Amendments waived; most FDA-cleared rapid influenza molecular assays are Clinical Laboratory Improvement Amendments waived depending on the specimen. RT, reverse transcriptase. Adapted from Uyeki T, Bernstein H, Bradley JS, et al. Clinical practice guidelines by the Infectious Diseases Society of America (IDSA): 2018 update: diagnosis, treatment, chemoprophylaxis, and institutional outbreak management of seasonal influenza. Clin Infect Dis. 2018;67: in press.

improve patient safety, especially because HCP frequently come into contact with patients at high risk of influenza illness in their clinical settings. For the prevention and control of influenza, all HCP must continue to prioritize the health and safety of patients; and

- people with influenza-associated encephalopathy (IAE). One complication associated with influenza observed in young children is encephalopathy, the most severe category being acute necrotizing encephalopathy (ANE). During the 2009 pandemic, a large increase in pediatric IAE was observed in Japan, and there have been sporadic cases of influenza A(H1N1)pdm09–associated IAE in children reported in the United States and worldwide.[42] Studies support annual influenza vaccination for all children ≥6 months of age in the United States, and it might be especially important in survivors of ANE, their household contacts, and their caregivers. Because of the potential for ANE recurrence, it also is important to closely monitor children with a history of neurologic complications

associated with respiratory illnesses and to promptly initiate antiviral treatment along with influenza testing.

CONTRAINDICATIONS AND PRECAUTIONS

An anaphylactic or serious allergic reaction to any component of the vaccine is the only medical contraindication to influenza vaccination. Children who have had a previous allergic reaction to any component of the influenza vaccine, for any reason, should be evaluated by an allergist to determine whether future receipt of the vaccine is appropriate. Minor illnesses, with or without fever, are not contraindications to the use of influenza vaccines, particularly among children with mild upper respiratory infection symptoms or allergic rhinitis. Children with a moderate-to-severe febrile illness, based on the judgment of the clinician, should not be vaccinated until resolution of the illness.

Specific to influenza vaccination, a history of Guillain-Barre syndrome

(GBS) is considered to be a precaution for the administration of influenza vaccine. The estimated risk for GBS is low, especially in children. Although influenza infection is recognized to be associated with GBS, there is no elevated risk of GBS from influenza vaccination in children. As a precaution, people who are not at high risk for severe influenza and who are known to have experienced GBS within 6 weeks of influenza vaccination generally should not be vaccinated. However, the benefits of influenza vaccination might outweigh the risks for certain people who have a history of GBS (particularly if not associated with previous influenza vaccination) and who also are at high risk for severe complications from influenza.

CHILDREN WHO SHOULD NOT BE VACCINATED WITH LAIV

The following should not be vaccinated with LAIV:

- children younger than 2 years;

- children who have a moderate-to-severe febrile illness as judged by the clinician;

- children with an amount of nasal congestion that would notably impede vaccine delivery;

- children 2 through 4 years of age with a history of recurrent wheezing or a medically attended wheezing episode in the previous 12 months because of the potential for increased wheezing after immunization. In this age range, many children have a history of wheezing with respiratory tract illnesses and are eventually diagnosed with asthma. Therefore, when offering LAIV to children 24 through 59 months of age, pediatricians should screen them by asking the parents or guardians, "In the previous 12 months, has a health care professional ever told you that your child had wheezing?" If a parent answers "yes" to this question, an IIV, rather than LAIV, is recommended;

- children with a diagnosis of asthma;

- children who have received other live-virus vaccines within the previous 4 weeks; however, LAIV can be administered on the same day as other live-virus vaccines if necessary;

- children who have a known or suspected immunodeficiency disease or who are receiving immunosuppressive or immunomodulatory therapies;

- children who are receiving aspirin or other salicylates;

- women who are pregnant or considering pregnancy;

- children with any condition that can compromise respiratory function or the handling of secretions or can increase the risk for aspiration, such as neurodevelopmental disorders, spinal cord injuries, seizure disorders, or neuromuscular abnormalities;

- children taking an influenza antiviral medication (oseltamivir, zanamivir, or peramivir) until 48 hours after stopping the influenza antiviral therapy. If a child recently received LAIV but has an influenza illness for which antiviral agents are appropriate, the antiviral agents should be given. If antiviral agents are necessary for treatment within 5 to 7 days of LAIV immunization, reimmunization may be indicated because of the potential effects of antiviral medications on LAIV replication and immunogenicity; and

- children with chronic underlying medical conditions that may predispose them to complications after wild-type influenza infection, including metabolic disease, diabetes mellitus, other chronic disorders of the pulmonary or cardiovascular systems, renal dysfunction, or hemoglobinopathies. The safety of LAIV in these populations has not been established. These conditions are not contraindications but are listed under the warnings and precautions section of the LAIV package insert. A precaution is a condition in a recipient that might increase the risk or seriousness of an adverse reaction or complicate making another diagnosis because of a possible vaccine-related reaction. A precaution also may exist for conditions that might compromise the ability of the vaccine to produce immunity. Vaccination may be recommended in the presence of a precaution if the benefit of protection from the vaccine outweighs any risk.

An IIV is the vaccine of choice for anyone in close contact with a subset of severely immunocompromised people (ie, those in a protected environment). An IIV is preferred over LAIV for contacts of people who are severely immunocompromised because of a theoretical risk of infection attributable to the LAIV strain in an immunocompromised contact of a person who is LAIV immunized. Available data indicate a low risk of transmission of the virus in both children and adults vaccinated with LAIV. HCP immunized with LAIV may continue to work in most units of a hospital, including the NICU and general oncology ward, using standard infection control techniques. As a precautionary measure, people recently vaccinated with LAIV should restrict contact with patients who are severely immunocompromised for 7 days after immunization, although there have been no reports of LAIV transmission from a person who is vaccinated to a person who is immunocompromised. In the theoretical scenario in which symptomatic LAIV infection develops in an immunocompromised host, oseltamivir or zanamivir could be prescribed because LAIV strains are susceptible to these antiviral medications.

SURVEILLANCE

Information about influenza surveillance is available through the CDC Voice Information System (for influenza updates, call 1-800-232-4636) or at www.cdc.gov/flu/index.htm.[29] Although current influenza season data on circulating strains can not necessarily be used to predict which and in what proportion strains will circulate in the subsequent season, it is instructive to be aware of 2018–2019 influenza surveillance data and use them as a guide for empirical therapy until current seasonal data are available from the CDC. Information is posted weekly on the CDC Web site (www.cdc.gov/flu/weekly/fluactivitysurv.htm).[43] The AAP offers "What's the Latest with the Flu" (www.aap.org/disasters/flu) messages[44] to highlight those details most relevant to AAP members and child care providers on a monthly basis during influenza season.

VACCINE IMPLEMENTATION

The AAP Partnership for Policy Implementation has developed a series of definitions using accepted health information technology standards to assist in the implementation of these recommendations in computer systems and quality measurement efforts. This document is available at https://www.aap.org/en-us/advocacy-and-policy/aap-health-initiatives/immunizations/Influenza-Implementation-Guidance/Pages/default.aspx.[45] In addition, the AAP has developed implementation guidance on supply, payment, coding, and liability issues; these documents can be found in the *Red Book Online*.[28]

USE OF ANTIVIRAL MEDICATIONS

Oral oseltamivir remains the antiviral drug of choice for the management of influenza infections. Although more difficult to administer, inhaled zanamivir is an equally acceptable alternative for patients who do not have chronic respiratory disease. Options are limited for children who cannot absorb orally or enterally administered oseltamivir or tolerate inhaled zanamivir. Intravenous peramivir (Rapivab), a third NAI, was approved in September 2017 as treatment of acute uncomplicated influenza in children 2 years and older who are not hospitalized and have been symptomatic for no more than 2 days. Intravenous zanamivir is not approved in the United States. A prospective, open-label pediatric clinical trial was conducted to investigate pharmacokinetics and the clinical and/or virologic response to treatment with intravenous zanamivir for children 6 months or older with a serious influenza infection and who could not tolerate oral or inhaled NAIs.[25]

Compassionate use was not available for the 2017–2018 season and is not likely to be available during the 2018–2019 influenza season.

Antiviral resistance to any drug can emerge, necessitating continuous population-based assessment that is conducted by the CDC. If local or national influenza surveillance data indicate emergence of an influenza strain with a known antiviral resistance profile, then according to the CDC, empirical treatment can be directed toward that strain with an effective antiviral agent. During the 2017–2018 season, 99% of the influenza A(H1N1)pdm09 viruses tested were susceptible to oseltamivir and peramivir, and all of the tested influenza strains were susceptible to zanamivir. All tested influenza A(H3N2) and influenza B viruses were susceptible to oseltamivir, zanamivir, and peramivir. In contrast, high levels of resistance to amantadine and rimantadine persist among the influenza A viruses currently circulating. Adamantane drugs are not recommended for use against influenza at this time unless resistance patterns change significantly.[1]

Current treatment guidelines for antiviral medications (Table 4) are unchanged for the 2018–2019 season and are applicable to both infants and children with suspected influenza when strains are known to be circulating in the community or when infants or children are tested and confirmed to have influenza.

Oseltamivir is available in capsule and oral suspension formulations. The available capsule doses are 30 mg, 45 mg, and 75 mg, and the commercially manufactured liquid formulation has a concentration of 6 mg/mL in a 60 mL bottle. If the commercially manufactured oral suspension is not available, the capsule may be opened and the contents mixed with simple syrup or Ora-Sweet SF (sugar free) by retail

pharmacies for a final concentration of 6 mg/mL (Table 5).

Continuous monitoring of the epidemiology, change in severity, and resistance patterns of influenza strains by the CDC may lead to new guidance.

Regardless of influenza vaccination status, antiviral treatment should be offered as early as possible to the following individuals (Table 4):

- Children hospitalized with suspected influenza;
- Children hospitalized for severe, complicated, or progressive illness attributable to influenza, regardless of duration of symptoms; and
- Children with suspected influenza (of any severity) and at high risk of complications (Table 2).

Efforts should be made to minimize treatment in patients who are not infected with influenza.

Treatment may be considered for the following individuals (Table 4):

- any otherwise healthy child suspected of having influenza disease. The greatest effect on outcome is expected to occur if treatment can be initiated within 48 hours of illness onset, but it still should be considered if later in the course of a progressive, symptomatic illness; and
- children suspected of having influenza disease and whose siblings or household contacts either are younger than 6 months or have underlying medical conditions that predispose them to complications of influenza.

Studies conducted to date to evaluate the efficacy of NAIs have revealed that timely treatment can reduce the duration of influenza symptoms and fever as well as the risk of certain complications, including hospitalization and death, in pediatric and adult populations.[24,46-51] The number of published randomized, controlled clinical (RCT) studies in children is limited, and interpretation of the results of these studies needs to take into consideration the size of the study (the number of events might not be sufficient to assess specific outcomes in small studies), the variations in the case definition of influenza illness (clinical versus laboratory confirmed), the time of treatment administration in relation to the onset of illness, and the child's age and health status as important variables. A Cochrane review of 6 RCTs of treatment involving 2356 children with clinical influenza, 1255 of whom had laboratory-confirmed influenza, revealed that in children with laboratory-confirmed influenza, oseltamivir and zanamivir reduced the median duration of illness by 36 hours (26%; *P* < .001) and 1.3 days (24%; *P* < .001), respectively.[52] Among the studies reviewed, 1 trial of oseltamivir in children with asthma who had laboratory-confirmed influenza revealed only a nonsignificant reduction in illness duration (10.4 hours [8%]; *P* = .542). Oseltamivir significantly reduced acute otitis media in children aged 1 to 5 years with laboratory-confirmed influenza (risk difference −0.14; 95% CI −0.24 to −0.04).[52] Another Cochrane review of RCTs of adult and children, which included 20 oseltamivir (9623 participants) and 26 zanamivir trials (14 628 participants),[53] revealed no effect of oseltamivir in reducing the duration of illness in children with asthma; but in otherwise healthy children, there was a reduction by a mean difference of 29 hours (95% CI 12 to 47 hours; *P* = .001). No significant effect was observed with zanamivir. Regarding complications, the authors of this review did not find a significant effect of NAIs on reducing hospitalizations, pneumonia, bronchitis, otitis media, or sinusitis in children.[53] More recently, in a meta-analysis of 5 new RCTs that included 1598 children with laboratory-confirmed

influenza, treatment with oseltamivir significantly reduced the duration of illness in this population by 17.6 hours (95% CI −34.7 to −0.62 hours), and when children with asthma were excluded, this difference was larger (−29.9 hours; 95% CI −53.9 to −5.8 hours). The risk of otitis media was 34% lower in this group as well.[47] Overall, efficacy outcomes are best demonstrated in patients with laboratory-confirmed influenza. Researchers in all these studies confirmed vomiting as a frequent side effect of oseltamivir, occurring in approximately 5% of treated patients. The balance between benefits and harms should be considered when making decisions about the use of NAIs for either the treatment or prophylaxis of influenza.

Although prospective comparative studies to determine the efficacy of NAIs in patients who are hospitalized or pediatric patients with comorbidities have not been conducted and prospectively collected data to determine the role of NAIs in treating severe influenza are limited, on the basis of information obtained from retrospective observational studies and meta-analyses conducted to date in both adults and children, most experts support the use of NAIs to treat pediatric patients with severe influenza, including patients who are hospitalized.

Importantly, treatment with oseltamivir for children with serious, complicated, or progressive diseases presumptively or definitively caused by influenza, irrespective of influenza vaccination status or whether illness began greater than 48 hours before admission, continues to be recommended by the AAP, CDC, Infectious Diseases Society of America, and Pediatric Infectious Diseases Society. Earlier treatment provides better clinical responses. However, treatment after 48 hours

of symptoms in adults and children with a moderate-to-severe disease or progressive disease has been shown to provide some benefit and should be offered. No benefit exists for double-dose NAI therapy compared with standard-dose therapy based on published data from a randomized prospective trial enrolling 75% of subjects younger than 15 years.[1,54]

Dosages of antiviral agents for both treatment and chemoprophylaxis in children can be found in Table 5 (for children of all ages, including doses for preterm infants that have not been evaluated by the FDA) and on the CDC Web site (www.cdc.gov/flu/professionals/antivirals/index.htm).[55] Children younger than 2 years are at an increased risk of hospitalization and complications attributable to influenza. The FDA has approved oseltamivir for the treatment of children as young as 2 weeks. Given preliminary pharmacokinetic data and limited safety data, the AAP supports the use of oseltamivir to treat influenza in both term and preterm infants from birth because the benefits of therapy for neonatal influenza are likely to outweigh the possible risks of treatment.

In adverse event data collected systematically in prospective trials, vomiting was the only adverse effect seen more often with oseltamivir compared with a placebo when studied in children 1 through 12 years of age (ie, 15% of treated children versus 9% receiving a placebo). In addition, following reports from Japan of oseltamivir-attributable neuropsychiatric adverse effects, reviewers of controlled clinical trial data and ongoing surveillance have failed to establish a link between this drug and neurologic or psychiatric events. Information is available through the FDA Web site.[56]

Clinical judgment (on the basis of underlying conditions, disease severity, time since symptom onset, and local influenza activity) is an important factor in treatment decisions for pediatric patients who present with ILI. Antiviral treatment should be started as soon as possible after illness onset and should not be delayed while waiting for a definitive influenza test result because early therapy provides the best outcomes. Influenza diagnostic tests vary by method, availability, processing time, sensitivity, and cost (Table 6), all of which should be considered in making the best clinical judgment. Positive and negative predictive values of influenza test results are influenced by the level of influenza activity in the population being tested, the characteristics of a test compared with a gold standard, pretest probability, whether the influenza virus is actively replicating in the person, proper collection and transport of specimens, and proper test procedures. Testing should be performed when timely results will be available to influence clinical management or infection control measures. Although decisions on treatment and infection control can be made on the basis of positive rapid antigen test results, negative results should not always be used in a similar fashion because of the suboptimal sensitivity and potential for false-negative results. Positive results of rapid influenza tests are helpful because they may reduce additional testing to identify the cause of a child's ILI and promote appropriate antimicrobial stewardship. Available FDA-approved rapid molecular assays are highly sensitive and specific diagnostic tests performed in less than 20 minutes by using RNA detection. These molecular assays and polymerase chain reaction (PCR) test confirmation are preferred in patients who are hospitalized because they are more sensitive compared with antigen detection. Immunofluorescence assays may be an alternative to PCR testing,

although the sensitivity is lower. Early detection, prompt antiviral treatment, and infection control interventions can lead to improved individual patient outcomes and allow for effective cohorting and disease containment.

People with suspected influenza who present with an uncomplicated febrile illness should be offered treatment with antiviral medications if they are at higher risk of influenza complications (Table 2). Efforts should be made to minimize treatment in patients who are not infected with influenza. Otherwise healthy children who have suspected influenza with an uncomplicated presentation should be considered for antiviral medication, particularly if they are in contact with other children who either are younger than 6 months or have underlying medical conditions that predispose them to complications of influenza. If there is a local shortage of antiviral medications, local public health authorities should be consulted to provide additional guidance about testing and treatment. In past years, local shortages of oseltamivir suspension have occurred because of uneven local drug distribution, although national shortages have not occurred since 2009, particularly given the availability of the capsule formulation that can be made into a suspension for young children if needed (Table 5).

Randomized placebo-controlled studies revealed that oral oseltamivir and inhaled zanamivir were efficacious when administered as chemoprophylaxis to household contacts after a family member had laboratory-confirmed influenza.[1, 24] During the 2009 pandemic, the emergence of oseltamivir resistance was noted rarely among people receiving postexposure prophylaxis, highlighting the need to be aware of the possibility of emerging resistance in this population. Decisions on

whether to administer antiviral chemoprophylaxis should take into account the exposed person's risk of influenza complications, vaccination status, the type and duration of contact, recommendations from local or public health authorities, and clinical judgment. Optimally, postexposure chemoprophylaxis should only be used when antiviral agents can be started within 48 hours of exposure; the lower dose for prophylaxis should not be used for the treatment of children symptomatic with influenza. Early, full treatment doses (rather than prophylaxis doses) provided to patients who are at high-risk and symptomatic without waiting for laboratory confirmation is an alternate strategy.

Although vaccination is the preferred approach to the prevention of infection, chemoprophylaxis during an influenza outbreak, as defined by the CDC (http://www.cdc.gov/ophss/csels/dsepd/ss1978/lesson1/section11.html),[57] is recommended in the following situations:

- for children at high risk of complications from influenza for whom an influenza vaccine is contraindicated;

- for children at high risk during the 2 weeks after influenza vaccination, before optimal immunity is achieved;

- for family members or HCP who are unimmunized and are likely to have ongoing, close exposure to unimmunized children at high risk or unimmunized infants and toddlers who are younger than 24 months;

- for control of influenza outbreaks for unimmunized staff and children in a closed institutional setting with children at high risk (eg, extended-care facilities);

- as a supplement to vaccination among children at high risk, including children who are immunocompromised and may not respond with sufficient protective immune responses after vaccination;

- as postexposure prophylaxis for family members and close contacts of an infected person if those people are at high risk for complications from influenza; and

- for children at high risk of complications and their family members and close contacts, as well as HCP, when circulating strains of influenza virus in the community are not matched with seasonal influenza vaccine strains on the basis of current data from the CDC and local health departments.

These recommendations apply to routine circumstances, but it should be noted that guidance may be changed on the basis of updated recommendations from the CDC in concert with antiviral availability, local resources, clinical judgment, recommendations from local or public health authorities, risk of influenza complications, type and duration of exposure contact, and change in epidemiology (resistance and antigenic shift) or severity of influenza. Chemoprophylaxis is not routinely recommended for infants younger than 3 months given limited safety and efficacy data in this age group.

CHEMOPROPHYLAXIS SHOULD NOT BE CONSIDERED AS A SUBSTITUTE FOR VACCINATION

An influenza vaccine should always be offered before and during the influenza season when not contraindicated even after the influenza virus has been circulating in the community. Antiviral medications currently licensed are important adjuncts to influenza vaccination for the control and prevention of influenza disease. Toxicities are associated with antiviral agents,

and indiscriminate use might limit availability. Pediatricians should inform recipients of antiviral chemoprophylaxis that risk of influenza is lowered but still remains while taking the medication, and susceptibility to influenza returns when medication is discontinued. Oseltamivir use is not a contraindication to vaccination with an IIV, although LAIV effectiveness will be decreased for the children receiving oseltamivir. No data are available on the impact of inhaled zanamivir on the effectiveness of LAIV. For recommendations about treatment and chemoprophylaxis against influenza, see Table 5. Among some people at high risk, both vaccination and antiviral chemoprophylaxis may be considered. Updates will be available in the *Red Book Online*[58] and the CDC Web site.[55]

FUTURE DIRECTIONS

For the 2018–2019 season, the safety and effectiveness of influenza vaccines will be analyzed as they become available and reported by the CDC as it is each season.[59] The manufacturer of LAIV4 reported that it will employ additional vaccine virus evaluation techniques in its selection of candidate vaccine viruses for inclusion in LAIV4 with the expectation that this will result in improved effectiveness of the formulation for the 2018–2019 season. Continued evaluation of the safety, immunogenicity, and effectiveness of the influenza vaccine, especially for young children and pregnant women, is important. The potential role of previous influenza vaccination on overall vaccine effectiveness by vaccine formulation, virus strain, and subject age in preventing outpatient medical visits, hospitalizations, and deaths continues to be evaluated. Furthermore, complete analysis of quadrivalent vaccines is needed

as the number of formulations of IIV4 increase. Additionally, with limited data on the use of NAIs in children who are hospitalized or in children with comorbid conditions, prospective randomized clinical trials in this population are warranted.

Immunizing all HCP, which is a crucial step in efforts to reduce health care–associated influenza infections, serves as an example to patients, highlighting the safety and effectiveness of annual vaccination. Ongoing efforts should include broader implementation and evaluation of mandatory vaccination programs in both inpatient and outpatient settings. Further investigation into the extent of offering to immunize parents and adult child care providers in the pediatric office setting; the level of family contact satisfaction with this practice; how practices handle the logistic, liability, legal, and financial barriers that limit or complicate this service; and most importantly, how this practice will affect disease rates in children and adults is needed. There is also a need for more systematic health services research on influenza vaccine uptake and refusal as well as for an identification of methods to enhance uptake.

Efforts should be made to create adequate outreach and infrastructure to facilitate the optimal distribution of vaccines so that more people are immunized. Pediatricians also might consider becoming more involved in pandemic preparedness and disaster planning efforts. A bidirectional partner dialogue between pediatricians and public health decision-makers assists efforts to address children's issues during the initial state, regional, and local plan development stages. Pandemic influenza preparedness of directors of child care centers also needs to improve. Additional information can be found in the Pediatric Preparedness Resource Kit.[60]

Pandemic influenza preparedness is of particular interest because of the increase in the number of human infections with Asian lineage avian influenza A(H7N9) reported in China (updates are available at https://www.cdc.gov/flu/avianflu/h7n9-virus.htm). A few human infections of Asian lineage avian influenza A(H7N9) have been reported outside of mainland China, but most of these infections have occurred among people who had traveled to China before becoming ill. These Asian lineage avian influenza A(H7N9) viruses have not been detected in people or birds in the United States. Although the current risk to the public's health from this virus is low, Asian lineage avian influenza A(H7N9) virus is among the nonhuman influenza viruses that are most concerning to public health officials because of their pandemic potential and ability to cause severe disease in infected humans. The current risk to the public's health from the virus remains low; however, the CDC is monitoring the situation carefully and taking routine preparedness measures, including testing candidate vaccines.

With the increased demand for vaccination during each influenza season, the AAP and the CDC recommend vaccine administration at any visit to the medical home during influenza season when it is not contraindicated, at specially arranged vaccine-only sessions, and through cooperation with community sites, schools, and Head Start and child care facilities to provide the influenza vaccine. It is important that the annual delivery of influenza vaccines to primary care medical homes should be timely to avoid missed opportunities. If alternative venues, including pharmacies and other retail-based clinics, are used for vaccination, a system of patient record transfer is beneficial in maintaining the accuracy of immunization records. Immunization information systems should be used whenever available and prioritized to document influenza vaccination. Two-dimensional barcodes have been used to facilitate more efficient and accurate documentation of vaccine administration with limited experience to date. Additional information concerning current vaccines shipped with 2-dimensional barcodes can be found on the CDC Web site.[61]

Access to care issues, a lack of immunization records, and questions regarding who can provide consent may be addressed by linking children (eg, those in foster care and/or the juvenile justice system or who are refugees, immigrants, or homeless) with a medical home, using all health care encounters as vaccination opportunities, and more consistently using immunization registry data. One new strategy of interest is an IIV delivered by a dissolvable microneedle patch, which has the potential to improve vaccine acceptability and coverage and reduce costs. Data from the first phase 1 human clinical trial ($n = 100$) found that the microneedle patch immunization was well tolerated and generated robust antibody responses.[62]

Development efforts continue for a universal influenza vaccine that induces broader protection and eliminates the need for annual vaccination. In addition, the development of a safe, immunogenic vaccine for infants younger than 6 months is essential. Studies on the effectiveness and safety of influenza vaccines containing adjuvants that enhance immune responses to influenza vaccines are ongoing. Efforts to improve the vaccine development process to allow for a shorter interval between the identification of vaccine strains and vaccine production continue. Lastly, many antiviral drugs are in various development phases given the need to improve options for the treatment and chemoprophylaxis of influenza. One recent example, baloxavir marboxil, a new antiviral for influenza that works by a different mechanism than NAIs and requires only a single dose for the treatment of infection, has recently been approved in Japan for adults and children. The FDA recently granted a priority review of this new drug, for which impact on the treatment of influenza will be followed closely.[63] Finally, pediatricians should remain informed during the influenza season by following the CDC influenza page[64] (www.cdc/gov/flu) and the AAP *Red Book Online* influenza resource page (www.aapredbook.org/flu)[58].

ACKNOWLEDGMENTS

This AAP Policy Statement was prepared in parallel with CDC recommendations and reports. Much of this statement is based on literature reviews, analyses of unpublished data, and deliberations of CDC staff in collaboration with the ACIP Influenza Working Group with liaison from the AAP.

COMMITTEE ON INFECTIOUS DISEASES, 2018–2019

Yvonne A. Maldonado, MD, FAAP, Chairperson
Theoklis E. Zaoutis, MD, MSCE, FAAP, Vice Chairperson
Ritu Banerjee, MD, PhD, FAAP
Elizabeth D. Barnett, MD, FAAP
James D. Campbell, MD, MS, FAAP
Jeffrey S. Gerber, MD, PhD, FAAP
Athena P. Kourtis, MD, PhD, MPH
Ruth Lynfield, MD, FAAP
Flor M. Munoz, MD, MSc, FAAP
Dawn Nolt, MD, MPH, FAAP
Ann-Christine Nyquist, MD, MSPH, FAAP
Sean T. O'Leary, MD, MPH, FAAP
Mark H. Sawyer, MD, FAAP
William J. Steinbach, MD, FAAP
Tina Q. Tan, MD, FAAP

FORMER COMMITTEE MEMBERS

Carrie L. Byington, MD, FAAP

EX OFFICIO

Henry H. Bernstein, DO, MHCM, FAAP — *Red Book* Online Associate Editor

Michael T. Brady, MD, FAAP, *Red Book* Associate Editor

Mary Anne Jackson, MD, FAAP, *Red Book* Associate Editor

David W. Kimberlin, MD, FAAP — *Red Book* Editor

Sarah S. Long, MD, FAAP — *Red Book* Associate Editor

H. Cody Meissner, MD, FAAP — Visual *Red Book* Associate Editor

CONTRIBUTORS

Stuart T. Weinberg, MD, FAAP — Partnership for Policy Implementation

Angie Lee, BA — Research Assistant, Cohen Children's Medical Center

Shannon Cleary, BA — Research Assistant, Cohen Children's Medical Center

Victoria Chi, BA — Research Assistant, Cohen Children's Medical Center

Tiffany Wang, BA — Second-year Medical Student, Donald and Barbara Zucker School of Medicine at Hofstra/Northwell, Hofstra University

Yingna Wang, BA — Research Assistant, Cohen Children's Medical Center

Irene Song, BA — Research Assistant, Cohen Children's Medical Center

John M. Kelso, MD, FAAP — Division of Allergy, Asthma, and Immunology, Scripps Clinic

John S. Bradley, MD, FAAP — Rady Children's Hospital

Caroline Braun, BA — Research Assistant, Cohen Children's Medical Center

Y. Amanda Wang, BA — Research Assistant, Cohen Children's Medical Center

LIAISONS

Amanda C. Cohn, MD, FAAP — *Centers for Disease Control and Prevention*

Jamie Deseda-Tous, MD — *Sociedad Latinoamericana de Infectologia Pediatrica*

Karen M. Farizo, MD — *US Food and Drug Administration*

Marc Fischer, MD, FAAP — *Centers for Disease Control and Prevention*

Natasha B. Halasa, MD, MPH, FAAP — *Pediatric Infectious Diseases Society*

Nicole Le Saux, MD, FRCPC — *Canadian Paediatric Society*

Scot Moore, MD, FAAP — *Committee on Practice Ambulatory Medicine*

Angela K. Shen, ScD, MPH — *National Vaccine Program Office*

James J. Stevermer, MD, MSPH, FAAFP — *American Academy of Family Physicians*

Jeffrey R. Starke, MD, FAAP — *American Thoracic Society*

Kay M. Tomashek, MD, MPH, DTM — *National Institutes of Health*

STAFF

Jennifer M. Frantz, MPH

ABBREVIATIONS

AAP: American Academy of Pediatrics

ACIP: Advisory Committee on Immunization Practices

ANE: acute necrotizing encephalopathy

CDC: Centers for Disease Control and Prevention

CI: confidence interval

FDA: Food and Drug Administration

GBS: Guillain-Barre syndrome

HCP: health care personnel

IAE: influenza-associated encephalopathy

IIV: inactivated influenza vaccine

IIV3: trivalent inactivated influenza vaccine

IIV4: quadrivalent inactivated influenza vaccine

ILI: influenza-like illness

LAIV: live attenuated influenza vaccine

LAIV3: trivalent live attenuated influenza vaccine

LAIV4: quadrivalent live attenuated influenza vaccine

NAI: neuraminidase inhibitor

PCR: polymerase chain reaction

PCV13: 13-valent pneumococcal conjugate vaccine

RCT: randomized controlled trial

RIV4: quadrivalent recombinant influenza vaccine

REFERENCES

1. Centers for Disease Control and Prevention. Prevention and control of influenza with vaccines: recommendations of the Advisory Committee on Immunization Practices, United States, 2018–19 influenza season. *MMWR Morb Mortal Wkly Rep.* 2018;67(22):643–645

2. Shope TR, Walker BH, Aird LD, Southward L, McCown JS, Martin JM. Pandemic influenza preparedness among child care center directors in 2008 and 2016. *Pediatrics.* 2017;139(6):e20163690

3. Garten R, Blanton L, Elal AIA, et al. Update: influenza activity in the United States during the 2017–18 season and composition of the 2018–19 influenza vaccine. *MMWR Morb Mortal Wkly Rep.* 2018;67(22):634–642

4. Biggerstaff M, Kniss K, Jernigan DB, et al. Systematic assessment of multiple routine and near real-time indicators to classify the severity of influenza seasons and pandemics in the United States, 2003-2004 through 2015-2016. *Am J Epidemiol.* 2018;187(5):1040–1050

5. Flannery B, Reynolds SB, Blanton L, et al. Influenza vaccine effectiveness against pediatric deaths: 2010-2014. *Pediatrics.* 2017;139(5):e20164244

6. Ferdinands JM, Olsho LE, Agan AA, et al; Pediatric Acute Lung Injury and Sepsis Investigators (PALISI) Network. Effectiveness of influenza vaccine against life-threatening RT-PCR-confirmed influenza illness in US children, 2010-2012. *J Infect Dis.* 2014;210(5):674–683

7. Tran D, Vaudry W, Moore D, et al; Members of the Canadian Immunization Monitoring Program Active. Hospitalization for influenza A versus B. *Pediatrics.* 2016;138(3):e20154643

8. Robison SG, Osborn AW. The concordance of parent and child immunization. *Pediatrics.* 2017;139(5):e2016883

9. Lessin HR, Edwards KM; Committee on Practice and Ambulatory Medicine; Committee on Infectious Diseases. Immunizing parents and other close family contacts in the pediatric office setting. *Pediatrics.* 2012;129(1). Available at: www.pediatrics.org/cgi/content/full/129/1/e247

10. ACOG Committee Opinion No. 732 summary: influenza vaccination during pregnancy. *Obstet Gynecol.* 2018;131(4):752–753

11. Zaman K, Roy E, Arifeen SE, et al. Effectiveness of maternal influenza immunization in mothers and infants [published correction appears in *N Engl J Med.* 2009;360(6):648]. *N Engl J Med.* 2008;359(15):1555–1564

12. Tapia MD, Sow SO, Tamboura B, et al. Maternal immunisation with trivalent inactivated influenza

vaccine for prevention of influenza in infants in Mali: a prospective, active-controlled, observer-blind, randomised phase 4 trial. *Lancet Infect Dis.* 2016;16(9):1026–1035

13. Madhi SA, Cutland CL, Kuwanda L, et al; Maternal Flu Trial (Matflu) Team. Influenza vaccination of pregnant women and protection of their infants. *N Engl J Med.* 2014;371(10):918–931

14. Steinhoff MC, Katz J, Englund JA, et al. Year-round influenza immunisation during pregnancy in Nepal: a phase 4, randomised, placebo-controlled trial. *Lancet Infect Dis.* 2017;17(9):981–989

15. Shakib JH, Korgenski K, Presson AP, et al. Influenza in infants born to women vaccinated during pregnancy. *Pediatrics.* 2016;137(6):e20152360

16. Nunes MC, Madhi SA. Prevention of influenza-related illness in young infants by maternal vaccination during pregnancy. *F1000Res.* 2018;7:122

17. Omer SB, Clark DR, Aqil AR, et al; BMGF Supported Maternal Influenza Immunization Trials Investigators Group. Maternal influenza immunization and prevention of severe clinical pneumonia in young infants: analysis of randomized controlled trials conducted in Nepal, Mali and South Africa. *Pediatr Infect Dis J.* 2018;37(5):436–440

18. Nunes MC, Madhi SA. Influenza vaccination during pregnancy for prevention of influenza confirmed illness in the infants: a systematic review and meta-analysis. *Hum Vaccin Immunother.* 2018;14(3):758–766

19. Sheffield JS, Greer LG, Rogers VL, et al. Effect of influenza vaccination in the first trimester of pregnancy. *Obstet Gynecol.* 2012;120(3):532–537

20. Chambers CD, Johnson DL, Xu R, et al; OTIS Collaborative Research Group. Safety of the 2010-11, 2011-12, 2012-13, and 2013-14 seasonal influenza vaccines in pregnancy: birth defects, spontaneous abortion, preterm delivery, and small for gestational age infants, a study from the cohort arm of VAMPSS. *Vaccine.* 2016;34(37):4443–4449

21. Donahue JG, Kieke BA, King JP, et al. Association of spontaneous abortion with receipt of inactivated influenza vaccine containing H1N1pdm09 in 2010-11 and 2011-12. *Vaccine.* 2017;35(40):5314–5322

22. Ferdinands JM, Fry AM, Reynolds S, et al. Intraseason waning of influenza vaccine protection: evidence from the US Influenza Vaccine Effectiveness Network, 2011-12 through 2014-15. *Clin Infect Dis.* 2017;64(5):544–550

23. American Academy of Pediatrics Committee on Infectious Diseases. Red Book online influenza resource page. Available at: https://redbook.solutions.aap.org/selfserve/ssPage.aspx?SelfServeContentId=influenza-resources. Accessed June 20, 2018

24. Fiore AE, Fry A, Shay D, Gubareva L, Bresee JS, Uyeki TM; Centers for Disease Control and Prevention (CDC). Antiviral agents for the treatment and chemoprophylaxis of influenza — recommendations of the Advisory Committee on Immunization Practices (ACIP). *MMWR Recomm Rep.* 2011;60(1):1–24

25. Bradley JS, Blumer JL, Romero JR, et al. Intravenous zanamivir in hospitalized patients with influenza. *Pediatrics.* 2017;140(5):e20162727

26. Chan-Tack KM, Kim C, Moruf A, Birnkrant DB. Clinical experience with intravenous zanamivir under an Emergency IND program in the United States (2011-2014). *Antivir Ther.* 2015;20(5):561–564

27. Centers for Disease Control and Prevention. Influenza (flu). Available at: https://www.cdc.gov/flu/. Accessed June 20, 2018

28. American Academy of Pediatrics. Implementation Guidance for AAP Vaccine Policy Statements. Available at: https://redbook.solutions.aap.org/ss/vaccine-policy-guidance.aspx. Accessed August 11, 2018

29. Vesikari T, Kirstein J, Devota Go G, et al. Efficacy, immunogenicity, and safety evaluation of an MF59-adjuvanted quadrivalent influenza virus vaccine compared with non-adjuvanted influenza vaccine in children: a multicentre, randomised controlled, observer-blinded, phase 3 trial. *Lancet Respir Med.* 2018;6(5):345–356

30. Duffy J, Weintraub E, Hambidge SJ, et al; Vaccine Safety Datalink. Febrile seizure risk after vaccination in children 6 to 23 months. *Pediatrics.* 2016;138(1):e20160320

31. Thompson CA. Vaccine safety signal from spontaneous system not supported by active surveillance. *Am J Health Syst Pharm.* 2014;71(17):1432–1433

32. Sentinel; CBER. Influenza vaccines and febrile seizures in the 2013-2014 and 2014-2015 influenza seasons. 2017. Available at: https://www.sentinelinitiative.org/sites/default/files/vaccines-blood-biologics/assessments/Influenza-Vaccines-Febrile-Seizures-Final-Report.pdf. Accessed June 20, 2018

33. Grohskopf LA, Sokolow LZ, Fry AM, Walter EB, Jernigan DB. Update: ACIP recommendations for the use of quadrivalent live attenuated influenza vaccine (LAIV4) - United States, 2018-19 influenza season. *MMWR Morb Mortal Wkly Rep.* 2018;67(22):643–645

34. Kelso JM, Greenhawt MJ, Li JT; Joint Task Force on Practice Parameters (JTFPP). Update on influenza vaccination of egg allergic patients. *Ann Allergy Asthma Immunol.* 2013;111(4):301–302

35. Greenhawt M, Turner PJ, Kelso JM. Administration of influenza vaccines to egg allergic recipients: a practice parameter update 2017. *Ann Allergy Asthma Immunol.* 2018;120(1):49–52

36. American Academy of Pediatrics. AAP immunization resources storage and handling series disaster planning. Available at: https://www.aap.org/en-us/Documents/immunization_disasterplanning.pdf. Accessed June 20, 2018

37. American Academy of Pediatrics. Children and disasters. Available at: www.aap.org/disasters. Accessed June 20, 2018

38. Polyzos KA, Konstantelias AA, Pitsa CE, Falagas ME. Maternal influenza vaccination and risk for congenital malformations: a systematic review and meta-analysis. *Obstet Gynecol.* 2015;126(5):1075–1084

39. Schlaudecker EP, Steinhoff MC, Omer SB, et al. IgA and neutralizing antibodies to influenza a virus in human milk: a randomized trial of

antenatal influenza immunization. *PLoS One.* 2013;8(8):e70867

40. Centers for Disease Control and Prevention. Breastfeeding and special circumstances: influenza (flu). Available at: https://www.cdc.gov/breastfeeding/breastfeeding-special-circumstances/maternal-or-infant-illnesses/influenza.html. Accessed June 20, 2018

41. Centers for Disease Control and Prevention. Guidance for the prevention and control of influenza in the peri- and postpartum settings. Available at: https://www.cdc.gov/flu/professionals/infectioncontrol/peri-post-settings.htm. Accessed June 20, 2018

42. Howard A, Uyeki TM, Fergie J. Influenza-associated acute necrotizing encephalopathy in siblings [published online ahead of print May 4, 2018]. *J Pediatric Infect Dis Soc.* doi:10.1093/jpids/piy033

43. Centers for Disease Control and Prevention. Flu activity and surveillance. Available at: www.cdc.gov/flu/weekly/fluactivitysurv.htm. Accessed June 20, 2018

44. American Academy of Pediatrics. What's the latest with the flu? Available at: https://www.aap.org/en-us/advocacy-and-policy/aap-health-initiatives/Pages/What's-the-Latest-with-the-Flu.aspx. Accessed June 20, 2018

45. American Academy of Pediatrics. Child Health Informatics Center: health information technology at the AAP. Available at: www2.aap.org/informatics/PPI.html. Accessed June 20, 2018

46. Dobson J, Whitley RJ, Pocock S, Monto AS. Oseltamivir treatment for influenza in adults: a meta-analysis of randomised controlled trials. *Lancet.* 2015;385(9979):1729–1737

47. Malosh RE, Martin ET, Heikkinen T, Brooks WA, Whitley RJ, Monto AS. Efficacy and safety of oseltamivir in children: systematic review and individual patient data meta-analysis of randomized controlled trials. *Clin Infect Dis.* 2018;66(10):1492–1500

48. Hsu J, Santesso N, Mustafa R, et al. Antivirals for treatment of influenza: a systematic review and meta-analysis of observational studies. *Ann Intern Med.* 2012;156(7):512–524

49. Doll MK, Winters N, Boikos C, Kraicer-Melamed H, Gore G, Quach C. Safety and effectiveness of neuraminidase inhibitors for influenza treatment, prophylaxis, and outbreak control: a systematic review of systematic reviews and/or meta-analyses. *J Antimicrob Chemother.* 2017;72(11):2990–3007

50. Venkatesan S, Myles PR, Leonardi-Bee J, et al. Impact of outpatient neuraminidase inhibitor treatment in patients infected with influenza A(H1N1)pdm09 at high risk of hospitalization: an individual participant data metaanalysis. *Clin Infect Dis.* 2017;64(10):1328–1334

51. Muthuri SG, Venkatesan S, Myles PR, et al; PRIDE Consortium Investigators. Effectiveness of neuraminidase inhibitors in reducing mortality in patients admitted to hospital with influenza A H1N1pdm09 virus infection: a meta-analysis of individual participant data. *Lancet Respir Med.* 2014;2(5):395–404

52. Wang K, Shun-Shin M, Gill P, Perera R, Harnden A. Neuraminidase inhibitors for preventing and treating influenza in children (published trials only). *Cochrane Database Syst Rev.* 2012;(4):CD002744

53. Jefferson T, Jones MA, Doshi P, et al. Neuraminidase inhibitors for preventing and treating influenza in healthy adults and children. *Cochrane Database Syst Rev.* 2014;(4):CD008965

54. South East Asia Infectious Disease Clinical Research Network. Effect of double dose oseltamivir on clinical and virological outcomes in children and adults admitted to hospital with severe influenza: double blind randomised controlled trial. *BMJ.* 2013;346:f3039

55. Centers for Disease Control and Prevention. Antiviral drugs: information for health care professionals. Available at: www.cdc.gov/flu/professionals/antivirals/index.htm. Accessed June 20, 2018

56. US Food and Drug Administration. Tamiflu Pediatric Adverse Events: Questions and Answers. Available at: https://www.fda.gov/Drugs/DrugSafety/PostmarketDrugSafetyInformationforPatientsandProviders/ucm107840.htm. Accessed August 21, 2018

57. Centers for Disease Control and Prevention. Lesson 1: introduction to epidemiology. Section 11: epidemic disease occurrence. Available at: http://www.cdc.gov/ophss/csels/dsepd/ss1978/lesson1/section11.html. Accessed June 20, 2018

58. American Academy of Pediatrics. Red Book Online Influenza Resource page. Available at: https://redbook.solutions.aap.org/chapter.aspx?sectionid=189640115&bookid=2205. Accessed June 20, 2018

59. Flannery B, Chung JR, Belongia EA, et al. Interim estimates of 2017-18 seasonal influenza vaccine effectiveness - United States, February 2018. *MMWR Morb Mortal Wkly Rep.* 2018;67(6):180–185

60. American Academy of Pediatrics. Pediatric Preparedness Resource Kit. Available at: www.aap.org/disasters/resourcekit. Accessed June 20, 2018

61. Centers for Disease Control and Prevention. Two-dimensional (2D) vaccine barcodes. Available at: www.cdc.gov/vaccines/programs/iis/2d-vaccine-barcodes/. Accessed June 20, 2018

62. Rouphael NG, Paine M, Mosley R, et al; TIV-MNP 2015 Study Group. The safety, immunogenicity, and acceptability of inactivated influenza vaccine delivered by microneedle patch (TIV-MNP 2015): a randomised, partly blinded, placebo-controlled, phase 1 trial. *Lancet.* 2017;390(10095):649–658

63. Heo YA. Baloxavir: first global approval. *Drugs.* 2018;78(6):693–697

64. Centers for Disease Control and Prevention. Influenza (Flu). Available at: www.cdc/gov/flu. Accessed August 11, 2018

ADDITIONAL RESOURCES

Committee on Infectious Diseases. Influenza immunization for all health care personnel: keep it mandatory. Pediatrics. 2015;136(4):809–818

Frush K; American Academy of Pediatrics Committee on Pediatric Emergency

Medicine. Preparation for emergencies in the offices of pediatricians and pediatric primary care providers. Pediatrics. 2007;120(1):200-212. Reaffirmed June 2011

Committee on Practice and Ambulatory Medicine; Committee on Infectious Diseases; Committee on State Government Affairs; Council on School Health; Section on Administration and Practice Management. Medical versus nonmedical immunization exemptions for child care and school attendance. Pediatrics. 2016;138(3):e20162145

Edwards KM, Hackell JM; Committee on Infectious Diseases, The Committee on Practice and Ambulatory Medicine. Countering vaccine hesitancy. Pediatrics. 2016;138(3):e20162146

Committee on Pediatric Emergency Medicine; Committee on Medical Liability; Task Force on Terrorism. The pediatrician and disaster preparedness. Pediatrics. 2006;117(2):560-565. Reaffirmed September 2013

American Academy of Pediatrics. Influenza. In: Kimberlin DW, Brady MT, Jackson MA, Long SS, eds. Red Book: 2018 Report of the Committee on Infectious Diseases.

31st ed. Elk Grove Village, IL: American Academy of Pediatrics; 2018:476–489

Uyeki T., Bernstein H., Bradley J.S. et al; Expert Panel of the Infectious Diseases Society of America. Seasonal influenza in adults and children-diagnosis, treatment, chemoprophylaxis, and institutional outbreak management: clinical practice guidelines of the Infectious Diseases Society of America. Clin Infect Dis. 2018;67 In Press.

Centers for Disease Control and Prevention. Antiviral Drugs. Available at: www.cdc. gov/flu/professionals/antivirals/antiviral-drug-resistance.htm.

Recommended Childhood and Adolescent Immunization Schedules: United States, 2019

•••••••••••••••••••••••••••••••••••••••

- *Policy Statement*

POLICY STATEMENT Organizational Principles to Guide and Define the Child Health
Care System and/or Improve the Health of all Children

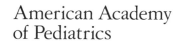

American Academy
of Pediatrics

DEDICATED TO THE HEALTH OF ALL CHILDREN™

Recommended Childhood and Adolescent Immunization Schedules: United States, 2019

COMMITTEE ON INFECTIOUS DISEASES

The 2019 recommended childhood and adolescent immunization schedules have been approved by the American Academy of Pediatrics (AAP), the Advisory Committee on Immunization Practices and the Centers for Disease Control and Prevention (CDC), the American Academy of Family Physicians, and the American College of Obstetricians and Gynecologists. The schedules are revised annually to reflect current recommendations for the use of vaccines licensed by the US Food and Drug Administration.

The 2019 childhood and adolescent immunization schedule has been updated to ensure consistency between the format of the childhood and adolescent and adult immunization schedules. Changes have been made to the cover page, including guidance for use of the schedule as well as a list of links to "Helpful information." Similar to last year, the cover page includes a table with alphabetical listing of vaccines, approved abbreviations for each vaccine, and vaccine trade names.

Table 1 contains the recommended immunization schedule from birth through 18 years of age. The influenza row has been modified to reflect current CDC recommendations for use of LAIV in age-appropriate and health status–appropriate children 24 months of age and older. A purple bar has been added to the hepatitis A vaccine row, indicating a recommendation for use of this vaccine among infants 6 through 11 months of age before departure to an international destination. A purple bar has been added to the Tdap row, indicating vaccine use for pregnant adolescents 13 through 18 years of age.

Table 2 is the catch-up immunization schedule for persons 4 months through 18 years of age who start late or who are more than 1 month behind the recommended age for vaccine administration. A change is noted in relation to administration of *Haemophilus influenzae* type b and pneumococcal conjugate vaccines. The criteria under which no further doses are needed are presented, followed by recommendations for those in whom additional doses are indicated.

DOI: https://doi.org/10.1542/peds.2019-0065

PEDIATRICS (ISSN Numbers: Print, 0031-4005; Online, 1098-4275).

To cite: COMMITTEE ON INFECTIOUS DISEASES. Recommended Childhood and Adolescent Immunization Schedules: United States, 2019. *Pediatrics.* 2019;143(3): e20190065

Table 3 lists the vaccines that may be indicated for children and adolescents 18 years of age or younger on the basis of medical conditions. A pink color has been added to the pregnancy column in the HPV row, indicating the need for a delay in vaccination for pregnant adolescents. The influenza vaccine row has been modified to separate LAIV from IIV and to include contraindications and precautions for LAIV.

A bullet directing providers to their state or local health departments for information regarding vaccination in the setting of a vaccine-preventable disease outbreak has been added to the "Additional Information" section of the notes.

This year, the notes are presented in alphabetical order. The following changes to individual footnotes have been made:

- Hepatitis A vaccine
  - Information regarding the use of combined HepA-HepB (Twinrix) vaccine in persons 18 years of age or older has been added.
  - A section for international travel has been added with recommendation for vaccination of those 6 through 11 months of age and unvaccinated persons 12 months of age or older.
  - Homelessness has been added as an indication for vaccination.
- Hepatitis B vaccine
  - The word "all" has been added to the vaccine recommendation for the birth dose for medically stable infants (≥2000 g) born to hepatitis B surface antigen-negative mothers. This was added to emphasize the recommendation for this population.
  - Information regarding the use of CPG–adjuvanted HepB (Heplisav-B) vaccine and combination Twinrix vaccine in persons 18 years or older has been added.

- Polio vaccine
  - A bullet has been added regarding the use of combination vaccines that contain IPV. This bullet mirrors similar information presented in the hepatitis B vaccine note.
- Influenza vaccines
  - LAIV has been added where appropriate.
  - A "special situations" section has been added with information regarding vaccination of persons with a history of egg allergy and information regarding when not to use LAIV.
- MMR and meningococcal vaccines
  - Language regarding use of the MMR vaccine in the setting of a mumps outbreak and Men-ACWY and MenB vaccine use in the setting of meningococcal outbreaks has been removed, and providers are now directed to local health departments for information regarding vaccination during an outbreak (see "Additional Information" section).
- Tdap vaccine
  - The catch-up vaccination section has been updated to indicate that those who received a dose of Tdap or DTaP at 7 through 10 years of age inadvertently or as part of the catch-up schedule should receive the routine dose of Tdap at 11 through 12 years of age.
  - A link to information regarding the use of Tdap/Td for wound prophylaxis has been added.

The 2019 version of tables 1 through 3 and the notes are available on the American Academy of Pediatrics Web site (https://redbook.solutions.aap. org/SS/Immunization_Schedules. aspx) and the CDC Web site (www. cdc.gov/vaccines/schedules/hcp/ child-adolescent.html). A parent-friendly vaccine schedule for children and adolescents is available at www. cdc.gov/vaccines/schedules/index. html. An adult immunization schedule

is published in February of each year and is available at www.cdc.gov/ vaccines/schedules/hcp/adult.html.

Clinically significant adverse events that follow immunization should be reported to the Vaccine Adverse Event Reporting System. Guidance about how to obtain and complete a Vaccine Adverse Event Reporting System form can be obtained at www.vaers.hhs.gov or by calling 800-822-7967. Additional information can be found in the *Red Book* and at *Red Book* Online (http:// aapredbook.aappublications.org/). Statements from the Advisory Committee on Immunization Practices and the CDC that contain detailed recommendations for individual vaccines, including recommendations for children with high-risk conditions, are available at www.cdc.gov/ vaccines/hcp/acip-recs/index.html. Information on new vaccine releases, vaccine supplies, and interim recommendations resulting from vaccine shortages and statements on specific vaccines can be found at www. aapredbook.org/news/vaccstatus. shtml.

COMMITTEE ON INFECTIOUS DISEASES, 2018–2019

Yvonne A. Maldonado, MD, FAAP, Chairperson
Theoklis E. Zaoutis, MD, MSCE, FAAP, Vice Chairperson
Ritu Banerjee, MD, PhD, FAAP
Elizabeth D. Barnett, MD, FAAP
James D. Campbell, MD, MS, FAAP
Jeffrey S. Gerber, MD, PhD, FAAP
Athena P. Kourtis, MD, PhD, MPH, FAAP
Ruth Lynfield, MD, FAAP
Flor M. Munoz, MD, MSc, FAAP
Dawn Nolt, MD, MPH, FAAP
Ann-Christine Nyquist, MD, MSPH, FAAP
Sean T. O'Leary, MD, MPH, FAAP
Mark H. Sawyer, MD, FAAP
William J. Steinbach, MD, FAAP
Tina Q. Tan, MD, FAAP

EX OFFICIO

David W. Kimberlin, MD, FAAP – *Red Book* Editor
Henry H. Bernstein, DO, MHCM, FAAP – *Red Book* Online Associate Editor
H. Cody Meissner, MD, FAAP – Visual *Red Book* Associate Editor

LIAISONS

Amanda C. Cohn, MD, FAAP – *Centers for Disease Control and Prevention*
Jamie Deseda-Tous, MD – *Sociedad Latinoamericana de Infectologia Pediatrica*
Karen M. Farizo, MD – *US Food and Drug Administration*
Marc Fischer, MD, FAAP – *Centers for Disease Control and Prevention*
Natasha B. Halasa, MD, MPH, FAAP – *Pediatric Infectious Diseases Society*

Nicole Le Saux, MD, FRCP(C) – *Canadian Paediatric Society*
Scot B. Moore, MD, FAAP – *Committee on Practice Ambulatory Medicine*
Neil S. Silverman, MD – *American College of Obstetricians and Gynecologists*
Jeffrey R. Starke, MD, FAAP – *American Thoracic Society*
James J. Stevermer, MD, MSPH, FAAFP – *American Academy of Family Physicians*
Kay M. Tomashek, MD, MPH, DTM – *National Institutes of Health*

STAFF

Jennifer M. Frantz, MPH

ABBREVIATIONS
AAP: American Academy of
   Pediatrics
CDC: Centers for Disease Control
   and Prevention

The Role of Integrated Care in a Medical Home for Patients With a Fetal Alcohol Spectrum Disorder

• *Clinical Report*

CLINICAL REPORT   Guidance for the Clinician in Rendering Pediatric Care

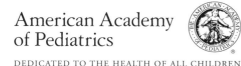

American Academy
of Pediatrics

DEDICATED TO THE HEALTH OF ALL CHILDREN™

The Role of Integrated Care in a Medical Home for Patients With a Fetal Alcohol Spectrum Disorder

Renee M. Turchi, MD, MPH, FAAP,[a] Vincent C. Smith, MD, MPH, FAAP,[b] COMMITTEE ON SUBSTANCE USE AND PREVENTION, COUNCIL ON CHILDREN WITH DISABILITIES

abstract

Fetal alcohol spectrum disorder (FASD) is an umbrella term used to describe preventable birth defects and intellectual and/or developmental disabilities resulting from prenatal alcohol exposure. The American Academy of Pediatrics has a previous clinical report in which diagnostic criteria for a child with an FASD are discussed and tools to assist pediatricians with its management can be found. This clinical report is intended to foster pediatrician awareness of approaches for screening for prenatal alcohol exposure in clinical practice, to guide management of a child with an FASD after the diagnosis is made, and to summarize available resources for FASD management.

[a]Department of Pediatrics, St. Christopher's Hospital for Children and Drexel Dornsife School of Public Health, Philadelphia, Pennsylvania; and [b]Department of Neonatology, Beth Israel Deaconess Medical Center and Harvard Medical School, Harvard University, Boston, Massachusetts

Drs Turchi and Smith shared the responsibility for writing and revising the manuscript and considering the input of reviewers; and all authors approve the final manuscript as submitted.

This document is copyrighted and is property of the American Academy of Pediatrics and its Board of Directors. All authors have filed conflict of interest statements with the American Academy of Pediatrics. Any conflicts have been resolved through a process approved by the Board of Directors. The American Academy of Pediatrics has neither solicited nor accepted any commercial involvement in the development of the content of this publication.

Clinical reports from the American Academy of Pediatrics benefit from expertise and resources of liaisons and internal (AAP) and external reviewers. However, clinical reports from the American Academy of Pediatrics may not reflect the views of the liaisons or the organizations or government agencies that they represent.

The guidance in this report does not indicate an exclusive course of treatment or serve as a standard of medical care. Variations, taking into account individual circumstances, may be appropriate.

All clinical reports from the American Academy of Pediatrics automatically expire 5 years after publication unless reaffirmed, revised, or retired at or before that time.

DOI: https://doi.org/10.1542/peds.2018-2333

To cite: Turchi RM, Smith VC, AAP COMMITTEE ON SUBSTANCE USE AND PREVENTION, AAP COUNCIL ON CHILDREN WITH DISABILITIES. The Role of Integrated Care in a Medical Home for Patients With a Fetal Alcohol Spectrum Disorder. *Pediatrics.* 2018;142(4):e20182333

INTRODUCTION

Prenatal alcohol exposure (PAE) is the most common preventable cause of intellectual and developmental delay and disabilities in the United States.[1] Fetal alcohol spectrum disorder (FASD) is an umbrella term used to describe preventable birth defects and intellectual and/or developmental disabilities that result from PAE. In 2010, the American Academy of Pediatrics (AAP) conducted a needs assessment of pediatricians and found that during training, many pediatric clinicians did not receive sufficient education about the hazards of PAE and the options for universal screening for prenatal alcohol use.[2] Addressing this knowledge gap in 2015, the AAP released a clinical report with the goals of aiding pediatricians with the diagnosis of a child with an FASD, stressing the importance of universal screening for PAE (www.aap.org/FASD).[3]

After the release of the AAP clinical report, pediatricians expressed a need for further clinical guidance regarding managing an individual with an FASD within the medical home beyond diagnosis. Many medical home providers are reluctant to screen for PAE when unsure of how to manage patients after a diagnosis of an FASD. For some pediatricians, it can seem like a daunting task to care for an individual with an FASD, but there are aspects of integrated care and providing a medical home that can be instituted as with all children with complex medical diagnoses.[4] In addition, not recognizing an FASD can lead to inadequate treatment and less-than-optimal outcomes for the patient and family. This clinical report provides an approach to caring for children with an FASD and their families.

The goal and scope of this clinical report is to support pediatric providers in managing patients after a diagnosis of an FASD. It emphasizes the lifelong effects of having an FASD and suggests strategies to support families who are interacting with early intervention services, the educational system, the behavioral and/or mental health system, other community resources, and the transition to adult-oriented heath care systems when appropriate.

EPIDEMIOLOGY

In a survey conducted between 2011 and 2013, approximately 1 in 10 pregnant women in the United States reported drinking alcohol in the past 30 days, and about 1 in 33 pregnant women report binge drinking (having 4 or more drinks at one time) in the past 30 days.[5,6] Studies of grade school children suggest that the rate of an FASD is estimated at 24 to 48 per 1000 children,[7] thus approaching the prevalence of other disorders, such as autism spectrum disorder (https://www.cdc.gov/ncbddd/autism/data.html). In addition, studies suggest the rates of FASDs are even higher in certain regions of the United States and among vulnerable populations, such as children in foster care, internationally adopted children, and/or some children of American Indian or Alaska Native descent.[8–10]

Alcohol is a known teratogen.[11] All drinks containing alcohol have the potential to harm a developing fetus, but not every developing fetus exposed to alcohol will develop an FASD. Harm may occur even before a woman recognizes she is pregnant, which is especially significant, because nearly half of all pregnancies in the United States are unplanned.[12] Currently, it is not possible to predict which fetuses will be affected. The safest choice is for women to completely refrain from alcohol consumption while pregnant or trying to get pregnant. The AAP endorsed the following message via the 2015 clinical report[3] (www.cdc.gov/ncbddd/fasd/facts.html):

- There is no amount of alcohol during pregnancy that is risk free.

- There is no kind of alcohol during pregnancy that is risk free.

- There is no time during pregnancy when alcohol consumption is risk free.

FASD TERMINOLOGY AND LIFE SPAN

FASD is not a specific diagnostic term; rather, it is an overarching expression covering a range of possible conditions resulting from PAE.[3,13–17] The signs and symptoms of an FASD vary by individual and can include physical stigmata as well as mental, behavioral, and learning problems. The term FASD includes all of the following conditions: fetal alcohol syndrome (FAS), partial FAS, alcohol-related birth defects, alcohol-related neurodevelopmental disorder, and neurobehavioral disorder associated with prenatal alcohol exposure (ND-PAE; Table 1).[3,16,17] FAS is often the condition associated with PAE under the FASD umbrella that individuals are familiar with.

Several FASD diagnostic frameworks are available. The AAP devised the "Flow Diagram for Medical Home Evaluation of Fetal Alcohol

Spectrum Disorders"[18] (see Fig 1) to facilitate greater clinical recognition of children with an FASD, acknowledging that FASD could and would be beneficial to recognize in individuals of any age (www.aap.org/FASD). For further detail about specific FASD diagnostic schema, please see other sources.[13–15,17]

ROLE OF THE MEDICAL HOME AND CARE INTEGRATION

For nearly 5 decades, the medical home concept has evolved from a place to store medical records for children with special care needs[19] to a setting in which high-quality care is delivered for all children, including those with an FASD.[20] Provision of a medical home includes continuity, care coordination, cultural competence, patient and family centeredness, compassion, and care consistency across the lifespan of children and their families.[20,21] The care provided in the medical home may facilitate the patient- and family-centered care necessary for children with special health care needs, and especially those children with an FASD, to optimize their potential and support their families and caregivers.[22] Providing a medical home for children and youth with an FASD optimizes their potential and supports their families and caregivers. This clinical report seeks to highlight the role of a medical home for children and youth with an FASD and describe key constructs and management of this important population of children.

Approach to Universal Screening and Documentation of PAE in the Pediatric Encounter

Early identification of developmental disorders, including FASDs, is critical to the well-being of children and their families. Screening for PAE is an important function of the medical home. Although potentially challenging, it is an appropriate and necessary responsibility

TABLE 1 Criteria for Diagnosis of FASD and Related Disorders

Terminology	Diagnostic Features
FAS	Explicit diagnostic criteria that include all of the following:
	Three facial abnormalities (ie, smooth philtrum, thin vermillion border, and small palpebral fissures). Also may see midface hypoplasia, micrognathia, microcephaly, epicanthal folds
	Growth deficiency (height and/or wt ≤10th percentile at any age)
	Structural, neurologic, or functional CNS abnormalities
	Prenatal exposure to alcohol[a]
Partial FAS	Some but not all of the physical features of full FAS (above)
	CNS damage (structural, neurologic, and/or functional impairment)
	Confirmed prenatal exposure to alcohol
Alcohol-related birth defects	Classification for individuals who do not have the facial characteristics of full FAS
	Significant birth defects affecting the heart, eyes, kidneys, and/or bones resulting from PAE
	Hearing may also be affected
	Usually do not meet criteria for CNS structural or functional abnormalities
	Confirmed prenatal exposure to alcohol
Alcohol-related neurodevelopmental disorder	Cluster of symptoms that may include intellectual disabilities as well as challenges with behavior and learning resulting from PAE
	May also have a CNS anomaly
	Often perform poorly in school and have difficulties with math, memory, attention, judgment, and impulse control
	Confirmed prenatal exposure to alcohol
ND-PAE	Have impairment of neurocognition, self-regulation, and adaptive functioning
	Combines deficits in these 3 areas in conjunction with evidence of PAE, childhood onset of symptoms, and significant distress or impairment in social, academic, occupational, or other important area of function
	Confirmed prenatal exposure to alcohol

CNS, central nervous system. Adapted from Hoyme HE, Kalberg WO, Elliott AJ, et al. Updated clinical guidelines for diagnosing fetal alcohol spectrum disorders. *Pediatrics.* 2016;138(2):e20154256 and Fetal Alcohol Spectrum Disorders Expert Panel. Flow Diagram for Medical Home Evaluation of Fetal Alcohol Spectrum Disorders. Elk Grove Village, IL: American Academy of Pediatrics; 2013. Available at: www.aap.org/en-us/advocacy-and-policy/aap-health-initiatives/fetal-alcohol-spectrum-disorders-toolkit/Pages/Algorithm-for-Evaluation.aspx. Accessed December 18, 2017.

[a] Confirming PAE is not necessary if the first 3 features are present.[17]

of all pediatric providers. Early identification of a child at risk for an FASD because of a positive screen result for PAE prompts careful monitoring followed by further evaluation, developmental or behavioral monitoring, and diagnosis and treatment, if warranted. Ideally, screening for PAE would be a component of a pediatrician's routine family assessment during a clinical encounter.

Pediatric providers, as well as obstetricians and gynecologists, have a unique opportunity to identify and engage families regarding alcohol consumption during pregnancy. Pediatric providers, collaborating with other interested partners, such as the American College of Obstetrics and Gynecology, can enhance practice and policy changes for women and children before and during pregnancy. Communication of PAE from the obstetric provider to the pediatrician would facilitate

screening and monitoring of (high-risk) infants and children. Ideally, pediatric primary care providers would adopt a "universal screening" approach of alcohol exposure in their patients. In practice, multiple opportunities already exist to incorporate this screening into office workflows. In fact, screening for PAE can be completed during any family interactions, especially the following times: in prenatal visits, in newborn or infant visits, at the time of adoption, and as new patients and families join the practice. For PAE screening resources, visit www.aap.org/pae.

- A prenatal encounter is an ideal time for a pediatric provider to engage with a family about prenatal substance exposure, including alcohol.

- In the newborn nursery setting, when a new mother typically has keen interest in discussing

health issues possibly affecting her infant, a provider can use this time to screen for PAE as part of the discussion about the newborn infant's health.

- In the office setting, this discussion could be part of the pregnancy history. It could be included in the discussion of maternal medical issues, medications, tobacco, and substance use during pregnancy.

- During the newborn period and first few months of infancy, pediatric providers generally inquire about any number of prenatal or pregnancy risk factors possibly affecting the infant's health history. This inquiry could include screening for PAE if screening has not already been performed. Some practices could also include this in their routine postpartum depression screening at 1, 2, and 4 months,[23] screening for maternal health, or while

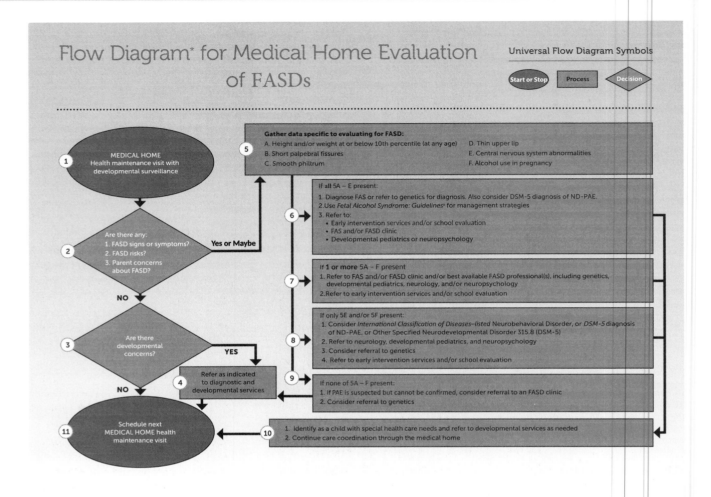

FIGURE 1

Flow diagram for medical home evaluation of FASDs. [a]Page 2: Flow diagram pathway details; FAS criteria; selected resources. The flow diagram was developed by the FASD Expert Panel of the AAP via cooperative agreement #5U380T000167 with the Centers for Disease Control and Prevention; does not necessarily represent the views of the Centers for Disease Control and Prevention.

screening for history of trauma using an Adverse Child Event Screener in practice.[24]

- All patients who are new to a practice benefit from screening for exposure to prenatal alcohol, regardless of the age of the child. In addition, patients who present with emerging behavioral issues at any age warrant rescreening for PAE, regardless of previous positive or negative screening results.

Once screening for PAE is completed and documented as positive, there is little need for repeated screening unless there is potential for a

change in answers. Using a standard script may ease potential physician discomfort and provide reassurance to the caregiver when discussing topics that may be sensitive. Incorporating the "universal screening" for PAE in either decision support prompts or electronic health record questions are key.

There is no uniformly accepted practice regarding documenting PAE. The tools available through the *Bright Futures Tool and Resource Kit* are compatible with, but do not require, an electronic health record. The main components of the *Bright Futures Tool and Resource Kit* are available

for review and reference at https://brightfutures.aap.org/materials-and-tools/tool-and-resource-kit. Pediatricians are encouraged to work with other members of their practice to develop a standard process for screening, documentation, and follow-up within their office and/or clinical setting and team.

As mandated reporters of child abuse and neglect, health care providers should be cognizant of their state's laws regarding prenatal and/or postnatal maternal substance use and understand obligatory child abuse reporting laws in their states and should know how to make a report to the responsible agency that investigates cases of alleged child abuse or neglect in their jurisdiction.[25,26] Under the federal Child Abuse Prevention and Treatment Act (CAPTA), health care providers are mandated reporters. CAPTA does not require clinicians to report to child protective services if a child has been exposed prenatally to alcohol (ie, for a positive PAE screening result). Referral to child protective services is required if the child has been diagnosed with an FASD in the period between birth and 3 years. The intent of this referral is to develop safe care and possible treatment plans for the infant and caregiver if needed, not to initiate punitive actions.

CAPTA mandates referral, not reporting, so states are able to establish their own definitions and practices related to reporting child abuse and neglect. A small number of states have included the presence of an FASD in their abuse and neglect codes. Physicians are encouraged to be aware of their respective state laws on this matter.

If a child is diagnosed with an FASD in a state where a mandatory referral or report to child protective services is necessary, health care providers can engage families in this process with a transparent and caring direct approach. To set the stage for a transparent interaction up front, a health care provider can discuss all of the following: (1) the risks of parental substance abuse and its effects on children; (2) the requirements for mandated reporting to child protective services; (3) the resources and services available to the family; and (4) how child welfare can be a support to the family.

States vary widely with respect to the reporting guidelines and requirements; as such, a discussion of these is beyond the scope of this clinical report. The practicing provider's specific state guidelines and knowledge will inform their

counseling. Additional information about the CAPTA Reauthorization Act of 2010 is available from the American Bar Association.[27] Additional information about referral requirements under CAPTA and Individuals with Disabilities Education Act are available from the Early Childhood Technical Assistance Center.[28]

Medical Home Management and Treatment Strategies

The primary care medical home plays a pivotal role in the continuity and integration of care for children with an FASD. Although there is no cure for FASDs, there are evidence-based treatment options that can improve outcomes for affected individuals. Treatment options are aimed at improving the symptoms and/or providing environmental modifications, as well as parenting strategies and educational interventions to optimally address the brain-based problems experienced by children with FASDs.[3] Studies suggest an increased odds of mitigating adverse life outcomes for individuals with an FASD when the diagnosis was made before 6 years of age and also being reared in a stable home environment with appropriate, integrated support services.[29,30] As such, screening and diagnosis of an FASD in childhood may benefit both patients and their families and allow pediatricians to link patients with an FASD to necessary resources.

Each person with an FASD is unique, so management needs to be tailored to the requirements of the individual. Some children with an FASD may experience growth issues and failure to thrive requiring follow-up and management that uses evidence-based practice guidelines. In addition, any significant congenital defects resulting from PAE affecting the heart, eyes, kidneys, and/or bones warrant evaluation, referral, and appropriate follow-up in the medical home. Fewer than 20% of

children with adverse effects from PAE will present with dysmorphic facial features, and the majority of pediatricians will encounter and need to manage behavioral issues related to PAE.[14,31]

Some children with an FASD may have typical intelligence and fail to qualify for services in the public school system, yet still have specific functional issues. Often when children with an FASD are further assessed by a developmental pediatrician or psychologist, they may receive another concomitant diagnosis, such as a specific learning disability or attention-deficit/hyperactivity disorder (ADHD), for which they could receive either accommodation or an individualized education program (IEP) from the school system.

Children with an FASD may exhibit signs and symptoms also observed in mood, anxiety, autism spectrum, and disruptive behavior disorders (eg, ADHD). These children are also at risk for a receptive or expressive language disorder.[32] Some of the parent-identified behavior challenges for children with an FASD include but are not limited to externalizing behaviors, cognitive difficulties, and social difficulties and/or maladjustment.[33] Some children with an FASD have behavioral issues, such as impulsivity, aggressiveness, and/or hyperactivity.[32] The effects of PAE can include impaired executive function, leading to poor judgment and organic brain dysfunction that can manifest as an inability to comprehend social rules and expectations, learning disabilities, academic and employment difficulties, and challenges navigating activities of daily living.[32] Often, a potential lack of stranger anxiety can put individuals with an FASD at risk for abuse and trauma.[33]

Pediatricians can use typical evidence-based diagnostic and standard screening approaches to diagnose comorbid conditions (eg, flow diagrams, the *Diagnostic and Statistical Manual of Mental Disorders, Fifth Edition* [*DSM-5*], referral to specialists).[34] If comorbid or co-occurring diagnoses are confirmed, pharmacologic treatment may begin as indicated. If the comorbid condition is ADHD, the 2011 clinical practice guidelines from the AAP recommend that doctors prescribe behavior therapy as the first line of treatment of preschool-aged children (4–5 years of age) with ADHD.[35] Parent training in behavior therapy has the most evidence of being effective, and teachers and early childhood caregivers can use behavior therapy in the classroom as well. However, traditional behavioral therapy that does not consider the child's neurobehavioral challenges does not work well for children with an FASD because they often do not respond to typical reward and consequence approaches. Efforts can be made to find behavioral therapists who have been trained in treating children with an FASD. Stimulants and/or atypical antipsychotic agents may be useful in treating the impulsivity, aggressiveness, and/or hyperactivity and oppositional defiant and conduct disorders that may co-occur in individuals with an FASD, especially if those are accurate co-occurring diagnoses and not merely symptoms of the brain damage attributable to PAE. Some pediatricians may be comfortable prescribing stimulants and/or atypical antipsychotic agents, but others may seek referrals to developmental and behavioral specialists, child and adolescent psychiatrists, and/or pediatric neurologists. Treatment approaches could include feedback and assessment from teachers, therapists, and families as well as administration of validated scales, including but not limited to such scales as the Vanderbilt (https://shop.aap.org/adhd-vanderbilt-assessment-forms-package/) and the Screen for Child Anxiety Related

Emotional Disorders for anxiety-related disorders.[36] A resource on pediatric psychopharmacology for the treatment of childhood ADHD, depression, and anxiety may be useful to medical practitioners when they treat these comorbid symptoms in children with FASDs.[37,38]

The heterogeneity of FASD manifestations calls for tailoring treatments to meet individual needs. Inattention, hyperactivity, and impulsivity afflict 50% to 90% of children with FASD and are 3 to 9 times more common than in the general population.[39,40] A large proportion of children with an FASD are affected by oppositional defiant disorder or conduct disorder, including lack of social judgment and failure to learn from experience. Moreover, it can be difficult to tease out the individual effects of ADHD and coexisting cognitive defects on learning in patients with an FASD.[41]

Research on the pharmacologic treatment of FASDs is lacking. Stimulants appear to be effective in managing hyperactivity and impulsivity but are less effective in managing inattention. Risperidone is widely used for aggression, but no controlled studies of risperidone in children with an FASD have been published.[41]

There is some evidence to suggest that virtual reality training, cognitive control therapy, language and literacy therapy, mathematics intervention, and rehearsal training for memory may be beneficial strategies. Three studies evaluating social communication and behavioral strategies (2 randomized controlled trials) suggest that social skills training may improve social skills and behavior at home and attention process training may improve attention.[42]

The nuances and overlap of symptoms of FASDs with other diagnoses make them challenging to distinguish. Children with an

FASD may also have been exposed to other drugs and toxins in utero, and the diagnostician may not always be able to determine what etiology is accounting for which deficit or challenge.[15,33] Not all children will fit neatly into *DSM-5* criteria for specific diagnoses,[34] including an FASD, but their clinical picture and symptomatology may still warrant treatment and support services. Although the response to medication management can be variable and unpredictable in this population of children with an FASD, approaches with typical stimulant, mood dysregulation prescribing practices can be used with the appropriate medications (eg, methylphenidate or amphetamine derivatives, guanfacine, risperidone, aripiprazole, selective serotonin reuptake inhibitors, etc). Variability in clinical profile and response to treatment can pose challenges for the primary care pediatrician caring for children with an FASD and supports the need for collaboration with mental health specialists such as neuropsychologists, clinical psychologists, developmental and/or behavioral pediatricians, child and adolescent psychiatrists, pediatric behavioral mental health clinicians, and developmental therapists (eg, speech, physical, and occupational therapists).[43]

Many children with an FASD are born to a parent(s) who has a substance use disorder including but not always limited to just alcohol. Children of parents with substance use disorders are also at greater risk of later mental health and behavioral problems, including developing a substance use disorder themselves. Exposure to a parent using substances is considered an adverse childhood experience.[44] Youth with an FASD should be screened for substance use, as should all youth in routine pediatric practice. Resources for substance use screening, brief interventions, and referrals to treatment are available for pediatricians.[45] Nearly 60% of individuals with an FASD in the criminal justice system have a history of substance use issues.[29]

At times, children with an FASD may be placed with a foster or adoptive family. A 2013 meta-analysis suggests the prevalence of FAS is 6% and the prevalence of an FASD is 16.9% in child welfare settings.[10] As a particularly vulnerable population, children in foster care and adoptive settings warrant special consideration. Pediatricians caring for youth in foster care may not have access to the biological mother or the pregnancy history, and prenatal substance exposure information is often missing, not available, or inaccurate. Still, this population is at increased risk of having PAE-related health and behavioral issues that are best addressed in a timely manner. Pediatricians partnering with foster and adoptive parents as well as child welfare agencies to proactively address issues have the potential to favorably impact outcomes in this population. Thus, pediatricians may have an opportunity to help disrupt multigenerational cycles of substance use by being informed about the effects of parental substance use on children, intervening when necessary, and collaborating with the family, other health care providers, and appropriate government agencies to address the issues involved.

Given the complex array of systems and services requiring navigation and coordination for children with an FASD and their families, a high-quality primary care medical home with partnerships with families, specialists, therapists, mental and/or behavioral health professionals, and community partners is critical, as it is for all children with special health care needs.

Supporting Families After the Diagnosis Is Made and Providing Patient- and/or Family-Centered Care

Supporting a patient and family after a diagnosis of an FASD is integral to a high-quality medical home. Often, families are distressed and need support and linkages to resources in the days after a diagnosis as they begin to process and begin their journey to support their child. Because the provision of patient- and family-centered care is ideal in practice,[46] actively involving patients and families in decision-making is also important. Patients and families should be part of goal setting and creating, implementing, and updating a formal, written plan of care with family and/or patient input that is sensitive to their language, values, and culture.[47,48] Linking families with other families or caregivers with shared experiences can be helpful in diagnosis and long-term support for families.[46,49] After the diagnosis of an FASD, patients may need referrals to neuropsychologists, clinical psychologists, developmental and/ or behavioral pediatricians, child and adolescent psychiatrists, pediatric developmental therapists (speech, physical, and occupational therapy), and behavioral mental health clinicians and partners. Patients will also often need help with education, coordination, integration, and navigation of the needed services and supports to maximize the potential of their child with an FASD.

Parenting a child with an FASD can prove challenging because a child with an FASD may not respond to typical parenting practices. This often creates stress and frustration for parents and caregivers. A child with an FASD is a child with special health care needs, and children with special health care needs are 4 times more likely to be victims of abuse than their typically developing peers.[50,51] To productively parent a child with an FASD, caregivers may benefit

from special training and education about the child's condition and parenting strategies and approaches that are more likely to be successful. Often, trying different approaches to parenting that exemplify understanding of the child's unique strengths and weaknesses can make a tremendous improvement in the child and his or her family's functioning. Traditional behavioral approaches may not work for children with an FASD because they may have impaired cause-and-effect reasoning as well as an inability to apply learning from one situation to another despite having a normal or low-average IQ.[7] It can be helpful for pediatricians to reframe difficult or challenging behaviors for parents or caregivers of children with an FASD. Reframing helps parents understand that behaviors or difficulties of a child with an FASD may result from prenatal brain damage rather than willful disobedience, thus avoiding the "can't versus won't" misinterpretation. A child with an FASD may have difficulty learning from his or her own experiences. For example, many things that other children pick up naturally (eg, playground rules) may need to be presented explicitly to a child with an FASD. Furthermore, a child with an FASD may benefit from having communication and consensus among caregivers about reasonable and consistent adjustments to expectations, rules, and models of discipline. Children with an FASD often thrive better in a structured environment where there are reasonable rules, routines, and supervision.[33] Structured environments help to provide calming techniques before learning activities or other stressful situations.[52] Picture schedules, visual cues, and repetitions all provide support for the mastery of concepts for a child with an FASD.

Some tools and evidence-based interventions have been shown to help families in which a child has an FASD. The cultural values, belief systems, and context of patients and families are relevant when recommending interventions. Resources, supports, and suggestions are available in the areas of parenting and education, attention and self-regulation, adaptive functioning, and nutrition and medication that also address potential cultural barriers and strategies for clinicians when making recommendations.[53]

All About Me is a downloadable manual for parenting strategies in the light of differences in brain function commonly observed in children with an FASD. It was developed by Kentucky's Prevention Enhancement Site for Fetal Alcohol Spectrum Disorders and is a helpful free resource available at http://www.fasdnetwork.org/uploads/9/5/1/1/9511748/all_about_me..pdf. Also, the following 8 Magic Keys are a set of strategies parents, teachers, and others can use when they care for and interact with children who have an FASD[54]:

- Concrete: Speak in concrete terms; do not use idioms, abstract language, or words with double meanings.

- Consistency: Use the same key words all the time.

- Repetition: Children with an FASD have chronic memory problems, so teach and reteach; repeat instructions multiple times.

- Routine: Keep the child's routine and environment calm, stable, and predictable, with few changes.

- Simplicity: Children with an FASD are literal thinkers, so euphemisms or abstractions can be confusing; give only 1 or 2 instructions at a time.

- Specific: Be explicit and say exactly what you mean.

- Structure: Provide an environment with clear structure and boundaries.

- Supervision: Provide constant supervision to keep the child safe and to help him or her develop appropriate behaviors.

Although these tools are clinically informed and anecdotally useful, they are not evidence based or specific for an FASD.

Role of Care Integration and Care Planning for Individuals With an FASD Over Time

Although the medical home is poised to provide care for children with medical and behavioral complexity such as those with an FASD, care coordination and integration is necessary to support families requiring multiple systems and services.[22] Care coordination is a "cross-cutting system intervention,"[55] which is "the deliberate organization of patient care activities between two or more participants (including the patient) involved in a patient's care to facilitate the appropriate delivery of health care services."[56] "Organizing care for children with an FASD involves the marshalling of personnel and other resources needed to carry out all necessary patient care activities and is often managed by the exchange of information among participants responsible for different aspects of care."[22] A framework for care coordination is provided (Fig 2) to foster high-quality care for children with an FASD.[57]

The myriad of lifelong problems resulting from PAE is extensive. Significant cognitive and behavioral issues ensue from the effects of alcohol on the brain, as well as physical abnormalities, including heart, lung, and kidney defects.[7] The neurobehavioral aspects of an FASD include hyperactivity and behavior problems, difficulty with judgment and social skills, attention and learning difficulties, and drug and alcohol issues.[7] This paradigm supports the need for a collaborating and integrated medical home for

children with an FASD consisting of neuropsychologists, developmental and/or behavioral pediatricians, child and adolescent psychiatrists, pediatric therapists (speech, physical, and occupational therapy), behavioral and mental health clinicians, and community partners all working together, effectively communicating, and coordinating care across systems.

Community Partnerships in Education, Mental, and Behavioral Health

People with an FASD are at increased risk for learning disabilities, mental illness, addiction, school failure, dropping out of school, and interactions with the criminal justice system. Over their lifetimes, people with an FASD may need a plethora of services to maintain and improve their functioning, including support in the medical, education, specialty care, vocational services, and behavioral health systems (Table 2).

Early intervention has been shown to be beneficial for children 0 to 3 years old with developmental delays, including children with an FASD.[58] Children with an FASD without significant delay (>25%) may still benefit from early intervention services and/or surveillance, given their risk for developmental delay and behavioral challenges. Appropriate early intervention services can favorably impact some common challenges experienced by children with an FASD, including word comprehension, learning, naming, academic skills, visual motor integration, and fine motor speed and/or coordination.[59,60]

Children with an FASD who are also 3 years old or older can receive services through the school system, local mental health agencies, or in private therapy under educational, physical, and/or mental health diagnoses. Care coordination across systems is a key construct that can help patients and families with an

PEDIATRIC CARE COORDINATION FRAMEWORK

Care Coordination Definition:
Pediatric care coordination is a patient- and family-centered, assessment-driven, team-based activity designed to meet the needs of children and youth while enhancing the caregiving capabilities of families. Care coordination addresses interrelated medical, social, developmental, behavioral, educational, and financial needs to achieve optimal health and wellness outcomes.

Defining Characteristics of Care Coordination

1. Patient- and family-centered
2. Proactive, planned, and comprehensive

3. Promotes self-care skills and independence
4. Emphasizes cross-organizational relationships

Care Coordination Competencies:

1) Develop partnerships
2) Communicate proficiently
3) Use assessments for intervention
4) Facile in care-planning skills (patient- and family-centered)
5) Integrate all resource knowledge
6) Possess goal and/or outcome orientation
7) Approach is adaptable and flexible
8) Desire continuous learning
9) Apply solid team-building skills
10) Adept with information technology

Care Coordination Functions:

1) Provide separate visits and care coordination interactions
2) Manage continuous communications
3) Complete and analyze assessments
4) Develop care plans (with family)
5) Manage and track tests, referrals, and outcomes
6) Coach patient and/or family skills learning
7) Integrate critical care information
8) Support and/or facilitate all care transitions
9) Facilitate patient- and family-centered team meetings
10) Use health information technology for care coordination

FIGURE 2
Pediatric care coordination framework. Adapted with permission from the Commonwealth Fund; Antonelli RC, McAllister JW, Popp J. Making Care Coordination a Critical Component of the Pediatric Health System: A Multidisciplinary Framework. New York, NY: Commonwealth Fund; 2009.

FASD navigate the complex array of services needed to support a child or youth with an FASD. A child with an FASD may receive early intervention until 3 years of age and, when appropriate, receive special education in local public schools until age 22. In addition, children with an FASD can receive services through local mental health agencies or in private therapy under educational, physical, and/or mental health diagnoses.[60] Some individuals with an FASD can receive adult services from various state agencies for life. Proper services often help individuals with an FASD maximize their long-term potential. Without proper services, treatment or supports, individuals with an FASD may be at higher risk for referrals to child welfare, juvenile justice facilities, adult prisons or jails, and homeless shelters.[29,44] Care coordination across systems is a key construct that can help to navigate the complex array of services needed to support a child or youth with an FASD.[22]

Partnering with families in addressing the developmental, behavioral, and educational concerns of children with an FASD is valuable in practice. Garnering appropriate educational supports

TABLE 2 Resources for Practitioners Caring for Children and Youth With FASDs in a Medical Home

	Resource
FASD general resources	AAP FASD toolkit: www.aap.org/fasd
	PAE screening resources: www.aap.org/pae
	Centers for Disease Control and Prevention: www.cdc.gov/fasd
	FAS Diagnostic and Prevention Network. FAS facial photography and measurement instruction using images and animations to teach accurate measurement of FAS facial features: http://depts.washington.edu/fasdpn/htmls/photo-face.htm
	National Institute on Alcohol Abuse and Alcoholism (NIAAA): www.niaaa.nih.gov
	NIAAA Collaborative Initiative on Fetal Alcohol Spectrum Disorders: www.cifasd.org
	Handouts easily downloaded for education: https://pubs.niaaa.nih.gov/publications/FASDFactsheet/FASD.pdf
	National Institute on Child Health and Human Development: www.nichd.nih.gov
	National Organization for Fetal Alcohol Syndrome: www.nofas.org; national and state resource directory: www.nofas.org/resource-directory
Mental health resources	National Association on Mental Illness: a grassroots organization with advocacy and educational resources with local and state chapters to support clinicians and families: http://www.nami.org/
	American Academy of Child and Adolescent Psychiatry: resources and support for primary care providers, families, and youth: https://www.aacap.org/
SAMHSA	Fetal Alcohol Spectrum Disorders Center for Excellence: https://www.samhsa.gov/fetal-alcohol-spectrum-disorders-fasd-center
	Substance Abuse and Mental Health Services Administration. Addressing Fetal Alcohol Spectrum Disorders. Treatment Improvement Protocol Series 58. HHS Publication No. (SMA) 13-4803. Rockville, MD: Substance Abuse and Mental Health Services Administration; 2014: https://store.samhsa.gov/shin/content//SMA13-4803/SMA13-4803.pdf
	SAMHSA treatment locator: www.samhsa.gov/treatment/index.aspx
Education and disability services	National Dissemination Center for Children with Disabilities
	http://www.parentcenterhub.org/disability-landing/
	All about the IEP: http://www.parentcenterhub.org/iep/
	Assistive Technology State Programs: connects users to programs that can help them find funding for assistive technology, which is any sort of device or service that allows a person with a disability to perform more difficult or unmanageable tasks: http://www.resnaprojects.org/allcontacts/statewidecontacts.html
	Learning Disabilities Association of America: provides parental support services, educates policy makers on legislation regarding learning disabilities, works with school programs that address learning disabilities, and publishes materials for adults with learning disabilities about workplace issues, adult literacy, parenting, and assistive technology: http://ldaamerica.org/
	National Center on Accessible Instructional Materials: serves as a resource to educate parents and teachers on accessible educational materials for children who are unable to use regular printed text: http://aem.cast.org/
	National Disability Navigator Resource Collaborative: informs people with disabilities about their health insurance options through the Affordable Care Act, helping them enroll in the best possible insurance available to them through the Marketplace: http://www.nationaldisabilitynavigator.org
Employment disability services	Job Accommodation Network: works with both potential job seekers and employers and helps people with disabilities market their skills and assists employers in understanding the requirements of the Americans with Disabilities Act: https://askjan.org/
	SourceAmerica: helps people with significant disabilities find jobs by networking with community nonprofit agencies to fulfill contracting needs for the federal government, offers training to people with disabilities who are trying to find employment, and helps them find the best work environment for their needs: http://www.sourceamerica.org/
	Think Beyond the Label: connects qualified candidates with disabilities to businesses looking to hire said candidates through a network of online tools, information, and training to help job seekers find suitable positions and works with businesses to ensure that 7% of their workforce consists of people with disabilities, as mandated by law. http://www.thinkbeyondthelabel.com/

TABLE 2 Continued

	Resource
Medical home and care coordination resources	AAP National Center for Medical Home Implementation: provides tools and resources for care coordination with specific supports, templates, and guides for pediatricians: http://www.medicalhomeinfo.org/
	Agency for Healthcare Research and Quality Care Coordination Accountability Measures for Primary Care Practice: a report that presents selected measures from the Care Coordination Measures Atlas that are well suited for primary care practice. The selected measures are divided into 2 sets: Care Coordination Accountability Measures (from the patient and/or family perspective) and Companion Measures (from the health care professional and system perspectives; ie, self-assessment): http://www.ahrq.gov/qual/pcpaccountability/pcpaccountability.pdf
	The Pediatric Care Coordination Curriculum: a 4-module core curriculum developed by physicians, nurses, social workers, family partner organizations, and family members demonstrating the principles, key concepts, and activities that are necessary to successfully provide care coordination and multidisciplinary, team-based care: http://www.childrenshospital.org/care-coordination-curriculum
	Care Mapping Tool User Guides: family driven tool to support family and/or professional partnerships in working on care mapping. http://www.childrenshospital.org/care-coordination-curriculum/care-mapping
	Jeanne W. McAllister and Lucile Packard Foundation for Children's Health. *Achieving a Shared Plan of Care with Children and Youth with Special Health Care Needs*, a tool that provides a set of recommendations and templates for shared care planning: https://www.lpfch.org/publication/achieving-shared-plan-care-children-and-youth-special-health-care-needs
	ADHD: Clinical Practice Guideline for the Diagnosis, Evaluation, and Treatment of Attention-Deficit/Hyperactivity Disorder in Children and Adolescents. *Pediatrics.* 2011; http://pediatrics.aappublications.org/content/early/2011/10/14/peds.2011-2654. This updates the AAP recommendations for day-to-day care of patients with ADHD. It is complemented by an interactive overview of the ADHD Care Process algorithm that provides step-by-step guidance for implementing the guideline recommendations. A toolkit is available at: http://shop.aap.org/Caring-for-Children-with-ADHD-A-Resource-Toolkit-for-Clinicians/
Transition to adult-oriented systems	The National Health Care Transition Center, Got Transition, also developed and published the Six Core Elements of Health Care Transition and created Web-based tools and resources to aid pediatric and adult providers in transition processes: www.GotTransition.org
Patient- and family-centered care	Family Voices: a national, nonprofit, family-led organization promoting quality health care for all children and youth, particularly those with special health care needs: www.familyvoices.org
	Institute for Patient- and Family-Centered Care: fosters the understanding of patient- and family-centered care for professionals, patients, and families seeking to integrate these concepts into all aspects of health care: http://www.ipfcc.org/
	Positioning the Family and Patient at the Center: A Guide to Family and Patient Partnership in the Medical Home. A comprehensive monograph with strategies for partnering with families as reported by practices, including offering peer and family support and providing information and education through written materials, programs, and events: https://medicalhomeinfo.aap.org/tools-resources/Documents/Positioning_FINAL_May24.pdf

HHS, Health and Human Services; NIAAA, National Institute on Alcohol Abuse and Alcoholism; SAMHSA, Substance Abuse and Mental Health Services Administration.

tailored to the child's needs as part of an Individual Family Service Plan (IFSP) or an IEP is paramount for all children with special health care needs experiencing developmental, behavioral, and educational challenges.[61] An IFSP is a plan for special services for young children with developmental delays and only applies to children from birth to 3 years of age. The IFSP focuses on the family because most young children spend most of their time with their family.

Once a child turns 3 years old, an IEP is put into place. An IEP is a plan for special services for children with developmental delays provided by the school system. The IEP is focused on the child more than the family. In addition, section 504 of the Rehabilitation Act requires that schools make "reasonable accommodations" to ensure that children are not denied a "free and appropriate public education because of a disability."[62] When supporting children with an FASD in their medical home, collaborating with early intervention services and educational systems maximizes their potential. As such, working collaboratively with educational partners, in the context of an IEP when relevant, encompassing the necessary emotional, cognitive, and behavioral supports for children with an FASD is important, as it is with all children with special health care needs experiencing developmental, behavioral, and educational challenges.[63]

To better educate a child with an FASD, teachers and educators may benefit from special training and education about the child's condition. Teaching caregivers about learning challenges, including the need for repetition, one-step commands, innovative training, and educational strategies for patients and families is imperative and an area that continues to evolve.[64] Challenges associated with disabilities that are not addressed early not only persist but also may become more severe and result in additional disabilities or problems as an individual ages. Training and understanding the specific needs of a child with an FASD in both home and school settings cannot be overemphasized. Resources, books, and support groups specific to FASDs are available for clinicians and families.[65,66]

Pediatricians may also need to support families in accessing mental health services for patients and families, including individual and/or family therapeutic services and possibly trauma-informed counseling services, depending on the circumstances. Mothers and families with substance use issues may also be in need of treatment resources for addiction or preventive services.[44] Partnerships with communities foster an understanding of available services and care integration for patients and families in the medical home.[22]

Legal Issues and the Criminal Justice System

Because individuals with an FASD often have additional concerns such as mental health problems, substance use disorders, an inability to comprehend social rules and expectations, learning disabilities, school and employment difficulties, behavioral issues (eg, impulsivity, aggressiveness, hyperactivity, and poor judgement), housing insecurity, and challenges navigating activities of daily living, they may be more vulnerable to having interactions with the criminal justice system, either as a victim or an offender.[16,67] Individuals with an FASD have been shown to have a higher rate of incarceration and arrest, with a significant portion of people with an FASD facing legal trouble at some point.[16,67,68] One study found that approximately 60% of the 415 adolescents and adults with FASDs who lived in the Pacific Northwest and were enrolled in the Fetal Alcohol Follow-up Study of the University of Washington's Fetal

Alcohol and Drug Unit had legal issues defined as being charged, arrested, convicted, or otherwise in trouble with the authorities.[30] The most common criminal complaint (45%) in these cases was crimes against persons.[30] Individuals in prison have much higher rates of FASDs than the general population, but it is not currently possible to estimate the exact number of individuals with an FASD that are in the American criminal justice system because of unavailability and/or limitations in available data.[16,29] In 2015, the total cost of FASDs in Canada was estimated to be a staggering $9.7 billion Canadian dollars, of which criminal justice systems accounted for 40%, health care 21%, education 17%, social services 13%, and others 9%.[69] Specifically, the total cost per person with an FASD per year was estimated at $27 000 Canadian dollars in 2015.[69]

Fast and Conry[67] found that individuals with an FASD have neurologic impairments including learning disabilities, impulsivity, weak executive function, poor judgment, and limited social skills, increasing their susceptibility to criminal behavior and victimization. Individuals with an FASD may not be able to advocate in their own defense because the court systems and law enforcement officials (eg, police, officers of the court) usually use advanced language and/or give directions possibly perceived as confusing and/or conflicting to a person with an FASD. Also, individuals with an FASD can have memory and learning deficits that prevent them from learning from their past experiences and applying those experiences to new situations.[67] Many crimes committed by people with an FASD may be related to their environmental and psychosocial issues, including permanent effects PAE had on their brain. For example, a person with an

FASD may steal because he or she has trouble understanding the abstract concept of ownership. Specifically, from the perspective of a person with an FASD, if the real owner is not there, then the object has no owner and is therefore available to be acquired.[70]

Law enforcement and other individuals in the criminal justice system are not always familiar with FASDs and their lifelong effects. This lack of experience can lead to misunderstanding and inappropriate treatment of the individual with an FASD during a law enforcement or legal encounter. In many cases, education targeting the law enforcement and legal system is needed for people with FASDs to have fair treatment and appropriate support. A medical information card explaining what an FASD represents can help affected individuals interact with law enforcement. When law enforcement officers understand that the individual they are dealing with has an FASD, they can call a designated support person as soon as possible. Sample content of the medical information card could include the following language:

"I have a medical diagnosis of Fetal Alcohol Spectrum Disorder (FASD). Because of this, I may not understand abstract concepts (such as legal rights). If you need my cooperation or I need help, please call the person listed on the back of this card."

Transitioning the Individual to Adult-Oriented Systems When Appropriate

Family-centered care in a patient-centered medical home model may greatly improve transition experiences for a youth with an FASD. Youth with special health care needs obtaining care within a medical home are more likely to receive transition services than those who do not receive care through a medical home.[71] Health care transition preparation is transdisciplinary and holistic, including resources for all aspects of life for youth with an FASD (health care, educational, social, vocational, and recreational). Providers, care coordinators, and system navigators promote participation and inclusion in the adult environment to the fullest extent possible for each patient with an FASD. Individualized case management, care coordination, guidance in navigating available resources and the complex social services system, and broad communication with patients and families extending beyond health care are valuable to help youth reach their full potential.[22] Most importantly, patients and families need to be included in transition planning to optimize success. There are several guidelines and resources available for those involved in transition planning.[71,72]

CONCLUSIONS

PAE can alter normal fetal brain development, leading to permanent structural and/or functional changes that may manifest as a host of significantly impairing emotional, neurologic, cognitive, learning, and behavioral problems. PAE remains one of the leading preventable causes of birth defects, intellectual disability, and neurodevelopmental disorders. The effects of having an FASD last a lifetime. Given the high prevalence, FASDs are as common as other well-known conditions, such as autism spectrum disorder and trisomy 21 (Down syndrome). As such, general and subspecialist pediatricians will care for patients with an FASD who need access to integrated care in a medical home. A health care provider can support the individual and family, integrate care and/or services, facilitate access to community resources, and assist with the transition to adult-oriented systems when appropriate. Proper services often help individuals with an FASD maximize their long-term potential. Without proper services,

treatment, or supports, individuals with an FASD may be at higher risk for referrals to child welfare, juvenile justice facilities, adult prisons or jails, and homeless shelters.

RECOMMENDATIONS FOR PEDIATRICIANS

1. Understand the epidemiology of FASDs and that its prevalence approaches, if not exceeds, that of more commonly known conditions.

2. Collaborate and communicate with obstetric providers regarding prenatal alcohol exposure and risk factors to optimize screening and monitoring of children.

3. Understand the various classifications and diagnostic criteria for FASDs and implications for screening, care, and management.

4. Universally screen all infants, children, and youth for PAE at the time of initial visits and when additional cognitive and behavioral concerns arise.

5. Become familiar with reporting laws and mandates in your practicing states and/or territories related to exposures and child outcomes.

6. Monitor children exposed to alcohol prenatally for physical, developmental, behavioral, and cognitive effects of such exposure.

7. Consider comorbid conditions in children with an FASD (ADHD, depression) and use evidence-based screening tools, medication management, and behavioral interventions, often in collaboration with neurobehavioral professionals.

8. Consider the need to reevaluate the diagnosis of ADHD, oppositional defiant disorder, or other diagnoses the child or

youth may have been given and refer when necessary.

9. Partner with the mental health community, therapists, educational professionals, and families to best meet the needs of children with an FASD and to foster understanding of the diagnosis, management, and interventions for an FASD.

10. Recognize that children with an FASD may have cognitive, behavioral, and physical manifestations of their condition warranting specific treatment strategies and interventions specific to the nuances of an FASD.

11. Proactively partner with foster parents, adoptive parents, and child welfare agencies to address issues such as obtaining accurate histories of prenatal alcohol or drug use.

12. Link patients and families with resources and supports for early intervention services, the educational system, the behavioral/mental health system, transition to adult-oriented heath care systems, and other community resources when appropriate.

13. Embrace a preventive approach to FASDs, as there is no amount of alcohol during pregnancy that is risk free, no kind of alcohol during pregnancy that is risk free, and no time during pregnancy when alcohol consumption is risk free; share this information with all families.

14. Provide a high-quality medical home for all children and youth, including those with an FASD, consisting of care coordination, care integration, transition planning, and patient- and family-centered care.

LEAD AUTHORS

Renee M. Turchi, MD, MPH, FAAP
Vincent C. Smith, MD, MPH, FAAP

COMMITTEE ON SUBSTANCE USE AND PREVENTION, 2017–2018

Sheryl A. Ryan, MD, FAAP, Chairperson
Deepa R. Camenga, MD, MHS, FAAP
Stephen W. Patrick, MD, MPH, MS, FAAP
Jennifer Plumb, MD, MPH, FAAP
Joanna Quigley, MD, FAAP
Leslie R. Walker-Harding, MD, FAAP

FORMER COMMITTEE ON SUBSTANCE USE AND PREVENTION MEMBERS

Lucien Gonzalez, MD, MS, FAAP
Vincent C. Smith, MD, MPH, FAAP

LIAISON

Gregory Tau, MD, PhD – *American Academy of Child and Adolescent Psychiatry*

STAFF

Renee Jarrett, MPH

COUNCIL ON CHILDREN WITH DISABILITIES EXECUTIVE COMMITTEE, 2017–2018

Dennis Z. Kuo, MD, MHS, FAAP, Chairperson
Susan Apkon, MD, FAAP
Timothy J. Brei, MD, FAAP
Lynn F. Davidson, MD, FAAP
Beth Ellen Davis, MD, MPH, FAAP
Kathryn A. Ellerbeck, MD, FAAP
Susan L. Hyman, MD, FAAP
Mary O'Connor Leppert, MD, FAAP

Garey H. Noritz, MD, FAAP
Christopher J. Stille, MD, MPH, FAAP
Larry Yin, MD, MSPH, FAAP

FORMER COUNCIL ON CHILDREN WITH DISABILITIES EXECUTIVE COMMITTEE MEMBERS

Amy J. Houtrow, MD, PhD, MPH, FAAP
Kenneth W. Norwood Jr, MD, FAAP, Immediate Past Chairperson
Renee M. Turchi, MD, MPH, FAAP

LIAISONS

Peter J. Smith, MD, MA, FAAP – *Section on Developmental and Behavioral Pediatrics*
Edwin Simpser, MD, FAAP – *Section on Home Care*
Georgina Peacock, MD, MPH – *Centers for Disease Control and Prevention*
Marie Mann, MD, MPH, FAAP – *Maternal and Child Health Bureau*
The Council on Children with Disabilities maintains a formal liaison relationship with Family Voices and would like to thank Family Voices for their continued partnership.

STAFF

Alexandra Kuznetsov, RD

ACKNOWLEDGMENT

The authors thank Dan Dubovsky, MSW, for his careful review and input.

ABBREVIATIONS

AAP: American Academy of Pediatrics
ADHD: attention-deficit/ hyperactivity disorder
CAPTA: Child Abuse Prevention and Treatment Act
DSM-5: *Diagnostic and Statistical Manual of Mental Disorders, Fifth Edition*
FAS: fetal alcohol syndrome
FASD: fetal alcohol spectrum disorder
IEP: individualized education program
IFSP: Individual Family Service Plan
ND-PAE: neurobehavioral disorder associated with prenatal alcohol exposure
PAE: prenatal alcohol exposure

Address correspondence to Renee M. Turchi, MD, MPH, FAAP. E-mail: rmt28@drexel.edu

PEDIATRICS (ISSN Numbers: Print, 0031-4005; Online, 1098-4275).

Copyright © 2018 by the American Academy of Pediatrics

FINANCIAL DISCLOSURE: The authors have indicated they have no financial relationships relevant to this article to disclose.

FUNDING: No external funding.

POTENTIAL CONFLICT OF INTEREST: The authors have indicated they have no potential conflicts of interest to disclose.

REFERENCES

1. Barry KL, Caetano R, Chang G, et al; National Task Force on Fetal Alcohol Syndrome and Fetal Alcohol Effect. *Reducing Alcohol-Exposed Pregnancies: A Report of the National Task Force on Fetal Alcohol Syndrome and Fetal Alcohol Effect.* Atlanta, GA: Centers for Disease Control and Prevention; 2009. Available at: www.cdc.gov/ncbddd/fasd/documents/redalcohpreg.pdf. Accessed December 18, 2017

2. Smith VC, Matthias P, Senturias YN, Turchi RM, Williams JF. Fetal alcohol research caring for patients with prenatal alcohol exposure: a needs assessment. *J Popul Ther Clin Pharmacol.* 2017;24(1):e25–e39

3. Williams JF, Smith VC; Committee on Substance Abuse. Fetal alcohol spectrum disorders. *Pediatrics.* 2015;136(5). Available at: www.pediatrics.org/cgi/content/full/136/5/e1395

4. Turchi RM, Berhane Z, Bethell C, Pomponio A, Antonelli R, Minkovitz CS. Care coordination for CSHCN: associations with family-provider relations and family/child outcomes. *Pediatrics.* 2009;124(suppl 4):S428–S434

5. Green PP, McKnight-Eily LR, Tan CH, Mejia R, Denny CH. Vital signs: alcohol-exposed pregnancies—United States, 2011-2013. *MMWR Morb Mortal Wkly Rep.* 2016;65(4):91–97

6. Tan CH, Denny CH, Cheal NE, Sniezek JE, Kanny D. Alcohol use and binge drinking among women of childbearing age - United States, 2011-2013. *MMWR Morb Mortal Wkly Rep.* 2015;64(37):1042–1046

7. May PA, Baete A, Russo J, et al. Prevalence and characteristics of fetal alcohol spectrum disorders. *Pediatrics.* 2014;134(5):855–866

8. Astley SJ, Stachowiak J, Clarren SK, Clausen C. Application of the fetal alcohol syndrome facial photographic screening tool in a foster care population. *J Pediatr.* 2002;141(5):712–717

9. Chasnoff IJ, Wells AM, King L. Misdiagnosis and missed diagnoses in foster and adopted children with prenatal alcohol exposure. *Pediatrics.* 2015;135(2):264–270

10. Lange S, Shield K, Rehm J, Popova S. Prevalence of fetal alcohol spectrum disorders in child care settings: a meta-analysis. *Pediatrics.* 2013;132(4). Available at: www.pediatrics.org/cgi/content/full/132/4/e980

11. Jones KL, Smith DW, Ulleland CN, Streissguth P. Pattern of malformation in offspring of chronic alcoholic mothers. *Lancet.* 1973;1(7815): 1267–1271

12. Finer LB, Zolna MR. Declines in unintended pregnancy in the United States, 2008–2011. *N Engl J Med.* 2016;374(9):843–852

13. Astley SJ, Clarren SK. Diagnosing the full spectrum of fetal alcohol-exposed individuals: introducing the 4-digit diagnostic code. *Alcohol Alcohol.* 2000;35(4):400–410

14. Centers for Disease Control and Prevention, National Center on Birth Defects and Developmental Disabilities, National Task Force on Fetal Alcohol Syndrome and Fetal Alcohol Effects. Fetal alcohol syndrome: guidelines for referral and diagnosis. Available at: www.cdc.gov/ncbddd/fasd/documents/fas_guidelines_accessible.pdf. Accessed December 18, 2017

15. Cook JL, Green CR, Lilley CM, et al; Canada Fetal Alcohol Spectrum Disorder Research Network. Fetal alcohol spectrum disorder: a guideline for diagnosis across the lifespan. *CMAJ.* 2016;188(3):191–197

16. Popova S, Lange S, Bekmuradov D, Mihic A, Rehm J. Fetal alcohol spectrum disorder prevalence estimates in correctional systems: a systematic literature review. *Can J Public Health.* 2011;102(5):336–340

17. Hoyme HE, Kalberg WO, Elliott AJ, et al. Updated clinical guidelines for diagnosing fetal alcohol spectrum disorders. *Pediatrics.* 2016;138(2):e20154256

18. Fetal Alcohol Spectrum Disorders Expert Panel. *Flow Diagram for Medical Home Evaluation of Fetal Alcohol Spectrum Disorders.* Elk Grove Village, IL: American Academy of Pediatrics; 2013. Available at: www.aap.org/en-us/advocacy-and-policy/aap-health-initiatives/fetal-alcohol-spectrum-disorders-toolkit/Pages/Algorithm-for-Evaluation.aspx. Accessed December 18, 2017

19. American Academy of Pediatrics, Council on Pediatric Practice. Pediatric records and a "medical home." In: *Standards of Child Health Care.* Evanston, IL: American Academy of Pediatrics; 1967:77–79

20. American Academy of Family Physicians; American Academy of Pediatrics; American College of Physicians; American Osteopathic Association. Joint principles of the patient-centered medical home. 2007. Available at: www.aafp.org/dam/AAFP/documents/practice_management/pcmh/initiatives/PCMHJoint.pdf. Accessed December 18, 2017

21. Medical Home Initiatives for Children With Special Needs Project Advisory Committee; American Academy of Pediatrics. The medical home. *Pediatrics.* 2002;110(1 pt 1):184–186

22. Council on Children With Disabilities and Medical Home Implementation Project Advisory Committee. Patient- and family-centered care coordination: a framework for integrating care for children and youth across multiple systems. *Pediatrics.* 2014;133(5). Available at: www.pediatrics.org/cgi/content/full/133/5/e1451

23. Earls MF; Committee on Psychosocial Aspects of Child and Family Health American Academy of Pediatrics. Incorporating recognition and management of perinatal and postpartum depression into pediatric practice. *Pediatrics.* 2010;126(5):1032–1039

24. Garner AS, Shonkoff JP, Siegel BS, et al; Committee on Psychosocial Aspects of Child and Family Health; Committee on Early Childhood, Adoption, and Dependent Care; Section on Developmental and Behavioral Pediatrics. Early childhood adversity, toxic stress, and the role of the pediatrician: translating developmental science into lifelong health. *Pediatrics.* 2012;129(1). Available at: www.pediatrics.org/cgi/content/full/129/1/e224

25. Christian CW; Committee on Child Abuse and Neglect, American Academy of Pediatrics. The evaluation of suspected child physical abuse [published correction appears in *Pediatrics.* 2015;136(3):583]. *Pediatrics.* 2015;135(5). Available at: www.pediatrics.org/cgi/content/full/135/5/e1337

26. Committee on Child Abuse and Neglect. Policy statement—child abuse, confidentiality, and the health insurance portability and accountability act. *Pediatrics.* 2010;125(1):197–201

27. American Bar Association. The CAPTA Reauthorization Act of 2010: what advocates should know. 2011. Available at: https://apps.americanbar.org/litigation/committees/childrights/content/articles/010311-capta-reauthorization.html. Accessed December 12, 2017

28. Early Identification; The Early Childhood Technical Assistance Center. Referral requirements under CAPTA and IDEA. Available at: http://ectacenter.org/topics/earlyid/capta.asp. Accessed December 12, 2017

29. Burd L, Selfridge R, Klug M, Bakko S. Fetal alcohol syndrome in the United States corrections system. *Addict Biol.* 2004;9(2):169–176; discussion 177–178

30. Streissguth AP, Bookstein FL, Barr HM, Sampson PD, O'Malley K, Young JK. Risk factors for adverse life outcomes in fetal alcohol syndrome and fetal alcohol effects. *J Dev Behav Pediatr.* 2004;25(4):228–238

31. American Academy of Pediatrics, Committee on Nutrition. Failure to thrive. In: Kleinman RE, Greer FR, eds. *Pediatric Nutrition.* 7th ed. Elk Grove Village, IL: American Academy of Pediatrics; 2014:663

32. Popova S, Lange S, Shield K, et al. Comorbidity of fetal alcohol spectrum disorder: a systematic review and meta-analysis. *Lancet.* 2016;387(10022):978–987

33. Green CR, Roane J, Hewitt A, et al. Frequent behavioural challenges in children with fetal alcohol spectrum disorder: a needs-based assessment reported by caregivers and clinicians. *J Popul Ther Clin Pharmacol.* 2014;21(3):e405–e420

34. American Psychiatric Association. *Diagnostic and Statistical Manual of Mental Disorders: (DSM-5).* 5th ed. Washington, DC: American Psychiatric Association; 2013

35. Wolraich M, Brown L, Brown RT, et al; Subcommittee on Attention-Deficit/Hyperactivity Disorder; Steering Committee on Quality Improvement and Management. ADHD: clinical practice guideline for the diagnosis, evaluation, and treatment of attention-deficit/hyperactivity disorder in children and adolescents. *Pediatrics.* 2011;128(5):1007–1022

36. Birmaher B, Brent DA, Chiappetta L, Bridge J, Monga S, Baugher M. Psychometric properties of the Screen for Child Anxiety Related Emotional Disorders (SCARED): a replication study. *J Am Acad Child Adolesc Psychiatry.* 1999;38(10):1230–1236

37. Southammakosane C, Schmitz K. Pediatric psychopharmacology for treatment of ADHD, depression, and anxiety. *Pediatrics.* 2015;136(2):351–359

38. Center for Mental Health Services in Pediatric Primary Care. A guide to psychopharmacology for pediatricians. Available at: http://web.jhu.edu/pedmentalhealth/Psychopharmacolog%20use.html. Accessed December 12, 2017

39. Rasmussen C, Benz J, Pei J, et al. The impact of an ADHD co-morbidity on the diagnosis of FASD. *Can J Clin Pharmacol.* 2010;17(1):e165–e176

40. Peadon E, Elliott EJ. Distinguishing between attention-deficit hyperactivity and fetal alcohol spectrum disorders in children: clinical guidelines. *Neuropsychiatr Dis Treat.* 2010;6:509–515

41. Koren G. Pharmacological treatment of disruptive behavior in children with fetal alcohol spectrum disorder. *Paediatr Drugs.* 2015;17(3):179–184

42. Peadon E, Rhys-Jones B, Bower C, Elliott EJ. Systematic review of interventions for children with Fetal Alcohol Spectrum Disorders. *BMC Pediatr.* 2009;9:35

43. Daley D, van der Oord S, Ferrin M, et al; European ADHD Guidelines Group. Behavioral interventions in attention-deficit/hyperactivity disorder: a meta-analysis of randomized controlled trials across multiple outcome domains. *J Am Acad Child Adolesc Psychiatry.* 2014;53(8):835–847, 847.e1–847.e5

44. Bailey JA, Hill KG, Oesterle S, Hawkins JD. Linking substance use and problem behavior across three generations. *J Abnorm Child Psychol.* 2006;34(3):263–292

45. Hunt L, Srinivas G. Newborn with a perineal lesion. *Pediatrics.* 2016;37(1). Available at: www.pediatrics.org/cgi/content/full/37/1/e1

46. Cené CW, Johnson BH, Wells N, Baker B, Davis R, Turchi R. A narrative review of patient and family engagement: the "foundation" of the medical "home". *Med Care.* 2016;54(7):697–705

47. Malouin RA. *Positioning the Family and Patient at the Center: A Guide to Family and Patient Partnership in the Medical Home.* Elk Grove Village, IL: American Academy of Pediatrics, National Center for Medical Home Implementation; 2013. Available at: https://medicalhomeinfo.aap.org/tools-resources/Documents/Positioning_FINAL_May24.pdf. Accessed December 14, 2017

48. McAllister JW; Lucile Packard Foundation for Children's Health. Achieving a shared plan of care with children and youth with special health care needs. 2014. Available at: https://www.lpfch.org/publication/achieving-shared-plan-care-children-and-youth-special-health-care-needs. Accessed August 20, 2018

49. Murphy NA, Carbone PS; Council on Children With Disabilities; American Academy of Pediatrics. Parent-provider-community partnerships: optimizing outcomes for children with disabilities. *Pediatrics.* 2011;128(4):795–802

50. Sullivan PM, Knutson JF. Maltreatment and disabilities: a population-based epidemiological study. *Child Abuse Negl.* 2000;24(10):1257–1273

51. Brodie N, McColgan MD, Spector ND, Turchi RM. Child abuse in children and youth with special health care needs. *Pediatr Rev.* 2017;38(10):463–470

52. Zarnegar Z, Hambrick EP, Perry BD, Azen SP, Peterson C. Clinical improvements in adopted children with fetal alcohol spectrum disorders through neurodevelopmentally informed clinical intervention: a pilot study. *Clin Child Psychol Psychiatry.* 2016;21(4):551–567

53. Petrenko CL, Alto ME. Interventions in fetal alcohol spectrum disorders: an international perspective. *Eur J Med Genet.* 2017;60(1):79–91

54. Evensen D, Lutke J. Eight magic keys: developing successful interventions for students with FAS. 1997. Available at: www.faslink.org/EightMagicKeys.pdf. Accessed December 14, 2017

55. Institute of Medicine, Committee on Quality of Health Care in America. *Crossing the Quality Chasm: A New Health System for the 21st Century.* Washington, DC: National Academies Press; 2001

56. McDonald KM, Sundaram V, Bravata DM, et al. Care coordination. In: Shojania KG, McDonald KM, Wachter RM, Owens DK, eds. *Closing the Quality Gap: A Critical Analysis of Quality Improvement Strategies.* Vol 7. Rockville, MD: Agency for Healthcare Research and Quality; 2007

57. Antonelli R, McAllister J, Popp J. *Making Care Coordination a Critical Component of the Pediatric Health System: A Multidisciplinary Framework.* New York, NY: The Commonwealth Fund; 2009

58. Karoly LA, Kilburn R, Cannon JS. *Early Childhood Interventions: Proven Results, Future Promise.* Santa Monica, CA: Monograph, RAND Corporation; 2005

59. Mattson SN, Riley EP, Gramling L, Delis DC, Jones KL. Neuropsychological comparison of alcohol-exposed children with or without physical features of fetal alcohol syndrome. *Neuropsychology.* 1998;12(1):146–153

60. Petrenko CL, Davis AS. Neuropsychological aspects of

prevention and intervention for FASD: international perspectives. *J Pediatr Neuropsychol.* 2017;3(1):1–6

61. Adams RC, Tapia C; Council on Children With Disabilities. Early intervention, IDEA part C services, and the medical home: collaboration for best practice and best outcomes. *Pediatrics.* 2013;132(4). Available at: www.pediatrics.org/cgi/content/full/132/4/e1073

62. Section 504 of the Rehabilitation Act of 1973. 29USC §701 et seq (1973)

63. Lipkin PH, Okamoto J; Council on Children With Disabilities; Council on School Health. The Individuals with Disabilities Education Act (IDEA) for children with special educational needs. *Pediatrics.* 2015;136(6). Available at: www.pediatrics.org/cgi/content/full/136/6/e1650

64. Hundert AS, Huguet A, Green CR, et al. Usability testing of guided internet-based parent training for challenging behavior in children with fetal alcohol spectrum disorder (strongest families FASD). *J Popul Ther Clin Pharmacol.* 2016;23(1):e60–e76

65. Kleinfeld J, Wescott S. *Fantastic Antone Succeeds! Experiences in Educating Children With Fetal Alcohol Syndrome.* Fairbanks, AK: University of Alaska Press; 1993

66. Zevenbergen AA, Ferraro FR. Assessment and treatment of fetal alcohol syndrome in children and adolescents. *J Dev Phys Disabil.* 2001;13(2):123–136

67. Fast DK, Conry J. Fetal alcohol spectrum disorders and the criminal justice system. *Dev Disabil Res Rev.* 2009;15(3):250–257

68. Currie BA, Hoy J, Legge L, Temple VK, Tahir M. Adults with fetal alcohol spectrum disorder: factors associated with positive outcomes and contact with the criminal justice system. *J Popul Ther Clin Pharmacol.* 2016;23(1):e37–e52

69. Thanh NX, Jonsson E. Costs of fetal alcohol spectrum disorder in the Canadian criminal justice system. *J Popul Ther Clin Pharmacol.* 2015;22(1):e125–e131

70. Momino W, Félix TM, Abeche AM, et al. Maternal drinking behavior and Fetal Alcohol Spectrum Disorders in adolescents with criminal behavior in southern Brazil. *Genet Mol Biol.* 2012; 35(4 (suppl)):960–965

71. McManus MA, Pollack LR, Cooley WC, et al. Current status of transition preparation among youth with special needs in the United States. *Pediatrics.* 2013;131(6):1090–1097

72. Got Transition. Available at: http://gottransition.org. Accessed December 18, 2017

The Role of Pediatricians in Global Health

• *Policy Statement*

POLICY STATEMENT Organizational Principles to Guide and Define the Child Health Care System and/or Improve the Health of all Children

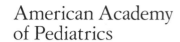

DEDICATED TO THE HEALTH OF ALL CHILDREN™

The Role of Pediatricians in Global Health

Parminder S. Suchdev, MD, MPH, FAAP,[a] Cynthia R. Howard, MD, MPHTM, FAAP,[b] SECTION ON INTERNATIONAL CHILD HEALTH

abstract

Ninety percent of the world's children live in low- and middle-income countries, where barriers to health contribute to significant child morbidity and mortality. The American Academy of Pediatrics is dedicated to the health and well-being of *all* children. To fulfill this promise, this policy statement defines the role of the pediatrician in global health and provides a specific set of recommendations directed to all pediatricians, emphasizing the importance of global health as an integral function of the profession of pediatrics.

[a]Department of Pediatrics, Hubert Department of Global Health, and Emory Global Health Institute, Emory University, Atlanta, Georgia; and [b]Department of Pediatrics and Center for Global Health and Responsibility, University of Minnesota, Minneapolis, Minnesota

Dr Suchdev served as the lead author for the manuscript, organized the writing team, drafted the initial manuscript, and finalized the manuscript; Dr Howard contributed to writing the manuscript and reviewed and revised subsequent versions of the manuscript; and all authors approved the final manuscript as submitted and agree to be accountable for all aspects of the work.

Policy statements from the American Academy of Pediatrics benefit from expertise and resources of liaisons and internal (AAP) and external reviewers. However, policy statements from the American Academy of Pediatrics may not reflect the views of the liaisons or the organizations or government agencies that they represent.

The guidance in this statement does not indicate an exclusive course of treatment or serve as a standard of medical care. Variations, taking into account individual circumstances, may be appropriate.

All policy statements from the American Academy of Pediatrics automatically expire 5 years after publication unless reaffirmed, revised, or retired at or before that time.

DOI: https://doi.org/10.1542/peds.2018-2997

Address correspondence to Parminder S. Suchdev, MD, MPH, FAAP. E-mail: psuchde@emory.edu

PEDIATRICS (ISSN Numbers: Print, 0031-4005; Online, 1098-4275).

Although its definition may vary, we define global health as a discipline that prioritizes equity in health care and stresses the commonality of health issues that require collective, interdisciplinary action both within and across national borders.[1] The American Academy of Pediatrics (AAP) declares that pediatricians are "dedicated to the health of *all* children." To fulfill this promise, pediatricians can work domestically and collaboratively across international borders to improve the health of children throughout the world, regardless of the nationality, culture, language, religion, or socioeconomic status of those children.

Under this broad definition of global health, it is clear that AAP members may engage in global health both within the United States—for example, by caring for children from different cultures—as well as outside US borders. Disparities in health and its determinants are often striking across ethnic and cultural groups, both in the United States and abroad, and warrant a global health framework. For example, pediatricians in the United States routinely care for immigrants, refugees, non–English speakers, and international adoptees who often have specialized health needs similar to those of children in other countries.[2] In addition, a record number of US citizens (87.7 million), many of whom are children, traveled abroad in 2017,[3] resulting in exposure to health conditions and communicable diseases prevalent in foreign countries. Finally, emerging global pathogens, such as Ebola and Zika viruses, have arrived in the United States. Thus, global health is local health and comprises both domestic and cross-border issues.

To cite: Suchdev PS, Howard CR, AAP SECTION ON INTERNATIONAL CHILD HEALTH. The Role of Pediatricians in Global Health. *Pediatrics.* 2018;142(6):e20182997

Ninety percent of the world's children live in low- and middle-income countries (LMICs), where barriers to health, including poor control of infectious diseases, insufficient chronic disease prevention, malnutrition, health care worker shortages, armed conflict, injuries and surgical diseases, mental health, and environmental health issues, contribute to significantly increased child morbidity and mortality.[4–6] Although the number of childhood deaths in LMICs has been cut by more than half in the last 2 decades, approximately 5.4 million deaths among children younger than 5 years still occur each year.[7] Furthermore, the burden of risk for poor developmental outcomes remains extremely high; in fact, approximately 250 million or 43% of children younger than 5 years in LMICs are at risk for not attaining their developmental potential because of extreme poverty or poor nutrition.[8] To underscore shared commitment and to establish a universal global agenda, leaders from 193 countries created the Sustainable Development Goals (SDGs), an ambitious set of 17 goals meant to be achieved by 2030.[9] The SDGs provide a global framework for eliminating poverty and improving health and well-being. Meeting the SDGs will require an emphasis on the health and well-being of all children and their right to both survive and thrive in an equitable and sustainable world.[9,10]

ROLE OF THE PEDIATRICIAN IN GLOBAL HEALTH

Global health is an increasingly valued dimension of medical education, and more than 25% of pediatric residency programs in the United States now offer formal global health tracks.[11] The American Board of Pediatrics, AAP, and their academic partners, represented by the Federation of Pediatric Organizations, have called for

global health training for all pediatricians,[12–14] and as a result, standardized curricula for residency training in global child health have been published and implemented.[15–17] This policy statement, by contrast, focuses on practicing pediatricians—all pediatricians, not just those who may pursue a global health career or more extended global health experiences. The intent of this statement is to describe the collective role of pediatricians in the evolving field of global health. Recommendations may also be relevant to other health professionals working with children.

Pediatricians may engage in global health activities in multiple domains, including but not limited to direct patient care, teaching and training, research, and advocacy. Examples of patient care include US pediatricians who provide medical homes for children from other countries, as well as pediatricians who travel internationally to provide clinical care for children in LMICs. Pediatrician educators trained in global health may teach young physicians in the United States to be globally minded and clinically prepared to care for children from diverse socioeconomic and cultural backgrounds. Pediatricians with the requisite background may also train physicians and health care workers in LMICs.[6] Participation in global health research is an opportunity for pediatricians from all countries; it can be a means to address emerging challenges in medicine, including low-cost technologies, social determinants of health, and implementation science.[18] Finally, examples of global health advocacy include efforts to deepen or sustain investment in global childhood vaccines, research, pharmaceuticals, and supporting policies that aim to fulfill achievement of the SDGs.[19,20]

Engagement in global health is not without challenges or risks, so efforts to address ethics, safety,

medical liability, and legal and fiscal considerations are essential, along with adequate preparation and supervision.[11] Regardless of the domain in which pediatricians may engage in global health and regardless of personal interest, global health has clearly become integral to the profession of pediatrics. Implementation of the following recommendations has the potential to advance global health and the profession of pediatrics.

RECOMMENDATIONS

1. Pediatric continuing medical education (CME) providers and departments of pediatrics are encouraged to make training in global health available to pediatricians and trainees. Topics include the global burden of disease; immigrant and refugee health; patient communication through interpreters; social determinants of health; cultural humility; global child health disparities; disaster management; travel and tropical medicine; population health, including strategies for prevention and treatment of common diseases; and ethical considerations, including the ethics of short-term international medical missions and international research. Although some topics are regularly included in courses offered by CME providers, gaps exist, and topics are frequently addressed without a global health framework.

2. As part of their CME training, pediatricians are encouraged to recognize the enormous differences that exist throughout the world in access to and quality of health care for children and to examine how different models of care variably affect health outcomes for children.

3. Before volunteering for short-term trips or accepting long-term

positions abroad, pediatricians should become knowledgeable of best practices (eg, pre-travel preparation, coordination with local partners, language study, cultural sensitivity, and attention to ethics).[17]

4. As described in the AAP Blueprint for Children,[21] pediatricians are encouraged to advocate for government policies that support global child health, including promotion of the growth and development of every child to his or her full potential; access to education; equitable distribution of immunizations and life-saving medicines; prevention of child abuse and neglect; tobacco control; health equity and disaster preparedness; access to essential surgery, safe anesthesia, and perioperative care; and protection of children from violence. The United Nations' Convention on the Rights of the Child can serve as an effective advocacy tool.[20]

5. Pediatricians working in global health should work collaboratively with international partners to achieve shared goals, whether broad (eg, fulfillment of SDGs) or context specific.

6. Pediatricians working in global health are encouraged to incorporate the use of telemedicine as a viable option for enhancing knowledge transfer and increasing access to patient care.[22]

7. Pediatricians are encouraged not only to use skills learned at home to benefit children abroad but also to use knowledge and innovation gained abroad, such as the use of cost-effective diagnostic and treatment strategies, to improve medical and surgical care for children domestically (reciprocal innovation).

8. AAP chapters are encouraged to play a role in coordinating and offering global health training and service opportunities within their regions.

9. Pediatric organizations are encouraged to consider a global health perspective in their missions and activities, including addressing global health disparities and supporting young pediatricians and trainees in becoming globally minded.

10. Pediatric societies and organizations around the world are invited to collaborate with the AAP to promote long-term partnerships that support global health training, advocacy, and leadership.

SUGGESTED RESOURCES

American Academy of Pediatrics, Section on International Child Health: http://www2.aap.org/sections/ich/

Association of Pediatric Program Directors, Global Health Pediatric Education Group: http://appdgh.wordpress.com/

Global Pediatric Education Consortium: http://www.globalpediatrics.org/

Consortium of Universities for Global Health educational modules: http://www.cugh.org/resources/educational-modules

Johns Hopkins Berman Institute of Bioethics, Ethical Challenges in Short-term Global Health Training: http://ethicsandglobalhealth.org

Boston University, The Practitioner's Guide to Global Health Course: http://www.edx.org/course/the-practitioners-guide-to-global-health

American Academy of Pediatrics, Immigrant Child Health Toolkit: https://www.aap.org/en-us/about-the-aap/Committees-Councils-Sections/Council-on-Community-Pediatrics/Pages/Immigrant-Child-Health-Toolkit.aspx

World Health Organization: http://www.who.int/en/

Global Initiative for Children's Surgery: http://www.globalchildrenssurgery.org/

LEAD AUTHORS

Parminder S. Suchdev, MD, MPH, FAAP
Cynthia R. Howard, MD, MPHTM, FAAP

SECTION ON INTERNATIONAL CHILD HEALTH EXECUTIVE COMMITTEE, 2017–2018

Parminder S. Suchdev, MD, MPH, FAAP, Chairperson
Kevin J. Chan, MD, MPH, FAAP
Cynthia R. Howard, MD, MPH, FAAP
Patrick McGann, MD, FAAP
Nicole E. St Clair, MD, FAAP
Katherine Yun, MD, MHS, FAAP
Linda D. Arnold, MD, FAAP, Immediate Past Chairperson

ABBREVIATIONS

AAP: American Academy of Pediatrics
CDC: Centers for Disease Control and Prevention
LMIC: low- and middle-income country
SDGs: Sustainable Development Goals
WHO: World Health Organization

FINANCIAL DISCLOSURE: The authors have indicated they have no financial relationships relevant to this article to disclose.

FUNDING: No external funding.

POTENTIAL CONFLICT OF INTEREST: The authors have indicated they have no potential conflicts of interest to disclose.

REFERENCES

1. Koplan JP, Bond TC, Merson MH, et al; Consortium of Universities for Global Health Executive Board. Towards a common definition of global health. *Lancet*. 2009;373(9679):1993–1995

2. Chilton LA, Handal GA, Paz-Soldan GJ; Council on Community Pediatrics. Providing care for immigrant, migrant, and border children. *Pediatrics*. 2013;131(6). Available at: www.pediatrics.org/cgi/content/full/131/6/e2028

3. National Travel & Tourism Office. US citizen international outbound travel up nine percent in 2017. Available at: https://travel.trade.gov/tinews/archive/tinews2018/20180327.asp. Accessed August 13, 2018

4. Denno D. Global child health. *Pediatr Rev*. 2011;32(2):e25–e38

5. United Nations Children's Fund. *The State of the World's Children 2016: A Fair Chance for Every Child*. New York, NY: United Nations Children's Fund; 2016

6. Frenk J, Chen L, Bhutta ZA, et al. Health professionals for a new century: transforming education to strengthen health systems in an interdependent world. *Lancet*. 2010;376(9756):1923–1958

7. World Health Organization. *World Health Statistics 2018: Monitoring Health for the SDGs, Sustainable Development Goals*. Geneva: World Health Organization; 2018

8. Black MM, Walker SP, Fernald LCH, et al; Lancet Early Childhood Development Series Steering Committee. Early childhood development coming of age: science through the life course. *Lancet*. 2017;389(10064):77–90

9. United Nations. *The Sustainable Development Goals Report 2017*. New York, NY: United Nations; 2017

10. Chan M. Linking child survival and child development for health, equity, and sustainable development. *Lancet*. 2013;381(9877):1514–1515

11. Butteris SM, Schubert CJ, Batra M, et al. Global health education in US pediatric residency programs. *Pediatrics*. 2015;136(3):458–465

12. Stanton B, Huang CC, Armstrong RW, et al. Global health training for pediatric residents. *Pediatr Ann*. 2008;37(12):786–787, 792–796

13. Gladding SP, McGann PT, Summer A, et al. The collaborative role of North American departments of pediatrics in global child health. *Pediatrics*. 2018;142(1):e20172966

14. Arora G, Esmaili E, Pitt MB, et al; Global Health Task Force of the American Board of Pediatrics. Pediatricians and global health: opportunities and considerations for meaningful engagement. *Pediatrics*. 2018;142(2):e20172964

15. Suchdev PS, Shah A, Derby KS, et al. A proposed model curriculum in global child health for pediatric residents. *Acad Pediatr*. 2012;12(3):229–237

16. Pitt MB, Gladding SP, Suchdev PS, Howard CR. Pediatric global health education: past, present, and future. *JAMA Pediatr*. 2016;170(1):78–84

17. St Clair NE, Pitt MB, Bakeera-Kitaka S, et al. Global health: preparation for working in resource-limited settings. *Pediatrics*. 2017;140(5):e20163783

18. Glass RI. What the United States has to gain from global health research. *JAMA*. 2013;310(9):903–904

19. Suchdev PS, Breiman RF, Stoll BJ. Global child health: a call to collaborative action for academic health centers. *JAMA Pediatr*. 2014;168(11):983–984

20. Armstrong RW. The global pediatrician: is there such a person, or can there be? *J Pediatr*. 2010;156(4):517–518

21. American Academy of Pediatrics. *Blueprint for Children: How the Next President Can Build a Foundation for a Healthy Future*. Washington, DC: American Academy of Pediatrics; 2016

22. Marcin JP, Rimsza ME, Moskowitz WB; Committee on Pediatric Workforce. The use of telemedicine to address access and physician workforce shortages. *Pediatrics*. 2015;136(1):202–209

School Bus Transportation of Children With Special Health Care Needs

- *Policy Statement*

POLICY STATEMENT   Organizational Principles to Guide and Define the Child Health Care System and/or Improve the Health of all Children

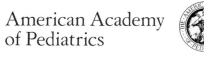

American Academy
of Pediatrics

DEDICATED TO THE HEALTH OF ALL CHILDREN™

School Bus Transportation of Children With Special Health Care Needs

Joseph O'Neil, MD, MPH, FAAP,[a] Benjamin D. Hoffman, MD, FAAP,[b] COUNCIL ON INJURY, VIOLENCE, AND POISON PREVENTION

School systems are responsible for ensuring that children with special needs are safely transported on all forms of federally approved transportation provided by the school system. A plan to provide the most current and proper support to children with special transportation needs should be developed by the Individualized Education Program team, including the parent, school transportation director, and school nurse, in conjunction with physician orders and recommendations. With this statement, we provide current guidance for the protection of child passengers with specific health care needs. Guidance that applies to general school transportation should be followed, inclusive of staff training, provision of nurses or aides if needed, and establishment of a written emergency evacuation plan as well as a comprehensive infection control program. Researchers provide the basis for recommendations concerning occupant securement for children in wheelchairs and children with other special needs who are transported on a school bus. Pediatricians can help their patients by being aware of guidance for restraint systems for children with special needs and by remaining informed of new resources. Pediatricians can also play an important role at the state and local level in the development of school bus specifications.

abstract

[a]Department of Pediatrics, Indiana University School of Medicine and Riley Hospital for Children, Indiana University Health, Indianapolis, Indiana; and [b]Department of Pediatrics, Oregon Health and Science University, Portland, Oregon

Dr O'Neil wrote and revised the draft with the help of chair-elect Dr Hoffman; and all authors approved the final manuscript as submitted.

This document is copyrighted and is property of the American Academy of Pediatrics and its Board of Directors. All authors have filed conflict of interest statements with the American Academy of Pediatrics. Any conflicts have been resolved through a process approved by the Board of Directors. The American Academy of Pediatrics has neither solicited nor accepted any commercial involvement in the development of the content of this publication.

Policy statements from the American Academy of Pediatrics benefit from expertise and resources of liaisons and internal (AAP) and external reviewers. However, policy statements from the American Academy of Pediatrics may not reflect the views of the liaisons or the organizations or government agencies that they represent.

The guidance in this statement does not indicate an exclusive course of treatment or serve as a standard of medical care. Variations, taking into account individual circumstances, may be appropriate.

All policy statements from the American Academy of Pediatrics automatically expire 5 years after publication unless reaffirmed, revised, or retired at or before that time.

DOI: https://doi.org/10.1542/peds.2018-0513

Address correspondence to Joseph O'Neil, MD, MPH, FAAP. E-mail: joeoneil@iu.edu

PEDIATRICS (ISSN Numbers: Print, 0031-4005; Online, 1098-4275).

To cite: O'Neil J, Hoffman BD, AAP COUNCIL ON INJURY, VIOLENCE, AND POISON PREVENTION. School Bus Transportation of Children With Special Health Care Needs. *Pediatrics.* 2018;141(5):e20180513

INTRODUCTION

Many preschool and school-aged children with special health care needs are transported in school buses. These children have the same need for safe transportation as all children. According to the US Department of Education, approximately 13.1% of all students have some disability.[1] The authors of a detailed review of the issues associated with school bus transportation of students seated in wheelchairs using data from the US Department of Transportation, US Department of Education, and a survey from *School Bus Fleet* magazine estimated that approximately 300 000 students travel seated in wheelchairs on school buses in the United States daily.[2] In addition, innumerable children ride in child safety restraint systems (CSRSs), which include conventional car seats, safety vests and/or harnesses, school bus–only devices, and 5-point harnesses integrated into bus seating. In 2007, the American Academy of Pediatrics (AAP) published the policy statement "School Transportation Safety," in which they recommended that all guidelines for safe transportation of all passengers be applied during all school and school-related trips, regardless of the hours of operation.[3]

Established in the Individuals with Disabilities Education Act (IDEA) is the right for children with qualifying disabilities from birth to 21 years of age to a "free and appropriate public education."[4] As needed, these students are entitled to school-provided transportation as a "related service" to access school and health services (for example, audiology and occupational therapy). For qualifying families of children ages 0 to 3 years, early intervention needs are addressed in an Individualized Family Service Plan (IFSP) (IDEA 2004, Part C). Older children ages 3 through 21 years with qualifying special needs receive special education that is guided by an Individualized Education Program (IEP). Whether the child should receive transportation as a related service is determined by the team that develops the child's IFSP and/or IEP.[4] Most children with special needs who are entitled to transportation should consider an Individual Transportation Plan as part of the IFSP and/or IEP document that specifies whether a seat belt, CSRS, or wheelchair is recommended.

Any time a child's special need affects transportation, representatives of school transportation services and other school staff with appropriate knowledge and expertise should be included in the meeting to help develop the transportation plan. The safe transportation of students seated in CSRSs or wheelchairs on school buses requires planning, selection, and procedures developed in collaboration with the parent by a team of transportation professionals, including occupational and physical therapists, school nurses, and certified child passenger safety technicians with the specialized training to ensure the appropriate device is selected, installed, and used properly. Transportation staff who work with children with special needs can effectively conduct their daily responsibilities when provided with appropriate, documented training from the team of professionals. The strategies described in this policy can also be used in disaster situations. Pediatricians should work collaboratively with educators, school personnel, and emergency management teams to effectively meet children's needs in the context of disasters.

Special transportation considerations are required for children with many different conditions. Children with respiratory problems, tracheostomies, thermoregulatory difficulty, seizures, and feeding tubes all require special thought and planning for transportation. Additionally, children with neuromuscular problems in which sitting posture is affected and children with developmental, behavioral, and cognitive problems require special resources to ensure safety during transportation. Children with intellectual disability, autism, or emotional problems may exhibit behaviors that are impulsive, hyperactive, aggressive, or noncompliant. If a child on the school bus has a behavior problem that will affect passenger safety, a school psychologist and other qualified personnel should attempt behavioral interventions. If these interventions are insufficient, a CSRS may be recommended to ensure the safety of all passengers on the school bus. The IEP team should specify which equipment is required, depending on the child's individual needs.

In addition to IDEA, other federal laws protect the educational rights of children with special needs.

Transportation is specifically addressed in the Americans with Disabilities Act (Public Law 110–325, as amended in 2008),[5] which protects the civil rights of Americans with disabilities. In it are requirements established for federal agencies, such as local educational agencies, to address the needs of students who have disabilities, including students with conditions that do not qualify under IDEA. In addition, the Head Start Act, which was established to serve low-income preschoolers through the program Early Head Start, has been expanded to include infants, toddlers, and preschoolers and requires that a minimum 10% of program enrollment be available to children with special needs.[6] It is required by federal law that children in Head Start who receive transportation services be properly restrained in an appropriate occupant restraint because these children are too small to be protected by the compartmentalization approach used in a regular school bus (Head Start Transportation Regulation, 45 CFR 1310, Subpart B). Guidance on the proper use of child safety restraints on school buses is also provided by the National Highway Traffic Safety Administration.[7]

Occupant protection on school buses has been based on the concept of compartmentalization. Compartmentalization is provided by seats that are closely spaced with high energy-absorbing seat backs. In certain crash scenarios, optimal protection is not offered by compartmentalization, which is not consistent with current technology and messages for children and families regarding the use of car safety seats and seat belts in all vehicles.[3] The AAP further recommends that all newly manufactured school buses be equipped with lap/shoulder restraint systems in which car safety seats and harness systems can also be accommodated. The AAP also recommends that all school buses used for school and all school-related activities be in compliance with all applicable federal regulations.[3]

School buses that transport children with special needs, including both small and full-size buses, are regulated through several federal standards. In Federal Motor Vehicle Safety Standard (FMVSS) 222, School Bus Passenger Seating and Crash Protection, adopted January 1976 and last amended April 2009, safety requirements for school bus interiors are established.[8] These regulations mainly apply to school bus features intended to protect able-bodied children. However, added in a 1992 amendment to FMVSS 222 were the basic requirements for wheelchair tiedowns and occupant restraint systems (WTORSs), including a requirement that there must be at least 4 adjustable securement anchorages (2 at the front and 2 at the rear) to secure the wheelchair facing forward and separate torso and pelvis restraints for the occupant. Also added were strength-testing procedures of all securement devices (meeting the seat belt standards of FMVSS 209).[9] Other FMVSSs that pertain to the transportation of children with special needs include FMVSS 403 and 404 in which platform lift performance standards and installation requirements are specified.[10,11] FMVSS 213, in which all safety restraints for use by children are regulated, also applies to CSRSs used on school buses.[12] Per FMVSS 225, it is required that 2 seating positions be equipped with Lower Anchors and Tethers for Children for the installation of CSRSs on buses weighing 10 000 lb or less.[13]

In addition to federal regulations, the school bus industry has established voluntary guidelines via the National School Transportation Specifications and Procedures (NSTSP), which include some guidance on the safe transportation of students with special needs.[14] The purpose of the NSTSP is to help establish national best practices and provide guidelines for state rules and procedures for school transportation. The document is in alignment with all FMVSSs relevant to the transportation of pupils and provides additional procedures and specifications. Wheelchair-related guidelines in the NSTSP specify that buses for wheelchair-seated students be "specially equipped" with a power lift or ramp, if preferable, depending on the student's medical condition, and outline specific loading and securement procedures. The use of CSRSs is also discussed, with emphasis on following manufacturers' instructions and providing necessary training to on-bus personnel. Stated in the NSTSP is the guideline that a child's IFSP and/or IEP team should determine when it is appropriate to transfer a child from a wheelchair to a CSRS for transport.

WHEELCHAIRS USED IN VEHICLE TRANSPORT

Using a CSRS on a bench seat provides the best protection in a crash and should be selected for every child who can be transferred out of a wheelchair for travel.[15] However, for children who must remain in a wheelchair for travel, using a system that meets the voluntary industry standards of the American National Standards Institute and Rehabilitation Engineering Society of North America greatly enhances safety. A certified transit-ready wheelchair system is one that meets these voluntary design and performance requirements for use as a seat by its occupant when traveling in a motor vehicle.[16] These standards are designated as WC 18, 19, and 20. WC 18 (formerly SAE International J2249) is a voluntary standard for the securement of wheelchairs and occupant restraints for wheelchair-seated children and adults in the forward-facing orientation. The standard applies to the system or device that both secures the wheelchair (tiedowns) and the system of belts that restrains the wheelchair-seated occupant used in motor vehicles, including school buses.[16] Collectively, these systems and devices are called WTORSs. Addressed in the WC 18 standard is the securement of the wheelchair to the vehicle floor, typically accompanied by a 4-point, strap-type system that includes 2 straps at the rear of the wheelchair to bear most of the crash load, and 2 straps at the front to provide stability. Heavier wheelchairs, specifically when the wheelchair and occupant's combined weight exceeds 250 lb, require 1 or 2 additional securement straps at the rear of the wheelchair.[16]

Although a wheelchair's built-in postural support device helps the occupant maintain an upright position, in most cases, these supports are not crash-tested and cannot be used for occupant restraint. Unless a postural support harness is clearly marked as being crash tested successfully, it should not be used in place of the vehicle's lap and shoulder belt system. An occupant restraint system that has been tested at force conditions of 30 mph and 20 g for upper torso restraint provides necessary safety for each wheelchair-seated occupant. This may be accomplished in 1 of 3 ways:

1. The most common method is to use bus-mounted lap and shoulder belts that cross the hips and shoulder of the occupant and anchor to the wall and floor of the school bus;

2. Newer wheelchairs that meet voluntary standards may include some transit-ready belts that replace all or some of the bus-mounted occupant restraint system. To provide comparable occupant protection, these

wheelchair-based occupant restraints should comply with current industry standards and provide the same degree of protection that the vehicle seat belt system provides; and

3. Some wheelchairs made for children weighing from 25 to 50 pounds have the option to be equipped with a crashworthy 5-point harness system that is anchored to the wheelchair frame.

WC 19 is a voluntary industry standard for designing, testing, and labeling a wheelchair used as a seat in a motor vehicle certified as "transit-ready."[17] WC 20 is a standard for specialized seating devices for use in motor vehicles.[18] Established in WC 20 is the design and performance criteria for a wheelchair seating system that is added to a WC 19 frame. WC 20 allows for independent testing of a seating system using a surrogate wheelchair base, which is important because an individual's seating and position needs may require a pairing of a specialized seating system and wheelchair frame that have not been crash tested together as a unit.

Whenever possible, a wheelchair used for school bus transportation should be certified as such. A transit option wheelchair system should meet the WTORS criteria of WC 18 and be used with a complete WC 19 wheelchair or with a wheelchair frame that satisfies WC 19 paired with a specialized aftermarket seating system that meets WC 20. Rehabilitation therapists can help identify products that are certified by the wheelchair manufacturer to meet this standard.

The safe transportation of students seated in CSRSs or wheelchairs on school buses requires planning, selection, and procedures developed by a team of transportation professionals, including occupational and physical therapists and a child

passenger safety technician with the specialized training to apply the safety principles of these devices. There is no certification or standard for training of bus operators or attendants who transport students who ride in wheelchairs, although training is regularly offered by manufacturers of WTORSs and lifts. In addition, there is generally no monitoring of procedures to enforce compliance with proper installation and use of WTORSs in practice. For the proper installation of CSRSs, specially trained child passenger safety technicians are available in most communities. An 8-hour national training course for transportation personnel has been developed by the National Highway Traffic Safety Administration and is frequently offered at national conferences or can be taught locally. Training standards for bus operators and attendants would improve the quality of transportation safety among children with special health care needs and should be developed in each state.

RECOMMENDATIONS

These recommendations are provided for the primary care provider within the medical home. This information is intended to assist the family in understanding important issues for the safe transportation of a child with special health care needs for appropriate securement on a school bus. The responsibility for these specific recommendations may vary among school districts and should be discussed at the time of IEP and transportation planning.

1. Any child who can assist with transfer or be reasonably moved from a wheelchair, stroller, or special seating device to a seat belt or CSRS complying with FMVSS 213 should be transferred for transportation. If a child is transferred to a CSRS,

the CSRS should face forward unless the child is younger than 2 years.[19] Children weighing less than 80 lb (36.3 kg) and who can safely transfer or who need the additional support of a harness should ride in a properly used CSRS, which may be integrated or added to bus seating. School-aged children who are able to ride properly in a seat belt should use a lap-shoulder belt that was manufactured specifically for the vehicle. The unoccupied wheelchair should also be secured adequately in the vehicle to prevent it from becoming a dangerous projectile in the event of a sudden stop or crash;

2. Passenger seats that have a seat belt or that are used to attach a CSRS must have a reinforced frame meeting the requirements of FMVSS 208 (Occupant Crash Protection),[20] FMVSS 209 (Seat Belt Assemblies),[9] and FMVSS 210 (Seatbelt Assembly Anchorages).[21] The manufacturer of the school bus should be consulted regarding the noted requirements when ordering or retrofitting an existing school bus;

3. If possible, all children weighing less than 80 lb (36.3 kg) should be secured in an appropriate CSRS meeting the requirements of FMVSS 213[12];

4. CSRSs must be secured to the bus seat in a manner prescribed and approved by the manufacturer of the safety device. The CSRS should not be secured on a school bus seat adjacent to an emergency exit or in a seating position that blocks the evacuation route for other passengers;

5. CSRSs for which weight, length, and harness requirements are specified by the seat's manufacturer for rear facing should be used to transport

children who are younger than 2 years or whose weight and length meet the seat's requirements. CSRSs for these children should be attached, whenever possible, to the school bus seat in a rear-facing position. School districts should check with the school bus manufacturer to verify that a rear-facing CSRS may be used[3];

6. Three-wheeled, cart-, or stroller-type wheelchair devices should not be permitted for occupied transport in a school bus unless the results of impact tests reveal that the device can be secured under impact loading conditions as specified in the voluntary standards of WC 19;

7. Occupied wheelchairs aboard buses should be secured with 4 tiedown devices that are attached to the floor. If the combined weight of the chair and occupant exceeds 250 lb (113.4 kg), additional tiedowns may be required.[16] The wheelchair occupant must be restrained with a separate device;

8. An occupant restraint system that meets the FMVSS for upper torso restraint (shoulder harness) and lower torso restraint (lap belt over pelvis) should be provided for each wheelchair-seated occupant;

9. Lap boards and metal or plastic trays attached to the wheelchair or to adaptive equipment should be removed before loading and should be secured separately for transport. If necessary for the health or well-being of the child, a foam tray may be substituted during travel; and

10. Any medical equipment needed to support the child during school bus transport needs to be secured to prevent it from becoming a potentially lethal projectile during a crash, sudden braking, or a sudden stop. Any

liquid oxygen transported in a school bus should be securely mounted and fastened to prevent damage and exposure to intense heat. An appropriate sign indicating that oxygen is in use should be placed in the school bus.

ADDITIONAL CONSIDERATIONS FOR PASSENGER TRANSPORTATION

The following considerations should be incorporated into the school system plan for the transportation requirements of children with special needs:

1. A school nurse or an aide with appropriate medical training or a specially trained individual to accompany the patient is necessary to provide onboard assistance and support to children with certain special conditions, such as tracheostomies, who may require suctioning or emergency care during school bus transport. School systems should provide a school nurse or trained aide when medically necessary to help ensure health-related problems occurring while children with special needs are on the school bus are properly managed;

2. Children with special health care needs may need rescue medications for acute exacerbations of their medical condition. These medications and a school nurse or trained individual to administer them should be available at all times on board the vehicle. The child's primary care provider should know the local and state regulations and the local school limitations and resources for administering rescue medications and how to help with the development of emergency action plans. Although the school nurse is

responsible for the development of the student's individualized health care plan, including transportation plans, assistance from the student's primary care provider in the form of signed health care provider's orders should be included in the child's IEP or the family's IFSP. If provision of trained personnel or administration of rescue medicines is not possible during transport, the vehicle route should be designed to provide rapid access to emergency medical personnel. The family, school nurse, school administration, and prescribing provider should establish criteria for contacting emergency medical services. Guidance should be provided for onboard personnel to render support while waiting for emergency medical personnel to arrive. In the action plan, there should be provisions for rapid access of emergency medical services such as cell phone or radio use;

3. School transportation staff, in conjunction with the school nurse, should participate in the development of the transportation portion of the IEP or IFSP for children who have special transportation requirements. On-bus personnel should be apprised of aspects of a child's medical condition and potential medical emergencies that are relevant to the child's safety while on the bus. The Family Educational Rights and Privacy Act authorizes such information to be shared with school officials as well as the bus driver, aides, and substitutes[22];

4. School bus transportation staff should participate in training programs annually and have resource materials available on the subject of transportation of children with special needs to ensure that they can provide

the most current and proper services to children with special transportation requirements;

5. The caregiver (family, guardian, or foster parent) of a child with special needs must be invited to meetings regarding the child's IEP and/or IFSP. Caregivers, primary care providers, and school personnel should be informed of the importance of incorporating and maintaining appropriate and safe transportation specifications as part of these documents. It is also important to know that a caregiver and/or the transportation department representative can reconvene the IEP and/or IFSP team should important changes to the documentation become necessary for the child's continued safety;

6. The caregiver of a child with special needs, in conjunction with the school nurse and the designated bus driver for the child's bus route, should share information addressing the specific medical, developmental, and behavioral needs of the child before and during the school year, which should be reflected in the student's transportation plan, while maintaining adherence to specifications of the child's IEP and/or IFSP. An emergency medical information card or care plan should be available for the bus drivers for each student with special health care needs being transported. Substitute bus drivers also need to be aware of this information. Transportation personnel must adhere to the school district's policy regarding confidentiality of student information;

7. In addition to safe transportation on the school bus, the transportation plan should include safe procedures for embarking to and disembarking from the school bus. Standard policy for school bus drivers should include procedures to ensure no child is left on the bus;

8. Preparation for emergency evacuation should include the particular procedures required to evacuate each child with special needs. A written plan that outlines procedures for emergency evacuation of each child should be maintained. The plans (IEP and/or IFSP) should include detailed information on contacting the parent or caregiver in case of an emergency. At a minimum, 1 evacuation drill should be conducted for each school year to enable the transportation staff to practice evacuating the children under their care. Local emergency response personnel should be invited to participate in evacuation drills;

9. In the event of a medical emergency on the bus during transport, the driver should pull to the side of the road as quickly and safely as possible. The driver should then call 911 and summon emergency personnel. If a school nurse or trained aide is on the bus, he or she will provide supportive care until emergency assistance arrives. If there is no other school staff support on the bus, the driver may provide supportive care until emergency assistance arrives; and

10. Children who are supported by technology may be at increased risk of acquiring infectious diseases. All caregivers should cleanse their hands thoroughly before and after providing direct care for students, including toileting and tracheostomy or gastrostomy care. Standard (universal) precautions should be used when caring for all children when exposed to blood or blood-containing body fluids. Schools should follow the legal requirements of their states or the Occupational Safety and Health Administration with respect to all immunizations, including hepatitis B immunization. Children and adults who are in the recommended categories should receive yearly influenza immunization. Transportation staff should be provided with training and supplies that prepare them to conduct universal precaution practices and procedures.[23]

The AAP encourages states to address and support the transportation requirements of children with special needs. Pediatricians can help their patients and their families through awareness of general principles and guidance for restraint systems for children with special needs and remaining informed of new resources as they become available.[24] Periodically updated information on specific restraint systems for children with special needs can be obtained through the AAP at www.healthychildren. org. Resources are also available through the National Center for the Safe Transportation of Children With Special Health Care Needs at http://www.preventinjury.org/ Special-Needs-Transportation. For pediatricians involved in early intervention, including Head Start, a joint publication from the AAP, American Public Health Association, and the Maternal Child Health Bureau titled *Caring For Our Children: National Health and Safety Performance Standards; Guidelines for Early Care and Education Programs, Third Edition*, is helpful for developing written policies for safe transportation.[25]

Pediatricians can play important roles at the state and local levels as advocates for children through collaboration with their community leaders and services in the evaluation and development of school bus specifications responsive to the safe transportation requirements of children with special needs.

ACKNOWLEDGMENT

We thank Denise Donaldson of *Safe Ride News* for her contribution in the review and drafting of this article.

LEAD AUTHORS

Joseph O'Neil, MD, MPH, FAAP
Benjamin D. Hoffman, MD, FAAP

COUNCIL ON INJURY, VIOLENCE, AND POISON PREVENTION EXECUTIVE COMMITTEE, 2014–2015

Kyran P. Quinlan, MD, MPH, FAAP, Chairperson
Michele Burns, MD, FAAP
Sarah Denny, MD, FAAP
Beth Ebel, MD, MSc, MPH, FAAP
Michael Hirsh, MD, FAAP

Marlene Melzer-Lange, MD, FAAP
Joseph O'Neil, MD, MPH, FAAP
Elizabeth Powell, MD, FAAP
Judith Schaechter, MD, FAAP
Mark R. Zonfrillo, MD, MSCE, FAAP

EX OFFICIO

Benjamin D. Hoffman, MD, FAAP
Eliot Nelson, MD, FAAP

LIAISONS

Elizabeth Edgerton, MD, MPH, FAAP – *Health Resources and Services Administration*
Julie Gilchrist, MD, FAAP – *Centers for Disease Control and Prevention*
Lynne J. Haverkos, MD, MPH – *National Institute of Child Health and Human Development*
Jonathan D. Midgett, PhD – *Consumer Product Safety Commission*
Alexander W. (Sandy) Sinclair – *National Highway Traffic Safety Administration*

STAFF

Bonnie Kozial

ABBREVIATIONS

AAP: American Academy of
    Pediatrics
CSRS: child safety restraint
    system
FMVSS: Federal Motor Vehicle
    Safety Standard
IDEA: Individuals with
    Disabilities Education Act
IEP: Individualized Education
    Program
IFSP: Individualized Family
    Service Plan
NSTSP: National School
    Transportation
    Specifications and
    Procedures
WTORS: wheelchair tiedown
    and occupant restraint
    system

FUNDING: No external funding.

POTENTIAL CONFLICT OF INTEREST: The authors have indicated they have no potential conflicts of interest to disclose.

REFERENCES

1. National Center for Educational Statistics; Institute of Educational Sciences; US Department of Education. Children and youth with disabilities. 2017. Available at: https://nces.ed.gov/programs/coe/indicator_cgg.asp. Accessed March 28, 2018

2. Buning ME, Karg PE. School bus transportation for students seated in wheelchairs. *J Pediatr Rehabil Med*. 2011;4(4):259–268

3. Agran PF; American Academy of Pediatrics Committee on Injury, Violence, and Poison Prevention; American Academy of Pediatrics Council on School Health. School transportation safety. *Pediatrics*. 2007;120(1):213–220

4. Individuals With Disabilities Education Improvement Act of 2004. Pub L No. 108-446, volume 118, Stat 2647–2808

5. US Department of Justice. Americans With Disabilities Act Title II Regulations: nondiscrimination on the basis of disability in state and local government services. 2010. Available at: https://www.ada.gov/regs2010/titleII_2010/titleII_2010_regulations.pdf. Accessed February 1, 2018

6. US Department of Health and Human Services; Administration for Children and Families Office of Head Start. Head Start Act, 42 USC §9801 et. seq (2017). Available at: https://eclkc.ohs.acf.hhs.gov/hslc/standards/law/HS_Act_2007.pdf. Accessed January 5, 2017

7. Department of Transportation; National Highway Traffic Safety Administration. *Proper Use of Child Safety Restraint Systems on School Buses.* Washington, DC: US Department of Transportation, National Highway Traffic Safety Administration. Available at: www.nhtsa.gov/people/injury/buses/busseatbelt/index.html. Accessed January 5, 2017

8. Department of Transportation; National Highway Traffic Safety Administration. *Standard No. 222. School Bus Passenger Seating and Crash Protection.* Washington, DC: US Department of Transportation,

Federal Motor Vehicle Carrier Safety Administration; 1977. Available at: https://www.gpo.gov/fdsys/pkg/CFR-2016-title49-vol6/pdf/CFR-2016-title49-vol6-sec571-222.pdf. Accessed December 8, 2017

9. US Department of Transportation; National Highway Traffic Safety Administration. Standard No. 209; Seat Belt Assemblies. Available at: https://www.gpo.gov/fdsys/pkg/CFR-2016-title49-vol6/pdf/CFR-2016-title49-vol6-sec571-209.pdf. Accessed December 8, 2017

10. US Department of Transportation; National Highway Traffic Safety Administration. Standard No. 403; Platform lift systems for motor vehicles. Available at: https://www.federalregister.gov/documents/2012/04/05/2012-8138/federal-motor-vehicle-safety-standards-platform-lifts-for-motor-vehicles-platform-lift-installations. Accessed January 5, 2017

11. US Department of Transportation; National Highway Traffic Safety

Administration. Standard No. 404; Platform lift installation for motor vehicles. Available at: https://www.gpo.gov/fdsys/granule/CFR-2011-title49-vol6/CFR-2011-title49-vol6-sec571-404. Accessed January 5, 2017

12. US Department of Transportation; National Highway Traffic Safety Administration. Standard No. 213; Child restraint systems. Available at: https://www.gpo.gov/fdsys/pkg/CFR-2016-title49-vol6/pdf/CFR-2016-title49-vol6-sec571-213.pdf. Accessed December 8, 2017

13. US Department of Transportation; National Highway Traffic Safety Administration. Federal Motor Vehicle Safety Standard 225; Child Restraint Systems; Child Restraint Anchorage Systems. Available at: https://www.gpo.gov/fdsys/pkg/CFR-2016-title49-vol6/pdf/CFR-2016-title49-vol6-sec571-225.pdf. Accessed December 8, 2017

14. University of Central Missouri. *National School Transportation Specifications and Procedures: Adopted by the Fifteenth National Congress on School Transportation*. 2010 Revised Edition. Warrensburg, MO: University of Central Missouri; 2010

15. University of Michigan Transportation Research Institute. Ride safe brochure. Available at: http://wc-transportation-safety.umtri.umich.edu/ridesafe-brochure. Accessed January 5, 2017

16. Rehabilitation Engineering and Assistive Technology Society of North America. *Section 18: Wheelchair Tiedown and Occupant Restraint Systems for Use in Motor Vehicles*. Vol

20. Arlington, VA: American National Standards Institute/Rehabilitation Engineering and Assistive Technology Society of North America; 2013

17. Rehabilitation Engineering and Assistive Technology Society of North America. *Wheelchairs Used as Seats in Motor Vehicles*. Vol 1. Arlington, VA: American National Standards Institute/ Rehabilitation Engineering and Assistive Technology Society of North America; 2000

18. Rehabilitation Engineering and Assistive Technology Society of North America. *Section 20: Seating Systems Used in Motor Vehicles*. Vol 4. Arlington, VA: RESNA Committee on Wheelchairs and Transportation; American National Standards Institute/ Rehabilitation Engineering and Assistive Technology Society of North America; 2008

19. Durbin DR; Committee on Injury, Violence, and Poison Prevention. Child passenger safety. *Pediatrics*. 2011;127(4):788–793

20. US Department of Transportation; National Highway Traffic Safety Administration. Standard No. 208; Occupant crash protection. Available at: https://www.gpo.gov/fdsys/pkg/CFR-2016-title49-vol6/pdf/CFR-2016-title49-vol6-sec571-208.pdf. Accessed December 8, 2017

21. US Department of Transportation; National Highway Traffic Safety Administration. Standard No. 210; Seat belt assembly anchorages. Available at: https://www.gpo.gov/fdsys/pkg/CFR-2016-title49-vol6/pdf/

CFR-2016-title49-vol6-sec571-210.pdf. Accessed December 8, 2017

22. US Department of Education. Family Policy Compliance Office. Available at: https://www.ed.gov/category/keyword/family-policy-compliance-office-fpco. Accessed January 5, 2017

23. American Academy of Pediatrics. School health. In: Kimberlin DW, Brady MT, Jackson MA, Long SS, eds. *Red Book: 2015 Report of the Committee on Infectious Diseases*. 30th ed. Elk Grove Village, IL: American Academy of Pediatrics; 2015:152–161

24. US Department of Transportation; National Highway Traffic Safety Administration. *Child Passenger Safety Restraint Systems on School Buses National Training Participant Manual*. Washington, DC: National Highway Traffic Safety Administration; 2007. Available at: http://cpsboard.org/cps/wp-content/uploads/2013/03/Participant-Manual-with-Covers.pdf. Accessed January 5, 2017

25. American Academy of Pediatrics; American Public Health Administration; National Resource Center for Health and Safety in Childcare and Early Education. *Caring for Our Children: National Health and Safety Performance Standards; Guidelines for Early Care and Education Programs*. 3rd ed.Elk Grove Village, IL: American Academy of Pediatrics; Washington DC: American Public Health Association; 2011. Available at: http://cfoc.nrckids.org/WebFiles/CFOC3_updated_final.pdf. Accessed January 5, 2017

Screening Examination of Premature Infants for Retinopathy of Prematurity

- *Policy Statement*

POLICY STATEMENT Organizational Principles to Guide and Define the Child Health Care System and/or Improve the Health of all Children

American Academy of Pediatrics

DEDICATED TO THE HEALTH OF ALL CHILDREN™

Screening Examination of Premature Infants for Retinopathy of Prematurity

Walter M. Fierson, MD, FAAP, AMERICAN ACADEMY OF PEDIATRICS Section on Ophthalmology, AMERICAN ACADEMY OF OPHTHALMOLOGY, AMERICAN ASSOCIATION FOR PEDIATRIC OPHTHALMOLOGY AND STRABISMUS, AMERICAN ASSOCIATION OF CERTIFIED ORTHOPTISTS

abstract

This policy statement revises a previous statement on screening of preterm infants for retinopathy of prematurity (ROP) that was published in 2013. ROP is a pathologic process that occurs in immature retinal tissue and can progress to a tractional retinal detachment, which may then result in visual loss or blindness. For more than 3 decades, treatment of severe ROP that markedly decreases the incidence of this poor visual outcome has been available. However, severe, treatment-requiring ROP must be diagnosed in a timely fashion to be treated effectively. The sequential nature of ROP requires that infants who are at-risk and preterm be examined at proper times and intervals to detect the changes of ROP before they become destructive. This statement presents the attributes of an effective program to detect and treat ROP, including the timing of initial and follow-up examinations.

Dr Fierson was responsible for writing and revising the policy statement and responding to reviewers' concerns and has approved the final manuscript as submitted.

This document is copyrighted and is property of the American Academy of Pediatrics and its Board of Directors. All authors have filed conflict of interest statements with the American Academy of Pediatrics. Any conflicts have been resolved through a process approved by the Board of Directors. The American Academy of Pediatrics has neither solicited nor accepted any commercial involvement in the development of the content of this publication.

Policy statements from the American Academy of Pediatrics benefit from expertise and resources of liaisons and internal (AAP) and external reviewers. However, policy statements from the American Academy of Pediatrics may not reflect the views of the liaisons or the organizations or government agencies that they represent.

The guidance in this statement does not indicate an exclusive course of treatment or serve as a standard of medical care. Variations, taking into account individual circumstances, may be appropriate.

All policy statements from the American Academy of Pediatrics automatically expire 5 years after publication unless reaffirmed, revised, or retired at or before that time.

DOI: https://doi.org/10.1542/peds.2018-3061

Address correspondence to Walter M. Fierson, MD, FAAP. E-mail: wfierson@yahoo.com

PEDIATRICS (ISSN Numbers: Print, 0031-4005; Online, 1098-4275).

Copyright © 2018 by the American Academy of Pediatrics

To cite: Fierson WM, AAP AMERICAN ACADEMY OF PEDIATRICS Section on Ophthalmology, AAP AMERICAN ACADEMY OF OPHTHALMOLOGY, AAP AMERICAN ASSOCIATION FOR PEDIATRIC OPHTHALMOLOGY AND STRABISMUS, AAP AMERICAN ASSOCIATION OF CERTIFIED ORTHOPTISTS. Screening Examination of Premature Infants for Retinopathy of Prematurity. *Pediatrics.* 2018;142(6):e20183061

INTRODUCTION

Retinopathy of prematurity (ROP) is a disorder of the developing retinal blood vessels in preterm infants who are low birth weight and is a leading cause of childhood blindness. In almost all term infants, the retina and retinal vasculature are fully developed, and, therefore, ROP cannot occur; however, in preterm infants, the development of the retina, which proceeds peripherally from the optic nerve head during the course of gestation, is incomplete, with the extent of the immaturity of the retina depending mainly on the degree of prematurity at birth, thus creating the possibility for abnormal development.

In the Multicenter Trial of Cryotherapy for Retinopathy of Prematurity, researchers demonstrated the efficacy of peripheral retinal cryotherapy (ie, cryoablation of the immature, avascular peripheral retina) in reducing unfavorable outcomes for threshold ROP, defined as morphologic changes beyond which the incidence of unfavorable outcome was >50%.[1] In the study's 15-year follow-up report,[2] authors confirmed the following lasting benefits: unfavorable structural outcomes were reduced from 48% to 27%, and unfavorable visual outcomes (ie, best corrected visual acuity worse than 20/200) were reduced from 62% to 44%. Subsequently, laser photocoagulation has been used for peripheral retinal ablation with at least equal success and is now the preferred method of ablation.[3–6] More recently, in the Early Treatment of Retinopathy of Prematurity Randomized Trial (ETROP), researchers confirmed the efficacy of treatment of high-risk prethreshold ROP (recategorized as type 1 ROP), redefined the indications for treatment, and replaced the terms "prethreshold ROP" and "threshold ROP" with "type 1 ROP" (aggressive, treatment-requiring) and "type 2 ROP" (more indolent, less aggressive), respectively.[7]

Because of the usually predictable and sequential nature of ROP progression and the proven benefits of timely treatment in reducing the risk of visual loss, efficacious care now requires that infants who are at risk receive carefully timed retinal examinations to identify treatment-requiring ROP in time for that treatment to be effective. These examinations should be performed by an ophthalmologist who is experienced in the examination of preterm infants for ROP using a binocular indirect ophthalmoscope. The examinations should be scheduled according to the preterm infant's gestational age at birth and subsequent disease presence and severity, with all pediatricians or other primary care providers who care for the at-risk preterm infant aware of this schedule. When implemented properly, telemedicine systems using wide-angle retinal images and clinical data may be used for preliminary ROP screening or as an adjunct to binocular indirect ophthalmoscopy for ROP screening.

This statement outlines the principles on which a program to detect, follow, and treat ROP in infants who are at risk might be based. The goal of an effective ROP screening program is to identify infants who could benefit from treatment and make appropriate recommendations on the timing of future screening and treatment interventions. Because undiagnosed or treatment-delayed ROP can lead to permanent blindness, it is important that all infants who are at risk be screened in a timely fashion, recognizing that not all infants require treatment. On the basis of information published thus far, the sponsoring organizations of this statement suggest the following recommendations for the United States. It is important to recognize that other locations around the world could have different screening parameters.[8,9] It is also important to note that despite appropriate timing of examinations and treatment, a small number of at-risk infants with ROP still progress to blindness.[3–6]

RECOMMENDATIONS

1. All infants with a birth weight of ≤1500 g or a gestational age of 30 weeks or less (as defined by the attending neonatologist) and selected infants with a birth weight between 1500 and 2000 g or a gestational age of >30 weeks who are believed by their attending pediatrician or neonatologist to be at risk for ROP (such as infants with hypotension requiring inotropic support, infants who received oxygen supplementation for more than a few days, or infants who received oxygen without saturation monitoring) should be screened for ROP. Retinal screening examinations should be performed after pupillary dilation by using binocular indirect ophthalmoscopy with

a lid speculum and scleral depression (as needed) to detect ROP. Dilating drops should be sufficient to allow adequate examination of the fundi, but care should be taken in using multiple drops if the pupil fails to dilate because poor pupillary dilation can occur in advanced ROP, and administering multiple doses of dilating drops can adversely affect the cardiorespiratory and gastrointestinal status of the infant. Separate sterile instruments or instruments cleaned in accord with the anti-infective protocol for metal instruments for each NICU should be used to examine each infant to avoid possible cross-contamination by infectious agents. One examination is sufficient only if it unequivocally reveals the retina to be fully vascularized in both eyes. Effort should be made to minimize the discomfort and systemic effect of this examination. In recent literature, authors suggest that a carefully organized program of remotely interpreted wide-angle fundus camera ROP screening may initially be used in place of binocular indirect ophthalmoscope examinations up to the point at which treatment of ROP is believed to be indicated; at this point, indirect ophthalmoscopy is required. This possibility is further discussed in recommendation 6.

2. Retinal examinations in preterm infants should be performed by an ophthalmologist who has sufficient knowledge and experience to accurately identify the location and sequential retinal changes of ROP. The International Classification of Retinopathy of Prematurity Revisited (ICROP)[10] should be used to classify, diagram, and record these retinal findings at the time of examination.

The initiation of acute-phase ROP screening should be based on the infant's postmenstrual age because the onset of serious ROP correlates better with postmenstrual age (gestational age at birth plus chronologic age) than with postnatal age.[11] That is, the more preterm an infant is at birth, the longer the time to develop serious ROP. This knowledge has been used previously in developing a screening schedule.[12,13] Table 1 was developed from an evidence-based analysis of the Multicenter Trial of Cryotherapy for Retinopathy of Prematurity natural history data and confirmed by the Light Reduction in ROP Study, which was conducted a decade later.[14] It represents a suggested schedule for the timing of the initial eye examinations based on postmenstrual age and chronologic (postnatal) age to detect ROP before it becomes severe enough to result in retinal detachment while minimizing the number of potentially traumatic examinations.[15] In Table 1, a rigorously tested schedule is provided for detecting treatable ROP with high confidence in infants with gestational ages of 24 to 30 weeks. However, its recommendations are extrapolated for gestational ages of 22 and 23 weeks. Although there is little evidence that initiating earlier screening is beneficial, some practitioners have advocated for earlier screening on the basis of speculation that treatable aggressive posterior retinopathy of prematurity (AP-ROP) (a severe form of ROP that is characterized by rapid progression to advanced stages in posterior ROP) could occur before 31 weeks' postmenstrual age. Because there is no significant body of evidence to support either practice, each practitioner and NICU will have to rely on clinical

TABLE 1 Timing of First Eye Examination Based on Gestational Age at Birth

Gestational Age at Birth, wk	Age at Initial Examination, wk	
	Postmenstrual	Chronologic
22[a]	31	9
23[a]	31	8
24	31	7
25	31	6
26	31	5
27	31	4
28	32	4
29	33	4
30	34	4
Older gestational age, high-risk factors[b]	—	4

Shown is a schedule for detecting prethreshold ROP with 99% confidence, usually before any required treatment. —, not applicable.

[a] This guideline should be considered tentative rather than evidence based for infants with a gestational age of 22 to 23 wk because of the small number of survivors in these postmenstrual age categories.

[b] Consider timing on the basis of the severity of comorbidities.

judgment as to the initiation of screening in preterm infants of 22 and 23 weeks' gestational age.

3. Authors of recent reports of neonatal algorithms, such as WIN-ROP,[16] Co-ROP,[17] and CHOP-ROP,[18] take factors into account other than birth weight, postmenstrual age, or gestational age. These factors include rapid postnatal weight gain and may be helpful in selecting infants at risk for ROP who should be screened and in eliminating some infants from the need for screening despite their meeting the previously mentioned screening criteria. Substitution of these algorithms for the screening measures described in this article is not justified by current literature, and it is not clear that these criteria apply to international populations.

4. Follow-up examinations should be recommended by the examining ophthalmologist on the basis of retinal findings classified according to the "International classification of retinopathy of prematurity revisited" (see Fig 1).[8] The following schedule is suggested as an acceptable one for most infants, but certain infants may require an altered frequency of examinations, remembering that the goal of examinations is to

offer treatment at the time when it is most likely to succeed.

One-Week-or-Less Follow-up

- Zone I: immature vascularization, no ROP;
- Zone I: stage 1 or stage 2 ROP;
- Immature retina extending into posterior zone II, near the boundary of zone I–zone II;
- Suspected presence of AP-ROP; and
- Stage 3 ROP, zone I requires treatment, not observation.

One- to 2-Week Follow-up

- Posterior zone II: immature vascularization;
- Zone II: stage 2 ROP; and
- Zone I: unequivocally regressing ROP.

Two-Week Follow-up

- Zone II: stage 1 ROP;
- Zone II: no ROP, immature vascularization; and
- Zone II: unequivocally regressing ROP.

Two- to 3-Week Follow-up

- Zone III: stage 1 or 2 ROP; and
- Zone III: regressing ROP.

5. The termination of acute retinal screening examinations should

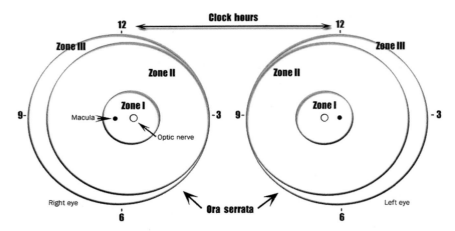

FIGURE 1
Scheme of retina of the right and left eyes showing zone borders and clock hours used to describe the location and extent of ROP. Diagrammatic representation of the potential total area of the premature retina, with zone I (the most posterior) symmetrically surrounding the optic nerve head (the earliest to develop) is shown. A larger retinal area is present temporally (laterally) rather than nasally (medially) (zone III). Only zones I and II are present nasally. The retinal changes discussed in recommendation 4 are usually recorded on a diagram such as this one.

be based on age and retinal ophthalmoscopic findings.[13] Findings in which is it suggested that examinations can be terminated include the following:

- Full retinal vascularization in close proximity to the ora serrata for 360°, that is, the normal distance found in mature retina between the end of vascularization and the ora serrata. This criterion should also be used for all cases treated for ROP solely with anti–vascular endothelial growth factor (VEGF) injectable medications.

- Zone III retinal vascularization attained without previous zone I or II ROP (if there is examiner doubt about the zone or if the postmenstrual age is less than 35 weeks, confirmatory examinations may be warranted).

- Postmenstrual age of 45 weeks and no type 1 ROP (previously called "prethreshold") disease (defined as stage 3 ROP in zone II, any ROP in zone I) or worse ROP is present.

- If anti-VEGF injectable medications were used to cause regression of the ROP, postmenstrual age of at least 65 weeks, because this treatment alters the natural history of this disease. Very late recurrences of proliferative ROP have been reported,[19–21] so caution and clinical judgment are required to determine when surveillance can be safely terminated in individual cases. Infants treated with anti-VEGF medications need particularly close follow-up during the time of highest risk for disease reactivation, between postmenstrual age 45 to 55 weeks.

- Regression of ROP[22] (care must be taken to be sure that there is no abnormal vascular tissue present that is capable of reactivation and progression in zone II or III).

6. The use of digital photographic retinal images that are captured and sent for remote interpretation is a developing alternative approach to ophthalmoscopic ROP screening[23,24]; however, few outcome comparisons between

large-scale operational digital-imaging systems with remote interpretation versus binocular indirect ophthalmoscopy have been published.[25] Nevertheless, some neonatal centers are conducting remote ROP screening for infants still in the hospital.[23,24] At a minimum, programs that use this method should comply with the timing and other recommendations outlined in the preceding guidelines as well as have capacity for timely bedside examinations if images are ambiguous or be able to promptly transfer to a hospital that can provide this examination. Protocol modifications may be required to allow for additional time for communication, processing, transportation, or other logistical issues,[26,27] with no time added to the timing noted below for treatment. Captured images and their interpretations should be incorporated into the permanent medical record. It is also recommended that indirect ophthalmoscopy be performed at least once by a qualified ophthalmologist before treatment or termination of acute-phase screening of ROP for infants at risk for ROP. A technical report in which authors have outlined the requirements for a safe program of remote photo screening for ROP has been published by the sponsoring organizations of this policy statement.[23]

Digital image capture (taking of retinal photographs) requires skill, experience, broad understanding of the infant eye, and knowledge of ROP (zone, stage, and plus). Ophthalmologists who perform remote interpretation of screening photos for ROP should have the same training requirements as bedside examiners as well as experience in the interpretation of digital images for ROP. Interpretation requires not only expert knowledge about ROP but also understanding of the limitations of interpreting static images and the special care that must be taken to schedule more frequent imaging sessions that may be required because of those limitations. Remote ophthalmologist interpreters must provide timely clinical input on the timing of follow-up imaging sessions and ophthalmoscopic examinations using appropriate methodology. These findings must be communicated in a manner that is compliant with rules of the Health Insurance Portability and Accountability Act (HIPAA) and other federal and state legal requirements.

Digital retinal imaging may also be a useful tool for objective documentation of retinal findings and for teaching NICU staff and parents about examination results, even if it is not the primary method used for ROP screening in the NICU.[28]

ROP care that includes off-site image interpretation by ophthalmologists requires close collaboration among neonatologists, imaging staff, and examining ophthalmologists. As with all ROP screening programs, specific responsibilities of each individual must be carefully delineated in a protocol written in advance so that repeat imaging and/or confirmatory examinations and required treatments can be performed without delay.

Treatment

- The presence of plus disease (defined as abnormal dilation and tortuosity of the posterior retinal blood vessels in 2 or more quadrants of the retina meeting or exceeding the degree of abnormality represented in reference photographs[1,8]; see below) in zones I or II indicates

that treatment, rather than observation, is appropriate.[7,13]

  o Treatment should be initiated for the following retinal findings that characterize Type 1 ROP:

    · Zone I ROP: any stage with plus disease;

    · Zone I ROP: stage 3, no plus disease; and

    · Zone II: stage 2 or 3 with plus disease.

- Practitioners involved in the ophthalmologic care of preterm infants should be aware that the presence of the retinal findings requiring strong consideration of ablative treatment were revised according to the Early Treatment of Retinopathy of Prematurity Randomized Trial study.[7] This recommendation is based on the findings of improved visual outcomes with earlier treatment recommended by the Final Visual Acuity Results in the Early Treatment of Retinopathy of Prematurity Study.[29] "Threshold ROP," a term that refers to specific morphologic features defined in the Multicenter Trial of Cryotherapy for Retinopathy of Prematurity, is no longer the least severe ROP for which intervention should be considered. "Threshold ROP," as defined in the Multicenter Trial of Cryotherapy for Retinopathy of Prematurity study, is now included in type 1 ROP, as are certain levels of what was previously known as prethreshold disease that also respond better to ablative treatment than to observation.[7]

  o Special care must be used in determining the zone of disease. The authors of the "International classification of retinopathy of prematurity revisited" provide specific examples on how to identify zone I and zone II disease by using binocular indirect ophthalmoscopy;

  o As noted previously, the presence of plus disease, rather than the number of clock hours of disease, is the better determining factor in recommending ablative treatment;

  o Treatment should generally be accomplished as soon as possible, at least within 72 hours of determination of the presence of treatable disease, in order to minimize the risk of retinal detachment; and

  o Follow-up is recommended in 3 to 7 days after laser photocoagulation or anti-VEGF injection to ensure that there is no need for additional laser treatment in areas where ablative treatment was not complete or additional anti-VEGF injection.

- Anti-VEGF treatment may hold great promise in the treatment of type 1 ROP. Recently published data[30] indicate that intravitreal bevacizumab monotherapy, as compared with conventional laser therapy, in infants with stage 3+ ROP is effective in and may offer significantly improved structural results compared with laser ablation for zone I but not for zone II disease. Development of peripheral retinal vessels continues after treatment with intravitreal bevacizumab, whereas conventional laser therapy led to permanent ablation of the peripheral retina, although authors of published studies indicate that this apparent destruction was associated with only a modest visual field loss. This trial[30] was too small to assess the safety and effects on future development of the brain and other tissues. Additional studies are also currently being conducted with other anti-VEGF agents, including ranibizumab (Lucentis). Consideration may be given to treatment of infants with zone I, stage 3+ ROP with intravitreal injection of bevacizumab. However, practitioners using this therapy should be aware that neither bevacizumab nor other anti-VEGF substances is currently approved by the US Food and Drug Administration for the treatment of ROP.

o If intravitreal injection of bevacizumab or other anti-VEGF agents for zone I stage 3+ ROP is contemplated, it is essential that treatment be administered only after obtaining a detailed informed consent because there remain unanswered questions involving dosage, timing, safety, and visual and systemic outcomes. Whether there are neurodevelopmental complications related to this treatment remains to be seen. To date, studies have yielded contrary findings, with 1 publication[31–33] reporting increased incidence of neurodevelopmental problems, including severe cerebral palsy, hearing loss, and bilateral blindness, in preterm infants treated with bevacizumab compared with infants whose ROP was treated with laser peripheral ablation alone, but another publication revealed no such effect.[34] In addition, reports indicate that there might be less myopic progression in infants treated with bevacizumab compared with infants treated with laser ablation, although long-term comparisons between laser and bevacizumab therapy are lacking.[35,36]

• Infants treated with bevacizumab injection should be monitored closely after injection by using techniques in accord with these ROP examination guidelines until retinal vascularization is completed or, if not completed,

until the examiner can be assured that reactivation of proliferative ROP will not occur. In the BEAT-ROP study,[30] recurrence of ROP after bevacizumab injection tended to occur considerably later than after conventional laser peripheral retinal ablative treatment (16 ± 4.6 vs 6.2 ± 5.7 weeks); therefore, longer follow-up is required for infants treated with bevacizumab to ensure that ROP requiring treatment does not recur. Long-term follow-up of the BEAT-ROP cohort revealed the time frame of highest disease reactivation was between 45 and 55 weeks' postmenstrual age, with 1 AP-ROP case reactivating at 64 weeks' postmenstrual age.[31,37] There are additional reports[25,31,35,36,38] of recurrence requiring retreatment as late as 65 to 70 weeks' postmenstrual age.

o Infants treated with intravitreal injection of bevacizumab or ranibizumab alone, therefore, require special caution in the decision to conclude regular retinal examinations. Because of the propensity for late reactivation of significant proliferative disease, one cannot rely on the findings of initial ROP regression or the achievement of 45 weeks' postmenstrual age. Full retinal vascularization is the only criterion listed above that can be relied on as a valid conclusion point. However, full retinal vascularization is not always achieved in infants treated with these agents alone. Under these circumstances, the examiner will have to rely on prolonged observation, clinical judgment, and evolving criteria in the literature for termination of examinations or a need for further treatment.[3]

• Communication with parents by members of the care team is important, as is documentation of those communications.

Parents should be aware of ROP examinations and should be informed if their child has ROP, with subsequent updates on ROP progression, and should be aware of the possibility of blindness if they do not adhere to the examination schedule after discharge. The possible consequences of serious ROP should be discussed at the time that a significant risk of poor visual outcome develops. Documentation of such conversations with parents in the nurse or physician notes is highly recommended, as is the use of standardized parental educational materials.

• Responsibility for examination and follow-up of infants at risk for ROP must be carefully defined by the staff and consultants of each NICU. Unit-specific criteria with respect to birth weight and gestational age for examination for ROP should be established for each NICU by consultation and agreement between neonatology and ophthalmology services. These criteria should be recorded and should automatically trigger ophthalmologic examinations or photographic documentation with transmission for reading if remote digital camera screening for ROP is used.

Follow-up and Transition of Care

• If hospital discharge or transfer to another neonatal unit or hospital is contemplated before retinal development into anterior zone III has taken place, or if the infant has been treated for ROP and there is either incomplete regression or incomplete retinal healing or maturation, follow-up must be arranged before the infant's departure from the hospital, including ensuring the availability of appropriate ophthalmologic follow-up; specific arrangement for that examination must be made before such discharge or transfer occurs. The transferring or discharging pediatrician, after consultation with the examining ophthalmologist, has the responsibility for communicating to the receiving physician what eye examinations are needed and their required timing. By review of the medical record and communication with the transferring and/ or discharging pediatrician, as appropriate, the receiving physician should ascertain the current ocular examination status of the infant. This period of review and communication before discharge or transfer provides the opportunity for any necessary examinations by an ophthalmologist with ongoing experience and expertise in examination of preterm infants for ROP to be arranged at the appropriate time at the receiving facility or on an outpatient basis if discharge is contemplated before the need for continued examination has ceased, as outlined in recommendation 5 and in the section above on treatment with anti-VEGF agents. For infants managed by using remote photo screening, especially those treated with anti-VEGF agents, outpatient remote photo screening is not currently available. In these cases, examination with indirect ophthalmoscopy is the only option available, and these follow-up examinations must be arranged before discharge.

- It is strongly recommended that the hospital staff arrange and schedule the first postdischarge outpatient ophthalmology appointment with a physician trained in ROP care before the infant's discharge from

the hospital. If responsibility for arranging follow-up ophthalmologic care after discharge is delegated to the parents, they must be made to understand the potential for severe visual loss, including blindness; that there is a critical examination time schedule to be met if treatment is to be successful; and that timely follow-up examination is essential to successful treatment. This information should be communicated both verbally and in writing and should be carefully documented in the infant's medical record. If such arrangements for communication and follow-up after transfer or discharge cannot be made, the infant should not be discharged until appropriate follow-up examination can be arranged by the unit staff who are discharging the infant.

- Regardless of whether infants at risk develop treatment-requiring ROP, pediatricians and other physicians who care for infants who have had ROP should be aware that these infants are at increased risk for other seemingly unrelated visual disorders, such as strabismus, amblyopia, high refractive errors, cataracts, and glaucoma. Ophthalmologic follow-up for these potential problems after discharge from the NICU is indicated within 4 to 6 months after discharge.

This statement replaces the previous statement on ROP from the American Academy of Pediatrics, American Academy of Ophthalmology, American Association for Pediatric Ophthalmology and Strabismus, and American Association of Certified Orthoptists[39]; ROP care is evolving, and recommendations may be

modified as additional data about ROP risk factors, treatments, and long-term outcomes are published.

LEAD AUTHOR

Walter M. Fierson, MD, FAAP

SUBCOMMITTEE ON RETINOPATHY OF PREMATURITY, 2015–2018

Walter M. Fierson, MD, FAAP, Chairperson
Michael F. Chiang, MD, FAAP
William Good, MD, FAAP
Dale Phelps, MD, FAAP
James Reynolds, MD, FAAP
Shira L. Robbins, MD, FAAP

SECTION ON OPHTHALMOLOGY EXECUTIVE COMMITTEE, 2017–2018

Daniel J. Karr, MD, FAAP, Chairperson
Geoffrey E. Bradford, MD, FAAP, Chairperson-Elect
Kanwal Nischal, MD, FAAP
John Roarty, MD, FAAP
Steven E. Rubin, MD, FAAP
Donny Won Suh, MD, FAAP
Sharon S. Lehman, MD, FAAP, Immediate Past Chair
George S. Ellis, Jr, MD, FAAP, Section Historian

LIAISONS

Pamela Erskine Williams, MD, FAAP – *American Academy of Ophthalmology*
Gregg T. Lueder, MD, FAAP – *American Academy of Ophthalmology Council*
Christie L. Morse, MD, FAAP – *American Association for Pediatric Ophthalmology and Strabismus*
Sarah MacKinnon, MSc, OC(C), COMT – *American Association of Certified Orthoptists*

STAFF

Jennifer G. Riefe, MEd

ABBREVIATIONS

AP-ROP: aggressive posterior retinopathy of prematurity
HIPAA: Health Insurance Portability and Accountability Act
ICROP: International Classification of Retinopathy of Prematurity Revisited
ROP: retinopathy of prematurity
VEGF: vascular endothelial growth factor

FINANCIAL DISCLOSURE: The lead author has indicated he has no financial relationships relevant to this article to disclose. Committee member Dr Chiang has disclosed the following: a research relationship with the National Institutes of Health, a research relationship with the National Science Foundation, a consulting relationship with Novartis (member of the Steering Committee for the RAINBOW study, which is an international, multicenter, Novartis-sponsored trial involving anti–vascular endothelial growth factor for retinopathy of prematurity treatment), and stock ownership relationship with Inteleretina, a company that is beginning to provide telemedicine services for diabetic retinopathy in Hawaii.

FUNDING: No external funding.

POTENTIAL CONFLICT OF INTEREST: The lead author has indicated he has no potential conflicts of interest to disclose. Committee member Dr Chiang has disclosed the following: an advisory board relationship with Clarity Medical Systems (unpaid).

REFERENCES

1. Cryotherapy for Retinopathy of Prematurity Cooperative Group. Multicenter trial of cryotherapy for retinopathy of prematurity. Preliminary results. *Arch Ophthalmol.* 1988;106(4):471–479

2. Palmer EA, Hardy RJ, Dobson V, et al; Cryotherapy for Retinopathy of Prematurity Cooperative Group. 15-year outcomes following threshold retinopathy of prematurity: final results from the multicenter trial of cryotherapy for retinopathy of prematurity. *Arch Ophthalmol.* 2005;123(3):311–318

3. McNamara JA, Tasman W, Brown GC, Federman JL. Laser photocoagulation for stage 3+ retinopathy of prematurity. *Ophthalmology.* 1991;98(5):576–580

4. Hunter DG, Repka MX. Diode laser photocoagulation for threshold retinopathy of prematurity. A randomized study. *Ophthalmology.* 1993;100(2):238–244

5. Laser ROP Study Group. Laser therapy for retinopathy of prematurity. *Arch Ophthalmol.* 1994;112(2):154–156

6. Iverson DA, Trese MT, Orgel IK, Williams GA. Laser photocoagulation for threshold retinopathy of prematurity. *Arch Ophthalmol.* 1991;109(10):1342–1343

7. Early Treatment for Retinopathy of Prematurity Cooperative Group. Revised indications for the treatment of retinopathy of prematurity: results of the early treatment for retinopathy of prematurity randomized trial. *Arch Ophthalmol.* 2003;121(12):1684–1694

8. Gilbert C, Fielder A, Gordillo L, et al; International NO-ROP Group. Characteristics of infants with severe retinopathy of prematurity in countries with low, moderate, and high levels of development: implications for screening programs. *Pediatrics.* 2005;115(5). Available at: www.pediatrics.org/cgi/content/full/115/5/e518

9. Gilbert C. Retinopathy of prematurity: a global perspective of the epidemics, population of babies at risk and implications for control. *Early Hum Dev.* 2008;84(2):77–82

10. International Committee for the Classification of Retinopathy of Prematurity. The international classification of retinopathy of prematurity revisited. *Arch Ophthalmol.* 2005;123(7):991–999

11. Palmer EA, Flynn JT, Hardy RJ, et al; The Cryotherapy for Retinopathy of Prematurity Cooperative Group. Incidence and early course of retinopathy of prematurity. *Ophthalmology.* 1991;98(11):1628–1640

12. LIGHT-ROP Cooperative Group. The design of the multicenter study of light reduction in retinopathy of prematurity (LIGHT-ROP). *J Pediatr Ophthalmol Strabismus.* 1999;36(5):257–263

13. Hutchinson AK, Saunders RA, O'Neil JW, Lovering A, Wilson ME. Timing of initial screening examinations for retinopathy of prematurity. *Arch Ophthalmol.* 1998;116(5):608–612

14. Reynolds JD, Hardy RJ, Kennedy KA, Spencer R, van Heuven WA, Fielder AR; Light Reduction in Retinopathy of Prematurity (LIGHT-ROP) Cooperative Group. Lack of efficacy of light reduction in preventing retinopathy of prematurity. *N Engl J Med.* 1998;338(22):1572–1576

15. Reynolds JD, Dobson V, Quinn GE, et al; CRYO-ROP and LIGHT-ROP Cooperative Study Groups. Evidence-based screening criteria for retinopathy of prematurity: natural history data from the CRYO-ROP and LIGHT-ROP studies. *Arch Ophthalmol.* 2002;120(11):1470–1476

16. Löfqvist C, Andersson E, Sigurdsson J, et al. Longitudinal postnatal weight and insulin-like growth factor I measurements in the prediction of retinopathy of prematurity. *Arch Ophthalmol.* 2006;124(12):1711–1718

17. Cao JH, Wagner BD, Cerda A, et al. Colorado retinopathy of prematurity model: a multi-institutional validation study. *J AAPOS.* 2016;20(3):220–225

18. Binenbaum G, Ying GS, Quinn GE, et al. The CHOP postnatal weight gain, birth weight, and gestational age retinopathy of prematurity risk model. *Arch Ophthalmol.* 2012;130(12):1560–1565

19. Snyder LL, Garcia-Gonzalez JM, Shapiro MJ, Blair MP. Very late reactivation of retinopathy of prematurity after monotherapy with intravitreal bevacizumab. *Ophthalmic Surg Lasers Imaging Retina.* 2016;47(3):280–283

20. Mehta S, Hubbard GB III. Delayed recurrent neovascularization and persistent avascular retina following intravitreal bevacizumab for retinopathy of prematurity. *Retin Cases Brief Rep.* 2013;7(3):206–209

21. Hajrasouliha AR, Garcia-Gonzales JM, Shapiro MJ, Yoon H, Blair MP. Reactivation of retinopathy of prematurity three years after treatment with bevacizumab. *Ophthalmic Surg Lasers Imaging Retina.* 2017;48(3):255–259

22. Repka MX, Palmer EA, Tung B; Cryotherapy for Retinopathy of Prematurity Cooperative Group. Involution of retinopathy of prematurity. *Arch Ophthalmol.* 2000;118(5):645–649

23. Fierson WM, Capone A Jr; American Academy of Pediatrics Section on Ophthalmology; American Academy of Ophthalmology, American Association of Certified Orthoptists. Telemedicine for evaluation of retinopathy of

prematurity. *Pediatrics*. 2015;135(1). Available at: www.pediatrics.org/cgi/content/full/135/1/e238

24. Lorenz B, Spasovska K, Elflein H, Schneider N. Wide-field digital imaging based telemedicine for screening for acute retinopathy of prematurity (ROP). Six-year results of a multicentre field study. *Graefes Arch Clin Exp Ophthalmol*. 2009;247(9):1251–1262

25. Quinn GE, Ying GS, Daniel E, et al; e-ROP Cooperative Group. Validity of a telemedicine system for the evaluation of acute-phase retinopathy of prematurity. *JAMA Ophthalmol*. 2014;132(10):1178–1184

26. Silva RA, Murakami Y, Lad EM, Moshfeghi DM. Stanford University network for diagnosis of retinopathy of prematurity (SUNDROP): 36-month experience with telemedicine screening. *Ophthalmic Surg Lasers Imaging*. 2011;42(1):12–19

27. Chiang MF, Wang L, Busuioc M, et al. Telemedical retinopathy of prematurity diagnosis: accuracy, reliability, and image quality. *Arch Ophthalmol*. 2007;125(11):1531–1538

28. Scott KE, Kim DY, Wang L, et al. Telemedical diagnosis of retinopathy of prematurity intraphysician agreement between ophthalmoscopic examination and image-based interpretation. *Ophthalmology*. 2008;115(7):1222–1228.e3

29. Good WV, Hardy RJ, Dobson V, et al; Early Treatment for Retinopathy of Prematurity Cooperative Group. Final visual acuity results in the early treatment for retinopathy of prematurity study. *Arch Ophthalmol*. 2010;128(6):663–671

30. Mintz-Hittner HA, Kennedy KA, Chuang AZ; BEAT-ROP Cooperative Group. Efficacy of intravitreal bevacizumab for stage 3+ retinopathy of prematurity. *N Engl J Med*. 2011;364(7):603–615

31. Honda S, Hirabayashi H, Tsukahara Y, Negi A. Acute contraction of the proliferative membrane after an intravitreal injection of bevacizumab for advanced retinopathy of prematurity. *Graefes Arch Clin Exp Ophthalmol*. 2008;246(7):1061–1063

32. Morin J, Luu TM, Superstein R, et al; Canadian Neonatal Network and the Canadian Neonatal Follow-Up Network Investigators. Neurodevelopmental outcomes following bevacizumab injections for retinopathy of prematurity. *Pediatrics*. 2016;137(4):e20153218

33. Quinn GE, Darlow BA. Concerns for development after bevacizumab treatment of ROP. *Pediatrics*. 2016;137(4):e20160057

34. Araz-Ersan B, Kir N, Tuncer S, et al. Preliminary anatomical and neurodevelopmental outcomes of intravitreal bevacizumab as adjunctive treatment for retinopathy of prematurity. *Curr Eye Res*. 2015;40(6):585–591

35. Geloneck MM, Chuang AZ, Clark WL, et al; BEAT-ROP Cooperative Group. Refractive outcomes following bevacizumab monotherapy compared with conventional laser treatment: a randomized clinical trial. *JAMA Ophthalmol*. 2014;132(11):1327–1333

36. Hu J, Blair MP, Shapiro MJ, Lichtenstein SJ, Galasso JM, Kapur R. Reactivation of retinopathy of prematurity after bevacizumab injection. *Arch Ophthalmol*. 2012;130(8):1000–1006

37. Mintz-Hittner HA, Geloneck MM, Chuang AZ. Clinical management of recurrent retinopathy of prematurity after intravitreal bevacizumab monotherapy. *Ophthalmology*. 2016;123(9):1845–1855

38. Zepeda-Romero LC, Liera-Garcia JA, Gutiérrez-Padilla JA, Valtierra-Santiago CI, Avila-Gómez CD. Paradoxical vascular-fibrotic reaction after intravitreal bevacizumab for retinopathy of prematurity [published correction appears in *Eye (Lond)*. 2010;24(1):202]. *Eye (Lond)*. 2010;24(5):931–933

39. Fierson WM; American Academy of Pediatrics Section on Ophthalmology; American Academy of Ophthalmology; American Association for Pediatric Ophthalmology and Strabismus; American Association of Certified Orthoptists. Screening examination of premature infants for retinopathy of prematurity. *Pediatrics*. 2013;131(1):189–195

Sport-Related Concussion in Children and Adolescents

• *Clinical Report*

CLINICAL REPORT Guidance for the Clinician in Rendering Pediatric Care

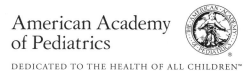

American Academy
of Pediatrics
DEDICATED TO THE HEALTH OF ALL CHILDREN™

Sport-Related Concussion in Children and Adolescents

Mark E. Halstead, MD, FAAP,[a] Kevin D. Walter, MD, FAAP,[b] Kody Moffatt, MD, FAAP,[c] COUNCIL ON SPORTS MEDICINE AND FITNESS

Sport-related concussion is an important topic in nearly all sports and at all levels of sport for children and adolescents. Concussion knowledge and approaches to management have progressed since the American Academy of Pediatrics published its first clinical report on the subject in 2010. Concussion's definition, signs, and symptoms must be understood to diagnose it and rule out more severe intracranial injury. Pediatric health care providers should have a good understanding of diagnostic evaluation and initial management strategies. Effective management can aid recovery and potentially reduce the risk of long-term symptoms and complications. Because concussion symptoms often interfere with school, social life, family relationships, and athletics, a concussion may affect the emotional well-being of the injured athlete. Because every concussion has its own unique spectrum and severity of symptoms, individualized management is appropriate. The reduction, not necessarily elimination, of physical and cognitive activity is the mainstay of treatment. A full return to activity and/ or sport is accomplished by using a stepwise program while evaluating for a return of symptoms. An understanding of prolonged symptoms and complications will help the pediatric health care provider know when to refer to a specialist. Additional research is needed in nearly all aspects of concussion in the young athlete. This report provides education on the current state of sport-related concussion knowledge, diagnosis, and management in children and adolescents.

abstract

[a]Washington University School of Medicine, St Louis, Missouri;
[b]Department of Orthopaedic Surgery, Pediatric Sports Medicine,
Medical College of Wisconsin, Milwaukee, Wisconsin; and [c]Creighton
University School of Medicine, Omaha, Nebraska

Drs Halstead, Walter, and Moffatt served as coauthors of the
manuscript and provided substantial input into its content and
revision; and all authors approved the final manuscript as submitted.

Clinical reports from the American Academy of Pediatrics benefit from
expertise and resources of liaisons and internal (AAP) and external
reviewers. However, clinical reports from the American Academy of
Pediatrics may not reflect the views of the liaisons or the organizations
or government agencies that they represent.

The guidance in this report does not indicate an exclusive course of
treatment or serve as a standard of medical care. Variations, taking
into account individual circumstances, may be appropriate.

All clinical reports from the American Academy of Pediatrics
automatically expire 5 years after publication unless reaffirmed,
revised, or retired at or before that time.

DOI: https://doi.org/10.1542/peds.2018-3074

Address correspondence to Mark E. Halstead, MD, FAAP. E-mail:
mehalstead@wustl.edu

PEDIATRICS (ISSN Numbers: Print, 0031-4005; Online, 1098-4275).

To cite: Halstead ME, Walter KD, Moffatt K. Sport-Related
Concussion in Children and Adolescents. *Pediatrics.* 2018;
142(6):e20183074

INTRODUCTION

Over the last several decades, sport-related concussions (SRCs) have been recognized as a major health concern in young athletes. Exposure to contact sports at younger ages, long-term exposure to repetitive head trauma, and consequences of the immediate effect on an athlete's daily life are continued concerns among parents, athletes, and health care providers.[1,2] Research about SRCs is being published at a robust pace with the hope of identifying the best ways to diagnose, treat, and (ideally) prevent SRCs.

Many organizations have published position statements or clinical reports on SRCs, including the American Academy of Pediatrics (AAP), National Athletic Trainers' Association, American Medical Society for Sports Medicine, American College of Sports Medicine, American Academy of Neurology, and National Academy of Medicine (formerly Institute of Medicine).[3–8] Despite these publications as well as existing legislation throughout the United States mandating education about concussions, knowledge of concussions by athletes, parents, coaches, and health care providers can be improved.[9–17] This report serves as an update the 2010 AAP clinical report for pediatric health care providers on the current state of knowledge and guidance for the diagnosis and management of pediatric and adolescent SRC.

DEFINITION

There is currently no universally accepted definition of SRC. A universally accepted definition is important when discussing the injury with patients and their parents, for health care providers in making the diagnosis correctly, and for researchers to have uniform standards when conducting studies about SRCs. Debate still exists as to whether the term concussion or mild traumatic brain injury (mTBI) should be used to describe the injury. Often, concussion is considered to be a subset of mTBI and will be considered as such for this report.

Several international symposia on concussion in sport have been held since 2001.[18,19] In the Concussion in Sport Group, a consensus of experts defined SRC as "a traumatic brain injury induced by biomechanical forces." This consensus statement also includes 5 common features of concussive head injury:

1. SRC may be caused by a direct blow to the head, face, neck, or elsewhere on the body with an impulsive force transmitted to the head.

2. SRC typically results in the rapid onset of short-lived impairment of neurologic function that resolves spontaneously. However, in some cases, signs and symptoms may evolve over a number of minutes to hours.

3. SRC may result in neuropathologic changes, but the acute clinical signs and symptoms largely reflect a functional disturbance rather than a structural injury, and as such, no abnormality is seen on standard neuroimaging studies.

4. SRC results in a range of clinical signs and symptoms that may or may not involve loss of consciousness. Resolution of the clinical and cognitive symptoms typically follows a sequential course. However, in some cases, symptoms may be prolonged.

5. The clinical signs and symptoms cannot be explained by drug, alcohol, or medication use; other injuries (such as cervical injuries, peripheral vestibular dysfunction, etc); or other comorbidities (eg, psychological factors or coexisting medical conditions).

In 2014, a systematic review was published by an expert panel attempting to develop an evidence-based definition of concussion.[20] This study found the following prevalent and consistent indicators of a concussion:

- observed and documented disorientation or confusion immediately after the event;

- impaired balance within 1 day after injury;

- slower reaction time within 2 days after injury; and/or

- impaired verbal learning and memory within 2 days after injury.

GRADING SCALES

More than 25 grading scales for SRC and mTBI have been published.[21] Because these grading scales are based on expert opinion alone, the 2001 Vienna Concussion in Sport Group recommended the discontinuation of their use in describing SRC or guiding return to play. Current recommendations are to diagnose the SRC without labels such as mild, moderate, or severe or as simple versus complex and to use current consensus protocols to guide return to play.

PATHOPHYSIOLOGY

The biokinetics that induce SRC consist of forces of acceleration, deceleration, and rotation of the head.[22–24] SRCs are usually caused by a direct blow to the head; however, SRCs may also be caused by a blow elsewhere on the body with a secondary force transmitted to the head.[18,19] Weaker neck muscles, which are more frequently seen in the pediatric population, may impair the attenuation of force to the head and increase SRC risk.[25,26]

Neurologic signs and symptoms of SRCs are not related to macroscopic neural damage; they are believed to be a functional or microstructural injury.[18,19,27] The pathophysiology of concussion, as described in animal models and some recent human studies, involves a neurometabolic cascade of events.[27–29]

After the biomechanical injury to the brain, there is potassium efflux from the neurons and a dramatic increase in extracellular glutamate.[29,30] Glutamate, an excitatory neurotransmitter, activates the N-methyl-D-aspartate receptor. This leads to neuronal depolarization with further potassium efflux and calcium and sodium influx, which depresses neuronal activity.[27,29] In an attempt to restore homeostasis, there is upregulation of the sodium-potassium ion pumps, which depletes intracellular energy reserves as a result of the increased use of adenosine triphosphate and hyperglycolysis.[27,30] Pediatric and adolescent studies have revealed reduced cerebral blood flow after SRC, which, when coupled with the increased energy demand, leads to a proposed "energy crisis."[27,30–32] In an attempt to normalize increased intracellular calcium levels, neurons sequester calcium into mitochondria, leading to mitochondrial dysfunction and impaired oxidative metabolism, worsening the energy crisis.[27] After the increase in glucose metabolism, there is an ensuing hypometabolic state that may persist for up to 4 weeks.[33,34]

Structurally, the intracellular calcium flux can damage the cytoskeleton and also cause axonal injury; however, axonal injury primarily occurs from shear and tensile forces of trauma.[27,30] This damage can reduce conductive velocity through the neuron and could be correlated with the cognitive impairments seen in SRC. Findings suggest that the young brain may be more vulnerable to axonal injury because myelination is an ongoing maturational change throughout brain development.[27,35–37] Although all the postinjury changes can lead to cell death, there appears to be little cell death after a concussion.[27–30] Currently, it is unclear how chronic structural changes and cognitive dysfunction may evolve over time.

EPIDEMIOLOGY

Historically, it is reported that up to 3.8 million recreational and SRCs occur annually at all ages in the United States.[38–42] Because of the large number of participants in youth and high school sports, concussions in the pediatric and adolescent age groups account for the majority of SRCs. A recent study that evaluated 3 national injury databases

estimated that 1.1 million to 1.9 million recreational concussions and SRCs occur annually in the United States in children 18 years of age or younger.[43] This large range highlights the challenges of understanding the true epidemiology of SRCs: variable definitions used in research, the lack of a widespread injury surveillance system, different entry points for athletes with concussion into the health care system, and underreporting of the injury.[8,44–46] Many epidemiologic studies are based on emergency department visits, but a recent study showed that 75% of 5- to 17-year-old patients with SRCs entered the health care system through their primary care provider.[47] To further complicate finding the true epidemiology, some patients may never seek medical care for their injuries. A pediatric study estimated that between 511 590 and 1 240 972 (45%–65%) patients with concussion were not seen in health care settings, and an adult-based study revealed that 42% of patients with an mTBI did not seek medical care.[43,48]

Concussion incidence and reporting have increased over the last 2 decades. Many studies report SRC rates using athletic exposures (AEs). An AE means that an athlete has participated in some or all of 1 practice or 1 game. Studies of high school athletes show an overall increase in SRCs from 0.12 in 1000 AEs in 1997–1998 to 0.51 in 1000 AEs in 2011–2012.[40,49] Studies have also demonstrated increased emergency department visits over the last decade for recreational concussions and SRCs ranging from increases of 57% to more than 200% in the 8- to 19-year-old age group.[50,51] This increasing rate is likely explained by increased overall awareness because of medical, coaching, and lay public education and increased media exposure, leading to improved reporting and diagnosis. There may also be

an increase in the true incidence with more opportunity for sport participation, leading to increased injury exposure risk, and with the increasing size, strength, and speed of young athletes over the years.[40,49,51,52]

Underreporting by athletes with SRCs remains a large concern, especially because in most cases, SRC is not a visible injury to an observer, so identification relies on self-reporting. When surveyed in 2013, 70.6% of high school athletes indicated they would report their SRC, which is an increase from 2002 data indicating that only 47.3% indicated they would report their injury.[44,45] Unfortunately, athletes still attempt to hide their injury.[16] A recent study of high school athletes found only 40% to 45% of high school athletes reported their SRC.[53] A study of youth rugby players revealed that 80% of athletes either did not report a concussion or returned to play before full recovery.[54] Other surveys indicate that 66% of high school athletes would play through their SRC, with the primary reasons being that they did not want to be removed from play and that they were fearful of approaching their coach, in addition to a lack of recognition by coaches, athletes, and parents.[55,56] There is evidence that female high school athletes are more likely than male athletes to report concussive symptoms to an authority figure despite having similar knowledge about SRC symptoms.[57]

On the basis of a compilation of several large epidemiologic studies, the high school sport with the highest risk of concussion remains American tackle football (Table 1).[49,58–60] The high-contact boys' sports of lacrosse, ice hockey, and wrestling also carry high concussion risk. In girls' sports, soccer carries the highest risk of concussion, followed by lacrosse, field hockey, and basketball.

In comparable sports played by those of both sexes, such as basketball and

TABLE 1 Concussion Rates in High School Sports

Sport	Concussions per 1000 AEs
Boys' tackle football	0.54–0.94
Girls' soccer	0.30–0.73
Boys' lacrosse	0.30–0.67
Boys' ice hockey	0.54–0.62
Boys' wrestling	0.17–0.58
Girls' lacrosse	0.20–0.55
Girls' field hockey	0.10–0.44
Girls' basketball	0.16–0.44
Boys' soccer	0.17–0.44
Girls' softball	0.10–0.36
Boys' basketball	0.07–0.25
Girls' volleyball	0.05–0.25
Cheerleading	0.06–0.22
Boys' baseball	0.04–0.14
Girls' gymnastics	0.07
Boys' and girls' track and/or field	0.02
Boys' and girls' swimming and/or diving	0.01–0.02

Data compiled from Gessel et al,[39] Lincoln et al,[40] Rosenthal et al,[49] Marar et al,[58] Meehan et al,[59] O'Connor et al,[60] Currie et al,[61] and Castile et al.[62]

soccer, girls have a higher concussion risk when compared with boys.[49,58–60] Girls' ice hockey data specific to high school are limited, but in college-aged female ice hockey players, the concussion rate is higher than in male ice hockey players and is similar to football rates.[8,63] The reason behind the sex differences in concussion rates remains unclear, although some have theorized that female athletes have weaker neck musculature or that estrogen may play a role.[25] It has also been suggested that female athletes may report symptoms more frequently than male athletes.[64]

Most studies classify youth athletes as anyone younger than 18 years, but the majority of these include only high school athletes. Recent research has shown that middle school tackle football has the highest concussion rate (2.6–2.9 in 1000 AEs), followed by girls' soccer (1.2–2.2 in 1000 AEs).[65–67] Cheerleading (0.68–1.1 in 1000 AEs) and girls' basketball (0.88 in 1000 AEs) had the next-highest rates. A study of youth tackle football players 8 to 12 years of age revealed concussion rates that were

higher (1.76 in 1000 AEs) than in high school athletes, with a nearly 2.5 times higher concussion risk in 11- to 12-year-olds when compared with 8- to 10-year-olds.[68] A study of youth ice hockey players 12 to 18 years of age revealed a similar concussion rate to that in the tackle football study (1.58 in 1000 AEs), but in contrast to the pattern seen in other contact sports, the younger athletes (12–14 years) had a 2.4 times higher concussion risk than the older athletes (15–18 years).[69] No studies of young children that reported SRC incidence by AE were identified; however, a study evaluating athletes ages 4 to 13 years seen in the emergency department revealed tackle football to be the most likely sport to cause athletes to sustain a concussion, followed by basketball, soccer, and baseball.[70] The youngest athletes in this study, 4- to 7-year-olds, were also found to be more likely to sustain SRC from player–to–other-object contact than were their older counterparts.[70]

In general, the concussion incidence is higher in competition than practice for both male and female athletes across nearly all sports.[8,58,60] For boys, the concussion rate in competition when compared with practice is more than 7 times higher in lacrosse and soccer, about 3 times higher in tackle football, and over twice as high in wrestling.[60,71] In girls, the concussion rate in competition when compared with practice is about 5 times higher in lacrosse, soccer, and basketball.[60,71] The exception to this is cheerleading, which showed a higher concussion rate in practice (0.14 in 1000 AEs) than in competition and/or performance (0.12 in 1000 AEs).[58,61]

SIGNS AND SYMPTOMS

Signs and symptoms of SRCs can be classified into 5 categories, including somatic, vestibular, oculomotor, cognitive, and emotional and sleep (Table 2). Headache (86%

TABLE 2 Signs and Symptoms of a Concussion

Category	Symptoms
Somatic	Headache
	Nausea and/or vomiting
	Neck pain
	Light sensitivity
	Noise sensitivity
Vestibular and/or oculomotor	Vision problems
	Hearing problems and/or tinnitus
	Balance problems
	Dizziness
Cognitive	Confusion
	Feeling mentally "foggy"
	Difficulty concentrating
	Difficulty remembering
	Answers questions slowly
	Repeats questions
	Loss of consciousness
Emotional	Irritable
	More emotional than usual
	Sadness
	Nervous and/or anxious
Sleep	Drowsiness and/or fatigue
	Feeling slowed down
	Trouble falling asleep
	Sleeping too much
	Sleeping too little

to 96%) is the most frequently reported SRC symptom, followed by dizziness (65% to 75%), difficulty concentrating (48% to 61%), and confusion (40% to 46%).[60,62,72] Loss of consciousness is not a requirement to diagnose concussion and is reported to occur in less than 5% of SRCs.[62,72] Recent studies have also demonstrated high rates of vestibular and oculomotor dysfunction in athletes after SRC, including accommodative disorders, convergence insufficiency, and saccadic dysfunction.[73,74]

It is important for the clinician to recognize that symptoms of a concussion are not specific to that diagnosis and may mimic preexisting problems of an athlete. Specific attention to athletes with migraine and/or headache disorders, learning disorders, attention-deficit/hyperactivity disorder (ADHD), mental health conditions (such as depression or anxiety), and sleep disorders is critical to not falsely attributing those symptoms to the concussion, although it is important to realize that an SRC may temporarily worsen the symptoms the athlete experiences with these conditions.

A postconcussion symptom checklist is useful in assessing an athlete after an SRC and often is a component of sideline assessment tools (Table 3). Several variations are available, and it is helpful to use an age-appropriate symptom questionnaire in athletes younger than 12 years (Table 4). These tools typically use a 7-point Likert scale graded from 0 (no symptoms) to 6 (severe symptoms) for athletes older than 12 years, although tools for athletes 5 to 12 years of age often use 4-point Likert scales. A graded scale permits the assessment of the severity of symptom burden and may minimize the reluctance of an athlete to admit symptoms if asked verbally about the presence or absence of specific symptoms. Parental questionnaires may also be of benefit.[19,75,76] Athletes have been found to report a greater number and severity of symptoms than their parents, with better agreement observed if they are asked within 1 week of the injury.[75]

Multiple studies have found that girls typically report a higher symptom burden than boys.[77–79] The presence of a higher overall initial symptom burden, and especially a higher burden of somatic symptoms, has been found to be the most consistent predictor of a prolonged (>28 days) recovery after a concussion.[80–83] This underscores the importance of symptom monitoring with a postconcussion symptoms checklist. The presence of ADHD, female sex, a high cognitive symptom load, loss of consciousness, dizziness, and early pubertal stage have been suggested to increase the risk for a prolonged recovery after SRC in some studies; however, other studies have revealed no increased risk.[81,82,84–87]

TABLE 3 Postconcussion Symptom Scale (Ages 13 and Older)

Symptoms	No Symptoms	Mild		Moderate		Severe	
Headache	0	1	2	3	4	5	6
"Pressure in head"	0	1	2	3	4	5	6
Neck pain	0	1	2	3	4	5	6
Nausea or vomiting	0	1	2	3	4	5	6
Dizziness	0	1	2	3	4	5	6
Blurred vision	0	1	2	3	4	5	6
Balance problems	0	1	2	3	4	5	6
Sensitivity to light	0	1	2	3	4	5	6
Sensitivity to noise	0	1	2	3	4	5	6
Feeling slowed down	0	1	2	3	4	5	6
Feeling "in a fog"	0	1	2	3	4	5	6
"Don't feel right"	0	1	2	3	4	5	6
Difficulty concentrating	0	1	2	3	4	5	6
Difficulty remembering	0	1	2	3	4	5	6
Fatigue and/or low energy	0	1	2	3	4	5	6
Confusion	0	1	2	3	4	5	6
Drowsiness	0	1	2	3	4	5	6
More emotional	0	1	2	3	4	5	6
Irritability	0	1	2	3	4	5	6
Sadness	0	1	2	3	4	5	6
Nervous or anxious	0	1	2	3	4	5	6
Trouble falling asleep	0	1	2	3	4	5	6

Use of the Postconcussion Symptom Scale: The athlete should fill out the form, on his or her own, to give a subjective value for each symptom. This form can be used with each encounter to track the athlete's progress toward the resolution of symptoms. Many athletes may have some of these reported symptoms at baseline, such as concentration difficulties in a patient with ADHD or sadness in an athlete with underlying depression, and this must be taken into consideration when interpreting the score. Athletes do not have to be at a total score of 0 to return to play if they had similar symptoms before the concussion. There are currently no guidelines that determine the severity of a concussion on the basis of these scores.

TABLE 4 Postconcussion Symptom Scale (Ages 5–12 Years)

	Not at All or Never	A Little or Rarely	Somewhat or Sometimes	A Lot or Often
I have headaches	0	1	2	3
I feel dizzy	0	1	2	3
I feel like the room is spinning	0	1	2	3
I feel like I'm going to faint	0	1	2	3
Things are blurry when I look at them	0	1	2	3
I see double	0	1	2	3
I feel sick to my stomach	0	1	2	3
My neck hurts	0	1	2	3
I get tired a lot	0	1	2	3
I get tired easily	0	1	2	3
I have trouble paying attention	0	1	2	3
I get distracted easily	0	1	2	3
I have a hard time concentrating	0	1	2	3
I have problems remembering what people tell me	0	1	2	3
I have problems following directions	0	1	2	3
I daydream too much	0	1	2	3
I get confused	0	1	2	3
I forget things	0	1	2	3
I have problems finishing things	0	1	2	3
I have trouble figuring things out	0	1	2	3
It's hard for me to learn new things	0	1	2	3

ACUTE ASSESSMENT

On the Field and/or Sideline

Ideally, initial evaluation of a conscious athlete who is suspected of having an SRC involves a neurologic examination and an assessment of current symptoms, cognition, balance, and vision. It is highly preferred that this assessment is performed by a health care provider who is knowledgeable in the assessment of SRC. It would also be ideal if this assessment is conducted by a health care provider who already knows the athlete because he or she may be better suited to identify subtle changes in his or her function or demeanor. If available, a quiet area (such as a locker room) would be a preferable place to assess the athlete instead of on a field and/or sideline or in a loud gymnasium.

If an athlete is unconscious after a head injury, initial assessment includes the "ABCs": airway, breathing, and circulation. If the athlete remains unconscious, the athlete must be assumed to have an associated cervical spine injury, and appropriate measures of stabilizing the cervical spine and transportation to an emergency facility should occur. If the athlete regains consciousness, the cervical spine can be adequately assessed, and if there is normal function and sensation in all 4 extremities, further assessment may be conducted on the sideline or, preferably, in a quiet location.

Various sideline assessment tools are readily available. The most frequently used concussion assessment tool is the Sport Concussion Assessment Tool (SCAT), which is available in both child (ages 5–12 years; Child SCAT 5) and adolescent and/or adult (13 years and older; SCAT 5) versions.[76,88] These tools are updated with each Concussion in Sport Group meeting on the basis of research published in previous versions between meetings.[19,76,88] To complete a full assessment using the entire tool requires a minimum of 10 minutes. The Acute Concussion Evaluation is an additional history-taking and assessment tool produced by the Centers for Disease Control and Prevention that may be useful to pediatricians.[89]

The SCAT 5 begins with the observable signs of SRC, which include lying motionless on the playing surface, balance and/or gait abnormalities or stumbling movements, inability to appropriately respond to questions or disorientation, blank and/or vacant look, and facial injury. Memory is assessed regarding the current event through the use of the Maddocks questions. The Child SCAT 5 no longer includes the Maddocks questions because they have not yet been determined to be valid in children younger than 13 years.[76] The SCAT 5 and Child SCAT 5 also include the Glasgow Coma Scale (GCS), a cervical spine assessment, and demographic and symptom assessments. The Child SCAT 5 also includes parental assessment of the child. The Standardized Assessment of Concussion (which assesses cognition), a brief neurologic examination, and a modified version of the Balance Error Scoring System (BESS) are also components of the SCAT 5 and Child SCAT 5.

Studies of previous versions of the SCAT revealed significant differences in performance on testing between younger and older athletes, which led to the development of the Child SCAT 3 in 2013 with revision to the SCAT 5 in 2017.[90–92] Younger athletes perform worse on components of the Standardized Assessment of Concussion, including ability to perform months of the year in reverse and digits in reverse, as well as the BESS.[91,93] Female athletes, in general, perform better than their male counterparts on most components of the SCAT.[90,93–95] Several studies have published normative data and reliability assessments for the BESS in young athletes, although the BESS has not been demonstrated to consistently reveal balance deficits greater than 3 days after SRC.[93,96–99]

The assessment of visual deficits after SRC is drawing more interest. Tools

such as the King-Devick Test and vestibular/ocular motor screening have demonstrated some usefulness in the evaluation of SRC.[100–103] At this time, there are not enough studies of adequate quality to recommend their inclusion in the SCAT.[76,88]

Sideline assessment tools can assist health care providers in the evaluation of SRC but are not intended to be used in isolation for making the diagnosis of SRC. These tools can provide additional information, along with the clinical judgement of the assessor, in making the diagnosis of SRC. However, these tools, particularly in younger athletes, have not be studied adequately to recommend widespread use. Despite the availability of limited normative data on the SCAT and Child SCAT, it is preferable to be able to compare an athlete's performance with his or her own preinjury status. It is noted that preinjury assessments are often not obtained or are not available at the time of assessment immediately after injury.

Because an athlete may not always present immediately with symptoms or deficits on his or her cognitive or balance assessments, repeat assessments are crucial for the athlete after head trauma. If an assessment for a concussion has been initiated, it is better to err on the side of caution and keep an athlete from returning to play on that day, while continuing serial assessments, unless the assessor is confident that SRC has not occurred.

When evaluating an athlete after suspected head trauma, there are several red flags that warrant urgent referral to an emergency department. These red flags include weakness or tingling in the arms or legs, severe or progressively increasing headache, loss of consciousness, deteriorating level of consciousness, repeated episodes of vomiting, a combative state, and seizures or convulsions. These findings may indicate that a more serious and potentially life-threatening head injury has occurred and may require further evaluation with neuroimaging. Tonic posturing and convulsive movements may immediately follow a concussion. Fortunately, these are often benign and self-limited and do not portend long-term deficits and generally can be addressed through routine SRC management. If seizure or seizure-like activity has occurred minutes to hours following head trauma, further evaluation in an emergency department is warranted.[104]

In-Office and/or Emergency Department Assessment

When assessing a patient in the office after an SRC, obtaining a history of the injury as well as relevant past history, including previous head injuries and any preexisting conditions (eg, ADHD, depression, anxiety, migraine headaches, and learning disabilities), is important.[89] The use of a postconcussion symptom checklist is helpful in facilitating the history taking and reminding the health care provider to ask about all relevant symptoms. A physical examination may include a neurologic examination, a head-and-neck evaluation, an ocular evaluation (such as the vestibular and/or ocular motor screening assessment), a balance assessment (which may include the BESS, Romberg test, and/or tandem gait), and an assessment of cognitive function. It is currently unclear whether the use of sideline tools, such as the SCAT, are as useful after SRC when assessed multiple days after the original injury.[19] If evaluation occurs immediately after the injury, monitoring the athlete for deterioration may be needed. It is important to also assess for findings on the history or physical examination that may be concerning for a structural injury (eg, cervical spine injury, skull fracture, or intracranial hemorrhage) that would require further evaluation with neuroimaging. Even if an

athlete becomes symptom free or is minimally symptomatic after his or her injury, return to play on the day of injury is not permissible if the diagnosis of SRC has been made. All 50 states and the District of Columbia have enacted laws requiring an individual who is suspected of sustaining a concussion to be removed from play and evaluated by a medical provider before returning to play.

NEUROIMAGING

Results of conventional neuroimaging are typically normal in SRC. Computed tomography (CT) or MRI of the brain contribute little to concussion evaluation and management except when there is suspicion of a more severe intracranial injury or structural lesion (eg, skull fracture or hemorrhage).[19,105,106] Despite a decrease in reported injury severity and conventional neuroimaging often yielding normal results, emergency department head CT use for concussions increased 36% from 2006 to 2011.[107]

Concussion may be associated with a significant cervical spine injury, skull fracture, or any of the 4 types of intracranial hemorrhage (subdural, epidural, intracerebral, or subarachnoid).[106] Signs and symptoms that increase the index of suspicion for more serious intracranial injury include severe headache, seizures, focal neurologic deficits, loss of consciousness for over 30 seconds, significant mental status impairment, repeated emesis, significant irritability, and worsening symptoms.[19,108] Normal neuroimaging in the acute phase of injury may not absolutely rule out a chronic subdural hematoma, nor does it help predict subsequent neurobehavioral dysfunction or recovery time.[109]

Recent literature has shown that the likelihood of finding clinically

significant intracranial hemorrhaging after 6 hours without deterioration in level of consciousness is extremely rare: 0.03% of patients.[110] Therefore, CT for delayed diagnosis of intracranial hemorrhage in patients without deterioration in level of consciousness after 6 hours is unlikely to be helpful, although past studies have recommended CT to be performed in the first 48 hours after injury.[105,111] CT is easier to perform and more cost-effective to obtain when compared with MRI. However, CT exposes children to the potentially harmful effects of ionizing radiation, which increases the risk for benign and malignant neoplasm.[112–115] Therefore, criteria to guide neuroimaging decisions have been developed, but none are sensitive enough to diagnose all intracranial pathology.[116–119]

In a 2009 prospective study, more than 42 000 patients were evaluated regarding who may be at high risk of structural brain injury and had a CT scan performed through the emergency department.[118] In patients older than 2 years, approximately 7% of the injuries were sport related. Patients with a GCS score less than 15, signs of basilar skull fracture, or signs of altered mental status (agitation, somnolence, repetitive questioning, slow response to verbal communication) were found to be at the highest risk for structural brain injury, and CT scanning was recommended. Patients with a GCS of 15 in the emergency department but with a history of loss of consciousness, history of vomiting, severe headache, or severe mechanism of injury (falls >3 feet, motor vehicle or bicycle crash, or head struck by high-impact object) carried a 0.9% risk of structural brain injury, and the authors recommended CT instead of observation. In this study population, 58% did not fall into those categories, and CT was not recommended because the structural brain injury risk was less than

0.05%. A 2010 Canadian study came to similar conclusions and found that acutely worsening headaches elevated the risk of structural brain injury, and CT was recommended.[119]

MRI is superior to CT in the detection of cerebral contusion, petechial hemorrhage, and white matter injury.[120] MRI is believed to be the test of choice if neuroimaging is needed outside of the emergency period. Patients who are clinically worsening or not improving over time may benefit from MRI to assess for other structural problems that may cause a similar symptom profile (eg, Chiari malformation or tumor). These findings may have implications for long-term outcomes and return-to-play decisions. However, only 0.5% of pediatric patients with persistent symptoms after SRC had findings on an MRI that were compatible with traumatic injury, whereas another 14.3% were found to have abnormal findings unrelated to trauma, with the majority of those findings being benign.[121]

Emerging neuroimaging modalities hold promise for identifying imaging biomarkers that may improve diagnosis, management, and prognosis; however, further research is needed before these modalities can be recommended for clinical care.[105,122,123] These modalities include diffusion tensor imaging with tractography, magnetic resonance spectroscopy, functional MRI, positron emission tomography, and single-photon emission CT. Research has shown postinjury changes using these modalities.[32,122–124] The identification of biomarkers through neuroimaging and the measurement of metabolic and hemodynamic changes in the brain through functional imaging will likely provide a more accurate picture of the injury and provide a biologic basis for concussion symptoms while potentially improving management strategies and recovery predictions.[8,122] Currently, these modalities are best

used for research purposes to expand knowledge about concussion and validate management strategies.

NEUROCOGNITIVE TESTING

Neurocognitive testing may be performed in the assessment of an athlete with SRC to help provide objective information about recovery from the injury. Traditional pencil-and-paper neurocognitive testing often takes several hours to administer and requires interpretation by a neuropsychologist. Several computerized neurocognitive tests (CNTs) are available that allow for rapid and uniform testing of large numbers of athletes. There have been numerous studies evaluating the reliability of various CNT platforms; however, studies conducted independently of the developers of the tests have questioned the overall reliability of testing from year to year.[125–138] The reliability of pencil-and-paper testing has also been questioned.[139]

It is important for the individual interpreting the results of baseline and postinjury CNTs to be knowledgeable about the modifiers that may affect performance on the test. Sleep has frequently been cited as a modifier for performance on baseline and postinjury CNTs.[140–143] History of concussion, regardless of sex, did not affect performance on CNTs.[144,145] Individuals with ADHD tend to have lower baseline scores on CNTs than those without and perform worse on CNTs if they do not take their medication before testing.[146,147] Athletes with musculoskeletal injuries were found to have impaired CNT results similar to those of athletes with concussion.[148] The mechanism of the hit that produces an SRC has not been shown to alter performance on CNTs.[149] Athletes found to be more severely depressed performed worse than those who were considered mildly depressed.[150]

To be efficient when baseline testing multiple teams at a school, many schools use a group setting. It has been demonstrated that performance in a group setting will result in lower baseline scores than performance in those tested individually, although 1 study revealed an elimination of these differences when standardized test instructions were used and a trained administrator was present.[151–153] A baseline CNT is ideally performed in a quiet environment, free of distractions, before the athlete's season, while the athlete is well rested, and following the recommendations of the test manufacturers. Repeating invalid baseline tests more than once has been shown not to be beneficial because the individual has a low likelihood of obtaining a valid test result.[154]

Concerns have been raised about athletes "sandbagging" their baseline CNTs, which means intentionally performing poorly to be able to have an easier goal to reach on their testing after an SRC. Although there was initial concern about this possibility, the majority of these sandbagging results can be detected.[155–157] Studies have demonstrated that 11% to 35% of athletes could successfully avoid detection when intentionally performing poorly on CNTs, but experience in test interpretation can help identify those who may be sandbagging.[155–157]

It must be acknowledged that when using a group setting for baseline testing, most schools and organizations will have great difficulty in creating the proper testing environment with administrators who have the time and are appropriately trained to review all baseline results individually. The ideal methodology for baseline and postinjury testing may be impractical for most schools and organizations. Careful consideration is necessary when schools or organizations are considering using CNTs as part of their concussion program. Providing baseline and postinjury CNT results in isolation for athletes is not considered to be an adequate concussion program for the school or organization seeking to use these tools. If a school chooses to implement CNTs as part of its concussion program, a plan should be in place to include proper administration and interpretation of the baseline and postinjury test results.

There is no agreed-on time at which to conduct CNTs after SRCs. Given that CNTs cannot be used to predict the length of recovery, it is likely prudent to perform postinjury testing on an athlete when he or she is free of concussion symptoms. Ideally, comparison is with an athlete's own baseline because several studies demonstrate improved identification of cognitive impairment when an athlete's own baseline is used for comparison rather than population-based norms.[158,159]

Ideally, neurocognitive testing is performed and interpreted by a neuropsychologist. However, given the large number of athletes participating in sports and the relative scarcity of and limited access to neuropsychologists, a widespread CNT program would not be practical or possible.[160] Ideally, if a nonneuropsychologist is using CNTs, collaboration with a neuropsychologist to aid in test administration and interpretation may be beneficial.[161]

Currently, it is not recommended that routine mandatory baseline and postinjury CNTs be conducted.[19] CNTs, when used, should be conducted by individuals with appropriate training in the administration, interpretation, and limitations of the specific test. Ideally, the tests should be interpreted against a patient's individual baseline. These tests should not be

used as the sole determining factor in return-to-play decisions. If an athlete is suffering from prolonged symptoms over several months or has had multiple concussions with cognitive or emotional concerns believed to be related to the concussion, a formal assessment by a neuropsychologist may be beneficial.

ACUTE MANAGEMENT

The management of an athlete with concussion involves the education of the athlete and his or her family about concussions and expectations for recovery, assessing for injuries or deficits that may benefit from rehabilitation, and guiding the athlete back to school and physical activity. Because each patient and concussion is unique, it is important to proceed with an individualized approach to managing the athlete.

Athletes who are suspected to have a concussion should be removed from play and not be allowed to return the same day. Athletes who continued to play immediately after a SRC were found to have worse symptoms and CNT scores than those who were removed immediately from play.[162] The athletes who continued to play were also 8.8 times more likely to have a recovery longer than 21 days.[162] Another study demonstrated that athletes who sustained an additional head impact within 24 hours of the first had a greater symptom burden and a longer recovery time (52.3 vs 36.9 days) than those who did not sustain an additional head injury.[163] These studies reinforce the importance of immediate removal from play to reduce the likelihood of a longer recovery and worse symptoms or exposure to additional head trauma.

The previous clinical report emphasized the role of physical and cognitive rest.[3] Although there is a role for reducing physical and cognitive activity after an SRC, recent research has revealed that

there may be negative consequences of extremes of rest in an athlete's recovery from SRC. Several recent studies have demonstrated that athletes who are recommended periods of strict rest, regardless of symptom severity, typically take longer to recover and often continue to report higher symptom burdens than athletes who rest for only a few days.[164–169] A study of the role of cognitive rest after an SRC demonstrated that athletes who did not reduce their cognitive load at all after injury did take the longest to improve, but even mild reductions in their cognitive load resulted in similar recovery times as in those who had extreme rest.[170]

In light of recent research, a reasonable approach to physical rest includes immediate removal from play and, while the athlete is having consistent symptoms, limiting physical exertion to brisk walking but avoiding complete inactivity. Allowing some light cardiovascular activity, such as brisk walking, although not allowing a return to full sports participation, seems prudent and is supported by recent research.[171] This exercise is intended to be subsymptom exercise, meaning the intensity of the exercise is limited to a level that does not increase or provoke symptoms. This may be self-monitored or through a formal physical therapy program. Further research is needed to determine the optimal time to initiate this type of exercise after an SRC as well as the most beneficial type and duration of exercise.

When returning an athlete to school after a concussion, it is beneficial for the student to receive academic adjustments to reduce his or her workload and environmental triggers that may exacerbate symptoms. Communication with teachers and working with school staff who will be implementing these adjustments is important for a smooth transition back into school. Prolonged school removal or absence is discouraged. A more detailed discussion of returning to learning after a concussion can be found in the AAP clinical report "Returning to Learning Following a Concussion."[172]

Because many young athletes are highly socially connected through their electronics and social media, blanket recommendations to have athletes with SRCs completely avoid the use of electronics, computers, television, video games, and texting is discouraged. To date, no research has documented any detrimental effect of electronic use in SRC recovery. Individuals with light sensitivity or oculomotor dysfunction may find their symptoms worsen while using electronics and may need to limit their overall screen time, adjust brightness levels, or increase font sizes to reduce episodes of symptom worsening. A complete elimination of electronics may result in feeling socially isolated from friends, which may lead to depressive or anxious symptoms.[8]

Several studies have demonstrated deficits in the reaction time to and judgment of road hazards in adults with concussion attempting a driving simulator in the first 24 hours after injury.[173,174] Similar deficits likely exist in adolescent athletes after an SRC, so it is worthwhile to avoid driving for the first few days after an SRC.

Reported recommendations for the use of medications after a concussion are common among primary care, emergency department, and sports medicine physicians.[175–177] Acetaminophen and nonsteroidal anti-inflammatory medications were the most commonly used.[175–177] Emergency department physicians reported high rates of use of ondansetron.[176] Primary care physicians also report a frequent recommendation of melatonin and amitriptyline.[175,177] The chronic use of acetaminophen or nonsteroidal anti-inflammatory medications

is discouraged because they may contribute to medication overuse headaches.[178] There are currently no medications that are specific to treat concussion. Despite the widespread prescription of medications by physicians caring for patients with SRCs, there is no evidence-based research to support their use in the management of SRCs.

Because many SRCs occur through a whiplash-type mechanism, cervical strains are commonly associated with a concussion. A cervical strain may also lead to cervicogenic headaches. If a cervical strain is diagnosed, physical therapy can be considered to help facilitate recovery.[179]

Athletes may also experience vestibular injuries or oculomotor dysfunction after an SRC. Rehabilitation of these injuries may also be of benefit, although it is unclear when the appropriate time is to initiate therapy for these problems because many cases are mild and may resolve spontaneously. Persistent symptoms of dizziness and balance problems may benefit from vestibular rehabilitation by appropriately trained physical therapists.[179]

It is important to counsel patients regarding their expected recovery and provide reassurance that they are expected to improve. Each concussion is unique, and there are currently no diagnostic tests, physical examination findings, or historical elements that can definitively predict how long it will take for a patient to recover. Studies on recovery time have reported that the majority of pediatric and adolescent athletes with SRCs recover between 1 and 4 weeks.[180–186] Not all athletes with SRCs will recover within that time frame, however. Athletes who sustain a second concussion within 1 year after recovery from the first concussion were not found to have a longer recovery time than that of the initial concussion.[180]

RETURN TO SPORT AND/OR PLAY

Determining when an athlete returns to play after a concussion should follow an individualized course, because each athlete recovers at a different pace. Return to sport after an SRC is best accomplished by following a graduated stepwise program updated by the Berlin Concussion in Sport Group (Table 5).[19] Return-to-sport recommendations for children have been extrapolated from adult consensus guidelines, and further research is required to refine a pediatric- and adolescent-specific program. Studies reveal a longer recovery period for adolescents and younger athletes compared with college-aged athletes; therefore, a more conservative approach to deciding when pediatric and adolescent athletes can return to full sport is warranted.[181–186]

No athlete should be allowed to return to play on the same day as the injury.[162,163] The phrase, "When in doubt, sit them out!" is paramount in the management of pediatric and adolescent concussion.[18] Despite the existence of state laws and the AAP, American Medical Society for Sports Medicine, American Academy of Neurology, and Concussion in Sport Group all having published statements recommending not returning to play on the same day of the injury, literature reveals that 10% to 38% of young athletes reported returning to play on the same day as the injury.[187,188] Additional education of all stakeholders in SRCs remains an important task.

Athletes should not be allowed to return to contact, collision, or high-risk activities until symptoms of the concussion have resolved and a return-to-sport progression has been completed. Premature return to contact increases the risk of more severe injury, repeat injury, and prolonged recovery.[189,190] Cognitive and noncontact physical exertion might increase symptoms, but it

TABLE 5 Graduated Return-to-Sport Program

Stage	Aim	Activity	Goal of Step
1	Symptom-limited activity	Daily activities that do not provoke symptoms	Gradual reintroduction of work and/or school activities
2	Light aerobic exercise	Walking or stationary cycling at slow-to-medium pace; no resistance training	Increase heart rate
3	Sport-specific exercise	Running or skating drills; no activities with risk of head impact	Add movement
4	Noncontact training drills	Harder drills (eg, passing drills and team drills); may begin progressive resistance training	Exercise, coordination, and increased thinking during sport
5	Full-contact practice	After medical clearance, participate in full, normal training activities	Restore confidence and allow coaching staff to assess functional skills
6	Return to sport	Normal game play	Full clearance/participation

Recommend 48 h of relative physical and cognitive rest before beginning the program. No more than 1 step should be completed per day. If any symptoms worsen during exercise, the athlete should return to the previous step. Consider prolonging and/or altering the return-to-sport program for any pediatric and/or adolescent patient with symptoms over 4 wk.

is unlikely to worsen the injury or outcomes, whereas prolonged inactivity is known to result in a higher symptom level and prolonged recovery.[164,168,191] Although beginning symptom-limited aerobic activity may be appropriate in some young athletes with a concussion, children and adolescents should not fully return to sports until they have also successfully returned to full academics.

The graded return-to-sports program was initially proposed by the Canadian Academy of Sport and Exercise Medicine in 2000 and endorsed by the first meeting of the Vienna Concussion in Sport Group in 2001.[18,192] Children and adolescents should not advance beyond step 2 until they return to their preinjury symptom levels and are fully participating in school. Ideally, the progression is monitored by a licensed health care professional who is knowledgeable in concussion management; however, a parent or coach may monitor the progression through the return-to-sport program if he or she is given proper instructions and can monitor for the return of symptoms. Athletic trainers are also licensed health care professionals who can supervise a return-to-sport program once they are instructed to do so. Each step should take at least 24 hours, and it may take the athlete just under a week to resume full game participation, provided that

symptoms do not return. A return of symptoms may indicate incomplete recovery from the concussion. If symptoms return while the athlete is in the program, the athlete should wait 24 hours, and if the symptoms have resolved, he or she may then attempt the previous step that was completed without symptoms and continue the progression if symptoms do not recur. Reevaluation by a health care provider is indicated for any athlete who has a continued return of symptoms with exertion. An athlete who has a history of multiple concussions or who had a prolonged recovery (over 4 weeks) may need a longer period of time to progress through each step of the program. A specialist with experience in concussion management may be needed to create an appropriate return-to-activity program.

LEGISLATION

By 2014, every state and the District of Columbia had passed youth sports concussion laws.[193] Most laws consist of the 3 key components found in Washington state's 2009 Zackery Lystedt Act[193]:

1. Organizations operating sports programs for athletes younger than 18 years, both schools and youth sports organizations, must provide educational materials and/or programs to inform coaches, athletes, and parents about the nature and risks of

concussion. These materials should be provided on an annual basis, and all stakeholders should sign the forms acknowledging their participation and understanding.

2. Any athlete suspected of sustaining a concussion should be immediately removed from play and cannot return to play on the same day.

3. Any athlete with a suspected concussion cannot return to participation until written medical clearance is received from a health care provider who is trained in the evaluation and management of concussion.

States may vary on the type of education, frequency of signed certification, return-to-play content, and type of health care provider who can provide written clearance.[194,195] Every health care provider should understand his or her state's law and how it affects the patients and practice.

Research indicates that concussion laws have had a positive impact by increasing the reporting of symptoms by athletes and decreasing instances in which coaches allow athletes who are symptomatic to return to play.[195–197] Before all states passed concussion legislation, states that had laws had a 10% higher concussion-related health care use rate compared with states that did not have laws, indicating a positive effect.[198] However, education does not seem to be spread evenly across the athletic community. A study performed 3 years after the passage of the Washington state law revealed that although nearly all high school football and soccer coaches received education through 2 or more modalities (written, in-person, video, and slide presentation), only 34.7% of the athletes and 16.2% of parents were exposed to that much education.[199] In addition, a recent study in Illinois showed that although pediatricians had good knowledge about concussion diagnosis and initial management, only 26.6% were "somewhat familiar" or "very familiar" with a recently passed state law.[12] A pediatric health care provider can have a positive impact by incorporating concussion education for both parents and athletes into the young athlete annual examination.

PROLONGED SYMPTOMS AND/OR LONG-TERM ISSUES

Although the vast majority of young athletes will have a resolution of their symptoms within 4 weeks, some will have symptoms that linger beyond that time. In athletes with persistent symptoms, it is important to evaluate for associated injuries that may benefit from rehabilitation or other treatments, including cervical strains; vestibular injuries; oculomotor disorders; sleep cycle disturbances; and developing depression, anxiety, or problems with attention.[8] Because the majority of these possible coexisting conditions can mimic symptoms of concussion, providers may attribute persistent symptoms to the concussive injury itself and miss an opportunity to potentially improve a treatable problem. Several studies have also demonstrated young athletes with prolonged symptoms have a higher likelihood of high preinjury somatization.[87,200] It is reasonable to consider referral of patients with prolonged symptoms

to a concussion specialist for further evaluation.

There is still no consensus agreement on the definition of postconcussion syndrome (PCS). The World Health Organization's definition of PCS includes the presence of 3 or more of the following symptoms after a head injury: headache; dizziness; fatigue; irritability; difficulty with concentrating and performing mental tasks; impairment of memory; insomnia; and reduced tolerance to stress, emotional excitement, or alcohol.[201] There was no minimum time frame for these symptoms provided by the World Health Organization to diagnose PCS. The *Diagnostic and Statistical Manual of Mental Disorders, Fourth Edition* included a definition of PCS, but this was removed in the fifth edition because of confusion and a lack of consensus regarding the disorder.[202]

Long-term Effects

Significant attention in the medical community and media has been given to the concern of potential long-term effects of SRC and repetitive head trauma. The most emphasis is on the condition known as chronic traumatic encephalopathy (CTE). There is currently not a way to conclusively diagnose CTE in a living individual; this is exclusively a postmortem pathologic diagnosis. In a recent convenience sample study of former football players who donated their brains for evaluation after their deaths, 3 of 14 high school (21%) and 0 of 2 pre–high school players were found to have CTE on analysis.[203] The 3 athletes who only played in high school were noted to have stage 1, the mildest form of CTE. Nearly all of the professional athletes were found to have evidence of CTE, the majority of them with evidence of severe pathology. Further research is necessary to correlate pathologic findings with clinical manifestations, including larger-scale evaluations of the brains of contact-sport athletes

with no clinical problems to reduce the bias of convenience samples. Two studies revealed no increased risk of dementia, Parkinson disease, amyotrophic lateral sclerosis, or cognitive or depressive problems in former high school football players compared with classmates who did not play football.[204,205]

Second-impact syndrome is a condition that is still contested in the medical community.[206] This injury is believed to be the result of an individual sustaining a second head injury before fully recovering from the first, which can result in cerebral vascular congestion, progressing to diffuse cerebral edema and death.[207] Particular attention to this condition in the young athlete is important because the vast majority of cases have been reported in individuals of high school age and younger.[208] Fortunately, this is believed to be a rare phenomenon but lends support to the recommendation to immediately remove an athlete from play after a suspected SRC and to not allow premature return to play, particularly while symptomatic.

Retirement

The decision to retire an athlete from a particular sport or sports after an SRC is often a difficult decision. No evidence-based criteria exist to help guide the clinician in making a decision concerning the appropriate time to retire. Several expert opinion publications have offered some considerations for retirement.[209,210] It is likely prudent to refer an athlete to a specialist with expertise in SRC if a clinician is contemplating retiring an athlete from a particular sport. There is no "magic number" of concussions that an individual has sustained that can be used to determine when an athlete should no longer be allowed to participate in a particular sport.

PREVENTION

The prevention of all concussions is highly unlikely, and expectations should be focused on efforts to reduce the risk and minimize any potential long-term outcomes. Concussion prevention efforts have historically been focused on protective equipment, educational efforts, rule changes, evaluating for increased risk, and dietary supplements.

Mouth Guards

The use of mouth guards in sports has been described since 1930.[211] The potential for mouth guards to prevent concussion was initially suggested in 1954, with data supporting this notion being published a decade later.[212,213] Since then, several larger studies with varying designs have refuted this assertion.[214–218] Evidence of an advantage in concussion prevention between athletes wearing custom-made versus noncustom-made mouth guards remains inconclusive.[215,216,219–221] However, the use of mouth guards is paramount in reducing maxillofacial and dental trauma.[214,217,222]

Helmets

Football helmets have evolved significantly over the past 50 years. Current football helmets are larger, heavier, and designed to absorb and dissipate impact forces to a greater extent than earlier models.[223] Since the 1970s, football helmets have been designed to reduce severe injuries, such as skull fractures, subdural hematomas, and brainstem contusion or hemorrhage.[224] The current goal of reducing concussions through helmet design remains elusive. Several studies have not demonstrated a difference in concussion symptom severity, time to recovery, or incidence of concussion among various brands and models of football helmets, whether new or refurbished.[220,225]

In terms of concussion prevention, football helmet improvements may be reaching a point of diminishing returns and are not likely to be the solution to the issue of concussions.[226] Properly fitted football helmets may decrease the likelihood of sustaining more significant intracranial injury and are recommended.[227,228] Helmet fit is best assessed by individuals with proper training in this area, such as athletic trainers.

There are several after-market helmet attachments, such as bumpers, pads, and sensors. No studies demonstrate that helmets or third-party attachments prevent or reduce the severity of concussions. These attachments have not been tested by the National Operating Committee on Standards for Athletic Equipment and may void the helmet certification and manufacturer's warranty. Data suggesting an impact threshold for injury are not supported, and the use of helmet impact indicators has a low positive predictive value and may generate unnecessary evaluations.[229,230] The use of these sensors does not appear to have a role in clinical decision-making but may have a role in research regarding rule changes or improved helmet design.[229–231] The use of helmet-based or other sensor systems to clinically diagnose or assess SRC cannot be supported at this time.[19]

Studies in the sports of skiing, snowboarding, lacrosse, equestrianism, rodeo, and recreational bicycling have demonstrated a protective effect of helmet use in limiting impact forces causing head injury overall but none regarding concussion specifically.[232–241] Hockey helmets have been shown to reduce the impact force from elbow collisions and low-velocity puck impacts but not from shoulder collisions, falls, or high-velocity puck impacts.[242]

Headgear

Soccer headgear has been marketed to help reduce the impact associated with heading and head hits and ultimately the risk for concussion. Headgear has not been demonstrated to have a benefit for head-to-ball impact or neurocognitive performance.[243–245] Soccer headgear may increase the risk of injury attributable to possibly increased rotational forces to the head and an increased risk for a more aggressive style of play.[246–248] Headgear has also not been found to provide significant protection from SRC in rugby.[249–251] Given the lack of evidence-based research conclusively demonstrating benefit, the use or mandating of headgear for reducing concussion risk cannot be supported at this time.

Education

Education and awareness of concussion are also important when trying to reduce SRC as well as improve diagnosis and management. Several studies have demonstrated the benefit of education efforts in improving concussion knowledge, reducing referrals for neuroimaging, and increasing the likelihood of reporting SRCs.[252–255] Although these particular education efforts may not directly reduce SRCs alone, understanding how concussions occur through education may result in rule changes as well as changes in behaviors and attitudes toward SRC.

Biomarkers

Several different biomarkers have been investigated as playing a potential role in concussion evaluation, including S100β, glial fibrillary acidic protein, neuron-specific enolase, τ, neurofilament light protein, amyloid β, brain-derived neurotrophic factor, creatine kinase and heart-type fatty acid binding protein, prolactin, cortisol, and albumin.[256] Additionally, apolipoprotein E ε4, apolipoprotein E ε4 promoter G-219T-TT genotype, and $\tau^{Ser}53^{Pro}$ polymorphism have been suggested as possible risk factors for a predisposition to concussion, potential delayed recovery, or increased risk for catastrophic injury.[257,258] These investigations are preliminary, and none of these potential biomarkers have advanced to use in the clinical setting.[259]

Supplements

Similar to biomarkers, numerous nutritional supplements have been investigated as having potential preventive and/or therapeutic roles in concussion management, including Ω-3 fatty acids, eicosapentaenoic acid, docosahexaenoic acid, curcumin, resveratrol, melatonin, creatine, *Scutellaria baicalensis*, green tea, caffeine, and vitamins C, D, and E.[260,261] There are some animal studies to support their possible benefit, but there is currently no evidence that these supplements can help in the prevention or treatment of concussions in humans.[260–263]

Neck Strengthening

A simple and somewhat promising form of prevention may come from a cervical muscle strengthening program. Poor neck strength was found to be a predictor of concussion, and for each additional pound of strength a player had, the overall risk of SRC was reduced by 5%.[25] Improved neck strength, as well as the ability to anticipate and activate the neck muscles, was found to mitigate the kinematic forces from head impact.[264]

Rule Changes

Rule changes and a proper enforcement of rules by officials may help reduce the likelihood of concussion. The AAP has addressed the benefits of reducing concussion risk by eliminating body checking in youth hockey.[265] The AAP policy statement on tackling in youth football reviewed the literature regarding rule changes in American football and provided recommendations for reducing SRC risk.[266] Increasing the age at which heading is initiated may provide some reductions in SRCs in soccer in younger age groups, although greater reductions may be achieved through limiting player-to-player contact.[267] There is likely a benefit of encouraging athletes to play by the rules and discouraging aggressive playing styles, which may be influenced by coaching.

FUTURE DIRECTIONS

Since the original clinical report in 2010, there has been an exponential increase in the amount of published research on SRCs. This research has advanced the knowledge base and understanding of the injury and has helped guide the evolution in evaluation and management of SRC. There continue to be large gaps in research, particularly in the middle school and younger-aged populations. The need exists for furthering our knowledge in the area of diagnosis, especially in terms of finding tests or imaging studies to help increase sensitivity and specificity in truly determining what is and is not an SRC. Agreement on a definition of SRC would also further the field. Refining our approaches to the management of the injury will only benefit athletes as they recover. Much work is needed to clarify the confusing information the general public receives regarding the absolute risk of CTE, what the pathologic findings mean in relation to the clinical picture, what dose response may exist, and what modifying factors may also contribute to the development of CTE. Continuing to make and enforce rule changes that reduce the risk of contact, modifying practices to eliminate unnecessary or extra contact, and determining if equipment modifications may help mitigate the SRC risk are all important SRC reduction goals.

CONCLUSIONS

Our conclusions are as follows:

1. SRCs remain common in youth and high school sports. Further research continues to be needed, especially in middle school and younger athletes.

2. Each concussion is unique and has a spectrum of severity and types of symptoms. These symptoms may overlap with other medical conditions.

3. Conventional neuroimaging is generally normal after an SRC. Following evidence-based guidelines may significantly reduce unnecessary imaging.

4. Various tools exist to evaluate the athlete after an SRC. Familiarity with these tools and their limitations can aid clinicians in appropriate evaluation after a suspected SRC.

5. The majority of pediatric athletes with SRCs will have a resolution of the symptoms within 4 weeks of the time of injury.

6. After a concussion, initial reductions in physical and cognitive activity can be beneficial to recovery, but prolonged restrictions on physical exertion or removal from school can have negative effects on recovery and symptoms.

7. The long-term effects of a single concussion or multiple concussions has still not been conclusively determined. Prolonged exposure over many years to repetitive brain trauma has been associated with pathologic changes in the brain in collegiate and professional athletes but is notably less in younger athletes. The exact correlation of clinical symptoms

with pathologic findings has not yet been established.

8. Currently, no medications have been developed to specifically prevent or treat the symptoms of SRCs. There are no quality studies at this time that demonstrate benefit in concussion recovery.

9. Retirement from sports after an SRC is an individualized decision that may benefit from consultation with a physician who has experience in recommendations for retirement after SRC.

RECOMMENDATIONS

Our recommendations are as follows:

1. Neurocognitive testing after an SRC is only 1 tool that may be used in assessing an athlete for recovery and should not be used as a sole determining factor to determine when return to play is appropriate. Testing should be performed and conducted by providers who have been trained in the proper administration and interpretation of the tests.

2. Athletes who remain unconscious after a head injury should be assumed to have a cervical spine injury. Appropriate stabilization of the cervical spine should occur, and the patient should be transported to an emergency facility for further evaluation.

3. Athletes with prolonged symptoms after an SRC should be evaluated for coexisting problems that may be contributing to the lack of symptom resolution and may benefit from referral to an appropriate health care provider who can evaluate and treat these problems.

4. All athletes with a suspected SRC should be immediately removed from play and not returned to full sports participation until they have returned to their baseline level of symptoms and functioning and completed a full stepwise return-to-sport progression without a return of concussion symptoms. If injury recovery occurs during the academic year, a return to the full academic workload is expected before a return to full sports participation.

5. Although all concussions cannot be prevented, reducing the risk through rule changes, educational programs, equipment design, and cervical strengthening programs may be of benefit. Prevention efforts should be focused on reducing the risk of long-term injury after a concussion.

6. Health care providers should have an understanding of their individual state's laws regarding return to play after a concussion.

LEAD AUTHORS

Mark E. Halstead, MD, FAAP
Kevin D. Walter, MD, FAAP
Kody Moffatt, MD, FAAP

COUNCIL ON SPORTS MEDICINE AND FITNESS EXECUTIVE COMMITTEE, 2017–2018

Cynthia R. LaBella, MD, FAAP, Chairperson

M. Alison Brooks, MD, FAAP
Greg Canty, MD, FAAP
Alex B. Diamond, DO, MPH, FAAP
William Hennrikus, MD, FAAP
Kelsey Logan, MD, MPH, FAAP
Kody Moffatt, MD, FAAP
Blaise A. Nemeth, MD, MS, FAAP
K. Brooke Pengel, MD, FAAP
Andrew R. Peterson, MD, MSPH, FAAP
Paul R. Stricker, MD, FAAP

LIAISONS

Donald W. Bagnall, LAT, ATC — *National Athletic Trainers' Association*

CONSULTANTS

Joel Brenner, MD, FAAP
Gregory Landry MD, FAAP

STAFF

Anjie Emanuel, MPH

ABBREVIATIONS

AAP: American Academy of Pediatrics
ADHD: attention-deficit/hyperactivity disorder
AE: athletic exposure
BESS: Balance Error Scoring System
CNT: computerized neurocognitive test
CT: computed tomography
CTE: chronic traumatic encephalopathy
GCS: Glasgow Coma Scale
mTBI: mild traumatic brain injury
PCS: postconcussion syndrome
SCAT: Sport Concussion Assessment Tool
SRC: sport-related concussion

FINANCIAL DISCLOSURE: The authors have indicated they have no financial relationships relevant to this article to disclose.

FUNDING: No external funding.

POTENTIAL CONFLICT OF INTEREST: The authors have indicated they have no potential conflicts of interest to disclose.

REFERENCES

1. Stein CJ, MacDougall R, Quatman-Yates CC, et al. Young athletes' concerns about sport-related concussion: the patient's perspective. *Clin J Sport Med.* 2016;26(5):386–390

2. Fishman M, Taranto E, Perlman M, Quinlan K, Benjamin HJ, Ross LF. Attitudes and counseling practices of pediatricians regarding youth sports participation and concussion risks. *J Pediatr.* 2017;184:19–25

3. Halstead ME, Walter KD; Council on Sports Medicine and Fitness. American Academy of Pediatrics. Clinical report—sport-related concussion in children and adolescents. *Pediatrics.* 2010;126(3):597–615

4. Broglio SP, Cantu RC, Gioia GA, et al; National Athletic Trainer's Association. National Athletic Trainers' Association position statement: management of sport concussion. *J Athl Train.* 2014;49(2):245–265

5. Harmon KG, Drezner JA, Gammons M, et al. American Medical Society for Sports Medicine position statement: concussion in sport. *Br J Sports Med.* 2013;47(1):15–26

6. Herring SA, Cantu RC, Guskiewicz KM, et al; American College of Sports Medicine. Concussion (mild traumatic brain injury) and the team physician: a consensus statement–2011 update. *Med Sci Sports Exerc.* 2011;43(12):2412–2422

7. Giza CC, Kutcher JS, Ashwal S, et al. Summary of evidence-based guideline update: evaluation and management of concussion in sports: report of the guideline development Subcommittee of the American Academy of Neurology. *Neurology.* 2013;80(24):2250–2257

8. Graham R, Rivara FP, Ford MA, Spicer CM, eds. *Sports-Related Concussions in Youth: Improving the Science, Changing the Culture.* Washington, DC: The National Academies Press; 2014

9. Mannings C, Kalynych C, Joseph MM, Smotherman C, Kraemer DF. Knowledge assessment of sports-related concussion among parents of children aged 5 years to 15 years enrolled in recreational tackle football. *J Trauma Acute Care Surg.* 2014;77(3, suppl 1):S18–S22

10. Mrazik M, Perra A, Brooks BL, Naidu D. Exploring minor hockey players' knowledge and attitudes toward concussion: implications for prevention. *J Head Trauma Rehabil.* 2015;30(3):219–227

11. Stoller J, Carson JD, Garel A, et al. Do family physicians, emergency department physicians, and pediatricians give consistent sport-related concussion management advice? *Can Fam Physician.* 2014;60(6):548, 550–552

12. Carl RL, Kinsella SB. Pediatricians' knowledge of current sports concussion legislation and guidelines and comfort with sports concussion management: a cross-sectional study. *Clin Pediatr (Phila).* 2014;53(7):689–697

13. Lebrun CM, Mrazik M, Prasad AS, et al. Sport concussion knowledge base, clinical practises and needs for continuing medical education: a survey of family physicians and cross-border comparison. *Br J Sports Med.* 2013;47(1):54–59

14. Lin AC, Salzman GA, Bachman SL, et al. Assessment of parental knowledge and attitudes toward pediatric sports-related concussions. *Sports Health.* 2015;7(2):124–129

15. Zemek R, Eady K, Moreau K, et al. Knowledge of paediatric concussion among front-line primary care providers. *Paediatr Child Health.* 2014;19(9):475–480

16. Register-Mihalik JK, Guskiewicz KM, McLeod TC, Linnan LA, Mueller FO, Marshall SW. Knowledge, attitude, and concussion-reporting behaviors among high school athletes: a preliminary study. *J Athl Train.* 2013;48(5):645–653

17. Zonfrillo MR, Master CL, Grady MF, Winston FK, Callahan JM, Arbogast KB. Pediatric providers' self-reported knowledge, practices, and attitudes about concussion. *Pediatrics.* 2012;130(6):1120–1125

18. Aubry M, Cantu R, Dvorak J, et al; Concussion in Sport (CIS) Group. Summary and agreement statement of the 1st international symposium on concussion in sport, Vienna 2001. *Clin J Sport Med.* 2002;12(1):6–11

19. McCrory P, Meeuwisse W, Dvořák J, et al. Consensus statement on concussion in sport-the 5th international conference on concussion in sport held in Berlin, October 2016. *Br J Sports Med.* 2017;51(11):838–847

20. Carney N, Ghajar J, Jagoda A, et al. Concussion guidelines step 1: systematic review of prevalent indicators. *Neurosurgery.* 2014;75(suppl 1):S3–S15

21. Johnston KM, McCrory P, Mohtadi NG, Meeuwisse W. Evidence-based review of sport-related concussion: clinical science. *Clin J Sport Med.* 2001;11(3):150–159

22. Barth JT, Freeman JR, Broshek DK, Varney RN. Acceleration-deceleration sport-related concussion: the gravity of it all. *J Athl Train.* 2001;36(3):253–256

23. Denny-Brown DE, Russell WR. Experimental concussion: (section of neurology). *Proc R Soc Med.* 1941;34(11):691–692

24. Ommaya AK, Gennarelli TA. Cerebral concussion and traumatic unconsciousness. Correlation of experimental and clinical observations of blunt head injuries. *Brain.* 1974;97(4):633–654

25. Collins CL, Fletcher EN, Fields SK, et al. Neck strength: a protective factor reducing risk for concussion in high school sports. *J Prim Prev.* 2014;35(5):309–319

26. Buzzini SR, Guskiewicz KM. Sport-related concussion in the young athlete. *Curr Opin Pediatr.* 2006;18(4):376–382

27. Giza CC, Hovda DA. The new neurometabolic cascade of concussion. *Neurosurgery.* 2014;75(suppl 4):S24–S33

28. Barkhoudarian G, Hovda DA, Giza CC. The molecular pathophysiology of concussive brain injury. *Clin Sports Med.* 2011;30(1):33–48, vii–iii

29. Giza CC, Hovda DA. The neurometabolic cascade of concussion. *J Athl Train.* 2001;36(3):228–235

30. Choe MC, Babikian T, DiFiori J, Hovda DA, Giza CC. A pediatric perspective on concussion pathophysiology. *Curr Opin Pediatr.* 2012;24(6):689–695

31. Katayama Y, Becker DP, Tamura T, Hovda DA. Massive increases in extracellular potassium and the indiscriminate release of glutamate following concussive brain injury. *J Neurosurg.* 1990;73(6):889–900

32. Maugans TA, Farley C, Altaye M, Leach J, Cecil KM. Pediatric sports-related concussion produces cerebral blood flow alterations. *Pediatrics.* 2012;129(1):28–37

33. Yoshino A, Hovda DA, Kawamata T, Katayama Y, Becker DP. Dynamic changes in local cerebral glucose utilization following cerebral conclusion in rats: evidence of a hyper- and subsequent hypometabolic state. *Brain Res.* 1991;561(1):106–119

34. Sunami K, Nakamura T, Ozawa Y, Kubota M, Namba H, Yamaura A. Hypermetabolic state following

experimental head injury. *Neurosurg Rev.* 1989;12(suppl 1):400–411

35. Creed JA, DiLeonardi AM, Fox DP, Tessler AR, Raghupathi R. Concussive brain trauma in the mouse results in acute cognitive deficits and sustained impairment of axonal function. *J Neurotrauma.* 2011;28(4):547–563

36. Ajao DO, Pop V, Kamper JE, et al. Traumatic brain injury in young rats leads to progressive behavioral deficits coincident with altered tissue properties in adulthood. *J Neurotrauma.* 2012;29(11):2060–2074

37. Prins ML, Hales A, Reger M, Giza CC, Hovda DA. Repeat traumatic brain injury in the juvenile rat is associated with increased axonal injury and cognitive impairments. *Dev Neurosci.* 2010;32(5–6):510–518

38. Comstock D, Logan K. *Epidemiology and Prevention in Mild Traumatic Brain Injury in Children and Adolescents: From Basic Science to Clinical Management.* New York, NY: Guilford Press; 2012

39. Gessel LM, Fields SK, Collins CL, Dick RW, Comstock RD. Concussions among United States high school and collegiate athletes. *J Athl Train.* 2007;42(4):495–503

40. Lincoln AE, Caswell SV, Almquist JL, Dunn RE, Norris JB, Hinton RY. Trends in concussion incidence in high school sports: a prospective 11-year study. *Am J Sports Med.* 2011;39(5):958–963

41. Langlois JA, Rutland-Brown W, Wald MM. The epidemiology and impact of traumatic brain injury: a brief overview. *J Head Trauma Rehabil.* 2006;21(5):375–378

42. Thurman DJ, Branche CM, Sniezek JE. The epidemiology of sports-related traumatic brain injuries in the United States: recent developments. *J Head Trauma Rehabil.* 1998;13(2):1–8

43. Bryan MA, Rowhani-Rahbar A, Comstock RD, Rivara F; Seattle Sports Concussion Research Collaborative. Sports- and recreation-related concussions in US youth. *Pediatrics.* 2016;138(1):e20154635

44. McCrea M, Hammeke T, Olsen G, Leo P, Guskiewicz K. Unreported concussion in high school football players:

implications for prevention. *Clin J Sport Med.* 2004;14(1):13–17

45. LaRoche AA, Nelson LD, Connelly PK, Walter KD, McCrea MA. Sport-related concussion reporting and state legislative effects. *Clin J Sport Med.* 2016;26(1):33–39

46. Daneshvar DH, Nowinski CJ, McKee AC, Cantu RC. The epidemiology of sport-related concussion. *Clin Sports Med.* 2011;30(1):1–17, vii

47. Arbogast KB, Curry AE, Pfeiffer MR, et al. Point of health care entry for youth with concussion within a large pediatric care network. *JAMA Pediatr.* 2016;170(7):e160294

48. Setnik L, Bazarian JJ. The characteristics of patients who do not seek medical treatment for traumatic brain injury. *Brain Inj.* 2007;21(1):1–9

49. Rosenthal JA, Foraker RE, Collins CL, Comstock RD. National high school athlete concussion rates from 2005-2006 to 2011-2012. *Am J Sports Med.* 2014;42(7):1710–1715

50. Gilchrist J, Thomas KE, Xu L, et al; Centers for Disease Control and Prevention. Nonfatal traumatic brain injuries related to sports and recreation activities among persons aged ≤19 years—United States, 2001-2009. *MMWR Morb Mortal Wkly Rep.* 2011;60(39):1337–1342

51. Bakhos LL, Lockhart GR, Myers R, Linakis JG. Emergency department visits for concussion in young child athletes. *Pediatrics.* 2010;126(3). Available at: www.pediatrics.org/cgi/content/full/126/3/e550

52. Guerriero RM, Proctor MR, Mannix R, Meehan WP III. Epidemiology, trends, assessment and management of sport-related concussion in United States high schools. *Curr Opin Pediatr.* 2012;24(6):696–701

53. Wallace J, Covassin T, Nogle S, Gould D, Kovan J. Knowledge of concussion and reporting behaviors in high school athletes with or without access to an athletic trainer. *J Athl Train.* 2017;52(3):228–235

54. Sye G, Sullivan SJ, McCrory P. High school rugby players' understanding of concussion and return to play

guidelines. *Br J Sports Med.* 2006;40(12):1003–1005

55. Chrisman SP, Quitiquit C, Rivara FP. Qualitative study of barriers to concussive symptom reporting in high school athletics. *J Adolesc Health.* 2013;52(3):330–335.e3

56. Pfister T, Pfister K, Hagel B, Ghali WA, Ronksley PE. The incidence of concussion in youth sports: a systematic review and meta-analysis. *Br J Sports Med.* 2016;50(5):292–297

57. Wallace J, Covassin T, Beidler E. Sex differences in high school athletes' knowledge of sport-related concussion symptoms and reporting behaviors. *J Athl Train.* 2017;52(7):682–688

58. Marar M, McIlvain NM, Fields SK, Comstock RD. Epidemiology of concussions among United States high school athletes in 20 sports. *Am J Sports Med.* 2012;40(4):747–755

59. Meehan WP III, d'Hemecourt P, Collins CL, Comstock RD. Assessment and management of sport-related concussions in United States high schools. *Am J Sports Med.* 2011;39(11):2304–2310

60. O'Connor KL, Baker MM, Dalton SL, Dompier TP, Broglio SP, Kerr ZY. Epidemiology of sport-related concussions in high school athletes: national athletic treatment, injury and outcomes network (NATION), 2011-2012 through 2013-2014. *J Athl Train.* 2017;52(3):175–185

61. Currie DW, Fields SK, Patterson MJ, Comstock RD. Cheerleading injuries in United States high schools. *Pediatrics.* 2016;137(1):e20152447

62. Castile L, Collins CL, McIlvain NM, Comstock RD. The epidemiology of new versus recurrent sports concussions among high school athletes, 2005-2010. *Br J Sports Med.* 2012;46(8):603–610

63. Agel J, Harvey EJ. A 7-year review of men's and women's ice hockey injuries in the NCAA. *Can J Surg.* 2010;53(5):319–323

64. Covassin T, Elbin RJ. The female athlete: the role of gender in the assessment and management of sport-related concussion. *Clin Sports Med.* 2011;30(1):125–131, x

65. Kerr ZY, Cortes N, Caswell AM, et al. Concussion rates in U.S. middle school athletes, 2015-2016 school year. *Am J Prev Med*. 2017;53(6):914–918

66. Caswell S, Prebble M, Romm K, Ambegaonkar J, Caswell A, Cortes N. Epidemiology of sports injuries among middle school students. *Br J Sports Med*. 2017;51(4):305

67. O'Kane JW, Spieker A, Levy MR, Neradilek M, Polissar NL, Schiff MA. Concussion among female middle-school soccer players. *JAMA Pediatr*. 2014;168(3):258–264

68. Kontos AP, Elbin RJ, Fazio-Sumrock VC, et al. Incidence of sports-related concussion among youth football players aged 8-12 years. *J Pediatr*. 2013;163(3):717–720

69. Kontos AP, Elbin RJ, Sufrinko A, et al. Incidence of concussion in youth ice hockey players. *Pediatrics*. 2016;137(2):e20151633

70. Buzas D, Jacobson NA, Morawa LG. Concussions from 9 youth organized sports: results from NEISS hospitals over an 11-year time frame, 2002-2012. *Orthop J Sports Med*. 2014;2(4):2325967114528460

71. Xiang J, Collins CL, Liu D, McKenzie LB, Comstock RD. Lacrosse injuries among high school boys and girls in the United States: academic years 2008-2009 through 2011-2012. *Am J Sports Med*. 2014;42(9):2082–2088

72. Meehan WP III, d'Hemecourt P, Comstock RD. High school concussions in the 2008-2009 academic year: mechanism, symptoms, and management. *Am J Sports Med*. 2010;38(12):2405–2409

73. Master CL, Scheiman M, Gallaway M, et al. Vision diagnoses are common after concussion in adolescents. *Clin Pediatr (Phila)*. 2016;55(3):260–267

74. Ellis MJ, Cordingley DM, Vis S, Reimer KM, Leiter J, Russell K. Clinical predictors of vestibulo-ocular dysfunction in pediatric sports-related concussion. *J Neurosurg Pediatr*. 2017;19(1):38–45

75. Rowhani-Rahbar A, Chrisman SP, Drescher S, Schiff MA, Rivara FP. Agreement between high school athletes and their parents on reporting athletic events and concussion symptoms. *J Neurotrauma*. 2016;33(8):784–791

76. Davis GA, Purcell L, Schneider KJ, et al. The child sport concussion assessment tool 5th edition (Child SCAT5): background and rationale. *Br J Sports Med*. 2017;51(11):859–861

77. Ono KE, Burns TG, Bearden DJ, McManus SM, King H, Reisner A. Sex-based differences as a predictor of recovery trajectories in young athletes after a sports-related concussion. *Am J Sports Med*. 2016;44(3):748–752

78. Zuckerman SL, Apple RP, Odom MJ, Lee YM, Solomon GS, Sills AK. Effect of sex on symptoms and return to baseline in sport-related concussion. *J Neurosurg Pediatr*. 2014;13(1):72–81

79. Brown DA, Elsass JA, Miller AJ, Reed LE, Reneker JC. Differences in symptom reporting between males and females at baseline and after a sports-related concussion: a systematic review and meta-analysis. *Sports Med*. 2015;45(7):1027–1040

80. Gibson S, Nigrovic LE, O'Brien M, Meehan WP III. The effect of recommending cognitive rest on recovery from sport-related concussion. *Brain Inj*. 2013;27(7–8):839–842

81. Heyer GL, Schaffer CE, Rose SC, Young JA, McNally KA, Fischer AN. Specific factors influence postconcussion symptom duration among youth referred to a sports concussion clinic. *J Pediatr*. 2016;174:33–38.e2

82. Meehan WP III, Mannix RC, Stracciolini A, Elbin RJ, Collins MW. Symptom severity predicts prolonged recovery after sport-related concussion, but age and amnesia do not. *J Pediatr*. 2013;163(3):721–725

83. Meehan WP III, Mannix R, Monuteaux MC, Stein CJ, Bachur RG. Early symptom burden predicts recovery after sport-related concussion. *Neurology*. 2014;83(24):2204–2210

84. Biederman J, Feinberg L, Chan J, et al. Mild traumatic brain injury and attention-deficit hyperactivity disorder in young student athletes. *J Nerv Ment Dis*. 2015;203(11):813–819

85. Lau BC, Kontos AP, Collins MW, Mucha A, Lovell MR. Which on-field signs/symptoms predict protracted recovery from sport-related concussion among high school football players? *Am J Sports Med*. 2011;39(11):2311–2318

86. Kriz PK, Stein C, Kent J, et al. Physical maturity and concussion symptom duration among adolescent ice hockey players. *J Pediatr*. 2016;171:234–239.e1–e2

87. Grubenhoff JA, Currie D, Comstock RD, Juarez-Colunga E, Bajaj L, Kirkwood MW. Psychological factors associated with delayed symptom resolution in children with concussion. *J Pediatr*. 2016;174:27–32.e1

88. Echemendia RJ, Meeuwisse W, McCrory P, et al. The sport concussion assessment tool 5th edition (SCAT5): background and rationale. *Br J Sports Med*. 2017;51(11):848–850

89. Giola G, Collins M; Centers for Disease Control and Prevention. Acute Concussion Evaluation (ACE): physician/clinician office evaluation. 2006. Available at: https://www.cdc.gov/headsup/pdfs/providers/ace-a.pdf. Accessed May 14, 2018

90. Glaviano NR, Benson S, Goodkin HP, Broshek DK, Saliba S. Baseline SCAT2 assessment of healthy youth student-athletes: preliminary evidence for the use of the Child-SCAT3 in children younger than 13 years. *Clin J Sport Med*. 2015;25(4):373–379

91. Jinguji TM, Bompadre V, Harmon KG, et al. Sport concussion assessment tool-2: baseline values for high school athletes. *Br J Sports Med*. 2012;46(5):365–370

92. Brooks MA, Snedden TR, Mixis B, Hetzel S, McGuine TA. Establishing baseline normative values for the child sport concussion assessment tool. *JAMA Pediatr*. 2017;171(7):670–677

93. Hansen C, Cushman D, Anderson N, et al. A normative dataset of the balance error scoring system in children aged between 5 and 14. *Clin J Sport Med*. 2016;26(6):497–501

94. Schneider KJ, Emery CA, Kang J, Schneider GM, Meeuwisse WH. Examining sport concussion assessment tool ratings for male and female youth hockey players with and without a history of concussion. *Br J Sports Med*. 2010;44(15):1112–1117

95. Snedden TR, Brooks MA, Hetzel S, McGuine T. Normative values of the sport concussion assessment tool 3 (SCAT3) in high school athletes. *Clin J Sport Med.* 2017;27(5):462–467

96. Khanna NK, Baumgartner K, LaBella CR. Balance error scoring system performance in children and adolescents with no history of concussion. *Sports Health.* 2015;7(4):341–345

97. Alsalaheen B, McClafferty A, Haines J, Smith L, Yorke A. Reference values for the balance error scoring system in adolescents. *Brain Inj.* 2016;30(7):914–918

98. Murray N, Salvatore A, Powell D, Reed-Jones R. Reliability and validity evidence of multiple balance assessments in athletes with a concussion. *J Athl Train.* 2014;49(4):540–549

99. Hansen C, Cushman D, Chen W, Bounsanga J, Hung M. Reliability testing of the balance error scoring system in children between the ages of 5 and 14. *Clin J Sport Med.* 2017;27(1):64–68

100. Tjarks BJ, Dorman JC, Valentine VD, et al. Comparison and utility of King-Devick and ImPACT® composite scores in adolescent concussion patients. *J Neurol Sci.* 2013;334(1–2):148–153

101. Mucha A, Collins MW, Elbin RJ, et al. A brief Vestibular/Ocular Motor Screening (VOMS) assessment to evaluate concussions: preliminary findings. *Am J Sports Med.* 2014;42(10):2479–2486

102. Pearce KL, Sufrinko A, Lau BC, Henry L, Collins MW, Kontos AP. Near point of convergence after a sport-related concussion: measurement reliability and relationship to neurocognitive impairment and symptoms. *Am J Sports Med.* 2015;43(12):3055–3061

103. Vernau BT, Grady MF, Goodman A, et al. Oculomotor and neurocognitive assessment of youth ice hockey players: baseline associations and observations after concussion. *Dev Neuropsychol.* 2015;40(1):7–11

104. McCrory PR, Berkovic SF. Video analysis of acute motor and convulsive manifestations in sport-related concussion. *Neurology.* 2000;54(7):1488–1491

105. Pulsipher DT, Campbell RA, Thoma R, King JH. A critical review of neuroimaging applications in sports concussion. *Curr Sports Med Rep.* 2011;10(1):14–20

106. Davis GA, Iverson GL, Guskiewicz KM, Ptito A, Johnston KM. Contributions of neuroimaging, balance testing, electrophysiology and blood markers to the assessment of sport-related concussion. *Br J Sports Med.* 2009;43(suppl 1):i36–i45

107. Zonfrillo MR, Kim KH, Arbogast KB. Emergency department visits and head computed tomography utilization for concussion patients from 2006 to 2011. *Acad Emerg Med.* 2015;22(7):872–877

108. Fung M, Willer B, Moreland D, Leddy JJ. A proposal for an evidenced-based emergency department discharge form for mild traumatic brain injury. *Brain Inj.* 2006;20(9):889–894

109. Kirkwood MW, Yeates KO, Wilson PE. Pediatric sport-related concussion: a review of the clinical management of an oft-neglected population. *Pediatrics.* 2006;117(4):1359–1371

110. Hamilton M, Mrazik M, Johnson DW. Incidence of delayed intracranial hemorrhage in children after uncomplicated minor head injuries. *Pediatrics.* 2010;126(1). Available at: www.pediatrics.org/cgi/content/full/126/1/e33

111. Johnston KM, Ptito A, Chankowsky J, Chen JK. New frontiers in diagnostic imaging in concussive head injury. *Clin J Sport Med.* 2001;11(3):166–175

112. Huang WY, Muo CH, Lin CY, et al. Paediatric head CT scan and subsequent risk of malignancy and benign brain tumour: a nation-wide population-based cohort study. *Br J Cancer.* 2014;110(9):2354–2360

113. Pearce MS, Salotti JA, Little MP, et al. Radiation exposure from CT scans in childhood and subsequent risk of leukaemia and brain tumours: a retrospective cohort study. *Lancet.* 2012;380(9840):499–505

114. Brenner DJ. Estimating cancer risks from pediatric CT: going from the qualitative to the quantitative. *Pediatr Radiol.* 2002;32(4):228–231; discussion 242–244

115. Brenner DJ, Hall EJ. Computed tomography—an increasing source of radiation exposure. *N Engl J Med.* 2007;357(22):2277–2284

116. Haydel MJ, Preston CA, Mills TJ, Luber S, Blaudeau E, DeBlieux PM. Indications for computed tomography in patients with minor head injury. *N Engl J Med.* 2000;343(2):100–105

117. Stiell IG, Lesiuk H, Wells GA, et al; Canadian CT Head and C-Spine Study Group. The Canadian CT Head Rule Study for patients with minor head injury: rationale, objectives, and methodology for phase I (derivation). *Ann Emerg Med.* 2001;38(2):160–169

118. Kuppermann N, Holmes JF, Dayan PS, et al; Pediatric Emergency Care Applied Research Network (PECARN). Identification of children at very low risk of clinically-important brain injuries after head trauma: a prospective cohort study. *Lancet.* 2009;374(9696):1160–1170

119. Osmond MH, Klassen TP, Wells GA, et al; Pediatric Emergency Research Canada (PERC) Head Injury Study Group. CATCH: a clinical decision rule for the use of computed tomography in children with minor head injury. *CMAJ.* 2010;182(4):341–348

120. Lee B, Newberg A. Neuroimaging in traumatic brain imaging. *NeuroRx.* 2005;2(2):372–383

121. Bonow RH, Friedman SD, Perez FA, et al. Prevalence of abnormal magnetic resonance imaging findings in children with persistent symptoms after pediatric sports-related concussion. *J Neurotrauma.* 2017;34(19):2706–2712

122. Toledo E, Lebel A, Becerra L, et al. The young brain and concussion: imaging as a biomarker for diagnosis and prognosis. *Neurosci Biobehav Rev.* 2012;36(6):1510–1531

123. Eierud C, Craddock RC, Fletcher S, et al. Neuroimaging after mild traumatic brain injury: review and meta-analysis. *Neuroimage Clin.* 2014;4:283–294

124. Shenton ME, Hamoda HM, Schneiderman JS, et al. A review of

magnetic resonance imaging and diffusion tensor imaging findings in mild traumatic brain injury. *Brain Imaging Behav.* 2012;6(2):137–192

125. Cernich A, Reeves D, Sun W, Bleiberg J. Automated neuropsychological assessment metrics sports medicine battery. *Arch Clin Neuropsychol.* 2007;22(suppl 1):S101–S114

126. Collie A, Maruff P, Makdissi M, McCrory P, McStephen M, Darby D. CogSport: reliability and correlation with conventional cognitive tests used in postconcussion medical evaluations. *Clin J Sport Med.* 2003;13(1):28–32

127. Erlanger D, Feldman D, Kutner K, et al. Development and validation of a web-based neuropsychological test protocol for sports-related return-to-play decision-making. *Arch Clin Neuropsychol.* 2003;18(3):293–316

128. Schatz P, Pardini JE, Lovell MR, Collins MW, Podell K. Sensitivity and specificity of the ImPACT test battery for concussion in athletes. *Arch Clin Neuropsychol.* 2006;21(1):91–99

129. Segalowitz SJ, Mahaney P, Santesso DL, MacGregor L, Dywan J, Willer B. Retest reliability in adolescents of a computerized neuropsychological battery used to assess recovery from concussion. *NeuroRehabilitation.* 2007;22(3):243–251

130. Van Kampen DA, Lovell MR, Pardini JE, Collins MW, Fu FH. The "value added" of neurocognitive testing after sports-related concussion. *Am J Sports Med.* 2006;34(10):1630–1635

131. Fazio VC, Lovell MR, Pardini JE, Collins MW. The relation between post concussion symptoms and neurocognitive performance in concussed athletes. *NeuroRehabilitation.* 2007;22(3):207–216

132. Collins MW, Field M, Lovell MR, et al. Relationship between postconcussion headache and neuropsychological test performance in high school athletes. *Am J Sports Med.* 2003;31(2):168–173

133. Erlanger D, Saliba E, Barth J, Almquist J, Webright W, Freeman J. Monitoring resolution of postconcussion symptoms in athletes: preliminary results of a web-based

neuropsychological test protocol. *J Athl Train.* 2001;36(3):280–287

134. Broglio SP, Ferrara MS, Macciocchi SN, Baumgartner TA, Elliott R. Test-retest reliability of computerized concussion assessment programs. *J Athl Train.* 2007;42(4):509–514

135. Randolph C, McCrea M, Barr WB. Is neuropsychological testing useful in the management of sport-related concussion? *J Athl Train.* 2005;40(3):139–152

136. MacDonald J, Duerson D. Reliability of a computerized neurocognitive test in baseline concussion testing of high school athletes. *Clin J Sport Med.* 2015;25(4):367–372

137. Elbin RJ, Schatz P, Covassin T. One-year test-retest reliability of the online version of ImPACT in high school athletes. *Am J Sports Med.* 2011;39(11):2319–2324

138. Brett BL, Smyk N, Solomon G, Baughman BC, Schatz P. Long-term stability and reliability of baseline cognitive assessments in high school athletes using ImPACT at 1-, 2-, and 3-year test-retest intervals [published online ahead of print August 18, 2016]. *Arch Clin Neuropsychol.* doi:10.1093/arclin/acw055

139. Barr WB. Neuropsychological testing of high school athletes. Preliminary norms and test-retest indices. *Arch Clin Neuropsychol.* 2003;18(1):91–101

140. McClure DJ, Zuckerman SL, Kutscher SJ, Gregory AJ, Solomon GS. Baseline neurocognitive testing in sports-related concussions: the importance of a prior night's sleep. *Am J Sports Med.* 2014;42(2):472–478

141. Kostyun RO, Milewski MD, Hafeez I. Sleep disturbance and neurocognitive function during the recovery from a sport-related concussion in adolescents. *Am J Sports Med.* 2015;43(3):633–640

142. Sufrinko A, Johnson EW, Henry LC. The influence of sleep duration and sleep-related symptoms on baseline neurocognitive performance among male and female high school athletes. *Neuropsychology.* 2016;30(4):484–491

143. Stocker RPJ, Khan H, Henry L, Germain A. Effects of sleep loss on

subjective complaints and objective neurocognitive performance as measured by the immediate post-concussion assessment and cognitive testing. *Arch Clin Neuropsychol.* 2017;32(3):349–368

144. Brooks BL, Mrazik M, Barlow KM, McKay CD, Meeuwisse WH, Emery CA. Absence of differences between male and female adolescents with prior sport concussion. *J Head Trauma Rehabil.* 2014;29(3):257–264

145. Mannix R, Iverson GL, Maxwell B, Atkins JE, Zafonte R, Berkner PD. Multiple prior concussions are associated with symptoms in high school athletes. *Ann Clin Transl Neurol.* 2014;1(6):433–438

146. Zuckerman SL, Lee YM, Odom MJ, Solomon GS, Sills AK. Baseline neurocognitive scores in athletes with attention deficit-spectrum disorders and/or learning disability. *J Neurosurg Pediatr.* 2013;12(2):103–109

147. Littleton AC, Schmidt JD, Register-Mihalik JK, et al. Effects of attention deficit hyperactivity disorder and stimulant medication on concussion symptom reporting and computerized neurocognitive test performance. *Arch Clin Neuropsychol.* 2015;30(7):683–693

148. Hutchison M, Comper P, Mainwaring L, Richards D. The influence of musculoskeletal injury on cognition: implications for concussion research. *Am J Sports Med.* 2011;39(11):2331–2337

149. Broglio SP, Eckner JT, Surma T, Kutcher JS. Post-concussion cognitive declines and symptomatology are not related to concussion biomechanics in high school football players. *J Neurotrauma.* 2011;28(10):2061–2068

150. Covassin T, Elbin RJ III, Larson E, Kontos AP. Sex and age differences in depression and baseline sport-related concussion neurocognitive performance and symptoms. *Clin J Sport Med.* 2012;22(2):98–104

151. Moser RS, Schatz P, Neidzwski K, Ott SD. Group versus individual administration affects baseline neurocognitive test performance. *Am J Sports Med.* 2011;39(11):2325–2330

152. Lichtenstein JD, Moser RS, Schatz P. Age and test setting affect the prevalence of invalid baseline scores

on neurocognitive tests. *Am J Sports Med.* 2014;42(2):479–484

153. Vaughan CG, Gerst EH, Sady MD, Newman JB, Gioia GA. The relation between testing environment and baseline performance in child and adolescent concussion assessment. *Am J Sports Med.* 2014;42(7):1716–1723

154. Schatz P, Kelley T, Ott SD, et al. Utility of repeated assessment after invalid baseline neurocognitive test performance. *J Athl Train.* 2014;49(5):659–664

155. Erdal K. Neuropsychological testing for sports-related concussion: how athletes can sandbag their baseline testing without detection. *Arch Clin Neuropsychol.* 2012;27(5):473–479

156. Schatz P, Glatts C. "Sandbagging" baseline test performance on ImPACT, without detection, is more difficult than it appears. *Arch Clin Neuropsychol.* 2013;28(3):236–244

157. Higgins KL, Denney RL, Maerlender A. Sandbagging on the immediate post-concussion assessment and cognitive testing (ImPACT) in a high school athlete population. *Arch Clin Neuropsychol.* 2017;32(3):259–266

158. Schmidt JD, Register-Mihalik JK, Mihalik JP, Kerr ZY, Guskiewicz KM. Identifying impairments after concussion: normative data versus individualized baselines. *Med Sci Sports Exerc.* 2012;44(9):1621–1628

159. Schatz P, Robertshaw S. Comparing post-concussive neurocognitive test data to normative data presents risks for under-classifying "above average" athletes. *Arch Clin Neuropsychol.* 2014;29(7):625–632

160. Pleacher MD, Dexter WW. Concussion management by primary care providers. *Br J Sports Med.* 2006;40(1):e2, discussion e2

161. Echemendia RJ, Herring S, Bailes J. Who should conduct and interpret the neuropsychological assessment in sports-related concussion? *Br J Sports Med.* 2009;43(suppl 1):i32–i35

162. Elbin RJ, Sufrinko A, Schatz P, et al. Removal from play after concussion and recovery time. *Pediatrics.* 2016;138(3):e202160910

163. Terwilliger VK, Pratson L, Vaughan CG, Gioia GA. Additional post-concussion impact exposure may affect recovery in adolescent athletes. *J Neurotrauma.* 2016;33(8):761–765

164. Thomas DG, Apps JN, Hoffmann RG, McCrea M, Hammeke T. Benefits of strict rest after acute concussion: a randomized controlled trial. *Pediatrics.* 2015;135(2):213–223

165. Moor HM, Eisenhauer RC, Killian KD, et al. The relationship between adherence behaviors and recovery time in adolescents after a sports-related concussion: an observational study. *Int J Sports Phys Ther.* 2015;10(2):225–233

166. Buckley TA, Munkasy BA, Clouse BP. Acute cognitive and physical rest may not improve concussion recovery time. *J Head Trauma Rehabil.* 2016;31(4):233–241

167. Sufrinko AM, Kontos AP, Apps JN, et al. The effectiveness of prescribed rest depends on initial presentation after concussion. *J Pediatr.* 2017;185:167–172

168. Grool AM, Aglipay M, Momoli F, et al; Pediatric Emergency Research Canada (PERC) Concussion Team. Association between early participation in physical activity following acute concussion and persistent postconcussive symptoms in children and adolescents. *JAMA.* 2016;316(23):2504–2514

169. Howell DR, Mannix RC, Quinn B, Taylor JA, Tan CO, Meehan WP III. Physical activity level and symptom duration are not associated after concussion. *Am J Sports Med.* 2016;44(4):1040–1046

170. Brown NJ, Mannix RC, O'Brien MJ, Gostine D, Collins MW, Meehan WP III. Effect of cognitive activity level on duration of post-concussion symptoms. *Pediatrics.* 2014;133(2). Available at: www.pediatrics.org/cgi/content/full/133/2/e299

171. Leddy J, Hinds A, Sirica D, Willer B. The role of controlled exercise in concussion management. *PM R.* 2016;8(suppl 3):S91–S100

172. Halstead ME, McAvoy K, Devore CD, Carl R, Lee M, Logan K; Council on Sports Medicine and Fitness; Council on School Health. Returning to learning following a concussion. *Pediatrics.* 2013;132(5):948–957

173. Baker A, Unsworth CA, Lannin NA. Fitness-to-drive after mild traumatic brain injury: mapping the time trajectory of recovery in the acute stages post injury. *Accid Anal Prev.* 2015;79:50–55

174. Preece MH, Horswill MS, Geffen GM. Driving after concussion: the acute effect of mild traumatic brain injury on drivers' hazard perception. *Neuropsychology.* 2010;24(4):493–503

175. Kinnaman KA, Mannix RC, Comstock RD, Meehan WP III. Management strategies and medication use for treating paediatric patients with concussions. *Acta Paediatr.* 2013;102(9):e424–e428

176. Kinnaman KA, Mannix RC, Comstock RD, Meehan WP III. Management of pediatric patients with concussion by emergency medicine physicians. *Pediatr Emerg Care.* 2014;30(7):458–461

177. Stache S, Howell D, Meehan WP III. Concussion management practice patterns among sports medicine physicians. *Clin J Sport Med.* 2016;26(5):381–385

178. Heyer GL, Idris SA. Does analgesic overuse contribute to chronic post-traumatic headaches in adolescent concussion patients? *Pediatr Neurol.* 2014;50(5):464–468

179. Schneider KJ, Meeuwisse WH, Nettel-Aguirre A, et al. Cervicovestibular rehabilitation in sport-related concussion: a randomised controlled trial. *Br J Sports Med.* 2014;48(17):1294–1298

180. Taubman B, McHugh J, Rosen F, Elci OU. Repeat concussion and recovery time in a primary care pediatric office. *J Child Neurol.* 2016;31(14):1607–1610

181. Nelson LD, Guskiewicz KM, Barr WB, et al. Age differences in recovery after sport-related concussion: a comparison of high school and collegiate athletes. *J Athl Train.* 2016;51(2):142–152

182. Williams RM, Puetz TW, Giza CC, Broglio SP. Concussion recovery time among high school and collegiate athletes: a systematic review and meta-analysis. *Sports Med.* 2015;45(6):893–903

183. Erlanger D, Kaushik T, Cantu R, et al. Symptom-based assessment of the severity of a concussion. *J Neurosurg.* 2003;98(3):477–484

184. Lee YM, Odom MJ, Zuckerman SL, Solomon GS, Sills AK. Does age affect symptom recovery after sports-related concussion? A study of high school and college athletes. *J Neurosurg Pediatr.* 2013;12(6):537–544

185. Purcell L, Harvey J, Seabrook JA. Patterns of recovery following sport-related concussion in children and adolescents. *Clin Pediatr (Phila).* 2016;55(5):452–458

186. McClincy MP, Lovell MR, Pardini J, Collins MW, Spore MK. Recovery from sports concussion in high school and collegiate athletes. *Brain Inj.* 2006;20(1):33–39

187. Sabatino M, Zynda A, Miller S. Same-day return to play after pediatric athletes sustain concussions. In: *American Academy of Pediatrics National Conference and Exhibition*; October 22–25, 2016; San Francisco, CA. Abstract

188. Kerr ZY, Zuckerman SL, Wasserman EB, Covassin T, Djoko A, Dompier TP. Concussion symptoms and return to play time in youth, high school, and college American football athletes. *JAMA Pediatr.* 2016;170(7):647–653

189. Boden BP, Tacchetti RL, Cantu RC, Knowles SB, Mueller FO. Catastrophic head injuries in high school and college football players. *Am J Sports Med.* 2007;35(7):1075–1081

190. Bey T, Ostick B. Second impact syndrome. *West J Emerg Med.* 2009;10(1):6–10

191. DiFazio M, Silverberg ND, Kirkwood MW, Bernier R, Iverson GL. Prolonged activity restriction after concussion: are we worsening outcomes? *Clin Pediatr (Phila).* 2016;55(5):443–451

192. Canadian Academy of Sport Medicine Concussion Committee. Guidelines for assessment and management of sport-related concussion. *Clin J Sport Med.* 2000;10(3):209–211

193. Green L; National Federation of State High School Associations. Legal perspectives, recommendations on state concussion laws. 2014. Available at: https://www.nfhs.org/articles/legal-perspectives-recommendations-on-state-concussion-laws/. Accessed March 28, 2017

194. Simon LM, Mitchell CN. Youth concussion laws across the nation: implications for the traveling team physician. *Curr Sports Med Rep.* 2016;15(3):161–167

195. Concannon LG. Effects of legislation on sports-related concussion. *Phys Med Rehabil Clin N Am.* 2016;27(2):513–527

196. Pfaller AY, Nelson LD, Apps JN, Walter KD, McCrea MA. Frequency and outcomes of a symptom-free waiting period after sport-related concussion. *Am J Sports Med.* 2016;44(11):2941–2946

197. Shenouda C, Hendrickson P, Davenport K, Barber J, Bell KR. The effects of concussion legislation one year later— what have we learned: a descriptive pilot survey of youth soccer player associates. *PM R.* 2012;4(6):427–435

198. Gibson TB, Herring SA, Kutcher JS, Broglio SP. Analyzing the effect of state legislation on health care utilization for children with concussion. *JAMA Pediatr.* 2015;169(2):163–168

199. Chrisman SP, Schiff MA, Chung SK, Herring SA, Rivara FP. Implementation of concussion legislation and extent of concussion education for athletes, parents, and coaches in Washington State. *Am J Sports Med.* 2014;42(5):1190–1196

200. Root JM, Zuckerbraun NS, Wang L, et al. History of somatization is associated with prolonged recovery from concussion. *J Pediatr.* 2016;174:39–44. e1

201. World Health Organization. *The ICD-10 Classification of Mental and Behavioural Disorders: Clinical Descriptions and Diagnostic Guidelines.* Geneva, Switzerland: World Health Organization; 1992

202. American Psychiatric Association. *Diagnostic and Statistical Manual of Mental Disorders.* 4th ed. Washington, DC: American Psychiatric Association; 2000

203. Mez J, Daneshvar DH, Kiernan PT, et al. Clinicopathological evaluation of chronic traumatic encephalopathy in players of American football. *JAMA.* 2017;318(4):360–370

204. Savica R, Parisi JE, Wold LE, Josephs KA, Ahlskog JE. High school football and risk of neurodegeneration: a community-based study. *Mayo Clin Proc.* 2012;87(4):335–340

205. Deshpande SK, Hasegawa RB, Rabinowitz AR, et al. Association of playing high school football with cognition and mental health later in life. *JAMA Neurol.* 2017;74(8):909–918

206. McLendon LA, Kralik SF, Grayson PA, Golomb MR. The controversial second impact syndrome: a review of the literature. *Pediatr Neurol.* 2016;62:9–17

207. Cantu RC, Voy R. Second impact syndrome. *Phys Sportsmed.* 1995;23(6):27–34

208. Mueller FO. Catastrophic head injuries in high school and collegiate sports. *J Athl Train.* 2001;36(3):312–315

209. Cantu RC, Register-Mihalik JK. Considerations for return-to-play and retirement decisions after concussion. *PM R.* 2011;3(10, suppl 2):S440–S444

210. Concannon LG, Kaufman MS, Herring SA. The million dollar question: when should an athlete retire after concussion? *Curr Sports Med Rep.* 2014;13(6):365–369

211. Mayer C. Tooth protectors for boxers. *Oral Hyg.* 1930;20:298–299

212. Watts G, Woolard A, Singer CE. Functional mouth protectors for contact sports. *J Am Dent Assoc.* 1954;49(1):7–11

213. Stenger JM, Lawson EA, Wright JM, Ricketts J. Mouthguards: protection against shock to head, neck and teeth. *J Am Dent Assoc.* 1964;69:273–281

214. Labella CR, Smith BW, Sigurdsson A. Effect of mouthguards on dental injuries and concussions in college basketball. *Med Sci Sports Exerc.* 2002;34(1):41–44

215. Wisniewski JF, Guskiewicz K, Trope M, Sigurdsson A. Incidence of cerebral concussions associated with type of mouthguard used in college football. *Dent Traumatol.* 2004;20(3):143–149

216. Finch C, Braham R, McIntosh A, McCrory P, Wolfe R. Should football players wear custom fitted mouthguards? Results from a group randomised controlled trial. *Inj Prev.* 2005;11(4):242–246

217. Mihalik JP, McCaffrey MA, Rivera EM, et al. Effectiveness of mouthguards in reducing neurocognitive deficits following sports-related cerebral concussion. *Dent Traumatol.* 2007;23(1):14–20

218. Viano DC, Withnall C, Wonnacott M. Effect of mouthguards on head responses and mandible forces in football helmet impacts. *Ann Biomed Eng.* 2012;40(1):47–69

219. Singh GD, Maher GJ, Padilla RR. Customized mandibular orthotics in the prevention of concussion/mild traumatic brain injury in football players: a preliminary study. *Dent Traumatol.* 2009;25(5):515–521

220. McGuine TA, Hetzel S, McCrea M, Brooks MA. Protective equipment and player characteristics associated with the incidence of sport-related concussion in high school football players: a multifactorial prospective study. *Am J Sports Med.* 2014;42(10):2470–2478

221. Winters J, DeMont R. Role of mouthguards in reducing mild traumatic brain injury/concussion incidence in high school football athletes. *Gen Dent.* 2014;62(3):34–38

222. Section on Oral Health. Maintaining and improving the oral health of young children. *Pediatrics.* 2014;134(6):1224–1229

223. Viano DC, Withnall C, Halstead D. Impact performance of modern football helmets. *Ann Biomed Eng.* 2012;40(1):160–174

224. Levy ML, Ozgur BM, Berry C, Aryan HE, Apuzzo ML. Birth and evolution of the football helmet. *Neurosurgery.* 2004;55(3):656–661; discussion 661–662

225. Collins CL, McKenzie LB, Ferketich AK, Andridge R, Xiang H, Comstock RD. Concussion characteristics in high school football by helmet age/recondition status, manufacturer, and model: 2008-2009 through 2012-2013 academic years in the United States. *Am J Sports Med.* 2016;44(6):1382–1390

226. Schneider DK, Grandhi RK, Bansal P, et al. Current state of concussion prevention strategies: a systematic review and meta-analysis of prospective, controlled studies. *Br J Sports Med.* 2017;51(20):1473–1482

227. McGuine T, Nass S. Football helmet fitting errors in Wisconsin high school players. In: Hoerner EF, ed. *Safety in American Football. ASTM STP 1305.* West Conshohocken, PA: American Society for Testing and Materials; 1996:83–88

228. Greenhill DA, Navo P, Zhao H, Torg J, Comstock RD, Boden BP. Inadequate helmet fit increases concussion severity in American high school football players. *Sports Health.* 2016;8(3):238–243

229. Mihalik JP, Bell DR, Marshall SW, Guskiewicz KM. Measurement of head impacts in collegiate football players: an investigation of positional and event-type differences. *Neurosurgery.* 2007;61(6):1229–1235; discussion 1235

230. Mihalik JP, Lynall RC, Wasserman EB, Guskiewicz KM, Marshall SW. Evaluating the "Threshold theory": can head impact indicators help? *Med Sci Sports Exerc.* 2017;49(2): 247–253

231. Siegmund GP, Guskiewicz KM, Marshall SW, DeMarco AL, Bonin SJ. Laboratory validation of two wearable sensor systems for measuring head impact severity in football players. *Ann Biomed Eng.* 2016;44(4):1257–1274

232. McCrory P. The role of helmets in skiing and snowboarding. *Br J Sports Med.* 2002;36(5):314

233. Sulheim S, Holme I, Ekeland A, Bahr R. Helmet use and risk of head injuries in alpine skiers and snowboarders. *JAMA.* 2006;295(8):919–924

234. Fukuda O, Hirashima Y, Origasa H, Endo S. Characteristics of helmet or knit cap use in head injury of snowboarders. *Neurol Med Chir (Tokyo).* 2007;47(11):491–494; discussion 494

235. Mueller BA, Cummings P, Rivara FP, Brooks MA, Terasaki RD. Injuries of the head, face, and neck in relation to ski helmet use. *Epidemiology.* 2008;19(2):270–276

236. Cusimano MD, Kwok J. The effectiveness of helmet wear in skiers and snowboarders: a systematic review. *Br J Sports Med.* 2010;44(11):781–786

237. Caswell SV, Deivert RG. Lacrosse helmet designs and the effects of impact forces. *J Athl Train.* 2002;37(2):164–171

238. Bond GR, Christoph RA, Rodgers BM. Pediatric equestrian injuries: assessing the impact of helmet use. *Pediatrics.* 1995;95(4):487–489

239. Brandenburg MA, Archer P. Survey analysis to assess the effectiveness of the bull tough helmet in preventing head injuries in bull riders: a pilot study. *Clin J Sport Med.* 2002;12(6):360–366

240. Downey DJ. Rodeo injuries and prevention. *Curr Sports Med Rep.* 2007;6(5):328–332

241. Wasserman RC, Buccini RV. Helmet protection from head injuries among recreational bicyclists. *Am J Sports Med.* 1990;18(1):96–97

242. Clark JM, Post A, Hoshizaki TB, Gilchrist MD. Protective capacity of ice hockey helmets against different impact events. *Ann Biomed Eng.* 2016;44(12):3693–3704

243. Withnall C, Shewchenko N, Gittens R, Dvorak J. Biomechanical investigation of head impacts in football. *Br J Sports Med.* 2005;39(suppl 1):i49–i57

244. Elbin RJ, Beatty A, Covassin T, Schatz P, Hydeman A, Kontos AP. A preliminary examination of neurocognitive performance and symptoms following a bout of soccer heading in athletes wearing protective soccer headbands. *Res Sports Med.* 2015;23(2):203–214

245. McIntosh AS, McCrory P. Impact energy attenuation performance of football headgear. *Br J Sports Med.* 2000;34(5):337–341

246. Guskiewicz KM, Marshall SW, Broglio SP, Cantu RC, Kirkendall DT. No evidence of impaired neurocognitive performance in collegiate soccer players. *Am J Sports Med.* 2002;30(2):157–162

247. Withnall C, Shewchenko N, Wonnacott M, Dvorak J. Effectiveness of headgear in football. *Br J Sports Med.* 2005;39(suppl 1):i40–i48; discussion i48

248. Tierney RT, Higgins M, Caswell SV, et al. Sex differences in head acceleration during heading while

wearing soccer headgear. *J Athl Train.* 2008;43(6):578–584

249. McIntosh AS, McCrory P. Effectiveness of headgear in a pilot study of under 15 rugby union football. *Br J Sports Med.* 2001;35(3):167–169

250. McIntosh AS, McCrory P, Finch CF, Best JP, Chalmers DJ, Wolfe R. Does padded headgear prevent head injury in rugby union football? *Med Sci Sports Exerc.* 2009;41(2):306–313

251. Marshall SW, Loomis DP, Waller AE, et al. Evaluation of protective equipment for prevention of injuries in rugby union. *Int J Epidemiol.* 2005;34(1):113–118

252. Glang AE, Koester MC, Chesnutt JC, et al. The effectiveness of a web-based resource in improving postconcussion management in high schools. *J Adolesc Health.* 2015;56(1):91–97

253. Reisner A, Burns TG, Hall LB, et al. Quality improvement in concussion care: influence of guideline-based education. *J Pediatr.* 2017;184:26–31

254. Parker EM, Gilchrist J, Schuster D, Lee R, Sarmiento K. Reach and knowledge change among coaches and other participants of the online course: "concussion in sports: what you need to know". *J Head Trauma Rehabil.* 2015;30(3):198–206

255. Bramley H, Patrick K, Lehman E, Silvis M. High school soccer players with concussion education are more likely to notify their coach of a suspected concussion. *Clin Pediatr (Phila).* 2012;51(4):332–336

256. Papa L, Ramia MM, Edwards D, Johnson BD, Slobounov SM. Systematic review of clinical studies examining biomarkers of brain injury in athletes after sports-related concussion. *J Neurotrauma.* 2015;32(10):661–673

257. Moran LM, Taylor HG, Ganesalingam K, et al. Apolipoprotein E4 as a predictor of outcomes in pediatric mild traumatic brain injury. *J Neurotrauma.* 2009;26(9):1489–1495

258. Kutner KC, Erlanger DM, Tsai J, Jordan B, Relkin NR. Lower cognitive performance of older football players possessing apolipoprotein E epsilon4. *Neurosurgery.* 2000;47(3):651–657; discussion 657–658

259. Kawata K, Liu CY, Merkel SF, Ramirez SH, Tierney RT, Langford D. Blood biomarkers for brain injury: what are we measuring? *Neurosci Biobehav Rev.* 2016;68:460–473

260. Petraglia AL, Winkler EA, Bailes JE. Stuck at the bench: potential natural neuroprotective compounds for concussion. *Surg Neurol Int.* 2011;2:146

261. Ashbaugh A, McGrew C. The role of nutritional supplements in sports concussion treatment. *Curr Sports Med Rep.* 2016;15(1):16–19

262. Trojian TH, Jackson E. Ω-3 polyunsaturated fatty acids and concussions: treatment or not? *Curr Sports Med Rep.* 2011;10(4):180–185

263. Barrett EC, McBurney MI, Ciappio ED. ω-3 fatty acid supplementation as a potential therapeutic aid for the recovery from mild traumatic brain injury/concussion. *Adv Nutr.* 2014;5(3):268–277

264. Eckner JT, Oh YK, Joshi MS, Richardson JK, Ashton-Miller JA. Effect of neck muscle strength and anticipatory cervical muscle activation on the kinematic response of the head to impulsive loads. *Am J Sports Med.* 2014;42(3):566–576

265. Brooks A, Loud KJ, Brenner JS, et al; Council on Sports Medicine and Fitness. Reducing injury risk from body checking in boys' youth ice hockey. *Pediatrics.* 2014;133(6):1151–1157

266. Council on Sports Medicine and Fitness. Tackling in youth football. *Pediatrics.* 2015;136(5). Available at: www.pediatrics.org/cgi/content/full/136/5/e1419

267. Comstock RD, Currie DW, Pierpoint LA, Grubenhoff JA, Fields SK. An evidence-based discussion of heading the ball and concussions in high school soccer. *JAMA Pediatr.* 2015;169(9):830–837

Supporting the Health Care Transition From Adolescence to Adulthood in the Medical Home

- *Clinical Report*

CLINICAL REPORT Guidance for the Clinician in Rendering Pediatric Care

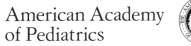

American Academy
of Pediatrics

DEDICATED TO THE HEALTH OF ALL CHILDREN™

Supporting the Health Care Transition From Adolescence to Adulthood in the Medical Home

Patience H. White, MD, MA, FAAP, FACP,[a] W. Carl Cooley, MD, FAAP,[b] TRANSITIONS CLINICAL REPORT AUTHORING GROUP, AMERICAN ACADEMY OF PEDIATRICS, AMERICAN ACADEMY OF FAMILY PHYSICIANS, AMERICAN COLLEGE OF PHYSICIANS

abstract

Risk and vulnerability encompass many dimensions of the transition from adolescence to adulthood. Transition from pediatric, parent-supervised health care to more independent, patient-centered adult health care is no exception. The tenets and algorithm of the original 2011 clinical report, "Supporting the Health Care Transition from Adolescence to Adulthood in the Medical Home," are unchanged. This updated clinical report provides more practice-based quality improvement guidance on key elements of transition planning, transfer, and integration into adult care for all youth and young adults. It also includes new and updated sections on definition and guiding principles, the status of health care transition preparation among youth, barriers, outcome evidence, recommended health care transition processes and implementation strategies using quality improvement methods, special populations, education and training in pediatric onset conditions, and payment options. The clinical report also includes new recommendations pertaining to infrastructure, education and training, payment, and research.

[a]Got Transition/The National Alliance to Advance Adolescent Health and Department of Medicine and Pediatrics, School of Medicine and Health Sciences, George Washington University, Washington, District of Columbia; and [b]Department of Pediatrics, Geisel School of Medicine, Dartmouth College, Hanover, New Hampshire

Dr White conceptualized and drafted the initial clinical report manuscript and led the reviews and revisions from the authoring group and the American Academy of Pediatrics, American Academy of Family Physicians, and American College of Physicians; Dr Cooley assisted in the drafting of the manuscript and in addressing reviews and revisions by the authoring group and the American Academy of Pediatrics, American Academy of Family Physicians, and the American College of Physicians; and all authors approved the final manuscript as submitted.

Clinical reports from the American Academy of Pediatrics benefit from expertise and resources of liaisons and internal (AAP) and external reviewers. However, clinical reports from the American Academy of Pediatrics may not reflect the views of the liaisons or the organizations or government agencies that they represent.

The guidance in this report does not indicate an exclusive course of treatment or serve as a standard of medical care. Variations, taking into account individual circumstances, may be appropriate.

Risk and vulnerability encompass many dimensions of the transition from adolescence to adulthood, and the transition from pediatric, parent-supervised health care to more independent, patient-centered adult health care is no exception. Twenty years of national child health surveys and state and community studies continue to demonstrate that most youth and young adults with special health care needs (SHCN) and families do not receive the support they need in the transition from pediatric to adult health care. In 2011, the American Academy of Pediatrics (AAP), with the endorsement of the American Academy of Family Physicians (AAFP) and the American College of Physicians (ACP), and the authoring group published a clinical report on health care transition (HCT) that included a process for transition preparation, planning, tracking, and follow-through for all youth and young adults beginning in early adolescence and continuing into young adulthood.[1]

To cite: White PH, Cooley WC, TRANSITIONS CLINICAL REPORT AUTHORING GROUP, AMERICAN ACADEMY OF PEDIATRICS, AMERICAN ACADEMY OF FAMILY PHYSICIANS, AMERICAN COLLEGE OF PHYSICIANS. Supporting the Health Care Transition From Adolescence to Adulthood in the Medical Home. *Pediatrics.* 2018;142(5):e20182587

After the release of that original clinical report, new research and several US and international professional societies' statements on the topic have been published.[2–20] This update of the AAP, AAFP, and ACP clinical report draws on this recent work and presents the latest implementation experience and refinements of the 2011 transition algorithm. It also reviews new transition research, provides more explicit attention to the role of adult medical and behavioral health clinicians in transition, and makes recommendations pertaining to transition infrastructure, training, payment, and research.

HCT has evolved from a focus on pediatric care responsibility to a shared responsibility by pediatric and adult care clinicians (eg, physicians, nurses, social workers, and others who work together to provide patient care). The crucial role of adult care clinicians in accepting and partnering with young adults has emerged as both a delivery system and a professional education and training challenge.[21–23] Young adults are increasingly recognized as a vulnerable population not only in terms of high rates of behavioral health risks but also susceptibility to emerging or worsening chronic health conditions and traditionally low use of health care.[24–26] In addition, many young adults regard health care as a low priority compared with other dimensions of their adult transition (education, employment, housing, relationships, and recreation).[27,28] Successful HCT efforts are needed to raise awareness among youth, young adults, and their families that maintaining health and continuity of care are central to attainment of broader adult goals.

DEFINITION AND GUIDING PRINCIPLES

HCT is the process of moving from a child to an adult model of health care with or without a transfer to a new clinician. Transition from pediatric to adult health care is part of a larger theoretical framework for transition affecting all youth, young adults, and families, as outlined by Meleis,[29] Geary and Schumacher,[30] and Schwartz et al.[31] Transition theory informs the following overarching principles for this HCT clinical report:

1. Importance of youth- and/or young adult–centered, strength-based focus;

2. Emphasis on self-determination, self-management, and family and/or caregiver engagement;

3. Acknowledgment of individual differences and complexities;

4. Recognition of vulnerabilities and need for a distinct population health approach for youth and young adults;

5. Need for early and ongoing preparation, including the integration into an adult model of care;

6. Importance of shared accountability, effective communication, and care coordination between pediatric and adult clinicians and systems of care;

7. Recognition of the influences of cultural beliefs and attitudes as well as socioeconomic status;

8. Emphasis on achieving health equity and elimination of disparities; and

9. Need for parents and caregivers to support youth and young adults in building knowledge regarding their own health and skills in making health decisions and using health care.

The Transitions Clinical Report Authoring Group, cochaired by Drs Patience White and Carl Cooley, included representatives from the AAP, AAFP, and ACP, the medicine and pediatrics (med-peds) and family medicine community, the nursing profession, and family and young adult transition experts. A draft of this clinical report underwent extensive peer review by committees, councils, sections, and others within the AAP and by the AAFP and ACP.

STATUS OF TRANSITION PREPARATION AND OUTCOME AMONG US YOUTH

The vast majority of US youth are not receiving transition preparation, according to the 2016 National Survey of Children's Health, a nationally representative survey of parents.[32] New estimates of transition preparation for youth (ages 12 through 17) with and, for the first time, without SHCN reveal that 83% of youth with SHCN and 86% of youth without special needs do not meet the national HCT performance measure. This composite measure examines the extent to which (1) youth had time alone to speak with the doctor or other health care clinician during his or her last preventive visit; (2) the doctor or other health care clinician worked with youth to gain self-care skills or understand the changes in health care that happen at 18 years of age; and (3) the doctor or other health care clinician talked with youth about eventually seeing doctors who treat adults. These estimates are lower than past national studies of youth with SHCN[33–37] because the previous National Survey of Children with Special Needs (in 2009–2010) assessed whether parents perceived a need for discussion of specific transition topics, and many did not. Consequently, those parents were not counted in the overall estimate. Lack of preparation has also been reported in hospitalized adolescents[38] and among children's hospitals.[39]

Published studies continue to reveal the adverse effects associated with lack of structured HCT interventions in terms of medical complications,[40–43] limitations in health and well-being,[44,45] problems with treatment

TABLE 1 Youth, Young Adult, and Family Transition[27,28,37,59,63–84]

Fear of a new health care system and/or hospital
Not wanting to leave their pediatric clinician and pediatric institution
Anxiety about how to relinquish control around managing their youth condition
Anxiety of not knowing the adult clinicians, adult health care system, and logistical issues (ie, finding parking, making appointments, finding a physician who is taking new patients, inadequate transferring patient records, and insurance issues)
Changing and/or different therapies recommended in adult health care
Families' fear that adult clinicians will not listen to and value their expertise
Negative beliefs about adult health care
Inadequate planning
Inadequate preparation and support from clinicians on the transition process and adult model of care
Not having seen clinician alone
Youth and young adults less interested in health compared with broader life circumstances
Adolescents' age, sex, and race and/or ethnicity and their parents' socioeconomic status can affect transition preparation
System difficulties
Lack of communication and coordination and transfer of medical records between adult and pediatric clinician or system
Limited availability of adult primary and specialty clinicians
Difficulty in locating adult clinicians who have specialized knowledge about and community resources for youth with pediatric-onset chronic diseases
Loss of insurance coverage among young adults and cost of care barriers

and medication adherence,[46] discontinuity of care,[47–51] patient dissatisfaction, higher emergency department and hospital use,[52,53] and higher costs of care.[54–57] An additional challenge is that parents often do not appreciate their role in giving youth ways to increase their independence in seeking and managing their health care.[58] Other barriers to transition for youth with various chronic conditions are unstable living conditions, lack of a high school degree, low parental education, lack of insurance, distance from adult clinicians, low income, poor psychosocial functioning, and age.[59]

PEDIATRIC TO ADULT HCT BARRIERS AND PREFERENCES

To inform the updated clinical report, a literature search was conducted of peer-reviewed articles published between January 2010 and December 2017. Many transition barriers are experienced by youth, young adults, and parents (Table 1). These barriers mainly are measured among youth and young adults with SHCN. The most prominent barrier mentioned by youth with SHCN and parents and/or caregivers is difficulty in leaving their pediatric clinicians with whom they have had a long-standing relationship. Although youth with

SHCN have limited preparation, they appear to have greater transition readiness skills and demonstrate more independence in completing medical tasks than their peers without special needs.[60] Clinicians also identify many transition barriers (Table 2). The most common obstacles reported by pediatric and adult care clinicians are the lack of communication and coordination and the different practice styles between health professionals. Also, both pediatric and adult clinicians find the transition of youth with medical complexity more difficult.[61,62]

Studies of pediatric clinicians on barriers to HCT often mention the lack of adult clinicians to care for youth with pediatric-onset conditions. Yet, recent surveys of adult clinicians in 3 large integrated care systems and in a national survey of adult endocrinologists[85,110] indicate an increased willingness to accept new young adult patients. To care for young adults, especially those with pediatric-onset conditions, adult clinicians request improved infrastructure (care coordination, links to community resources, lists of subspecialists interested in caring for young adults with SHCN, and availability of pediatric consultation support) and education and training about specific disease processes and

the physical and behavioral stages of youth and young adult development.

OUTCOME EVIDENCE FOR PEDIATRIC TO ADULT HCT INTERVENTION

Although the evidence base on HCT outcomes remains limited, there have been several evaluation studies published in the United States and internationally that document beneficial outcomes of a structured transition approach in terms of quality of care and, to a lesser extent, in terms of service use and patient and family experience. A recent systematic literature review of studies published between January 1995 and April 2016 identified 43 (out of 3844 articles) that met rigorous evaluation criteria.[111] Two-thirds of the included studies revealed statistically significant positive outcomes. The most commonly reported quality of care outcome was improvement in adherence to care followed by improved perceived health status, quality of life, and self-care skills. The most common positive outcomes for service use were increased adult visit attendance and less time between the last pediatric visit and the initial adult visit. Decreased hospitalization rates were also found, although not as often. Unfortunately, in Gabriel et al's[111] systematic

TABLE 2 Adult and Pediatric Clinician Transition Barriers[22,82,85–109]

Communication and/or consultation gaps
    Lack of communication, coordination, guidelines, and protocols between the pediatric and adult systems
    Inadequate communication from pediatric clinicians, often with a lack of medical records and follow-up recommendations
    Lack of long-term follow-up guidelines with care information for youth with SHCN
    Gap in consultation with pediatric clinicians
    Adult clinicians' concerns about not enough adult subspecialty or mental health care clinicians to care for young adults
Training limitations
    Lack of knowledge and/or training in pediatric-onset conditions and adolescent development and behavior
    Difficulty meeting psychosocial needs of young adults with pediatric-onset conditions
    Caring for adult patients reliant on caregivers
Care delivery, care coordination, and/or staff support gaps
    Lack of care coordination and follow-up
    Lack of mental health and supportive services
    Unfamiliarity with local and regional resources for young adults with chronic conditions
    Lack of adequate infrastructure and training
    Administrative constraints and lack of time and reimbursement
    Lack of coverage for young adults
Lack of patient knowledge and engagement
    Young adults' lack of knowledge about disease treatments, medications, and medical history
    Lack of information about community resources and/or support groups
    Dependency on parents or guardians
    Lack of self-advocacy, decision-making skills, and self-care skills
    Poor adherence to care
    Unrealistic expectations of youth or young adult knowledge of adult medical system and lack of readiness for adult care
Lack of comfort with adult care
    Unrealistic youth, young adult, and family expectations of time and attention
    Concerns regarding loss of strong relationships with previous clinicians (patient, parent, and/or staff)
    Pediatric clinician's lack of confidence in adult clinician and in the stylistic differences between pediatric and adult care, particularly for some youth and
        young adults with intellectual or developmental disabilities or behavioral health conditions
    Parents' reluctance to relinquish responsibility
    Parents unaware of changes in privacy issues

---

review, few studies examined costs, and no study revealed significant cost savings. Positive effects on the experience of care most often cited pertained to the general transition or transfer process. Of the 43 studies in this systematic review, all but 5 addressed youth with a single chronic condition; there were no studies that met inclusion criteria that examined youth with mental health conditions or common chronic conditions (eg, asthma) or of youth without chronic conditions. The systematic review concluded that because of the lack of detailed descriptions of transition interventions, it was not possible to link specific transition interventions to outcomes, as was found in earlier reviews on transition.[112,113] Since the publication of the systematic review by Gabriel et al,[111] 2 articles reporting transition cost savings have been published.[114,115]

Other systematic literature reviews on transition for youth with SHCN have revealed that transition evaluation studies often fail to incorporate conceptual frameworks,[111,116] clinical recommendations,[1,18] and international consensus statements.[117,118] Studies have identified a variety of transition outcome variables,[86,117–123] and to date, there is no common agreement on which outcome variables should be measured.[124] The Agency for Healthcare Research and Quality,[125] the Institute of Medicine,[24] and others[126–129] have identified the need for more robust and consistent measurement of transition. Using the triple aim approach that includes quality of care, patient and clinician experience, and use/cost measures can offer a framework for evaluating transition outcomes.[128] Patients who are more activated (eg, willingness to take independent actions to manage

their own health) have better health outcomes and care experiences.[130] There are several ways to measure patient activation, such as through the Patient Activation Measure[131] or through the assessment of health confidence[132] and motivation.[133] There are readiness and self-care assessment tools modeled after motivational interviewing that include scorable questions on transition and health confidence that lead to improved patient activation.[134] Care coordination is a common feature associated with increased transition planning activities.[135]

UPDATED HCT PROCESSES AND IMPLEMENTATION

Updated HCT Processes

The tenets of the original AAP, AAFP, and ACP transition clinical report and algorithm are unchanged and still include transition guidance for all youth and young adults.[1] This update provides more specificity and practical guidance on key elements of transition planning, transfer, and integration into adult care. The 2011 clinical report provided guidance for primary and specialty care clinicians on practice-based transition supports for all youth using an age-based algorithm with a component for youth with SHCN. The algorithm contained action steps (discussion of a transition policy, initiation of a transition plan, and review and/or update of the transition plan) for specific age ranges. It also incorporated an assessment of transition readiness or self-care skills to build a youth's independence and preparation for an adult model of care in anticipation of legally becoming an adult at age 18 years, unless alternative decision-making supports are in place. The algorithm recommended the identification of an adult care clinician, communication between pediatric and adult clinicians, and timely exchange of current medical information. The 2011 clinical report also acknowledged that caring for transitioning young adults can present certain challenges, including a need for adult practices to clarify the following issues for the young adult: (1) medical decision-making responsibilities; (2) continued support for developing self-management skills; (3) adult consent and confidentiality policies; (4) how their practice operates; and (5) how to access routine and after-hours care. Recommendations for clinicians to use an adult model of care for youth in either pediatric or adult clinical settings over 18 years of age was not discussed but now is a key part of transition preparation. An adult model of care places the young adult in the center of their care with primary responsibility for their own health care decisions. They have the option to authorize

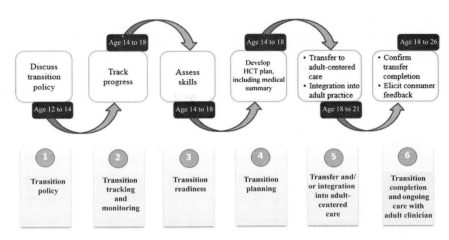

FIGURE 1
Timeline for introducing the Six Core Elements into pediatric practices.

other individuals to be involved in their health care on the basis of Health Insurance Portability and Accountability Act privacy rules and other applicable law. In addition, consistent with Bright Futures,[136] clinicians should incorporate one-on-one time with youth during the medical visit to better prepare youth for managing their own health and health care. One-on-one time has been shown to increase adherence to care, engagement in care, and the likelihood of sharing health risks with their clinician.[136–139]

After the publication of the 2011 clinical report, a structured clinical approach with sample tools, called the "Six Core Elements of Health Care Transition," was developed for all youth. From 2011 to 2013, 5 learning collaboratives with both pediatric and adult care clinicians from rural, suburban, and urban sites across the country tested the Six Core Elements. The collaboratives used quality improvement (QI) methodologies developed by the Institute for Healthcare Improvement[140] to pilot the original Six Core Elements. One of the HCT learning collaboratives was in the District of Columbia and involved teams (pediatric and adult physicians, nurses, social workers, family navigators, young adults, and parents) from both pediatric and adult practices (representing

both family medicine and internal medicine programs) from 3 academic health centers. This work demonstrated the effectiveness of an organized transition process for youth, young adults, and families as well as for primary care pediatric, family medicine, and internal medicine practices.[141] In 2014, the Six Core Elements were updated on the basis of the experiences of these multisite QI projects, a literature review, and input from pediatric and adult clinicians and youth, young adult, and family transition experts (Figs 1 and 2).

The Six Core Elements is not a model of care but a structured process that can be customized for use in a busy practice and applied to many different types of transition care models[142] and settings such as transition and young adult clinics and programs. The intensity of the HCT intervention can be guided by several aspects, such as the complexity of the health condition, the social determinants of health,[143] and adverse childhood experiences[144] of the youth and young adult. For example, if the youth has many comorbidities and/or there is poor adherence to care before the transition, more supports are likely to be needed during and after the transition process.[145–147] The Six Core Element tools are meant to be

Practice or provider	#1 Transition and/or care policy	#2 Tracking and monitoring	#3 Transition readiness and/or orientation to adult practice	#4 Transition planning and/or integration into adult approach to care or practice	#5 Transfer of care and/or initial visit	#6 Transition completion or ongoing care
Pediatric[a]	Create and discuss with youth and/or family	Track progress of youth and/or family transition preparation and transfer	Conduct transition readiness assessments	Develop transition plan, including needed readiness assessment skills and medical summary, prepare youth for adult approach to care, and communicate with new clinician	Transfer of care with information and communication including residual pediatric clinician's responsibility	Obtain feedback on the transition process and confirm young adult has been seen by the new clincian
Adult[a]	Create and discuss with young adult and guardian, if needed	Track progress of young adult's integration into adult care	Share and discuss welcome and FAQs with young adult and guardian, if needed	Communicate with previous clinician, ensure receipt of transfer package	Review transfer package, address young adult's needs and concerns at initial visit, update self-care assessment and medical summary	Confirm transfer completion with previous clinician, provide ongoing care with self-care skill building and link to needed specialists

FIGURE 2
Summary of Six Core Elements approach for pediatric and adult practices.
[a]Providers that care for youth and/or young adults throughout the life span can use both the pediatric and adult sets of core elements without the transfer process components.

customized for the youth, young adults, and families being served and the transition care model being used by the practice, system, or hospital.[148] They have been shown to facilitate an effective transition process in subspecialty practices,[149] a managed care plan,[150] a children's hospital,[151] and a med-peds residency program.[152]

Figure 2 outlines the Six Core Elements. All 3 phases of transition support (preparation, transfer, and integration into adult health care) are included in this approach. The Six Core Elements contain a set of customizable sample tools for use in primary and specialty care practices, 2 process measurement tools[153] (the Current Assessment of HCT Activities and the HCT Process Measurement Tool)[154] and a feedback measurement tool that can be customized for feedback from youth, young adults, or family on their transition experience (the Transition Feedback Survey for Youth, Young Adults, and Parents and/or Caregivers). In addition, there is a recently validated transition experience tool (Adolescent Assessment of

Preparation for Transition survey) for 16- and 17-year-olds with chronic conditions.[155]

The Six Core Elements are packaged into 3 different versions[154]:

- For pediatric practices, the Six Core Elements consist of a transition policy, tracking and monitoring, readiness assessment, transition planning (including patient education to fill the gaps in knowledge identified by the readiness assessment), transfer of care, and transfer completion.

- For adult practices, the Six Core Elements include a transition and young adult care policy, tracking and monitoring, orientation to adult practice, initial visit, and ongoing care including a self-management skills assessment and continued self-care education.

- For clinicians who care for youth throughout their life span, such as family medicine physicians, physicians dually trained in internal med-peds, and family nurse practitioners, the Six Core Elements of HCT define ways to transition to an adult approach to care by age 18 years and, if needed,

to transfer to a new adult clinician. This version includes a transition policy, tracking and monitoring, transition readiness, transition planning and/or integration into adult approach to care, transfer to adult approach to care, and transfer completion with ongoing care including continued self-management skills assessment and self-care education.

Figure 3 offers 3 examples of customizable tools available for the first core element (creating a transition policy) for pediatric, family medicine, med-peds, and internal medicine practices.

Implementation of HCT Process

Experience implementing a successful transition process underscores the importance of support of key decision makers from both pediatric and adult practices and/or health systems, hospitals and the early and ongoing engagement of parents and/or caregivers and young adults. Along with physicians, other implementation team members to consider are social workers, nurses, clinic administrators, information technology staff, home

A

For Practices Transitioning Youth to Adult Health Care Clinicians

[Practice Name] wants to help our patients make a smooth transition from pediatric to adult health care. This process involves working with youth, beginning at ages 12 to 14 years, and their families to prepare for the change. The change is from a "pediatric" model of care where parents make most health choices to an "adult" model of care where youth make their own health choices. This means that we will spend time during the visit with the teen without the parent present. This will help youth to be more independent with their own health care.

At age 18 years, most youth legally become adults.[a] We respect that many of our young adult patients choose to continue to involve their families in health care decisions. Only with the young adult's consent will we be able to discuss any personal health information with family members. If the youth has a condition that keeps him/her from making health care choices, we ask parents/caregivers to consider options for supported decision making.

We will work with youth and families about the age for moving to an adult provider and suggest that this transfer occur before the age of (insert age [b]). We will assist with this transfer process, including helping to identify an adult clinician, sending medical records, and work with the adult clinician about the unique needs of our patients.

As always, if you have any questions, please feel free to contact us.

B

Practices Transitioning Youth to an Adult Model of Care Without Changing Clinicians

[Practice Name] wants to help our pediatric patients become better prepared for an adult model of health care to stay with our practice as young adults. At about age 14 years, we will begin to spend time during the visit without the parent present to help you to answer questions, set health goals, and support more independence with health care choices. At age 18 years, most youth legally become adults.[a] We respect that many of our young adult patients choose to continue to involve their families in their health care choices. Yet, we will no longer be able to discuss your health care with parents or share any personal health information without the young adult's written approval. To allow others to be involved in health care decisions requires that a signed form be completed. We have the form at the clinic. If a youth has a condition that prevents him/her from making decisions, we encourage families to consider options for supported decision-making. Your health is important to us. If you have any questions or concerns, please feel free to contact us.

C

For Practices Integrating Young Adults into Adult Health Care

[Practice Name] welcomes young adults, including those with special health care needs, to our practice. We aim to provide high-quality, complete, and confidential health care to meet young adults' unique needs.

At age 18, most youth legally become adults.[a] The health care clinician is a partner in supporting your health goals. This means that adult clinicians do not discuss any aspects of your care with anyone else unless you ask that we do. We know that some young adults involve family and close friends in their health care decisions and would like their clinician to share information with those close to them. To allow others to be involved in your health care decisions requires that a signed consent form be completed. The form is available at the clinic. For young adults unable to provide consent, we will need legal documentation about decision-making arrangements.

We ask that new patients moving to our practice call their previous clinicians(s) to have a medical summary or medical record sent to us before the first visit. We make every effort to coordinate the transfer of care with previous clinicians, including speaking with your pediatric clinician and assisting with transfer of specialty care, as needed. Having your medical information before the visit helps with your continuity of care and a better experience for you.

Your health is important to us, and we look forward to having you as a new patient. If you have any questions or concerns, please feel free to contact us.

FIGURE 3

Examples of customizable tools for Core Element No. 1: creating an HCT policy. [a]Although most states have set the age of majority at 18 years, it is greater in some states. For this clinical report, we chose consistently to use the age 18 years out of economy but recommend that readers consult appropriate laws and regulations in their jurisdiction to assist in determining the appropriate age

care clinicians, and insurers. With the teams identified, defining the HCT QI project's goals, strategies, outcomes, measures, and timeline at the start and allowing the time needed to test and implement the transition improvements are key. In addition, utilizing a plan-do-study-act rapid cycle improvement approach[140,157,158] promotes a process that is efficient and well-tested.

Teamwork is key to improving coordination and communication in the HCT process.[159] In the ideal situation, the availability of care coordination support to guide the transition process and team-based care[160] in both the pediatric and adult settings increases chances of success.[135,161] Clinicians from nursing and social work professions often fill this important role and often drive the HCT QI process.[162–164] Families also need assistance with their new role in the health care of their young adult.[165] For youth with multiple pediatric clinicians (primary, subspecialty, behavioral) involved in their care, transfers to adult clinicians are best planned sequentially rather than at the same time.

Transferring to adult primary care clinicians[126,166] could be the initial transfer so the adult care clinicians can assist in locating and/or coordinating adult subspecialty or behavioral care clinicians, as needed. In transitioning youth with certain chronic conditions, the interplay between pediatric subspecialists and the transfer to adult primary care and/or subspecialty clinicians can vary according to the youth's needs and availability of adult care clinicians with appropriate specialty knowledge. In the absence of a particular adult subspecialty clinician, transitioning the young adult to an adult primary care clinician with consultation to the pediatric subspecialist could occur until adult clinicians are comfortable with the needed subspecialty knowledge or appropriate adult subspecialists are available.[167] In addition, transfer to adult care is best conducted when the youth's health condition is stable.[168] For patients receiving pediatric palliative care or end-of-life care, timing of transition to adult health care depends on the youth's anticipated disease trajectory and overall goals of care.

A growing number of pediatric and adult practices/systems and public health programs in the United States are customizing and implementing the Six Core Elements to establish a structured process for transition to adult care. In 2016, the Council of Subspecialty Societies of the ACP identified pediatric to adult HCT as a priority initiative as part of its High Value Care Initiative.[21] Several of the adult medical specialty societies created customized transition readiness and self-care assessments and medical summary templates from the Six Core Elements for young adults with selected conditions that include sickle cell disease, type 1 diabetes mellitus, juvenile idiopathic arthritis, systemic lupus erythematosus, epilepsy and other neurologic conditions, and, in conjunction with the Society of Internal Medicine and the Society of Adolescent Health and Medicine, developmental disabilities and physical disabilities.[169]

In 2014, the US Maternal and Child Health Bureau articulated HCT as 1 of its top 15 national priorities for state Title V programs.[170,171] A total of 32 states and the District of Columbia have chosen to focus on transition and are adopting components of the Six Core Elements approach in activities related to practice and care coordination improvements, health care professional and family and youth education, interagency transition planning, and outreach and communications.[172]

SPECIAL POPULATIONS

Youth and young adults between the ages of 12 and 26 years represent 20% of the population in the United States.[173] This stage of life is characterized by change as well as growing independence and self-determination.[147] It is also a period when health risk behaviors peak, chronic conditions are often exacerbated, and general health care use, particularly among the male sex, is low, while emergency department use is high.[174] In addition, it is a time when many leave home for college, employment, or military service and begin to use a new system of health care. Although pediatric medical training programs recognize that adolescents are special populations warranting distinct, proactive care and monitoring,[136] adult medical training programs are just beginning to recognize young adults as a special population.[175] The Institute of Medicine (now the National Academy of Medicine) and the National Research Council acknowledged the young adult population as a particularly vulnerable population and called for improving the transition process with innovative approaches for engaging and communicating with young adults about their own health care and adapting adult care services to better meet their unique needs.[24,25] Studies have recently suggested a role for digital communication, telemedicine, and shared medical appointments in health communication strategies in HCT with youth and young adults.[176–181]

Although all youth and young adults need a safe and seamless HCT to adult health care, some youth (those with complex medical conditions, developmental and/or intellectual disabilities, mental and/or behavioral health conditions, and social complexity) may pose additional challenges to the transition process. These individuals often experience multiple transitions in services and supports from pediatric care and special education to much less resource-rich adult systems. For these special populations, refinements in the transition process may be necessary, including flexibility in the age of transfer to adult care,[182] delayed scheduling of specialist transfers, condition-specific protocols, greater care coordination support, pediatric consultation arrangements, use of peer and/or community health workers, and strong linkages to nonhealth support systems such as education, independent living, community, and employment. System supports like care coordination, care planning, and social services found in many pediatric clinical settings may be less available in adult clinical settings.[87–89]

Youth with developmental and/or intellectual disabilities, including autism spectrum disorders, often face challenges in transitioning to self-directed care because systemic supports for their preparation and training and accommodations in the health care delivery process are not widely available.[183–187] The presence of intellectual disability or intellectual impairment attributable to brain injury may affect an individual's ability to fully participate in health-related decision-making and to independently navigate the adult health care system. Although these youth and/or young adults aspire to the highest possible level of independence and community inclusion, many will require decision supports, including those formalized

---

FIGURE 3 Continued

of majority. It is also important to note that there are nuances in the care of adolescents regarding consent and privacy triggered by emancipation, mature minor doctrine, and for specific health services such as reproductive health and substance abuse treatment. These issues are beyond the scope of this report. Consultation with a lawyer in your state may be appropriate. [b]At the discretion of the practice. Adapted from Got Transition.[156]

through a legal process, such as guardianship or custodianship. Planning for decision-making support is best started at least by age 17 years, and the resulting modifications need to be documented in the medical record and communicated to new adult care clinicians.

Youth with mental or behavioral health conditions also face substantial adversity during the transition period for several reasons.[188-193] Mental health conditions often peak during young adulthood and impair one's ability for self-care and participation in routine medical or mental health care or decision-making. Shortages of mental and/or behavioral health clinicians are pervasive, and many youth and young adults with psychiatric conditions have no access to a regular source of either mental health or medical care. Consequently, they are at higher risk of dropping out of care as well as employment, education, stable housing, and relationships. Transition planning for this special population is most helpful when the clinic incorporates active preparation, outreach, and support for effective self-advocacy as well as partnerships with family members, medical and mental health and/or behavioral clinicians, and community supports to bridge service gaps.[194]

Youth with medical complexity represent approximately 1% of all US children and are a subset of youth with SHCN.[195,196] These youth have multiple significant chronic health problems that affect multiple organ systems and result in functional limitations, high care need or use, and often use of medical technology.[197] Many youth with SHCN have frequent hospitalizations. Youth and their families have become familiar with the nursing staff, ancillary staff, routines, expectations, and services that are available in children's hospitals or on children's units within hospitals. In addition to their outpatient care sites and

their clinicians, transitioning to adult hospitals represent a unique set of challenges. Youth and families with frequent admissions should have transition planning discussions with both their children's hospital team and the new adult hospital staff about the upcoming hospital, facility, or transition. In both pediatric and adult hospitals, complex care centers and transition clinics and programs have been established to provide both outpatient and inpatient coordination and management for youth and young adults with medical complexity, recognizing their needs for more individualized planning and collaborative care partnerships between pediatric and adult clinicians or practices.[196]

Social complexity, either in isolation or in combination with chronic medical conditions, is the source of many disparities in care for ethnic and racial minorities; immigrant and refugee populations; those with linguistic and cultural differences; lesbian, gay, bisexual, transgender, and queer youth and families[198]; and youth affected by poverty,[63,199,200] homelessness, and foster care.[201,202] Specific resources that may enhance the transition process include engagement of culturally similar peers, use of family navigators and community health workers, and involvement of schools and community centers. Special populations may not represent the majority of youth transitioning to adulthood, but in the aggregate, they include those most vulnerable to poor outcomes and higher health care costs.

EDUCATION AND TRAINING IN THE CARE OF YOUTH AND/OR YOUNG ADULTS WITH PEDIATRIC-ONSET CONDITIONS

Training of adult clinicians in pediatric-onset diseases and youth and young adult development is a recognized need to improve

transition and improved outcomes for youth and young adults moving to the adult health care system.[88,90,91,203] Studies of internal medicine residents' exposure and preferences around transition from pediatric to adult health care have shown that internal medicine residents receive little exposure to transition issues or young adult patients in their training[91] and that they want to receive this education mainly through clinical exposure and case discussions.[204]

HCT is already included in the training of family medicine and med-peds clinicians who care for people throughout the life span. To make transition training more explicit, the Medicine-Pediatrics Program Directors Association developed a special transition curriculum for primary care med-peds residents incorporating training around HCT.[203] Recently, several academic medical centers have started joint pediatric and adult residency training sessions that address transition and caring for young adults with congenital or childhood-onset conditions. Other training approaches include introducing internal medicine residents to young adult patients in continuity clinics and offering electives in college and university health clinics or in transition clinics for youth with SHCN or medical complexity.[205]

A few pediatric and adult professional societies also have developed HCT training modules for residents in pediatrics and internal medicine, but more training is needed, particularly for adult clinicians during residency and for practicing clinicians through continuing medical education (CME) options and maintenance of certification requirements. Similarly, both pediatric and adult residency training programs could have more training in adolescent and young adult health.[206,207] The AAP offers a series of case-based, educational modules designed for pediatric residency program directors and faculty. These modules focus on the patient- and family-centered medical home, care coordination, care planning, transition to adult care, and team-based care.[208] In addition, the Association of American Medical Colleges has a transition case scenario, called *But Tommy Likes It Here: Moving to Adult Medicine*, available on its Web site.[209]

The Society of General Internal Medicine in 2016 published the *Care of Adults With Chronic Childhood Conditions: A Practical Guide*, which provides an overview of HCTs, strategies for primary care clinicians caring for young adults, condition-specific medical information, and sociolegal issues that can assist adult clinicians in caring for young adults.[210]

Two options are available for maintenance of certification Part IV credit for pediatric clinicians from the American Board of Pediatrics: The University of California San Diego and Rady Children's Hospital with the North American Society for Pediatric Gastroenterology, Hepatology and Nutrition[211] and the Illinois Transition Care Project.[212] CME training on transition is becoming more available, especially at national meetings for primary care and subspecialty clinicians.

PAYMENT OPPORTUNITIES FOR HCT

Current payment mechanisms address professional services through traditional fee-for-service reporting or various types of performance-based and alternative models of payment. In recent years, the American Medical Association's Current Procedural Terminology (CPT), along with the Centers for Medicare and Medicaid Services (CMS), have addressed the importance of care management and coordination services through code development for vulnerable care

scenarios such as hospital-to-home transition, chronic care coordination, and behavioral health. These types of codes acknowledge the role that clinical staff play in coordinating the care for vulnerable patients. Although there is currently not a code specifically defined as pediatric-to-adult transition, as called for in the AAP "Principles of Child Health Care Financing,"[213] newly developed care management services offer an opportunity to report fee-for-service for many of the elements of transitional care.

Although alternative payment options for transition (eg, using pay-for-performance, capitation, or shared savings) have not yet been incorporated into existing medical home, health home, care coordination, or accountable care payment innovations, collaboration continues to occur among major payers and with CPT to address current voids. CMS recently noted that "…we have sought to recognize significant changes in health care practice, especially innovations in the active management and ongoing care of chronically ill patients. We have been engaged in an ongoing incremental effort to identify gaps in appropriate coding and payment for care management/coordination, cognitive services and primary care within the physician fee schedule."[214]

As billing options for these services continue to evolve, several coding options are currently available to support transition services in both pediatric and adult care settings. For example, in addition to evaluation and management codes for face-to-face visits, CPT includes services that address the following categories: prolonged services with (or without) direct patient contact, medical team conferences, care plan oversight, preventive medicine counseling and behavior change interventions, interprofessional Internet and/or telephone consultations, and

chronic and complex chronic care management.

In addition, CPT includes codes that represent administration of health risk assessment instruments can be used to report transition readiness assessments conducted with youth and parents and self-care assessments conducted with young adults. As a prerequisite for billing, the assessment tools[215] must be scorable and standardized. Some examples of standardized scorable tools include the Transition Readiness Assessment Questionnaire,[216] Am I ON TRAC for Adult Care Questionnaire (ON TRAC),[217] University of North Carolina TR(x) ANSITION Scale,[218] Self-Management and Transition for Adulthood with Rx = Treatment (STARx Questionnaire),[219,220] Transition Q,[221] an electronic medical record–based transition planning tool,[222] California Healthy and Ready to Work,[223] Got Transition's Transition Readiness and Self-Care assessment tools,[134] and the Patient Activation Measure.[131,224] More information about transition-related codes and case scenarios can be found in the AAP and Got Transition Coding and Reimbursement Tip Sheet[225] as well as a report on value-based payment options.[226]

RECOMMENDATIONS

Infrastructure

Since the 2011 clinical report, system infrastructure needs are becoming increasingly apparent as more youth, especially those with pediatric-onset conditions and others included as special populations, enter the transition period. To address these gaps, the following recommendations are called for:

- Clinicians and systems of care (eg, pediatric and adult hospitals including emergency departments, integrated delivery systems, accountable care organizations, community health centers, health plans, public health programs, behavioral health programs, and school and college health centers) are essential in preparing youth for needed transition preparation, transfer with current medical information, and facilitating integration into adult care. The following actions can support safe and effective transition:

○ Integrate HCTs into routine preventive,[227] primary, specialty and subspecialty, and mental and/or behavioral health care.

○ Support QI processes within health care systems and pediatric and adult practices to implement the Six Core Element approach with active youth, young adult, and family engagement and feedback. Work directly with their electronic health record support team and/or vendor representative to integrate the Six Core Elements (transition policy, registry, readiness and self-care assessments, transition plan of care, medical summary, transition and/or transfer checklists, and feedback surveys) in a way that supports their own workflow and practice needs.

○ Incorporate HCT support as a recommended element in all medical home[228] and health home recognition and certification programs, including standards developed by the National Committee for Quality Assurance, The Joint Commission, and the Utilization Review Accreditation Commission.

○ Articulate specific HCT roles and responsibilities among pediatric and adult health care clinicians and systems to facilitate the provision and coordination of recommended transition support.

○ Increase the availability and quality of care coordination support, particularly for adult

practices and systems serving young adults with chronic medical, developmental, and behavioral conditions and social complexity.

○ Integrate HCT support into other life course systems such as changes in education, guardianship, and power of attorney as needed.[146,147]

• Expand the availability of pediatric consultation for adult clinicians caring for youth with pediatric-onset conditions.

• Incorporate HCTs into the transition policies and plans of other public program systems (eg, special education, foster care).

• Create up-to-date listings of community resources (eg, adult disability programs) and adult clinicians interested in caring for young adults with pediatric-onset conditions and other special populations.

Education and Training

• In partnership with families and youth, increase education and training opportunities for pediatric and adult health care clinicians in HCTs, youth and young adult development, pediatric-onset diseases, interprofessional practice, and team-based care by adding:

○ CME opportunities[229] (eg, learning modules such as focusing on young adult health and pediatric onset conditions, clinical experiences, curriculum, and interprofessional training opportunities);

○ Enhanced training opportunities during residency and subspecialty training, including joint pediatric and adult training; and

○ HCT processes and support into education systems such as school-based health centers, colleges, and universities.

Payment

To align HCT delivery system innovations with payment incentives, public and private payors and their contracted plans should:

• Compensate clinicians and systems of care for the provision of recommended HCT support related to planning, transfer, and integration into a new adult practice.

• Recognize and pay for CPT and Healthcare Common Procedure Coding System codes important to transition to adult care.

• Develop a CPT Category II code that can be used as a quality measure for tracking the use of transition services by pediatric and adult clinicians.

• Develop innovative payment approaches to encourage collaboration between pediatric and adult care clinicians in the adoption of the HCT process, including the following:

○ Financial incentives for collaboration between pediatric and adult practices around HCT;

○ A per-member, per-month additional payment involved in preparing youth and young adults for transfer out of pediatric care and for outreach and follow-up of young adults coming into a new adult care setting;

○ Performance-based incentives to encourage pediatric practices to transfer their patients at a certain age with a current medical summary, readiness assessment, and evidence of communication with the new practice and to encourage adult practices to accept a certain volume of new young adults with SHCN with pediatric consultation support; and

○ Payment rates for transition as well as future related research and evaluation studies should stratify for patient risk,[230] taking into consideration not only disease complexity but also social determinants of health, adverse childhood experiences, and availability of family and community supports.

Research

To promote a stronger evidence base for HCTs, funders and researchers should:

- Incorporate all 3 components of HCTs (preparation, transfer, and integration into adult care) in their study design and evaluate HCT processes and outcomes.

- Examine transition outcomes in terms of population health (eg, adherence to care, self-care skill development); experience of youth, young adults, and families; and use (eg, time between last pediatric and first adult visit, adherence to initial and follow-up adult clinician appointments, decreased emergency department use,

and urgent care visits) and cost savings.

- Develop pediatric to adult HCT measures as a part of the CMS Child and Adult Core Measure Set and the National Quality Forum measures.

- Study the impact of HCTs from pediatric to adult health care in terms of long-term outcomes of young adults.

- Encourage national health surveys to include HCT questions for young adults.

LEAD AUTHORS

Patience H. White, MD, MA, FAAP, FACP
W. Carl Cooley, MD, FAAP

TRANSITIONS CLINICAL REPORT REVISION AUTHORING GROUP

Patience White, MD, MA, FAAP, FACP
W. Carl Cooley, MD, FAAP
Alexy D. Arauz Boudreau, MD, MPH, FAAP
Mallory Cyr, MPH
Beth Ellen Davis, MD, MPH, FAAP
Deborah E. Dreyfus, MD, MSc
Eileen Forlenza, BS
Allen Friedland, MD, FACP, FAAP
Carol Greenlee, MD, FACE, FACP
Marie Mann, MD, MPH, FAAP
Margaret McManus, MHS
Afaf I. Meleis, PhD, Dr PS(hon), FAAN
Laura Pickler, MD, MPH

AAP STAFF

Dana Bright, MSW
Christina Boothby, MPA

ABBREVIATIONS

AAFP: American Academy of Family Physicians
AAP: American Academy of Pediatrics
ACP: American College of Physicians
CME: continuing medical education
CMS: Centers for Medicare and Medicaid Services
CPT: Current Procedural Terminology
HCT: health care transition
med-peds: medicine and pediatrics
QI: quality improvement
SHCN: special health care needs

All clinical reports from the American Academy of Pediatrics automatically expire 5 years after publication unless reaffirmed, revised, or retired at or before that time.

DOI: https://doi.org/10.1542/peds.2018-2587

Address correspondence to Patience H. White, MD, MA, FAAP, FACP. E-mail: pwhite@thenationalalliance.org

PEDIATRICS (ISSN Numbers: Print, 0031-4005; Online, 1098-4275).

Copyright © 2018 by the American Academy of Pediatrics

FINANCIAL DISCLOSURE: The authors have indicated they have no financial relationships relevant to this article to disclose.

FUNDING: No external funding.

POTENTIAL CONFLICT OF INTEREST: The authors have indicated they have no potential conflicts of interest to disclose.

REFERENCES

1. Cooley WC, Sagerman PJ; American Academy of Pediatrics; American Academy of Family Physicians; American College of Physicians; Transitions Clinical Report Authoring Group. Supporting the health care transition from adolescence to adulthood in the medical home. *Pediatrics.* 2011;128(1):182–200

2. Canadian Pediatric Society. Transition to adult care for youth with special health care needs. *Paediatr Child Health.* 2007;12(9):785–793

3. American College of Obstetricians and Gynecologists. The transition from pediatric to adult health care: preventative care for young women aged 18-26 years. 2015. Available at: https://www.acog.org/-/media/Committee-Opinions/Committee-on-Adolescent-Health-Care/co626.pdf?dmc=1&ts=20170719T1757289470. Accessed July 21, 2017

4. Andrade DM, Bassett AS, Bercovici E, et al. Epilepsy: transition from pediatric to adult care. Recommendations of the Ontario epilepsy implementation task force. *Epilepsia.* 2017;58(9):1502–1517

5. Betz CL. SPN position statement: transition of pediatric patients into adult care. *J Pediatr Nurs.* 2017;35:160–164

6. Brooks AJ, Smith PJ, Cohen R, et al. UK guideline on transition of adolescent and young persons with chronic digestive diseases from paediatric to adult care. *Gut.* 2017;66(6):988–1000

7. Brown LW, Camfield P, Capers M, et al. The neurologist's role in supporting transition to adult health care: a consensus statement. *Neurology*. 2016;87(8):835–840

8. Bryant R, Porter JS, Sobota A; Association of Pediatric Hematology/Oncology Nurses; American Society of Pediatri Hematology Oncology. APHON/ASPHO policy statement for the transition of patients with sickle cell disease from pediatric to adult health care. *J Pediatr Oncol Nurs*. 2015;32(6):355–359

9. Committee on Adolescence. Achieving quality health services for adolescents. *Pediatrics*. 2016;138(2):e20161347

10. Committee on Pediatric Aids. Transitioning HIV-infected youth into adult health care. *Pediatrics*. 2013;132(1):192–197

11. Crane S; Autistic Self Advocacy Network (ASAN). The transition to adulthood for youth with ID/DD: a review of research, policy and next steps. 2013. Available at: http://autisticadvocacy.org/wp-content/uploads/2013/12/HealthCareTransit ion_ASAN_PolicyBrief_r2.pdf. Accessed January 17, 2018

12. Escherich G, Bielack S, Maier S, et al. Building a national framework for adolescent and young adult hematology and oncology and transition from pediatric to adult care: report of the inaugural meeting of the "AjET" working group of the German Society for Pediatric Oncology and Hematology. *J Adolesc Young Adult Oncol*. 2017;6(2):194–199

13. Foster HE, Minden K, Clemente D, et al. EULAR/PReS standards and recommendations for the transitional care of young people with juvenile-onset rheumatic diseases. *Ann Rheum Dis*. 2017;76(4):639–646

14. Mazur A, Dembinski L, Schrier L, Hadjipanayis A, Michaud PA. European Academy of Paediatric consensus statement on successful transition from paediatric to adult care for adolescents with chronic conditions. *Acta Paediatr*. 2017;106(8):1354–1357

15. Peters A, Laffel L; American Diabetes Association Transitions Working Group. Diabetes care for emerging adults: recommendations for transition from pediatric to adult diabetes care systems: a position statement of the American Diabetes Association, with representation by the American College of Osteopathic Family Physicians, the American Academy of Pediatrics, the American Association of Clinical Endocrinologists, the American Osteopathic Association, the Centers for Disease Control and Prevention, Children with Diabetes, The Endocrine Society, the International Society for Pediatric and Adolescent Diabetes, Juvenile Diabetes Research Foundation International, the National Diabetes Education Program, and the Pediatric Endocrine Society (formerly Lawson Wilkins Pediatric Endocrine Society) [published correction appears in *Diabetes Care*. 2012;35(1):191]. *Diabetes Care*. 2011;34(11):2477–2485

16. Royal College of Nursing. Lost in transition: moving young people between child and adult health services. Available at: https://www.rcn.org.uk/professional-development/publications/pub-003227. Accessed January 16, 2018

17. Sable C, Foster E, Uzark K, et al; American Heart Association Congenital Heart Defects Committee of the Council on Cardiovascular Disease in the Young, Council on Cardiovascular Nursing, Council on Clinical Cardiology, and Council on Peripheral Vascular Disease. Best practices in managing transition to adulthood for adolescents with congenital heart disease: the transition process and medical and psychosocial issues: a scientific statement from the American Heart Association. *Circulation*. 2011;123(13):1454–1485

18. UK National Institute for Health Care Excellence (NICE). Transition from children's to adults' services for young people using health or social care services. 2016. Available at: https://www.nice.org.uk/guidance/ng43. Accessed July 21, 2017

19. Watson AR, Harden P, Ferris M, Kerr PG, Mahan J, Ramzy MF. Transition from pediatric to adult renal services: a consensus statement by the International Society of Nephrology (ISN) and the International Pediatric Nephrology Association (IPNA). *Pediatr Nephrol*. 2011;26(10):1753–1757

20. Young S, Adamou M, Asherson P, et al. Recommendations for the transition of patients with ADHD from child to adult healthcare services: a consensus statement from the UK adult ADHD network. *BMC Psychiatry*. 2016;16:301

21. Greenlee MC, D'Angelo L, Harms SR, et al; American College of Physicians Council of Subspecialty Societies Pediatric to Adult Care Transitions Initiative Steering Committee. Enhancing the role of internists in the transition from pediatric to adult health care. *Ann Intern Med*. 2017;166(4):299–300

22. Tanner AE, Philbin MM, Ma A, et al; Adolescent Trials Network for HIV/AIDS Interventions. Adolescent to adult HIV health care transition from the perspective of adult providers in the United States. *J Adolesc Health*. 2017;61(4):434–439

23. Zuckerman AL. Transition of care to an adult provider. *Curr Opin Obstet Gynecol*. 2017;29(5):295–300

24. Institute of Medicine; National Research Council of the National Academies. *Investing in the Health and Well-Being of Young Adults*. Washington, DC: The National Academies Press; 2015

25. Society for Adolescent Health and Medicine. Young adult health and well-being: a position statement of the Society for Adolescent Health and Medicine. *J Adolesc Health*. 2017;60(6):758–759

26. Spencer DL, McManus M, Call KT, et al. Health care coverage and access among children, adolescents, and young adults, 2010-2016: implications for future health reforms. *J Adolesc Health*. 2018;62(6):667–673

27. Junge N, Migal K, Goldschmidt I, Baumann U. Transition after pediatric liver transplantation - perceptions of adults, adolescents and parents. *World J Gastroenterol*. 2017;23(13):2365–2375

28. Pyatak EA, Sequeira PA, Whittemore R, Vigen CP, Peters AL, Weigensberg MJ. Challenges contributing to disrupted transition from paediatric to adult diabetes care in young adults with type 1 diabetes. *Diabet Med*. 2014;31(12):1615–1624

29. Meleis AI, ed. *Transitions Theory: Middle Range and Situation Specific Theories in Nursing Research and Practice.* New York, NY: Springer Publishing Company; 2010

30. Geary CR, Schumacher KL. Care transitions: integrating transition theory and complexity science concepts. *ANS Adv Nurs Sci.* 2012;35(3):236–248

31. Schwartz LA, Brumley LD, Tuchman LK, et al. Stakeholder validation of a model of readiness for transition to adult care. *JAMA Pediatr.* 2013;167(10):939–946

32. Lebrun-Harris LA, McManus MA, Ilango SM, et al. Transition Planning Among US Youth With and Without Special Health Care Needs. *Pediatrics.* 2018;142(4):e20180194

33. Downing KF, Oster ME, Farr SL. Preparing adolescents with heart problems for transition to adult care, 2009-2010 national survey of children with special health care needs. *Congenit Heart Dis.* 2017;12(4):497–506

34. Lotstein DS, Ghandour R, Cash A, McGuire E, Strickland B, Newacheck P. Planning for health care transitions: results from the 2005-2006 national survey of children with special health care needs. *Pediatrics.* 2009;123(1). Available at: www.pediatrics.org/cgi/content/full/123/1/e145

35. McManus MA, Pollack LR, Cooley WC, et al. Current status of transition preparation among youth with special needs in the United States. *Pediatrics.* 2013;131(6):1090–1097

36. Sawicki GS, Whitworth R, Gunn L, Butterfield R, Lukens-Bull K, Wood D. Receipt of health care transition counseling in the national survey of adult transition and health. *Pediatrics.* 2011;128(3). Available at: www.pediatrics.org/cgi/content/full/128/3/e521

37. Syverson EP, McCarter R, He J, D'Angelo L, Tuchman LK. Adolescents' perceptions of transition importance, readiness, and likelihood of future success: the role of anticipatory guidance. *Clin Pediatr (Phila).* 2016;55(11):1020–1025

38. Dwyer-Matzky K, Blatt A, Asselin BL, Wood DL. Lack of preparedness for pediatric to adult-oriented health care transition in hospitalized adolescents and young adults. *Acad Pediatr.* 2018;18(1):102–110

39. Coller RJ, Ahrens S, Ehlenbach ML, et al. Transitioning from general pediatric to adult-oriented inpatient care: National Survey of US Children's Hospitals. *J Hosp Med.* 2018;13(1):13–20

40. Foster BJ. Heightened graft failure risk during emerging adulthood and transition to adult care. *Pediatr Nephrol.* 2015;30(4):567–576

41. Majumdar S. The adolescent with sickle cell disease. *Adolesc Med State Art Rev.* 2013;24(1):295–306, xv

42. Wafa S, Nakhla M. Improving the transition from pediatric to adult diabetes healthcare: a literature review. *Can J Diabetes.* 2015;39(6):520–528

43. Yeung E, Kay J, Roosevelt GE, Brandon M, Yetman AT. Lapse of care as a predictor for morbidity in adults with congenital heart disease. *Int J Cardiol.* 2008;125(1):62–65

44. Chaudhry SR, Keaton M, Nasr SZ. Evaluation of a cystic fibrosis transition program from pediatric to adult care. *Pediatr Pulmonol.* 2013;48(7):658–665

45. Maslow G, Adams C, Willis M, et al. An evaluation of a positive youth development program for adolescents with chronic illness. *J Adolesc Health.* 2013;52(2):179–185

46. Annunziato RA, Baisley MC, Arrato N, et al. Strangers headed to a strange land? A pilot study of using a transition coordinator to improve transfer from pediatric to adult services. *J Pediatr.* 2013;163(6):1628–1633

47. Bohun CM, Woods P, Winter C, et al. Challenges of intra-institutional transfer of care from paediatric to adult congenital cardiology: the need for retention as well as transition. *Cardiol Young.* 2016;26(2):327–333

48. Luque Ramos A, Hoffmann F, Albrecht K, Klotsche J, Zink A, Minden K. Transition to adult rheumatology care is necessary to maintain DMARD therapy in young people with juvenile idiopathic arthritis. *Semin Arthritis Rheum.* 2017;47(2):269–275

49. Montano CB, Young J. Discontinuity in the transition from pediatric to adult health care for patients with attention-deficit/hyperactivity disorder. *Postgrad Med.* 2012;124(5):23–32

50. Szymanski KM, Cain MP, Hardacker TJ, Misseri R. How successful is the transition to adult urology care in spina bifida? A single center 7-year experience. *J Pediatr Urol.* 2017;13(1):40.e1–40.e6

51. Wojciechowski EA, Hurtig A, Dorn L. A natural history study of adolescents and young adults with sickle cell disease as they transfer to adult care: a need for case management services. *J Pediatr Nurs.* 2002;17(1):18–27

52. Shaw KL, Southwood TR, McDonagh JE; British Society of Paediatric and Adolescent Rheumatology. Young people's satisfaction of transitional care in adolescent rheumatology in the UK. *Child Care Health Dev.* 2007;33(4):368–379

53. Shepard CL, Doerge EJ, Eickmeyer AB, Kraft KH, Wan J, Stoffel JT. Ambulatory care use among patients with Spina Bifida: change in care from childhood to adulthood. *J Urol.* 2018;199(4):1050–1055

54. Barr NG, Longo CJ, Embrett MG, Mulvale GM, Nguyen T, Randall GE. The transition from youth to adult mental health services and the economic impact on youth and their families. *Healthc Manage Forum.* 2017;30(6):283–288

55. Cohen E, Gandhi S, Toulany A, et al. Health care use during transfer to adult care among youth with chronic conditions. *Pediatrics.* 2016;137(3):e20152734

56. Lochridge J, Wolff J, Oliva M, O'Sullivan-Oliveira J. Perceptions of solid organ transplant recipients regarding self-care management and transitioning. *Pediatr Nurs.* 2013;39(2):81–89

57. Mosquera RA, Avritscher EB, Samuels CL, et al. Effect of an enhanced medical home on serious illness and cost of care among high-risk children with chronic illness: a randomized clinical trial. *JAMA.* 2014;312(24):2640–2648

58. C.S. Mott Children's Hospital. Back off: parents impeding teens' healthcare independence? 2015. Available at:

https://mottpoll.org/sites/default/files/documents/121415_teenhealthcare.pdf. Accessed November 21, 2017

59. Gray WN, Schaefer MR, Resmini-Rawlinson A, Wagoner ST. Barriers to transition from pediatric to adult care: a systematic review. *J Pediatr Psychol.* 2018;43(5):488–502

60. Eaton CK, Davis MF, Gutierrez-Colina AM, LaMotte J, Blount RL, Suveg C. Different demands, same goal: promoting transition readiness in adolescents and young adults with and without medical conditions. *J Adolesc Health.* 2017;60(6):727–733

61. de Silva PSA, Fishman LN. The transition of the gastrointestinal patient from pediatric to adult care. *Pediatr Clin North Am.* 2017;64(3):707–720

62. Stehouwer N, Edge P, Katie Park B, Piccone C, Little J. Acute pain in adolescents and young adults with sickle cell disease: delayed and increased opioid dosing following transition to adult care. *Am J Hematol.* 2017;92(4):E40–E42

63. Sawicki GS, Garvey KC, Toomey SL, et al. Preparation for transition to adult care among Medicaid-insured adolescents. *Pediatrics.* 2017;140(1):e20162768

64. Betz CL, Nehring WM, Lobo ML. Transition needs of parents of adolescents and emerging adults with special health care needs and disabilities. *J Fam Nurs.* 2015;21(3):362–412

65. Bindels-de Heus KG, van Staa A, van Vliet I, Ewals FV, Hilberink SR. Transferring young people with profound intellectual and multiple disabilities from pediatric to adult medical care: parents' experiences and recommendations. *Intellect Dev Disabil.* 2013;51(3):176–189

66. Cheak-Zamora NC, Teti M, Maurer-Batjer A, Koegler E. Exploration and comparison of adolescents with autism spectrum disorder and their caregiver's perspectives on transitioning to adult health care and adulthood. *J Pediatr Psychol.* 2017;42(9):1028–1039

67. Fernandes SM, O'Sullivan-Oliveira J, Landzberg MJ, et al. Transition and transfer of adolescents and young adults with pediatric onset chronic disease: the patient and parent perspective. *J Pediatr Rehabil Med.* 2014;7(1):43–51

68. Frederick NN, Bober SL, Berwick L, Tower M, Kenney LB. Preparing childhood cancer survivors for transition to adult care: the young adult perspective. *Pediatr Blood Cancer.* 2017;64(10)

69. Garvey KC, Foster NC, Agarwal S, et al. Health care transition preparation and experiences in a U.S. national sample of young adults with type 1 diabetes. *Diabetes Care.* 2017;40(3):317–324

70. Geerlings RP, Aldenkamp AP, de With PH, Zinger S, Gottmer-Welschen LM, de Louw AJ. Transition to adult medical care for adolescents with epilepsy. *Epilepsy Behav.* 2015;44:127–135

71. Gray WN, Resmini AR, Baker KD, et al. Concerns, barriers, and recommendations to improve transition from pediatric to adult IBD care: perspectives of patients, parents, and health professionals. *Inflamm Bowel Dis.* 2015;21(7):1641–1651

72. Heath G, Farre A, Shaw K. Parenting a child with chronic illness as they transition into adulthood: a systematic review and thematic synthesis of parents' experiences. *Patient Educ Couns.* 2017;100(1):76–92

73. Kuhlthau KA, Delahaye J, Erickson-Warfield M, Shui A, Crossman M, van der Weerd E. Health care transition services for youth with autism spectrum disorders: perspectives of caregivers. *Pediatrics.* 2016;137(suppl 2):S158–S166

74. Nieboer AP, Cramm JM, Sonneveld HM, Roebroeck ME, van Staa A, Strating MM. Reducing bottlenecks: professionals' and adolescents' experiences with transitional care delivery. *BMC Health Serv Res.* 2014;14:47

75. Raina R, Wang J, Sethi SK, Ferris M. Survey on health care transition services in pediatric nephrology. *Clin Exp Nephrol.* 2018;22(1):206–207

76. Rutishauser C, Sawyer SM, Ambresin AE. Transition of young people with chronic conditions: a cross-sectional study of patient perceptions before and after transfer from pediatric to adult health care. *Eur J Pediatr.* 2014;173(8):1067–1074

77. Sheehan AM, While AE, Coyne I. The experiences and impact of transition from child to adult healthcare services for young people with type 1 diabetes: a systematic review. *Diabet Med.* 2015;32(4):440–458

78. Tuchman LK, Slap GB, Britto MT. Transition to adult care: experiences and expectations of adolescents with a chronic illness. *Child Care Health Dev.* 2008;34(5):557–563

79. Timmer A, Peplies J, Westphal M, et al. Transition from pediatric to adult medical care - a survey in young persons with inflammatory bowel disease. *PLoS One.* 2017;12(5):e0177757

80. Bregnballe V, Boisen KA, Schiøtz PO, Pressler T, Lomborg K. Flying the nest: a challenge for young adults with cystic fibrosis and their parents. *Patient Prefer Adherence.* 2017;11:229–236

81. Lopez KN, Karlsten M, Bonaduce De Nigris F, et al. Understanding age-based transition needs: perspectives from adolescents and adults with congenital heart disease. *Congenit Heart Dis.* 2015;10(6):561–571

82. Philbin MM, Tanner AE, Chambers BD, et al; The Adolescent Trials Network. Transitioning HIV-infected adolescents to adult care at 14 clinics across the United States: using adolescent and adult providers' insights to create multi-level solutions to address transition barriers. *AIDS Care.* 2017;29(10):1227–1234

83. Porter JS, Wesley KM, Zhao MS, Rupff RJ, Hankins JS. Pediatric to adult care transition: perspectives of young adults with sickle cell disease. *J Pediatr Psychol.* 2017;42(9):1016–1027

84. Davidson LF, Doyle M, Silver EJ. Discussing future goals and legal aspects of health care: essential steps in transitioning youth to adult-oriented care. *Clin Pediatr (Phila).* 2017;56(10):902–908

85. Garvey KC, Telo GH, Needleman JS, Forbes P, Finkelstein JA, Laffel LM. Health care transition in young adults with type 1 diabetes: perspectives of adult endocrinologists in the U.S. *Diabetes Care.* 2016;39(2):190–197

86. Sobota AE, Shah N, Mack JW. Development of quality indicators for transition from pediatric to adult care in sickle cell disease: a modified Delphi survey of adult providers. *Pediatr Blood Cancer.* 2017;64(6)

87. Okumura MJ, Kerr EA, Cabana MD, Davis MM, Demonner S, Heisler M. Physician views on barriers to primary care for young adults with childhood-onset chronic disease. *Pediatrics.* 2010;125(4). Available at: www.pediatrics.org/cgi/content/full/125/4/e748

88. Peter NG, Forke CM, Ginsburg KR, Schwarz DF. Transition from pediatric to adult care: internists' perspectives. *Pediatrics.* 2009;123(2):417–423

89. Suh E, Daugherty CK, Wroblewski K, et al. General internists' preferences and knowledge about the care of adult survivors of childhood cancer: a cross-sectional survey. *Ann Intern Med.* 2014;160(1):11–17

90. Hunt S, Sharma N. Pediatric to adult-care transitions in childhood-onset chronic disease: hospitalist perspectives. *J Hosp Med.* 2013;8(11):627–630

91. Patel MS, O'Hare K. Residency training in transition of youth with childhood-onset chronic disease. *Pediatrics.* 2010;126(suppl 3):S190–S193

92. O'Sullivan-Oliveira J, Fernandes SM, Borges LF, Fishman LN. Transition of pediatric patients to adult care: an analysis of provider perceptions across discipline and role. *Pediatr Nurs.* 2014;40(3):113–120, 142

93. Heldman MR, Sohn MW, Gordon EJ, et al. National survey of adult transplant hepatologists on the pediatric-to-adult care transition after liver transplantation. *Liver Transpl.* 2015;21(2):213–223

94. McLaughlin SE, Machan J, Fournier P, Chang T, Even K, Sadof M. Transition of adolescents with chronic health conditions to adult primary care: factors associated with physician acceptance. *J Pediatr Rehabil Med.* 2014;7(1):63–70

95. Nakhla M, Bell LE, Wafa S, Dasgupta K. Improving the transition from pediatric to adult diabetes care: the pediatric care provider's perspective in Quebec, Canada. *BMJ Open Diabetes Res Care.* 2017;5(1):e000390

96. Nathan PC, Daugherty CK, Wroblewski KE, et al. Family physician preferences and knowledge gaps regarding the care of adolescent and young adult survivors of childhood cancer. *J Cancer Surviv.* 2013;7(3):275–282

97. Nehring WM, Betz CL, Lobo ML. Uncharted territory: systematic review of providers' roles, understanding, and views pertaining to health care transition. *J Pediatr Nurs.* 2015;30(5):732–747

98. Okumura MJ, Heisler M, Davis MM, Cabana MD, Demonner S, Kerr EA. Comfort of general internists and general pediatricians in providing care for young adults with chronic illnesses of childhood. *J Gen Intern Med.* 2008;23(10):1621–1627

99. Oskoui M, Wolfson C. Current practice and views of neurologists on the transition from pediatric to adult care. *J Child Neurol.* 2012;27(12):1553–1558

100. Sebastian S, Jenkins H, McCartney S, et al. The requirements and barriers to successful transition of adolescents with inflammatory bowel disease: differing perceptions from a survey of adult and paediatric gastroenterologists. *J Crohn's Colitis.* 2012;6(8):830–844

101. Sparud-Lundin C, Berghammer M, Moons P, Bratt EL. Health care providers' attitudes towards transfer and transition in young persons with long term illness- a web-based survey. *BMC Health Serv Res.* 2017;17(1):260

102. Szalda DE, Jimenez ME, Long JE, Ni A, Shea JA, Jan S. Healthcare system supports for young adult patients with pediatric onset chronic conditions: a qualitative study. *J Pediatr Nurs.* 2015;30(1):126–132

103. Telfair J, Alexander LR, Loosier PS, Alleman-Velez PL, Simmons J. Providers' perspectives and beliefs regarding transition to adult care for adolescents with sickle cell disease. *J Health Care Poor Underserved.* 2004;15(3):443–461

104. Wright EK, Williams J, Andrews JM, et al. Perspectives of paediatric and adult gastroenterologists on transfer and transition care of adolescents with inflammatory bowel disease. *Intern Med J.* 2014;44(5):490–496

105. Durkin ET, Zurakowski D, Rangel SJ, Lillehei CW, Fishman LN. Passing the baton: the pediatric surgical perspective on transition. *J Pediatr Surg.* 2015;50(7):1196–1200

106. Essig S, Steiner C, Kuehni CE, Weber H, Kiss A. Improving communication in adolescent cancer care: a multiperspective study. *Pediatr Blood Cancer.* 2016;63(8):1423–1430

107. Fishman LN, DiFazio R, Miller P, Shanske S, Waters PM. Pediatric orthopaedic providers' views on transition from pediatric to adult care. *J Pediatr Orthop.* 2016;36(6):e75–e80

108. Rothstein DH, Li V. Transitional care in pediatric neurosurgical patients. *Semin Pediatr Surg.* 2015;24(2):79–82

109. Ekim A, Kolay M, Ocakci AF. Readiness for transition from pediatric to adult care for adolescents with chronic heart disease. *J Spec Pediatr Nurs.* 2018;23(1)

110. White P, Cuomo C, Johnson-Hooper T, Harwood C, McManus M. Adult provider willingness to accept young adults into their practice: results from three integrated delivery systems. In: *Healthcare Transition Research Consortium Meeting*; October 26, 2016; Houston, TX

111. Gabriel P, McManus M, Rogers K, White P. Outcome evidence for structured pediatric to adult health care transition interventions: a systematic review. *J Pediatr.* 2017;188:263–269.e15

112. Campbell F, Biggs K, Aldiss SK, et al. Transition of care for adolescents from paediatric services to adult health services. *Cochrane Database Syst Rev.* 2016;4:CD009794

113. Chu PY, Maslow GR, von Isenburg M, Chung RJ. Systematic review of the impact of transition interventions for adolescents with chronic illness on transfer from pediatric to adult healthcare. *J Pediatr Nurs.* 2015;30(5):e19–e27

114. Burns K, Farrell K, Myszka R, Park K, Holmes-Walker DJ. Access to a youth-specific service for young adults with type 1 diabetes mellitus is associated with decreased hospital length of stay

for diabetic ketoacidosis. *Intern Med J.* 2018;48(4):396–402

115. Maeng DD, Snyder SR, Davis TW, Tomcavage JF. Impact of a complex care management model on cost and utilization among adolescents and young adults with special care and health needs. *Popul Health Manag.* 2017;20(6):435–441

116. Betz CL, Ferris ME, Woodward JF, Okumura MJ, Jan S, Wood DL. The health care transition research consortium health care transition model: a framework for research and practice. *J Pediatr Rehabil Med.* 2014;7(1):3–15

117. Fair C, Cuttance J, Sharma N, et al; International and Interdisciplinary Health Care Transition Research Consortium. International and interdisciplinary identification of health care transition outcomes. *JAMA Pediatr.* 2016;170(3):205–211

118. Suris JC, Akre C. Key elements for, and indicators of, a successful transition: an international Delphi study. *J Adolesc Health.* 2015;56(6):612–618

119. Coyne B, Hallowell SC, Thompson M. Measurable outcomes after transfer from pediatric to adult providers in youth with chronic illness. *J Adolesc Health.* 2017;60(1):3–16

120. Philbin MM, Tanner AE, Ma A, et al. Adolescent and adult HIV providers' definitions of HIV-infected youths' successful transition to adult care in the United States. *AIDS Patient Care STDS.* 2017;31(10):421–427

121. Pierce JS, Aroian K, Schifano E, et al. Health care transition for young adults with type 1 diabetes: stakeholder engagement for defining optimal outcomes. *J Pediatr Psychol.* 2017;42(9):970–982

122. Rachas A, Lefeuvre D, Meyer L, et al. Evaluating continuity during transfer to adult care: a systematic review. *Pediatrics.* 2016;138(1):e20160256

123. Sattoe JNT, Hilberink SR, van Staa A. How to define successful transition? An exploration of consensus indicators and outcomes in young adults with chronic conditions. *Child Care Health Dev.* 2017;43(5):768–773

124. Sharma N, O'Hare K, Antonelli RC, Sawicki GS. Transition care: future

directions in education, health policy, and outcomes research. *Acad Pediatr.* 2014;14(2):120–127

125. Davis AM, Brown RF, Taylor JL, Epstein RA, McPheeters M. Transition Care for Children With Special Health Needs. *Pediatrics.* 2014;134(5):900–908

126. Bhawra J, Toulany A, Cohen E, Moore Hepburn C, Guttmann A. Primary care interventions to improve transition of youth with chronic health conditions from paediatric to adult healthcare: a systematic review. *BMJ Open.* 2016;6(5):e011871

127. Le Roux E, Mellerio H, Guilmin-Crépon S, et al. Methodology used in comparative studies assessing programmes of transition from paediatrics to adult care programmes: a systematic review. *BMJ Open.* 2017;7(1):e012338

128. Prior M, McManus M, White P, Davidson L. Measuring the "triple aim" in transition care: a systematic review. *Pediatrics.* 2014;134(6). Available at: www.pediatrics.org/cgi/content/full/134/6/e1648

129. Vaks Y, Bensen R, Steidtmann D, et al. Better health, less spending: redesigning the transition from pediatric to adult healthcare for youth with chronic illness. *Healthc (Amst).* 2016;4(1):57–68

130. Hibbard JH, Greene J. What the evidence shows about patient activation: better health outcomes and care experiences; fewer data on costs. *Health Aff (Millwood).* 2013;32(2):207–214

131. Hibbard JH, Mahoney ER, Stockard J, Tusler M. Development and testing of a short form of the patient activation measure. *Health Serv Res.* 2005; 40(6 pt 1):1918–1930

132. Wasson J, Coleman EA. Health confidence: an essential measure for patient engagement and better practice. *Fam Pract Manag.* 2014;21(5):8–12

133. Wigfield A, Eccles JS. Expectancy-value theory of achievement motivation. *Contemp Educ Psychol.* 2000;25(1):68–81

134. Got Transition. Transition readiness. Available at: www.gottransition.org/

providers/staying-3.cfm. Accessed July 21, 2017

135. Sharma N, O'Hare K, O'Connor KG, Nehal U, Okumura MJ. Care coordination and comprehensive electronic health records are associated with increased transition planning activities. *Acad Pediatr.* 2018;18(1):111–118

136. Hagan JF, Shaw JS, Duncan PM, eds. *Bright Futures: Guidelines for Health Supervision of Infants, Children, and Adolescents.* 4th ed. Elk Grove Village, IL: American Academy of Pediatrics; 2017

137. American Academy of Family Physicians. Adolescent and young adult health. Available at: https://www.aafp.org/patient-care/public-health/adolescent-young-adult.html. Accessed March 23, 2018

138. Edman JC, Adams SH, Park MJ, Irwin CE Jr. Who gets confidential care? Disparities in a national sample of adolescents. *J Adolesc Health.* 2010;46(4):393–395

139. Ford CA. Which adolescents have opportunities to talk to doctors alone? *J Adolesc Health.* 2010;46(4): 307–308

140. Institute for Healthcare Improvement. *The Breakthrough Series: IHI's Collaborative Model for Achieving Breakthrough Improvement.* Boston, MA: Institute for Healthcare Improvement; 2003

141. McManus M, White P, Barbour A, et al. Pediatric to adult transition: a quality improvement model for primary care. *J Adolesc Health.* 2015;56(1):73–78

142. Wright C, Steinway C, Jan S. The genesis of systems of care for transition to adulthood services: emerging models in primary and subspecialty care. *Curr Opin Pediatr.* 2018;30(2):303–310

143. Byhoff E, Freund KM, Garg A. Accelerating the implementation of social determinants of health interventions in internal medicine. *J Gen Intern Med.* 2018;33(2):223–225

144. Chartier MJ, Walker JR, Naimark B. Separate and cumulative effects of adverse childhood experiences in predicting adult health and health care utilization. *Child Abuse Negl.* 2010;34(6):454–464

145. Alassaf A, Gharaibeh L, Grant C, Punthakee Z. Predictors of type 1 diabetes mellitus outcomes in young adults after transition from pediatric care. *J Diabetes*. 2017;9(12):1058–1064

146. Nguyen T, Stewart D, Gorter JW. Looking back to move forward: reflections and lessons learned about transitions to adulthood for youth with disabilities. *Child Care Health Dev*. 2018;44(1):83–88

147. Wood D, Crapnell T, Lau L, et al. In: Halfon N, Forrest CB, Lerner RM, Faustman EM, eds. *Handbook of Life Course Health Development*. Basel, Switzerland: Springer International Publishing; 2018:123–144

148. Farre A, McDonagh JE. Helping health services to meet the needs of young people with chronic conditions: towards a developmental model for transition. *Healthcare (Basel)*. 2017;5(4):E77

149. Jones MR, Robbins BW, Augustine M, et al. Transfer from pediatric to adult endocrinology. *Endocr Pract*. 2017;23(7):822–830

150. McManus M, White P, Pirtle R, Hancock C, Ablan M, Corona-Parra R. Incorporating the six core elements of health care transition into a Medicaid managed care plan: lessons learned from a pilot project. *J Pediatr Nurs*. 2015;30(5):700–713

151. Hickam T, White PH, Modrcin A, McManus M, Cox K. Implementing a nationally recognized pediatric-to-adult transitional care approach in a major children's hospital. *Health Soc Work*. 2018;43(1):3–6

152. Volertas SD, Rossi-Foulkes R. Using quality improvement in resident education to improve transition care. *Pediatr Ann*. 2017;46(5):e203–e206

153. Bilimoria KY. Facilitating quality improvement: pushing the pendulum back toward process measures. *JAMA*. 2015;314(13):1333–1334

154. Got Transition. Six core elements of health care transition. 2014. Available at: www.gottransition.org/resources/index.cfm. Accessed June 29, 2017

155. Sawicki GS, Garvey KC, Toomey SL, et al. Development and validation of the adolescent assessment of preparation for transition: a novel patient experience measure. *J Adolesc Health*. 2015;57(3):282–287

156. Got Transition. Home page. Available at: www.gottransition.org/. Accessed July 25, 2017

157. Fredericks EM, Magee JC, Eder SJ, et al. Quality improvement targeting adherence during the transition from a pediatric to adult liver transplant clinic. *J Clin Psychol Med Settings*. 2015;22(2–3):150–159

158. Langley GL, Moen R, Nolan KM, Nolan TW, Norman CL, Provost LP. *The Improvement Guide: A Practical Approach to Enhancing Organizational Performance*. 2nd ed. San Francisco, CA: Jossey-Bass; 2009

159. Mahan JD, Betz CL, Okumura MJ, Ferris ME. Self-management and transition to adult health care in adolescents and young adults: a team process. *Pediatr Rev*. 2017;38(7):305–319

160. Bolen SD, Stange KC. Investing in relationships and teams to support managing complexity. *J Gen Intern Med*. 2017;32(3):241–242

161. Katkin JP, Kressly SJ, Edwards AR, et al; Task Force on Pediatric Practice Change. Guiding principles for team-based pediatric care. *Pediatrics*. 2017:e20171489

162. Davidson LF, Chhabra R, Cohen HW, Lechuga C, Diaz P, Racine A. Pediatricians transitioning practices, youth with special health care needs in New York State. *Clin Pediatr (Phila)*. 2015;54(11):1051–1058

163. Gold JI, Boudos R, Shah P, Rossi-Foulkes R. Transition consultation models in two academic medical centers. *Pediatr Ann*. 2017;46(6):e235–e241

164. Zoni S, Verga ME, Hauschild M, et al. Patient perspectives on nurse-led consultations within a pilot structured transition program for young adults moving from an academic tertiary setting to community-based type 1 diabetes care. *J Pediatr Nurs*. 2018;38:99–105

165. Suris JC, Larbre JP, Hofer M, et al. Transition from paediatric to adult care: what makes it easier for parents? *Child Care Health Dev*. 2017;43(1):152–155

166. Kerr H, Price J, Nicholl H, O'Halloran P. Transition from children's to adult services for young adults with life-limiting conditions: a realist review of the literature. *Int J Nurs Stud*. 2017;76:1–27

167. Shah P, Boudos R. Transitions from adolescent to adult care. *Pediatr Ann*. 2012;41(2):73–78

168. Klostermann NR, McAlpine L, Wine E, Goodman KJ, Kroeker KI. Assessing the transition intervention needs of young adults with inflammatory bowel diseases. *J Pediatr Gastroenterol Nutr*. 2018;66(2):281–285

169. American College of Physicians. Homepage. Available at: https://www.acponline.org/. Accessed July 21, 2017

170. Association of Maternal & Child Health Programs, National Academy for State Health Policy, Lucile Packard Foundation for Children's Health. *Standards for Systems of Care for Children and Youth With Special Health Care Needs, Version 2.0*. Washington, DC: Association of Maternal & Child Health Programs; 2017

171. Lu MC, Lauver CB, Dykton C, et al. Transformation of the title V maternal and child health services block grant. *Matern Child Health J*. 2015;19(5):927–931

172. McManus M, Beck D. *Transition to Adult Health Care and State Title V Program Directions: A Review of 2017 Block Grant Applications*. Washington, DC: The National Alliance to Advance Adolescent Health; 2017

173. US Census Bureau. Annual estimates of the resident population: April 1, 2010 to July 1, 2016. 2016. Available at: https://factfinder.census.gov/faces/tableservices/jsf/pages/productview.xhtml?src=bkmk. Accessed September 20, 2018

174. Hemker BG, Brousseau DC, Yan K, Hoffmann RG, Panepinto JA. When children with sickle-cell disease become adults: lack of outpatient care leads to increased use of the emergency department. *Am J Hematol*. 2011;86(10):863–865

175. Ozer EM, Urquhart JT, Brindis CD, Park MJ, Irwin CE Jr. Young adult preventive health care guidelines: there but can't be found. *Arch Pediatr Adolesc Med*. 2012;166(3):240–247

176. Badawy SM, Kuhns LM. Economic evaluation of text-messaging and smartphone-based interventions to improve medication adherence in adolescents with chronic health conditions: a systematic review. *JMIR Mhealth Uhealth*. 2016;4(4):e121

177. Coyne I, Prizeman G, Sheehan A, Malone H, While AE. An e-health intervention to support the transition of young people with long-term illnesses to adult healthcare services: design and early use. *Patient Educ Couns*. 2016;99(9):1496–1504

178. Griffiths F, Bryce C, Cave J, et al. Timely digital patient-clinician communication in specialist clinical services for young people: a mixed-methods study (the LYNC study). *J Med Internet Res*. 2017;19(4):e102

179. Hausmann JS, Touloumtzis C, White MT, Colbert JA, Gooding HC. Adolescent and young adult use of social media for health and its implications. *J Adolesc Health*. 2017;60(6):714–719

180. Los E, Ulrich J, Guttmann-Bauman I. Technology use in transition-age patients with type 1 diabetes: reality and promises. *J Diabetes Sci Technol*. 2016;10(3):662–668

181. Raymond JK. Models of care for adolescents and young adults with type 1 diabetes in transition: shared medical appointments and telemedicine. *Pediatr Ann*. 2017;46(5):e193–e197

182. Hardin AP, Hackell JM; Committee on Practice and Ambulatory Medicine. Age limit of pediatrics. *Pediatrics*. 2017;140(3):e20172151

183. US Government Accountability Office. *Youth With Autism: Roundtable Views of Services Needed During the Transition Into Adulthood*. Washington, DC: US Government Accountability Office; 2016

184. Anderson KA, Sosnowy C, Kuo AA, Shattuck PT. Transition of individuals with autism to adulthood: a review of qualitative studies. *Pediatrics*. 2018;141(suppl 4):S318–S327

185. Nathenson RA, Zablotsky B. The transition to the adult health care system among youths with autism spectrum disorder. *Psychiatr Serv*. 2017;68(7):735–738

186. van Schalkwyk GI, Volkmar FR. Autism spectrum disorders: challenges and opportunities for transition to adulthood. In: Martel A, Fuchs DC, eds. *Transitional Age Youth and Mental Illness: Influences on Young Adult Outcomes*. Philadelphia, PA: Elsevier; 2017:329–340

187. Walsh C, Jones B, Schonwald A. Health care transition planning among adolescents with autism spectrum disorder. *J Autism Dev Disord*. 2017;47(4):980–991

188. Abidi S. Paving the way to change for youth at the gap between child and adolescent and adult mental health services. *Can J Psychiatry*. 2017;62(6):388–392

189. McConachie H, Hoole S, Le Couteur AS. Improving mental health transitions for young people with autism spectrum disorder. *Child Care Health Dev*. 2011;37(6):764–766

190. Nguyen T, Embrett MG, Barr NG, et al. Preventing youth from falling through the cracks between child/adolescent and adult mental health services: a systematic review of models of care. *Community Ment Health J*. 2017;53(4):375–382

191. Paul M, Street C, Wheeler N, Singh SP. Transition to adult services for young people with mental health needs: a systematic review. *Clin Child Psychol Psychiatry*. 2015;20(3):436–457

192. Signorini G, Singh SP, Marsanic VB, et al; MILESTONE Consortium. The interface between child/adolescent and adult mental health services: results from a European 28-country survey. *Eur Child Adolesc Psychiatry*. 2018;27(4):501–511

193. Singh SP, Tuomainen H. Transition from child to adult mental health services: needs, barriers, experiences and new models of care. *World Psychiatry*. 2015;14(3):358–361

194. McManus M, White P. Transition to adult health care services for young adults with chronic medical illness and psychiatric comorbility. In: Martel A, Fuchs DC, eds. *Transitional Age Youth and Mental Illness: Influences on Young Adult Outcomes*. Philadelphia, PA: Elsevier; 2017:367–380

195. Cohen E, Berry JG, Sanders L, Schor EL, Wise PH. Status complexicus? The emergence of pediatric complex care. *Pediatrics*. 2018;141(suppl 3):S202–S211

196. Kuo DZ, Houtrow AJ; Council on Children With Disabilities. Recognition and management of medical complexity. *Pediatrics*. 2016;138(6):e20163021

197. Cohen E, Kuo DZ, Agrawal R, et al. Children with medical complexity: an emerging population for clinical and research initiatives. *Pediatrics*. 2011;127(3):529–538

198. Rogers SM. Transitional age lesbian, gay, bisexual, transgender, and questioning youth: issues of diversity, integrated identities, and mental health. In: Martel A, Fuchs DC, eds. *Transitional Age Youth and Mental Illness: Influences on Young Adult Outcomes*. Philadelphia, PA: Elsevier; 2017:297–310

199. Bisgaier J, Rhodes KV. Auditing access to specialty care for children with public insurance. *N Engl J Med*. 2011;364(24):2324–2333

200. DeBaun MR, Telfair J. Transition and sickle cell disease. *Pediatrics*. 2012;130(5):926–935

201. Kang-Yi CD, Adams DR. Youth with behavioral health disorders aging out of foster care: a systematic review and implications for policy, research, and practice. *J Behav Health Serv Res*. 2017;44(1):25–51

202. Lee T, Morgan W. Transitioning to adulthood from foster care. In: Martel A, Fuchs DC, eds. *Transitional Age Youth and Mental Illness: Influences on Young Adult Outcomes*. Philadelphia, PA: Elsevier; 2017:283–296

203. Kuo AA, Ciccarelli MR, Sharma N, Lotstein DS. A health care transition curriculum for primary care residents: identifying goals and objectives. *Pediatrics*. 2018;141(suppl 4):S346–S354

204. Mennito S. Resident preferences for a curriculum in healthcare transitions for young adults. *South Med J*. 2012;105(9):462–466

205. Chung RJ, Jasien J, Maslow GR. Resident dyads providing transition care to adolescents and young

adults with chronic illnesses and neurodevelopmental disabilities. *J Grad Med Educ.* 2017;9(2):222–227

206. Coles MS, Greenberg KB. The time is here: a comprehensive curriculum for adolescent health teaching and learning from the Society for Adolescent Health and Medicine. *J Adolesc Health.* 2017;61(2):129–130

207. Michaud PA, Schrier L, Ross-Russel R, et al. Paediatric departments need to improve residents' training in adolescent medicine and health: a position paper of the European Academy of Paediatrics. *Eur J Pediatr.* 2018;177(4):479–487

208. American Academy of Pediatrics. Homepage. Available at: https://www. aap.org/. Accessed July 21, 2017

209. Fishman L. But Tommy likes it here: moving to adult medicine. 2012. Available at: www.mededportal.org/ publication/9190. Accessed July 21, 2017

210. Pilapil M, DeLaet DE, Kuo AA, Peacock C, Sharma N, eds. *Care of Adults With Chronic Childhood Conditions: A Practical Guide.* Basel, Switzerland: Springer International Publishing; 2016

211. North American Society for Pediatric Gastroenterology, Hepatology, and Nutrition (NASPGHAN). Home page. Available at: www.naspghan.org. Accessed July 21, 2017

212. American Academy of Pediatrics. Illinois chapter. Welcome to ICAAP online. Available at: https://icaap. remote-learner.net/. Accessed July 27, 2017

213. Hudak ML, Helm ME, White PH; Committee on Child Health Financing. Principles of child health care financing. *Pediatrics.* 2017;140(3):e20172098

214. Centers for Medicare & Medicaid Services; US Department of Health and Human Services. Medicare program; revisions to payment policies under the physician fee schedule and other revisions to part B for CY 2018; Medicare shared savings program

requirements; and Medicare diabetes prevention program. Final rule. *Fed Regist.* 2017;82(219):52976–53371

215. Stinson J, Kohut SA, Spiegel L, et al. A systematic review of transition readiness and transfer satisfaction measures for adolescents with chronic illness. *Int J Adolesc Health Med.* 201426;159–174

216. Wood DL, Sawicki GS, Miller DM, et al. Factor structure, reliability and validity of the Transition Readiness Assessment Questionnaire (TRAQ). *Acad Pediatr.* 2014:14:415–422

217. Moynihan M, Saewyc E, Whitehouse S, Paone M, McPherson G. Assessing readiness for transition from paediatric to adult health care: revision and psychometric evaluation of the Am I ON TRAC for Adult Care questionnaire. *J Adv Nurs.* 2015;71(6):1324–1335

218. Ferris ME, Harward DH, Bickford K, et al. A clinical tool to measure the components of health-care transition from pediatric care to adult care: the UNC TR(x)ANSITION scale. *Ren Fail.* 2012;34(6):744–753

219. Cohen SE, Hooper SR, Javalkar K, et al. Self-management and transition readiness assessment: concurrent, predictive and discriminant validation of the STARx questionnaire. *J Pediatr Nurs.* 2015;30(5):668–676

220. Nazareth M, Hart L, Ferris M, Rak E, Hooper S, van Tilburg MAL. A parental report of youth transition readiness: the parent STARx questionnaire (STARx-P) and re-evaluation of the STARx child report. *J Pediatr Nurs.* 2018;38:122–126

221. Klassen AF, Grant C, Barr R, et al. Development and validation of a generic scale for use in transition programmes to measure self-management skills in adolescents with chronic health conditions: the TRANSITION-Q. *Child Care Health Dev.* 2015;41(4):547–558

222. Wiemann CM, Hergenroeder AC, Bartley KA, et al. Integrating an EMR-based transition planning tool for CYSHCN

at a children's hospital: a quality improvement project to increase provider use and satisfaction. *J Pediatr Nurs.* 2015;30(5):776–787

223. Betz CL. California healthy and ready to work transition health care guide: developmental guidelines for teaching health care self-care skills to children. *Issues Compr Pediatr Nurs.* 2000;23(4):203–244

224. Bomba F, Markwart H, Muhlan H, et al. Adaptation and validation of the German Patient Activation Measure for adolescents with chronic conditions in transitional care: PAM® 13 for adolescents. *Res Nurs Health.* 2018;41(1):78–87

225. McManus M, White P, Harwood C, Molteni R, Kanter D, Salus T. 2018 coding and reimbursement tip sheet for transition from pediatric to adult health care. 2018. Available at: www. gottransition.org/resourceGet.cfm?id= 353. Accessed October 1, 2018

226. McManus M, White P, Schmidt A. *Recommendations for Value-Based Transition Payment for Pediatric and Adult Health Care Systems: A Leadership Roundtable Report.* Washington, DC: The National Alliance to Advance Adolescent Health; 2018

227. White P, Schmidt A, McManus M, Irwin CE Jr. *Incorporating Health Care Transition Services Into Preventive Care for Adolescents and Young Adults: A Toolkit for Clinicians.* Washington, DC: Got Transition; 2018

228. Harwood C, McManus M, White P. *Incorporating Pediatric-to-Adult Transition Into NCQA Patient-Centered Medical Home Recognition.* Washington, DC: Got Transition; 2017

229. Stevenson R, Moore DE Jr. Ascent to the summit of the CME pyramid. *JAMA.* 2018;319(6):543–544

230. Stille CJ, Antonelli RC, Spencer K, et al. *Aligning Services With Needs: Characterizing the Pyramid of Complexity Tiering for Children With Chronic and Complex Conditions.* Palo Alto, CA: Lucile Packard Foundation for Children's Health; 2018

Targeted Reforms in Health Care Financing to Improve the Care of Adolescents and Young Adults

- *Policy Statement*

POLICY STATEMENT Organizational Principles to Guide and Define the Child Health Care System and/or Improve the Health of all Children

American Academy
of Pediatrics

DEDICATED TO THE HEALTH OF ALL CHILDREN™

Targeted Reforms in Health Care Financing to Improve the Care of Adolescents and Young Adults

Arik V. Marcell, MD, MPH, FAAP,[a] Cora C. Breuner, MD, MPH, FAAP,[b] Lawrence Hammer, MD, FAAP,[c] Mark L. Hudak, MD, FAAP,[d] COMMITTEE ON ADOLESCENCE, COMMITTEE ON CHILD HEALTH FINANCING

abstract

Significant changes have occurred in the commercial and government insurance marketplace after the passage of 2 federal legislation acts, the Patient Protection and Affordable Care Act of 2010 and the Paul Wellstone and Pete Domenici Mental Health Parity and Addiction Equity Act of 2008. Despite the potential these 2 acts held to improve the health care of adolescents and young adults (AYAs), including the financing of care, there are barriers to achieving this goal. In the first quarter of 2016, 13.7% of individuals 18 to 24 years of age still lacked health insurance. Limitations in the scope of benefits coverage and inadequate provider payment can curtail access to health care for AYAs, particularly care related to sexual and reproductive health and mental and behavioral health. Some health plans impose financial barriers to access because they require families to absorb high cost-sharing expenses (eg, deductibles, copayments, and coinsurance). Finally, challenges of confidentiality inherent in the billing and insurance claim practices of some health insurance plans can discourage access to health care in the absence of other obstacles and interfere with provision of confidential care. This policy statement summarizes the current state of impediments that AYA, including those with special health care needs, face in accessing timely and appropriate health care and that providers face in serving these patients. These impediments include limited scope of benefits, high cost sharing, inadequate provider payment, and insufficient confidentiality protections. With this statement, we aim to improve both access to health care by AYAs and providers' delivery of developmentally appropriate health care for these patients through the presentation of an overview of the issues, specific recommendations for reform of health care financing for AYAs, and practical actions that pediatricians and other providers can take to advocate for appropriate payments for providing health care to AYAs.

Departments of [a]Pediatrics and Population, Family and Reproductive Health, Johns Hopkins University, Baltimore, Maryland; [b]Division of Adolescent Medicine, Department of Pediatrics, Seattle Children's Hospital and University of Washington, Seattle, Washington; [c]Department of Pediatrics, School of Medicine, Stanford University, Stanford, California; and [d]Department of Pediatrics, College of Medicine – Jacksonville, University of Florida, Jacksonville, Florida

Drs Marcell and Hammer wrote the initial draft and contributed to subsequent revisions; Drs Breuner and Hudak amplified the draft by adding sections, details, and footnotes and by revising draft text; Members of the Committee on Adolescence and the Committee on Child Health Financing provided guidance on content and key edits; Dr Hudak revised the statement to reflect input from American Academy of Pediatrics committees, sections, and councils and from the American Academy of Pediatrics Board of Directors; and all authors reviewed and approved the final manuscript as submitted.

To cite: Marcell AV, Breuner CC, Hammer L, et al AAP COMMITTEE ON ADOLESCENCE, AAP COMMITTEE ON CHILD HEALTH FINANCING. Targeted Reforms in Health Care Financing to Improve the Care of Adolescents and Young Adults. *Pediatrics.* 2018;142(6):e20182998

INTRODUCTION

Adolescence and young adulthood are critical developmental periods characterized by distinct physical, psychological, cognitive, and social changes. Primary care providers can play important roles in promoting healthy behaviors and lifestyles for adolescents and young adults (AYAs) and their families. During this transition into adulthood, AYAs develop autonomy and may adopt high-risk behaviors that can cause serious and preventable morbidity and even mortality.[1,2] Timely prevention and treatment of these problems during this transition can change the trajectory of health into adulthood and reduce unnecessary costs to the patient, family, and health care system.

Provider-initiated screening for physical and mental health conditions, early disease identification and prevention, health promotion, and anticipatory guidance are critical components of routine care for AYAs.[3,4] The cornerstone of clinical prevention is the periodic health supervision visit, the elements of which are detailed by *Bright Futures: Guidelines for Health Supervision of Infants, Children, and Adolescents, Fourth Edition.*[5] The National Committee for Quality Assurance, through its Health Employer Data and Information System, continues to affirm the importance of well-care visits for patients 12 to 21 years of age in its 2019 metrics.[6] Delivery of routine clinical preventive services to all AYAs, including those with special health care needs, encompasses screening for physical and mental health conditions and risk behaviors and has been shown to identify individuals who are more likely to engage in high-risk behaviors.[7,8] Payment reform can eliminate barriers to providers' delivery of such care by paying fairly for services provided and by covering benefits that are critical for AYAs. In addition, payers should eliminate

patient barriers to seeking care, such as concerns about breaches of confidentiality or excessive cost sharing for preventive services.

There have been significant changes in the commercial and government insurance marketplace after the passage of 2 important pieces of federal legislation. The Patient Protection and Affordable Care Act of 2010 (ACA) (Pub L No. 111-148) created substantial improvements in insurance coverage for AYAs by allowing parents to extend coverage for their dependent children until their 26th birthday, precluding denials for preexisting conditions, eliminating copays and deductibles for certain preventive health maintenance services, and setting a framework for extending Medicaid to thousands of previously uninsured individuals. The ACA exempted some health plans from some key ACA reforms, including certain governmental plans and many individual and group plans that were in effect before the law was enacted on March 23, 2010 (so-called "grandfathered" plans), as long as specific features of these plans did not change.* The Paul Wellstone

---

* The ACA treated "grandfathered" plans differently than any new individual or group plan that became effective after March 23, 2010. The ACA required grandfathered plans to cover adult children up to the age of 26 but did not require free preventive care, coverage of all the essential health benefits outlined in the ACA, or coverage of preexisting conditions. New plans that became effective after March 23, 2010, but before October 1, 2013 (so-called "grandmothered" plans), were required to provide preventive care without cost sharing but still had no mandate to cover all essential health benefits or to insure preexisting conditions. Grandmothered plans initially were required to terminate by December 31, 2013, with a pathway to transition to a fully compliant ACA plan. This date was later extended by 4 years to December 31, 2017. Enrollment in grandfathered plans has been decreasing over time. By 2015, only 25% of workers with employee-sponsored insurance were enrolled in a grandfathered plan. By 1 estimate, only 400 000 enrollees will continue to be covered by grandfathered non-ACA individual plans. Some insurance carriers have terminated grandfathered plans in various states.

and Pete Domenici Mental Health Parity and Addiction Equity Act of 2008 (Part C of Pub L No. 110-343) implemented parity in payments for medical and behavioral health services, the latter of which has often been covered at lower payment rates.

This policy statement discusses improvements in health care financing for AYAs aimed at mitigating the following existing barriers: (1) continued uninsurance; (2) variability in benefit structures across insurance plans; (3) adverse impact of cost sharing; (4) inadequate provider payment for health care services; and (5) insufficient confidentiality protections for billing and insurance claims.

CONTINUED UNINSURANCE AMONG AYAs

Comprehensive and affordable health insurance for AYAs is vital. According to data reported by the Centers for Disease Control and Prevention, in 2015, the rate of uninsurance among children and adolescents from birth to 18 years of age was 5%, and the rate of uninsurance among young adults between 18 and 24 years of age was 14.1%.[9] Although these rates are an improvement over the previous 3-year period, a significant number of AYAs remain uninsured. Uninsurance rates also vary from state to state, with substantially higher rates for individuals 18 to 64 years of age in states that have not accepted Medicaid expansion under the ACA.† In addition, young men

---

† As of February 2016, 19 states had chosen not to take advantage of the ACA Medicaid expansion, thereby excluding many eligible uninsured adults 18 to 64 years of age from Medicaid coverage, after the 2012 Supreme Court's ruling that allowed states to opt out of this federally funded opportunity.[22] As a result, the percentage of uninsured adults fell by ~50% (from 18.4% to 9.4%) between 2013 and the first half of 2016 in Medicaid expansion states, whereas a more modest decline from 22.7% to 17.5% ensued in nonexpansion states.[51]

are more likely to be uninsured than young women.[10]

In states that have opted to expand Medicaid, many uninsured young adults obtained their initial health insurance in this program. A recent study has revealed that children in families in which young adult parents have enrolled in Medicaid are 29% more likely to receive preventive annual well-child visits.[11]

VARIABILITY IN BENEFIT STRUCTURES ACROSS INSURANCE PLANS

Provisions to improve preventive and other health care benefits for AYAs are vital, especially with mandates that employer-based plans insure dependents up to 26 years of age (variably interpreted to mean the 26th birthday or the end of the calendar year in which the 26th birthday falls). The latter provision addressed the phenomenon of "aging out" of coverage after age 18 or 19 that was a primary reason for lack of insurance coverage during the young adult years before passage of the ACA.[12] The ACA also states that all nonexempt health plans (ie, grandfathered and grandmothered plans) cover 10 essential health benefit classes for all enrollees:

1. ambulatory services;

2. emergency services;

3. hospitalization;

4. maternity and newborn care;

5. mental health and substance use disorder services, including behavioral health treatment;

6. prescription drugs;

7. rehabilitative and habilitative services and devices;

8. laboratory services;

9. preventive and wellness services and chronic disease management; and

10. pediatric services.

The last category of pediatrics services is incompletely defined but does include a prescription to cover oral and vision care.[13]

The ACA mandates coverage of clinical preventive services for AYAs on the basis of recommendations in *Bright Futures: Guidelines for Health Supervision of Infants, Children, and Adolescents*, including immunizations for children younger than 18 years and, as recommended by the US Preventive Services Task Force, for young adults 18 years and older. The ACA also mandates coverage for women's reproductive services, including contraception, without copays or deductibles, as recommended by the Institute of Medicine (now the National Academy of Medicine) in its report "Clinical Preventive Services for Women: Closing the Gaps"[14] and adopted by the US Health Resources and Services Administration.[15]

Despite recommendations to adopt a single, comprehensive, preemptive federal standard in implementing the essential health benefit statute,[16] the US Department of Health and Human Services elected to use a variation of the Children's Health Insurance Program (CHIP) benchmark strategy.[17] The authors of 1 study reported that no state specified a distinct pediatric services benefit class.[18] Although some benchmark plans explicitly included multiple pediatric conditions, many plans also exclude services on which children with special health care needs may rely, thereby leading to a state-by-state patchwork of coverage with exclusions.[18]

Although the ACA offered the potential to reduce barriers to the delivery and receipt of clinical preventive services if screening were to be incorporated into health supervision visits,[12] disparities in coverage across all health care plans persist and contribute to disparities in access to care as well as care delivery. In addition, some states legally offer only a "minimal health benefit" (excluding benefits available in Medicaid and some commercial health care plans) through their own ACA exchanges. For behavioral health services, use of carve-out arrangements continues to limit access to and thus receipt of behavioral health services because of insufficient numbers of appropriate providers in the contracted networks (see discussion of behavioral health services, below, for more details).

ADVERSE IMPACT OF COST SHARING

The ACA established rules regarding cost sharing and the actuarial value of health plans (the percent of medical costs an average person can expect the plan to cover versus the percent of costs the patient must cover through a combination of deductibles, copayments, and coinsurance); however, it can still be difficult for patients to predict how much they are expected to pay for health supervision visits (ie, well-child visits). Although all ACA-compliant plans must provide certain preventive care services at no cost to the beneficiary, ACA-exempt plans may require substantial cost sharing for preventive care,[19] thereby discouraging access to these services.

Although health care use highly correlates with insurance coverage,[20] having insurance does not necessarily guarantee use of health care services.[21] Publicly and privately insured AYAs may not have certain benefits in categories that the ACA labels as "essential" (including behavioral health benefits) or may have difficulty paying deductible, copay, and coinsurance costs. As an extreme example, "catastrophic" health insurance plans that are available on the federal healthcare. gov marketplace exchanges can be purchased at low premiums but carry a high individual out-of-pocket maximum (currently $6850). These catastrophic plans were selected by almost 30 000 AYAs during the enrollment period of November 2015 through February 2016, thereby leaving these AYAs or their parents with almost complete financial responsibility beyond certain preventive services and 3 primary care visits per year.[22]

Over the last decade, the number of high-deductible health plans (HDHPs) has also steadily increased. HDHPs decrease the insurance policy premium costs for purchasers and shift the risk of further payments to the individual subscriber. The high deductibles and other out-of-pocket expenses associated with these plans result in the inability to access care or delays in needed care because of a prohibitive cost to the insured and generate high medical debt for families when care has been accessed.[23] Although HDHPs are designed to reduce use and total medical costs in the short-term, out-of-pocket costs for primary care and other outpatient services may increase total health care costs in the long-term.[24]

INADEQUATE PROVIDER PAYMENT FOR AYA SERVICES

Despite the fact that Medicaid, CHIP, and ACA plans are now mandated to pay for the full *Current Procedural Terminology* (CPT) expense of some number of preventive visits per year with no cost sharing, they are not required to pay separately for other potential components of the visit. Indeed, a plan may require that these separate components are bundled with the visit code, thereby not paying the provider/practice for the expenses of these additional services. Grandfathered non-ACA plans may impose deductibles and copays for well visits and all of their components (including vaccines) and can still charge copays for any individual component (such as vaccines) or even exclude specific components from coverage. In addition, payments to different providers for the same services by a given payer will vary depending on

the leverage the provider can bring to bear during contract negotiations. Providers with smaller patient panels, with higher cost attribution, or with lower quality metrics are disadvantaged with respect to payment schedules.

Payment levels by many governmental and private health care plans do not appropriately pay for the time and effort providers need to deliver services to AYAs.[25] For example, Medicaid payments for evaluation and management services average less than 80% of Medicare's payment.[26] An increase in Medicaid payment to office-based primary care pediatricians to Medicare levels, as was transiently achieved as mandated by the ACA in 2013–2014, did increase physician participation.[27] The American Academy of Pediatrics (AAP) Committee on Coding and Nomenclature recommends that the Resource-Based Relative Value Scale, a system of valuing physician services by using relative value units, should accurately reflect the resources expended in providing recommended care, including consideration of the complexity of both cognitive and procedural physician work, comprehensive practice expense, and professional liability insurance expense.[28] Policy makers and payers need to ensure that payment for AYA preventive care services are appropriately covered and paid for adequately.

Other issues further complicate payment for providers' delivery of preventive services. Some plans do not adhere to CPT guidelines, do not pay individually for specific services (eg, they may bundle separate procedure codes into 1), do not cover CPT billing codes for health education or chronic care management, may restrict coverage of certain diagnostic codes, or have complex and variable coding requirements. Payment for non–face-to-face services, such as telephone calls and e-mails,

for nonchronic conditions is also variable or nonexistent.

Providers should become familiar, if not already, with best billing and coding practices for adolescent care.[29] Importantly, providers may choose to bill for added time spent on specific identified problems (eg, an acute condition or a condition identified during a screening) during a health maintenance visit using a −25 modifier and the pertinent diagnostic codes as part of the billing process. However, this may subject patients to unexpected copays and higher out-of-pocket costs.

At some point, providers face the challenge of transitioning some or all aspects of the care of AYA to other providers who care for adults. Recommendations for best coding and payment procedures for these activities are available at http://www.gottransition.org/resourceGet.cfm?id=352.

Specific challenges to the delivery of behavioral health and sexual and reproductive health services remain for providers of care to AYAs. These specific aspects of care merit in-depth discussion, including the delivery of behavioral health services (including care for mental health problems, eating disorders, and substance use disorder) and the delivery of sexual and reproductive health services.

For behavioral health services, the Paul Wellstone and Pete Dominici Mental Health Parity and Addiction Equity Act of 2008 (Pub L No. 110-343), further expanded in 2013, requires that qualifying financial requirements and coverage limitations be no more restrictive for mental health benefits than any other health benefits, that no separate qualifying criteria may be applied, and that the same level of out-of-network coverage must be available for mental health, substance use, and medical or surgical benefits. As of yet, not all states have implemented full parity of coverage for mental health disorders or only require limited parity linked to severity of illness or a limited range of disorders, thereby allowing discrepancies in the form of visit limits, copays, deductibles, annual and lifetime limits, treatment caps, or more stringent medical necessity standards to be placed on mental health than on other aspects of health care.[30] Plans are often not clear about which inpatient and outpatient mental health services are covered. Patients may not learn that a service is not covered until a submitted charge is denied after initiation of treatment.[30]

Eligibility for new enrollees under Medicaid expansion may not be equivalent to traditional Medicaid benefits, yet it can include a lower level of "benchmark-equivalent" coverage, which translates to gaps in coverage for newly insured individuals with mental illness conditions and substance use disorders.[31] Low payment rates and service carve-out arrangements further limit mental health and substance use disorder treatment access and care. People with mental health disorders have been more likely to be covered by public than private insurance.[32] However, inadequate payment for these services by many Medicaid and CHIP plans reduces the number of mental health clinicians who participate.[33]

Insurers also "carve out" services that are included in the benefit package to a contracted third party, especially in the area of behavioral health. Plans may carve out specific diagnoses (eg, depression, substance use disorder) or a class of patients (eg, patients with "serious mental illness"). This can occur at the payer (primary carve-out) or health plan (secondary carve-out) level. Patients may be placed under highly restrictive, managed care programs for behavioral health. These arrangements can

limit access to appropriate care, both because members may have difficulty in understanding how to achieve access and because the number of appropriate contracted providers may be insufficient. According to a report published online by Open Minds in 2014, 14 states contracted with managed care organizations (MCOs) for fully integrated behavioral and physical health benefits; 11 states contracted with MCOs for fully integrated behavioral and physical health benefits but carved out 1 behavioral health benefit category, such as substance use disorder or psychiatric inpatient care; 16 states carved out all behavioral health benefits from their MCO contracts or fee-for-service systems; and 10 states operated primarily fee-for-service systems of coverage with minimal managed care or primary care case management.[34] Children and youth with special health care needs enrolled in state Medicaid plans that carve out behavioral health coverage experienced greater unmet behavioral health care needs than children in plans that did not.[33]

In recognition of the need for primary care clinicians' expanded role in the identification and management of behavioral health disorders, the AAP published extensive guidance in a supplement to *Pediatrics* in 2010.[35] The AAP has developed recommendations that help practices to overcome the significant administrative and financial barriers to providing behavioral health care in the primary care setting.[36] The AAP has also issued a call to action for the payer community for all children and AYAs to have access to mental health services, insurance coverage for mental health care, and payment systems that ensure appropriate payment to pediatricians.[37]

For sexual and reproductive health services, after passage of the ACA,

women's access to a full range of contraception methods has improved and expenses related to cost-sharing have decreased. Many female AYAs now have increased access to preventive sexual and reproductive health services[38] under the ACA, which should include provision of the full range of contraception methods without cost sharing. Initial data indicate that after ACA implementation, the mean and median per prescription out-of-pocket expenses have decreased for almost all reversible contraceptive methods on the market.[37] Out-of-pocket spending for oral contraceptive pill prescriptions and intrauterine device insertions by women using those methods has decreased by 20%.[39]

Even after implementation of the ACA's coverage expansions, safety-net family planning clinics continue to see millions of women, men, and adolescents.[40] Research by the National Women's Law Center has reported that insurance companies are (1) not providing coverage for methods of birth control approved by the Food and Drug Administration or are imposing out-of-pocket costs for them; (2) providing payment only for generic oral contraceptives; and (3) failing to cover the services associated with birth control without out-of-pocket costs, including counseling or follow-up visits.[41] Other violations of the ACA's birth control benefit included plans not having a required waiver process, failing to cover sterilization for dependents, imposing age limits on coverage, and adopting other policies that in effect deny or restrict coverage of birth control.

Finally, contraceptive methods used by males, especially condoms, were excluded from the ACA's guarantee of contraceptive coverage without out-of-pocket costs, despite their proven health benefits.[42]

INSUFFICIENT CONFIDENTIALITY PROTECTIONS FOR BILLING AND INSURANCE CLAIMS PRACTICES

Few insurers have adjusted their administrative and billing systems to protect adolescent confidentiality. Regulations governing those systems may vary from state to state, with some states now mandating changes in explanations of benefits (EOBs) to protect confidentiality.[43,44] Historically, a number of barriers prevent or limit confidentiality in billing practices of insured adolescents.[44,45] With ACA insurance expansion covering dependents through the age of 26 years, issues regarding confidential care now affect young adults 18 years and older, who have traditionally been protected by Health Insurance Portability and Accountability Act privacy laws.[44,46]

Inadvertent breaches of confidentiality for AYAs covered by their parents' private insurance plans occurs commonly because of information available via patient portals that link with electronic medical records, EOBs sent to the primary policy holder (including parents), requests for additional information about a claim, actual payment of claims, and claims made in cases of divorce and child custody disputes.[46] Some of the issues contributing to these breaches include (1) use of protected health information under the Health Insurance Portability and Accountability Act to secure payment, even in the absence of specific authorization from the patient; (2) disclosures contained in EOBs that make it impossible for an individual covered as a dependent to obtain care confidentially; and (3) the standard industry practice for insurers to communicate solely, or primarily, with the designated policy holder, thereby permitting access to all information about claims filed via the insurer's Web site.

Some states have fee-for-service payment mechanisms or carve-outs to reimburse providers for confidential care, although most do not.[41] Use of such an approach can allow for compensation of providers of care to AYAs seeking services, including services related to sexual and reproductive health, behavioral health, substance use, pregnancy, and abortion.

CONCLUSIONS

Significant health care needs of all AYAs, including those with disabilities, may not be met because of a number of factors, including continued uninsurance, deficiencies in scope of benefits, high cost sharing, inadequate provider payments, and insufficient confidentiality protections despite passage of 2 important pieces of federal legislation, the Paul Wellstone and Pete Dominici Mental Health Parity and Addiction Equity Act and the ACA. Clear definition of broader essential health benefits for AYAs and better alignment of provider payments with the cost of services will catalyze increased availability of key clinical care and preventive services that may improve the overall current and future health and well-being of AYAs. Reducing cost sharing for key services other than an annual preventive visit, as well as implementation of effective billing and claims procedures that maintain confidentiality, will encourage AYAs to obtain needed care. These interventions work to improve financing for health care that can lead to improving AYAs' access to and receipt of health care, to achieving better compliance and lessen financial challenges for providers delivering recommended AAP care guidelines, and to alleviating the hardship of high out-of-pocket expenses that may ration essential care.[5,47–50]

RECOMMENDATIONS

The AAP recommends the following strategies targeted at improving financing for the health care of AYAs:

1. Federal and state agencies should increase their efforts to further reduce the number of AYAs who are not insured or who lack comprehensive and affordable health insurance. An important fact that AAP members can use during advocacy activities with policy makers is that states that have adopted Medicaid expansion have witnessed, on average, a greater reduction in uninsurance rates for young adults ages 19 to 26 years than have states that have chosen not to participate.

2. The Centers for Medicare and Medicaid Services should implement its regulatory authority to update its standards for essential health benefits, as defined in the ACA, in the 2 categories of mental and behavioral health services and pediatric services. These essential health benefits should be consistent with the full scope of benefits outlined in *Bright Futures: Guidelines for Health Supervision of Infants, Children, and Adolescents, Fourth Edition* (including health supervision visits, nationally recommended immunizations, screening for high-risk conditions, and adequate counseling and treatment of conditions related to sexual and reproductive health, mental and behavioral health, and substance use disorder). In this way, all AYAs can access the full range of services needed during this developmentally critical period to secure optimal physical and mental health as they enter middle adulthood.

3. All health plans should provide preventive services without member cost sharing. In addition, to reduce financial barriers to care for AYAs, payers should limit the

burden on families by reducing or eliminating copayments and eliminating coinsurance for visits related to anticipatory guidance and/or treatment of sexual and reproductive health, behavioral health, and immunization visits.

4. To provide sufficient payment to physicians and other health care providers for medical services to AYAs, insurers' claims systems should recognize and pay for all preventive medicine CPT codes related to services for health and behavior assessment, counseling, risk screening, and/or appropriate interventions as recommended in *Bright Futures*. These services should not be bundled under a single health maintenance CPT code.

5. Government and private insurance payers should increase the relative value unit allocation and level of payment for practitioners delivering care and clinical preventive services to AYAs to a level that is commensurate with the time and effort expended, including health maintenance services, screening, and counseling.

6. The Centers for Medicare and Medicaid Services should mandate that payers provide enhanced access to cost effective and clinically sound behavioral health services for AYAs, ensure that payment for all mental health services is more equitable with payment provided for medical or surgical services, and ensure that primary care providers

are paid for mental health services provided during health maintenance and follow-up visits.

7. There is an ethical and regulatory imperative that private and government insurance plans develop and implement unique billing and claims strategies that ensure AYAs can obtain care with full protection of their confidentiality for appropriate services.

8. The Centers for Medicare and Medicaid Services, together with state agencies, should invest in tracking the impact of the ACA on care of AYAs by monitoring insurance rates, access and delivery of services, coverage, costs, payment, and confidentiality protections, especially those related to billing and insurance claims practices for medically sensitive services.

LEAD AUTHORS

Arik V. Marcell, MD, MPH, FAAP
Cora C. Breuner, MD, MPH, FAAP
Lawrence Hammer, MD, FAAP
Mark L. Hudak, MD, FAAP

COMMITTEE ON ADOLESCENCE, 2017–2018

Cora C. Breuner, MD, MPH, FAAP, Chairperson
Elizabeth M. Alderman, MD, FAAP, FSHAM
Laura K. Grubb, MD, FAAP
Makia E. Powers, MD, MPH, FAAP
Krishna Upadhya, MD, FAAP
Stephenie Wallace, MD, FAAP

LIAISONS

Laurie Hornberger, MD, MPH, FAAP — *Section on Adolescent Health*
Liwei Hua, MD, PhD — *American Academy of Child and Adolescent Psychiatry*
Margo Lane, MD, FRCPC, FAAP — *Canadian Paediatric Society*
Meredith Loveless, MD, FACOG — *American College of Obstetricians and Gynecologists*
Seema Menon, MD — *North American Society for Pediatric and Adolescent Gynecology*
Lauren Zapata, PhD, MSPH — *Centers for Disease Control and Prevention*

STAFF

Karen Smith
James Baumberger

COMMITTEE ON CHILD HEALTH FINANCING, 2017–2018

Mark L. Hudak, MD, FAAP, Chairperson
Suzanne K. Berman, MD, FAAP
Mary L. Brandt, MD, FACS, FAAP
Kenneth M. Carlson, MD, FAAP
Angelo P. Giardino, MD, FAAP
Lawrence Hammer, MD, FAAP
Stephen A. Pearlman, MD, MS, FAAP
Jonathan Price, MD, FAAP
Beena Gaind Sood, MD, MS, FAAP

LIAISON

Peter G. Szilagyi, MD, MPH, FAAP — *Medicaid and CHIP Payment and Access Commission*

STAFF

Lou Terranova, MHA

ABBREVIATIONS

AAP: American Academy of Pediatrics
ACA: Patient Protection and Affordable Care Act of 2010
AYA: adolescent and young adult
CHIP: Children's Health Insurance Program
CPT: *Current Procedural Terminology*
EOB: explanation of benefits
HDHP: high-deductible health plan
MCO: managed care organization

DOI: https://doi.org/10.1542/peds.2018-2998

Address correspondence to Arik V. Marcell, MD, MPH, FAAP. E-mail: amarcell@jhu.edu

PEDIATRICS (ISSN Numbers: Print, 0031-4005; Online, 1098-4275).

FINANCIAL DISCLOSURE: The authors have indicated they have no financial relationships relevant to this article to disclose.

FUNDING: No external funding.

POTENTIAL CONFLICT OF INTEREST: The authors have indicated they have no potential conflicts of interest to disclose.

REFERENCES

1. Sawyer SM, Afifi RA, Bearinger LH, et al. Adolescence: a foundation for future health. *Lancet.* 2012;379(9826):1630–1640

2. Kann L, Kinchen S, Shanklin SL, et al; Centers for Disease Control and Prevention (CDC). Youth risk behavior surveillance–United States, 2013 [published correction appears in *MMWR Morb Wkly Rep.* 2014;63(26):576]. *MMWR Suppl.* 2014;63(4):1–168

3. Olfson M, Druss BG, Marcus SC. Trends in mental health care among children and adolescents. *N Engl J Med.* 2015;372(21):2029–2038

4. Hargreaves DS, Elliott MN, Viner RM, Richmond TK, Schuster MA. Unmet health care need in US adolescents and adult health outcomes. *Pediatrics.* 2015;136(3):513–520

5. Hagan JF Jr, Shaw JS, Duncan P, eds. *Bright Futures: Guidelines for Health Supervision of Infants, Children, and Adolescents.* 4th ed. Elk Grove Village, IL: American Academy of Pediatrics; 2017

6. National Committee for Quality Assurance. *2019 HEDIS Summary Table of Measures, Product Lines and Changes.* Washington, DC: 1996. Available at: https://www.ncqa.org/wp-content/uploads/2018/08/20190000_ HEDIS_Measures_SummaryofChanges. pdf. Accessed October 12, 2018

7. Ozer EM, Adams SH, Orrell-Valente JK, et al. Does delivering preventive services in primary care reduce adolescent risky behavior? *J Adolesc Health.* 2011;49(5):476–482

8. Knight JR, Shrier LA, Bravender TD, Farrell M, Vander Bilt J, Shaffer HJ. A new brief screen for adolescent substance abuse. *Arch Pediatr Adolesc Med.* 1999;153(6):591–596

9. National Center for Health Statistics. Early release of selected estimates based on data from the National Health Interview Survey, January–June, 2016. Available at: https://www.cdc. gov/nchs/data/nhis/earlyrelease/ earlyrelease201611_01.pdf. Accessed September 3, 2017

10. Smith JC, Medalia M. *US Census Bureau, Current Population Reports, P60-253, Health Insurance Coverage in the United States: 2014.* Washington, DC: US Government Printing Office; 2015. Available at: https://www.census. gov/content/dam/Census/library/ publications/2015/demo/p60-253.pdf. Accessed October 18, 2018

11. Venkataramani M, Pollack CE, Roberts ET. Spillover effects of adult Medicaid expansions on children's use of preventive services. *Pediatrics.* 2017;140(6):e20170953

12. Monaghan M. The Affordable Care Act and implications for young adult health. *Transl Behav Med.* 2014;4(2):170–174

13. 42 USC Sect. 18022(b)(1)(J). Available at: https://www.gpo.gov/fdsys/pkg/ USCODE-2011-title42/pdf/USCODE-2011-title42-chap157-subchapIII-partA-sec18022.pdf. Accessed October 18, 2018

14. Institute of Medicine. *Clinical Preventive Services for Women: Closing the Gaps. Report Brief.* Washington, DC: The National Academies Press; 2011. Available at: http://nationalacademies.org/hmd/ Reports/2011/Clinical-Preventive-Services-for-Women-Closing-the-Gaps. aspx. Accessed October 12, 2018

15. Health Resources and Services Administration. *Women's Preventive Services Guidelines.* Washington, DC: US Department of Health and Human Services; 2016. Available at: www.hrsa. gov/womens-guidelines-2016/index. html. Accessed October 12, 2018

16. Institute of Medicine. *Essential Health Benefits: Balancing Coverage and Cost.* Washington, DC: National Academies Press; 2012. Available at: https://doi. org/10.17226/13234. Accessed October 12, 2018

17. Centers for Medicare and Medicaid Services; Center for Consumer Information and Insurance Oversight. Essential health benefits bulletin. Available at: www.cms.gov/CCIIO/ Resources/Files/Downloads/essential_ health_benefits_bulletin.pdf. Accessed September 3, 2017

18. Grace AM, Noonan KG, Cheng TL, et al. The ACA's pediatric essential health benefit has resulted in a state-by-state patchwork of coverage with exclusions. *Health Aff (Millwood).* 2014;33(12):2136–2143

19. Center for Consumer Information and Insurance Oversight. Limitations on cost sharing under the Affordable Care Act. 2017. Available at: https:// www.cms.gov/CCIIO/Resources/Fact-Sheets-and-FAQs/aca_implementation_ faqs12.html#Limitations%20on%20 Cost-Sharing%20under%20the%20 Affordable%20Care%20Act. Accessed August 30, 2017

20. Wong CA, Ford CA, French B, Rubin DM. Changes in young adult primary care under the affordable care act. *Am J Public Health.* 2015;105(suppl 5):S680–S685

21. Zuvekas SH, Weinick RM. Changes in access to care, 1977-1996: the role of health insurance. *Health Serv Res.* 1999;34(1, pt 2):271–279

22. Department of Health and Human Services, Office of the Assistant Secretary for Planning and Evaluation. Health insurance marketplace 2015 open enrollment period: March enrollment report for the period: November 15, 2014 – February 15, 2015 (including additional special enrollment period activity reported through 2-22-15). 2015. Available at: https://aspe.hhs.gov/sites/default/ files/pdf/83656/ib_2015mar_ enrollment.pdf. Accessed September 3, 2017

23. Collins SR, Rasmussen PW, Beutel S, Doty MM. The problem of underinsurance and how rising deductibles will make it worse. Findings from the Commonwealth Fund Biennial Health Insurance Survey, 2014. *Issue Brief (Commonw Fund).* 2015;13:1–20

24. Committee on Child Health Financing. High-deductible health plans. *Pediatrics.* 2014;133(5). Available at: www.pediatrics.org/cgi/content/full/ 133/5/e1461

25. McManus MA, Shejavali KI, Fox HB. *Is the Health Care System Working for Adolescents? Perspectives From Providers in Boston, Denver, Houston, and San Francisco.* Washington, DC: Maternal and Child Health Policy

Research Center; 2003. Available at: https://www.issuelab.org/resources/9938/9938.pdf. Accessed October 12, 2018

26. Tang SF; American Academy of Pediatrics. Medicaid payment for commonly used pediatrics services, 2004/05. Available at: https://www.aap.org/en-us/professional-resources/Research/Medicaid%20Reimbursement%20Reports/2004-2005_MedicaidPayments45StatesandDC.pdf. Accessed September 3, 2017

27. Tang SS, Hudak ML, Cooley DM, Shenkin BN, Racine AD. Increased Medicaid payment and participation by office-based primary care pediatricians. Pediatrics. 2018;141(1):e20172570

28. Gerstle RS, Molteni RA, Andreae MC, et al; Committee on Coding and Nomenclature. Application of the resource-based relative value scale system to pediatrics. Pediatrics. 2014;133(6):1158–1162

29. American Academy of Pediatrics. Adolescent health services coding. Available at: https://www.aap.org/en-us/Documents/coding_factsheet_adolescenthealth.pdf. Accessed February 20, 2018

30. National Alliance on Mental Illness. State mental health legislation 2015: trends, themes and effective practices. Available at: www.nami.org/About-NAMI/Publications-Reports/Public-Policy-Reports/State-Mental-Health-Legislation-2015/NAMI-StateMentalHealthLegislation2015.pdf. Accessed September 3, 2017

31. Garfield RL, Lave JR, Donohue JM. Health reform and the scope of benefits for mental health and substance use disorder services. Psychiatr Serv. 2010;61(11):1081–1086

32. Rowan K, McAlpine DD, Blewett LA. Access and cost barriers to mental health care, by insurance status, 1999-2010. Health Aff (Millwood). 2013;32(10):1723–1730

33. Tang MH, Hill KS, Boudreau AA, Yucel RM, Perrin JM, Kuhlthau KA. Medicaid managed care and the unmet need for mental health care among children with special health care needs. Health Serv Res. 2008;43(3):882–900

34. Open Minds. Update on behavioral health carve-outs from Medicaid MCOs. Available at: https://www.openminds.com/market-intelligence/executive-briefings/update-behavioral-health-carve-outs-medicaid-mcos.html. Accessed September 3, 2017

35. Foy JM, Kelleher KJ, Laraque D; American Academy of Pediatrics Task Force on Mental Health. Enhancing pediatric mental health care: strategies for preparing a primary care practice. Pediatrics. 2010;125(suppl 3):S87–S108

36. American Academy of Child and Adolescent Psychiatry Committee on Health Care Access and Economics Task Force on Mental Health. Improving mental health services in primary care: reducing administrative and financial barriers to access and collaboration [published correction appears in Pediatrics. 2009;123(6):1611]. Pediatrics. 2009;123(4):1248–1251

37. American Academy of Pediatrics. Improving mental health services in primary care: a call to action for the payer community - August 2016. Available at: https://www.aap.org/en-us/Documents/payeradvocacy_business_case.pdf. Accessed September 3, 2017

38. Kelly A; The Council of State Governments; Capitol Research. Health reform coverage for prevention: sexual health services. 2011. Available at: http://knowledgecenter.csg.org/kc/content/health-reform-coverage-prevention-sexual-health-services. Accessed October 12, 2018

39. Becker NV, Polsky D. Women saw large decrease in out-of-pocket spending for contraceptives after ACA mandate removed cost sharing. Health Aff (Millwood). 2015;34(7):1204–1211

40. Hasstedt K, Vierboom Y, Gold RB. Still needed: the family planning safety net under health reform. Guttmacher Policy Rev. 2015;18(3):56–61

41. National Women's Law Center. State of birth control coverage: health plan violations of the Affordable Care Act. 2015. Available at: https://nwlc.org/resources/state-birth-control-coverage-health-plan-violations-affordable-care-act/. Accessed October 12, 2018

42. Sonfield A. Rounding out the contraceptive coverage guarantee: why 'male' contraceptive methods matter for everyone. Guttmacher Policy Rev. 2015;18(2):34–39

43. English A, Lewis J. Privacy protection in billing and health insurance communications. AMA J Ethics. 2016;18(3):279–287

44. Society for Adolescent Health and Medicine; American Academy of Pediatrics. Confidentiality protections for adolescents and young adults in the health care billing and insurance claims process. J Adolesc Health. 2016;58(3):374–377

45. English A, Ford CA. The HIPAA privacy rule and adolescents: legal questions and clinical challenges. Perspect Sex Reprod Health. 2004;36(2):80–86

46. English A, Gold RB, Nash E, Levine J; Guttmacher Institute and Public Health Solutions. Confidentiality for individuals insured as dependents: a review of state laws and policies. 2012. Available at: www.guttmacher.org/pubs/confidentiality-review.pdf. Accessed October 12, 2018

47. Committee on Child Health Financing. Scope of health care benefits for children from birth through age 26. Pediatrics. 2012;129(1):185–189

48. Hammer LD, Curry ES, Harlor AD, et al; Committee on Practice and Ambulatory Medicine; Council on Community Pediatrics. Increasing immunization coverage. Pediatrics. 2010;125(6):1295–1304

49. Hudak ML, Helm ME, White PH; Committee on Child Health Financing. Principles of child health care financing. Pediatrics. 2017;140(3):e20172098

50. Lee GM, Santoli JM, Hannan C, et al. Gaps in vaccine financing for underinsured children in the United States. JAMA. 2007;298(6):638–643

51. National Center for Health Statistics. Health insurance coverage: early release of estimates from the National Health Interview Survey, January–June 2016. Available at: https://www.cdc.gov/nchs/data/nhis/earlyrelease/insur201611.pdf. Accessed October 12, 2018

The Teen Driver

. . . .

- *Policy Statement*

POLICY STATEMENT Organizational Principles to Guide and Define the Child Health Care System and/or Improve the Health of all Children

American Academy of Pediatrics

DEDICATED TO THE HEALTH OF ALL CHILDREN™

The Teen Driver

Elizabeth M. Alderman, MD, FAAP, FSAHM,[a] Brian D. Johnston, MD, MPH, FAAP,[b] COMMITTEE ON ADOLESCENCE, COUNCIL ON INJURY, VIOLENCE, AND POISON PREVENTION

abstract

For many teenagers, obtaining a driver's license is a rite of passage, conferring the ability to independently travel to school, work, or social events. However, immaturity, inexperience, and risky behavior put newly licensed teen drivers at risk. Motor vehicle crashes are the most common cause of mortality and injury for adolescents and young adults in developed countries. Teen drivers (15–19 years of age) have the highest rate of motor vehicle crashes among all age groups in the United States and contribute disproportionately to traffic fatalities. In addition to the deaths of teen drivers, more than half of 8- to 17-year-old children who die in car crashes are killed as passengers of drivers younger than 20 years of age. This policy statement, in which we update the previous 2006 iteration of this policy statement, is used to reflect new research on the risks faced by teen drivers and offer advice for pediatricians counseling teen drivers and their families.

[a]Division of Adolescent Medicine, Department of Pediatrics, Children's Hospital at Montefiore, Albert Einstein College of Medicine, Bronx, New York; and [b]Division of General Pediatrics, Department of Pediatrics, University of Washington, Seattle, Washington

Drs Alderman and Johnston together conceptualized, wrote, and revised this policy statement. They are jointly responsible for its content.

This document is copyrighted and is property of the American Academy of Pediatrics and its Board of Directors. All authors have filed conflict of interest statements with the American Academy of Pediatrics. Any conflicts have been resolved through a process approved by the Board of Directors. The American Academy of Pediatrics has neither solicited nor accepted any commercial involvement in the development of the content of this publication.

Policy statements from the American Academy of Pediatrics benefit from expertise and resources of liaisons and internal (AAP) and external reviewers. However, policy statements from the American Academy of Pediatrics may not reflect the views of the liaisons or the organizations or government agencies that they represent.

The guidance in this statement does not indicate an exclusive course of treatment or serve as a standard of medical care. Variations, taking into account individual circumstances, may be appropriate.

All policy statements from the American Academy of Pediatrics automatically expire 5 years after publication unless reaffirmed, revised, or retired at or before that time.

DOI: https://doi.org/10.1542/peds.2018-2163

Address correspondence to Elizabeth M. Alderman, MD, FAAP. E-mail: ealderma@montefiore.org

PEDIATRICS (ISSN Numbers: Print, 0031-4005; Online, 1098-4275).

Copyright © 2018 by the American Academy of Pediatrics

FINANCIAL DISCLOSURE: The authors have indicated they have no financial relationships relevant to this article to disclose.

To cite: Alderman EM, Johnston BD, AAP COMMITTEE ON ADOLESCENCE, AAP COUNCIL ON INJURY, VIOLENCE, AND POISON PREVENTION. The Teen Driver. *Pediatrics.* 2018;142(4):e20182163

BACKGROUND

The transition to independent mobility is a milestone in personal development, but learning to drive is a challenging neurocognitive task. Adolescents have many modes of transportation available to them, with differing relative costs, convenience, and safety. Options include active transport (walking, cycling), mass transit, and ride-sharing services. For many teenagers, however, driving a vehicle is a skill that enables them to work, access education, and exert their growing autonomy. Parents are often relieved when adolescents can drive themselves to activities, alleviating carpool burdens. Driving has particular significance in rural areas and regions where public transportation systems or other options are unavailable or limited.

Novice adolescent drivers (those with <18 months of driving experience) are at 4 times the overall risk of crash or near-crash events.[1] Adolescents are at risk for crashing because of their inexperience, their poorly developed skills, and for some, their engagement in risk behaviors. Age and associated neurocognitive maturity also contribute. Per mile driven, drivers 16 through 17 years of age have the highest rates of crash involvement, of injuries to themselves or others in their car, and of death to people outside the car in a crash.[2] For these reasons, motor vehicle crashes (MVCs) are among the most common cause of mortality and injury for adolescents and young adults in industrialized countries.[3] Adolescent drivers have the highest rate of MVCs among all age groups in the United States and contribute disproportionately to traffic fatalities. In addition to the deaths of teen drivers, more than half of 8- to 17-year-old children who die in car crashes are killed as passengers of drivers younger than 20 years of age.[4]

Nevertheless, the number of teenagers killed in MVCs has decreased by almost 50% over the last decade,[5] in parallel with overall reductions in traffic deaths. This reduction in teen traffic deaths reflects vehicle safety advances, improvements in seat belt use and impaired driving enforcement, and the impact of graduated driver's licensing (GDL) laws, which have been used to promote skills development through behind-the-wheel supervised experience and reduced exposure to risky driving situations. Although there is no national licensing standard in the United States, all 50 states and the District of Columbia have implemented GDL programs.[6]

Another reason for the reduction in motor vehicle mortality is that fewer teenagers are driving. Over the 15 years from 1996 to 2010, the proportion of US high school seniors licensed to drive declined from 85% to 73%,[7] and the proportion who reported driving did not rebound with the economic recovery.[8] Nevertheless, data from 2014 to 2016 can be used to suggest that teen motor vehicle fatalities are again on the rise.[5,9] In 2015, among 15- to 20-year-old individuals, 1886 young drivers died in MVCs, which is an increase of 9% from 2014 (see Fig 1). Another 195 000 young drivers were

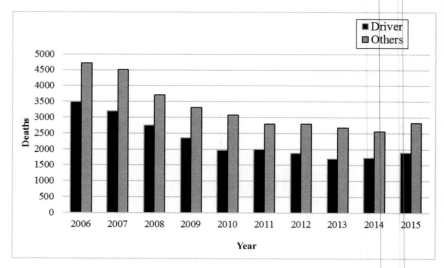

FIGURE 1

Trends in motor vehicle fatalities in crashes involving young drivers (15–20-year-olds); US data by person type ("others" are passengers of young drivers, occupants of other vehicles, and nonoccupants). (Adapted from National Highway Traffic Safety Administration; US Department of Transportation. Young drivers: 2015 data. Traffic safety facts. Report No. DOT HS 812 363. 2017. Available at: https://crashstats.nhtsa.dot.gov/Api/Public/ViewPublication/812363. Accessed December 14, 2017.)

injured in MVCs, which is up 14% from 2014.[10]

With this policy statement, we outline the unique risks faced by teen drivers and passengers that contribute to MVC mortality, describe promising interventions to curb this significant public health risk, and provide recommendations to guide pediatricians in counseling teenagers and families. We also describe the responsibilities of schools, community organizations, and governments in supporting programs and policies that can be used to mitigate the risks adolescents face on the road to support their development into competent and safe drivers. Other private-sector entities, such as automakers and insurers, are highly engaged in this effort, but their activities are beyond the scope of this statement. This policy statement, in which we update the previous 2006 iteration of this policy statement, is used to reflect new research on the risks faced by teen drivers and offer advice for pediatricians counseling teen drivers and their families.[11]

RISK FACTORS FOR ADOLESCENT DRIVERS

Inexperience

Driving is a complex skill, and inexperience is a common source of error. New drivers are less skilled at recognizing risks than are experienced drivers.[12] A common problem is that adolescents tend to fix their attention on nearby individual hazards rather than looking ahead and anticipating hazards. The best way for teenagers to reduce the risk of inexperience-related crash and injury is to practice driving, ideally under circumstances suited to promote learning while maintaining safety.[13]

Teen Passengers

Transporting peers can increase the crash risk for adolescent drivers.[14] Teen passengers may contribute to risk through distraction or negative peer influence on driving norms.[15] The likelihood of a teenager being involved in a fatal car crash is directly related to the number of teen passengers, an effect that is stronger in male drivers than in female drivers.[16] Compared with adult drivers, 16-year-old solo drivers have a 2.3-fold increased risk of crash. The presence of multiple passengers can increase the risk of a crash for a variety of reasons, including driver distraction, speeding, or alcohol use.[17]

Speed and Risky Driving

For all drivers, speed is an independent risk for crashing and for death or injury in the event of a crash. Teen drivers are more likely to drive at unsafe speeds and to maintain shorter following distances, especially with young passengers in the vehicle.[18] Among fatal crashes involving 15- to 20-year-olds, speed was implicated in 36%.[19] The availability of in-vehicle cameras and data recording has allowed researchers to better measure and understand "kinematic" risky driving behaviors, defined as excessive gravitational force events (eg, stops, starts, swerving) detected by the accelerometer. On the basis of kinematic events, adolescents can be classified as having higher or lower risk driving profiles that are relatively stable, even with increased driving experience, and that are correlated with self-reported driving behaviors.[20]

Distraction

Distraction is a risk for all drivers. Distracting events can include visual distraction (having one's eyes off the road), manual distraction (removing one's hands from the vehicle controls), or cognitive distraction (having one's attention diverted from driving).[21] Electronic devices, such as cell phones, can present all 3 modes of distraction in combination and are increasingly recognized as a major threat to driver safety.[22]

In 2015, 42% of US teen drivers reported the use of e-mail or text messaging while driving in the previous month,[23] and data from 2013 revealed that 58% of teenagers 16 to 18 years of age had used cell phones while driving.[24] Researchers in cross-sectional observations estimate that at any point in time, nearly 5% of teen drivers were holding a cell phone to their ear and talking, and an additional 5% were manipulating the phone.[25] In fatal crashes, teenagers represent 7% of the drivers but comprise 10% of distracted drivers and 13% of drivers distracted by cell phones at the time of the crash.[26]

The strongest predictor of distraction-associated crash risk among novice drivers may be the duration of glances away from the road, regardless of the nature of the distracting secondary task.[27] In-vehicle recordings of teen drivers revealed that eye glances away from the road for longer than 2 seconds were associated with a 5.5-fold increased risk of a crash or near-crash event.[27]

Alcohol, Marijuana, and Medication Use

Impaired driving is a serious risk factor for MVCs, injuries, and fatalities among all age groups. Alcohol-impaired drivers of all ages were identified in 16% of fatal traffic crashes involving children younger than 14 years old, with more than half of these drivers having a blood alcohol content (BAC) greater than 0.08 g/dL.[28] Teen drivers have a higher risk of involvement in MVCs at any BAC compared with older drivers.[29]

In the United States, the National Minimum Drinking Age Act of 1984 required states to increase the minimum age for alcohol purchase to 21 years. This resulted in a downward trend in the use of alcohol by adolescent and young adult drivers. This trend has continued. According to the Youth Risk Behavior Survey of high school students, the percentage of high school drivers who drank alcohol and drove within 30 days of the survey decreased from 10.0% in 2013 to 5.5% in 2017.[23] Older students had higher rates of impaired driving relative to younger students. Over the past 16 years, among high school students, the 30-day prevalence of riding in a car with a driver who had been drinking alcohol decreased from almost 40% to 16.5%.[23]

Despite improvements, the use of alcohol by an adolescent driver remains a serious risk factor for MVC and resultant fatalities. For 2015, the National Highway Traffic Safety Administration reported that 16% of drivers 16 to 20 years of age involved in fatal MVCs had a BAC level of 0.08% or higher,[28] and 64% of teen drivers who were killed in alcohol-involved crashes were not wearing seat belts.[30]

Drug-impaired driving is a growing concern for drivers and road users of all ages. From 1999 to 2010, 24.8% of drivers in fatal crashes tested positive for drugs of abuse, and 39.7% tested positive for alcohol. In the 11 years studied, the prevalence of drugs increased from 16.6% to 28.3%, whereas the prevalence of alcohol remained stable.[31] Cannabinoids were most commonly detected, and the prevalence increased from 4.2% to 12.2% over the study period.[31] Although there is increased detection of drugs other than alcohol in drivers involved in MVCs, the specific impact of these substances on crash risk is being studied by multiple investigators. Many drugs are used with alcohol, and detection can be challenging, making acute intoxication or impairment difficult to define or to detect in a rigorous manner.[32] In a recent case-control study, crash risk was 1.21 times higher for drivers who tested positive for illegal drugs and 1.25 times higher in those who tested positive for tetrahydrocannabinol. But when analyses were adjusted for demographic variables, such as age, sex, ethnicity, and concurrent alcohol use, the increase in crash risk was not associated solely with marijuana use.[33]

Other substances that may impair driving include prescription and over-the-counter medications. Many over-the-counter liquid medications contain alcohol or other ingredients that can cause drowsiness, including antihistamines (eg, diphenhydramine), antidiarrheals (eg, loperamide), and antiemetics.[34] For the adolescent driver, the effect of these medications on crash risk may depend on individual factors and the coingestion of other drugs or medications.

Drowsiness and Nighttime Driving

Most US teenagers do not get enough sleep[35] and, as a result, have altered circadian rhythms, which contribute to risk of fatigue.[36] Lack of sleep influences attention, learning, and judgment. Eliminating early high school start times to promote sleep is associated with reductions in teen driver crashes.[37,38] For all ages, driving at night is more dangerous than during the day, but adolescents are at particular risk during nighttime driving.[39] The independent effect of drowsiness on nighttime driving is compounded by the presence of other crash risk factors. For teenagers, nighttime driving is more likely to be "recreational" and is associated with having teen passengers, alcohol and drug use, and speeding.[40] Risk may also reflect the novice driver's inexperience with specific nighttime driving conditions.

Seat Belts

Lap and shoulder seat belts reduce the risk of death for front-seat occupants in a crash by 45% and the risk of moderate-to-critical injury by 50%.[41] Nationwide, front seat belt use for all drivers exceeded 90% in 2016 and was higher in states with primary enforcement laws (92%) than in those with only secondary enforcement laws (83%).[42] However,

in 2011, only 54% of US high school students reported always wearing a seat belt, and seat belt use varied by state from 32% to 65%.[43]

Unlicensed Driving

A small but important proportion of adolescents engage in driving while unlicensed. These teenagers miss out on any type of instruction, skill validation, or graduated supervision afforded to those completing traditional driver's education and licensure. By 1 estimate, although 6% of 9th through 11th grade students had engaged in unlicensed driving, 18% of 14- to 18-year-olds involved in fatal crashes were unlicensed.[44]

Biological Risk

The human brain does not achieve complete development until after adolescence.[45,46] Puberty is a time of physical growth and sexual maturation accompanied by development and change in the adolescent brain, particularly the regions that control behavior, emotions, decision-making, and self-regulation.[47] Adolescent cognitive immaturity, including deficits in self-control, attention, and executive function, may also contribute to teen driving behaviors but have not been independently associated with crash risk.[47] Many behaviors and motivations related to driving, such as risk and sensation seeking, are neurobiological in origin, are less related to age than to stage of puberty,[48,49] and are exacerbated when coupled with normative psychosocial changes of adolescence related to limit testing. Developmental demands present unique challenges for novice drivers, as they master skills that require knowledge, experience, and judgment at a time when risk-taking behaviors and the influence of peer pressure are at their peak.[50]

Other Medical Concerns

Adolescents with attention-deficit/hyperactivity disorder (ADHD) are at higher risk for MVCs and injury. Teen drivers with ADHD experience a risk of crash 36% higher than their peers,[51] a risk that does not vary by sex, by age, or over time. Drivers with ADHD may be less attentive to driving tasks at baseline and at least as susceptible to distraction caused by technology, passengers, and external factors.[52,53] The benefit of medication is uncertain. Although data for teenagers are inconsistent, adults with ADHD for whom medication was prescribed in a given month experienced a 40% reduction in emergency visits for injuries sustained in MVCs, compared with months when they did not receive ADHD medication.[54] However, medication effectiveness varies over the course of the day, and even if treated, adolescents may be functionally unmedicated in the late afternoon or night, which are times of the highest risk of crash. Moreover, adherence can be challenging, and many teenagers with ADHD are not treated with medication. In a recent cohort, only 12% of adolescents with ADHD were prescribed medication in the 30 days before licensure.[51]

In 2009, sport-related concussions were diagnosed in almost 250 000 teenagers,[55] a number generally thought to be an underestimate. Acute concussion symptoms are associated with impairments in standard driving performance,[56] and data from adult studies suggest that these impairments may persist after the resolution of other concussive symptoms.[57] More research is needed to assist families and physicians with the decision to allow a teenager to return to driving after having a concussion.

Additional medical concerns may affect driving ability and outcome. These include conditions for which the risk is well recognized, such as epilepsy,[58] but also sleep apnea, diabetes mellitus, depression, autism spectrum disorders, and other developmental disabilities that might require special training, assessment, or accommodation before a young person begins to drive.[59–61] Only a few states, however, require a physician visit or any form of physical health assessment (aside from visual acuity testing) before initial or subsequent noncommercial driver's licensing. Prelicensing medical evaluations for teen drivers have not been studied, although there is evidence in older drivers that even a simple statement of physician concern related to driving safety has a measurable and sustained effect on subsequent crash risk.[62]

INTERVENTIONS

Any policy, program, or design enhancement used to improve the safety of all drivers provides the greatest benefits to drivers at greatest risk, such as novice young drivers. Therefore, improved road designs, signage, separation of vehicles, and removal of objects near roadways provide great safety advantages to those who are most likely to crash. Similarly, policies regarding seat belt use and impaired driving or programs used to discourage cell phone use or aggressive driving behavior may be particularly important for young drivers. Given their high risk, young age, and inexperience, special policies and programs for young drivers are needed.

GDL

Perhaps the most important advance in teen driver safety over the last 25 years has been the development and implementation of GDL used to improve teen driving safety. Now present in all 50 states, GDL is a set of policies or regulations enacted variably at the state level and designed to introduce driving in a staged manner of increasing risk and responsibility.[63] Recognizing that driving is a skill that benefits from supervised practice and a stepwise increase in exposure and that certain driving exposures, such as driving at night, are more dangerous than other exposures, most GDL plans include a period of monitored driving before licensure, a term of probationary driving or intermediate licensure (in which certain high-risk situations, like night driving or driving with peers in the vehicle, are limited), and progression to full licensure that is contingent on performance during the probationary period.[63]

Studies of the effectiveness of GDL are encouraging. The strongest effect is observed with reduction in crashes among 16-year-old novice drivers, with a smaller effect for 17-year-old drivers.[64] In some states, a 25% or greater reduction in crashes among novice teen drivers has been reported.[65–67] GDL may reduce risk by reducing exposure if teenagers postpone licensing or drive fewer miles under GDL provisions.[68,69] Population-based data have revealed an association between GDL (for novice drivers <18 years old) and increased risk of crashing and fatal crashes among 18-year-old drivers.[67] It is unclear whether the involved 18-year-olds were novice drivers who postponed licensure or drivers who matured under GDL but with limited independent experience. Nevertheless, it suggests that GDL might be productively extended to 18- to 19-year-old novice drivers.[70] Indeed, some states now extend GDL to include novice drivers younger than 20 years old, but data are limited on the effectiveness, acceptability, and feasibility of extended GDL programs.[71]

The aspects of GDL responsible for its safety benefit are not firmly established. The provisions of GDL laws most strongly associated with lowering teen fatal crash rates are (1) strong nighttime driving restrictions, (2) restriction on teen passengers, and (3) increases in the minimum age at which a learner's permit or license can be obtained.[72] Enforcement of these selective licensing restrictions is difficult. However, New Jersey has required the use of decals on vehicles to identify novice drivers under its GDL program. Implementation of these decals was associated with a significant increase in citations to teen drivers for the violation of GDL provisions, including for the use of wireless technology,[73] and a sustained 2-year decrease of 9.5% in MVCs among young intermediate-licensed drivers.[74]

Driver Education

Formal driver education is a curriculum of didactic and basic in-car instruction designed to prepare students for a licensing examination. States vary in their requirement for formal driver's education before licensure. Driver training, by contrast, refers to behind-the-wheel instruction for novice or more experienced drivers and is often focused on specific skills.[75] Although driver education increases the proportion of students who can pass a licensing examination, there is little evidence that the program produces safer drivers, as measured by their risk of citations, crashes, injuries, or death. Studies consistently reveal no safety effect (or, in some cases, reveal an increase in risk) associated with traditional driver education.[76–80]

These counterintuitive findings that driver education may not be effective have been examined in detail elsewhere.[75,80,81] The most likely explanation of these findings is that driver education is focused on learning the rules of the road and basic vehicle handling. Unfortunately, the knowledge required to pass licensing examinations is seldom related to an evidence-based understanding of the behaviors and skills associated with novice driver crash risk.[75,81,82] Although some newer driver training programs have shown promise in improving hazard anticipation, hazard mitigation, and maintenance of attention,[83,84] there is still little evidence that these programs translate to safety in real-world settings or that they can be effectively scaled into a driver education curriculum.[85,86] In the meantime, harm can result if completion of training allows exposure to driving or release from GDL restrictions at a younger age or with less formal experience.[80]

Parent Interventions

Parents wield considerable ability to influence teen driving exposure, behavior, and risk. Parents can set positive examples well before children begin to drive by discussing expectations and parental roles as teenagers move into driver training and by monitoring and enforcing those expectations during the supervised driving phase. Parental monitoring and guidance are associated with a reduction in traffic violations and crash rates,[87–90] and teenagers whose parents have an authoritative parenting style, have high standards, but are supportive and instructive are less likely to drink or use cell phones while driving and experience fewer crashes.[91] There is, however, substantial variation in parental involvement and little empirical evidence on how best to influence parents to provide optimal monitoring.[92] A number of formal programs built around parent–teen driving agreements (or contracts) are aimed to encourage parents to honor and support GDL policies, monitor the early driving experience, and generally treat driving as the dangerous activity it is, requiring parents to manage their children's exposure and performance. Authors of a recent review of parent-directed teen driving interventions suggest that passive dissemination of program materials is ineffective.[93] However, more intensive programs,

including active parental engagement or the use of in-vehicle data recorders, reveal modest beneficial effects in the quality of risk-related communication, parental supervision in early driving, and reductions in self-reported teen risky driving.[93,94]

Winston et al[95] have called for a "precision prevention" approach to teen driving safety. In this tiered approach, a robust universal prevention strategy (eg, GDL) is paired with tools and support for parents to optimize the effect of GDL on their teen driver. For example, the Checkpoints program, which uses a parent–teen driving agreement used to assist parents in monitoring teen driving, has been used to bolster parental restrictions on teen driving behavior and reduced risky driving.[87] Similarly, a randomized trial of the Teen Driving Plan, which was used to address the quality and variety of parent-supervised teen driving, suggested that the program improved the supervised practice and the driving performance of prelicensed teen drivers.[96] The Centers for Disease Control and Prevention maintains a useful Web page for parents of teen drivers that includes a sample parent–teen driving agreement (see Resources).

Beyond universal interventions, selected interventions for subgroups of teenagers at predictably higher driving risk may be required.[95] For example, teenagers with ADHD might benefit from additional behind-the-wheel training, longer periods of restriction or supervision, and medication optimization. Most of these interventions call for increased parental involvement. Family-focused interventions for these young drivers seek to improve parental communication and monitoring.[97]

Winston et al[95] noted that some adolescents will require individualized interventions on the basis of their personal history of risk taking or demonstrated difficulties in driving tasks. These

drivers might benefit from in-vehicle technological monitoring, coupled with interventions used to strengthen parental monitoring. In-vehicle data recorders can be triggered by sudden changes in speed or erratic driving. Feedback provided to teenagers and parents has been associated with a reduction in risky driving behaviors.[98,99] Parental involvement is important; however, as revealed in many studies, it is difficult to secure.

Seat Belt Laws

All states have enacted laws that require teen drivers and vehicle occupants to use seat belts. The efficacy of these laws depends on the type of enforcement and the existence of exemptions (such as for back seat passengers); there is considerable room for improvement to save lives and prevent injury. As of May 2018, 34 states and the District of Columbia have a primary enforcement seat belt law, meaning that law enforcement officials may stop and ticket a passenger or driver solely for not wearing a seat belt, independent of any other violation.[100] Secondary enforcement seat belt laws allow law enforcement to give a ticket for not wearing a seat belt only if another violation has occurred. Seat belt use is consistently higher in primary enforcement states. Episodic, intensive enforcement campaigns have also been associated with an increase in seat belt use by up to 25% and a reduction in fatalities between 7% and 15%. For details about current specific state laws, refer to the resources at the end of this statement.

Alcohol and Drug Laws

Minimum legal drinking age laws played a role in decreasing the incidence of teen involvement in fatal crashes when they were instituted in the 1980s.[101] In addition, all states have passed "zero tolerance" laws designating a BAC of 0.02% or more for young drivers as indicative of driving under the influence of alcohol. Offenders face automatic or administrative suspension or revocation of their license. These laws have also decreased the incidence of fatal crashes.[101]

A number of states have legalized cannabis for medical use, decriminalized possession, and legalized recreational use. Although every state has laws regarding impaired driving, there remains significant variability in substance and enforcement of the laws. As of 2017, 16 states have zero tolerance laws for the use of 1 or more drugs while driving, and 6 states have "per se" laws that specify limits that cannot be exceeded for 1 or more drugs.[102]

Efforts to increase the knowledge of teenagers and parents about the potential effect of marijuana and illicit drugs on the risk of motor vehicle fatalities are needed, particularly in states where the use and/or possession of cannabis has been legalized, because teenagers may be a passenger in a car where the adult, who has obtained the cannabis legally, is driving. Moreover, the effect of prescribed medications and over-the-counter drugs needs to be conveyed to teenagers and their parents.

Many states and municipalities are examining their laws around drug-impaired driving. At the federal level, bills have been proposed to require states that have legalized cannabis use to also have laws prohibiting an individual from driving while impaired by marijuana and specifying methods for determining cognitive or physical marijuana impairment.[103] Effective models and programs used to help teenagers and parents comply with existing and ever-changing laws around drug-impaired driving must be developed, studied, and disseminated.

Laws Related to Distraction or Technology

Laws pertaining to electronic distraction are variably written and inconsistently enforced. Most states prohibit texting while driving; although some states prohibit handheld cell phone use, others ban all cell phone use. In many jurisdictions, teen drivers under a GDL program are prohibited from using any technology. Studies have been used to suggest that all-age bans reduce the frequency of observed cell phone use[104] and crash rates for young drivers.[72] Bans on the use of electronic communication devices specifically by teen drivers have not been shown to change driver behavior or safety outcomes.[105] Similarly, the effect of laws that are focused on texting is less clear.[106]

On the basis of accumulating evidence about enforceability and efficacy, experts advocate for laws that apply to the use of all handheld devices, laws that apply to all drivers in all driving environments, and laws that make distracted driving violations offenses reportable to insurance companies.[107]

Technological Interventions

Technological advances not only contribute to driver risk and distraction, but can be used to make driving safer as well. Newer model automobiles have safety features that are available to all drivers, including electronic stability control, rear vision cameras, automatic braking, blind spot threat detection, and lane-maintenance alerts.[108,109] In the near future, advanced driver assistance systems may be tailored to teen drivers, guiding them toward less hazardous routes, restricting their car speed via intelligent speed adaptation, and locking out potentially distracting on-board technologies.[110] Parents can be referred to updated lists of new and used vehicles with safety ratings for novice drivers based on the availability of key technologies.[111]

Technologies used to block electronic distraction in the car are available but are not highly regarded by consumers.[112,113] Cellular phone service can be integrated with vehicular controls, reducing the need for handling the device but increasing access to other wireless applications; the risks and benefits of this integration have yet to be adequately studied. Some vehicles now feature teen-specific driving modes or key fobs that limit speed and block access to specific electronic distractions. Similar parental control applications can be added to teen phones to report or to limit access to distracting technologies while in a moving vehicle.[114,115] Finally, some insurers provide client families with in-vehicle monitoring and feedback technology used to assist new teen drivers.[116]

CONCLUSIONS

Driving is a skill, and driver licensure is a rite of passage for adolescents that signals newfound independence. However, the special risks teen drivers face are many. These risks reflect their inexperience, vulnerability to distraction, high prevalence of speeding and kinematic risky driving, lower-than-average use of seat belts, and sensitivity to driving impairment caused by alcohol and other substances. The biological and cognitive substrate of adolescence magnifies these specific challenges as well as the social and emotional imperatives that influence so many aspects of teen behavior, risk appraisal, and decision-making. Policies, programs, and technologies exist to help mitigate these risks but, in most cases, depend on active participation by the teenager and parents. Pediatricians, communities, and governments need to take action to better educate teen drivers and their parents around these risks and strategies to reduce them.

RECOMMENDATIONS

Anticipatory Guidance

Pediatricians can do the following:

- Remind parents that their driving and behavior, including seat belt use and use of wireless technology in the car, serve as a powerful role model for their children and, ultimately, will shape the behavior of their teen drivers.

- Assist parents in identifying adolescents with acute or chronic medical or behavioral risk factors for especially high driving risk.

- Become familiar with components of their state's specific GDL laws to better counsel teen drivers.

- Discuss avoidance of distracted driving and responsible use of technology as components of teen driving safety.

- Continue to counsel adolescents on seat belt use and the risk of alcohol-, illicit substance-, and medication-impaired driving, both as a driver and a passenger.

- Promote the use of active and alternative transport modes (including ride-sharing services) to reduce total teen driving exposure, where this is feasible.

- Encourage parents to practice driving with their teenagers in a variety of environments and for more than the state-required minimum number of hours.

Professional Practice

Pediatricians, their professional organizations, and research funders can do the following:

- Explore with patients and payers the creation of a standardized prelicensure medical visit to promote thoughtful interaction between teenagers, parents, and health care providers around issues related to driving safety. This visit could include the assessment of individual risks, review of the provisions of local GDL laws, and tailored recommendations for specific monitoring or instruction.

- Study the effect of concussion on teen driving to develop, test, and disseminate guidelines for a safe return to driving after a minor traumatic brain injury.

- Advocate for the revision and rigorous testing of driver's education curricula to address the risks and behaviors associated with novice driver crashes and to be evaluated in terms of important outcomes (crashes, near crashes, injury, or death) for durability of effect and application to higher-risk subpopulations.

- Recognize the increased challenges experienced by teenagers with developmental or acquired disabilities and define the role of driving rehabilitation specialists with these individuals.

Community Advocacy

As community experts in child and adolescent health, pediatricians can do the following:

- Advocate for policies and practices that generally improve road safety for all users, including vulnerable novice drivers.

- Promote the availability and use of safe and active alternative routes to school for teenagers to reduce exposure to driving.

- Support later high school start times to help address adolescent chronobiology and associated safety risks.

- Advocate for the availability of nonpunitive and free sober–ride home programs in their community.

- Remind parents, schools, and community organizations that traditional driver education is not sufficient to reduce teen motor vehicle citations, crashes, injury, or death. Although needed to learn the basic operation of a vehicle and the rules of the road, these courses have never been shown to produce "safer" teen drivers.

Legislative Advocacy

Pediatricians can work with local, state, or federal lawmakers to do the following:

- Pass primary enforcement laws for seat belt use, electronic distraction prevention, and GDL compliance.

- Advocate for enactment and enforcement of strong, evidence-based GDL laws.

- Advocate for standards and safety for teenagers who drive as part of their jobs.

- Adopt the use of standard decals or plates to identify learner and intermediate drivers.

- Study the effectiveness, acceptability, and feasibility of extending GDL provisions to novice drivers 18 to 19 years of age.

- Maintain and enforce the minimum legal drinking age and zero tolerance laws for teen drivers.

- Support the improvement and enforcement of other laws designed to limit the underage purchase, possession, and consumption of alcohol, as well as cannabis (in states where it is legalized) and other drugs.

RESOURCES

HealthyChildren

Teen driving safety tips and resources for parents from the American Academy of Pediatrics can be found at https://www.healthychildren.org/English/ages-stages/teen/safety/.

Parents Are the Key to Safe Teen Drivers

https://www.cdc.gov/parentsarethekey/

A Campaign From the Centers for Disease Control and Prevention to Help Parents, Pediatricians, and Communities Keep Teen Drivers Safe on the Road

Teen driving education and resources from the American Automobile Association, including a parent-teen driving agreement can be found at Keys2Drive (http://teendriving.aaa.com).

Teen Driver Source

Free teen driver safety information and downloadable information can be found at http://www.teendriversource.org/.

Prevent Child Injury

A toolkit for injury prevention campaign that is focused on teen driving safety can be found at https://www.preventchildinjury.org/toolkits//teen-driving.

Drive It Home

Lesson plans and tips for parents to help them supervise new teen drivers can be found at http://driveithome.org/.

Association for Driver Rehabilitation Specialists

Help for finding driver rehabilitation specialists that includes fact sheets on driving and specific disabilities can be found at ww.aded.net.

Governors Highway Safety Association

State-by-state listing and comparison of relevant motor vehicle laws, including those applicable to teen or novice drivers can be found at http://www.ghsa.org/state-laws/issues.

Insurance Institute for Highway Safety

An up-to-date reference resource for traffic safety laws, by state and by topic can be found at http://www.iihs.org/iihs/topics#statelaws.

National Highway Traffic Safety Administration

A teen driving information site with links to Parents Central for resources can be found at https://www.nhtsa.gov/road-safety/teen-driving.

Potential Content for Prelicensure Medical Visits

- Review general driving risks by age and experience.
- Review health and safety implications of alternatives to driving, including active transportation, ride-sharing, and public transit.
- Review state-specific graduated licensing provisions.
- Discuss biological risk factors, including but not limited to the following:
  o Chronic conditions
  o Developmental disabilities
  o Sleep
  o Seizure disorder
  o Diabetes
  o Visual acuity or other perceptual challenges
- Discuss cognitive concerns, including but not limited to the following:
  o Role of distraction
  o ADHD
  o Depression
  o Concussion
- Review medications, alcohol use, and other drug use.
- Discuss whether this teenager would benefit from an additional period of supervised driving or use of in-vehicle data recording technology.

- Facilitate a discussion of parent expectations and restrictions on teen driving.
- Discuss and promote the use of a parent–teen driving contract.
- Provide advice or references on selecting the safest family vehicle for the teenager to drive.

LEAD AUTHORS

Elizabeth M. Alderman, MD, FAAP, FSAHM
Brian D. Johnston, MD, MPH, FAAP

COMMITTEE ON ADOLESCENCE, 2017–2018

Cora Breuner, MD, MPH, FAAP, Chairperson
Elizabeth M. Alderman, MD, FAAP, FSHAM
Laura K. Grubb, MD, MPH, FAAP
Makia Powers, MD, MPH, FAAP
Krishna Upadhya, MD, FAAP
Stephenie Wallace, MD, FAAP

LIAISONS

Laurie Hornberger, MD, MPH, FAAP – *Section on Adolescent Health*
Liwei Hua, MD, PhD – *American Academy of Child and Adolescent Psychiatry*
Margo Lane, MD, FRCPC, FAAP – *Canadian Paediatric Society*
Meredith Loveless, MD, FACOG – *American College of Obstetricians and Gynecologists*
Seema Menon, MD – *North American Society for Pediatric and Adolescent Gynecology*
Lauren Zapata, PhD, MSPH – *Centers for Disease Control and Prevention*

STAFF

Karen Smith
James Baumberger

COUNCIL ON INJURY, VIOLENCE, AND POISON PREVENTION, 2017–2018

Benjamin D. Hoffman, MD, FAAP, Chairperson
Kyran Quinlan, MD, MPH, FAAP, Immediate Past Chairperson
Phyllis Agran, MD, MPH, FAAP
Sarah Denny, MD, FAAP
Michael Hirsh, MD, FAAP
Brian Johnston, MD, MPH, FAAP
Lois Lee, MD, MPH, FAAP
Kathy Monroe, MD, FAAP
Judy Schaechter, MD, MBA, FAAP
Milton Tenenbein, MD, FAAP
Mark R. Zonfrillo, MD, MSCE, FAAP

LIAISONS

Elizabeth Edgerton, MD, MPH, FAAP – *Health Resources and Services Administration*
Julie Gilchrist, MD, FAAP – *Centers for Disease Control and Prevention*

Jonathan Midgett, PhD — *Consumer Product Safety Commission*
Alexander (Sandy) Sinclair — *National Highway Traffic Safety Administration*

STAFF

Bonnie Kozial
Ami Gadhia

Zachary Laris
Katie Matlin

CONSULTANTS

Beth E. Ebel, MD, MScE, MPH, FAAP — *District VIII*
Michael Gittelman, MD, FAAP — *District V*
Suzan Mazor, MD, FAAP — *District VIII*
Eliot Nelson, MD, FAAP — *District I*
Joseph O'Neil, MD, MPH, FAAP — *District V*
Karen Sheehan, MD, MPH, FAAP — *District VI*

ABBREVIATIONS

ADHD: attention-deficit/hyperactivity disorder
BAC: blood alcohol content
GDL: graduated driver's licensing
MVC: motor vehicle crash

FUNDING: No external funding.

POTENTIAL CONFLICT OF INTEREST: The authors have indicated they have no potential conflicts of interest to disclose.

REFERENCES

1. Simons-Morton BG, Klauer SG, Ouimet MC, et al. Naturalistic teenage driving study: findings and lessons learned. *J Safety Res*. 2015;54:41–44

2. Tefft BC. *Rates of Motor Vehicle Crashes, Injuries, and Deaths in Relation to Driver Age, United States, 2014-2015. (Research Brief)*. Washington, DC: American Automobile Association Foundation for Traffic Safety; 2017. Available at: http://newsroom.aaa.com/download/10260/. Accessed December 14, 2017

3. Haagsma JA, Graetz N, Bolliger I, et al. The global burden of injury: incidence, mortality, disability-adjusted life years and time trends from the Global Burden of Disease study 2013. *Inj Prev*. 2016;22(1):3–18

4. Winston FK, Kallan MJ, Senserrick TM, Elliott MR. Risk factors for death among older child and teenaged motor vehicle passengers. *Arch Pediatr Adolesc Med*. 2008;162(3):253–260

5. US Department of Transportation; National Highway Traffic Safety Administration. Traffic safety facts. 2015 motor vehicle crashes: overview. 2016. Available at: https://crashstats.nhtsa.dot.gov/Api/Public/ViewPublication/812318. Accessed December 14, 2017

6. Insurance Institute for Highway Safety; Highway Loss Data Institute. Teenagers. Graduated driver licensing introduction. 2017. Available at: www.iihs.org/iihs/topics/laws/graduatedlicenseintro?topicName=teenagers. Accessed December 14, 2017

7. Shults RA, Olsen E, Williams AF; Centers for Disease Control and Prevention (CDC). Driving among high school students - United States, 2013. *MMWR Morb Mortal Wkly Rep*. 2015;64(12):313–317

8. Shults RA, Williams AF. Trends in teen driver licensure, driving patterns and crash involvement in the United States, 2006-2015. *J Safety Res*. 2017;62:181–184

9. National Center for Statistics and Analysis. Early estimate of motor vehicle traffic fatalities for the first half (Jan–Jun) of 2016. In: *Crash-Stats Brief Statistical Summary*. Report No. DOT HS 812 332. Washington, DC: National Highway Traffic Safety Administration; 2016:1–2

10. National Highway Traffic Safety Administration; US Department of Transportation. Young drivers: 2015 data. Traffic safety facts. Report No. DOT HS 812 363. 2017. Available at: https://crashstats.nhtsa.dot.gov/Api/Public/ViewPublication/812363. Accessed December 14, 2017

11. Weiss JC; Committee on Injury, Violence, and Poison Prevention, American Academy of Pediatrics; Committee on Adolescence, American Academy of Pediatrics. The teen driver. *Pediatrics*. 2006;118(6):2570–2581

12. McKnight AJ, McKnight AS. Young novice drivers: careless or clueless? *Accid Anal Prev*. 2003;35(6):921–925

13. Lam LT. Factors associated with young drivers' car crash injury: comparisons among learner, provisional, and full licensees. *Accid Anal Prev*. 2003;35(6):913–920

14. Simons-Morton BG, Ouimet MC, Zhang Z, et al. The effect of passengers and risk-taking friends on risky driving and crashes/near crashes among novice teenagers. *J Adolesc Health*. 2011;49(6):587–593

15. Chen LH, Baker SP, Braver ER, Li G. Carrying passengers as a risk factor for crashes fatal to 16- and 17-year-old drivers. *JAMA*. 2000;283(12):1578–1582

16. Ouimet MC, Pradhan AK, Brooks-Russell A, Ehsani JP, Berbiche D, Simons-Morton BG. Young drivers and their passengers: a systematic review of epidemiological studies on crash risk. *J Adolesc Health*. 2015;57(suppl 1):S24–S35.e6

17. Graham R, Gootman JA. Preventing teen motor crashes: contributions from the behavioral and social sciences and summary of the report of the National Research Council and Institute of Medicine. *Am J Prev Med*. 2008;35(suppl 3):S253–S257

18. Simons-Morton B, Lerner N, Singer J. The observed effects of teenage passengers on the risky driving behavior of teenage drivers. *Accid Anal Prev*. 2005;37(6):973–982

19. National Center for Statistics and Analysis. Speeding: 2014 data. *Traffic Safety Facts*. Report No. DOT HS 812 265. Washington, DC: US Department of Transportation; 2016:1–7

20. Simons-Morton BG, Cheon K, Guo F, Albert P. Trajectories of kinematic risky driving among novice teenagers. *Accid Anal Prev.* 2013;51:27–32

21. National Highway Traffic Safety Administration. Distraction. Available at: https://one.nhtsa.gov/Research/Human-Factors/Distraction. Accessed December 14, 2017

22. Klauer SG, Guo F, Simons-Morton BG, Ouimet MC, Lee SE, Dingus TA. Distracted driving and risk of road crashes among novice and experienced drivers. *N Engl J Med.* 2014;370(1):54–59

23. Kann L, McManus T, Harris WA, et al. Youth risk behavior surveillance - United States, 2015. *MMWR Surveill Summ.* 2016;65(6):1–174

24. American Automobile Association Foundation for Traffic Safety. 2015 traffic safety culture index. 2015. Available at: https://aaafoundation.org/2015-traffic-safety-culture-index/. Accessed December 14, 2017

25. US Department of Transportation; National Highway Traffic Safety Administration. Driver electronic device use in 2015. *Traffic Safety Facts Research Note.* Report No. DOT HS 812 326. Washington, DC: National Highway Traffic Safety Administration; 2016:1–9

26. US Department of Transportation; National Highway Traffic Safety Administration. Research note: distracted driving 2014. 2016. Available at: https://crashstats.nhtsa.dot.gov/Api/Public/ViewPublication/812260. Accessed December 14, 2017

27. Simons-Morton BG, Guo F, Klauer SG, Ehsani JP, Pradhan AK. Keep your eyes on the road: young driver crash risk increases according to duration of distraction. *J Adolesc Health.* 2014;54(suppl 5):S61–S67

28. National Center for Statistics and Analysis. Alcohol impaired driving: 2015 data. In: *Traffic Safety Facts.* DOT HS 812 350. Washington, DC: National Highway Traffic Safety Administration; 2016:1–7

29. Voas RB, Torres P, Romano E, Lacey JH. Alcohol-related risk of driver fatalities: an update using 2007 data. *J Stud Alcohol Drugs.* 2012;73(3):341–350

30. US Department of Transportation; National Highway Traffic Safety Administration. 2014 data: young drivers. 2016. Available at: https://crashstats.nhtsa.dot.gov/Api/Public/ViewPublication/812278. Accessed December 14, 2017

31. Brady JE, Li G. Trends in alcohol and other drugs detected in fatally injured drivers in the United States, 1999-2010. *Am J Epidemiol.* 2014;179(6):692–699

32. US Department of Transportation; National Highway Traffic Safety Administration. *Traffic Safety Facts: Understanding the Limitations of Drug Test Information, Reporting, and Testing Practices in Fatal Crashes.* Washington, DC: National Highway Traffic Safety Administration; 2014

33. US Department of Transportation; National Highway Traffic Safety Administration. *Traffic Safety Facts: Drug and Alcohol Crash Risk.* Washington, DC: National Highway Traffic Safety Administration; 2015

34. US Food and Drug Administration. FDA consumer health information. Caution: some over-the-counter medicines may affect your driving. 2014. Available at: alternative URL https://sleepfoundation.org/sites/default/files/2006_summary_of_findings.pdf. Accessed December 14, 2017

35. National Sleep Foundation. 2006 sleep in America poll – teens and sleep. *Sleep Health.* 2015;1(2):e5

36. Owens J; Adolescent Sleep Working Group; Committee on Adolescence. Insufficient sleep in adolescents and young adults: an update on causes and consequences. *Pediatrics.* 2014;134(3). Available at: www.pediatrics.org/cgi/content/full/134/3/e921

37. Danner F, Phillips B. Adolescent sleep, school start times, and teen motor vehicle crashes. *J Clin Sleep Med.* 2008;4(6):533–535

38. Wahlstrom KL, Dretzke BJ, Gordon MF, et al. *Examining the Impact of Later High School Start Times on the Health and Academic Performance of High School Students: A Multi-Site Study.* St Paul, MN: Center for Applied Research and Educational Improvement; 2014. Available at: https://conservancy.umn.edu/handle/11299/162769. Accessed December 14, 2017

39. Rice TM, Peek-Asa C, Kraus JF. Nighttime driving, passenger transport, and injury crash rates of young drivers. *Inj Prev.* 2003;9(3):245–250

40. Williams AF, Preusser DF. Night driving restrictions for youthful drivers: a literature review and commentary. *J Public Health Policy.* 1997;18(3):334–345

41. National Highway Traffic Safety Administration; US Department of Transportation. Traffic safety facts. 2013 data. Occupant protection. 2015. Available at: https://crashstats.nhtsa.dot.gov/Api/Public/ViewPublication/812153. Accessed December 14, 2017

42. Pickrell T, Li R. *Seat Belt Use in 2016—Overall Results (Traffic Safety Facts Research Note. Report No. DOT HS 812 351).* Washington, DC: National Highway Traffic Safety Administration; 2016. Available at: https://crashstats.nhtsa.dot.gov/Api/Public/ViewPublication/812351. Accessed December 14, 2017

43. Shults RA, Haegerich TM, Bhat G, Zhang X. Teens and seat belt use: what makes them click? *J Safety Res.* 2016;57:19–25

44. Winston FK, Durbin DR, Ginsburg KR. *Driving Through the Eyes of Teens: A Closer Look.* Philadelphia, PA: Children's Hospital of Philadelphia/State Farm Insurance Co; 2009

45. Giedd JN, Blumenthal J, Jeffries NO, et al. Brain development during childhood and adolescence: a longitudinal MRI study. *Nat Neurosci.* 1999;2(10):861–863

46. Shaw P, Kabani NJ, Lerch JP, et al. Neurodevelopmental trajectories of the human cerebral cortex. *J Neurosci.* 2008;28(14):3586–3594

47. Dahl RE. Biological, developmental, and neurobehavioral factors relevant to adolescent driving risks. *Am J Prev Med.* 2008;35(suppl 3):S278–S284

48. Spear LP. The adolescent brain and age-related behavioral manifestations. *Neurosci Biobehav Rev.* 2000;24(4):417–463

49. Martin CA, Kelly TH, Rayens MK, et al. Sensation seeking, puberty, and nicotine, alcohol, and marijuana use in adolescence. *J Am Acad Child Adolesc Psychiatry.* 2002;41(12):1495–1502

50. Shope JT, Bingham CR. Teen driving: motor-vehicle crashes and factors that contribute. *Am J Prev Med*. 2008;35(suppl 3):S261–S271

51. Curry AE, Metzger KB, Pfeiffer MR, Elliott MR, Winston FK, Power TJ. Motor vehicle crash risk among adolescents and young adults with attention-deficit/hyperactivity disorder. *JAMA Pediatr*. 2017;171(8):756–763

52. Reimer B, Mehler B, D'Ambrosio LA, Fried R. The impact of distractions on young adult drivers with attention deficit hyperactivity disorder (ADHD). *Accid Anal Prev*. 2010;42(3):842–851

53. Narad M, Garner AA, Brassell AA, et al. Impact of distraction on the driving performance of adolescents with and without attention-deficit/hyperactivity disorder. *JAMA Pediatr*. 2013;167(10):933–938

54. Chang Z, Quinn PD, Hur K, et al. Association between medication use for attention-deficit/hyperactivity disorder and risk of motor vehicle crashes. *JAMA Psychiatry*. 2017;74(6):597–603

55. Centers for Disease Control and Prevention. Nonfatal traumatic brain injuries related to sports and recreation activities among persons aged ≤19 years–United States, 2001-2009. *MMWR Morb Mortal Wkly Rep*. 2011;60(39):1337–1342

56. Preece MH, Horswill MS, Geffen GM. Driving after concussion: the acute effect of mild traumatic brain injury on drivers' hazard perception. *Neuropsychology*. 2010;24(4):493–503

57. Schmidt JD, Hoffman NL, Ranchet M, et al. Driving after concussion: is it safe to drive after symptoms resolve? *J Neurotrauma*. 2017;34(8):1571–1578

58. Chen WC, Chen EY, Gebre RZ, et al. Epilepsy and driving: potential impact of transient impaired consciousness. *Epilepsy Behav*. 2014;30:50–57

59. Rizzo D, Libman E, Creti L, et al. Determinants of policy decisions for non-commercial drivers with OSA: an integrative review. *Sleep Med Rev*. 2018;37:130–137

60. Wickens CM, Smart RG, Mann RE. The impact of depression on driver performance. *Int J Ment Health Addict*. 2014;12(4):524–537

61. Daly BP, Nicholls EG, Patrick KE, Brinckman DD, Schultheis MT. Driving behaviors in adults with autism spectrum disorders. *J Autism Dev Disord*. 2014;44(12):3119–3128

62. Redelmeier DA, Yarnell CJ, Thiruchelvam D, Tibshirani RJ. Physicians' warnings for unfit drivers and the risk of trauma from road crashes. *N Engl J Med*. 2012;367(13):1228–1236

63. Williams AF, McCartt AT, Sims LB. History and current status of state graduated driver licensing (GDL) laws in the United States. *J Safety Res*. 2016;56:9–15

64. Zhu M, Cummings P, Chu H, Coben JH, Li G. Graduated driver licensing and motor vehicle crashes involving teenage drivers: an exploratory age-stratified meta-analysis. *Inj Prev*. 2013;19(1):49–57

65. Shope JT, Molnar LJ. Graduated driver licensing in the United States: evaluation results from the early programs. *J Safety Res*. 2003;34(1):63–69

66. Foss RD, Feaganes JR, Rodgman EA. Initial effects of graduated driver licensing on 16-year-old driver crashes in North Carolina. *JAMA*. 2001;286(13):1588–1592

67. Masten SV, Foss RD, Marshall SW. Graduated driver licensing and fatal crashes involving 16- to 19-year-old drivers. *JAMA*. 2011;306(10):1098–1103

68. Zhu M, Zhao S, Long DL. Brief report: the association of graduated driver licensing with nondriver transport-related injuries among adolescents. *Epidemiology*. 2016;27(5):620–623

69. Zhu M, Cummings P, Zhao S, Coben JH, Smith GS. The association of graduated driver licensing with miles driven and fatal crash rates per miles driven among adolescents. *Inj Prev*. 2015;21(e1):e23–e27

70. Curry AE, Metzger KB, Williams AF, Tefft BC. Comparison of older and younger novice driver crash rates: informing the need for extended graduated driver licensing restrictions. *Accid Anal Prev*. 2017;108:66–73

71. Curry AE, Foss RD, Williams AF. Graduated driver licensing for older novice drivers: critical analysis of the issues. *Am J Prev Med*. 2017;53(6):923–927

72. McCartt AT, Teoh ER, Fields M, Braitman KA, Hellinga LA. Graduated licensing laws and fatal crashes of teenage drivers: a national study. *Traffic Inj Prev*. 2010;11(3):240–248

73. Curry AE, Pfeiffer MR, Localio R, Durbin DR. Graduated driver licensing decal law: effect on young probationary drivers. *Am J Prev Med*. 2013;44(1):1–7

74. Curry AE, Elliott MR, Pfeiffer MR, Kim KH, Durbin DR. Long-term changes in crash rates after introduction of a graduated driver licensing decal provision. *Am J Prev Med*. 2015;48(2):121–127

75. Lonero LP. Trends in driver education and training. *Am J Prev Med*. 2008;35(suppl 3):S316–S323

76. Stock JR, Weaver JK, Ray HW, Brink JR, Sadof MG. *Evaluation of Safe Performance Secondary School Driver Education Curriculum Demonstration Project. DOT HS-806 568*. Washington, DC: US Department of Transportation; 1983

77. Vernick JS, Li G, Ogaitis S, MacKenzie EJ, Baker SP, Gielen AC. Effects of high school driver education on motor vehicle crashes, violations, and licensure. *Am J Prev Med*. 1999;16(suppl 1):40–46

78. Vaa T, Elvik R. *The Handbook of Road Safety Measures*. 1st ed. Amsterdam, Netherlands: Elsevier; 2004

79. Ian R, Irene K; Cochrane Injuries Group Driver Education Reviewers. School based driver education for the prevention of traffic crashes. *Cochrane Database Syst Rev*. 2001;(3):CD003201

80. Mayhew DR. Driver education and graduated licensing in North America: past, present, and future. *J Safety Res*. 2007;38(2):229–235

81. Lonero L, Mayhew D. *Teen Driver Safety. Review of the Literature on Driver Education Evaluation, 2010 Update*. Washington, DC: American Automobile Association Foundation for Traffic Safety; 2010

82. Durbin DR, Mirman JH, Curry AE, et al. Driving errors of learner teens: frequency, nature and their association with practice. *Accid Anal Prev*. 2014;72:433–439

83. Taylor TG, Masserang KM, Pradhan AK, et al. Long term effects of hazard anticipation training on novice drivers measured on the open road. In: *Proceedings of the Driving Symposium on Human Factors Driver Assessment, Training, and Vehicle Design*; June 27–30, 2011; Lake Tahoe, CA

84. Yamani Y, Samuel S, Knodler MA, Fisher DL. Evaluation of the effectiveness of a multi-skill program for training younger drivers on higher cognitive skills. *Appl Ergon*. 2016;52:135–141

85. McDonald CC, Goodwin AH, Pradhan AK, Romoser MR, Williams AF. A review of hazard anticipation training programs for young drivers. *J Adolesc Health*. 2015;57(suppl 1):S15–S23

86. McDonald CC, Kandadai V, Loeb H, et al. Evaluation of a risk awareness perception training program on novice teen driver behavior at left-turn intersections. *Transp Res Rec*. 2015;2516(2516):15–21

87. Simons-Morton BG, L Hartos J, Leaf WA, Preusser DF. The effect on teen driving outcomes of the Checkpoints Program in a state-wide trial. *Accid Anal Prev*. 2006;38(5):907–912

88. Hartos J, Eitel P, Simons-Morton B. Parenting practices and adolescent risky driving: a three-month prospective study. *Health Educ Behav*. 2002;29(2):194–206

89. Hartos JL, Eitel P, Haynie DL, Simons-Morton BG. Can I take the car? Relations among parenting practices and adolescent problem-driving practices. *J Adolesc Res*. 2000;15(3):352–367

90. McCartt AT, Shabanova VI, Leaf WA. Driving experience, crashes and traffic citations of teenage beginning drivers. *Accid Anal Prev*. 2003;35(3):311–320

91. Ginsburg KR, Durbin DR, García-España JF, Kalicka EA, Winston FK. Associations between parenting styles and teen driving, safety-related behaviors and attitudes. *Pediatrics*. 2009;124(4):1040–1051

92. Simons-Morton B, Ouimet MC. Parent involvement in novice teen driving: a review of the literature. *Inj Prev*. 2006;12(suppl 1):i30–i37

93. Curry AE, Peek-Asa C, Hamann CJ, Mirman JH. Effectiveness of parent-focused interventions to increase teen driver safety: a critical review. *J Adolesc Health*. 2015;57(suppl 1):S6–S14

94. Peek-Asa C, Cavanaugh JE, Yang J, Chande V, Young T, Ramirez M. Steering teens safe: a randomized trial of a parent-based intervention to improve safe teen driving. *BMC Public Health*. 2014;14:777

95. Winston FK, Puzino K, Romer D. Precision prevention: time to move beyond universal interventions. *Inj Prev*. 2016;22(2):87–91

96. Mirman JH, Curry AE, Winston FK, et al. Effect of the teen driving plan on the driving performance of teenagers before licensure: a randomized clinical trial. *JAMA Pediatr*. 2014;168(8):764–771

97. Fabiano GA, Schatz NK, Morris KL, et al. Efficacy of a family-focused intervention for young drivers with attention-deficit hyperactivity disorder. *J Consult Clin Psychol*. 2016;84(12):1078–1093

98. McGehee DV, Raby M, Carney C, Lee JD, Reyes ML. Extending parental mentoring using an event-triggered video intervention in rural teen drivers. *J Safety Res*. 2007;38(2):215–227

99. Farmer CM, Kirley BB, McCartt AT. Effects of in-vehicle monitoring on the driving behavior of teenagers. *J Safety Res*. 2010;41(1):39–45

100. Governors Highway Safety Association. Seat belts. 2018. Available at: www.ghsa.org/html/stateinfo/laws/seatbelt_laws.html. Accessed August 10, 2018

101. Shults RA, Elder RW, Sleet DA, et al; Task Force on Community Preventive Services. Reviews of evidence regarding interventions to reduce alcohol-impaired driving. *Am J Prev Med*. 2001;21(suppl 4):66–88

102. Governors Highway Safety Association. Drug impaired driving. 2016. Available at: www.ghsa.org/state-laws/issues/drug impaired driving. Accessed December 14, 2017

103. US House of Representatives. Lucid Act of 2015, HR 2598, 114th Cong, (2015-2016). 2015. Available at: https://www.congress.gov/bill/114th-congress/house-bill/2598. Accessed December 14, 2017

104. McCartt AT, Hellinga LA, Strouse LM, Farmer CM. Long-term effects of handheld cell phone laws on driver handheld cell phone use. *Traffic Inj Prev*. 2010;11(2):133–141

105. Goodwin AH, O'Brien NP, Foss RD. Effect of North Carolina's restriction on teenage driver cell phone use two years after implementation. *Accid Anal Prev*. 2012;48:363–367

106. Ferdinand AO, Menachemi N, Blackburn JL, Sen B, Nelson L, Morrisey M. The impact of texting bans on motor vehicle crash-related hospitalizations. *Am J Public Health*. 2015;105(5):859–865

107. Nevin PE, Blanar L, Kirk AP, et al. "I wasn't texting; I was just reading an email …": a qualitative study of distracted driving enforcement in Washington State. *Inj Prev*. 2017;23(3):165–170

108. Caird JK, Johnston KA, Willness CR, Asbridge M, Steel P. A meta-analysis of the effects of texting on driving. *Accid Anal Prev*. 2014;71:311–318

109. Mehler B, Reimer B, Lavallière M, Dobres J, Coughlin JF. *Evaluating Technologies Relevant to the Enhancement of Driver Safety*. Washington, DC: American Automobile Association Foundation for Traffic Safety; 2014:25–29

110. Lee JD. Technology and teen drivers. *J Safety Res*. 2007;38(2):203–213

111. Insurance Institute for Highway Safety; Highway Loss Data Institute. Choosing the best vehicles for your teen. Available at: www.iihs.org/iihs/ratings/vehicles-for-teens. Accessed December 14, 2017

112. Funkhouser D, Sayer JR. *Cell Phone Filter/Blocker Technology Field Test. Report No. DOT HS 811 863*. Washington, DC: National Highway Traffic Safety Administration; 2013. Available at: https://one.nhtsa.gov/DOT/NHTSA/NVS/Crash%20Avoidance/Technical%20Publications/2013/Cell_Phone_Filter_Blocker_Technology_Field_Test_811863.pdf. Accessed December 14, 2017

113. McDonald AB, McGehee DV, Chrysler ST, Askelson NM, Angell LS, Seppelt BD. National consumer survey of driving safety technologies. *Transportation*

& *Vehicle Safety Policy.* 2015. Available at: http://ir.uiowa.edu/ppc_ transportation/32. Accessed December 14, 2017

114. Delgado MK, Wanner KJ, McDonald C. Adolescent cellphone use while

driving: an overview of the literature and promising future directions for prevention. *Media Commun.* 2016;4(3):79–89

115. Creaser JI, Edwards CJ, Morris NL, Donath M. Are cellular phone blocking

applications effective for novice teen drivers? *J Safety Res.* 2015;54:75–78

116. American Family Insurance. Teen safe driver program. Available at: www.teensafedriver.com/. Accessed December 14, 2017

Section 5

Current Policies

From the American Academy of Pediatrics

• •

(Through December 31, 2018)

- *Policy Statements*
  ORGANIZATIONAL PRINCIPLES TO GUIDE AND DEFINE THE CHILD HEALTH CARE SYSTEM
  AND TO IMPROVE THE HEALTH OF ALL CHILDREN

- *Clinical Reports*
  GUIDANCE FOR THE CLINICIAN IN RENDERING PEDIATRIC CARE

- *Technical Reports*
  BACKGROUND INFORMATION TO SUPPORT AMERICAN ACADEMY OF PEDIATRICS POLICY

American Academy of Pediatrics

Policy Statements, Clinical Reports, Technical Reports

Current through December 31, 2018
The companion *Pediatric Clinical Practice Guidelines & Policies* eBook
points to the full text of all titles listed herein.

2017 RECOMMENDATIONS FOR PREVENTIVE PEDIATRIC HEALTH CARE

Committee on Practice and Ambulatory Medicine and Bright Futures Periodicity Schedule Workgroup

ABSTRACT. The 2017 Recommendations for Preventive Pediatric Health Care (Periodicity Schedule) has been approved by the American Academy of Pediatrics (AAP) and represents a consensus of AAP and the Bright Futures Periodicity Schedule Workgroup. Each child and family is unique; therefore, these recommendations are designed for the care of children who are receiving competent parenting, have no manifestations of any important health problems, and are growing and developing in a satisfactory fashion. Developmental, psychosocial, and chronic disease issues for children and adolescents may require frequent counseling and treatment visits separate from preventive care visits. Additional visits also may become necessary if circumstances suggest variations from normal. (2/17)
http://pediatrics.aappublications.org/content/139/4/e20170254

AAP DIVERSITY AND INCLUSION STATEMENT

American Academy of Pediatrics

ABSTRACT. The vision of the American Academy of Pediatrics (AAP) is that all children have optimal health and well-being and are valued by society and that AAP members practice the highest quality health care and experience professional satisfaction and personal well-being. From the founding of the AAP, pursuing this vision has included treasuring the uniqueness of each child and fostering a profession, health care system, and communities that celebrate all aspects of the diversity of each child and family. (3/18)

See full text on page 499.
http://pediatrics.aappublications.org/content/141/4/e20180193

ABUSIVE HEAD TRAUMA IN INFANTS AND CHILDREN

Cindy W. Christian, MD; Robert Block, MD; and Committee on Child Abuse and Neglect

ABSTRACT. Shaken baby syndrome is a term often used by physicians and the public to describe abusive head trauma inflicted on infants and young children. Although the term is well known and has been used for a number of decades, advances in the understanding of the mechanisms and clinical spectrum of injury associated with abusive head trauma compel us to modify our terminology to keep pace with our understanding of pathologic mechanisms. Although shaking an infant has the potential to cause neurologic injury, blunt impact or a combination of shaking and blunt impact cause injury as well. Spinal cord injury and secondary hypoxic ischemic injury can contribute to poor outcomes of victims. The use of broad medical terminology that is inclusive of all mechanisms of injury, including shaking, is required. The American Academy of Pediatrics recommends that pediatricians develop skills in the recognition of signs and symptoms of abusive head injury, including those caused by both shaking and blunt impact, consult with pediatric subspecialists when necessary, and embrace a less mechanistic term, abusive head trauma, when describing an inflicted injury to the head and its contents. (4/09, reaffirmed 3/13, 4/17)
http://pediatrics.aappublications.org/content/123/5/1409

ACCESS TO OPTIMAL EMERGENCY CARE FOR CHILDREN

Committee on Pediatric Emergency Medicine

ABSTRACT. Millions of pediatric patients require some level of emergency care annually, and significant barriers limit access to appropriate services for large numbers of children. The American Academy of Pediatrics has a strong commitment to identifying barriers to access to emergency care, working to surmount these obstacles, and encouraging, through education and system changes, improved levels of emergency care available to all children. (1/07, reaffirmed 8/10, 7/14)
http://pediatrics.aappublications.org/content/119/1/161

ACHIEVING QUALITY HEALTH SERVICES FOR ADOLESCENTS

Committee on Adolescence

ABSTRACT. This update of the 2008 statement from the American Academy of Pediatrics redirects the discussion of quality health care from the theoretical to the practical within the medical home. This statement reviews the evolution of the medical home concept and challenges the provision of quality adolescent health care within the patient-centered medical home. Areas of attention for quality adolescent health care are reviewed, including developmentally appropriate care, confidentiality, location of adolescent care, providers who offer such care, the role of research in advancing care, and the transition to adult care. (7/16)
http://pediatrics.aappublications.org/content/138/2/e20161347

ADDRESSING EARLY CHILDHOOD EMOTIONAL AND BEHAVIORAL PROBLEMS

Council on Early Childhood, Committee on Psychosocial Aspects of Child and Family Health, and Section on Developmental and Behavioral Pediatrics

ABSTRACT. Emotional, behavioral, and relationship problems can develop in very young children, especially those living in high-risk families or communities. These early problems interfere with the normative activities of young children and their families and predict long-lasting problems across multiple domains. A growing evidence base demonstrates the efficacy of specific family-focused therapies in reducing the symptoms of emotional, behavioral, and relationship symptoms, with effects lasting years after the therapy has ended. Pediatricians are usually the primary health care providers for children with emotional or behavioral difficulties, and awareness of emerging research about evidence-based treatments will enhance this care. In most communities, access to these interventions is insufficient. Pediatricians can improve the care of young children with emotional, behavioral, and relationship problems by calling for the following: increased access to care; increased research identifying alternative approaches, including primary care delivery of treatments; adequate payment for pediatric providers who serve these young children; and improved education for pediatric providers about the principles of evidence-based interventions. (11/16)

http://pediatrics.aappublications.org/content/138/6/e20163023

ADDRESSING EARLY CHILDHOOD EMOTIONAL AND BEHAVIORAL PROBLEMS (TECHNICAL REPORT)

Mary Margaret Gleason, MD, FAAP; Edward Goldson, MD, FAAP; Michael W. Yogman, MD, FAAP; Council on Early Childhood; Committee on Psychosocial Aspects of Child and Family Health; and Section on Developmental and Behavioral Pediatrics

ABSTRACT. More than 10% of young children experience clinically significant mental health problems, with rates of impairment and persistence comparable to those seen in older children. For many of these clinical disorders, effective treatments supported by rigorous data are available. On the other hand, rigorous support for psychopharmacologic interventions is limited to 2 large randomized controlled trials. Access to psychotherapeutic interventions is limited. The pediatrician has a critical role as the leader of the medical home to promote well-being that includes emotional, behavioral, and relationship health. To be effective in this role, pediatricians promote the use of safe and effective treatments and recognize the limitations of psychopharmacologic interventions. This technical report reviews the data supporting treatments for young children with emotional, behavioral, and relationship problems and supports the policy statement of the same name. (11/16)

http://pediatrics.aappublications.org/content/138/6/e20163025

ADMISSION AND DISCHARGE GUIDELINES FOR THE PEDIATRIC PATIENT REQUIRING INTERMEDIATE CARE (CLINICAL REPORT)

Committee on Hospital Care and Section on Critical Care (joint with Society of Critical Care Medicine)

ABSTRACT. During the past 3 decades, the specialty of pediatric critical care medicine has grown rapidly, leading to a number of pediatric intensive care units opening across the country. Many patients who are admitted to the hospital require a higher level of care than routine inpatient general pediatric care, yet not to the degree of intensity of pediatric critical care; therefore, an intermediate care level has been developed in institutions providing multidisciplinary subspecialty pediatric care. These patients may require frequent monitoring of vital signs and nursing interventions, but usually they do not require invasive monitoring. The admission of the pediatric intermediate care patient is guided by physiologic parameters depending on the respective organ system involved relative to an institution's resources and capacity to care for a patient in a general care environment. This report provides admission and discharge guidelines for intermediate pediatric care. Intermediate care promotes greater flexibility in patient triage and provides a cost-effective alternative to admission to a pediatric intensive care unit. This level of care may enhance the efficiency of care and make health care more affordable for patients receiving intermediate care. (5/04, reaffirmed 2/08, 5/17)

http://pediatrics.aappublications.org/content/113/5/1430

ADOLESCENT AND YOUNG ADULT TATTOOING, PIERCING, AND SCARIFICATION (CLINICAL REPORT)

Cora C. Breuner, MD, MPH; David A. Levine, MD; and Committee on Adolescence

ABSTRACT. Tattoos, piercing, and scarification are now commonplace among adolescents and young adults. This first clinical report from the American Academy of Pediatrics on voluntary body modification will review the methods used to perform the modifications. Complications resulting from body modification methods, although not common, are discussed to provide the pediatrician with management information. Body modification will be contrasted with nonsuicidal self-injury. When available, information also is presented on societal perceptions of body modification. (9/17)

http://pediatrics.aappublications.org/content/140/4/e20163494

ADOLESCENT DRUG TESTING POLICIES IN SCHOOLS

Sharon Levy, MD, MPH, FAAP; Miriam Schizer, MD, MPH, FAAP; and Committee on Substance Abuse

ABSTRACT. School-based drug testing is a controversial approach to preventing substance use by students. Although school drug testing has hypothetical benefits, and studies have noted modest reductions in self-reported student drug use, the American Academy of Pediatrics opposes widespread implementation of these programs because of the lack of solid evidence for their effectiveness. (3/15)

http://pediatrics.aappublications.org/content/135/4/782

ADOLESCENT DRUG TESTING POLICIES IN SCHOOLS (TECHNICAL REPORT)

Sharon Levy, MD, MPH, FAAP; Miriam Schizer, MD, MPH, FAAP; and Committee on Substance Abuse

ABSTRACT. More than a decade after the US Supreme Court established the legality of school-based drug testing, these programs remain controversial, and the evidence evaluating efficacy and risks is inconclusive. The objective of this technical report is to review the relevant literature that explores the benefits, risks, and costs of these programs. (3/15)

http://pediatrics.aappublications.org/content/135/4/e1107

ADOLESCENT PREGNANCY: CURRENT TRENDS AND ISSUES (CLINICAL REPORT)

Jonathan D. Klein, MD, MPH, and Committee on Adolescence

ABSTRACT. The prevention of unintended adolescent pregnancy is an important goal of the American Academy of Pediatrics and our society. Although adolescent pregnancy and birth rates have been steadily decreasing, many adolescents still become pregnant. Since the last statement on adolescent pregnancy was issued by the Academy in 1998, efforts to prevent adolescent pregnancy have increased, and new observations, technologies, and prevention effectiveness data have emerged. The purpose of this clinical report is to review current trends and issues related to adolescent pregnancy, update practitioners on this topic, and review legal and policy implications of concern to pediatricians. (7/05)

http://pediatrics.aappublications.org/content/116/1/281

ADOLESCENT PREGNANCY: CURRENT TRENDS AND ISSUES—ADDENDUM

Committee on Adolescence

INTRODUCTION. The purpose of this addendum is to update pediatricians and other professionals on recent research and data regarding adolescent sexuality, contraceptive use, and childbearing since publication of the original 2005 clinical report, "Adolescent Pregnancy: Current Trends and Issues." There has been a trend of decreasing sexual activity and teen births and pregnancies since 1991, except between the years of 2005 and 2007, when there was a 5% increase in birth rates. Currently, teen birth rates in the United States are at a record low secondary to increased use of contraception at first intercourse and use of dual methods of condoms and hormonal contraception among sexually active teenagers. Despite these data, the United States continues to lead other industrialized countries in having unacceptably high rates of adolescent pregnancy, with over 700 000 pregnancies per year, the direct health consequence of unprotected intercourse. Importantly, the 2006–2010 National Survey of Family Growth (NSFG) revealed that less than one-third of

15- to 19-year-old female subjects consistently used contraceptive methods at last intercourse. (4/14)

http://pediatrics.aappublications.org/content/133/5/954

ADOLESCENTS AND HIV INFECTION: THE PEDIATRICIAN'S ROLE IN PROMOTING ROUTINE TESTING

Committee on Pediatric AIDS

ABSTRACT. Pediatricians can play a key role in preventing and controlling HIV infection by promoting risk-reduction counseling and offering routine HIV testing to adolescent and young adult patients. Most sexually active youth do not feel that they are at risk of contracting HIV and have never been tested. Obtaining a sexual history and creating an atmosphere that promotes nonjudgmental risk counseling is a key component of the adolescent visit. In light of increasing numbers of people with HIV/AIDS and missed opportunities for HIV testing, the Centers for Disease Control and Prevention recommends universal and routine HIV testing for all patients seen in health care settings who are 13 to 64 years of age. There are advances in diagnostics and treatment that help support this recommendation. This policy statement reviews the epidemiologic data and recommends that routine screening be offered to all adolescents at least once by 16 to 18 years of age in health care settings when the prevalence of HIV in the patient population is more than 0.1%. In areas of lower community HIV prevalence, routine HIV testing is encouraged for all sexually active adolescents and those with other risk factors for HIV. This statement addresses many of the real and perceived barriers that pediatricians face in promoting routine HIV testing for their patients. (10/11, reaffirmed 9/15)

http://pediatrics.aappublications.org/content/128/5/1023

THE ADOLESCENT'S RIGHT TO CONFIDENTIAL CARE WHEN CONSIDERING ABORTION

Committee on Adolescence

ABSTRACT. In this statement, the American Academy of Pediatrics reaffirms its position that the rights of adolescents to confidential care when considering abortion should be protected. Adolescents should be encouraged to involve their parents and other trusted adults in decisions regarding pregnancy termination, and most do so voluntarily. The majority of states require that minors have parental consent for an abortion. However, legislation mandating parental involvement does not achieve the intended benefit of promoting family communication, and it increases the risk of harm to the adolescent by delaying access to appropriate medical care. This statement presents a summary of pertinent current information related to the benefits and risks of legislation requiring mandatory parental involvement in an adolescent's decision to obtain an abortion. (1/17)

http://pediatrics.aappublications.org/content/139/2/e20163861

ADVANCED PRACTICE IN NEONATAL NURSING

Committee on Fetus and Newborn

ABSTRACT. The participation of advanced practice registered nurses in neonatal care continues to be accepted and supported by the American Academy of Pediatrics. Recognized categories of advanced practice neonatal nursing are the neonatal clinical nurse specialist and the neonatal nurse practitioner. (5/09, reaffirmed 1/14)

http://pediatrics.aappublications.org/content/123/6/1606

ADVOCACY FOR IMPROVING NUTRITION IN THE FIRST 1000 DAYS TO SUPPORT CHILDHOOD DEVELOPMENT AND ADULT HEALTH

Sarah Jane Schwarzenberg, MD, FAAP; Michael K. Georgieff, MD, FAAP; and Committee on Nutrition

ABSTRACT. Maternal prenatal nutrition and the child's nutrition in the first 2 years of life (1000 days) are crucial factors in a child's neurodevelopment and lifelong mental health. Child and adult health risks, including obesity, hypertension, and diabetes, may be programmed by nutritional status during this period. Calories are essential for growth of both fetus and child but are not sufficient for normal brain development. Although all nutrients are necessary for brain growth, key nutrients that support neurodevelopment include protein; zinc; iron; choline; folate; iodine; vitamins A, D, B_6, and B_{12}; and long-chain polyunsaturated fatty acids. Failure to provide key nutrients during this critical period of brain development may result in lifelong deficits in brain function despite subsequent nutrient repletion. Understanding the complex interplay of micro- and macronutrients and neurodevelopment is key to moving beyond simply recommending a "good diet" to optimizing nutrient delivery for the developing child. Leaders in pediatric health and policy makers must be aware of this research given its implications for public policy at the federal and state level. Pediatricians should refer to existing services for nutrition support for pregnant and breastfeeding women, infants, and toddlers. Finally, all providers caring for children can advocate for healthy diets for mothers, infants, and young children in the first 1000 days. Prioritizing public policies that ensure the provision of adequate nutrients and healthy eating during this crucial time would ensure that all children have an early foundation for optimal neurodevelopment, a key factor in long-term health. (1/18)

See full text on page 503.

http://pediatrics.aappublications.org/content/141/2/e20173716

ADVOCATING FOR LIFE SUPPORT TRAINING OF CHILDREN, PARENTS, CAREGIVERS, SCHOOL PERSONNEL, AND THE PUBLIC

James M. Callahan, MD, FAAP; Susan M. Fuchs, MD, FAAP; and Committee on Pediatric Emergency Medicine

ABSTRACT. Out-of-hospital cardiac arrest occurs frequently among people of all ages, including more than 6000 children annually. Pediatric cardiac arrest in the out-of-hospital setting is a stressful event for family, friends, caregivers, classmates, school personnel, and witnesses. Immediate bystander cardiopulmonary resuscitation and the use of automated external defibrillators are associated with improved survival in adults. There is some evidence in which improved survival in children who receive immediate bystander cardiopulmonary resuscitation is shown. Pediatricians, in their role as advocates to improve the health of all children, are uniquely positioned to strongly encourage the training of children, parents, caregivers, school personnel, and the lay public in the provision of basic life support, including pediatric basic life support, as well as the appropriate use of automated external defibrillators. (5/18)

See full text on page 515.

http://pediatrics.aappublications.org/content/141/6/e20180704

ADVOCATING FOR LIFE SUPPORT TRAINING OF CHILDREN, PARENTS, CAREGIVERS, SCHOOL PERSONNEL, AND THE PUBLIC (TECHNICAL REPORT)

Susan M. Fuchs, MD, FAAP, and Committee on Pediatric Emergency Medicine

ABSTRACT. Pediatric cardiac arrest in the out-of-hospital setting is a traumatic event for family, friends, caregivers, classmates, and school personnel. Immediate bystander cardiopulmonary resuscitation and the use of automatic external defibrillators have been shown to improve survival in adults. There is some evidence to show improved survival in children who receive immediate bystander cardiopulmonary resuscitation. Pediatricians, in their role as advocates to improve the health of all children, are uniquely positioned to strongly encourage the training of children, parents, caregivers, school personnel, and the lay public in the provision of basic life support, including pediatric basic life support, as well as the appropriate use of automated external defibrillators. (5/18)

See full text on page 521.

http://pediatrics.aappublications.org/content/141/6/e20180705

AGE LIMIT OF PEDIATRICS

Amy Peykoff Hardin, MD, FAAP; Jesse M. Hackell, MD, FAAP; and Committee on Practice and Ambulatory Medicine

ABSTRACT. Pediatrics is a multifaceted specialty that encompasses children's physical, psychosocial, developmental, and mental health. Pediatric care may begin periconceptionally and continues through gestation, infancy, childhood, adolescence, and young adulthood. Although adolescence and young adulthood are recognizable phases of life, an upper age limit is not easily demarcated and varies depending on the individual patient. The establishment of arbitrary age limits on pediatric care by health care providers should be discouraged. The decision to continue care with a pediatrician or pediatric medical or surgical subspecialist should be made solely by the patient (and family, when appropriate) and the physician and must take into account the physical and psychosocial needs of the patient and the abilities of the pediatric provider to meet these needs. (8/17)

http://pediatrics.aappublications.org/content/140/3/e20172151

AGE TERMINOLOGY DURING THE PERINATAL PERIOD

Committee on Fetus and Newborn

ABSTRACT. Consistent definitions to describe the length of gestation and age in neonates are needed to compare neurodevelopmental, medical, and growth outcomes. The purposes of this policy statement are to review conventional definitions of age during the perinatal period and to recommend use of standard terminology including gestational age, postmenstrual age, chronological age, corrected age, adjusted age, and estimated date of delivery. (11/04, reaffirmed 10/07, 11/08, 7/14)

http://pediatrics.aappublications.org/content/114/5/1362

ALCOHOL USE BY YOUTH AND ADOLESCENTS: A PEDIATRIC CONCERN

Committee on Substance Abuse

ABSTRACT. Alcohol use continues to be a major problem from preadolescence through young adulthood in the United States. Results of recent neuroscience research have substantiated the deleterious effects of alcohol on adolescent brain development and added even more evidence to support the call to prevent and reduce underaged drinking. Pediatricians should be knowledgeable about substance abuse to be able to recognize risk factors for alcohol and other substance abuse among youth, screen for use, provide appropriate brief interventions, and refer to treatment. The integration of alcohol use prevention programs in the community and our educational system from elementary school through college should be promoted by pediatricians and the health care community. Promotion of media responsibility to connect alcohol consumption with realistic consequences should be supported by pediatricians. Additional research into the prevention, screening and identification, brief intervention, and management and treatment of alcohol and other substance use by adolescents continues to be needed to improve evidence-based practices. (4/10, reaffirmed 12/14)

http://pediatrics.aappublications.org/content/125/5/1078

ALLERGY TESTING IN CHILDHOOD: USING ALLERGEN-SPECIFIC IGE TESTS (CLINICAL REPORT)

Scott H. Sicherer, MD; Robert A. Wood, MD; and Section on Allergy and Immunology

ABSTRACT. A variety of triggers can induce common pediatric allergic diseases which include asthma, allergic rhinitis, atopic dermatitis, food allergy, and anaphylaxis. Allergy testing serves to confirm an allergic trigger suspected on the basis of history. Tests for allergen-specific immunoglobulin E (IgE) are performed by in vitro assays or skin tests. The tests are excellent for identifying a sensitized state in which allergen-specific IgE is present, and may identify triggers to be eliminated and help guide immunotherapy treatment. However, a positive test result does not always equate with clinical allergy. Newer enzymatic assays based on anti-IgE antibodies have supplanted the radioallergosorbent test (RAST). This clinical report focuses on allergen-specific IgE testing, emphasizing that the medical history and knowledge of disease characteristics are crucial for rational test selection and interpretation. (12/11)

http://pediatrics.aappublications.org/content/129/1/193

ALL-TERRAIN VEHICLE INJURY PREVENTION: TWO-, THREE-, AND FOUR-WHEELED UNLICENSED MOTOR VEHICLES

Committee on Injury and Poison Prevention

ABSTRACT. Since 1987, the American Academy of Pediatrics (AAP) has had a policy about the use of motorized cycles and all-terrain vehicles (ATVs) by children. The purpose of this policy statement is to update and strengthen previous policy. This statement describes the various kinds of motorized cycles and ATVs and outlines the epidemiologic characteristics of deaths and injuries related to their use by children in light of the 1987 consent decrees entered into by the US Consumer Product Safety Commission and the manufacturers of ATVs. Recommendations are made for public, patient, and parent education by pediatricians; equipment modifications; the use of safety equipment; and the development and improvement of safer off-road trails and responsive emergency medical systems. In addition, the AAP strengthens its recommendation for passage of legislation in all states prohibiting the use of 2- and 4-wheeled off-road vehicles by children younger than 16 years, as well as a ban on the sale of new and used 3-wheeled ATVs, with a recall of all used 3-wheeled ATVs. (6/00, reaffirmed 5/04, 1/07, 5/13)

http://pediatrics.aappublications.org/content/105/6/1352

AMBIENT AIR POLLUTION: HEALTH HAZARDS TO CHILDREN

Committee on Environmental Health

ABSTRACT. Ambient (outdoor) air pollution is now recognized as an important problem, both nationally and worldwide. Our scientific understanding of the spectrum of health effects of air pollution has increased, and numerous studies are finding important health effects from air pollution at levels once considered safe. Children and infants are among the most susceptible to many of the air pollutants. In addition to associations between air pollution and respiratory symptoms, asthma exacerbations, and asthma hospitalizations, recent studies have found links between air pollution and preterm birth, infant mortality, deficits in lung growth, and possibly, development of asthma. This policy statement summarizes the recent literature linking ambient air pollution to adverse health outcomes in children and includes a perspective on the current regulatory process. The statement provides advice to pediatricians on how to integrate issues regarding air quality and health into patient education and children's environmental health advocacy and concludes with recommendations to the government on promotion of effective air-pollution policies to ensure protection of children's health. (12/04, reaffirmed 4/09)

http://pediatrics.aappublications.org/content/114/6/1699

ANTENATAL COUNSELING REGARDING RESUSCITATION AND INTENSIVE CARE BEFORE 25 WEEKS OF GESTATION (CLINICAL REPORT)

James Cummings, MD, FAAP, and Committee on Fetus and Newborn

ABSTRACT. The anticipated birth of an extremely low gestational age (<25 weeks) infant presents many difficult questions, and variations in practice continue to exist. Decisions regarding care of periviable infants should ideally be well informed, ethically sound, consistent within medical teams, and consonant with the parents' wishes. Each health care institution should consider having policies and procedures for antenatal counseling in these situations. Family counseling may be aided by the use of visual materials, which should take into consideration the intellectual, cultural, and other characteristics of the family members. Although general recommendations can guide practice, each situation is unique; thus, decision-making should be individualized. In most cases, the approach should be shared decision-making with the family, guided by considering both the likelihood of death or morbidity and the parents' desires for their unborn child. If a decision is made not to resuscitate, providing comfort care, encouraging family bonding, and palliative care support are appropriate. (8/15)
http://pediatrics.aappublications.org/content/136/3/588

ANTERIOR CRUCIATE LIGAMENT INJURIES: DIAGNOSIS, TREATMENT, AND PREVENTION (CLINICAL REPORT)

Cynthia R. LaBella, MD, FAAP; William Hennrikus, MD, FAAP; Timothy E. Hewett, PhD, FACSM; Council on Sports Medicine and Fitness; and Section on Orthopaedics

ABSTRACT. The number of anterior cruciate ligament (ACL) injuries reported in athletes younger than 18 years has increased over the past 2 decades. Reasons for the increasing ACL injury rate include the growing number of children and adolescents participating in organized sports, intensive sports training at an earlier age, and greater rate of diagnosis because of increased awareness and greater use of advanced medical imaging. ACL injury rates are low in young children and increase sharply during puberty, especially for girls, who have higher rates of non-contact ACL injuries than boys do in similar sports. Intrinsic risk factors for ACL injury include higher BMI, subtalar joint overpronation, generalized ligamentous laxity, and decreased neuromuscular control of knee motion. ACL injuries often require surgery and/or many months of rehabilitation and substantial time lost from school and sports participation. Unfortunately, regardless of treatment, athletes with ACL injuries are up to 10 times more likely to develop degenerative arthritis of the knee. Safe and effective surgical techniques for children and adolescents continue to evolve. Neuromuscular training can reduce risk of ACL injury in adolescent girls. This report outlines the current state of knowledge on epidemiology, diagnosis, treatment, and prevention of ACL injuries in children and adolescents. (4/14, reaffirmed 7/18)
http://pediatrics.aappublications.org/content/133/5/e1437

THE APGAR SCORE

Committee on Fetus and Newborn (joint with American College of Obstetricians and Gynecologists Committee on Obstetric Practice)

ABSTRACT. The Apgar score provides an accepted and convenient method for reporting the status of the newborn infant immediately after birth and the response to resuscitation if needed. The Apgar score alone cannot be considered as evidence of, or a consequence of, asphyxia; does not predict individual neonatal mortality or neurologic outcome; and should not be used for that purpose. An Apgar score assigned during resuscitation is not equivalent to a score assigned to a spontaneously breathing infant. The American Academy of Pediatrics and the American College of Obstetricians and Gynecologists encourage use of an expanded Apgar score reporting form that accounts for concurrent resuscitative interventions. (9/15)
http://pediatrics.aappublications.org/content/136/4/819

APNEA OF PREMATURITY (CLINICAL REPORT)

Eric C. Eichenwald, MD, FAAP, and Committee on Fetus and Newborn

ABSTRACT. Apnea of prematurity is one of the most common diagnoses in the NICU. Despite the frequency of apnea of prematurity, it is unknown whether recurrent apnea, bradycardia, and hypoxemia in preterm infants are harmful. Research into the development of respiratory control in immature animals and preterm infants has facilitated our understanding of the pathogenesis and treatment of apnea of prematurity. However, the lack of consistent definitions, monitoring practices, and consensus about clinical significance leads to significant variation in practice. The purpose of this clinical report is to review the evidence basis for the definition, epidemiology, and treatment of apnea of prematurity as well as discharge recommendations for preterm infants diagnosed with recurrent apneic events. (12/15)
http://pediatrics.aappublications.org/content/137/1/e20153757

APPLICATION OF THE RESOURCE-BASED RELATIVE VALUE SCALE SYSTEM TO PEDIATRICS

Committee on Coding and Nomenclature

ABSTRACT. The majority of public and private payers in the United States currently use the Medicare Resource-Based Relative Value Scale as the basis for physician payment. Many large group and academic practices have adopted this objective system of physician work to benchmark physician productivity, including using it, wholly or in part, to determine compensation. The Resource-Based Relative Value Scale survey instrument, used to value physician services, was designed primarily for procedural services, leading to current concerns that American Medical Association/Specialty Society Relative Value Scale Update Committee (RUC) surveys may undervalue nonprocedural evaluation and management services. The American Academy of Pediatrics is represented on the RUC, the committee charged with maintaining accurate physician work values across specialties and age groups. The Academy, working closely with other primary care and subspecialty societies, actively pursues a balanced RUC membership and a survey instrument that will ensure appropriate work relative value unit assignments, thereby allowing pediatricians to receive appropriate payment for their services relative to other services. (5/14)
http://pediatrics.aappublications.org/content/133/6/1158

ASSESSMENT AND MANAGEMENT OF INGUINAL HERNIA IN INFANTS (CLINICAL REPORT)

Kasper S. Wang, MD; Committee on Fetus and Newborn; and Section on Surgery

ABSTRACT. Inguinal hernia repair in infants is a routine surgical procedure. However, numerous issues, including timing of the repair, the need to explore the contralateral groin, use of laparoscopy, and anesthetic approach, remain unsettled. Given the lack of compelling data, consideration should be given to large, prospective, randomized controlled trials to determine best practices for the management of inguinal hernias in infants. (9/12)
http://pediatrics.aappublications.org/content/130/4/768

ATOPIC DERMATITIS: SKIN-DIRECTED MANAGEMENT (CLINICAL REPORT)

Megha M. Tollefson, MD; Anna L. Bruckner, MD, FAAP; and Section on Dermatology

ABSTRACT. Atopic dermatitis is a common inflammatory skin condition characterized by relapsing eczematous lesions in a typical distribution. It can be frustrating for pediatric patients, parents, and health care providers alike. The pediatrician will

treat the majority of children with atopic dermatitis as many patients will not have access to a pediatric medical subspecialist, such as a pediatric dermatologist or pediatric allergist. This report provides up-to-date information regarding the disease and its impact, pathogenesis, treatment options, and potential complications. The goal of this report is to assist pediatricians with accurate and useful information that will improve the care of patients with atopic dermatitis. (11/14)
http://pediatrics.aappublications.org/content/134/6/e1735

ATTENTION-DEFICIT/HYPERACTIVITY DISORDER AND SUBSTANCE ABUSE (CLINICAL REPORT)

Elizabeth Harstad, MD, MPH, FAAP; Sharon Levy, MD, MPH, FAAP; and Committee on Substance Abuse

ABSTRACT. Attention-deficit/hyperactivity disorder (ADHD) and substance use disorders are inextricably intertwined. Children with ADHD are more likely than peers to develop substance use disorders. Treatment with stimulants may reduce the risk of substance use disorders, but stimulants are a class of medication with significant abuse and diversion potential. The objectives of this clinical report were to present practical strategies for reducing the risk of substance use disorders in patients with ADHD and suggestions for safe stimulant prescribing. (6/14)
http://pediatrics.aappublications.org/content/134/1/e293

BASEBALL AND SOFTBALL

Council on Sports Medicine and Fitness

ABSTRACT. Baseball and softball are among the most popular and safest sports in which children and adolescents participate. Nevertheless, traumatic and overuse injuries occur regularly, including occasional catastrophic injury and even death. Safety of the athlete is a constant focus of attention among those responsible for modifying rules. Understanding the stresses placed on the arm, especially while pitching, led to the institution of rules controlling the quantity of pitches thrown in youth baseball and established rest periods between pitching assignments. Similarly, field maintenance and awareness of environmental conditions as well as equipment maintenance and creative prevention strategies are critically important in minimizing the risk of injury. This statement serves as a basis for encouraging safe participation in baseball and softball. This statement has been endorsed by the Canadian Paediatric Society. (2/12, reaffirmed 7/15)
http://pediatrics.aappublications.org/content/129/3/e842

BEST PRACTICES FOR IMPROVING FLOW AND CARE OF PEDIATRIC PATIENTS IN THE EMERGENCY DEPARTMENT (TECHNICAL REPORT)

Isabel Barata, MD; Kathleen M. Brown, MD; Laura Fitzmaurice, MD; Elizabeth Stone Griffin, RN; Sally K. Snow, BSN, RN; and Committee on Pediatric Emergency Medicine (joint with American College of Emergency Physicians Pediatric Emergency Medicine Committee and Emergency Nurses Association Pediatric Committee)

ABSTRACT. This report provides a summary of best practices for improving flow, reducing waiting times, and improving the quality of care of pediatric patients in the emergency department. (12/14)
http://pediatrics.aappublications.org/content/135/1/e273

BICYCLE HELMETS

Committee on Injury and Poison Prevention

ABSTRACT. Bicycling remains one of the most popular recreational sports among children in America and is the leading cause of recreational sports injuries treated in emergency departments. An estimated 23 000 children younger than 21 years sustained head injuries (excluding the face) while bicycling in 1998.
The bicycle helmet is a very effective device that can prevent the occurrence of up to 88% of serious brain injuries. Despite this, most children do not wear a helmet each time they ride a bicycle, and adolescents are particularly resistant to helmet use. Recently, a group of national experts and government agencies renewed the call for all bicyclists to wear helmets. This policy statement describes the role of the pediatrician in helping attain universal helmet use among children and teens for each bicycle ride. (10/01, reaffirmed 1/05, 2/08, 11/11)
http://pediatrics.aappublications.org/content/108/4/1030

BINGE DRINKING (CLINICAL REPORT)

Lorena Siqueira, MD, MSPH, FAAP; Vincent C. Smith, MD, MPH, FAAP; and Committee on Substance Abuse

ABSTRACT. Alcohol is the substance most frequently abused by children and adolescents in the United States, and its use is associated with the leading causes of death and serious injury at this age (ie, motor vehicle accidents, homicides, and suicides). Among youth who drink, the proportion who drink heavily is higher than among adult drinkers, increasing from approximately 50% in those 12 to 14 years of age to 72% among those 18 to 20 years of age. In this clinical report, the definition, epidemiology, and risk factors for binge drinking; the neurobiology of intoxication, blackouts, and hangovers; genetic considerations; and adverse outcomes are discussed. The report offers guidance for the pediatrician. As with any high-risk behavior, prevention plays a more important role than later intervention and has been shown to be more effective. In the pediatric office setting, it is important to ask every adolescent about alcohol use. (8/15)
http://pediatrics.aappublications.org/content/136/3/e718

BONE DENSITOMETRY IN CHILDREN AND ADOLESCENTS (CLINICAL REPORT)

Laura K. Bachrach, MD; Catherine M. Gordon, MD, MS; and Section on Endocrinology

ABSTRACT. Concerns about bone health and potential fragility in children and adolescents have led to a high interest in bone densitometry. Pediatric patients with genetic and acquired chronic diseases, immobility, and inadequate nutrition may fail to achieve expected gains in bone size, mass, and strength, leaving them vulnerable to fracture. In older adults, bone densitometry has been shown to predict fracture risk and reflect response to therapy. The role of densitometry in the management of children at risk of bone fragility is less clear. This clinical report summarizes current knowledge about bone densitometry in the pediatric population, including indications for its use, interpretation of results, and risks and costs. The report emphasizes updated consensus statements generated at the 2013 Pediatric Position Development Conference of the International Society of Clinical Densitometry by an international panel of bone experts. Some of these recommendations are evidence-based, whereas others reflect expert opinion, because data are sparse on many topics. The statements from this and other expert panels provide general guidance to the pediatrician, but decisions about ordering and interpreting bone densitometry still require clinical judgment. The interpretation of bone densitometry results in children differs from that in older adults. The terms "osteopenia" and "osteoporosis" based on bone densitometry findings alone should not be used in younger patients; instead, bone mineral content or density that falls >2 SDs below expected is labeled "low for age." Pediatric osteoporosis is defined by the Pediatric Position Development Conference by using 1 of the following criteria: ≥1 vertebral fractures occurring in the absence of local disease or high-energy trauma (without or with densitometry measurements) or low bone density for age and a significant fracture history (defined as ≥2 long bone fractures before 10 years of age or ≥3 long bone fractures before 19 years of age).

Ongoing research will help define the indications and best methods for assessing bone strength in children and the clinical factors that contribute to fracture risk. The Pediatric Endocrine Society affirms the educational value of this publication. (9/16)
http://pediatrics.aappublications.org/content/138/4/e20162398

BOXING PARTICIPATION BY CHILDREN AND ADOLESCENTS
Council on Sports Medicine and Fitness (joint with Canadian Paediatric Society Healthy Active Living and Sports Medicine Committee)
ABSTRACT. Thousands of boys and girls younger than 19 years participate in boxing in North America. Although boxing provides benefits for participants, including exercise, self-discipline, and self-confidence, the sport of boxing encourages and rewards deliberate blows to the head and face. Participants in boxing are at risk of head, face, and neck injuries, including chronic and even fatal neurologic injuries. Concussions are one of the most common injuries that occur with boxing. Because of the risk of head and facial injuries, the American Academy of Pediatrics and the Canadian Paediatric Society oppose boxing as a sport for children and adolescents. These organizations recommend that physicians vigorously oppose boxing in youth and encourage patients to participate in alternative sports in which intentional head blows are not central to the sport. (8/11, reaffirmed 2/15)
http://pediatrics.aappublications.org/content/128/3/617

BREASTFEEDING AND THE USE OF HUMAN MILK
Section on Breastfeeding
ABSTRACT. Breastfeeding and human milk are the normative standards for infant feeding and nutrition. Given the documented short- and long-term medical and neurodevelopmental advantages of breastfeeding, infant nutrition should be considered a public health issue and not only a lifestyle choice. The American Academy of Pediatrics reaffirms its recommendation of exclusive breastfeeding for about 6 months, followed by continued breastfeeding as complementary foods are introduced, with continuation of breastfeeding for 1 year or longer as mutually desired by mother and infant. Medical contraindications to breastfeeding are rare. Infant growth should be monitored with the World Health Organization (WHO) Growth Curve Standards to avoid mislabeling infants as underweight or failing to thrive. Hospital routines to encourage and support the initiation and sustaining of exclusive breastfeeding should be based on the American Academy of Pediatrics-endorsed WHO/UNICEF "Ten Steps to Successful Breastfeeding." National strategies supported by the US Surgeon General's Call to Action, the Centers for Disease Control and Prevention, and The Joint Commission are involved to facilitate breastfeeding practices in US hospitals and communities. Pediatricians play a critical role in their practices and communities as advocates of breastfeeding and thus should be knowledgeable about the health risks of not breastfeeding, the economic benefits to society of breastfeeding, and the techniques for managing and supporting the breastfeeding dyad. The "Business Case for Breastfeeding" details how mothers can maintain lactation in the workplace and the benefits to employers who facilitate this practice. (2/12)
http://pediatrics.aappublications.org/content/129/3/e827

THE BREASTFEEDING-FRIENDLY PEDIATRIC OFFICE PRACTICE (CLINICAL REPORT)
Joan Younger Meek, MD, MS, RD, FAAP, IBCLC; Amy J. Hatcher, MD, FAAP; and Section on Breastfeeding
ABSTRACT. The landscape of breastfeeding has changed over the past several decades as more women initiate breastfeeding in the postpartum period and more hospitals are designated as Baby-Friendly Hospitals by following the evidence-based Ten Steps to Successful Breastfeeding. The number of births in such facilities has increased more than sixfold over the past decade. With more women breastfeeding and stays in the maternity facilities lasting only a few days, the vast majority of continued breastfeeding support occurs in the community. Pediatric care providers evaluate breastfeeding infants and their mothers in the office setting frequently during the first year of life. The office setting should be conducive to providing ongoing breastfeeding support. Likewise, the office practice should avoid creating barriers for breastfeeding mothers and families or unduly promoting infant formula. This clinical report aims to review practices shown to support breastfeeding that can be implemented in the outpatient setting, with the ultimate goal of increasing the duration of exclusive breastfeeding and the continuation of any breastfeeding. (4/17)
http://pediatrics.aappublications.org/content/139/5/e20170647

THE BUILT ENVIRONMENT: DESIGNING COMMUNITIES TO PROMOTE PHYSICAL ACTIVITY IN CHILDREN
Committee on Environmental Health
ABSTRACT. An estimated 32% of American children are overweight, and physical inactivity contributes to this high prevalence of overweight. This policy statement highlights how the built environment of a community affects children's opportunities for physical activity. Neighborhoods and communities can provide opportunities for recreational physical activity with parks and open spaces, and policies must support this capacity. Children can engage in physical activity as a part of their daily lives, such as on their travel to school. Factors such as school location have played a significant role in the decreased rates of walking to school, and changes in policy may help to increase the number of children who are able to walk to school. Environment modification that addresses risks associated with automobile traffic is likely to be conducive to more walking and biking among children. Actions that reduce parental perception and fear of crime may promote outdoor physical activity. Policies that promote more active lifestyles among children and adolescents will enable them to achieve the recommended 60 minutes of daily physical activity. By working with community partners, pediatricians can participate in establishing communities designed for activity and health. (5/09, reaffirmed 1/13)
http://pediatrics.aappublications.org/content/123/6/1591

CALCIUM AND VITAMIN D REQUIREMENTS OF ENTERALLY FED PRETERM INFANTS (CLINICAL REPORT)
Steven A. Abrams, MD, and Committee on Nutrition
ABSTRACT. Bone health is a critical concern in managing preterm infants. Key nutrients of importance are calcium, vitamin D, and phosphorus. Although human milk is critical for the health of preterm infants, it is low in these nutrients relative to the needs of the infants during growth. Strategies should be in place to fortify human milk for preterm infants with birth weight <1800 to 2000 g and to ensure adequate mineral intake during hospitalization and after hospital discharge. Biochemical monitoring of very low birth weight infants should be performed during their hospitalization. Vitamin D should be provided at 200 to 400 IU/day both during hospitalization and after discharge from the hospital. Infants with radiologic evidence of rickets should have efforts made to maximize calcium and phosphorus intake by using available commercial products and, if needed, direct supplementation with these minerals. (4/13)
http://pediatrics.aappublications.org/content/131/5/e1676

CARDIOVASCULAR MONITORING AND STIMULANT DRUGS FOR ATTENTION-DEFICIT/HYPERACTIVITY DISORDER

James M. Perrin, MD; Richard A. Friedman, MD; Timothy K. Knilans, MD; Black Box Working Group; and Section on Cardiology and Cardiac Surgery

ABSTRACT. A recent American Heart Association (AHA) statement recommended electrocardiograms (ECGs) routinely for children before they start medications to treat attention-deficit/hyperactivity disorder (ADHD). The AHA statement reflected the thoughtful work of a group committed to improving the health of children with heart disease. However, the recommendation to obtain an ECG before starting medications for treating ADHD contradicts the carefully considered and evidence-based recommendations of the American Academy of Child and Adolescent Psychiatry and the American Academy of Pediatrics (AAP). These organizations have concluded that sudden cardiac death (SCD) in persons taking medications for ADHD is a very rare event, occurring at rates no higher than those in the general population of children and adolescents. Both of these groups also noted the lack of any evidence that the routine use of ECG screening before beginning medication for ADHD treatment would prevent sudden death. The AHA statement pointed out the importance of detecting silent but clinically important cardiac conditions in children and adolescents, which is a goal that the AAP shares. The primary purpose of the AHA statement is to prevent cases of SCD that may be related to stimulant medications. The recommendations of the AAP and the rationale for these recommendations are the subject of this statement. (8/08)
http://pediatrics.aappublications.org/content/122/2/451

CARE OF ADOLESCENT PARENTS AND THEIR CHILDREN (CLINICAL REPORT)

Jorge L. Pinzon, MD; Veronnie F. Jones, MD; Committee on Adolescence; and Committee on Early Childhood

ABSTRACT. Teen pregnancy and parenting remain an important public health issue in the United States and the world, and many children live with their adolescent parents alone or as part of an extended family. A significant proportion of teen parents reside with their family of origin, significantly affecting the multigenerational family structure. Repeated births to teen parents are also common. This clinical report updates a previous policy statement on care of the adolescent parent and their children and addresses medical and psychosocial risks specific to this population. Challenges unique to teen parents and their children are reviewed, along with suggestions for the pediatrician on models for intervention and care. (11/12, reaffirmed 7/16)
http://pediatrics.aappublications.org/content/130/6/e1743

THE CARE OF CHILDREN WITH CONGENITAL HEART DISEASE IN THEIR PRIMARY MEDICAL HOME

M. Regina Lantin-Hermoso, MD, FAAP, FACC; Stuart Berger, MD, FAAP; Ami B. Bhatt, MD, FACC; Julia E. Richerson, MD, FAAP; Robert Morrow, MD, FAAP; Michael D. Freed, MD, FAAP, FACC; Robert H. Beekman III, MD, FAAP, FACC; and Section on Cardiology and Cardiac Surgery

ABSTRACT. Congenital heart disease (CHD) is the most common birth anomaly. With advances in repair and palliation of these complex lesions, more and more patients are surviving and are discharged from the hospital to return to their families. Patients with CHD have complex health care needs that often must be provided for or coordinated for by the primary care provider (PCP) and medical home. This policy statement aims to provide the PCP with general guidelines for the care of the child with congenital heart defects and outlines anticipated problems, serving as a repository of current knowledge in a practical, readily accessible format. A timeline approach is used, emphasizing the role of the PCP and medical home in the management of patients with CHD in their various life stages. (10/17)
http://pediatrics.aappublications.org/content/140/5/e20172607

CARE OF THE ADOLESCENT AFTER AN ACUTE SEXUAL ASSAULT (CLINICAL REPORT)

James E. Crawford-Jakubiak, MD, FAAP; Elizabeth M. Alderman, MD, FAAP, SAHM; John M. Leventhal, MD, FAAP; Committee on Child Abuse and Neglect; and Committee on Adolescence

ABSTRACT. *Sexual violence* is a broad term that encompasses a wide range of sexual victimizations. Since the American Academy of Pediatrics published its last policy statement on sexual assault in 2008, additional information and data have emerged about sexual violence affecting adolescents and the treatment and management of the adolescent who has been a victim of sexual assault. This report provides new information to update physicians and focuses on the acute assessment and care of adolescent victims who have experienced a recent sexual assault. Follow-up of the acute assault, as well as prevention of sexual assault, are also discussed. (2/17)
http://pediatrics.aappublications.org/content/139/3/e20164243

CAREGIVER-FABRICATED ILLNESS IN A CHILD: A MANIFESTATION OF CHILD MALTREATMENT (CLINICAL REPORT)

Emalee G. Flaherty, MD; Harriet L. MacMillan, MD; and Committee on Child Abuse and Neglect

ABSTRACT. Caregiver-fabricated illness in a child is a form of child maltreatment caused by a caregiver who falsifies and/or induces a child's illness, leading to unnecessary and potentially harmful medical investigations and/or treatment. This condition can result in significant morbidity and mortality. Although caregiver-fabricated illness in a child has been widely known as Munchausen syndrome by proxy, there is ongoing discussion about alternative names, including pediatric condition falsification, factitious disorder (illness) by proxy, child abuse in the medical setting, and medical child abuse. Because it is a relatively uncommon form of maltreatment, pediatricians need to have a high index of suspicion when faced with a persistent or recurrent illness that cannot be explained and that results in multiple medical procedures or when there are discrepancies between the history, physical examination, and health of a child. This report updates the previous clinical report "Beyond Munchausen Syndrome by Proxy: Identification and Treatment of Child Abuse in the Medical Setting." The authors discuss the need to agree on appropriate terminology, provide an update on published reports of new manifestations of fabricated medical conditions, and discuss approaches to assessment, diagnosis, and management, including how best to protect the child from further harm. (8/13, reaffirmed 8/18)
http://pediatrics.aappublications.org/content/132/3/590

CHEERLEADING INJURIES: EPIDEMIOLOGY AND RECOMMENDATIONS FOR PREVENTION

Council on Sports Medicine and Fitness

ABSTRACT. Over the last 30 years, cheerleading has increased dramatically in popularity and has evolved from leading the crowd in cheers at sporting events into a competitive, year-round sport involving complex acrobatic stunts and tumbling. Consequently, cheerleading injuries have steadily increased over the years in both number and severity. Sprains and strains to the lower extremities are the most common injuries. Although the overall injury rate remains relatively low, cheerleading has accounted for approximately 66% of all catastrophic injuries in high school girl athletes over the past 25 years. Risk factors for injuries in cheerleading include higher BMI, previous injury, cheering on harder surfaces, performing stunts, and supervision

by a coach with low level of training and experience. This policy statement describes the epidemiology of cheerleading injuries and provides recommendations for injury prevention. (10/12, reaffirmed 7/15)
http://pediatrics.aappublications.org/content/130/5/966

CHEMICAL-BIOLOGICAL TERRORISM AND ITS IMPACT ON CHILDREN

Committee on Environmental Health and Committee on Infectious Diseases

ABSTRACT. Children remain potential victims of chemical or biological terrorism. In recent years, children have even been specific targets of terrorist acts. Consequently, it is necessary to address the needs that children would face after a terrorist incident. A broad range of public health initiatives have occurred since September 11, 2001. Although the needs of children have been addressed in many of them, in many cases, these initiatives have been inadequate in ensuring the protection of children. In addition, public health and health care system preparedness for terrorism has been broadened to the so-called all-hazards approach, in which response plans for terrorism are blended with plans for a public health or health care system response to unintentional disasters (eg, natural events such as earthquakes or pandemic flu or manmade catastrophes such as a hazardous-materials spill). In response to new principles and programs that have appeared over the last 5 years, this policy statement provides an update of the 2000 policy statement. The roles of both the pediatrician and public health agencies continue to be emphasized; only a coordinated effort by pediatricians and public health can ensure that the needs of children, including emergency protocols in schools or child care centers, decontamination protocols, and mental health interventions, will be successful. (9/06, reaffirmed 12/16)
http://pediatrics.aappublications.org/content/118/3/1267

CHEMICAL-MANAGEMENT POLICY: PRIORITIZING CHILDREN'S HEALTH

Council on Environmental Health

ABSTRACT. The American Academy of Pediatrics recommends that chemical-management policy in the United States be revised to protect children and pregnant women and to better protect other populations. The Toxic Substance Control Act (TSCA) was passed in 1976. It is widely recognized to have been ineffective in protecting children, pregnant women, and the general population from hazardous chemicals in the marketplace. It does not take into account the special vulnerabilities of children in attempting to protect the population from chemical hazards. Its processes are so cumbersome that in its more than 30 years of existence, the TSCA has been used to regulate only 5 chemicals or chemical classes of the tens of thousands of chemicals that are in commerce. Under the TSCA, chemical companies have no responsibility to perform premarket testing or post-market follow-up of the products that they produce; in fact, the TSCA contains disincentives for the companies to produce such data. Voluntary programs have been inadequate in resolving problems. Therefore, chemical-management policy needs to be rewritten in the United States. Manufacturers must be responsible for developing information about chemicals before marketing. The US Environmental Protection Agency must have the authority to demand additional safety data about a chemical and to limit or stop the marketing of a chemical when there is a high degree of suspicion that the chemical might be harmful to children, pregnant women, or other populations. (4/11, reaffirmed 9/16)
http://pediatrics.aappublications.org/content/127/5/983

CHILD ABUSE, CONFIDENTIALITY, AND THE HEALTH INSURANCE PORTABILITY AND ACCOUNTABILITY ACT

Committee on Child Abuse and Neglect

ABSTRACT. The federal Health Insurance Portability and Accountability Act (HIPAA) of 1996 has significantly affected clinical practice, particularly with regard to how patient information is shared. HIPAA addresses the security and privacy of patient health data, ensuring that information is released appropriately with patient or guardian consent and knowledge. However, when child abuse or neglect is suspected in a clinical setting, the physician may determine that release of information without consent is necessary to ensure the health and safety of the child. This policy statement provides an overview of HIPAA regulations with regard to the role of the pediatrician in releasing or reviewing patient health information when the patient is a child who is a suspected victim of abuse or neglect. This statement is based on the most current regulations provided by the US Department of Health and Human Services and is subject to future changes and clarifications as updates are provided. (12/09, reaffirmed 1/14)
http://pediatrics.aappublications.org/content/125/1/197

CHILD FATALITY REVIEW

Cindy W. Christian, MD; Robert D. Sege, MD, PhD; Committee on Child Abuse and Neglect; Committee on Injury, Violence, and Poison Prevention; and Council on Community Pediatrics

ABSTRACT. Injury remains the leading cause of pediatric mortality and requires public health approaches to reduce preventable deaths. Child fatality review teams, first established to review suspicious child deaths involving abuse or neglect, have expanded toward a public health model of prevention of child fatality through systematic review of child deaths from birth through adolescence. Approximately half of all states report reviewing child deaths from all causes, and the process of fatality review has identified effective local and state prevention strategies for reducing child deaths. This expanded approach can be a powerful tool in understanding the epidemiology and preventability of child death locally, regionally, and nationally; improving accuracy of vital statistics data; and identifying public health and legislative strategies for reducing preventable child fatalities. The American Academy of Pediatrics supports the development of federal and state legislation to enhance the child fatality review process and recommends that pediatricians become involved in local and state child death reviews. (8/10, reaffirmed 5/14)
http://pediatrics.aappublications.org/content/126/3/592

CHILD LIFE SERVICES

Committee on Hospital Care and Child Life Council

ABSTRACT. Child life programs are an important component of pediatric hospital–based care to address the psychosocial concerns that accompany hospitalization and other health care experiences. Child life specialists focus on the optimal development and well-being of infants, children, adolescents, and young adults while promoting coping skills and minimizing the adverse effects of hospitalization, health care, and/or other potentially stressful experiences. Using therapeutic play, expressive modalities, and psychological preparation as primary tools, in collaboration with the entire health care team and family, child life interventions facilitate coping and adjustment at times and under circumstances that might otherwise prove overwhelming for the child. Play and developmentally appropriate communication are used to: (1) promote optimal development; (2) educate children and families about health conditions; (3) prepare children and families for medical events or procedures; (4) plan and rehearse useful coping and pain management strategies; (5) help children work through feelings about past or impending experiences; and (6) establish therapeutic relationships with patients, siblings, and parents to support family involvement in each child's care. (4/14, reaffirmed 2/18)

http://pediatrics.aappublications.org/content/133/5/e1471

CHILD PASSENGER SAFETY

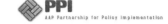

Dennis R. Durbin, MD,
  MSCE, FAAP; Benjamin D.
  Hoffman, MD, FAAP; and Council on Injury, Violence, and
  Poison Prevention

ABSTRACT. Child passenger safety has dramatically evolved over the past decade; however, motor vehicle crashes continue to be the leading cause of death for children 4 years and older. This policy statement provides 4 evidence-based recommendations for best practices in the choice of a child restraint system to optimize safety in passenger vehicles for children from birth through adolescence: (1) rear-facing car safety seats as long as possible; (2) forward-facing car safety seats from the time they outgrow rear-facing seats for most children through at least 4 years of age; (3) belt-positioning booster seats from the time they outgrow forward-facing seats for most children through at least 8 years of age; and (4) lap and shoulder seat belts for all who have outgrown booster seats. In addition, a fifth evidence-based recommendation is for all children younger than 13 years to ride in the rear seats of vehicles. It is important to note that every transition is associated with some decrease in protection; therefore, parents should be encouraged to delay these transitions for as long as possible. These recommendations are presented in the form of an algorithm that is intended to facilitate implementation of the recommendations by pediatricians to their patients and families and should cover most situations that pediatricians will encounter in practice. The American Academy of Pediatrics urges all pediatricians to know and promote these recommendations as part of child passenger safety anticipatory guidance at every health supervision visit. (10/18)

See full text on page 533.

http://pediatrics.aappublications.org/content/142/5/e20182460

CHILD PASSENGER SAFETY (TECHNICAL REPORT)

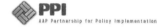

Dennis R. Durbin, MD, MSCE,
  FAAP; Benjamin D. Hoffman, MD, FAAP; and Council on
  Injury, Violence, and Poison Prevention

ABSTRACT. Despite significant reductions in the number of children killed in motor vehicle crashes over the past decade, crashes continue to be the leading cause of death to children 4 years and older. Therefore, the American Academy of Pediatrics continues to recommend the inclusion of child passenger safety anticipatory guidance at every health supervision visit. This technical report provides a summary of the evidence in support of 5 recommendations for best practices to optimize safety in passenger vehicles for children from birth through adolescence that all pediatricians should know and promote in their routine practice. These recommendations are presented in the revised policy statement on child passenger safety in the form of an algorithm that is intended to facilitate their implementation by pediatricians with their patients and families. The algorithm is designed to cover the majority of situations that pediatricians will encounter in practice. In addition, a summary of evidence on a number of additional issues affecting the safety of children in motor vehicles, including the proper use and installation of child restraints, exposure to air bags, travel in pickup trucks, children left in or around vehicles, and the importance of restraint laws, is provided. Finally, this technical report provides pediatricians with a number of resources for additional information to use when providing anticipatory guidance to families. (10/18)

See full text on page 541.

http://pediatrics.aappublications.org/content/142/5/e20182461

CHILD SEX TRAFFICKING AND COMMERCIAL SEXUAL EXPLOITATION: HEALTH CARE NEEDS OF VICTIMS (CLINICAL REPORT)

*Jordan Greenbaum, MD; James E. Crawford-Jakubiak, MD, FAAP;
  and Committee on Child Abuse and Neglect*

ABSTRACT. Child sex trafficking and commercial sexual exploitation of children (CSEC) are major public health problems in the United States and throughout the world. Despite large numbers of American and foreign youth affected and a plethora of serious physical and mental health problems associated with CSEC, there is limited information available to pediatricians regarding the nature and scope of human trafficking and how pediatricians and other health care providers may help protect children. Knowledge of risk factors, recruitment practices, possible indicators of CSEC, and common medical and behavioral health problems experienced by victims will help pediatricians recognize potential victims and respond appropriately. As health care providers, educators, and leaders in child advocacy, pediatricians play an essential role in addressing the public health issues faced by child victims of CSEC. Their roles can include working to increase recognition of CSEC, providing direct care and anticipatory guidance related to CSEC, engaging in collaborative efforts with medical and nonmedical colleagues to provide for the complex needs of youth, and educating child-serving professionals and the public. (2/15)

http://pediatrics.aappublications.org/content/135/3/566

THE CHILD WITNESS IN THE COURTROOM

*Robert H. Pantell, MD, FAAP, and Committee on Psychosocial
  Aspects of Child and Family Health*

ABSTRACT. Beginning in the 1980s, children have increasingly served as witnesses in the criminal, civil, and family courts; currently, >100000 children appear in court each year. This statement updates the 1992 American Academy of Pediatrics (AAP) policy statement "The Child as a Witness" and the subsequent 1999 "The Child in Court: A Subject Review." It also builds on existing AAP policy on adverse life events affecting children and resources developed to understand and address childhood trauma. The purpose of this policy statement is to provide background information on some of the legal issues involving children testifying in court, including the accuracy and psychological impact of child testimony; to provide suggestions for how pediatricians can support patients who will testify in court; and to make recommendations for policy improvements to minimize the adverse psychological consequences for child witnesses. These recommendations are, for the most part, based on studies on the psychological and physiologic consequences of children witnessing and experiencing violence, as well as appearing in court, that have emerged since the previous AAP publications on the subject. The goal is to reduce the secondary traumatization of and long-term consequences for children providing testimony about violence they have experienced or witnessed. This statement primarily addresses children appearing in court as victims of physical or sexual abuse or as witnesses of violent acts; most of the scientific literature addresses these specific situations. It may apply, in certain situations, to children required to provide testimony in custody disputes, child welfare proceedings, or immigration court. It does not address children appearing in court as offenders or as part of juvenile justice proceedings. (2/17)

http://pediatrics.aappublications.org/content/139/3/e20164008

CHILDREN, ADOLESCENTS, AND ADVERTISING

Committee on Communications

ABSTRACT. Advertising is a pervasive influence on children and adolescents. Young people view more than 40 000 ads per year on television alone and increasingly are being exposed to

advertising on the Internet, in magazines, and in schools. This exposure may contribute significantly to childhood and adolescent obesity, poor nutrition, and cigarette and alcohol use. Media education has been shown to be effective in mitigating some of the negative effects of advertising on children and adolescents. (12/06, reaffirmed 3/10, 11/17)
http://pediatrics.aappublications.org/content/118/6/2563

CHILDREN, ADOLESCENTS, AND THE MEDIA
Council on Communications and Media
ABSTRACT. Media, from television to the "new media" (including cell phones, iPads, and social media), are a dominant force in children's lives. Although television is still the predominant medium for children and adolescents, new technologies are increasingly popular. The American Academy of Pediatrics continues to be concerned by evidence about the potential harmful effects of media messages and images; however, important positive and prosocial effects of media use should also be recognized. Pediatricians are encouraged to take a media history and ask 2 media questions at every well-child visit: How much recreational screen time does your child or teenager consume daily? Is there a television set or Internet-connected device in the child's bedroom? Parents are encouraged to establish a family home use plan for all media. Media influences on children and teenagers should be recognized by schools, policymakers, product advertisers, and entertainment producers. (10/13)
http://pediatrics.aappublications.org/content/132/5/958

CHILDREN AND ADOLESCENTS AND DIGITAL MEDIA (TECHNICAL REPORT)
Yolanda (Linda) Reid Chassiakos, MD, FAAP; Jenny Radesky, MD, FAAP; Dimitri Christakis, MD, FAAP; Megan A. Moreno, MD, MSEd, MPH, FAAP; Corinn Cross, MD, FAAP; and Council on Communications and Media
ABSTRACT. Today's children and adolescents are immersed in both traditional and new forms of digital media. Research on traditional media, such as television, has identified health concerns and negative outcomes that correlate with the duration and content of viewing. Over the past decade, the use of digital media, including interactive and social media, has grown, and research evidence suggests that these newer media offer both benefits and risks to the health of children and teenagers. Evidence-based benefits identified from the use of digital and social media include early learning, exposure to new ideas and knowledge, increased opportunities for social contact and support, and new opportunities to access health promotion messages and information. Risks of such media include negative health effects on sleep, attention, and learning; a higher incidence of obesity and depression; exposure to inaccurate, inappropriate, or unsafe content and contacts; and compromised privacy and confidentiality. This technical report reviews the literature regarding these opportunities and risks, framed around clinical questions, for children from birth to adulthood. To promote health and wellness in children and adolescents, it is important to maintain adequate physical activity, healthy nutrition, good sleep hygiene, and a nurturing social environment. A healthy Family Media Use Plan (www.healthychildren.org/MediaUsePlan) that is individualized for a specific child, teenager, or family can identify an appropriate balance between screen time/online time and other activities, set boundaries for accessing content, guide displays of personal information, encourage age-appropriate critical thinking and digital literacy, and support open family communication and implementation of consistent rules about media use. (10/16)
http://pediatrics.aappublications.org/content/138/5/e20162593

CHILDREN'S HEALTH INSURANCE PROGRAM (CHIP): ACCOMPLISHMENTS, CHALLENGES, AND POLICY RECOMMENDATIONS
Committee on Child Health Financing
ABSTRACT. Sixteen years ago, the 105th Congress, responding to the needs of 10 million children in the United States who lacked health insurance, created the State Children's Health Insurance Program (SCHIP) as part of the Balanced Budget Act of 1997. Enacted as Title XXI of the Social Security Act, the Children's Health Insurance Program (CHIP; or SCHIP as it has been known at some points) provided states with federal assistance to create programs specifically designed for children from families with incomes that exceeded Medicaid thresholds but that were insufficient to enable them to afford private health insurance. Congress provided $40 billion in block grants over 10 years for states to expand their existing Medicaid programs to cover the intended populations, to erect new stand-alone SCHIP programs for these children, or to effect some combination of both options. Congress reauthorized CHIP once in 2009 under the Children's Health Insurance Program Reauthorization Act and extended its life further within provisions of the Patient Protection and Affordable Care Act of 2010. The purpose of this statement is to review the features of CHIP as it has evolved over the 16 years of its existence; to summarize what is known about the effects that the program has had on coverage, access, health status, and disparities among participants; to identify challenges that remain with respect to insuring this group of vulnerable children, including the impact that provisions of the new Affordable Care Act will have on the issue of health insurance coverage for near-poor children after 2015; and to offer recommendations on how to expand and strengthen the national commitment to provide health insurance to all children regardless of means. (2/14)
http://pediatrics.aappublications.org/content/133/3/e784

CHRONIC ABDOMINAL PAIN IN CHILDREN (CLINICAL REPORT)
Steering Committee on Quality Improvement and Management and Subcommittee on Chronic Abdominal Pain (joint with North American Society for Pediatric Gastroenterology, Hepatology, and Nutrition)
ABSTRACT. Children and adolescents with chronic abdominal pain pose unique challenges to their caregivers. Affected children and their families experience distress and anxiety that can interfere with their ability to perform regular daily activities. Although chronic abdominal pain in children is usually attributable to a functional disorder rather than organic disease, numerous misconceptions, insufficient knowledge among health care professionals, and inadequate application of knowledge may contribute to a lack of effective management. This clinical report accompanies a technical report (see page e370 in this issue) on childhood chronic abdominal pain and provides guidance for the clinician in the evaluation and treatment of children with chronic abdominal pain. The recommendations are based on the evidence reviewed in the technical report and on consensus achieved among subcommittee members. (3/05)
http://pediatrics.aappublications.org/content/115/3/812

CHRONIC ABDOMINAL PAIN IN CHILDREN (TECHNICAL REPORT)
Steering Committee on Quality Improvement and Management and Subcommittee on Chronic Abdominal Pain (joint with North American Society for Pediatric Gastroenterology, Hepatology, and Nutrition)
ABSTRACT. Chronic abdominal pain, defined as long-lasting intermittent or constant abdominal pain, is a common pediatric problem encountered by primary care physicians, medical

subspecialists, and surgical specialists. Chronic abdominal pain in children is usually functional, that is, without objective evidence of an underlying organic disorder. The Subcommittee on Chronic Abdominal Pain of the American Academy of Pediatrics and the North American Society for Pediatric Gastroenterology, Hepatology, and Nutrition has prepared this report based on a comprehensive, systematic review and rating of the medical literature. This report accompanies a clinical report based on the literature review and expert opinion.

The subcommittee examined the diagnostic and therapeutic value of a medical and psychological history, diagnostic tests, and pharmacologic and behavioral therapy. The presence of alarm symptoms or signs (such as weight loss, gastrointestinal bleeding, persistent fever, chronic severe diarrhea, and significant vomiting) is associated with a higher prevalence of organic disease. There was insufficient evidence to state that the nature of the abdominal pain or the presence of associated symptoms (such as anorexia, nausea, headache, and joint pain) can discriminate between functional and organic disorders. Although children with chronic abdominal pain and their parents are more often anxious or depressed, the presence of anxiety, depression, behavior problems, or recent negative life events does not distinguish between functional and organic abdominal pain. Most children who are brought to the primary care physician's office for chronic abdominal pain are unlikely to require diagnostic testing. Pediatric studies of therapeutic interventions were examined and found to be limited or inconclusive. (3/05)
http://pediatrics.aappublications.org/content/115/3/e370

CIRCUMCISION POLICY STATEMENT
Task Force on Circumcision
ABSTRACT. Male circumcision is a common procedure, generally performed during the newborn period in the United States. In 2007, the American Academy of Pediatrics (AAP) formed a multidisciplinary task force of AAP members and other stakeholders to evaluate the recent evidence on male circumcision and update the Academy's 1999 recommendations in this area. Evaluation of current evidence indicates that the health benefits of newborn male circumcision outweigh the risks and that the procedure's benefits justify access to this procedure for families who choose it. Specific benefits identified included prevention of urinary tract infections, penile cancer, and transmission of some sexually transmitted infections, including HIV. The American College of Obstetricians and Gynecologists has endorsed this statement. (8/12)
http://pediatrics.aappublications.org/content/130/3/585

CLIMATIC HEAT STRESS AND EXERCISING CHILDREN AND ADOLESCENTS
Council on Sports Medicine and Fitness and Council on School Health
ABSTRACT. Results of new research indicate that, contrary to previous thinking, youth do not have less effective thermoregulatory ability, insufficient cardiovascular capacity, or lower physical exertion tolerance compared with adults during exercise in the heat when adequate hydration is maintained. Accordingly, besides poor hydration status, the primary determinants of reduced performance and exertional heat-illness risk in youth during sports and other physical activities in a hot environment include undue physical exertion, insufficient recovery between repeated exercise bouts or closely scheduled same-day training sessions or rounds of sports competition, and inappropriately wearing clothing, uniforms, and protective equipment that play a role in excessive heat retention. Because these known contributing risk factors are modifiable, exertional heat illness is usually preventable. With appropriate preparation, modifications, and monitoring, most healthy children and adolescents can safely participate in outdoor sports and other physical activities through a wide range of challenging warm to hot climatic conditions. (8/11, reaffirmed 2/15)
http://pediatrics.aappublications.org/content/128/3/e741

CLINICAL CONSIDERATIONS RELATED TO THE BEHAVIORAL MANIFESTATIONS OF CHILD MALTREATMENT (CLINICAL REPORT)
Robert D. Sege, MD, PhD, FAAP; Lisa Amaya-Jackson, MD, MPH, FAACAP; Committee on Child Abuse and Neglect; and Council on Foster Care, Adoption, and Kinship Care (joint with American Academy of Child and Adolescent Psychiatry Committee on Child Maltreatment and Violence and National Center for Child Traumatic Stress)
ABSTRACT. Children who have suffered early abuse or neglect may later present with significant health and behavior problems that may persist long after the abusive or neglectful environment has been remediated. Neurobiological research suggests that early maltreatment may result in an altered psychological and physiologic response to stressful stimuli, a response that deleteriously affects the child's subsequent development. Pediatricians can assist caregivers by helping them recognize the abused or neglected child's emotional and behavioral responses associated with child maltreatment and guide them in the use of positive parenting strategies, referring the children and families to evidence-based therapeutic treatment and mobilizing available community resources. (3/17)
http://pediatrics.aappublications.org/content/139/4/e20170100

CLINICAL GENETIC EVALUATION OF THE CHILD WITH MENTAL RETARDATION OR DEVELOPMENTAL DELAYS (CLINICAL REPORT)
John B. Moeschler, MD; Michael Shevell, MD; and Committee on Genetics
ABSTRACT. This clinical report describes the clinical genetic evaluation of the child with developmental delays or mental retardation. The purpose of this report is to describe the optimal clinical genetics diagnostic evaluation to assist pediatricians in providing a medical home for children with developmental delays or mental retardation and their families. The literature supports the benefit of expert clinical judgment by a consulting clinical geneticist in the diagnostic evaluation. However, it is recognized that local factors may preclude this particular option. No single approach to the diagnostic process is supported by the literature. This report addresses the diagnostic importance of clinical history, 3-generation family history, dysmorphologic examination, neurologic examination, chromosome analysis (≥650 bands), fragile X molecular genetic testing, fluorescence in situ hybridization studies for subtelomere chromosome rearrangements, molecular genetic testing for typical and atypical presentations of known syndromes, computed tomography and/or magnetic resonance brain imaging, and targeted studies for metabolic disorders. (6/06, reaffirmed 5/12)
http://pediatrics.aappublications.org/content/117/6/2304

CLINICAL PRACTICE POLICY TO PROTECT CHILDREN FROM TOBACCO, NICOTINE, AND TOBACCO SMOKE
Section on Tobacco Control
ABSTRACT. Tobacco dependence starts in childhood. Tobacco exposure of children is common and causes illness and premature death in children and adults, with adverse effects starting in the womb. There is no safe level of tobacco smoke exposure. Pediatricians should screen for use of tobacco and other nicotine delivery devices and provide anticipatory guidance to prevent smoking initiation and reduce tobacco smoke exposure. Pediatricians need to be aware of the different nicotine delivery systems marketed and available.

Parents and caregivers are important sources of children's tobacco smoke exposure. Because tobacco dependence is a severe addiction, to protect children's health, caregiver tobacco dependence treatment should be offered or referral for treatment should be provided (such as referral to the national smoker's quitline at 1-800-QUIT-NOW). If the source of tobacco exposure cannot be eliminated, counseling about reducing exposure to children should be provided.

Health care delivery systems should facilitate the effective prevention, identification, and treatment of tobacco dependence in children and adolescents, their parents, and other caregivers. Health care facilities should protect children from tobacco smoke exposure and tobacco promotion. Tobacco dependence prevention and treatment should be part of medical education, with knowledge assessed as part of board certification examinations. (10/15)
http://pediatrics.aappublications.org/content/136/5/1008

CLINICAL TOOLS TO ASSESS ASTHMA CONTROL IN CHILDREN (CLINICAL REPORT)

Chitra Dinakar, MD, FAAP; Bradley E. Chipps, MD, FAAP; Section on Allergy and Immunology; and Section on Pediatric Pulmonology and Sleep Medicine

ABSTRACT. Asthma affects an estimated 7 million children and causes significant health care and disease burden. The most recent iteration of the National Heart, Lung and Blood Institute asthma guidelines, the Expert Panel Report 3, emphasizes the assessment and monitoring of asthma control in the management of asthma. Asthma control refers to the degree to which the manifestations of asthma are minimized by therapeutic interventions and the goals of therapy are met. Although assessment of asthma severity is used to guide initiation of therapy, monitoring of asthma control helps determine whether therapy should be maintained or adjusted. The nuances of estimation of asthma control include understanding concepts of current impairment and future risk and incorporating their measurement into clinical practice. Impairment is assessed on the basis of frequency and intensity of symptoms, variations in lung function, and limitations of daily activities. "Risk" refers to the likelihood of exacerbations, progressive loss of lung function, or adverse effects from medications. Currently available ambulatory tools to measure asthma control range are subjective measures, such as patient-reported composite asthma control score instruments or objective measures of lung function, airway hyperreactivity, and biomarkers. Because asthma control exhibits short- and long-term variability, health care providers need to be vigilant regarding the fluctuations in the factors that can create discordance between subjective and objective assessment of asthma control. Familiarity with the properties, application, and relative value of these measures will enable health care providers to choose the optimal set of measures that will adhere to national standards of care and ensure delivery of high-quality care customized to their patients. (12/16)
http://pediatrics.aappublications.org/content/139/1/e20163438

COCHLEAR IMPLANTS IN CHILDREN: SURGICAL SITE INFECTIONS AND PREVENTION AND TREATMENT OF ACUTE OTITIS MEDIA AND MENINGITIS

Lorry G. Rubin, MD; Blake Papsin, MD; Committee on Infectious Diseases; and Section on Otolaryngology—Head and Neck Surgery

ABSTRACT. The use of cochlear implants is increasingly common, particularly in children younger than 3 years. Bacterial meningitis, often with associated acute otitis media, is more common in children with cochlear implants than in groups of control children. Children with profound deafness who are candidates for cochlear implants should receive all age-appropriate doses of pneumococcal conjugate and Haemophilus influenzae type b conjugate vaccines and appropriate annual immunization against influenza. In addition, starting at 24 months of age, a single dose of 23-valent pneumococcal polysaccharide vaccine should be administered. Before implant surgery, primary care providers and cochlear implant teams should ensure that immunizations are up-to-date, preferably with completion of indicated vaccines at least 2 weeks before implant surgery. Imaging of the temporal bone/inner ear should be performed before cochlear implantation in all children with congenital deafness and all patients with profound hearing impairment and a history of bacterial meningitis to identify those with inner-ear malformations/cerebrospinal fluid fistulas or ossification of the cochlea. During the initial months after cochlear implantation, the risk of complications of acute otitis media may be higher than during subsequent time periods. Therefore, it is recommended that acute otitis media diagnosed during the first 2 months after implantation be initially treated with a parenteral antibiotic (eg, ceftriaxone or cefotaxime). Episodes occurring 2 months or longer after implantation can be treated with a trial of an oral antimicrobial agent (eg, amoxicillin or amoxicillin/clavulanate at a dose of approximately 90 mg/kg per day of amoxicillin component), provided the child does not appear toxic and the implant does not have a spacer/positioner, a wedge that rests in the cochlea next to the electrodes present in certain implant models available between 1999 and 2002. "Watchful waiting" without antimicrobial therapy is inappropriate for children with implants with acute otitis media. If feasible, tympanocentesis should be performed for acute otitis media, and the material should be sent for culture, but performance of this procedure should not result in an undue delay in initiating antimicrobial therapy. For patients with suspected meningitis, cerebrospinal fluid as well as middle-ear fluid, if present, should be sent for culture. Empiric antimicrobial therapy for meningitis occurring within 2 months of implantation should include an agent with broad activity against Gram-negative bacilli (eg, meropenem) plus vancomycin. For meningitis occurring 2 months or longer after implantation, standard empiric antimicrobial therapy for meningitis (eg, ceftriaxone plus vancomycin) is indicated. For patients with meningitis, urgent evaluation by an otolaryngologist is indicated for consideration of imaging and surgical exploration. (7/10, reaffirmed 1/18)
http://pediatrics.aappublications.org/content/126/2/381

CODEINE: TIME TO SAY "NO" (CLINICAL REPORT)

Joseph D. Tobias, MD; Thomas P. Green, MD; Charles J. Coté, MD; Section on Anesthesiology and Pain Medicine; and Committee on Drugs

ABSTRACT. Codeine has been prescribed to pediatric patients for many decades as both an analgesic and an antitussive agent. Codeine is a prodrug with little inherent pharmacologic activity and must be metabolized in the liver into morphine, which is responsible for codeine's analgesic effects. However, there is substantial genetic variability in the activity of the responsible hepatic enzyme, *CYP2D6*, and, as a consequence, individual patient response to codeine varies from no effect to high sensitivity. Drug surveillance has documented the occurrence of unanticipated respiratory depression and death after receiving codeine in children, many of whom have been shown to be ultrarapid metabolizers. Patients with documented or suspected obstructive sleep apnea appear to be at particular risk because of opioid sensitivity, compounding the danger among rapid metabolizers in this group. Recently, various organizations and regulatory bodies, including the World Health Organization, the US Food and Drug Administration, and the European Medicines Agency, have promulgated stern warnings regarding the occurrence of adverse effects of codeine in children. These and other groups have or are considering a declaration of a contraindication for the use of codeine for children as either an analgesic or an antitussive. Additional clinical research must extend the understanding of the risks and benefits of both opioid and

nonopioid alternatives for orally administered, effective agents for acute and chronic pain. (9/16)
http://pediatrics.aappublications.org/content/138/4/e20162396

COLLABORATIVE ROLE OF THE PEDIATRICIAN IN THE DIAGNOSIS AND MANAGEMENT OF BIPOLAR DISORDER IN ADOLESCENTS (CLINICAL REPORT)

Benjamin N. Shain, MD, PhD, and Committee on Adolescence
ABSTRACT. Despite the complexity of diagnosis and management, pediatricians have an important collaborative role in referring and partnering in the management of adolescents with bipolar disorder. This report presents the classification of bipolar disorder as well as interviewing and diagnostic guidelines. Treatment options are described, particularly focusing on medication management and rationale for the common practice of multiple, simultaneous medications. Medication adverse effects may be problematic and better managed with collaboration between mental health professionals and pediatricians. Case examples illustrate a number of common diagnostic and management issues. (11/12)
http://pediatrics.aappublications.org/content/130/6/e1725

COMMUNICATING WITH CHILDREN AND FAMILIES: FROM EVERYDAY INTERACTIONS TO SKILL IN CONVEYING DISTRESSING INFORMATION (TECHNICAL REPORT)

Marcia Levetown, MD, and Committee on Bioethics
ABSTRACT. Health care communication is a skill that is critical to safe and effective medical practice; it can and must be taught. Communication skill influences patient disclosure, treatment adherence and outcome, adaptation to illness, and bereavement. This article provides a review of the evidence regarding clinical communication in the pediatric setting, covering the spectrum from outpatient primary care consultation to death notification, and provides practical suggestions to improve communication with patients and families, enabling more effective, efficient, and empathic pediatric health care. (5/08, reaffirmed 12/16)
http://pediatrics.aappublications.org/content/121/5/e1441

COMMUNITY PEDIATRICS: NAVIGATING THE INTERSECTION OF MEDICINE, PUBLIC HEALTH, AND SOCIAL DETERMINANTS OF CHILDREN'S HEALTH

Council on Community Pediatrics
ABSTRACT. This policy statement provides a framework for the pediatrician's role in promoting the health and well-being of all children in the context of their families and communities. It offers pediatricians a definition of community pediatrics, emphasizes the importance of recognizing social determinants of health, and delineates the need to partner with public health to address population-based child health issues. It also recognizes the importance of pediatric involvement in child advocacy at local, state, and federal levels to ensure all children have access to a high-quality medical home and to eliminate child health disparities. This statement provides a set of specific recommendations that underscore the critical nature of this dimension of pediatric practice, teaching, and research. (2/13, reaffirmed 10/16)
http://pediatrics.aappublications.org/content/131/3/623

COMPREHENSIVE EVALUATION OF THE CHILD WITH INTELLECTUAL DISABILITY OR GLOBAL DEVELOPMENTAL DELAYS (CLINICAL REPORT)

John B. Moeschler, MD, MS, FAAP, FACMG; Michael Shevell, MDCM, FRCP; and Committee on Genetics
ABSTRACT. Global developmental delay and intellectual disability are relatively common pediatric conditions. This report describes the recommended clinical genetics diagnostic approach. The report is based on a review of published reports, most consisting of medium to large case series of diagnostic tests used, and the proportion of those that led to a diagnosis in such patients. Chromosome microarray is designated as a first-line test and replaces the standard karyotype and fluorescent in situ hybridization subtelomere tests for the child with intellectual disability of unknown etiology. Fragile X testing remains an important first-line test. The importance of considering testing for inborn errors of metabolism in this population is supported by a recent systematic review of the literature and several case series recently published. The role of brain MRI remains important in certain patients. There is also a discussion of the emerging literature on the use of whole-exome sequencing as a diagnostic test in this population. Finally, the importance of intentional comanagement among families, the medical home, and the clinical genetics specialty clinic is discussed. (8/14)
http://pediatrics.aappublications.org/content/134/3/e903

COMPREHENSIVE HEALTH EVALUATION OF THE NEWLY ADOPTED CHILD (CLINICAL REPORT)

Veronnie F. Jones, MD, PhD, MSPH, and Committee on Early Childhood, Adoption, and Dependent Care
ABSTRACT. Children who join families through the process of adoption often have multiple health care needs. After placement in an adoptive home, it is essential that these children have a timely comprehensive health evaluation. This evaluation should include a review of all available medical records and a complete physical examination. Evaluation should also include diagnostic testing based on the findings from the history and physical examination as well as the risks presented by the child's previous living conditions. Age-appropriate screens should be performed, including, for example, newborn screening panels, hearing, vision, dental, and formal behavioral/developmental screens. The comprehensive assessment can occur at the time of the initial visit to the physician after adoptive placement or can take place over several visits. Adopted children should be referred to other medical specialists as deemed appropriate. The Section on Adoption and Foster Care is a resource within the American Academy of Pediatrics for physicians providing care for children who are being adopted. (12/11, reaffirmed 9/15)
http://pediatrics.aappublications.org/content/129/1/e214

CONDOM USE BY ADOLESCENTS

Committee on Adolescence
ABSTRACT. Rates of sexual activity, pregnancies, and births among adolescents have continued to decline during the past decade to historic lows. Despite these positive trends, many adolescents remain at risk for unintended pregnancy and sexually transmitted infections (STIs). This policy statement has been developed to assist the pediatrician in understanding and supporting the use of condoms by their patients to prevent unintended pregnancies and STIs and address barriers to their use. When used consistently and correctly, male latex condoms reduce the risk of pregnancy and many STIs, including HIV. Since the last policy statement published 12 years ago, there is an increased evidence base supporting the protection provided by condoms against STIs. Rates of acquisition of STIs/HIV among adolescents remain unacceptably high. Interventions that increase availability or accessibility to condoms are most efficacious when combined with additional individual, small-group, or community-level activities that include messages about safer sex. Continued research is needed to inform public health interventions for adolescents that increase the consistent and correct use of condoms and promote dual protection of condoms for STI prevention with other effective methods of contraception. (10/13)
http://pediatrics.aappublications.org/content/132/5/973

CONFLICTS BETWEEN RELIGIOUS OR SPIRITUAL BELIEFS AND PEDIATRIC CARE: INFORMED REFUSAL, EXEMPTIONS, AND PUBLIC FUNDING

Committee on Bioethics

ABSTRACT. Although respect for parents' decision-making authority is an important principle, pediatricians should report suspected cases of medical neglect, and the state should, at times, intervene to require medical treatment of children. Some parents' reasons for refusing medical treatment are based on their religious or spiritual beliefs. In cases in which treatment is likely to prevent death or serious disability or relieve severe pain, children's health and future autonomy should be protected. Because religious exemptions to child abuse and neglect laws do not equally protect all children and may harm some children by causing confusion about the duty to provide medical treatment, these exemptions should be repealed. Furthermore, public health care funds should not cover alternative unproven religious or spiritual healing practices. Such payments may inappropriately legitimize these practices as appropriate medical treatment. (10/13, reaffirmed 12/16, 11/17)
http://pediatrics.aappublications.org/content/132/5/962

CONGENITAL BRAIN AND SPINAL CORD MALFORMATIONS AND THEIR ASSOCIATED CUTANEOUS MARKERS (CLINICAL REPORT)

Mark Dias, MD, FAANS, FAAP; Michael Partington, MD, FAANS, FAAP; and Section on Neurologic Surgery

ABSTRACT. The brain, spinal cord, and skin are all derived from the embryonic ectoderm; this common derivation leads to a high association between central nervous system dysraphic malformations and abnormalities of the overlying skin. A myelomeningocele is an obvious open malformation, the identification of which is not usually difficult. However, the relationship between congenital spinal cord malformations and other cutaneous malformations, such as dimples, vascular anomalies (including infantile hemangiomata and other vascular malformations), congenital pigmented nevi or other hamartomata, or midline hairy patches may be less obvious but no less important. Pediatricians should be aware of these associations, recognize the cutaneous markers associated with congenital central nervous system malformations, and refer children with such markers to the appropriate specialist in a timely fashion for further evaluation and treatment. (9/15)
http://pediatrics.aappublications.org/content/136/4/e1105

A CONSENSUS STATEMENT ON HEALTH CARE TRANSITIONS FOR YOUNG ADULTS WITH SPECIAL HEALTH CARE NEEDS

American Academy of Pediatrics, American Academy of Family Physicians, and American College of Physicians-American Society of Internal Medicine

ABSTRACT. This policy statement represents a consensus on the critical first steps that the medical profession needs to take to realize the vision of a family-centered, continuous, comprehensive, coordinated, compassionate, and culturally competent health care system that is as developmentally appropriate as it is technically sophisticated. The goal of transition in health care for young adults with special health care needs is to maximize lifelong functioning and potential through the provision of high-quality, developmentally appropriate health care services that continue uninterrupted as the individual moves from adolescence to adulthood. This consensus document has now been approved as policy by the boards of the American Academy of Pediatrics, the American Academy of Family Physicians, and the American College of Physicians-American Society of Internal Medicine. (12/02)
http://pediatrics.aappublications.org/content/110/Supplement_3/1304

CONSENT BY PROXY FOR NONURGENT PEDIATRIC CARE (CLINICAL REPORT)

Jonathan M. Fanaroff, MD, JD, FAAP, FCLM, and Committee on Medical Liability and Risk Management

ABSTRACT. Minor-aged patients are often brought to the pediatrician for nonurgent acute medical care, physical examinations, or health supervision visits by someone other than their legally authorized representative, which, in most situations, is a parent. These surrogates or proxies can be members of the child's extended family, such as a grandparent, adult sibling, or aunt/uncle; a noncustodial parent or stepparent in cases of divorce and remarriage; an adult who lives in the home but is not biologically or legally related to the child; or even a child care provider (eg, au pair, nanny, private-duty nurse/nurse's aide, group home supervisor). This report identifies common situations in which pediatricians may encounter "consent by proxy" for nonurgent medical care for minors, including physical examinations, and explains the potential for liability exposure associated with these circumstances. The report suggests practical steps that balance the need to minimize the physician's liability exposure with the patient's access to health care. Key issues to be considered when creating or updating office policies for obtaining and documenting consent by proxy are offered. (1/17)
http://pediatrics.aappublications.org/content/139/2/e20163911

CONSENT FOR EMERGENCY MEDICAL SERVICES FOR CHILDREN AND ADOLESCENTS

Committee on Pediatric Emergency Medicine and Committee on Bioethics

ABSTRACT. Parental consent generally is required for the medical evaluation and treatment of minor children. However, children and adolescents might require evaluation of and treatment for emergency medical conditions in situations in which a parent or legal guardian is not available to provide consent or conditions under which an adolescent patient might possess the legal authority to provide consent. In general, a medical screening examination and any medical care necessary and likely to prevent imminent and significant harm to the pediatric patient with an emergency medical condition should not be withheld or delayed because of problems obtaining consent. The purpose of this policy statement is to provide guidance in those situations in which parental consent is not readily available, in which parental consent is not necessary, or in which parental refusal of consent places a child at risk of significant harm. (7/11, reaffirmed 9/15)
http://pediatrics.aappublications.org/content/128/2/427

CONSUMPTION OF RAW OR UNPASTEURIZED MILK AND MILK PRODUCTS BY PREGNANT WOMEN AND CHILDREN

Committee on Infectious Diseases and Committee on Nutrition

ABSTRACT. Sales of raw or unpasteurized milk and milk products are still legal in at least 30 states in the United States. Raw milk and milk products from cows, goats, and sheep continue to be a source of bacterial infections attributable to a number of virulent pathogens, including *Listeria monocytogenes, Campylobacter jejuni, Salmonella* species, *Brucella* species, and *Escherichia coli* O157. These infections can occur in both healthy and immunocompromised individuals, including older adults, infants, young children, and pregnant women and their unborn fetuses, in whom life-threatening infections and fetal miscarriage can occur. Efforts to limit the sale of raw milk products have met with opposition from those who are proponents of the purported health benefits of consuming raw milk products, which contain natural or unprocessed factors not inactivated by pasteurization. However, the benefits of these natural factors have not been clearly demonstrated in evidence-based studies and, therefore, do not outweigh the risks of raw milk consumption. Substantial data suggest that pasteurized milk confers equivalent health benefits compared with raw milk, without the additional risk of bacterial infections. The purpose of this policy statement was to review the risks of raw milk consumption in the United States and to provide evidence of the risks of infectious complications associated with consumption of unpasteurized milk and milk products, especially among pregnant women, infants, and children. (12/13)

http://pediatrics.aappublications.org/content/133/1/175

CONTRACEPTION FOR ADOLESCENTS
Committee on Adolescence
ABSTRACT. Contraception is a pillar in reducing adolescent pregnancy rates. The American Academy of Pediatrics recommends that pediatricians develop a working knowledge of contraception to help adolescents reduce risks of and negative health consequences related to unintended pregnancy. Over the past 10 years, a number of new contraceptive methods have become available to adolescents, newer guidance has been issued on existing contraceptive methods, and the evidence base for contraception for special populations (adolescents who have disabilities, are obese, are recipients of solid organ transplants, or are HIV infected) has expanded. The Academy has addressed contraception since 1980, and this policy statement updates the 2007 statement on contraception and adolescents. It provides the pediatrician with a description and rationale for best practices in counseling and prescribing contraception for adolescents. It is supported by an accompanying technical report. (9/14)

http://pediatrics.aappublications.org/content/134/4/e1244

CONTRACEPTION FOR ADOLESCENTS (TECHNICAL REPORT)
Mary A. Ott, MD, MA, FAAP; Gina S. Sucato, MD, MPH, FAAP; and Committee on Adolescence
ABSTRACT. A working knowledge of contraception will assist the pediatrician in both sexual health promotion as well as treatment of common adolescent gynecologic problems. Best practices in adolescent anticipatory guidance and screening include a sexual health history, screening for pregnancy and sexually transmitted infections, counseling, and if indicated, providing access to contraceptives. Pediatricians' long-term relationships with adolescents and families allow them to help promote healthy sexual decision-making, including abstinence and contraceptive use. Additionally, medical indications for contraception, such as acne, dysmenorrhea, and heavy menstrual bleeding, are frequently uncovered during adolescent visits. This technical report provides an evidence base for the accompanying policy statement and addresses key aspects of adolescent contraceptive use, including the following: (1) sexual history taking, confidentiality, and counseling; (2) adolescent data on the use and side effects of newer contraceptive methods; (3) new data on older contraceptive methods; and (4) evidence supporting the use of contraceptives in adolescent patients with complex medical conditions. (9/14)

http://pediatrics.aappublications.org/content/134/4/e1257

CONTRACEPTION FOR HIV-INFECTED ADOLESCENTS (CLINICAL REPORT)
Athena P. Kourtis, MD, PhD, MPH, FAAP; Ayesha Mirza, MD, FAAP; and Committee on Pediatric AIDS
ABSTRACT. Access to high-quality reproductive health care is important for adolescents and young adults with HIV infection to prevent unintended pregnancies, sexually transmitted infections, and secondary transmission of HIV to partners and children. As perinatally HIV-infected children mature into adolescence and adulthood and new HIV infections among adolescents and young adults continue to occur in the United States, medical providers taking care of such individuals often face issues related to sexual and reproductive health. Challenges including drug interactions between several hormonal methods and antiretroviral agents make decisions regarding contraceptive options more complex for these adolescents. Dual protection, defined as the use of an effective contraceptive along with condoms, should be central to ongoing discussions with HIV-infected young women and couples wishing to avoid pregnancy. Last, reproductive health discussions need to be integrated with discussions on HIV care, because a reduction in plasma HIV viral load below the level of detection (an "undetectable viral load") is essential for the individual's health as well as for a reduction in HIV transmission to partners and children. (8/16)

http://pediatrics.aappublications.org/content/138/3/e20161892

CONTROVERSIES CONCERNING VITAMIN K AND THE NEWBORN
Committee on Fetus and Newborn
ABSTRACT. Prevention of early vitamin K deficiency bleeding (VKDB) of the newborn, with onset at birth to 2 weeks of age (formerly known as classic hemorrhagic disease of the newborn), by oral or parenteral administration of vitamin K is accepted practice. In contrast, late VKDB, with onset from 2 to 12 weeks of age, is most effectively prevented by parenteral administration of vitamin K. Earlier concern regarding a possible causal association between parenteral vitamin K and childhood cancer has not been substantiated. This revised statement presents updated recommendations for the use of vitamin K in the prevention of early and late VKDB. (7/03, reaffirmed 5/06, 5/09, 9/14)

http://pediatrics.aappublications.org/content/112/1/191

CORD BLOOD BANKING FOR POTENTIAL FUTURE TRANSPLANTATION
William T. Shearer, MD, PhD, FAAP; Bertram H. Lubin, MD, FAAP; Mitchell S. Cairo, MD, FAAP; Luigi D. Notarangelo, MD; Section on Hematology/Oncology; and Section on Allergy and Immunology
ABSTRACT. This policy statement is intended to provide information to guide pediatricians, obstetricians, and other medical specialists and health care providers in responding to parents' questions about cord blood donation and banking as well as the types (public versus private) and quality of cord blood banks. Cord blood is an excellent source of stem cells for hematopoietic stem cell transplantation in children with some fatal diseases. Cord blood transplantation offers another method of definitive therapy for infants, children, and adults with certain hematologic malignancies, hemoglobinopathies, severe forms of T-lymphocyte and other immunodeficiencies, and metabolic diseases. The development of universal screening for severe immunodeficiency assay in a growing number of states is likely to increase the number of cord blood transplants. Both public and private cord blood banks worldwide hold hundreds of thousands of cord blood units designated for the treatment of fatal or debilitating illnesses. The procurement, characterization, and cryopreservation of cord blood is free for families who choose public banking. However, the family cost for private banking is significant and not covered by insurance, and the unit may never be used. Quality-assessment reviews by several national and international accrediting bodies show private cord blood banks to be underused for treatment, less regulated for quality control, and more expensive for the family than public cord blood banks. There is an unquestionable need to study the use of cord blood banking to make new and important alternative means of reconstituting the hematopoietic blood system in patients with malignancies and blood disorders and possibly regenerating tissue systems in the future. Recommendations regarding appropriate ethical and operational standards (including informed consent policies, financial disclosures, and conflict-of-interest policies) are provided for physicians, institutions, and organizations that operate or have a relationship with cord blood banking programs. The information on all aspects of cord blood banking

gathered in this policy statement will facilitate parental choice for public or private cord blood banking. (10/17)
http://pediatrics.aappublications.org/content/140/5/e20172695

CORPORAL PUNISHMENT IN SCHOOLS
Committee on School Health
ABSTRACT. The American Academy of Pediatrics recommends that corporal punishment in schools be abolished in all states by law and that alternative forms of student behavior management be used. (8/00, reaffirmed 6/03, 5/06, 2/12)
http://pediatrics.aappublications.org/content/106/2/343

COUNSELING IN PEDIATRIC POPULATIONS AT RISK FOR INFERTILITY AND/OR SEXUAL FUNCTION CONCERNS (CLINICAL REPORT)
Leena Nahata, MD, FAAP; Gwendolyn P. Quinn, PhD; Amy C. Tishelman, PhD; and Section on Endocrinology
ABSTRACT. Reproductive health is an important yet often overlooked topic in pediatric health care; when addressed, the focus is generally on prevention of sexually transmitted infections and unwanted pregnancy. Two aspects of reproductive health counseling that have received minimal attention in pediatrics are fertility and sexual function for at-risk pediatric populations, and youth across many disciplines are affected. Although professional organizations, such as the American Academy of Pediatrics and the American Society of Clinical Oncology, have published recommendations about fertility preservation discussions, none of these guidelines address how to have ongoing conversations with at-risk youth and their families about the potential for future infertility and sexual dysfunction in developmentally appropriate ways. Researchers suggest many pediatric patients at risk for reproductive problems remain uncertain and confused about their fertility or sexual function status well into young adulthood. Potential infertility may cause distress and anxiety, has been shown to affect formation of romantic relationships, and may lead to unplanned pregnancy in those who incorrectly assumed they were infertile. Sexual dysfunction is also common and may lead to problems with intimacy and self-esteem; survivors of pediatric conditions consistently report inadequate guidance from clinicians in this area. Health care providers and parents report challenges in knowing how and when to discuss these issues. In this context, the goal of this clinical report is to review evidence and considerations for providers related to information sharing about impaired fertility and sexual function in pediatric patients attributable to congenital and acquired conditions or treatments. (7/18)
See full text on page 561.
http://pediatrics.aappublications.org/content/142/2/e20181435

COUNSELING PARENTS AND TEENS ABOUT MARIJUANA USE IN THE ERA OF LEGALIZATION OF MARIJUANA (CLINICAL REPORT)
Sheryl A. Ryan, MD, FAAP; Seth D. Ammerman, MD, FAAP; and Committee on Substance Use and Prevention
ABSTRACT. Many states have recently made significant changes to their legislation making recreational and/or medical marijuana use by adults legal. Although these laws, for the most part, have not targeted the adolescent population, they have created an environment in which marijuana increasingly is seen as acceptable, safe, and therapeutic. This clinical report offers guidance to the practicing pediatrician based on existing evidence and expert opinion/consensus of the American Academy of Pediatrics regarding anticipatory guidance and counseling to teenagers and their parents about marijuana and its use. The recently published technical report provides the detailed evidence and references regarding the research on which the information in this clinical report is based. (2/17)
http://pediatrics.aappublications.org/content/139/3/e20164069

COUNTERING VACCINE HESITANCY (CLINICAL REPORT)
Kathryn M. Edwards, MD; Jesse M. Hackell, MD; Committee on Infectious Diseases; and Committee on Practice and Ambulatory Medicine
ABSTRACT. Immunizations have led to a significant decrease in rates of vaccine-preventable diseases and have made a significant impact on the health of children. However, some parents express concerns about vaccine safety and the necessity of vaccines. The concerns of parents range from hesitancy about some immunizations to refusal of all vaccines. This clinical report provides information about addressing parental concerns about vaccination. (8/16)
http://pediatrics.aappublications.org/content/138/3/e20162146

CREATING HEALTHY CAMP EXPERIENCES
Council on School Health
ABSTRACT. The American Academy of Pediatrics has created recommendations for health appraisal and preparation of young people before participation in day or resident camps and to guide health and safety practices for children at camp. These recommendations are intended for parents, primary health care providers, and camp administration and health center staff. Although camps have diverse environments, there are general guidelines that apply to all situations and specific recommendations that are appropriate under special conditions. This policy statement has been reviewed and is supported by the American Camp Association. (3/11)
http://pediatrics.aappublications.org/content/127/4/794

CRITICAL ELEMENTS FOR THE PEDIATRIC PERIOPERATIVE ANESTHESIA ENVIRONMENT
Section on Anesthesiology and Pain Medicine
ABSTRACT. The American Academy of Pediatrics proposes guidance for the pediatric perioperative anesthesia environment. Essential components are identified to optimize the perioperative environment for the anesthetic care of infants and children. Such an environment promotes the safety and well-being of infants and children by reducing the risk of adverse events. (11/15)
http://pediatrics.aappublications.org/content/136/6/1200

THE CRUCIAL ROLE OF RECESS IN SCHOOL
Council on School Health
ABSTRACT. Recess is at the heart of a vigorous debate over the role of schools in promoting the optimal development of the whole child. A growing trend toward reallocating time in school to accentuate the more academic subjects has put this important facet of a child's school day at risk. Recess serves as a necessary break from the rigors of concentrated, academic challenges in the classroom. But equally important is the fact that safe and well-supervised recess offers cognitive, social, emotional, and physical benefits that may not be fully appreciated when a decision is made to diminish it. Recess is unique from, and a complement to, physical education—not a substitute for it. The American Academy of Pediatrics believes that recess is a crucial and necessary component of a child's development and, as such, it should not be withheld for punitive or academic reasons. (12/12, reaffirmed 8/16)
http://pediatrics.aappublications.org/content/131/1/183

DEALING WITH THE PARENT WHOSE JUDGMENT IS IMPAIRED BY ALCOHOL OR DRUGS: LEGAL AND ETHICAL CONSIDERATIONS (CLINICAL REPORT)
Committee on Medical Liability
ABSTRACT. An estimated 11 to 17.5 million children are being raised by a substance-abusing parent or guardian. The importance of this statistic is undeniable, particularly when a patient is brought to a pediatric office by a parent or guardian exhibiting

symptoms of judgment impairment. Although the physician-patient relationship exists between the pediatrician and the minor patient, other obligations (some perceived and some real) should be considered as well. In managing encounters with impaired parents who may become disruptive or dangerous, pediatricians should be aware of their responsibilities before acting. In addition to fulfilling the duty involved with an established physician-patient relationship, the pediatrician should take reasonable care to safeguard patient confidentiality; protect the safety of the patient and other patients, visitors, and employees; and comply with reporting mandates. This clinical report identifies and discusses the legal and ethical concepts related to these circumstances. The report offers implementation suggestions when establishing anticipatory office procedures and training programs for staff on what to do (and not do) in such situations to maximize the patient's well-being and safety and minimize the liability of the pediatrician. (9/04, reaffirmed 9/10)
http://pediatrics.aappublications.org/content/114/3/869

DEATH OF A CHILD IN THE EMERGENCY DEPARTMENT

Committee on Pediatric Emergency Medicine (joint with American College of Emergency Physicians Pediatric Emergency Medicine Committee and Emergency Nurses Association Pediatric Committee)

ABSTRACT. The American Academy of Pediatrics, American College of Emergency Physicians, and Emergency Nurses Association have collaborated to identify practices and principles to guide the care of children, families, and staff in the challenging and uncommon event of the death of a child in the emergency department in this policy statement and in an accompanying technical report. (6/14)
http://pediatrics.aappublications.org/content/134/1/198

DEATH OF A CHILD IN THE EMERGENCY DEPARTMENT (TECHNICAL REPORT)

Patricia O'Malley, MD; Isabel Barata, MD; Sally Snow, RN; and Committee on Pediatric Emergency Medicine (joint with American College of Emergency Physicians Pediatric Emergency Medicine Committee and Emergency Nurses Association Pediatric Committee)

ABSTRACT. The death of a child in the emergency department (ED) is one of the most challenging problems facing ED clinicians. This revised technical report and accompanying policy statement reaffirm principles of patient- and family-centered care. Recent literature is examined regarding family presence, termination of resuscitation, bereavement responsibilities of ED clinicians, support of child fatality review efforts, and other issues inherent in caring for the patient, family, and staff when a child dies in the ED. Appendices are provided that offer an approach to bereavement activities in the ED, carrying out forensic responsibilities while providing compassionate care, communicating the news of the death of a child in the acute setting, providing a closing ritual at the time of terminating resuscitation efforts, and managing the child with a terminal condition who presents near death in the ED. (6/14)
http://pediatrics.aappublications.org/content/134/1/e313

DEFINITION OF A PEDIATRICIAN

Committee on Pediatric Workforce

POLICY. The American Academy of Pediatrics (AAP) has developed the following definition of pediatrics and a pediatrician:

Pediatrics is the specialty of medical science concerned with the physical, mental, and social health of children from birth to young adulthood. Pediatric care encompasses a broad spectrum of health services ranging from preventive health care to the diagnosis and treatment of acute and chronic diseases.

Pediatrics is a discipline that deals with biological, social, and environmental influences on the developing child and with the impact of disease and dysfunction on development. Children differ from adults anatomically, physiologically, immunologically, psychologically, developmentally, and metabolically.

The pediatrician, a term that includes primary care pediatricians, pediatric medical subspecialists, and pediatric surgical specialists, understands this constantly changing functional status of his or her patients' incident to growth and development and the consequent changing standards of "normal" for age. A pediatrician is a physician who is concerned primarily with the health, welfare, and development of children and is uniquely qualified for these endeavors by virtue of interest and initial training. This training includes 4 years of medical school education, plus an additional year or years (usually at least 3) of intensive training devoted solely to all aspects of medical care for children, adolescents, and young adults. Maintenance of these competencies is achieved by experience, training, continuous education, self-assessment, and practice improvement.

A pediatrician is able to define accurately the child's health status and to serve as a consultant and make use of other specialists as consultants as needed, ideally in the context of, or in conjunction with, the physician-led medical home. Because the child's welfare is heavily dependent on the home and family, the pediatrician supports efforts to create a nurturing environment. Such support includes education about healthful living and anticipatory guidance for both patients and parents.

A pediatrician participates at the community level in preventing or solving problems in child health care and publicly advocates the causes of children. (3/15)
http://pediatrics.aappublications.org/content/135/4/780

DETENTION OF IMMIGRANT CHILDREN

Julie M. Linton, MD, FAAP; Marsha Griffin, MD, FAAP; Alan J. Shapiro, MD, FAAP; and Council on Community Pediatrics

ABSTRACT. Immigrant children seeking safe haven in the United States, whether arriving unaccompanied or in family units, face a complicated evaluation and legal process from the point of arrival through permanent resettlement in communities. The conditions in which children are detained and the support services that are available to them are of great concern to pediatricians and other advocates for children. In accordance with internationally accepted rights of the child, immigrant and refugee children should be treated with dignity and respect and should not be exposed to conditions that may harm or traumatize them. The Department of Homeland Security facilities do not meet the basic standards for the care of children in residential settings. The recommendations in this statement call for limited exposure of any child to current Department of Homeland Security facilities (ie, Customs and Border Protection and Immigration and Customs Enforcement facilities) and for longitudinal evaluation of the health consequences of detention of immigrant children in the United States. From the moment children are in the custody of the United States, they deserve health care that meets guideline-based standards, treatment that mitigates harm or traumatization, and services that support their health and well-being. This policy statement also provides specific recommendations regarding postrelease services once a child is released into communities across the country, including a coordinated system that facilitates access to a medical home and consistent access to education, child care, interpretation services, and legal services. (4/17)
http://pediatrics.aappublications.org/content/139/5/e20170483

DEVELOPMENTAL DYSPLASIA OF THE HIP PRACTICE GUIDELINE (TECHNICAL REPORT)

Harold P. Lehmann, MD, PhD; Richard Hinton, MD, MPH; Paola Morello, MD; Jeanne Santoli, MD; in conjunction with Steering Committee on Quality Improvement and Subcommittee on Developmental Dysplasia of the Hip Detention of Immigrant Children

ABSTRACT. *Objective.* To create a recommendation for pediatricians and other primary care providers about their role as screeners for detecting developmental dysplasia of the hip (DDH) in children.

Patients. Theoretical cohorts of newborns.

Method. Model-based approach using decision analysis as the foundation. Components of the approach include the following:

Perspective: Primary care provider.

Outcomes: DDH, avascular necrosis of the hip (AVN).

Options: Newborn screening by pediatric examination; orthopaedic examination; ultrasonographic examination; orthopaedic or ultrasonographic examination by risk factors. Intercurrent health supervision-based screening.

Preferences: 0 for bad outcomes, 1 for best outcomes.

Model: Influence diagram assessed by the Subcommittee and by the methodology team, with critical feedback from the Subcommittee.

Evidence Sources: Medline and EMBASE search of the research literature through June 1996. Hand search of sentinel journals from June 1996 through March 1997. Ancestor search of accepted articles.

Evidence Quality: Assessed on a custom subjective scale, based primarily on the fit of the evidence to the decision model.

Results. After discussion, explicit modeling, and critique, an influence diagram of 31 nodes was created. The computer-based and the hand literature searches found 534 articles, 101 of which were reviewed by 2 or more readers. Ancestor searches of these yielded a further 17 articles for evidence abstraction. Articles came from around the globe, although primarily Europe, British Isles, Scandinavia, and their descendants. There were 5 controlled trials, each with a sample size less than 40. The remainder were case series. Evidence was available for 17 of the desired 30 probabilities. Evidence quality ranged primarily between one third and two thirds of the maximum attainable score (median: 10–21; interquartile range: 8–14). Based on the raw evidence and Bayesian hierarchical meta-analyses, our estimate for the incidence of DDH revealed by physical examination performed by pediatricians is 8.6 per 1000; for orthopaedic screening, 11.5; for ultrasonography, 25. The odds ratio for DDH, given breech delivery, is 5.5; for female sex, 4.1; for positive family history, 1.7, although this last factor is not statistically significant. Postneonatal cases of DDH were divided into mid-term (younger than 6 months of age) and late-term (older than 6 months of age). Our estimates for the mid-term rate for screening by pediatricians is 0.34/1000 children screened; for orthopaedists, 0.1; and for ultrasonography, 0.28. Our estimates for late-term DDH rates are 0.21/1000 newborns screened by pediatricians; 0.08, by orthopaedists; and 0.2 for ultrasonography. The rates of AVN for children referred before 6 months of age is estimated at 2.5/1000 infants referred. For those referred after 6 months of age, our estimate is 109/1000 referred infants. The decision model (reduced, based on available evidence) suggests that orthopaedic screening is optimal, but because orthopaedists in the published studies and in practice would differ, the supply of orthopaedists is relatively limited, and the difference between orthopaedists and pediatricians is statistically insignificant, we conclude that pediatric screening is to be recommended. The place of ultrasonography in the screening process remains to be defined because there are too few data about postneonatal diagnosis by ultrasonographic screening to permit definitive recommendations. These data could be used by others to refine the conclusions based on costs, parental preferences, or physician style. Areas for research are well defined by our model-based approach. (4/00)

http://pediatrics.aappublications.org/content/105/4/e57

DIAGNOSIS, EVALUATION, AND MANAGEMENT OF HIGH BLOOD PRESSURE IN CHILDREN AND ADOLESCENTS (TECHNICAL REPORT)

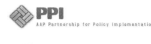

Carissa M. Baker-Smith, MD, MS, MPH, FAAP, FAHA; Susan K. Flinn, MA; Joseph T. Flynn, MD, MS, FAAP; David C. Kaelber, MD, PhD, MPH, FAAP, FACP, FACMI; Douglas Blowey, MD; Aaron E. Carroll, MD, MS, FAAP; Stephen R. Daniels, MD, PhD, FAAP; Sarah D. de Ferranti, MD, MPH, FAAP; Janis M. Dionne, MD, FRCPC; Bonita Falkner, MD; Samuel S. Gidding, MD; Celeste Goodwin; Michael G. Leu, MD, MS, MHS, FAAP; Makia E. Powers, MD, MPH, FAAP; Corinna Rea, MD, MPH, FAAP; Joshua Samuels, MD, MPH, FAAP; Madeline Simasek, MD, MSCP, FAAP; Vidhu V. Thaker, MD, FAAP; Elaine M. Urbina, MD, MS, FAAP; and Subcommittee on Screening and Management of High BP in Children

ABSTRACT. Systemic hypertension is a major cause of morbidity and mortality in adulthood. High blood pressure (HBP) and repeated measures of HBP, hypertension (HTN), begin in youth. Knowledge of how best to diagnose, manage, and treat systemic HTN in children and adolescents is important for primary and subspecialty care providers.

Objectives: To provide a technical summary of the methodology used to generate the 2017 "Clinical Practice Guideline for Screening and Management of High Blood Pressure in Children and Adolescents," an update to the 2004 "Fourth Report on the Diagnosis, Evaluation, and Treatment of High Blood Pressure in Children and Adolescents."

Data Sources: Medline, Cochrane Central Register of Controlled Trials, and Excerpta Medica Database references published between January 2003 and July 2015 followed by an additional search between August 2015 and July 2016.

Study Selection: English-language observational studies and randomized trials.

Methods: Key action statements (KASs) and additional recommendations regarding the diagnosis, management, and treatment of HBP in youth were the product of a detailed systematic review of the literature. A content outline establishing the breadth and depth was followed by the generation of 4 patient, intervention, comparison, outcome, time questions. Key questions addressed: (1) diagnosis of systemic HTN, (2) recommended work-up of systemic HTN, (3) optimal blood pressure (BP) goals, and (4) impact of high BP on indirect markers of cardiovascular disease in youth. Once selected, references were subjected to a 2-person review of the abstract and title followed by a separate 2-person full-text review. Full citation information, population data, findings, benefits and harms of the findings, as well as other key reference information were archived. Selected primary references were then used for KAS generation. Level of evidence (LOE) scoring was assigned for each reference and then in aggregate. Appropriate language was used to generate each KAS based on the LOE and the balance of benefit versus harm of the findings. Topics that could not be researched via the stated approach were (1) definition of HTN in youth, and (2) definition of left ventricular hypertrophy. KASs related to these stated topics were generated via expert opinion.

Results: Nearly 15 000 references were identified during an initial literature search. After a deduplication process, 14 382 references were available for title and abstract review, and 1379 underwent full text review. One hundred twenty-four experimental and observational studies published between 2003 and 2016 were selected as primary references for KAS generation, followed by an additional 269 primary references selected between August 2015 and July 2016. The LOE for the majority of references was C. In total, 30 KASs and 27 additional recommendations were generated; 12 were related to the diagnosis of HTN, 13 were related to management and additional diagnostic testing, 3 to treatment goals, and 2 to treatment options. Finally, special additions to the clinical practice guideline included creation of new BP tables based on BP values obtained solely from children with normal weight, creation of a simplified table to enhance screening and recognition of abnormal BP, and a revision of the criteria for diagnosing left ventricular hypertrophy.

Conclusions: An extensive and detailed systematic approach was used to generate evidence-based guidelines for the diagnosis, management, and treatment of youth with systemic HTN. (8/18)

See full text on page 571.

http://pediatrics.aappublications.org/content/142/3/e20182096

DIAGNOSIS, TREATMENT, AND PREVENTION OF CONGENITAL TOXOPLASMOSIS IN THE UNITED STATES (TECHNICAL REPORT)

Yvonne A. Maldonado, MD, FAAP; Jennifer S. Read, MD, MS, MPH, DTM&H, FAAP; and Committee on Infectious Diseases

ABSTRACT. Congenital toxoplasmosis (CT) is a parasitic disease that can cause significant fetal and neonatal harm. Coordinated efforts by pregnant women, researchers, physicians, and health policy makers regarding potential primary and secondary preventive measures for CT and their implementation may lead to a lower incidence of CT as well as lower morbidity and mortality rates associated with CT. The purpose of this technical report is to summarize available information regarding the diagnosis, treatment, and prevention of CT. (1/17)

http://pediatrics.aappublications.org/content/139/2/e20163860

DIAGNOSIS AND MANAGEMENT OF AN INITIAL UTI IN FEBRILE INFANTS AND YOUNG CHILDREN (TECHNICAL REPORT)

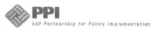

PPI
AAP Partnership for Policy Implementation

S. Maria E. Finnell, MD, MS; Aaron E. Carroll, MD, MS; Stephen M. Downs, MD, MS; Steering Committee on Quality Improvement and Management; and Subcommittee on Urinary Tract Infection

ABSTRACT. *Objectives.* The diagnosis and management of urinary tract infections (UTIs) in young children are clinically challenging. This report was developed to inform the revised, evidence-based, clinical guideline regarding the diagnosis and management of initial UTIs in febrile infants and young children, 2 to 24 months of age, from the American Academy of Pediatrics Subcommittee on Urinary Tract Infection.

Methods. The conceptual model presented in the 1999 technical report was updated after a comprehensive review of published literature. Studies with potentially new information or with evidence that reinforced the 1999 technical report were retained. Meta-analyses on the effectiveness of antimicrobial prophylaxis to prevent recurrent UTI were performed.

Results. Review of recent literature revealed new evidence in the following areas. Certain clinical findings and new urinalysis methods can help clinicians identify febrile children at very low risk of UTI. Oral antimicrobial therapy is as effective as parenteral therapy in treating UTI. Data from published, randomized controlled trials do not support antimicrobial prophylaxis to prevent febrile UTI when vesicoureteral reflux is found through voiding cystourethrography. Ultrasonography of the urinary tract after the first UTI has poor sensitivity. Early antimicrobial treatment may decrease the risk of renal damage from UTI.

Conclusions. Recent literature agrees with most of the evidence presented in the 1999 technical report, but meta-analyses of data from recent, randomized controlled trials do not support antimicrobial prophylaxis to prevent febrile UTI. This finding argues against voiding cystourethrography after the first UTI. (8/11)

http://pediatrics.aappublications.org/content/128/3/e749

DIAGNOSIS AND MANAGEMENT OF CHILDHOOD OBSTRUCTIVE SLEEP APNEA SYNDROME (TECHNICAL REPORT)

Carole L. Marcus, MBBCh; Lee J. Brooks, MD; Sally Davidson Ward, MD; Kari A. Draper, MD; David Gozal, MD; Ann C. Halbower, MD; Jacqueline Jones, MD; Christopher Lehmann, MD; Michael S. Schechter, MD, MPH; Stephen Sheldon, MD; Richard N. Shiffman, MD, MCIS; Karen Spruyt, PhD; Steering Committee on Quality Improvement and Management; and Subcommittee on Obstructive Sleep Apnea Syndrome

ABSTRACT. *Objective.* This technical report describes the procedures involved in developing recommendations on the management of childhood obstructive sleep apnea syndrome (OSAS).

Methods. The literature from 1999 through 2011 was evaluated.

Results and Conclusions. A total of 3166 titles were reviewed, of which 350 provided relevant data. Most articles were level II through IV. The prevalence of OSAS ranged from 0% to 5.7%, with obesity being an independent risk factor. OSAS was associated with cardiovascular, growth, and neurobehavioral abnormalities and possibly inflammation. Most diagnostic screening tests had low sensitivity and specificity. Treatment of OSAS resulted in improvements in behavior and attention and likely improvement in cognitive abilities. Primary treatment is adenotonsillectomy (AT). Data were insufficient to recommend specific surgical techniques; however, children undergoing partial tonsillectomy should be monitored for possible recurrence of OSAS. Although OSAS improved postoperatively, the proportion of patients who had residual OSAS ranged from 13% to 29% in low-risk populations to 73% when obese children were included and stricter polysomnographic criteria were used. Nevertheless, OSAS may improve after AT even in obese children, thus supporting surgery as a reasonable initial treatment. A significant number of obese patients required intubation or continuous positive airway pressure (CPAP) postoperatively, which reinforces the need for inpatient observation. CPAP was effective in the treatment of OSAS, but adherence is a major barrier. For this reason, CPAP is not recommended as first-line therapy for OSAS when AT is an option. Intranasal steroids may ameliorate mild OSAS, but follow-up is needed. Data were insufficient to recommend rapid maxillary expansion. (8/12)

http://pediatrics.aappublications.org/content/130/3/e714

DIAGNOSIS AND MANAGEMENT OF GASTROESOPHAGEAL REFLUX IN PRETERM INFANTS (CLINICAL REPORT)

Eric C. Eichenwald, MD, FAAP, and Committee on Fetus and Newborn

ABSTRACT. Gastroesophageal reflux (GER), generally defined as the passage of gastric contents into the esophagus, is an almost universal phenomenon in preterm infants. It is a common diagnosis in the NICU; however, there is large variation in its treatment across NICU sites. In this clinical report, the physiology, diagnosis, and symptomatology in preterm infants as well as currently used treatment strategies in the NICU are examined. Conservative measures to control reflux, such as left lateral body position, head elevation, and feeding regimen manipulation, have not been shown to reduce clinically assessed signs of GER in the preterm infant. In addition, preterm infants with clinically diagnosed GER are often treated with pharmacologic agents; however, a lack of evidence of efficacy together with emerging evidence of significant harm (particularly with gastric acid blockade) strongly suggest that these agents should be used sparingly, if at all, in preterm infants. (6/18)

See full text on page 589.

http://pediatrics.aappublications.org/content/142/1/e20181061

DIAGNOSIS AND MANAGEMENT OF INFANTILE HEMANGIOMA (CLINICAL REPORT)

David H. Darrow, MD, DDS; Arin K. Greene, MD; Anthony J. Mancini, MD; Amy J. Nopper, MD; Section on Dermatology; Section on Otolaryngology—Head & Neck Surgery; and Section on Plastic Surgery

ABSTRACT. Infantile hemangiomas (IHs) are the most common tumors of childhood. Unlike other tumors, they have the unique ability to involute after proliferation, often leading primary care providers to assume they will resolve without intervention or consequence. Unfortunately, a subset of IHs rapidly develop complications, resulting in pain, functional impairment, or permanent disfigurement. As a result, the primary clinician has the task of determining which lesions require early consultation with a specialist. Although several recent reviews have been published, this clinical report is the first based on input from individuals representing the many specialties involved in the treatment of IH. Its purpose is to update the pediatric community regarding recent discoveries in IH pathogenesis, treatment, and clinical associations and to provide a basis for clinical decision-making in the management of IH. (9/15)

http://pediatrics.aappublications.org/content/136/4/e1060

DIAGNOSIS AND MANAGEMENT OF INFANTILE HEMANGIOMA: EXECUTIVE SUMMARY

David H. Darrow, MD, DDS; Arin K. Greene, MD; Anthony J. Mancini, MD; Amy J. Nopper, MD; Section on Dermatology; Section on Otolaryngology—Head & Neck Surgery; and Section on Plastic Surgery

ABSTRACT. Infantile hemangiomas (IHs) are the most common tumors of childhood. Unlike other tumors, they have the capacity to involute after proliferation, often leading primary care providers to assume they will resolve without intervention or consequence. However, a subset of IHs may be associated with complications, resulting in pain, functional impairment, or permanent disfigurement. As a result, the primary care provider is often called on to decide which lesions should be referred for early consultation with a specialist.

This document provides a summary of the guidance contained in the clinical report "Diagnosis and Management of Infantile Hemangioma," published concurrently in the online version of *Pediatrics* (*Pediatrics*. 2015;136[4]:e1060–e1104, available at: www.pediatrics.org/content/136/4/e1060). The report is uniquely based on input from the many specialties involved in the treatment of IH. Its purpose is to update the pediatric community about recent discoveries in IH pathogenesis, clinical associations, and treatment and to provide a knowledge base and framework for clinical decision-making in the management of IH. (9/15)

http://pediatrics.aappublications.org/content/136/4/786

DIAGNOSIS AND PREVENTION OF IRON DEFICIENCY AND IRON-DEFICIENCY ANEMIA IN INFANTS AND YOUNG CHILDREN (0–3 YEARS OF AGE) (CLINICAL REPORT)

Robert D. Baker, MD, PhD; Frank R. Greer, MD; and Committee on Nutrition

ABSTRACT. This clinical report covers diagnosis and prevention of iron deficiency and iron-deficiency anemia in infants (both breastfed and formula fed) and toddlers from birth through 3 years of age. Results of recent basic research support the concerns that iron-deficiency anemia and iron deficiency without anemia during infancy and childhood can have long-lasting detrimental effects on neurodevelopment. Therefore, pediatricians and other health care providers should strive to eliminate iron deficiency and iron-deficiency anemia. Appropriate iron intakes for infants and toddlers as well as methods for screening for iron deficiency and iron-deficiency anemia are presented. (10/10)

http://pediatrics.aappublications.org/content/126/5/1040

DIAGNOSIS OF HIV-1 INFECTION IN CHILDREN YOUNGER THAN 18 MONTHS IN THE UNITED STATES (TECHNICAL REPORT)

Jennifer S. Read, MD, MS, MPH, DTM&H, and Committee on Pediatric AIDS

ABSTRACT. The objectives of this technical report are to describe methods of diagnosis of HIV-1 infection in children younger than 18 months in the United States and to review important issues that must be considered by clinicians who care for infants and young children born to HIV-1–infected women. Appropriate HIV-1 diagnostic testing for infants and children younger than 18 months differs from that for older children, adolescents, and adults because of passively transferred maternal HIV-1 antibodies, which may be detectable in the child's bloodstream until 18 months of age. Therefore, routine serologic testing of these infants and young children is generally only informative before the age of 18 months if the test result is negative. Virologic assays, including HIV-1 DNA or RNA assays, represent the gold standard for diagnostic testing of infants and children younger than 18 months. With such testing, the diagnosis of HIV-1 infection (as well as the presumptive exclusion of HIV-1 infection) can be established within the first several weeks of life among nonbreastfed infants. Important factors that must be considered when selecting HIV-1 diagnostic assays for pediatric patients and when choosing the timing of such assays include the age of the child, potential timing of infection of the child, whether the infection status of the child's mother is known or unknown, the antiretroviral exposure history of the mother and of the child, and characteristics of the virus. If the mother's HIV-1 serostatus is unknown, rapid HIV-1 antibody testing of the newborn infant to identify HIV-1 exposure is essential so that antiretroviral prophylaxis can be initiated within the first 12 hours of life if test results are positive. For HIV-1–exposed infants (identified by positive maternal test results or positive antibody results for the infant shortly after birth), it has been recommended that diagnostic testing with HIV-1 DNA or RNA assays be performed within the first 14 days of life, at 1 to 2 months of age, and at 3 to 6 months of age. If any of these test results are positive, repeat testing is recommended to confirm the diagnosis of HIV-1 infection. A diagnosis of HIV-1 infection can be made on the basis of 2 positive HIV-1 DNA or RNA assay results. In nonbreastfeeding children younger than 18 months with no positive HIV-1 virologic test results, presumptive exclusion of HIV-1 infection can be based on 2 negative virologic test results (1 obtained at ≥2 weeks and 1 obtained at ≥4 weeks of age); 1 negative virologic test result obtained at ≥8 weeks of age; or 1 negative HIV-1 antibody test result obtained at ≥6 months of age. Alternatively, presumptive exclusion of HIV-1 infection can be based on 1 positive HIV-1 virologic test with at least 2 subsequent negative virologic test results (at least 1 of which is performed at ≥8 weeks of age) or negative HIV-1 antibody test results (at least 1 of which is performed at ≥6 months of age). Definitive exclusion of HIV-1 infection is based on 2 negative virologic test results, 1 obtained at ≥1 month of age and 1 obtained at ≥4 months of age, or 2 negative HIV-1 antibody test results from separate specimens obtained at ≥6 months of age. For both presumptive and definitive exclusion of infection, the child should have no other laboratory (eg, no positive virologic test results) or clinical (eg, no AIDS-defining conditions) evidence of HIV-1 infection. Many clinicians confirm the absence of HIV-1 infection with a negative HIV-1 antibody assay result at 12 to 18 months of age. For breastfeeding infants, a similar testing algorithm can be followed, with timing of testing

starting from the date of complete cessation of breastfeeding instead of the date of birth. (12/07, reaffirmed 4/10, 2/15)
http://pediatrics.aappublications.org/content/120/6/e1547

DIAGNOSIS OF PREGNANCY AND PROVIDING OPTIONS COUNSELING FOR THE ADOLESCENT PATIENT (CLINICAL REPORT)

Laurie L. Hornberger, MD, MPH, FAAP, and Committee on Adolescence

ABSTRACT. The American Academy of Pediatrics policy statement "Options Counseling for the Pregnant Adolescent Patient" recommends the basic content of the pediatrician's counseling for an adolescent facing a new diagnosis of pregnancy. However, options counseling is just one aspect of what may be one of the more challenging scenarios in the pediatric office. Pediatricians must remain alert to the possibility of pregnancy among their adolescent female patients. When discovering symptoms suggestive of pregnancy, pediatricians must obtain a relevant history, perform diagnostic testing and properly interpret the results, and understand the significance of the results from the patient perspective and reveal them to the patient in a sensitive manner. If the patient is indeed pregnant, the pediatrician, in addition to providing comprehensive options counseling, may need to help recruit adult support for the patient and should offer continued assistance to the adolescent and her family after the office visit. All pediatricians should be aware of the legal aspects of adolescent reproductive care and the resources for pregnant adolescents in their communities. This clinical report presents a more comprehensive view of the evaluation and management of pregnancy in the adolescent patient and a context for options counseling. (8/17)
http://pediatrics.aappublications.org/content/140/3/e20172273

DIAGNOSTIC IMAGING OF CHILD ABUSE

Section on Radiology

ABSTRACT. The role of imaging in cases of child abuse is to identify the extent of physical injury when abuse is present and to elucidate all imaging findings that point to alternative diagnoses. Effective diagnostic imaging of child abuse rests on high-quality technology as well as a full appreciation of the clinical and pathologic alterations occurring in abused children. This statement is a revision of the previous policy published in 2000. (4/09)
http://pediatrics.aappublications.org/content/123/5/1430

DISASTER PLANNING FOR SCHOOLS

Council on School Health

ABSTRACT. Community awareness of the school district's disaster plan will optimize a community's capacity to maintain the safety of its school-aged population in the event of a school-based or greater community crisis. This statement is intended to stimulate awareness of the disaster-preparedness process in schools as a part of a global, community-wide preparedness plan. Pediatricians, other health care professionals, first responders, public health officials, the media, school nurses, school staff, and parents all need to be unified in their efforts to support schools in the prevention of, preparedness for, response to, and recovery from a disaster. (10/08, reaffirmed 9/11)
http://pediatrics.aappublications.org/content/122/4/895

DISASTER PREPAREDNESS IN NEONATAL INTENSIVE CARE UNITS (CLINICAL REPORT)

Wanda D. Barfield, MD, MPH, FAAP, RADM USPHS; Steven E. Krug, MD, FAAP; Committee on Fetus and Newborn; and Disaster Preparedness Council

ABSTRACT. Disasters disproportionally affect vulnerable, technology-dependent people, including preterm and critically ill newborn infants. It is important for health care providers to be aware of and prepared for the potential consequences of disasters for the NICU. Neonatal intensive care personnel can provide specialized expertise for their hospital, community, and regional emergency preparedness plans and can help develop institutional surge capacity for mass critical care, including equipment, medications, personnel, and facility resources. (4/17)
http://pediatrics.aappublications.org/content/139/5/e20170507

DISCLOSURE OF ADVERSE EVENTS IN PEDIATRICS

Committee on Medical Liability and Risk Management and Council on Quality Improvement and Patient Safety

ABSTRACT. Despite increasing attention to issues of patient safety, preventable adverse events (AEs) continue to occur, causing direct and consequential injuries to patients, families, and health care providers. Pediatricians generally agree that there is an ethical obligation to inform patients and families about preventable AEs and medical errors. Nonetheless, barriers, such as fear of liability, interfere with disclosure regarding preventable AEs. Changes to the legal system, improved communications skills, and carefully developed disclosure policies and programs can improve the quality and frequency of appropriate AE disclosure communications. (11/16)
http://pediatrics.aappublications.org/content/138/6/e20163215

DISPENSING MEDICATIONS AT THE HOSPITAL UPON DISCHARGE FROM AN EMERGENCY DEPARTMENT (TECHNICAL REPORT)

Loren G. Yamamoto, MD, MPH, MBA; Shannon Manzi, PharmD; and Committee on Pediatric Emergency Medicine

ABSTRACT. Although most health care services can and should be provided by their medical home, children will be referred or require visits to the emergency department (ED) for emergent clinical conditions or injuries. Continuation of medical care after discharge from an ED is dependent on parents or caregivers' understanding of and compliance with follow-up instructions and on adherence to medication recommendations. ED visits often occur at times when the majority of pharmacies are not open and caregivers are concerned with getting their ill or injured child directly home. Approximately one-third of patients fail to obtain priority medications from a pharmacy after discharge from an ED. The option of judiciously dispensing ED discharge medications from the ED's outpatient pharmacy within the facility is a major convenience that overcomes this obstacle, improving the likelihood of medication adherence. Emergency care encounters should be routinely followed up with primary care provider medical homes to ensure complete and comprehensive care. (1/12, reaffirmed 9/15)
http://pediatrics.aappublications.org/content/129/2/e562

DISTINGUISHING SUDDEN INFANT DEATH SYNDROME FROM CHILD ABUSE FATALITIES (CLINICAL REPORT)

Kent P. Hymel, MD, and Committee on Child Abuse and Neglect (joint with National Association of Medical Examiners)

ABSTRACT. Fatal child abuse has been mistaken for sudden infant death syndrome. When a healthy infant younger than 1 year dies suddenly and unexpectedly, the cause of death may be certified as sudden infant death syndrome. Sudden infant death syndrome is more common than infanticide. Parents of sudden infant death syndrome victims typically are anxious to provide unlimited information to professionals involved in death investigation or research. They also want and deserve to be approached in a nonaccusatory manner. This clinical report provides professionals with information and suggestions for procedures to help avoid stigmatizing families of sudden infant death syndrome victims while allowing accumulation of appropriate evidence in potential cases of infanticide. This clinical report addresses deficiencies and updates recommendations in the 2001 American

Academy of Pediatrics policy statement of the same name. (7/06, reaffirmed 4/09, 3/13, 7/17)
http://pediatrics.aappublications.org/content/118/1/421

DONOR HUMAN MILK FOR THE HIGH-RISK INFANT: PREPARATION, SAFETY, AND USAGE OPTIONS IN THE UNITED STATES

Committee on Nutrition, Section on Breastfeeding, and Committee on Fetus and Newborn

ABSTRACT. The use of donor human milk is increasing for high-risk infants, primarily for infants born weighing <1500 g or those who have severe intestinal disorders. Pasteurized donor milk may be considered in situations in which the supply of maternal milk is insufficient. The use of pasteurized donor milk is safe when appropriate measures are used to screen donors and collect, store, and pasteurize the milk and then distribute it through established human milk banks. The use of nonpasteurized donor milk and other forms of direct, Internet-based, or informal human milk sharing does not involve this level of safety and is not recommended. It is important that health care providers counsel families considering milk sharing about the risks of bacterial or viral contamination of nonpasteurized human milk and about the possibilities of exposure to medications, drugs, or herbs in human milk. Currently, the use of pasteurized donor milk is limited by its availability and affordability. The development of public policy to improve and expand access to pasteurized donor milk, including policies that support improved governmental and private financial support for donor milk banks and the use of donor milk, is important. (12/16)
http://pediatrics.aappublications.org/content/139/1/e20163440

DRINKING WATER FROM PRIVATE WELLS AND RISKS TO CHILDREN

Committee on Environmental Health and Committee on Infectious Diseases

ABSTRACT. Drinking water for approximately one sixth of US households is obtained from private wells. These wells can become contaminated by pollutant chemicals or pathogenic organisms and cause illness. Although the US Environmental Protection Agency and all states offer guidance for construction, maintenance, and testing of private wells, there is little regulation. With few exceptions, well owners are responsible for their own wells. Children may also drink well water at child care or when traveling. Illness resulting from children's ingestion of contaminated water can be severe. This policy statement provides recommendations for inspection, testing, and remediation for wells providing drinking water for children. (5/09, reaffirmed 1/13)
http://pediatrics.aappublications.org/content/123/6/1599

DRINKING WATER FROM PRIVATE WELLS AND RISKS TO CHILDREN (TECHNICAL REPORT)

Walter J. Rogan, MD; Michael T. Brady, MD; Committee on Environmental Health; and Committee on Infectious Diseases

ABSTRACT. Drinking water for approximately one sixth of US households is obtained from private wells. These wells can become contaminated by pollutant chemicals or pathogenic organisms, leading to significant illness. Although the US Environmental Protection Agency and all states offer guidance for construction, maintenance, and testing of private wells, there is little regulation, and with few exceptions, well owners are responsible for their own wells. Children may also drink well water at child care or when traveling. Illness resulting from children's ingestion of contaminated water can be severe. This report reviews relevant aspects of groundwater and wells; describes the common chemical and microbiologic contaminants; gives an algorithm with recommendations for inspection, testing, and remediation for wells providing drinking water for children; reviews the definitions and uses of various bottled waters; provides current estimates of costs for well testing; and provides federal, national, state, and, where appropriate, tribal contacts for more information. (5/09, reaffirmed 1/13)
http://pediatrics.aappublications.org/content/123/6/e1123

EARLY CHILDHOOD ADVERSITY, TOXIC STRESS, AND THE ROLE OF THE PEDIATRICIAN: TRANSLATING DEVELOPMENTAL SCIENCE INTO LIFELONG HEALTH

Committee on Psychosocial Aspects of Child and Family Health; Committee on Early Childhood, Adoption, and Dependent Care; and Section on Developmental and Behavioral Pediatrics

ABSTRACT. Advances in a wide range of biological, behavioral, and social sciences are expanding our understanding of how early environmental influences (the ecology) and genetic predispositions (the biologic program) affect learning capacities, adaptive behaviors, lifelong physical and mental health, and adult productivity. A supporting technical report from the American Academy of Pediatrics (AAP) presents an integrated ecobiodevelopmental framework to assist in translating these dramatic advances in developmental science into improved health across the life span. Pediatricians are now armed with new information about the adverse effects of toxic stress on brain development, as well as a deeper understanding of the early life origins of many adult diseases. As trusted authorities in child health and development, pediatric providers must now complement the early identification of developmental concerns with a greater focus on those interventions and community investments that reduce external threats to healthy brain growth. To this end, AAP endorses a developing leadership role for the entire pediatric community—one that mobilizes the scientific expertise of both basic and clinical researchers, the family-centered care of the pediatric medical home, and the public influence of AAP and its state chapters—to catalyze fundamental change in early childhood policy and services. AAP is committed to leveraging science to inform the development of innovative strategies to reduce the precipitants of toxic stress in young children and to mitigate their negative effects on the course of development and health across the life span. (12/11, reaffirmed 7/16)
http://pediatrics.aappublications.org/content/129/1/e224

EARLY CHILDHOOD CARIES IN INDIGENOUS COMMUNITIES

Committee on Native American Child Health (joint with Canadian Paediatric Society First Nations, Inuit, and Métis Committee)

ABSTRACT. The oral health of Indigenous children of Canada (First Nations, Inuit, and Métis) and the United States (American Indian, Alaska Native) is a major child health issue: there is a high prevalence of early childhood caries (ECC) and resulting adverse health effects in this community, as well as high rates and costs of restorative and surgical treatments under general anesthesia. ECC is an infectious disease that is influenced by multiple factors, including socioeconomic determinants, and requires a combination of approaches for improvement. This statement includes recommendations for preventive oral health and clinical care for young infants and pregnant women by primary health care providers, community-based health-promotion initiatives, oral health workforce and access issues, and advocacy for community water fluoridation and fluoride-varnish program access. Further community-based research on the epidemiology, prevention, management, and microbiology of ECC in Indigenous communities would be beneficial. (5/11)
http://pediatrics.aappublications.org/content/127/6/1190

EARLY CHILDHOOD HOME VISITING

James H. Duffee, MD, MPH, FAAP; Alan L. Mendelsohn, MD, FAAP; Alice A. Kuo, MD, PhD, FAAP; Lori A. Legano, MD, FAAP; Marian F. Earls, MD, MTS, FAAP; Council on Community Pediatrics; Council on Early Childhood; and Committee on Child Abuse and Neglect

ABSTRACT. High-quality home-visiting services for infants and young children can improve family relationships, advance school readiness, reduce child maltreatment, improve maternal-infant health outcomes, and increase family economic self-sufficiency. The American Academy of Pediatrics supports unwavering federal funding of state home-visiting initiatives, the expansion of evidence-based programs, and a robust, coordinated national evaluation designed to confirm best practices and cost-efficiency. Community home visiting is most effective as a component of a comprehensive early childhood system that actively includes and enhances a family-centered medical home. (8/17)

http://pediatrics.aappublications.org/content/140/3/e20172150

EARLY INTERVENTION, IDEA PART C SERVICES, AND THE MEDICAL HOME: COLLABORATION FOR BEST PRACTICE AND BEST OUTCOMES (CLINICAL REPORT)

Richard C. Adams, MD; Carl Tapia, MD; and Council on Children With Disabilities

ABSTRACT. The medical home and the Individuals With Disabilities Education Act Part C Early Intervention Program share many common purposes for infants and children ages 0 to 3 years, not the least of which is a family-centered focus. Professionals in pediatric medical home practices see substantial numbers of infants and toddlers with developmental delays and/or complex chronic conditions. Economic, health, and family-focused data each underscore the critical role of timely referral for relationship-based, individualized, accessible early intervention services and the need for collaborative partnerships in care. The medical home process and Individuals With Disabilities Education Act Part C policy both support nurturing relationships and family-centered care; both offer clear value in terms of economic and health outcomes. Best practice models for early intervention services incorporate learning in the natural environment and coaching models. Proactive medical homes provide strategies for effective developmental surveillance, family-centered resources, and tools to support high-risk groups, and comanagement of infants with special health care needs, including the monitoring of services provided and outcomes achieved. (9/13, reaffirmed 5/17)

http://pediatrics.aappublications.org/content/132/4/e1073

ECHOCARDIOGRAPHY IN INFANTS AND CHILDREN

Section on Cardiology

ABSTRACT. It is the intent of this statement to inform pediatric providers on the appropriate use of echocardiography. Although on-site consultation may be impossible, methods should be established to ensure timely review of echocardiograms by a pediatric cardiologist. With advances in data transmission, echocardiography information can be exchanged, in some cases eliminating the need for a costly patient transfer. By cooperating through training, education, and referral, complete and cost-effective echocardiographic services can be provided to all children. (6/97, reaffirmed 3/03, 3/07)

http://pediatrics.aappublications.org/content/99/6/921

EFFECTIVE DISCIPLINE TO RAISE HEALTHY CHILDREN

Robert D. Sege, MD, PhD, FAAP; Benjamin S. Siegel, MD, FAAP; Council on Child Abuse and Neglect; and Committee on Psychosocial Aspects of Child and Family Health

ABSTRACT. Pediatricians are a source of advice for parents and guardians concerning the management of child behavior, including discipline strategies that are used to teach appropriate behavior and protect their children and others from the adverse effects of challenging behavior. Aversive disciplinary strategies, including all forms of corporal punishment and yelling at or shaming children, are minimally effective in the short-term and not effective in the long-term. With new evidence, researchers link corporal punishment to an increased risk of negative behavioral, cognitive, psychosocial, and emotional outcomes for children. In this Policy Statement, the American Academy of Pediatrics provides guidance for pediatricians and other child health care providers on educating parents about positive and effective parenting strategies of discipline for children at each stage of development as well as references to educational materials. This statement supports the need for adults to avoid physical punishment and verbal abuse of children. (11/18)

See full text on page 601.

http://pediatrics.aappublications.org/content/142/6/e20183112

THE EFFECTS OF ARMED CONFLICT ON CHILDREN

Sherry Shenoda, MD, FAAP; Ayesha Kadir, MD, MSc, FAAP; Shelly Pitterman, PhD; Jeffrey Goldhagen, MD, MPH, FAAP; and Section on International Child Health

ABSTRACT. Children are increasingly exposed to armed conflict and targeted by governmental and nongovernmental combatants. Armed conflict directly and indirectly affects children's physical, mental, and behavioral health. It can affect every organ system, and its impact can persist throughout the life course. In addition, children are disproportionately impacted by morbidity and mortality associated with armed conflict. A children's rights–based approach provides a framework for collaboration by the American Academy of Pediatrics, child health professionals, and national and international partners to respond in the domains of clinical care, systems development, and policy formulation. The American Academy of Pediatrics and child health professionals have critical and synergistic roles to play in the global response to the impact of armed conflict on children. (11/18)

See full text on page 613.

http://pediatrics.aappublications.org/content/142/6/e20182585

THE EFFECTS OF ARMED CONFLICT ON CHILDREN (TECHNICAL REPORT)

Ayesha Kadir, MD, MSc, FAAP; Sherry Shenoda, MD, FAAP; Jeffrey Goldhagen, MD, MPH, FAAP; Shelly Pitterman, PhD; and Section on International Child Health

ABSTRACT. More than 1 in 10 children worldwide are affected by armed conflict. The effects are both direct and indirect and are associated with immediate and long-term harm. The direct effects of conflict include death, physical and psychological trauma, and displacement. Indirect effects are related to a large number of factors, including inadequate and unsafe living conditions, environmental hazards, caregiver mental health, separation from family, displacement-related health risks, and the destruction of health, public health, education, and economic infrastructure. Children and health workers are targeted by combatants during attacks, and children are recruited or forced to take part in combat in a variety of ways. Armed conflict is both a toxic stress and a significant social determinant of child health. In this Technical Report, we review the available knowledge on the effects of armed conflict on children and support the recommendations in the accompanying Policy Statement on children and armed conflict. (11/18)

See full text on page 625.

http://pediatrics.aappublications.org/content/142/6/e20182586

EFFECTS OF EARLY NUTRITIONAL INTERVENTIONS ON THE DEVELOPMENT OF ATOPIC DISEASE IN INFANTS AND CHILDREN: THE ROLE OF MATERNAL DIETARY RESTRICTION, BREASTFEEDING, TIMING OF INTRODUCTION OF COMPLEMENTARY FOODS, AND HYDROLYZED FORMULAS (CLINICAL REPORT)

Frank R. Greer, MD; Scott H. Sicherer, MD; A. Wesley Burks, MD;
Committee on Nutrition; and Section on Allergy and Immunology

ABSTRACT. This clinical report reviews the nutritional options during pregnancy, lactation, and the first year of life that may affect the development of atopic disease (atopic dermatitis, asthma, food allergy) in early life. It replaces an earlier policy statement from the American Academy of Pediatrics that addressed the use of hypoallergenic infant formulas and included provisional recommendations for dietary management for the prevention of atopic disease. The documented benefits of nutritional intervention that may prevent or delay the onset of atopic disease are largely limited to infants at high risk of developing allergy (ie, infants with at least 1 first-degree relative [parent or sibling] with allergic disease). Current evidence does not support a major role for maternal dietary restrictions during pregnancy or lactation. There is evidence that breastfeeding for at least 4 months, compared with feeding formula made with intact cow milk protein, prevents or delays the occurrence of atopic dermatitis, cow milk allergy, and wheezing in early childhood. In studies of infants at high risk of atopy and who are not exclusively breastfed for 4 to 6 months, there is modest evidence that the onset of atopic disease may be delayed or prevented by the use of hydrolyzed formulas compared with formula made with intact cow milk protein, particularly for atopic dermatitis. Comparative studies of the various hydrolyzed formulas also indicate that not all formulas have the same protective benefit. There is also little evidence that delaying the timing of the introduction of complementary foods beyond 4 to 6 months of age prevents the occurrence of atopic disease. At present, there are insufficient data to document a protective effect of any dietary intervention beyond 4 to 6 months of age for the development of atopic disease. (1/08)
http://pediatrics.aappublications.org/content/121/1/183

ELECTRONIC NICOTINE DELIVERY SYSTEMS

Section on Tobacco Control

ABSTRACT. Electronic nicotine delivery systems (ENDS) are rapidly growing in popularity among youth. ENDS are hand-held devices that produce an aerosolized mixture from a solution typically containing concentrated nicotine, flavoring chemicals, and propylene glycol to be inhaled by the user. ENDS are marketed under a variety of names, most commonly electronic cigarettes and e-cigarettes. In 2014, more youth reported using ENDS than any other tobacco product. ENDS pose health risks to both users and nonusers. Nicotine, the major psychoactive ingredient in ENDS solutions, is both highly addictive and toxic. In addition to nicotine, other toxicants, carcinogens, and metal particles have been detected in solutions and aerosols of ENDS. Nonusers are involuntarily exposed to the emissions of these devices with secondhand and thirdhand aerosol. The concentrated and often flavored nicotine in ENDS solutions poses a poisoning risk for young children. Reports of acute nicotine toxicity from US poison control centers have been increasing, with at least 1 child death reported from unintentional exposure to a nicotine-containing ENDS solution. With flavors, design, and marketing that appeal to youth, ENDS threaten to renormalize and glamorize nicotine and tobacco product use. There is a critical need for ENDS regulation, legislative action, and counter promotion to protect youth. ENDS have the potential to addict a new generation of youth to nicotine and reverse more than 50 years of progress in tobacco control. (10/15)
http://pediatrics.aappublications.org/content/136/5/1018

ELECTRONIC PRESCRIBING IN PEDIATRICS: TOWARD SAFER AND MORE EFFECTIVE MEDICATION MANAGEMENT

Council on Clinical Information Technology

ABSTRACT. This policy statement identifies the potential value of electronic prescribing (e-prescribing) systems in improving quality and reducing harm in pediatric health care. On the basis of limited but positive pediatric data and on the basis of federal statutes that provide incentives for the use of e-prescribing systems, the American Academy of Pediatrics recommends the adoption of e-prescribing systems with pediatric functionality. The American Academy of Pediatrics also recommends a set of functions that technology vendors should provide when e-prescribing systems are used in environments in which children receive care. (3/13)
http://pediatrics.aappublications.org/content/131/4/824

ELECTRONIC PRESCRIBING IN PEDIATRICS: TOWARD SAFER AND MORE EFFECTIVE MEDICATION MANAGEMENT (TECHNICAL REPORT)

Kevin B. Johnson, MD, MS; Christoph U. Lehmann, MD; and
Council on Clinical Information Technology

ABSRACT. This technical report discusses recent advances in electronic prescribing (e-prescribing) systems, including the evidence base supporting their limitations and potential benefits. Specifically, this report acknowledges that there are limited but positive pediatric data supporting the role of e-prescribing in mitigating medication errors, improving communication with dispensing pharmacists, and improving medication adherence. On the basis of these data and on the basis of federal statutes that provide incentives for the use of e-prescribing systems, the American Academy of Pediatrics recommends the adoption of e-prescribing systems with pediatric functionality. This report supports the accompanying policy statement from the American Academy of Pediatrics recommending the adoption of e-prescribing by pediatric health care providers. (3/13)
http://pediatrics.aappublications.org/content/131/4/e1350

ELIMINATION OF PERINATAL HEPATITIS B: PROVIDING THE FIRST VACCINE DOSE WITHIN 24 HOURS OF BIRTH

Committee on Infectious Diseases and Committee on Fetus and Newborn

ABSTRACT. After the introduction of the hepatitis B vaccine in the United States in 1982, a greater than 90% reduction in new infections was achieved. However, approximately 1000 new cases of perinatal hepatitis B infection are still identified annually in the United States. Prevention of perinatal hepatitis B relies on the proper and timely identification of infants born to mothers who are hepatitis B surface antigen positive and to mothers with unknown status to ensure administration of appropriate postexposure immunoprophylaxis with hepatitis B vaccine and immune globulin. To reduce the incidence of perinatal hepatitis B transmission further, the American Academy of Pediatrics endorses the recommendation of the Advisory Committee on Immunization Practices of the Centers for Disease Control and Prevention that all newborn infants with a birth weight of greater than or equal to 2000 g receive hepatitis B vaccine by 24 hours of age. (8/17)
http://pediatrics.aappublications.org/content/140/3/e20171870

EMERGENCY CONTRACEPTION

Committee on Adolescence

ABSTRACT. Despite significant declines over the past 2 decades, the United States continues to have teen birth rates that are significantly higher than other industrialized nations. Use of emergency contraception can reduce the risk of pregnancy if used up to 120 hours after unprotected intercourse or contraceptive failure and is most effective if used in the first 24 hours. Indications

for the use of emergency contraception include sexual assault, unprotected intercourse, condom breakage or slippage, and missed or late doses of hormonal contraceptives, including the oral contraceptive pill, contraceptive patch, contraceptive ring (ie, improper placement or loss/expulsion), and injectable contraception. Adolescents younger than 17 years must obtain a prescription from a physician to access emergency contraception in most states. In all states, both males and females 17 years or older can obtain emergency contraception without a prescription. Adolescents are more likely to use emergency contraception if it has been prescribed in advance of need. The aim of this updated policy statement is to (1) educate pediatricians and other physicians on available emergency contraceptive methods; (2) provide current data on safety, efficacy, and use of emergency contraception in teenagers; and (3) encourage routine counseling and advance emergency-contraception prescription as 1 part of a public health strategy to reduce teen pregnancy. This policy focuses on pharmacologic methods of emergency contraception used within 120 hours of unprotected or underprotected coitus for the prevention of unintended pregnancy. Emergency contraceptive medications include products labeled and dedicated for use as emergency contraception by the US Food and Drug Administration (levonorgestrel and ulipristal) and the "off-label" use of combination oral contraceptives. (11/12, reaffirmed 7/16)
http://pediatrics.aappublications.org/content/130/6/1174

EMERGENCY CONTRACEPTION: ADDENDUM
Committee on Adolescence
This is an addendum to the American Academy of Pediatrics Policy Statement "Emergency Contraception" (*Pediatrics.* 2012;130(6):1174–1182).

In April 2013, Judge Edward Korman of the US District Court of Eastern New York directed the Food and Drug Administration (FDA) to lift the ban on over-the-counter availability of levonorgestrel-based emergency contraceptives without a prescription and without point-of-sale or age restrictions. In June 2013, the Obama administration withdrew its appeal to the Korman ruling, and the FDA allowed the 1-pill formulation Plan B One-Step (Teva Women's Health Inc, Frazer, PA) to be made available on the shelf without age restriction in the United States. The FDA granted Plan B One-Step 3 years of exclusive rights to sell the product without an age restriction. One-pill generic versions will likely be allowed to be sold on the shelf next to Plan B One-Step, but these products will require age verification and will not be sold to those younger than 17 years without a prescription. The 2-pill formulations of levonorgestrel-based emergency contraceptives will remain behind the pharmacy counter and will also not be sold to those younger than 17 years without a prescription. (2/14)
http://pediatrics.aappublications.org/content/133/3/e798

EMERGENCY INFORMATION FORMS AND EMERGENCY PREPAREDNESS FOR CHILDREN WITH SPECIAL HEALTH CARE NEEDS
Committee on Pediatric Emergency Medicine and Council on
  Clinical Information Technology (joint with American College of
  Emergency Physicians Pediatric Emergency Medicine Committee)
ABSTRACT. Children with chronic medical conditions rely on complex management plans for problems that cause them to be at increased risk for suboptimal outcomes in emergency situations. The emergency information form (EIF) is a medical summary that describes medical condition(s), medications, and special health care needs to inform health care providers of a child's special health conditions and needs so that optimal emergency medical care can be provided. This statement describes updates to EIFs, including computerization of the EIF, expanding the potential benefits of the EIF, quality-improvement programs using the EIF, the EIF as a central repository, and facilitating emergency preparedness in disaster management and drills by using the EIF. (3/10, reaffirmed 7/14, 10/14)
http://pediatrics.aappublications.org/content/125/4/829

ENDORSEMENT OF HEALTH AND HUMAN SERVICES RECOMMENDATION FOR PULSE OXIMETRY SCREENING FOR CRITICAL CONGENITAL HEART DISEASE
Section on Cardiology and Cardiac Surgery Executive Committee
ABSTRACT. Incorporation of pulse oximetry to the assessment of the newborn infant can enhance detection of critical congenital heart disease (CCHD). Recently, the Secretary of Health and Human Services (HHS) recommended that screening for CCHD be added to the uniform screening panel. The American Academy of Pediatrics (AAP) has been a strong advocate of early detection of CCHD and fully supports the decision of the Secretary of HHS.

The AAP has published strategies for the implementation of pulse oximetry screening, which addressed critical issues such as necessary equipment, personnel, and training, and also provided specific recommendations for assessment of saturation by using pulse oximetry as well as appropriate management of a positive screening result. The AAP is committed to the safe and effective implementation of pulse oximetry screening and is working with other advocacy groups and governmental agencies to promote pulse oximetry and to support widespread surveillance for CCHD.

Going forward, AAP chapters will partner with state health departments to implement the new screening strategy for CCHD and will work to ensure that there is an adequate system for referral for echocardiographic/pediatric cardiac evaluation after a positive screening result. It is imperative that AAP members engage their respective policy makers in adopting and funding the recommendations made by the Secretary of HHS. (12/11)
http://pediatrics.aappublications.org/content/129/1/190

ENHANCING PEDIATRIC WORKFORCE DIVERSITY AND PROVIDING CULTURALLY EFFECTIVE PEDIATRIC CARE: IMPLICATIONS FOR PRACTICE, EDUCATION, AND POLICY MAKING
Committee on Pediatric Workforce
ABSTRACT. This policy statement serves to combine and update 2 previously independent but overlapping statements from the American Academy of Pediatrics (AAP) on culturally effective health care (CEHC) and workforce diversity. The AAP has long recognized that with the ever-increasing diversity of the pediatric population in the United States, the health of all children depends on the ability of all pediatricians to practice culturally effective care. CEHC can be defined as the delivery of care within the context of appropriate physician knowledge, understanding, and appreciation of all cultural distinctions, leading to optimal health outcomes. The AAP believes that CEHC is a critical social value and that the knowledge and skills necessary for providing CEHC can be taught and acquired through focused curricula across the spectrum of lifelong learning.

This statement also addresses workforce diversity, health disparities, and affirmative action. The discussion of diversity is broadened to include not only race, ethnicity, and language but also cultural attributes such as gender, religious beliefs, sexual orientation, and disability, which may affect the quality of health care. The AAP believes that efforts must be supported through health policy and advocacy initiatives to promote the delivery of CEHC and to overcome educational, organizational, and other barriers to improving workforce diversity. (9/13, reaffirmed 10/15)
http://pediatrics.aappublications.org/content/132/4/e1105

ENSURING COMPREHENSIVE CARE AND SUPPORT FOR TRANSGENDER AND GENDER-DIVERSE CHILDREN AND ADOLESCENTS

Jason Rafferty, MD, MPH, EdM, FAAP; Committee on Psychosocial Aspects of Child and Family Health; Committee on Adolescence; and Section on Lesbian, Gay, Bisexual, and Transgender Health and Wellness

ABSTRACT. As a traditionally underserved population that faces numerous health disparities, youth who identify as transgender and gender diverse (TGD) and their families are increasingly presenting to pediatric providers for education, care, and referrals. The need for more formal training, standardized treatment, and research on safety and medical outcomes often leaves providers feeling ill equipped to support and care for patients that identify as TGD and families. In this policy statement, we review relevant concepts and challenges and provide suggestions for pediatric providers that are focused on promoting the health and positive development of youth that identify as TGD while eliminating discrimination and stigma. (9/18)

See full text on page 643.

http://pediatrics.aappublications.org/content/142/4/e20182162

ENSURING THE HEALTH OF CHILDREN IN DISASTERS

Disaster Preparedness Advisory Council and Committee on Pediatric Emergency Medicine

ABSTRACT. Infants, children, adolescents, and young adults have unique physical, mental, behavioral, developmental, communication, therapeutic, and social needs that must be addressed and met in all aspects of disaster preparedness, response, and recovery. Pediatricians, including primary care pediatricians, pediatric medical subspecialists, and pediatric surgical specialists, have key roles to play in preparing and treating families in cases of disasters. Pediatricians should attend to the continuity of practice operations to provide services in time of need and stay abreast of disaster and public health developments to be active participants in community planning efforts. Federal, state, tribal, local, and regional institutions and agencies that serve children should collaborate with pediatricians to ensure the health and well-being of children in disasters. (10/15)

http://pediatrics.aappublications.org/content/136/5/e1407

EPIDEMIOLOGY AND DIAGNOSIS OF HEALTH CARE–ASSOCIATED INFECTIONS IN THE NICU (TECHNICAL REPORT)

Committee on Fetus and Newborn and Committee on Infectious Diseases

ABSTRACT. Health care–associated infections in the NICU are a major clinical problem resulting in increased morbidity and mortality, prolonged length of hospital stays, and increased medical costs. Neonates are at high risk for health care–associated infections because of impaired host defense mechanisms, limited amounts of protective endogenous flora on skin and mucosal surfaces at time of birth, reduced barrier function of neonatal skin, the use of invasive procedures and devices, and frequent exposure to broad-spectrum antibiotics. This statement will review the epidemiology and diagnosis of health care–associated infections in newborn infants. (3/12, reaffirmed 2/16)

http://pediatrics.aappublications.org/content/129/4/e1104

EPINEPHRINE FOR FIRST-AID MANAGEMENT OF ANAPHYLAXIS (CLINICAL REPORT)

Scott H. Sicherer, MD, FAAP; F. Estelle R. Simons, MD, FAAP; and Section on Allergy and Immunology

ABSTRACT. Anaphylaxis is a severe, generalized allergic or hypersensitivity reaction that is rapid in onset and may cause death. Epinephrine (adrenaline) can be life-saving when administered as rapidly as possible once anaphylaxis is recognized. This clinical report from the American Academy of Pediatrics is an update of the 2007 clinical report on this topic. It provides information to help clinicians identify patients at risk of anaphylaxis and new information about epinephrine and epinephrine autoinjectors (EAs). The report also highlights the importance of patient and family education about the recognition and management of anaphylaxis in the community. Key points emphasized include the following: (1) validated clinical criteria are available to facilitate prompt diagnosis of anaphylaxis; (2) prompt intramuscular epinephrine injection in the mid-outer thigh reduces hospitalizations, morbidity, and mortality; (3) prescribing EAs facilitates timely epinephrine injection in community settings for patients with a history of anaphylaxis and, if specific circumstances warrant, for some high-risk patients who have not previously experienced anaphylaxis; (4) prescribing epinephrine for infants and young children weighing <15 kg, especially those who weigh 7.5 kg and under, currently presents a dilemma, because the lowest dose available in EAs, 0.15 mg, is a high dose for many infants and some young children; (5) effective management of anaphylaxis in the community requires a comprehensive approach involving children, families, preschools, schools, camps, and sports organizations; and (6) prevention of anaphylaxis recurrences involves confirmation of the trigger, discussion of specific allergen avoidance, allergen immunotherapy (eg, with stinging insect venom, if relevant), and a written, personalized anaphylaxis emergency action plan; and (7) the management of anaphylaxis also involves education of children and supervising adults about anaphylaxis recognition and first-aid treatment. (2/17)

http://pediatrics.aappublications.org/content/139/3/e20164006

EQUIPMENT FOR GROUND AMBULANCES

American Academy of Pediatrics (joint with American College of Emergency Physicians, American College of Surgeons Committee on Trauma, Emergency Medical Services for Children, Emergency Nurses Association, National Association of EMS Physicians, and National Association of State EMS Officials)

On January 1, 2014, the American Academy of Pediatrics, American College of Emergency Physicians, American College of Surgeons Committee on Trauma, Emergency Medical Services for Children, Emergency Nurses Association, National Association of EMS Physicians, and National Association of State EMS Officials coauthored a joint policy statement, "Equipment for Ground Ambulances" (*Prehosp Emerg Care*. 2014;19[1]:92–97). The full text of the joint policy statement is available at: http://informahealthcare.com/doi/full/10.3109/10903127.2013.851312. Copyright © 2014 Informa Plc. (8/14)

http://pediatrics.aappublications.org/content/134/3/e919

ERADICATING POLIO: HOW THE WORLD'S PEDIATRICIANS CAN HELP STOP THIS CRIPPLING ILLNESS FOREVER (CLINICAL REPORT)

Walter A. Orenstein, MD, FAAP, and Committee on Infectious Diseases

ABSTRACT. The American Academy of Pediatrics strongly supports the Polio Eradication and Endgame Strategic Plan of the Global Polio Eradication Initiative. This plan was endorsed in November 2012 by the Strategic Advisory Group of Experts on Immunization of the World Health Organization and published by the World Health Organization in April 2013. As a key component of the plan, it will be necessary to stop oral polio vaccine (OPV) use globally to achieve eradication, because the attenuated viruses in the vaccine rarely can cause polio. The plan includes procedures for elimination of vaccine-associated paralytic polio and circulating vaccine-derived polioviruses (cVDPVs). cVDPVs can proliferate when vaccine viruses are transmitted among susceptible people, resulting in mutations conferring both the neurovirulence and transmissibility characteristics of wild polioviruses. Although there are 3 different

types of wild poliovirus strains, the polio eradication effort has already resulted in the global elimination of type 2 poliovirus for more than a decade. Type 3 poliovirus may be eliminated because the wild type 3 poliovirus was last detected in 2012. Thus, of the 3 wild types, only wild type 1 poliovirus is still known to be circulating and causing disease. OPV remains the key vaccine for eradicating wild polioviruses in polio-infected countries because it induces high levels of systemic immunity to prevent paralysis and intestinal immunity to reduce transmission. However, OPV is a rare cause of paralysis and the substantial decrease in wild-type disease has resulted in estimates that the vaccine is causing more polio-related paralysis annually in recent years than the wild virus. The new endgame strategic plan calls for stepwise removal of the type 2 poliovirus component from trivalent oral vaccines, because type 2 wild poliovirus appears to have been eradicated (since 1999) and yet is the main cause of cVDPV outbreaks and approximately 40% of vaccine-associated paralytic polio cases. The Endgame and Strategic Plan will be accomplished by shifting from trivalent OPV to bivalent OPV (containing types 1 and 3 poliovirus only). It will be necessary to introduce trivalent inactivated poliovirus vaccine (IPV) into routine immunization programs in all countries using OPV to provide population immunity to type 2 before the switch from trivalent OPV to bivalent OPV. The Global Polio Eradication Initiative hopes to achieve global eradication of polio by 2018 with this strategy, after which all OPV use will be stopped. Challenges expected for adding IPV into routine immunization schedules include higher cost of IPV compared with OPV, cold-chain capacity limits, more complex administration of vaccine because IPV requires injections as opposed to oral administration, and inferior intestinal immunity conferred by IPV. The goal of this report is to help pediatricians understand the change in strategy and outline ways that pediatricians can help global polio eradication efforts, including advocating for the resources needed to accomplish polio eradication and for incorporation of IPV into routine immunization programs in all countries. (12/14)
http://pediatrics.aappublications.org/content/135/1/196

ESSENTIAL CONTRACTUAL LANGUAGE FOR MEDICAL NECESSITY IN CHILDREN

Committee on Child Health Financing

ABSTRACT. The previous policy statement from the American Academy of Pediatrics, "Model Language for Medical Necessity in Children," was published in July 2005. Since that time, there have been new and emerging delivery and payment models. The relationship established between health care providers and health plans should promote arrangements that are beneficial to all who are affected by these contractual arrangements. Pediatricians play an important role in ensuring that the needs of children are addressed in these emerging systems. It is important to recognize that health care plans designed for adults may not meet the needs of children. Language in health care contracts should reflect the health care needs of children and families. Informed pediatricians can make a difference in the care of children and influence the role of primary care physicians in the new paradigms. This policy highlights many of the important elements pediatricians should assess as providers develop a role in emerging care models. (7/13, reaffirmed 9/17)
http://pediatrics.aappublications.org/content/132/2/398

ESTABLISHING A STANDARD PROTOCOL FOR THE VOIDING CYSTOURETHROGRAPHY (CLINICAL REPORT)

Dominic Frimberger, MD; Maria-Gisela Mercado-Deane, MD, FAAP; Section on Urology; and Section on Radiology

ABSTRACT. The voiding cystourethrogram (VCUG) is a frequently performed test to diagnose a variety of urologic conditions, such as vesicoureteral reflux. The test results determine whether continued observation or an interventional procedure is indicated. VCUGs are ordered by many specialists and primary care providers, including pediatricians, family practitioners, nephrologists, hospitalists, emergency department physicians, and urologists. Current protocols for performing and interpreting a VCUG are based on the International Reflux Study in 1985. However, more recent information provided by many national and international institutions suggests a need to refine those recommendations. The lead author of the 1985 study, R.L. Lebowitz, agreed to and participated in the current protocol. In addition, a recent survey directed to the chairpersons of pediatric radiology of 65 children's hospitals throughout the United States and Canada showed that VCUG protocols vary substantially. Recent guidelines from the American Academy of Pediatrics (AAP) recommend a VCUG for children between 2 and 24 months of age with urinary tract infections but did not specify how this test should be performed. To improve patient safety and to standardize the data obtained when a VCUG is performed, the AAP Section on Radiology and the AAP Section on Urology initiated the current VCUG protocol to create a consensus on how to perform this test. (10/16)
http://pediatrics.aappublications.org/content/138/5/e20162590

ETHICAL AND POLICY ISSUES IN GENETIC TESTING AND SCREENING OF CHILDREN

Committee on Bioethics and Committee on Genetics (joint with American College of Medical Genetics and Genomics)

ABSTRACT. The genetic testing and genetic screening of children are commonplace. Decisions about whether to offer genetic testing and screening should be driven by the best interest of the child. The growing literature on the psychosocial and clinical effects of such testing and screening can help inform best practices. This policy statement represents recommendations developed collaboratively by the American Academy of Pediatrics and the American College of Medical Genetics and Genomics with respect to many of the scenarios in which genetic testing and screening can occur. (2/13, reaffirmed 6/18)
http://pediatrics.aappublications.org/content/131/3/620

ETHICAL CONSIDERATIONS IN RESEARCH WITH SOCIALLY IDENTIFIABLE POPULATIONS

Committee on Native American Child Health and Committee on Community Health Services

ABSTRACT. Community-based research raises ethical issues not normally encountered in research conducted in academic settings. In particular, conventional risk-benefits assessments frequently fail to recognize harms that can occur in socially identifiable populations as a result of research participation. Furthermore, many such communities require more stringent measures of beneficence that must be applied directly to the participating communities. In this statement, the American Academy of Pediatrics sets forth recommendations for minimizing harms that may result from community-based research by emphasizing community involvement in the research process. (1/04, reaffirmed 10/07, 1/13)
http://pediatrics.aappublications.org/content/113/1/148

ETHICAL CONTROVERSIES IN ORGAN DONATION AFTER CIRCULATORY DEATH

Committee on Bioethics

ABSTRACT. The persistent mismatch between the supply of and need for transplantable organs has led to efforts to increase the supply, including controlled donation after circulatory death (DCD). Controlled DCD involves organ recovery after the planned withdrawal of life-sustaining treatment and the declaration of death according to the cardiorespiratory criteria. Two central ethical issues in DCD are when organ recovery can

begin and how to manage conflicts of interests. The "dead donor rule" should be maintained, and donors in cases of DCD should only be declared dead after the permanent cessation of circulatory function. Permanence is generally established by a 2- to 5-minute waiting period. Given ongoing controversy over whether the cessation must also be irreversible, physicians should not be required to participate in DCD. Because the preparation for organ recovery in DCD begins before the declaration of death, there are potential conflicts between the donor's and recipient's interests. These conflicts can be managed in a variety of ways, including informed consent and separating the various participants' roles. For example, informed consent should be sought for premortem interventions to improve organ viability, and organ procurement organization personnel and members of the transplant team should not be involved in the discontinuation of life-sustaining treatment or the declaration of death. It is also important to emphasize that potential donors in cases of DCD should receive integrated interdisciplinary palliative care, including sedation and analgesia. (4/13, reaffirmed 12/16)
http://pediatrics.aappublications.org/content/131/5/1021

EVALUATING CHILDREN WITH FRACTURES FOR CHILD PHYSICAL ABUSE (CLINICAL REPORT)

Emalee G. Flaherty, MD; Jeannette M. Perez-Rossello, MD; Michael A. Levine, MD; William L. Hennrikus, MD; Committee on Child Abuse and Neglect; Section on Radiology; Section on Endocrinology; and Section on Orthopaedics (joint with Society for Pediatric Radiology)

ABSTRACT. Fractures are common injuries caused by child abuse. Although the consequences of failing to diagnose an abusive injury in a child can be grave, incorrectly diagnosing child abuse in a child whose fractures have another etiology can be distressing for a family. The aim of this report is to review recent advances in the understanding of fracture specificity, the mechanism of fractures, and other medical diseases that predispose to fractures in infants and children. This clinical report will aid physicians in developing an evidence-based differential diagnosis and performing the appropriate evaluation when assessing a child with fractures. (1/14)
http://pediatrics.aappublications.org/content/133/2/e477

EVALUATING FOR SUSPECTED CHILD ABUSE: CONDITIONS THAT PREDISPOSE TO BLEEDING (TECHNICAL REPORT)

Shannon L. Carpenter, MD, MS; Thomas C. Abshire, MD; James D. Anderst, MD, MS; Section on Hematology/Oncology; and Committee on Child Abuse and Neglect

ABSTRACT. Child abuse might be suspected when children present with cutaneous bruising, intracranial hemorrhage, or other manifestations of bleeding. In these cases, it is necessary to consider medical conditions that predispose to easy bleeding/bruising. When evaluating for the possibility of bleeding disorders and other conditions that predispose to hemorrhage, the pediatrician must consider the child's presenting history, medical history, and physical examination findings before initiating a laboratory investigation. Many medical conditions can predispose to easy bleeding. Before ordering laboratory tests for a disease, it is useful to understand the biochemical basis and clinical presentation of the disorder, condition prevalence, and test characteristics. This technical report reviews the major medical conditions that predispose to bruising/bleeding and should be considered when evaluating for abusive injury. (3/13, reaffirmed 7/16)
http://pediatrics.aappublications.org/content/131/4/e1357

EVALUATION AND MANAGEMENT OF CHILDREN AND ADOLESCENTS WITH ACUTE MENTAL HEALTH OR BEHAVIORAL PROBLEMS. PART I: COMMON CLINICAL CHALLENGES OF PATIENTS WITH MENTAL HEALTH AND/OR BEHAVIORAL EMERGENCIES (CLINICAL REPORT)

Thomas H. Chun, MD, MPH, FAAP; Sharon E. Mace, MD, FAAP, FACEP; Emily R. Katz, MD, FAAP; and Committee on Pediatric Emergency Medicine (joint with American College of Emergency Physicians Pediatric Emergency Medicine Committee)

INTRODUCTION. Mental health problems are among the leading contributors to the global burden of disease. Unfortunately, pediatric populations are not spared of mental health problems. In the United States, 21% to 23% of children and adolescents have a diagnosable mental health or substance use disorder. Among patients of emergency departments (EDs), 70% screen positive for at least 1 mental health disorder, 23% meet criteria for 2 or more mental health concerns, 45% have a mental health problem resulting in impaired psychosocial functioning, and 10% of adolescents endorse significant levels of psychiatric distress at the time of their ED visit. In pediatric primary care settings, the reported prevalence of mental health and behavioral disorders is between 12% to 22% of children and adolescents.

Although the American Academy of Pediatrics (AAP) has published a policy statement on mental health competencies and a Mental Health Toolkit for pediatric primary care providers, no such guidelines or resources exist for clinicians who care for pediatric mental health emergencies. This clinical report supports the 2006 joint policy statement of the AAP and American College of Emergency Physicians (ACEP) on pediatric mental health emergencies, with the goal of addressing the knowledge gaps in this area. The report is written primarily from the perspective of ED clinicians, but it is intended for all clinicians who care for children and adolescents with acute mental health and behavioral problems.

Recent epidemiologic studies of mental health visits have revealed a rapid burgeoning of both ED and primary care visits. An especially problematic trend is the increase in "boarding" of psychiatric patients in the ED and inpatient pediatric beds (ie, extended stays lasting days or even weeks). Although investigation of boarding practices is still in its infancy, the ACEP and the American Medical Association have both expressed concern about it, because it significantly taxes the functioning and efficiency of both the ED and hospital, and mental health services may not be available in the ED.

In addition, compared with other pediatric care settings, ED patients are known to be at higher risk of mental health disorders, including depression, anxiety, posttraumatic stress disorder, and substance abuse. These mental health conditions may be unrecognized not only by treating clinicians but also by the child/adolescent and his or her parents. A similar phenomenon has been described with suicidal patients. Individuals who have committed suicide frequently visited a health care provider in the months preceding their death. Although a minority of suicidal patients present with some form of self-harm, many have vague somatic complaints (eg, headache, gastrointestinal tract distress, back pain, concern for a sexually transmitted infection) masking their underlying mental health condition.

Despite studies demonstrating moderate agreement between emergency physicians and psychiatrists in the assessment and management of patients with mental health problems, ED clinicians frequently cite lack of training and confidence in their abilities as barriers to caring for patients with mental health emergencies. Another study of emergency medicine and pediatric emergency medicine training programs found that formal training in psychiatric problems is not required nor offered by most programs. Pediatric primary care providers report similar barriers to caring for their patients with mental health problems.

Part I of this clinical report focuses on the issues relevant to patients presenting to the ED with a mental health chief complaint and covers the following topics:

- Medical clearance of pediatric psychiatric patients
- Suicidal ideation and suicide attempts
- Involuntary hospitalization
- Restraint of the agitated patient
  — Verbal restraint
  — Chemical restraint
  — Physical restraint
- Coordination with the medical home

Part II discusses challenging patients with primarily medical or indeterminate presentations, in which the contribution of an underlying mental health condition may be unclear or a complicating factor, including:

- Somatic symptom and related disorders
- Adverse effects to psychiatric medications
  — Antipsychotic adverse effects
  — Neuroleptic malignant syndrome
  — Serotonin syndrome
- Children with special needs in the ED (autism spectrum and developmental disorders)
- Mental health screening in the ED

An executive summary of this clinical report can be found at www.pediatrics.org/cgi/doi/10.1542/peds.2016-1571. (8/16)
http://pediatrics.aappublications.org/content/138/3/e20161570

EVALUATION AND MANAGEMENT OF CHILDREN AND ADOLESCENTS WITH ACUTE MENTAL HEALTH OR BEHAVIORAL PROBLEMS. PART I: COMMON CLINICAL CHALLENGES OF PATIENTS WITH MENTAL HEALTH AND/OR BEHAVIORAL EMERGENCIES—EXECUTIVE SUMMARY (CLINICAL REPORT)

Thomas H. Chun, MD, MPH, FAAP; Sharon E. Mace, MD, FAAP, FACEP; Emily R. Katz, MD, FAAP; and Committee on Pediatric Emergency Medicine (joint with American College of Emergency Physicians Pediatric Emergency Medicine Committee)

ABSTRACT. The number of children and adolescents seen in emergency departments (EDs) and primary care settings for mental health problems has skyrocketed in recent years, with up to 23% of patients in both settings having diagnosable mental health conditions. Even when a mental health problem is not the focus of an ED or primary care visit, mental health conditions, both known and occult, may challenge the treating clinician and complicate the patient's care.

Although the American Academy of Pediatrics has published a policy statement on mental health competencies and a Mental Health Toolkit for pediatric primary care providers, no such guidelines or resources exist for clinicians who care for pediatric mental health emergencies. Many ED and primary care physicians report a paucity of training and lack of confidence in caring for pediatric psychiatry patients. The 2 clinical reports (www.pediatrics.org/cgi/doi/10.1542/peds.2016-1570 and www.pediatrics.org/cgi/doi/10.1542/peds.2016-1573) support the 2006 joint policy statement of the American Academy of Pediatrics and the American College of Emergency Physicians on pediatric mental health emergencies, with the goal of addressing the knowledge gaps in this area. Although written primarily from the perspective of ED clinicians, they are intended for all clinicians who care for children and adolescents with acute mental health and behavioral problems.

The clinical reports are organized around the common clinical challenges pediatric caregivers face, both when a child or adolescent presents with a psychiatric chief complaint or emergency (part I) and also when a mental health condition may be an unclear or complicating factor in a non–mental health clinical presentation (part II). Part II of the clinical reports (www.pediatrics.org/cgi/doi/10.1542/peds.2016-1573) includes discussions of somatic symptom and related disorders, adverse effects of psychiatric medications including neuroleptic malignant syndrome and serotonin syndrome, caring for children with special needs such as autism and developmental disorders, and mental health screening. This executive summary is an overview of part I of the clinical reports. The full text of the below topics can be accessed online at (www.pediatrics.org/cgi/doi/10.1542/peds.2016-1570). (8/16)
http://pediatrics.aappublications.org/content/138/3/e20161571

EVALUATION AND MANAGEMENT OF CHILDREN WITH ACUTE MENTAL HEALTH OR BEHAVIORAL PROBLEMS. PART II: RECOGNITION OF CLINICALLY CHALLENGING MENTAL HEALTH RELATED CONDITIONS PRESENTING WITH MEDICAL OR UNCERTAIN SYMPTOMS (CLINICAL REPORT)

Thomas H. Chun, MD, MPH, FAAP; Sharon E. Mace, MD, FAAP, FACEP; Emily R. Katz, MD, FAAP; and Committee on Pediatric Emergency Medicine (joint with American College of Emergency Physicians Pediatric Emergency Medicine Committee)

INTRODUCTION. Part I of this clinical report (http://www.pediatrics.org/cgi/doi/10.1542/peds.2016-1570) discusses the common clinical issues that may be encountered in caring for children and adolescents presenting to the emergency department (ED) or primary care setting with a mental health condition or emergency and includes the following:

- Medical clearance of pediatric psychiatric patients
- Suicidal ideation and suicide attempts
- Involuntary hospitalization
- Restraint of the agitated patient
  — Verbal restraint
  — Chemical restraint
  — Physical restraint
- Coordination with the medical home

Part II discusses the challenges a pediatric clinician may face when evaluating patients with a mental health condition, which may be contributing to or a complicating factor for a medical or indeterminate clinical presentation. Topics covered include the following:

- Somatic symptom and related disorders
- Adverse effects of psychiatric medications
  — Antipsychotic adverse effects
  — Neuroleptic malignant syndrome
  — Serotonin syndrome
- Children with special needs (autism spectrum disorders [ASDs] and developmental disorders [DDs])
- Mental health screening

The report is written primarily from the perspective of ED clinicians, but it is intended for all clinicians who care for children and adolescents with acute mental health and behavioral problems. An executive summary of this clinical report can be found at http://www.pediatrics.org/cgi/doi/10.1542/peds.2016-1574. (8/16)
http://pediatrics.aappublications.org/content/138/3/e20161573

EVALUATION AND MANAGEMENT OF CHILDREN WITH ACUTE MENTAL HEALTH OR BEHAVIORAL PROBLEMS. PART II: RECOGNITION OF CLINICALLY CHALLENGING MENTAL HEALTH RELATED CONDITIONS PRESENTING WITH MEDICAL OR UNCERTAIN SYMPTOMS—EXECUTIVE SUMMARY (CLINICAL REPORT)

Thomas H. Chun, MD, MPH, FAAP; Sharon E. Mace, MD, FAAP, FACEP; Emily R. Katz, MD, FAAP; and Committee on Pediatric Emergency Medicine (joint with American College of Emergency Physicians Pediatric Emergency Medicine Committee)

ABSTRACT. The number of children and adolescents seen in emergency departments (EDs) and primary care settings for mental health problems has skyrocketed in recent years, with up to 23% of patients in both settings having diagnosable mental health conditions. Even when a mental health problem is not the focus of an ED or primary care visit, mental health conditions, both known and occult, may challenge the treating clinician and complicate the patient's care.

Although the American Academy of Pediatrics (AAP) has published a policy statement on mental health competencies and a Mental Health Toolkit for pediatric primary care providers, no such guidelines or resources exist for clinicians who care for pediatric mental health emergencies. Many ED and primary care physicians report paucity of training and lack of confidence in caring for pediatric psychiatry patients. The 2 clinical reports support the 2006 joint policy statement of the AAP and the American College of Emergency Physicians on pediatric mental health emergencies, with the goal of addressing the knowledge gaps in this area. Although written primarily from the perspective of ED clinicians, it is intended for all clinicians who care for children and adolescents with acute mental health and behavioral problems. They are organized around the common clinical challenges pediatric caregivers face, both when a child or adolescent presents with a psychiatric chief complaint or emergency (part I) and when a mental health condition may be an unclear or complicating factor in a non-mental health ED presentation (part II). Part I of the clinical reports includes discussions of Medical Clearance of Pediatric Psychiatric Patients; Suicide and Suicidal Ideation; Restraint of the Agitated Patient Including Verbal, Chemical, and Physical Restraint; and Coordination of Care With the Medical Home, and it can be accessed online at www.pediatrics.org/cgi/doi/10.1542/peds.2016-1570. This executive summary is an overview of part II of the clinical reports. Full text of the following topics can be accessed online at www.pediatrics.org/cgi/doi/10.1542/peds.2016-1573. (8/16)

http://pediatrics.aappublications.org/content/138/3/e20161574

EVALUATION AND MANAGEMENT OF THE INFANT EXPOSED TO HIV-1 IN THE UNITED STATES (CLINICAL REPORT)

Peter L. Havens, MD; Lynne M. Mofenson, MD; and Committee on Pediatric AIDS

ABSTRACT. The pediatrician plays a key role in the prevention of mother-to-child transmission of HIV-1 infection. For infants born to women with HIV-1 infection identified during pregnancy, the pediatrician ensures that antiretroviral prophylaxis is provided to the infant to decrease the risk of acquiring HIV-1 infection and promotes avoidance of postnatal HIV-1 transmission by advising HIV-1–infected women not to breastfeed. The pediatrician should perform HIV-1 antibody testing for infants born to women whose HIV-1 infection status was not determined during pregnancy or labor. For HIV-1–exposed infants, the pediatrician monitors the infant for early determination of HIV-1 infection status and for possible short- and long-term toxicity from antiretroviral exposures. Provision of chemoprophylaxis for *Pneumocystis jiroveci* pneumonia and support of families living with HIV-1 by providing counseling to parents or

caregivers are also important components of care. (12/08, reaffirmed 8/15)

http://pediatrics.aappublications.org/content/123/1/175

EVALUATION AND MANAGEMENT OF THE INFANT EXPOSED TO HIV-1 IN THE UNITED STATES—ADDENDUM

Peter L. Havens, MD; Lynne M. Mofenson, MD; and Committee on Pediatric AIDS

The following paragraph is an addendum to the clinical report "Evaluation and Management of the Infant Exposed to HIV-1 in the United States" (*Pediatrics* 2009;123[1]:175–187). It pertains to the section with the heading "HIV-1 Testing of the Infant if the Mother's HIV-1 Infection Status Is Unknown":

For newborn infants whose mother's HIV-1 serostatus is unknown, the newborn infant's health care provider should perform rapid HIV-1 antibody testing on the mother or the infant as soon as possible after birth with appropriate consent as required by state and local law. These test results should be available as early as possible and certainly within 12 hours after birth and can be used to guide initiation of infant antiretroviral prophylaxis. Rapid HIV-1 antibody testing, by using either blood or saliva, is licensed for the diagnosis of HIV infection in adults. Rapid HIV-1 antibody testing of women in labor and delivery units at 16 US hospitals identified a prevalence of undiagnosed HIV infection of 7 of 1000 women and demonstrated a sensitivity of 100% and specificity of 99.9% by using several rapid test kits. Positive predictive value was 90% compared with 76% for enzyme immunoassay. However, the use of these tests in infants is neither well described nor licensed. Sherman et al evaluated 7 HIV-1 rapid tests on stored samples from 116 HIV-exposed infants and compared the findings to standard HIV enzyme immunoassay testing. In the youngest cohort tested (median age, 1.5 months; range, 3–7 weeks), sensitivity of rapid testing was greater than 99%. In a subsequent study using whole blood, sensitivities ranged between 93.3% and 99.3% in infants younger than 3 months by using 5 rapid tests. In both of these studies, rapid HIV-1 rapid tests failed to identify some HIV-infected infants. Oral fluid testing has been demonstrated to have a negative predictive value of >99% in HIV-exposed children older than 12 months. However, when used for screening infants with a median age of 1.5 months (range, birth to 6 months), oral fluid testing had a sensitivity less than 90% and failed to detect 14 of 63 HIV-infected infants (22.2%). On the basis of these findings, only blood should be used to perform rapid HIV-1 antibody testing in newborn infants. Furthermore, rapid testing of the mother, by using either blood or saliva, is preferred over rapid testing in her infant (blood only) because of increased sensitivity in identifying HIV-1 infection. (11/12, reaffirmed 8/15)

http://pediatrics.aappublications.org/content/130/6/64

EVALUATION AND REFERRAL FOR DEVELOPMENTAL DYSPLASIA OF THE HIP IN INFANTS (CLINICAL REPORT)

Brian A. Shaw, MD, FAAOS, FAAP; Lee S. Segal, MD, FAAOS, FAAP; and Section on Orthopaedics

ABSTRACT. Developmental dysplasia of the hip (DDH) encompasses a wide spectrum of clinical severity, from mild developmental abnormalities to frank dislocation. Clinical hip instability occurs in 1% to 2% of full-term infants, and up to 15% have hip instability or hip immaturity detectable by imaging studies. Hip dysplasia is the most common cause of hip arthritis in women younger than 40 years and accounts for 5% to 10% of all total hip replacements in the United States. Newborn and periodic screening have been practiced for decades, because DDH is clinically silent during the first year of life, can be treated more effectively if detected early, and can have severe consequences if left untreated. However, screening programs and techniques are not uniform, and there is little evidence-based literature to support current practice, leading to controversy. Recent literature shows that many mild forms of DDH resolve without treatment, and there is a lack of agreement on ultrasonographic diagnostic criteria for DDH as a disease versus developmental variations. The American Academy of Pediatrics has not published any policy statements on DDH since its 2000 clinical practice guideline and accompanying technical report. Developments since then include a controversial US Preventive Services Task Force "inconclusive" determination regarding usefulness of DDH screening, several prospective studies supporting observation over treatment of minor ultrasonographic hip variations, and a recent evidence-based clinical practice guideline from the American Academy of Orthopaedic Surgeons on the detection and management of DDH in infants 0 to 6 months of age. The purpose of this clinical report was to provide literature-based updated direction for the clinician in screening and referral for DDH, with the primary goal of preventing and/or detecting a dislocated hip by 6 to 12 months of age in an otherwise healthy child, understanding that no screening program has eliminated late development or presentation of a dislocated hip and that the diagnosis and treatment of milder forms of hip dysplasia remain controversial. (11/16)

http://pediatrics.aappublications.org/content/138/6/e20163107

EVALUATION AND REFERRAL OF CHILDREN WITH SIGNS OF EARLY PUBERTY (CLINICAL REPORT)

Paul Kaplowitz, MD, PhD, FAAP; Clifford Bloch, MD, FAAP; and Section on Endocrinology

ABSTRACT. Concerns about possible early pubertal development are a common cause for referral to pediatric medical subspecialists. Several recent studies have suggested that onset of breast and/or pubic hair development may be occurring earlier than in the past. Although there is a chance of finding pathology in girls with signs of puberty before 8 years of age and in boys before 9 years of age, the vast majority of these children with signs of apparent puberty have variations of normal growth and physical development and do not require laboratory testing, bone age radiographs, or intervention. The most common of these signs of early puberty are premature adrenarche (early onset of pubic hair and/or body odor), premature thelarche (nonprogressive breast development, usually occurring before 2 years of age), and lipomastia, in which girls have apparent breast development which, on careful palpation, is determined to be adipose tissue. Indicators that the signs of sexual maturation may represent true, central precocious puberty include progressive breast development over a 4- to 6-month period of observation or progressive penis and testicular enlargement, especially if accompanied by rapid linear growth. Children exhibiting these true indicators of early puberty need prompt evaluation by the appropriate pediatric medical subspecialist. Therapy with a gonadotropin-releasing hormone agonist may be indicated, as discussed in this report. (12/15)

http://pediatrics.aappublications.org/content/137/1/e20153732

EVALUATION FOR BLEEDING DISORDERS IN SUSPECTED CHILD ABUSE (CLINICAL REPORT)

James D. Anderst, MD, MS; Shannon L. Carpenter, MD, MS; Thomas C. Abshire, MD; Section on Hematology/Oncology; and Committee on Child Abuse and Neglect

ABSTRACT. Bruising or bleeding in a child can raise the concern for child abuse. Assessing whether the findings are the result of trauma and/or whether the child has a bleeding disorder is critical. Many bleeding disorders are rare, and not every child with bruising/bleeding concerning for abuse requires an evaluation for bleeding disorders. In some instances, however, bleeding disorders can present in a manner similar to child abuse. The history and clinical evaluation can be used to determine the necessity of an evaluation for a possible bleeding disorder, and prevalence and known clinical presentations of individual bleeding disorders can be used to guide the extent of the laboratory testing. This clinical report provides guidance to pediatricians and other clinicians regarding the evaluation for bleeding disorders when child abuse is suspected. (3/13, reaffirmed 7/16)

http://pediatrics.aappublications.org/content/131/4/e1314

THE EVALUATION OF CHILDREN IN THE PRIMARY CARE SETTING WHEN SEXUAL ABUSE IS SUSPECTED (CLINICAL REPORT)

Carole Jenny, MD, MBA; James E. Crawford-Jakubiak, MD; and Committee on Child Abuse and Neglect

ABSTRACT. This clinical report updates a 2005 report from the American Academy of Pediatrics on the evaluation of sexual abuse in children. The medical assessment of suspected child sexual abuse should include obtaining a history, performing a physical examination, and obtaining appropriate laboratory tests. The role of the physician includes determining the need to report suspected sexual abuse; assessing the physical, emotional, and behavioral consequences of sexual abuse; providing information to parents about how to support their child; and coordinating with other professionals to provide comprehensive treatment and follow-up of children exposed to child sexual abuse. (7/13, reaffirmed 8/18)

http://pediatrics.aappublications.org/content/132/2/e558

THE EVALUATION OF SEXUAL BEHAVIORS IN CHILDREN (CLINICAL REPORT)

Nancy D. Kellogg, MD, and Committee on Child Abuse and Neglect

ABSTRACT. Most children will engage in sexual behaviors at some time during childhood. These behaviors may be normal but can be confusing and concerning to parents or disruptive or intrusive to others. Knowledge of age-appropriate sexual behaviors that vary with situational and environmental factors can assist the clinician in differentiating normal sexual behaviors from sexual behavior problems. Most situations that involve sexual behaviors in young children do not require child protective services intervention; for behaviors that are age-appropriate and transient, the pediatrician may provide guidance in supervision and monitoring of the behavior. If the behavior is intrusive, hurtful, and/or age-inappropriate, a more comprehensive assessment is warranted. Some children with sexual behavior problems may reside or have resided in homes characterized by inconsistent parenting, violence, abuse, or neglect and may require more immediate intervention and referrals. (8/09, reaffirmed 3/13)

http://pediatrics.aappublications.org/content/124/3/992

THE EVALUATION OF SUSPECTED CHILD PHYSICAL ABUSE (CLINICAL REPORT)

Cindy W. Christian, MD, FAAP, and Committee on Child Abuse and Neglect

ABSTRACT. Child physical abuse is an important cause of pediatric morbidity and mortality and is associated with major physical and mental health problems that can extend into adulthood. Pediatricians are in a unique position to identify and prevent child abuse, and this clinical report provides guidance to the practitioner regarding indicators and evaluation of suspected physical abuse of children. The role of the physician may include identifying abused children with suspicious injuries who present for care, reporting suspected abuse to the child protection agency for investigation, supporting families who are affected by child abuse, coordinating with other professionals and community agencies to provide immediate and long-term treatment to victimized children, providing court testimony when necessary, providing preventive care and anticipatory guidance in the office, and advocating for policies and programs that support families and protect vulnerable children. (4/15)

http://pediatrics.aappublications.org/content/135/5/e1337

EVIDENCE FOR THE DIAGNOSIS AND TREATMENT OF ACUTE UNCOMPLICATED SINUSITIS IN CHILDREN: A SYSTEMATIC REVIEW (TECHNICAL REPORT)

Michael J. Smith, MD, MSCE

ABSTRACT. In 2001, the American Academy of Pediatrics published clinical practice guidelines for the management of acute bacterial sinusitis (ABS) in children. The technical report accompanying those guidelines included 21 studies that assessed the diagnosis and management of ABS in children. This update to that report incorporates studies of pediatric ABS that have been performed since 2001. Overall, 17 randomized controlled trials of the treatment of sinusitis in children were identified and analyzed. Four randomized, double-blind, placebo-controlled trials of antimicrobial therapy have been published. The results of these studies varied, likely due to differences in inclusion and exclusion criteria. Because of this heterogeneity, formal meta-analyses were not performed. However, qualitative analysis of these studies suggests that children with greater severity of illness at presentation are more likely to benefit from antimicrobial therapy. An additional 5 trials compared different antimicrobial therapies but did not include placebo groups. Six trials assessed a variety of ancillary treatments for ABS in children, and 3 focused on subacute sinusitis. Although the number of pediatric trials has increased since 2001, there are still limited data to guide the diagnosis and management of ABS in children. Diagnostic and treatment guidelines focusing on severity of illness at the time of presentation have the potential to identify those children most likely to benefit from antimicrobial therapy and at the same time minimize unnecessary use of antibiotics. (6/13)
http://pediatrics.aappublications.org/content/132/1/e284

AN EVIDENCE-BASED REVIEW OF IMPORTANT ISSUES CONCERNING NEONATAL HYPERBILIRUBINEMIA (TECHNICAL REPORT)

Stanley Ip, MD; Mei Chung, MPH; John Kulig, MD, MPH; Rebecca O'Brien, MD; Robert Sege, MD, PhD; Stephan Glicken, MD; M. Jeffrey Maisels, MB, BCh; Joseph Lau, MD; Steering Committee on Quality and Improvement; and Subcommittee on Hyperbilirubinemia

ABSTRACT. This article is adapted from a published evidence report concerning neonatal hyperbilirubinemia with an added section on the risk of blood exchange transfusion (BET). Based on a summary of multiple case reports that spanned more than 30 years, we conclude that kernicterus, although infrequent, has at least 10% mortality and at least 70% long-term morbidity. It is evident that the preponderance of kernicterus cases occurred in infants with a bilirubin level higher than 20 mg/dL. Given the diversity of conclusions on the relationship between peak bilirubin levels and behavioral and neurodevelopmental outcomes, it is apparent that the use of a single total serum bilirubin level to predict long-term outcomes is inadequate and will lead to conflicting results. Evidence for efficacy of treatments for neonatal hyperbilirubinemia was limited. Overall, the 4 qualifying studies showed that phototherapy had an absolute risk-reduction rate of 10% to 17% for prevention of serum bilirubin levels higher than 20 mg/dL in healthy infants with jaundice. There is no evidence to suggest that phototherapy for neonatal hyperbilirubinemia has any long-term adverse neurodevelopmental effects. Transcutaneous measurements of bilirubin have a linear correlation to total serum bilirubin and may be useful as screening devices to detect clinically significant jaundice and decrease the need for serum bilirubin determinations. Based on our review of the risks associated with BETs from 15 studies consisting mainly of infants born before 1970, we conclude that the mortality within 6 hours of BET ranged from 3 per 1000 to 4 per 1000 exchanged infants who were term and without serious hemolytic diseases. Regardless of the definitions and rates of BET-associated morbidity and the various pre-exchange clinical states of the exchanged infants, in many cases the morbidity was minor (eg, postexchange anemia). Based on the results from the most recent study to report BET morbidity, the overall risk of permanent sequelae in 25 sick infants who survived BET was from 5% to 10%. (7/04)
http://pediatrics.aappublications.org/content/114/1/e130

EXPERT WITNESS PARTICIPATION IN CIVIL AND CRIMINAL PROCEEDINGS

Stephan R. Paul, MD, JD, FAAP; Sandeep K. Narang, MD, JD, FAAP; and Committee on Medical Liability and Risk Management

ABSTRACT. The interests of the public and both the medical and legal professions are best served when scientifically sound and unbiased expert witness testimony is readily available in civil and criminal proceedings. As members of the medical community, patient advocates, and private citizens, pediatricians have ethical and professional obligations to assist in the civil and criminal judicial processes. This policy statement offers recommendations on advocacy, education, research, qualifications, standards, and ethical business practices all aimed at improving expert testimony. (2/17)
http://pediatrics.aappublications.org/content/139/3/e20163862

EXPERT WITNESS PARTICIPATION IN CIVIL AND CRIMINAL PROCEEDINGS (TECHNICAL REPORT)

Sandeep K. Narang, MD, JD, FAAP; Stephan R. Paul, MD, JD, FAAP; and Committee on Medical Liability and Risk Management

ABSTRACT. The interests of the public and both the medical and legal professions are best served when scientifically sound and unbiased expert witness testimony is readily available in civil and criminal proceedings. As members of the medical community, patient advocates, and private citizens, pediatricians have ethical and professional obligations to assist in the civil and criminal judicial processes. This technical report explains how the role of the expert witness differs in civil and criminal proceedings, legal and ethical standards for expert witnesses, and strategies that have been employed to deter unscientific and irresponsible testimony. A companion policy statement offers recommendations on advocacy, education, research, qualifications, standards, and ethical business practices all aimed at improving expert testimony. (2/17)
http://pediatrics.aappublications.org/content/139/3/e20164122

EXPOSURE TO NONTRADITIONAL PETS AT HOME AND TO ANIMALS IN PUBLIC SETTINGS: RISKS TO CHILDREN (CLINICAL REPORT)

Larry K. Pickering, MD; Nina Marano, DVM, MPH; Joseph A. Bocchini, MD; Frederick J. Angulo, DVM, PhD; and Committee on Infectious Diseases

ABSTRACT. Exposure to animals can provide many benefits during the growth and development of children. However, there are potential risks associated with animal exposures, including exposure to nontraditional pets in the home and animals in public settings. Educational materials, regulations, and guidelines have been developed to minimize these risks. Pediatricians, veterinarians, and other health care professionals can provide advice on selection of appropriate pets as well as prevention of disease transmission from nontraditional pets and when children contact animals in public settings. (10/08, reaffirmed 12/11, 1/15, 6/15)
http://pediatrics.aappublications.org/content/122/4/876

THE EYE EXAMINATION IN THE EVALUATION OF CHILD ABUSE (CLINICAL REPORT)

Cindy W. Christian, MD, FAAP; Alex V. Levin, MD, MHSc, FAAO, FRCSC, FAAP; Council on Child Abuse and Neglect; and Section on Ophthalmology (joint with American Association of Certified Orthoptists, American Association for Pediatric Ophthalmology and Strabismus, and American Academy of Ophthalmology)

ABSTRACT. Child abuse can cause injury to any part of the eye. The most common manifestations are retinal hemorrhages (RHs) in infants and young children with abusive head trauma (AHT). Although RHs are an important indicator of possible AHT, they are also found in other conditions. Distinguishing the number, type, location, and pattern of RHs is important in evaluating a differential diagnosis. Eye trauma can be seen in cases of physical abuse or AHT and may prompt referral for ophthalmologic assessment. Physicians have a responsibility to consider abuse in the differential diagnosis of pediatric eye trauma. Identification and documentation of inflicted ocular trauma requires a thorough examination by an ophthalmologist, including indirect ophthalmoscopy, most optimally through a dilated pupil, especially for the evaluation of possible RHs. An eye examination is helpful in detecting abnormalities that can help identify a medical or traumatic etiology for previously well young children who experience unexpected and unexplained mental status changes with no obvious cause, children with head trauma that results in significant intracranial hemorrhage and brain injury, and children with unexplained death. (7/18)

See full text on page 659.

http://pediatrics.aappublications.org/content/142/2/e20181411

FACILITIES AND EQUIPMENT FOR THE CARE OF PEDIATRIC PATIENTS IN A COMMUNITY HOSPITAL (CLINICAL REPORT)

Committee on Hospital Care

ABSTRACT. Many children who require hospitalization are admitted to community hospitals that are more accessible for families and their primary care physicians but vary substantially in their pediatric resources. The intent of this clinical report is to provide basic guidelines for furnishing and equipping a pediatric area in a community hospital. (5/03, reaffirmed 5/07, 8/13, 1/17)

http://pediatrics.aappublications.org/content/111/5/1120

FALLS FROM HEIGHTS: WINDOWS, ROOFS, AND BALCONIES

Committee on Injury and Poison Prevention

ABSTRACT. Falls of all kinds represent an important cause of child injury and death. In the United States, approximately 140 deaths from falls occur annually in children younger than 15 years. Three million children require emergency department care for fall-related injuries. This policy statement examines the epidemiology of falls from heights and recommends preventive strategies for pediatricians and other child health care professionals. Such strategies involve parent counseling, community programs, building code changes, legislation, and environmental modification, such as the installation of window guards and balcony railings. (5/01, reaffirmed 10/04, 5/07, 6/10)

http://pediatrics.aappublications.org/content/107/5/1188

FAMILIES AFFECTED BY PARENTAL SUBSTANCE USE (CLINICAL REPORT)

Vincent C. Smith, MD, MPH, FAAP; Celeste R. Wilson, MD, FAAP; and Committee on Substance Use and Prevention

ABSTRACT. Children whose parents or caregivers use drugs or alcohol are at increased risk of short- and long-term sequelae ranging from medical problems to psychosocial and behavioral challenges. In the course of providing health care services to children, pediatricians are likely to encounter families affected by parental substance use and are in a unique position to intervene. Therefore, pediatricians need to know how to assess a child's risk in the context of a parent's substance use. The purposes of this clinical report are to review some of the short-term effects of maternal substance use during pregnancy and long-term implications of fetal exposure; describe typical medical, psychiatric, and behavioral symptoms of children and adolescents in families affected by substance use; and suggest proficiencies for pediatricians involved in the care of children and adolescents of families affected by substance use, including screening families, mandated reporting requirements, and directing families to community, regional, and state resources that can address needs and problems. (7/16)

http://pediatrics.aappublications.org/content/138/2/e20161575

FATHERS' ROLES IN THE CARE AND DEVELOPMENT OF THEIR CHILDREN: THE ROLE OF PEDIATRICIANS (CLINICAL REPORT)

Michael Yogman, MD, FAAP; Craig F. Garfield, MD, FAAP; and Committee on Psychosocial Aspects of Child and Family Health

ABSTRACT. Fathers' involvement in and influence on the health and development of their children have increased in a myriad of ways in the past 10 years and have been widely studied. The role of pediatricians in working with fathers has correspondingly increased in importance. This report reviews new studies of the epidemiology of father involvement, including nonresidential as well as residential fathers. The effects of father involvement on child outcomes are discussed within each phase of a child's development. Particular emphasis is placed on (1) fathers' involvement across childhood ages and (2) the influence of fathers' physical and mental health on their children. Implications and advice for all child health providers to encourage and support father involvement are outlined. (6/16)

http://pediatrics.aappublications.org/content/138/1/e20161128

THE FEMALE ATHLETE TRIAD (CLINICAL REPORT)

Amanda K. Weiss Kelly, MD, FAAP; Suzanne Hecht, MD, FACSM; and Council on Sports Medicine and Fitness

ABSTRACT. The number of girls participating in sports has increased significantly since the introduction of Title XI in 1972. As a result, more girls have been able to experience the social, educational, and health-related benefits of sports participation. However, there are risks associated with sports participation, including the female athlete triad. The triad was originally recognized as the interrelationship of amenorrhea, osteoporosis, and disordered eating, but our understanding has evolved to recognize that each of the components of the triad exists on a spectrum from optimal health to disease. The triad occurs when energy intake does not adequately compensate for exercise-related energy expenditure, leading to adverse effects on reproductive, bone, and cardiovascular health. Athletes can present with a single component or any combination of the components. The triad can have a more significant effect on the health of adolescent athletes than on adults because adolescence is a critical time for bone mass accumulation. This report outlines the current state of knowledge on the epidemiology, diagnosis, and treatment of the triad conditions. (7/16)

http://pediatrics.aappublications.org/content/138/2/e20160922

FETAL ALCOHOL SPECTRUM DISORDERS (CLINICAL REPORT)

Janet F. Williams, MD, FAAP; Vincent C. Smith, MD, MPH, FAAP; and Committee on Substance Abuse

ABSTRACT. Prenatal exposure to alcohol can damage the developing fetus and is the leading preventable cause of birth defects and intellectual and neurodevelopmental disabilities. In 1973, fetal alcohol syndrome was first described as a specific cluster of birth defects resulting from alcohol exposure in utero. Subsequently, research unequivocally revealed that prenatal alcohol exposure causes a broad range of adverse developmental effects. Fetal alcohol spectrum disorder (FASD) is the general term that encompasses the range of adverse effects associated with prenatal alcohol exposure. The diagnostic criteria for fetal alcohol syndrome are specific, and comprehensive efforts are ongoing to establish definitive criteria for diagnosing the other FASDs. A large and growing body of research has led to evidence-based FASD education of professionals and the public, broader prevention initiatives, and recommended treatment approaches based on the following premises:

- Alcohol-related birth defects and developmental disabilities are completely preventable when pregnant women abstain from alcohol use.

- Neurocognitive and behavioral problems resulting from prenatal alcohol exposure are lifelong.

- Early recognition, diagnosis, and therapy for any condition along the FASD continuum can result in improved outcomes.

- During pregnancy:

   — no amount of alcohol intake should be considered safe;

   — there is no safe trimester to drink alcohol;

   — all forms of alcohol, such as beer, wine, and liquor, pose similar risk; and

   — binge drinking poses dose-related risk to the developing fetus. (10/15)

http://pediatrics.aappublications.org/content/136/5/e1395

FEVER AND ANTIPYRETIC USE IN CHILDREN (CLINICAL REPORT)

Janice E. Sullivan, MD; Henry C. Farrar, MD; Section on Clinical Pharmacology and Therapeutics; and Committee on Drugs

ABSTRACT. Fever in a child is one of the most common clinical symptoms managed by pediatricians and other health care providers and a frequent cause of parental concern. Many parents administer antipyretics even when there is minimal or no fever, because they are concerned that the child must maintain a "normal" temperature. Fever, however, is not the primary illness but is a physiologic mechanism that has beneficial effects in fighting infection. There is no evidence that fever itself worsens the course of an illness or that it causes long-term neurologic complications. Thus, the primary goal of treating the febrile child should be to improve the child's overall comfort rather than focus on the normalization of body temperature. When counseling the parents or caregivers of a febrile child, the general well-being of the child, the importance of monitoring activity, observing for signs of serious illness, encouraging appropriate fluid intake, and the safe storage of antipyretics should be emphasized. Current evidence suggests that there is no substantial difference in the safety and effectiveness of acetaminophen and ibuprofen in the care of a generally healthy child with fever. There is evidence that combining these 2 products is more effective than the use of a single agent alone; however, there are concerns that combined treatment may be more complicated and contribute to the unsafe use of these drugs. Pediatricians should also promote patient safety by advocating for simplified formulations, dosing instructions, and dosing devices. (2/11, reaffirmed 7/16)

http://pediatrics.aappublications.org/content/127/3/580

FINANCING GRADUATE MEDICAL EDUCATION TO MEET THE NEEDS OF CHILDREN AND THE FUTURE PEDIATRICIAN WORKFORCE

Committee on Pediatric Workforce

ABSTRACT. The American Academy of Pediatrics (AAP) believes that an appropriately financed graduate medical education (GME) system is critical to ensuring that sufficient numbers of trained pediatricians are available to provide optimal health care to all children. A shortage of pediatric medical subspecialists and pediatric surgical specialists currently exists in the United States, and this shortage is likely to intensify because of the growing numbers of children with chronic health problems and special health care needs. It is equally important to maintain the supply of primary care pediatricians. The AAP, therefore, recommends that children's hospital GME positions funded by the Health Resources and Services Administration be increased to address this escalating demand for pediatric health services. The AAP also recommends that GME funding for pediatric physician training provide full financial support for all years of training necessary to meet program requirements. In addition, all other entities that gain from GME training should participate in its funding in a manner that does not influence curriculum, requirements, or outcomes. Furthermore, the AAP supports funding for training innovations that improve the health of children. Finally, the AAP recommends that all institutional recipients of GME funding allocate these funds directly to the settings where training occurs in a transparent manner. (3/16)

http://pediatrics.aappublications.org/content/137/4/e20160211

FINANCING OF PEDIATRIC HOME HEALTH CARE

Edwin Simpser, MD, FAAP; Mark L. Hudak, MD, FAAP; Section on Home Care; and Committee on Child Health Financing

ABSTRACT. Pediatric home health care is an effective and holistic venue of treatment of children with medical complexity or developmental disabilities who otherwise may experience frequent and/or prolonged hospitalizations or who may enter chronic institutional care. Demand for pediatric home health care is increasing while the provider base is eroding, primarily because of inadequate payment or restrictions on benefits. As a result, home care responsibilities assumed by family caregivers have increased and imposed financial, physical, and psychological burdens on the family. The Patient Protection and Affordable Care Act set forth 10 mandated essential health benefits. Home care should be considered as an integral component of the habilitative and rehabilitative services and devices benefit, even though it is not explicitly recognized as a specific category of service. Pediatric-specific home health care services should be defined clearly as components of pediatric services, the 10th essential benefit, and recognized by all payers. Payments for home health care services should be sufficient to maintain an adequate provider work force with the pediatric-specific expertise and skills to care for children with medical complexity or developmental disability. Furthermore, coordination of care among various providers and the necessary direct patient care from which these care coordination plans are developed should be required and enabled by adequate payment. The American Academy of Pediatrics advocates for high-quality care by calling for development of pediatric-specific home health regulations and the licensure and certification of pediatric home health providers. (2/17)

http://pediatrics.aappublications.org/content/139/3/e20164202

FIREARM-RELATED INJURIES AFFECTING THE PEDIATRIC POPULATION

Council on Injury, Violence, and Poison Prevention Executive Committee

ABSTRACT. The absence of guns from children's homes and communities is the most reliable and effective measure to prevent firearm-related injuries in children and adolescents. Adolescent suicide risk is strongly associated with firearm availability. Safe gun storage (guns unloaded and locked, ammunition locked separately) reduces children's risk of injury. Physician counseling of parents about firearm safety appears to be effective, but firearm safety education programs directed at children are ineffective. The American Academy of Pediatrics continues to

support a number of specific measures to reduce the destructive effects of guns in the lives of children and adolescents, including the regulation of the manufacture, sale, purchase, ownership, and use of firearms; a ban on semiautomatic assault weapons; and the strongest possible regulations of handguns for civilian use. (10/12, reaffirmed 12/16)
http://pediatrics.aappublications.org/content/130/5/e1416

FIREWORKS-RELATED INJURIES TO CHILDREN
Committee on Injury and Poison Prevention
ABSTRACT. An estimated 8500 individuals, approximately 45% of them children younger than 15 years, were treated in US hospital emergency departments during 1999 for fireworks-related injuries. The hands (40%), eyes (20%), and head and face (20%) are the body areas most often involved. Approximately one third of eye injuries from fireworks result in permanent blindness. During 1999, 16 people died as a result of injuries associated with fireworks. Every type of legally available consumer (so-called "safe and sane") firework has been associated with serious injury or death. In 1997, 20,100 fires were caused by fireworks, resulting in $22.7 million in direct property damage. Fireworks typically cause more fires in the United States on the Fourth of July than all other causes of fire combined on that day. Pediatricians should educate parents, children, community leaders, and others about the dangers of fireworks. Fireworks for individual private use should be banned. Children and their families should be encouraged to enjoy fireworks at public fireworks displays conducted by professionals rather than purchase fireworks for home or private use. (7/01, reaffirmed 1/05, 2/08, 10/11, 11/14)
http://pediatrics.aappublications.org/content/108/1/190

FLUORIDE USE IN CARIES PREVENTION IN THE PRIMARY CARE SETTING (CLINICAL REPORT)
Melinda B. Clark, MD, FAAP; Rebecca L. Slayton, DDS, PhD; and Section on Oral Health
ABSTRACT. Dental caries remains the most common chronic disease of childhood in the United States. Caries is a largely preventable condition, and fluoride has proven effectiveness in the prevention of caries. The goals of this clinical report are to clarify the use of available fluoride modalities for caries prevention in the primary care setting and to assist pediatricians in using fluoride to achieve maximum protection against dental caries while minimizing the likelihood of enamel fluorosis. (8/14)
http://pediatrics.aappublications.org/content/134/3/626

FOLIC ACID FOR THE PREVENTION OF NEURAL TUBE DEFECTS
Committee on Genetics
ABSTRACT. The American Academy of Pediatrics endorses the US Public Health Service (USPHS) recommendation that all women capable of becoming pregnant consume 400 µg of folic acid daily to prevent neural tube defects (NTDs). Studies have demonstrated that periconceptional folic acid supplementation can prevent 50% or more of NTDs such as spina bifida and anencephaly. For women who have previously had an NTD-affected pregnancy, the Centers for Disease Control and Prevention (CDC) recommends increasing the intake of folic acid to 4000 µg per day beginning at least 1 month before conception and continuing through the first trimester. Implementation of these recommendations is essential for the primary prevention of these serious and disabling birth defects. Because fewer than 1 in 3 women consume the amount of folic acid recommended by the USPHS, the Academy notes that the prevention of NTDs depends on an urgent and effective campaign to close this prevention gap. (8/99, reaffirmed 9/16)
http://pediatrics.aappublications.org/content/104/2/325

FOLLOW-UP MANAGEMENT OF CHILDREN WITH TYMPANOSTOMY TUBES
Section on Otolaryngology and Bronchoesophagology
ABSTRACT. The follow-up care of children in whom tympanostomy tubes have been placed is shared by the pediatrician and the otolaryngologist. Guidelines are provided for routine follow-up evaluation, perioperative hearing assessment, and the identification of specific conditions and complications that warrant urgent otolaryngologic consultation. These guidelines have been developed by a consensus of expert opinions. (2/02)
http://pediatrics.aappublications.org/content/109/2/328

FOOD ADDITIVES AND CHILD HEALTH
Leonardo Trasande, MD, MPP, FAAP; Rachel M. Shaffer, MPH; Sheela Sathyanarayana, MD, MPH; and Council on Environmental Health
ABSTRACT. Our purposes with this policy statement and its accompanying technical report are to review and highlight emerging child health concerns related to the use of colorings, flavorings, and chemicals deliberately added to food during processing (direct food additives) as well as substances in food contact materials, including adhesives, dyes, coatings, paper, paperboard, plastic, and other polymers, which may contaminate food as part of packaging or manufacturing equipment (indirect food additives); to make reasonable recommendations that the pediatrician might be able to adopt into the guidance provided during pediatric visits; and to propose urgently needed reforms to the current regulatory process at the US Food and Drug Administration (FDA) for food additives. Concern regarding food additives has increased in the past 2 decades, in part because of studies in which authors document endocrine disruption and other adverse health effects. In some cases, exposure to these chemicals is disproportionate among minority and low-income populations. Regulation and oversight of many food additives is inadequate because of several key problems in the Federal Food, Drug, and Cosmetic Act. Current requirements for a "generally recognized as safe" (GRAS) designation are insufficient to ensure the safety of food additives and do not contain sufficient protections against conflict of interest. Additionally, the FDA does not have adequate authority to acquire data on chemicals on the market or reassess their safety for human health. These are critical weaknesses in the current regulatory system for food additives. Data about health effects of food additives on infants and children are limited or missing; however, in general, infants and children are more vulnerable to chemical exposures. Substantial improvements to the food additives regulatory system are urgently needed, including greatly strengthening or replacing the "generally recognized as safe" (GRAS) determination process, updating the scientific foundation of the FDA's safety assessment program, retesting all previously approved chemicals, and labeling direct additives with limited or no toxicity data. (7/18)
See full text on page 669.
http://pediatrics.aappublications.org/content/142/2/e20181408

FOOD ADDITIVES AND CHILD HEALTH (TECHNICAL REPORT)
Leonardo Trasande, MD, MPP, FAAP; Rachel M. Shaffer, MPH; Sheela Sathyanarayana, MD, MPH; and Council on Environmental Health
ABSTRACT. Increasing scientific evidence suggests potential adverse effects on children's health from synthetic chemicals used as food additives, both those deliberately added to food during processing (direct) and those used in materials that may contaminate food as part of packaging or manufacturing (indirect). Concern regarding food additives has increased in the past 2 decades in part because of studies that increasingly document endocrine disruption and other adverse health effects. In some

cases, exposure to these chemicals is disproportionate among minority and low-income populations. This report focuses on those food additives with the strongest scientific evidence for concern. Further research is needed to study effects of exposure over various points in the life course, and toxicity testing must be advanced to be able to better identify health concerns prior to widespread population exposure. The accompanying policy statement describes approaches policy makers and pediatricians can take to prevent the disease and disability that are increasingly being identified in relation to chemicals used as food additives, among other uses. (7/18)

See full text on page 679.

http://pediatrics.aappublications.org/content/142/2/e20181410

FORGOING MEDICALLY PROVIDED NUTRITION AND HYDRATION IN CHILDREN (CLINICAL REPORT)

Douglas S. Diekema, MD, MPH; Jeffrey R. Botkin, MD, MPH; and Committee on Bioethics

ABSTRACT. There is broad consensus that withholding or withdrawing medical interventions is morally permissible when requested by competent patients or, in the case of patients without decision-making capacity, when the interventions no longer confer a benefit to the patient or when the burdens associated with the interventions outweigh the benefits received. The withdrawal or withholding of measures such as attempted resuscitation, ventilators, and critical care medications is common in the terminal care of adults and children. In the case of adults, a consensus has emerged in law and ethics that the medical administration of fluid and nutrition is not fundamentally different from other medical interventions such as use of ventilators; therefore, it can be forgone or withdrawn when a competent adult or legally authorized surrogate requests withdrawal or when the intervention no longer provides a net benefit to the patient. In pediatrics, forgoing or withdrawing medically administered fluids and nutrition has been more controversial because of the inability of children to make autonomous decisions and the emotional power of feeding as a basic element of the care of children. This statement reviews the medical, ethical, and legal issues relevant to the withholding or withdrawing of medically provided fluids and nutrition in children. The American Academy of Pediatrics concludes that the withdrawal of medically administered fluids and nutrition for pediatric patients is ethically acceptable in limited circumstances. Ethics consultation is strongly recommended when particularly difficult or controversial decisions are being considered. (7/09, reaffirmed 1/14)
http://pediatrics.aappublications.org/content/124/2/813

FRUIT JUICE IN INFANTS, CHILDREN, AND ADOLESCENTS: CURRENT RECOMMENDATIONS

Melvin B. Heyman, MD, FAAP; Steven A. Abrams, MD, FAAP; Section on Gastroenterology, Hepatology, and Nutrition; and Committee on Nutrition

ABSTRACT. Historically, fruit juice was recommended by pediatricians as a source of vitamin C and as an extra source of water for healthy infants and young children as their diets expanded to include solid foods with higher renal solute load. It was also sometimes recommended for children with constipation. Fruit juice is marketed as a healthy, natural source of vitamins and, in some instances, calcium. Because juice tastes good, children readily accept it. Although juice consumption has some benefits, it also has potential detrimental effects. High sugar content in juice contributes to increased calorie consumption and the risk of dental caries. In addition, the lack of protein and fiber in juice can predispose to inappropriate weight gain (too much or too little). Pediatricians need to be knowledgeable about juice to inform parents and patients on its appropriate uses. (5/17)
http://pediatrics.aappublications.org/content/139/6/e20170967

THE FUTURE OF PEDIATRICS: MENTAL HEALTH COMPETENCIES FOR PEDIATRIC PRIMARY CARE

Committee on Psychosocial Aspects of Child and Family Health and Task Force on Mental Health

ABSTRACT. Pediatric primary care clinicians have unique opportunities and a growing sense of responsibility to prevent and address mental health and substance abuse problems in the medical home. In this report, the American Academy of Pediatrics proposes competencies requisite for providing mental health and substance abuse services in pediatric primary care settings and recommends steps toward achieving them. Achievement of the competencies proposed in this statement is a goal, not a current expectation. It will require innovations in residency training and continuing medical education, as well as a commitment by the individual clinician to pursue, over time, educational strategies suited to his or her learning style and skill level. System enhancements, such as collaborative relationships with mental health specialists and changes in the financing of mental health care, must precede enhancements in clinical practice. For this reason, the proposed competencies begin with knowledge and skills for systems-based practice. The proposed competencies overlap those of mental health specialists in some areas; for example, they include the knowledge and skills to care for children with attention-deficit/hyperactivity disorder, anxiety, depression, and substance abuse and to recognize psychiatric and social emergencies. In other areas, the competencies reflect the uniqueness of the primary care clinician's role: building resilience in all children; promoting healthy lifestyles; preventing or mitigating mental health and substance abuse problems; identifying risk factors and emerging mental health problems in children and their families; and partnering with families, schools, agencies, and mental health specialists to plan assessment and care. Proposed interpersonal and communication skills reflect the primary care clinician's critical role in overcoming barriers (perceived and/or experienced by children and families) to seeking help for mental health and substance abuse concerns. (6/09, reaffirmed 8/13)
http://pediatrics.aappublications.org/content/124/1/410

GASTROESOPHAGEAL REFLUX: MANAGEMENT GUIDANCE FOR THE PEDIATRICIAN (CLINICAL REPORT)

Jenifer R. Lightdale, MD, MPH; David A. Gremse, MD; and Section on Gastroenterology, Hepatology, and Nutrition

ABSTRACT. Recent comprehensive guidelines developed by the North American Society for Pediatric Gastroenterology, Hepatology, and Nutrition define the common entities of gastroesophageal reflux (GER) as the physiologic passage of gastric contents into the esophagus and gastroesophageal reflux disease (GERD) as reflux associated with troublesome symptoms or complications. The ability to distinguish between GER and GERD is increasingly important to implement best practices in the management of acid reflux in patients across all pediatric age groups, as children with GERD may benefit from further evaluation and treatment, whereas conservative recommendations are the only indicated therapy in those with uncomplicated physiologic reflux. This clinical report endorses the rigorously developed, well-referenced North American Society for Pediatric Gastroenterology, Hepatology, and Nutrition guidelines and likewise emphasizes important concepts for the general pediatrician. A key issue is distinguishing between clinical manifestations of GER and GERD in term infants, children, and adolescents to identify patients who can be managed with conservative treatment by the pediatrician and to refer patients who require consultation with the gastroenterologist. Accordingly, the evidence basis presented by the guidelines for diagnostic approaches as well as treatments is discussed. Lifestyle changes are emphasized as first-line therapy in both GER and GERD, whereas medications are explicitly indicated only for patients

with GERD. Surgical therapies are reserved for children with intractable symptoms or who are at risk for life-threatening complications of GERD. Recent black box warnings from the US Food and Drug Administration are discussed, and caution is underlined when using promoters of gastric emptying and motility. Finally, attention is paid to increasing evidence of inappropriate prescriptions for proton pump inhibitors in the pediatric population. (4/13)
http://pediatrics.aappublications.org/content/131/5/e1684

GENERIC PRESCRIBING, GENERIC SUBSTITUTION, AND THERAPEUTIC SUBSTITUTION

Committee on Drugs (5/87, reaffirmed 6/93, 5/96, 6/99, 5/01, 5/05, 10/08, 10/12)
http://pediatrics.aappublications.org/content/79/5/835

GLOBAL CLIMATE CHANGE AND CHILDREN'S HEALTH

Council on Environmental Health
ABSTRACT. Rising global temperatures are causing major physical, chemical, and ecological changes in the planet. There is wide consensus among scientific organizations and climatologists that these broad effects, known as "climate change," are the result of contemporary human activity. Climate change poses threats to human health, safety, and security, and children are uniquely vulnerable to these threats. The effects of climate change on child health include: physical and psychological sequelae of weather disasters; increased heat stress; decreased air quality; altered disease patterns of some climate-sensitive infections; and food, water, and nutrient insecurity in vulnerable regions. The social foundations of children's mental and physical health are threatened by the specter of far-reaching effects of unchecked climate change, including community and global instability, mass migrations, and increased conflict. Given this knowledge, failure to take prompt, substantive action would be an act of injustice to all children. A paradigm shift in production and consumption of energy is both a necessity and an opportunity for major innovation, job creation, and significant, immediate associated health benefits. Pediatricians have a uniquely valuable role to play in the societal response to this global challenge. (10/15)
http://pediatrics.aappublications.org/content/136/5/992

GLOBAL CLIMATE CHANGE AND CHILDREN'S HEALTH (TECHNICAL REPORT)

Samantha Ahdoot, MD, FAAP; Susan E. Pacheco, MD, FAAP; and Council on Environmental Health
ABSTRACT. Rising global temperature is causing major physical, chemical, and ecological changes across the planet. There is wide consensus among scientific organizations and climatologists that these broad effects, known as climate change, are the result of contemporary human activity. Climate change poses threats to human health, safety, and security. Children are uniquely vulnerable to these threats. The effects of climate change on child health include physical and psychological sequelae of weather disasters, increased heat stress, decreased air quality, altered disease patterns of some climate-sensitive infections, and food, water, and nutrient insecurity in vulnerable regions. Prompt implementation of mitigation and adaptation strategies will protect children against worsening of the problem and its associated health effects. This technical report reviews the nature of climate change and its associated child health effects and supports the recommendations in the accompanying policy statement on climate change and children's health. (10/15)
http://pediatrics.aappublications.org/content/136/5/e1468

GLOBAL HUMAN TRAFFICKING AND CHILD VICTIMIZATION

Jordan Greenbaum, MD; Nia Bodrick, MD, MPH, FAAP; Committee on Child Abuse and Neglect; and Section on International Child Health
ABSTRACT. Trafficking of children for labor and sexual exploitation violates basic human rights and constitutes a major global public health problem. Pediatricians and other health care professionals may encounter victims who present with infections, injuries, posttraumatic stress disorder, suicidality, or a variety of other physical or behavioral health conditions. Preventing child trafficking, recognizing victimization, and intervening appropriately require a public health approach that incorporates rigorous research on the risk factors, health impact, and effective treatment options for child exploitation as well as implementation and evaluation of primary prevention programs. Health care professionals need training to recognize possible signs of exploitation and to intervene appropriately. They need to adopt a multidisciplinary, outward-focused approach to service provision, working with nonmedical professionals in the community to assist victims. Pediatricians also need to advocate for legislation and policies that promote child rights and victim services as well as those that address the social determinants of health, which influence the vulnerability to human trafficking. This policy statement outlines major issues regarding public policy, medical education, research, and collaboration in the area of child labor and sex trafficking and provides recommendations for future work. (11/17)
http://pediatrics.aappublications.org/content/140/6/e20173138

GUIDANCE FOR EFFECTIVE DISCIPLINE

Committee on Psychosocial Aspects of Child and Family Health
ABSTRACT. When advising families about discipline strategies, pediatricians should use a comprehensive approach that includes consideration of the parent-child relationship, reinforcement of desired behaviors, and consequences for negative behaviors. Corporal punishment is of limited effectiveness and has potentially deleterious side effects. The American Academy of Pediatrics recommends that parents be encouraged and assisted in the development of methods other than spanking for managing undesired behavior. (4/98, reaffirmed 4/14)
http://pediatrics.aappublications.org/content/101/4/723

GUIDANCE FOR THE ADMINISTRATION OF MEDICATION IN SCHOOL

Council on School Health
ABSTRACT. Many children who take medications require them during the school day. This policy statement is designed to guide prescribing health care professionals, school physicians, and school health councils on the administration of medications to children at school. All districts and schools need to have policies and plans in place for safe, effective, and efficient administration of medications at school. Having full-time licensed registered nurses administering all routine and emergency medications in schools is the best situation. When a licensed registered nurse is not available, a licensed practical nurse may administer medications. When a nurse cannot administer medication in school, the American Academy of Pediatrics supports appropriate delegation of nursing services in the school setting. Delegation is a tool that may be used by the licensed registered school nurse to allow unlicensed assistive personnel to provide standardized, routine health services under the supervision of the nurse and on the basis of physician guidance and school nursing assessment of the unique needs of the individual child and the suitability of delegation of specific nursing tasks. Any delegation of nursing duties must be consistent with the requirements of state nurse practice acts, state regulations, and guidelines provided by professional

nursing organizations. Long-term, emergency, and short-term medications; over-the-counter medications; alternative medications; and experimental drugs that are administered as part of a clinical trial are discussed in this statement. This statement has been endorsed by the American School Health Association. (9/09, reaffirmed 2/13)
http://pediatrics.aappublications.org/content/124/4/1244

GUIDANCE ON COMPLETING A WRITTEN ALLERGY AND ANAPHYLAXIS EMERGENCY PLAN (CLINICAL REPORT)

Julie Wang, MD, FAAP; Scott H. Sicherer, MD, FAAP; and Section on Allergy and Immunology

ABSTRACT. Anaphylaxis is a potentially life-threatening, severe allergic reaction. The immediate assessment of patients having an allergic reaction and prompt administration of epinephrine, if criteria for anaphylaxis are met, promote optimal outcomes. National and international guidelines for the management of anaphylaxis, including those for management of allergic reactions at school, as well as several clinical reports from the American Academy of Pediatrics, recommend the provision of written emergency action plans to those at risk of anaphylaxis, in addition to the prescription of epinephrine autoinjectors. This clinical report provides information to help health care providers understand the role of a written, personalized allergy and anaphylaxis emergency plan to enhance the care of children at risk of allergic reactions, including anaphylaxis. This report offers a comprehensive written plan, with advice on individualizing instructions to suit specific patient circumstances. (2/17)
http://pediatrics.aappublications.org/content/139/3/e20164005

GUIDANCE ON FORGOING LIFE-SUSTAINING MEDICAL TREATMENT

Kathryn L. Weise, MD, MA, FAAP; Alexander L. Okun, MD, FAAP; Brian S. Carter, MD, FAAP; Cindy W. Christian, MD, FAAP; Committee on Bioethics; Section on Hospice and Palliative Medicine; and Committee on Child Abuse and Neglect

ABSTRACT. Pediatric health care is practiced with the goal of promoting the best interests of the child. Treatment generally is rendered under a presumption in favor of sustaining life. However, in some circumstances, the balance of benefits and burdens to the child leads to an assessment that forgoing life-sustaining medical treatment (LSMT) is ethically supportable or advisable. Parents are given wide latitude in decision-making concerning end-of-life care for their children in most situations. Collaborative decision-making around LSMT is improved by thorough communication among all stakeholders, including medical staff, the family, and the patient, when possible, throughout the evolving course of the patient's illness. Clear communication of overall goals of care is advised to promote agreed-on plans, including resuscitation status. Perceived disagreement among the team of professionals may be stressful to families. At the same time, understanding the range of professional opinions behind treatment recommendations is critical to informing family decision-making. Input from specialists in palliative care, ethics, pastoral care, and other disciplines enhances support for families and medical staff when decisions to forgo LSMT are being considered. Understanding specific applicability of institutional, regional, state, and national regulations related to forgoing LSMT is important to practice ethically within existing legal frameworks. This guidance represents an update of the 1994 statement from the American Academy of Pediatrics on forgoing LSMT. (8/17)
http://pediatrics.aappublications.org/content/140/3/e20171905

GUIDANCE ON MANAGEMENT OF ASYMPTOMATIC NEONATES BORN TO WOMEN WITH ACTIVE GENITAL HERPES LESIONS (CLINICAL REPORT)

Committee on Infectious Diseases and Committee on Fetus and Newborn

ABSTRACT. Herpes simplex virus (HSV) infection of the neonate is uncommon, but genital herpes infections in adults are very common. Thus, although treating an infant with neonatal herpes is a relatively rare occurrence, managing infants potentially exposed to HSV at the time of delivery occurs more frequently. The risk of transmitting HSV to an infant during delivery is determined in part by the mother's previous immunity to HSV. Women with primary genital HSV infections who are shedding HSV at delivery are 10 to 30 times more likely to transmit the virus to their newborn infants than are women with recurrent HSV infection who are shedding virus at delivery. With the availability of commercial serological tests that reliably can distinguish type-specific HSV antibodies, it is now possible to determine the type of maternal infection and, thus, further refine management of infants delivered to women who have active genital HSV lesions. The management algorithm presented herein uses both serological and virological studies to determine the risk of HSV transmission to the neonate who is delivered to a mother with active herpetic genital lesions and tailors management accordingly. The algorithm does not address the approach to asymptomatic neonates delivered to women with a history of genital herpes but no active lesions at delivery. (1/13, reaffirmed 9/16)
http://pediatrics.aappublications.org/content/131/2/e635

GUIDELINES FOR DEVELOPING ADMISSION AND DISCHARGE POLICIES FOR THE PEDIATRIC INTENSIVE CARE UNIT (CLINICAL REPORT)

Committee on Hospital Care and Section on Critical Care (joint with Society of Critical Care Medicine Pediatric Section Admission Criteria Task Force)

ABSTRACT. These guidelines were developed to provide a reference for preparing policies on admission to and discharge from pediatric intensive care units. They represent a consensus opinion of physicians, nurses, and allied health care professionals. By using this document as a framework for developing multidisciplinary admission and discharge policies, use of pediatric intensive care units can be optimized and patients can receive the level of care appropriate for their condition. (4/99, reaffirmed 5/17)
http://pediatrics.aappublications.org/content/103/4/840

GUIDELINES FOR MONITORING AND MANAGEMENT OF PEDIATRIC PATIENTS BEFORE, DURING, AND AFTER SEDATION FOR DIAGNOSTIC AND THERAPEUTIC PROCEDURES: UPDATE 2016 (CLINICAL REPORT)

Charles J. Coté, MD, FAAP; Stephen Wilson, DMD, MA, PhD; and American Academy of Pediatrics (joint with American Academy of Pediatric Dentistry)

ABSTRACT. The safe sedation of children for procedures requires a systematic approach that includes the following: no administration of sedating medication without the safety net of medical/dental supervision, careful presedation evaluation for underlying medical or surgical conditions that would place the child at increased risk from sedating medications, appropriate fasting for elective procedures and a balance between the depth of sedation and risk for those who are unable to fast because of the urgent nature of the procedure, a focused airway examination for large (kissing) tonsils or anatomic airway abnormalities that might increase the potential for airway obstruction, a clear understanding of the medication's pharmacokinetic and pharmacodynamic effects and drug interactions, appropriate training

and skills in airway management to allow rescue of the patient, age- and size-appropriate equipment for airway management and venous access, appropriate medications and reversal agents, sufficient numbers of staff to both carry out the procedure and monitor the patient, appropriate physiologic monitoring during and after the procedure, a properly equipped and staffed recovery area, recovery to the presedation level of consciousness before discharge from medical/dental supervision, and appropriate discharge instructions. This report was developed through a collaborative effort of the American Academy of Pediatrics and the American Academy of Pediatric Dentistry to offer pediatric providers updated information and guidance in delivering safe sedation to children. (6/16)
http://pediatrics.aappublications.org/content/138/1/e20161212

GUIDELINES FOR PEDIATRIC CANCER CENTERS

Section on Hematology/Oncology

ABSTRACT. Since the American Academy of Pediatrics published guidelines for pediatric cancer centers in 1986 and 1997, significant changes in the delivery of health care have prompted a review of the role of tertiary medical centers in the care of pediatric patients. The potential effect of these changes on the treatment and survival rates of children with cancer led to this revision. The intent of this statement is to delineate personnel and facilities that are essential to provide state-of-the-art care for children and adolescents with cancer. This statement emphasizes the importance of board-certified pediatric hematologists/oncologists, pediatric subspecialty consultants, and appropriately qualified pediatric medical subspecialists and pediatric surgical specialists overseeing the care of all pediatric and adolescent cancer patients and the need for facilities available only at a tertiary center as essential for the initial management and much of the follow-up for pediatric and adolescent cancer patients. (6/04, reaffirmed 10/08)
http://pediatrics.aappublications.org/content/113/6/1833

GUIDELINES FOR THE DETERMINATION OF BRAIN DEATH IN INFANTS AND CHILDREN: AN UPDATE OF THE 1987 TASK FORCE RECOMMENDATIONS (CLINICAL REPORT)

Thomas A. Nakagawa, MD; Stephen Ashwal, MD; Mudit Mathur, MD; Mohan Mysore, MD; Section on Critical Care; and Section on Neurology (joint with Society of Critical Care Medicine and Child Neurology Society)

ABSTRACT. *Objective.* To review and revise the 1987 pediatric brain death guidelines.

Methods. Relevant literature was reviewed. Recommendations were developed using the GRADE system.

Conclusions and Recommendations.

1. Determination of brain death in term newborns, infants and children is a clinical diagnosis based on the absence of neurologic function with a known irreversible cause of coma. Because of insufficient data in the literature, recommendations for preterm infants less than 37 weeks' gestational age are not included in this guideline.

2. Hypotension, hypothermia, and metabolic disturbances should be treated and corrected and medications that can interfere with the neurologic examination and apnea testing should be discontinued allowing for adequate clearance before proceeding with these evaluations.

3. Two examinations including apnea testing with each examination separated by an observation period are required. Examinations should be performed by different attending physicians. Apnea testing may be performed by the same physician. An observation period of 24 hours for term newborns (37 weeks' gestational age) to 30 days of age, and 12 hours for infants and children (> 30 days to 18 years) is recommended. The first examination determines the child has met the accepted neurologic examination criteria for brain death. The second examination confirms brain death based on an unchanged and irreversible condition. Assessment of neurologic function following cardiopulmonary resuscitation or other severe acute brain injuries should be deferred for 24 hours or longer if there are concerns or inconsistencies in the examination.

4. Apnea testing to support the diagnosis of brain death must be performed safely and requires documentation of an arterial $Paco_2$ 20 mm Hg above the baseline and ≥60 mm Hg with no respiratory effort during the testing period. If the apnea test cannot be safely completed, an ancillary study should be performed.

5. Ancillary studies (electroencephalogram and radionuclide cerebral blood flow) are not required to establish brain death and are not a substitute for the neurologic examination. Ancillary studies may be used to assist the clinician in making the diagnosis of brain death (1) when components of the examination or apnea testing cannot be completed safely due to the underlying medical condition of the patient; (2) if there is uncertainty about the results of the neurologic examination; (3) if a medication effect may be present; or (4) to reduce the inter-examination observation period. When ancillary studies are used, a second clinical examination and apnea test should be performed and components that can be completed must remain consistent with brain death. In this instance the observation interval may be shortened and the second neurologic examination and apnea test (or all components that are able to be completed safely) can be performed at any time thereafter.

6. Death is declared when the above criteria are fulfilled. (8/11, reaffirmed 1/15)
http://pediatrics.aappublications.org/content/128/3/e720

GUIDELINES FOR THE ETHICAL CONDUCT OF STUDIES TO EVALUATE DRUGS IN PEDIATRIC POPULATIONS (CLINICAL REPORT)

Robert E. Shaddy, MD; Scott C. Denne, MD; Committee on Drugs; and Committee on Pediatric Research

ABSTRACT. The proper ethical conduct of studies to evaluate drugs in children is of paramount importance to all those involved in these types of studies. This report is an updated revision to the previously published guidelines from the American Academy of Pediatrics in 1995. Since the previous publication, there have been great strides made in the science and ethics of studying drugs in children. There have also been numerous legislative and regulatory advancements that have promoted the study of drugs in children while simultaneously allowing for the protection of this particularly vulnerable group. This report summarizes these changes and advances and provides a framework from which to guide and monitor the ethical conduct of studies to evaluate drugs in children. (3/10, reaffirmed 1/14, 2/18)
http://pediatrics.aappublications.org/content/125/4/850

GUIDING PRINCIPLES FOR MANAGED CARE ARRANGEMENTS FOR THE HEALTH CARE OF NEWBORNS, INFANTS, CHILDREN, ADOLESCENTS, AND YOUNG ADULTS

Committee on Child Health Financing

ABSTRACT. By including the precepts of primary care and the medical home in the delivery of services, managed care can be effective in increasing access to a full range of health care services and clinicians. A carefully designed and administered managed care plan can minimize patient under- and overutilization of services, as well as enhance quality of care. Therefore, the American Academy of Pediatrics urges the use of the key

principles outlined in this statement in designing and implementing managed care programs for newborns, infants, children, adolescents, and young adults to maximize the positive potential of managed care for pediatrics. (10/13)
http://pediatrics.aappublications.org/content/132/5/e1452

GUIDING PRINCIPLES FOR PEDIATRIC HOSPITAL MEDICINE PROGRAMS

Section on Hospital Medicine

ABSTRACT. Pediatric hospital medicine programs have an established place in pediatric medicine. This statement speaks to the expanded roles and responsibilities of pediatric hospitalists and their integrated role among the community of pediatricians who care for children within and outside of the hospital setting. (9/13)
http://pediatrics.aappublications.org/content/132/4/782

GUIDING PRINCIPLES FOR TEAM-BASED PEDIATRIC CARE

Julie P. Katkin, MD, FAAP; Susan J. Kressly, MD, FAAP; Anne R. Edwards, MD, FAAP; James M. Perrin, MD, FAAP; Colleen A. Kraft, MD, FAAP; Julia E. Richerson, MD, FAAP; Joel S. Tieder, MD, MPH, FAAP; Liz Wall; and Task Force on Pediatric Practice Change

ABSTRACT. The American Academy of Pediatrics (AAP) recognizes that children's unique and ever-changing needs depend on a variety of support systems. Key components of effective support systems address the needs of the child and family in the context of their home and community and are dynamic so that they reflect, monitor, and respond to changes as the needs of the child and family change. The AAP believes that team-based care involving medical providers and community partners (eg, teachers and state agencies) is a crucial and necessary component of providing high-quality care to children and their families. Team-based care builds on the foundation of the medical home by reaching out to a potentially broad array of participants in the life of a child and incorporating them into the care provided. Importantly, the AAP believes that a high-functioning team includes children and their families as essential partners. The overall goal of team-based care is to enhance communication and cooperation among the varied medical, social, and educational partners in a child's life to better meet the global needs of children and their families, helping them to achieve their best potential. In support of the team-based approach, the AAP urges stakeholders to invest in infrastructure, education, and privacy-secured technology to meet the needs of children. This statement includes limited specific examples of potential team members, including health care providers and community partners, that are meant to be illustrative and in no way represent a complete or comprehensive listing of all team members who may be of importance for a specific child and family. (7/17)
http://pediatrics.aappublications.org/content/140/2/e20171489

GYNECOLOGIC EXAMINATION FOR ADOLESCENTS IN THE PEDIATRIC OFFICE SETTING (CLINICAL REPORT)

Paula K. Braverman, MD; Lesley Breech, MD; and Committee on Adolescence

ABSTRACT. The American Academy of Pediatrics promotes the inclusion of the gynecologic examination in the primary care setting within the medical home. Gynecologic issues are commonly seen by clinicians who provide primary care to adolescents. Some of the most common concerns include questions related to pubertal development; menstrual disorders such as dysmenorrhea, amenorrhea, oligomenorrhea, and abnormal uterine bleeding; contraception; and sexually transmitted and non–sexually transmitted infections. The gynecologic examination is a key element in assessing pubertal status and documenting physical findings. Most adolescents do not need an internal examination involving a speculum or bimanual examination. However, for cases in which more extensive examination is needed, the primary care office with the primary care clinician who has established rapport and trust with the patient is often the best setting for pelvic examination. This report reviews the gynecologic examination, including indications for the pelvic examination in adolescents and the approach to this examination in the office setting. Indications for referral to a gynecologist are included. The pelvic examination may be successfully completed when conducted without pressure and approached as a normal part of routine young women's health care. (8/10, reaffirmed 5/13)
http://pediatrics.aappublications.org/content/126/3/583

HANDOFFS: TRANSITIONS OF CARE FOR CHILDREN IN THE EMERGENCY DEPARTMENT

Committee on Pediatric Emergency Medicine (joint with American College of Emergency Physicians Pediatric Emergency Medicine Committee and Emergency Nurses Association Pediatric Committee)

ABSTRACT. Transitions of care (ToCs), also referred to as handoffs or sign-outs, occur when the responsibility for a patient's care transfers from 1 health care provider to another. Transitions are common in the acute care setting and have been noted to be vulnerable events with opportunities for error. Health care is taking ideas from other high-risk industries, such as aerospace and nuclear power, to create models of structured transition processes. Although little literature currently exists to establish 1 model as superior, multiorganizational consensus groups agree that standardization is warranted and that additional work is needed to establish characteristics of ToCs that are associated with clinical or practice outcomes. The rationale for structuring ToCs, specifically those related to the care of children in the emergency setting, and a description of identified strategies are presented, along with resources for educating health care providers on ToCs. Recommendations for development, education, and implementation of transition models are included. (10/16)
http://pediatrics.aappublications.org/content/138/5/e20162680

HEAD LICE (CLINICAL REPORT)

Cynthia D. Devore, MD, FAAP; Gordon E. Schutze, MD, FAAP; Council on School Health; and Committee on Infectious Diseases

ABSTRACT. Head lice infestation is associated with limited morbidity but causes a high level of anxiety among parents of school-aged children. Since the 2010 clinical report on head lice was published by the American Academy of Pediatrics, newer medications have been approved for the treatment of head lice. This revised clinical report clarifies current diagnosis and treatment protocols and provides guidance for the management of children with head lice in the school setting. (4/15)
http://pediatrics.aappublications.org/content/135/5/e1355

HEALTH AND MENTAL HEALTH NEEDS OF CHILDREN IN US MILITARY FAMILIES (CLINICAL REPORT)

Benjamin S. Siegel, MD; Beth Ellen Davis, MD, MPH; Committee on Psychosocial Aspects of Child and Family Health; and Section on Uniformed Services

ABSTRACT. The wars in Afghanistan and Iraq have been challenging for US uniformed service families and their children. Almost 60% of US service members have family responsibilities. Approximately 2.3 million active duty, National Guard, and Reserve service members have been deployed since the beginning of the wars in Afghanistan and Iraq (2001 and 2003, respectively), and almost half have deployed more than once, some for up to 18 months' duration. Up to 2 million US children have been exposed to a wartime deployment of a loved one in the past 10 years. Many service members have returned from combat deployments with symptoms of posttraumatic stress disorder, depression, anxiety, substance abuse, and traumatic brain injury. The mental health and well-being of spouses, significant others, children (and their friends), and extended family members of deployed service members continues to be significantly challenged by the experiences of wartime deployment as well as by combat mortality and morbidity. The medical system of the Department of Defense provides health and mental health services for active duty service members and their families as well as activated National Guard and Reserve service members and their families. In addition to military pediatricians and civilian pediatricians employed by military treatment facilities, nonmilitary general pediatricians care for >50% of children and family members before, during, and after wartime deployments. This clinical report is for all pediatricians, both active duty and civilian, to aid in caring for children whose loved ones have been, are, or will be deployed. (5/13)

http://pediatrics.aappublications.org/content/131/6/e2002

HEALTH CARE FOR YOUTH IN THE JUVENILE JUSTICE SYSTEM

Committee on Adolescence

ABSTRACT. Youth in the juvenile correctional system are a high-risk population who, in many cases, have unmet physical, developmental, and mental health needs. Multiple studies have found that some of these health issues occur at higher rates than in the general adolescent population. Although some youth in the juvenile justice system have interfaced with health care providers in their community on a regular basis, others have had inconsistent or nonexistent care. The health needs of these youth are commonly identified when they are admitted to a juvenile custodial facility. Pediatricians and other health care providers play an important role in the care of these youth, and continuity between the community and the correctional facility is crucial. This policy statement provides an overview of the health needs of youth in the juvenile correctional system, including existing resources and standards for care, financing of health care within correctional facilities, and evidence-based interventions. Recommendations are provided for the provision of health care services to youth in the juvenile correctional system as well as specific areas for advocacy efforts. (11/11, reaffirmed 5/15)

http://pediatrics.aappublications.org/content/128/6/1219

HEALTH CARE ISSUES FOR CHILDREN AND ADOLESCENTS IN FOSTER CARE AND KINSHIP CARE

Council on Foster Care, Adoption, and Kinship Care; Committee on Adolescence; and Council on Early Childhood

ABSTRACT. Children and adolescents who enter foster care often do so with complicated and serious medical, mental health, developmental, oral health, and psychosocial problems rooted in their history of childhood trauma. Ideally, health care for this population is provided in a pediatric medical home by physicians who are familiar with the sequelae of childhood trauma and adversity. As youth with special health care needs, children and adolescents in foster care require more frequent monitoring of their health status, and pediatricians have a critical role in ensuring the well-being of children in out-of-home care through the provision of high-quality pediatric health services, health care coordination, and advocacy on their behalves. (9/15)

http://pediatrics.aappublications.org/content/136/4/e1131

HEALTH CARE ISSUES FOR CHILDREN AND ADOLESCENTS IN FOSTER CARE AND KINSHIP CARE (TECHNICAL REPORT)

Moira A. Szilagyi, MD, PhD; David S. Rosen, MD, MPH; David Rubin, MD, MSCE; Sarah Zlotnik, MSW, MSPH; Council on Foster Care, Adoption, and Kinship Care; Committee on Adolescence; and Council on Early Childhood

ABSTRACT. Children and adolescents involved with child welfare, especially those who are removed from their family of origin and placed in out-of-home care, often present with complex and serious physical, mental health, developmental, and psychosocial problems rooted in childhood adversity and trauma. As such, they are designated as children with special health care needs. There are many barriers to providing high-quality comprehensive health care services to children and adolescents whose lives are characterized by transience and uncertainty. Pediatricians have a critical role in ensuring the well-being of children in out-of-home care through the provision of high-quality pediatric health services in the context of a medical home, and health care coordination and advocacy on their behalf. This technical report supports the policy statement of the same title. (9/15)

http://pediatrics.aappublications.org/content/136/4/e1142

HEALTH CARE OF YOUTH AGING OUT OF FOSTER CARE

Council on Foster Care, Adoption, and Kinship Care and Committee on Early Childhood

ABSTRACT. Youth transitioning out of foster care face significant medical and mental health care needs. Unfortunately, these youth rarely receive the services they need because of lack of health insurance. Through many policies and programs, the federal government has taken steps to support older youth in foster care and those aging out. The Fostering Connections to Success and Increasing Adoptions Act of 2008 (Pub L No. 110-354) requires states to work with youth to develop a transition plan that addresses issues such as health insurance. In addition, beginning in 2014, the Patient Protection and Affordable Care Act of 2010 (Pub L No. 111-148) makes youth aging out of foster care eligible for Medicaid coverage until age 26 years, regardless of income. Pediatricians can support youth aging out of foster care by working collaboratively with the child welfare agency in their state to ensure that the ongoing health needs of transitioning youth are met. (11/12, reaffirmed 7/17)

http://pediatrics.aappublications.org/content/130/6/1170

HEALTH CARE SUPERVISION FOR CHILDREN WITH WILLIAMS SYNDROME

Committee on Genetics

ABSTRACT. This set of guidelines is designed to assist the pediatrician to care for children with Williams syndrome diagnosed by clinical features and with regional chromosomal microdeletion confirmed by fluorescence in situ hybridization. (5/01, reaffirmed 5/05, 1/09)

http://pediatrics.aappublications.org/content/107/5/1192

HEALTH EQUITY AND CHILDREN'S RIGHTS

Council on Community Pediatrics and Committee on Native American Child Health

ABSTRACT. Many children in the United States fail to reach their full health and developmental potential. Disparities in their health and well-being result from the complex interplay of multiple social and environmental determinants that are not adequately addressed by current standards of pediatric practice or public policy. Integrating the principles and practice of child health equity—children's rights, social justice, human capital investment, and health equity ethics—into pediatrics will address the root causes of child health disparities.

Promoting the principles and practice of equity-based clinical care, child advocacy, and child- and family-centered public policy will help to ensure that social and environmental determinants contribute positively to the health and well-being of children. The American Academy of Pediatrics and pediatricians can move the national focus from documenting child health disparities to advancing the principles and practice of child health equity and, in so doing, influence the worldwide practice of pediatrics and child health. All pediatricians, including primary care practitioners and medical and surgical subspecialists, can

incorporate these principles into their practice of pediatrics and child health. Integration of these principles into competency-based training and board certification will secure their assimilation into all levels of pediatric practice. (3/10, reaffirmed 10/13)
http://pediatrics.aappublications.org/content/125/4/838

HEALTH INFORMATION TECHNOLOGY AND THE MEDICAL HOME

Council on Clinical Information Technology

ABSTRACT. The American Academy of Pediatrics (AAP) supports development and universal implementation of a comprehensive electronic infrastructure to support pediatric information functions of the medical home. These functions include (1) timely and continuous management and tracking of health data and services over a patient's lifetime for all providers, patients, families, and guardians, (2) comprehensive organization and secure transfer of health data during patient-care transitions between providers, institutions, and practices, (3) establishment and maintenance of central coordination of a patient's health information among multiple repositories (including personal health records and information exchanges), (4) translation of evidence into actionable clinical decision support, and (5) reuse of archived clinical data for continuous quality improvement. The AAP supports universal, secure, and vendor-neutral portability of health information for all patients contained within the medical home across all care settings (ambulatory practices, inpatient settings, emergency departments, pharmacies, consultants, support service providers, and therapists) for multiple purposes including direct care, personal health records, public health, and registries. The AAP also supports financial incentives that promote the development of information tools that meet the needs of pediatric workflows and that appropriately recognize the added value of medical homes to pediatric care. (4/11, reaffirmed 7/15)
http://pediatrics.aappublications.org/content/127/5/978

HEALTH SUPERVISION FOR CHILDREN WITH ACHONDROPLASIA (CLINICAL REPORT)

Tracy L. Trotter, MD; Judith G. Hall, OC, MD; and Committee on Genetics

ABSTRACT. Achondroplasia is the most common condition associated with disproportionate short stature. Substantial information is available concerning the natural history and anticipatory health supervision needs in children with this dwarfing disorder. Most children with achondroplasia have delayed motor milestones, problems with persistent or recurrent middle-ear dysfunction, and bowing of the lower legs. Less often, infants and children may have serious health consequences related to hydrocephalus, craniocervical junction compression, upper-airway obstruction, or thoracolumbar kyphosis. Anticipatory care should be directed at identifying children who are at high risk and intervening to prevent serious sequelae. This report is designed to help the pediatrician care for children with achondroplasia and their families. (9/05, reaffirmed 5/12)
http://pediatrics.aappublications.org/content/116/3/771

HEALTH SUPERVISION FOR CHILDREN WITH DOWN SYNDROME (CLINICAL REPORT)

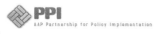

Marilyn J. Bull, MD, and Committee on Genetics

ABSTRACT. These guidelines are designed to assist the pediatrician in caring for the child in whom a diagnosis of Down syndrome has been confirmed by chromosome analysis. Although a pediatrician's initial contact with the child is usually during infancy, occasionally the pregnant woman who has been given a prenatal diagnosis of Down syndrome will be referred for review of the condition and the genetic counseling provided.

Therefore, this report offers guidance for this situation as well. (7/11, reaffirmed 9/16, 1/18)
http://pediatrics.aappublications.org/content/128/2/393

HEALTH SUPERVISION FOR CHILDREN WITH FRAGILE X SYNDROME (CLINICAL REPORT)

Joseph H. Hersh, MD; Robert A. Saul, MD; and Committee on Genetics

ABSTRACT. Fragile X syndrome (an *FMR1*–related disorder) is the most commonly inherited form of mental retardation. Early physical recognition is difficult, so boys with developmental delay should be strongly considered for molecular testing. The characteristic adult phenotype usually does not develop until the second decade of life. Girls can also be affected with developmental delay. Because multiple family members can be affected with mental retardation and other conditions (premature ovarian failure and tremor/ataxia), family history information is of critical importance for the diagnosis and management of affected patients and their families. This report summarizes issues for fragile X syndrome regarding clinical diagnosis, laboratory diagnosis, genetic counseling, related health problems, behavior management, and age-related health supervision guidelines. The diagnosis of fragile X syndrome not only involves the affected children but also potentially has significant health consequences for multiple generations in each family. (4/11)
http://pediatrics.aappublications.org/content/127/5/994

HEALTH SUPERVISION FOR CHILDREN WITH MARFAN SYNDROME (CLINICAL REPORT)

Brad T. Tinkle, MD, PhD; Howard M. Saal, MD; and Committee on Genetics

ABSTRACT. Marfan syndrome is a systemic, heritable connective tissue disorder that affects many different organ systems and is best managed by using a multidisciplinary approach. The guidance in this report is designed to assist the pediatrician in recognizing the features of Marfan syndrome as well as caring for the individual with this disorder. (9/13)
http://pediatrics.aappublications.org/content/132/4/e1059

HEALTH SUPERVISION FOR CHILDREN WITH NEUROFIBROMATOSIS (CLINICAL REPORT)

Joseph H. Hersh, MD, and Committee on Genetics

ABSTRACT. Neurofibromatosis 1 is a multisystem disorder that primarily involves the skin and nervous system. Its population prevalence is 1 in 3500. The condition usually is recognized in early childhood, when cutaneous manifestations are apparent. Although neurofibromatosis 1 is associated with marked clinical variability, most affected children do well from the standpoint of their growth and development. Some features of neurofibromatosis 1 are present at birth, and others are age-related abnormalities of tissue proliferation, which necessitate periodic monitoring to address ongoing health and developmental needs and to minimize the risk of serious medical complications. This clinical report provides a review of the clinical criteria needed to establish a diagnosis, the inheritance pattern of neurofibromatosis 1, its major clinical and developmental manifestations, and guidelines for monitoring and providing intervention to maximize the growth, development, and health of an affected child. (3/08, reaffirmed 9/16)
http://pediatrics.aappublications.org/content/121/3/633

HEALTH SUPERVISION FOR CHILDREN WITH PRADER-WILLI SYNDROME (CLINICAL REPORT)

Shawn E. McCandless, MD, and Committee on Genetics

ABSTRACT. This set of guidelines was designed to assist the pediatrician in caring for children with Prader-Willi syndrome diagnosed by clinical features and confirmed by molecular testing. Prader-Willi syndrome provides an excellent example

of how early diagnosis and management can improve the long-term outcome for some genetic disorders. (12/10)
http://pediatrics.aappublications.org/content/127/1/195

HEALTH SUPERVISION FOR CHILDREN WITH SICKLE CELL DISEASE

Section on Hematology/Oncology and Committee on Genetics

ABSTRACT. Sickle cell disease (SCD) is a group of complex genetic disorders with multisystem manifestations. This statement provides pediatricians in primary care and subspecialty practice with an overview of the genetics, diagnosis, clinical manifestations, and treatment of SCD. Specialized comprehensive medical care decreases morbidity and mortality during childhood. The provision of comprehensive care is a time-intensive endeavor that includes ongoing patient and family education, periodic comprehensive evaluations and other disease-specific health maintenance services, psychosocial care, and genetic counseling. Timely and appropriate treatment of acute illness is critical, because life-threatening complications develop rapidly. It is essential that every child with SCD receive comprehensive care that is coordinated through a medical home with appropriate expertise. (3/02, reaffirmed 1/06, 1/11, 2/16)
http://pediatrics.aappublications.org/content/109/3/526

HEARING ASSESSMENT IN INFANTS AND CHILDREN: RECOMMENDATIONS BEYOND NEONATAL SCREENING (CLINICAL REPORT)

PPI
AAP Partnership for Policy Implementation

Allen D. "Buz" Harlor Jr, MD; Charles Bower, MD; Committee on Practice and Ambulatory Medicine; and Section on Otolaryngology–Head and Neck Surgery

ABSTRACT. Congenital or acquired hearing loss in infants and children has been linked with lifelong deficits in speech and language acquisition, poor academic performance, personal-social maladjustments, and emotional difficulties. Identification of hearing loss through neonatal hearing screening, regular surveillance of developmental milestones, auditory skills, parental concerns, and middle-ear status and objective hearing screening of all infants and children at critical developmental stages can prevent or reduce many of these adverse consequences. This report promotes a proactive, consistent, and explicit process for the early identification of children with hearing loss in the medical home. An algorithm of the recommended approach has been developed to assist in the detection and documentation of, and intervention for, hearing loss. (9/09)
http://pediatrics.aappublications.org/content/124/4/1252

HELPING CHILDREN AND FAMILIES DEAL WITH DIVORCE AND SEPARATION (CLINICAL REPORT)

George J. Cohen, MD, FAAP; Carol C. Weitzman, MD, FAAP; Committee on Psychosocial Aspects of Child and Family Health; and Section on Developmental and Behavioral Pediatrics

ABSTRACT. For the past several years in the United States, there have been more than 800 000 divorces and parent separations annually, with over 1 million children affected. Children and their parents can experience emotional trauma before, during, and after a separation or divorce. Pediatricians can be aware of their patients' behavior and parental attitudes and behaviors that may indicate family dysfunction and that can indicate need for intervention. Age-appropriate explanation and counseling for the child and advice and guidance for the parents, as well as recommendation of reading material, may help reduce the potential negative effects of divorce. Often, referral to professionals with expertise in the social, emotional, and legal aspects of the separation and its aftermath may be helpful for these families. (11/16)
http://pediatrics.aappublications.org/content/138/6/e20163020

HIGH-DEDUCTIBLE HEALTH PLANS

Committee on Child Health Financing

ABSTRACT. High-deductible health plans (HDHPs) are insurance policies with higher deductibles than conventional plans. The Medicare Prescription Drug Improvement and Modernization Act of 2003 linked many HDHPs with tax-advantaged spending accounts. The 2010 Patient Protection and Affordable Care Act continues to provide for HDHPs in its lower-level plans on the health insurance marketplace and provides for them in employer-offered plans. HDHPs decrease the premium cost of insurance policies for purchasers and shift the risk of further payments to the individual subscriber. HDHPs reduce utilization and total medical costs, at least in the short term. Because HDHPs require out-of-pocket payment in the initial stages of care, primary care and other outpatient services as well as elective procedures are the services most affected, whereas higher-cost services in the health care system, incurred after the deductible is met, are unaffected. HDHPs promote adverse selection because healthier and wealthier patients tend to opt out of conventional plans in favor of HDHPs. Because the ill pay more than the healthy under HDHPs, families with children with special health care needs bear an increased cost burden in this model. HDHPs discourage use of nonpreventive primary care and thus are at odds with most recommendations for improving the organization of health care, which focus on strengthening primary care.

This policy statement provides background information on HDHPs, discusses the implications for families and pediatric care providers, and suggests courses of action. (4/14)
http://pediatrics.aappublications.org/content/133/5/e1461

HIV TESTING AND PROPHYLAXIS TO PREVENT MOTHER-TO-CHILD TRANSMISSION IN THE UNITED STATES

Committee on Pediatric AIDS

ABSTRACT. Universal HIV testing of pregnant women in the United States is the key to prevention of mother-to-child transmission of HIV. Repeat testing in the third trimester and rapid HIV testing at labor and delivery are additional strategies to further reduce the rate of perinatal HIV transmission. Prevention of mother-to-child transmission of HIV is most effective when antiretroviral drugs are received by the mother during her pregnancy and continued through delivery and then administered to the infant after birth. Antiretroviral drugs are effective in reducing the risk of mother-to-child transmission of HIV even when prophylaxis is started for the infant soon after birth. New rapid testing methods allow identification of HIV-infected women or HIV-exposed infants in 20 to 60 minutes. The American Academy of Pediatrics recommends documented, routine HIV testing for all pregnant women in the United States after notifying the patient that testing will be performed, unless the patient declines HIV testing ("opt-out" consent or "right of refusal"). For women in labor with undocumented HIV-infection status during the current pregnancy, immediate maternal HIV testing with opt-out consent, using a rapid HIV antibody test, is recommended. Positive HIV antibody screening test results should be confirmed with immunofluorescent antibody or Western blot assay. For women with a positive rapid HIV antibody test result, antiretroviral prophylaxis should be administered promptly to the mother and newborn infant on the basis of the positive result of the rapid antibody test without waiting for results of confirmatory HIV testing. If the confirmatory test result is negative, then prophylaxis should be discontinued. For a newborn infant whose mother's HIV serostatus is unknown, the health care professional should perform rapid HIV antibody testing on the mother or on the newborn infant, with results reported to the health care professional no later than 12 hours after the infant's birth. If the rapid HIV antibody test result is positive,

antiretroviral prophylaxis should be instituted as soon as possible after birth but certainly by 12 hours after delivery, pending completion of confirmatory HIV testing. The mother should be counseled not to breastfeed the infant. Assistance with immediate initiation of hand and pump expression to stimulate milk production should be offered to the mother, given the possibility that the confirmatory test result may be negative. If the confirmatory test result is negative, then prophylaxis should be stopped and breastfeeding may be initiated. If the confirmatory test result is positive, infants should receive antiretroviral prophylaxis for 6 weeks after birth, and the mother should not breastfeed the infant. (11/08, reaffirmed 6/11, 11/14)
http://pediatrics.aappublications.org/content/122/5/1127

HOME, HOSPITAL, AND OTHER NON–SCHOOL-BASED INSTRUCTION FOR CHILDREN AND ADOLESCENTS WHO ARE MEDICALLY UNABLE TO ATTEND SCHOOL
Committee on School Health
ABSTRACT. The American Academy of Pediatrics recommends that school-aged children and adolescents obtain their education in school in the least restrictive setting, that is, the setting most conducive to learning for the particular student. However, at times, acute illness or injury and chronic medical conditions preclude school attendance. This statement is meant to assist evaluation and planning for children to receive non–school-based instruction and to return to school at the earliest possible date. (11/00, reaffirmed 6/03, 5/06)
http://pediatrics.aappublications.org/content/106/5/1154

HOME CARE OF CHILDREN AND YOUTH WITH COMPLEX HEALTH CARE NEEDS AND TECHNOLOGY DEPENDENCIES (CLINICAL REPORT)
Ellen Roy Elias, MD; Nancy A. Murphy, MD; and Council on Children With Disabilities
ABSTRACT. Children and youth with complex medical issues, especially those with technology dependencies, experience frequent and often lengthy hospitalizations. Hospital discharges for these children can be a complicated process that requires a deliberate, multistep approach. In addition to successful discharges to home, it is essential that pediatric providers develop and implement an interdisciplinary and coordinated plan of care that addresses the child's ongoing health care needs. The goal is to ensure that each child remains healthy, thrives, and obtains optimal medical home and developmental supports that promote ongoing care at home and minimize recurrent hospitalizations. This clinical report presents an approach to discharging the child with complex medical needs with technology dependencies from hospital to home and then continually addressing the needs of the child and family in the home environment. (4/12, reaffirmed 5/17)
http://pediatrics.aappublications.org/content/129/5/996

HONORING DO-NOT-ATTEMPT-RESUSCITATION REQUESTS IN SCHOOLS
Council on School Health and Committee on Bioethics
ABSTRACT. Increasingly, children and adolescents with complex chronic conditions are living in the community. Federal legislation and regulations facilitate their participation in school. Some of these children and adolescents and their families may wish to forego life-sustaining medical treatment, including cardiopulmonary resuscitation, because they would be ineffective or because the risks outweigh the benefits. Honoring these requests in the school environment is complex because of the limited availability of school nurses and the frequent lack of supporting state legislation and regulations. Understanding and collaboration on the part of all parties is essential. Pediatricians have an important role in helping school nurses incorporate a specific action plan into the student's individualized health care plan. The action plan should include both communication and comfort-care plans. Pediatricians who work directly with schools can also help implement policies, and professional organizations can advocate for regulations and legislation that enable students and their families to effectuate their preferences. (4/10, reaffirmed 7/13, 8/16)
http://pediatrics.aappublications.org/content/125/5/1073

HOSPITAL DISCHARGE OF THE HIGH-RISK NEONATE
Committee on Fetus and Newborn
ABSTRACT. This policy statement updates the guidelines on discharge of the high-risk neonate first published by the American Academy of Pediatrics in 1998. As with the earlier document, this statement is based, insofar as possible, on published, scientifically derived information. This updated statement incorporates new knowledge about risks and medical care of the high-risk neonate, the timing of discharge, and planning for care after discharge. It also refers to other American Academy of Pediatrics publications that are relevant to these issues. This statement draws on the previous classification of high-risk infants into 4 categories: (1) the preterm infant; (2) the infant with special health care needs or dependence on technology; (3) the infant at risk because of family issues; and (4) the infant with anticipated early death. The issues of deciding when discharge is appropriate, defining the specific needs for follow-up care, and the process of detailed discharge planning are addressed as they apply in general to all 4 categories; in addition, special attention is directed to the particular issues presented by the 4 individual categories. Recommendations are given to aid in deciding when discharge is appropriate and to ensure that all necessary care will be available and well coordinated after discharge. The need for individualized planning and physician judgment is emphasized. (11/08, reaffirmed 5/11)
http://pediatrics.aappublications.org/content/122/5/1119

THE HOSPITAL RECORD OF THE INJURED CHILD AND THE NEED FOR EXTERNAL CAUSE-OF-INJURY CODES
Committee on Injury and Poison Prevention
ABSTRACT. Proper record-keeping of emergency department visits and hospitalizations of injured children is vital for appropriate patient management. Determination and documentation of the circumstances surrounding the injury event are essential. This information not only is the basis for preventive counseling, but also provides clues about how similar injuries in other youth can be avoided. The hospital records have an important secondary purpose; namely, if sufficient information about the cause and mechanism of injury is documented, it can be subsequently coded, electronically compiled, and retrieved later to provide an epidemiologic profile of the injury, the first step in prevention at the population level. To be of greatest use, hospital records should indicate the "who, what, when, where, why, and how" of the injury occurrence and whether protective equipment (eg, a seat belt) was used. The pediatrician has two important roles in this area: to document fully the injury event and to advocate the use of standardized external cause-of-injury codes, which allow such data to be compiled and analyzed. (2/99, reaffirmed 5/02, 5/05, 10/08, 10/13)
http://pediatrics.aappublications.org/content/103/2/524

HOSPITAL STAY FOR HEALTHY TERM NEWBORN INFANTS
William E. Benitz, MD, FAAP, and Committee on Fetus and Newborn
ABSTRACT. The hospital stay of the mother and her healthy term newborn infant should be long enough to allow identification of problems and to ensure that the mother is sufficiently recovered and prepared to care for herself and her newborn at

home. The length of stay should be based on the unique characteristics of each mother-infant dyad, including the health of the mother, the health and stability of the newborn, the ability and confidence of the mother to care for herself and her newborn, the adequacy of support systems at home, and access to appropriate follow-up care in a medical home. Input from the mother and her obstetrical care provider should be considered before a decision to discharge a newborn is made, and all efforts should be made to keep a mother and her newborn together to ensure simultaneous discharge. (4/15)
http://pediatrics.aappublications.org/content/135/5/948

HUMAN EMBRYONIC STEM CELL (HESC) AND HUMAN EMBRYO RESEARCH
Committee on Pediatric Research and Committee on Bioethics
ABSTRACT. Human embryonic stem cell research has emerged as an important platform for the understanding and treatment of pediatric diseases. From its inception, however, it has raised ethical concerns based not on the use of stem cells themselves but on objections to the source of the cells—specifically, the destruction of preimplantation human embryos. Despite differences in public opinion on this issue, a large majority of the public supports continued research using embryonic stem cells. Given the possible substantial benefit of stem cell research on child health and development, the American Academy of Pediatrics believes that funding and oversight for human embryo and embryonic stem cell research should continue. (10/12, reaffirmed 7/17)
http://pediatrics.aappublications.org/content/130/5/972

HUMAN IMMUNODEFICIENCY VIRUS AND OTHER BLOOD-BORNE VIRAL PATHOGENS IN THE ATHLETIC SETTING
Committee on Sports Medicine and Fitness
ABSTRACT. Because athletes and the staff of athletic programs can be exposed to blood during athletic activity, they have a very small risk of becoming infected with human immunodeficiency virus, hepatitis B virus, or hepatitis C virus. This statement, which updates a previous position statement of the American Academy of Pediatrics, discusses sports participation for athletes infected with these pathogens and the precautions needed to reduce the risk of infection to others in the athletic setting. Each of the recommendations in this statement is dependent upon and intended to be considered with reference to the other recommendations in this statement and not in isolation. (12/99, reaffirmed 1/05, 1/09, 11/11, 2/15)
http://pediatrics.aappublications.org/content/104/6/1400

HYPOTHERMIA AND NEONATAL ENCEPHALOPATHY (CLINICAL REPORT)
Committee on Fetus and Newborn
ABSTRACT. Data from large randomized clinical trials indicate that therapeutic hypothermia, using either selective head cooling or systemic cooling, is an effective therapy for neonatal encephalopathy. Infants selected for cooling must meet the criteria outlined in published clinical trials. The implementation of cooling needs to be performed at centers that have the capability to manage medically complex infants. Because the majority of infants who have neonatal encephalopathy are born at community hospitals, centers that perform cooling should work with their referring hospitals to implement education programs focused on increasing the awareness and identification of infants at risk for encephalopathy, and the initial clinical management of affected infants. (5/14)
http://pediatrics.aappublications.org/content/133/6/1146

IDENTIFICATION AND CARE OF HIV-EXPOSED AND HIV-INFECTED INFANTS, CHILDREN, AND ADOLESCENTS IN FOSTER CARE
Committee on Pediatric AIDS
ABSTRACT. As a consequence of the expanding human immunodeficiency virus (HIV) epidemic and major advances in medical management of HIV-exposed and HIV-infected persons, revised recommendations are provided for HIV testing of infants, children, and adolescents in foster care. Updated recommendations also are provided for the care of HIV-exposed and HIV-infected persons who are in foster care. (7/00, reaffirmed 12/16)
http://pediatrics.aappublications.org/content/106/1/149

IDENTIFICATION AND EVALUATION OF CHILDREN WITH AUTISM SPECTRUM DISORDERS (CLINICAL REPORT)

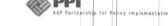

Chris Plauché Johnson, MD, MEd; Scott M. Myers, MD; and Council on Children With Disabilities
ABSTRACT. Autism spectrum disorders are not rare; many primary care pediatricians care for several children with autism spectrum disorders. Pediatricians play an important role in early recognition of autism spectrum disorders, because they usually are the first point of contact for parents. Parents are now much more aware of the early signs of autism spectrum disorders because of frequent coverage in the media; if their child demonstrates any of the published signs, they will most likely raise their concerns to their child's pediatrician. It is important that pediatricians be able to recognize the signs and symptoms of autism spectrum disorders and have a strategy for assessing them systematically. Pediatricians also must be aware of local resources that can assist in making a definitive diagnosis of, and in managing, autism spectrum disorders. The pediatrician must be familiar with developmental, educational, and community resources as well as medical subspecialty clinics. This clinical report is 1 of 2 documents that replace the original American Academy of Pediatrics policy statement and technical report published in 2001. This report addresses background information, including definition, history, epidemiology, diagnostic criteria, early signs, neuropathologic aspects, and etiologic possibilities in autism spectrum disorders. In addition, this report provides an algorithm to help the pediatrician develop a strategy for early identification of children with autism spectrum disorders. The accompanying clinical report addresses the management of children with autism spectrum disorders and follows this report on page 1162 [available at www.pediatrics.org/cgi/content/full/120/5/1162]. Both clinical reports are complemented by the toolkit titled "Autism: Caring for Children With Autism Spectrum Disorders: A Resource Toolkit for Clinicians," which contains screening and surveillance tools, practical forms, tables, and parent handouts to assist the pediatrician in the identification, evaluation, and management of autism spectrum disorders in children. (11/07, reaffirmed 9/10, 8/14)
http://pediatrics.aappublications.org/content/120/5/1183

IDENTIFICATION AND MANAGEMENT OF EATING DISORDERS IN CHILDREN AND ADOLESCENTS (CLINICAL REPORT)
David S. Rosen, MD, MPH, and Committee on Adolescence
ABSTRACT. The incidence and prevalence of eating disorders in children and adolescents has increased significantly in recent decades, making it essential for pediatricians to consider these disorders in appropriate clinical settings, to evaluate patients suspected of having these disorders, and to manage (or refer) patients in whom eating disorders are diagnosed. This clinical report includes a discussion of diagnostic criteria and

outlines the initial evaluation of the patient with disordered eating. Medical complications of eating disorders may affect any organ system, and careful monitoring for these complications is required. The range of treatment options, including pharmacotherapy, is described in this report. Pediatricians are encouraged to advocate for legislation and policies that ensure appropriate services for patients with eating disorders, including medical care, nutritional intervention, mental health treatment, and care coordination. (11/10, reaffirmed 11/14)
http://pediatrics.aappublications.org/content/126/6/1240

IDENTIFYING INFANTS AND YOUNG CHILDREN WITH DEVELOPMENTAL DISORDERS IN THE MEDICAL HOME: AN ALGORITHM FOR DEVELOPMENTAL SURVEILLANCE AND SCREENING

PPI
AAP Partnership for Policy Implementation

Council on Children With Disabilities, Section on Developmental and Behavioral Pediatrics, Bright Futures Steering Committee, and Medical Home Initiatives for Children With Special Needs Project Advisory Committee

ABSTRACT. Early identification of developmental disorders is critical to the well-being of children and their families. It is an integral function of the primary care medical home and an appropriate responsibility of all pediatric health care professionals. This statement provides an algorithm as a strategy to support health care professionals in developing a pattern and practice for addressing developmental concerns in children from birth through 3 years of age. The authors recommend that developmental surveillance be incorporated at every well-child preventive care visit. Any concerns raised during surveillance should be promptly addressed with standardized developmental screening tests. In addition, screening tests should be administered regularly at the 9-, 18-, and 30-month visits. (Because the 30-month visit is not yet a part of the preventive care system and is often not reimbursable by third-party payers at this time, developmental screening can be performed at 24 months of age. In addition, because the frequency of regular pediatric visits decreases after 24 months of age, a pediatrician who expects that his or her patients will have difficulty attending a 30-month visit should conduct screening during the 24-month visit.) The early identification of developmental problems should lead to further developmental and medical evaluation, diagnosis, and treatment, including early developmental intervention. Children diagnosed with developmental disorders should be identified as children with special health care needs, and chronic-condition management should be initiated. Identification of a developmental disorder and its underlying etiology may also drive a range of treatment planning, from medical treatment of the child to family planning for his or her parents. (7/06, reaffirmed 12/09, 8/14)
http://pediatrics.aappublications.org/content/118/1/405

IMMERSION IN WATER DURING LABOR AND DELIVERY (CLINICAL REPORT)

Committee on Fetus and Newborn (joint with American College of Obstetricians and Gynecologists Committee on Obstetric Practice)

ABSTRACT. Immersion in water has been suggested as a beneficial alternative for labor, delivery, or both and over the past decades has gained popularity in many parts of the world. Immersion in water during the first stage of labor may be associated with decreased pain or use of anesthesia and decreased duration of labor. However, there is no evidence that immersion in water during the first stage of labor otherwise improves perinatal outcomes, and it should not prevent or inhibit other elements of care. The safety and efficacy of immersion in water during the second stage of labor have not been established, and immersion in water during the second stage of labor has not been associated with maternal or fetal benefit. Given these facts and case reports of rare but serious adverse effects in the

newborn, the practice of immersion in the second stage of labor (underwater delivery) should be considered an experimental procedure that only should be performed within the context of an appropriately designed clinical trial with informed consent. Facilities that plan to offer immersion in the first stage of labor need to establish rigorous protocols for candidate selection, maintenance and cleaning of tubs and immersion pools, infection control procedures, monitoring of mothers and fetuses at appropriate intervals while immersed, and immediately and safely moving women out of the tubs if maternal or fetal concerns develop. (3/14)
http://pediatrics.aappublications.org/content/133/4/758

IMMUNIZATION FOR *STREPTOCOCCUS PNEUMONIAE* INFECTIONS IN HIGH-RISK CHILDREN

Committee on Infectious Diseases

ABSTACT. Routine use of the pneumococcal conjugate vaccines (PCV7 and PCV13), beginning in 2000, has resulted in a dramatic reduction in the incidence of invasive pneumococcal disease (IPD) attributable to serotypes of *Streptococcus pneumoniae* contained in the vaccines. The Advisory Committee on Immunization Practices of the Centers for Disease Control and Prevention and the American Academy of Pediatrics recommend the expanded use of PCV13 in children 6 through 18 years of age with certain conditions that place them at elevated risk of IPD. This statement provides recommendations for the use of PCV13 in children 6 through 18 years. A single dose of PCV13 should be administered to certain children in this age group who are at elevated risk of IPD. Recommendations for the use of PCV13 in healthy children and for pneumococcal polysaccharide vaccine (PPSV23) remain unchanged. (11/14)
http://pediatrics.aappublications.org/content/134/6/1230

IMMUNIZATION INFORMATION SYSTEMS

Committee on Practice and Ambulatory Medicine

ABSTRACT. The American Academy of Pediatrics continues to support the development and implementation of immunization information systems, previously referred to as immunization registries, and other systems for the benefit of children, pediatricians, and their communities. Pediatricians and others must be aware of the value that immunization information systems have for society, the potential fiscal influences on their practice, the costs and benefits, and areas for future improvement. (9/06, reaffirmed 10/11)
http://pediatrics.aappublications.org/content/118/3/1293

IMMUNIZING PARENTS AND OTHER CLOSE FAMILY CONTACTS IN THE PEDIATRIC OFFICE SETTING (TECHNICAL REPORT)

Herschel R. Lessin, MD; Kathryn M. Edwards, MD; Committee on Practice and Ambulatory Medicine; and Committee on Infectious Diseases

ABSTRACT. Additional strategies are needed to protect children from vaccine-preventable diseases. In particular, very young infants, as well as children who are immunocompromised, are at especially high risk for developing the serious consequences of vaccine-preventable diseases and cannot be immunized completely. There is some evidence that children who become infected with these diseases are exposed to pathogens through household contacts, particularly from parents or other close family contacts. Such infections likely are attributable to adults who are not fully protected from these diseases, either because their immunity to vaccine-preventable diseases has waned over time or because they have not received a vaccine. There are many challenges that have added to low adult immunization rates in the United States. One option to increase immunization coverage for parents and close family contacts of infants and vulnerable children is to provide alternative locations for these adults to be immunized, such as the pediatric office setting. Ideally, adults should receive immunizations in their medical homes; however, to provide greater protection to these adults and reduce the exposure of children to pathogens, immunizing parents or other adult family contacts in the pediatric office setting could increase immunization coverage for this population to protect themselves as well as children to whom they provide care. (12/11, reaffirmed 8/16)

http://pediatrics.aappublications.org/content/129/1/e247

THE IMPACT OF MARIJUANA POLICIES ON YOUTH: CLINICAL, RESEARCH, AND LEGAL UPDATE

Committee on Substance Abuse and Committee on Adolescence

ABSTRACT. This policy statement is an update of the American Academy of Pediatrics policy statement "Legalization of Marijuana: Potential Impact on Youth," published in 2004. Pediatricians have special expertise in the care of children and adolescents and may be called on to advise legislators about the potential impact of changes in the legal status of marijuana on adolescents. Parents also may look to pediatricians for advice as they consider whether to support state-level initiatives that propose to legalize the use of marijuana for medical and nonmedical purposes or to decriminalize the possession of small amounts of marijuana. This policy statement provides the position of the American Academy of Pediatrics on the issue of marijuana legalization. The accompanying technical report reviews what is currently known about the relationships of marijuana use with health and the developing brain and the legal status of marijuana and adolescents' use of marijuana to better understand how change in legal status might influence the degree of marijuana use by adolescents in the future. (2/15)

http://pediatrics.aappublications.org/content/135/3/584

THE IMPACT OF MARIJUANA POLICIES ON YOUTH: CLINICAL, RESEARCH, AND LEGAL UPDATE (TECHNICAL REPORT)

Seth Ammerman, MD, FAAP; Sheryl Ryan, MD, FAAP; William P. Adelman, MD, FAAP; Committee on Substance Abuse; and Committee on Adolescence

ABSTRACT. This technical report updates the 2004 American Academy of Pediatrics technical report on the legalization of marijuana. Current epidemiology of marijuana use is presented, as are definitions and biology of marijuana compounds, side effects of marijuana use, and effects of use on adolescent brain development. Issues concerning medical marijuana specifically are also addressed. Concerning legalization of marijuana, 4 different approaches in the United States are discussed: legalization of marijuana solely for medical purposes, decriminalization of recreational use of marijuana, legalization of recreational use of marijuana, and criminal prosecution of recreational (and medical) use of marijuana. These approaches are compared, and the latest available data are presented to aid in forming public policy. The effects on youth of criminal penalties for marijuana use and possession are also addressed, as are the effects or potential effects of the other 3 policy approaches on adolescent marijuana use. Recommendations are included in the accompanying policy statement. (2/15)

http://pediatrics.aappublications.org/content/135/3/e769

THE IMPACT OF SOCIAL MEDIA ON CHILDREN, ADOLESCENTS, AND FAMILIES (CLINICAL REPORT)

Gwenn Schurgin O'Keeffe, MD; Kathleen Clarke-Pearson, MD; and Council on Communications and Media

ABSTRACT. Using social media Web sites is among the most common activity of today's children and adolescents. Any Web site that allows social interaction is considered a social media site, including social networking sites such as Facebook, MySpace, and Twitter; gaming sites and virtual worlds such as Club Penguin, Second Life, and the Sims; video sites such as YouTube; and blogs. Such sites offer today's youth a portal for entertainment and communication and have grown exponentially in recent years. For this reason, it is important that parents become aware of the nature of social media sites, given that not all of them are healthy environments for children and adolescents. Pediatricians are in a unique position to help families understand these sites and to encourage healthy use and urge parents to monitor for potential problems with cyberbullying, "Facebook depression," sexting, and exposure to inappropriate content. (3/11)

http://pediatrics.aappublications.org/content/127/4/800

THE IMPORTANCE OF PLAY IN PROMOTING HEALTHY CHILD DEVELOPMENT AND MAINTAINING STRONG PARENT-CHILD BOND: FOCUS ON CHILDREN IN POVERTY (CLINICAL REPORT)

Regina M. Milteer, MD; Kenneth R. Ginsburg, MD, MSEd; Council on Communications and Media; and Committee on Psychosocial Aspects of Child and Family Health

ABSTRACT. Play is essential to the social, emotional, cognitive, and physical well-being of children beginning in early childhood. It is a natural tool for children to develop resiliency as they learn to cooperate, overcome challenges, and negotiate with others. Play also allows children to be creative. It provides time for parents to be fully engaged with their children, to bond with their children, and to see the world from the perspective of their child. However, children who live in poverty often face socioeconomic obstacles that impede their rights to have playtime, thus affecting their healthy social-emotional development. For children who are underresourced to reach their highest potential, it is essential that parents, educators, and pediatricians recognize the importance of lifelong benefits that children gain from play. (12/11, reaffirmed 9/15)

http://pediatrics.aappublications.org/content/129/1/e204

INCIDENTAL FINDINGS ON BRAIN AND SPINE IMAGING IN CHILDREN (CLINICAL REPORT)

Cormac O. Maher, MD, FAAP; Joseph H. Piatt Jr, MD, FAAP; and Section on Neurologic Surgery

ABSTRACT. In recent years, the utilization of diagnostic imaging of the brain and spine in children has increased dramatically, leading to a corresponding increase in the detection of incidental findings of the central nervous system. Patients with unexpected findings on imaging are often referred for subspecialty evaluation. Even with rational use of diagnostic imaging and subspecialty consultation, the diagnostic process will always generate unexpected findings that must be explained and managed. Familiarity with the most common findings that are discovered incidentally on diagnostic imaging of the brain and spine will assist the pediatrician in providing counseling to families and in making recommendations in conjunction with a neurosurgeon, when needed, regarding additional treatments and prognosis. (3/15)

http://pediatrics.aappublications.org/content/135/4/e1084

INCORPORATING RECOGNITION AND MANAGEMENT OF PERINATAL AND POSTPARTUM DEPRESSION INTO PEDIATRIC PRACTICE (CLINICAL REPORT)

Marian F. Earls, MD, and Committee on Psychosocial Aspects of Child and Family Health

ABSTRACT. Every year, more than 400 000 infants are born to mothers who are depressed, which makes perinatal depression the most underdiagnosed obstetric complication in America. Postpartum depression leads to increased costs of medical care, inappropriate medical care, child abuse and neglect, discontinuation of breastfeeding, and family dysfunction and adversely affects early brain development. Pediatric practices, as medical

homes, can establish a system to implement postpartum depression screening and to identify and use community resources for the treatment and referral of the depressed mother and support for the mother-child (dyad) relationship. This system would have a positive effect on the health and well-being of the infant and family. State chapters of the American Academy of Pediatrics, working with state Early Periodic Screening, Diagnosis, and Treatment (EPSDT) and maternal and child health programs, can increase awareness of the need for perinatal depression screening in the obstetric and pediatric periodicity of care schedules and ensure payment. Pediatricians must advocate for workforce development for professionals who care for very young children and for promotion of evidence-based interventions focused on healthy attachment and parent-child relationships. (10/10, reaffirmed 12/14)
http://pediatrics.aappublications.org/content/126/5/1032

INCREASING ANTIRETROVIRAL DRUG ACCESS FOR CHILDREN WITH HIV INFECTION

Committee on Pediatric AIDS and Section on International Child Health
ABSTRACT. Although there have been great gains in the prevention of pediatric HIV infection and provision of antiretroviral therapy for children with HIV infection in resource-rich countries, many barriers remain to scaling up HIV prevention and treatment for children in resource-limited areas of the world. Appropriate testing technologies need to be made more widely available to identify HIV infection in infants. Training of practitioners in the skills required to care for children with HIV infection is required to increase the number of children receiving antiretroviral therapy. Lack of availability of appropriate antiretroviral drug formulations that are easily usable and inexpensive is a major impediment to optimal care for children with HIV. The time and energy spent trying to develop liquid antiretroviral formulations might be better used in the manufacture of smaller pill sizes or crushable tablets, which are easier to dispense, transport, store, and administer to children. (4/07, reaffirmed 4/10, 4/16)
http://pediatrics.aappublications.org/content/119/4/838

INCREASING IMMUNIZATION COVERAGE

Committee on Practice and Ambulatory Medicine and Council on Community Pediatrics
ABSTRACT. In 1977, the American Academy of Pediatrics issued a statement calling for universal immunization of all children for whom vaccines are not contraindicated. In 1995, the policy statement "Implementation of the Immunization Policy" was published by the American Academy of Pediatrics, followed in 2003 with publication of the first version of this statement, "Increasing Immunization Coverage." Since 2003, there have continued to be improvements in immunization coverage, with progress toward meeting the goals set forth in *Healthy People 2010*. Data from the 2007 National Immunization Survey showed that 90% of children 19 to 35 months of age have received recommended doses of each of the following vaccines: inactivated poliovirus (IPV), measles-mumps-rubella (MMR), varicella-zoster virus (VZB), hepatitis B virus (HBV), and *Haemophilus influenzae* type b (Hib). For diphtheria and tetanus and acellular pertussis (DTaP) vaccine, 84.5% have received the recommended 4 doses by 35 months of age. Nevertheless, the *Healthy People 2010* goal of at least 80% coverage for the full series (at least 4 doses of DTaP, 3 doses of IPV, 1 dose of MMR, 3 doses of Hib, 3 doses of HBV, and 1 dose of varicella-zoster virus vaccine) has not yet been met, and immunization coverage of adolescents continues to lag behind the goals set forth in *Healthy People 2010*. Despite these encouraging data, a vast number of new challenges that threaten continued success toward the goal of universal immunization coverage have emerged. These challenges include an increase in new vaccines and new vaccine combinations as well as a significant

number of vaccines currently under development; a dramatic increase in the acquisition cost of vaccines, coupled with a lack of adequate payment to practitioners to buy and administer vaccines; unanticipated manufacturing and delivery problems that have caused significant shortages of various vaccine products; and the rise of a public antivaccination movement that uses the Internet as well as standard media outlets to advance a position, wholly unsupported by any scientific evidence, linking vaccines with various childhood conditions, particularly autism. Much remains to be accomplished by physician organizations; vaccine manufacturers; third-party payers; the media; and local, state, and federal governments to ensure dependable vaccine supply and payments that are sufficient to continue to provide immunizations in public and private settings and to promote effective strategies to combat unjustified misstatements by the antivaccination movement.

Pediatricians should work individually and collectively at the local, state, and national levels to ensure that all children without a valid contraindication receive all childhood immunizations on time. Pediatricians and pediatric organizations, in conjunction with government agencies such as the Centers for Disease Control and Prevention, must communicate effectively with parents to maximize their understanding of the overall safety and efficacy of vaccines. Most parents and children have not experienced many of the vaccine-preventable diseases, and the general public is not well informed about the risks and sequelae of these conditions. A number of recommendations are included for pediatricians, individually and collectively, to support further progress toward the goal of universal immunization coverage of all children for whom vaccines are not contraindicated. (5/10)
http://pediatrics.aappublications.org/content/125/6/1295

THE INDIVIDUALS WITH DISABILITIES EDUCATION ACT (IDEA) FOR CHILDREN WITH SPECIAL EDUCATIONAL NEEDS (CLINICAL REPORT)

Paul H. Lipkin, MD, FAAP; Jeffrey Okamoto, MD, FAAP; Council on Children With Disabilities; and Council on School Health
ABSTRACT. The pediatric health care provider has a critical role in supporting the health and well-being of children and adolescents in all settings, including early intervention (EI), preschool, and school environments. It is estimated that 15% of children in the United States have a disability. The Individuals with Disabilities Education Act entitles every affected child in the United States from infancy to young adulthood to a free appropriate public education through EI and special education services. These services bolster development and learning of children with various disabilities. This clinical report provides the pediatric health care provider with a summary of key components of the most recent version of this law. Guidance is also provided to ensure that every child in need receives the EI and special education services to which he or she is entitled. (11/15)
http://pediatrics.aappublications.org/content/136/6/e1650

INDOOR ENVIRONMENTAL CONTROL PRACTICES AND ASTHMA MANAGEMENT (CLINICAL REPORT)

Elizabeth C. Matsui, MD, MHS, FAAP; Stuart L. Abramson, MD, PhD, AE-C, FAAP; Megan T. Sandel, MD, MPH, FAAP; Section on Allergy and Immunology; and Council on Environmental Health
ABSTRACT. Indoor environmental exposures, particularly allergens and pollutants, are major contributors to asthma morbidity in children; environmental control practices aimed at reducing these exposures are an integral component of asthma management. Some individually tailored environmental control practices that have been shown to reduce asthma symptoms and exacerbations are similar in efficacy and cost to controller medications. As a part of developing tailored strategies regarding environmental control measures, an environmental history can

be obtained to evaluate the key indoor environmental exposures that are known to trigger asthma symptoms and exacerbations, including both indoor pollutants and allergens. An environmental history includes questions regarding the presence of pets or pests or evidence of pests in the home, as well as knowledge regarding whether the climatic characteristics in the community favor dust mites. In addition, the history focuses on sources of indoor air pollution, including the presence of smokers who live in the home or care for children and the use of gas stoves and appliances in the home. Serum allergen-specific immunoglobulin E antibody tests can be performed or the patient can be referred for allergy skin testing to identify indoor allergens that are most likely to be clinically relevant. Environmental control strategies are tailored to each potentially relevant indoor exposure and are based on knowledge of the sources and underlying characteristics of the exposure. Strategies include source removal, source control, and mitigation strategies, such as high-efficiency particulate air purifiers and allergen-proof mattress and pillow encasements, as well as education, which can be delivered by primary care pediatricians, allergists, pediatric pulmonologists, other health care workers, or community health workers trained in asthma environmental control and asthma education. (10/16)
http://pediatrics.aappublications.org/content/138/5/e20162589

INFANT FEEDING AND TRANSMISSION OF HUMAN IMMUNODEFICIENCY VIRUS IN THE UNITED STATES
Committee on Pediatric AIDS
ABSTRACT. Physicians caring for infants born to women infected with HIV are likely to be involved in providing guidance to HIV-infected mothers on appropriate infant feeding practices. It is critical that physicians are aware of the HIV transmission risk from human milk and the current recommendations for feeding HIV-exposed infants in the United States. Because the only intervention to completely prevent HIV transmission via human milk is not to breastfeed, in the United States, where clean water and affordable replacement feeding are available, the American Academy of Pediatrics recommends that HIV-infected mothers not breastfeed their infants, regardless of maternal viral load and antiretroviral therapy. (1/13, reaffirmed 4/16)
http://pediatrics.aappublications.org/content/131/2/391

INFANT METHEMOGLOBINEMIA: THE ROLE OF DIETARY NITRATE IN FOOD AND WATER (CLINICAL REPORT)
Frank R. Greer, MD; Michael Shannon, MD; Committee on Nutrition; and Committee on Environmental Health
ABSTRACT. Infants for whom formula may be prepared with well water remain a high-risk group for nitrate poisoning. This clinical report reinforces the need for testing of well water for nitrate content. There seems to be little or no risk of nitrate poisoning from commercially prepared infant foods in the United States. However, reports of nitrate poisoning from home-prepared vegetable foods for infants continue to occur. Breastfeeding infants are not at risk of methemoglobinemia even when mothers ingest water with very high concentrations of nitrate nitrogen (100 ppm). (9/05, reaffirmed 4/09)
http://pediatrics.aappublications.org/content/116/3/784

INFECTION PREVENTION AND CONTROL IN PEDIATRIC AMBULATORY SETTINGS
Mobeen H. Rathore, MD, FAAP; Mary Anne Jackson, MD, FAAP; and Committee on Infectious Diseases
ABSTRACT. Since the American Academy of Pediatrics published its statement titled "Infection Prevention and Control in Pediatric Ambulatory Settings" in 2007, there have been significant changes that prompted this updated statement. Infection prevention and control is an integral part of pediatric practice in ambulatory medical settings as well as in hospitals. Infection prevention and control practices should begin at the time the ambulatory visit is scheduled. All health care personnel should be educated regarding the routes of transmission and techniques used to prevent the transmission of infectious agents. Policies for infection prevention and control should be written, readily available, updated every 2 years, and enforced. Many of the recommendations for infection control and prevention from the Centers for Disease Control and Prevention for hospitalized patients are also applicable in the ambulatory setting. These recommendations include requirements for pediatricians to take precautions to identify and protect employees likely to be exposed to blood or other potentially infectious materials while on the job. In addition to emphasizing the key principles of infection prevention and control in this policy, we update those that are relevant to the ambulatory care patient. These guidelines emphasize the role of hand hygiene and the implementation of diagnosis- and syndrome-specific isolation precautions, with the exemption of the use of gloves for routine diaper changes and wiping a well child's nose or tears for most patient encounters. Additional topics include respiratory hygiene and cough etiquette strategies for patients with a respiratory tract infection, including those relevant for special populations like patients with cystic fibrosis or those in short-term residential facilities; separation of infected, contagious children from uninfected children when feasible; safe handling and disposal of needles and other sharp medical devices; appropriate use of personal protective equipment, such as gloves, gowns, masks, and eye protection; and appropriate use of sterilization, disinfection, and antisepsis. Lastly, in this policy, we emphasize the importance of public health interventions, including vaccination for patients and health care personnel, and outline the responsibilities of the health care provider related to prompt public health notification for specific reportable diseases and communication with colleagues who may be providing subsequent care of an infected patient to optimize the use of isolation precautions and limit the spread of contagions. (10/17)
http://pediatrics.aappublications.org/content/140/5/e20172857

INFECTIOUS COMPLICATIONS WITH THE USE OF BIOLOGIC RESPONSE MODIFIERS IN INFANTS AND CHILDREN (CLINICAL REPORT)
H. Dele Davies, MD, FAAP, and Committee on Infectious Diseases
ABSTRACT. Biologic response modifiers (BRMs) are substances that interact with and modify the host immune system. BRMs that dampen the immune system are used to treat conditions such as juvenile idiopathic arthritis, psoriatic arthritis, or inflammatory bowel disease and often in combination with other immunosuppressive agents, such as methotrexate and corticosteroids. Cytokines that are targeted include tumor necrosis factor α; interleukins (ILs) 6, 12, and 23; and the receptors for IL-1α (IL-1A) and IL-1β (IL-1B) as well as other molecules. Although the risk varies with the class of BRM, patients receiving immune-dampening BRMs generally are at increased risk of infection or reactivation with mycobacterial infections (*Mycobacterium tuberculosis* and nontuberculous mycobacteria), some viral (herpes simplex virus, varicella-zoster virus, Epstein-Barr virus, hepatitis B) and fungal (histoplasmosis, coccidioidomycosis) infections, as well as other opportunistic infections. The use of BRMs warrants careful determination of infectious risk on the basis of history (including exposure, residence, and travel and immunization history) and selected baseline screening test results. Routine immunizations should be given at least 2 weeks (inactivated or subunit vaccines) or 4 weeks (live vaccines) before initiation of BRMs whenever feasible, and inactivated influenza vaccine should be given annually. Inactivated and subunit vaccines should be given when needed while taking BRMs, but live vaccines should be avoided unless under special circumstances in consultation with an infectious diseases specialist. If the patient develops a febrile or serious respiratory illness during BRM

therapy, consideration should be given to stopping the BRM while actively searching for and treating possible infectious causes. (7/16)
http://pediatrics.aappublications.org/content/138/2/e20161209

INFECTIOUS DISEASES ASSOCIATED WITH ORGANIZED SPORTS AND OUTBREAK CONTROL (CLINICAL REPORT)

H. Dele Davies, MD, MS, MHCM, FAAP; Mary Anne Jackson, MD, FAAP; Stephen G. Rice, MD, PhD, MPH, FAAP; Committee on Infectious Diseases; and Council on Sports Medicine and Fitness

ABSTRACT. Participation in organized sports has a variety of health benefits but also has the potential to expose the athlete to a variety of infectious diseases, some of which may produce outbreaks. Major risk factors for infection include skin-to-skin contact with athletes who have active skin infections, environmental exposures and physical trauma, and sharing of equipment and contact with contaminated fomites. Close contact that is intrinsic to team sports and psychosocial factors associated with adolescence are additional risks. Minimizing risk requires leadership by the organized sports community (including the athlete's primary care provider) and depends on outlining key hygiene behaviors, recognition, diagnosis, and treatment of common sports-related infections, and the implementation of preventive interventions. (9/17)
http://pediatrics.aappublications.org/content/140/4/e20172477

INFLUENZA IMMUNIZATION FOR ALL HEALTH CARE PERSONNEL: KEEP IT MANDATORY

Committee on Infectious Diseases

ABSTRACT. The purpose of this statement is to reaffirm the American Academy of Pediatrics' support for a mandatory influenza immunization policy for all health care personnel. With an increasing number of organizations requiring influenza vaccination, coverage among health care personnel has risen to 75% in the 2013 to 2014 influenza season but still remains below the Healthy People 2020 objective of 90%. Mandatory influenza immunization for all health care personnel is ethical, just, and necessary to improve patient safety. It is a crucial step in efforts to reduce health care–associated influenza infections. (9/15)
http://pediatrics.aappublications.org/content/136/4/809

INFORMED CONSENT IN DECISION-MAKING IN PEDIATRIC PRACTICE

Committee on Bioethics

ABSTRACT. Informed consent should be seen as an essential part of health care practice; parental permission and childhood assent is an active process that engages patients, both adults and children, in health care. Pediatric practice is unique in that developmental maturation allows, over time, for increasing inclusion of the child's and adolescent's opinion in medical decision-making in clinical practice and research. (7/16)
http://pediatrics.aappublications.org/content/138/2/e20161484

INFORMED CONSENT IN DECISION-MAKING IN PEDIATRIC PRACTICE (TECHNICAL REPORT)

Aviva L. Katz, MD, FAAP; Sally A. Webb, MD, FAAP; and Committee on Bioethics

ABSTRACT. Informed consent should be seen as an essential part of health care practice; parental permission and childhood assent is an active process that engages patients, both adults and children, in their health care. Pediatric practice is unique in that developmental maturation allows, over time, for increasing inclusion of the child's and adolescent's opinion in medical decision-making in clinical practice and research. This technical report, which accompanies the policy statement "Informed Consent in Decision-Making in Pediatric Practice," was written to provide a broader background on the nature of informed

consent, surrogate decision-making in pediatric practice, information on child and adolescent decision-making, and special issues in adolescent informed consent, assent, and refusal. It is anticipated that this information will help provide support for the recommendations included in the policy statement. (7/16)
http://pediatrics.aappublications.org/content/138/2/e20161485

INJURIES ASSOCIATED WITH INFANT WALKERS

Committee on Injury and Poison Prevention

ABSTRACT. In 1999, an estimated 8800 children younger than 15 months were treated in hospital emergency departments in the United States for injuries associated with infant walkers. Thirty-four infant walker-related deaths were reported from 1973 through 1998. The vast majority of injuries occur from falls down stairs, and head injuries are common. Walkers do not help a child learn to walk; indeed, they can delay normal motor and mental development. The use of warning labels, public education, adult supervision during walker use, and stair gates have all been demonstrated to be insufficient strategies to prevent injuries associated with infant walkers. To comply with the revised voluntary standard (ASTM F977-96), walkers manufactured after June 30, 1997, must be wider than a 36-in doorway or must have a braking mechanism designed to stop the walker if 1 or more wheels drop off the riding surface, such as at the top of a stairway. Because data indicate a considerable risk of major and minor injury and even death from the use of infant walkers, and because there is no clear benefit from their use, the American Academy of Pediatrics recommends a ban on the manufacture and sale of mobile infant walkers. If a parent insists on using a mobile infant walker, it is vital that they choose a walker that meets the performance standards of ASTM F977-96 to prevent falls down stairs. Stationary activity centers should be promoted as a safer alternative to mobile infant walkers. (9/01, reaffirmed 1/05, 2/08, 10/11, 11/14)
http://pediatrics.aappublications.org/content/108/3/790

INJURIES IN YOUTH SOCCER (CLINICAL REPORT)

Chris G. Koutures, MD; Andrew J. M. Gregory, MD; and Council on Sports Medicine and Fitness

ABSTRACT. Injury rates in youth soccer, known as football outside the United States, are higher than in many other contact/collision sports and have greater relative numbers in younger, preadolescent players. With regard to musculoskeletal injuries, young females tend to suffer more knee injuries, and young males suffer more ankle injuries. Concussions are fairly prevalent in soccer as a result of contact/collision rather than purposeful attempts at heading the ball. Appropriate rule enforcement and emphasis on safe play can reduce the risk of soccer-related injuries. This report serves as a basis for encouraging safe participation in soccer for children and adolescents. (1/10, reaffirmed 5/13, 4/17)
http://pediatrics.aappublications.org/content/125/2/410

INJURY RISK OF NONPOWDER GUNS (TECHNICAL REPORT)

Committee on Injury, Violence, and Poison Prevention

ABSTRACT. Nonpowder guns (ball-bearing [BB] guns, pellet guns, air rifles, paintball guns) continue to cause serious injuries to children and adolescents. The muzzle velocity of these guns can range from approximately 150 ft/second to 1200 ft/second (the muzzle velocities of traditional firearm pistols are 750 ft/second to 1450 ft/second). Both low- and high-velocity nonpowder guns are associated with serious injuries, and fatalities can result from high-velocity guns. A persisting problem is the lack of medical recognition of the severity of injuries that can result from these guns, including penetration of the eye, skin, internal organs, and bone. Nationally, in 2000, there were an estimated 21840 (coefficient of variation: 0.0821) injuries related to nonpowder guns, with approximately 4% resulting in hospital-ization. Between 1990 and 2000, the US Consumer Product Safety Commission reported 39 nonpowder gun–related deaths, of which 32 were children younger than 15 years. The introduction of high-powered air rifles in the 1970s has been associated with approximately 4 deaths per year. The advent of war games and the use of paintball guns have resulted in a number of reports of injuries, especially to the eye. Injuries associated with nonpow-der guns should receive prompt medical management similar to the management of firearm-related injuries, and nonpowder guns should never be characterized as toys. (11/04, reaffirmed 2/08, 10/11)

http://pediatrics.aappublications.org/content/114/5/1357

IN-LINE SKATING INJURIES IN CHILDREN AND ADOLESCENTS

Committee on Injury and Poison Prevention and Committee on Sports Medicine and Fitness

ABSTRACT. In-line skating has become one of the fastest-growing recreational sports in the United States. Recent studies emphasize the value of protective gear in reducing the incidence of injuries. Recommendations are provided for parents and pedi-atricians, with special emphasis on the novice or inexperienced skater. (4/98, reaffirmed 1/02, 1/06, 1/09, 11/11)

http://pediatrics.aappublications.org/content/101/4/720

INSTITUTIONAL ETHICS COMMITTEES

Committee on Bioethics

ABSTRACT. In hospitals throughout the United States, institu-tional ethics committees (IECs) have become a standard vehicle for the education of health professionals about biomedical ethics, for the drafting and review of hospital policy, and for clinical ethics case consultation. In addition, there is increasing interest in a role for the IEC in organizational ethics. Recommendations are made about the membership and structure of an IEC, and guidelines are provided for those serving on an ethics commit-tee. (1/01, reaffirmed 1/04, 1/09, 10/12, 7/14)

http://pediatrics.aappublications.org/content/107/1/205

INSTRUMENT-BASED PEDIATRIC VISION SCREENING POLICY STATEMENT

Section on Ophthalmology and Committee on Practice and Ambulatory Medicine (joint with American Academy of Ophthalmology, American Association for Pediatric Ophthalmology and Strabismus, and American Association of Certified Orthoptists)

ABSTRACT. A policy statement describing the use of automated vision screening technology (instrument-based vision screen-ing) is presented. Screening for amblyogenic refractive error with instrument-based screening is not dependent on behav-ioral responses of children, as when visual acuity is measured. Instrument-based screening is quick, requires minimal coopera-tion of the child, and is especially useful in the preverbal, prelit-erate, or developmentally delayed child. Children younger than 4 years can benefit from instrument-based screening, and visual acuity testing can be used reliably in older children. Adoption of this new technology is highly dependent on third-party payment policies, which could present a significant barrier to adoption. (10/12)

http://pediatrics.aappublications.org/content/130/5/983

INSUFFICIENT SLEEP IN ADOLESCENTS AND YOUNG ADULTS: AN UPDATE ON CAUSES AND CONSEQUENCES (TECHNICAL REPORT)

Judith Owens, MD, MPH, FAAP; Adolescent Sleep Working Group; and Committee on Adolescence

ABSTRACT. Chronic sleep loss and associated sleepiness and daytime impairments in adolescence are a serious threat to the academic success, health, and safety of our nation's youth and an important public health issue. Understanding the extent and potential short- and long-term repercussions of sleep restric-tion, as well as the unhealthy sleep practices and environmental factors that contribute to sleep loss in adolescents, is key in set-ting public policies to mitigate these effects and in counseling patients and families in the clinical setting. This report reviews the current literature on sleep patterns in adolescents, factors contributing to chronic sleep loss (ie, electronic media use, caf-feine consumption), and health-related consequences, such as depression, increased obesity risk, and higher rates of drowsy driving accidents. The report also discusses the potential role of later school start times as a means of reducing adolescent sleepi-ness. (8/14)

http://pediatrics.aappublications.org/content/134/3/e921

INSURANCE COVERAGE OF MENTAL HEALTH AND SUBSTANCE ABUSE SERVICES FOR CHILDREN AND ADOLESCENTS: A CONSENSUS STATEMENT

American Academy of Pediatrics and Others (10/00)

http://pediatrics.aappublications.org/content/106/4/860

INTENSIVE TRAINING AND SPORTS SPECIALIZATION IN YOUNG ATHLETES

Committee on Sports Medicine and Fitness

ABSTRACT. Children involved in sports should be encouraged to participate in a variety of different activities and develop a wide range of skills. Young athletes who specialize in just one sport may be denied the benefits of varied activity while facing additional physical, physiologic, and psychologic demands from intense training and competition.

This statement reviews the potential risks of high-intensity training and sports specialization in young athletes. Pediatricians who recognize these risks can have a key role in monitoring the health of these young athletes and helping reduce risks associ-ated with high-level sports participation. (7/00, reaffirmed 11/04, 1/06, 5/09, 10/14)

http://pediatrics.aappublications.org/content/106/1/154

INTERFERON-γ RELEASE ASSAYS FOR DIAGNOSIS OF TUBERCULOSIS INFECTION AND DISEASE IN CHILDREN (TECHNICAL REPORT)

Jeffrey R. Starke, MD, FAAP, and Committee on Infectious Diseases

ABSTRACT. Tuberculosis (TB) remains an important prob-lem among children in the United States and throughout the world. Although diagnosis and treatment of infection with *Mycobacterium tuberculosis* (also referred to as latent tuberculosis infection [LTBI] or TB infection) remain the lynchpins of TB pre-vention, there is no diagnostic reference standard for LTBI. The tuberculin skin test (TST) has many limitations, including diffi-culty in administration and interpretation, the need for a return visit by the patient, and false-positive results caused by signifi-cant cross-reaction with *Mycobacterium bovis*–bacille Calmette-Guérin (BCG) vaccines and many nontuberculous mycobacteria. Interferon-γ release assays (IGRAs) are blood tests that measure ex vivo T-lymphocyte release of interferon-γ after stimulation by antigens specific for *M tuberculosis*. Because these antigens are not found on *M bovis*–BCG or most nontuberculous mycobacte-ria, IGRAs are more specific tests than the TST, yielding fewer false-positive results. However, IGRAs have little advantage over the TST in sensitivity, and both methods have reduced sensitivity in immunocompromised children, including children with severe TB disease. Both methods have a higher positive predictive value when applied to children with risk factors for LTBI. Unfortunately, neither method distinguishes between TB infection and TB disease. The objective of this technical report is to review what IGRAs are most useful for: (1) increasing test specificity in children who have received a BCG vaccine and

may have a false-positive TST result; (2) using with the TST to increase sensitivity for finding LTBI in patients at high risk of developing progression from LTBI to disease; and (3) helping to diagnose TB disease. (11/14)
http://pediatrics.aappublications.org/content/134/6/e1763

INTERPRETATION OF DO NOT ATTEMPT RESUSCITATION ORDERS FOR CHILDREN REQUIRING ANESTHESIA AND SURGERY (CLINICAL REPORT)

Mary E. Fallat, MD, FAAP; Courtney Hardy, MD, MBA, FAAP; Section on Surgery; Section on Anesthesiology and Pain Medicine; and Committee on Bioethics

ABSTRACT. This clinical report addresses the topic of pre-existing do not attempt resuscitation or limited resuscitation orders for children and adolescents undergoing anesthesia and surgery. Pertinent considerations for the clinician include the rights of children, decision-making by parents or legally approved representatives, the process of informed consent, and the roles of surgeon and anesthesiologist. A process of re-evaluation of the do not attempt resuscitation orders, called "required reconsideration," should be incorporated into the process of informed consent for surgery and anesthesia, distinguishing between goal-directed and procedure-directed approaches. The child's individual needs are best served by allowing the parent or legally approved representative and involved clinicians to consider whether full resuscitation, limitations based on procedures, or limitations based on goals is most appropriate. (4/18)
See full text on page 693.
http://pediatrics.aappublications.org/content/141/5/e20180598

INTIMATE PARTNER VIOLENCE: THE ROLE OF THE PEDIATRICIAN (CLINICAL REPORT)

Jonathan D. Thackeray, MD; Roberta Hibbard, MD; M. Denise Dowd, MD, MPH; Committee on Child Abuse and Neglect; and Committee on Injury, Violence, and Poison Prevention

ABSTRACT. The American Academy of Pediatrics and its members recognize the importance of improving the physician's ability to recognize intimate partner violence (IPV) and understand its effects on child health and development and its role in the continuum of family violence. Pediatricians are in a unique position to identify abused caregivers in pediatric settings and to evaluate and treat children raised in homes in which IPV may occur. Children exposed to IPV are at increased risk of being abused and neglected and are more likely to develop adverse health, behavioral, psychological, and social disorders later in life. Identifying IPV, therefore, may be one of the most effective means of preventing child abuse and identifying caregivers and children who may be in need of treatment and/or therapy. Pediatricians should be aware of the profound effects of exposure to IPV on children. (4/10, reaffirmed 1/14)
http://pediatrics.aappublications.org/content/125/5/1094

IODINE DEFICIENCY, POLLUTANT CHEMICALS, AND THE THYROID: NEW INFORMATION ON AN OLD PROBLEM

Council on Environmental Health

ABSTRACT. Many women of reproductive age in the United States are marginally iodine deficient, perhaps because the salt in processed foods is not iodized. Iodine deficiency, per se, can interfere with normal brain development in their offspring; in addition, it increases vulnerability to the effects of certain environmental pollutants, such as nitrate, thiocyanate, and perchlorate. Although pregnant and lactating women should take a supplement containing adequate iodide, only about 15% do so. Such supplements, however, may not contain enough iodide and may not be labeled accurately. The American Thyroid Association recommends that pregnant and lactating women take a supplement with adequate iodide. The American Academy of Pediatrics recommends that pregnant and lactating

women also avoid exposure to excess nitrate, which would usually occur from contaminated well water, and thiocyanate, which is in cigarette smoke. Perchlorate is currently a candidate for regulation as a water pollutant. The Environmental Protection Agency should proceed with appropriate regulation, and the Food and Drug Administration should address the mislabeling of the iodine content of prenatal/lactation supplements. (5/14)
http://pediatrics.aappublications.org/content/133/6/1163

LACTOSE INTOLERANCE IN INFANTS, CHILDREN, AND ADOLESCENTS (CLINICAL REPORT)

Melvin B. Heyman, MD, MPH, for Committee on Nutrition

ABSTRACT. The American Academy of Pediatrics Committee on Nutrition presents an updated review of lactose intolerance in infants, children, and adolescents. Differences between primary, secondary, congenital, and developmental lactase deficiency that may result in lactose intolerance are discussed. Children with suspected lactose intolerance can be assessed clinically by dietary lactose elimination or by tests including noninvasive hydrogen breath testing or invasive intestinal biopsy determination of lactase (and other disaccharidase) concentrations. Treatment consists of use of lactase-treated dairy products or oral lactase supplementation, limitation of lactose-containing foods, or dairy elimination. The American Academy of Pediatrics supports use of dairy foods as an important source of calcium for bone mineral health and of other nutrients that facilitate growth in children and adolescents. If dairy products are eliminated, other dietary sources of calcium or calcium supplements need to be provided. (9/06, reaffirmed 8/12)
http://pediatrics.aappublications.org/content/118/3/1279

"LATE-PRETERM" INFANTS: A POPULATION AT RISK (CLINICAL REPORT)

William A. Engle, MD; Kay M. Tomashek, MD; Carol Wallman, MSN; and Committee on Fetus and Newborn

ABSTRACT. Late-preterm infants, defined by birth at $34^6/_7$ through $36^6/_7$ weeks' gestation, are less physiologically and metabolically mature than term infants. Thus, they are at higher risk of morbidity and mortality than term infants. The purpose of this report is to define "late preterm," recommend a change in terminology from "near term" to "late preterm," present the characteristics of late-preterm infants that predispose them to a higher risk of morbidity and mortality than term infants, and propose guidelines for the evaluation and management of these infants after birth. (12/07, reaffirmed 5/10, 6/18)
http://pediatrics.aappublications.org/content/120/6/1390

LAWN MOWER-RELATED INJURIES TO CHILDREN

Committee on Injury and Poison Prevention

ABSTRACT. Lawn mower-related injuries to children are relatively common and can result in severe injury or death. Many amputations during childhood are caused by power mowers. Pediatricians have an important role as advocates and educators to promote the prevention of these injuries. (6/01, reaffirmed 10/04, 5/07, 6/10)
http://pediatrics.aappublications.org/content/107/6/1480

LAWN MOWER-RELATED INJURIES TO CHILDREN (TECHNICAL REPORT)

Committee on Injury and Poison Prevention

ABSTRACT. In the United States, approximately 9400 children younger than 18 years receive emergency treatment annually for lawn mower-related injuries. More than 7% of these children require hospitalization, and power mowers cause a large proportion of the amputations during childhood. Prevention of lawn mower-related injuries can be achieved by design changes of lawn mowers, guidelines for mower operation, and education of parents, child caregivers, and children. Pediatricians have

an important role as advocates and educators to promote the prevention of these injuries. (6/01, reaffirmed 10/04, 5/07, 6/10)
http://pediatrics.aappublications.org/content/107/6/e106

LEARNING DISABILITIES, DYSLEXIA, AND VISION

Section on Ophthalmology and Council on Children With Disabilities (joint with American Academy of Ophthalmology, American Association for Pediatric Ophthalmology and Strabismus, and American Association of Certified Orthoptists)

ABSTRACT. Learning disabilities, including reading disabilities, are commonly diagnosed in children. Their etiologies are multifactorial, reflecting genetic influences and dysfunction of brain systems. Learning disabilities are complex problems that require complex solutions. Early recognition and referral to qualified educational professionals for evidence-based evaluations and treatments seem necessary to achieve the best possible outcome. Most experts believe that dyslexia is a language-based disorder. Vision problems can interfere with the process of learning; however, vision problems are not the cause of primary dyslexia or learning disabilities. Scientific evidence does not support the efficacy of eye exercises, behavioral vision therapy, or special tinted filters or lenses for improving the long-term educational performance in these complex pediatric neurocognitive conditions. Diagnostic and treatment approaches that lack scientific evidence of efficacy, including eye exercises, behavioral vision therapy, or special tinted filters or lenses, are not endorsed and should not be recommended. (7/09, reaffirmed 7/14)
http://pediatrics.aappublications.org/content/124/2/837

LEARNING DISABILITIES, DYSLEXIA, AND VISION (TECHNICAL REPORT)

Sheryl M. Handler, MD; Walter M. Fierson, MD; and Section on Ophthalmology and Council on Children With Disabilities (joint with American Academy of Ophthalmology, American Association for Pediatric Ophthalmology and Strabismus, and American Association of Certified Orthoptists)

ABSTRACT. Learning disabilities constitute a diverse group of disorders in which children who generally possess at least average intelligence have problems processing information or generating output. Their etiologies are multifactorial and reflect genetic influences and dysfunction of brain systems. Reading disability, or dyslexia, is the most common learning disability. It is a receptive language-based learning disability that is characterized by difficulties with decoding, fluent word recognition, rapid automatic naming, and/or reading-comprehension skills. These difficulties typically result from a deficit in the phonologic component of language that makes it difficult to use the alphabetic code to decode the written word. Early recognition and referral to qualified professionals for evidence-based evaluations and treatments are necessary to achieve the best possible outcome. Because dyslexia is a language-based disorder, treatment should be directed at this etiology. Remedial programs should include specific instruction in decoding, fluency training, vocabulary, and comprehension. Most programs include daily intensive individualized instruction that explicitly teaches phonemic awareness and the application of phonics. Vision problems can interfere with the process of reading, but children with dyslexia or related learning disabilities have the same visual function and ocular health as children without such conditions. Currently, there is inadequate scientific evidence to support the view that subtle eye or visual problems cause or increase the severity of learning disabilities. Because they are difficult for the public to understand and for educators to treat, learning disabilities have spawned a wide variety of scientifically unsupported vision-based diagnostic and treatment procedures. Scientific evidence does not support the claims that visual training, muscle exercises, ocular pursuit-and-tracking exercises, behavioral/perceptual vision therapy, "training" glasses, prisms, and colored lenses and filters are effective direct or indirect treatments for learning disabilities. There is no valid evidence that children who participate in vision therapy are more responsive to educational instruction than children who do not participate. (3/11)
http://pediatrics.aappublications.org/content/127/3/e818

LEVELS OF NEONATAL CARE

Committee on Fetus and Newborn

ABSTRACT. Provision of risk-appropriate care for newborn infants and mothers was first proposed in 1976. This updated policy statement provides a review of data supporting evidence for a tiered provision of care and reaffirms the need for uniform, nationally applicable definitions and consistent standards of service for public health to improve neonatal outcomes. Facilities that provide hospital care for newborn infants should be classified on the basis of functional capabilities, and these facilities should be organized within a regionalized system of perinatal care. (8/12, reaffirmed 9/15)
http://pediatrics.aappublications.org/content/130/3/587

THE LIFELONG EFFECTS OF EARLY CHILDHOOD ADVERSITY AND TOXIC STRESS (TECHNICAL REPORT)

Jack P. Shonkoff, MD; Andrew S. Garner, MD, PhD; Committee on Psychosocial Aspects of Child and Family Health; Committee on Early Childhood, Adoption, and Dependent Care; and Section on Developmental and Behavioral Pediatrics

ABSTRACT. Advances in fields of inquiry as diverse as neuroscience, molecular biology, genomics, developmental psychology, epidemiology, sociology, and economics are catalyzing an important paradigm shift in our understanding of health and disease across the lifespan. This converging, multidisciplinary science of human development has profound implications for our ability to enhance the life prospects of children and to strengthen the social and economic fabric of society. Drawing on these multiple streams of investigation, this report presents an ecobiodevelopmental framework that illustrates how early experiences and environmental influences can leave a lasting signature on the genetic predispositions that affect emerging brain architecture and long-term health. The report also examines extensive evidence of the disruptive impacts of toxic stress, offering intriguing insights into causal mechanisms that link early adversity to later impairments in learning, behavior, and both physical and mental well-being. The implications of this framework for the practice of medicine, in general, and pediatrics, specifically, are potentially transformational. They suggest that many adult diseases should be viewed as developmental disorders that begin early in life and that persistent health disparities associated with poverty, discrimination, or maltreatment could be reduced by the alleviation of toxic stress in childhood. An ecobiodevelopmental framework also underscores the need for new thinking about the focus and boundaries of pediatric practice. It calls for pediatricians to serve as both front-line guardians of healthy child development and strategically positioned, community leaders to inform new science-based strategies that build strong foundations for educational achievement, economic productivity, responsible citizenship, and lifelong health. (12/11, reaffirmed 7/16)
http://pediatrics.aappublications.org/content/129/1/e232

LITERACY PROMOTION: AN ESSENTIAL COMPONENT OF PRIMARY CARE PEDIATRIC PRACTICE

Council on Early Childhood

ABSTRACT. Reading regularly with young children stimulates optimal patterns of brain development and strengthens parent-child relationships at a critical time in child development, which, in turn, builds language, literacy, and social-emotional skills that last a lifetime. Pediatric providers have a unique opportunity to encourage parents to engage in this important and enjoyable

activity with their children beginning in infancy. Research has revealed that parents listen and children learn as a result of literacy promotion by pediatricians, which provides a practical and evidence-based opportunity to support early brain development in primary care practice. The American Academy of Pediatrics (AAP) recommends that pediatric providers promote early literacy development for children beginning in infancy and continuing at least until the age of kindergarten entry by (1) advising all parents that reading aloud with young children can enhance parent-child relationships and prepare young minds to learn language and early literacy skills; (2) counseling all parents about developmentally appropriate shared-reading activities that are enjoyable for children and their parents and offer language-rich exposure to books, pictures, and the written word; (3) providing developmentally appropriate books given at health supervision visits for all high-risk, low-income young children; (4) using a robust spectrum of options to support and promote these efforts; and (5) partnering with other child advocates to influence national messaging and policies that support and promote these key early shared-reading experiences. The AAP supports federal and state funding for children's books to be provided at pediatric health supervision visits to children at high risk living at or near the poverty threshold and the integration of literacy promotion, an essential component of pediatric primary care, into pediatric resident education. This policy statement is supported by the AAP technical report "School Readiness" and supports the AAP policy statement "Early Childhood Adversity, Toxic Stress, and the Role of the Pediatrician: Translating Developmental Science Into Lifelong Health." (7/14)
http://pediatrics.aappublications.org/content/134/2/404

LONG-TERM FOLLOW-UP CARE FOR PEDIATRIC CANCER SURVIVORS (CLINICAL REPORT)

Section on Hematology/Oncology (joint with Children's Oncology Group)

ABSTRACT. Progress in therapy has made survival into adulthood a reality for most children, adolescents, and young adults diagnosed with cancer today. Notably, this growing population remains vulnerable to a variety of long-term therapy-related sequelae. Systematic ongoing follow-up of these patients, therefore, is important for providing for early detection of and intervention for potentially serious late-onset complications. In addition, health counseling and promotion of healthy lifestyles are important aspects of long-term follow-up care to promote risk reduction for health problems that commonly present during adulthood. Both general and subspecialty pediatric health care providers are playing an increasingly important role in the ongoing care of childhood cancer survivors, beyond the routine preventive care, health supervision, and anticipatory guidance provided to all patients. This report is based on the guidelines that have been developed by the Children's Oncology Group to facilitate comprehensive long-term follow-up of childhood cancer survivors (www.survivorshipguidelines.org). (3/09, reaffirmed 4/13, 8/17)
http://pediatrics.aappublications.org/content/123/3/906

MAINTAINING AND IMPROVING THE ORAL HEALTH OF YOUNG CHILDREN

Section on Oral Health

ABSTRACT. Oral health is an integral part of the overall health of children. Dental caries is a common and chronic disease process with significant short- and long-term consequences. The prevalence of dental caries for the youngest of children has not decreased over the past decade, despite improvements for older children. As health care professionals responsible for the overall health of children, pediatricians frequently confront morbidity associated with dental caries. Because the youngest children visit the pediatrician more often than they visit the dentist, it is important that pediatricians be knowledgeable about the disease process of dental caries, prevention of the disease, and interventions available to the pediatrician and the family to maintain and restore health. (11/14)
http://pediatrics.aappublications.org/content/134/6/1224

MALE ADOLESCENT SEXUAL AND REPRODUCTIVE HEALTH CARE (CLINICAL REPORT)

Arik V. Marcell, MD, MPH; Charles Wibbelsman, MD; Warren M. Seigel, MD; and Committee on Adolescence

ABSTRACT. Male adolescents' sexual and reproductive health needs often go unmet in the primary care setting. This report discusses specific issues related to male adolescents' sexual and reproductive health care in the context of primary care, including pubertal and sexual development, sexual behavior, consequences of sexual behavior, and methods of preventing sexually transmitted infections (including HIV) and pregnancy. Pediatricians are encouraged to address male adolescent sexual and reproductive health on a regular basis, including taking a sexual history, performing an appropriate examination, providing patient-centered and age-appropriate anticipatory guidance, and delivering appropriate vaccinations. Pediatricians should provide these services to male adolescent patients in a confidential and culturally appropriate manner, promote healthy sexual relationships and responsibility, and involve parents in age-appropriate discussions about sexual health with their sons. (11/11, reaffirmed 5/15)
http://pediatrics.aappublications.org/content/128/6/e1658

MALE CIRCUMCISION (TECHNICAL REPORT)

Task Force on Circumcision

ABSTRACT. Male circumcision consists of the surgical removal of some, or all, of the foreskin (or prepuce) from the penis. It is one of the most common procedures in the world. In the United States, the procedure is commonly performed during the newborn period. In 2007, the American Academy of Pediatrics (AAP) convened a multidisciplinary workgroup of AAP members and other stakeholders to evaluate the evidence regarding male circumcision and update the AAP's 1999 recommendations in this area. The Task Force included AAP representatives from specialty areas as well as members of the AAP Board of Directors and liaisons representing the American Academy of Family Physicians, the American College of Obstetricians and Gynecologists, and the Centers for Disease Control and Prevention. The Task Force members identified selected topics relevant to male circumcision and conducted a critical review of peer-reviewed literature by using the American Heart Association's template for evidence evaluation.

Evaluation of current evidence indicates that the health benefits of newborn male circumcision outweigh the risks; furthermore, the benefits of newborn male circumcision justify access to this procedure for families who choose it. Specific benefits from male circumcision were identified for the prevention of urinary tract infections, acquisition of HIV, transmission of some sexually transmitted infections, and penile cancer. Male circumcision does not appear to adversely affect penile sexual function/sensitivity or sexual satisfaction. It is imperative that those providing circumcision are adequately trained and that both sterile techniques and effective pain management are used. Significant acute complications are rare. In general, untrained providers who perform circumcisions have more complications than well-trained providers who perform the procedure, regardless of whether the former are physicians, nurses, or traditional religious providers.

Parents are entitled to factually correct, nonbiased information about circumcision and should receive this information from clinicians before conception or early in pregnancy, which is when parents typically make circumcision decisions. Parents should determine what is in the best interest of their child. Physicians who counsel families about this decision should provide assistance by explaining the potential benefits and risks and ensuring that parents understand that circumcision is an elective procedure. The Task Force strongly recommends the creation, revision, and enhancement of educational materials to assist parents of male infants with the care of circumcised and uncircumcised penises. The Task Force also strongly recommends the development of educational materials for providers to enhance practitioners' competency in discussing circumcision's benefits and risks with parents.

The Task Force made the following recommendations:

- Evaluation of current evidence indicates that the health benefits of newborn male circumcision outweigh the risks, and the benefits of newborn male circumcision justify access to this procedure for those families who choose it.

- Parents are entitled to factually correct, nonbiased information about circumcision that should be provided before conception and early in pregnancy, when parents are most likely to be weighing the option of circumcision of a male child.

- Physicians counseling families about elective male circumcision should assist parents by explaining, in a nonbiased manner, the potential benefits and risks and by ensuring that they understand the elective nature of the procedure.

- Parents should weigh the health benefits and risks in light of their own religious, cultural, and personal preferences, as the medical benefits alone may not outweigh these other considerations for individual families.

- Parents of newborn boys should be instructed in the care of the penis, regardless of whether the newborn has been circumcised or not.

- Elective circumcision should be performed only if the infant's condition is stable and healthy.

- Male circumcision should be performed by trained and competent practitioners, by using sterile techniques and effective pain management.

- Analgesia is safe and effective in reducing the procedural pain associated with newborn circumcision; thus, adequate analgesia should be provided whenever newborn circumcision is performed.

  — Nonpharmacologic techniques (eg, positioning, sucrose pacifiers) alone are insufficient to prevent procedural and postprocedural pain and are not recommended as the sole method of analgesia. They should be used only as analgesic adjuncts to improve infant comfort during circumcision.

  — If used, topical creams may cause a higher incidence of skin irritation in low birth weight infants, compared with infants of normal weight; penile nerve block techniques should therefore be chosen for this group of newborns.

- Key professional organizations (AAP, the American Academy of Family Physicians, the American College of Obstetricians and Gynecologists, the American Society of Anesthesiologists, the American College of Nurse Midwives, and other midlevel clinicians such as nurse practitioners) should work collaboratively to:

  — Develop standards of trainee proficiency in the performance of anesthetic and procedure techniques, including suturing;

  — Teach the procedure and analgesic techniques during postgraduate training programs;

  — Develop educational materials for clinicians to enhance their own competency in discussing the benefits and risks of circumcision with parents;

  — Offer educational materials to assist parents of male infants with the care of both circumcised and uncircumcised penises.

- The preventive and public health benefits associated with newborn male circumcision warrant third-party reimbursement of the procedure.

The American College of Obstetricians and Gynecologists has endorsed this technical report. (8/12)
http://pediatrics.aappublications.org/content/130/3/e756

MALTREATMENT OF CHILDREN WITH DISABILITIES (CLINICAL REPORT)

Roberta A. Hibbard, MD; Larry W. Desch, MD; Committee on Child Abuse and Neglect; and Council on Children With Disabilities

ABSTRACT. Widespread efforts are being made to increase awareness and provide education to pediatricians regarding risk factors of child abuse and neglect. The purpose of this clinical report is to ensure that children with disabilities are recognized as a population that is also at risk of maltreatment. Some conditions related to a disability can be confused with maltreatment. The need for early recognition and intervention of child abuse and neglect in this population, as well as the ways that a medical home can facilitate the prevention and early detection of child maltreatment, are the subject of this report. (5/07, reaffirmed 1/11, 4/16)
http://pediatrics.aappublications.org/content/119/5/1018

MANAGEMENT OF CHILDREN WITH AUTISM SPECTRUM DISORDERS (CLINICAL REPORT)

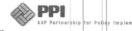

Scott M. Myers, MD; Chris Plauché Johnson, MD, MEd; and Council on Children With Disabilities

ABSTRACT. Pediatricians have an important role not only in early recognition and evaluation of autism spectrum disorders but also in chronic management of these disorders. The primary goals of treatment are to maximize the child's ultimate functional independence and quality of life by minimizing the core autism spectrum disorder features, facilitating development and learning, promoting socialization, reducing maladaptive behaviors, and educating and supporting families. To assist pediatricians in educating families and guiding them toward empirically supported interventions for their children, this report reviews the educational strategies and associated therapies that are the primary treatments for children with autism spectrum disorders. Optimization of health care is likely to have a positive effect on habilitative progress, functional outcome, and quality of life; therefore, important issues, such as management of associated medical problems, pharmacologic and nonpharmacologic intervention for challenging behaviors or coexisting mental health conditions, and use of complementary and alternative medical treatments, are also addressed. (11/07, reaffirmed 9/10, 8/14)
http://pediatrics.aappublications.org/content/120/5/1162

MANAGEMENT OF DENTAL TRAUMA IN A PRIMARY CARE SETTING (CLINICAL REPORT)

Martha Ann Keels, DDS, PhD, and Section on Oral Health

ABSTRACT. The American Academy of Pediatrics and its Section on Oral Health have developed this clinical report for pediatricians and primary care physicians regarding the diagnosis, evaluation, and management of dental trauma in children aged 1 to 21 years. This report was developed through a comprehensive search and analysis of the medical and dental literature and expert consensus. Guidelines published and updated by the International Association of Dental Traumatology (www.dentaltraumaguide.com) are an excellent resource for both dental and nondental health care providers. (1/14)
http://pediatrics.aappublications.org/content/133/2/e466

MANAGEMENT OF FOOD ALLERGY IN THE SCHOOL SETTING (CLINICAL REPORT)

Scott H. Sicherer, MD; Todd Mahr, MD; and Section on Allergy and Immunology

ABSTRACT. Food allergy is estimated to affect approximately 1 in 25 school-aged children and is the most common trigger of anaphylaxis in this age group. School food-allergy management requires strategies to reduce the risk of ingestion of the allergen as well as procedures to recognize and treat allergic reactions and anaphylaxis. The role of the pediatrician or pediatric health care provider may include diagnosing and documenting a potentially life-threatening food allergy, prescribing selfinjectable epinephrine, helping the child learn how to store and use the medication in a responsible manner, educating the parents of their responsibility to implement prevention strategies within and outside the home environment, and working with families, schools, and students in developing written plans to reduce the risk of anaphylaxis and to implement emergency treatment in the event of a reaction. This clinical report highlights the role of the pediatrician and pediatric health care provider in managing students with food allergies. (11/10)
http://pediatrics.aappublications.org/content/126/6/1232

MANAGEMENT OF NEONATES BORN AT ≥35 0/7 WEEKS' GESTATION WITH SUSPECTED OR PROVEN EARLY-ONSET BACTERIAL SEPSIS (CLINICAL REPORT)

Karen M. Puopolo, MD, PhD, FAAP; William E. Benitz, MD, FAAP; Theoklis E. Zaoutis, MD, MSCE, FAAP; Committee on Fetus and Newborn; and Committee on Infectious Diseases

ABSTRACT. The incidence of neonatal early-onset sepsis (EOS) has declined substantially over the last 2 decades, primarily because of the implementation of evidence-based intrapartum antimicrobial therapy. However, EOS remains a serious and potentially fatal illness. Laboratory tests alone are neither sensitive nor specific enough to guide EOS management decisions. Maternal and infant clinical characteristics can help identify newborn infants who are at risk and guide the administration of empirical antibiotic therapy. The incidence of EOS, the prevalence and implications of established risk factors, the predictive value of commonly used laboratory tests, and the uncertainties in the risk/benefit balance of antibiotic exposures all vary significantly with gestational age at birth. Our purpose in this clinical report is to provide a summary of the current epidemiology of neonatal sepsis among infants born at ≥35 0/7 weeks' gestation and a framework for the development of evidence-based approaches to sepsis risk assessment among these infants. (11/18)
See full text on page 705.
http://pediatrics.aappublications.org/content/142/6/e20182894

MANAGEMENT OF NEONATES BORN AT ≤34 6/7 WEEKS' GESTATION WITH SUSPECTED OR PROVEN EARLY-ONSET BACTERIAL SEPSIS (CLINICAL REPORT)

Karen M. Puopolo, MD, PhD, FAAP; William E. Benitz, MD, FAAP; Theoklis E. Zaoutis, MD, MSCE, FAAP; Committee on Fetus and Newborn; and Committee on Infectious Diseases

ABSTRACT. Early-onset sepsis (EOS) remains a serious and often fatal illness among infants born preterm, particularly among newborn infants of the lowest gestational age. Currently, most preterm infants with very low birth weight are treated empirically with antibiotics for risk of EOS, often for prolonged periods, in the absence of a culture-confirmed infection. Retrospective studies have revealed that antibiotic exposures after birth are associated with multiple subsequent poor outcomes among preterm infants, making the risk/benefit balance of these antibiotic treatments uncertain. Gestational age is the strongest single predictor of EOS, and the majority of preterm births occur in the setting of other factors associated with risk

of EOS, making it difficult to apply risk stratification strategies to preterm infants. Laboratory tests alone have a poor predictive value in preterm EOS. Delivery characteristics of extremely preterm infants present an opportunity to identify those with a lower risk of EOS and may inform decisions to initiate or extend antibiotic therapies. Our purpose for this clinical report is to provide a summary of the current epidemiology of preterm neonatal sepsis and provide guidance for the development of evidence-based approaches to sepsis risk assessment among preterm newborn infants. (11/18)
See full text on page 717.
http://pediatrics.aappublications.org/content/142/6/e20182896

MANAGEMENT OF PEDIATRIC TRAUMA

Committee on Pediatric Emergency Medicine; Council on Injury, Violence, and Poison Prevention; Section on Critical Care; Section on Orthopaedics; Section on Surgery; and Section on Transport Medicine (joint with Pediatric Trauma Society and Society of Trauma Nurses Pediatric Committee)

ABSTRACT. Injury is still the number 1 killer of children ages 1 to 18 years in the United States (http://www.cdc.gov/nchs/fastats/children.htm). Children who sustain injuries with resulting disabilities incur significant costs not only for their health care but also for productivity lost to the economy. The families of children who survive childhood injury with disability face years of emotional and financial hardship, along with a significant societal burden. The entire process of managing childhood injury is enormously complex and varies by region. Only the comprehensive cooperation of a broadly diverse trauma team will have a significant effect on improving the care of injured children. (7/16)
http://pediatrics.aappublications.org/content/138/2/e20161569

MANAGEMENT OF TYPE 2 DIABETES MELLITUS IN CHILDREN AND ADOLESCENTS (TECHNICAL REPORT)

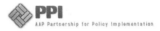

Shelley C. Springer, MD, MBA, MSc, JD; Janet Silverstein, MD; Kenneth Copeland, MD; Kelly R. Moore, MD; Greg E. Prazar, MD; Terry Raymer, MD, CDE; Richard N. Shiffman, MD; Vidhu V. Thaker, MD; Meaghan Anderson, MS, RD, LD, CDE; Stephen J. Spann, MD, MBA; and Susan K. Flinn, MA

ABSTRACT. *Objective.* Over the last 3 decades, the prevalence of childhood obesity has increased dramatically in North America, ushering in a variety of health problems, including type 2 diabetes mellitus (T2DM), which previously was not typically seen until much later in life. This technical report describes, in detail, the procedures undertaken to develop the recommendations given in the accompanying clinical practice guideline, "Management of Type 2 Diabetes Mellitus in Children and Adolescents," and provides in-depth information about the rationale for the recommendations and the studies used to make the clinical practice guideline's recommendations.

Methods. A primary literature search was conducted relating to the treatment of T2DM in children and adolescents, and a secondary literature search was conducted relating to the screening and treatment of T2DM's comorbidities in children and adolescents. Inclusion criteria were prospectively and unanimously agreed on by members of the committee. An article was eligible for inclusion if it addressed treatment (primary search) or 1 of 4 comorbidities (secondary search) of T2DM, was published in 1990 or later, was written in English, and included an abstract. Only primary research inquiries were considered; review articles were considered if they included primary data or opinion. The research population had to constitute children and/or adolescents with an existing diagnosis of T2DM; studies of adult patients were considered if at least 10% of the study population was younger than 35 years. All retrieved titles, abstracts, and articles were reviewed by the consulting epidemiologist.

Results. Thousands of articles were retrieved and considered in both searches on the basis of the aforementioned criteria. From those, in the primary search, 199 abstracts were identified for possible inclusion, 58 of which were retained for systematic review. Five of these studies were classified as grade A studies, 1 as grade B, 20 as grade C, and 32 as grade D. Articles regarding treatment of T2DM selected for inclusion were divided into 4 major subcategories on the basis of type of treatment being discussed: (1) medical treatments (32 studies); (2) nonmedical treatments (9 studies); (3) provider behaviors (8 studies); and (4) social issues (9 studies). From the secondary search, an additional 336 abstracts relating to comorbidities were identified for possible inclusion, of which 26 were retained for systematic review. These articles included the following: 1 systematic review of literature regarding comorbidities of T2DM in adolescents; 5 expert opinions presenting global recommendations not based on evidence; 5 cohort studies reporting natural history of disease and comorbidities; 3 with specific attention to comorbidity patterns in specific ethnic groups (case-control, cohort, and clinical report using adult literature); 3 reporting an association between microalbuminuria and retinopathy (2 case-control, 1 cohort); 3 reporting the prevalence of nephropathy (cohort); 1 reporting peripheral vascular disease (case series); 2 discussing retinopathy (1 case-control, 1 position statement); and 3 addressing hyperlipidemia (American Heart Association position statement on cardiovascular risks; American Diabetes Association consensus statement; case series). A breakdown of grade of recommendation shows no grade A studies, 10 grade B studies, 6 grade C studies, and 10 grade D studies. With regard to screening and treatment recommendations for comorbidities, data in children are scarce, and the available literature is conflicting. Therapeutic recommendations for hypertension, dyslipidemia, retinopathy, microalbuminuria, and depression were summarized from expert guideline documents and are presented in detail in the guideline. The references are provided, but the committee did not independently assess the supporting evidence. Screening tools are provided in the Supplemental Information. (1/13)

http://pediatrics.aappublications.org/content/131/2/e648

MARIJUANA USE DURING PREGNANCY AND BREASTFEEDING: IMPLICATIONS FOR NEONATAL AND CHILDHOOD OUTCOMES (CLINICAL REPORT)

Sheryl A. Ryan, MD, FAAP; Seth D. Ammerman, MD, FAAP, FSAHM, DABAM; Mary E. O'Connor, MD, MPH, FAAP; Committee on Substance Use and Prevention; and Section on Breastfeeding

ABSTRACT. Marijuana is one of the most widely used substances during pregnancy in the United States. Emerging data on the ability of cannabinoids to cross the placenta and affect the development of the fetus raise concerns about both pregnancy outcomes and long-term consequences for the infant or child. Social media is used to tout the use of marijuana for severe nausea associated with pregnancy. Concerns have also been raised about marijuana use by breastfeeding mothers. With this clinical report, we provide data on the current rates of marijuana use among pregnant and lactating women, discuss what is known about the effects of marijuana on fetal development and later neurodevelopmental and behavioral outcomes, and address implications for education and policy. (8/18)

See full text on page 729.

http://pediatrics.aappublications.org/content/142/3/e20181889

MATERNAL PHENYLKETONURIA

Committee on Genetics

ABSTRACT. Elevated maternal phenylalanine concentrations during pregnancy are teratogenic and may result in growth retardation, microcephaly, significant developmental delays, and birth defects in the offspring of women with poorly controlled phenylketonuria during pregnancy. Women of childbearing age with all forms of phenylketonuria, including mild variants such as mild hyperphenylalaninemia, should receive counseling concerning their risks for adverse fetal effects, optimally before conceiving. The best outcomes occur when strict control of maternal phenylalanine concentration is achieved before conception and continued throughout pregnancy. Included are brief descriptions of novel treatments for phenylketonuria. (8/08, reaffirmed 1/13)

http://pediatrics.aappublications.org/content/122/2/445

MATERNAL-FETAL INTERVENTION AND FETAL CARE CENTERS (CLINICAL REPORT)

Committee on Bioethics (joint with American College of Obstetricians and Gynecologists Committee on Ethics)

ABSTRACT. The past 2 decades have yielded profound advances in the fields of prenatal diagnosis and fetal intervention. Although fetal interventions are driven by a beneficence-based motivation to improve fetal and neonatal outcomes, advancement in fetal therapies raises ethical issues surrounding maternal autonomy and decision-making, concepts of innovation versus research, and organizational aspects within institutions in the development of fetal care centers. To safeguard the interests of both the pregnant woman and the fetus, the American College of Obstetricians and Gynecologists and the American Academy of Pediatrics make recommendations regarding informed consent, the role of research subject advocates and other independent advocates, the availability of support services, the multidisciplinary nature of fetal intervention teams, the oversight of centers, and the need to accumulate maternal and fetal outcome data. (7/11, reaffirmed 2/18)

http://pediatrics.aappublications.org/content/128/2/e473

MEDIA AND YOUNG MINDS

Council on Communications and Media

ABSTRACT. Infants, toddlers, and preschoolers are now growing up in environments saturated with a variety of traditional and new technologies, which they are adopting at increasing rates. Although there has been much hope for the educational potential of interactive media for young children, accompanied by fears about their overuse during this crucial period of rapid brain development, research in this area still remains limited. This policy statement reviews the existing literature on television, videos, and mobile/interactive technologies; their potential for educational benefit; and related health concerns for young children (0 to 5 years of age). The statement also highlights areas in which pediatric providers can offer specific guidance to families in managing their young children's media use, not only in terms of content or time limits, but also emphasizing the importance of parent-child shared media use and allowing the child time to take part in other developmentally healthy activities. (10/16)

http://pediatrics.aappublications.org/content/138/5/e20162591

MEDIA EDUCATION

Committee on Communications and Media

ABSTRACT. The American Academy of Pediatrics recognizes that exposure to mass media (eg, television, movies, video and computer games, the Internet, music lyrics and videos, newspapers, magazines, books, advertising) presents health risks for children and adolescents but can provide benefits as well.

Media education has the potential to reduce the harmful effects of media and accentuate the positive effects. By understanding and supporting media education, pediatricians can play an important role in reducing harmful effects of media on children and adolescents. (9/10)
http://pediatrics.aappublications.org/content/126/5/1012

MEDIA USE IN SCHOOL-AGED CHILDREN AND ADOLESCENTS
Council on Communications and Media
ABSTRACT. This policy statement focuses on children and adolescents 5 through 18 years of age. Research suggests both benefits and risks of media use for the health of children and teenagers. Benefits include exposure to new ideas and knowledge acquisition, increased opportunities for social contact and support, and new opportunities to access health-promotion messages and information. Risks include negative health effects on weight and sleep; exposure to inaccurate, inappropriate, or unsafe content and contacts; and compromised privacy and confidentiality. Parents face challenges in monitoring their children's and their own media use and in serving as positive role models. In this new era, evidence regarding healthy media use does not support a one-size-fits-all approach. Parents and pediatricians can work together to develop a Family Media Use Plan (www.healthychildren.org/MediaUsePlan) that considers their children's developmental stages to individualize an appropriate balance for media time and consistent rules about media use, to mentor their children, to set boundaries for accessing content and displaying personal information, and to implement open family communication about media. (10/16)
http://pediatrics.aappublications.org/content/138/5/e20162592

MEDIATORS AND ADVERSE EFFECTS OF CHILD POVERTY IN THE UNITED STATES (TECHNICAL REPORT)
John M. Pascoe, MD, MPH, FAAP; David L. Wood, MD, MPH, FAAP; James H. Duffee, MD, MPH, FAAP; Alice Kuo, MD, PhD, MEd, FAAP; Committee on Psychosocial Aspects of Child and Family Health; and Council on Community Pediatrics
ABSTRACT. The link between poverty and children's health is well recognized. Even temporary poverty may have an adverse effect on children's health, and data consistently support the observation that poverty in childhood continues to have a negative effect on health into adulthood. In addition to childhood morbidity being related to child poverty, epidemiologic studies have documented a mortality gradient for children aged 1 to 15 years (and adults), with poor children experiencing a higher mortality rate than children from higher-income families. The global great recession is only now very slowly abating for millions of America's children and their families. At this difficult time in the history of our nation's families and immediately after the 50th anniversary year of President Lyndon Johnson's War on Poverty, it is particularly germane for the American Academy of Pediatrics, which is "dedicated to the health of all children," to publish a research-supported technical report that examines the mediators associated with the long-recognized adverse effects of child poverty on children and their families. This technical report draws on research from a number of disciplines, including physiology, sociology, psychology, economics, and epidemiology, to describe the present state of knowledge regarding poverty's negative impact on children's health and development. Children inherit not only their parents' genes but also the family ecology and its social milieu. Thus, parenting skills, housing, neighborhood, schools, and other factors (eg, medical care) all have complex relations to each other and influence how each child's genetic canvas is expressed. Accompanying this technical report is a policy statement that describes specific actions that pediatricians and other child advocates can take to attenuate the negative effects of the mediators identified in this technical report and improve the well-being of our nation's children and their families. (3/16)
http://pediatrics.aappublications.org/content/137/4/e20160340

MEDICAID POLICY STATEMENT
Committee on Child Health Financing
ABSTRACT. Medicaid insures 39% of the children in the United States. This revision of the 2005 Medicaid Policy Statement of the American Academy of Pediatrics reflects opportunities for changes in state Medicaid programs resulting from the 2010 Patient Protection and Affordable Care Act as upheld in 2012 by the Supreme Court. Policy recommendations focus on the areas of benefit coverage, financing and payment, eligibility, outreach and enrollment, managed care, and quality improvement. (4/13)
http://pediatrics.aappublications.org/content/131/5/e1697

MEDICAL COUNTERMEASURES FOR CHILDREN IN PUBLIC HEALTH EMERGENCIES, DISASTERS, OR TERRORISM
Disaster Preparedness Advisory Council
ABSTRACT. Significant strides have been made over the past 10 to 15 years to develop medical countermeasures (MCMs) to address potential disaster hazards, including chemical, biological, radiologic, and nuclear threats. Significant and effective collaboration between the pediatric health community, including the American Academy of Pediatrics, and federal partners, such as the Office of the Assistant Secretary for Preparedness and Response, Centers for Disease Control and Prevention, Federal Emergency Management Agency, National Institutes of Health, Food and Drug Administration, and other federal agencies, over the past 5 years has resulted in substantial gains in addressing the needs of children related to disaster preparedness in general and MCMs in particular. Yet, major gaps still remain related to MCMs for children, a population highly vulnerable to the effects of exposure to such threats, because many vaccines and pharmaceuticals approved for use by adults as MCMs do not yet have pediatric formulations, dosing information, or safety information. As a result, the nation's stockpiles and other caches (designated supply of MCMs) where pharmacotherapeutic and other MCMs are stored are less prepared to address the needs of children compared with those of adults in the event of a disaster. This policy statement provides recommendations to close the remaining gaps for the development and use of MCMs in children during public health emergencies or disasters. The progress made by federal agencies to date to address the needs of children and the shared commitment of collaboration that characterizes the current relationship between the pediatric health community and the federal agencies responsible for MCMs should encourage all child advocates to invest the necessary energy and resources now to complete the process of remedying the remaining significant gaps in preparedness. (1/16)
http://pediatrics.aappublications.org/content/137/2/e20154273

MEDICAL EMERGENCIES OCCURRING AT SCHOOL
Council on School Health
ABSTRACT. Children and adults might experience medical emergency situations because of injuries, complications of chronic health conditions, or unexpected major illnesses that occur in schools. In February 2001, the American Academy of Pediatrics issued a policy statement titled "Guidelines for Emergency Medical Care in Schools" (available at: http://aappolicy.aappublications.org/cgi/content/full/pediatrics;107/2/435). Since the release of that statement, the spectrum of potential individual student emergencies has changed significantly. The increase in the number of children with special health care needs and chronic medical conditions attending schools and the challenges associated with ensuring that schools have access to

on-site licensed health care professionals on an ongoing basis have added to increasing the risks of medical emergencies in schools. The goal of this statement is to increase pediatricians' awareness of schools' roles in preparing for individual student emergencies and to provide recommendations for primary care and school physicians on how to assist and support school personnel. (10/08, reaffirmed 9/11, 4/17)
http://pediatrics.aappublications.org/content/122/4/887

THE MEDICAL HOME

Medical Home Initiatives for Children With Special Needs Project Advisory Committee

ABSTRACT. The American Academy of Pediatrics proposed a definition of the medical home in a 1992 policy statement. Efforts to establish medical homes for all children have encountered many challenges, including the existence of multiple interpretations of the "medical home" concept and the lack of adequate reimbursement for services provided by physicians caring for children in a medical home. This new policy statement contains an expanded and more comprehensive interpretation of the concept and an operational definition of the medical home. (7/02, reaffirmed 5/08)
http://pediatrics.aappublications.org/content/110/1/184

MEDICAL STAFF APPOINTMENT AND DELINEATION OF PEDIATRIC PRIVILEGES IN HOSPITALS (CLINICAL REPORT)

Daniel A. Rauch, MD; Committee on Hospital Care; and Section on Hospital Medicine

ABSTRACT. The review and verification of credentials and the granting of clinical privileges are required of every hospital to ensure that members of the medical staff are competent and qualified to provide specified levels of patient care. The credentialing process involves the following: (1) assessment of the professional and personal background of each practitioner seeking privileges; (2) assignment of privileges appropriate for the clinician's training and experience; (3) ongoing monitoring of the professional activities of each staff member; and (4) periodic reappointment to the medical staff on the basis of objectively measured performance. We examine the essential elements of a credentials review for initial and renewed medical staff appointments along with suggested criteria for the delineation of clinical privileges. Sample forms for the delineation of privileges can be found on the American Academy of Pediatrics Committee on Hospital Care Web site (http://www.aap.org/visit/cmte19.htm). Because of differences among individual hospitals, no 1 method for credentialing is universally applicable. The medical staff of each hospital must, therefore, establish its own process based on the general principles reviewed in this report. The issues of medical staff membership and credentialing have become very complex, and institutions and medical staffs are vulnerable to legal action. Consequently, it is advisable for hospitals and medical staffs to obtain expert legal advice when medical staff bylaws are constructed or revised. (3/12, reaffirmed 2/16)
http://pediatrics.aappublications.org/content/129/4/797

MEDICAL VERSUS NONMEDICAL IMMUNIZATION EXEMPTIONS FOR CHILD CARE AND SCHOOL ATTENDANCE

Committee on Practice and Ambulatory Medicine, Committee on Infectious Diseases, Committee on State Government Affairs, Council on School Health, and Section on Administration and Practice Management

ABSTRACT. Routine childhood immunizations against infectious diseases are an integral part of our public health infrastructure. They provide direct protection to the immunized individual and indirect protection to children and adults unable to be immunized via the effect of community immunity. All 50 states, the District of Columbia, and Puerto Rico have regulations requiring proof of immunization for child care and school attendance as a public health strategy to protect children in these settings and to secondarily serve as a mechanism to promote timely immunization of children by their caregivers. Although all states and the District of Columbia have mechanisms to exempt school attendees from specific immunization requirements for medical reasons, the majority also have a heterogeneous collection of regulations and laws that allow nonmedical exemptions from childhood immunizations otherwise required for child care and school attendance. The American Academy of Pediatrics (AAP) supports regulations and laws requiring certification of immunization to attend child care and school as a sound means of providing a safe environment for attendees and employees of these settings. The AAP also supports medically indicated exemptions to specific immunizations as determined for each individual child. The AAP views nonmedical exemptions to school-required immunizations as inappropriate for individual, public health, and ethical reasons and advocates for their elimination. (8/16)
http://pediatrics.aappublications.org/content/138/3/e20162145

MEDICATION-ASSISTED TREATMENT OF ADOLESCENTS WITH OPIOID USE DISORDERS

Committee on Substance Use and Prevention

ABSTRACT. Opioid use disorder is a leading cause of morbidity and mortality among US youth. Effective treatments, both medications and substance use disorder counseling, are available but underused, and access to developmentally appropriate treatment is severely restricted for adolescents and young adults. Resources to disseminate available therapies and to develop new treatments specifically for this age group are needed to save and improve lives of youth with opioid addiction. (8/16)
http://pediatrics.aappublications.org/content/138/3/e20161893

MENSTRUAL MANAGEMENT FOR ADOLESCENTS WITH DISABILITIES (CLINICAL REPORT)

Elisabeth H. Quint, MD; Rebecca F. O'Brien, MD; and Committee on Adolescence (joint with the North American Society for Pediatric and Adolescent Gynecology)

ABSTRACT. The onset of menses for adolescents with physical or intellectual disabilities can affect their independence and add additional concerns for families at home, in schools, and in other settings. The pediatrician is the primary health care provider to explore and assist with the pubertal transition and menstrual management. Menstrual management of both normal and abnormal cycles may be requested to minimize hygiene issues, premenstrual symptoms, dysmenorrhea, heavy or irregular bleeding, contraception, and conditions exacerbated by the menstrual cycle. Several options are available for menstrual management, depending on the outcome that is desired, ranging from cycle regulation to complete amenorrhea. The use of medications or the request for surgeries to help with the menstrual cycles in teenagers with disabilities has medical, social, legal, and ethical implications. This clinical report is designed to help guide pediatricians in assisting adolescent females with intellectual and/or physical disabilities and their families in making decisions related to successfully navigating menarche and subsequent menstrual cycles. (6/16)
http://pediatrics.aappublications.org/content/138/1/e20160295

THE METABOLIC SYNDROME IN CHILDREN AND ADOLESCENTS: SHIFTING THE FOCUS TO CARDIOMETABOLIC RISK FACTOR CLUSTERING (CLINICAL REPORT)

Sheela N. Magge, MD, MSCE, FAAP; Elizabeth Goodman, MD, MBA, FAAP; Sarah C. Armstrong, MD, FAAP; Committee on Nutrition; Section on Endocrinology; and Section on Obesity

ABSTRACT. Metabolic syndrome (MetS) was developed by the National Cholesterol Education Program Adult Treatment Panel III, identifying adults with at least 3 of 5 cardiometabolic risk factors (hyperglycemia, increased central adiposity, elevated triglycerides, decreased high-density lipoprotein cholesterol, and elevated blood pressure) who are at increased risk of diabetes and cardiovascular disease. The constellation of MetS component risk factors has a shared pathophysiology and many common treatment approaches grounded in lifestyle modification. Several attempts have been made to define MetS in the pediatric population. However, in children, the construct is difficult to define and has unclear implications for clinical care. In this Clinical Report, we focus on the importance of screening for and treating the individual risk factor components of MetS. Focusing attention on children with cardiometabolic risk factor clustering is emphasized over the need to define a pediatric MetS. (7/17)
http://pediatrics.aappublications.org/content/140/2/e20171603

METRIC UNITS AND THE PREFERRED DOSING OF ORALLY ADMINISTERED LIQUID MEDICATIONS

Committee on Drugs

ABSTRACT. Medication overdoses are a common, but preventable, problem among children. Volumetric dosing errors and the use of incorrect dosing delivery devices are 2 common sources of these preventable errors for orally administered liquid medications. To reduce errors and increase precision of drug administration, milliliter-based dosing should be used exclusively when prescribing and administering liquid medications. Teaspoon- and tablespoon-based dosing should not be used. Devices that allow for precise dose administration (preferably syringes with metric markings) should be used instead of household spoons and should be distributed with the medication. (3/15)
http://pediatrics.aappublications.org/content/135/4/784

MIND-BODY THERAPIES IN CHILDREN AND YOUTH (CLINICAL REPORT)

Section on Integrative Medicine

ABSTRACT. Mind-body therapies are popular and are ranked among the top 10 complementary and integrative medicine practices reportedly used by adults and children in the 2007–2012 National Health Interview Survey. A growing body of evidence supports the effectiveness and safety of mind-body therapies in pediatrics. This clinical report outlines popular mind-body therapies for children and youth and examines the best-available evidence for a variety of mind-body therapies and practices, including biofeedback, clinical hypnosis, guided imagery, meditation, and yoga. The report is intended to help health care professionals guide their patients to nonpharmacologic approaches to improve concentration, help decrease pain, control discomfort, or ease anxiety. (8/16)
http://pediatrics.aappublications.org/content/138/3/e20161896

MINORS AS LIVING SOLID-ORGAN DONORS (CLINICAL REPORT)

Lainie Friedman Ross, MD, PhD; J. Richard Thistlethwaite Jr, MD, PhD; and Committee on Bioethics

ABSTRACT. In the past half-century, solid-organ transplantation has become standard treatment for a variety of diseases in children and adults. The major limitation for all transplantation is the availability of donors, and the gap between demand and supply continues to grow despite the increase in living donors. Although rare, children do serve as living donors, and these donations raise serious ethical issues. This clinical report includes a discussion of the ethical considerations regarding minors serving as living donors, using the traditional benefit/burden calculus from the perspectives of both the donor and the recipient. The report also includes an examination of the circumstances under which a minor may morally participate as a living donor, how to minimize risks, and what the informed-consent process should entail. The American Academy of Pediatrics holds that minors can morally serve as living organ donors but only in exceptional circumstances when specific criteria are fulfilled. (8/08, reaffirmed 5/11)
http://pediatrics.aappublications.org/content/122/2/454

MODEL CONTRACTUAL LANGUAGE FOR MEDICAL NECESSITY FOR CHILDREN

Committee on Child Health Financing

ABSTRACT. The term "medical necessity" is used by Medicare and Medicaid and in insurance contracts to refer to medical services that are generally recognized as appropriate for the diagnosis, prevention, or treatment of disease and injury. There is no consensus on how to define and apply the term and the accompanying rules and regulations, and as a result there has been substantial variation in medical-necessity definitions and interpretations. With this policy statement, the American Academy of Pediatrics hopes to encourage insurers to adopt more consistent medical-necessity definitions that take into account the needs of children. (7/05, reaffirmed 10/11)
http://pediatrics.aappublications.org/content/116/1/261

MOTOR DELAYS: EARLY IDENTIFICATION AND EVALUATION (CLINICAL REPORT)

Garey H. Noritz, MD; Nancy A. Murphy, MD; and Neuromotor Screening Expert Panel

ABSTRACT. Pediatricians often encounter children with delays of motor development in their clinical practices. Earlier identification of motor delays allows for timely referral for developmental interventions as well as diagnostic evaluations and treatment planning. A multidisciplinary expert panel developed an algorithm for the surveillance and screening of children for motor delays within the medical home, offering guidance for the initial workup and referral of the child with possible delays in motor development. Highlights of this clinical report include suggestions for formal developmental screening at the 9-, 18-, 30-, and 48-month well-child visits; approaches to the neurologic examination, with emphasis on the assessment of muscle tone; and initial diagnostic approaches for medical home providers. Use of diagnostic tests to evaluate children with motor delays are described, including brain MRI for children with high muscle tone, and measuring serum creatine kinase concentration of those with decreased muscle tone. The importance of pursuing diagnostic tests while concurrently referring patients to early intervention programs is emphasized. (5/13, reaffirmed 5/17)
http://pediatrics.aappublications.org/content/131/6/e2016

THE NEED TO OPTIMIZE ADOLESCENT IMMUNIZATION (CLINICAL REPORT)

Henry H. Bernstein, DO, MHCM, FAAP; Joseph A. Bocchini Jr, MD, FAAP; and Committee on Infectious Diseases

ABSTRACT. The adolescent period heralds the pediatric patient's transition into adulthood. It is a time of dynamic development during which effective preventive care measures can promote safe behaviors and the development of lifelong health habits. One of the foundations of preventive adolescent health care is timely vaccination, and every visit can be viewed as an opportunity to update and complete an adolescent's immunizations.

In the past decade, the adolescent immunization schedule has expanded to include 2 doses of quadrivalent meningococcal conjugate vaccine; 1 dose of tetanus, diphtheria, acellular pertussis, absorbed vaccine; 2 or 3 doses of human papillomavirus vaccine, depending on the child's age; and an annual influenza vaccine. In addition, during adolescent visits, health care providers can determine whether catch-up vaccination is needed to meet early childhood recommendations for hepatitis B; hepatitis A; measles, mumps, rubella; poliovirus; and varicella vaccines. New serogroup B meningococcal vaccines are now available for those at increased risk for meningococcal disease; in addition, these serogroup B meningococcal vaccines received a Category B recommendation for healthy adolescents, where individual counseling and risk–benefit evaluation based on health care provider judgements and patient preferences are indicated. This clinical report focuses on the epidemiology of adolescent vaccine-preventable diseases by reviewing the rationale for the annual universally recommended adolescent immunization schedule of the American Academy of Pediatrics, the American Academy of Family Physicians, the Centers for Disease Control and Prevention, and the American Congress of Obstetricians and Gynecologists. In addition, the barriers that negatively influence adherence to this current adolescent immunization schedule will be highlighted. (2/17)

http://pediatrics.aappublications.org/content/139/3/e20164186

NEEDS OF KINSHIP CARE FAMILIES AND PEDIATRIC PRACTICE

David Rubin, MD, FAAP; Sarah H. Springer, MD, FAAP; Sarah Zlotnik, MSW, MSPH; Christina D. Kang-Yi, PhD; and Council on Foster Care, Adoption, and Kinship Care

ABSTRACT. As many as 3% of children in the United States live in kinship care arrangements with caregivers who are relatives but not the biological parents of the child. A growing body of evidence suggests that children who cannot live with their biological parents fare better, overall, when living with extended family than with nonrelated foster parents. Acknowledging this, federal laws and public policies increasingly favor kinship care over nonrelative foster care when children are unable to live with their biological parents. Despite overall better outcomes, families providing kinship care experience many hardships, and the children experience many of the same adversities of children in traditional foster care. This policy statement reviews both the strengths and vulnerabilities of kinship families and suggests strategies for pediatricians to use to address the needs of individual patients and families. Strategies are also outlined for community, state, and federal advocacy on behalf of these children and their families. (3/17)

http://pediatrics.aappublications.org/content/139/4/e20170099

NEONATAL DRUG WITHDRAWAL (CLINICAL REPORT)

Mark L. Hudak, MD; Rosemarie C. Tan, MD, PhD; Committee on Drugs; and Committee on Fetus and Newborn

ABSTRACT. Maternal use of certain drugs during pregnancy can result in transient neonatal signs consistent with withdrawal or acute toxicity or cause sustained signs consistent with a lasting drug effect. In addition, hospitalized infants who are treated with opioids or benzodiazepines to provide analgesia or sedation may be at risk for manifesting signs of withdrawal. This statement updates information about the clinical presentation of infants exposed to intrauterine drugs and the therapeutic options for treatment of withdrawal and is expanded to include evidence-based approaches to the management of the hospitalized infant who requires weaning from analgesics or sedatives. (1/12, reaffirmed 2/16)

http://pediatrics.aappublications.org/content/129/2/e540

A NEW ERA IN QUALITY MEASUREMENT: THE DEVELOPMENT AND APPLICATION OF QUALITY MEASURES

Terry Adirim, MD, MPH, FAAP; Kelley Meade, MD, FAAP; Kamila Mistry, PhD, MPH; Council on Quality Improvement and Patient Safety; and Committee on Practice and Ambulatory Medicine

ABSTRACT. Quality measures are used for a variety of purposes in health care, including clinical care improvement, regulation, accreditation, public reporting, surveillance, and maintenance of certification. Most quality measures are 1 of 3 types: structure, process, or outcome. Health care quality measures should address the domains of quality across the continuum of care and reflect patient and family experience. Measure development for pediatric health care has a number of important challenges, including gaps in the evidence base; the fact that measures for most conditions must be age-specific; the long, resourceintensive development process; and the national focus on measure development for adult conditions. Numerous national organizations focus on the development and application of quality measures, including the Pediatric Quality Measures Program, which is focused solely on the development and implementation of pediatric-specific measures. Once a quality measure is developed for use in national measurement programs, the organization that develops and/or "stewards" the measure may submit the measure or set of measures for endorsement, which is recognition of the scientific soundness, usability, and relevance of the measure. Quality measures must then be disseminated and applied to improve care. Although pediatric health care providers and child health care institutions alike must continually balance time and resources needed to address multiple reporting requirements, quality measurement is an important tool for advancing high-quality and safe health care for children. This policy statement provides an overview of quality measurement and describes the opportunities for pediatric health care providers to apply quality measures to improve clinical quality and performance in the delivery of pediatric health care services. (12/16)

http://pediatrics.aappublications.org/content/139/1/e20163442

NEWBORN SCREENING EXPANDS: RECOMMENDATIONS FOR PEDIATRICIANS AND MEDICAL HOMES—IMPLICATIONS FOR THE SYSTEM (CLINICAL REPORT)

PPI
AAP Partnership for Policy Implementation

Newborn Screening Authoring Committee

ABSTRACT. Advances in newborn screening technology, coupled with recent advances in the diagnosis and treatment of rare but serious congenital conditions that affect newborn infants, provide increased opportunities for positively affecting the lives of children and their families. These advantages also pose new challenges to primary care pediatricians, both educationally and in response to the management of affected infants. Primary care pediatricians require immediate access to clinical and diagnostic information and guidance and have a proactive role to play in supporting the performance of the newborn screening system. Primary care pediatricians must develop office policies and procedures to ensure that newborn screening is conducted and that results are transmitted to them in a timely fashion; they must also develop strategies to use should these systems fail. In addition, collaboration with local, state, and national partners is essential for promoting actions and policies that will optimize the function of the newborn screening systems and ensure that families receive the full benefit of them. (1/08, reaffirmed 9/16)

http://pediatrics.aappublications.org/content/121/1/192

NEWBORN SCREENING FOR BILIARY ATRESIA (TECHNICAL REPORT)

Kasper S. Wang, MD, FAAP, FACS; Section on Surgery; and Committee on Fetus and Newborn (joint with Childhood Liver Disease Research Network)

ABSTRACT. Biliary atresia is the most common cause of pediatric end-stage liver disease and the leading indication for pediatric liver transplantation. Affected infants exhibit evidence of biliary obstruction within the first few weeks after birth. Early diagnosis and successful surgical drainage of bile are associated with greater survival with the child's native liver. Unfortunately, because noncholestatic jaundice is extremely common in early infancy, it is difficult to identify the rare infant with cholestatic jaundice who has biliary atresia. Hence, the need for timely diagnosis of this disease warrants a discussion of the feasibility of screening for biliary atresia to improve outcomes. Herein, newborn screening for biliary atresia in the United States is assessed by using criteria established by the Discretionary Advisory Committee on Heritable Disorders in Newborns and Children. Published analyses indicate that newborn screening for biliary atresia by using serum bilirubin concentrations or stool color cards is potentially life-saving and cost-effective. Further studies are necessary to evaluate the feasibility, effectiveness, and costs of potential screening strategies for early identification of biliary atresia in the United States. (11/15)
http://pediatrics.aappublications.org/content/136/6/e1663

NICOTINE AND TOBACCO AS SUBSTANCES OF ABUSE IN CHILDREN AND ADOLESCENTS (TECHNICAL REPORT)

Lorena M. Siqueira, MD, MSPH, FAAP, FSAHM, and Committee on Substance Use and Prevention

ABSTRACT. Nicotine is the primary pharmacologic component of tobacco, and users of tobacco products seek out its effects. The highly addictive nature of nicotine is responsible for its widespread use and difficulty with quitting. This technical report focuses on nicotine and discusses the stages of use in progression to dependence on nicotine-containing products; the physiologic characteristics, neurobiology, metabolism, pharmacogenetics, and health effects of nicotine; and acute nicotine toxicity. Finally, some newer approaches to cessation are noted. (12/16)
http://pediatrics.aappublications.org/content/139/1/e20163436

NONDISCRIMINATION IN PEDIATRIC HEALTH CARE

Committee on Pediatric Workforce

ABSTRACT. This policy statement is a revision of a 2001 statement and articulates the positions of the American Academy of Pediatrics on nondiscrimination in pediatric health care. It addresses both pediatricians who provide health care and the infants, children, adolescents, and young adults whom they serve. (10/07, reaffirmed 6/11, 1/15)
http://pediatrics.aappublications.org/content/120/4/922

NONEMERGENCY ACUTE CARE: WHEN IT'S NOT THE MEDICAL HOME

Gregory P. Conners, MD, MPH, MBA, FAAP; Susan J. Kressly, MD, FAAP; James M. Perrin, MD, FAAP; Julia E. Richerson, MD, FAAP; Usha M. Sankrithi, MBBS, MPH, FAAP; Committee on Practice and Ambulatory Medicine; Committee on Pediatric Emergency Medicine; Section on Telehealth Care; Section on Emergency Medicine; Subcommittee on Urgent Care; and Task Force on Pediatric Practice Change

ABSTRACT. The American Academy of Pediatrics (AAP) affirms that the optimal location for children to receive care for acute, nonemergency health concerns is the medical home. The medical home is characterized by the AAP as a care model that "must be accessible, family centered, continuous, comprehensive, coordinated, compassionate, and culturally effective." However, some children and families use acute care services outside the medical home because there is a perceived or real benefit related to accessibility, convenience, or cost of care. Examples of such acute care entities include urgent care facilities, retail-based clinics, and commercial telemedicine services. Children deserve high-quality, appropriate, and safe acute care services wherever they access the health care system, with timely and complete communication with the medical home, to ensure coordinated and continuous care. Treatment of children under established, new, and evolving practice arrangements in acute care entities should adhere to the core principles of continuity of care and communication, best practices within a defined scope of services, pediatric-trained staff, safe transitions of care, and continuous improvement. In support of the medical home, the AAP urges stakeholders, including payers, to avoid any incentives (eg, reduced copays) that encourage visits to external entities for acute issues as a preference over the medical home. (4/17)
http://pediatrics.aappublications.org/content/139/5/e20170629

NONINITIATION OR WITHDRAWAL OF INTENSIVE CARE FOR HIGH-RISK NEWBORNS

Committee on Fetus and Newborn

ABSTRACT. Advances in medical technology have led to dilemmas in initiation and withdrawal of intensive care of newborn infants with a very poor prognosis. Physicians and parents together must make difficult decisions guided by their understanding of the child's best interest. The foundation for these decisions consists of several key elements: (1) direct and open communication between the health care team and the parents of the child with regard to the medical status, prognosis, and treatment options; (2) inclusion of the parents as active participants in the decision process; (3) continuation of comfort care even when intensive care is not being provided; and (4) treatment decisions that are guided primarily by the best interest of the child. (2/07, reaffirmed 5/10, 6/15)
http://pediatrics.aappublications.org/content/119/2/401

NONINVASIVE RESPIRATORY SUPPORT (CLINICAL REPORT)

James J. Cummings, MD, FAAP; Richard A. Polin, MD, FAAP; and Committee on Fetus and Newborn

ABSTRACT. Mechanical ventilation is associated with increased survival of preterm infants but is also associated with an increased incidence of chronic lung disease (bronchopulmonary dysplasia) in survivors. Nasal continuous positive airway pressure (nCPAP) is a form of noninvasive ventilation that reduces the need for mechanical ventilation and decreases the combined outcome of death or bronchopulmonary dysplasia. Other modes of noninvasive ventilation, including nasal intermittent positive pressure ventilation, biphasic positive airway pressure, and high-flow nasal cannula, have recently been introduced into the NICU setting as potential alternatives to mechanical ventilation or nCPAP. Randomized controlled trials suggest that these newer modalities may be effective alternatives to nCPAP and may offer some advantages over nCPAP, but efficacy and safety data are limited. (12/15)
http://pediatrics.aappublications.org/content/137/1/e20153758

NONORAL FEEDING FOR CHILDREN AND YOUTH WITH DEVELOPMENTAL OR ACQUIRED DISABILITIES (CLINICAL REPORT)

Richard C. Adams, MD, FAAP; Ellen Roy Elias, MD, FAAP; and Council on Children With Disabilities

ABSTRACT. The decision to initiate enteral feedings is multifaceted, involving medical, financial, cultural, and emotional considerations. Children who have developmental or acquired disabilities are at risk for having primary and secondary conditions that affect growth and nutritional well-being. This clinical report provides (1) an overview of clinical issues in children who have developmental or acquired disabilities that may prompt a need to consider nonoral feedings, (2) a systematic way to support the child and family in clinical decisions related to initiating nonoral feeding, (3) information on surgical options that the family may need to consider in that decision-making process, and (4) pediatric guidance for ongoing care after initiation of nonoral feeding intervention, including care of the gastrostomy tube and skin site. Ongoing medical and psychosocial support is needed after initiation of nonoral feedings and is best provided through the collaborative efforts of the family and a team of professionals that may include the pediatrician, dietitian, social worker, and/or therapists. (11/14)

http://pediatrics.aappublications.org/content/134/6/e1745

NONTHERAPEUTIC USE OF ANTIMICROBIAL AGENTS IN ANIMAL AGRICULTURE: IMPLICATIONS FOR PEDIATRICS (TECHNICAL REPORT)

Jerome A. Paulson, MD, FAAP; Theoklis E. Zaoutis, MD, MSCE, FAAP; Council on Environmental Health; and Committee on Infectious Diseases

ABSTRACT. Antimicrobial resistance is one of the most serious threats to public health globally and threatens our ability to treat infectious diseases. Antimicrobial-resistant infections are associated with increased morbidity, mortality, and health care costs. Infants and children are affected by transmission of susceptible and resistant food zoonotic pathogens through the food supply, direct contact with animals, and environmental pathways. The overuse and misuse of antimicrobial agents in veterinary and human medicine is, in large part, responsible for the emergence of antibiotic resistance. Approximately 80% of the overall tonnage of antimicrobial agents sold in the United States in 2012 was for animal use, and approximately 60% of those agents are considered important for human medicine. Most of the use involves the addition of low doses of antimicrobial agents to the feed of healthy animals over prolonged periods to promote growth and increase feed efficiency or at a range of doses to prevent disease. These nontherapeutic uses contribute to resistance and create new health dangers for humans. This report describes how antimicrobial agents are used in animal agriculture, reviews the mechanisms of how such use contributes to development of resistance, and discusses US and global initiatives to curb the use of antimicrobial agents in agriculture. (11/15)

http://pediatrics.aappublications.org/content/136/6/e1670

OFFICE-BASED CARE FOR LESBIAN, GAY, BISEXUAL, TRANSGENDER, AND QUESTIONING YOUTH

Committee on Adolescence

ABSTRACT. The American Academy of Pediatrics issued its last statement on homosexuality and adolescents in 2004. Although most lesbian, gay, bisexual, transgender, and questioning (LGBTQ) youth are quite resilient and emerge from adolescence as healthy adults, the effects of homophobia and heterosexism can contribute to health disparities in mental health with higher rates of depression and suicidal ideation, higher rates of substance abuse, and more sexually transmitted and HIV infections. Pediatricians should have offices that are teen-friendly and welcoming to sexual minority youth. Obtaining a comprehensive, confidential, developmentally appropriate adolescent psychosocial history allows for the discovery of strengths and assets as well as risks. Referrals for mental health or substance abuse may be warranted. Sexually active LGBTQ youth should have sexually transmitted infection/HIV testing according to recommendations of the Sexually Transmitted Diseases Treatment Guidelines of the Centers for Disease Control and Prevention based on sexual behaviors. With appropriate assistance and care, sexual minority youth should live healthy, productive lives while transitioning through adolescence and young adulthood. (6/13)

http://pediatrics.aappublications.org/content/132/1/198

OFFICE-BASED CARE FOR LESBIAN, GAY, BISEXUAL, TRANSGENDER, AND QUESTIONING YOUTH (TECHNICAL REPORT)

David A. Levine, MD, and Committee on Adolescence

ABSTRACT. The American Academy of Pediatrics issued its last statement on homosexuality and adolescents in 2004. This technical report reflects the rapidly expanding medical and psychosocial literature about sexual minority youth. Pediatricians should be aware that some youth in their care may have concerns or questions about their sexual orientation or that of siblings, friends, parents, relatives, or others and should provide factual, current, nonjudgmental information in a confidential manner. Although most lesbian, gay, bisexual, transgender, and questioning (LGBTQ) youth are quite resilient and emerge from adolescence as healthy adults, the effects of homophobia and heterosexism can contribute to increased mental health issues for sexual minority youth. LGBTQ and MSM/WSW (men having sex with men and women having sex with women) adolescents, in comparison with heterosexual adolescents, have higher rates of depression and suicidal ideation, higher rates of substance abuse, and more risky sexual behaviors. Obtaining a comprehensive, confidential, developmentally appropriate adolescent psychosocial history allows for the discovery of strengths and assets as well as risks. Pediatricians should have offices that are teen-friendly and welcoming to sexual minority youth. This includes having supportive, engaging office staff members who ensure that there are no barriers to care. For transgender youth, pediatricians should provide the opportunity to acknowledge and affirm their feelings of gender dysphoria and desires to transition to the opposite gender. Referral of transgender youth to a qualified mental health professional is critical to assist with the dysphoria, to educate them, and to assess their readiness for transition. With appropriate assistance and care, sexual minority youth should live healthy, productive lives while transitioning through adolescence and young adulthood. (6/13)

http://pediatrics.aappublications.org/content/132/1/e297

OFFICE-BASED COUNSELING FOR UNINTENTIONAL INJURY PREVENTION (CLINICAL REPORT)

H. Garry Gardner, MD, and Committee on Injury, Violence, and Poison Prevention

ABSTRACT. Unintentional injuries are the leading cause of death for children older than 1 year. Pediatricians should include unintentional injury prevention as a major component of anticipatory guidance for infants, children, and adolescents. The content of injury-prevention counseling varies for infants, preschool-aged children, school-aged children, and adolescents. This report provides guidance on the content of unintentional injury-prevention counseling for each of those age groups. (1/07)

http://pediatrics.aappublications.org/content/119/1/202

OFF-LABEL USE OF DRUGS IN CHILDREN

Committee on Drugs

ABSTRACT. The passage of the Best Pharmaceuticals for Children Act and the Pediatric Research Equity Act has collectively resulted in an improvement in rational prescribing for children, including more than 500 labeling changes. However, off-label drug use remains an important public health issue for infants, children, and adolescents, because an overwhelming number of drugs still have no information in the labeling for use in pediatrics. The purpose of off-label use is to benefit the individual patient. Practitioners use their professional judgment to determine these uses. As such, the term "off-label" does not imply an improper, illegal, contraindicated, or investigational use. Therapeutic decision-making must always rely on the best available evidence and the importance of the benefit for the individual patient. (2/14)

http://pediatrics.aappublications.org/content/133/3/563

OFF-LABEL USE OF MEDICAL DEVICES IN CHILDREN

*Section on Cardiology and Cardiac Surgery and Section on
    Orthopaedics*

ABSTRACT. Despite widespread therapeutic needs, the majority of medical and surgical devices used in children do not have approval or clearance from the Food and Drug Administration (FDA) for use in pediatric populations. The clinical need for devices to diagnose and treat diseases or conditions occurring in children has led to the widespread and necessary practice in pediatric medicine and surgery of using approved devices for "off-label" or "physician-directed" applications that are not included in FDA-approved labeling. This practice is common and often appropriate, even with the highest-risk (class III) devices. The legal and regulatory framework used by the FDA for devices is complex, and economic or market barriers to medical and surgical device development for children are significant. Given the need for pediatric medical and surgical devices and the challenges to pediatric device development, off-label use is a necessary and appropriate part of care. In addition, because of the relatively uncommon nature of pediatric conditions, FDA clearance or approval often requires other regulatory pathways (eg, Humanitarian Device Exemption), which can cause confusion among pediatricians and payers about whether a specific use, even of an approved device, is considered experimental. This policy statement describes the appropriateness of off-label use of devices in children; the use of devices approved or cleared through the FDA regulatory processes, including through the Humanitarian Device Exemption; and the important need to increase pediatric device labeling information for all devices and especially those that pose the highest risk to children. (12/16)
http://pediatrics.aappublications.org/content/139/1/e20163439

OPHTHALMOLOGIC EXAMINATIONS IN CHILDREN WITH JUVENILE RHEUMATOID ARTHRITIS (CLINICAL REPORT)

*James Cassidy, MD; Jane Kivlin, MD; Carol Lindsley, MD;
    James Nocton, MD; Section on Rheumatology; and Section on
    Ophthalmology*

ABSTRACT. Unlike the joints, ocular involvement with juvenile rheumatoid arthritis is most often asymptomatic; yet, the inflammation can cause serious morbidity with loss of vision. Scheduled slit-lamp examinations by an ophthalmologist at specific intervals can detect ocular disease early, and prompt treatment can prevent vision loss. (5/06, reaffirmed 10/12, 7/18)
http://pediatrics.aappublications.org/content/117/5/1843

OPTIMIZING BONE HEALTH IN CHILDREN AND ADOLESCENTS (CLINICAL REPORT)

*Neville H. Golden, MD; Steven A. Abrams, MD; and Committee on
    Nutrition*

ABSTRACT. The pediatrician plays a major role in helping optimize bone health in children and adolescents. This clinical report reviews normal bone acquisition in infants, children, and adolescents and discusses factors affecting bone health in this age group. Previous recommended daily allowances for calcium and vitamin D are updated, and clinical guidance is provided regarding weight-bearing activities and recommendations for calcium and vitamin D intake and supplementation. Routine calcium supplementation is not recommended for healthy children and adolescents, but increased dietary intake to meet daily requirements is encouraged. The American Academy of Pediatrics endorses the higher recommended dietary allowances for vitamin D advised by the Institute of Medicine and supports testing for vitamin D deficiency in children and adolescents with conditions associated with increased bone fragility. Universal screening for vitamin D deficiency is not routinely recommended in healthy children or in children with dark skin or obesity because there is insufficient evidence of the cost–benefit of such a practice in reducing fracture risk. The preferred test to assess bone health is dual-energy x-ray absorptiometry, but caution is advised when interpreting results in children and adolescents who may not yet have achieved peak bone mass. For analyses, z scores should be used instead of T scores, and corrections should be made for size. Office-based strategies for the pediatrician to optimize bone health are provided. This clinical report has been endorsed by American Bone Health. (9/14)
http://pediatrics.aappublications.org/content/134/4/e1229

OPTIONS COUNSELING FOR THE PREGNANT ADOLESCENT PATIENT

*Laurie L. Hornberger, MD, MPH, FAAP, and Committee on
    Adolescence*

ABSTRACT. Each year, more than 500 000 girls and young women younger than 20 years become pregnant. It is important for pediatricians to have the ability and the resources in their offices to make a timely pregnancy diagnosis in their adolescent patients and provide them with nonjudgmental pregnancy options counseling. Counseling includes an unbiased discussion of the adolescent's legal options to either continue or terminate her pregnancy, supporting the adolescent in the decision-making process, and referring the adolescent to appropriate resources and services. Pediatricians who choose not to provide such discussions should promptly refer pregnant adolescent patients to a health care professional who will offer developmentally appropriate pregnancy options counseling. This approach to pregnancy options counseling has not changed since the original 1989 American Academy of Pediatrics statement on this issue. (8/17)
http://pediatrics.aappublications.org/content/140/3/e20172274

ORAL AND DENTAL ASPECTS OF CHILD ABUSE AND NEGLECT (CLINICAL REPORT)

*Susan A. Fisher-Owens, MD, MPH, FAAP; James L. Lukefahr, MD,
    FAAP; Anupama Rao Tate, DMD, MPH; Section on Oral Health;
    and Committee on Child Abuse and Neglect (joint with American
    Academy of Pediatric Dentistry Council on Clinical Affairs,
    Council on Scientific Affairs, and Ad Hoc Work Group on Child
    Abuse and Neglect)*

ABSTRACT. In all 50 states, health care providers (including dentists) are mandated to report suspected cases of abuse and neglect to social service or law enforcement agencies. The purpose of this report is to review the oral and dental aspects of physical and sexual abuse and dental neglect in children and the role of pediatric care providers and dental providers in evaluating such conditions. This report addresses the evaluation of bite marks as well as perioral and intraoral injuries, infections, and diseases that may raise suspicion for child abuse or neglect. Oral health issues can also be associated with bullying and are commonly seen in human trafficking victims. Some medical providers may receive less education pertaining to oral health and dental injury and disease and may not detect the mouth and gum findings that are related to abuse or neglect as readily as they detect those involving other areas of the body. Therefore, pediatric care providers and dental providers are encouraged to collaborate to increase the prevention, detection, and treatment of these conditions in children. (7/17)
http://pediatrics.aappublications.org/content/140/2/e20171487

ORAL HEALTH CARE FOR CHILDREN WITH DEVELOPMENTAL DISABILITIES (CLINICAL REPORT)

*Kenneth W. Norwood Jr, MD; Rebecca L. Slayton, DDS,
    PhD; Council on Children With Disabilities; and Section on
    Oral Health*

ABSTRACT. Children with developmental disabilities often have unmet complex health care needs as well as significant physical and cognitive limitations. Children with more severe conditions and from low-income families are particularly at risk

with high dental needs and poor access to care. In addition, children with developmental disabilities are living longer, requiring continued oral health care. This clinical report describes the effect that poor oral health has on children with developmental disabilities as well as the importance of partnerships between the pediatric medical and dental homes. Basic knowledge of the oral health risk factors affecting children with developmental disabilities is provided. Pediatricians may use the report to guide their incorporation of oral health assessments and education into their well-child examinations for children with developmental disabilities. This report has medical, legal, educational, and operational implications for practicing pediatricians. (2/13)
http://pediatrics.aappublications.org/content/131/3/614

ORGANIC FOODS: HEALTH AND ENVIRONMENTAL ADVANTAGES AND DISADVANTAGES (CLINICAL REPORT)

Joel Forman, MD; Janet Silverstein, MD; Committee on Nutrition; and Council on Environmental Health

ABSTRACT. The US market for organic foods has grown from $3.5 billion in 1996 to $28.6 billion in 2010, according to the Organic Trade Association. Organic products are now sold in specialty stores and conventional supermarkets. Organic products contain numerous marketing claims and terms, only some of which are standardized and regulated.

In terms of health advantages, organic diets have been convincingly demonstrated to expose consumers to fewer pesticides associated with human disease. Organic farming has been demonstrated to have less environmental impact than conventional approaches. However, current evidence does not support any meaningful nutritional benefits or deficits from eating organic compared with conventionally grown foods, and there are no well-powered human studies that directly demonstrate health benefits or disease protection as a result of consuming an organic diet. Studies also have not demonstrated any detrimental or disease-promoting effects from an organic diet. Although organic foods regularly command a significant price premium, well-designed farming studies demonstrate that costs can be competitive and yields comparable to those of conventional farming techniques. Pediatricians should incorporate this evidence when discussing the health and environmental impact of organic foods and organic farming while continuing to encourage all patients and their families to attain optimal nutrition and dietary variety consistent with the US Department of Agriculture's MyPlate recommendations.

This clinical report reviews the health and environmental issues related to organic food production and consumption. It defines the term "organic," reviews organic food-labeling standards, describes organic and conventional farming practices, and explores the cost and environmental implications of organic production techniques. It examines the evidence available on nutritional quality and production contaminants in conventionally produced and organic foods. Finally, this report provides guidance for pediatricians to assist them in advising their patients regarding organic and conventionally produced food choices. (10/12)
http://pediatrics.aappublications.org/content/130/5/e1406

ORGANIZED SPORTS FOR CHILDREN AND PREADOLESCENTS

Committee on Sports Medicine and Fitness and Committee on School Health

ABSTRACT. Participation in organized sports provides an opportunity for young people to increase their physical activity and develop physical and social skills. However, when the demands and expectations of organized sports exceed the maturation and readiness of the participant, the positive aspects of participation can be negated. The nature of parental or adult involvement can also influence the degree to which participation in organized sports is a positive experience for preadolescents. This updates a previous policy statement on athletics for preadolescents and incorporates guidelines for sports participation for preschool children. Recommendations are offered on how pediatricians can help determine a child's readiness to participate, how risks can be minimized, and how child-oriented goals can be maximized. (6/01, reaffirmed 8/16)
http://pediatrics.aappublications.org/content/107/6/1459

OUT-OF-HOME PLACEMENT FOR CHILDREN AND ADOLESCENTS WITH DISABILITIES (CLINICAL REPORT)

Sandra L. Friedman, MD, MPH; Miriam A. Kalichman, MD; and Council on Children With Disabilities

ABSTRACT. The vast majority of children and youth with chronic and complex health conditions who also have intellectual and developmental disabilities are cared for in their homes. Social, legal, policy, and medical changes through the years have allowed for an increase in needed support within the community. However, there continues to be a relatively small group of children who live in various types of congregate care settings. This clinical report describes these settings and the care and services that are provided in them. The report also discusses reasons families choose out-of-home placement for their children, barriers to placement, and potential effects of this decision on family members. We examine the pediatrician's role in caring for children with severe intellectual and developmental disabilities and complex medical problems in the context of responding to parental inquiries about out-of-home placement and understanding factors affecting these types of decisions. Common medical problems and care issues for children residing outside the family home are reviewed. Variations in state and federal regulations, challenges in understanding local systems, and access to services are also discussed. (9/14)
http://pediatrics.aappublications.org/content/134/4/836

OUT-OF-HOME PLACEMENT FOR CHILDREN AND ADOLESCENTS WITH DISABILITIES—ADDENDUM: CARE OPTIONS FOR CHILDREN AND ADOLESCENTS WITH DISABILITIES AND MEDICAL COMPLEXITY (CLINICAL REPORT)

Sandra L. Friedman, MD, MPH, FAAP; Kenneth W. Norwood Jr, MD, FAAP; and Council on Children With Disabilities

ABSTRACT. Children and adolescents with significant intellectual and developmental disabilities and complex medical problems require safe and comprehensive care to meet their medical and psychosocial needs. Ideally, such children and youth should be cared for by their families in their home environments. When this type of arrangement is not possible, there should be exploration of appropriate, alternative noncongregate community-based settings, especially alternative family homes. Government funding sources exist to support care in the community, although there is variability among states with regard to the availability of community programs and resources. It is important that families are supported in learning about options of care. Pediatricians can serve as advocates for their patients and their families to access community-based services and to increase the availability of resources to ensure that the option to live in a family home is available to all children with complex medical needs. (11/16)
http://pediatrics.aappublications.org/content/138/6/e20163216

OUT-OF-SCHOOL SUSPENSION AND EXPULSION

Council on School Health

ABSTRACT. The primary mission of any school system is to educate students. To achieve this goal, the school district must maintain a culture and environment where all students feel safe, nurtured, and valued and where order and civility are expected standards of behavior. Schools cannot allow unacceptable behavior to interfere with the school district's primary

mission. To this end, school districts adopt codes of conduct for expected behaviors and policies to address unacceptable behavior. In developing these policies, school boards must weigh the severity of the offense and the consequences of the punishment and the balance between individual and institutional rights and responsibilities. Out-of-school suspension and expulsion are the most severe consequences that a school district can impose for unacceptable behavior. Traditionally, these consequences have been reserved for offenses deemed especially severe or dangerous and/or for recalcitrant offenders. However, the implications and consequences of out-of-school suspension and expulsion and "zero-tolerance" are of such severity that their application and appropriateness for a developing child require periodic review. The indications and effectiveness of exclusionary discipline policies that demand automatic or rigorous application are increasingly questionable. The impact of these policies on offenders, other children, school districts, and communities is broad. Periodic scrutiny of policies should be placed not only on the need for a better understanding of the educational, emotional, and social impact of out-of-school suspension and expulsion on the individual student but also on the greater societal costs of such rigid policies. Pediatricians should be prepared to assist students and families affected by out-of-school suspension and expulsion and should be willing to guide school districts in their communities to find more effective and appropriate alternatives to exclusionary discipline policies for the developing child. A discussion of preventive strategies and alternatives to out-of-school suspension and expulsion, as well as recommendations for the role of the physician in matters of out-of-school suspension and expulsion are included. School-wide positive behavior support/positive behavior intervention and support is discussed as an effective alternative. (2/13)
http://pediatrics.aappublications.org/content/131/3/e1000

OVERCROWDING CRISIS IN OUR NATION'S EMERGENCY DEPARTMENTS: IS OUR SAFETY NET UNRAVELING?

Committee on Pediatric Emergency Medicine

ABSTRACT. Emergency departments (EDs) are a vital component in our health care safety net, available 24 hours a day, 7 days a week, for all who require care. There has been a steady increase in the volume and acuity of patient visits to EDs, now with well over 100 million Americans (30 million children) receiving emergency care annually. This rise in ED utilization has effectively saturated the capacity of EDs and emergency medical services in many communities. The resulting phenomenon, commonly referred to as ED overcrowding, now threatens access to emergency services for those who need them the most. As managers of the pediatric medical home and advocates for children and optimal pediatric health care, there is a very important role for pediatricians and the American Academy of Pediatrics in guiding health policy decision-makers toward effective solutions that promote the medical home and timely access to emergency care. (9/04, reaffirmed 5/07, 6/11, 7/16)
http://pediatrics.aappublications.org/content/114/3/878

OVERUSE INJURIES, OVERTRAINING, AND BURNOUT IN CHILD AND ADOLESCENT ATHLETES (CLINICAL REPORT)

Joel S. Brenner, MD, MPH, and Council on Sports Medicine and Fitness

ABSTRACT. Overuse is one of the most common etiologic factors that lead to injuries in the pediatric and adolescent athlete. As more children are becoming involved in organized and recreational athletics, the incidence of overuse injuries is increasing. Many children are participating in sports year-round and sometimes on multiple teams simultaneously. This overtraining can lead to burnout, which may have a detrimental effect on the

child participating in sports as a lifelong healthy activity. One contributing factor to overtraining may be parental pressure to compete and succeed. The purpose of this clinical report is to assist pediatricians in identifying and counseling at-risk children and their families. This report supports the American Academy of Pediatrics policy statement on intensive training and sport specialization. (6/07, reaffirmed 3/11, 6/14)
http://pediatrics.aappublications.org/content/119/6/1242

OXYGEN TARGETING IN EXTREMELY LOW BIRTH WEIGHT INFANTS (CLINICAL REPORT)

James J. Cummings, MD, FAAP; Richard A. Polin, MD, FAAP; and Committee on Fetus and Newborn

ABSTRACT. The use of supplemental oxygen plays a vital role in the care of the critically ill preterm infant, but the unrestricted use of oxygen can lead to unintended harms, such as chronic lung disease and retinopathy of prematurity. An overly restricted use of supplemental oxygen may have adverse effects as well. Ideally, continuous monitoring of tissue and cellular oxygen delivery would allow clinicians to better titrate the use of supplemental oxygen, but such monitoring is not currently feasible in the clinical setting. The introduction of pulse oximetry has greatly aided the clinician by providing a relatively easy and continuous estimate of arterial oxygen saturation, but pulse oximetry has several practical, technical, and physiologic limitations. Recent randomized clinical trials comparing different pulse oximetry targets have been conducted to better inform the practice of supplemental oxygen use. This clinical report discusses the benefits and limitations of pulse oximetry for assessing oxygenation, summarizes randomized clinical trials of oxygen saturation targeting, and addresses implications for practice. (7/16)
http://pediatrics.aappublications.org/content/138/2/e20161576

PAIN ASSESSMENT AND TREATMENT IN CHILDREN WITH SIGNIFICANT IMPAIRMENT OF THE CENTRAL NERVOUS SYSTEM (CLINICAL REPORT)

Julie Hauer, MD, FAAP; Amy J. Houtrow, MD, PhD, MPH, FAAP; Section on Hospice and Palliative Medicine; and Council on Children With Disabilities

ABSTRACT. Pain is a frequent and significant problem for children with impairment of the central nervous system, with the highest frequency and severity occurring in children with the greatest impairment. Despite the significance of the problem, this population remains vulnerable to underrecognition and undertreatment of pain. Barriers to treatment may include uncertainty in identifying pain along with limited experience and fear with the use of medications for pain treatment. Behavioral pain-assessment tools are reviewed in this clinical report, along with other strategies for monitoring pain after an intervention. Sources of pain in this population include acute-onset pain attributable to tissue injury or inflammation resulting in nociceptive pain, with pain then expected to resolve after treatment directed at the source. Other sources can result in chronic intermittent pain that, for many, occurs on a weekly to daily basis, commonly attributed to gastroesophageal reflux, spasticity, and hip subluxation. Most challenging are pain sources attributable to the impaired central nervous system, requiring empirical medication trials directed at causes that cannot be identified by diagnostic tests, such as central neuropathic pain. Interventions reviewed include integrative therapies and medications, such as gabapentinoids, tricyclic antidepressants, α-agonists, and opioids. This clinical report aims to address, with evidence-based guidance, the inherent challenges with the goal to improve comfort throughout life in this vulnerable group of children. (5/17)
http://pediatrics.aappublications.org/content/139/6/e20171002

PARENTAL LEAVE FOR RESIDENTS AND PEDIATRIC TRAINING PROGRAMS

Section on Medical Students, Residents, and Fellowship Trainees and Committee on Early Childhood

ABSTRACT. The American Academy of Pediatrics (AAP) is committed to the development of rational, equitable, and effective parental leave policies that are sensitive to the needs of pediatric residents, families, and developing infants and that enable parents to spend adequate and good-quality time with their young children. It is important for each residency program to have a policy for parental leave that is written, that is accessible to residents, and that clearly delineates program practices regarding parental leave. At a minimum, a parental leave policy for residents and fellows should conform legally with the Family Medical Leave Act as well as with respective state laws and should meet institutional requirements of the Accreditation Council for Graduate Medical Education for accredited programs. Policies should be well formulated and communicated in a culturally sensitive manner. The AAP advocates for extension of benefits consistent with the Family Medical Leave Act to all residents and interns beginning at the time that pediatric residency training begins. The AAP recommends that regardless of gender, residents who become parents should be guaranteed 6 to 8 weeks, at a minimum, of parental leave with pay after the infant's birth. In addition, in conformance with federal law, the resident should be allowed to extend the leave time when necessary by using paid vacation time or leave without pay. Coparenting, adopting, or fostering of a child should entitle the resident, regardless of gender, to the same amount of paid leave (6–8 weeks) as a person who takes maternity/paternity leave. Flexibility, creativity, and advanced planning are necessary to arrange schedules that optimize resident education and experience, cultivate equity in sharing workloads, and protect pregnant residents from overly strenuous work experiences at critical times of their pregnancies. (1/13)

http://pediatrics.aappublications.org/content/131/2/387

PARENTAL PRESENCE DURING TREATMENT OF EBOLA OR OTHER HIGHLY CONSEQUENTIAL INFECTION (CLINICAL REPORT)

H. Dele Davies, MD, MS, MHCM, FAAP; Carrie L. Byington, MD, FAAP; and Committee on Infectious Diseases

ABSTRACT. This clinical report offers guidance to health care providers and hospitals on options to consider regarding parental presence at the bedside while caring for a child with suspected or proven Ebola virus disease (Ebola) or other highly consequential infection. Options are presented to help meet the needs of the patient and the family while also posing the least risk to providers and health care organizations. The optimal way to minimize risk is to limit contact between the person under investigation or treatment and family members/caregivers whenever possible while working to meet the emotional support needs of both patient and family. At times, caregiver presence may be deemed to be in the best interest of the patient, and in such situations, a strong effort should be made to limit potential risks of exposure to the caregiver, health care providers, and the community. The decision to allow parental/caregiver presence should be made in consultation with a team including an infectious diseases expert and state and/or local public health authorities and should involve consideration of many factors, depending on the stage of investigation and management, including (1) a careful history, physical examination, and investigations to elucidate the likelihood of the diagnosis of Ebola or other highly consequential infection; (2) ability of the facility to offer appropriate isolation for the person under investigation and family members and to manage Ebola; (3) ability to recognize and exclude people at increased risk of worse outcomes (eg, pregnant women); and (4) ability of parent/caregiver to follow instructions, including appropriate donning and doffing of personal protective equipment. (8/16)

http://pediatrics.aappublications.org/content/138/3/e20161891

PARENT-PROVIDER-COMMUNITY PARTNERSHIPS: OPTIMIZING OUTCOMES FOR CHILDREN WITH DISABILITIES (CLINICAL REPORT)

Nancy A. Murphy, MD; Paul S. Carbone, MD; and Council on Children With Disabilities

ABSTRACT. Children with disabilities and their families have multifaceted medical, developmental, educational, and habilitative needs that are best addressed through strong partnerships among parents, providers, and communities. However, traditional health care systems are designed to address acute rather than chronic conditions. Children with disabilities require high-quality medical homes that provide care coordination and transitional care, and their families require social and financial supports. Integrated community systems of care that promote participation of all children are needed. The purpose of this clinical report is to explore the challenges of developing effective community-based systems of care and to offer suggestions to pediatricians and policy-makers regarding the development of partnerships among children with disabilities, their families, and health care and other providers to maximize health and well-being of these children and their families. (9/11, reaffirmed 5/17)

http://pediatrics.aappublications.org/content/128/4/795

PATENT DUCTUS ARTERIOSUS IN PRETERM INFANTS

William E. Benitz, MD, FAAP, and Committee on Fetus and Newborn

ABSTRACT. Despite a large body of basic science and clinical research and clinical experience with thousands of infants over nearly 6 decades, there is still uncertainty and controversy about the significance, evaluation, and management of patent ductus arteriosus in preterm infants, resulting in substantial heterogeneity in clinical practice. The purpose of this clinical report is to summarize the evidence available to guide evaluation and treatment of preterm infants with prolonged ductal patency in the first few weeks after birth. (12/15)

http://pediatrics.aappublications.org/content/137/1/e20153730

PATIENT- AND FAMILY-CENTERED CARE AND THE PEDIATRICIAN'S ROLE

Committee on Hospital Care and Institute for Patient- and Family-Centered Care

ABSTRACT. Drawing on several decades of work with families, pediatricians, other health care professionals, and policy makers, the American Academy of Pediatrics provides a definition of patient- and family-centered care. In pediatrics, patient- and family-centered care is based on the understanding that the family is the child's primary source of strength and support. Further, this approach to care recognizes that the perspectives and information provided by families, children, and young adults are essential components of high-quality clinical decision-making, and that patients and family are integral partners with the health care team. This policy statement outlines the core principles of patient- and family-centered care, summarizes some of the recent literature linking patient- and family-centered care to improved health outcomes, and lists various other benefits to be expected when engaging in patient- and family-centered pediatric practice. The statement concludes with specific recommendations for how pediatricians can integrate patient- and family-centered care in hospitals, clinics, and community settings, and in broader systems of care, as well. (1/12, reaffirmed 2/18)

http://pediatrics.aappublications.org/content/129/2/394

PATIENT- AND FAMILY-CENTERED CARE AND THE ROLE OF THE EMERGENCY PHYSICIAN PROVIDING CARE TO A CHILD IN THE EMERGENCY DEPARTMENT

Committee on Pediatric Emergency Medicine (joint with American College of Emergency Physicians)

ABSTRACT. Patient- and family-centered care is an approach to health care that recognizes the role of the family in providing medical care; encourages collaboration between the patient, family, and health care professionals; and honors individual and family strengths, cultures, traditions, and expertise. Although there are many opportunities for providing patient- and family-centered care in the emergency department, there are also challenges to doing so. The American Academy of Pediatrics and the American College of Emergency Physicians support promoting patient dignity, comfort, and autonomy; recognizing the patient and family as key decision-makers in the patient's medical care; recognizing the patient's experience and perspective in a culturally sensitive manner; acknowledging the interdependence of child and parent as well as the pediatric patient's evolving independence; encouraging family-member presence; providing information to the family during interventions; encouraging collaboration with other health care professionals; acknowledging the importance of the patient's medical home; and encouraging institutional policies for patient- and family-centered care. (11/06, reaffirmed 6/09, 10/11, 9/15)
http://pediatrics.aappublications.org/content/118/5/2242

PATIENT- AND FAMILY-CENTERED CARE COORDINATION: A FRAMEWORK FOR INTEGRATING CARE FOR CHILDREN AND YOUTH ACROSS MULTIPLE SYSTEMS

Council on Children With Disabilities and Medical Home Implementation Project Advisory Committee

ABSTRACT. Understanding a care coordination framework, its functions, and its effects on children and families is critical for patients and families themselves, as well as for pediatricians, pediatric medical subspecialists/surgical specialists, and anyone providing services to children and families. Care coordination is an essential element of a transformed American health care delivery system that emphasizes optimal quality and cost outcomes, addresses family-centered care, and calls for partnership across various settings and communities. High-quality, cost-effective health care requires that the delivery system include elements for the provision of services supporting the coordination of care across settings and professionals. This requirement of supporting coordination of care is generally true for health systems providing care for all children and youth but especially for those with special health care needs. At the foundation of an efficient and effective system of care delivery is the patient-/family-centered medical home. From its inception, the medical home has had care coordination as a core element. In general, optimal outcomes for children and youth, especially those with special health care needs, require interfacing among multiple care systems and individuals, including the following: medical, social, and behavioral professionals; the educational system; payers; medical equipment providers; home care agencies; advocacy groups; needed supportive therapies/services; and families. Coordination of care across settings permits an integration of services that is centered on the comprehensive needs of the patient and family, leading to decreased health care costs, reduction in fragmented care, and improvement in the patient/family experience of care. (4/14, reaffirmed 4/18)
http://pediatrics.aappublications.org/content/133/5/e1451

PATIENT- AND FAMILY-CENTERED CARE OF CHILDREN IN THE EMERGENCY DEPARTMENT (TECHNICAL REPORT)

Nanette Dudley, MD; Alice Ackerman, MD, MBA; Kathleen M. Brown, MD; Sally K. Snow, BSN, RN; and Committee on Pediatric Emergency Medicine (joint with American College of Emergency Physicians Pediatric Emergency Medicine Committee and Emergency Nurses Association Pediatric Committee)

ABSTRACT. Patient- and family-centered care is an approach to the planning, delivery, and evaluation of health care that is grounded in a mutually beneficial partnership among patients, families, and health care professionals. Providing patient- and family-centered care to children in the emergency department setting presents many opportunities and challenges. This revised technical report draws on previously published policy statements and reports, reviews the current literature, and describes the present state of practice and research regarding patient- and family-centered care for children in the emergency department setting as well as some of the complexities of providing such care. (12/14)
http://pediatrics.aappublications.org/content/135/1/e255

PATIENT SAFETY IN THE PEDIATRIC EMERGENCY CARE SETTING

Committee on Pediatric Emergency Medicine

ABSTRACT. Patient safety is a priority for all health care professionals, including those who work in emergency care. Unique aspects of pediatric care may increase the risk of medical error and harm to patients, especially in the emergency care setting. Although errors can happen despite the best human efforts, given the right set of circumstances, health care professionals must work proactively to improve safety in the pediatric emergency care system. Specific recommendations to improve pediatric patient safety in the emergency department are provided in this policy statement. (12/07, reaffirmed 6/11, 7/14)
http://pediatrics.aappublications.org/content/120/6/1367

PEDESTRIAN SAFETY

Committee on Injury, Violence, and Poison Prevention

ABSTRACT. Each year, approximately 900 pediatric pedestrians younger than 19 years are killed. In addition, 51000 children are injured as pedestrians, and 5300 of them are hospitalized because of their injuries. Parents should be warned that young children often do not have the cognitive, perceptual, and behavioral abilities to negotiate traffic independently. Parents should also be informed about the danger of vehicle back-over injuries to toddlers playing in driveways. Because posttraumatic stress syndrome commonly follows even minor pedestrian injury, pediatricians should screen and refer for this condition as necessary. The American Academy of Pediatrics supports community- and school-based strategies that minimize a child's exposure to traffic, especially to high-speed, high-volume traffic. Furthermore, the American Academy of Pediatrics supports governmental and industry action that would lead to improvements in vehicle design, driver manuals, driver education, and data collection for the purpose of reducing pediatric pedestrian injury. (7/09, reaffirmed 8/13)
http://pediatrics.aappublications.org/content/124/2/802

PEDIATRIC AND ADOLESCENT MENTAL HEALTH EMERGENCIES IN THE EMERGENCY MEDICAL SERVICES SYSTEM (TECHNICAL REPORT)

Margaret A. Dolan, MD; Joel A. Fein, MD, MPH; and Committee on Pediatric Emergency Medicine

ABSTRACT. Emergency department (ED) health care professionals often care for patients with previously diagnosed psychiatric illnesses who are ill, injured, or having a behavioral crisis. In addition, ED personnel encounter children with psychiatric illnesses who may not present to the ED with overt mental health symptoms. Staff education and training regarding identification and management of pediatric mental health illness can help EDs overcome the perceived limitations of the setting that influence timely and comprehensive evaluation. In addition, ED physicians can inform and advocate for policy changes at local, state, and national levels that are needed to ensure comprehensive care of children with mental health illnesses. This report addresses the roles that the ED and ED health care professionals play in emergency mental health care of children and adolescents in the United States, which includes the stabilization and management of patients in mental health crisis, the discovery of mental illnesses and suicidal ideation in ED patients, and approaches to advocating for improved recognition and treatment of mental illnesses in children. The report also addresses special issues related to mental illness in the ED, such as minority populations, children with special health care needs, and children's mental health during and after disasters and trauma. (4/11, reaffirmed 7/14)

http://pediatrics.aappublications.org/content/127/5/e1356

PEDIATRIC ANTHRAX CLINICAL MANAGEMENT (CLINICAL REPORT)

John S. Bradley, MD, FAAP, FIDSA, FPIDS; Georgina Peacock, MD, MPH, FAAP; Steven E. Krug, MD, FAAP; William A. Bower, MD, FIDSA; Amanda C. Cohn, MD; Dana Meaney-Delman, MD, MPH, FACOG; Andrew T. Pavia, MD, FAAP, FIDSA; Committee on Infectious Diseases; and Disaster Preparedness Advisory Council

ABSTRACT. Anthrax is a zoonotic disease caused by *Bacillus anthracis,* which has multiple routes of infection in humans, manifesting in different initial presentations of disease. Because *B anthracis* has the potential to be used as a biological weapon and can rapidly progress to systemic anthrax with high mortality in those who are exposed and untreated, clinical guidance that can be quickly implemented must be in place before any intentional release of the agent. This document provides clinical guidance for the prophylaxis and treatment of neonates, infants, children, adolescents, and young adults up to the age of 21 (referred to as "children") in the event of a deliberate *B anthracis* release and offers guidance in areas where the unique characteristics of children dictate a different clinical recommendation from adults. (4/14)

http://pediatrics.aappublications.org/content/133/5/e1411

PEDIATRIC ANTHRAX CLINICAL MANAGEMENT: EXECUTIVE SUMMARY

John S. Bradley, MD, FAAP, FIDSA, FPIDS; Georgina Peacock, MD, MPH, FAAP; Steven E. Krug, MD, FAAP; William A. Bower, MD, FIDSA; Amanda C. Cohn, MD; Dana Meaney-Delman, MD, MPH, FACOG; Andrew T. Pavia, MD, FAAP, FIDSA; Committee on Infectious Diseases; and Disaster Preparedness Advisory Council

The use of *Bacillus anthracis* as a biological weapon is considered a potential national security threat by the US government. *B anthracis* has the ability to be used as a biological weapon and to cause anthrax, which can rapidly progress to systemic disease with high mortality in those who are untreated. Therefore, clear plans for managing children after a *B anthracis* bioterror exposure event must be in place before any intentional release of the agent. This document provides a summary of the guidance contained in the clinical report (appendices cited in this executive summary refer to those in the clinical report) for diagnosis and management of anthrax, including antimicrobial treatment and postexposure prophylaxis (PEP), use of antitoxin, and recommendations for use of anthrax vaccine in neonates, infants, children, adolescents, and young adults up to the age of 21 years (referred to as "children"). (4/14)

http://pediatrics.aappublications.org/content/133/5/940

PEDIATRIC ASPECTS OF INPATIENT HEALTH INFORMATION TECHNOLOGY SYSTEMS (TECHNICAL REPORT)

Christoph U. Lehmann, MD, FAAP, FACMI, and Council on Clinical Information Technology

ABSTRACT. In the past 3 years, the Health Information Technology for Economic and Clinical Health Act accelerated the adoption of electronic health records (EHRs) with providers and hospitals, who can claim incentive monies related to meaningful use. Despite the increase in adoption of commercial EHRs in pediatric settings, there has been little support for EHR tools and functionalities that promote pediatric quality improvement and patient safety, and children remain at higher risk than adults for medical errors in inpatient environments. Health information technology (HIT) tailored to the needs of pediatric health care providers can improve care by reducing the likelihood of errors through information assurance and minimizing the harm that results from errors. This technical report outlines pediatric-specific concepts, child health needs and their data elements, and required functionalities in inpatient clinical information systems that may be missing in adult-oriented HIT systems with negative consequences for pediatric inpatient care. It is imperative that inpatient (and outpatient) HIT systems be adapted to improve their ability to properly support safe health care delivery for children. (2/15)

http://pediatrics.aappublications.org/content/135/3/e756

PEDIATRIC CONSIDERATIONS BEFORE, DURING, AND AFTER RADIOLOGICAL OR NUCLEAR EMERGENCIES

Jerome A. Paulson, MD, FAAP and AAP Council on Environmental Health

ABSTRACT. Infants, children, and adolescents can be exposed unexpectedly to ionizing radiation from nuclear power plant events, improvised nuclear or radiologic dispersal device explosions, or inappropriate disposal of radiotherapy equipment. Children are likely to experience higher external and internal radiation exposure levels than adults because of their smaller body and organ size and other physiologic characteristics, by picking up contaminated items, and through consumption of contaminated milk or foodstuffs. This policy statement and accompanying technical report update the 2003 American Academy of Pediatrics policy statement on pediatric radiation emergencies by summarizing newer scientific knowledge from studies of the Chernobyl and Fukushima Daiichi nuclear power plant events, use of improvised radiologic dispersal devices, exposures from inappropriate disposal of radiotherapy equipment, and potential health effects from residential proximity to nuclear plants. Policy recommendations are made for providers and governments to improve future responses to these types of events. (11/18)

See full text on page 747.

http://pediatrics.aappublications.org/content/142/6/e20183000

PEDIATRIC CONSIDERATIONS BEFORE, DURING, AND AFTER RADIOLOGICAL OR NUCLEAR EMERGENCIES (TECHNICAL REPORT)

Martha S. Linet, MD, MPH; Ziad Kazzi, MD; Jerome A. Paulson, MD, FAAP; AAP Council on Environmental Health

ABSTRACT. Infants, children, and adolescents can be exposed unexpectedly to ionizing radiation from nuclear power plant events, improvised nuclear or radiologic dispersal device explosions, or inappropriate disposal of radiotherapy equipment. Children are likely to experience higher external and internal radiation exposure levels than adults because of their smaller body and organ size and other physiologic characteristics as well as their tendency to pick up contaminated items and consume contaminated milk or foodstuffs. This technical report accompanies the revision of the 2003 American Academy of Pediatrics policy statement on pediatric radiation emergencies by summarizing newer scientific data from studies of the Chernobyl and the Fukushima Daiichi nuclear power plant events, use of improvised radiologic dispersal devices, exposures from inappropriate disposal of radiotherapy equipment, and potential health effects from residential proximity to nuclear plants. Also included are recommendations from epidemiological studies and biokinetic models to address mitigation efforts. The report includes major emphases on acute radiation syndrome, acute and long-term psychological effects, cancer risks, and other late tissue reactions after low-to-high levels of radiation exposure. Results, along with public health and clinical implications, are described from studies of the Japanese atomic bomb survivors, nuclear plant accidents (eg, Three Mile Island, Chernobyl, and Fukushima), improper disposal of radiotherapy equipment in Goiania, Brazil, and residence in proximity to nuclear plants. Measures to reduce radiation exposure in the immediate aftermath of a radiologic or nuclear disaster are described, including the diagnosis and management of external and internal contamination, use of potassium iodide, and actions in relation to breastfeeding. (11/18)

See full text on page 755.
http://pediatrics.aappublications.org/content/142/6/e20183001

PEDIATRIC FELLOWSHIP TRAINING
Federation of Pediatric Organizations
ABSTRACT. In 1996, the Federation of Pediatric Organizations revised its 1990 statement on pediatric fellowship training. The following statement represents the current (2004) position of the federation regarding the purpose and objectives of fellowship training. (7/04)
http://pediatrics.aappublications.org/content/114/1/295

PEDIATRIC INTEGRATIVE MEDICINE (CLINICAL REPORT)
Hilary McClafferty, MD, FAAP; Sunita Vohra, MD, FAAP; Michelle Bailey, MD, FAAP; Melanie Brown, MD, MSE, FAAP; Anna Esparham, MD, FAAP; Dana Gerstbacher, MD, FAAP; Brenda Golianu, MD, FAAP; Anna-Kaisa Niemi, MD, PhD, FAAP, FACMG; Erica Sibinga, MD, FAAP; Joy Weydert, MD, FAAP; Ann Ming Yeh, MD; and Section on Integrative Medicine
ABSTRACT. The American Academy of Pediatrics is dedicated to optimizing the well-being of children and advancing family-centered health care. Related to this mission, the American Academy of Pediatrics recognizes the increasing use of complementary and integrative therapies for children and the subsequent need to provide reliable information and high-quality clinical resources to support pediatricians. This Clinical Report serves as an update to the original 2008 statement on complementary medicine. The range of complementary therapies is both extensive and diverse. Therefore, in-depth discussion of each therapy or product is beyond the scope of this report. Instead, our intentions are to define terms; describe epidemiology of use; outline common types of complementary therapies; review medicolegal, ethical, and research implications; review education and training for select providers of complementary therapies; provide educational resources; and suggest communication strategies for discussing complementary therapies with patients and families. (8/17)
http://pediatrics.aappublications.org/content/140/3/e20171961

PEDIATRIC MEDICATION SAFETY IN THE EMERGENCY DEPARTMENT
Lee Benjamin, MD, FAAP, FACEP; Karen Frush, MD, FAAP; Kathy Shaw, MD, MSCE, FAAP; Joan E. Shook, MD, MBA, FAAP; Sally K. Snow, BSN, RN, CPEN, FAEN; and Committee on Pediatric Emergency Medicine (joint with American College of Emergency Physicians Pediatric Emergency Medicine Committee and Emergency Nurses Association Pediatric Emergency Medicine Committee)
ABSTRACT. Pediatric patients cared for in emergency departments (EDs) are at high risk of medication errors for a variety of reasons. A multidisciplinary panel was convened by the Emergency Medical Services for Children program and the American Academy of Pediatrics Committee on Pediatric Emergency Medicine to initiate a discussion on medication safety in the ED. Top opportunities identified to improve medication safety include using kilogram-only weight-based dosing, optimizing computerized physician order entry by using clinical decision support, developing a standard formulary for pediatric patients while limiting variability of medication concentrations, using pharmacist support within EDs, enhancing training of medical professionals, systematizing the dispensing and administration of medications within the ED, and addressing challenges for home medication administration before discharge. (2/18)
See full text on page 775.
http://pediatrics.aappublications.org/content/141/3/e20174066

PEDIATRIC MENTAL HEALTH EMERGENCIES IN THE EMERGENCY MEDICAL SERVICES SYSTEM
Committee on Pediatric Emergency Medicine (joint with American College of Emergency Physicians)
ABSTRACT. Emergency departments are vital in the management of pediatric patients with mental health emergencies. Pediatric mental health emergencies are an increasing part of emergency medical practice because emergency departments have become the safety net for a fragmented mental health infrastructure that is experiencing critical shortages in services in all sectors. Emergency departments must safely, humanely, and in a culturally and developmentally appropriate manner manage pediatric patients with undiagnosed and known mental illnesses, including those with mental retardation, autistic spectrum disorders, and attention-deficit/hyperactivity disorder and those experiencing a behavioral crisis. Emergency departments also manage patients with suicidal ideation, depression, escalating aggression, substance abuse, posttraumatic stress disorder, and maltreatment and those exposed to violence and unexpected deaths. Emergency departments must address not only the physical but also the mental health needs of patients during and after mass-casualty incidents and disasters. The American Academy of Pediatrics and the American College of Emergency Physicians support advocacy for increased mental health resources, including improved pediatric mental health tools for the emergency department, increased mental health insurance coverage, and adequate reimbursement at all levels; acknowledgment of the importance of the child's medical home; and promotion of education and research for mental health emergencies. (10/06, reaffirmed 6/09, 4/13)
http://pediatrics.aappublications.org/content/118/4/1764

PEDIATRIC OBSERVATION UNITS (CLINICAL REPORT)
Gregory P. Conners, MD, MPH, MBA; Sanford M. Melzer, MD, MBA; Committee on Hospital Care; and Committee on Pediatric Emergency Medicine
ABSTRACT. Pediatric observation units (OUs) are hospital areas used to provide medical evaluation and/or management for health-related conditions in children, typically for a well-defined, brief period. Pediatric OUs represent an emerging alternative site of care for selected groups of children who historically may have received their treatment in an ambulatory setting, emergency department, or hospital-based inpatient unit. This clinical report provides an overview of pediatric OUs, including the definitions and operating characteristics of different types of OUs, quality considerations and coding for observation services, and the effect of OUs on inpatient hospital utilization. (6/12, reaffirmed 9/15)
http://pediatrics.aappublications.org/content/130/1/172

PEDIATRIC ORGAN DONATION AND TRANSPLANTATION

Committee on Hospital Care, Section on Surgery, and Section on Critical Care

ABSTRACT. Pediatric organ donation and organ transplantation can have a significant life-extending benefit to the young recipients of these organs and a high emotional impact on donor and recipient families. Pediatricians, pediatric medical specialists, and pediatric transplant surgeons need to be better acquainted with evolving national strategies that involve organ procurement and organ transplantation to help acquaint families with the benefits and risks of organ donation and transplantation. Efforts of pediatric professionals are needed to shape public policies to provide a system in which procurement, distribution, and cost are fair and equitable to children and adults. Major issues of concern are availability of and access to donor organs; oversight and control of the process; pediatric medical and surgical consultation and continued care throughout the organ-donation and transplantation process; ethical, social, financial, and follow-up issues; insurance-coverage issues; and public awareness of the need for organ donors of all ages. (3/10, reaffirmed 3/14)
http://pediatrics.aappublications.org/content/125/4/822

PEDIATRIC PALLIATIVE CARE AND HOSPICE CARE COMMITMENTS, GUIDELINES, AND RECOMMENDATIONS

Section on Hospice and Palliative Medicine and Committee on Hospital Care

ABSTRACT. Pediatric palliative care and pediatric hospice care (PPC-PHC) are often essential aspects of medical care for patients who have life-threatening conditions or need end-of-life care. PPC-PHC aims to relieve suffering, improve quality of life, facilitate informed decision-making, and assist in care coordination between clinicians and across sites of care. Core commitments of PPC-PHC include being patient centered and family engaged; respecting and partnering with patients and families; pursuing care that is high quality, readily accessible, and equitable; providing care across the age spectrum and life span, integrated into the continuum of care; ensuring that all clinicians can provide basic palliative care and consult PPC-PHC specialists in a timely manner; and improving care through research and quality improvement efforts. PPC-PHC guidelines and recommendations include ensuring that all large health care organizations serving children with life-threatening conditions have dedicated interdisciplinary PPC-PHC teams, which should develop collaborative relationships between hospital- and community-based teams; that PPC-PHC be provided as integrated multimodal care and practiced as a cornerstone of patient safety and quality for patients with life-threatening conditions; that PPC-PHC teams should facilitate clear, compassionate, and forthright discussions about medical issues and the goals of care and support families, siblings, and health care staff; that PPC-PHC be part of all pediatric education and training curricula, be an active area of research and quality improvement, and exemplify the highest ethical standards; and that PPC-PHC services be supported by financial and regulatory arrangements to ensure access to high-quality PPC-PHC by all patients with life-threatening and life-shortening diseases. (10/13)
http://pediatrics.aappublications.org/content/132/5/966

PEDIATRIC PRIMARY HEALTH CARE

Committee on Pediatric Workforce

ABSTRACT. Primary health care is described as accessible and affordable, first contact, continuous and comprehensive, and coordinated to meet the health needs of the individual and the family being served.

Pediatric primary health care encompasses health supervision and anticipatory guidance; monitoring physical and psychosocial growth and development; age-appropriate screening; diagnosis and treatment of acute and chronic disorders; management of serious and life-threatening illness and, when appropriate, referral of more complex conditions; and provision of first contact care as well as coordinated management of health problems requiring multiple professional services.

Pediatric primary health care for children and adolescents is family centered and incorporates community resources and strengths, needs and risk factors, and sociocultural sensitivities into strategies for care delivery and clinical practice. Pediatric primary health care is best delivered within the context of a "medical home," where comprehensive, continuously accessible and affordable care is available and delivered or supervised by qualified child health specialists.

The pediatrician, because of training (which includes 4 years of medical school education, plus an additional 3 or more years of intensive training devoted solely to all aspects of medical care for children and adolescents), coupled with the demonstrated interest in and total professional commitment to the health care of infants, children, adolescents, and young adults, is the most appropriate provider of pediatric primary health care. (1/11, reaffirmed 10/13)
http://pediatrics.aappublications.org/content/127/2/397

PEDIATRIC READINESS IN THE EMERGENCY DEPARTMENT

Katherine Remick, MD, FAAP, FACEP, FAEMS; Marianne Gausche-Hill, MD, FAAP, FACEP, FAEMS; Madeline M. Joseph, MD, FAAP, FACEP; Kathleen Brown, MD, FAAP, FACEP; Sally K. Snow, BSN, RN, CPEN; Joseph L. Wright, MD, MPH, FAAP; Committee on Pediatric Emergency Medicine; and Section on Surgery (joint with American College of Emergency Physicians Pediatric Emergency Medicine Committee and Emergency Nurses Association Pediatric Committee)

ABSTRACT. This is a revision of the previous joint Policy Statement titled "Guidelines for Care of Children in the Emergency Department." Children have unique physical and psychosocial needs that are heightened in the setting of serious or life-threatening emergencies. The majority of children who are ill and injured are brought to community hospital emergency departments (EDs) by virtue of proximity. It is therefore imperative that all EDs have the appropriate resources (medications, equipment, policies, and education) and capable staff to provide effective emergency care for children. In this Policy Statement, we outline the resources necessary for EDs to stand ready to care for children of all ages. These recommendations are consistent with the recommendations of the Institute of Medicine (now called the National Academy of Medicine) in its report "The Future of Emergency Care in the US Health System." Although resources within emergency and trauma care systems vary locally, regionally, and nationally, it is essential that ED staff, administrators, and medical directors seek to meet or exceed these recommendations to ensure that high-quality emergency care is available for all children. These updated recommendations are intended to serve as a resource for clinical and administrative leadership in EDs as they strive to improve their readiness for children of all ages. (10/18)

See full text on page 785.
http://pediatrics.aappublications.org/content/142/5/e20182459

PEDIATRIC SUDDEN CARDIAC ARREST

Section on Cardiology and Cardiac Surgery

ABSTRACT. Pediatric sudden cardiac arrest (SCA), which can cause sudden cardiac death if not treated within minutes, has a profound effect on everyone: children, parents, family members, communities, and health care providers. Preventing the tragedy of pediatric SCA, defined as the abrupt and unexpected loss of heart function, remains a concern to all. The goal of this statement is to increase the knowledge of pediatricians (including primary care providers and specialists) of the incidence of

pediatric SCA, the spectrum of causes of pediatric SCA, disease-specific presentations, the role of patient and family screening, the rapidly evolving role of genetic testing, and finally, important aspects of secondary SCA prevention. This statement is not intended to address sudden infant death syndrome or sudden unexplained death syndrome, nor will specific treatment of individual cardiac conditions be discussed. This statement has been endorsed by the American College of Cardiology, the American Heart Association, and the Heart Rhythm Society. (3/12)
http://pediatrics.aappublications.org/content/129/4/e1094

THE PEDIATRICIAN AND CHILDHOOD BEREAVEMENT
Committee on Psychosocial Aspects of Child and Family Health
ABSTRACT. Pediatricians should understand and evaluate children's reactions to the death of a person important to them by using age-appropriate and culturally sensitive guidance while being alert for normal and complicated grief responses. Pediatricians also should advise and assist families in responding to the child's needs. Sharing, family support, and communication have been associated with positive long-term bereavement adjustment. (2/00, reaffirmed 1/04, 3/13)
http://pediatrics.aappublications.org/content/105/2/445

THE PEDIATRICIAN WORKFORCE: CURRENT STATUS AND FUTURE PROSPECTS (TECHNICAL REPORT)
David C. Goodman, MD, MS, and Committee on Pediatric Workforce
ABSTRACT. The effective and efficient delivery of children's health care depends on the pediatrician workforce. The number, composition, and distribution of pediatricians necessary to deliver this care have been the subject of long-standing policy and professional debate. This technical report reviews current characteristics and recent trends in the pediatric workforce and couples the workforce to a conceptual model of improvement in children's health and well-being. Important recent changes in the workforce include (1) the growth in the number of pediatricians in relation to the child population, (2) increased numbers of female pediatricians and their attainment of majority gender status in the specialty, (3) the persistence of a large number of international medical graduates entering training programs, (4) a lack of ethnic and racial diversity in pediatricians compared with children, and (5) the persistence of marked regional variation in pediatrician supply. Supply models projecting the pediatric workforce are reviewed and generally indicate that the number of pediatricians per child will increase by 50% over the next 20 years. The differing methods of assessing workforce requirements are presented and critiqued. The report finds that the pediatric workforce is undergoing fundamental changes that will have important effects on the professional lives of pediatricians and children's health care delivery. (7/05)
http://pediatrics.aappublications.org/content/116/1/e156

PEDIATRICIAN WORKFORCE POLICY STATEMENT
Committee on Pediatric Workforce
ABSTRACT. This policy statement reviews important trends and other factors that affect the pediatrician workforce and the provision of pediatric health care, including changes in the pediatric patient population, pediatrician workforce, and nature of pediatric practice. The effect of these changes on pediatricians and the demand for pediatric care are discussed. The American Academy of Pediatrics (AAP) concludes that there is currently a shortage of pediatric medical subspecialists in many fields, as well as a shortage of pediatric surgical specialists. In addition, the AAP believes that the current distribution of primary care pediatricians is inadequate to meet the needs of children living in rural and other underserved areas, and more primary care pediatricians will be needed in the future because of the increasing number of children who have significant chronic health problems, changes in physician work hours, and implementation

of current health reform efforts that seek to improve access to comprehensive patient- and family-centered care for all children in a medical home. The AAP is committed to being an active participant in physician workforce policy development with both professional organizations and governmental bodies to ensure a pediatric perspective on health care workforce issues. The overall purpose of this statement is to summarize policy recommendations and serve as a resource for the AAP and other stakeholders as they address pediatrician workforce issues that ultimately influence the quality of pediatric health care provided to children in the United States. (7/13)
http://pediatrics.aappublications.org/content/132/2/390

PEDIATRICIAN-FAMILY-PATIENT RELATIONSHIPS: MANAGING THE BOUNDARIES
Committee on Bioethics
ABSTRACT. All professionals are concerned about maintaining the appropriate limits in their relationships with those they serve. Pediatricians should be aware that, under normal circumstances, caring for one's own children presents significant ethical issues. Pediatricians also must strive to maintain appropriate professional boundaries in their relationships with the family members of their patients. Pediatricians should avoid behavior that patients and parents might misunderstand as having sexual or inappropriate social meaning. Romantic and sexual involvement between physicians and patients is unacceptable. The acceptance of gifts or nonmonetary compensation for medical services has the potential to affect the professional relationship adversely. (11/09, reaffirmed 1/14)
http://pediatrics.aappublications.org/content/124/6/1685

THE PEDIATRICIAN'S ROLE IN CHILD MALTREATMENT PREVENTION (CLINICAL REPORT)
Emalee G. Flaherty, MD; John Stirling Jr, MD; and Committee on Child Abuse and Neglect
ABSTRACT. It is the pediatrician's role to promote the child's well-being and to help parents raise healthy, well-adjusted children. Pediatricians, therefore, can play an important role in the prevention of child maltreatment. Previous clinical reports and policy statements from the American Academy of Pediatrics have focused on improving the identification and management of child maltreatment. This clinical report outlines how the pediatrician can help to strengthen families and promote safe, stable, nurturing relationships with the aim of preventing maltreatment. After describing some of the triggers and factors that place children at risk for maltreatment, the report describes how pediatricians can identify family strengths, recognize risk factors, provide helpful guidance, and refer families to programs and other resources with the goal of strengthening families, preventing child maltreatment, and enhancing child development. (9/10, reaffirmed 1/14)
http://pediatrics.aappublications.org/content/126/4/833

THE PEDIATRICIAN'S ROLE IN FAMILY SUPPORT AND FAMILY SUPPORT PROGRAMS
Committee on Early Childhood, Adoption, and Dependent Care
ABSTRACT. Children's social, emotional, and physical health; their developmental trajectory; and the neurocircuits that are being created and reinforced in their developing brains are all directly influenced by their relationships during early childhood. The stresses associated with contemporary American life can challenge families' abilities to promote successful developmental outcomes and emotional health for their children. Pediatricians are positioned to serve as partners with families and other community providers in supporting the well-being of children and their families. The structure and support of families involve forces that are often outside the agenda of the usual pediatric health supervision visits. Pediatricians must ensure

that their medical home efforts promote a holistically healthy family environment for all children. This statement recommends opportunities for pediatricians to develop their expertise in assessing the strengths and stresses in families, in counseling families about strategies and resources, and in collaborating with others in their communities to support family relationships. (11/11, reaffirmed 12/16)

http://pediatrics.aappublications.org/content/128/6/e1680

THE PEDIATRICIAN'S ROLE IN OPTIMIZING SCHOOL READINESS

Council on Early Childhood and Council on School Health

ABSTRACT. School readiness includes not only the early academic skills of children but also their physical health, language skills, social and emotional development, motivation to learn, creativity, and general knowledge. Families and communities play a critical role in ensuring children's growth in all of these areas and thus their readiness for school. Schools must be prepared to teach all children when they reach the age of school entry, regardless of their degree of readiness. Research on early brain development emphasizes the effects of early experiences, relationships, and emotions on creating and reinforcing the neural connections that are the basis for learning. Pediatricians, by the nature of their relationships with families and children, may significantly influence school readiness. Pediatricians have a primary role in ensuring children's physical health through the provision of preventive care, treatment of illness, screening for sensory deficits, and monitoring nutrition and growth. They can promote and monitor the social-emotional development of children by providing anticipatory guidance on development and behavior, by encouraging positive parenting practices, by modeling reciprocal and respectful communication with adults and children, by identifying and addressing psychosocial risk factors, and by providing community-based resources and referrals when warranted. Cognitive and language skills are fostered through timely identification of developmental problems and appropriate referrals for services, including early intervention and special education services; guidance regarding safe and stimulating early education and child care programs; and promotion of early literacy by encouraging language-rich activities such as reading together, telling stories, and playing games. Pediatricians are also well positioned to advocate not only for children's access to health care but also for high-quality early childhood education and evidence-based family supports such as home visits, which help provide a foundation for optimal learning. (8/16)

http://pediatrics.aappublications.org/content/138/3/e20162293

THE PEDIATRICIAN'S ROLE IN SUPPORTING ADOPTIVE FAMILIES (CLINICAL REPORT)

Veronnie F. Jones, MD, PhD; Elaine E. Schulte, MD, MPH; Committee on Early Childhood; and Council on Foster Care, Adoption, and Kinship Care

ABSTRACT. Each year, more children join families through adoption. Pediatricians have an important role in assisting adoptive families in the various challenges they may face with respect to adoption. The acceptance of the differences between families formed through birth and those formed through adoption is essential in promoting positive emotional growth within the family. It is important for pediatricians to be aware of the adoptive parents' need to be supported in their communication with their adopted children. (9/12, reaffirmed 12/16)

http://pediatrics.aappublications.org/content/130/4/e1040

THE PEDIATRICIAN'S ROLE IN THE EVALUATION AND PREPARATION OF PEDIATRIC PATIENTS UNDERGOING ANESTHESIA

Section on Anesthesiology and Pain Medicine

ABSTRACT. Pediatricians play a key role in helping prepare patients and families for anesthesia and surgery. The questions to be answered by the pediatrician fall into 2 categories. The first involves preparation: is the patient in optimal medical condition for surgery, and are the patient and family emotionally and cognitively ready for surgery? The second category concerns logistics: what communication and organizational needs are necessary to enable safe passage through the perioperative process? This revised statement updates the recommendations for the pediatrician's role in the preoperative preparation of patients. (8/14)

http://pediatrics.aappublications.org/content/134/3/634

THE PEDIATRICIAN'S ROLE IN THE PREVENTION OF MISSING CHILDREN (CLINICAL REPORT)

Committee on Psychosocial Aspects of Child and Family Health

ABSTRACT. In 2002, the *Second National Incidence Studies of Missing, Abducted, Runaway, and Thrownaway Children* report was released by the US Department of Justice, providing new data on a problem that our nation continues to face. This clinical report describes the categories of missing children, the prevalence of each, and prevention strategies that primary care pediatricians can share with parents to increase awareness and education about the safety of their children. (10/04, reaffirmed 1/15)

http://pediatrics.aappublications.org/content/114/4/1100

PEDIATRICIANS AND PUBLIC HEALTH: OPTIMIZING THE HEALTH AND WELL-BEING OF THE NATION'S CHILDREN

Alice A. Kuo, MD, PhD, FAAP; Pauline A. Thomas, MD, FAAP; Lance A. Chilton, MD, FAAP; Laurene Mascola, MD, MPH; Council on Community Pediatrics; and Section on Epidemiology, Public Health, and Evidence

ABSTRACT. Ensuring optimal health for children requires a population-based approach and collaboration between pediatrics and public health. The prevention of major threats to children's health (such as behavioral health issues) and the control and management of chronic diseases, obesity, injury, communicable diseases, and other problems cannot be managed solely in the pediatric office. The integration of clinical practice with public health actions is necessary for multiple levels of disease prevention that involve the child, family, and community. Although pediatricians and public health professionals interact frequently to the benefit of children and their families, increased integration of the 2 disciplines is critical to improving child health at the individual and population levels. Effective collaboration is necessary to ensure that population health activities include children and that the child health priorities of the American Academy of Pediatrics (AAP), such as poverty and child health, early brain and child development, obesity, and mental health, can engage federal, state, and local public health initiatives. In this policy statement, we build on the 2013 AAP Policy Statement on community pediatrics by identifying specific opportunities for collaboration between pediatricians and public health professionals that are likely to improve the health of children in communities. In the statement, we provide recommendations for pediatricians, public health professionals, and the AAP and its chapters. (1/18)

See full text on page 801.

http://pediatrics.aappublications.org/content/141/2/e20173848

PERSONAL WATERCRAFT USE BY CHILDREN AND ADOLESCENTS
Committee on Injury and Poison Prevention

ABSTRACT. The use of personal watercraft (PWC) has increased dramatically during the past decade as have the speed and mobility of the watercraft. A similar dramatic increase in PWC-related injury and death has occurred simultaneously. No one younger than 16 years should operate a PWC. The operator and all passengers must wear US Coast Guard-approved personal flotation devices. Other safety recommendations are suggested for parents and pediatricians. (2/00, reaffirmed 5/04, 1/07, 6/10)

http://pediatrics.aappublications.org/content/105/2/452

PESTICIDE EXPOSURE IN CHILDREN
Council on Environmental Health

ABSTRACT. This statement presents the position of the American Academy of Pediatrics on pesticides. Pesticides are a collective term for chemicals intended to kill unwanted insects, plants, molds, and rodents. Children encounter pesticides daily and have unique susceptibilities to their potential toxicity. Acute poisoning risks are clear, and understanding of chronic health implications from both acute and chronic exposure are emerging. Epidemiologic evidence demonstrates associations between early life exposure to pesticides and pediatric cancers, decreased cognitive function, and behavioral problems. Related animal toxicology studies provide supportive biological plausibility for these findings. Recognizing and reducing problematic exposures will require attention to current inadequacies in medical training, public health tracking, and regulatory action on pesticides. Ongoing research describing toxicologic vulnerabilities and exposure factors across the life span are needed to inform regulatory needs and appropriate interventions. Policies that promote integrated pest management, comprehensive pesticide labeling, and marketing practices that incorporate child health considerations will enhance safe use. (11/12)

http://pediatrics.aappublications.org/content/130/6/e1757

PESTICIDE EXPOSURE IN CHILDREN (TECHNICAL REPORT)
James R. Roberts, MD, MPH; Catherine J. Karr, MD, PhD; and Council on Environmental Health

ABSTRACT. Pesticides are a collective term for a wide array of chemicals intended to kill unwanted insects, plants, molds, and rodents. Food, water, and treatment in the home, yard, and school are all potential sources of children's exposure. Exposures to pesticides may be overt or subacute, and effects range from acute to chronic toxicity. In 2008, pesticides were the ninth most common substance reported to poison control centers, and approximately 45% of all reports of pesticide poisoning were for children. Organophosphate and carbamate poisoning are perhaps the most widely known acute poisoning syndromes, can be diagnosed by depressed red blood cell cholinesterase levels, and have available antidotal therapy. However, numerous other pesticides that may cause acute toxicity, such as pyrethroid and neonicotinoid insecticides, herbicides, fungicides, and rodenticides, also have specific toxic effects; recognition of these effects may help identify acute exposures. Evidence is increasingly emerging about chronic health implications from both acute and chronic exposure. A growing body of epidemiological evidence demonstrates associations between parental use of pesticides, particularly insecticides, with acute lymphocytic leukemia and brain tumors. Prenatal, household, and occupational exposures (maternal and paternal) appear to be the largest risks. Prospective cohort studies link early-life exposure to organophosphates and organochlorine pesticides (primarily DDT) with adverse effects on neurodevelopment and behavior. Among the findings associated with increased pesticide levels are poorer mental development by using the Bayley index and increased scores on measures assessing pervasive developmental disorder, inattention, and attention-deficit/hyperactivity disorder. Related animal toxicology studies provide supportive biological plausibility for these findings. Additional data suggest that there may also be an association between parental pesticide use and adverse birth outcomes including physical birth defects, low birth weight, and fetal death, although the data are less robust than for cancer and neurodevelopmental effects. Children's exposures to pesticides should be limited as much as possible. (11/12)

http://pediatrics.aappublications.org/content/130/6/e1765

PHOTOTHERAPY TO PREVENT SEVERE NEONATAL HYPERBILIRUBINEMIA IN THE NEWBORN INFANT 35 OR MORE WEEKS OF GESTATION (TECHNICAL REPORT)
Vinod K. Bhutani, MD, and Committee on Fetus and Newborn

ABSTRACT. *Objective.* To standardize the use of phototherapy consistent with the American Academy of Pediatrics clinical practice guideline for the management of hyperbilirubinemia in the newborn infant 35 or more weeks of gestation.

Methods. Relevant literature was reviewed. Phototherapy devices currently marketed in the United States that incorporate fluorescent, halogen, fiber-optic, or blue light-emitting diode light sources were assessed in the laboratory.

Results. The efficacy of phototherapy units varies widely because of differences in light source and configuration. The following characteristics of a device contribute to its effectiveness: (1) emission of light in the blue-to-green range that overlaps the in vivo plasma bilirubin absorption spectrum (~460–490 nm); (2) irradiance of at least 30 μW·cm–2·nm–1 (confirmed with an appropriate irradiance meter calibrated over the appropriate wavelength range); (3) illumination of maximal body surface; and (4) demonstration of a decrease in total bilirubin concentrations during the first 4 to 6 hours of exposure.

Recommendations. The intensity and spectral output of phototherapy devices is useful in predicting potential effectiveness in treating hyperbilirubinemia (group B recommendation). Clinical effectiveness should be evaluated before and monitored during use (group B recommendation). Blocking the light source or reducing exposed body surface should be avoided (group B recommendation). Standardization of irradiance meters, improvements in device design, and lower-upper limits of light intensity for phototherapy units merit further study. Comparing the in vivo performance of devices is not practical, in general, and alternative procedures need to be explored. (9/11, reaffirmed 7/14)

http://pediatrics.aappublications.org/content/128/4/e1046

PHYSICIAN HEALTH AND WELLNESS (CLINICAL REPORT)
Hilary McClafferty, MD, FAAP; Oscar W. Brown, MD, FAAP; Section on Integrative Medicine; and Committee on Practice and Ambulatory Medicine

ABSTRACT. Physician health and wellness is a critical issue gaining national attention because of the high prevalence of physician burnout. Pediatricians and pediatric trainees experience burnout at levels equivalent to other medical specialties, highlighting a need for more effective efforts to promote health and well-being in the pediatric community. This report will provide an overview of physician burnout, an update on work in the field of preventive physician health and wellness, and a discussion of emerging initiatives that have potential to promote health at all levels of pediatric training.

Pediatricians are uniquely positioned to lead this movement nationally, in part because of the emphasis placed on wellness in the Pediatric Milestone Project, a joint collaboration between the Accreditation Council for Graduate Medical Education and the American Board of Pediatrics. Updated core competencies calling for a balanced approach to health, including focus on nutrition, exercise, mindfulness, and effective stress management, signal a paradigm shift and send the message that it is time for pediatricians to cultivate a culture of wellness better aligned with their responsibilities as role models and congruent with advances in pediatric training.

Rather than reviewing programs in place to address substance abuse and other serious conditions in distressed physicians, this article focuses on forward progress in the field, with an emphasis on the need for prevention and anticipation of predictable stressors related to burnout in medical training and practice. Examples of positive progress and several programs designed to promote physician health and wellness are reviewed. Areas where more research is needed are highlighted. (9/14)

http://pediatrics.aappublications.org/content/134/4/830

PHYSICIAN REFUSAL TO PROVIDE INFORMATION OR TREATMENT ON THE BASIS OF CLAIMS OF CONSCIENCE

Committee on Bioethics

ABSTRACT. Health care professionals may have moral objections to particular medical interventions. They may refuse to provide or cooperate in the provision of these interventions. Such objections are referred to as conscientious objections. Although it may be difficult to characterize or validate claims of conscience, respecting the individual physician's moral integrity is important. Conflicts arise when claims of conscience impede a patient's access to medical information or care. A physician's conscientious objection to certain interventions or treatments may be constrained in some situations. Physicians have a duty to disclose to prospective patients treatments they refuse to perform. As part of informed consent, physicians also have a duty to inform their patients of all relevant and legally available treatment options, including options to which they object. They have a moral obligation to refer patients to other health care professionals who are willing to provide those services when failing to do so would cause harm to the patient, and they have a duty to treat patients in emergencies when referral would significantly increase the probability of mortality or serious morbidity. Conversely, the health care system should make reasonable accommodations for physicians with conscientious objections. (11/09, reaffirmed 1/14, 6/18)

http://pediatrics.aappublications.org/content/124/6/1689

PHYSICIAN'S ROLE IN COORDINATING CARE OF HOSPITALIZED CHILDREN (CLINICAL REPORT)

Daniel A. Rauch, MD, FAAP; Committee on Hospital Care; and Section on Hospital Medicine

ABSTRACT. The hospitalization of a child is a stressful event for the child and family. The physician responsible for the admission has an important role in directing the care of the child, communicating with the child's providers (medical and primary caregivers), and advocating for the safety of the child during the hospitalization and transition out of the hospital. These challenges remain constant across the varied facilities in which children are hospitalized. The purpose of this revised clinical report is to update pediatricians about principles to improve the coordination of care and review expectations and practice. (7/18)

See full text on page 813.

http://pediatrics.aappublications.org/content/142/2/e20181503

PLANNED HOME BIRTH

Committee on Fetus and Newborn

ABSTRACT. The American Academy of Pediatrics concurs with the recent statement of the American College of Obstetricians and Gynecologists affirming that hospitals and birthing centers are the safest settings for birth in the United States while respecting the right of women to make a medically informed decision about delivery. This statement is intended to help pediatricians provide supportive, informed counsel to women considering home birth while retaining their role as child advocates and to summarize the standards of care for newborn infants born at home, which are consistent with standards for infants born in a medical care facility. Regardless of the circumstances of his or her birth, including location, every newborn infant deserves health care that adheres to the standards highlighted in this statement, more completely described in other publications from the American Academy of Pediatrics, including *Guidelines for Perinatal Care*. The goal of providing high-quality care to all newborn infants can best be achieved through continuing efforts by all participating health care providers and institutions to develop and sustain communications and understanding on the basis of professional interaction and mutual respect throughout the health care system. (4/13, reaffirmed 12/16)

http://pediatrics.aappublications.org/content/131/5/1016

POINT-OF-CARE ULTRASONOGRAPHY BY PEDIATRIC EMERGENCY MEDICINE PHYSICIANS

Committee on Pediatric Emergency Medicine (joint with Society for Academic Emergency Medicine Academy of Emergency Ultrasound, American College of Emergency Physicians Pediatric Emergency Medicine Committee, and World Interactive Network Focused on Critical Ultrasound)

ABSTRACT. Point-of-care ultrasonography is increasingly being used to facilitate accurate and timely diagnoses and to guide procedures. It is important for pediatric emergency medicine (PEM) physicians caring for patients in the emergency department to receive adequate and continued point-of-care ultrasonography training for those indications used in their practice setting. Emergency departments should have credentialing and quality assurance programs. PEM fellowships should provide appropriate training to physician trainees. Hospitals should provide privileges to physicians who demonstrate competency in point-of-care ultrasonography. Ongoing research will provide the necessary measures to define the optimal training and competency assessment standards. Requirements for credentialing and hospital privileges will vary and will be specific to individual departments and hospitals. As more physicians are trained and more research is completed, there should be one national standard for credentialing and privileging in point-of-care ultrasonography for PEM physicians. (3/15)

http://pediatrics.aappublications.org/content/135/4/e1097

POINT-OF-CARE ULTRASONOGRAPHY BY PEDIATRIC EMERGENCY MEDICINE PHYSICIANS (TECHNICAL REPORT)

Jennifer R. Marin, MD, MSc; Resa E. Lewiss, MD; and Committee on Pediatric Emergency Medicine (joint with Society for Academic Emergency Medicine Academy of Emergency Ultrasound, American College of Emergency Physicians Pediatric Emergency Medicine Committee, and World Interactive Network Focused on Critical Ultrasound)

ABSTRACT. Emergency physicians have used point-of-care ultrasonography since the 1990s. Pediatric emergency medicine physicians have more recently adopted this technology. Point-of-care ultrasonography is used for various scenarios, particularly the evaluation of soft tissue infections or blunt abdominal trauma and procedural guidance. To date, there are no published statements from national organizations specifically for pediatric emergency physicians describing the incorporation of point-of-care ultrasonography into their practice. This document outlines how pediatric emergency departments may establish a formal point-of-care ultrasonography program. This task includes appointing leaders with expertise in point-of-care ultrasonography, effectively training and credentialing physicians in the department, and providing ongoing quality assurance reviews.

Point-of-care ultrasonography (US) is a bedside technology that enables clinicians to integrate clinical examination findings with real-time sonographic imaging. General emergency physicians and other specialists have used point-of-care US for many years, and more recently, pediatric emergency medicine (PEM) physicians have adopted point-of-care US as a diagnostic and procedural adjunct. This technical report and accompanying policy statement provide a framework for point-of-care US training and point-of-care US integration into pediatric care by PEM physicians. (3/15)

http://pediatrics.aappublications.org/content/135/4/e1113

POSTDISCHARGE FOLLOW-UP OF INFANTS WITH CONGENITAL DIAPHRAGMATIC HERNIA (CLINICAL REPORT)

Section on Surgery and Committee on Fetus and Newborn

ABSTRACT. Infants with congenital diaphragmatic hernia often require intensive treatment after birth, have prolonged hospitalizations, and have other congenital anomalies. After discharge from the hospital, they may have long-term sequelae such as respiratory insufficiency, gastroesophageal reflux, poor growth, neurodevelopmental delay, behavior problems, hearing loss, hernia recurrence, and orthopedic deformities. Structured follow-up for these patients facilitates early recognition and treatment of these complications. In this report, follow-up of infants with congenital diaphragmatic hernia is outlined. (3/08, reaffirmed 5/11)

http://pediatrics.aappublications.org/content/121/3/627

POSTNATAL CORTICOSTEROIDS TO PREVENT OR TREAT BRONCHOPULMONARY DYSPLASIA

Kristi L. Watterberg, MD, and Committee on Fetus and Newborn

ABSTRACT. The purpose of this revised statement is to review current information on the use of postnatal glucocorticoids to prevent or treat bronchopulmonary dysplasia in the preterm infant and to make updated recommendations regarding their use. High-dose dexamethasone (0.5 mg/kg per day) does not seem to confer additional therapeutic benefit over lower doses and is not recommended. Evidence is insufficient to make a recommendation regarding other glucocorticoid doses and preparations. The clinician must use clinical judgment when attempting to balance the potential adverse effects of glucocorticoid treatment with those of bronchopulmonary dysplasia. (9/10, reaffirmed 1/14)

http://pediatrics.aappublications.org/content/126/4/800

POSTNATAL GLUCOSE HOMEOSTASIS IN LATE-PRETERM AND TERM INFANTS (CLINICAL REPORT)

David H. Adamkin, MD, and Committee on Fetus and Newborn

ABSTRACT. This report provides a practical guide and algorithm for the screening and subsequent management of neonatal hypoglycemia. Current evidence does not support a specific concentration of glucose that can discriminate normal from abnormal or can potentially result in acute or chronic irreversible neurologic damage. Early identification of the at-risk infant and institution of prophylactic measures to prevent neonatal hypoglycemia are recommended as a pragmatic approach despite the absence of a consistent definition of hypoglycemia in the literature. (3/11, reaffirmed 6/15)

http://pediatrics.aappublications.org/content/127/3/575

POVERTY AND CHILD HEALTH IN THE UNITED STATES

Council on Community Pediatrics

ABSTRACT. Almost half of young children in the United States live in poverty or near poverty. The American Academy of Pediatrics is committed to reducing and ultimately eliminating child poverty in the United States. Poverty and related social determinants of health can lead to adverse health outcomes in childhood and across the life course, negatively affecting physical health, socioemotional development, and educational achievement. The American Academy of Pediatrics advocates for programs and policies that have been shown to improve the quality of life and health outcomes for children and families living in poverty. With an awareness and understanding of the effects of poverty on children, pediatricians and other pediatric health practitioners in a family-centered medical home can assess the financial stability of families, link families to resources, and coordinate care with community partners. Further research, advocacy, and continuing education will improve the ability of pediatricians to address the social determinants of health when caring for children who live in poverty. Accompanying this policy statement is a technical report that describes current knowledge on child poverty and the mechanisms by which poverty influences the health and well-being of children. (3/16)

http://pediatrics.aappublications.org/content/137/4/e20160339

THE POWER OF PLAY: A PEDIATRIC ROLE IN ENHANCING DEVELOPMENT IN YOUNG CHILDREN (CLINICAL REPORT)

Michael Yogman, MD, FAAP; Andrew Garner, MD, PhD, FAAP; Jeffrey Hutchinson, MD, FAAP; Kathy Hirsh-Pasek, PhD; Roberta Michnick Golinkoff, PhD; Committee on Psychosocial Aspects of Child and Family Health; and Council on Communications and Media

ABSTRACT. Children need to develop a variety of skill sets to optimize their development and manage toxic stress. Research demonstrates that developmentally appropriate play with parents and peers is a singular opportunity to promote the social-emotional, cognitive, language, and self-regulation skills that build executive function and a prosocial brain. Furthermore, play supports the formation of the safe, stable, and nurturing relationships with all caregivers that children need to thrive.

Play is not frivolous: it enhances brain structure and function and promotes executive function (ie, the process of learning, rather than the content), which allow us to pursue goals and ignore distractions.

When play and safe, stable, nurturing relationships are missing in a child's life, toxic stress can disrupt the development of executive function and the learning of prosocial behavior; in the presence of childhood adversity, play becomes even more important. The mutual joy and shared communication and attunement (harmonious serve and return interactions) that parents and children can experience during play regulate the body's stress response. This clinical report provides pediatric providers with the information they need to promote the benefits of play and to write a prescription for play at well visits to complement reach out and read. At a time when early childhood programs are pressured to add more didactic components and less playful learning, pediatricians can play an important role in emphasizing the role of a balanced curriculum that includes the importance of playful learning for the promotion of healthy child development. (8/18)

See full text on page 821.

http://pediatrics.aappublications.org/content/142/3/e20182058

PRACTICAL APPROACHES TO OPTIMIZE ADOLESCENT IMMUNIZATION (CLINICAL REPORT)

Henry H. Bernstein, DO, MHCM, FAAP; Joseph A. Bocchini Jr, MD, FAAP; and Committee on Infectious Diseases

ABSTRACT. With the expansion of the adolescent immunization schedule during the past decade, immunization rates notably vary by vaccine and by state. Addressing barriers to improving adolescent vaccination rates is a priority. Every visit can be viewed as an opportunity to update and complete an adolescent's immunizations. It is essential to continue to focus and refine the appropriate techniques in approaching the adolescent patient and parent in the office setting. Health care providers must continuously strive to educate their patients and develop skills that can help parents and adolescents overcome vaccine hesitancy. Research on strategies to achieve higher vaccination rates is ongoing, and it is important to increase the knowledge and implementation of these strategies. This clinical report focuses on increasing adherence to the universally recommended vaccines in the annual adolescent immunization schedule of the American Academy of Pediatrics, the American Academy of Family Physicians, the Centers for Disease Control and Prevention, and the American Congress of Obstetricians and Gynecologists. This will be accomplished by (1) examining strategies that heighten confidence in immunizations and address patient and parental concerns to promote adolescent immunization and (2) exploring how best to approach the adolescent and family to improve immunization rates. (2/17)

http://pediatrics.aappublications.org/content/139/3/e20164187

PREMEDICATION FOR NONEMERGENCY ENDOTRACHEAL INTUBATION IN THE NEONATE (CLINICAL REPORT)

Praveen Kumar, MD; Susan E. Denson, MD; Thomas J. Mancuso, MD; Committee on Fetus and Newborn; and Section on Anesthesiology and Pain Medicine

ABSTRACT. Endotracheal intubation is a common procedure in newborn care. The purpose of this clinical report is to review currently available evidence on use of premedication for intubation, identify gaps in knowledge, and provide guidance for making decisions about the use of premedication. (2/10, reaffirmed 8/13, 5/18)

http://pediatrics.aappublications.org/content/125/3/608

PRENATAL SUBSTANCE ABUSE: SHORT- AND LONG-TERM EFFECTS ON THE EXPOSED FETUS (TECHNICAL REPORT)

Marylou Behnke, MD; Vincent C. Smith, MD; Committee on Substance Abuse; and Committee on Fetus and Newborn

ABSTRACT. Prenatal substance abuse continues to be a significant problem in this country and poses important health risks for the developing fetus. The primary care pediatrician's role in addressing prenatal substance exposure includes prevention, identification of exposure, recognition of medical issues for the exposed newborn infant, protection of the infant, and follow-up of the exposed infant. This report will provide information for the most common drugs involved in prenatal exposure: nicotine, alcohol, marijuana, opiates, cocaine, and methamphetamine. (2/13)

http://pediatrics.aappublications.org/content/131/3/e1009

THE PRENATAL VISIT (CLINICAL REPORT)

Michael Yogman, MD, FAAP; Arthur Lavin, MD, FAAP; George Cohen, MD, FAAP; and Committee on Psychosocial Aspects of Child and Family Health

ABSTRACT. A pediatric prenatal visit during the third trimester is recommended for all expectant families as an important first step in establishing a child's medical home, as recommended by *Bright Futures: Guidelines for Health Supervision of Infants, Children, and Adolescents, Fourth Edition*. As advocates for children and their families, pediatricians can support and guide expectant parents in the prenatal period. Prenatal visits allow general pediatricians to establish a supportive and trusting relationship with both parents, gather basic information from expectant parents, offer information and advice regarding the infant, and may identify psychosocial risks early and high-risk conditions that may require special care. There are several possible formats for this first visit. The one used depends on the experience and preference of the parents, the style of the pediatrician's practice, and pragmatic issues of payment. (6/18)

See full text on page 839.

http://pediatrics.aappublications.org/content/142/1/e20181218

PREPARATION FOR EMERGENCIES IN THE OFFICES OF PEDIATRICIANS AND PEDIATRIC PRIMARY CARE PROVIDERS

Committee on Pediatric Emergency Medicine

ABSTRACT. High-quality pediatric emergency care can be provided only through the collaborative efforts of many health care professionals and child advocates working together throughout a continuum of care that extends from prevention and the medical home to prehospital care, to emergency department stabilization, to critical care and rehabilitation, and finally to a return to care in the medical home. At times, the office of the pediatric primary care provider will serve as the entry site into the emergency care system, which comprises out-of-hospital emergency medical services personnel, emergency department nurses and physicians, and other emergency and critical care providers. Recognizing the important role of pediatric primary care providers in the emergency care system for children and understanding the capabilities and limitations of that system are essential if pediatric primary care providers are to offer the best chance at intact survival for every child who is brought to the office with an emergency. Optimizing pediatric primary care provider office readiness for emergencies requires consideration of the unique aspects of each office practice, the types of patients and emergencies that might be seen, the resources on site, and the resources of the larger emergency care system of which the pediatric primary care provider's office is a part. Parent education regarding prevention, recognition, and response to emergencies, patient triage, early recognition and stabilization of pediatric emergencies in the office, and timely transfer to an appropriate facility for definitive care are important responsibilities of every pediatric primary care provider. In addition, pediatric primary care providers can collaborate with out-of-hospital and hospital-based providers and advocate for the best-quality emergency care for their patients. (7/07, reaffirmed 6/11)

http://pediatrics.aappublications.org/content/120/1/200

PREPARING FOR PEDIATRIC EMERGENCIES: DRUGS TO CONSIDER (CLINICAL REPORT)

Mary A. Hegenbarth, MD, and Committee on Drugs

ABSTRACT. This clinical report provides current recommendations regarding the selection and use of drugs in preparation for pediatric emergencies. It is not intended to be a comprehensive list of all medications that may be used in all emergencies. When possible, dosage recommendations are consistent with those used in current emergency references such as the *Advanced Pediatric Life Support and Pediatric Advanced Life Support* textbooks and the recently revised American Heart Association resuscitation guidelines. (2/08, reaffirmed 10/11, 2/16)

http://pediatrics.aappublications.org/content/121/2/433

PRESCRIBING ASSISTIVE-TECHNOLOGY SYSTEMS: FOCUS ON CHILDREN WITH IMPAIRED COMMUNICATION (CLINICAL REPORT)

Larry W. Desch, MD; Deborah Gaebler-Spira, MD; and Council on Children With Disabilities

ABSTRACT. This clinical report defines common terms of use and provides information on current practice, research, and limitations of assistive technology that can be used in systems for communication. The assessment process to determine the best devices for use with a particular child (ie, the best fit of a device) is also reviewed. The primary care pediatrician, as part of the medical home, plays an important role in the interdisciplinary effort to provide appropriate assistive technology and may be asked to make a referral for assessment or prescribe a particular device. This report provides resources to assist pediatricians in this role and reviews the interdisciplinary team functional evaluation using standardized assessments; the multiple funding opportunities available for obtaining devices and ways in which

pediatricians can assist families with obtaining them; the training necessary to use these systems once the devices are procured; the follow-up evaluation to ensure that the systems are meeting their goals; and the leadership skills needed to advocate for this technology. The American Academy of Pediatrics acknowledges the need for key resources to be identified in the community and recognizes that these resources are a shared medical, educational, therapeutic, and family responsibility. Although this report primarily deals with assistive technology specific for communication impairments, many of the details in this report also can aid in the acquisition and use of other types of assistive technology. (6/08, reaffirmed 1/12, 6/18)
http://pediatrics.aappublications.org/content/121/6/1271

PRESCRIBING THERAPY SERVICES FOR CHILDREN WITH MOTOR DISABILITIES (CLINICAL REPORT)

Committee on Children With Disabilities

ABSTRACT. Pediatricians often are called on to prescribe physical, occupational, and speech-language therapy services for children with motor disabilities. This report defines the context in which rehabilitation therapies should be prescribed, emphasizing the evaluation and enhancement of the child's function and abilities and participation in age-appropriate life roles. The report encourages pediatricians to work with teams including the parents, child, teachers, therapists, and other physicians to ensure that their patients receive appropriate therapy services. (6/04, reaffirmed 12/16)
http://pediatrics.aappublications.org/content/113/6/1836

PRESERVATION OF FERTILITY IN PEDIATRIC AND ADOLESCENT PATIENTS WITH CANCER (TECHNICAL REPORT)

Mary E. Fallat, MD; John Hutter, MD; Committee on Bioethics; Section on Hematology/Oncology; and Section on Surgery

ABSTRACT. Many cancers that present in children and adolescents are curable with surgery, chemotherapy, and/or radiation therapy. Potential adverse consequences of treatment include sterility, infertility, or subfertility as a result of either gonad removal or damage to germ cells from adjuvant therapy. In recent years, treatment of solid tumors and hematologic malignancies has been modified in an attempt to reduce damage to the gonads. Simultaneously, advances in assisted reproductive techniques have led to new possibilities for the prevention and treatment of infertility. This technical report reviews the topic of fertility preservation in pediatric and adolescent patients with cancer, including ethical considerations. (5/08, reaffirmed 2/12)
http://pediatrics.aappublications.org/content/121/5/e1461

PREVENTING OBESITY AND EATING DISORDERS IN ADOLESCENTS (CLINICAL REPORT)

Neville H. Golden, MD, FAAP; Marcie Schneider, MD, FAAP; Christine Wood, MD, FAAP; Committee on Nutrition; Committee on Adolescence; and Section on Obesity

ABSTRACT. Obesity and eating disorders (EDs) are both prevalent in adolescents. There are concerns that obesity prevention efforts may lead to the development of an ED. Most adolescents who develop an ED did not have obesity previously, but some teenagers, in an attempt to lose weight, may develop an ED. This clinical report addresses the interaction between obesity prevention and EDs in teenagers, provides the pediatrician with evidence-informed tools to identify behaviors that predispose to both obesity and EDs, and provides guidance about obesity and ED prevention messages. The focus should be on a healthy lifestyle rather than on weight. Evidence suggests that obesity prevention and treatment, if conducted correctly, do not predispose to EDs. (8/16)
http://pediatrics.aappublications.org/content/138/3/e20161649

PREVENTION AND MANAGEMENT OF PROCEDURAL PAIN IN THE NEONATE: AN UPDATE

Committee on Fetus and Newborn and Section on Anesthesiology and Pain Medicine

ABSTRACT. The prevention of pain in neonates should be the goal of all pediatricians and health care professionals who work with neonates, not only because it is ethical but also because repeated painful exposures have the potential for deleterious consequences. Neonates at greatest risk of neurodevelopmental impairment as a result of preterm birth (ie, the smallest and sickest) are also those most likely to be exposed to the greatest number of painful stimuli in the NICU. Although there are major gaps in knowledge regarding the most effective way to prevent and relieve pain in neonates, proven and safe therapies are currently underused for routine minor, yet painful procedures. Therefore, every health care facility caring for neonates should implement (1) a pain-prevention program that includes strategies for minimizing the number of painful procedures performed and (2) a pain assessment and management plan that includes routine assessment of pain, pharmacologic and non-pharmacologic therapies for the prevention of pain associated with routine minor procedures, and measures for minimizing pain associated with surgery and other major procedures. (1/16)
http://pediatrics.aappublications.org/content/137/2/e20154271

PREVENTION OF AGRICULTURAL INJURIES AMONG CHILDREN AND ADOLESCENTS

Committee on Injury and Poison Prevention and Committee on Community Health Services

ABSTRACT. Although the annual number of farm deaths to children and adolescents has decreased since publication of the 1988 American Academy of Pediatrics statement, "Rural Injuries," the rate of nonfatal farm injuries has increased. Approximately 100 unintentional injury deaths occur annually to children and adolescents on US farms, and an additional 22 000 injuries to children younger than 20 years occur on farms. Relatively few adolescents are employed on farms compared with other types of industry, yet the proportion of fatalities in agriculture is higher than that for any other type of adolescent employment. The high mortality and severe morbidity associated with farm injuries require continuing and improved injury-control strategies. This statement provides recommendations for pediatricians regarding patient and community education as well as public advocacy related to agricultural injury prevention in childhood and adolescence. (10/01, reaffirmed 1/07, 11/11)
http://pediatrics.aappublications.org/content/108/4/1016

PREVENTION OF CHILDHOOD LEAD TOXICITY

Council on Environmental Health

ABSTRACT. Blood lead concentrations have decreased dramatically in US children over the past 4 decades, but too many children still live in housing with deteriorated lead-based paint and are at risk for lead exposure with resulting lead-associated cognitive impairment and behavioral problems. Evidence continues to accrue that commonly encountered blood lead concentrations, even those below 5 µg/dL (50 ppb), impair cognition; there is no identified threshold or safe level of lead in blood. From 2007 to 2010, approximately 2.6% of preschool children in the United States had a blood lead concentration ≥5 µg/dL (≥50 ppb), which represents about 535 000 US children 1 to 5 years of age. Evidence-based guidance is available for managing increased lead exposure in children, and reducing sources of lead in the environment, including lead in housing, soil, water, and consumer products, has been shown to be cost-beneficial. Primary prevention should be the focus of policy on childhood lead toxicity. (6/16)
http://pediatrics.aappublications.org/content/138/1/e20161493

PREVENTION OF CHOKING AMONG CHILDREN

Committee on Injury, Violence, and Poison Prevention

ABSTRACT. Choking is a leading cause of morbidity and mortality among children, especially those aged 3 years or younger. Food, coins, and toys are the primary causes of choking-related injury and death. Certain characteristics, including shape, size, and consistency, of certain toys and foods increase their potential to cause choking among children. Childhood choking hazards should be addressed through comprehensive and coordinated prevention activities. The US Consumer Product Safety Commission (CPSC) should increase efforts to ensure that toys that are sold in retail store bins, vending machines, or on the Internet have appropriate choking-hazard warnings; work with manufacturers to improve the effectiveness of recalls of products that pose a choking risk to children; and increase efforts to prevent the resale of these recalled products via online auction sites. Current gaps in choking-prevention standards for children's toys should be reevaluated and addressed, as appropriate, via revisions to the standards established under the Child Safety Protection Act, the Consumer Product Safety Improvement Act, or regulation by the CPSC. Prevention of food-related choking among children in the United States has been inadequately addressed at the federal level. The US Food and Drug Administration should establish a systematic, institutionalized process for examining and addressing the hazards of food-related choking. This process should include the establishment of the necessary surveillance, hazard evaluation, enforcement, and public education activities to prevent food-related choking among children. While maintaining its highly cooperative arrangements with the CPSC and the US Department of Agriculture, the Food and Drug Administration should have the authority to address choking-related risks of all food products, including meat products that fall under the jurisdiction of the US Department of Agriculture. The existing National Electronic Injury Surveillance System–All Injury Program of the CPSC should be modified to conduct more-detailed surveillance of choking on food among children. Food manufacturers should design new foods and redesign existing foods to avoid shapes, sizes, textures, and other characteristics that increase choking risk to children, to the extent possible. Pediatricians, dentists, and other infant and child health care providers should provide choking-prevention counseling to parents as an integral part of anticipatory guidance activities. (2/10)

http://pediatrics.aappublications.org/content/125/3/601

PREVENTION OF DROWNING

Committee on Injury, Violence, and Poison Prevention

ABSTRACT. Drowning is a leading cause of injury-related death in children. In 2006, fatal drowning claimed the lives of approximately 1100 US children younger than 20 years. A number of strategies are available to prevent these tragedies. As educators and advocates, pediatricians can play an important role in the prevention of drowning. (5/10)

http://pediatrics.aappublications.org/content/126/1/178

PREVENTION OF DROWNING (TECHNICAL REPORT)

Jeffrey Weiss, MD, and Committee on Injury, Violence, and Poison Prevention

ABSTRACT. Drowning is a leading cause of injury-related death in children. In 2006, approximately 1100 US children younger than 20 years died from drowning. A number of strategies are available to prevent these tragedies. As educators and advocates, pediatricians can play an important role in the prevention of drowning. (5/10)

http://pediatrics.aappublications.org/content/126/1/e253

PREVENTION OF SEXUAL HARASSMENT IN THE WORKPLACE AND EDUCATIONAL SETTINGS

Committee on Pediatric Workforce

ABSTRACT. The American Academy of Pediatrics is committed to working to ensure that workplaces and educational settings in which pediatricians spend time are free of sexual harassment. The purpose of this statement is to heighten awareness and sensitivity to this important issue, recognizing that institutions, clinics, and office-based practices may have existing policies. (10/06, reaffirmed 5/09, 1/12, 10/14)

http://pediatrics.aappublications.org/content/118/4/1752

THE PREVENTION OF UNINTENTIONAL INJURY AMONG AMERICAN INDIAN AND ALASKA NATIVE CHILDREN: A SUBJECT REVIEW (CLINICAL REPORT)

Committee on Native American Child Health and Committee on Injury and Poison Prevention

ABSTRACT. Among ethnic groups in the United States, American Indian and Alaska Native (AI/AN) children experience the highest rates of injury mortality and morbidity. Injury mortality rates for AI/AN children have decreased during the past quarter century, but remain almost double the rate for all children in the United States. The Indian Health Service (IHS), the federal agency with the primary responsibility for the health care of AI/AN people, has sponsored an internationally recognized injury prevention program designed to reduce the risk of injury death by addressing community-specific risk factors. Model programs developed by the IHS and tribal governments have led to successful outcomes in motor vehicle occupant safety, drowning prevention, and fire safety. Injury prevention programs in tribal communities require special attention to the sovereignty of tribal governments and the unique cultural aspects of health care and communication. Pediatricians working with AI/AN children on reservations or in urban environments are strongly urged to collaborate with tribes and the IHS to create community-based coalitions and develop programs to address highly preventable injury-related mortality and morbidity. Strong advocacy also is needed to promote childhood injury prevention as an important priority for federal agencies and tribes. (12/99, reaffirmed 12/02 COIVPP, 5/03 CONACH, 1/06, 9/08)

http://pediatrics.aappublications.org/content/104/6/1397

THE PRIMARY CARE PEDIATRICIAN AND THE CARE OF CHILDREN WITH CLEFT LIP AND/OR CLEFT PALATE (CLINICAL REPORT)

PPI
AAP Partnership for Policy Implementation

Charlotte W. Lewis, MD, MPH, FAAP; Lisa S. Jacob, DDS, MS; Christoph U. Lehmann, MD, FAAP, FACMI; and Section on Oral Health

ABSTRACT. Orofacial clefts, specifically cleft lip and/or cleft palate (CL/P), are among the most common congenital anomalies. CL/P vary in their location and severity and comprise 3 overarching groups: cleft lip (CL), cleft lip with cleft palate (CLP), and cleft palate alone (CP). CL/P may be associated with one of many syndromes that could further complicate a child's needs. Care of patients with CL/P spans prenatal diagnosis into adulthood. The appropriate timing and order of specific cleft-related care are important factors for optimizing outcomes; however, care should be individualized to meet the specific needs of each patient and family. Children with CL/P should receive their specialty cleft-related care from a multidisciplinary cleft or craniofacial team with sufficient patient and surgical volume to promote successful outcomes. The primary care pediatrician at the child's medical home has an essential role in making a timely diagnosis and referral; providing ongoing health care maintenance, anticipatory guidance, and acute care; and functioning as an advocate for the patient and a liaison between the family and the craniofacial/cleft team. This document provides background

on CL/P and multidisciplinary team care, information about typical timing and order of cleft-related care, and recommendations for cleft/craniofacial teams and primary care pediatricians in the care of children with CL/P. (4/17)
http://pediatrics.aappublications.org/content/139/5/e20170628

PRINCIPLES OF CHILD HEALTH CARE FINANCING

Mark L. Hudak, MD, FAAP; Mark E. Helm, MD, MBA, FAAP; Patience H. White, MD, MA, FAAP, FACP; and Committee on Child Health Financing

ABSTRACT. After passage of the Patient Protection and Affordable Care Act, more children and young adults have become insured and have benefited from health care coverage than at any time since the creation of the Medicaid program in 1965. From 2009 to 2015, the uninsurance rate for children younger than 19 years fell from 9.7% to 5.3%, whereas the uninsurance rate for young adults 19 to 25 years of age declined from 31.7% to 14.5%. Nonetheless, much work remains to be done. The American Academy of Pediatrics (AAP) believes that the United States can and should ensure that all children, adolescents, and young adults from birth through the age of 26 years who reside within its borders have affordable access to high-quality and comprehensive health care, regardless of their or their families' incomes. Public and private health insurance should safeguard existing benefits for children and take further steps to cover the full array of essential health care services recommended by the AAP. Each family should be able to afford the premiums, deductibles, and other cost-sharing provisions of the plan. Health plans providing these benefits should ensure, insofar as possible, that families have a choice of professionals and facilities with expertise in the care of children within a reasonable distance of their residence. Traditional and innovative payment methodologies by public and private payers should be structured to guarantee the economic viability of the pediatric medical home and of other pediatric specialty and subspecialty practices to address developing shortages in the pediatric specialty and subspecialty workforce, to promote the use of health information technology, to improve population health and the experience of care, and to encourage the delivery of evidence-based and quality health care in the medical home, as well as in other outpatient, inpatient, and home settings. All current and future health care insurance plans should incorporate the principles for child health financing outlined in this statement. Espousing the core principle to do no harm, the AAP believes that the United States must not sacrifice any of the hard-won gains for our children. Medicaid, as the largest single payer of health care for children and young adults, should remain true to its origins as an entitlement program; in other words, future fiscal or regulatory reforms of Medicaid should not reduce the eligibility and scope of benefits for children and young adults below current levels nor jeopardize children's access to care. Proposed Medicaid funding "reforms" (eg, institution of block grant, capped allotment, or per-capita capitation payments to states) will achieve their goal of securing cost savings but will inevitably compel states to reduce enrollee eligibility, trim existing benefits (such as Early and Periodic Screening, Diagnostic, and Treatment), and/or compromise children's access to necessary and timely care through cuts in payments to providers and delivery systems. In fact, the AAP advocates for increased Medicaid funding to improve access to essential care for existing enrollees, fund care for eligible but uninsured children once they enroll, and accommodate enrollment growth that will occur in states that choose to expand Medicaid eligibility. The AAP also calls for Congress to extend funding for the Children's Health Insurance Program, a plan vital to the 8.9 million children it covered in fiscal year 2016, for a minimum of 5 years. (8/17)
http://pediatrics.aappublications.org/content/140/3/e20172098

PRINCIPLES OF PEDIATRIC PATIENT SAFETY: REDUCING HARM DUE TO MEDICAL CARE

Steering Committee on Quality Improvement and Management and Committee on Hospital Care

ABSTRACT. Pediatricians are rendering care in an environment that is increasingly complex, which results in multiple opportunities to cause unintended harm. National awareness of patient safety risks has grown in the 10 years since the Institute of Medicine published its report To Err Is Human, and patients and society as a whole continue to challenge health care providers to examine their practices and implement safety solutions. The depth and breadth of harm incurred by the practice of medicine is still being defined as reports continue to uncover a variety of avoidable errors, from those that involve specific high-risk medications to those that are more generalizable, such as patient misidentification. Pediatricians in all venues must have a working knowledge of patient-safety language, advocate for best practices that attend to risks that are unique to children, identify and support a culture of safety, and lead efforts to eliminate avoidable harm in any setting in which medical care is rendered to children. (5/11)
http://pediatrics.aappublications.org/content/127/6/1199

PROBIOTICS AND PREBIOTICS IN PEDIATRICS (CLINICAL REPORT)

Dan W. Thomas, MD; Frank R. Greer, MD; Committee on Nutrition; and Section on Gastroenterology, Hepatology, and Nutrition

ABSTRACT. This clinical report reviews the currently known health benefits of probiotic and prebiotic products, including those added to commercially available infant formula and other food products for use in children. Probiotics are supplements or foods that contain viable microorganisms that cause alterations of the microflora of the host. Use of probiotics has been shown to be modestly effective in randomized clinical trials (RCTs) in (1) treating acute viral gastroenteritis in healthy children; and (2) preventing antibiotic-associated diarrhea in healthy children. There is some evidence that probiotics prevent necrotizing enterocolitis in very low birth weight infants (birth weight between 1000 and 1500 g), but more studies are needed. The results of RCTs in which probiotics were used to treat childhood Helicobacter pylori gastritis, irritable bowel syndrome, chronic ulcerative colitis, and infantile colic, as well as in preventing childhood atopy, although encouraging, are preliminary and require further confirmation. Probiotics have not been proven to be beneficial in treating or preventing human cancers or in treating children with Crohn disease. There are also safety concerns with the use of probiotics in infants and children who are immunocompromised, chronically debilitated, or seriously ill with indwelling medical devices.

Prebiotics are supplements or foods that contain a nondigestible food ingredient that selectively stimulates the favorable growth and/or activity of indigenous probiotic bacteria. Human milk contains substantial quantities of prebiotics. There is a paucity of RCTs examining prebiotics in children, although there may be some long-term benefit of prebiotics for the prevention of atopic eczema and common infections in healthy infants. Confirmatory well-designed clinical research studies are necessary. (11/10)
http://pediatrics.aappublications.org/content/126/6/1217

PROCEDURES FOR THE EVALUATION OF THE VISUAL SYSTEM BY PEDIATRICIANS (CLINICAL REPORT)

Sean P. Donahue, MD, PhD, FAAP; Cynthia N. Baker, MD, FAAP; Committee on Practice and Ambulatory Medicine; and Section on Ophthalmology (joint with American Association of Certified Orthoptists, American Association for Pediatric Ophthalmology and Strabismus, and American Academy of Ophthalmology)

ABSTRACT. Vision screening is crucial for the detection of visual and systemic disorders. It should begin in the newborn nursery and continue throughout childhood. This clinical report provides details regarding methods for pediatricians to use for screening. (12/15)
http://pediatrics.aappublications.org/content/137/1/e20153597

PROFESSIONAL LIABILITY INSURANCE AND MEDICOLEGAL EDUCATION FOR PEDIATRIC RESIDENTS AND FELLOWS

Committee on Medical Liability and Risk Management

ABSTRACT. The American Academy of Pediatrics believes that pediatric residents and fellows should be fully informed of the scope and limitations of their professional liability insurance coverage while in training. The academy states that residents and fellows should be educated by their training institutions on matters relating to medical liability and the importance of maintaining adequate and continuous professional liability insurance coverage throughout their careers in medicine. (8/11)
http://pediatrics.aappublications.org/content/128/3/624

PROFESSIONALISM IN PEDIATRICS (TECHNICAL REPORT)

Mary E. Fallat, MD; Jacqueline Glover, PhD; and Committee on Bioethics

ABSTRACT. The purpose of this report is to provide a concrete overview of the ideal standards of behavior and professional practice to which pediatricians should aspire and by which students and residents can be evaluated. Recognizing that the ideal is not always achievable in the practical sense, this document details the key components of professionalism in pediatric practice with an emphasis on core professional values for which pediatricians should strive and that will serve as a moral compass needed to provide quality care for children and their families. (10/07, reaffirmed 5/11)
http://pediatrics.aappublications.org/content/120/4/e1123

PROFESSIONALISM IN PEDIATRICS: STATEMENT OF PRINCIPLES

Committee on Bioethics

ABSTRACT. The purpose of this statement is to delineate the concept of professionalism within the context of pediatrics and to provide a brief statement of principles to guide the behavior and professional practice of pediatricians. (10/07, reaffirmed 5/11)
http://pediatrics.aappublications.org/content/120/4/895

PROMOTING EDUCATION, MENTORSHIP, AND SUPPORT FOR PEDIATRIC RESEARCH

Committee on Pediatric Research

ABSTRACT. Pediatricians play a key role in advancing child health research to best attain and improve the physical, mental, and social health and well-being of all infants, children, adolescents, and young adults. Child health presents unique issues that require investigators who specialize in pediatric research. In addition, the scope of the pediatric research enterprise is transdisciplinary and includes the full spectrum of basic science, translational, community-based, health services, and child health policy research. Although most pediatricians do not directly engage in research, knowledge of research methodologies and approaches promotes critical evaluation of scientific literature, the practice of evidence-based medicine, and advocacy for evidence-based child health policy. This statement includes specific recommendations to promote further research education and support at all levels of pediatric training, from premedical to continuing medical education, as well as recommendations to increase support and mentorship for research activities. Pediatric research is crucial to the American Academy of Pediatrics' goal of improving the health of all children. The American Academy of Pediatrics continues to promote and encourage efforts to facilitate the creation of new knowledge and ways to reduce barriers experienced by trainees, practitioners, and academic faculty pursuing research. (4/14, reaffirmed 2/18)
http://pediatrics.aappublications.org/content/133/5/943

PROMOTING FOOD SECURITY FOR ALL CHILDREN

Council on Community Pediatrics and Committee on Nutrition

ABSTRACT. Sixteen million US children (21%) live in households without consistent access to adequate food. After multiple risk factors are considered, children who live in households that are food insecure, even at the lowest levels, are likely to be sick more often, recover from illness more slowly, and be hospitalized more frequently. Lack of adequate healthy food can impair a child's ability to concentrate and perform well in school and is linked to higher levels of behavioral and emotional problems from preschool through adolescence. Food insecurity can affect children in any community, not only traditionally underserved ones. Pediatricians can play a central role in screening and identifying children at risk for food insecurity and in connecting families with needed community resources. Pediatricians should also advocate for federal and local policies that support access to adequate healthy food for an active and healthy life for all children and their families. (10/15)
http://pediatrics.aappublications.org/content/136/5/e1431

PROMOTING OPTIMAL DEVELOPMENT: SCREENING FOR BEHAVIORAL AND EMOTIONAL PROBLEMS (CLINICAL REPORT)

Carol Weitzman, MD, FAAP; Lynn Wegner, MD, FAAP; Section on Developmental and Behavioral Pediatrics; Committee on Psychosocial Aspects of Child and Family Health; and Council on Early Childhood (joint with Society for Developmental and Behavioral Pediatrics)

ABSTRACT. By current estimates, at any given time, approximately 11% to 20% of children in the United States have a behavioral or emotional disorder, as defined in the *Diagnostic and Statistical Manual of Mental Disorders, Fifth Edition*. Between 37% and 39% of children will have a behavioral or emotional disorder diagnosed by 16 years of age, regardless of geographic location in the United States. Behavioral and emotional problems and concerns in children and adolescents are not being reliably identified or treated in the US health system. This clinical report focuses on the need to increase behavioral screening and offers potential changes in practice and the health system, as well as the research needed to accomplish this. This report also (1) reviews the prevalence of behavioral and emotional disorders, (2) describes factors affecting the emergence of behavioral and emotional problems, (3) articulates the current state of detection of these problems in pediatric primary care, (4) describes barriers to screening and means to overcome those barriers, and (5) discusses potential changes at a practice and systems level that are needed to facilitate successful behavioral and emotional screening. Highlighted and discussed are the many factors at the level of the pediatric practice, health system, and society contributing to these behavioral and emotional problems. (1/15)
http://pediatrics.aappublications.org/content/135/2/384

PROMOTING THE PARTICIPATION OF CHILDREN WITH DISABILITIES IN SPORTS, RECREATION, AND PHYSICAL ACTIVITIES (CLINICAL REPORT)

Nancy A. Murphy, MD; Paul S. Carbone, MD; and Council on Children With Disabilities

ABSTRACT. The benefits of physical activity are universal for all children, including those with disabilities. The participation of children with disabilities in sports and recreational activities promotes inclusion, minimizes deconditioning, optimizes physical functioning, and enhances overall well-being. Despite these benefits, children with disabilities are more restricted in their participation, have lower levels of fitness, and have higher levels of obesity than their peers without disabilities. Pediatricians and parents may overestimate the risks or overlook the benefits of physical activity in children with disabilities. Well-informed decisions regarding each child's participation must consider overall health status, individual activity preferences, safety precautions, and availability of appropriate programs and equipment. Health supervision visits afford pediatricians, children with disabilities, and parents opportunities to collaboratively generate goal-directed activity "prescriptions." Child, family, financial, and societal barriers to participation need to be directly identified and addressed in the context of local, state, and federal laws. The goal is inclusion for all children with disabilities in appropriate activities. This clinical report discusses the importance of physical activity, recreation, and sports participation for children with disabilities and offers practical suggestions to pediatric health care professionals for the promotion of participation. (5/08, reaffirmed 1/12, 6/18)
http://pediatrics.aappublications.org/content/121/5/1057

PROMOTING THE WELL-BEING OF CHILDREN WHOSE PARENTS ARE GAY OR LESBIAN

Committee on Psychosocial Aspects of Child and Family Health

ABSTRACT. To promote optimal health and well-being of all children, the American Academy of Pediatrics (AAP) supports access for all children to (1) civil marriage rights for their parents and (2) willing and capable foster and adoptive parents, regardless of the parents' sexual orientation. The AAP has always been an advocate for, and has developed policies to support, the optimal physical, mental, and social health and well-being of all infants, children, adolescents, and young adults. In so doing, the AAP has supported families in all their diversity, because the family has always been the basic social unit in which children develop the supporting and nurturing relationships with adults that they need to thrive. Children may be born to, adopted by, or cared for temporarily by married couples, nonmarried couples, single parents, grandparents, or legal guardians, and any of these may be heterosexual, gay or lesbian, or of another orientation. Children need secure and enduring relationships with committed and nurturing adults to enhance their life experiences for optimal social-emotional and cognitive development. Scientific evidence affirms that children have similar developmental and emotional needs and receive similar parenting whether they are raised by parents of the same or different genders. If a child has 2 living and capable parents who choose to create a permanent bond by way of civil marriage, it is in the best interests of their child(ren) that legal and social institutions allow and support them to do so, irrespective of their sexual orientation. If 2 parents are not available to the child, adoption or foster parenting remain acceptable options to provide a loving home for a child and should be available without regard to the sexual orientation of the parent(s). (3/13)
http://pediatrics.aappublications.org/content/131/4/827

PROMOTING THE WELL-BEING OF CHILDREN WHOSE PARENTS ARE GAY OR LESBIAN (TECHNICAL REPORT)

Ellen C. Perrin, MD, MA; Benjamin S. Siegel, MD; and Committee on Psychosocial Aspects of Child and Family Health

ABSTRACT. Extensive data available from more than 30 years of research reveal that children raised by gay and lesbian parents have demonstrated resilience with regard to social, psychological, and sexual health despite economic and legal disparities and social stigma. Many studies have demonstrated that children's well-being is affected much more by their relationships with their parents, their parents' sense of competence and security, and the presence of social and economic support for the family than by the gender or the sexual orientation of their parents. Lack of opportunity for same-gender couples to marry adds to families' stress, which affects the health and welfare of all household members. Because marriage strengthens families and, in so doing, benefits children's development, children should not be deprived of the opportunity for their parents to be married. Paths to parenthood that include assisted reproductive techniques, adoption, and foster parenting should focus on competency of the parents rather than their sexual orientation. (3/13)
http://pediatrics.aappublications.org/content/131/4/e1374

PROMOTION OF HEALTHY WEIGHT-CONTROL PRACTICES IN YOUNG ATHLETES (CLINICAL REPORT)

Rebecca L. Carl, MD, MS, FAAP; Miriam D. Johnson, MD, FAAP; Thomas J. Martin, MD, FAAP; and Council on Sports Medicine and Fitness

ABSTRACT. Children and adolescents may participate in sports that favor a particular body type. Some sports, such as gymnastics, dance, and distance running, emphasize a slim or lean physique for aesthetic or performance reasons. Participants in weight-class sports, such as wrestling and martial arts, may attempt weight loss so they can compete at a lower weight class. Other sports, such as football and bodybuilding, highlight a muscular physique; young athletes engaged in these sports may desire to gain weight and muscle mass. This clinical report describes unhealthy methods of weight loss and gain as well as policies and approaches used to curb these practices. The report also reviews healthy strategies for weight loss and weight gain and provides recommendations for pediatricians on how to promote healthy weight control in young athletes. (8/17)
http://pediatrics.aappublications.org/content/140/3/e20171871

PROTECTING CHILDREN FROM SEXUAL ABUSE BY HEALTH CARE PROVIDERS

Committee on Child Abuse and Neglect

ABSTRACT. Sexual abuse or exploitation of children is never acceptable. Such behavior by health care providers is particularly concerning because of the trust that children and their families place on adults in the health care profession. The American Academy of Pediatrics strongly endorses the social and moral prohibition against sexual abuse or exploitation of children by health care providers. The academy opposes any such sexual abuse or exploitation by providers, particularly by the academy's members. Health care providers should be trained to recognize and abide by appropriate provider-patient boundaries. Medical institutions should screen staff members for a history of child abuse issues, train them to respect and maintain appropriate boundaries, and establish policies and procedures to receive and investigate concerns about patient abuse. Each person has a responsibility to ensure the safety of children in health care settings and to scrupulously follow appropriate legal and ethical reporting and investigation procedures. (6/11, reaffirmed 10/14)
http://pediatrics.aappublications.org/content/128/2/407

PROTECTING CHILDREN FROM TOBACCO, NICOTINE, AND TOBACCO SMOKE (TECHNICAL REPORT)

Harold J. Farber, MD, MSPH, FAAP; Judith Groner, MD, FAAP; Susan Walley, MD, FAAP; Kevin Nelson, MD, PhD, FAAP; and Section on Tobacco Control

ABSTRACT. This technical report serves to provide the evidence base for the American Academy of Pediatrics' policy statements "Clinical Practice Policy to Protect Children From Tobacco, Nicotine, and Tobacco Smoke" and "Public Policy to Protect Children From Tobacco, Nicotine, and Tobacco Smoke." Tobacco use and involuntary exposure are major preventable causes of morbidity and premature mortality in adults and children. Tobacco dependence almost always starts in childhood or adolescence. Electronic nicotine delivery systems are rapidly gaining popularity among youth, and their significant harms are being documented. In utero tobacco smoke exposure, in addition to increasing the risk of preterm birth, low birth weight, stillbirth, placental abruption, and sudden infant death, has been found to increase the risk of obesity and neurodevelopmental disorders. Actions by pediatricians can help to reduce children's risk of developing tobacco dependence and reduce children's involuntary tobacco smoke exposure. Public policy actions to protect children from tobacco are essential to reduce the toll that the tobacco epidemic takes on our children. (10/15)
http://pediatrics.aappublications.org/content/136/5/e1439

PROTECTIVE EYEWEAR FOR YOUNG ATHLETES

Committee on Sports Medicine and Fitness (joint with American Academy of Ophthalmology)

ABSTRACT. The American Academy of Pediatrics and American Academy of Ophthalmology strongly recommend protective eyewear for all participants in sports in which there is risk of eye injury. Protective eyewear should be mandatory for athletes who are functionally 1-eyed and for athletes whose ophthalmologists recommend eye protection after eye surgery or trauma. (3/04, reaffirmed 2/08, 6/11, 2/15)
http://pediatrics.aappublications.org/content/113/3/619

PROVIDING A PRIMARY CARE MEDICAL HOME FOR CHILDREN AND YOUTH WITH CEREBRAL PALSY (CLINICAL REPORT)

Gregory S. Liptak, MD, MPH; Nancy A. Murphy, MD; and Council on Children With Disabilities

ABSTRACT. All primary care providers will care for children with cerebral palsy in their practice. In addition to well-child and acute illness care, the role of the medical home in the management of these children includes diagnosis, planning for interventions, authorizing treatments, and follow-up. Optimizing health and well-being for children with cerebral palsy and their families entails family-centered care provided in the medical home; comanagement is the most common model. This report reviews the aspects of care specific to cerebral palsy that a medical home should provide beyond the routine health care needed by all children. (10/11, reaffirmed 11/14)
http://pediatrics.aappublications.org/content/128/5/e1321

PROVIDING A PRIMARY CARE MEDICAL HOME FOR CHILDREN AND YOUTH WITH SPINA BIFIDA (CLINICAL REPORT)

Robert Burke, MD, MPH; Gregory S. Liptak, MD, MPH; and Council on Children With Disabilities

ABSTRACT. The pediatric primary care provider in the medical home has a central and unique role in the care of children with spina bifida. The primary care provider addresses not only the typical issues of preventive and acute health care but also the needs specific to these children. Optimal care requires communication and comanagement with pediatric medical and developmental subspecialists, surgical specialists, therapists, and community providers. The medical home provider is essential in supporting the family and advocating for the child from the time of entry into the practice through adolescence, which includes transition and transfer to adult health care. This report reviews aspects of care specific to the infant with spina bifida (particularly myelomeningocele) that will facilitate optimal medical, functional, and developmental outcomes. (11/11, reaffirmed 2/15)
http://pediatrics.aappublications.org/content/128/6/e1645

PROVIDING CARE FOR CHILDREN AND ADOLESCENTS FACING HOMELESSNESS AND HOUSING INSECURITY

Council on Community Pediatrics

ABSTRACT. Child health and housing security are closely intertwined, and children without homes are more likely to suffer from chronic disease, hunger, and malnutrition than are children with homes. Homeless children and youth often have significant psychosocial development issues, and their education is frequently interrupted. Given the overall effects that homelessness can have on a child's health and potential, it is important for pediatricians to recognize the factors that lead to homelessness, understand the ways that homelessness and its causes can lead to poor health outcomes, and when possible, help children and families mitigate some of the effects of homelessness. Through practice change, partnership with community resources, awareness, and advocacy, pediatricians can help optimize the health and well-being of children affected by homelessness. (5/13, reaffirmed 10/16)
http://pediatrics.aappublications.org/content/131/6/1206

PROVIDING CARE FOR IMMIGRANT, MIGRANT, AND BORDER CHILDREN

Council on Community Pediatrics

ABSTRACT. This policy statement, which recognizes the large changes in immigrant status since publication of the 2005 statement "Providing Care for Immigrant, Homeless, and Migrant Children," focuses on strategies to support the health of immigrant children, infants, adolescents, and young adults. Homeless children will be addressed in a forthcoming separate statement ("Providing Care for Children and Adolescents Facing Homelessness and Housing Insecurity"). While recognizing the diversity across and within immigrant, migrant, and border populations, this statement provides a basic framework for serving and advocating for all immigrant children, with a particular focus on low-income and vulnerable populations. Recommendations include actions needed within and outside the health care system, including expansion of access to high-quality medical homes with culturally and linguistically effective care as well as education and literacy programs. The statement recognizes the unique and special role that pediatricians can play in the lives of immigrant children and families. Recommendations for policies that support immigrant child health are included. (5/13)
http://pediatrics.aappublications.org/content/131/6/e2028

PROVIDING PSYCHOSOCIAL SUPPORT TO CHILDREN AND FAMILIES IN THE AFTERMATH OF DISASTERS AND CRISES (CLINICAL REPORT)

David J. Schonfeld, MD, FAAP; Thomas Demaria, PhD; Disaster Preparedness Advisory Council; and Committee on Psychosocial Aspects of Child and Family Health

ABSTRACT. Disasters have the potential to cause short- and long-term effects on the psychological functioning, emotional adjustment, health, and developmental trajectory of children. This clinical report provides practical suggestions on how to identify common adjustment difficulties in children in the aftermath of a disaster and to promote effective coping strategies to mitigate the impact of the disaster as well as any associated

bereavement and secondary stressors. This information can serve as a guide to pediatricians as they offer anticipatory guidance to families or consultation to schools, child care centers, and other child congregate care sites. Knowledge of risk factors for adjustment difficulties can serve as the basis for mental health triage. The importance of basic supportive services, psychological first aid, and professional self-care are discussed. Stress is intrinsic to many major life events that children and families face, including the experience of significant illness and its treatment. The information provided in this clinical report may, therefore, be relevant for a broad range of patient encounters, even outside the context of a disaster. Most pediatricians enter the profession because of a heartfelt desire to help children and families most in need. If adequately prepared and supported, pediatricians who are able to draw on their skills to assist children, families, and communities to recover after a disaster will find the work to be particularly rewarding. (9/15)
http://pediatrics.aappublications.org/content/136/4/e1120

PSYCHOLOGICAL MALTREATMENT (CLINICAL REPORT)

Roberta Hibbard, MD; Jane Barlow, DPhil; Harriet MacMillan, MD; Committee on Child Abuse and Neglect (joint with American Academy of Child and Adolescent Psychiatry Child Maltreatment and Violence Committee)

ABSTRACT. Psychological or emotional maltreatment of children may be the most challenging and prevalent form of child abuse and neglect. Caregiver behaviors include acts of omission (ignoring need for social interactions) or commission (spurning, terrorizing); may be verbal or nonverbal, active or passive, and with or without intent to harm; and negatively affect the child's cognitive, social, emotional, and/or physical development. Psychological maltreatment has been linked with disorders of attachment, developmental and educational problems, socialization problems, disruptive behavior, and later psychopathology. Although no evidence-based interventions that can prevent psychological maltreatment have been identified to date, it is possible that interventions shown to be effective in reducing overall types of child maltreatment, such as the Nurse Family Partnership, may have a role to play. Furthermore, prevention before occurrence will require both the use of universal interventions aimed at promoting the type of parenting that is now recognized to be necessary for optimal child development, alongside the use of targeted interventions directed at improving parental sensitivity to a child's cues during infancy and later parent-child interactions. Intervention should, first and foremost, focus on a thorough assessment and ensuring the child's safety. Potentially effective treatments include cognitive behavioral parenting programs and other psychotherapeutic interventions. The high prevalence of psychological abuse in advanced Western societies, along with the serious consequences, point to the importance of effective management. Pediatricians should be alert to the occurrence of psychological maltreatment and identify ways to support families who have risk indicators for, or evidence of, this problem. (7/12, reaffirmed 4/16)
http://pediatrics.aappublications.org/content/130/2/372

PSYCHOSOCIAL IMPLICATIONS OF DISASTER OR TERRORISM ON CHILDREN: A GUIDE FOR THE PEDIATRICIAN (CLINICAL REPORT)

Joseph F. Hagan Jr, MD; Committee on Psychosocial Aspects of Child and Family Health; and Task Force on Terrorism

ABSTRACT. During and after disasters, pediatricians can assist parents and community leaders not only by accommodating the unique needs of children but also by being cognizant of the psychological responses of children to reduce the possibility of long-term psychological morbidity. The effects of disaster on children are mediated by many factors including personal experience, parental reaction, developmental competency, gender, and the stage of disaster response. Pediatricians can be effective advocates for the child and family and at the community level and can affect national policy in support of families. In this report, specific children's responses are delineated, risk factors for adverse reactions are discussed, and advice is given for pediatricians to ameliorate the effects of disaster on children. (9/05, reaffirmed 11/14)
http://pediatrics.aappublications.org/content/116/3/787

PSYCHOSOCIAL SUPPORT FOR YOUTH LIVING WITH HIV (CLINICAL REPORT)

Jaime Martinez, MD, FAAP; Rana Chakraborty, MD, FAAP; and Committee on Pediatric AIDS

ABSTRACT. This clinical report provides guidance for the pediatrician in addressing the psychosocial needs of adolescents and young adults living with HIV, which can improve linkage to care and adherence to life-saving antiretroviral (ARV) therapy. Recent national case surveillance data for youth (defined here as adolescents and young adults 13 to 24 years of age) revealed that the burden of HIV/AIDS fell most heavily and disproportionately on African American youth, particularly males having sex with males. To effectively increase linkage to care and sustain adherence to therapy, interventions should address the immediate drivers of ARV compliance and also address factors that provide broader social and structural support for HIV-infected adolescents and young adults. Interventions should address psychosocial development, including lack of future orientation, inadequate educational attainment and limited health literacy, failure to focus on the long-term consequences of near-term risk behaviors, and coping ability. Associated challenges are closely linked to the structural environment. Individual case management is essential to linkage to and retention in care, ARV adherence, and management of associated comorbidities. Integrating these skills into pediatric and adolescent HIV practice in a medical home setting is critical, given the alarming increase in new HIV infections in youth in the United States. (2/14)
http://pediatrics.aappublications.org/content/133/3/558

A PUBLIC HEALTH RESPONSE TO OPIOID USE IN PREGNANCY

Stephen W. Patrick, MD, MPH, MS, FAAP; Davida M. Schiff, MD, FAAP; and Committee on Substance Use and Prevention

ABSTRACT. The use of opioids during pregnancy has grown rapidly in the past decade. As opioid use during pregnancy increased, so did complications from their use, including neonatal abstinence syndrome. Several state governments responded to this increase by prosecuting and incarcerating pregnant women with substance use disorders; however, this approach has no proven benefits for maternal or infant health and may lead to avoidance of prenatal care and a decreased willingness to engage in substance use disorder treatment programs. A public health response, rather than a punitive approach to the opioid epidemic and substance use during pregnancy, is critical, including the following: a focus on preventing unintended pregnancies and improving access to contraception; universal screening for alcohol and other drug use in women of childbearing age; knowledge and informed consent of maternal drug testing and reporting practices; improved access to comprehensive obstetric care, including opioid-replacement therapy; gender-specific substance use treatment programs; and improved funding for social services and child welfare systems. The American College of Obstetricians and Gynecologists supports the value of this clinical document as an educational tool (December 2016). (2/17)
http://pediatrics.aappublications.org/content/139/3/e20164070

PUBLIC POLICY TO PROTECT CHILDREN FROM TOBACCO, NICOTINE, AND TOBACCO SMOKE

Section on Tobacco Control

ABSTRACT. Tobacco use and tobacco smoke exposure are among the most important health threats to children, adolescents, and adults. There is no safe level of tobacco smoke exposure. The developing brains of children and adolescents are particularly vulnerable to the development of tobacco and nicotine dependence. Tobacco is unique among consumer products in that it causes disease and death when used exactly as intended. Tobacco continues to be heavily promoted to children and young adults. Flavored and alternative tobacco products, including little cigars, chewing tobacco, and electronic nicotine delivery systems, are gaining popularity among youth. This statement describes important evidence-based public policy actions that, when implemented, will reduce tobacco product use and tobacco smoke exposure among youth and, by doing so, improve the health of children and young adults. (10/15)
http://pediatrics.aappublications.org/content/136/5/998

QUALITY EARLY EDUCATION AND CHILD CARE FROM BIRTH TO KINDERGARTEN

Elaine A. Donoghue, MD, FAAP, and Council on Early Childhood

ABSTRACT. High-quality early education and child care for young children improves physical and cognitive outcomes for the children and can result in enhanced school readiness. Preschool education can be viewed as an investment (especially for at-risk children), and studies show a positive return on that investment. Barriers to high-quality early childhood education include inadequate funding and staff education as well as variable regulation and enforcement. Steps that have been taken to improve the quality of early education and child care include creating multidisciplinary, evidence-based child care practice standards; establishing state quality rating and improvement systems; improving federal and state regulations; providing child care health consultation; and initiating other innovative partnerships. Pediatricians have a role in promoting quality early education and child care for all children not only in the medical home but also at the community, state, and national levels. (7/17)
http://pediatrics.aappublications.org/content/140/2/e20171488

RACE, ETHNICITY, AND SOCIOECONOMIC STATUS IN RESEARCH ON CHILD HEALTH

Tina L. Cheng, MD, MPH, FAAP; Elizabeth Goodman, MD, FAAP; and Committee on Pediatric Research

ABSTRACT. An extensive literature documents the existence of pervasive and persistent child health, development, and health care disparities by race, ethnicity, and socioeconomic status (SES). Disparities experienced during childhood can result in a wide variety of health and health care outcomes, including adult morbidity and mortality, indicating that it is crucial to examine the influence of disparities across the life course. Studies often collect data on the race, ethnicity, and SES of research participants to be used as covariates or explanatory factors. In the past, these variables have often been assumed to exert their effects through individual or genetically determined biologic mechanisms. However, it is now widely accepted that these variables have important social dimensions that influence health. SES, a multidimensional construct, interacts with and confounds analyses of race and ethnicity. Because SES, race, and ethnicity are often difficult to measure accurately, leading to the potential for misattribution of causality, thoughtful consideration should be given to appropriate measurement, analysis, and interpretation of such factors. Scientists who study child and adolescent health and development should understand the multiple measures used to assess race, ethnicity, and SES, including their validity and shortcomings and potential confounding of race and ethnicity with SES. The American Academy of Pediatrics (AAP) recommends that research on eliminating health and health care disparities related to race, ethnicity, and SES be a priority. Data on race, ethnicity, and SES should be collected in research on child health to improve their definitions and increase understanding of how these factors and their complex interrelationships affect child health. Furthermore, the AAP believes that researchers should consider both biological and social mechanisms of action of race, ethnicity, and SES as they relate to the aims and hypothesis of the specific area of investigation. It is important to measure these variables, but it is not sufficient to use these variables alone as explanatory for differences in disease, morbidity, and outcomes without attention to the social and biologic influences they have on health throughout the life course. The AAP recommends more research, both in the United States and internationally, on measures of race, ethnicity, and SES and how these complex constructs affect health care and health outcomes throughout the life course. (12/14)
http://pediatrics.aappublications.org/content/135/1/e225

RACIAL AND ETHNIC DISPARITIES IN THE HEALTH AND HEALTH CARE OF CHILDREN (TECHNICAL REPORT)

Glenn Flores, MD, and Committee on Pediatric Research

ABSTRACT. *Objective.* This technical report reviews and synthesizes the published literature on racial/ethnic disparities in children's health and health care.

Methods. A systematic review of the literature was conducted for articles published between 1950 and March 2007. Inclusion criteria were peer-reviewed, original research articles in English on racial/ethnic disparities in the health and health care of US children. Search terms used included "child," "disparities," and the Index Medicus terms for each racial/ethnic minority group.

Results. Of 781 articles initially reviewed, 111 met inclusion criteria and constituted the final database. Review of the literature revealed that racial/ethnic disparities in children's health and health care are quite extensive, pervasive, and persistent. Disparities were noted across the spectrum of health and health care, including in mortality rates, access to care and use of services, prevention and population health, health status, adolescent health, chronic diseases, special health care needs, quality of care, and organ transplantation. Mortality-rate disparities were noted for children in all 4 major US racial/ethnic minority groups, including substantially greater risks than white children of all-cause mortality; death from drowning, from acute lymphoblastic leukemia, and after congenital heart defect surgery; and an earlier median age at death for those with Down syndrome and congenital heart defects. Certain methodologic flaws were commonly observed among excluded studies, including failure to evaluate children separately from adults (22%), combining all nonwhite children into 1 group (9%), and failure to provide a white comparison group (8%). Among studies in the final database, 22% did not perform multivariable or stratified analyses to ensure that disparities persisted after adjustment for potential confounders.

Conclusions. Racial/ethnic disparities in children's health and health care are extensive, pervasive, and persistent, and occur across the spectrum of health and health care. Methodologic flaws were identified in how such disparities are sometimes documented and analyzed. Optimal health and health care for all children will require recognition of disparities as pervasive problems, methodologically sound disparities studies, and rigorous evaluation of disparities interventions. (3/10, reaffirmed 5/13)
http://pediatrics.aappublications.org/content/125/4/e979

RADIATION DISASTERS AND CHILDREN

Committee on Environmental Health

ABSTRACT. The special medical needs of children make it essential that pediatricians be prepared for radiation disasters, including (1) the detonation of a nuclear weapon; (2) a nuclear power plant event that unleashes a radioactive cloud; and (3) the dispersal of radionuclides by conventional explosive or the crash of a transport vehicle. Any of these events could occur unintentionally or as an act of terrorism. Nuclear facilities (eg, power plants, fuel processing centers, and food irradiation facilities) are often located in highly populated areas, and as they age, the risk of mechanical failure increases. The short- and long-term consequences of a radiation disaster are significantly greater in children for several reasons. First, children have a disproportionately higher minute ventilation, leading to greater internal exposure to radioactive gases. Children have a significantly greater risk of developing cancer even when they are exposed to radiation in utero. Finally, children and the parents of young children are more likely than are adults to develop enduring psychologic injury after a radiation disaster. The pediatrician has a critical role in planning for radiation disasters. For example, potassium iodide is of proven value for thyroid protection but must be given before or soon after exposure to radioiodines, requiring its placement in homes, schools, and child care centers. Pediatricians should work with public health authorities to ensure that children receive full consideration in local planning for a radiation disaster. (6/03, reaffirmed 1/07)
http://pediatrics.aappublications.org/content/111/6/1455

RADIATION RISK TO CHILDREN FROM COMPUTED TOMOGRAPHY (CLINICAL REPORT)

Alan S. Brody, MD; Donald P. Frush, MD; Walter Huda, PhD; Robert L. Brent, MD, PhD; and Section on Radiology

ABSTRACT. Imaging studies that use ionizing radiation are an essential tool for the evaluation of many disorders of childhood. Ionizing radiation is used in radiography, fluoroscopy, angiography, and computed tomography scanning. Computed tomography is of particular interest because of its relatively high radiation dose and wide use. Consensus statements on radiation risk suggest that it is reasonable to act on the assumption that low-level radiation may have a small risk of causing cancer. The medical community should seek ways to decrease radiation exposure by using radiation doses as low as reasonably achievable and by performing these studies only when necessary. There is wide agreement that the benefits of an indicated computed tomography scan far outweigh the risks. Pediatric health care professionals' roles in the use of computed tomography on children include deciding when a computed tomography scan is necessary and discussing the risk with patients and families. Radiologists should be a source of consultation when forming imaging strategies and should create specific protocols with scanning techniques optimized for pediatric patients. Families and patients should be encouraged to ask questions about the risks and benefits of computed tomography scanning. The information in this report is provided to aid in decision-making and discussions with the health care team, patients, and families. (9/07)
http://pediatrics.aappublications.org/content/120/3/677

RECOGNITION AND MANAGEMENT OF IATROGENICALLY INDUCED OPIOID DEPENDENCE AND WITHDRAWAL IN CHILDREN (CLINICAL REPORT)

Jeffrey Galinkin, MD, FAAP; Jeffrey Lee Koh, MD, FAAP; Committee on Drugs; and Section on Anesthesiology and Pain Medicine

ABSTRACT. Opioids are often prescribed to children for pain relief related to procedures, acute injuries, and chronic conditions. Round-the-clock dosing of opioids can produce opioid dependence within 5 days. According to a 2001 consensus paper from the American Academy of Pain Medicine, American Pain Society, and American Society of Addiction Medicine, dependence is defined as "a state of adaptation that is manifested by a drug class specific withdrawal syndrome that can be produced by abrupt cessation, rapid dose reduction, decreasing blood level of the drug, and/or administration of an antagonist." Although the experience of many children undergoing iatrogenically induced withdrawal may be mild or goes unreported, there is currently no guidance for recognition or management of withdrawal for this population. Guidance on this subject is available only for adults and primarily for adults with substance use disorders. The guideline will summarize existing literature and provide readers with information currently not available in any single source specific for this vulnerable pediatric population. (12/13)
http://pediatrics.aappublications.org/content/133/1/152

RECOGNITION AND MANAGEMENT OF MEDICAL COMPLEXITY (CLINICAL REPORT)

Dennis Z. Kuo, MD, MHS, FAAP; Amy J. Houtrow, MD, PhD, MPH, FAAP; and Council on Children With Disabilities

ABSTRACT. Children with medical complexity have extensive needs for health services, experience functional limitations, and are high resource utilizers. Addressing the needs of this population to achieve high-value health care requires optimizing care within the medical home and medical neighborhood. Opportunities exist for health care providers, payers, and policy makers to develop strategies to enhance care delivery and to decrease costs. Important outcomes include decreasing unplanned hospital admissions, decreasing emergency department use, ensuring access to health services, limiting out-of-pocket expenses for families, and improving patient and family experiences, quality of life, and satisfaction with care. This report describes the population of children with medical complexity and provides strategies to optimize medical and health outcomes. (11/16)
http://pediatrics.aappublications.org/content/138/6/e20163021

RECOGNIZING AND RESPONDING TO MEDICAL NEGLECT (CLINICAL REPORT)

Carole Jenny, MD, MBA, and Committee on Child Abuse and Neglect

ABSTRACT. A caregiver may fail to recognize or respond to a child's medical needs for a variety of reasons. An effective response by a health care professional to medical neglect requires a comprehensive assessment of the child's needs, the parents' resources, the parents' efforts to provide for the needs of the child, and options for ensuring optimal health for the child. Such an assessment requires clear, 2-way communication between the family and the health care professional. Physicians should consider the least intrusive options for managing cases of medical neglect that ensure the health and safety of the child. (12/07, reaffirmed 1/11, 2/16)
http://pediatrics.aappublications.org/content/120/6/1385

RECOMMENDATIONS FOR PREVENTION AND CONTROL OF INFLUENZA IN CHILDREN, 2018–2019

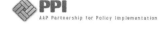

Committee on Infectious Diseases

ABSTRACT. The authors of this statement update the recommendations of the American Academy of Pediatrics for the routine use of influenza vaccine and antiviral medications in the prevention and treatment of influenza in children. Highlights for the upcoming 2018–2019 season include the following:

1. Annual influenza immunization is recommended for everyone 6 months and older, including children and adolescents.

2. The American Academy of Pediatrics recommends an inactivated influenza vaccine (IIV), trivalent or quadrivalent, as the primary choice for influenza vaccination in children because the effectiveness of a live attenuated influenza vaccine against influenza A(H1N1) was inferior during past influenza seasons and is unknown for this upcoming season.

3. A live attenuated influenza vaccine may be used for children who would not otherwise receive an influenza vaccine (eg, refusal of an IIV) and for whom it is appropriate because of age (2 years of age and older) and health status (ie, healthy and without any underlying chronic medical condition).

4. All 2018–2019 seasonal influenza vaccines contain an influenza A(H1N1) vaccine strain similar to that included in the 2017–2018 seasonal vaccines. In contrast, the influenza A(H3N2) and influenza B (Victoria lineage) vaccine strains included in the 2018–2019 trivalent and quadrivalent vaccines differ from those in the 2017–2018 seasonal vaccines.

   a. Trivalent vaccines contain an influenza A(Michigan/45/2015[H1N1])pdm09–like virus, an influenza A(Singapore/INFIMH-16-0019/2016[H3N2])–like virus (updated), and an influenza B (Colorado/60/2017)–like virus (B/Victoria lineage; updated).

   b. Quadrivalent vaccines contain an additional B virus (Phuket/3073/2013–like virus; B/Yamagata lineage).

5. All children with egg allergy of any severity can receive an influenza vaccine without any additional precautions beyond those recommended for all vaccines.

6. Pregnant women may receive an influenza vaccine (IIV only) at any time during pregnancy to protect themselves as well as their infants, who benefit from the transplacental transfer of antibodies. Postpartum women who did not receive vaccination during pregnancy should be encouraged to receive an influenza vaccine before discharge from the hospital. Influenza vaccination during breastfeeding is safe for mothers and their infants.

7. The vaccination of health care workers is a crucial step in preventing influenza and reducing health care–associated influenza infections because health care personnel often care for individuals at high risk for influenza-related complications.

8. Pediatricians should attempt to promptly identify their patients who are suspected of having an influenza infection for timely initiation of antiviral treatment when indicated and on the basis of shared decision-making between each pediatrician and child caregiver to reduce morbidity and mortality. Although best results are seen when a child is treated within 48 hours of symptom onset, antiviral therapy should still be considered beyond 48 hours of symptom onset in children with severe disease or those at high risk of complications (see Table 2 in the full policy statement). (9/18)
See full text on page 851.
http://pediatrics.aappublications.org/content/142/4/e20182367

RECOMMENDATIONS FOR SEROGROUP B MENINGOCOCCAL VACCINE FOR PERSONS 10 YEARS AND OLDER

Committee on Infectious Diseases

ABSTRACT. This policy statement provides recommendations for the prevention of serogroup B meningococcal disease through the use of 2 newly licensed serogroup B meningococcal vaccines: MenB-FHbp (Trumenba; Wyeth Pharmaceuticals, a subsidiary of Pfizer, Philadelphia, PA) and MenB-4C (Bexsero; Novartis Vaccines, Siena, Italy). Both vaccines are approved for use in persons 10 through 25 years of age. MenB-FHbp is licensed as a 2- or 3-dose series, and MenB-4C is licensed as a 2-dose series for all groups. Either vaccine is recommended for routine use in persons 10 years and older who are at increased risk of serogroup B meningococcal disease (category A recommendation). Persons at increased risk of meningococcal serogroup B disease include the following: (1) persons with persistent complement component diseases, including inherited or chronic deficiencies in C3, C5–C9, properdin, factor D, or factor H, or persons receiving eculizumab (Soliris; Alexion Pharmaceuticals, Cheshire, CT), a monoclonal antibody that acts as a terminal complement inhibitor by binding C5 and inhibiting cleavage of C5 to C5A; (2) persons with anatomic or functional asplenia, including sickle cell disease; and (3) healthy persons at increased risk because of a serogroup B meningococcal disease outbreak. Both serogroup B meningococcal vaccines have been shown to be safe and immunogenic and are licensed by the US Food and Drug Administration for individuals between the ages of 10 and 25 years. On the basis of epidemiologic and antibody persistence data, the American Academy of Pediatrics agrees with the Advisory Committee on Immunization Practices of the Centers for Disease Control and Prevention that either vaccine may be administered to healthy adolescents and young adults 16 through 23 years of age (preferred ages are 16 through 18 years) to provide short-term protection against most strains of serogroup B meningococcal disease (category B recommendation). (8/16)
http://pediatrics.aappublications.org/content/138/3/e20161890

RECOMMENDED CHILDHOOD AND ADOLESCENT IMMUNIZATION SCHEDULES: UNITED STATES, 2019

Committee on Infectious Diseases (2/19)
   See full text on page 879.
http://pediatrics.aappublications.org/content/early/2019/02/01/peds.2019-0065

REDUCING INJURY RISK FROM BODY CHECKING IN BOYS' YOUTH ICE HOCKEY

Council on Sports Medicine and Fitness

ABSTRACT. Ice hockey is an increasingly popular sport that allows intentional collision in the form of body checking for males but not for females. There is a two- to threefold increased risk of all injury, severe injury, and concussion related to body checking at all levels of boys' youth ice hockey. The American Academy of Pediatrics reinforces the importance of stringent enforcement of rules to protect player safety as well as educational interventions to decrease unsafe tactics. To promote ice hockey as a lifelong recreational pursuit for boys, the American Academy of Pediatrics recommends the expansion of nonchecking programs and the restriction of body checking to elite levels of boys' youth ice hockey, starting no earlier than 15 years of age. (5/14, reaffirmed 7/18)
http://pediatrics.aappublications.org/content/133/6/1151

REDUCING THE NUMBER OF DEATHS AND INJURIES FROM RESIDENTIAL FIRES

Committee on Injury and Poison Prevention

ABSTRACT. Smoke inhalation, severe burns, and death from residential fires are devastating events, most of which are preventable. In 1998, approximately 381 500 residential structure fires resulted in 3250 non-firefighter deaths, 17 175 injuries, and approximately $4.4 billion in property loss. This statement reviews important prevention messages and intervention strategies related to residential fires. It also includes recommendations for pediatricians regarding office anticipatory guidance, work in the community, and support of regulation and legislation that could result in a decrease in the number of fire-related injuries and deaths to children. (6/00)
http://pediatrics.aappublications.org/content/105/6/1355

REFERRAL TO PEDIATRIC SURGICAL SPECIALISTS

Surgical Advisory Panel

ABSTRACT. The American Academy of Pediatrics, with the collaboration of the Surgical Sections of the American Academy of Pediatrics, has created referral recommendations intended to serve as voluntary practice parameters to assist general pediatricians in determining when and to whom to refer their patients for pediatric surgical specialty care. It is recognized that these recommendations may be difficult to implement, because communities vary in terms of access to major pediatric medical centers. Limited access does not negate the value of the recommendations, however, because the child who needs specialized surgical and anesthetic care is best served by the skills of the appropriate pediatric surgical team. Major congenital anomalies, malignancies, major trauma, and chronic illnesses (including those associated with preterm birth) in infants and children should be managed by pediatric medical subspecialists and pediatric surgical specialists at pediatric referral centers that can provide expertise in many areas, including the pediatric medical subspecialties and surgical specialties of pediatric radiology, pediatric anesthesiology, pediatric pathology, and pediatric intensive care. The optimal management of the child with complex problems, chronic illness, or disabilities requires coordination, communication, and cooperation of the pediatric surgical specialist with the child's primary care pediatrician or physician. (1/14)

http://pediatrics.aappublications.org/content/133/2/350

REIMBURSEMENT FOR FOODS FOR SPECIAL DIETARY USE

Committee on Nutrition

ABSTRACT. Foods for special dietary use are recommended by physicians for chronic diseases or conditions of childhood, including inherited metabolic diseases. Although many states have created legislation requiring reimbursement for foods for special dietary use, legislation is now needed to mandate consistent coverage and reimbursement for foods for special dietary use and related support services with accepted medical benefit for children with designated medical conditions. (5/03, reaffirmed 1/06)

http://pediatrics.aappublications.org/content/111/5/1117

RELIEF OF PAIN AND ANXIETY IN PEDIATRIC PATIENTS IN EMERGENCY MEDICAL SYSTEMS (CLINICAL REPORT)

Joel A. Fein, MD, MPH; William T. Zempsky, MD, MPH; Joseph P. Cravero, MD; Committee on Pediatric Emergency Medicine; and Section on Anesthesiology and Pain Medicine

ABSTRACT. Control of pain and stress for children is a vital component of emergency medical care. Timely administration of analgesia affects the entire emergency medical experience and can have a lasting effect on a child's and family's reaction to current and future medical care. A systematic approach to pain management and anxiolysis, including staff education and protocol development, can provide comfort to children in the emergency setting and improve staff and family satisfaction. (10/12, reaffirmed 9/15)

http://pediatrics.aappublications.org/content/130/5/e1391

RESCUE MEDICINE FOR EPILEPSY IN EDUCATION SETTINGS (CLINICAL REPORT)

Adam L. Hartman, MD, FAAP; Cynthia Di Laura Devore, MD; Section on Neurology; and Council on School Health

ABSTRACT. Children and adolescents with epilepsy may experience prolonged seizures in school-associated settings (eg, during transportation, in the classroom, or during sports activities). Prolonged seizures may evolve into status epilepticus. Administering a seizure rescue medication can abort the seizure and may obviate the need for emergency medical services and subsequent care in an emergency department. In turn, this may save patients from the morbidity of more invasive interventions and the cost of escalated care. There are significant variations in prescribing practices for seizure rescue medications, partly because of inconsistencies between jurisdictions in legislation and professional practice guidelines among potential first responders (including school staff). There also are potential liability issues for prescribers, school districts, and unlicensed assistive personnel who might administer the seizure rescue medications. This clinical report highlights issues that providers may consider when prescribing seizure rescue medications and creating school medical orders and/or action plans for students with epilepsy. Collaboration among prescribing providers, families, and schools may be useful in developing plans for the use of seizure rescue medications. (12/15)

http://pediatrics.aappublications.org/content/137/1/e20153876

RESPIRATORY SUPPORT IN PRETERM INFANTS AT BIRTH

Committee on Fetus and Newborn

ABSTRACT. Current practice guidelines recommend administration of surfactant at or soon after birth in preterm infants with respiratory distress syndrome. However, recent multicenter randomized controlled trials indicate that early use of continuous positive airway pressure with subsequent selective surfactant administration in extremely preterm infants results in lower rates of bronchopulmonary dysplasia/death when compared with treatment with prophylactic or early surfactant therapy. Continuous positive airway pressure started at or soon after birth with subsequent selective surfactant administration may be considered as an alternative to routine intubation with prophylactic or early surfactant administration in preterm infants. (12/13)

http://pediatrics.aappublications.org/content/133/1/171

RESPONDING TO PARENTAL REFUSALS OF IMMUNIZATION OF CHILDREN (CLINICAL REPORT)

Douglas S. Diekema, MD, MPH, and Committee on Bioethics

ABSTRACT. The American Academy of Pediatrics strongly endorses universal immunization. However, for childhood immunization programs to be successful, parents must comply with immunization recommendations. The problem of parental refusal of immunization for children is an important one for pediatricians. The goal of this report is to assist pediatricians in understanding the reasons parents may have for refusing to immunize their children, review the limited circumstances under which parental refusals should be referred to child protective services agencies or public health authorities, and provide practical guidance to assist the pediatrician faced with a parent who is reluctant to allow immunization of his or her child. (5/05, reaffirmed 1/09, 11/12)

http://pediatrics.aappublications.org/content/115/5/1428

RESPONSIBLE INNOVATION IN CHILDREN'S SURGICAL CARE

Section on Surgery and Committee on Bioethics (joint with American Pediatric Surgical Association New Technology Committee)

ABSTRACT. Advances in medical care may occur when a change in practice incorporates a new treatment or methodology. In surgery, this may involve the translation of a completely novel concept into a new procedure or device or the adaptation of existing treatment approaches or technology to a new clinical application. Regardless of the specifics, innovation should have, as its primary goal, the enhancement of care leading to improved outcomes from the patient's perspective. This policy statement examines innovation as it pertains to surgical care, focusing on some of the definitions that help differentiate applied innovation or innovative therapy from research. The ethical challenges and the potential for conflict of interest for surgeons or institutions

seeking to offer innovative surgical therapy are examined. The importance of engaging patients and families as "innovation partners" to ensure complete transparency of expectations from the patient's and provider's perspectives is also examined, with specific emphasis on cultural competence and mutually respectful approaches. A framework for identifying, evaluating, and safely implementing innovative surgical therapy in children is provided. (12/16)
http://pediatrics.aappublications.org/content/139/1/e20163437

RETURNING TO LEARNING FOLLOWING A CONCUSSION (CLINICAL REPORT)

Mark E. Halstead, MD, FAAP; Karen McAvoy, PsyD; Cynthia D. Devore, MD, FAAP; Rebecca Carl, MD, FAAP; Michael Lee, MD, FAAP; Kelsey Logan, MD, FAAP; Council on Sports Medicine and Fitness; and Council on School Health

ABSTRACT. Following a concussion, it is common for children and adolescents to experience difficulties in the school setting. Cognitive difficulties, such as learning new tasks or remembering previously learned material, may pose challenges in the classroom. The school environment may also increase symptoms with exposure to bright lights and screens or noisy cafeterias and hallways. Unfortunately, because most children and adolescents look physically normal after a concussion, school officials often fail to recognize the need for academic or environmental adjustments. Appropriate guidance and recommendations from the pediatrician may ease the transition back to the school environment and facilitate the recovery of the child or adolescent. This report serves to provide a better understanding of possible factors that may contribute to difficulties in a school environment after a concussion and serves as a framework for the medical home, the educational home, and the family home to guide the student to a successful and safe return to learning. (10/13, reaffirmed 7/18)
http://pediatrics.aappublications.org/content/132/5/948

RITUAL GENITAL CUTTING OF FEMALE MINORS

Board of Directors (6/10)
http://pediatrics.aappublications.org/content/126/1/191

THE ROLE OF INTEGRATED CARE IN A MEDICAL HOME FOR PATIENTS WITH A FETAL ALCOHOL SPECTRUM DISORDER (CLINICAL REPORT)

Renee M. Turchi, MD, MPH, FAAP; Vincent C. Smith, MD, MPH, FAAP; Committee on Substance Use and Prevention; and Council on Children With Disabilities

ABSTRACT. Fetal alcohol spectrum disorder (FASD) is an umbrella term used to describe preventable birth defects and intellectual and/or developmental disabilities resulting from prenatal alcohol exposure. The American Academy of Pediatrics has a previous clinical report in which diagnostic criteria for a child with an FASD are discussed and tools to assist pediatricians with its management can be found. This clinical report is intended to foster pediatrician awareness of approaches for screening for prenatal alcohol exposure in clinical practice, to guide management of a child with an FASD after the diagnosis is made, and to summarize available resources for FASD management. (9/18)
See full text on page 885.
http://pediatrics.aappublications.org/content/142/4/e20182333

ROLE OF PEDIATRICIANS IN ADVOCATING LIFE SUPPORT TRAINING COURSES FOR PARENTS AND THE PUBLIC

Committee on Pediatric Emergency Medicine

ABSTRACT. Available literature suggests a need for both initial cardiopulmonary resuscitation basic life support training and refresher courses for parents and the public as well as health care professionals. The promotion of basic life support training courses that establish a pediatric chain of survival spanning from prevention of cardiac arrest and trauma to rehabilitative and follow-up care for victims of cardiopulmonary arrest is advocated in this policy statement and is the focus of an accompanying technical report. Immediate bystander cardiopulmonary resuscitation for victims of cardiac arrest improves survival for out-of-hospital cardiac arrest. Pediatricians will improve the chance of survival of children and adults who experience cardiac arrest by advocating for cardiopulmonary resuscitation training and participating in basic life support training courses as participants and instructors. (12/04, reaffirmed 5/07, 8/10, 8/13, 7/16)
http://pediatrics.aappublications.org/content/114/6/1676

ROLE OF PEDIATRICIANS IN ADVOCATING LIFE SUPPORT TRAINING COURSES FOR PARENTS AND THE PUBLIC (TECHNICAL REPORT)

Lee A. Pyles, MD; Jane Knapp, MD; and Committee on Pediatric Emergency Medicine

ABSTRACT. Available literature suggests a need for both initial cardiopulmonary resuscitation training and refresher courses. The establishment of a pediatric chain of survival for victims of cardiopulmonary arrest is the focus of this technical report and is advocated in the accompanying policy statement. Immediate bystander cardiopulmonary resuscitation for victims of cardiac arrest improves survival for out-of-hospital cardiac arrest. Pediatricians will improve the chance of survival of children and adults who experience cardiac arrest by advocating for basic life support training and participating in basic life support courses as participants and teachers. (12/04, reaffirmed 5/07, 8/10, 1/14)
http://pediatrics.aappublications.org/content/114/6/e761

THE ROLE OF PEDIATRICIANS IN GLOBAL HEALTH

Parminder S. Suchdev, MD, MPH, FAAP; Cynthia R. Howard, MD, MPHTM, FAAP; Section on International Child Health

ABSTRACT. Ninety percent of the world's children live in low- and middle-income countries, where barriers to health contribute to significant child morbidity and mortality. The American Academy of Pediatrics is dedicated to the health and well-being of *all* children. To fulfill this promise, this policy statement defines the role of the pediatrician in global health and provides a specific set of recommendations directed to all pediatricians, emphasizing the importance of global health as an integral function of the profession of pediatrics. (11/18)
See full text on page 905.
http://pediatrics.aappublications.org/content/142/6/e20182997

ROLE OF PULSE OXIMETRY IN EXAMINING NEWBORNS FOR CONGENITAL HEART DISEASE: A SCIENTIFIC STATEMENT FROM THE AHA AND AAP

William T. Mahle, MD; Jane W. Newburger, MD, MPH; G. Paul Matherne, MD; Frank C. Smith, MD; Tracey R. Hoke, MD; Robert Koppel, MD; Samuel S. Gidding, MD; Robert H. Beekman III, MD; Scott D. Grosse, PhD; on behalf of Section on Cardiology and Cardiac Surgery and Committee of Fetus and Newborn (joint with American Heart Association Congenital Heart Defects Committee of the Council on Cardiovascular Disease in the Young, Council on Cardiovascular Nursing, and Interdisciplinary Council on Quality of Care and Outcomes Research)

ABSTRACT. *Background.* The purpose of this statement is to address the state of evidence on the routine use of pulse oximetry in newborns to detect critical congenital heart disease (CCHD).

Methods and Results. A writing group appointed by the American Heart Association and the American Academy of Pediatrics reviewed the available literature addressing current detection methods for CCHD, burden of missed and/or delayed diagnosis of CCHD, rationale of oximetry screening, and clinical studies of oximetry in otherwise asymptomatic newborns. MEDLINE database searches from 1966 to 2008 were done for

English-language papers using the following search terms: congenital heart disease, pulse oximetry, physical examination, murmur, echocardiography, fetal echocardiography, and newborn screening. The reference lists of identified papers were also searched. Published abstracts from major pediatric scientific meetings in 2006 to 2008 were also reviewed. The American Heart Association classification of recommendations and levels of evidence for practice guidelines were used. In an analysis of pooled studies of oximetry assessment performed after 24 hours of life, the estimated sensitivity for detecting CCHD was 69.6%, and the positive predictive value was 47.0%; however, sensitivity varied dramatically among studies from 0% to 100%. False-positive screens that required further evaluation occurred in only 0.035% of infants screened after 24 hours.

Conclusions. Currently, CCHD is not detected in some newborns until after their hospital discharge, which results in significant morbidity and occasional mortality. Furthermore, routine pulse oximetry performed on asymptomatic newborns after 24 hours of life, but before hospital discharge, may detect CCHD. Routine pulse oximetry performed after 24 hours in hospitals that have on-site pediatric cardiovascular services incurs very low cost and risk of harm. Future studies in larger populations and across a broad range of newborn delivery systems are needed to determine whether this practice should become standard of care in the routine assessment of the neonate. (8/09)
http://pediatrics.aappublications.org/content/124/2/823

THE ROLE OF THE PEDIATRICIAN IN PRIMARY PREVENTION OF OBESITY (CLINICAL REPORT)
Stephen R. Daniels, MD, PhD, FAAP; Sandra G. Hassink, MD, FAAP; and Committee on Nutrition
ABSTRACT. The adoption of healthful lifestyles by individuals and families can result in a reduction in many chronic diseases and conditions of which obesity is the most prevalent. Obesity prevention, in addition to treatment, is an important public health priority. This clinical report describes the rationale for pediatricians to be an integral part of the obesity-prevention effort. In addition, the 2012 Institute of Medicine report "Accelerating Progress in Obesity Prevention" includes health care providers as a crucial component of successful weight control. Research on obesity prevention in the pediatric care setting as well as evidence-informed practical approaches and targets for prevention are reviewed. Pediatricians should use a longitudinal, developmentally appropriate life-course approach to help identify children early on the path to obesity and base prevention efforts on family dynamics and reduction in high-risk dietary and activity behaviors. They should promote a diet free of sugar-sweetened beverages, of fewer foods with high caloric density, and of increased intake of fruits and vegetables. It is also important to promote a lifestyle with reduced sedentary behavior and with 60 minutes of daily moderate to vigorous physical activity. This report also identifies important gaps in evidence that need to be filled by future research. (6/15)
http://pediatrics.aappublications.org/content/136/1/e275

THE ROLE OF THE PEDIATRICIAN IN RURAL EMERGENCY MEDICAL SERVICES FOR CHILDREN
Committee on Pediatric Emergency Medicine
ABSTRACT. In rural America, pediatricians can play a key role in the development, implementation, and ongoing supervision of emergency medical services for children (EMSC). Pediatricians may represent the only source of pediatric expertise for a large region and are a vital resource for rural physicians (eg, general and family practice, emergency medicine) and other rural health care professionals (physician assistants, nurse practitioners, and emergency medical technicians), providing education about management and prevention of pediatric illness and injury; appropriate equipment for the acutely ill or injured child; and acute, chronic, and rehabilitative care. In addition to providing clinical expertise, the pediatrician may be involved in quality assurance, clinical protocol development, and advocacy, and may serve as a liaison between emergency medical services and other entities working with children (eg, school nurses, child care centers, athletic programs, and programs for children with special health care needs). (10/12, reaffirmed 9/15)
http://pediatrics.aappublications.org/content/130/5/978

ROLE OF THE PEDIATRICIAN IN YOUTH VIOLENCE PREVENTION
Committee on Injury, Violence, and Poison Prevention
ABSTRACT. Youth violence continues to be a serious threat to the health of children and adolescents in the United States. It is crucial that pediatricians clearly define their role and develop the appropriate skills to address this threat effectively. From a clinical perspective, pediatricians should become familiar with *Connected Kids: Safe, Strong, Secure,* the American Academy of Pediatrics' primary care violence prevention protocol. Using this material, practices can incorporate preventive education, screening for risk, and linkages to community-based counseling and treatment resources. As advocates, pediatricians may bring newly developed information regarding key risk factors such as exposure to firearms, teen dating violence, and bullying to the attention of local and national policy makers. This policy statement refines the developing role of pediatricians in youth violence prevention and emphasizes the importance of this issue in the strategic agenda of the American Academy of Pediatrics. (6/09)
http://pediatrics.aappublications.org/content/124/1/393

ROLE OF THE SCHOOL NURSE IN PROVIDING SCHOOL HEALTH SERVICES
Council on School Health
ABSTRACT. The American Academy of Pediatrics recognizes the important role school nurses play in promoting the optimal biopsychosocial health and well-being of school-aged children in the school setting. Although the concept of a school nurse has existed for more than a century, uniformity among states and school districts regarding the role of a registered professional nurse in schools and the laws governing it are lacking. By understanding the benefits, roles, and responsibilities of school nurses working as a team with the school physician, as well as their contributions to school-aged children, pediatricians can collaborate with, support, and promote school nurses in their own communities, thus improving the health, wellness, and safety of children and adolescents. (5/16)
http://pediatrics.aappublications.org/content/137/6/e20160852

ROLE OF THE SCHOOL PHYSICIAN
Council on School Health
ABSTRACT. The American Academy of Pediatrics recognizes the important role physicians play in promoting the optimal biopsychosocial well-being of children in the school setting. Although the concept of a school physician has existed for more than a century, uniformity among states and school districts regarding physicians in schools and the laws governing it are lacking. By understanding the roles and contributions physicians can make to schools, pediatricians can support and promote school physicians in their communities and improve health and safety for children. (12/12)
http://pediatrics.aappublications.org/content/131/1/178

SAFE SLEEP AND SKIN-TO-SKIN CARE IN THE NEONATAL PERIOD FOR HEALTHY TERM NEWBORNS (CLINICAL REPORT)

Lori Feldman-Winter, MD, MPH, FAAP; Jay P. Goldsmith, MD, FAAP; Committee on Fetus and Newborn; and Task Force on Sudden Infant Death Syndrome

ABSTRACT. Skin-to-skin care (SSC) and rooming-in have become common practice in the newborn period for healthy newborns with the implementation of maternity care practices that support breastfeeding as delineated in the World Health Organization's "Ten Steps to Successful Breastfeeding." SSC and rooming-in are supported by evidence that indicates that the implementation of these practices increases overall and exclusive breastfeeding, safer and healthier transitions, and improved maternal-infant bonding. In some cases, however, the practice of SSC and rooming-in may pose safety concerns, particularly with regard to sleep. There have been several recent case reports and case series of severe and sudden unexpected postnatal collapse in the neonatal period among otherwise healthy newborns and near fatal or fatal events related to sleep, suffocation, and falls from adult hospital beds. Although these are largely case reports, there are potential dangers of unobserved SSC immediately after birth and throughout the postpartum hospital period as well as with unobserved rooming-in for at-risk situations. Moreover, behaviors that are modeled in the hospital after birth, such as sleep position, are likely to influence sleeping practices after discharge. Hospitals and birthing centers have found it difficult to develop policies that will allow SSC and rooming-in to continue in a safe manner. This clinical report is intended for birthing centers and delivery hospitals caring for healthy newborns to assist in the establishment of appropriate SSC and safe sleep policies. (8/16)

http://pediatrics.aappublications.org/content/138/3/e20161889

SAFE TRANSPORTATION OF NEWBORNS AT HOSPITAL DISCHARGE

Committee on Injury and Poison Prevention

ABSTRACT. All hospitals should set policies that require the discharge of every newborn in a car safety seat that is appropriate for the infant's maturity and medical condition. Discharge policies for newborns should include a parent education component, regular review of educational materials, and periodic in-service education for responsible staff. Appropriate child restraint systems should become a benefit of coverage by Medicaid, managed care organizations, and other third-party insurers. (10/99, reaffirmed 1/03, 1/06, 10/08)

http://pediatrics.aappublications.org/content/104/4/986

SAFE TRANSPORTATION OF PRETERM AND LOW BIRTH WEIGHT INFANTS AT HOSPITAL DISCHARGE (CLINICAL REPORT)

Marilyn J. Bull, MD; William A. Engle, MD; Committee on Injury, Violence, and Poison Prevention; and Committee on Fetus and Newborn

ABSTRACT. Safe transportation of preterm and low birth weight infants requires special considerations. Both physiologic immaturity and low birth weight must be taken into account to properly position such infants. This clinical report provides guidelines for pediatricians and other caregivers who counsel parents of preterm and low birth weight infants about car safety seats. (4/09, reaffirmed 8/13)

http://pediatrics.aappublications.org/content/123/5/1424

SCHOOL BUS TRANSPORTATION OF CHILDREN WITH SPECIAL HEALTH CARE NEEDS

Joseph O'Neil, MD, MPH, FAAP; Benjamin D. Hoffman, MD, FAAP; and Council on Injury, Violence, and Poison Prevention

ABSTRACT. School systems are responsible for ensuring that children with special needs are safely transported on all forms of federally approved transportation provided by the school system. A plan to provide the most current and proper support to children with special transportation needs should be developed by the Individualized Education Program team, including the parent, school transportation director, and school nurse, in conjunction with physician orders and recommendations. With this statement, we provide current guidance for the protection of child passengers with specific health care needs. Guidance that applies to general school transportation should be followed, inclusive of staff training, provision of nurses or aides if needed, and establishment of a written emergency evacuation plan as well as a comprehensive infection control program. Researchers provide the basis for recommendations concerning occupant securement for children in wheelchairs and children with other special needs who are transported on a school bus. Pediatricians can help their patients by being aware of guidance for restraint systems for children with special needs and by remaining informed of new resources. Pediatricians can also play an important role at the state and local level in the development of school bus specifications. (4/18)

See full text on page 911.

http://pediatrics.aappublications.org/content/141/5/e20180513

SCHOOL HEALTH ASSESSMENTS

Committee on School Health

ABSTRACT. Comprehensive health assessments often are performed in school-based clinics or public health clinics by health professionals other than pediatricians. Pediatricians or other physicians skilled in child health care should participate in such evaluations. This statement provides guidance on the scope of in-school health assessments and the roles of the pediatrician, school nurse, school, and community. (4/00, reaffirmed 6/03, 5/06, 10/11)

http://pediatrics.aappublications.org/content/105/4/875

SCHOOL READINESS (TECHNICAL REPORT)

Pamela C. High, MD; Committee on Early Childhood, Adoption, and Dependent Care; and Council on School Health

ABSTRACT. School readiness includes the readiness of the individual child, the school's readiness for children, and the ability of the family and community to support optimal early child development. It is the responsibility of schools to be ready for all children at all levels of readiness. Children's readiness for kindergarten should become an outcome measure for community-based programs, rather than an exclusion criterion at the beginning of the formal educational experience. Our new knowledge of early brain and child development has revealed that modifiable factors in a child's early experience can greatly affect that child's learning trajectory. Many US children enter kindergarten with limitations in their social, emotional, cognitive, and physical development that might have been significantly diminished or eliminated through early identification of and attention to child and family needs. Pediatricians have a role in promoting school readiness for all children, beginning at birth, through their practices and advocacy. The American Academy of Pediatrics affords pediatricians many opportunities to promote the physical, social-emotional, and educational health of young children, with other advocacy groups. This technical report supports American Academy of Pediatrics policy statements "Quality Early Education and Child Care From

Birth to Kindergarten" and "The Inappropriate Use of School 'Readiness' Tests." (4/08, reaffirmed 9/13)
http://pediatrics.aappublications.org/content/121/4/e1008

SCHOOL START TIMES FOR ADOLESCENTS

Adolescent Sleep Working Group, Committee on Adolescence, and Council on School Health

ABSTRACT. The American Academy of Pediatrics recognizes insufficient sleep in adolescents as an important public health issue that significantly affects the health and safety, as well as the academic success, of our nation's middle and high school students. Although a number of factors, including biological changes in sleep associated with puberty, lifestyle choices, and academic demands, negatively affect middle and high school students' ability to obtain sufficient sleep, the evidence strongly implicates earlier school start times (ie, before 8:30 AM) as a key modifiable contributor to insufficient sleep, as well as circadian rhythm disruption, in this population. Furthermore, a substantial body of research has now demonstrated that delaying school start times is an effective countermeasure to chronic sleep loss and has a wide range of potential benefits to students with regard to physical and mental health, safety, and academic achievement. The American Academy of Pediatrics strongly supports the efforts of school districts to optimize sleep in students and urges high schools and middle schools to aim for start times that allow students the opportunity to achieve optimal levels of sleep (8.5–9.5 hours) and to improve physical (eg, reduced obesity risk) and mental (eg, lower rates of depression) health, safety (eg, drowsy driving crashes), academic performance, and quality of life. (8/14)
http://pediatrics.aappublications.org/content/134/3/642

SCHOOL TRANSPORTATION SAFETY

Committee on Injury, Violence, and Poison Prevention and Council on School Health

ABSTRACT. This policy statement replaces the previous version published in 1996. It provides new information, studies, regulations, and recommendations related to the safe transportation of children to and from school and school-related activities. Pediatricians can play an important role at the patient/family, community, state, and national levels as child advocates and consultants to schools and early education programs about transportation safety. (7/07, reaffirmed 10/11)
http://pediatrics.aappublications.org/content/120/1/213

SCHOOL-BASED HEALTH CENTERS AND PEDIATRIC PRACTICE

Council on School Health

ABSTRACT. School-based health centers (SBHCs) have become an important method of health care delivery for the youth of our nation. Although they only represent 1 aspect of a coordinated school health program approach, SBHCs have provided access to health care services for youth confronted with age, financial, cultural, and geographic barriers. A fundamental principle of SBHCs is to create an environment of service coordination and collaboration that addresses the health needs and well-being of youth with health disparities or poor access to health care services. Some pediatricians have concerns that these centers are in conflict with the primary care provider's medical home. This policy provides an overview of SBHCs and some of their documented benefits, addresses the issue of potential conflict with the medical home, and provides recommendations that support the integration and coordination of SBHCs and the pediatric medical home practice. (1/12)
http://pediatrics.aappublications.org/content/129/2/387

SCOPE OF HEALTH CARE BENEFITS FOR CHILDREN FROM BIRTH THROUGH AGE 26

Committee on Child Health Financing

ABSTRACT. The optimal health of all children is best achieved with access to appropriate and comprehensive health care benefits. This policy statement outlines and defines the recommended set of health insurance benefits for children through age 26. The American Academy of Pediatrics developed a set of recommendations concerning preventive care services for children, adolescents, and young adults. These recommendations are compiled in the publication *Bright Futures: Guidelines for Health Supervision of Infants, Children, and Adolescents,* third edition. The Bright Futures recommendations were referenced as a standard for access and design of age-appropriate health insurance benefits for infants, children, adolescents, and young adults in the Patient Protection and Affordable Care Act of 2010 (Pub L No. 114–148). (11/11)
http://pediatrics.aappublications.org/content/129/1/185

SCOPE OF PRACTICE ISSUES IN THE DELIVERY OF PEDIATRIC HEALTH CARE

Committee on Pediatric Workforce

ABSTRACT. The American Academy of Pediatrics (AAP) believes that optimal pediatric health care depends on a team-based approach with supervision by a physician leader, preferably a pediatrician. The pediatrician, here defined to include not only pediatric generalists but all pediatric medical subspecialists, all surgical specialists, and internal medicine/pediatric physicians, is uniquely qualified to manage, coordinate, and supervise the entire spectrum of pediatric care, from diagnosis through all stages of treatment, in all practice settings. The AAP recognizes the valuable contributions of nonphysician clinicians, including nurse practitioners and physician assistants, in delivering optimal pediatric care. However, the expansion of the scope of practice of nonphysician pediatric clinicians raises critical public policy and child health advocacy concerns. Pediatricians should serve as advocates for optimal pediatric care in state legislatures, public policy forums, and the media and should pursue opportunities to resolve scope of practice conflicts outside state legislatures. The AAP affirms the importance of appropriate documentation and standards in pediatric education, training, skills, clinical competencies, examination, regulation, and patient care to ensure safety and quality health care for all infants, children, adolescents, and young adults. (5/13, reaffirmed 10/15)
http://pediatrics.aappublications.org/content/131/6/1211

SCREENING EXAMINATION OF PREMATURE INFANTS FOR RETINOPATHY OF PREMATURITY

Walter M. Fierson, MD, FAAP, and Section on Ophthalmology (joint with American Academy of Ophthalmology, American Association for Pediatric Ophthalmology and Strabismus, and American Association of Certified Orthoptists)

ABSTRACT. This policy statement revises a previous statement on screening of preterm infants for retinopathy of prematurity (ROP) that was published in 2013. ROP is a pathologic process that occurs in immature retinal tissue and can progress to a tractional retinal detachment, which may then result in visual loss or blindness. For more than 3 decades, treatment of severe ROP that markedly decreases the incidence of this poor visual outcome has been available. However, severe, treatment-requiring ROP must be diagnosed in a timely fashion to be treated effectively. The sequential nature of ROP requires that infants who are at-risk and preterm be examined at proper times and intervals to detect the changes of ROP before they become destructive. This statement presents the attributes of an effective program to detect and treat ROP, including the timing of initial and follow-up examinations. (11/18)

See full text on page 921.

http://pediatrics.aappublications.org/content/142/6/e20183061

SCREENING FOR NONVIRAL SEXUALLY TRANSMITTED INFECTIONS IN ADOLESCENTS AND YOUNG ADULTS

Committee on Adolescence (joint with Society for Adolescent Health and Medicine)

ABSTRACT. Prevalence rates of many sexually transmitted infections (STIs) are highest among adolescents. If nonviral STIs are detected early, they can be treated, transmission to others can be eliminated, and sequelae can be averted. The US Preventive Services Task Force and the Centers for Disease Control and Prevention have published chlamydia, gonorrhea, and syphilis screening guidelines that recommend screening those at risk on the basis of epidemiologic and clinical outcomes data. This policy statement specifically focuses on these curable, nonviral STIs and reviews the evidence for nonviral STI screening in adolescents, communicates the value of screening, and outlines recommendations for routine nonviral STI screening of adolescents. (6/14)

http://pediatrics.aappublications.org/content/134/1/e302

SCREENING FOR RETINOPATHY IN THE PEDIATRIC PATIENT WITH TYPE 1 DIABETES MELLITUS (CLINICAL REPORT)

Gregg T. Lueder, MD; Janet Silverstein, MD; Section on Ophthalmology; and Section on Endocrinology (joint with American Association for Pediatric Ophthalmology and Strabismus)

ABSTRACT. Diabetic retinopathy (DR) is the leading cause of blindness in young adults in the United States. Early identification and treatment of DR can decrease the risk of vision loss in affected patients. This clinical report reviews the risk factors for the development of DR and screening guidance for pediatric patients with type 1 diabetes mellitus. (7/05, reaffirmed 1/09, 7/14)

http://pediatrics.aappublications.org/content/116/1/270

SECONDHAND AND PRENATAL TOBACCO SMOKE EXPOSURE (TECHNICAL REPORT)

Dana Best, MD, MPH; Committee on Environmental Health; Committee on Native American Child Health; and Committee on Adolescence

ABSTRACT. Secondhand tobacco smoke (SHS) exposure of children and their families causes significant morbidity and mortality. In their personal and professional roles, pediatricians have many opportunities to advocate for elimination of SHS exposure of children, to counsel tobacco users to quit, and to counsel children never to start. This report discusses the harms of tobacco use and SHS exposure, the extent and costs of tobacco use and SHS exposure, and the evidence that supports counseling and other clinical interventions in the cycle of tobacco use. Recommendations for future research, policy, and clinical practice change are discussed. To improve understanding and provide support for these activities, the harms of SHS exposure are discussed, effective ways to eliminate or reduce SHS exposure are presented, and policies that support a smoke-free environment are outlined. (10/09, reaffirmed 5/14)

http://pediatrics.aappublications.org/content/124/5/e1017

SELECTING APPROPRIATE TOYS FOR YOUNG CHILDREN: THE PEDIATRICIAN'S ROLE (CLINICAL REPORT)

Committee on Early Childhood, Adoption, and Dependent Care

ABSTRACT. Play is essential for learning in children. Toys are the tools of play. Which play materials are provided and how they are used are equally important. Adults caring for children can be reminded that toys facilitate but do not substitute for the most important aspect of nurture—warm, loving, dependable relationships. Toys should be safe, affordable, and developmentally appropriate. Children do not need expensive toys. Toys should be appealing to engage the child over a period of time. Information and resources are provided in this report so pediatricians can give parents advice about selecting toys. (4/03, reaffirmed 10/06, 5/11)

http://pediatrics.aappublications.org/content/111/4/911

SENSORY INTEGRATION THERAPIES FOR CHILDREN WITH DEVELOPMENTAL AND BEHAVIORAL DISORDERS

Section on Complementary and Integrative Medicine and Council on Children With Disabilities

ABSTRACT. Sensory-based therapies are increasingly used by occupational therapists and sometimes by other types of therapists in treatment of children with developmental and behavioral disorders. Sensory-based therapies involve activities that are believed to organize the sensory system by providing vestibular, proprioceptive, auditory, and tactile inputs. Brushes, swings, balls, and other specially designed therapeutic or recreational equipment are used to provide these inputs. However, it is unclear whether children who present with sensory-based problems have an actual "disorder" of the sensory pathways of the brain or whether these deficits are characteristics associated with other developmental and behavioral disorders. Because there is no universally accepted framework for diagnosis, sensory processing disorder generally should not be diagnosed. Other developmental and behavioral disorders must always be considered, and a thorough evaluation should be completed. Difficulty tolerating or processing sensory information is a characteristic that may be seen in many developmental behavioral disorders, including autism spectrum disorders, attention-deficit/hyperactivity disorder, developmental coordination disorders, and childhood anxiety disorders.

Occupational therapy with the use of sensory-based therapies may be acceptable as one of the components of a comprehensive treatment plan. However, parents should be informed that the amount of research regarding the effectiveness of sensory integration therapy is limited and inconclusive. Important roles for pediatricians and other clinicians may include discussing these limitations with parents, talking with families about a trial period of sensory integration therapy, and teaching families how to evaluate the effectiveness of a therapy. (5/12)

http://pediatrics.aappublications.org/content/129/6/1186

SEXUAL AND REPRODUCTIVE HEALTH CARE SERVICES IN THE PEDIATRIC SETTING (CLINICAL REPORT)

Arik V. Marcell, MD, MPH; Gale R. Burstein, MD, MPH; and Committee on Adolescence

ABSTRACT. Pediatricians are an important source of health care for adolescents and young adults and can play a significant role in addressing their patients' sexual and reproductive health needs, including preventing unintended pregnancies and sexually transmitted infections (STIs), including HIV, and promoting healthy relationships. STIs, HIV, and unintended pregnancy are all preventable health outcomes with potentially serious permanent sequelae; the highest rates of STIs, HIV, and unintended pregnancy are reported among adolescents and young adults. Office visits present opportunities to provide comprehensive education and health care services to adolescents and young adults to prevent STIs, HIV, and unintended pregnancies. The American Academy of Pediatrics, other professional medical organizations, and the government have guidelines and recommendations regarding the provision of sexual and reproductive health information and services. However, despite these recommendations, recent studies have revealed that there is substantial room for improvement in actually delivering the recommended services. The purpose of this clinical report is

to assist pediatricians to operationalize the provision of various aspects of sexual and reproductive health care into their practices and to provide guidance on overcoming barriers to providing this care routinely while maximizing opportunities for confidential health services delivery in their offices. (10/17)
http://pediatrics.aappublications.org/content/140/5/e20172858

SEXUALITY EDUCATION FOR CHILDREN AND ADOLESCENTS (CLINICAL REPORT)

Cora C. Breuner, MD, MPH; Gerri Mattson, MD, MSPH;
Committee on Adolescence; and Committee on Psychosocial
Aspects of Child and Family Health

ABSTRACT. The purpose of this clinical report is to provide pediatricians updated research on evidence-based sexual and reproductive health education conducted since the original clinical report on the subject was published by the American Academy of Pediatrics in 2001. Sexuality education is defined as teaching about human sexuality, including intimate relationships, human sexual anatomy, sexual reproduction, sexually transmitted infections, sexual activity, sexual orientation, gender identity, abstinence, contraception, and reproductive rights and responsibilities. Developmentally appropriate and evidence-based education about human sexuality and sexual reproduction over time provided by pediatricians, schools, other professionals, and parents is important to help children and adolescents make informed, positive, and safe choices about healthy relationships, responsible sexual activity, and their reproductive health. Sexuality education has been shown to help to prevent and reduce the risks of adolescent pregnancy, HIV, and sexually transmitted infections for children and adolescents with and without chronic health conditions and disabilities in the United States. (7/16)
http://pediatrics.aappublications.org/content/138/2/e20161348

SEXUALITY OF CHILDREN AND ADOLESCENTS WITH DEVELOPMENTAL DISABILITIES (CLINICAL REPORT)

Nancy A. Murphy, MD; Ellen Roy Elias, MD; for Council on
Children With Disabilities

ABSTRACT. Children and adolescents with developmental disabilities, like all children, are sexual persons. However, attention to their complex medical and functional issues often consumes time that might otherwise be invested in addressing the anatomic, physiologic, emotional, and social aspects of their developing sexuality. This report discusses issues of puberty, contraception, psychosexual development, sexual abuse, and sexuality education specific to children and adolescents with disabilities and their families. Pediatricians, in the context of the medical home, are encouraged to discuss issues of sexuality on a regular basis, ensure the privacy of each child and adolescent, promote self-care and social independence among persons with disabilities, advocate for appropriate sexuality education, and provide ongoing education for children and adolescents with developmental disabilities and their families. (7/06, reaffirmed 12/09, 7/13, 11/17)
http://pediatrics.aappublications.org/content/118/1/398

SHARED DECISION-MAKING AND CHILDREN WITH DISABILITIES: PATHWAYS TO CONSENSUS (CLINICAL REPORT)

Richard C. Adams, MD, FAAP; Susan E. Levy, MD, MPH, FAAP;
and Council on Children With Disabilities

ABSTRACT. Shared decision-making (SDM) promotes family and clinician collaboration, with ultimate goals of improved health and satisfaction. This clinical report provides a basis for a systematic approach to the implementation of SDM by clinicians for children with disabilities. Often in the discussion of treatment plans, there are gaps between the child's/family's values, priorities, and understanding of perceived "best choices" and those of the clinician. When conducted well, SDM affords an appropriate balance incorporating voices of all stakeholders, ultimately supporting both the child/family and clinician. With increasing knowledge of and functional use of SDM skills, the clinician will become an effective partner in the decision-making process with families, providing family-centered care. The outcome of the process will support the beneficence of the physician, the authority of the family, and the autonomy and well-being of the child. (5/17)
http://pediatrics.aappublications.org/content/139/6/e20170956

SHOPPING CART–RELATED INJURIES TO CHILDREN

Committee on Injury, Violence, and Poison Prevention

ABSTRACT. Shopping cart–related injuries to children are common and can result in severe injury or even death. Most injuries result from falls from carts or cart tip-overs, and injuries to the head and neck represent three fourths of cases. The current US standard for shopping carts should be revised to include clear and effective performance criteria to prevent falls from carts and cart tip-overs. Pediatricians have an important role as educators, researchers, and advocates to promote the prevention of these injuries. (8/06, reaffirmed 4/09, 8/13)
http://pediatrics.aappublications.org/content/118/2/825

SHOPPING CART–RELATED INJURIES TO CHILDREN (TECHNICAL REPORT)

Gary A. Smith, MD, DrPH, for Committee on Injury, Violence, and
Poison Prevention

ABSTRACT. An estimated 24 200 children younger than 15 years, 20 700 (85%) of whom were younger than 5 years, were treated in US hospital emergency departments in 2005 for shopping cart–related injuries. Approximately 4% of shopping cart–related injuries to children younger than 15 years require admission to the hospital. Injuries to the head and neck represent three fourths of all injuries. Fractures account for 45% of all hospitalizations. Deaths have occurred from falls from shopping carts and cart tip-overs. Falls are the most common mechanism of injury and account for more than half of injuries associated with shopping carts. Cart tip-overs are the second most common mechanism, responsible for up to one fourth of injuries and almost 40% of shopping cart–related injuries among children younger than 2 years. Public-awareness initiatives, education programs, and parental supervision, although important, are not enough to prevent these injuries effectively. European Standard EN 1929-1:1998 and joint Australian/New Zealand Standard AS/NZS 3847.1:1999 specify requirements for the construction, performance, testing, and safety of shopping carts and have been implemented as national standards in 21 countries. A US performance standard for shopping carts (ASTM [American Society for Testing and Materials] F2372-04) was established in July 2004; however, it does not adequately address falls and cart tip-overs, which are the leading mechanisms of shopping cart–related injuries to children. The current US standard for shopping carts should be revised to include clear and effective performance criteria for shopping cart child-restraint systems and cart stability to prevent falls from carts and cart tip-overs. This is imperative to decrease the number and severity of shopping cart–related injuries to children. Recommendations from the American Academy of Pediatrics regarding prevention of shopping cart–related injuries are included in the accompanying policy statement. (8/06, reaffirmed 4/09, 8/13)
http://pediatrics.aappublications.org/content/118/2/e540

SIDS AND OTHER SLEEP-RELATED INFANT DEATHS: UPDATED 2016 RECOMMENDATIONS FOR A SAFE INFANT SLEEPING ENVIRONMENT

Task Force on Sudden Infant Death Syndrome

ABSTRACT. Approximately 3500 infants die annually in the United States from sleep-related infant deaths, including sudden infant death syndrome (SIDS; International Classification of Diseases, 10th Revision [ICD-10], R95), ill-defined deaths (ICD-10 R99), and accidental suffocation and strangulation in bed (ICD-10 W75). After an initial decrease in the 1990s, the overall death rate attributable to sleep-related infant deaths has not declined in more recent years. Many of the modifiable and nonmodifiable risk factors for SIDS and other sleep-related infant deaths are strikingly similar. The American Academy of Pediatrics recommends a safe sleep environment that can reduce the risk of all sleep-related infant deaths. Recommendations for a safe sleep environment include supine positioning, the use of a firm sleep surface, room-sharing without bed-sharing, and the avoidance of soft bedding and overheating. Additional recommendations for SIDS reduction include the avoidance of exposure to smoke, alcohol, and illicit drugs; breastfeeding; routine immunization; and use of a pacifier. New evidence is presented for skin-to-skin care for newborn infants, use of bedside and in-bed sleepers, sleeping on couches/armchairs and in sitting devices, and use of soft bedding after 4 months of age. The recommendations and strength of evidence for each recommendation are included in this policy statement. The rationale for these recommendations is discussed in detail in the accompanying technical report (www.pediatrics.org/cgi/doi/10.1542/peds.2016-2940). (10/16)
http://pediatrics.aappublications.org/content/138/5/e20162938

SIDS AND OTHER SLEEP-RELATED INFANT DEATHS: EVIDENCE BASE FOR 2016 UPDATED RECOMMENDATIONS FOR A SAFE INFANT SLEEPING ENVIRONMENT (TECHNICAL REPORT)

Rachel Y. Moon, MD, FAAP, and Task Force on Sudden Infant Death Syndrome

ABSTRACT. Approximately 3500 infants die annually in the United States from sleep-related infant deaths, including sudden infant death syndrome (SIDS), ill-defined deaths, and accidental suffocation and strangulation in bed. After an initial decrease in the 1990s, the overall sleep-related infant death rate has not declined in more recent years. Many of the modifiable and nonmodifiable risk factors for SIDS and other sleep-related infant deaths are strikingly similar. The American Academy of Pediatrics recommends a safe sleep environment that can reduce the risk of all sleep-related infant deaths. Recommendations for a safe sleep environment include supine positioning, use of a firm sleep surface, room-sharing without bed-sharing, and avoidance of soft bedding and overheating. Additional recommendations for SIDS risk reduction include avoidance of exposure to smoke, alcohol, and illicit drugs; breastfeeding; routine immunization; and use of a pacifier. New evidence and rationale for recommendations are presented for skin-to-skin care for newborn infants, bedside and in-bed sleepers, sleeping on couches/armchairs and in sitting devices, and use of soft bedding after 4 months of age. In addition, expanded recommendations for infant sleep location are included. The recommendations and strength of evidence for each recommendation are published in the accompanying policy statement, "SIDS and Other Sleep-Related Infant Deaths: Updated 2016 Recommendations for a Safe Infant Sleeping Environment," which is included in this issue. (10/16)
http://pediatrics.aappublications.org/content/138/5/e20162940

SKATEBOARD AND SCOOTER INJURIES

Committee on Injury, Violence, and Poison Prevention

ABSTRACT. Skateboard-related injuries account for an estimated 50 000 emergency department visits and 1500 hospitalizations among children and adolescents in the United States each year. Nonpowered scooter-related injuries accounted for an estimated 9400 emergency department visits between January and August 2000, and 90% of these patients were children younger than 15 years. Many such injuries can be avoided if children and youth do not ride in traffic, if proper protective gear is worn, and if, in the absence of close adult supervision, skateboards and scooters are not used by children younger than 10 and 8 years, respectively. (3/02, reaffirmed 5/05, 10/08, 10/13)
http://pediatrics.aappublications.org/content/109/3/542

SKIN-TO-SKIN CARE FOR TERM AND PRETERM INFANTS IN THE NEONATAL ICU (CLINICAL REPORT)

Jill Baley, MD, and Committee on Fetus and Newborn

ABSTRACT. "Kangaroo mother care" was first described as an alternative method of caring for low birth weight infants in resource-limited countries, where neonatal mortality and infection rates are high because of overcrowded nurseries, inadequate staffing, and lack of equipment. Intermittent skin-to-skin care (SSC), a modified version of kangaroo mother care, is now being offered in resource-rich countries to infants needing neonatal intensive care, including those who require ventilator support or are extremely premature. SSC significantly improves milk production by the mother and is associated with a longer duration of breastfeeding. Increased parent satisfaction, better sleep organization, a longer duration of quiet sleep, and decreased pain perception during procedures have also been reported in association with SSC. Despite apparent physiologic stability during SSC, it is prudent that infants in the NICU have continuous cardiovascular monitoring and that care be taken to verify correct head positioning for airway patency as well as the stability of the endotracheal tube, arterial and venous access devices, and other life support equipment. (8/15)
http://pediatrics.aappublications.org/content/136/3/596

SNACKS, SWEETENED BEVERAGES, ADDED SUGARS, AND SCHOOLS

Council on School Health and Committee on Nutrition

ABSTRACT. Concern over childhood obesity has generated a decade-long reformation of school nutrition policies. Food is available in school in 3 venues: federally sponsored school meal programs; items sold in competition to school meals, such as a la carte, vending machines, and school stores; and foods available in myriad informal settings, including packed meals and snacks, bake sales, fundraisers, sports booster sales, in-class parties, or other school celebrations. High-energy, low-nutrient beverages, in particular, contribute substantial calories, but little nutrient content, to a student's diet. In 2004, the American Academy of Pediatrics recommended that sweetened drinks be replaced in school by water, white and flavored milks, or 100% fruit and vegetable beverages. Since then, school nutrition has undergone a significant transformation. Federal, state, and local regulations and policies, along with alternative products developed by industry, have helped decrease the availability of nutrient-poor foods and beverages in school. However, regular access to foods of high energy and low quality remains a school issue, much of it attributable to students, parents, and staff. Pediatricians, aligning with experts on child nutrition, are in a position to offer a perspective promoting nutrient-rich foods within calorie guidelines to improve those foods brought into or sold in schools. A positive emphasis on nutritional value, variety, appropriate portion, and encouragement for a steady improvement in quality will be a more effective approach for improving nutrition

and health than simply advocating for the elimination of added sugars. (2/15)
http://pediatrics.aappublications.org/content/135/3/575

SNOWMOBILING HAZARDS
Committee on Injury and Poison Prevention
ABSTRACT. Snowmobiles continue to pose a significant risk to children younger than 15 years and adolescents and young adults 15 through 24 years of age. Head injuries remain the leading cause of mortality and serious morbidity, arising largely from snowmobilers colliding, falling, or overturning during operation. Children also were injured while being towed in a variety of conveyances by snowmobiles. No uniform code of state laws governs the use of snowmobiles by children and youth. Because evidence is lacking to support the effectiveness of operator safety certification and because many children and adolescents do not have the required strength and skills to operate a snowmobile safely, the recreational operation of snowmobiles by persons younger than 16 years is not recommended. Snowmobiles should not be used to tow persons on a tube, tire, sled, or saucer. Furthermore, a graduated licensing program is advised for snowmobilers 16 years and older. Both active and passive snowmobile injury prevention strategies are suggested, as well as recommendations for manufacturers to make safer equipment for snowmobilers of all ages. (11/00, reaffirmed 5/04, 1/07, 6/10)
http://pediatrics.aappublications.org/content/106/5/1142

SPECIAL REQUIREMENTS OF ELECTRONIC HEALTH RECORD SYSTEMS IN PEDIATRICS (CLINICAL REPORT)
S. Andrew Spooner, MD, MS, and Council on Clinical Information Technology
ABSTRACT. Some functions of an electronic health record system are much more important in providing pediatric care than in adult care. Pediatricians commonly complain about the absence of these "pediatric functions" when they are not available in electronic health record systems. To stimulate electronic health record system vendors to recognize and incorporate pediatric functionality into pediatric electronic health record systems, this clinical report reviews the major functions of importance to child health care providers. Also reviewed are important but less critical functions, any of which might be of major importance in a particular clinical context. The major areas described here are immunization management, growth tracking, medication dosing, data norms, and privacy in special pediatric populations. The American Academy of Pediatrics believes that if the functions described in this document are supported in all electronic health record systems, these systems will be more useful for patients of all ages. (3/07, reaffirmed 5/12, 5/16)
http://pediatrics.aappublications.org/content/119/3/631

SPECTRUM OF NONINFECTIOUS HEALTH EFFECTS FROM MOLDS
Committee on Environmental Health
ABSTRACT. Molds are eukaryotic (possessing a true nucleus) nonphotosynthetic organisms that flourish both indoors and outdoors. For humans, the link between mold exposure and asthma exacerbations, allergic rhinitis, infections, and toxicities from ingestion of mycotoxin-contaminated foods are well known. However, the cause-and-effect relationship between inhalational exposure to mold and other untoward health effects (eg, acute idiopathic pulmonary hemorrhage in infants and other illnesses and health complaints) requires additional investigation. Pediatricians play an important role in the education of families about mold, its adverse health effects, exposure prevention, and remediation procedures. (12/06, reaffirmed 9/16)
http://pediatrics.aappublications.org/content/118/6/2582

SPECTRUM OF NONINFECTIOUS HEALTH EFFECTS FROM MOLDS (TECHNICAL REPORT)
Lynnette J. Mazur, MD, MPH; Janice Kim, MD, PhD, MPH; and Committee on Environmental Health
ABSTRACT. Molds are multicellular fungi that are ubiquitous in outdoor and indoor environments. For humans, they are both beneficial (for the production of antimicrobial agents, chemotherapeutic agents, and vitamins) and detrimental. Exposure to mold can occur through inhalation, ingestion, and touching moldy surfaces. Adverse health effects may occur through allergic, infectious, irritant, or toxic processes. The cause-and-effect relationship between mold exposure and allergic and infectious illnesses is well known. Exposures to toxins via the gastrointestinal tract also are well described. However, the cause-and-effect relationship between inhalational exposure to mold toxins and other untoward health effects (eg, acute idiopathic pulmonary hemorrhage in infants and other illnesses and health complaints) is controversial and requires additional investigation. In this report we examine evidence of fungal-related illnesses and the unique aspects of mold exposure to children. Mold-remediation procedures are also discussed. (12/06, reaffirmed 9/16)
http://pediatrics.aappublications.org/content/118/6/e1909

SPORT-RELATED CONCUSSION IN CHILDREN AND ADOLESCENTS (CLINICAL REPORT)
Mark E. Halstead, MD, FAAP; Kevin D. Walter, MD, FAAP; Kody Moffatt, MD, FAAP; and Council on Sports Medicine and Fitness
ABSTRACT. Sport-related concussion is an important topic in nearly all sports and at all levels of sport for children and adolescents. Concussion knowledge and approaches to management have progressed since the American Academy of Pediatrics published its first clinical report on the subject in 2010. Concussion's definition, signs, and symptoms must be understood to diagnose it and rule out more severe intracranial injury. Pediatric health care providers should have a good understanding of diagnostic evaluation and initial management strategies. Effective management can aid recovery and potentially reduce the risk of long-term symptoms and complications. Because concussion symptoms often interfere with school, social life, family relationships, and athletics, a concussion may affect the emotional well-being of the injured athlete. Because every concussion has its own unique spectrum and severity of symptoms, individualized management is appropriate. The reduction, not necessarily elimination, of physical and cognitive activity is the mainstay of treatment. A full return to activity and/or sport is accomplished by using a stepwise program while evaluating for a return of symptoms. An understanding of prolonged symptoms and complications will help the pediatric health care provider know when to refer to a specialist. Additional research is needed in nearly all aspects of concussion in the young athlete. This report provides education on the current state of sport-related concussion knowledge, diagnosis, and management in children and adolescents. (11/18)
See full text on page 933.
http://pediatrics.aappublications.org/content/142/6/e20183074

SPORTS DRINKS AND ENERGY DRINKS FOR CHILDREN AND ADOLESCENTS: ARE THEY APPROPRIATE? (CLINICAL REPORT)
Committee on Nutrition and Council on Sports Medicine and Fitness
ABSTRACT. Sports and energy drinks are being marketed to children and adolescents for a wide variety of inappropriate uses. Sports drinks and energy drinks are significantly different products, and the terms should not be used interchangeably. The primary objectives of this clinical report are to define the ingredients of sports and energy drinks, categorize the similarities and differences between the products, and discuss misuses and abuses. Secondary objectives are to encourage screening during

annual physical examinations for sports and energy drink use, to understand the reasons why youth consumption is widespread, and to improve education aimed at decreasing or eliminating the inappropriate use of these beverages by children and adolescents. Rigorous review and analysis of the literature reveal that caffeine and other stimulant substances contained in energy drinks have no place in the diet of children and adolescents. Furthermore, frequent or excessive intake of caloric sports drinks can substantially increase the risk for overweight or obesity in children and adolescents. Discussion regarding the appropriate use of sports drinks in the youth athlete who participates regularly in endurance or high-intensity sports and vigorous physical activity is beyond the scope of this report. (5/11, reaffirmed 7/17)

http://pediatrics.aappublications.org/content/127/6/1182

SPORTS SPECIALIZATION AND INTENSIVE TRAINING IN YOUNG ATHLETES (CLINICAL REPORT)

Joel S. Brenner, MD, MPH, FAAP, and Council on Sports Medicine and Fitness

ABSTRACT. Sports specialization is becoming the norm in youth sports for a variety of reasons. When sports specialization occurs too early, detrimental effects may occur, both physically and psychologically. If the timing is correct and sports specialization is performed under the correct conditions, the athlete may be successful in reaching specific goals. Young athletes who train intensively, whether specialized or not, can also be at risk of adverse effects on the mind and body. The purpose of this clinical report is to assist pediatricians in counseling their young athlete patients and their parents regarding sports specialization and intensive training. This report supports the American Academy of Pediatrics clinical report "Overuse Injuries, Overtraining, and Burnout in Child and Adolescent Athletes." (8/16)

http://pediatrics.aappublications.org/content/138/3/e20162148

STANDARD TERMINOLOGY FOR FETAL, INFANT, AND PERINATAL DEATHS (CLINICAL REPORT)

Wanda D. Barfield, MD, MPH, and Committee on Fetus and Newborn

ABSTRACT. Accurately defining and reporting perinatal deaths (ie, fetal and infant deaths) is a critical first step in understanding the magnitude and causes of these important events. In addition to obstetric health care providers, neonatologists and pediatricians should have easy access to current and updated resources that clearly provide US definitions and reporting requirements for live births, fetal deaths, and infant deaths. Correct identification of these vital events will improve local, state, and national data so that these deaths can be better addressed and prevented. (4/16)

http://pediatrics.aappublications.org/content/137/5/e20160551

STANDARDIZATION OF INPATIENT HANDOFF COMMUNICATION (CLINICAL REPORT)

Jennifer A. Jewell, MD, FAAP, and Committee on Hospital Care

ABSTRACT. Handoff communication is identified as an integral part of hospital care. Throughout medical communities, inadequate handoff communication is being highlighted as a significant risk to patients. The complexity of hospitals and the number of providers involved in the care of hospitalized patients place inpatients at high risk of communication lapses. This miscommunication and the potential resulting harm make effective handoffs more critical than ever. Although hospitalized patients are being exposed to many handoffs each day, this report is limited to describing the best handoff practices between providers at the time of shift change. (10/16)

http://pediatrics.aappublications.org/content/138/5/e20162681

STANDARDS FOR HEALTH INFORMATION TECHNOLOGY TO ENSURE ADOLESCENT PRIVACY

Committee on Adolescence and Council on Clinical Information Technology

ABSTRACT. Privacy and security of health information is a basic expectation of patients. Despite the existence of federal and state laws safeguarding the privacy of health information, health information systems currently lack the capability to allow for protection of this information for minors. This policy statement reviews the challenges to privacy for adolescents posed by commercial health information technology systems and recommends basic principles for ideal electronic health record systems. This policy statement has been endorsed by the Society for Adolescent Health and Medicine. (10/12)

http://pediatrics.aappublications.org/content/130/5/987

STANDARDS FOR PEDIATRIC CANCER CENTERS

Section on Hematology/Oncology

ABSTRACT. Since the American Academy of Pediatrics– published guidelines for pediatric cancer centers in 1986, 1997, and 2004, significant changes in the delivery of health care have prompted a review of the role of medical centers in the care of pediatric patients. The potential effect of these changes on the treatment and survival rates of children with cancer led to this revision. The intent of this statement is to delineate personnel, capabilities, and facilities that are essential to provide state-of-the-art care for children, adolescents, and young adults with cancer. This statement emphasizes the importance of board-certified pediatric hematologists/oncologists and appropriately qualified pediatric medical subspecialists and pediatric surgical specialists overseeing patient care and the need for specialized facilities as essential for the initial management and much of the follow-up for pediatric, adolescent, and young adult patients with cancer. For patients without practical access to a pediatric cancer center, care may be provided locally by a primary care physician or adult oncologist but at the direction of a pediatric oncologist. (7/14)

http://pediatrics.aappublications.org/content/134/2/410

STIGMA EXPERIENCED BY CHILDREN AND ADOLESCENTS WITH OBESITY

Stephen J. Pont, MD, MPH, FAAP; Rebecca Puhl, PhD, FTOS; Stephen R. Cook, MD, MPH, FAAP, FTOS; Wendelin Slusser, MD, MS, FAAP; Section on Obesity; and The Obesity Society

ABSTRACT. The stigmatization of people with obesity is widespread and causes harm. Weight stigma is often propagated and tolerated in society because of beliefs that stigma and shame will motivate people to lose weight. However, rather than motivating positive change, this stigma contributes to behaviors such as binge eating, social isolation, avoidance of health care services, decreased physical activity, and increased weight gain, which worsen obesity and create additional barriers to healthy behavior change. Furthermore, experiences of weight stigma also dramatically impair quality of life, especially for youth. Health care professionals continue to seek effective strategies and resources to address the obesity epidemic; however, they also frequently exhibit weight bias and stigmatizing behaviors. This policy statement seeks to raise awareness regarding the prevalence and negative effects of weight stigma on pediatric patients and their families and provides 6 clinical practice and 4 advocacy recommendations regarding the role of pediatricians in addressing weight stigma. In summary, these recommendations include improving the clinical setting by modeling best practices for non-biased behaviors and language; using empathetic and empowering counseling techniques, such as motivational interviewing, and addressing weight stigma and bullying in the clinic visit; advocating for inclusion of training and education about weight stigma in medical schools, residency programs, and continuing

medical education programs; and empowering families to be advocates to address weight stigma in the home environment and school setting. (11/17)
http://pediatrics.aappublications.org/content/140/6/e20173034

STRATEGIES FOR PREVENTION OF HEALTH CARE–ASSOCIATED INFECTIONS IN THE NICU (CLINICAL REPORT)

Richard A. Polin, MD; Susan Denson, MD; Michael T. Brady, MD; Committee on Fetus and Newborn; and Committee on Infectious Diseases

ABSTRACT. Health care–associated infections in the NICU result in increased morbidity and mortality, prolonged lengths of stay, and increased medical costs. Neonates are at high risk of acquiring health care–associated infections because of impaired host-defense mechanisms, limited amounts of protective endogenous flora on skin and mucosal surfaces at time of birth, reduced barrier function of their skin, use of invasive procedures and devices, and frequent exposure to broad-spectrum antibiotic agents. This clinical report reviews management and prevention of health care–associated infections in newborn infants. (3/12, reaffirmed 2/16)
http://pediatrics.aappublications.org/content/129/4/e1085

STRENGTH TRAINING BY CHILDREN AND ADOLESCENTS

Council on Sports Medicine and Fitness

ABSTRACT. Pediatricians are often asked to give advice on the safety and efficacy of strength-training programs for children and adolescents. This statement, which is a revision of a previous American Academy of Pediatrics policy statement, defines relevant terminology and provides current information on risks and benefits of strength training for children and adolescents. (4/08, reaffirmed 6/11, 12/16)
http://pediatrics.aappublications.org/content/121/4/835

SUBSTANCE USE SCREENING, BRIEF INTERVENTION, AND REFERRAL TO TREATMENT

Committee on Substance Use and Prevention

ABSTRACT. The enormous public health impact of adolescent substance use and its preventable morbidity and mortality show the need for the health care sector, including pediatricians and the medical home, to increase its capacity related to substance use prevention, detection, assessment, and intervention. The American Academy of Pediatrics published its policy statement "Substance Use Screening, Brief Intervention, and Referral to Treatment for Pediatricians" in 2011 to introduce the concepts and terminology of screening, brief intervention, and referral to treatment (SBIRT) and to offer clinical guidance about available substance use screening tools and intervention procedures. This policy statement is a revision of the 2011 SBIRT statement. An accompanying clinical report updates clinical guidance for adolescent SBIRT. (6/16)
http://pediatrics.aappublications.org/content/138/1/e20161210

SUBSTANCE USE SCREENING, BRIEF INTERVENTION, AND REFERRAL TO TREATMENT (CLINICAL REPORT)

Sharon J. L. Levy, MD, MPH, FAAP; Janet F. Williams, MD, FAAP; and Committee on Substance Use and Prevention

ABSTRACT. The enormous public health impact of adolescent substance use and its preventable morbidity and mortality highlight the need for the health care sector, including pediatricians and the medical home, to increase its capacity regarding adolescent substance use screening, brief intervention, and referral to treatment (SBIRT). The American Academy of Pediatrics first published a policy statement on SBIRT and adolescents in 2011 to introduce SBIRT concepts and terminology and to offer clinical guidance about available substance use screening tools and intervention procedures. This clinical report provides a simplified adolescent SBIRT clinical approach that, in combination with the accompanying updated policy statement, guides pediatricians in implementing substance use prevention, detection, assessment, and intervention practices across the varied clinical settings in which adolescents receive health care. (6/16)
http://pediatrics.aappublications.org/content/138/1/e20161211

SUICIDE AND SUICIDE ATTEMPTS IN ADOLESCENTS (CLINICAL REPORT)

Benjamin Shain, MD, PhD, and Committee on Adolescence

ABSTRACT. Suicide is the second leading cause of death for adolescents 15 to 19 years old. This report updates the previous statement of the American Academy of Pediatrics and is intended to assist pediatricians, in collaboration with other child and adolescent health care professionals, in the identification and management of the adolescent at risk for suicide. Suicide risk can only be reduced, not eliminated, and risk factors provide no more than guidance. Nonetheless, care for suicidal adolescents may be improved with the pediatrician's knowledge, skill, and comfort with the topic, as well as ready access to appropriate community resources and mental health professionals. (6/16)
http://pediatrics.aappublications.org/content/138/1/e20161420

SUPPLEMENTAL SECURITY INCOME (SSI) FOR CHILDREN AND YOUTH WITH DISABILITIES

Council on Children With Disabilities

ABSTRACT. The Supplemental Security Income (SSI) program remains an important source of financial support for low-income families of children with special health care needs and disabling conditions. In most states, SSI eligibility also qualifies children for the state Medicaid program, providing access to health care services. The Social Security Administration (SSA), which administers the SSI program, considers a child disabled under SSI if there is a medically determinable physical or mental impairment or combination of impairments that results in marked and severe functional limitations. The impairment(s) must be expected to result in death or have lasted or be expected to last for a continuous period of at least 12 months. The income and assets of families of children with disabilities are also considered when determining financial eligibility. When an individual with a disability becomes an adult at 18 years of age, the SSA considers only the individual's income and assets. The SSA considers an adult to be disabled if there is a medically determinable impairment (or combination of impairments) that prevents substantial gainful activity for at least 12 continuous months. SSI benefits are important for youth with chronic conditions who are transitioning to adulthood. The purpose of this statement is to provide updated information about the SSI medical and financial eligibility criteria and the disability-determination process. This statement also discusses how pediatricians can help children and youth when they apply for SSI benefits. (11/09, reaffirmed 2/15)
http://pediatrics.aappublications.org/content/124/6/1702

SUPPORTING THE FAMILY AFTER THE DEATH OF A CHILD (CLINICAL REPORT)

Esther Wender, MD, and Committee on Psychosocial Aspects of Child and Family Health

ABSTRACT. The death of a child can have a devastating effect on the family. The pediatrician has an important role to play in supporting the parents and any siblings still in his or her practice after such a death. Pediatricians may be poorly prepared to provide this support. Also, because of the pain of confronting the grief of family members, they may be reluctant to become involved. This statement gives guidelines to help the pediatrician provide such support. It describes the grief reactions that can be expected in family members after the death of a child. Ways of supporting family members are suggested, and other helpful resources in the community are described. The goal of this guidance is to prevent outcomes that may impair the health and development of affected parents and children. (11/12, reaffirmed 12/16)

http://pediatrics.aappublications.org/content/130/6/1164

SUPPORTING THE GRIEVING CHILD AND FAMILY (CLINICAL REPORT)

David J. Schonfeld, MD, FAAP; Thomas Demaria, PhD; Committee on Psychosocial Aspects of Child and Family Health; and Disaster Preparedness Advisory Council

ABSTRACT. The death of someone close to a child often has a profound and lifelong effect on the child and results in a range of both short- and long-term reactions. Pediatricians, within a patient-centered medical home, are in an excellent position to provide anticipatory guidance to caregivers and to offer assistance and support to children and families who are grieving. This clinical report offers practical suggestions on how to talk with grieving children to help them better understand what has happened and its implications and to address any misinformation, misinterpretations, or misconceptions. An understanding of guilt, shame, and other common reactions, as well an appreciation of the role of secondary losses and the unique challenges facing children in communities characterized by chronic trauma and cumulative loss, will help the pediatrician to address factors that may impair grieving and children's adjustment and to identify complicated mourning and situations when professional counseling is indicated. Advice on how to support children's participation in funerals and other memorial services and to anticipate and address grief triggers and anniversary reactions is provided so that pediatricians are in a better position to advise caregivers and to offer consultation to schools, early education and child care facilities, and other child congregate care sites. Pediatricians often enter their profession out of a profound desire to minimize the suffering of children and may find it personally challenging when they find themselves in situations in which they are asked to bear witness to the distress of children who are acutely grieving. The importance of professional preparation and self-care is therefore emphasized, and resources are recommended. (8/16)

http://pediatrics.aappublications.org/content/138/3/e20162147

SUPPORTING THE HEALTH CARE TRANSITION FROM ADOLESCENCE TO ADULTHOOD IN THE MEDICAL HOME (CLINICAL REPORT)

Patience H. White, MD, MA, FAAP, FACP; W. Carl Cooley, MD, FAAP; American Academy of Pediatrics (joint with Transitions Clinical Report Authoring Group, American Academy of Family Physicians, and American College of Physicians)

ABSTRACT. Risk and vulnerability encompass many dimensions of the transition from adolescence to adulthood. Transition from pediatric, parent-supervised health care to more independent, patient-centered adult health care is no exception. The tenets and algorithm of the original 2011 clinical report, "Supporting the Health Care Transition from Adolescence to Adulthood in the Medical Home," are unchanged. This updated clinical report provides more practice-based quality improvement guidance on key elements of transition planning, transfer, and integration into adult care for all youth and young adults. It also includes new and updated sections on definition and guiding principles, the status of health care transition preparation among youth, barriers, outcome evidence, recommended health care transition processes and implementation strategies using quality improvement methods, special populations, education and training in pediatric onset conditions, and payment options. The clinical report also includes new recommendations pertaining to infrastructure, education and training, payment, and research. (10/18)

See full text on page 959.

http://pediatrics.aappublications.org/content/142/5/e20182587

SURFACTANT REPLACEMENT THERAPY FOR PRETERM AND TERM NEONATES WITH RESPIRATORY DISTRESS (CLINICAL REPORT)

Richard A. Polin, MD, FAAP; Waldemar A. Carlo, MD, FAAP; and Committee on Fetus and Newborn

ABSTRACT. Respiratory failure secondary to surfactant deficiency is a major cause of morbidity and mortality in preterm infants. Surfactant therapy substantially reduces mortality and respiratory morbidity for this population. Secondary surfactant deficiency also contributes to acute respiratory morbidity in late-preterm and term neonates with meconium aspiration syndrome, pneumonia/sepsis, and perhaps pulmonary hemorrhage; surfactant replacement may be beneficial for these infants. This statement summarizes the evidence regarding indications, administration, formulations, and outcomes for surfactant-replacement therapy. The clinical strategy of intubation, surfactant administration, and extubation to continuous positive airway pressure and the effect of continuous positive airway pressure on outcomes and surfactant use in preterm infants are also reviewed. (12/13)

http://pediatrics.aappublications.org/content/133/1/156

TACKLING IN YOUTH FOOTBALL

Council on Sports Medicine and Fitness

ABSTRACT. American football remains one of the most popular sports for young athletes. The injuries sustained during football, especially those to the head and neck, have been a topic of intense interest recently in both the public media and medical literature. The recognition of these injuries and the potential for long-term sequelae have led some physicians to call for a reduction in the number of contact practices, a postponement of tackling until a certain age, and even a ban on high school football. This statement reviews the literature regarding injuries in football, particularly those of the head and neck, the relationship between tackling and football-related injuries, and the potential effects of limiting or delaying tackling on injury risk. (10/15)

http://pediatrics.aappublications.org/content/136/5/e1419

TARGETED REFORMS IN HEALTH CARE FINANCING TO IMPROVE THE CARE OF ADOLESCENTS AND YOUNG ADULTS

Arik V. Marcell, MD, MPH, FAAP; Cora C. Breuner, MD, MPH, FAAP; Lawrence Hammer, MD, FAAP; Mark L. Hudak, MD, FAAP; Committee on Adolescence; and Committee on Child Health Financing

ABSTRACT. Significant changes have occurred in the commercial and government insurance marketplace after the passage of 2 federal legislation acts, the Patient Protection and Affordable Care Act of 2010 and the Paul Wellstone and Pete Domenici Mental Health Parity and Addiction Equity Act of 2008. Despite the potential these 2 acts held to improve the health care of adolescents and young adults (AYAs), including the financing of care, there are barriers to achieving this goal. In the first quarter of 2016, 13.7% of individuals 18 to 24 years of age still lacked health insurance. Limitations in the scope of benefits coverage and inadequate provider payment can curtail access to health care for AYAs, particularly care related to sexual and reproductive health and mental and behavioral health. Some health plans impose financial barriers to access because they require families to absorb high cost-sharing expenses (eg, deductibles, copayments, and coinsurance). Finally, challenges of confidentiality inherent in the billing and insurance claim practices of some health insurance plans can discourage access to health care in the absence of other obstacles and interfere with provision of confidential care. This policy statement summarizes the current state of impediments that AYA, including those with special health care needs, face in accessing timely and appropriate health care and that providers face in serving these patients.

These impediments include limited scope of benefits, high cost sharing, inadequate provider payment, and insufficient confidentiality protections. With this statement, we aim to improve both access to health care by AYAs and providers' delivery of developmentally appropriate health care for these patients through the presentation of an overview of the issues, specific recommendations for reform of health care financing for AYAs, and practical actions that pediatricians and other providers can take to advocate for appropriate payments for providing health care to AYAs. (11/18)

See full text on page 981.

http://pediatrics.aappublications.org/content/142/6/e20182998

THE TEEN DRIVER

Elizabeth M. Alderman, MD, FAAP, FSAHM; Brian D. Johnston, MD, MPH, FAAP; Committee on Adolescence; and Council on Injury, Violence, and Poison Prevention

ABSTRACT. For many teenagers, obtaining a driver's license is a rite of passage, conferring the ability to independently travel to school, work, or social events. However, immaturity, inexperience, and risky behavior put newly licensed teen drivers at risk. Motor vehicle crashes are the most common cause of mortality and injury for adolescents and young adults in developed countries. Teen drivers (15–19 years of age) have the highest rate of motor vehicle crashes among all age groups in the United States and contribute disproportionately to traffic fatalities. In addition to the deaths of teen drivers, more than half of 8- to 17-year-old children who die in car crashes are killed as passengers of drivers younger than 20 years of age. This policy statement, in which we update the previous 2006 iteration of this policy statement, is used to reflect new research on the risks faced by teen drivers and offer advice for pediatricians counseling teen drivers and their families. (9/18)

See full text on page 993.

http://pediatrics.aappublications.org/content/142/4/e20182163

TELEMEDICINE FOR EVALUATION OF RETINOPATHY OF PREMATURITY (TECHNICAL REPORT)

Walter M. Fierson, MD, FAAP; Antonio Capone Jr, MD; and Section on Ophthalmology (joint with American Academy of Ophthalmology and American Association of Certified Orthoptists)

ABSTRACT. Retinopathy of prematurity (ROP) remains a significant threat to vision for extremely premature infants despite the availability of therapeutic modalities capable, in most cases, of managing this disorder. It has been shown in many controlled trials that application of therapies at the appropriate time is essential to successful outcomes in premature infants affected by ROP. Bedside binocular indirect ophthalmoscopy has been the standard technique for diagnosis and monitoring of ROP in these patients. However, implementation of routine use of this screening method for at-risk premature infants has presented challenges within our existing care systems, including relative local scarcity of qualified ophthalmologist examiners in some locations and the remote location of some NICUs. Modern technology, including the development of wide-angle ocular digital fundus photography, coupled with the ability to send digital images electronically to remote locations, has led to the development of telemedicine-based remote digital fundus imaging (RDFI-TM) evaluation techniques. These techniques have the potential to allow the diagnosis and monitoring of ROP to occur in lieu of the necessity for some repeated on-site examinations in NICUs. This report reviews the currently available literature on RDFI-TM evaluations for ROP and outlines pertinent practical and risk management considerations that should be used when including RDFI-TM in any new or existing ROP care structure. (12/14)

http://pediatrics.aappublications.org/content/135/1/e238

TELEMEDICINE: PEDIATRIC APPLICATIONS (TECHNICAL REPORT)

Bryan L. Burke Jr, MD, FAAP; R. W. Hall, MD, FAAP; and Section on Telehealth Care

ABSTRACT. Telemedicine is a technological tool that is improving the health of children around the world. This report chronicles the use of telemedicine by pediatricians and pediatric medical and surgical specialists to deliver inpatient and outpatient care, educate physicians and patients, and conduct medical research. It also describes the importance of telemedicine in responding to emergencies and disasters and providing access to pediatric care to remote and underserved populations. Barriers to telemedicine expansion are explained, such as legal issues, inadequate payment for services, technology costs and sustainability, and the lack of technology infrastructure on a national scale. Although certain challenges have constrained more widespread implementation, telemedicine's current use bears testimony to its effectiveness and potential. Telemedicine's widespread adoption will be influenced by the implementation of key provisions of the Patient Protection and Affordable Care Act, technological advances, and growing patient demand for virtual visits. (6/15)

http://pediatrics.aappublications.org/content/136/1/e293

TESTING FOR DRUGS OF ABUSE IN CHILDREN AND ADOLESCENTS (CLINICAL REPORT)

Sharon Levy, MD, MPH, FAAP; Lorena M. Siqueira, MD, MSPH, FAAP; and Committee on Substance Abuse

ABSTRACT. Drug testing is often used as part of an assessment for substance use in children and adolescents. However, the indications for drug testing and guidance on how to use this procedure effectively are not clear. The complexity and invasiveness of the procedure and limitations to the information derived from drug testing all affect its utility. The objective of this clinical report is to provide guidance to pediatricians and other clinicians on the efficacy and efficient use of drug testing on the basis of a review of the nascent scientific literature, policy guidelines, and published clinical recommendations. (5/14)

http://pediatrics.aappublications.org/content/133/6/e1798

TOWARD TRANSPARENT CLINICAL POLICIES

Steering Committee on Quality Improvement and Management

ABSTRACT. Clinical policies of professional societies such as the American Academy of Pediatrics are valued highly, not only by clinicians who provide direct health care to children but also by many others who rely on the professional expertise of these organizations, including parents, employers, insurers, and legislators. The utility of a policy depends, in large part, on the degree to which its purpose and basis are clear to policy users, an attribute known as the policy's transparency. This statement describes the critical importance and special value of transparency in clinical policies, guidelines, and recommendations; helps identify obstacles to achieving transparency; and suggests several approaches to overcome these obstacles. (3/08, reaffirmed 2/14)

http://pediatrics.aappublications.org/content/121/3/643

TRAMPOLINE SAFETY IN CHILDHOOD AND ADOLESCENCE

Council on Sports Medicine and Fitness

ABSTRACT. Despite previous recommendations from the American Academy of Pediatrics discouraging home use of trampolines, recreational use of trampolines in the home setting continues to be a popular activity among children and adolescents. This policy statement is an update to previous statements, reflecting the current literature on prevalence, patterns, and mechanisms of trampoline-related injuries. Most trampoline injuries occur with multiple simultaneous users on the mat. Cervical spine injuries often occur with falls off the trampoline

or with attempts at somersaults or flips. Studies on the efficacy of trampoline safety measures are reviewed, and although there is a paucity of data, current implementation of safety measures have not appeared to mitigate risk substantially. Therefore, the home use of trampolines is strongly discouraged. The role of trampoline as a competitive sport and in structured training settings is reviewed, and recommendations for enhancing safety in these environments are made. (9/12, reaffirmed 7/15)
http://pediatrics.aappublications.org/content/130/4/774

THE TRANSFER OF DRUGS AND THERAPEUTICS INTO HUMAN BREAST MILK: AN UPDATE ON SELECTED TOPICS (CLINICAL REPORT)

Hari Cheryl Sachs, MD, FAAP, and Committee on Drugs
ABSTRACT. Many mothers are inappropriately advised to discontinue breastfeeding or avoid taking essential medications because of fears of adverse effects on their infants. This cautious approach may be unnecessary in many cases, because only a small proportion of medications are contraindicated in breastfeeding mothers or associated with adverse effects on their infants. Information to inform physicians about the extent of excretion for a particular drug into human milk is needed but may not be available. Previous statements on this topic from the American Academy of Pediatrics provided physicians with data concerning the known excretion of specific medications into breast milk. More current and comprehensive information is now available on the Internet, as well as an application for mobile devices, at LactMed (http://toxnet.nlm.nih.gov). Therefore, with the exception of radioactive compounds requiring temporary cessation of breastfeeding, the reader will be referred to LactMed to obtain the most current data on an individual medication. This report discusses several topics of interest surrounding lactation, such as the use of psychotropic therapies, drugs to treat substance abuse, narcotics, galactagogues, and herbal products, as well as immunization of breastfeeding women. A discussion regarding the global implications of maternal medications and lactation in the developing world is beyond the scope of this report. The World Health Organization offers several programs and resources that address the importance of breastfeeding (see http://www.who.int/topics/breastfeeding/en/). (8/13, reaffirmed 5/18)
http://pediatrics.aappublications.org/content/132/3/e796

TRANSITIONING HIV-INFECTED YOUTH INTO ADULT HEALTH CARE

Committee on Pediatric AIDS
ABSTRACT. With advances in antiretroviral therapy, most HIV-infected children survive into adulthood. Optimal health care for these youth includes a formal plan for the transition of care from primary and/or subspecialty pediatric/adolescent/family medicine health care providers (medical home) to adult health care provider(s). Successful transition involves the early engagement and participation of the youth and his or her family with the pediatric medical home and adult health care teams in developing a formal plan. Referring providers should have a written policy for the transfer of HIV-infected youth to adult care, which will guide in the development of an individualized plan for each youth. The plan should be introduced to the youth in early adolescence and modified as the youth approaches transition. Assessment of developmental milestones is important to define the readiness of the youth in assuming responsibility for his or her own care before initiating the transfer. Communication among all providers is essential and should include both personal contact and a written medical summary. Progress toward the transition should be tracked and, once completed, should be documented and assessed. (6/13, reaffirmed 4/16)
http://pediatrics.aappublications.org/content/132/1/192

TRANSPORTING CHILDREN WITH SPECIAL HEALTH CARE NEEDS

Committee on Injury and Poison Prevention
ABSTRACT. Children with special health care needs should have access to proper resources for safe transportation. This statement reviews important considerations for transporting children with special health care needs and provides current guidelines for the protection of children with specific health care needs, including those with a tracheostomy, a spica cast, challenging behaviors, or muscle tone abnormalities as well as those transported in wheelchairs. (10/99, reaffirmed 1/03, 1/06, 3/13)
http://pediatrics.aappublications.org/content/104/4/988

THE TREATMENT OF NEUROLOGICALLY IMPAIRED CHILDREN USING PATTERNING

Committee on Children With Disabilities
ABSTRACT. This statement reviews patterning as a treatment for children with neurologic impairments. This treatment is based on an outmoded and oversimplified theory of brain development. Current information does not support the claims of proponents that this treatment is efficacious, and its use continues to be unwarranted. (11/99, reaffirmed 11/02, 1/06, 8/10, 4/14, 5/18)
http://pediatrics.aappublications.org/content/104/5/1149

ULTRAVIOLET RADIATION: A HAZARD TO CHILDREN AND ADOLESCENTS

Council on Environmental Health and Section on Dermatology
ABSTRACT. Ultraviolet radiation (UVR) causes the 3 major forms of skin cancer: basal cell carcinoma; squamous cell carcinoma; and cutaneous malignant melanoma. Public awareness of the risk is not optimal, overall compliance with sun protection is inconsistent, and melanoma rates continue to rise. The risk of skin cancer increases when people overexpose themselves to sun and intentionally expose themselves to artificial sources of UVR. Yet, people continue to sunburn, and teenagers and adults alike remain frequent visitors to tanning parlors. Pediatricians should provide advice about UVR exposure during health-supervision visits and at other relevant times. Advice includes avoiding sunburning, wearing clothing and hats, timing activities (when possible) before or after periods of peak sun exposure, wearing protective sunglasses, and applying and reapplying sunscreen. Advice should be framed in the context of promoting outdoor physical activity. Adolescents should be strongly discouraged from visiting tanning parlors. Sun exposure and vitamin D status are intertwined. Cutaneous vitamin D production requires sunlight exposure, and many factors, such as skin pigmentation, season, and time of day, complicate efficiency of cutaneous vitamin D production that results from sun exposure. Adequate vitamin D is needed for bone health. Accumulating information suggests a beneficial influence of vitamin D on many health conditions. Although vitamin D is available through the diet, supplements, and incidental sun exposure, many children have low vitamin D concentrations. Ensuring vitamin D adequacy while promoting sun-protection strategies will require renewed attention to children's use of dietary and supplemental vitamin D. (2/11, reaffirmed 9/16)
http://pediatrics.aappublications.org/content/127/3/588

ULTRAVIOLET RADIATION: A HAZARD TO CHILDREN AND ADOLESCENTS (TECHNICAL REPORT)

Sophie J. Balk, MD; Council on Environmental Health; and Section on Dermatology
ABSTRACT. Sunlight sustains life on earth. Sunlight is essential for vitamin D synthesis in the skin. The sun's ultraviolet rays can be hazardous, however, because excessive exposure causes skin cancer and other adverse health effects. Skin cancer is a major

public health problem; more than 2 million new cases are diagnosed in the United States each year. Ultraviolet radiation (UVR) causes the 3 major forms of skin cancer: basal cell carcinoma; squamous cell carcinoma; and cutaneous malignant melanoma. Exposure to UVR from sunlight and artificial sources early in life elevates the risk of developing skin cancer. Approximately 25% of sun exposure occurs before 18 years of age. The risk of skin cancer is increased when people overexpose themselves to sun and intentionally expose themselves to artificial sources of UVR. Public awareness of the risk is not optimal, compliance with sun protection is inconsistent, and skin-cancer rates continue to rise in all age groups including the younger population. People continue to sunburn, and teenagers and adults are frequent visitors to tanning parlors. Sun exposure and vitamin D status are intertwined. Adequate vitamin D is needed for bone health in children and adults. In addition, there is accumulating information suggesting a beneficial influence of vitamin D on various health conditions. Cutaneous vitamin D production requires sunlight, and many factors complicate the efficiency of vitamin D production that results from sunlight exposure. Ensuring vitamin D adequacy while promoting sun-protection strategies, therefore, requires renewed attention to evaluating the adequacy of dietary and supplemental vitamin D. Daily intake of 400 IU of vitamin D will prevent vitamin D deficiency rickets in infants. The vitamin D supplementation amounts necessary to support optimal health in older children and adolescents are less clear. This report updates information on the relationship of sun exposure to skin cancer and other adverse health effects, the relationship of exposure to artificial sources of UVR and skin cancer, sun-protection methods, vitamin D, community skin-cancer–prevention efforts, and the pediatrician's role in preventing skin cancer. In addition to pediatricians' efforts, a sustained public health effort is needed to change attitudes and behaviors regarding UVR exposure. (2/11, reaffirmed 9/16)
http://pediatrics.aappublications.org/content/127/3/e791

UMBILICAL CORD CARE IN THE NEWBORN INFANT (CLINICAL REPORT)

*Dan Stewart, MD, FAAP; William Benitz, MD, FAAP; and
Committee on Fetus and Newborn*

ABSTRACT. Postpartum infections remain a leading cause of neonatal morbidity and mortality worldwide. A high percentage of these infections may stem from bacterial colonization of the umbilicus, because cord care practices vary in reflection of cultural traditions within communities and disparities in health care practices globally. After birth, the devitalized umbilical cord often proves to be an ideal substrate for bacterial growth and also provides direct access to the bloodstream of the neonate. Bacterial colonization of the cord not infrequently leads to omphalitis and associated thrombophlebitis, cellulitis, or necrotizing fasciitis. Various topical substances continue to be used for cord care around the world to mitigate the risk of serious infection. More recently, particularly in high-resource countries, the treatment paradigm has shifted toward dry umbilical cord care. This clinical report reviews the evidence underlying recommendations for care of the umbilical cord in different clinical settings. (8/16)
http://pediatrics.aappublications.org/content/138/3/e20162149

UNDERINSURANCE OF ADOLESCENTS: RECOMMENDATIONS FOR IMPROVED COVERAGE OF PREVENTIVE, REPRODUCTIVE, AND BEHAVIORAL HEALTH CARE SERVICES

Committee on Adolescence and Committee on Child Health Financing

ABSTRACT. The purpose of this policy statement is to address the serious underinsurance (ie, insurance that exists but is inadequate) problems affecting insured adolescents' access to needed preventive, reproductive, and behavioral health care. In addition, the statement addresses provider payment problems that disproportionately affect clinicians who care for adolescents.

Among adolescents with insurance, particularly private health insurance, coverage of needed services is often inadequate. Benefits are typically limited in scope and amount; certain diagnoses are often excluded; and cost-sharing requirements are often too high. As a result, underinsurance represents a substantial problem among adolescents and adversely affects their health and well-being.

In addition to underinsurance problems, payment problems in the form of inadequate payment, uncompensated care for confidential reproductive services, and the failure of insurers to recognize and pay for certain billing and diagnostic codes are widespread among both private and public insurers. Payment problems negatively affect clinicians' ability to offer needed services to adolescents, especially publicly insured adolescents. (12/08, reaffirmed 8/12, 5/15)
http://pediatrics.aappublications.org/content/123/1/191

UNDERSTANDING THE BEHAVIORAL AND EMOTIONAL CONSEQUENCES OF CHILD ABUSE (CLINICAL REPORT)

*John Stirling Jr, MD; Committee on Child Abuse and Neglect; and
Section on Adoption and Foster Care (joint with Lisa Amaya-
Jackson, MD, MPH; American Academy of Child and Adolescent
Psychiatry; and National Center for Child Traumatic Stress)*

ABSTRACT. Children who have suffered early abuse or neglect may later present with significant behavior problems including emotional instability, depression, and a tendency to be aggressive or violent with others. Troublesome behaviors may persist long after the abusive or neglectful environment has changed or the child has been in foster care placement. Neurobiological research has shown that early abuse results in an altered physiological response to stressful stimuli, a response that deleteriously affects the child's subsequent socialization. Pediatricians can assist caregivers by helping them recognize the abused or neglected child's altered responses, formulate more effective coping strategies, and mobilize available community resources. (9/08, reaffirmed 8/12)
http://pediatrics.aappublications.org/content/122/3/667

UPDATE OF NEWBORN SCREENING AND THERAPY FOR CONGENITAL HYPOTHYROIDISM (CLINICAL REPORT)

*Susan R. Rose, MD; Section on Endocrinology; and Committee on
Genetics (joint with Rosalind S. Brown, MD; American Thyroid
Association; and Lawson Wilkins Pediatric Endocrine Society)*

ABSTRACT. Unrecognized congenital hypothyroidism leads to mental retardation. Newborn screening and thyroid therapy started within 2 weeks of age can normalize cognitive development. The primary thyroid-stimulating hormone screening has become standard in many parts of the world. However, newborn thyroid screening is not yet universal in some countries. Initial dosage of 10 to 15 µg/kg levothyroxine is recommended. The goals of thyroid hormone therapy should be to maintain frequent evaluations of total thyroxine or free thyroxine in the upper half of the reference range during the first 3 years of life and to normalize the serum thyroid-stimulating hormone concentration to ensure optimal thyroid hormone dosage and compliance.

Improvements in screening and therapy have led to improved developmental outcomes in adults with congenital hypothyroidism who are now in their 20s and 30s. Thyroid hormone regimens used today are more aggressive in targeting early correction of thyroid-stimulating hormone than were those used 20 or even 10 years ago. Thus, newborn infants with congenital hypothyroidism today may have an even better intellectual and neurologic prognosis. Efforts are ongoing to establish the optimal therapy that leads to maximum potential for normal development for infants with congenital hypothyroidism.

Remaining controversy centers on infants whose abnormality in neonatal thyroid function is transient or mild and on optimal care of very low birth weight or preterm infants. Of note, thyroid-stimulating hormone is not elevated in central hypothyroidism. An algorithm is proposed for diagnosis and management.

Physicians must not relinquish their clinical judgment and experience in the face of normal newborn thyroid test results. Hypothyroidism can be acquired after the newborn screening. When clinical symptoms and signs suggest hypothyroidism, regardless of newborn screening results, serum free thyroxine and thyroid-stimulating hormone determinations should be performed. (6/06, reaffirmed 12/11)
http://pediatrics.aappublications.org/content/117/6/2290

UPDATED GUIDANCE FOR PALIVIZUMAB PROPHYLAXIS AMONG INFANTS AND YOUNG CHILDREN AT INCREASED RISK OF HOSPITALIZATION FOR RESPIRATORY SYNCYTIAL VIRUS INFECTION

Committee on Infectious Diseases and Bronchiolitis Guidelines Committee

ABSTRACT. Palivizumab was licensed in June 1998 by the Food and Drug Administration for the reduction of serious lower respiratory tract infection caused by respiratory syncytial virus (RSV) in children at increased risk of severe disease. Since that time, the American Academy of Pediatrics has updated its guidance for the use of palivizumab 4 times as additional data became available to provide a better understanding of infants and young children at greatest risk of hospitalization attributable to RSV infection. The updated recommendations in this policy statement reflect new information regarding the seasonality of RSV circulation, palivizumab pharmacokinetics, the changing incidence of bronchiolitis hospitalizations, the effect of gestational age and other risk factors on RSV hospitalization rates, the mortality of children hospitalized with RSV infection, the effect of prophylaxis on wheezing, and palivizumab-resistant RSV isolates. (7/14)
http://pediatrics.aappublications.org/content/134/2/415

UPDATED GUIDANCE FOR PALIVIZUMAB PROPHYLAXIS AMONG INFANTS AND YOUNG CHILDREN AT INCREASED RISK OF HOSPITALIZATION FOR RESPIRATORY SYNCYTIAL VIRUS INFECTION (TECHNICAL REPORT)

Committee on Infectious Diseases and Bronchiolitis Guidelines Committee

ABSTRACT. Guidance from the American Academy of Pediatrics (AAP) for the use of palivizumab prophylaxis against respiratory syncytial virus (RSV) was first published in a policy statement in 1998. Guidance initially was based on the result from a single randomized, placebo-controlled clinical trial conducted in 1996–1997 describing an overall reduction in RSV hospitalization rate from 10.6% among placebo recipients to 4.8% among children who received prophylaxis. The results of a second randomized, placebo-controlled trial of children with hemodynamically significant heart disease were published in 2003 and revealed a reduction in RSV hospitalization rate from 9.7% in control subjects to 5.3% among prophylaxis recipients. Because no additional controlled trials regarding efficacy were published, AAP guidance has been updated periodically to reflect the most recent literature regarding children at greatest risk of severe disease. Since the last update in 2012, new data have become available regarding the seasonality of RSV circulation, palivizumab pharmacokinetics, the changing incidence of bronchiolitis hospitalizations, the effects of gestational age and other risk factors on

RSV hospitalization rates, the mortality of children hospitalized with RSV infection, and the effect of prophylaxis on wheezing and palivizumab-resistant RSV isolates. These data enable further refinement of AAP guidance to most clearly focus on those children at greatest risk. (7/14)
http://pediatrics.aappublications.org/content/134/2/e620

THE USE AND MISUSE OF FRUIT JUICE IN PEDIATRICS

Committee on Nutrition

ABSTRACT. Historically, fruit juice was recommended by pediatricians as a source of vitamin C and an extra source of water for healthy infants and young children as their diets expanded to include solid foods with higher renal solute. Fruit juice is marketed as a healthy, natural source of vitamins and, in some instances, calcium. Because juice tastes good, children readily accept it. Although juice consumption has some benefits, it also has potential detrimental effects. Pediatricians need to be knowledgeable about juice to inform parents and patients on its appropriate uses. (5/01, reaffirmed 10/06, 8/13)
http://pediatrics.aappublications.org/content/107/5/1210

USE OF CHAPERONES DURING THE PHYSICAL EXAMINATION OF THE PEDIATRIC PATIENT

Committee on Practice and Ambulatory Medicine

ABSTRACT. Physicians should always communicate the scope and nature of the physical examination to be performed to the pediatric patient and his or her parent. This statement addresses the use of chaperones and issues of patient comfort, confidentiality, and privacy. The use of a chaperone should be a shared decision between the patient and physician. In some states, the use of a chaperone is mandated by state regulations. (4/11, 11/17)
http://pediatrics.aappublications.org/content/127/5/991

USE OF INHALED NITRIC OXIDE IN PRETERM INFANTS (CLINICAL REPORT)

Praveen Kumar, MD, FAAP, and Committee on Fetus and Newborn

ABSTRACT. Nitric oxide, an important signaling molecule with multiple regulatory effects throughout the body, is an important tool for the treatment of full-term and late-preterm infants with persistent pulmonary hypertension of the newborn and hypoxemic respiratory failure. Several randomized controlled trials have evaluated its role in the management of preterm infants ≤34 weeks' gestational age with varying results. The purpose of this clinical report is to summarize the existing evidence for the use of inhaled nitric oxide in preterm infants and provide guidance regarding its use in this population. (12/13)
http://pediatrics.aappublications.org/content/133/1/164

USE OF PERFORMANCE-ENHANCING SUBSTANCES (CLINICAL REPORT)

Michele LaBotz, MD, FAAP; Bernard A. Griesemer, MD, FAAP; and Council on Sports Medicine and Fitness

ABSTRACT. Performance-enhancing substances (PESs) are used commonly by children and adolescents in attempts to improve athletic performance. More recent data reveal that these same substances often are used for appearance-related reasons as well. PESs include both legal over-the-counter dietary supplements and illicit pharmacologic agents. This report reviews the current epidemiology of PES use in the pediatric population, as well as information on those PESs in most common use. Concerns regarding use of legal PESs include high rates of product contamination, correlation with future use of anabolic androgenic steroids, and adverse effects on the focus and experience of youth sports participation. The physical maturation and endogenous hormone production that occur in adolescence are associated with large improvements in strength and athletic performance. For most young athletes, PES use does not produce significant

gains over those seen with the onset of puberty and adherence to an appropriate nutrition and training program. (6/16)
http://pediatrics.aappublications.org/content/138/1/e20161300

USE OF SOY PROTEIN-BASED FORMULAS IN INFANT FEEDING (CLINICAL REPORT)

Jatinder Bhatia, MD; Frank Greer, MD; and Committee on Nutrition
ABSTRACT. Soy protein-based formulas have been available for almost 100 years. Since the first use of soy formula as a milk substitute for an infant unable to tolerate a cow milk protein-based formula, the formulation has changed to the current soy protein isolate. Despite very limited indications for its use, soy protein-based formulas in the United States may account for nearly 25% of the formula market. This report reviews the limited indications and contraindications of soy formulas. It will also review the potential harmful effects of soy protein-based formulas and the phytoestrogens contained in these formulas. (5/08)
http://pediatrics.aappublications.org/content/121/5/1062

THE USE OF SYSTEMIC AND TOPICAL FLUOROQUINOLONES (CLINICAL REPORT)

Mary Anne Jackson, MD, FAAP; Gordon E. Schutze, MD, FAAP; and Committee on Infectious Diseases
ABSTRACT. Appropriate prescribing practices for fluoroquinolones, as well as all antimicrobial agents, are essential as evolving resistance patterns are considered, additional treatment indications are identified, and the toxicity profile of fluoroquinolones in children has become better defined. Earlier recommendations for systemic therapy remain; expanded uses of fluoroquinolones for the treatment of certain infections are outlined in this report. Prescribing clinicians should be aware of specific adverse reactions associated with fluoroquinolones, and their use in children should continue to be limited to the treatment of infections for which no safe and effective alternative exists or in situations in which oral fluoroquinolone treatment represents a reasonable alternative to parenteral antimicrobial therapy. (10/16)
http://pediatrics.aappublications.org/content/138/5/e20162706

THE USE OF TELEMEDICINE TO ADDRESS ACCESS AND PHYSICIAN WORKFORCE SHORTAGES

Committee on Pediatric Workforce
ABSTRACT. The use of telemedicine technologies by primary care pediatricians, pediatric medical subspecialists, and pediatric surgical specialists (henceforth referred to as "pediatric physicians") has the potential to transform the practice of pediatrics. The purpose of this policy statement is to describe the expected and potential impact that telemedicine will have on pediatric physicians' efforts to improve access and physician workforce shortages. The policy statement also describes how the American Academy of Pediatrics can advocate for its members and their patients to best use telemedicine technologies to improve access to care, provide more patient- and family-centered care, increase efficiencies in practice, enhance the quality of care, and address projected shortages in the clinical workforce. As the use of telemedicine increases, it is likely to impact health care access, quality, and education and costs of care. Telemedicine technologies, applied to the medical home and its collaborating providers, have the potential to improve current models of care by increasing communication among clinicians, resulting in more efficient, higher quality, and less expensive care. Such a model can serve as a platform for providing more continuous care, linking primary and specialty care to support management of the needs of complex patients. In addition, telemedicine technologies can be used to efficiently provide pediatric physicians working in remote locations with ongoing medical education, increasing their ability to care for more complex patients in their community, reducing the burdens of travel on patients and families, and supporting the medical home. On the other hand, telemedicine technologies used for episodic care by nonmedical home providers have the potential to disrupt continuity of care and to create redundancy and imprudent use of health care resources. Fragmentation should be avoided, and telemedicine, like all primary and specialty services, should be coordinated through the medical home. (6/15)
http://pediatrics.aappublications.org/content/136/1/202

VENTRICULAR FIBRILLATION AND THE USE OF AUTOMATED EXTERNAL DEFIBRILLATORS ON CHILDREN

Committee on Pediatric Emergency Medicine and Section on Cardiology and Cardiac Surgery
ABSTRACT. The use of automated external defibrillators (AEDs) has been advocated in recent years as one part of the chain of survival to improve outcomes for adult cardiac arrest victims. When AEDs first entered the market, they had not been tested for pediatric usage and rhythm interpretation. In addition, the presumption was that children do not experience ventricular fibrillation, so they would not benefit from the use of AEDs. Recent literature has shown that children do experience ventricular fibrillation, which has a better outcome than do other cardiac arrest rhythms. At the same time, the arrhythmia software on AEDs has become more extensive and validated for children, and attenuation devices have become available to downregulate the energy delivered by AEDs to allow their use on children. Pediatricians are now being asked whether AED programs should be implemented, and where they are being implemented, pediatricians are being asked to provide guidance on the use of them on children. As AED programs expand, pediatricians must advocate on behalf of children so that their needs are accounted for. For pediatricians to be able to provide guidance and ensure that children are included in AED programs, it is important for pediatricians to know how AEDs work, be up-to-date on the literature regarding pediatric fibrillation and energy delivery, and understand the role of AEDs as life-saving interventions for children. (11/07, reaffirmed 6/11, 7/14)
http://pediatrics.aappublications.org/content/120/5/1159

VIRTUAL VIOLENCE

Council on Communications and Media
ABSTRACT. In the United States, exposure to media violence is becoming an inescapable component of children's lives. With the rise in new technologies, such as tablets and new gaming platforms, children and adolescents increasingly are exposed to what is known as "virtual violence." This form of violence is not experienced physically; rather, it is experienced in realistic ways via new technology and ever more intense and realistic games. The American Academy of Pediatrics continues to be concerned about children's exposure to virtual violence and the effect it has on their overall health and well-being. This policy statement aims to summarize the current state of scientific knowledge regarding the effects of virtual violence on children's attitudes and behaviors and to make specific recommendations for pediatricians, parents, industry, and policy makers. (7/16)
http://pediatrics.aappublications.org/content/138/2/e20161298

VISUAL SYSTEM ASSESSMENT IN INFANTS, CHILDREN, AND YOUNG ADULTS BY PEDIATRICIANS

Committee on Practice and Ambulatory Medicine and Section on Ophthalmology (joint with American Association of Certified Orthoptists, American Association for Pediatric Ophthalmology and Strabismus, and American Academy of Ophthalmology)
ABSTRACT. Appropriate visual assessments help identify children who may benefit from early interventions to correct or improve vision. Examination of the eyes and visual system should begin in the nursery and continue throughout both childhood and adolescence during routine well-child visits

in the medical home. Newborn infants should be examined using inspection and red reflex testing to detect structural ocular abnormalities, such as cataract, corneal opacity, and ptosis. Instrument-based screening, if available, should be first attempted between 12 months and 3 years of age and at annual well-child visits until acuity can be tested directly. Direct testing of visual acuity can often begin by 4 years of age, using age-appropriate symbols (optotypes). Children found to have an ocular abnormality or who fail a vision assessment should be referred to a pediatric ophthalmologist or an eye care specialist appropriately trained to treat pediatric patients. (12/15)
http://pediatrics.aappublications.org/content/137/1/e20153596

WIC PROGRAM
Provisional Section on Breastfeeding
ABSTRACT. This policy statement highlights the important collaboration between pediatricians and local Special Supplemental Nutrition Program for Women, Infants, and Children (WIC) programs to ensure that infants and children receive high-quality, cost-effective health care and nutrition services. Specific recommendations are provided for pediatricians and WIC personnel to help children and their families receive optimum services through a medical home. (11/01)
http://pediatrics.aappublications.org/content/108/5/1216

WITHHOLDING OR TERMINATION OF RESUSCITATION IN PEDIATRIC OUT-OF-HOSPITAL TRAUMATIC CARDIOPULMONARY ARREST
Committee on Pediatric Emergency Medicine (joint with American College of Surgeons Committee on Trauma and National Association of EMS Physicians)
ABSTRACT. This multiorganizational literature review was undertaken to provide an evidence base for determining whether recommendations for out-of-hospital termination of resuscitation could be made for children who are victims of traumatic cardiopulmonary arrest. Although there is increasing acceptance of out-of-hospital termination of resuscitation for adult traumatic cardiopulmonary arrest when there is no expectation of a good outcome, children are routinely excluded from state termination-of-resuscitation protocols. The decision to withhold resuscitative efforts in a child under specific circumstances (decapitation or dependent lividity, rigor mortis, etc) is reasonable. If there is any doubt as to the circumstances or timing of the traumatic cardiopulmonary arrest, under the current status of limiting termination of resuscitation in the field to persons older than 18 years in most states, resuscitation should be initiated and continued until arrival to the appropriate facility. If the patient has arrested, resuscitation has already exceeded 30 minutes, and the nearest facility is more than 30 minutes away, involvement of parents and family of these children in the decision-making process with assistance and guidance from medical professionals should be considered as part of an emphasis on family-centered care because the evidence suggests that either death or a poor outcome is inevitable. (3/14)
http://pediatrics.aappublications.org/content/133/4/e1104

YEAR 2007 POSITION STATEMENT: PRINCIPLES AND GUIDELINES FOR EARLY HEARING DETECTION AND INTERVENTION PROGRAMS
Joint Committee on Infant Hearing
ABSTRACT. The Joint Committee on Infant Hearing (JCIH) endorses early detection of and intervention for infants with hearing loss. The goal of early hearing detection and intervention (EHDI) is to maximize linguistic competence and literacy development for children who are deaf or hard of hearing. Without appropriate opportunities to learn language, these children will fall behind their hearing peers in communication, cognition, reading, and social-emotional development. Such delays may result in lower educational and employment levels in adulthood. To maximize the outcome for infants who are deaf or hard of hearing, the hearing of all infants should be screened at no later than 1 month of age. Those who do not pass screening should have a comprehensive audiological evaluation at no later than 3 months of age. Infants with confirmed hearing loss should receive appropriate intervention at no later than 6 months of age from health care and education professionals with expertise in hearing loss and deafness in infants and young children. Regardless of previous hearing-screening outcomes, all infants with or without risk factors should receive ongoing surveillance of communicative development beginning at 2 months of age during well-child visits in the medical home. EHDI systems should guarantee seamless transitions for infants and their families through this process. (10/07)
http://pediatrics.aappublications.org/content/120/4/898

YOUTH PARTICIPATION AND INJURY RISK IN MARTIAL ARTS (CLINICAL REPORT)
Rebecca A. Demorest, MD, FAAP; Chris Koutures, MD, FAAP; and Council on Sports Medicine and Fitness
ABSTRACT. The martial arts can provide children and adolescents with vigorous levels of physical exercise that can improve overall physical fitness. The various types of martial arts encompass noncontact basic forms and techniques that may have a lower relative risk of injury. Contact-based sparring with competitive training and bouts have a higher risk of injury. This clinical report describes important techniques and movement patterns in several types of martial arts and reviews frequently reported injuries encountered in each discipline, with focused discussions of higher risk activities. Some of these higher risk activities include blows to the head and choking or submission movements that may cause concussions or significant head injuries. The roles of rule changes, documented benefits of protective equipment, and changes in training recommendations in attempts to reduce injury are critically assessed. This information is intended to help pediatric health care providers counsel patients and families in encouraging safe participation in martial arts. (11/16)
http://pediatrics.aappublications.org/content/138/6/e20163022

Section 6

Endorsed Policies

· · · · · · · · · · · · · · · · · · ·

The American Academy of Pediatrics endorses
and accepts as its policy the following
documents from other organizations.

AMERICAN ACADEMY OF PEDIATRICS
Endorsed Policies

2015 SPCTPD/ACC/AAP/AHA TRAINING GUIDELINES FOR PEDIATRIC CARDIOLOGY FELLOWSHIP PROGRAMS (REVISION OF THE 2005 TRAINING GUIDELINES FOR PEDIATRIC CARDIOLOGY FELLOWSHIP PROGRAMS)
Robert D. Ross, MD, FAAP, FACC; Michael Brook, MD; Jeffrey A. Feinstein, MD; et al (8/15)

INTRODUCTION
Robert D. Ross, MD, FAAP, FACC; Michael Brook, MD; Peter Koenig, MD, FACC, FASE; et al (8/15)

TASK FORCE 1: GENERAL CARDIOLOGY
Alan B. Lewis, MD, FAAP, FACC; Gerard R. Martin, MD, FAAP, FACC, FAHA; Peter J. Bartz, MD, FASE; et al (8/15)

TASK FORCE 2: NONINVASIVE CARDIAC IMAGING
Shubhika Srivastava, MBBS, FAAP, FACC, FASE; Beth F. Printz, MD, PhD, FAAP, FASE; Tal Geva, MD, FACC; et al (8/15)

TASK FORCE 3: CARDIAC CATHETERIZATION
Laurie B. Armsby, MD, FAAP, FSCAI; Robert N. Vincent, MD, CM, FACC, FSCAI; Susan R. Foerster, MD, FSCAI; et al (8/15)

TASK FORCE 4: ELECTROPHYSIOLOGY
Anne M. Dubin, MD, FHRS; Edward P. Walsh, MD, FHRS; Wayne Franklin, MD, FAAP, FACC, FAHA; et al (8/15)

TASK FORCE 5: CRITICAL CARE CARDIOLOGY
Timothy F. Feltes, MD, FAAP, FACC, FAHA; Stephen J. Roth, MD, MPH, FAAP; Melvin C. Almodovar, MD; et al (8/15)

TASK FORCE 6: ADULT CONGENITAL HEART DISEASE
Karen Stout, MD, FACC; Anne Marie Valente, MD, FACC; Peter J. Bartz, MD, FASE; et al (8/15)

TASK FORCE 7: PULMONARY HYPERTENSION, ADVANCED HEART FAILURE, AND TRANSPLANTATION
Steven A. Webber, MB, ChB; Daphne T. Hsu, MD, FAAP, FACC, FAHA; D. Dunbar Ivy, MD, FAAP, FACC; et al (8/15)

TASK FORCE 8: RESEARCH AND SCHOLARLY ACTIVITY
William T. Mahle, MD, FAAP, FACC, FAHA; Anne M. Murphy, MD, FACC, FAHA; Jennifer S. Li, MD; et al (8/15)

ADVANCED PRACTICE REGISTERED NURSE: ROLE, PREPARATION, AND SCOPE OF PRACTICE
National Association of Neonatal Nurses

ABSTRACT. In recent years, the National Association of Neonatal Nurses (NANN) and the National Association of Neonatal Nurse Practitioners (NANNP) have developed several policy statements on neonatal advanced practice registered nurse (APRN) workforce, education, competency, fatigue, safety, and scope of practice. This position paper is a synthesis of previous efforts and discusses the role, preparation, and scope of practice of the neonatal APRN. (1/14)

ANTENATAL CORTICOSTEROID THERAPY FOR FETAL MATURATION
American College of Obstetricians and Gynecologists

ABSTRACT. Corticosteroid administration before anticipated preterm birth is one of the most important antenatal therapies available to improve newborn outcomes. A single course of corticosteroids is recommended for pregnant women between 24 0/7 weeks and 33 6/7 weeks of gestation who are at risk of preterm delivery within 7 days, including for those with ruptured membranes and multiple gestations. It also may be considered for pregnant women starting at 23 0/7 weeks of gestation who are at risk of preterm delivery within 7 days, based on a family's decision regarding resuscitation, irrespective of membrane rupture status and regardless of fetal number. Administration of betamethasone may be considered in pregnant women between 34 0/7 weeks and 36 6/7 weeks of gestation who are at risk of preterm birth within 7 days, and who have not received a previous course of antenatal corticosteroids. A single repeat course of antenatal corticosteroids should be considered in women who are less than 34 0/7 weeks of gestation who are at risk of preterm delivery within 7 days, and whose prior course of antenatal corticosteroids was administered more than 14 days previously. Rescue course corticosteroids could be provided as early as 7 days from the prior dose, if indicated by the clinical scenario. Continued surveillance of long-term outcomes after in utero corticosteroid exposure should be supported. Quality improvement strategies to optimize appropriate and timely antenatal corticosteroid administration are encouraged. (8/17)

APPROPRIATE USE CRITERIA FOR INITIAL TRANSTHORACIC ECHOCARDIOGRAPHY IN OUTPATIENT PEDIATRIC CARDIOLOGY
American College of Cardiology Appropriate Use Task Force

ABSTRACT. The American College of Cardiology (ACC) participated in a joint project with the American Society of Echocardiography, the Society of Pediatric Echocardiography, and several other subspecialty societies and organizations to establish and evaluate Appropriate Use Criteria (AUC) for the initial use of outpatient pediatric echocardiography. Assumptions for the AUC were identified, including the fact that all indications assumed a first-time transthoracic echocardiographic study in an outpatient setting for patients without previously known heart disease. The definitions for frequently used terminology in outpatient pediatric cardiology were established using published guidelines and standards and expert opinion. These AUC serve as a guide to help clinicians in the care of children with possible heart disease, specifically in terms of when a transthoracic echocardiogram is warranted as an initial diagnostic modality in the outpatient setting. They are also a useful tool for education and provide the infrastructure for future quality improvement initiatives as well as research in healthcare delivery, outcomes, and resource utilization.

To complete the AUC process, the writing group identified 113 indications based on common clinical scenarios and/or published clinical practice guidelines, and each indication was classified into 1 of 9 categories of common clinical presentations, including palpitations, syncope, chest pain, and murmur. A separate, independent rating panel evaluated each indication using a scoring scale of 1 to 9, thereby designating each indication as "Appropriate" (median score 7 to 9), "May Be Appropriate" (median score 4 to 6), or "Rarely Appropriate" (median score 1 to 3). Fifty-three indications were identified as Appropriate, 28 as May Be Appropriate, and 32 as Rarely Appropriate. (11/14)

BEST PRACTICE FOR INFANT SURGERY: A POSITION STATEMENT FROM THE AMERICAN PEDIATRIC SURGICAL ASSOCIATION

American Pediatric Surgical Association (9/08)

CARDIOVASCULAR RISK REDUCTION IN HIGH-RISK PEDIATRIC PATIENTS

American Heart Association

ABSTRACT. Although for most children the process of atherosclerosis is subclinical, dramatically accelerated atherosclerosis occurs in some pediatric disease states, with clinical coronary events occurring in childhood and very early adult life. As with most scientific statements about children and the future risk for cardiovascular disease, there are no randomized trials documenting the effects of risk reduction on hard clinical outcomes. A growing body of literature, however, identifies the importance of premature cardiovascular disease in the course of certain pediatric diagnoses and addresses the response to risk factor reduction. For this scientific statement, a panel of experts reviewed what is known about very premature cardiovascular disease in 8 high-risk pediatric diagnoses and, from the science base, developed practical recommendations for management of cardiovascular risk. (*Circulation.* 2006;114:2710–2738.) (12/06)

CHILDREN'S SURGERY VERIFICATION PILOT DRAFT DOCUMENTS

OPTIMAL RESOURCES FOR CHILDREN'S SURGICAL CARE—DRAFT

American College of Surgeons

EXECUTIVE SUMMARY. The Task Force for Children's Surgical Care, an ad hoc multidisciplinary group of invited leaders in relevant disciplines, assembled in Rosemont, IL, initially April 30—May 1, 2012, and subsequently in 2013 and 2014 to consider approaches to optimize the delivery of children's surgical care in today's competitive national healthcare environment. Specifically, a mismatch between individual patient needs and available clinical resources for some infants and children receiving surgical care is recognized as a problem in the U.S. and elsewhere. While this phenomenon is apparent to most practitioners involved with children's surgical care, comprehensive data are not available and relevant data are imperfect. The scope of this problem is unknown at present. However, it does periodically, and possibly systematically result in suboptimal patient outcomes. The composition of the Task Force is detailed above. Support was provided by the Children's Hospital Association (CHA) and the American College of Surgeons (ACS). The group represented key disciplines and perspectives. Published literature and data were utilized when available and expert opinion when not, as the basis for these recommendations. The objective was to develop consensus recommendations that would be of use to relevant policy makers and to providers. Principles regarding resource standards, quality improvement and safety processes, data collection and a verification process were initially published in March 2014 [*J Am Coll Surg* 2014;218(3):479-487]. This document details those principles in a specific manner designed to inform and direct a verification process to be conducted by the American College of Surgeons and the ACS Committee on Children's Surgery. (11/14)

HOSPITAL PREREVIEW QUESTIONNAIRE (PRQ)—DRAFT

American College of Surgeons (11/14)

COLLABORATION IN PRACTICE: IMPLEMENTING TEAM-BASED CARE

American College of Obstetricians and Gynecologists Task Force on Collaborative Practice

INTRODUCTION. Quality, efficiency, and value are necessary characteristics of our evolving health care system. Team-based care will work toward the Triple Aim of 1) improving the experience of care of individuals and families; 2) improving the health of populations; and 3) lowering per capita costs. It also should respond to emerging demands and reduce undue burdens on health care providers. Team-based care has the ability to more effectively meet the core expectations of the health care system proposed by the Institute of Medicine. These expectations require that care be safe, effective, patient centered, timely, efficient, and equitable. This report outlines a mechanism that all specialties and practices can use to achieve these expectations.

The report was written by the interprofessional Task Force on Collaborative Practice and is intended to appeal to multiple specialties (eg, internal medicine, pediatrics, family medicine, and women's health) and professions (eg, nurse practitioners, certified nurse–midwives/certified midwives, physician assistants, physicians, clinical pharmacists, and advanced practice registered nurses). This document provides a framework for organizations or practices across all specialties to develop team-based care. In doing so, it offers a map to help practices navigate the increasingly complex and continuously evolving health care system. The guidance presented is a result of the task force's work and is based on current evidence and expert consensus. The task force challenges and welcomes all medical specialties to gather additional data on how and what types of team-based care best accomplish the Triple Aim and the Institute of Medicine's expectations of health care. (3/16)

CONFIDENTIALITY PROTECTIONS FOR ADOLESCENTS AND YOUNG ADULTS IN THE HEALTH CARE BILLING AND INSURANCE CLAIMS PROCESS

Society for Adolescent Health and Medicine

ABSTRACT. The importance of protecting confidential health care for adolescents and young adults is well documented. State and federal confidentiality protections exist for both minors and young adults, although the laws vary among states, particularly for minors. However, such confidentiality is potentially violated by billing practices and in the processing of health insurance claims. To address this problem, policies and procedures should be established so that health care billing and insurance claims processes do not impede the ability of providers to deliver essential health care services on a confidential basis to adolescents and young adults covered as dependents on a family's health insurance plan. (3/16)

CONSENSUS COMMUNICATION ON EARLY PEANUT INTRODUCTION AND THE PREVENTION OF PEANUT ALLERGY IN HIGH-RISK INFANTS

Primary contributors: David M. Fleischer, MD; Scott Sicherer, MD; Matthew Greenhawt, MD; Dianne Campbell, MB BS, FRACP, PhD; Edmond Chan, MD; Antonella Muraro, MD, PhD; Susanne Halken, MD; Yitzhak Katz, MD; Motohiro Ebisawa, MD, PhD; Lawrence Eichenfield, MD; Hugh Sampson, MD; Gideon Lack, MB, BCh; and George Du Toit, MB, BCh

INTRODUCTION AND RATIONALE. Peanut allergy is an increasingly troubling global health problem affecting between 1% and 3% of children in many westernized countries. Although multiple methods of measurement have been used and specific estimates differ, there appears to have been a sudden increase in the number of cases in the past 10- to 15-year period, suggesting that the prevalence might have tripled in some countries, such as the United States. Extrapolating the currently estimated prevalence, this translates to nearly 100 000 new cases annually (in the United States and United Kingdom), affecting some 1 in 50 primary school-aged children in the United States, Canada, the United Kingdom, and Australia. A similar increase in incidence is now being noted in developing countries, such as Ghana.

The purpose of this brief communication is to highlight emerging evidence for existing allergy prevention guidelines regarding potential benefits of supporting early rather than delayed peanut introduction during the period of complementary food introduction in infants. A recent study entitled "Randomized trial of peanut consumption in infants at risk for peanut allergy" demonstrated a successful 11% to 25% absolute reduction in the risk of peanut allergy in high-risk infants (and a relative risk reduction of up to 80%) if peanut was introduced between 4 and 11 months of age. In light of the significance of these findings, this document serves to better inform the decision-making process for health care providers regarding such potential benefits of early peanut introduction. More formal guidelines regarding early-life, complementary feeding practices and the risk of allergy development will follow in the next year from the National Institute of Allergy and Infectious Diseases (NIAID)–sponsored Working Group and the European Academy of Allergy and Clinical Immunology (EAACI), and thus this document should be considered interim guidance. (8/15)

CONSENSUS STATEMENT: ABUSIVE HEAD TRAUMA IN INFANTS AND YOUNG CHILDREN

Arabinda Kumar Choudhary; Sabah Servaes; Thomas L. Slovis; Vincent J. Palusci; Gary L. Hedlund; Sandeep K. Narang; Joëlle Anne Moreno; Mark S. Dias; Cindy W. Christian; Marvin D. Nelson Jr; V. Michelle Silvera; Susan Palasis; Maria Raissaki; Andrea Rossi; and Amaka C. Offiah

ABSTRACT. Abusive head trauma (AHT) is the leading cause of fatal head injuries in children younger than 2 years. A multidisciplinary team bases this diagnosis on history, physical examination, imaging and laboratory findings. Because the etiology of the injury is multifactorial (shaking, shaking and impact, impact, etc.) the current best and inclusive term is AHT. There is no controversy concerning the medical validity of the existence of AHT, with multiple components including subdural hematoma, intracranial and spinal changes, complex retinal hemorrhages, and rib and other fractures that are inconsistent with the provided mechanism of trauma. The workup must exclude medical diseases that can mimic AHT. However, the courtroom has become a forum for speculative theories that cannot be reconciled with generally accepted medical literature. There is no reliable medical evidence that the following processes are causative in the constellation of injuries of AHT: cerebral sinovenous thrombosis, hypoxic-ischemic injury, lumbar puncture or dysphagic choking/vomiting. There is no substantiation, at a time remote from birth, that an asymptomatic birth-related subdural hemorrhage can result in rebleeding and sudden collapse. Further, a diagnosis of AHT is a medical conclusion, not a legal determination of the intent of the perpetrator or a diagnosis of murder. We hope that this consensus document reduces confusion by recommending to judges and jurors the tools necessary to distinguish genuine evidence-based opinions of the relevant medical community from legal arguments or etiological speculations that are unwarranted by the clinical findings, medical evidence and evidence-based literature. (5/18)

CONSENSUS STATEMENT: DEFINITIONS FOR CONSISTENT EMERGENCY DEPARTMENT METRICS

American Academy of Emergency Medicine, American Association of Critical Care Nurses, American College of Emergency Physicians, Association of periOperative Registered Nurses, Emergency Department Practice Management Association, Emergency Nurses Association, and National Association of EMS Physicians (2/10)

CONSENSUS STATEMENT ON MANAGEMENT OF INTERSEX DISORDERS

International Consensus Conference on Intersex (Lawson Wilkins Pediatric Endocrine Society and European Society for Paediatric Endocrinology)

INTRODUCTION. The birth of an intersex child prompts a long-term management strategy that involves myriad professionals working with the family. There has been progress in diagnosis, surgical techniques, understanding psychosocial issues, and recognizing and accepting the place of patient advocacy. The Lawson Wilkins Pediatric Endocrine Society and the European Society for Paediatric Endocrinology considered it timely to review the management of intersex disorders from a broad perspective, review data on longer-term outcome, and formulate proposals for future studies. The methodology comprised establishing a number of working groups, the membership of which was drawn from 50 international experts in the field. The groups prepared previous written responses to a defined set of questions resulting from evidence-based review of the literature. At a subsequent gathering of participants, a framework for a consensus document was agreed. This article constitutes its final form. (8/06)

DEFINING PEDIATRIC MALNUTRITION: A PARADIGM SHIFT TOWARD ETIOLOGY-RELATED DEFINITIONS

American Society for Parenteral and Enteral Nutrition

ABSTRACT. Lack of a uniform definition is responsible for underrecognition of the prevalence of malnutrition and its impact on outcomes in children. A pediatric malnutrition definitions workgroup reviewed existing pediatric age group English-language literature from 1955 to 2011, for relevant references related to 5 domains of the definition of *malnutrition* that were *a priori* identified: anthropometric parameters, growth, chronicity of malnutrition, etiology and pathogenesis, and developmental/functional outcomes. Based on available evidence and an iterative process to arrive at multidisciplinary consensus in the group, these domains were included in the overall construct of a new definition. Pediatric malnutrition (undernutrition) is defined as an imbalance between nutrient requirements and intake that results in cumulative deficits of energy, protein, or micronutrients that may negatively affect growth, development, and other relevant outcomes. A summary of the literature is presented and a new classification scheme is proposed that incorporates chronicity, etiology, mechanisms of nutrient imbalance, severity of malnutrition, and its impact on outcomes. Based on its etiology, malnutrition is either *illness related* (secondary to 1 or more diseases/injury) or *non–illness related*, (caused by environmental/behavioral factors), or both. Future research must focus on the relationship between inflammation and illness-related malnutrition. We anticipate that the definition of malnutrition will continue to evolve with improved understanding of the processes that lead to and complicate the treatment of this condition. A uniform definition should permit future research to focus on the impact of pediatric malnutrition on functional outcomes and help solidify the scientific basis for evidence-based nutrition practices. (3/13)

DELAYED UMBILICAL CORD CLAMPING AFTER BIRTH

American College of Obstetricians and Gynecologists

ABSTRACT. Delayed umbilical cord clamping appears to be beneficial for term and preterm infants. In term infants, delayed umbilical cord clamping increases hemoglobin levels at birth and improves iron stores in the first several months of life, which may have a favorable effect on developmental outcomes. There is a small increase in jaundice that requires phototherapy in this group of infants. Consequently, health care providers adopting delayed umbilical cord clamping in term infants should ensure that mechanisms are in place to monitor for and treat neonatal jaundice. In preterm infants, delayed umbilical cord clamping is associated with significant neonatal benefits, including improved transitional circulation, better establishment of red blood cell volume, decreased need for blood transfusion, and lower incidence of necrotizing enterocolitis and intraventricular hemorrhage. Delayed umbilical cord clamping was not associated with an increased risk of postpartum hemorrhage or increased blood loss at delivery, nor was it associated with a difference in postpartum hemoglobin levels or the need for blood transfusion. Given the benefits to most newborns and concordant with other professional organizations, the American College of Obstetricians and Gynecologists now recommends a delay in umbilical cord clamping in vigorous term and preterm infants for at least 30–60 seconds after birth. The ability to provide delayed umbilical cord clamping may vary among institutions and settings; decisions in those circumstances are best made by the team caring for the mother–infant dyad. (1/17)

DIABETES CARE FOR EMERGING ADULTS: RECOMMENDATIONS FOR TRANSITION FROM PEDIATRIC TO ADULT DIABETES CARE SYSTEMS

American Diabetes Association (11/11)

DIAGNOSIS, TREATMENT, AND LONG-TERM MANAGEMENT OF KAWASAKI DISEASE: A STATEMENT FOR HEALTH PROFESSIONALS

American Heart Association (12/04)

DIETARY RECOMMENDATIONS FOR CHILDREN AND ADOLESCENTS: A GUIDE FOR PRACTITIONERS

American Heart Association (9/05)

DIETARY REFERENCE INTAKES FOR CALCIUM AND VITAMIN D

Institute of Medicine (2011)

EMERGENCY EQUIPMENT AND SUPPLIES IN THE SCHOOL SETTING

National Association of School Nurses (1/12)

ENHANCING THE WORK OF THE HHS NATIONAL VACCINE PROGRAM IN GLOBAL IMMUNIZATIONS

National Vaccine Advisory Committee (9/13)

EPIDEMIOLOGY IN FIREARM VIOLENCE PREVENTION

Amy B. Davis; James A. Gaudino; Colin L. Soskolne; Wael K. Al-Delaimy; and International Network for Epidemiology in Policy

INTRODUCTION. Firearm violence has reached pandemic levels, with some countries experiencing high injury and death rates from privately owned guns and firearms (hereinafter collectively referred to as 'firearms'). Significant factors in the increase in deaths and injuries from privately held firearms include the ease of obtaining these arms and, most importantly, the growing lethality of these weapons.

Society cannot be satisfied with reactive responses only in treating victims' physical and psychological wounds after these occurrences; more must be done proactively to prevent firearm violence and address societal circumstances that either facilitate or impede it. Where they exist, well-intended policies fail to adequately protect people from firearm violence, often because they mainly focus on the purchase and illegal uses of guns while neglecting underlying social determinants of the violent uses of firearms.

Laws intended to curb firearm violence are often not enforced, are inadequate or do not address local societal factors of crime, mental well-being, poverty or low education in the relevant communities. These considerations point to the need for a multisectoral approach in which the public health sciences would play a pivotal role in preventing harms relating to firearm violence with a greater focus on its causes. Evidence-based multicomponent interventions, often shown by systematic reviews to be the most effective to address complex, community-level health issues, are needed but are not well-defined to address firearm violence. To both advance understanding of and to guide community-level public health services and actions needed to prevent firearm violence, decision-makers need to rely more on surveillance, research and programme evaluation by public health organizations, schools and universities.

Epidemiologists have unique interdisciplinary tools for addressing the contributors and barriers to preventing and mitigating injury, including firearm violence. These include quantitative, qualitative and social epidemiological methods. Interventions to prevent and mitigate the problem are currently under-developed, under-funded and under-utilized, particularly in the USA. The problem could be addressed by putting in place a robust evidence base to inform policy decisions. Additionally, public health can create, scale up and evaluate interventions designed to address social and behavioural factors associated with firearm violence. We call on governments, community leaders and community members to take meaningful action to support public health in addressing the problem of firearm violence. (4/18)

ETHICAL CONSIDERATION FOR INCLUDING WOMEN AS RESEARCH PARTICIPANTS

American College of Obstetricians and Gynecologists

ABSTRACT. Inclusion of women in research studies is necessary for valid inferences about health and disease in women. The generalization of results from trials conducted in men may yield erroneous conclusions that fail to account for the biologic differences between men and women. Although significant changes in research design and practice have led to an increase in the proportion of women included in research trials, knowledge gaps remain because of a continued lack of inclusion of women, especially those who are pregnant, in premarketing research trials. This document provides a historical overview of issues surrounding women as participants in research trials, followed by an ethical framework and discussion of the issues of informed consent, contraception requirements, intimate partner consent, and the appropriate inclusion of pregnant women in research studies. (11/15)

EVIDENCE REPORT: GENETIC AND METABOLIC TESTING ON CHILDREN WITH GLOBAL DEVELOPMENTAL DELAY

American Academy of Neurology and Child Neurology Society

ABSTRACT. *Objective.* To systematically review the evidence concerning the diagnostic yield of genetic and metabolic evaluation of children with global developmental delay or intellectual disability (GDD/ID).

Methods. Relevant literature was reviewed, abstracted, and classified according to the 4-tiered American Academy of Neurology classification of evidence scheme.

Results and Conclusions. In patients with GDD/ID, microarray testing is diagnostic on average in 7.8% (Class III), G-banded karyotyping is abnormal in at least 4% (Class II and III), and sub-telomeric fluorescence in situ hybridization is positive in 3.5% (Class I, II, and III). Testing for X-linked ID genes has a yield of up to 42% in males with an appropriate family history (Class III). *FMR*1 testing shows full expansion in at least 2% of patients with mild to moderate GDD/ID (Class II and III), and *MeCP*2 testing is diagnostic in 1.5% of females with moderate to severe GDD/ID (Class III). Tests for metabolic disorders have a yield of up to 5%, and tests for congenital disorders of glycosylation and cerebral creatine disorders have yields of up to 2.8% (Class III). Several genetic and metabolic screening tests have been shown to have a better than 1% diagnostic yield in selected populations of children with GDD/ID. These values should be among the many factors considered in planning the laboratory evaluation of such children. (9/11)

EVIDENCE-BASED MANAGEMENT OF SICKLE CELL DISEASE: EXPERT PANEL REPORT, 2014
National Heart, Lung, and Blood Institute (2014)

EXECUTING JUVENILE OFFENDERS: A FUNDAMENTAL FAILURE OF SOCIETY
Society for Adolescent Medicine (10/04)

FACULTY COMPETENCIES FOR GLOBAL HEALTH
Academic Pediatric Association Global Health Task Force
International partnerships among medical professionals from different countries are an increasingly common form of clinical and academic collaboration. Global health partnerships can include a variety of activities and serve multiple purposes in the areas of research, medical education and training, health system improvement, and clinical care. Competency domains, introduced by the Accreditation Council for Graduate Medical Education and the American Board of Medical Specialties in 1999, are now widely accepted to provide an organized, structured set of interrelated competencies, mostly for medical trainees. Although there are now competency domains and specific competencies recommended for pediatric trainees pursuing further professional training in global child health, none of these addresses competencies for faculty in global health.

In 2010 the Academic Pediatric Association established a Global Health Task Force to provide a forum for communication and collaboration for diverse pediatric academic societies and groups to advance global child health. Given the burgeoning demand for global health training, and particularly in light of a new global perspective on health education, as outlined in a Lancet Commission Report: *Health Professionals for a New Century: Transforming Education to Strengthen Health Systems in an Interdependent World,* in 2012 the Global Health Task Force noted the lack of defined faculty competencies and decided to develop a set of global health competencies for pediatric faculty engaged in the teaching and practice of global health. Using some of the principles suggested by Milner, et al. to define a competency framework, four domains were chosen, adapted from existing collaborative practice competencies. A fifth domain was added to address some of the unique challenges of global health practice encountered when working outside of one's own culture and health system. The domains are described below and specific competencies are provided for faculty working in global health research, education, administration, and clinical practice. (6/14)

GENETIC BASIS FOR CONGENITAL HEART DEFECTS: CURRENT KNOWLEDGE
American Heart Association
ABSTRACT. The intent of this review is to provide the clinician with a summary of what is currently known about the contribution of genetics to the origin of congenital heart disease. Techniques are discussed to evaluate children with heart disease for genetic alterations. Many of these techniques are now available on a clinical basis. Information on the genetic and clinical evaluation of children with cardiac disease is presented, and several tables have been constructed to aid the clinician in the assessment of children with different types of heart disease. Genetic algorithms for cardiac defects have been constructed and are available in an appendix. It is anticipated that this summary will update a wide range of medical personnel, including pediatric cardiologists and pediatricians, adult cardiologists, internists, obstetricians, nurses, and thoracic surgeons, about the genetic aspects of congenital heart disease and will encourage an interdisciplinary approach to the child and adult with congenital heart disease. (*Circulation.* 2007;115:3015-3038.) (6/07)

GIFTS TO PHYSICIANS FROM INDUSTRY
American Medical Association (8/01)

GUIDELINES FOR FIELD TRIAGE OF INJURED PATIENTS
Centers for Disease Control and Prevention (1/12)

GUIDELINES FOR REFERRAL OF CHILDREN AND ADOLESCENTS TO PEDIATRIC RHEUMATOLOGISTS
American College of Rheumatology (6/02, reaffirmed 5/07)

HELPING THE STUDENT WITH DIABETES SUCCEED: A GUIDE FOR SCHOOL PERSONNEL
National Diabetes Education Program (6/03)

IMPORTANCE AND IMPLEMENTATION OF TRAINING IN CARDIOPULMONARY RESUSCITATION AND AUTOMATED EXTERNAL DEFIBRILLATION IN SCHOOLS
American Heart Association Emergency Cardiovascular Care Committee; Council on Cardiopulmonary, Critical Care, Perioperative and Resuscitation; Council on Cardiovascular Diseases in the Young; Council on Cardiovascular Nursing; Council on Clinical Cardiology; and Advocacy Coordinating Committee
ABSTRACT. In 2003, the International Liaison Committee on Resuscitation published a consensus document on education in resuscitation that strongly recommended that "…instruction in CPR [cardiopulmonary resuscitation] be incorporated as a standard part of the school curriculum." The next year the American Heart Association (AHA) recommended that schools "…establish a goal to train every teacher in CPR and first aid and train all students in CPR" as part of their preparation for a response to medical emergencies on campus.

Since that time, there has been an increased interest in legislation that would mandate that school curricula include training in CPR or CPR and automated external defibrillation. Laws or curriculum content standards in 36 states (as of the 2009–2010 school year) now encourage the inclusion of CPR training programs in school curricula. The language in those laws and standards varies greatly, ranging from a suggestion that students "recognize" the steps of CPR to a requirement for certification in CPR. Not surprisingly, then, implementation is not uniform among states, even those whose laws or standards encourage CPR training in schools in the strongest language. This statement recommends that training in CPR and familiarization with automated external defibrillators (AEDs) should be required elements of secondary school curricula and provides the rationale for implementation of CPR training, as well as guidance in overcoming barriers to implementation. (2/11)

INTER-ASSOCIATION CONSENSUS STATEMENT ON BEST PRACTICES FOR SPORTS MEDICINE MANAGEMENT FOR SECONDARY SCHOOLS AND COLLEGES

National Athletic Trainers Association, National Interscholastic Athletic Administrators Association, College Athletic Trainers' Society, National Federation of State High School Associations, American College Health Association, American Orthopaedic Society for Sports Medicine, National Collegiate Athletic Association, American Medical Society for Sports Medicine, National Association of Collegiate Directors of Athletics, and National Association of Intercollegiate Athletics (7/13)

LONG-TERM CARDIOVASCULAR TOXICITY IN CHILDREN, ADOLESCENTS, AND YOUNG ADULTS WHO RECEIVE CANCER THERAPY: PATHOPHYSIOLOGY, COURSE, MONITORING, MANAGEMENT, PREVENTION, AND RESEARCH DIRECTIONS; A SCIENTIFIC STATEMENT FROM THE AMERICAN HEART ASSOCIATION

American Heart Association (5/13)

THE MANAGEMENT OF HYPOTENSION IN THE VERY-LOW-BIRTH-WEIGHT INFANT: GUIDELINE FOR PRACTICE

National Association of Neonatal Nurses
ABSTRACT. This guideline, released in 2011, focuses on the clinical management of systemic hypotension in the very-low-birth-weight (VLBW) infant during the first 3 days of postnatal life. (2011)

MEETING OF THE STRATEGIC ADVISORY GROUP OF EXPERTS ON IMMUNIZATION, APRIL 2012–CONCLUSIONS AND RECOMMENDATIONS

World Health Organization (5/12) (The AAP endorses the recommendation pertaining to the use of thimerosal in vaccines.)

MENSTRUATION IN GIRLS AND ADOLESCENTS: USING THE MENSTRUAL CYCLE AS A VITAL SIGN

American College of Obstetricians and Gynecologists Committee on Adolescent Health Care
ABSTRACT. Despite variations worldwide and within the U.S. population, median age at menarche has remained relatively stable—between 12 years and 13 years—across well-nourished populations in developed countries. Environmental factors, including socioeconomic conditions, nutrition, and access to preventive health care, may influence the timing and progression of puberty. A number of medical conditions can cause abnormal uterine bleeding, characterized by unpredictable timing and variable amount of flow. Clinicians should educate girls and their caretakers (eg, parents or guardians) about what to expect of a first menstrual period and the range for normal cycle length of subsequent menses. Identification of abnormal menstrual patterns in adolescence may improve early identification of potential health concerns for adulthood. It is important for clinicians to have an understanding of the menstrual patterns of adolescent girls, the ability to differentiate between normal and abnormal menstruation, and the skill to know how to evaluate the adolescent girl patient. By including an evaluation of the menstrual cycle as an additional vital sign, clinicians reinforce its importance in assessing overall health status for patients and caretakers. (12/15)

MULTILINGUAL CHILDREN: BEYOND MYTHS AND TOWARD BEST PRACTICES

Society for Research in Child Development
ABSTRACT. Multilingualism is an international fact of life and increasing in the United States. Multilingual families are exceedingly diverse, and policies relevant to them should take this into account. The quantity and quality of a child's exposure to responsive conversation spoken by fluent adults predicts both monolingual and multilingual language and literacy achievement. Contexts supporting optimal multilingualism involve early exposure to high quality conversation in each language, along with continued support for speaking both languages. Parents who are not fluent in English should not be told to speak English instead of their native language to their children; children require fluent input, and fluent input in another language will transfer to learning a second or third language. Messages regarding optimal multilingual practices should be made available to families using any and all available methods for delivering such information, including home visitation programs, healthcare settings, center-based early childhood programs, and mass media. (2013)

NATIONAL ADOPTION CENTER: OPEN RECORDS

National Adoption Center
The National Adoption Center believes that it is an inalienable right of all citizens, including adopted adults, to have unencumbered access to their original birth certificates. In keeping with this position, we believe that copies of both the original and the amended birth certificate should be given to the adoptive family at the time of finalization unless specifically denied by the birthparents. In any case, the National Adoption Center advocates that the adoptee, at age 18, be granted access to his/her original birth certificate. (6/00)

NEONATAL ENCEPHALOPATHY AND NEUROLOGIC OUTCOME, SECOND EDITION

American College of Obstetricians and Gynecologists Task Force on Neonatal Encephalopathy
In the first edition of this report, the Task Force on Neonatal Encephalopathy and Cerebral Palsy outlined criteria deemed essential to establish a causal link between intrapartum hypoxic events and cerebral palsy. It is now known that there are multiple potential causal pathways that lead to cerebral palsy in term infants, and the signs and symptoms of neonatal encephalopathy may range from mild to severe, depending on the nature and timing of the brain injury. Thus, for the current edition, the Task Force on Neonatal Encephalopathy determined that a broader perspective may be more fruitful. This conclusion reflects the sober recognition that knowledge gaps still preclude a definitive test or set of markers that accurately identifies, with high sensitivity and specificity, an infant in whom neonatal encephalopathy is attributable to an acute intrapartum event. The information necessary for assessment of likelihood can be derived from a comprehensive evaluation of all potential contributing factors in cases of neonatal encephalopathy. This is the broader perspective championed in the current report. If a comprehensive etiologic evaluation is not possible, the term hypoxic–ischemic encephalopathy should best be replaced by neonatal encephalopathy because neither hypoxia nor ischemia can be assumed to have been the unique initiating causal mechanism. The title of this report has been changed from *Neonatal Encephalopathy and Cerebral Palsy: Defining the Pathogenesis and Pathophysiology* to *Neonatal Encephalopathy and Neurologic Outcome* to indicate that an array of developmental outcomes may arise after neonatal encephalopathy in addition to cerebral palsy. (4/14)

NEURODEVELOPMENTAL OUTCOMES IN CHILDREN WITH CONGENITAL HEART DISEASE: EVALUATION AND MANAGEMENT; A SCIENTIFIC STATEMENT FROM THE AMERICAN HEART ASSOCIATION

American Heart Association (7/12)

THE NEUROLOGIST'S ROLE IN SUPPORTING TRANSITION TO ADULT HEALTH CARE

Lawrence W. Brown, MD; Peter Camfield, MD, FRCPC; Melissa Capers, MA; Greg Cascino, MD; Mary Ciccarelli, MD; Claudio M. de Gusmao, MD; Stephen M. Downs, MD; Annette Majnemer, PhD, FCAHS; Amy Brin Miller, MSN; Christina SanInocencio, MS; Rebecca Schultz, PhD; Anne Tilton, MD; Annick Winokur, BS; and Mary Zupanc, MD

ABSTRACT. The child neurologist has a critical role in planning and coordinating the successful transition from the pediatric to adult health care system for youth with neurologic conditions. Leadership in appropriately planning a youth's transition and in care coordination among health care, educational, vocational, and community services providers may assist in preventing gaps in care, delayed entry into the adult care system, and/or health crises for their adolescent patients. Youth whose neurologic conditions result in cognitive or physical disability and their families may need additional support during this transition, given the legal and financial considerations that may be required. Eight common principles that define the child neurologist's role in a successful transition process have been outlined by a multidisciplinary panel convened by the Child Neurology Foundation are introduced and described. The authors of this consensus statement recognize the current paucity of evidence for successful transition models and outline areas for future consideration. *Neurology.* 2016;87:1–6. (7/16)

NONINHERITED RISK FACTORS AND CONGENITAL CARDIOVASCULAR DEFECTS: CURRENT KNOWLEDGE

American Heart Association

ABSTRACT. Prevention of congenital cardiovascular defects has been hampered by a lack of information about modifiable risk factors for abnormalities in cardiac development. Over the past decade, there have been major breakthroughs in the understanding of inherited causes of congenital heart disease, including the identification of specific genetic abnormalities for some types of malformations. Although relatively less information has been available on noninherited modifiable factors that may have an adverse effect on the fetal heart, there is a growing body of epidemiological literature on this topic. This statement summarizes the currently available literature on potential fetal exposures that might alter risk for cardiovascular defects. Information is summarized for periconceptional multivitamin or folic acid intake, which may reduce the risk of cardiac disease in the fetus, and for additional types of potential exposures that may increase the risk, including maternal illnesses, maternal therapeutic and nontherapeutic drug exposures, environmental exposures, and paternal exposures. Information is highlighted regarding definitive risk factors such as maternal rubella; phenylketonuria; pregestational diabetes; exposure to thalidomide, vitamin A cogeners, or retinoids; and indomethacin tocolysis. Caveats regarding interpretation of possible exposure-outcome relationships from case-control studies are given because this type of study has provided most of the available information. Guidelines for prospective parents that could reduce the likelihood that their child will have a major cardiac malformation are given. Issues related to pregnancy monitoring are discussed. Knowledge gaps and future sources of new information on risk factors are described. (*Circulation.* 2007;115:2995–3014.) (6/07)

ORTHOPTISTS AS PHYSICIAN EXTENDERS

American Association for Pediatric Ophthalmology and Strabismus
(5/15)

A PRACTICAL GUIDE FOR PRIMARY CARE PHYSICIANS: INSTRUMENT-BASED VISION SCREENING IN CHILDREN

Children's Eye Foundation

SUMMARY. In January 2016 a new joint policy statement from the American Academy of Pediatrics (AAP), American Academy of Ophthalmology (AAO), American Association for Pediatric Ophthalmology and Strabismus (AAPOS) and American Association of Certified Orthoptists (AACO) regarding the pediatric eye examination was published. The updated policy statement, published in the journal *Pediatrics,* incorporates earlier and routine visual assessments using instrument-based screening to help identify children who may benefit from early intervention to improve vision (or correct vision problems). Instrument-based screening technology is revolutionizing early detection and prevention of amblyopia by allowing screening of more children and at a younger age.

This guide for primary care physicians is produced by the Children's Eye Foundation of AAPOS to provide information regarding instrument-based screening. Early detection and treatment of amblyopia is key to preventing unnecessary blindness, and primary care physicians play a critical role in its detection through vision screening in the preschool and school age groups. (2016)

PREVENTION AND CONTROL OF MENINGOCOCCAL DISEASE: RECOMMENDATIONS OF THE ADVISORY COMMITTEE ON IMMUNIZATION PRACTICES (ACIP)

Centers for Disease Control and Prevention

SUMMARY. Meningococcal disease describes the spectrum of infections caused by *Neisseria meningitidis,* including meningitidis, bacteremia, and bacteremic pneumonia. Two quadrivalent meningococcal polysaccharide-protein conjugate vaccines that provide protection against meningococcal serogroups A, C, W, and Y (MenACWY-D [Menactra, manufactured by Sanofi Pasteur, Inc., Swiftwater, Pennsylvania] and MenACWY-CRM [Menveo, manufactured by Novartis Vaccines, Cambridge, Massachusetts]) are licensed in the United States for use among persons aged 2 through 55 years. MenACWY-D also is licensed for use among infants and toddlers aged 9 through 23 months. Quadrivalent meningococcal polysaccharide vaccine (MPSV4 [Menommune, manufactured by Sanofi Pasteur, Inc., Swiftwater, Pennsylvania]) is the only vaccine licensed for use among persons aged ≥56 years. A bivalent meningococcal polysaccharide protein conjugate vaccine that provides protection against meningococcal serogroups C and Y along with *Haemophilus influenzae* type b (Hib) (Hib-MenCY-TT [MenHibrix, manufactured by GlaxoSmithKline Biologicals, Rixensart, Belgium]) is licensed for use in children aged 6 weeks through 18 months.

This report compiles and summarizes all recommendations from CDC's Advisory Committee on Immunization Practices (ACIP) regarding prevention and control of meningococcal disease in the United States, specifically the changes in the recommendations published since 2005 (CDC. Prevention and control of meningococcal disease: recommendations of the Advisory Committee on Immunization Practices [ACIP]. *MMWR* 2005;54 Adobe PDF file [No. RR-7]). As a comprehensive summary of previously published recommendations, this report does not contain any new recommendations; it is intended for use by clinicians as a resource. ACIP recommends routine vaccination with a quadrivalent meningococcal conjugate vaccine (MenACWY) for adolescents aged 11 or 12 years, with a booster dose at age 16 years. ACIP also recommends routine vaccination for persons at increased risk for meningococcal disease (i.e., persons who have persistent complement component deficiencies, persons who have anatomic or functional asplenia, microbiologists who routinely are exposed to isolates of *N. meningitidis,* military recruits, and persons who travel to or reside in areas in which meningococcal disease is hyperendemic or epidemic). Guidelines for antimicrobial chemoprophylaxis and for evaluation and management of suspected outbreaks of meningococcal disease also are provided. (3/13)

PROTECTING ADOLESCENTS: ENSURING ACCESS TO CARE AND REPORTING SEXUAL ACTIVITY AND ABUSE

Society for Adolescent Medicine (11/04)

RECOMMENDED AMOUNT OF SLEEP FOR PEDIATRIC POPULATIONS: A CONSENSUS STATEMENT OF THE AMERICAN ACADEMY OF SLEEP MEDICINE

Shalini Paruthi, MD; Lee J. Brooks, MD; Carolyn D'Ambrosio, MD; Wendy A. Hall, PhD, RN; Suresh Kotagal, MD; Robin M. Lloyd, MD; Beth A. Malow, MD, MS; Kiran Maski, MD; Cynthia Nichols, PhD; Stuart F. Quan, MD; Carol L. Rosen, MD; Matthew M. Troester, DO; and Merrill S. Wise, MD

Background and Methodology. Healthy sleep requires adequate duration, appropriate timing, good quality, regularity, and the absence of sleep disturbances or disorders. Sleep duration is a frequently investigated sleep measure in relation to health. A panel of 13 experts in sleep medicine and research used a modified RAND Appropriateness Method to develop recommendations regarding the sleep duration range that promotes optimal health in children aged 0–18 years. The expert panel reviewed published scientific evidence addressing the relationship between sleep duration and health using a broad set of National Library of Medicine Medical Subject Headings (MeSH) terms and no date restrictions, which resulted in a total of 864 scientific articles. The process was further guided by the Oxford grading system. The panel focused on seven health categories with the best available evidence in relation to sleep duration: general health, cardiovascular health, metabolic health, mental health, immunologic function, developmental health, and human performance. Consistent with the RAND Appropriateness Method, multiple rounds of evidence review, discussion, and voting were conducted to arrive at the final recommendations. The process to develop these recommendations was conducted over a 10-month period and concluded with a meeting held February 19–21, 2016, in Chicago, Illinois. (6/16)

REPORT OF THE NATIONAL CONSENSUS CONFERENCE ON FAMILY PRESENCE DURING PEDIATRIC CARDIO-PULMONARY RESUSCITATION AND PROCEDURES

Ambulatory Pediatric Association

INTRODUCTION. The National Consensus Conference on Family Presence during Pediatric Cardiopulmonary Resuscitation and Procedures was held in Washington, DC, on September 7–8, 2003. The concept, funding, planning and organization for the conference were the Ambulatory Pediatric Association (APA) Presidential Project of James Seidel, M.D., Ph.D. Dr. Seidel was in the final stages of preparation for chairing the conference when he died on July 25, 2003. In Dr. Seidel's absence, the conference was chaired by Deborah Parkman Henderson R.N., PhD, his co-investigator, and Jane F. Knapp, M.D., a colleague.

The National Consensus Conference on Family Presence during Pediatric Procedures and Cardiopulmonary Resuscitation was funded by a grant to the APA from the Maternal Child Health Bureau (MCHB) Partnership for Children. This meeting brought together a panel of over 20 appointed representatives from a multidisciplinary, diverse group of national organizations interested in the emergency care of children. The conference was part of a multiphase process designed with the goal of publishing consensus guidelines useful for defining policy regarding family presence (FP) during pediatric procedures and CPR in the Emergency Department (ED). It is also possible that the consensus panel recommendations could be applied to other settings.

Panel members completed a review of the literature prior to attending the conference. This review, along with results of a pre-conference questionnaire, formed the basis of the discussion during the conference. During the two day conference the participants completed the outline of the guidelines presented here. We believe these recommendations are a powerful testimony to Dr. Seidel's vision for promoting FP through multidisciplinary consensus building. Beyond that vision, however, we hope that the guidelines will make a difference in improving the quality of children's health care. (9/03)

RESPONSE TO CARDIAC ARREST AND SELECTED LIFE-THREATENING MEDICAL EMERGENCIES: THE MEDICAL EMERGENCY RESPONSE PLAN FOR SCHOOLS. A STATEMENT FOR HEALTHCARE PROVIDERS, POLICYMAKERS, SCHOOL ADMINISTRATORS, AND COMMUNITY LEADERS

American Heart Association (1/04)

SCREENING CHILDREN AT RISK FOR RETINOBLASTOMA: CONSENSUS REPORT FROM THE AMERICAN ASSOCIATION OF OPHTHALMIC ONCOLOGISTS AND PATHOLOGISTS

Alison H. Skalet, MD, PhD; Dan S. Gombos, MD; Brenda L. Gallie, MD; Jonathan W. Kim, MD; Carol L. Shields, MD; Brian P. Marr, MD; Sharon E. Plon, MD, PhD; and Patricia Chévez-Barrios, MD

Purpose: To provide a set of surveillance guidelines for children at risk for development of retinoblastoma.

Design: Consensus panel.

Participants: Expert panel of ophthalmic oncologists, pathologists, and geneticists.

Methods: A group of members of the American Association of Ophthalmic Oncologists and Pathologists (AAOOP) with support of the American Association for Pediatric Ophthalmology and Strabismus and the American Academy of Pediatrics (AAP) was convened. The panel included representative ophthalmic oncologists, pathologists, and geneticists from retinoblastoma referral centers located in various geographic regions who met and discussed screening approaches for retinoblastoma. A patient "at risk" was defined as a person with a family history of retinoblastoma in a parent, sibling, or first- or second-degree relative.

Main Outcome Measures: Screening recommendations for children at risk for retinoblastoma.

Results: Consensus statement from the panel: (1) Dedicated ophthalmic screening is recommended for all children at risk for retinoblastoma above the population risk. (2) Frequency of examinations is adjusted on the basis of expected risk for *RB1* mutation. (3) Genetic counseling and testing clarify the risk for retinoblastoma in children with a family history of the disease. (4) Examination schedules are stratified on the basis of high-, intermediate-, and low-risk children. (5) Children at high risk for retinoblastoma require more frequent screening, which may preferentially be examinations under anesthesia.

Conclusions: Risk stratification including genetic testing and counseling serves as the basis for screening of children at elevated risk for development of retinoblastoma. (10/17)

SCREENING FOR IDIOPATHIC SCOLIOSIS IN ADOLESCENTS—POSITION STATEMENT

American Academy of Orthopedic Surgeons, Scoliosis Research Society, and Pediatric Orthopedic Society of North America

ABSTRACT. The Scoliosis Research Society (SRS), American Academy of Orthopedic Surgeons (AAOS), Pediatric Orthopedic Society of North America (POSNA), and American Academy of Pediatrics (AAP) believe that there has been additional useful research in the early detection and management of adolescent idiopathic scoliosis (AIS) since the review performed by the United States Preventive Services Task Force (USPSTF) in 2004. This information should be available for use by patients, treating health care providers, and policy makers in assessing the relative risks and benefits of the early identification and management of AIS.

The AAOS, SRS, POSNA, and AAP believe that there are documented benefits of earlier detection and non-surgical management of AIS, earlier identification of severe deformities that are surgically treated, and of incorporating screening of children for AIS by knowledgeable health care providers as a part of their care. (9/15)

SKIING AND SNOWBOARDING INJURY PREVENTION
Canadian Paediatric Society

ABSTRACT. Skiing and snowboarding are popular recreational and competitive sport activities for children and youth. Injuries associated with both activities are frequent and can be serious. There is new evidence documenting the benefit of wearing helmets while skiing and snowboarding, as well as data refuting suggestions that helmet use may increase the risk of neck injury. There is also evidence to support using wrist guards while snowboarding. There is poor uptake of effective preventive measures such as protective equipment use and related policy. Physicians should have the information required to counsel children, youth and families regarding safer snow sport participation, including helmet use, wearing wrist guards for snowboarding, training and supervision, the importance of proper equipment fitting and binding adjustment, sun safety and avoiding substance use while on the slopes. (1/12)

SUPPLEMENT TO THE JCIH 2007 POSITION STATEMENT: PRINCIPLES AND GUIDELINES FOR EARLY INTERVENTION AFTER CONFIRMATION THAT A CHILD IS DEAF OR HARD OF HEARING
Joint Committee on Infant Hearing

PREFACE. This document is a supplement to the recommendations in the year 2007 position statement of the Joint Committee on Infant Hearing (JCIH) and provides comprehensive guidelines for early hearing detection and intervention (EHDI) programs on establishing strong early intervention (EI) systems with appropriate expertise to meet the needs of children who are deaf or hard of hearing (D/HH).

EI services represent the purpose and goal of the entire EHDI process. Screening and confirmation that a child is D/HH are largely meaningless without appropriate, individualized, targeted and high-quality intervention. For the infant or young child who is D/HH to reach his or her full potential, carefully designed individualized intervention must be implemented promptly, utilizing service providers with optimal knowledge and skill levels and providing services on the basis of research, best practices, and proven models.

The delivery of EI services is complex and requires individualization to meet the identified needs of the child and family. Because of the diverse needs of the population of children who are D/HH and their families, well-controlled intervention studies are challenging. At this time, few comparative effectiveness studies have been conducted. Randomized controlled trials are particularly difficult for ethical reasons, making it challenging to establish causal links between interventions and outcomes. EI systems must partner with colleagues in research to document what works for children and families and to strengthen the evidence base supporting practices.

Despite limitations and gaps in the evidence, the literature does contain research studies in which all children who were D/HH had access to the same well-defined EI service. These studies indicate that positive outcomes are possible, and they provide guidance about key program components that appear to promote these outcomes. This EI services document, drafted by teams of professionals with extensive expertise in EI programs for children who are D/HH and their families, relied on literature searches, existing systematic reviews, and recent professional consensus statements in developing this set of guidelines.

Terminology presented a challenge throughout document development. The committee noted that many of the frequently occurring terms necessary within the supplement may not reflect the most contemporary understanding and/or could convey inaccurate meaning. Rather than add to the lack of clarity or consensus and to avoid introducing new terminology to stakeholders, the committee opted to use currently recognized terms consistently herein and will monitor the emergence and/or development of new descriptors before the next JCIH consensus statement.

For purposes of this supplement:

- *Language* refers to all spoken and signed languages.
- *Early intervention* (EI), according to part C of the Individuals with Disabilities Education Improvement Act (IDEA) of 2004, is the process of providing services, education, and support to young children who are deemed to have an established condition, those who are evaluated and deemed to have a diagnosed physical or mental condition (with a high probability of resulting in a developmental delay), those who have an existing delay, or those who are at risk of developing a delay or special need that may affect their development or impede their education.
- *Communication* is used in lieu of terms such as communication options, methods, opportunities, approaches, etc.
- *Deaf or hard of hearing* (D/HH) is intended to be inclusive of all children with congenital and acquired hearing loss, unilateral and bilateral hearing loss, all degrees of hearing loss from minimal to profound, and all types of hearing loss (sensorineural, auditory neuropathy spectrum disorder, permanent conductive, and mixed).
- *Core knowledge and skills* is used to describe the expertise needed to provide appropriate EI that will optimize the development and well-being of infants/children and their families. Core knowledge and skills will differ according to the roles of individuals within the EI system (eg, service coordinator or EI provider).

This supplement to JCIH 2007 focuses on the practices of EI providers outside of the primary medical care and specialty medical care realms, rather than including the full spectrum of necessary medical, audiologic, and educational interventions. For more information about the recommendations for medical follow-up, primary care surveillance for related medical conditions, and specialty medical care and monitoring, the reader is encouraged to reference the year 2007 position statement of the JCIH as well as any subsequent revision. When an infant is confirmed to be D/HH, the importance of ongoing medical and audiologic management and surveillance both in the medical home and with the hearing health professionals, the otolaryngologist and the audiologist, cannot be overstated. A comprehensive discussion of those services is beyond the scope of this document. (3/13)

SYSTEMATIC REVIEW AND EVIDENCE-BASED GUIDELINES FOR THE MANAGEMENT OF PATIENTS WITH POSITIONAL PLAGIOCEPHALY
Congress of Neurologic Surgeons

ABSTRACT. *Background.* Positional plagiocephaly is a common problem seen by pediatricians, pediatric neurologists, and pediatric neurosurgeons. Currently, there are no evidence-based guidelines on the management of positional plagiocephaly.

The topics addressed in subsequent chapters of this guideline include: diagnosis, repositioning, physical therapy, and orthotic devices.

Objective. To evaluate topics relevant to the diagnosis and management of patients with positional plagiocephaly. The rigorous systematic process in which this guideline was created is presented in this chapter.

Methods. This guideline was prepared by the Plagiocephaly Guideline Task Force, a multidisciplinary team comprised of physician volunteers (clinical experts), medical librarians, and clinical guidelines specialists. The task force conducted a series of systematic literature searches of the National Library of Medicine and the Cochrane Library, according to standard protocols described below, for each topic addressed in subsequent chapters of this guideline.

Results. The systematic literature searches returned 396 abstracts relative to the 4 main topics addressed in this guideline. The results were analyzed and are described in detail in each subsequent chapter included in this guideline.

Conclusion. Evidence-based guidelines for the management of infants with positional plagiocephaly will help practitioners manage this common disorder. (11/16)

TIMING OF UMBILICAL CORD CLAMPING AFTER BIRTH

American College of Obstetricians and Gynecologists Committee on Obstetric Practice (12/12)

WEIGHING ALL PATIENTS IN KILOGRAMS

Emergency Nurses Association (9/16)

APPENDIX 1

PPI: AAP Partnership for Policy Implementation

BACKGROUND

The American Academy of Pediatrics (AAP) develops policies that promote attainment of optimal physical, mental, and social health and well-being for all infants, children, adolescents, and young adults. These documents are valued highly not only by clinicians who provide direct health care to children but by members of other organizations who share similar goals and by parents, payers, and legislators. To increase clarity and action of AAP clinical guidance and recommendations for physicians at the point of care, the AAP formed the Partnership for Policy Implementation (PPI). The PPI is a group of pediatric medical informaticians who partner with authors of AAP clinical practice guidelines and clinical reports to help assure that clinical recommendations are stated with the precision needed to implement them in an electronic health record (EHR) system. Partnership for Policy Implementation volunteers focus on helping content experts develop clinical guidance that specifies exactly who is to do what, for whom, and under what circumstances.

VISION

The vision of the PPI is that all AAP clinical recommendations include clear guidance on how pediatricians can implement those recommendations into their patient care and that AAP clinical guidance can be easily incorporated within EHR decision-support systems.

MISSION

The mission of the PPI is to facilitate implementation of AAP recommendations at the point of care by ensuring that AAP documents are written in a practical, action-oriented fashion with unambiguous recommendations.

WHAT THE PPI IS

The PPI is a network of pediatric informaticians who work with AAP authors and clinical practice guideline subcommittees throughout the writing process.

Contributions of the PPI to the AAP writing process include disambiguation and specification; development of clear definitions; clearly defined logic; implementation techniques; action-oriented recommendations, including clinical algorithms; transparency of the evidence base for recommendations; and health information technology (HIT) standard development.

WHAT THE PPI HAS ACCOMPLISHED

Since inception of the PPI, more than 30 statements have been published using the PPI process, covering a wide variety of child health topics, including influenza prevention and control (*Pediatrics*. 2018;142[4]:e20182367), child passenger safety (*Pediatrics*. 2018;142[5]:e20182460), high blood pressure in children and adolescents (*Pediatrics*. 2017;140[3]:e20170017), brief resolved unexplained events (commonly known as BRUE) (*Pediatrics*. 2016;137[5]:e20160590), respiratory syncytial virus (*Pediatrics*. 2014;134[2]:415–420), bronchiolitis (*Pediatrics*. 2014; 134[5]:e1474–e1502), and type 2 diabetes (*Pediatrics*. 2013; 131[2]:364–382).

One example of how a statement developed using PPI process has gained broader acceptance is the AAP annual influenza statement. Since 2007, the Centers for Disease Control and Prevention has adopted components of the PPI statement (specifically, the clinical algorithm) within its own statement on the same topic.

WHAT THE PPI IS DOING NOW

In addition to creating practical, action-oriented guidance that pediatricians can use at the point of care, the PPI works to make it easier for these recommendations to be incorporated into electronic systems. To date, the PPI has focused its involvement on the statement development process. Involvement of the PPI during the writing process helps produce a clear, more concise document. As these standards of care become well-documented, the PPI can begin to focus on building or mapping pediatric vocabulary; once solidified, this vocabulary can be built into EHR systems. The standards of care can also be matched to various logical and functional HIT standards that already exist today. Through this work, the PPI improves AAP policy documents by providing specific guidance to pediatricians at the point of care, helping ensure that EHRs are designed to assist pediatricians in providing optimal care for children. The PPI developed a short video that provides an overview of its mission and process. This video is available on the PPI website (https://www.aap.org/en-us/professional-resources/quality-improvement/Pages/Partnership-for-Policy-Implementation.aspx) as well as the AAP YouTube channel at www.youtube.com/watch?v=woTfeoNcxn4.

The PPI recently began expanding and is mentoring new members. For more information on the application process and about the PPI, please visit its website (https://www.aap.org/en-us/professional-resources/quality-improvement/Pages/Partnership-for-Policy-Implementation.aspx) or contact Jeremiah Salmon (jsalmon@aap.org or 630/626-6260).

APPENDIX 2

American Academy of Pediatrics Acronyms

AACAP	American Academy of Child and Adolescent Psychiatry
AAFP	American Academy of Family Physicians
AAMC	Association of American Medical Colleges
AAOS	American Academy of Orthopaedic Surgeons
AAP	American Academy of Pediatrics
AAPD	American Academy of Pediatric Dentistry
ABM	Academy of Breastfeeding Medicine
ABMS	American Board of Medical Specialties
ABP	American Board of Pediatrics
ACCME	Accreditation Council for Continuing Medical Education
ACEP	American College of Emergency Physicians
ACGME	Accreditation Council for Graduate Medical Education
ACIP	Advisory Committee on Immunization Practices
ACMG	American College of Medical Genetics
ACO	Accountable Care Organization
ACOG	American College of Obstetricians and Gynecologists
ACOP	American College of Osteopathic Pediatricians
ACP	American College of Physicians
ADAMHA	Alcohol, Drug Abuse, and Mental Health Administration
AG-M	Action Group—Multidisciplinary (Section Forum)
AG-M1	Action Group—Medical 1 (Section Forum)
AG-M2	Action Group—Medical 2 (Section Forum)
AG-S	Action Group—Surgical (Section Forum)
AHA	American Heart Association
AHA	American Hospital Association
AHRQ	Agency for Healthcare Research and Quality
ALF	Annual Leadership Forum
AMA	American Medical Association
AMCHP	Association of Maternal and Child Health Programs
AMSA	American Medical Student Association
AMSPDC	Association of Medical School Pediatric Department Chairs
AMWA	American Medical Women's Association
APA	Academic Pediatric Association
APHA	American Public Health Association
APLS	Advanced Pediatric Life Support
APPD	Association of Pediatric Program Directors
APQ	Alliance for Pediatric Quality
APS	American Pediatric Society
AQA	Ambulatory Care Quality Alliance
ASHG	American Society of Human Genetics
ASTM	American Society of Testing and Materials
BHP	Bureau of Health Professions
BIA	Bureau of Indian Affairs
BLAST	Babysitter Lessons and Safety Training

BOD	Board of Directors
BPC	Breastfeeding Promotion Consortium
CAG	Corporate Advisory Group
CAMLWG	Children, Adolescents, and Media Leadership Workgroup
CAP	College of American Pathologists
CAQI	Chapter Alliance for Quality Improvement
CATCH	Community Access to Child Health
CDC	Centers for Disease Control and Prevention
CESP	Confederation of European Specialty Pediatrics
CFMC	Chapter Forum Management Committee
CFT	Cross Functional Team
CHA	Children's Hospital Association
CHIC	Child Health Informatics Center
CHIP	Children's Health Insurance Program
CISP	Childhood Immunization Support Program
CMC	Council Management Committee
CME	Continuing Medical Education
CMS	Centers for Medicare & Medicaid Services
CMSS	Council of Medical Specialty Societies
CnF	Council Forum
COA	Committee on Adolescence
COB	Committee on Bioethics
COCAN	Council on Child Abuse and Neglect
COCHF	Committee on Child Health Financing
COCIT	Council on Clinical Information Technology
COCM	Council on Communications and Media
COCME	Committee on Continuing Medical Education
COCN	Committee on Coding and Nomenclature
COCP	Council on Community Pediatrics
COCWD	Council on Children With Disabilities
COD	Committee on Drugs
CODe	Committee on Development
COEC	Council on Early Childhood
COEH	Council on Environmental Health
CoF	Committee Forum
COFCAKC	Council on Foster Care, Adoption, and Kinship Care
COFGA	Committee on Federal Government Affairs
CoFMC	Committee Forum Management Committee
COFN	Committee on Fetus and Newborn
COG	Committee on Genetics
COGME	Council on Graduate Medical Education (DHHS/HRSA)
COHC	Committee on Hospital Care
COID	Committee on Infectious Diseases
COIVPP	Committee on Injury, Violence, and Poison Prevention
COM	Committee on Membership
COMLRM	Committee on Medical Liability and Risk Management
COMSEP	Council on Medical Student Education in Pediatrics (AMSPDC)

CON	Committee on Nutrition
CONACH	Committee on Native American Child Health
COPA	Committee on Pediatric AIDS
COPACFH	Committee on Psychosocial Aspects of Child and Family Health
COPAM	Committee on Practice and Ambulatory Medicine
COPE	Committee on Pediatric Education
COPEM	Committee on Pediatric Emergency Medicine
COPR	Committee on Pediatric Research
COPW	Committee on Pediatric Workforce
COQIPS	Council on Quality Improvement and Patient Safety
CORS	Committee on Residency Scholarships
COSGA	Committee on State Government Affairs
COSH	Council on School Health
COSMF	Council on Sports Medicine and Fitness
COSUP	Committee on Substance Use and Prevention
CPS	Canadian Paediatric Society
CPTI	Community Pediatrics Training Initiative
CQN	Chapter Quality Network
CSHCN	Children With Special Health Care Needs
DHHS	Department of Health and Human Services
DOD	Department of Defense
DPAC	Disaster Preparedness Advisory Council
DVC	District Vice Chairperson
EBCDLWG	Early Brain and Child Development Leadership Workgroup
EC	Executive Committee
ECHO	Expanding Capacity for Health Outcomes
ELWG	Epigenetics Leadership Workgroup
EMSC	Emergency Medical Services for Children
EPA	Environmental Protection Agency
EQIPP	Education in Quality Improvement for Pediatric Practice
eTACC	Electronic Translation of Academy Clinical Content
FAAN	Federal Advocacy Action Network
FASD	Fetal Alcohol Spectrum Disorder
FCF	Friends of Children Fund
FDA	Food and Drug Administration
FERPA	Family Educational Rights and Privacy Act
FOPE II	Future of Pediatric Education II
FOPO	Federation of Pediatric Organizations
FPN	Family Partnerships Network
FTC	Federal Trade Commission
GME	Graduate Medical Education
HAAC	Historical Archives Advisory Committee
HBB	Helping Babies Breathe
HBSPG	Helping Babies Survive Planning Group
HCCA	Healthy Child Care America
HEDIS	Healthcare Effectiveness Data and Information Set
HHS	Health and Human Services
HIPAA	Health Insurance Portability and Accountability Act of 1996
HMO	Health Maintenance Organization
HOF	Headquarters of the Future
HQA	Hospital Quality Alliance
HRSA	Health Resources and Services Administration
HTC	Help the Children
HTPCP	Healthy Tomorrows Partnership for Children Program
IHS	Indian Health Service
IMG	International Medical Graduate
IPA	International Pediatric Association
IPC	International Pediatric Congress

IRB	Institutional Review Board
LLLI	La Leche League International
LWG	Leadership Workgroup
MCAN	Merck Childhood Asthma Network
MCH	Maternal and Child Health
MCHB	Maternal and Child Health Bureau
MCN	Migrant Clinicians Network
MHICSN-PAC	Medical Home Initiatives for Children With Special Needs Project Advisory Committee
MHLWG	Mental Health Leadership Work Group
MOC	Maintenance of Certification
MRT	Media Resource Team
MSAP	Medical Subspecialty Advisory Panel
NACHC	National Association of Community Health Centers
NAEMSP	National Association of EMS Physicians
NAEPP	National Asthma Education and Prevention Program
NAM	National Academy of Medicine
NAPNAP	National Association of Pediatric Nurse Practitioners
NASPGHAN	North American Society for Pediatric Gastroenterology, Hepatology, and Nutrition
NAWD	National Association of WIC Directors
NBME	National Board of Medical Examiners
NCBDDD	National Center on Birth Defects and Developmental Disabilities
NCEPG	National Conference & Exhibition Planning Group
NCQA	National Committee for Quality Assurance
NHLBI	National Heart, Lung, and Blood Institute
NHMA	National Hispanic Medical Association
NHTSA	National Highway Traffic Safety Administration
NIAAA	National Institute on Alcohol Abuse and Alcoholism
NICHD	National Institute of Child Health and Human Development
NICHQ	National Initiative for Children's Health Quality
NIDA	National Institute on Drug Abuse
NIH	National Institutes of Health
NIMH	National Institute of Mental Health
NMA	National Medical Association
NNC	National Nominating Committee
NQF	National Quality Forum
NRHA	National Rural Health Association
NRMP	National Resident Matching Program
NRP	Neonatal Resuscitation Program
NSC	National Safety Council
NVAC	National Vaccine Advisory Committee
ODPHP	Office of Disease Prevention and Health Promotion
OED	Office of the Executive Director
OHISC	Oral Health Initiative Steering Committee
OLWG	Obesity Leadership Workgroup
P4P	Pay for Performance
PAC	Project Advisory Committee
PAHO	Pan American Health Organization
PALS	Pediatric Advanced Life Support
PAS	Pediatric Academic Societies
PCO	*Pediatric Care Online*™
PCOC	Primary Care Organizations Consortium
PCPCC	Patient-Centered Primary Care Collaborative
PCPI	Physician Consortium on Performance Improvement
PEAC	Practice Expense Advisory Committee

PECOS	Pediatric Education in Community and Office Settings
PECS	Pediatric Education in Community Settings
PEPP	Pediatric Education for Prehospital Professionals
PIR	*Pediatrics in Review*
PLA	Pediatric Leadership Alliance
PPAAC	Private Payer Advocacy Advisory Committee (COCHF Subcommittee)
PPAC	Past President's Advisory Committee
PPC-PCMH	Physician Practice Connections—Patient-Centered Medical Home (NCQA)
PPI	Partnership for Policy Implementation
PPMA	Pediatric Practice Management Alliance
PREP	Pediatric Review and Education Program
PROS	Pediatric Research in Office Settings
PUPVS	Project Universal Preschool Vision Screening
QA	Quality Assurance
QI	Quality Improvement
QuIIN	Quality Improvement Innovation Network
RBPE	Resource-Based Practice Expense
RBRVS	Resource-Based Relative Value Scale
RCAC	Richmond Center Advisory Committee
RCE	Richmond Center of Excellence
RRC	Residency Review Committee (ACGME)
RUC	AMA/Specialty Society Relative Value Scale Update Committee
RVU	Relative Value Unit
SAM	Society for Adolescent Medicine
SAMHSA	Substance Abuse and Mental Health Services Administration
SAP	Surgical Advisory Panel
SCHIP	State Children's Health Insurance Program
SDBP	Society for Developmental and Behavioral Pediatrics
SF	Section Forum
SFMC	Section Forum Management Committee
SLGBTHW	Section on Lesbian, Gay, Bisexual, and Transgender Health and Wellness
SOA	Section on Anesthesiology and Pain Medicine
SOAC	Subcommittee on Access to Care
SOAH	Section on Adolescent Health
SOAI	Section on Allergy and Immunology
SOAPM	Section on Administration and Practice Management
SOATT	Section on Advances in Therapeutics and Technology
SOB	Section on Bioethics
SOBr	Section on Breastfeeding
SOCAN	Section on Child Abuse and Neglect
SOCC	Section on Critical Care
SOCCS	Section on Cardiology and Cardiac Surgery
SOCDRP	Section on Child Death Review and Prevention
SOCPT	Section on Clinical Pharmacology and Therapeutics
SOD	Section on Dermatology
SODBP	Section on Developmental and Behavioral Pediatrics
SOECP	Section on Early Career Physicians
SOEM	Section on Emergency Medicine
SOEn	Section on Endocrinology
SOEPHE	Section on Epidemiology, Public Health, and Evidence

SOGBD	Section on Genetics and Birth Defects
SOGHN	Section on Gastroenterology, Hepatology, and Nutrition
SOHC	Section on Home Care
SOHM	Section on Hospital Medicine
SOHO	Section on Hematology/Oncology
SOHPM	Section on Hospice and Palliative Medicine
SOICH	Section on International Child Health
SOID	Section on Infectious Diseases
SOIM	Section on Integrative Medicine
SOIMG	Section on International Medical Graduates
SOIMP	Section on Internal Medicine/Pediatrics
SOMHEI	Section on Minority Health, Equity, and Inclusion
SOMP	Section on Medicine-Pediatrics
SONp	Section on Nephrology
SONPM	Section on Neonatal-Perinatal Medicine
SONS	Section on Neurological Surgery
SONu	Section on Neurology
SOOb	Section on Obesity
SOOH	Section on Oral Health
SOOHNS	Section on Otolaryngology—Head and Neck Surgery
SOOp	Section on Ophthalmology
SOOPe	Section on Osteopathic Pediatricians
SOOr	Section on Orthopaedics
SOPPSM	Section on Pediatric Pulmonology and Sleep Medicine
SOPS	Section on Plastic Surgery
SOPT	Section on Pediatric Trainees
SORa	Section on Radiology
SORh	Section on Rheumatology
SOSILM	Section on Simulation and Innovative Learning Methods
SOSM	Section on Senior Members
SOSu	Section on Surgery
SOTC	Section on Telehealth Care
SOTCo	Section on Tobacco Control
SOTM	Section on Transport Medicine
SOU	Section on Urology
SOUS	Section on Uniformed Services
SPR	Society for Pediatric Research
SPWG	Strategic Planning Work Group
TA	Technical Assistance
TA	Technology Assessment
TFOA	Task Force on Access (also known as Task Force on Health Insurance Coverage and Access to Care)
TFOABD	Task Force on Addressing Bias and Discrimination
TFOC	Task Force on Circumcision
TFODI	Task Force on Diversity and Inclusion
TFOSIDS	Task Force on Sudden Infant Death Syndrome
TIPP	The Injury Prevention Program
TJC	The Joint Commission
UNICEF	United Nations Children's Fund
UNOS	United Network for Organ Sharing
USDA	US Department of Agriculture
VIP	Value in Inpatient Pediatrics
WHO	World Health Organization
WIC	Special Supplemental Nutrition Program for Women, Infants, and Children

Subject Index

• • • • • • • • • • • • • •

A

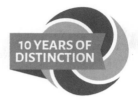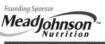
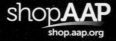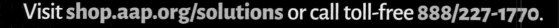